CTMA

Compendium of Therapeutics for Minor Ailments

Second Edition

Published by: Canadian Pharmacists Association, Ottawa, Ontario, Canada

Copyright

Electronic

The content in the *Compendium of Therapeutics for Minor Ailments (CTMA)* is available online as part of RxTx in English and French; to subscribe visit **www.pharmacists.ca/rxtx**. Licensed content is also available for data integration purposes. For more information on data licensing, please call 1-800-917-9489.

Publisher

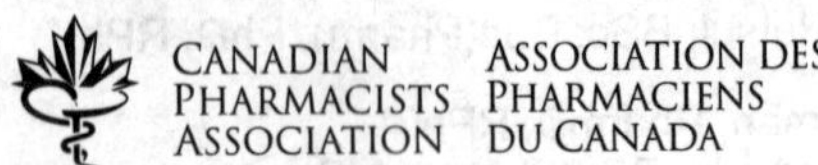

1785 Alta Vista Drive, Ottawa, ON K1G 3Y6 Canada

Comments/Inquiries

Tel: 613-523-7877, 1-800-917-9489 | Fax: 613-523-0445, 1-800-601-1904 | service@pharmacists.ca
Website: www.pharmacists.ca

Illustrations

Lianne Friesen

Printed in Canada

Webcom Inc., 3480 Pharmacy Avenue, Toronto, ON, M1W 2S7 Canada

Website: www.webcomlink.com

Compendium of Therapeutics for Minor Ailments, Second Edition
ISSN: 2368-0237
ISBN: 978-1-894402-96-5

Cataloguing data available from Library and Archives Canada

Table of Contents

Respiratory Conditions

Metabolic and Cardiovascular Conditions

Gastrointestinal Conditions

Nutrition

Musculoskeletal Conditions

Foot Conditions

Dermatologic Conditions

Reproductive, Gynecologic and Genitourinary Health

Dental Health

Mouth Conditions

General Appendices

Editorial Advisory Committee

Authors

Shirin Abadi, BSc(Pharm), ACPR, PharmD
Clinical Pharmacy Specialist & Pharmacy Education Coordinator, BC Cancer Agency
Clinical Associate Professor of Pharmacy & Associate Member of Medicine
University of British Columbia
Vancouver, BC

Manjit Bains, BScPharm
Pharmacist
Concordia Hospital
Winnipeg, MB

Alasdair M. Barr, PhD
Associate Professor
Department of Anesthesiology, Pharmacology & Therapeutics
University of British Columbia
Vancouver, BC

Marie Berry, BSc(Pharm), BA, LLB
Vimy Park Health
Winnipeg, MB

Michelle Bourassa, BPharm, MSc, DMD
Dental Surgeon, Quebec Heart and Lung Institute
Chargée d'enseignement, Faculté de Médecine dentaire
Université Laval
Québec, QC

Jane Bowles-Jordan, BScPhm, RPh, ACPR, CDE
MediLink Community Health Services
Hamilton, ON

Joan Brennan-Donnan, BASc, RD
Manager, Clinical Dietetics
Hospital for Sick Children
Toronto, ON

Thomas E.R. Brown, BScPhm, PharmD
Doctor of Pharmacy Program
University of Toronto
Toronto, ON

Joyce Chan, BScPhm, ACPR, MS, PharmD, BCPS(AQ Cardiology), CDE
Pharmacist, University Health Network
Adjunct Lecturer, Leslie Dan Faculty of Pharmacy
University of Toronto
Toronto, ON

James S. Conklin, BSc(Pharm), ACPR
BC Cancer Agency
Vancouver, BC

Shelita Dattani, BSc, BScPhm, PharmD
Associate Director, Professional Development
Canadian Pharmacists Association
Ottawa, ON

Carla Dillon, BScPharm, ACPR, PharmD
Assistant Professor, School of Pharmacy
Memorial University of Newfoundland
Pharmacist, Family Health Team
St. John's, NL

Lisa Dolovich, BScPhm, PharmD, MSc
Research Director & Associate Professor
Department of Family Medicine, McMaster University
Scientist & Associate Director
Centre for Evaluation of Medicines
Hamilton, ON

Barbara J. Farrell, BScPhm, PharmD, ACPR, FCSHP
Pharmacist, Bruyère Geriatric Day Hospital
Bruyère Continuing Care
Scientist, Bruyère Research Institute
Assistant Professor, Department of Family Medicine
University of Ottawa
Ottawa, ON
Adjunct Assistant Professor, School of Pharmacy
University of Waterloo
Waterloo, ON

Antonietta Forrester, BScPhm
Clinical Consultant Pharmacist, Smartmeds Pharmacy
Hamilton, ON

Anne M. Friesen, BSc(Pharm), MSc
Seven Oaks General Hospital
Winnipeg Regional Health Authority
Winnipeg, MB

Ken Gellatly, OD, FAAO
Downtown Vision Care
Calgary, AB

Kelly Grindrod, BScPharm, PharmD, MSc
Assistant Professor, School of Pharmacy
University of Waterloo
Waterloo, ON

L. Maria Gutschi, BScPhm, PharmD
Canada Chemists
Scientific Consultant, Patented Medicines Prices Review Board
Faculty of Dentistry and Faculty of Medicine
Canadian Forces Health Support Unit
Ottawa, ON

Shirley Heschuk, BScPharm, MSc(Pharmacology)
Adjunct Professor, Faculty of Pharmacy and Pharmaceutical Sciences
University of Alberta
Edmonton, AB

Christine Hughes, BScPharm, PharmD, FCSHP
Faculty of Pharmacy & Pharmaceutical Sciences
University of Alberta
Edmonton, AB

Mark Kearney, BScH, MSc(Pharmacology), BScPharm, Certificate in Travel Health
Clinical Pharmacist
Queensway Carleton Hospital
Ottawa, ON

Jennifer Kendrick, BScPharm, ACPR, PharmD
Pharmacist - Respirology and Cystic Fibrosis
St Paul's Hospital
Vancouver, BC

Jason Kielly, BSc(Pharm), PharmD
Assistant Professor, School of Pharmacy
Memorial University of Newfoundland
Clinical Pharmacist, Rheumatic Health Program, Eastern Health
St. John's, NL

Nancy Kleiman, BSP, MBA
Pharmacy Practice Liaison & Senior Instructor
Faculty of Pharmacy
University of Manitoba
Winnipeg, MB

Victoria Kletas, BScPharm, MSc
Oncology Drug Information Specialist
BC Cancer Agency
Vancouver, BC

Sandra Knowles, RPh, ACPR, BScPhm
Drug Safety Pharmacist
Drug Information Centre
Sunnybrook Health Sciences Centre
Toronto, ON

Lynette Kosar, BSP, MSc(Pharm)
Information Support Pharmacist
RxFiles Academic Detailing Program
Saskatoon, SK

Lily Lum, BScPharm, CSPI
Alberta Poison and Drug Information Service (PADIS)
Calgary, AB

Lori MacCallum, BScPhm, PharmD, RPh, CDE
Assistant Professor, Leslie Dan Faculty of Pharmacy
University of Toronto
Program Director, Knowledge Translation and Optimizing Care Models
Sun Life Financial Professor in Wellness and Diabetes Education
Banting and Best Diabetes Centre
Faculty of Medicine, University of Toronto
Toronto, ON

Anne Mallin, RPh, BScPhm, PharmD, CDE
Clinical Pharmacist
Hamilton Family Health Team
Hamilton, ON

Adeline T. Chau Markarian, BSc (Pharm), ACPR
BC Cancer Agency
Vancouver, BC

Carlo Marra, BSc(Pharm), ACPR, PharmD, PhD, FCSHP
Professor and Dean
School of Pharmacy
Memorial University of Newfoundland
St. John's, NL

Penny F. Miller, BSc (Pharm), MA
Senior Instructor, Faculty of Pharmaceutical Sciences and Pharmacotherapeutic Consultant
Department of Family Practice, Faculty of Medicine,
University of British Columbia
Vancouver, BC

Myla Moretti, MSc
Assistant Director, Motherisk Program
The Hospital for Sick Children
Toronto, ON

Nardine Nakhla, PharmD
Adjunct Clinical Assistant Professor, School of Pharmacy, Faculty of Science
University of Waterloo
Clinical Lecturer; CPD Education Coordinator
Leslie Dan Faculty of Pharmacy
University of Toronto
Mississauga, ON

Kristine Petrasko, BScPharm, CRE
Regional Pulmonary Educator
Winnipeg Regional Health Authority
Winnipeg, MB

Co Q. D. Pham, BSc, BA, BScPharm, ACPR, PharmD
Lecturing Professor and Pharmacology Longitudinal Expert
Faculty of Medicine, University of Ottawa
Scientific Manager, Marketed Health Products Directorate, Health Canada
Ottawa, ON

Laura-Lynn Pollock, BSc(Pharm), RPh, NARTC Dip AC
Clinical Pharmacist, Health Educator
Victoria, BC

Ric M. Procyshyn, BSc(Pharm), MSc, PharmD, PhD
Psychopharmacologist
Clinical Associate Professor, Psychiatry
University of British Columbia
Vancouver, BC

Lalitha Raman-Wilms, BSc(Phm), PharmD, FCSHP
Associate Professor, Leslie Dan Faculty of Pharmacy
University of Toronto
Pharmacist
The Anne Johnston Health Station
Toronto, ON

Cynthia Richard, BSc(Pharm), PhD
Clinical Lecturer, School of Pharmacy
University of Waterloo
Kitchener, ON

Cheryl A. Sadowski, BSc(Pharm), PharmD
Associate Professor, Faculty of Pharmacy and Pharmaceutical Sciences
University of Alberta
Edmonton, AB

Yvonne M. Shevchuk, BSP, PharmD, FCSHP
Professor, College of Pharmacy and Nutrition
Director, medSask Medication Information Service
University of Saskatchewan
Saskatoon, SK

Debra Sibbald, BScPhm, RPh, ACPR, MA (Adult Education), PhD (Curriculum, Teaching and Learning)
Senior Tutor, Division of Pharmacy Practice
Leslie Dan Faculty of Pharmacy
Toronto, ON

Ronald Silver, BSc, BScPharm
Pharmacist
Winnipeg, MB

Tom Smiley, BScPhm, PharmD
Pharmavision Health Consulting Inc.
Paris, ON

Richard Spagnuolo, PhD
Assistant Professor, School of Pharmacy
University of Waterloo
Kitchener, ON

Daniel Thirion, BPharm, MSc, PharmD, FCSHP
Pharmacien, Centre Universitaire de Santé McGill
Professeur agrégé de clinique, Faculté de pharmacie
Université de Montréal
Montreal, QC

Peter Thomson, BSc(Pharm), PharmD
Clinical Resource Pharmacist
Clinical Assistant Professor
Faculty of Pharmacy
University of Manitoba
Winnipeg Regional Authority
Winnipeg, MB

Dorothy Tscheng, BScPhm, CGP, RPh
Project Lead
Institute for Safe Medication Practices Canada
Toronto, ON

Anne Marie Whelan, BSc(Pharm), PharmD, FCSHP
College of Pharmacy, Dalhousie University
Pharmacy Consultant, Department of Family Medicine
Dalhousie University
Halifax, NS

David S. Wing, BSP, MS, MBA
Pharmacist
Calgary, AB

Karen Wlock, BScPharm
Clinical Pharmacist
BC Cancer Agency
Vancouver, BC

Irene Worthington, BScPhm, RPh
Coordinator, MetroDIS (retired)
Sunnybrook Health Sciences Centre
Toronto, ON

Reviewers

David R. Anderson, MD, FRCPC
Professor of Medicine
Pathology and Community Health & Epidemiology
Head, Department of Medicine
Dalhousie University and Capital Health
Halifax, NS

Gary Butterworth, BScPharm, OD
Optometrist
Winnipeg, MB

Roxane Carr, BSc(Pharm), PharmD, BCPS, FCSHP
Children's and Women's Health Centre of British Columbia
Assistant Professor, Faculty of Pharmaceutical Sciences
University of British Columbia
Vancouver, BC

Michel Cauchon, MD, FCMF
Professor of Family Medicine
Université Laval
Quebec, QC

Alice Yuk-Yan Cheng, MD, FRCPC
Department of Medicine
Trillium Health Partners
Mississauga, ON

Paul J. Daeninck, MD, MSc, FRCPC
Assistant Professor
Internal Medicine and Family Medicine
University of Manitoba
Consultant Medical Oncologist and Coordinator
CancerCare Manitoba
Consultant Palliative Medicine Specialist
Palliative Care Program
Winnipeg, MB

Linda Dresser, PharmD, FCSHP
Pharmacology Specialist, Antimicrobial Stewardship
University Health Network
Assistant Professor, Leslie Dan Faculty of Pharmacy
University of Toronto
Toronto, ON

Mary Feero, BSc(Pharm), RPh
Owner, The Medicine Shoppe Pharmacy
Fredericton, NB

David Gardner, BScPharm, ACPR, PharmD, MSc
Professor
Department of Psychiatry and College of Pharmacy
Dalhousie University
Halifax, NS

Alfred S. Gin, BScPharm, PharmD, FCSHP
Clinical Pharmacist, Infectious Diseases
Department of Pharmaceutical Services
Health Sciences Centre
Assistant Professor of Medicine (Medical Microbiology)
University of Manitoba
Winnipeg, MB

Gino Gizzarelli, BScPhm, DDS, MSc, (Medical Anesthesia)
University Health Network
Toronto, ON

L. Maria Gutschi, BScPhm, PharmD
Canada Chemists
Scientific Consultant, Patented Medicines Prices Review Board
Faculty of Dentistry and Faculty of Medicine
Canadian Forces Health Support Unit
Ottawa, ON

Jill Hall, BScPharm, ACPR, PharmD
Clinical Assistant Professor, Faculty of Pharmacy and Pharmaceutical Sciences
Pharmaceutical Sciences Consultant, Allergy & Immunology
University of Alberta
Edmonton, AB

Antony J. Ham Pong, MBBS, FRCPC
Consultant, Allergy & Immunology
Assistant Professor (VPT)
Children's Hospital of Eastern Ontario
Ottawa, ON

Brian G. Hardy, PharmD, FCSHP, FCCP
Coordinator, Education and Clinical Programs
Department of Pharmacy
Sunnybrook Health Sciences Centre
Associate Professor, Leslie Dan Faculty of Pharmacy
University of Toronto
Toronto, ON

Lyall Higginson, MD, FRCPC
Professor of Medicine
Clinical Cardiologist
University of Ottawa
Ottawa, ON

Shinya Ito, MD, FRCPC
Professor and Head
Division of Clinical Pharmacology & Toxicology
Department of Pediatrics
Hospital for Sick Children
University of Toronto
Toronto, ON

Derek Jorgenson, BSP, PharmD, FCSHP
Associate Professor
College of Pharmacy and Nutrition
University of Saskatchewan
West Winds Primary Health Centre
Saskatoon, SK

David N. Juurlink, BPhm, MD, PhD, FRCPC, FACMT, FAACT
Professor of Medicine (Pediatrics and Health Policy)
Divisions of General Internal Medicine and Clinical Pharmacology and Toxicology
Sunnybrook Health Sciences Centre
Institute for Clinical Evaluative Sciences
Ontario Poison Centre
Toronto, ON

Steven Katz, MD, FRCPC
Assistant Clinical Professor of Medicine (Rheumatology)
University of Alberta
Edmonton, AB

Heather Kertland, PharmD
Clinical Pharmacy Specialist/Leader
St. Michael's Hospital
Assistant Professor, Leslie Dan Faculty of Pharmacy
University of Toronto
Toronto, ON

Sandra Knowles, RPh, ACPR, BScPhm
Drug Safety Pharmacist
Sunnybrook Health Sciences Centre
University of Toronto
Toronto, ON

Gideon Koren, MD, FRCPC, FACMT
Professor & Director, Motherisk Program
The Hospital for Sick Children and University of Toronto
The Ivey Chair in Molecular Toxicology
The University of Western Ontario
Toronto, ON

Michael Libman, MD, FRCPC
Director, Division of Infectious Disease
Department of Microbiology
McGill University Health Centre
Associate Professor, McGill University
Montreal, QC

Mark J. Makowsky, BSP, PharmD, ACPR
Assistant Professor, Faculty of Pharmacy and Pharmaceutical Sciences
University of Alberta
Edmonton, AB

Anne Massicotte, BPharm, MSc
Drug Information Pharmacist
The Ottawa Hospital, Civic Campus
Ottawa, ON

Doreen Matsui, MD, FRCPC
Department of Pediatrics
Children's Hospital, London Health Sciences Centre
University of Western Ontario
London, ON

G. B. Meterissian, MD, FRCPC
Department of Psychiatry
Faculty of Medicine, McGill University
Montreal General Hospital Site
McGill University Health Centre
Montreal, QC

Katrina Mulherin, BScPharm, PharmD
Deputy Registrar, New Brunswick College of Pharmacists
Project Manager, Association of Faculties of Pharmacy of Canada
Associate Professor (Status), Leslie Dan Faculty of Pharmacy
University of Toronto
Lecturer, University of New Brunswick Faculty of Nursing
Clinical Pharmacist, Sunnybrook Health Science Centre, Neonatal Intensive Care
Toronto, ON

Scott J. Murray, MD, FRCPC
Division of Dermatology
Dalhousie University
Halifax, NS

Tania Mysak, BSP, PharmD
Clinical Practice Manager North Pharmacy Services
Alberta Health Services
Faculty of Pharmacy and Pharmaceutical Sciences
University of Alberta
Edmonton, AB

Richard W. Norman, MD, FRCSC
Chief Urologist
Tantallon Medical Clinics
Upper Tantallon, NS

Cynthia Richard, BSc(Pharm), PhD
Clinical Lecturer, School of Pharmacy
University of Waterloo
Kitchener, ON

Fraoch Shepherd, BSc(Pod)
Chiropodist
Total Foot Care
The Ottawa Hospital
Ottawa, ON

Robert Siemans, MD, FRCSC
Department of Urology
Kingston General Hospital
Queen's University
Kingston, ON

Jose Silveira, BSc, MD, FRCPC, Dip ABAM
Assistant Professor, Department of Psychiatry
University of Toronto
Medical Director, Mental Health and Addiction
Chief of Psychiatry, St. Joseph's Health Centre
Toronto, ON

Neil Skjodt, MD, MSc, FRCPC, FCCP, DABSM, FAASM
Specialist in Internal, Respiratory Critical Care & Sleep Medicine
Adjunct Associate Professor
Canadian Centre for Behavioural Neuroscience
Lethbridge, AB

Kathy Slayter, BScPharm, PharmD, FCSHP
Clinical Pharmacy Specialist, Division of Infectious Diseases
Department of Medicine
Clinical Coordinator, Department of Pharmacy
Capital District Health Authority
Canadian Centre for Vaccinology
Adjunct Assistant Professor, Faculties of Medicine and Health Professions
Dalhousie University
Halifax, NS

Penelope Smyth, BSc, MD, FRCPC
Assistant Professor, Department of Medicine
University of Alberta
Neurologist, MS Specialist
WMC Health Sciences Centre
Edmonton, AB

Laura Targownik, MD, FRCPC, MS(Health Services)
Associate Professor
Section of Gastroenterology
University of Manitoba
Winnipeg, MB

Peter Thomson, BSc(Pharm), PharmD
Clinical Resource Pharmacist, Medicine Program
Winnipeg Regional Health Authority
Clinical Assistant Professor, Faculty of Pharmacy
University of Manitoba
Winnipeg, MB

Deborah L. Thompson, BScPharm, PharmD, BCPP
Clinical Pharmacy Specialist
Fraser Health Mental Health and Substance Use Services
Langley, BC

Nese Yuksel, BScPharm, PharmD, ACPR, FCSHP, NCMP
Associate Professor
Faculty of Pharmacy and Pharmaceutical Sciences
University of Alberta
Edmonton, AB

Editor's Message

Welcome to the *Compendium of Therapeutics for Minor Ailments, Second Edition (CTMA 2)*. Since the first edition of *CTMA*, many exciting changes have taken place in the profession of pharmacy and other primary care disciplines. *CTMA* has been updated and enhanced to meet the growing needs of primary care practitioners. Language around triage and referral has been aligned with the evolution of primary healthcare delivery in recent years—no longer is there a clear line between physician and pharmacist practice with respect to prescriptive authority and the delivery of services such as vaccine administration. Each chapter describes the full spectrum of therapeutic recommendations for the condition, allowing practitioners to apply the information according to their professional and jurisdictional scopes of practice.

The information in these chapters and appendices is invaluable to pharmacists and other healthcare practitioners working on the front line of care delivery. Each chapter provides essential information on conditions that can be self-managed, at least initially, by patients. Sections include pathophysiology, nonpharmacologic and pharmacologic therapy, monitoring of therapy, assessment and treatment algorithms, drug tables and plain-language information for patients. For the second edition, drug tables have been completely reformatted in line with those in the *Compendium of Therapeutic Choices* (*CTC*). Brand names and comparative costs are now included, making these tables even more useful at the point of care. As the breadth of health services provided by pharmacists continues to evolve, it is increasingly important to rely on a dependable source of evidence-based therapeutic information that seamlessly spans the range of nonprescription and prescription therapy, helping pharmacists and patients work together to manage common conditions.

CTMA 2's companion publication, *Compendium of Products for Minor Ailments, Second Edition (CPMA 2)*, provides essential information on available products, organized by condition. Comparative product tables provide a unique source of information on formulations, ingredients and features of nonprescription drugs, natural health products, medical devices and aids to daily living. *CTMA* and *CPMA* are indispensable resources for the optimal management of minor ailments. Now that pharmacists are able to modify or initiate prescription therapy in many Canadian jurisdictions, *CTC* also plays a crucial role in providing complementary information on the management of common ailments. Together, these resources provide an unrivalled compilation of drug and therapeutic information for Canadian primary care practitioners. All are available online (visit pharmacists.ca/rxtx), where they are extensively interlinked—with each other and with CPS monographs.

CPhA is grateful for the expertise and dedication of the many authors and reviewers who contribute to this publication. The Editorial Advisory Committee provides valued strategic guidance on all of CPhA's publications. A skilled team of clinical and scientific editors contribute significantly to the quality of the content, working with authors and reviewers to ensure that it is current, clearly presented and informed by the best available evidence. The final product would not be possible without the talents of CPhA's graphic designers, editorial processing staff, senior product manager, product marketing manager, information technologists and content publishing specialists.

We encourage you to get in touch if you have any comments or questions about this book. Feedback helps us refine and improve our publications, and we welcome your thoughts and suggestions for optimizing the role of *CTMA* in helping you provide the best possible care to your patients.

Barbara Jovaisas

Editor-in-Chief

Editorial Policy, Description and Limitations of Information

Editorial Process

Chapters and appendices in the *Compendium of Therapeutics for Minor Ailments* (*CTMA*) are written by expert authors and are based on the best available evidence. The Canadian Pharmacists Association (CPhA) employs a rigorous review process to ensure that the information is accurate and unbiased. Content is extensively reviewed and validated by CPhA's clinical and scientific editors, and by reviewers who are recognized experts in the relevant clinical area.

CPhA asks authors and reviewers to disclose any potential conflicts of interest, and does not accept funding from pharmaceutical manufacturers for any content that we develop.

Description and Limitations of Information

Although based on the best available evidence, the *Compendium of Therapeutics for Minor Ailments* also contains selected information representing the opinions and experience of individual authors. The authors, editors and publisher have endeavored to ensure the accuracy of the information at the time of printing. Readers should be aware that the text may contain information, statements and drug dosages that differ from those approved by the Therapeutic Products Directorate, Health Canada. The information presented in this text is not intended to be comprehensive. Healthcare practitioners are encouraged to seek additional and confirmatory information to meet their practice requirements and standards.

Errata

In spite of the rigorous review process, should a major error be identified it will be corrected immediately on www.pharmacists.ca/errata and reflected in the electronic version on myrxtx.ca (formerly e-therapeutics.ca). All errors will be corrected in the next print edition.

How to Use the *Compendium of Therapeutics for Minor Ailments*

The *Compendium of Therapeutics for Minor Ailments Second Edition (CTMA 2)* contains 93 chapters and 6 appendices. Following the Communicating with Patients section, the book is organized according to body systems.

General appendices (Complementary and Alternative Therapies, Home Testing, Information for the Traveller, Medical Devices and Aids to Daily Living, Pregnancy and Breastfeeding: Self-care Therapy for Common Conditions and Nutritional Supplements) follow the therapeutic topics.

High-quality photographs, located in a separate section following Dermatologic Conditions, help you visually identify and distinguish certain conditions.

Each chapter is presented in a similar format: Pathophysiology, Patient Assessment, Goals of Therapy, Nonpharmacologic Therapy, Pharmacologic Therapy, Monitoring of Therapy, Assessment and Treatment Algorithms, Drug Tables, Resource Tips (for patients), Suggested Readings and References. Prevention and pregnancy/breastfeeding are also addressed when appropriate. Illustrations complement the text of the chapters. Nonprescription and prescription therapy and natural health products are described under Pharmacologic Therapy. References to corresponding chapters in CPhA's *Compendium of Therapeutic Choices* are included where applicable.

CTMA 2's companion publication, the *Compendium of Products for Minor Ailments Second Edition (CPMA 2)*, offers a unique compilation of comparative tables of nonprescription drugs and devices. Tables are organized by condition/purpose to facilitate product selection.

Patient Information sheets on self-care conditions (titled What You Need to Know) follow each therapeutic chapter, and we invite you to photocopy them for your patients. Additional sources of information designed for patients are provided as Resource Tips.

The entire text is referenced and based on the best available evidence.

Chapter 1
Effective Pharmacist-patient Interactions

Barbara J. Farrell, BScPhm, PharmD

Throughout an interaction, the participants (e.g., the pharmacist and the patient) alternate between the roles of "sender" and "receiver" of the message. Information should not be provided in a unidirectional manner. Rather, information is exchanged. As a receiver, the pharmacist has the responsibility of listening to what the patient is saying, understanding the issue and providing feedback on whether the message was understood. As the sender, the pharmacist has the responsibility of transmitting the message clearly, in language understood by the patient and in an environment conducive to clear transmission.

For effective patient interaction consider 2 major components—how the interaction is organized, and how well the pharmacist uses communication skills. Use of verbal and nonverbal communication skills throughout the interaction ensures that a full description of the presenting complaint and associated symptoms, as well as other relevant information, are gathered from the patient.

There are 3 major stages or types of patient interactions: assessment and triage, counselling, and follow up. The chapter provides guidance on how these interactions can be organized and examples of the topics and questions that could be included. Further detailed discussion of the process of assessment and triage can be found in Chapter 3: Pharmacist Assessment of the Self-treating Patient.

Assessment and Triage

The primary purposes of this stage of the interaction with a patient are to determine the nature of the patient's concerns or symptoms, and to help the patient determine whether self-treatment with a pharmacy product is appropriate or referral to another provider is necessary. A pharmacy technician or pharmacist may initially respond to a request from a patient in the pharmacy. The pharmacy technician will need to use these initial steps in greeting the patient—finding out in a general way about the problem and ensuring comfort and privacy, then engaging the pharmacist in conducting the patient interview and assessment process. The emphasis is on skillfully eliciting relevant information from the patient so that the pharmacist gains a complete picture of the patient's issue and does not jump to conclusions about what the patient needs. This is also the point at which the pharmacist begins to build rapport with patients and earn their trust.

How

- Introduce yourself or greet the patient by name if you know him or her
- Find out briefly what the patient needs
- Explain, in a general way, how you can help
- Ensure comfort and privacy to impress that you are concerned about how the patient is feeling and value the importance of confidentiality
- Proceed with questioning, listening and basic physical assessment (if required), for assessment and triage. Suggestions for the assessment process are found in Chapter 3: Pharmacist Assessment of the Self-treating Patient.

Examples of statements and questions that can be used at each stage are listed in Figure 1.

Figure 1: **What to Say when Assessing Patients**

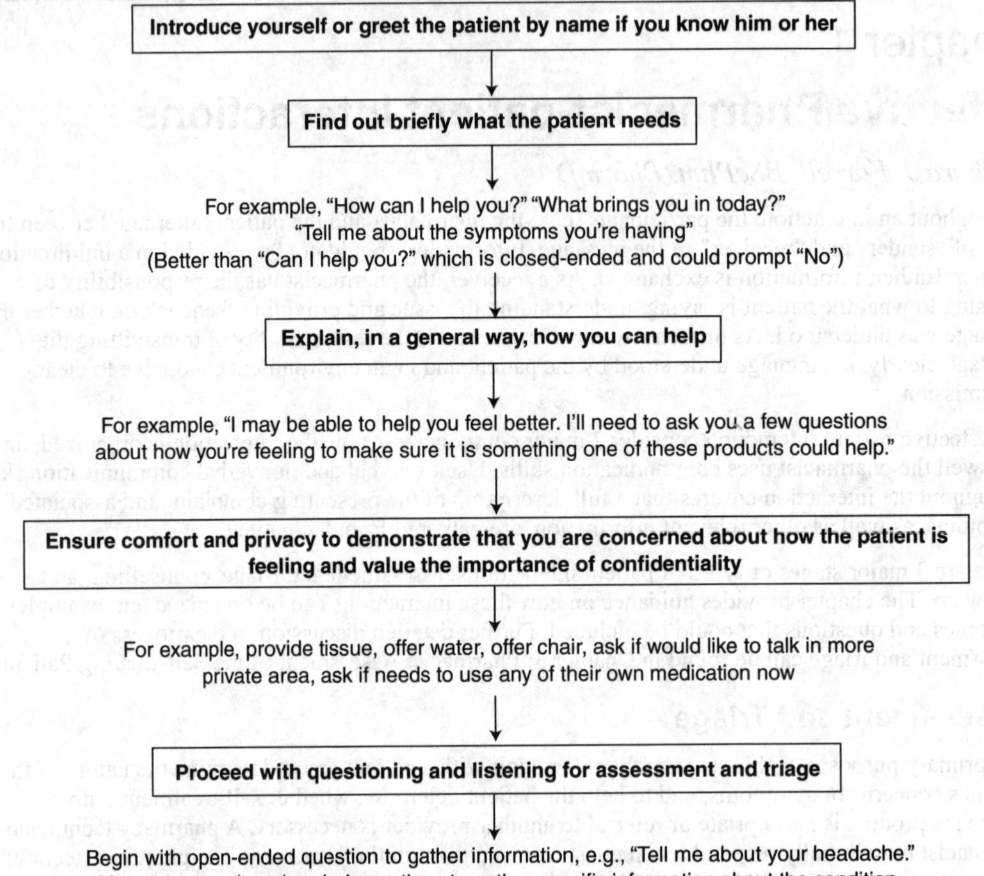

Use good communication skills. This will help you send messages in a manner that can be understood by the patient and will help you understand the messages that you receive. Both verbal and nonverbal communication skills are important and should reflect one another. Good verbal communication skills and poor or distracting nonverbal skills send conflicting messages, and the patient may lose confidence in the pharmacist. The reverse is also true.

Verbal communication skills include: the ability to question appropriately (Table 1), speaking in language that the patient can understand (Table 2), listening effectively (Table 3) and responding using empathy (Table 4).

Nonverbal communication transmits more than half of the messages that people send and receive. These skills must be practised when the pharmacist is both speaking and listening to the patient. Techniques to optimize nonverbal communication are outlined in Table 5.

The importance of listening and being empathetic, through effective verbal and nonverbal communication, cannot be underestimated. Spending time without being distracted, as well as understanding patient feelings and perspectives without judging, criticizing or blaming, builds acceptance and respect that creates a therapeutic alliance.

Table 1: **Question Appropriately**

Use open-ended questions:	Use closed-ended questions:	Avoid:
▪ When you need to gather symptom information that is uppermost in the patient's mind ▪ When you need to begin a line of questioning ▪ When you want to determine the patient's understanding, level of sophistication of their assessment of the problem and what level of vocabulary would be appropriate for you to use ▪ To convey a willingness to listen ▪ To promote rapport and trust Examples: ▪ Describe... (the feeling to me) ▪ Explain... (how the pain feels) ▪ Tell me about... (the heartburn) ▪ How... (does the headache feel?) ▪ What... (brings you in today?)	▪ When you want a yes, no or number response ▪ When you want to gather specific, focused information about the nature of the symptoms and treatment ▪ When you need to gather information quickly ▪ When you need to keep a talkative patient focused Examples: ▪ Do you... (have any discharge?) ▪ Have you... (ever had this before?) ▪ Will you... (be able to take this every 4 hours?) ▪ How many times... (do you wake up during the night?)	▪ Using only open-ended questions (will make the discussion much longer and unfocused) ▪ Using only closed-ended questions (will prevent discussion from moving to details of which you are unaware, may create passivity) ▪ Asking several questions in succession without patient input. For example asking, is the pain mostly in your stomach or is it more like heartburn? What does it feel like? Do you usually get it after you eat? (one after another without giving the patient a chance to answer) ▪ Asking leading or biased questions. For example, "There isn't any blood in your stool, is there?" ▪ Asking questions that start with "why" (can seem judgmental and cause defensiveness) ▪ Using slang or medical terminology

Table 2: **Speak at an Appropriate Language Level**

Use:	Not:	Use:	Not:
A lot of phlegm	Productive	Digestive system	Gastrointestinal
High blood pressure	Hypertension	Lower	Decrease
Painkiller	Analgesic	Raise	Increase or elevate
Cough suppressant	Antitussive	Condition	Diagnosis
Shooting pain	Radiating pain	How bad	Severity
Bum	Rectum	On the skin	Topically

Counselling

The main purposes of this stage of interaction are to assist with product selection and provide counselling that will enable the patient to gain the most benefit from the product. Again, the pharmacist acts as both "sender" and "receiver" of messages, but with more emphasis on sending messages to the patient. To ensure counselling is effective, pharmacists need to pay attention to transmitting their message clearly and explicitly without adhering to a strict monologue type of counselling routine. They need to continually check for understanding throughout and pay attention to new information that the patient may offer.

Table 3: **Listen Effectively**

You are listening when you:	You are not listening when you:
▪ Encourage talking (e.g., hmm, yes, go on) ▪ Wait during silence (allows the patient a chance to think and react) ▪ Repeat (so you're having difficulty sleeping) ▪ Reflect (why do you think that) ▪ Explore (could you say a bit more about that) ▪ Summarize accurately ▪ Ask questions ▪ Paraphrase	▪ Are in a hurry (looking at watch) ▪ Interrupt ▪ Change subject for no apparent reason ▪ Ask a question twice ▪ Don't ask any questions at all ▪ Are talking ▪ Don't allow the patient a chance to finish speaking ▪ Lecture ▪ Cut off expressions of feeling ▪ Give advice prematurely

Table 4: **Respond Effectively**[a]

Use empathy	Avoid automatically giving the following responses until you understand what the patient is feeling
▪ Make an effort to understand how the patient is feeling;[b] respond to that feeling ▪ Some of what the patient tells you involves their feelings about it; be sensitive to those feelings	▪ Judgmental or critical responses (You shouldn't be doing that) ▪ Advising/recommending responses ▪ Reassuring responses (You'll be fine) ▪ Generalizing responses (Everybody feels that way) ▪ Distracting responses, e.g., changing the subject

a *Some responses will be factual but always consider why the patient raised the point or asked the question.*
b *You can learn a lot about a patient's feelings by observing their nonverbal behaviour: do they look sad? frustrated? angry? weak or sick? worried? in pain?*

Table 5: **Nonverbal Communication**

Do	Do not
▪ Smile ▪ Demonstrate genuine interest and concern ▪ Maintain eye contact as culturally, socially and gender appropriate ▪ Use appropriate body language (show interest and concern in your facial expression, maintain appropriate distance from the patient, keep your body posture open, lean forward) ▪ Sit or squat if the patient is sitting, stand if the patient is standing ▪ Have a neat and clean personal appearance and a neat and clean physical environment	▪ Look down or away repeatedly ▪ Look at or play with other objects repeatedly ▪ Cross your arms or your legs ▪ Use distracting gestures ▪ Tilt to one side ▪ Slouch ▪ Stare ▪ Get so close that you are in the patient's "personal space" ▪ Have barriers between you and the patient (high counter)

How

- Establish goals
- Help with product selection
- Provide information (while continuing to listen to the patient for new information)
- Check for understanding
- Close

Examples of statements and questions that can be used at each stage are listed in Figure 2.

Use communication skills. The same skills highlighted in the Follow Up section apply.

Additional verbal skills that are useful in the counselling component of the interaction include the rate, volume, tone and pitch of speech. These are outlined in Table 6.

The nonverbal skills used in counselling are the same as those used in assessment and triage. You may need to use additional nonverbal skills to indicate the closure of the interaction. Examples are standing up (if sitting), changing stance, shaking hands and sometimes packing up papers or putting pen and paper away.

Figure 2: What to Say when Counselling Patients

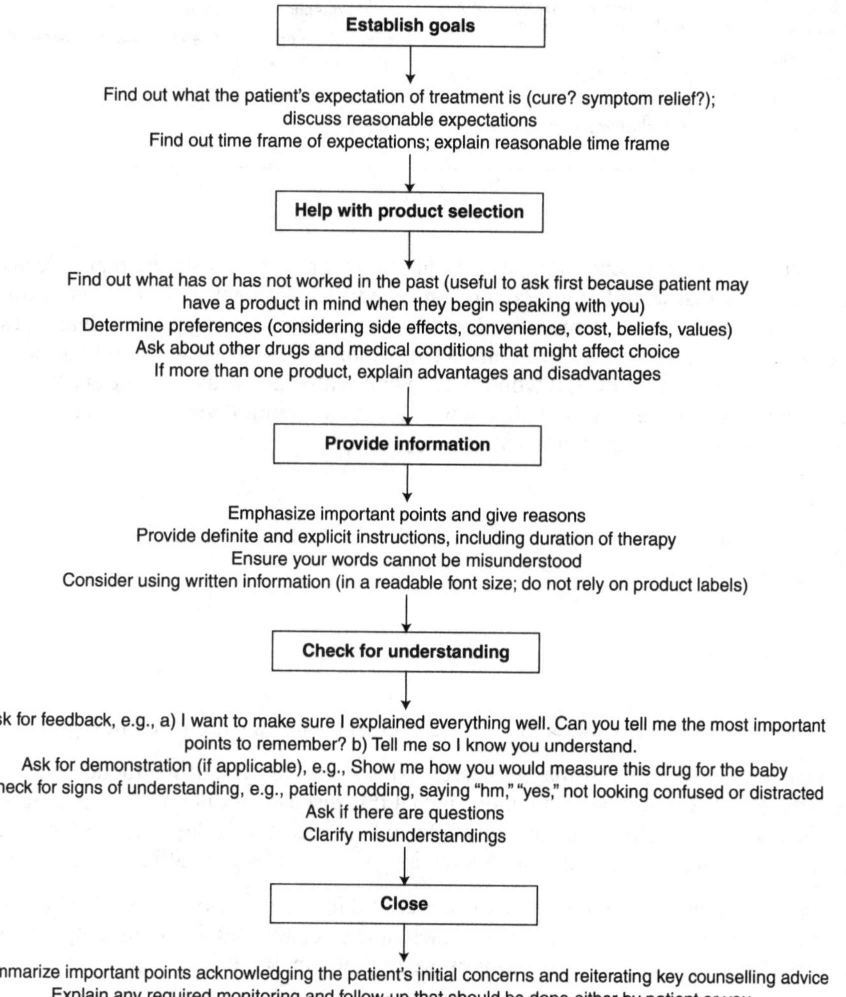

Establish goals
Find out what the patient's expectation of treatment is (cure? symptom relief?); discuss reasonable expectations
Find out time frame of expectations; explain reasonable time frame
Help with product selection
Find out what has or has not worked in the past (useful to ask first because patient may have a product in mind when they begin speaking with you)
Determine preferences (considering side effects, convenience, cost, beliefs, values)
Ask about other drugs and medical conditions that might affect choice
If more than one product, explain advantages and disadvantages
Provide information
Emphasize important points and give reasons
Provide definite and explicit instructions, including duration of therapy
Ensure your words cannot be misunderstood
Consider using written information (in a readable font size; do not rely on product labels)
Check for understanding
Ask for feedback, e.g., a) I want to make sure I explained everything well. Can you tell me the most important points to remember? b) Tell me so I know you understand.
Ask for demonstration (if applicable), e.g., Show me how you would measure this drug for the baby
Check for signs of understanding, e.g., patient nodding, saying "hm," "yes," not looking confused or distracted
Ask if there are questions
Clarify misunderstandings
Close
Summarize important points acknowledging the patient's initial concerns and reiterating key counselling advice
Explain any required monitoring and follow-up that should be done either by patient or you
Arrange time and date of follow-up call if necessary
End graciously

Challenge: Closing an interview with a patient who continues to talk once the product is selected and counselling is provided: try the nonverbal techniques listed above; try a closed-ended question like "Do you have any further questions?"

Table 6: **Speaking Skills**

Do	Do not
▪ Slow down; resist the temptation to "download" information quickly, e.g., learn to pause when there are periods or natural commas in your sentences. This helps the patient digest the information and provides an opportunity for them to speak if they have a question or another piece of information to provide ▪ Speak loudly enough so the patient can hear you ▪ Speak in a friendly tone ▪ Raise and lower the pitch of your voice appropriately (lower at the end of sentences; lower if patient is hard of hearing) ▪ Use precise language, e.g., "with an 8-oz glass of water," *not* "with plenty of water;" or "one hour before a meal," *not* "on an empty stomach" ▪ Write information down when verbal explanation is not sufficient	▪ Increase the rate of speech (tempting when you have a lot of information to provide) ▪ Speak so loudly that others in the pharmacy can also hear you (have another staff member tell you if your conversation was heard) ▪ Speak in a condescending or patronizing manner ▪ Speak in a monotonous voice pitch (boring) ▪ Raise your pitch at the end of a sentence (sounds like you are questioning yourself) ▪ Hand out printed written information without also providing verbal counselling

Follow Up

Use follow up to determine whether the patient's goals were achieved with the plan selected and that no red flag has arisen that would require referral for medical treatment. Follow up is similar in format to a combination of both the assessment/triage phase and the counselling phase. Ideally, it's best if the same person can provide the follow up as this is the person with whom the patient has developed a relationship. Let the patient know you would like to call within a few days to ensure that the plan is working and that no problems have developed with the medication. Patients appreciate this and are often happy to arrange a time for you to call.

How

- Introduce yourself
- Explain purpose of follow up
- Assess response
- Advise if necessary
- Close

Examples of statements and questions that can be used at each stage are listed in Figure 3.

Use good communication skills. A major difference between this type of interaction and the assessment/triage and counselling interactions is that this discussion often takes place over the telephone. Since neither you nor the patient will be able to read each other's nonverbal cues, particular attention must be paid to clear verbal communication. Verbal skills are outlined in Table 7.

The nonverbal messages you send will confirm your real interest in and concern for the patient. They will also make it easier for both of you to hear each other. Techniques for optimizing nonverbal communication during telephone conversations are outlined in Table 8.

Table 7: **Verbal Skills to Use Over the Telephone**

Do
▪ Start with a friendly greeting ▪ Speak more slowly than you would face to face ▪ Enunciate clearly ▪ Let the patient know if you need to stop talking to write something down or pause to think ▪ If you use a speaker phone confirm that the patient can hear you ▪ Hold the receiver an appropriate distance from your mouth so that your voice is not muffled or too soft

Table 8: **Nonverbal Skills to Use During Telephone Conversations**

Do	Do not
▪ Be prepared ▪ Give your full attention to the phone call ▪ Smile to help ensure your voice carries a friendly tone ▪ Listen carefully to the tone of the patient's voice and speech in order to determine concerns or misunderstanding	▪ Put the patient on hold ▪ Be interrupted ▪ Have background noise, e.g., voices, music, ringing telephones ▪ Be overheard by other people

Tips for Special Situations

Tips for interacting with the talkative patient who gets off topic:

- Minimize your contribution to the "off topic"
- Acknowledge but continue returning to the questioning or counselling; if possible, try to link the therapy discussion to the "off topic," e.g., patient starts talking about husband's death 10 years ago; ask "Is that when your stomach problems started?" then focus discussion back on today's presenting complaint
- Try referring back to the discussion about the presenting complaint and introducing a closed-ended question (e.g., "A few minutes ago, you said that you were having trouble sleeping; have you had this problem before?"), then continue with the line of questioning.

Tips for interacting with the angry patient:

- Remember that feelings of hostility are rarely personal; the patient may be under a great deal of stress
- Acknowledge anger
- Let patients vent their anger
- Stay calm
- Lower your voice, speak slowly and maintain eye contact
- If you are at fault, agree; agreeing often diffuses anger
- Avoid defensiveness (which can aggravate the situation).

Tips for interacting with the depressed/upset/crying patient:

- Offer privacy, tissues, time alone
- Offer to call someone
- Ask "Is it something you want to talk about?"

Figure 3: **What to Say at Follow Up**

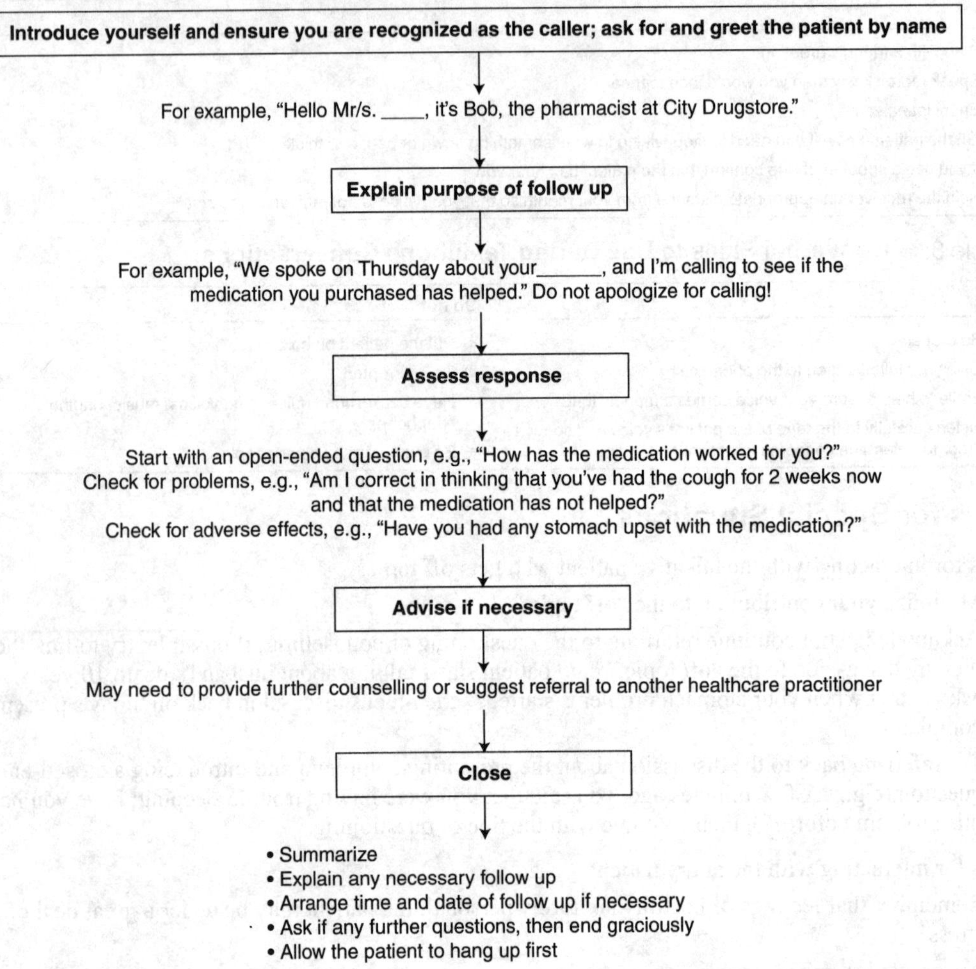

Introduce yourself and ensure you are recognized as the caller; ask for and greet the patient by name
For example, "Hello Mr/s. ____, it's Bob, the pharmacist at City Drugstore."
Explain purpose of follow up
For example, "We spoke on Thursday about your______, and I'm calling to see if the medication you purchased has helped." Do not apologize for calling!
Assess response
Start with an open-ended question, e.g., "How has the medication worked for you?"
Check for problems, e.g., "Am I correct in thinking that you've had the cough for 2 weeks now and that the medication has not helped?"
Check for adverse effects, e.g., "Have you had any stomach upset with the medication?"
Advise if necessary
May need to provide further counselling or suggest referral to another healthcare practitioner
Close
• Summarize
• Explain any necessary follow up
• Arrange time and date of follow up if necessary
• Ask if any further questions, then end graciously
• Allow the patient to hang up first

Tips for interacting with the patient who does not want to see their doctor:

- Explain your reasons for concern; be assertive, e.g., "When diarrhea goes on longer than 2 weeks, I worry that there could be something serious going on; it's important to see a doctor because they can tell if there are any serious problems."

Tips for interacting with the patient who does not want to take your advice:

- Determine preferences before recommending a product
- Explain advantages and disadvantages in terms of patient's medications and medical conditions
- Consider "rolling with it"; sometimes resistance is normal (think of products to help with smoking cessation); consider using techniques of motivational interviewing described in Chapter 2: Facilitating Behaviour Change, if behaviour change is challenging.

Tips for interacting with the patient with hearing impairment:

- Ask if the patient can hear you
- Ask if better to speak to one side

- Face the patient so they can read your lips
- Speak more slowly, enunciate clearly and lower your tone of voice to make it easier for the patient to differentiate words
- Increase your volume of speech but don't shout
- Use short, simple sentences
- Keep in mind that your facial expression, body posture and gesture are as important as lip movements for the patient to understand what you are saying.

Tips for interacting with the patient with vision impairment:

- Tell the patient what you are doing and if there is anyone else present, e.g., a student
- If writing information, use large print and pastel-coloured paper rather than white.

Tips for interacting with the patient with cognitive impairment:

- Speak slowly
- Allow time for patient to answer questions
- Write information down.

Tips for interacting with the noncommunicative patient:

- Wait during silence so the patient can respond
- Ask open-ended questions.

Tips for interacting with the patient with a potentially embarrassing complaint:

- Offer privacy
- Use closed-ended questions for assessment, e.g., "Do you have any discharge? Is it clear or white?" *not* "Tell me about the discharge."

Tips for interacting with the elderly patient:

- Slow down your rate of speech
- Decrease the amount of information given at one time.

Tips for interacting with the patient with speech impairment:

- Speak slowly
- Face the patient
- Let the patient finish speaking
- Provide writing pads
- Learn simple sign language if used by the patient.

Tips for interacting with the patient who does not speak your language:

- Speak slowly and simply
- Use an interpreter, e.g., caregiver.

Tips for interacting with the aphasic patient (patients who have perhaps suffered a stroke and have a decreased ability to understand what others are saying and to express themselves):

- Do not shout
- Avoid complex conversations
- Be patient
- Help patient select words by offering a few choices

- Talk to caregiver.

Tips for interacting with the caregiver:

- Provide written information for the patient
- Follow up by telephone (if possible) with the patient.

Evaluate Yourself

We can all improve our communication skills. There are some easy ways to evaluate your effectiveness. Try audio or video recording some patient interactions (with permission of course). You may find that you sound different and say things that are different from what you thought you said. Look for nonverbal cues in others: what do you like? what do you dislike? Think about the nonverbal cues that you send. Have a student or colleague watch you interact with a patient and then give you some feedback. Think about the patient: was he or she relaxed and open during your discussion? did you check for patient understanding? how did you do?

Suggested Readings

Kimberlin CL, Tindall WN. *Communication skills in pharmacy practice: a practical guide for students and practitioners*. 6th ed. Philadelphia: Wolters Kluwer/Lippincott Williams & Wilkins; 2011.

National Association of Pharmacy Regulatory Authorities. *Professional competencies for Canadian pharmacists at entry to practice*. 2nd rev. Ottawa: NAPRA; 2007. Available from: napra.ca/Content_Files/Files/Entry_to_Practice_Competencies_March2007_final_new_layout_2009.pdf.

Rantucci MJ. *Pharmacists talking with patients: a guide to patient counseling*. 2nd ed. Philadelphia: Lippincott Williams & Wilkins; 2007.

Chapter 2
Facilitating Behaviour Change

Lisa Dolovich, BSc Phm, PharmD, MSc

Changing behaviour is the culmination of a complex set of thoughts, beliefs, motivations and actions. Maintaining a new behaviour over time requires continued motivation, engagement and interest. Individuals are ultimately responsible for their own health. Healthcare practitioners cannot dictate behaviour; they can only help facilitate positive behaviours that would improve a person's health and well-being.

Effectively managing a medical condition almost always requires some type of short- or long-term behaviour change. This change could be to adhere to a medication regimen, exercise regularly, decrease dietary fat or salt, reduce body weight, stop smoking or monitor blood pressure or blood glucose.

It is vital that healthcare practitioners understand how to facilitate behaviour change so that people can be as successful as possible in initiating and maintaining change. The transtheoretical model of behaviour change is a well-accepted framework that can help healthcare practitioners understand decision making and change. It guides practitioners in individualizing strategies based on the patient, and explains that it takes varying amounts of time for patients to move through stages of change—a process that can continue throughout life.

Motivational interviewing, a directive counselling technique, can be used to help foster behaviour change. The transtheoretical model of behaviour change can help identify patient's specific stage of change, then motivational interviewing can be used to help move them from one stage to another.[1]

The Transtheoretical Model of Behaviour Change

The transtheoretical model of behaviour change is based on an extensive review of leading theories of psychotherapy and behaviour change.[2,3,4] It is called "transtheoretical" because it integrates many major theories of intervention in the psychotherapy and behaviour-change fields.

The model is an integrative framework for understanding how individuals and populations move towards initiating and maintaining health behaviour change. It deals with intentional behaviour change, i.e., when individuals intend to change their own behaviour or others intend to help them change.[5] It has been tested in multiple studies, mainly in patients who had problem behaviours such as smoking, poor diet and lack of exercise.

This theory encompasses and integrates 5 core components:

1. Stages of change
2. Processes of change
3. Decisional balance
4. Self-efficacy
5. Temptation

The best chance for successful movement through the stages of change incorporates aspects from all of these core constructs.

Stages of Change

There are 6 stages of change: precontemplation, contemplation, preparation, action, maintenance and termination (Figure 1).[4]

Precontemplation

People who are in this stage of change are not intending to change their behaviour in the foreseeable future (within the next 6 months). They are generally uninformed or underinformed about the consequences of their current behaviour.[4] They may be reluctant or resistant to change. They may have tried to change but became discouraged because they did not succeed.[4]

Contemplation

People in this stage are intending to change, at least within the next 6 months.[4] They are aware that there is a need for change and are open to information and education. They recognize the benefits (pros) of changing but are also very much aware of the disadvantages (cons). These opposing beliefs can prevent someone from moving on to the next stage. People in this stage are generally not ready for traditional action-oriented programs.[4]

Preparation

People who are in this stage are intending to take action in the immediate future (in the next month).[4] They are beginning to set goals and prepare emotionally for change. They are the most open to change.

Figure 1: **The Transtheoretical Model of Behaviour Change**[a,2,3,4]

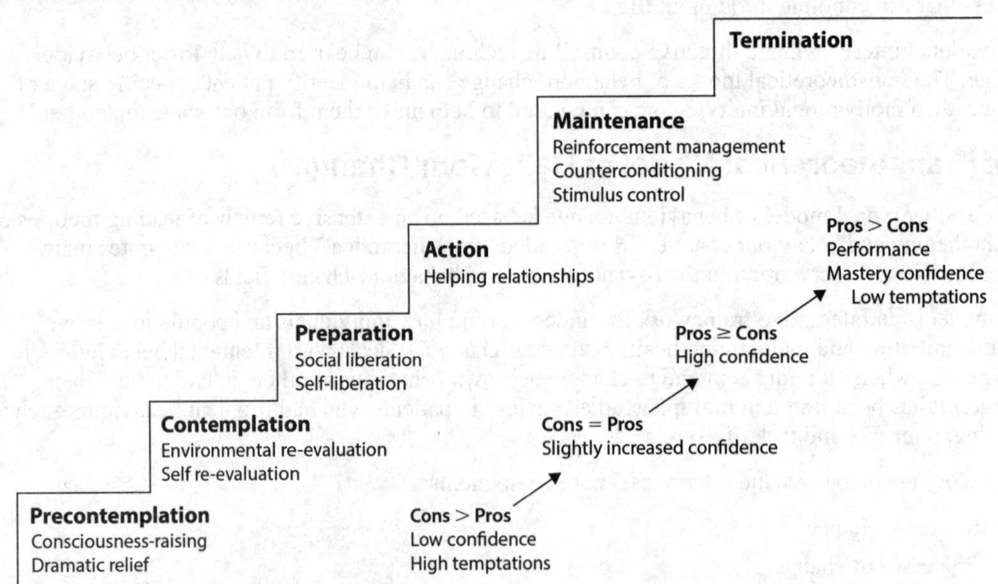

[a] The figure shows the stages of change (e.g., Action) in bold from left to right, the 10 processes of change (see Table 1) that can support individuals to varying degrees at each stage of change, and how pros and cons, self-efficacy (confidence) and temptations manifest across each of the stages of change.

Abbreviations: Cons = disadvantages; Pros = benefits

Action

People in this stage of change have actually engaged in new behaviours within the past 6 months.[4] They are carrying out plans, dealing with negative forces and developing a fledgling confidence in their ability to continue with their new behaviour. But they may also experience guilt, failure and limits to personal freedom.[6] Since a person's action is observable, the overall concept of behaviour change has often been equated with action, so it is useful to recognize that the action stage is only 1 of the 6 stages of change.[4]

Maintenance

People in the maintenance stage have been engaged in the new behaviour for at least 6 months. They are working to prevent relapse. This stage can last anywhere from 6 months to 5 years.[4]

Termination

This stage of change includes people who have completely integrated a new behaviour into their lifestyle.[4] The new behaviour is now a usual action. They are certain they will not return to their old behaviour.

Figure 2: **Identifying the Stages of Change[2,4,6,7]**

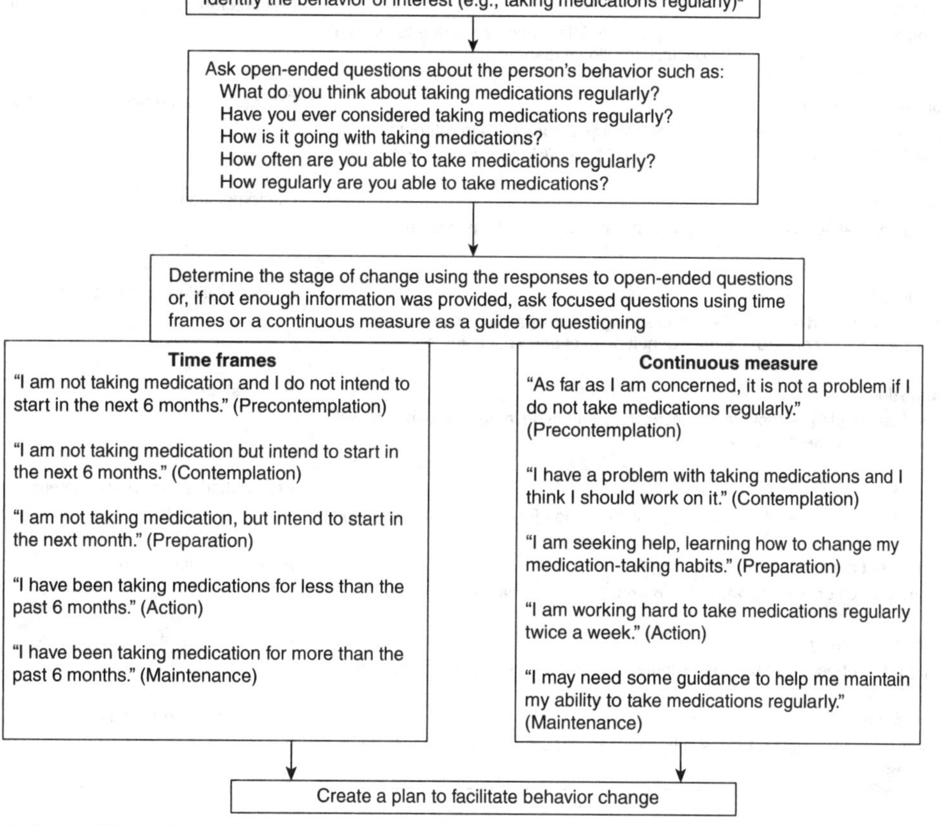

[a] Other behaviours could be exercising regularly, decreasing dietary fat or salt, reducing body weight, stopping smoking or monitoring blood pressure or blood glucose.

Patient Assessment to Identify Stages of Change

An assessment plan to identify what stage of change a person is in for a particular behaviour (in this case taking medications regularly) is shown in Figure 2.

Processes of Change

The processes of change are the covert and overt actions that people use to progress through the stages of change.[4] Different processes of change should be applied at different stages to help people move from stage to stage. This concept is an extremely useful one to consider when developing intervention programs.[4] The processes are listed, defined and matched to the stages of change in Table 1. Healthcare practitioners who recognize the need for a change to occur, and then design an intervention to help the person go through the specific process of change, will help them achieve success.

Table 1: **Characteristics of the Processes of Change Based on the Transtheoretical Model of Behaviour Change[4,6]**

Process	Applicable Stages
Consciousness-raising Gaining and thinking about the causes, consequences and cures for a particular health behaviour	Precontemplation and contemplation
Dramatic relief Experiencing or expressing feelings in response to information about the hazards of not changing, and then recovering from this emotional response	Precontemplation and contemplation
Environmental re-evaluation Assessing the differences in one's social environment compared to without a particular behaviour (e.g., the effect of smoking on others)	Precontemplation and contemplation
Self re-evaluation Evaluating one's attitudes and self-image compared to without a particular behaviour	Contemplation
Social liberation Recognizing, taking advantage of and supporting social opportunities that help others in the environment with a similar condition to change behaviours	Contemplation and preparation
Self-liberation Realizing that people are capable of successfully engaging in healthy behaviours if they make a commitment to do so	Preparation
Helping relationships The existence of meaningful others who provide support for one's efforts to change	Preparation, action and maintenance
Reinforcement management Rewarding oneself or being rewarded by others for healthy behaviours	Action and maintenance
Counterconditioning Developing and engaging in new behaviours to substitute for old, unhealthy ones	Action and maintenance
Stimulus control Removing cues that trigger relapses in behaviours and adding cues to facilitate healthy ones	Action and maintenance

Decisional Balance

Decisional balance encompasses the weighing of the pros and cons of behaviour change by an individual who is thinking about changing. When lists of pros and cons generated by participants in studies were assessed, it was found that the cons of changing were higher than the pros for people in precontemplation stage, and the pros were higher than the cons for people in the action stage.[2] It has also been shown that the pros must increase twice as much as the cons decrease for a person to move from precontemplation to action.[8] Therefore, a healthcare professional doing a patient assessment should recognize what a person's decisional balance is likely to be (depending on their stage of change) to help determine whether the predicted balance of a person's particular pros and cons has been detected. Interventions need to target reducing cons or increasing pros accordingly.

Self-efficacy

Self-efficacy is the situation-specific confidence that people have about their ability to cope with high-risk situations without relapsing to their unhealthy or high-risk habit.[4,9] The cognitive beliefs people have about their self-efficacy influence their activities, motivations, persistence, thought patterns and emotional responses to difficult situations.[9,10,11] Self-efficacy is low in the initial stage of change and progressively increases as people move through the stages.

Temptation

Temptation is the intensity of urges to engage in a specific habit when in the midst of difficult situations. Common tempting situations that can create difficulties in undertaking or maintaining behaviour change include positive social situations, emotional distress and cravings.[4]

Developing a Plan to Facilitate Behaviour Change

Once a person's at-risk behaviour and stage of change have been identified, a plan to facilitate a person's behaviour change can be developed and implemented (Table 2). People do not skip stages. Instead, success occurs when there is movement along the continuum of change.[5] Few people are in the preparation stage for more than one behaviour at a time, so it is more helpful to identify the highest-priority issue and work only on this behaviour. A study examining those who have at-risk behaviours (e.g., smokers) found the distribution to be the following: precontemplation (40%), contemplation (40%) and preparation (20%).[4] A group of patients with arthritis who were assessed for their willingness to adopt self-management strategies included 44% of people in the precontemplation stage and 11% of people in the contemplation stage.[12] Given that most people are not in the preparation or action stage for many at-risk behaviours, those who are intending to change will not be helped by conventional action-oriented approaches. Various strategies specific to each stage of change are provided in Table 3.

Table 2: **Steps to Facilitate Behaviour Change**

1. Complete an initial general patient assessment (medical and medication histories).
2. Identify at-risk behaviours.
3. Identify stages of change for each behaviour (Figure 1).
4. Determine priorities for change (focus on only one issue at a time).
5. Ensure these priorities are consistent with urgent health needs based on health consequences.
6. Complete a focused patient assessment for the targeted behaviour, including the patient's particular history, personal circumstances and personality.
7. Create appropriate strategies that are matched to patients' stage of change and their individual circumstances.
8. Monitor progress to facilitate movement through stages, respond to relapses and determine whether the termination stage occurs.

Table 3: **Stages of Change and Healthcare Professional Assessment and Strategies for Intervention**[4,6]

Stage	Characteristics	Sample Questions about Taking Medications	Strategies to Facilitate Behaviour Change
Precontemplation	Not intending to change within next 6 months; discouraged, uninformed, underinformed, has not tried anything; cons outweighs pros; low self-efficacy; temptations are high	"What do you see are the benefits of taking medications?" "What have people said to you about your medical condition?" "Would you like to read more about the benefits?" "What pressures do you have to take medications?" "What kind of help could you get to help you take your medications?"	▪ Educate to raise their consciousness. ▪ Create some uncertainty so people begin to question whether their current behaviour patterns are the best ones. ▪ Provide personalized information regarding benefits and risks. ▪ Give information about helpful services available when patients are ready. ▪ Identify barriers to change (e.g., what knowledge gaps or errors exist, what environmental or social issues exist?). ▪ Focus on increasing awareness of the pros of changing. ▪ Do not cheerlead, use persuasive strategies, be argumentative, suggest or expect change or let information overload occur. ▪ Do not use action-oriented strategies.
Contemplation	Intending to try something within 6 months; open to information, education; slightly higher self-efficacy than precontemplation stage; temptations are high; pros and cons are about equal	"What is difficult about taking your medications? How can I help?" "Who would help you to take your medications?" "How would taking your medications help your health?" "What is one small thing you could do to help you take your medications?"	▪ Help them accept ownership of the problem. ▪ Help identify advantages and try to soften the effect of the disadvantages. ▪ Use a pros vs. cons approach and try to eliminate cons (e.g., money, memory aids). ▪ Identify barriers and temptations (self- and environmental evaluations). ▪ Help bolster self-confidence. ▪ Help identify their own and others attitudes towards new vs. old behaviour. ▪ Encourage them to talk to you again when they are ready to begin taking their medications. ▪ Do not use action-oriented strategies.
Preparation	Ready to engage in behaviour(s) in the next month; beginning to set goals and get emotionally ready for change; pros and cons are about equal, or pros are greater than cons	"Have you decided whether you are going to start medications? When is that?" "Have you told your doctor you are going to continue to take the medications?"	▪ Help them commit to a course of action (e.g., suggest a date they start, tell them to tell other people they are starting, contract to make the change, set objective and realistic goals).

Stage	Characteristics	Sample Questions about Taking Medications	Strategies to Facilitate Behaviour Change
		"Have you thought about how you are going to change your schedule to make medication-taking easier?"	▪ Announce course of action to others. ▪ Identify and involve supportive others in the plan for change. ▪ Provide frequent encouragement. ▪ Increase awareness of social policies that support their new behaviour (e.g., smoking ban, Canada's Food Guide). ▪ Engage in action-focused education program.
Action	Actually trying to change behaviour; improved self-efficacy; pros outweigh cons; temptations are low	"How have you had to rearrange your life so that you can take your medications more easily?" "Who has been helping you stick to your plan?" "How have you been feeling about how to manage taking your medications?"	▪ Reinforce successes to increase self-efficacy. ▪ Assist with stimulus control (reminders, conduct encouraging follow-up calls). ▪ Support their use of helping relationships. ▪ Highlight decreasing the cons. ▪ Recognize and quickly address faltering behaviour change (e.g., frequent monitoring, work to problem-solve unanticipated issues).
Maintenance	Has been engaged in new behaviours for at least 6 months; working to prevent relapse; self-efficacy is high, temptations are low; taking responsibility for actions	"How is taking your medications going?" "What do you think has been the most helpful thing you did to achieve success?" (Reinforce this) "Have there been any difficulties with taking your medications over the last while?"	▪ Reinforcement of successes (notes, measurement of results, updates on benefits of activity). ▪ Assist with stimulus control (reminders, conduct encouraging follow-up calls). ▪ Suggest additional behaviours that can add to current success. ▪ Suggest alterations that remove cues that trigger relapses. ▪ Recognize relapses as part of process and assist with getting back on track.
Termination	Zero temptation and 100% self-efficacy; will not return to old habits	"How is taking your medications going?"	▪ Recognize that regular healthcare professional facilitation is no longer required.

Motivational Interviewing

Motivational interviewing (MI) is a patient-centred approach that is used to determine a patient's readiness to engage in a target behaviour such as taking a prescribed medication. The approach aims to respect the patient's autonomy and help patient decision making. In doing so, MI also helps develop a better relationship with the patient.[13] MI is a directive, client-centred counselling style used to bring about behaviour change by helping patients explore and resolve ambivalence.[14] It is not intended to be persuasive but instead aims to help patients understand their diagnosis as well as the risks and benefits of a course of action, and focuses the healthcare practitioner on the specifics of what is motivating patients not to follow a course of action.

The MI approach can be used to help a patient move from one stage of behaviour to another. The MI approach is a counselling style, not a treatment. It is more goal-directed and focused than nondirective counselling.[14,15] The characteristics of MI are summarized as follows:[16]

- Motivation to change is elicited from the client, and not imposed from without
- It is the client's task, not the counsellor's, to articulate and resolve his or her ambivalence
- Direct persuasion is not an effective method for resolving ambivalence
- The counselling style is generally a quiet and eliciting one
- The counsellor is directive in helping the client to examine and resolve ambivalence
- Readiness to change is not a client trait but a fluctuating product of interpersonal interaction
- The therapeutic relationship is more like a partnership or companionship than expert/recipient roles.

In MI, 5 principles are used along with a menu of strategies to assess how ready patients are to change their behaviour and to focus on their ambivalence and resistance.[13] Strategies focus on:

- Eliciting information from patients to understand their typical day and lifestyle, their perspective on their medical condition and treatments and the barriers to change
- Providing information based on their situation or concerns
- Eliciting further concerns and helping with decision making.

The combined first letters of each of the 5 principles form the acronym READS: roll with resistance, express empathy, avoid argumentation, develop discrepancies and support self-efficacy.[13]

An example of conventional paternalistic dialogue when talking to a female patient about taking ASA daily to prevent cardiovascular complications could be as follows: "If you do not take this medication, your risk of stroke increases by about 17%".[17] In contrast an MI based dialogue might include questions such as: "How important is reducing your risk of future heart disease or strokes?" and "What benefits do you think you might get from taking this drug?".

In a meta-analytic review, Rubak et al. found that the evoking style of MI outperformed advice giving in approximately 80% of randomized controlled trials and was not more time-consuming.[16] This was in a broad range of areas, including obesity, cholesterol and hypertension control. Healthcare practitioners in any setting can use this approach when patients may be hesitant about a behaviour change or treatment because it is a style instead of a specific and formal technique. Pharmacists report MI techniques are more successful in an environment and workflow that allowed for longer conversations with patients at times when fewer patients are in the store.[18] Evidence suggests that telephone-based motivational interviewing or combining interviewing with cognitive behavioural interventions may also be associated with improved medication adherence.[19,20]

Conclusions

Changing behaviour is often difficult. Healthcare practitioners have an essential role in providing education and guidance for patients at risk of unfavourable health outcomes. The transtheoretical model of behaviour change can be used to identify a patient's specific stage of change. Motivational interviewing can be employed to help a patient move from one stage to another stage to promote constructive behaviour change.

Resource Tips

Motivational Interviewing Network of Trainers (resources for clinicians, supervisors, program managers and trainers). Available from: www.motivationalinterviewing.org.

Suggested Readings

Berger BA, Hudmon KS. Readiness for change: implications for patient care. *J Am Pharm Assoc (Wash)* 1997;NS37:321-9.

Prochaska JO, Johnson S, Lee P. The transtheoretical model of behavior change. In: Shumacker SA et al., eds. *The handbook of health behavior change*. 3rd ed. New York: Springer Publishing Company; 2009. p. 59-84.

Rollnick S, Miller WR. What is motivational interviewing? *Behav Cogn Psychother* 1995;23:325-34.

Soderlund LL, Nilsen P. Feasibility of using motivational interviewing in a Swedish pharmacy setting. *Int J Pharm Pract* 2009;17:143-9.

References

1. Erol S, Erdogan S. Application of a stage based motivational interviewing approach to adolescent smoking cessation: the Transtheoretical Model-based study. *Patient Educ Couns* 2008;72:42-8.
2. Prochaska JO, Velicer WF, Rossi JS et al. Stages of change and decisional balance for 12 problem behaviors. *Health Psychol* 1994;13:39-46.
3. Prochaska JO, DiClemente CC. Transtheoretical therapy: toward a more integrative model of change. *Psychother Theory Res Pract* 1982;19:276-88.
4. Prochaska JO, Johnson S, Lee P. The transtheoretical model of behavior change. In: Shumacker SA et al., eds. *The handbook of health behavior change*. 3rd ed. New York: Springer Publishing Company; 2009. p. 59-84.
5. Prochaska JO, DiClemente CC, Velicer WF et al. Criticisms and concerns of the transtheoretical model in light of recent research. *Br J Addict* 1992;87:825-8.
6. Berger BA, Hudmon KS. Readiness for change: implications for patient care. *J Am Pharm Assoc (Wash)* 1997;NS37:321-9.
7. Jones H, Edwards L, Belton A et al. Helping people with diabetes change. *Lifescan Education Institute* 1998:1-29.
8. Prochaska JO. Strong and weak principles for progressing from precontemplation to action on the basis of twelve problem behaviors. *Health Psychol* 1994;13:47-51.
9. Bandura A. Self-efficacy: toward a unifying theory of behavioral change. *Psychol Rev* 1977;84:191-215.
10. Bandura A. Human agency in social cognitive theory. *Am Psychol* 1989;44:1175-84.
11. Bandura A. *Social foundations of thought and action*. Englewood Cliffs: Prentice Hall; 1986.
12. Keefe FJ, Lefebvre JC, Kerns RD et al. Understanding the adoption of arthritis self-management: stages of change profiles among arthritis patients. *Pain* 2000;87:303-13.
13. Villaume WA, Berger BA, Barker BN. Learning motivational interviewing: scripting a virtual patient. *Am J Pharm Educ* 2006;70:33.
14. Rollnick S, Miller WR. What is motivational interviewing? *Behav Cogn Psychother* 1995;23:325-34.
15. Miller WR, Rollnick S. *Motivational interviewing: preparing people for change*. New York: Guilford Press; 1991.
16. Rubak S, Sandbaek A, Lauritzen T et al. Motivational interviewing: a systematic review and meta-analysis. *Br J Gen Pract* 2005;55:305-12.
17. U.S. Preventive Services Task Force. Aspirin for the prevention of cardiovascular disease: U.S. Preventive Services Task Force recommendation statement. *Ann Intern Med* 2009;150:396-404.
18. Soderlund LL, Nilsen P. Feasibility of using motivational interviewing in a Swedish pharmacy setting. *Int J Pharm Pract* 2009;17:143-9.
19. Teeter BS, Kavookjian J. Telephone-based motivational interviewing for medication adherence: a systematic review. *Transl Behav Med* 2014;4:372-81.
20. Spoelstra SL, Schueller M, Hilton M et al. Interventions combining motivational interviewing and cognitive behaviour to promote medication adherence: a literature review. *J Clin Nurs* 2015;24:1163-73.

Chapter 3

Pharmacist Assessment of the Self-treating Patient

Nardine Nakhla, PharmD

CPhA acknowledges the contribution of J. D. Barry Power as a previous author of this chapter.

Nonprescription medications are readily available in many retail outlets and commonly self-selected by the public. Consultation with a pharmacist will ensure that self-treatment is both safe and effective. To help meet these goals, pharmacists must accurately determine the seriousness of the condition for which treatment is being sought, determine how the condition should be managed, and then assist with selection of suitable pharmacologic and nonpharmacologic therapies within their scope of practice. Systematic patient assessment and triage can help the busy pharmacist do this quickly and effectively.

Problem Solving Process

Advising patients on self-care activities carries great professional responsibility.[1] Patients requiring self-care may not have been assessed by or received any treatment from another healthcare practitioner. In addition to gathering patient information (including obtaining laboratory or diagnostic measurements) and, if needed, performing a physical exam (mainly inspection and palpation), pharmacists must assist patients in determining when and how to treat their condition(s), or when to access emergency services or seek care from another healthcare practitioner. Before making any recommendations, a thorough assessment is required to identify patients who require additional care or who have special needs that might influence product selection.

To determine which recommendation is most appropriate for a patient, the pharmacist must complete the following problem-solving steps:

1. Collect patient-specific information relative to each health problem/chief complaint/symptom
2. Perform assessment and triage
3. Create, implement, and counsel on a care plan
4. Evaluate the results of the care plan and make adjustments when the patient outcome is less than optimal.

A systematic approach to determining patients' self-care needs will result in consistent and comprehensive patient assessment, and lead to optimal therapeutic outcomes[2] (Figure 1). Several mnemonics have been developed to assist pharmacists in standardizing their approach to information gathering, patient assessment and triage. Two useful mnemonics are presented in Table 1. Evidence shows that the use of a structured interviewing framework improves user confidence, recommendations and counselling.[6] Also, patient assessment is more comprehensive and there is less opportunity for error.

Table 1: **Mnemonics to Assist with Information Gathering and Standardized Patient Assessment**[1,3,4,5]

Mnemonic	Interpretation
WWHAM	▪ **W**ho is the medicine for? ▪ **W**hat is the medicine for? ▪ **H**ow long have the symptoms been present? ▪ **A**ction(s) already taken? ▪ **M**edicines taken for other reasons, prescribed or otherwise?
QuEST SCHOLAR MAC(S)	▪ **Qu**ickly and accurately assess the patient using SCHOLAR MAC(S)[a] – **S**ymptoms-main and associated symptoms – **C**haracteristics-what is the situation like? Is it changing? – **H**istory-what has been done so far? – **O**nset-when did it start? – **L**ocation-where is the problem? – **A**ggravating factors-what makes it worse? – **R**emitting factors-what makes it better? – **MAC(S)**: Ask about other **M**edications, **A**llergies, **C**onditions, **S**ocial history[a] ▪ **E**stablish self-care appropriateness ▪ **S**uggest care ▪ **T**alk to patient

[a] S for social history is not part of the original published algorithm,[5] but was added by the author.

Step 1: Collecting Patient Information

- Determine why the patient is seeking help or looking for a nonprescription product.
- Ask the patient to explain the condition(s), symptom(s) or problem(s) they wish to treat.
- Enquire about the patient's history. The MAC(S) acronym (Table 1) is specific to an individual's medical history and is intended to prompt users to collect additional pieces of key patient information. If relevant, ask women about the possibility that they might be pregnant or planning a pregnancy.
- Perform physical assessment when appropriate. For example, a pharmacist may need to inspect a rash to be able to make an appropriate recommendation. Some patients may not be able to explain what their condition looks like, but may be able to show it. Warts, athlete's foot and minor cuts and burns are easily inspected.

Step 2: Patient Assessment and Triage

This step involves the assessment of the information gathered in Step 1 to identify the patient's problem, its severity, urgency and its most probable cause.[1] Clear articulation of the problem is critical to assist with differentiation among conditions with similar symptoms and to determine the goals of self-treatment. This is followed by triage to determine the most appropriate action:

- Referring to another healthcare practitioner
- Recommending self-care (nonpharmacologic or pharmacologic therapy)
- Recommending self-care until patient can see another healthcare practitioner
- Reassuring patient that no treatment is necessary at this time.

Patient-specific data should be assessed to identify exclusions for self-treatment. It may not be appropriate for an individual to self-treat for several reasons (see Table 2). To establish that the patient is an appropriate self-care candidate ask if the patient:

- has any severe symptoms?
- has any symptoms that persist or return repeatedly?
- is self-treating to avoid medical care?

A patient meeting any of these criteria is referred for further medical evaluation,[6,7] since most medical conditions that can be safely self-treated are characterized as having no severe symptoms, and no symptoms that are persistent or repeatedly return without an identifiable cause. Additionally, patients should not self-treat in an attempt to avoid evaluation and treatment by a healthcare practitioner.

Poisoning

Management of the patient who may have been accidentally or intentionally exposed to a poison requires a specific type of assessment and triage. Suggested management is shown in Figure 2. The likelihood of accidental poisoning is highest with children, especially between 1 and 3 years of age.[8] Common sources of poisoning in children are nonprescription medicines (cough and cold, analgesics), plants and cleaning agents. Determining the source of the poison, if possible, can be helpful in management.

Table 2: **Red Flags Warranting Referral for More Intensive/Urgent Care**[a]

Red Flag	Possible Significance of Red Flag
Change in level of consciousness, change in senses (vision, hearing, taste), seizures or difficulty breathing	Infection, concussion, stroke, hypoglycemia, poisoning or overdose
Paralysis of face, arms, legs; difficulty speaking	Transient ischemic attack, stroke
Severe headache ("Worst headache I've ever had.")	Cerebral aneurysm or stroke
Fever in infants <6 months	Infection, meningitis
Fever in those >6 months for >72 hours	Infection
Fever, vomiting, headache, confusion, difficulty bending neck	Meningitis
Diarrhea or vomiting in high-risk groups (e.g., infants, children, elderly)	Risk of dehydration. More intensive investigation may be required
Persistent bleeding	Clotting abnormalities
Spontaneous bleeding/bruising	Clotting abnormalities
Bleeding from any orifice	Internal bleeding
Discolored urine or feces (rule out drug causes)	Internal bleeding
Chest pain	Acute coronary syndromes
Increasing breathlessness	Pulmonary embolism, heart failure, bronchospasm
Partial- or full-thickness burns to the face or mouth	May cause airway obstruction
Localized redness, swelling, tenderness, heat or pus	Infection
Yellowing of skin and/or eyes	Jaundice or liver damage

[a] Other signs or symptoms may suggest less urgent referral for further investigation. Consult the relevant chapter for the body system involved e.g., Chapter 12: Assessment of Patients with Eye Conditions.

Step 3: Create, Implement and Counsel on a Care Plan

If self-treatment is deemed appropriate, the pharmacist can provide the patient with suitable products and provide education about relevant nonpharmacologic and preventive measures. Establishing patient goals and educating on realistic timeframes for outcomes is imperative and should be discussed first. It is also important to involve the patient in the decision-making process for product selection. Then clearly communicate the therapeutic plan: provide an explanation of the condition, treatment recommendations and rationale.[1] In some provinces the pharmacist care plan may be part of a recognized minor ailments prescribing program which may include a specified range of treatment options.

1. Establish the patient's goals:
   - Discuss and set realistic goals for therapy and realistic timelines for therapeutic outcomes. For example, "curing" a cold is not possible, but relief of symptoms is.
2. Involve the patient in the decision making process:
   - Provide patient with a choice of products if possible
   - When possible tailor the product selection to meet the patient's expectations
   - Provide additional information resources.
3. Select product and counsel:
   - Determine appropriate product(s) for the condition on the basis of patient- or therapy-specific variables[1]
   - Educate the patient on proper use, adverse effects and onset of action of each treatment selected
   - Advise the patient about what to expect from the treatment and what actions to take if symptoms do not resolve within the expected timeframe
   - Where applicable, the plan should include lifestyle changes and nonpharmacologic prevention and treatment measures.

Step 4: Evaluation and Follow Up

- Provide guidelines for follow up if necessary and encourage the patient to call or return if symptoms fail to resolve (e.g., "If your fever does not go away in 3 days, or if your temperature exceeds 40.5°C, contact your doctor.").
- For some cases, follow up is vital. For example, parents seeking a rehydration fluid for their child should be contacted within 24 hours to determine whether the child is displaying signs of dehydration.
- Follow up may not be possible in many cases.
- Use professional judgment in determining cases for follow up.
- Documentation will allow for more effective follow up and continuity of care.

Figure 1: **Self-care Problem-solving Process**

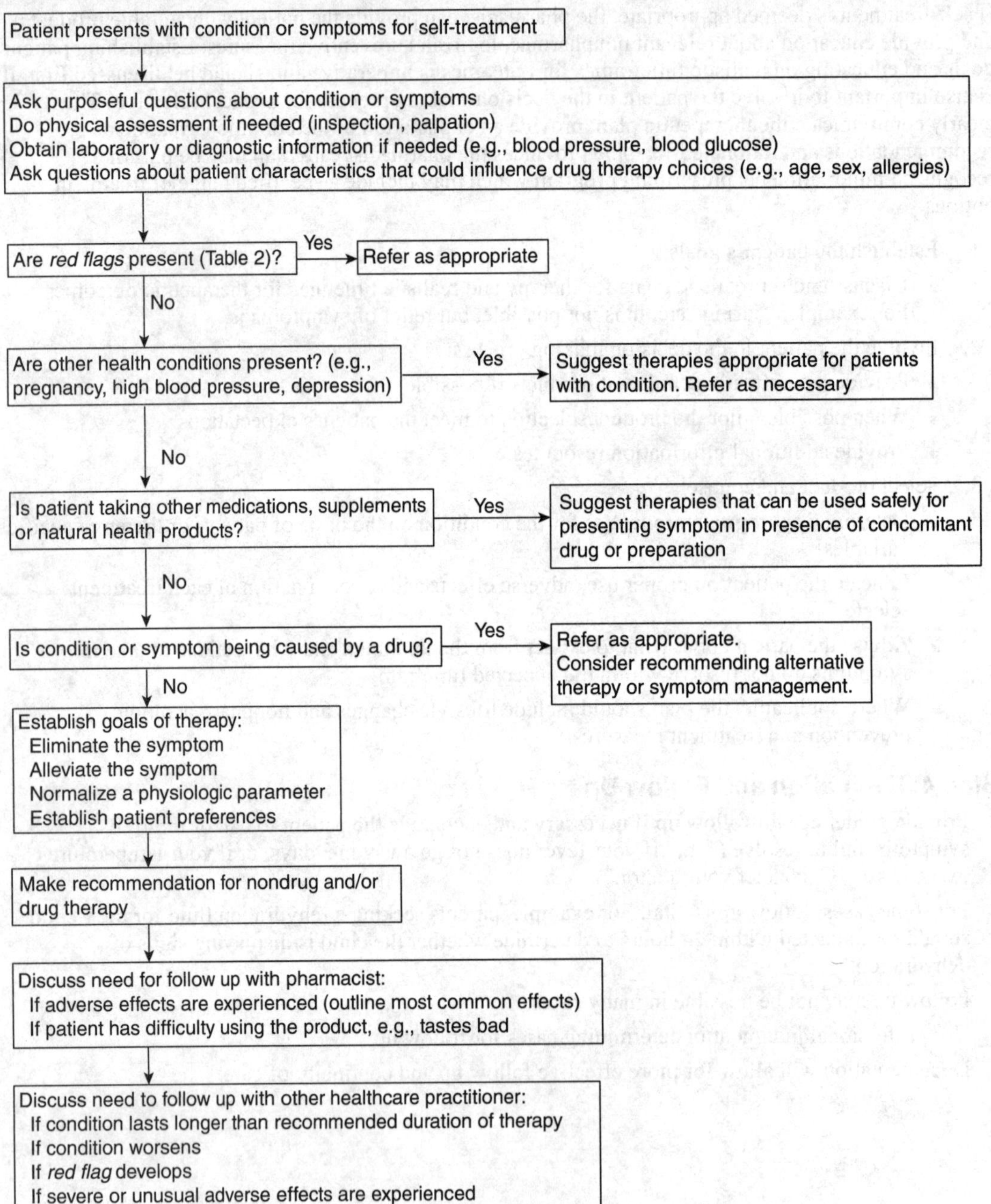

Figure 2: **Triage of the Poisoned Patient**

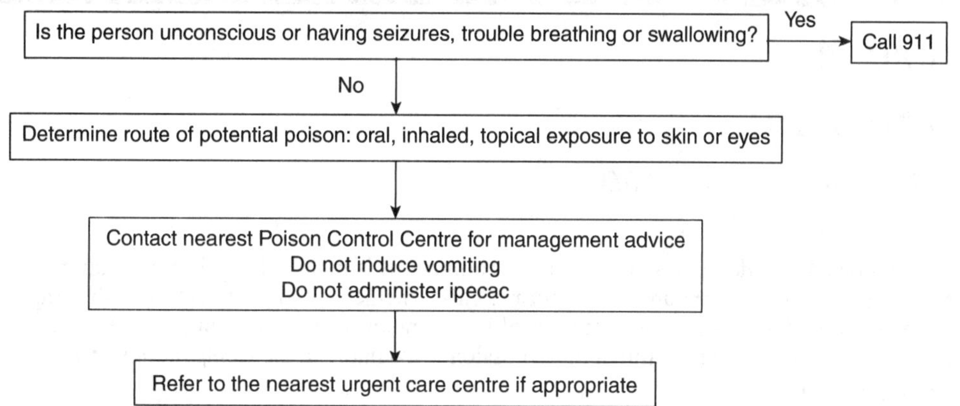

Suggested Readings

Dolovich L, Hudson A. Collecting the evidence. *Pharm Pract* 1997;13:68-77.

Jones RM *Patient assessment in pharmacy practice*. 3rd ed. Philadelphia: Wolters Kluwer; 2016.

Longe RL, Calvert JC, Young LY. *Physical assessment: a guide for evaluating drug therapy.* Vancouver: Applied Therapeutics; 1994.

Stein SM. *BOH's pharmacy practice manual: a guide to the clinical experience*. 4th ed. Philadelphia: Wolters Kluwer Health/Lippincott Williams & Wilkins; 2015.

References

1. Newton GD, Divine H. Patient assessment and consultation. In: *Handbook of nonprescription drugs*. 18th ed. Washington: American Pharmacists Association; 2015. p. 17-31.
2. Dinkins M. Patient counseling: a pharmacist in every OTC aisle. *US Pharm* 2010;35:9-12.
3. Addison B, Brown A, Edwards R et al. *Minor illness or major disease?* 5th ed. London: Pharmaceutical Press; 2012.
4. Rodgers R. PJ practice checklist: sale of medicines protocols. *Pharm J* 1996;178:34-6.
5. Leibowitz K, Ginsburg D. Counseling self-treating patients quickly and effectively. *Proceedings of the APhA Inaugural Self-Care Institute*; 2002 May 17-19; Chantilly, VA.
6. Buring SM, Kirby J, Conrad WF. A structured approach for teaching students to counsel self-care patients. *Am J Pharm Educ* 2007;71:8.
7. Jones R, Charlton J, Latinovic R et al. Alarm symptoms and identification of non-cancer diagnoses in primary care: cohort study. *BMJ* 2009;339:b3094.
8. British Columbia Drug and Poison Information Centre. *Fact sheet*. Vancouver: BC DPIC. Available from: dpic.org/bc-dpic-fact-sheets/british-columbia-poison-control-centre-fact-sheet.

Chapter 4
Depression

Ric M. Procyshyn, PharmD, PhD
Alasdair M. Barr, PhD

Even in its mildest form, depression is not a minor ailment. It is included in this compendium of conditions to support the continuum of care for patients, whether initially presenting with symptoms of depression or being followed by one or more healthcare practitioners at any stage of the disease. More detailed information regarding treatment of depression is available in the *Compendium of Therapeutic Choices*: Depression.

Pathophysiology

Although the exact mechanism underlying the etiology of depression is unknown, it is understood to be the result of complex interactions involving monoamine neurotransmitter function, gene products such as brain-derived neurotrophic factor (BDNF) that enhance postsynaptic neuronal function and other biological factors including neuroendocrine and neuroimmune regulation, sleep abnormalities and aberrant neuronal circuits.[1]

The signs and symptoms of depressive disorders described in DSM-5 are presented in Table 1.[2] It is important to recognize that an estimated one-third of patients who present with depressive symptoms may be experiencing depression in the context of bipolar disorder and will require a different treatment plan from those with primary depression.[3] Patients presenting with depression should be asked if there have been manic or hypomanic episodes in their past.

Depression that occurs in association with other medical conditions can negatively affect the prognosis of these conditions and the patient's adherence to treatment. For example, depression exhibits a bidirectional association with cardiovascular disease and can lead to poorer cardiovascular outcomes.[4,5] When assessing patients for depression, investigate for any association with other medical conditions.

Many medications (e.g., beta-blockers, corticosteroids, oral contraceptives) have been implicated in the etiology of depression, though good quality evidence of a causal link is often lacking. Nonetheless, in the differential diagnosis of depression, consider the patient's medication profile and make any adjustments that seem reasonable and appropriate.

Prevalence

Depressive disorders are common, with an annual and lifetime prevalence in Canada of 4% and 11% respectively.[6] The risk of major depressive disorder (MDD) is 1.5–3 times greater among those who have a first-degree relative with depression. The risk of recurrence in an individual who has experienced 1 previous major depressive episode is 60%; this risk increases to 70% following 2 episodes and 90% after 3. Depression is a leading cause of disability worldwide with significant impact on occupational functioning and quality of life.[7]

Goals of Therapy

- Relieve symptoms of depression
- Prevent suicide

- Return to optimal levels of psychosocial functioning
- Prevent relapse and recurrence

Patient Assessment

Clinical features of depressive disorders are presented in Table 1. Screening for depression can help to identify patients who would benefit from further assessment and, when indicated, appropriate treatment. The Patient Health Questionnaire-9 (PHQ-9)[8] is a 9-item depression module from a general health screening tool used in primary care assessments. A quick and effective tool to identify patients who may require further assessment is to ask the first 2 questions from the PHQ-9 (also referred to as the PHQ-2).[9,10] Patients should undergo further assessment if they answer "yes" to either of following PHQ-2 questions:

1. Over the past 2 weeks, have you been bothered by feeling down, depressed or hopeless nearly every day?
2. Over the past 2 weeks, have you had little interest or pleasure in doing things nearly every day?

The Edinburgh Postnatal Depression Scale is a useful screening tool for detecting postpartum depression.[11] Patient information on postpartum depression is included in Chapter 82: Prenatal and Postpartum Care.

Table 1: Clinical Features of Depressive Disorders[2]

Disorder	Diagnostic Features[a,b]
Major Depressive Disorder (MDD)	History of one or more major depressive episodes, with 5 or more of the following symptoms on most days for at least 2 weeks (at least 1 of the first 2 must be present): 1. Depressed mood 2. Markedly decreased interest or pleasure 3. Significant weight loss or gain 4. Insomnia or hypersomnia 5. Agitation/restlessness or lethargy 6. Fatigue or loss of energy 7. Feelings of worthlessness or excessive guilt 8. Decreased ability to think, concentrate, make decisions 9. Suicidal thoughts, plans or actions
Persistent Depressive Disorder (Dysthymia)	Characterized by depressed mood for most of the day, more days than not, for at least 2 years, plus at least 2 of the following: 1. Poor appetite or overeating 2. Insomnia or hypersomnia 3. Low energy or fatigue 4. Low self-esteem 5. Poor concentration or decision-making ability 6. Feelings of hopelessness Note: In children and adolescents, mood can be irritable and the duration must be at least 1 year.
Other Depressive Disorders listed in DSM-5	▪ Disruptive mood dysregulation disorder ▪ Premenstrual dysphoric disorder ▪ Substance/medication-induced depressive disorder ▪ Depressive disorder due to another medical condition ▪ Other specified depressive disorder ▪ Unspecified depressive disorder

[a] Not due to medically or drug-induced conditions or normal bereavement.
[b] Symptoms must be associated with impairment in social, occupational or other areas of functioning.

Nonpharmacologic Therapy

Psychotherapy involves the use of communication based on a psychological model of illness. Of the many different types, cognitive behavioural therapy (CBT) and interpersonal therapy (IPT) are the most studied and widely recommended forms.[12] Psychotherapy has traditionally involved a relationship between a patient and therapist but has evolved to include patient-managed psychotherapy options such as bibliotherapy (e.g., self-help books) and Internet-delivered CBT.[13] For depression, the combination of psychotherapy and pharmacotherapy has been shown to be superior to either modality alone, especially with respect to relapse prevention. Psychotherapy alone may be effective, particularly in mild-to-moderate depression, but is not recommended for suicidal patients or those with psychotic features.[12] Exercise as an adjunctive measure can be effective in ameliorating symptoms of depression[14,15] and should be encouraged because of its general health benefits. Patients may gain insight and learn useful strategies to self-manage their depressive symptoms from many resources available on the Internet (see Resource Tips).

Light therapy is considered a first-line option for seasonal MDD (seasonal affective disorder; "SAD") or as an adjunctive measure for nonseasonal MDD of mild to moderate severity.[14] A randomized controlled study showed that light therapy, both as monotherapy and in combination with fluoxetine, was effective and well tolerated in the treatment of adults with nonseasonal MDD; the combination treatment had the most consistent effects.[16] Patients are exposed to a 10 000-lux intensity light box slanted toward the face for 30 minutes per day, preferably in the early morning. Improvement in depressive symptoms usually occurs within 1–3 weeks. Adverse effects (e.g., headache, eye strain, irritability, insomnia) are usually mild and do not cause patients to discontinue light therapy. To minimize side effects, patients may begin with 10–15 minutes per day and gradually increase exposure to 30 minutes. Patients with eye conditions that make them more vulnerable to light should check with their eye care practitioner before beginning light therapy. Light boxes with UV filters are recommended.

Electroconvulsive therapy (ECT), a treatment that involves the electrical induction of seizures in an anesthetized patient, has the highest rate of response of any form of antidepressant therapy. It is generally reserved for use in patients with severe symptoms and functional impairment, comorbid psychotic symptoms or catatonia, acute suicidal ideation or treatment-resistant depression.[17] In a study designed to predict nonresponse to ECT in a cohort of patients with major depression who were resistant to pharmacologic treatment, a lack of response was associated with bipolar subtype, the presence of manic symptoms during depression, slightly less severe depressive symptomatology and protracted duration of the depressive episode.[18]

Repetitive transcranial magnetic stimulation (rTMS) is a noninvasive technique used in conscious patients. An electrical current is passed through a coil on the surface of the head to deliver a magnetic field through the skull to the brain, where it stimulates neuronal function. Though response rates are generally lower than with ECT, rTMS is considered to be a safe and well-tolerated option for patients who do not respond to initial treatment.[17] Although further studies are needed to determine the optimal duration of treatment and predictors of treatment response, a meta-analysis found rTMS to be an effective and safe technique for the treatment of medication-refractory depression.[19]

Pharmacologic Therapy

Pharmacotherapy combined with psychotherapy is recognized as having better efficacy in the treatment of depression than either modality alone. For an in-depth review of drug therapy for depression, consult the *Compendium of Therapeutic Choices*: Depression.

Antidepressants

First-, second- and third-line agents listed in the 2009 CANMAT guidelines are included in Table 2.[20] Between drug classes and within drug classes, the clinical effectiveness of antidepressants is generally comparable. When initiating therapy, select an antidepressant after considering the patient's concomitant medical problems, their response to any prior antidepressant and the drug's side effect profile, potential drug interactions and cost.[20]

Some general principles of antidepressant therapy include:[20]

- Many antidepressants can be used as first-line agents (Table 2).[20] Choice of therapy may be based on individual patient characteristics (comorbidities, concomitant medications, previous response to antidepressant, preference)
- Although clinical lore states that antidepressants take 2–4 weeks (or longer) to exert their therapeutic effects, meta-analyses have concluded that antidepressants begin to exhibit a beneficial effect within 1–2 weeks of initiation[21,22]
- When patients are starting or switching to a new antidepressant, monitor for response to treatment, adverse effects and improvement in target symptoms (Table 3)
- An antidepressant is considered effective if there is >20% improvement in depressive symptoms using a depression rating scale
- If there is little improvement after 2 weeks of antidepressant therapy, consider a change in treatment strategy, such as increasing the dose[20]
- If there is improvement, e.g., within 6 weeks, continue the antidepressant for another 2–4 weeks before considering a change in treatment strategy[20]
- Advise patients not to stop taking antidepressants suddenly as this can cause a withdrawal syndrome. Symptoms might include headache, dizziness, nausea, diarrhea, insomnia, mood lability, electric "shock-like" sensations, vivid dreams/nightmares. To prevent withdrawal symptoms, taper antidepressant doses gradually by 25% per week and monitor for a re-emergence of depressive symptoms.[26]

Table 2: **CANMAT Classification of Antidepressants[20]**

Classification	Antidepressants
First-line agents[a]	bupropion mirtazapine moclobemide SNRIs (desvenlafaxine, duloxetine, venlafaxine) SSRIs (citalopram, escitalopram, fluoxetine, fluvoxamine, paroxetine, sertraline)
Second-line agents[a]	quetiapine trazodone tricyclic antidepressants
Third-line agents[a]	irreversible MAOIs (phenelzine, tranylcypromine)

[a] Within each category, antidepressants are listed in alphabetical order rather than order of preference.

Abbreviations: MAOI = monoamine oxidase inhibitor; SNRI = serotonin norepinephrine reuptake inhibitor; SSRI = selective serotonin reuptake inhibitor

Duration of Antidepressant Therapy

There is no clear consensus on the recommended duration of antidepressant therapy. Factors to consider include the duration and severity of the current episode as well as the number of previous depressive episodes. Clinical guidelines recommend maintaining antidepressant therapy for at least

6–9 months after remission of symptoms in patients experiencing a first episode of depression.[20] The guidelines are less clear for patients with a history of multiple episodes or inadequate treatment response. Since these individuals are at a greater risk of a recurrence, treatment with an antidepressant longer than 1 year after remission of symptoms is not unreasonable.

Natural Health Products

It is estimated that more than half of patients with MDD will have used one or more complementary and alternative medicines in the last year, with or without the knowledge of their healthcare provider. Healthcare practitioners should routinely ask patients about their use of natural health products and provide guidance about the risks and benefits of these agents. Patients should know that these treatments do not normally replace standard medications for MDD. While better quality research is needed to evaluate the effect of natural health products on psychiatric illness, limited evidence has shown that some of these agents may be beneficial for patients with depression or for overall health. Some natural health products should not be combined with antidepressants. When patients are taking natural health products, carefully monitor for potential drug interactions. Several natural health products (Table 4) have shown some benefit in the treatment of depression.

For comparative ingredients of nonprescription products, consult the *Compendium of Products for Minor Ailments*—Herbal and Natural Health Products: Single Entity.

Monotherapy with **St. John's wort** is considered a potential first-line option for MDD of mild to moderate severity based on several studies and systematic reviews.[14,30,31,32,33] As an inducer of CYP3A4 and intestinal P-glycoprotein, St. John's wort can decrease the effectiveness of many medications by increasing their metabolism and reducing their systemic bioavailability.[34] Combined therapy with other serotonergic medications (particularly MAO inhibitors) is associated with an increased risk of serotonin syndrome, a potentially fatal reaction characterized by mental status changes, agitation and tremor, potentially progressing to malignant hyperthermia, rhabdomyolysis, seizures, arrhythmias and respiratory arrest. Evaluate potential drug interactions in patients who wish to take this herbal product.

S-adenosyl-L-methionine (SAMe), a synthetic form of a dietary amino acid, may be an effective second-line monotherapy option for the treatment of mild to moderate depression. SAMe has also been shown to be effective, well-tolerated and a safe adjunctive treatment for individuals showing nonresponse to serotonin reuptake inhibitors.[35] SAMe is well tolerated with few adverse effects, but may be associated with an increased risk of serotonin syndrome when combined with other serotonergic drugs.[14,27,36]

Omega-3 fatty acids are often recommended as second-line therapy for the treatment of mild to moderate depression.[14,27,37] However a meta-analysis suggests that the evidence to support their use is of low quality, and the benefits are not clinically significant.[38] Since they are nutritional compounds with established benefits for human health, including fetal and infant development, omega-3 fatty acids may be considered as an add-on option for perinatal depression.[39,40] Side effects such as fishy aftertaste, nausea and diarrhea are usually mild.

Folate is a naturally-occurring B vitamin found in leafy green vegetables, fruits, dried beans and peas whereas **folic acid** is the synthetic form of folate found in supplements and fortified foods. Evidence suggests that folate deficiency is associated with the symptoms of depression, symptom severity and treatment outcomes.[41,42] A trial funded by the NIHR Health Technology Assessment program (UK) failed to find evidence for the clinical- or cost-effectiveness of folic acid (5 mg po daily) as an adjunct to antidepressant medication.[43] This negative study further highlights that methylfolate, and not folic acid, may be a better candidate for augmenting antidepressants in patients with low folate levels. Methylfolate is not commercially available in Canada.

Vitamin D supplementation may have a beneficial effect on depression.[14] In a systematic review and meta-analysis, low serum levels of vitamin D were found to be associated with depression.[44] More randomized controlled trials with vitamin D are needed to determine whether this association is causal and to clarify its potential role in prevention and treatment of depression.

Monitoring of Therapy

Routine monitoring of patients with depression should be performed at regular intervals during treatment. In general, pediatric patients and those with more severe illness should be monitored more frequently (e.g., weekly for 4 weeks, then biweekly for 4 weeks, then at 3 months).[45,46] Table 3 provides examples of monitoring parameters that can be used by health professionals to gauge the patient's response to depression treatment. Because antidepressants can take some time to provide full benefit, support and education are important to help patients cope with symptoms of guilt, worthlessness, helplessness and hopelessness. Provide patients with resources to help them understand their symptoms, their medication and what they can do to help optimize their response to treatment and quality of life (see Resource Tips).

Table 3: **Monitoring of Therapy for Depression**[20]

Monitoring Parameter	Comments
Target symptoms	Symptoms such as anxiety, decreased appetite and insomnia usually begin to improve within the first week of treatment. Increased energy and libido are often seen within 1 month. Depressive symptoms may take up to 8 wk or longer to fully respond to antidepressant medication. Some improvement is usually seen within 3–4 wk.
Adverse effects of antidepressant therapy	Anticholinergic effects, e.g., constipation, dry mouth, urinary retention. Cardiovascular, e.g., dizziness, hypertension, tachycardia. For patients older than 40 y, an ECG is warranted prior to starting treatment with a TCA.[23] CNS, e.g., headaches, memory impairment, sedation, seizures. GI, e.g., diarrhea, nausea, vomiting, weight gain. Sexual dysfunction, e.g., anorgasmia, decreased libido, erectile/ejaculatory dysfunction. Withdrawal (abrupt), e.g., anxiety, confusion, crying, fever, headache, insomnia, irritability, lethargy, nausea, sweating, vivid dreams.
Emergence of suicidal ideation	Though untreated depression is associated with a higher overall risk of suicide, increased suicidality can occur during treatment, more often in pediatric patients and young adults. Patients should be asked about suicidal thinking, particularly during the initial phases of treatment.
Psychometric rating scales, e.g., BDI-II,[24] PHQ-9,[8] QIDS-SR[25]	Allows for rapid and reliable measurement of symptom severity.
Interviewing family member or friend	Can provide valuable information regarding depressive symptoms as well as daily, social and occupational functioning. Patient permission should be obtained.

Abbreviations: BDI-II = Beck Depression Inventory II; CNS = central nervous system; ECG = electrocardiogram; PHQ-9 = Patient Health Questionnaire-9; QIDS-SR = Quick Inventory of Depressive Symptomatology, Self-Rated; TCA = tricyclic antidepressant

Table 4: Natural Health Products for Depression[14,27,28,29]

Class	Drug	Dosage	Adverse Effects	Drug Interactions	Comments	Cost[a]
Natural Health Products	*omega-3 fatty acids*	1–2 g/day po of an EPA-DHA mixture	Mild side effects include fishy aftertaste, GI upset. Risk of bleeding documented (minimal with doses less than 3 g/day).	Potential additive bleeding risk with drugs such as ASA, warfarin, other antiplatelet agents.	Insufficient evidence for or against use during pregnancy or breastfeeding.	$
	S-adenosyl-L-methionine	400–1600 mg/day po in 2–3 divided doses	Infrequent: Constipation, dizziness, dry mouth, insomnia (mild), nausea, sweating. Case reports of increased anxiety, mania or hypomania in patients with bipolar disorder.	Avoid concurrent use with other serotonergic drugs such as antidepressants (possible serotonin syndrome).	Insufficient evidence for or against use during pregnancy or breastfeeding.	$$$
	St. John's wort	Usual: 300 mg TID po Range: 300–1800 mg/day, usually in 2–3 divided doses	Agitation, dizziness, insomnia, GI upset, photosensitivity (rare), restlessness. Case reports of mania or hypomania.	Avoid concurrent use with MAOIs (risk of severe, potentially fatal serotonin syndrome). Avoid concurrent use with SSRIs or other serotonergic drugs such as tricyclic antidepressants (possible serotonin syndrome). May decrease plasma concentration and effectiveness of several drugs including cyclosporine, digoxin, indinavir, oral contraceptives, theophylline, warfarin.	Avoid during pregnancy and breastfeeding.	$

[a] Cost of 30-day supply for mean usual dose; includes drug cost only.

Abbreviations: EPA-DHA = eicosapentaenoic acid-docosahexaenoic acid; GI = gastrointestinal; MAOI = monoamine oxidase inhibitor; SSRI = selective serotonin reuptake inhibitor

Legend: $ < $30 $$ $30–60 $$$ $60–90

Resource Tips

Canadian Network for Mood and Anxiety Treatments. Help & Resources. *Depression and anxiety.* Available from: www.canmat.org/help.php.

HeretoHelp. Available from: www.heretohelp.bc.ca.

Kutcher S. Teen Mental Health. Available from: www.teenmentalhealth.org.

MoodGYM Training Program. Available from: www.moodgym.anu.edu.au/welcome.

National Institute of Mental Health. *Depression.* Available from: www.nimh.nih.gov/health/topics/depression/index.shtml.

Patient Care Tools. *Getting started with antidepressants. Staying on track with antidepressants.* Available from: medicationinfoshare.com/tools.

Suggested Readings

Lam RW, Kennedy SH, Grigoriadis S et al. Canadian Network for Mood and Anxiety Treatments (CANMAT) clinical guidelines for the management of major depressive disorder in adults. III. Pharmacotherapy. *J Affect Disord* 2009;117:S26-43.

Parikh SV, Segal ZV, Grigoriadis S et al. Canadian Network for Mood and Anxiety Treatments (CANMAT) clinical guidelines for the management of major depressive disorder in adults. II. Psychotherapy alone or in combination with antidepressant medication. *J Affect Disord* 2009;117:S15-25.

Patten SB, Kennedy SH, Lam RW et al. Canadian Network for Mood and Anxiety Treatments (CANMAT) clinical guidelines for the management of major depressive disorder in adults. I. Classification, burden and principles of management. *J Affect Disord* 2009;117:S5-14.

Ravindran AV, Lam RW, Filteau MJ et al. Canadian Network for Mood and Anxiety Treatments (CANMAT) clinical guidelines for the management of major depressive disorder in adults. V. Complementary and alternative medicine treatments. *J Affect Disord* 2009;117:S54-64.

Teter CJ, Kando JC, Wells BG et al. Major depressive disorder. In: DiPiro JT, Talbert RL, Yee GC et al., eds. *Pharmacotherapy: a pathophysiologic approach.* 9th ed. New York: McGraw-Hill Medical; 2014. p. 1047-66.

References

1. Krishnan V, Nestler EJ. The molecular neurobiology of depression. *Nature* 2008;455:894-902.
2. American Psychiatric Association. *Diagnostic and statistical manual of mental disorders: DSM-5.* 5th ed. Washington: American Psychiatric Publishing; 2013.
3. Yatham LN, Kennedy SH, Parikh SV et al. Canadian Network for Mood and Anxiety Treatments (CANMAT) and International Society for Bipolar Disorders (ISBD) collaborative update of CANMAT guidelines for the management of patients with bipolar disorder: update 2013. *Bipolar Disord* 2013;15:1-44.
4. Lippi G, Montagnana M, Favaloro EJ et al. Mental depression and cardiovascular disease: a multifaceted, bidirectional association. *Semin Thromb Hemost* 2009;35:325-36.
5. Lesman-Leegte I, van Veldehuisen DJ, Hillege HL et al. Depressive symptoms and outcomes in patients with heart failure: data from the COACH study. *Eur J Heart Fail* 2009;11:1202-7.
6. Patten SB, Wang JL, Williams JV et al. Descriptive epidemiology of major depression in Canada. *Can J Psychiatry* 2006;51:84-90.
7. Patten SB, Kennedy SH, Lam RW et al. Canadian Network for Mood and Anxiety Treatments (CANMAT) clinical guidelines for the management of major depressive disorder in adults. I. Classification, burden and principles of management. *J Affect Disord* 2009;117:S5-14.
8. Kroenke K, Spitzer RL, Williams JB. The PHQ-9: validity of a brief depression severity measure. *J Gen Intern Med* 2001;16:606-13.
9. Whooley MA, Avins AL, Miranda J et al. Case-finding instruments for depression. Two questions are as good as many. *J Gen Intern Med* 1997;12:439-45.
10. Kroenke K, Spitzer RL, Williams JB. The Patient Health Questionnaire-2: validity of a two-item depression screener. *Med Care* 2003;41:1284-92.
11. Cox JL, Holden JM, Sagovsky R. Detection of postnatal depression. Development of the 10-item Edinburgh Postnatal Depression Scale. *Br J Psychiatry* 1987;150:782-6.
12. Parikh SV, Segal ZV, Grigoriadis S et al. Canadian Network for Mood and Anxiety Treatments (CANMAT) clinical guidelines for the management of major depressive disorder in adults. II. Psychotherapy alone or in combination with antidepressant medication. *J Affect Disord* 2009;117:S15-25.

13. Spek V, Cuijpers P, Nyklicek I et al. Internet-based cognitive behaviour therapy for symptoms of depression and anxiety: a meta-analysis. *Psychol Med* 2007;37:319-28.
14. Ravindran AV, Lam RW, Filteau MJ et al. Canadian Network for Mood and Anxiety Treatments (CANMAT) clinical guidelines for the management of major depressive disorder in adults. V. Complementary and alternative medicine treatments. *J Affect Disord* 2009;117:S54-64.
15. Rimer J, Dwan K, Lawlor DA et al. Exercise for depression. *Cochrane Database Syst Rev* 2012;7:CD004366.
16. Lam RW, Levitt AJ, Levitan RD et al. Efficacy of bright light treatment, fluoxetine, and the combination of patients with nonseasonal major depressive disorder: a randomized clinical trial. JAMA Psychiatry 2016;73:56-63.
17. Kennedy SH, Milev R, Giacobbe P et al. Canadian Network for Mood and Anxiety Treatments (CANMAT) clinical guidelines for the management of major depressive disorder in adults. IV. Neurostimulation therapies. *J Affect Disord* 2009;117:S44-53.
18. Perugi G, Medda P, Zanello S et al. Episode length and mixed features as predictors of ECT nonresponse in patients with medication-resistant major depression. *Brain Stimul* 2012;5:18-24.
19. Dell'osso B, Camuri G, Castellano F et al. Meta-review of metanalytic studies with repetitive transcranial magnetic stimulation (rTMS) for the treatment of major depression. *Clin Pract Epidemiol Ment Health* 2011;7:167-77.
20. Lam RW, Kennedy SH, Grigoriadis S et al. Canadian Network for Mood and Anxiety Treatments (CANMAT) clinical guidelines for the management of major depressive disorder in adults. III. Pharmacotherapy. *J Affect Disord* 2009;117:S26-43.
21. Posternak MA, Zimmerman M. Is there a delay in the antidepressant effect? A meta-analysis. *J Clin Psychiatry* 2005;66:148-58.
22. Papakostas GI, Perlis RH, Scalia MJ et al. A meta-analysis of early sustained response rates between antidepressants and placebo for the treatment of major depressive disorder. *J Clin Psychopharmacol* 2006;26:56-60.
23. Solvason HB, Debattista C. Antidepressant dosing for the acute treatment of unipolar depression. *Prim Psychiatry* 2009;16:30-6.
24. Beck AT. *Beck Depression Inventory-II (BDI-II)*. San Antonio: Harcourt Brace; 1996.
25. Rush AJ, Trivedi MH, Ibrahim HM et al. The 16-Item Quick Inventory of Depressive Symptomatology (QIDS), clinician rating (QIDS-C), and self-report (QIDS-SR): a psychometric evaluation in patients with chronic major depression. *Biol Psychiatry* 2003;54:573-83.
26. Warner CH, Bobo W, Warner C et al. Antidepressant discontinuation syndrome. *Am Fam Physician* 2006;74;449-56.
27. Mischoulon D. Update and critique of natural remedies as antidepressant treatments. *Psychiatr Clin North Am* 2007;30:51-68.
28. Bezchlibnyk-Butler KZ, Jeffries JJ, Procyshyn RM et al., eds. *Clinical handbook of psychotropic drugs*. 20th ed. Toronto: Hogrefe & Huber Publishers; 2012.
29. Natural Medicines Comprehensive Database. Stockton: Therapeutic Research Facility. Available from: naturaldatabase.therapeuticresearch.com. Accessed March 10, 2010. Subscription required.
30. Whiskey E, Werneke U, Taylor D. A systematic review and meta-analysis of Hypericum perforatum in depression: a comprehensive clinical review. *Int Clin Psychopharmacol* 2001;16:239-52.
31. De Smet PA. Herbal remedies. *N Engl J Med* 2002;347:2046-56.
32. Ernst E. Herbal remedies for depression and anxiety. *APT* 2007;13:312-6.
33. Van der Watt G, Laugharne J, Janca A. Complementary and alternative medicine in the treatment of anxiety and depression. *Curr Opin Psychiatry* 2008;21:37-42.
34. Borrelli F, Izzo AA. Herb-drug interactions with St. John's wort (Hypericum perforatum): an update on clinical observations. *AAPS J* 2009;11:710-27.
35. Papakostas GI, Mischoulon D, Shyu I et al. S-adenosyl methionine (SAMe) augmentation of serotonin reuptake inhibitors for antidepressant nonresponders with major depressive disorder: a double-blind, randomized clinical trial. *Am J Psychiatry* 2010;167:942-8.
36. Fetrow CW, Avila JR. Efficacy of the dietary supplement of S-adenosyl-L-methionine. *Ann Pharmacother* 2001;35:1414-25.
37. Parker G, Gibson NA, Brotchie H et al. Omega-3 fatty acids and mood disorders. *Am J Psychiatry* 2006;163:969-78.
38. Appleton KM, Sallis HM, Perry R et al. Omega-3 fatty acids for depression in adults. *Cochrane Database Syst Rev* 2015;11:CD004692.
39. Freeman MP. Complementary and alternative medicine for perinatal depression. *J Affect Disord* 2009;112:1-10.
40. Kaviani M, Saniee L, Azima S et al. The effect of omega-3 fatty acid supplementation on maternal depression during pregnancy: a double blind randomized controlled clinical trial. *Int J Community Based Nurs Midwifery* 2014;2:142-7.
41. Sánchez-Villegas A, Doreste J, Schlatter J et al. Association between folate, vitamin B(6) and vitamin B(12) intake and depression in the SUN cohort study. *J Hum Nutr Diet* 2009;22:122-33.
42. Skarupski KA, Tangney C, Li H et al. Longitudinal association of vitamin B-6, folate, and vitamin B-12 with depressive symptoms among older adults over time. *Am J Clin Nutr* 2010;92:330-5.
43. Bedson E, Bell D, Carr D et al. Folate Augmentation of Treatment—Evaluation for Depression (FolATED): randomized trial and economic evaluation. *Health Technol Assess* 2014:18:1-159.
44. Anglin RE, Samaan Z, Walter SD et al. Vitamin D deficiency and depression in adults: systematic review and meta-analysis. *Br J Psychiatry* 2013;202:100-7.
45. Morrato EH, Libby AM, Orton HD et al. Frequency of provider contact after FDA advisory on risk of pediatric suicidality with SSRIs. *Am J Psychiatry* 2008;165:42-50.
46. Gagne JJ, Patrick AR, Wang PS et al. Health advisories and patterns of patient monitoring among new users of antidepressant medications. *J Clin Psychopharmacol* 2009;29:590-4.

Depression—What You Need to Know

About 10% of people experience depression at some time in their life. It is not a sign of personal weakness. Depression is caused by biochemical changes in the brain. It is often referred to as a "chemical imbalance."

Depression can last weeks, months or even years before getting better on its own. But it will usually improve when treated with medication or other kinds of therapy. Most people who get treatment (3 out of 4) find it works for them. Early treatment reduces the chance of depression coming back.

How is depression treated?

- Antidepressants are used to shorten the length of time it takes to get over an episode of depression.
- You may start to feel better in 1–2 weeks, or it could take longer. Talk to your doctor if you don't notice any improvement in symptoms or mood after 2 weeks.
- Don't get discouraged if you don't feel better right away. Sometimes medications or dosages have to be adjusted to get the full benefit.
- Continue your medication even if you start to feel better. Taking your medication for the proper amount of time lowers the chances of your depression coming back.

How long do you have to take antidepressant medication?

- If you are being treated for depression for the first time, you may have to take medication for many months after you get better.
- If you have had depression more than once, you may have to take medication for 2 years or more.

What can you do to help your treatment?

- Avoid alcohol. Many patients with depression drink alcohol to help them sleep or to "calm their nerves." But alcohol alters brain chemistry and disrupts sleep the same way depression does. Talk to your healthcare provider to find out whether you can have an occasional alcoholic drink.
- **Do not** use illegal drugs, sedatives or stimulants.
- Tell your healthcare team if you take nonprescription medications, including herbal products. These products may affect how your medication works.
- Get plenty of rest.
- Exercise regularly.
- Eat regularly.
- Keep socially active.
- **Do not** make any major life changes. When you are feeling bad, it can be difficult to deal with problems. They will seem more manageable when you are feeling better.

What happens if you stop taking antidepressant medication too soon?

- **Do not** stop taking your antidepressant medication without consulting your healthcare practitioner.
- Your healthcare practitioner must supervise the process of gradually reducing your medication. It may take several weeks or several months to stop.
- If you stop your antidepressant suddenly you may experience withdrawal symptoms.
  You may have any of these symptoms:
  - flu-like symptoms
  - muscle aches

- fatigue (tiredness) and headache
- stomach or bowel upset
- anxiety, irritability and mood changes
- feelings like electric shocks throughout the body, especially in the arms and legs.

Does depression come back?

- Some people do have recurring episodes of depression. Whether your depression comes back will depend on:
  - how long you have been depressed
  - the number of times you have had depression before
  - whether you have a family history of depression.

Chapter 5
Insomnia

Ric M. Procyshyn, PharmD, PhD
Alasdair M. Barr, PhD

Insomnia disorder is the most prevalent of all sleep disorders. Although the term is used in a variety of ways, most often it is defined by an individual's report of difficulty with sleep.[1] From a medical perspective, insomnia can be defined by the following DSM-5 diagnostic criteria:[2]

A. Dissatisfaction with sleep quantity or quality, despite adequate opportunity for sleep, as the predominant complaint and ≥1 of the following symptoms:
   1. Difficulty with sleep initiation. (Children may have difficulty falling sleep without help from caregiver.)
   2. Difficulty with sleep maintenance including frequent awakenings or problems returning to sleep. (Children may have difficulty returning to sleep without help from caregiver.)
   3. Early-morning awakening and unable to return to sleep.

B. Clinically significant distress or impairment in social, occupational, educational, academic, behavioral or other important areas of functioning due to sleep disturbance.

C. Sleep difficulty occurs ≥3 nights per week and is present for ≥3 months.

D. Insomnia is not explained by, and does not occur exclusively during the course of, another sleep-wake disorder (e.g., narcolepsy, a breathing-related sleep disorder, a circadian rhythm sleep-wake disorder).

E. Insomnia is not due to the physiologic effects of a substance (e.g., a drug of abuse, a medication) and is not adequately explained by coexisting mental disorders and medical conditions.

Insomnia diagnosis is based on the patient's subjective complaints and does not always correlate with objective measures such as sleep architecture, i.e., cyclic phases of REM (rapid eye movement) and non-REM sleep, or with a specific number of hours of sleep each night.[3] For a description of specific types of insomnia disorder, see Table 1.

Apart from insomnia disorder, there are other common sleep-wake disorders that include the following:

- Situational/acute insomnia:
  - Often associated with life events or with changes in sleep schedules and lasts a few days to a few weeks
  - May result in significant distress and interfere with social, personal and occupational functioning
- Circadian rhythm sleep-wake disorders:
  - Insomnia occurs only when trying to sleep at socially normal times, but not when bed and rising times are delayed and coincide with their endogenous circadian rhythm
- Restless legs syndrome:
  - An urge to move the legs and any accompanying unpleasant leg sensations are features that differentiate this disorder from insomnia disorder

- Breathing-related sleep disorders:
  - Usually accompanied by a history of loud snoring, breathing pauses, and excessive daytime sleepiness
  - Up to 50% of individuals with sleep apnea may report symptoms of insomnia disorder
- Narcolepsy:
  - Distinguished from insomnia disorder by the predominance of symptoms of excessive daytime sleepiness, cataplexy, sleep paralysis, and sleep-related hallucinations
- Parasomnias:
  - Unusual behavior or events during sleep that may lead to intermittent awakenings and difficulty resuming sleep
- Substance/medication-induced sleep disorder:
  - Differs from insomnia disorder in that a substance is judged to be etiologically related to the insomnia.

Pathophysiology

Insomnia is believed to be a disorder of hyperarousal that is experienced throughout the entire day. Currently, there are 2 models that attempt to explain this hyperarousal state. The cognitive model suggests that life's stressors cause an individual to worry and ruminate to the point that they have difficulty falling asleep or going back to sleep once awakened.[4] After a period of time, the focus of worry and rumination shifts to the lack of sleep itself and its effect on functioning the next day.

Another model suggests that hyperarousal is due to physiologic factors, based on the significantly higher metabolic rates seen in patients with insomnia compared with healthy controls.[5] The neuroendocrine system may also play a role in hyperarousal as evidenced by increased levels of urinary and plasma cortisol and adrenocorticotropic hormone (ACTH) in persons suffering from insomnia.[6,7]

Prevalence

Depending on the diagnostic criteria used and population studied, widely variable prevalence rates of insomnia have been reported (5–50%). In epidemiologic studies assessing insomnia symptoms without restrictive criteria, the prevalence is approximately 33% in the general population.[8] If more stringent diagnostic criteria are applied, in which the symptoms of insomnia must persist for at least 1 month and not occur exclusively during the course of another sleep disorder, mental disorder or as the direct physiologic effects of a substance or medical condition, the estimated prevalence is approximately 6%.[9]

Insomnia is reportedly more common in women than men (ratio 1.4:1), in elderly patients (particularly those with health problems), and in patients with comorbid psychiatric or medical illness.[8,10] Use of certain medications has also been associated with insomnia (Table 2).

Insomnia is associated with more frequent use of healthcare services, more days with limited activity, more days spent in bed, impaired job performance, higher rates of absenteeism, increased risk of traffic and workplace accidents and reduced quality of life.[11,12] Insomnia appears to be a predictor of psychiatric and medical comorbidities including depression,[13] hypertension,[14] diabetes[15] and cardiac events,[16] all of which contribute to an increase in healthcare utilization.[17] The impact of insomnia on overall health and well-being highlights the importance of making treatment options available to affected individuals.

Classification

Insomnia is no longer classified as primary or secondary in DSM-5. The diagnosis of insomnia disorder is given whether it is an independent condition or a comorbidity with a mental disorder, a medical condition or a different sleep disorder.[1,2] The duration of symptoms can be episodic (1–2 months), persistent (≥3 months) or recurrent (2 or more episodes in 1 year).

Table 1: **Specifiers of Insomnia**

Specifier	Associated Factors
Independent condition (no identifiable medical cause)	Acute emotional or physical discomfort (acute illness; environmental disturbance such as noise, light and temperature; hospitalization; jet lag; life stress) Acute stressor usually related to work or family life (death or illness of a loved one, loss of job)
Comorbid with another mental disorder	Dementia, eating disorders, mood, anxiety or psychotic disorders, substance-use disorders
Comorbid with a medical condition	Cardiovascular disorders (e.g., cerebrovascular disease, heart disease, untreated hypertension); chronic pain; GI conditions (e.g., gastroesophageal reflux disease, stomach or gastric ulcer); hormonal changes (e.g., menopause, perimenopause, pregnancy); infection; neurologic conditions (e.g., epilepsy, head injury, Huntington's disease, migraine, Parkinson's disease); obstructive airway diseases; rheumatic diseases (e.g., arthritis)
Comorbid with another sleep disorder	Breathing-related sleep disorder (i.e., obstructive sleep apnea, hypoapnea, central sleep apnea, sleep-related hypoventilation); circadian rhythm sleep-wake disorders (i.e., delayed sleep phase type, advanced sleep phase type, irregular sleep-wake type, non-24–hour sleep-wake type, shift work type); parasomnias (i.e., non-rapid eye movement sleep arousal disorders, nightmare disorder, rapid eye movement sleep behavior disorder, restless legs syndrome)

Goals of Therapy

- Promote a sound and satisfying sleep (sleep initiation, quality, quantity and continuity) to prevent deterioration of daytime performance
- Resolve or mitigate underlying conditions that may be contributing to insomnia
- Prevent the progression from transient to chronic insomnia
- Promote healthy sleep hygiene practices
- Prevent excessive use of sedatives by recommending medication only when necessary

Patient Assessment

An assessment plan for patients suffering from insomnia is illustrated in Figure 1.

Table 2 lists medications that have been associated with insomnia.

Nonpharmacologic Therapy

A task force appointed by the American Academy of Sleep Medicine has reviewed and graded evidence regarding nonpharmacologic therapies for the treatment of chronic insomnia.[20] Their findings support both psychological and behavioural interventions, with the strongest evidence for stimulus control therapy, relaxation training and cognitive-behavioural therapy.[20,21,22] Sleep restriction therapy, multicomponent therapy (without cognitive therapy), biofeedback and paradoxical intention are also considered effective, but the evidence for their efficacy is not as strong. Sleep hygiene education is recommended as a general measure but has not been shown to be effective as monotherapy in the treatment of insomnia.[23,24]

Table 2: **Drugs Associated with Insomnia**[2,19]

Drug	Comments
Alcohol	Acute intoxication may produce increased wakefulness, restless sleep, and vivid and anxiety-laden dreams. Alcohol can aggravate breathing-related sleep disorders. With chronic use, alcohol has a short-lived sedative effect for the first half of the night, followed by sleep disruption in the second half.
Caffeine	Produces insomnia in a dose-dependent manner.
Cannabis	Acute use may shorten sleep latency though arousing effects with increments in sleep latency also occur. In chronic users, tolerance to the sleep-inducing effect develops. Upon withdrawal, sleep difficulties and unpleasant dreams may last for several weeks.
Opioids	With chronic use, tolerance to the sedative effects develops followed by complaints of insomnia.
Sedatives, hypnotics, or anxiolytics (e.g., benzodiazepines)	Acute intoxication produces the expected increase in sleepiness and decrease in wakefulness. Chronic use may cause tolerance with subsequent return of insomnia. Sedative-hypnotics can increase the frequency and severity of obstructive sleep apnea events. Parasomnias are associated with benzodiazepines. Abrupt discontinuation of chronic use can lead to withdrawal and rebound insomnia.
Amphetamines (or other stimulants, e.g., methylphenidate)	Acute intoxication characterized by insomnia whereas withdrawal results in excessive sleepiness. Drugs like ecstasy lead to restless and disturbed sleep within 48 hours of intake.
Nicotine	Chronic use associated with symptoms of insomnia, with a reduction of sleep efficiency, and increased daytime sleepiness. Withdrawal from tobacco can lead to impaired sleep. Heavy smokers may have regular nocturnal awakenings caused by tobacco craving.
Other non-psychotropic substances including: adrenergic agonists and antagonists (e.g., antihypertensives, bronchodilators) antihistamines cholinergic agonists and antagonists corticosteroids dopamine agonists and antagonists hormonal therapy (e.g., anabolic steroids, estrogen, medroxyprogesterone, oral contraceptives, progesterone, thyroid hormone) serotonergic modulators (e.g., bupropion, MAO inhibitors, SSRIs)	Related to various effects on the central or autonomic nervous system.

Cognitive-behavioural Therapy

Cognitive-behavioural therapy for insomnia (CBT-I) consists of any of the recommended behavioral therapies (e.g., stimulus-control, sleep hygiene education, sleep restriction) in combination with cognitive procedures, such as identifying dysfunctional beliefs and attitudes about sleep and replacing them with a more adaptive substitute. It is aimed at creating a new attitude to minimize anticipatory anxiety and arousal that can interfere with sleep. CBT-I has proven to be more effective than medication for the treatment of chronic and persistent insomnia, particularly in long-term maintenance.[25,26,27,28] The Canadian Toward Optimized Practice (TOP) 2015 guidelines recommend CBT-I as first-line treatment for both acute and chronic insomnia.[29] The following pamphlet provides information about on-line CBT-I resources for the treatment of chronic insomnia: www.medicationinfoshare.com/gallery/online-cbt-for-insomnia/.

Stimulus-control Therapy

Stimulus-control therapy is based on the concept that sleep is a conditioned response to temporal (bedtime) and environmental cues. The focus of stimulus-control therapy is to eliminate maladaptive behaviours, with the overall goal of associating the bedroom with sleep. These measures complement and are often included in general sleep hygiene recommendations.

- Go to bed only when tired.
- Use the bedroom only for sleep and sex.
- Get up at the same time in the morning regardless of sleep duration.
- Avoid napping during the day.
- If unable to sleep after 15–20 minutes, get out of bed and go to another room to read in a dimly lit environment. Avoid watching television or a computer screen as the light emitted from such devices may have an arousing effect. Return to bed when feeling sleepy.

Relaxation Techniques

Relaxation techniques may improve sleep latency times and sleep maintenance and may be particularly helpful in cases where hyperarousal is believed to be the cause of insomnia. These techniques include the following:

- Progressive muscle relaxation is based on the premise that mental relaxation will be a natural outcome of physical relaxation. Muscle groups are tightened and relaxed one at a time in a specific order. A greater degree of muscle tension is attempted in subsequent exercises as the patient becomes familiar with the technique
- Biofeedback is a therapeutic technique that teaches patients how to facilitate increased slow brain wave activity by using electroencephalographic (EEG) monitoring. Eventually the patient is able to apply this skill without the use of the EEG
- Imagery training is a relaxation technique that teaches the patient to substitute pleasant, calm and peaceful thoughts for unpleasant ones in order to reduce worry and stress.

Sleep Restriction

Sleep restriction involves controlling the amount of time spent in bed but increasing the percentage of time asleep. For example, a patient who sleeps for only 6 hours but stays in bed for 8 hours per night would be asked to decrease the time in bed to 7 hours (sleep time, plus 50% of nonsleep time). This would be accomplished by changing the bedtime while maintaining the wake-up time to establish a good sleep-wake cycle. The mild state of intentional sleep deprivation promotes more rapid sleep onset and more efficient sleep. The allowable time in bed is gradually lengthened by 30 minutes as sleep efficiency increases. In a randomized controlled trial, patients with insomnia independent of other specifiers reported improved sleep and reduced fatigue with sleep restriction therapy.[30]

Multicomponent Therapy

Multicomponent therapy combines several different interventions and may include cognitive, behavioural and sleep hygiene components.

Paradoxical Intention

Paradoxical intention focuses on removing performance anxiety by having the patient partake in their most feared behaviour (remaining awake). In the case of insomnia, patients try to remain awake as long as possible when in bed, with their eyes open and the room darkened. By changing the emphasis from falling asleep to staying awake, the performance anxiety associated with trying to fall asleep slowly disappears. Advise patients to avoid activities in the bedroom that are incompatible with sleep such as keeping the lights on, reading, watching television or using a computer device with a lighted screen.

Sleep Hygiene Education

General sleep hygiene education focuses on behavioural and environmental factors that precede sleep and that may interfere with sleep. Stimulus control measures (above) are often included in sleep hygiene recommendations.

- Personal habits:
  - Fix a bedtime and an awakening time
  - Avoid caffeine 4–6 hours before bedtime and minimize total daily intake
  - Avoid nicotine near bedtime and upon awakening at night
  - Avoid alcohol 4–6 hours before bedtime
  - Avoid heavy, spicy or sugary foods 4–6 hours before bedtime
  - Exercise regularly, but not right before bed
- Sleeping environment:
  - Use comfortable bedding
  - Find a comfortable temperature setting for sleeping and keep the room well ventilated
  - Block out all distracting noise
- Getting ready for bed:
  - Try a light snack before bed such as warm milk and foods high in the amino acid tryptophan (e.g., bananas)
  - Try relaxation techniques before bed
  - Don't take your worries to bed
  - Establish a pre-sleep ritual such as a warm bath or a few minutes of reading
  - Get into your favourite sleeping position

Pharmacologic Therapy

For comparative ingredients of nonprescription products, consult the *Compendium of Products for Minor Ailments*—Sleep Aid Products.

Diphenhydramine, an antihistamine with significant sedative effect,[31,32] is the mainstay of nonprescription pharmacotherapy for insomnia and is described in Table 4.

Principles for nonprescription therapy include:[33]

- Consider potential contraindications and adverse effects
- May not be suitable in the elderly because of anticholinergic side effects
- Use the lowest effective dose
- Use intermittent dosing (up to 4 times weekly)
- Use short term, no longer than 7 consecutive days
- Discontinue medication gradually if used long term.

Prescription therapy for insomnia includes primarily **benzodiazepines** (e.g., lorazepam, oxazepam, temazepam)[34,35] and **nonbenzodiazepine GABA agonists** (zolpidem, zopiclone).[36] Barbiturates and other hypnotics such as chloral hydrate are no longer recommended for the management of insomnia due to an unacceptable risk/benefit profile and rapid development of tolerance, respectively. Antidepressants have been used, particularly in patients with depressive symptoms, but with the exception of **trazodone**,[29] their use solely for insomnia is not generally supported.[37]

For further information on prescription therapy, consult the *Compendium of Therapeutic Choices*: Insomnia.

Pharmacotherapy for insomnia should be recommended with caution, as these agents are associated with cognitive impairment, increased risk of falls, work-related injuries, tolerance, dependence, withdrawal and rebound effects.[38] Nonbenzodiazepine GABA agonists are also associated with decreased mental alertness and driving impairment the morning after use, despite the patient feeling fully alert.[39,40] Nonpharmacologic treatment of insomnia (e.g., CBT-I) has proven to be a safe and effective alternative to pharmacotherapy,[25,26,27] and should be considered a first-line treatment option.

Natural Health Products

For comparative ingredients of nonprescription products, consult the *Compendium of Products for Minor Ailments*—Herbal and Natural Health Products: Combinations, Single Entity; Sleep Aid Products.

Valerian (*Valeriana officinalis*) is marketed as a nonprescription therapy for insomnia. A systematic review and meta-analysis reported subjective improvement in sleep quality when outcome was measured as a dichotomous variable (i.e., yes or no).[41] However, most of the studies had significant problems with methodology and considerable variation in the doses, preparations and treatment lengths. Cases of hepatotoxicity have been reported with valerian use. One case of severe withdrawal syndrome was reported after long-term, high-dose valerian therapy. Valerian is not recommended during pregnancy and breastfeeding.

Melatonin (N-acetyl-5-methoxytryptamine) is a neurohormone produced primarily by the pineal gland. Commercially available animal-sourced melatonin must be isolated only from the pineal glands of animals that are *not* susceptible to transmissible spongiform encephalopathy (TSE) diseases including bovine spongiform encephalopathy (BSE). Melatonin has been reported to increase total sleep time, relieve or prevent daytime fatigue associated with jet lag, reduce sleep latency and help reset the body's sleep-wake cycle.[42] A meta-analysis reported that melatonin decreases sleep onset latency, increases total sleep time and improves overall sleep quality.[43] However, it also found that the absolute benefit of melatonin compared with placebo is smaller than other pharmacological treatments for insomnia. The overall evidence for its use in insomnia is weak. Fatigue, headache, dizziness, irritability and abdominal cramps are possible side effects.

There is insufficient evidence to recommend use of herbals such as German **chamomile** (*Matricaria recutita*), **eleuthero** (*Siberian ginseng*), **passion flower** (*Passiflora*), **reishi** (*Ganoderma lucidum*), **lavender** (*Lavandula angustifolia*), **wild lettuce** (*Lactuca virosa*), **hops** (*Humulus lupulus*) and **St. John's wort** (*Hypericum perforatum*) for insomnia. **Kava kava** (*Piper methysticum*) may promote sleep but was removed from the Canadian market in 2002 because of reports of hepatotoxicity.

Monitoring of Therapy

Table 3 provides a framework for a monitoring plan that should be individualized.

Points to cover when counselling patients who choose nonprescription drug therapy for insomnia:

- Potential benefits of stimulus control and relaxation training; sleep hygiene education should also be reinforced (see Nonpharmacologic Therapy)
- Do not operate vehicles or machinery or engage in any potentially hazardous activities while under the influence of sedating medication
- Do not combine sedating drug therapy with alcohol
- Expected outcomes of drug therapy and management of side effects (Table 3).

Table 3: **Monitoring of Nonprescription Therapy for Insomnia[21,44]**

Symptoms/Side Effects	Therapeutic Goals	Frequency of Monitoring	Actions
Inability to fall asleep	Decrease in sleep latency to ≤30 min	Patient: Daily while on drug therapy Healthcare practitioner: After 3 and 7 days of therapy or next visit	If ineffective after 3 evenings of therapy and treatment still required, assess for further therapy or consultation. If drug therapy is required for more than 7 consecutive days, assess for further therapy or consultation.
Frequent nocturnal awakenings	Decrease in or no nocturnal awakenings		
Early morning awakening	Duration of sleep between 5–7 h per night		
Reduced overall quality of sleep	Improved subjective sleep quality with 3 nights of therapy		
Morning drowsiness, grogginess and/or dizziness (elderly are more at risk)	Minimal/acceptable morning drowsiness, grogginess and/or dizziness throughout therapy	Patient or family member: Daily Healthcare practitioner: After 3 and 7 days of therapy or next visit	Decrease dose by 50%. If still a problem after dosage adjustment and therapy still required, assess for further therapy or consultation.
Constipation (adverse effect of diphenhydramine; elderly are more at risk)	Minimal constipation throughout therapy	Patient: Every 3 days Healthcare practitioner: Within 1 wk or next visit	Discontinue therapy. Increase dietary fibre, water intake and exercise. If no improvement in bowel function, recommend a laxative.
Confusion (adverse effect of diphenhydramine; elderly are more at risk)	No confusion throughout therapy	Family: Daily Healthcare practitioner: Within 1 wk or next visit	Discontinue therapy immediately and assess for further therapy or consultation.

Figure 1: **Assessment of Patient with Insomnia**[18]

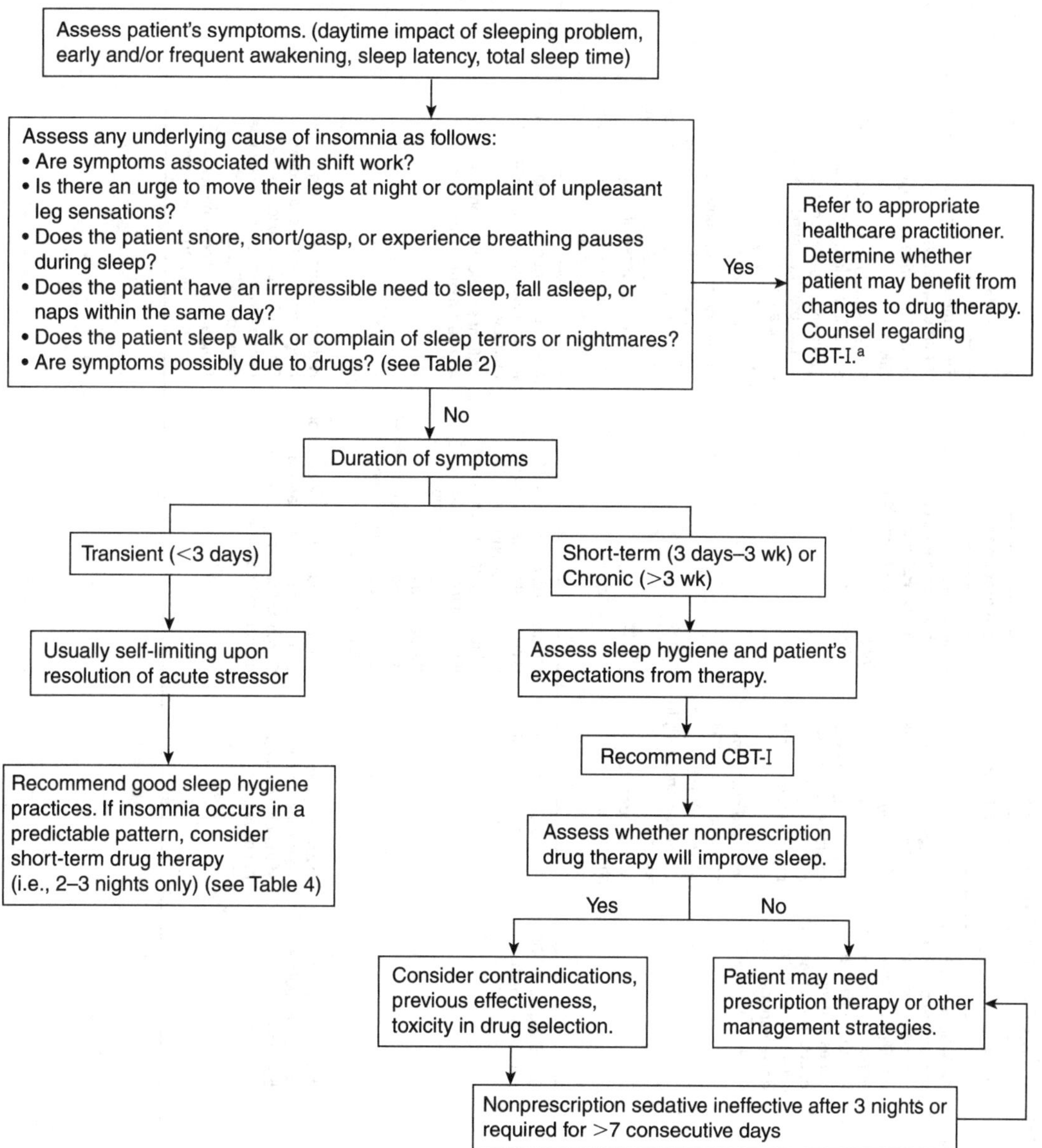
Assess patient's symptoms. (daytime impact of sleeping problem, early and/or frequent awakening, sleep latency, total sleep time)
Assess any underlying cause of insomnia as follows:
• Are symptoms associated with shift work?
• Is there an urge to move their legs at night or complaint of unpleasant leg sensations?
• Does the patient snore, snort/gasp, or experience breathing pauses during sleep?
• Does the patient have an irrepressible need to sleep, fall asleep, or naps within the same day?
• Does the patient sleep walk or complain of sleep terrors or nightmares?
• Are symptoms possibly due to drugs? (see Table 2)
Yes
Refer to appropriate healthcare practitioner. Determine whether patient may benefit from changes to drug therapy. Counsel regarding CBT-I.[a]
No
Duration of symptoms
Transient (<3 days)
Usually self-limiting upon resolution of acute stressor
Recommend good sleep hygiene practices. If insomnia occurs in a predictable pattern, consider short-term drug therapy (i.e., 2–3 nights only) (see Table 4)
Short-term (3 days–3 wk) or Chronic (>3 wk)
Assess sleep hygiene and patient's expectations from therapy.
Recommend CBT-I
Assess whether nonprescription drug therapy will improve sleep.
Yes
No
Consider contraindications, previous effectiveness, toxicity in drug selection.
Patient may need prescription therapy or other management strategies.
Nonprescription sedative ineffective after 3 nights or required for >7 consecutive days

[a] Ask patient to maintain a sleep diary. See Insomnia—What You Need to Know.

Table 4: Nonprescription Medications for Insomnia

Class	Drug	Dosage	Adverse Effects	Drug Interactions	Comments	Cost[a]
Antihistamines	*diphenhydramine* Nytol, Sleep-Eze, Unisom, ZzzQuil, generics	12.5–50 mg po 30–60 min before bedtime. Optimal dose: 50 mg po. Slight dose-dependent increase in hypnotic effect at doses ≤50 mg, especially in hypnotic-naïve patients; flat dose response with doses >50 mg	Dizziness (8%), grogginess (10–19%), morning drowsiness (10–15%). Anticholinergic side effects (e.g., urinary retention, dry mouth, constipation), of particular concern in elderly. Impaired psychomotor and cognitive function. Increased risk of delirium, particularly in elderly. May lower seizure threshold.	Additive sedation with alcohol or other sedating medications. Inhibits CYP2D6 and can increase serum levels of many drugs including antidepressants and cardiovascular drugs.	Recommend intermittent use only (≤4 times weekly). Limited evidence to support efficacy. Patient should seek professional advice if required for >7 days. Contraindicated in patients with benign prostatic hyperplasia, constipation, dementia/cognitive impairment, dry mouth, dry eyes, glaucoma, heart disease. Beers criteria recommends against use of diphenhydramine in the elderly due to increased risk of anticholinergic toxicity, delirium and CNS adverse effects. Dimenhydrinate contains 50–55% diphenhydramine.	$$
Natural Health Products	*melatonin*	0.3–5 mg po 30–60 min before bedtime	Fatigue, headache, dizziness, irritability and abdominal cramps	Melatonin is a substrate of CYP1A2; its metabolism may be affected by strong CYP1A2 inhibitors (e.g., ciprofloxacin, fluvoxamine) or inducers (e.g., carbamazepine, rifampin). Decreased efficacy of dihydropyridine calcium channel blockers (e.g., amlodipine, nifedipine, nicardipine).	May relieve insomnia related to jet lag. Limited evidence to support efficacy. Patient should seek professional advice if required for >7 days.	$
	valerian	400–900 mg po 30–60 min before bedtime	Dizziness, nausea, headache, upset stomach, morning hangover	Additive sedation with alcohol or other sedating medications. Combinations should be avoided or used with caution.	Not recommended during pregnancy and breastfeeding. Cases of hepatotoxicity have been reported. Limited evidence to support efficacy. Patient should seek professional advice if required for >7 days.	$$

[a] Cost of 7-day supply; includes drug cost only.
Legend: $ < $1 $$ $1–2

Resource Tips

Mayo Clinic. *Insomnia*. Available from: www.mayoclinic.com/health/insomnia/DS00187.

Sleepnet.com. Available from: www.sleepnet.com.

Sleepwell Nova Scotia. Available from: www.sleepwellns.ca

Suggested Readings

Benca RM. Diagnosis and treatment of chronic insomnia: a review. *Psychiatr Serv* 2005;56:332-43.

McMillan JM, Aitken E, Holroyd-Leduc JM. Management of insomnia and long-term use of sedative-hypnotic drugs in older patients. *CMAJ* 2013;185:1499-505.

Morin CM, Benca R. Chronic insomnia. *Lancet* 2012;379:1129-41.

Passarella S, Duong MT. Diagnosis and treatment of insomnia. *Am J Health Syst Pharm* 2008;65:927-34.

Roehrs T, Roth T. Insomnia pharmacotherapy. *Neurotherapeutics* 2012;9:728-38.

Toward Optimized Practice (TOP) Insomnia Group. *Assessment to management of adult insomnia: clinical practice guideline*. December 2015. Available from: www.topalbertadoctors.org/download/1920/Adult%20Insomnia%20CPG.pdf.

References

1. Roth T. Insomnia: definition, prevalence, etiology, and consequences. *J Clin Sleep Med* 2007;3:S7-10.
2. American Psychiatric Association. *Diagnostic and statistical manual of mental disorders: DSM-5*. 5th ed. Washington: American Psychiatric Publishing; 2013.
3. Erman MK. Sleep architecture and its relationship to insomnia. *J Clin Psychiatry* 2001;62:9-17.
4. Harvey AG. A cognitive model of insomnia. *Behav Res Ther* 2002;40:869-93.
5. Bonnet MH, Arand DL. 24-hour metabolic rate in insomniacs and matched normal sleepers. *Sleep* 1995;18:581-8.
6. Vgontzas AN, Bixler EO, Lin HM et al. Chronic insomnia is associated with nyctohemeral activation of the hypothalamic-pituitary-adrenal axis: clinical implications. *J Clin Endocrinol Metab* 2001;86:3787-94.
7. Riemann D, Klein T, Rodenbeck A et al. Nocturnal cortisol and melatonin secretion in primary insomnia. *Psychiatry Res* 2002;113:17-27.
8. Ohayon MM. Epidemiology of insomnia: what we know and what we still need to learn. *Sleep Med Rev* 2002;6:97-111.
9. Ohayon MM. Prevalence of DSM-IV diagnostic criteria of insomnia: distinguishing insomnia related to mental disorders from sleep disorders. *J Psychiatr Res* 1997;31:333-46.
10. Ohayon MM, Shapiro CM, Kennedy SH. Differentiating DSM-IV anxiety and depressive disorders in the general population: comorbidity and treatment consequences. *Can J Psychiatry* 2000;45:166-72.
11. Simon GE, VonKorff M. Prevalence, burden, and treatment of insomnia in primary care. *Am J Psychiatry* 1997;154:1417-23.
12. Bonnet MH, Arand DL. Consequences of insomnia. *Sleep Med Clin* 2006;1:351-8.
13. Breslau N, Roth T, Rosenthal L et al. Sleep disturbance and psychiatric disorders: a longitudinal epidemiological study of young adults. *Biol Psychiatry* 1996;39:411-8.
14. Suka M, Yoshida K, Sugimori H. Persistent insomnia is a predictor of hypertension in Japanese male workers. *J Occup Health* 2003;45:344-50.
15. Nilsson PM, Roost M, Engstrom G et al. Incidence of diabetes in middle-aged men is related to sleep disturbances. *Diabetes Care* 2004;27:2464-9.
16. Asplund R. Sleep and cardiac diseases amongst elderly people. *J Intern Med* 1994;236:65-71.
17. Walsh JK. Clinical and socioeconomic correlates of insomnia. *J Clin Psychiatry* 2004;65:13-9.
18. Schenck CH, Mahowald MW, Sack RL. Assessment and management of insomnia. *JAMA* 2003;289:2475-9.
19. Novak M, Shapiro CM. Drug-induced sleep disturbances. Focus on nonpsychotropic medications. *Drug Saf* 1997;16:133-49.
20. Morin CM, Bootzin RR, Buysse DJ et al. Psychological and behavioral treatment of insomnia: update of the recent evidence (1984-2004). *Sleep* 2006:29;1398-414.
21. Morgenthaler T, Kramer M, Alessi C et al. Practice parameters for the psychological and behavioral treatment of insomnia: an update. An American Academy of Sleep Medicine report. *Sleep* 2006;29:1415-9.
22. Morin CM, Hauri PJ, Espie CA et al. Nonpharmacologic treatment of chronic insomnia. An American Academy of Sleep Medicine review. *Sleep* 1999;22:1134-56.
23. University of Maryland Medical Center. Sleep Disorders Center. *Sleep hygiene: helpful hints to help you sleep*. Available from: www.ummidtown.org/programs/sleep/patients/sleep-hygiene. Accessed June 11, 2015.
24. Morin CM, Culbert JP, Schwartz SM. Nonpharmacological interventions for insomnia: a meta-analysis of treatment efficacy. *Am J Psychiatry* 1994;151:1172-80.
25. Siversten B, Omvik S, Pallesen S et al. Cognitive behavioral therapy vs zopiclone for treatment of chronic primary insomnia in older adults: a randomized controlled trial. *JAMA* 2006;295:2851-8.
26. Morin CM, Vallieres A, Guay B et al. Cognitive behavioral therapy, singly and combined with medication, for persistent insomnia: a randomized controlled trial. *JAMA* 2009;301:2005-15.
27. Mitchell MD, Gehrman P, Perlis M et al. Comparative effectiveness of cognitive behavioral therapy for insomnia: a systematic review. *BMC Fam Pract* 2012;13:40.

28. Brasure M, MacDonald R, Fuchs E et al. *Management of insomnia disorder* [Internet]. Rockville: Agency for Healthcare Research and Quality; 2015 Dec. Available from www.ncbi.nlm.nih.gov/books/NBK343503/.
29. Toward Optimized Practice (TOP) Insomnia Group. *Assessment to management of adult insomnia: clinical practice guideline*. December 2015. Available from: www.topalbertadoctors.org/download/1920/Adult%20Insomnia%20CPG.pdf. Accessed April 28, 2016.
30. Falloon K, Elley CR, Fernando A et al. Simplified sleep restriction for insomnia in general practice: a randomised controlled trial. *Br J Gen Pract* 2015;65:e508-15.
31. Kudo Y, Kurihara M. Clinical evaluation of diphenhydramine hydrochloride for the treatment of insomnia in psychiatric patients: a double-blind study. *J Clin Pharmacol* 1990;30:1041-8.
32. Roth T, Roehrs T, Koshorek G et al. Sedative effects of antihistamines. *J Allergy Clin Immunol* 1987;80:94-8.
33. NIH State of the Science Conference statement on manifestations and management of chronic insomnia and adults. *J Clin Sleep Med* 2005;1:412-21.
34. Holbrook AM, Crowther R, Lotter A et al. Meta-analysis of benzodiazepine use in the treatment of insomnia. *CMAJ* 2000;162:225-33.
35. Winkelman J, Pies R. Current patterns and future directions in the treatment of insomnia. *Ann Clin Psychiatry* 2005;17:31-40.
36. Goa KL, Heel RC. Zopiclone. A review of its pharmacodynamic and pharmacokinetic properties and therapeutic efficacy as an hypnotic. *Drugs* 1986;32:48-65.
37. Wiegand MH. Antidepressants for the treatment of insomnia: a suitable approach? *Drugs* 2008;68:2411-7.
38. Uehli K, Mehta AJ, Miedinger D et al. Sleep problems and work injuries: a systematic review and meta-analysis. *Sleep Med Rev* 2014;18:61-73.
39. U.S. Food and Drug Administration (FDA). *FDA Drug Safety Communication: FDA warns of next-day impairment with sleep aid Lunesta (eszopiclone) and lowers recommended dose.* Available from: www.fda.gov/Drugs/DrugSafety/ucm397260.htm. Accessed November 13, 2015.
40. U.S. Food and Drug Administration (FDA). *FDA Drug Safety Communication: FDA approves new label changes and dosing for zolpidem products and a recommendation to avoid driving the day after using Ambien CR.* Available from: www.fda.gov/Drugs/DrugSafety/ucm352085.htm. Accessed November 13, 2015.
41. Bent S, Padula A, Moore D et al. Valerian for sleep: a systematic review and meta-analysis. *Am J Med* 2006:119:1005-12.
42. Buscemi N, Vandermeer B, Pandya R et al. Melatonin for treatment of sleep disorders. *Evid Rep Technol Assess (Summ)* 2004;108:1-7.
43. Ferracioli-Oda E, Qawasmi A, Bloch MH. Meta-analysis: melatonin for the treatment of primary sleep disorders. *PLoS One* 2013;8:e63773.
44. Benca RM. Diagnosis and treatment of chronic insomnia: a review. *Psychiatr Serv* 2005;56:332-43.

Insomnia—What You Need to Know

Tips to help improve your sleep:

- Avoid napping during the day.
- Go to bed at a regular time and get up at a regular time every day (even on weekends).
- Develop a bedtime ritual to relax before going to bed (such as a warm bath, stretching or reading).
- Avoid watching the clock if you can't sleep.
- Go to bed only when you are sleepy. Sleep as much as you can to feel refreshed.
- Use the bedroom only for sleep and sex. Avoid watching television or a computer screen, listening to the radio or eating in the bedroom.
- Make the bedroom a good place to sleep—cut down on noise and light and make sure the room is not too hot or too cold.
- Select a mattress, pillows and bedding that are comfortable.
- If you cannot sleep after being in bed for 15–20 minutes, get up and go into another room to read. Keep the lights low. Avoid watching TV as the bright light may make you more alert. Return to bed only when you feel sleepy again.
- Regular exercise in the late afternoon may help you sleep. However, avoid exercising 2 hours prior to bedtime as this may interfere with sleep.
- Products containing caffeine (e.g., tea, coffee, chocolate, soft drinks) should not be consumed within 4 hours of going to bed. Caffeine is a stimulant and can keep you awake.
- Reduce the amount of fluid you drink before going to bed. It may help to decrease the number of times you have to go to the bathroom.
- Avoid nicotine (e.g., nicotine patches, chewing gum, lozenges) an hour before bedtime and when you wake up during the night. Nicotine is a stimulant, and can keep you awake.
- Avoid using alcohol to help you fall asleep. Although it can help you to get to sleep, it can disrupt sleep later in the night.
- Avoid eating heavy meals before going to bed. However, a light snack may be beneficial.

What about taking nonprescription medication?

Ask your pharmacist for advice about taking nonprescription medication to help you sleep. If your pharmacist recommends a medication, remember:

- **Do not** drive or operate machinery while under the influence of the medication.
- **Do not** take the medication with alcohol.

When should you seek advice from a healthcare practitioner?

You may need to seek advice from a healthcare practitioner if:

- the medication is not working after taking it for 3 nights
- you need the medication for more than 7 days in a row
- you feel confused, dizzy or drowsy in the morning after taking medication.

Before seeing your healthcare practitioner, keep a sleep diary for a few days. This will help find the best treatment for you. A sample sleep diary is provided below.

Table 1: **Sample Sleep Diary**

Enter the Weekday (Mon, Tues, etc.)	Day 1	Day 2	Day 3	Day 4	Day 5	Day 6
What time did you go to bed?						
How long did it take you to fall asleep?						
After falling asleep, how many times did you wake up in the night?						
What time did you finally wake up?						
How long did you spend in bed last night (from first getting in, to finally getting up in the morning)						
How many alcoholic drinks did you have that day? What time?						
If you smoke, what time did you have your last cigarette?						
How much time did you spend doing exercises? At what time of the day?						
What medications did you take for sleep?						
How would you rate the quality of your sleep last night? 1-very poor; 2-poor; 3-fair; 4-good; 5-very good						
List any daytime symptoms you may have experienced such as tiredness, irritability, lack of concentration, inability to stay alert, other						

Chapter 6
Smoking Cessation

Kristine Petrasko, BScPharm, CRE
Manjit Bains, BScPharm

Pathophysiology

Nicotine addiction involves a variety of physical, psychological and behavioural factors.[1,2,3] Nicotine acts as a stimulant, increasing alertness and sense of well-being and elevating heart rate and blood pressure. Due to rapid delivery (within 7–10 seconds) to the mesolimbic pleasure-reward system in the brain, nicotine is highly addictive. With continued use, chemical and biologic changes occur in the brain and tolerance develops very quickly. Nicotine addiction is characterized by cravings which promote continued smoking and the tendency to increase nicotine intake to counter the profound physical and psychological symptoms elicited by withdrawal. There are multiple ways to consume nicotine: smoking, chewing or snorting smokeless tobacco, vaping and others. Table 1 describes various factors that reinforce nicotine addiction.

Nicotine addiction is now classified in the Diagnostic and Statistical Manual of Mental Disorders 5th edition (DSM-5) as tobacco use disorder.[3]

Prevalence

About 4.6 million Canadians (16% of the population) currently smoke.[6] Smoking tobacco is the number one cause of preventable death in Canada, killing over 37 000 people every year, which is more than car accidents, suicides, homicides, AIDS and other substance abuse issues combined.[6] Now considered a chronic medical condition,[7] tobacco dependency is the inability to discontinue tobacco use despite awareness of the health consequences.[8] All forms of tobacco use have harmful effects. These include smokeless tobacco (chewing tobacco and "snuff"), pipe tobacco, cigars, hookahs and other nicotine delivery systems.[7,9]

Table 1: Factors Reinforcing Nicotine Addiction

Category	Reinforcing Factors[3,4,5]
Physical	Pleasure or "high" similar to other addictive psychomotor stimulants.
Psychological	Behavioural conditioning resulting from hand-to-mouth ritual repeated on average 250 times a day for a pack-a-day smoker. Fear of weight gain associated with quitting.
Social	Routine activities associated with smoking such as waking up, phone calls, meals, coffee, driving, break time at work, spending time with family or friends who smoke. Quitting does not eliminate these activities so they continue to act as triggers.
Withdrawal Symptoms	Dysphoric or depressed mood, irritability, anxiety, difficulty concentrating, restlessness, increased appetite/weight gain, GI symptoms, headaches and insomnia. Symptoms generally peak 24–72 h after the last cigarette and subside after about 2 wk. Cravings can continue for years, and are probably related to behavioural and psychological aspects of nicotine addiction.

Health Risks

On average, a cigarette delivers 1–3 mg of nicotine to the brain.[2,10] Light or ultralight cigarettes may deliver the same amount of nicotine as regular cigarettes, regardless of the reported nicotine content, and are not safer than regular cigarettes.[10] Many factors are involved, such as more intense inhalation ("compensation") or blocking of the vent holes on the cigarette filter by the lips or fingers.

The health risks associated with smoking (see Table 2) are attributable to at least 50 of the known carcinogens among the 4000 chemicals in tobacco smoke, including: tar, arsenic, formaldehyde, ammonia and nickel.

Table 2: **Health Risks Associated with Tobacco Use**

Category	Potential Health Effects
Cancer	Cancer of the lung, pancreas, kidney, bladder, lip, oral cavity and pharynx, esophagus and larynx are all increased 2–27 times for smokers compared with nonsmokers. Smoking accounts for about 30% of all cancer-related deaths.[17]
Cardiovascular	Smokers have 2–4 times higher risk of coronary artery disease, 1.5 times higher risk of cerebral thrombosis[18] and increased risk of arteriosclerotic peripheral vascular disease.[19] Smoking cessation is an effective means of cardiovascular risk reduction and should be assessed in addition to blood pressure, lipid and blood glucose control.
Delayed wound healing	Wounds resulting from trauma, disease, or surgical procedures heal slowly in smokers. Smokers experience a greater degree of complications as well as a higher incidence of unsatisfactory healing following reconstructive surgeries.[20]
Dermatologic effects	Premature aging of skin and wrinkling.[21]
Endocrine	Chronic smokers develop insulin resistance. There is also an increased risk of microvascular complications in smokers who develop insulin resistance.[22]
Musculoskeletal effects	Increased risk of lumbar disk disease and delayed bone healing. Decreased bone mineral density; though evidence of causality is lacking, bone loss associated with smoking could be expected to increase risk of hip fracture, especially in postmenopausal women.[23,24,25]
Oral contraceptive use	Cardiovascular events, including stroke and MI, are more common in women ≥35 y taking oral contraceptives.[26]
Oral diseases	Smoking increases the risk of oral diseases such as leukoplakia (white premalignant lesions on oral mucosa), gingival bleeding, periodontitis and ulcerative gingivitis, as well as lip, mouth and throat cancers that resulted in the deaths of 1108 Canadians in 2007.[27]
Peptic ulcer disease	Increased incidence of bleeding and perforated ulcers.
Pregnancy and postpartum	Smoking during pregnancy has been linked to increased risk of: intrauterine growth restriction (average 150 g lower birth weight at term); preterm and extremely preterm births; fetal and infant mortality; sudden infant death syndrome (SIDS); potential long-term effects such as increased risk of type 2 diabetes, obesity, asthma, certain childhood cancers.[28,29,30]
Respiratory	Smoking leads to chronic obstructive pulmonary disease (COPD) including chronic bronchitis and emphysema,[31] as well as a higher incidence of lung and throat infections.[32] Patients requiring inhaled corticosteroids have less of a response than nonsmokers.
Sexual function	Erectile dysfunction is twice as likely to occur in smokers than nonsmokers; exposure to second-hand smoke is also a significant risk factor for erectile dysfunction.[18]

Environmental tobacco smoke (ETS) or second-hand smoke puts nonsmokers at risk, accounting for over 1000 lung cancer or cardiac deaths each year.[6] Patients with chronic lung conditions may be most susceptible to ETS, with increased risk of asthma or COPD exacerbations. However, all nonsmokers are at risk of the effects of ETS, which also include eye and throat irritation, coughing, rhinitis, headaches and various types of cancer, particularly lung cancer. In children it has also been linked to asthma, recurrent acute otitis media and sudden infant death syndrome.[11]

For those who do quit, there are immediate and long-term health benefits: improved breathing and sense of taste, and reduced risk of heart disease, cancer, respiratory problems and infections. Long-term smoking cessation has also been associated with mental health benefits, including improvements in depression, anxiety and stress.[12] Quitting before the age of 50 results in a 50% reduction in risk of death in the next 15 years.[13] The younger a person is when quitting, the better their overall quality of life, with a significant decrease in mortality.[14,15] Compared with those who continue to smoke, people who stop smoking when aged 25–34, 35–44, 45–54 and 55–64 lived 10, 9, 6 and 4 years longer, respectively.[16] This highlights the importance of assisting younger smokers to quit, and more importantly, preventing them from starting in the first place. It is also important to emphasize to patients with a long history of smoking that it is never too late to quit.

Goals of Therapy

The foremost goal of therapy is to achieve lasting smoking cessation. Healthcare practitioners can help patients achieve this goal by:

- Supporting smokers in the pre-contemplative and contemplative stages of change to move to preparation and then action stages.
- Supporting smokers who successfully quit to achieve long-term abstinence (maintenance stage).
- These goals may be achieved by initiating dialogue, providing education and following up regularly with patients.

Patient Assessment

Healthcare practitioners are in an ideal position not only to help patients who have already decided to quit smoking, but also to identify smokers and assist them in making the decision to quit. An assessment plan for smoking cessation is presented in Figure 2.

Healthcare practitioners should take the initiative to provide, at minimum, a brief intervention (<20 minutes) to assess smoking status and readiness to quit. This type of intervention can increase unassisted quit rates of 2–3% by a further 1–3%.[33] Longer consultations (30–90 minutes) are even more effective.[7,34,35,36] Though effectiveness is higher with longer interviews, brief interventions of even 3–5 minutes have been shown to be beneficial.[33]

The following 3 main assessment questions can be used to initiate a brief intervention or discussion with a patient:

1. Do you smoke?

2. Have you ever considered quitting?

3. Is now a good time?

The patient's motivation to quit is assessed by the Stages of Change model of behavioural change (see Figure 2). The precontemplation stage describes the patient who is not even thinking about quitting. In the contemplation stage, the patient is considering quitting, typically in the next 6 months to a year. In the preparation stage, the patient has made the decision to quit and is preparing to begin the process. Next is the action stage where quitting actually occurs, followed by maintenance, where the patient has been abstinent for at least 6 months and is working at remaining smoke-free. See Figure 2 and Nonpharmacologic Therapy for intervention strategies for each stage of the process.

If the degree of physical dependence is low as assessed by the Modified Fagerström Nicotine Tolerance Scale (see Table 3), the chances of successful smoking cessation are good even with behavioural assistance alone. If the degree of physical dependence is high, e.g., Fagerström score ≥6, the patient will likely require some form of pharmacotherapy (with or without behavioural assistance) to achieve success.[7]

Table 3: **Modified Fagerström Nicotine Tolerance Scale**

Questions[a]	0 points	1 point	2 points	3 points	Score[b]
1. How soon after you wake up do you smoke your first cigarette?	After 60 min	Within 31–60 min	Within 6–30 min	Within 5 min	___
2. Do you find it difficult to refrain from smoking in places where it is forbidden?	No	Yes	–	–	___
3. Which of all the cigarettes you smoke in a day is the most satisfying one (the hardest one to give up)?	Any other than first one in the morning	First one in the morning	–	–	___
4. How many cigarettes per day do you smoke?	10 or less	11–20	21–30	31 or more	___
5. Do you smoke more during the morning than during the rest of the day?	No	Yes	–	–	___
6. Do you smoke when you are so ill that you are in bed most of the day?	No	Yes	–	–	___
				Total:	___

[a] For some nicotine replacement products, only question 1 or 4 is required to determine the appropriate initial dose.
[b] Initiate pharmacotherapy for scores ≥6.

Score: <5 = low nicotine dependence; 5 = moderate nicotine dependence; 6–7 = high nicotine dependence; 8–10 = very high nicotine dependence

Adapted with permission from Heatherton TF, Kozlowski LT, Frecker RC, Fagerström KO. The Fagerström Test for Nicotine Dependence: a revision of the Fagerström Tolerance Questionnaire. *Br J Addict* 1991;86:1119-27.

Nonpharmacologic Therapy

Nonpharmacologic therapy for smoking cessation includes various behavioural interventions and alternative therapies. Combining one or more of these methods may be sufficient for success in patients who are light smokers. It is also the most appropriate option for patients in whom pharmacologic therapy is contraindicated because of potential interaction with other medications or because of other physical conditions such as severe heart disease (see Cardiovascular Disease) or pregnancy (see Pregnancy).

Environmental changes can be made to assist a person in tobacco cessation. Smoking paraphernalia such as ash trays and lighters should be removed from the home, car and workspace. It may also be beneficial, especially in the first few weeks after the quit date, to avoid or limit interaction with friends or family members who smoke. To help deal with cravings, advise patients to take a walk, practise breathing techniques, or take up a new hobby or project. Suggest healthy, crunchy snacks such as carrot sticks or celery to help with cravings and the increased hunger that can be associated with tobacco cessation.

Counselling approaches for patients at various stages of change might include:

Precontemplation—Ask and Listen

- Encourage patients to discuss their smoking openly and to think about quitting, e.g., "What do you like and not like about smoking?"
- Reinforce relevant health consequences of smoking, but avoid confrontational or judgmental comments or body language.

- When possible, use a personalized approach to initiating a dialogue, e.g., "I am concerned about the effect smoking is having on your asthma. Would you be willing to discuss this at some point?"
- Empower patients with belief in their ability to quit. Help them to remember what successes they have had in the past, no matter how small, and focus on the positives, e.g., "During your last quit attempt, what went well for you?" or "What is the longest time you have been able to remain smoke-free?"
- Provide information and reassurance that you will be available to help when they are ready.

Contemplation—Motivate and Assist

- Encourage patients to think about their own pros and cons for smoking versus quitting. Help them understand that the benefits of quitting are well worth the challenge.
- Be understanding if patients express ambivalence about quitting or seem discouraged from failed attempts to quit in the past.
- Provide encouragement and positive reinforcement of their desire to quit and reassurance about any perceived deterrents, e.g., "It is great that you are thinking about quitting. That is the first step towards success. I know you are concerned about gaining weight, but this is something that can be prevented. I can certainly help you with this. Let me know when you are ready to talk more about it."

Preparation—Show and Tell

- Help patients set a quit date, ideally within the next 2 weeks. The patient may choose to quit abruptly on that day with NRT or to gradually reduce cigarettes smoked to help minimize withdrawal before the quit date.[37]
- Use the Modified Fagerström Nicotine Tolerance Scale (see Table 3) to assess nicotine dependence, then help select the most suitable smoking cessation method.
- Address questions/concerns about smoking cessation, e.g., nicotine withdrawal, nicotine replacement products, triggers, past quit attempts, weight gain.
- Prior to quitting, encourage patients to avoid smoking in places where a great deal of time will be spent such as in the car or at home to help minimize the behavioural and psychological aspects of smoking.[38]
- Suggest avoiding triggers by removing smoking paraphernalia, e.g., ashtrays and lighters from the home and vehicles, and cleaning areas to remove the smell of smoke.
- Suggest strategies to deal with cravings, e.g., remembering the reasons for quitting smoking, distractions such as exercise, relaxation, taking deep breaths, low calorie snacks and seeking social support.
- Encourage patients to identify and inform individuals they will count on for support during the quit process, e.g., family, friends, co-workers.
- Inform patients of community resources available to assist with smoking cessation such as quit lines (see Table 4).

Action—Congratulate

- Provide positive feedback and praise for taking the important step of quitting.
- Ask patient about progress since your last visit, e.g., "How are you dealing with cravings? Have you had any setbacks since we last spoke and if so how did they affect you?"
- Reinforce coping strategies that were successful or suggest new ones if necessary.
- Reassess medication use and suggest changes as appropriate.
- Continue to provide support and follow up periodically.

Maintenance—Support

- Continue to provide positive reinforcement.
- Work to prevent relapse and encourage long-term self-management.
- Remind patients of their own reasons for quitting and help demonstrate their success and progress, e.g., "You know, you have barely needed your blue inhaler in the last few months. This tells me that your asthma is under much better control since you quit smoking."

Relapse—Don't Give Up

- Remind patients that this situation should be considered a "learning experience" rather than a failure.
- Find out what stage of change they are currently in and assist them with getting back into the preparation stage.
- Identify triggers for relapse and discuss strategies for prevention.
- Help patients identify personal strengths and weaknesses and formulate a new plan of attack.
- Motivate and encourage them to try again no matter what, e.g., "Quitting smoking is one of the most difficult things to do and it often takes a few attempts before a person becomes completely smoke-free. With each attempt, you are getting that much closer to quitting permanently. If you are willing to try again, we can discuss. I am here to help."

Motivational Interviewing

Motivational interviewing is a goal-orientated method used to motivate a patient to change behaviour. Although there is a lack of evidence due to inconsistency and standardization issues, motivational interviewing can still be a valuable tool when properly used, to assist a patient in overcoming barriers and making a commitment to change.[39]

Some strategies and techniques in motivational interviewing include:

- Open-ended questions: Engage the patient in open-ended questions to encourage elaboration and discussion. For example, ask, "What do you like (or not like) about smoking?" or "What does your life look like to you 10 years from now. Are you still smoking?"
- Change talk: Engage patients in conversation that inquires about their own personal reasons for changing. For example, ask, "Tell me your reasons for changing or quitting smoking. Why are these reasons important to you?"
- Reflective listening: Listen to patients and paraphrase their responses back to them to gain understanding and perspective
- Normalizing: Communicate to patients that the difficulties and barriers they may be facing are common for someone at their stage of change
- Summarizing: Summarize points that have been discussed, specific plans of action, and personal reasons for taking that action.

For further information on motivational interviewing, see Resource Tips.

Behaviour Modification Programs

About 1 in 5 smokers preparing to stop smoking actually seeks formal help with quitting. Although smokers can become involved in self-help programs, healthcare practitioners should be providing information on behavioural interventions for all smokers, regardless of the patient's motivation to quit. For effective engagement strategies, see Suggested Readings.

Even brief advice to quit from a primary care physician during a routine consultation has been effective in increasing the number of smokers who remain abstinent for at least 6 months. Person-to-person counselling over 4 or more sessions is especially effective. In general, greater contact between the patient and the program provider leads to greater success.[7,40]

Regardless of their level of nicotine dependence, encourage patients to participate in a behaviour modification program. Light smokers may be able to achieve lasting abstinence using behaviour modification alone, while moderate to heavy smokers benefit from the addition of pharmacologic therapy. The combination of pharmacotherapy and behaviour modification increases success rates in smoking cessation compared with usual care.[41] This further validates the importance of behaviour modification programs in addition to pharmacotherapy.

Even the simplest type of behaviour modification programs may be beneficial. Self-help in the form of electronic aids such as internet sites and text messages designed to assist individuals to stop smoking may be effective in increasing the likelihood of long-term cessation.[42,43,44]

Support groups are more effective than self-help materials such as pamphlets or handouts, but more evidence is needed to compare support groups with one-on-one counselling.[45]

Many self-help materials, individual and group programs, and counselling programs are available to both healthcare practitioners and patients. A list of programs in each province is available on the Health Canada and the Lung Association web sites (see Table 4).

Table 4: **Smoking Cessation Programs and Resources**

Program Name	Description	Contact Information	Cost
Canadian Action Network for the Advancement, Dissemination and Adoption of Practice-informed Tobacco Treatment (CAN-ADAPTT)	Mainly for HCPs; user can post online questions to panel experts or colleagues. Quick reference to guideline updates	1-416-535-8501 (Ext. 7427) www.nicotinedependenceclinic.com/English/CANADAPTT/Pages/Home.aspx (affiliated with CAMH)	Free[a]
Centre for Addiction and Mental Health (CAMH)	Online information for the public on tobacco use. HCP education programs such as the TEACH project	www.camh.ca 1-416-535-8501 (Ext. 1600)	Free[a]
Lung Association	Tips for quitting and listings of local support groups	www.lung.ca/lung-health/smoking-and-tobacco/how-quit-smoking/choose-support	
On the Road to Quitting—Guide to Becoming a Non-smoker	A 40-page self-help guide and online program to assist smokers with the quitting process	Health Canada smoking cessation website www.hc-sc.gc.ca/hc-ps/pubs/tobac-tabac/road-voie-eng.php	Free[a]
One Step at a Time—A Smoker's Guide to Quitting	Self-help program for patients—includes books (*For Smokers Who Want to Quit* and *For Smokers Who Don't Want to Quit*) and a pamphlet for assisting others who wish to quit	Canadian Cancer Society 1-888-939-3333 www.cancer.ca (also available through the Smoker's Helpline service)	Free[a]
QUIT—Quit Using and Inhaling Tobacco	Training program that provides useful resources and tools for practising pharmacists. Live workshops and an online lesson are available	Canadian Pharmacists Association 1-800-917-9489 www.pharmacists.ca/quit	[b]
Smokers' Helpline	Service provided by trained counsellors to assist patients who are seeking help with smoking cessation. Telephone assistance, online and print materials available in French and English	www.smokershelpline.ca Toll-free telephone numbers provided for each province and territory	Free[a]

[a] Shipping costs may apply for large orders.
[b] Fee for live and online workshops; resources free for participants.

Abbreviations: HCP = healthcare practitioner; TEACH = Training Enhancement in Applied Cessation Counselling and Health

To provide optimum support for smoking cessation, healthcare practitioners need proper training.[46] The "5 A's Approach" is a universally adopted tool healthcare practitioners often use as part of a smoking cessation program. The 5 A's consist of: Ask, Advise, Assess, Assist and Arrange. Healthcare practitioners can be trained in this approach via several programs including QUIT and TEACH (see Table 4).

Acupuncture

Acupuncture therapy for smoking cessation is based on the Chinese concept of energy pathways in the body. It involves special needles placed at strategic points under the skin of the nose or ear. Evidence of effectiveness in smoking cessation is not available; most studies were poorly conducted, yielding unreliable results.[47,48,49]

Aversion Therapy

Aversion therapy is based on the concept that association of an unpleasant sensation with smoking can reduce the desire to smoke. Techniques have included mild electric shock, breath-holding, rapid smoking, unpleasant taste, noise or smell, and imagined stimuli. Good evidence to support aversion techniques is lacking; rapid or excessive smoking has shown the most promise; however, due to the potentially harmful effect on the heart and lungs, this method is not recommended as a smoking cessation strategy.[47,49]

Clove and Herbal Cigarettes

Imitation cigarettes containing ingredients such as cloves and various herbs are available. However, these products may also contain tar, carbon monoxide and various other toxins. Clove cigarettes may actually contain up to 70% tobacco, providing nicotine and the same toxins as all-tobacco cigarettes.[50,51]

Electronic Cigarettes

Electronic cigarettes contain a battery-powered mechanism to heat and vapourize a liquid chemical mixture composed of varying amounts of nicotine, propylene glycol, other chemicals and/or impurities. The vapour produced resembles the smoke of an actual cigarette, which may satisfy the behaviours associated with smoking (handling of cigarette, inhaling of smoke) in addition to nicotine addiction. Advocates of e-cigarettes praise them as a clean drug delivery device, although the chemical safety is unknown. For example, propylene glycol is a known irritant and the long-term effects on the lungs are unknown at this time.[52] Additionally, the FDA conducted a preliminary analysis on samples of e-cigarettes from leading brands and found known carcinogens and toxic chemicals.[53] Although the analysis conducted was preliminary, it illustrates the lack of research on these products and the need for additional data on safety and effectiveness.

Electronic cigarettes are currently sold in Canada and are also available via the internet. However, since the production is not regulated, some electronic cigarettes contain nicotine while others contain varying levels of other chemicals. It is important to note that only those products without nicotine or health claims can be legally imported and sold in Canada.[54] Over 400 brands of electronic cigarettes are available.[53] There is world-wide debate concerning electronic cigarettes, since the potential benefit of smoking cessation may outweigh the potential risks. Current evidence does not support the use of electronic cigarettes for smoking cessation.[55,56] Health Canada does not recommend using electronic cigarettes due to lack of safety information regarding exposure to vapourized propylene glycol (among other chemicals used in the products) and their unknown long-term effects.[54]

Financial Incentives

Financial incentives are being used more frequently to encourage people to quit smoking. Although there has been some success with improved abstinence rates in the short term, the long-term (>12 months) efficacy of these strategies is yet to be determined.[57] Further research is required.[58,59] One population that may respond to financial incentives is pregnant women. See Pregnancy for more information.

Hypnosis

Hypnosis is a deep, relaxed state of attention during which people are more responsive to suggestions. Hypnotherapy for smoking cessation attempts to change a person's habits and attitudes to cigarettes. The therapist's skill and experience are very important, as are the patient's susceptibility to hypnosis and desire to quit. Although there are reports of success with this method, a Cochrane review concluded there was insufficient evidence to consider hypnotherapy effective for smoking cessation.[48] If this method is tried, advise patients to combine it with behaviour modification or counselling. Follow-up counselling and support or combining the therapy with other smoking cessation methods may also improve the success of hypnotherapy.[47,49,60]

Laser Therapy

Similar to the application of acupuncture, laser therapy uses laser beams which are directed at certain key points on the body surface. This stimulation of key points purportedly triggers a release of endorphins and relieves nicotine cravings. No reliable studies support this therapy.[47,48,49]

Pharmacologic Therapy

Pharmacologic therapy for smoking cessation can be divided into 2 broad categories: nicotine replacement therapy and non-nicotine therapies.

The purpose of pharmacologic therapy is to reduce the physical effects of nicotine withdrawal (see Table 1), which peak within 72 hours and may continue intermittently for several weeks. In some patients, pharmacologic therapy is also needed to reduce the psychological effects of withdrawal (cravings), which can last up to several years, or as some ex-smokers will attest, indefinitely.[4,5] While many patients may benefit from pharmacologic therapy, patients who are only mildly addicted may not require it to quit successfully. Pharmacotherapy may be contraindicated for certain patients because of potential drug or disease interactions.

Determining the most effective therapy from published studies is difficult. Varenicline, NRT and combination NRT have been found to be comparable at increasing the likelihood of a successful quit attempt.[61] Other assessments have shown varenicline to be superior to the nicotine patch but comparable to combination NRT.[62] Bupropion is generally thought to be less effective than varenicline, but has been found to be comparable to the patch alone.[63] Some of the difficulty in interpreting results of studies is due to variations in study design and population, and differences in the definition of abstinence. All available therapeutic options increase the chances of a successful quit attempt. Recommend the form of therapy that is most appropriate and acceptable to the patient.

Alternative agents that are effective but with more side effects or less evidence are clonidine, nortriptyline and cytisine.[62]

Nicotine Replacement Therapy

Nicotine replacement therapy (NRT), designed to replace the nicotine found in cigarettes, is the mainstay of nonprescription therapy for smoking cessation. In Canada, NRT medications are considered unscheduled products and can be obtained from any retailer without a prescription.

Available dosage forms include chewing pieces (gum), lozenges, inhalers, mouth sprays and transdermal patches (see Table 8). Nasal sprays and sublingual tablets are not available in Canada.

Nicotine replacement therapy increases abstinence rates by 50–70 percent.[64] The success of NRT is independent of dosage form, concurrent therapy and setting.

In general, the incidence of adverse effects with NRT is low provided the patient receives adequate counselling on the appropriate use of the product. It is important to consider that some contraindications may be relative rather than absolute contraindications, requiring clinical judgment in the decision-making process. Given the significant risks of continued smoking, the risk/benefit ratio for pharmacotherapy may be favourable even in pregnant patients or those with heart disease. These patients can often be successfully and safely managed with NRT or other pharmacotherapy under guidance of their healthcare practitioner or specialist. See Special Considerations.[65]

For comparative ingredients of nonprescription products, consult the *Compendium of Products for Minor Ailments*—Smoking Cessation Products.

Combination NRT

The combination of nicotine patch with as-needed gum, inhaler or lozenges may be more effective than the individual products, possibly because it provides a steady baseline level of nicotine with "boluses" for flexibility and treatment of cravings.[7,63,64] One study comparing combination NRT to NRT patch alone and varenicline found no difference in long-term quit rates of about 20% for all therapies.[61]

For heavy smokers who continue to suffer withdrawal symptoms despite indicated doses, i.e., a single nicotine patch, it is common practice to increase the total daily nicotine doses by use of combinations of NRT products. Off-label uses include total daily doses of nicotine up to 35 mg per day for smokers previously using 21–40 cigarettes a day, and up to 40 mg per day for smokers previously using more than 40 cigarettes a day, with reported safety and improved efficacy.[66,67,68] These doses may be achieved by using additional patches or fast-acting nicotine, e.g., gum, inhaler, lozenge or spray, or a combination of patch and fast-acting products. Using more than 1 patch or total daily doses >30 mg requires appropriate healthcare practitioner supervision.

Further studies are needed to define the ideal candidates for combination therapy. In practice, it would be reasonable to provide combination NRT to smokers who have struggled with NRT patches or other single forms.

Non-nicotine Pharmacotherapy

A number of non-nicotine therapeutic agents have been investigated for use in smoking cessation.

Bupropion is effective for smoking cessation.[7,69] Contraindications include a history of seizures, anorexia or bulimia nervosa and concurrent MAOI therapy. More common adverse effects include dry mouth and insomnia. Less common are hypertension, arthralgia, myalgia, dizziness, tremor, somnolence, bronchitis, pruritus, rash and taste perversion.[70] Some patients may develop agitation-like behavioural or emotional changes, which may increase the rare risk of harm to themselves or to others. Close patient monitoring is advised for all patients, but especially in those with underlying psychiatric illness.[70]

As with other pharmacotherapeutic agents for smoking cessation, bupropion should be used in combination with behavioural programs to assist the quitting process, and can be used during pregnancy if benefit outweighs the risk.[70]

Varenicline is an $alpha_4beta_2$-nicotinic receptor partial agonist used to assist patients with smoking cessation.[7] It also may be an option for smokers who are unable to abruptly stop smoking. One study has shown that among cigarette smokers who are not willing or able to quit but are willing to reduce the number of cigarettes smoked, varenicline used for 24 weeks significantly increased cessation rates (27%) compared with placebo (9.9%).[71] Patients should be advised about common side effects such as nausea, vomiting, headache, insomnia, abnormal dreams and dizziness.

Concerns regarding potential cardiovascular risks of varenicline[72,73] prompted Health Canada to review its cardiovascular safety.[74] The review drew no firm conclusions due to small study populations available at the time.[75] Subsequent analyses, including a meta-analysis of 18 clinical trials, suggested no significant increase in cardiovascular adverse events associated with varenicline use.[76,77,78] It still may be prudent to cautiously assess patients before initiating therapy in those with cardiovascular concerns.

Safety concerns have also been raised regarding neuropsychiatric symptoms. Investigations into concerns regarding severe behavioural changes, e.g., suicidal ideation, depression or suicide attempt, have found no increase in these events in patients on varenicline compared with placebo.[79,80] One study confirmed the lack of association but found a small increase in anxiety and mood conditions only in persons with pre-existing psychiatric disorders.[81] Regardless of therapy being used for smoking cessation, psychological changes should be monitored with every patient.[82]

Varenicline is contraindicated during pregnancy as there is evidence of reproductive toxicity in animal studies, though no human pregnancy data are available.[83]

Nortriptyline is a treatment option that has been shown to aid long-term smoking cessation. As with bupropion, the mode of action of nortriptyline is independent of its antidepressant effects and it has similar efficacy to NRT.[69] **Clonidine** is somewhat effective but of limited use because of significant side effects.[7,62,84,85] See Table 9.

Although it is not currently available in Canada, **cytisine**, a partial agonist that binds the nicotinic acetylcholine receptor, has been found to be superior to NRT when combined with brief behavioural support. Its use is limited by frequently reported adverse events.[86]

Combination Therapy

Despite concerns over additive side effects, such as nausea, headache or dyspepsia when combining varenicline with NRT, the combination was found to be well tolerated in 2 separate studies.[87,88] These 2 studies yielded contradictory results. One study found the combination to be superior to varenicline alone for cessation rates;[88] the other found no benefit.[87] Further studies are needed to assess long-term efficacy and safety of the combination.

The combination of varenicline and bupropion was studied in a group of people who were unable to reduce their smoking by at least 50% after 1 week of NRT.[89] Compared with varenicline alone, subjects taking varenicline plus bupropion were more likely to be smoke free at 8–11 weeks. The combination was statistically superior in men, but not in women. Smokers with high nicotine dependence were also more likely to be successful on the combination. This study was of short duration, but suggests that the combination is safe and may be effective for select smokers. Further studies are needed to better define the role of this combination.

Bupropion combined with NRT has been studied with mixed results. One study found higher quit rates in the combination group, but the difference was not statistically significant.[90] Another study found no difference among bupropion monotherapy, NRT monotherapy or the combination.[91] A third study in patients with schizophrenia found the combination of bupropion and high-dose NRT had greater abstinence rates while using bupropion and high-dose NRT compared with placebo and high-dose NRT, but relapse rates were high and no difference in cessation rates was found at 1 year. This study was small and may have lacked statistical power to detect a true difference.[92] Based on the currently available evidence, the combination of bupropion and NRT cannot be recommended for routine use.

Special Considerations

Pregnancy

Nonpharmacologic choices are always first-line for pregnant patients, as behavioural therapy has proven effective for smoking cessation in pregnancy.[93] Financial incentives such as shopping vouchers demonstrated substantial evidence of efficacy for smoking cessation in pregnancy.[94] Psychosocial interventions such as social support and counselling can increase the proportion of pregnant women who stop smoking which will help reduce the risk of low birth weight and preterm birth.

Evidence is insufficient to determine whether NRT is effective or safe for smoking cessation in pregnancy.[95] Women with moderate to high nicotine dependence will likely require some form of pharmacotherapy.[7] One must balance the risks of continuing to smoke with the risks of using NRT. The products are not officially approved for use in pregnancy and NRT may have potential risks to the mother and fetus;[7,96] however, cigarette smoking during pregnancy may have far greater risks including exposure to the 4000 other chemicals in tobacco smoke. Most experts believe that if nonpharmacologic and/or behavioural strategies fail, interventions with NRT would be justified and can be attempted with close supervision by an appropriate healthcare practitioner. It is important to incorporate behavioural interventions and to use the lowest effective dose of NRT. Initiation of smoking cessation is important during the earlier stages of pregnancy, ideally within the first 16 weeks.

Evidence shows that nicotine patches do not have a lasting effect on smoking cessation in pregnancy compared with placebo; however, use of NRT patches during pregnancy resulted in lower incidence of developmental impairment in the offspring at 2 years, compared with placebo.[97,98] Further research is required to determine the safety and efficacy of NRT use in pregnancy.

If NRT is to be used in pregnancy, an immediate-release form of NRT such as the gum, lozenge or inhaler may be preferred over a continuous dosage form such as the patch. Use the lowest effective dose, for the shortest possible time, to reduce fetal exposure to nicotine. If a patient is highly addicted to nicotine, use of the patch may be necessary. In these cases, use of a patch during waking hours only (e.g., a 24-hour patch applied for 16 hours and removed at night) can reduce fetal nicotine exposure. Close supervision and monitoring is essential for all pregnant patients and should involve the patient's physician.

Breastfeeding

Nicotine is excreted in breast milk when NRT is used. The risk to the infant for NRT-related nicotine exposure is lower than the risk from second-hand smoke, such as increased risk of sudden infant death syndrome, respiratory infections or asthma.[7] Intermittent use of immediate-release forms of NRT are preferred in breastfeeding mothers. Encourage the mother to breastfeed just before using the NRT product, to minimize infant exposure to nicotine.[96]

Cardiovascular Disease

It is dangerous for patients with cardiovascular disease to continue to smoke. Smoking can activate coagulation pathways in the body, promoting thrombus formation and increasing the risk of myocardial infarction. Nicotine can also cause vasoconstriction as well as increased heart rate and contractility.[2] Despite this, many experts now believe that short-term use of NRT is safer than smoking, although there are risks involved with the use of NRT products. Evidence suggests that NRT is generally safe in patients with stable cardiovascular disease.[99,100] Caution and supervision by an appropriate healthcare practitioner are recommended, particularly within 2 weeks following myocardial infarction or in patients with unstable angina or serious arrhythmias.[7,101] The transdermal patch may be preferable to immediate-release dosage forms because of more consistent nicotine plasma concentrations.

Older Adults

Although damage to the lungs cannot be reversed, quitting smoking can extend the time to disability or death regardless of age or smoking history.[102] Even at older ages, smoking cessation is beneficial for reducing cardiovascular risk.[103] Improvements in health from smoking cessation are achievable in older adults, making it critical to emphasize to patients that it is never too late to quit. The loss of lung function is not reversed but it can be slowed with successful cessation. Even at advanced ages, smokers who quit can slow the decline in function and reduce morbidity. See Figure 1 for an illustration of the impact of smoking cessation on FEV_1 at various ages. NRT remains the therapy of choice in older adults due to experience and limited evidence showing efficacy.[104] Further research in this population is needed to compare NRT with other therapeutic options such as varenicline and bupropion.

Figure 1: **Impact of Smoking Status on Lung Function Over Lifetime**

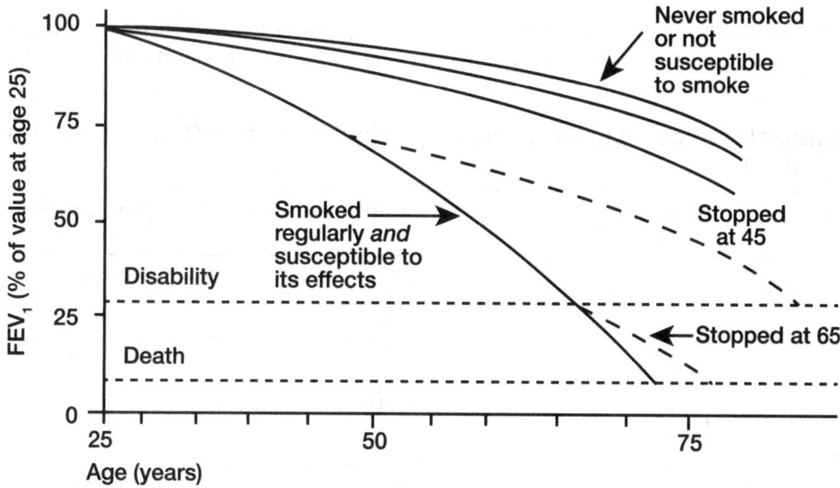

Adapted from Fletcher C, Peto R. The natural history of chronic airflow obstruction. *Br Med J* 1977;1(6077):1645-8, with permission of BMJ Publishing Group Limited.

Children and Adolescents

Tobacco use is a major concern in the pediatric population.[7] Experimentation with nicotine and drugs begins ages 11–17 years or earlier in some cases. Nicotine dependence can occur rapidly in this population. Primary prevention is key and healthcare practitioners must deliver strong messages of prevention and cessation to this group and their parents.[105] Adolescents are interested in quitting. A survey of about 5000 eleventh grade students revealed that approximately 79% would be willing to discuss or acknowledge their smoking habit if they were asked about it.[7] This sets the stage for healthcare practitioners to engage in tobacco use discussion—simply by asking the 3 main assessment questions (see Patient Assessment). Many patients may not be ready to quit at the first visit but a strong message from a healthcare practitioner regarding tobacco abstinence and/or cessation to young patients and their parents is important in the prevention of youth tobacco use.

The current recommendation for smoking cessation in adolescent smokers focuses on behavioural approaches. Recommend Health Canada's "Quit4Life" program to this age group (see Table 4). Avoid incentive programs that use prizes aimed at prevention of smoking. They are not effective in adolescents.[106] Although NRT has been shown to be safe in this population, it is generally not recommended. Counselling is the most effective approach. There is little evidence that pharmacotherapy is effective in promoting long-term abstinence rates in younger patients.[7] When pharmacologic therapy (including NRT) is required in patients under 18 years of age, it should be initiated and monitored by a healthcare practitioner.

Smokeless Tobacco

Discontinuation of smokeless tobacco products in post-MI patients was associated with an almost 50% reduction in mortality, similar to the benefit seen with smoking cessation.[107] This finding emphasizes the importance of encouraging users of smokeless tobacco to quit. Counselling is effective for treating patients who use smokeless tobacco products and should be considered first-line.[7,108] Bupropion and nicotine replacement therapy (NRT) have not demonstrated long-term abstinence rates for smokeless tobacco cessation; however, NRT can be used in the short-term to alleviate nicotine withdrawal symptoms. Varenicline is an effective pharmacologic choice for tobacco abstinence in smokeless tobacco users.[109] High-dose NRT and combination therapies have not yet been studied in these patients.[108]

Table 5 can be used to estimate the equivalent number of cigarettes to smokeless tobacco consumption. The healthcare practitioner can then recommend a trial dose of NRT therapy if that is the chosen pharmacotherapy.

Table 5: **Smokeless Tobacco, Cigarettes and Nicotine Patch: Conversion and Dosing Chart[110]**

Pinches of Smokeless Tobacco	Number of Cans of Tobacco/Week	Number of Cigarettes	Suggested Nicotine Patch Starting Dose
1		3–4	7 mg daily
2		6–8	
3	1	9–11	14 mg daily
4		12–14	
5		15–17	
6	2	18–20 (1 pack)	21 mg daily
13	4	39–41 (2 packs)	42 mg daily
20	6	60–62 (3 packs)	
26	8	78–80 (4 packs)	

Drug Interactions

Cigarette smoking can affect the metabolism of many drugs. A major carcinogen found in tobacco smoke, polycyclic aromatic hydrocarbons (PAH), is responsible for induction of hepatic enzymes CYP1A1, 1A2, and possibly 2E1.[111] CYP1A2 is the main pathway affected. Nicotine does not induce enzymes so drug interactions occur with tobacco smoke but not with NRT.

Induction of enzymes or changes in effects of drugs can take a couple of weeks to manifest so monitoring of therapy is essential. The clearance of drugs such as acetaminophen, caffeine, clozapine, diazepam, estrogens, fluvoxamine, methadone, nifedipine, olanzapine, opioid analgesics, rasagiline, theophylline, and warfarin may be increased in smokers. Consequently, when patients quit smoking, increased monitoring and dosage reduction may be required once drug metabolism is no longer affected by smoking.

Table 6: **Drug Interactions with Tobacco Smoke**[111,112,113]

Drug/Class	Suggested Clinical Management
acetaminophen caffeine clozapine diazepam estrogens fluvoxamine methadone nifedipine olanzapine opioid analgesics (e.g., oxycodone, codeine) rasagiline theophylline warfarin	**When patient stops smoking:** ▪ Consider decreasing dose based on clinical and adverse effects. Clinical management requires individualization of approach based on needs and response of the patient. ▪ Recommend decreasing caffeine intake by 50% upon initiation of cessation attempt. **When patient starts smoking:** ▪ Consider increasing dose if clinical effect appears to be lessened. Clinical management requires individualization of approach based on needs and response of the patient.

Assess for drug interactions or refer patients to an appropriate healthcare practitioner if they are taking drugs that may be affected by smoking and are planning to quit. Reduction of caffeine intake is advised to minimize caffeine-induced palpitations, agitation and other side effects during and after the quit attempt. Potential interactions involving tobacco smoke are listed in Table 6.

Monitoring of Therapy

Because of the large behavioural component of smoking cessation, monitoring of therapy is crucial to success. Ideally, the patient receives ongoing monitoring for a period of time by a clinician or therapist involved with a smoking cessation program (see Table 7). If monitoring is not available from the program, healthcare practitioners should offer it.

Relapse rates are high, particularly at the beginning of smoking cessation attempts, with 66% of patients reportedly relapsing within 48 hours and 76% within the first week of unassisted quit attempts.[7] Follow up should begin within the initial week following the quit date, particularly if the patient is receiving NRT, to avoid adverse effects from excessive nicotine levels. Follow-up counselling should be provided regularly, e.g., every month for 3 months, then at 6 and 12 months. In general, more counselling time yields higher abstinence rates.[7] Additional monitoring should be considered for patients who are at high risk, e.g., highly nicotine-addicted patients with history of many previous smoking cessation attempts, patients experiencing severe psychosocial stress, those with comorbid substance abuse disorders or history of depression or schizophrenia, patients taking concomitant medication that interacts with nicotine, or cases where smoking cessation is medically urgent. A suggested schedule for more intensive monitoring might involve follow up every 2 weeks for the first 3 months, then at 6, 9, 12, 18 and 24 months.

Table 7: **Monitoring of Therapy for Smoking Cessation[a]**

Parameter	Indicators/Goal/ Time Frame	Suggested Monitoring Frequency	Recommended Intervention
Smoking	Patient reports no smoking.	Patient: Daily Healthcare practitioner: Monthly × 3 months then at 6 and 12 months	Inquire about amount smoked; provide encouragement and support. If patient has a relapse, discontinue nicotine replacement therapy until patient is ready to quit again; encourage patient to reset a quit date; discuss possible reasons for relapse and help patient strategize about how to be more successful with the next quit attempt; be empathetic and avoid scolding the patient.
Desire to smoke	Patient reports level of desire decreasing to minimal (or none) by end of therapy (3–6 months); cravings may never completely end for some.	As above	Intense craving may require alternate treatment (see Table 8 and Table 9). Encourage behavioural changes to decrease desire; empathize with patient's difficulty and strongly encourage perseverance.
Nicotine withdrawal symptoms	Patient on NRT reports reduction in withdrawal symptoms (see Table 1) within 25 min to 24 h of initiating therapy.	As above	If symptoms are bothersome, consider increasing dose of NRT if using, switching to or adding an alternate therapy (see Table 8 and Table 9). Remind patients that the most difficult period is the first 2–14 days. Recommend additional behavioural interventions if necessary.
Medication adverse effects	Patient reports no adverse effects when questioned specifically throughout duration of pharmacotherapeutic treatment.	As above	If minor side effects occur, suggest ways to modify, e.g., for belching, hiccoughs and GI upset with gum, advise proper chewing technique, or consider switching to an alternative method of NRT. If serious adverse effects occur, (e.g., hypertension, nicotine toxicity, mood changes, seizures) consider reducing dose or discontinuing medication and/or switching to alternate therapy (see Table 8 and Table 9).
Weight gain[114,115]	Patient reports minimal or no weight gain over the 6–12 months following quitting.	Patient: Weekly Healthcare practitioner: 3, 6, 9, 12, 18 and 24 months	Encourage healthy eating habits, exercise, healthy snacks to deal with cravings, e.g., carrot sticks, to prevent or minimize weight gain. Reassure patient that slight weight gain is less harmful to their health than continued smoking.
Stress	Patient reports minimal additional stress due to smoking cessation over 6–12 months following quitting.	Patient: Daily Healthcare practitioner: 3, 6, 9, 12, 18 and 24 months	Assess for evidence of excessive stress, e.g., weight loss, nervous habits, GI symptoms, headache. Suggest behavioural therapy, e.g., deep breathing, muscle relaxation, positive self-talk, or refer to stress management program. Encourage exercise and other distracting activities. Treat stress-related symptoms as needed (recommend appropriate medication to reduce stress or treat stress-related physical symptoms).
Mood	Patient reports minimal mood changes due to smoking cessation.	Patient: daily Healthcare practitioner: 3, 6, 9, 12, 18 and 24 months	Assess for any signs of depression, severe agitation or mood changes. Family and/or caregivers should be informed and alerted to watch for these changes or symptoms.

a List of monitoring parameters is not exhaustive. Parameters should be tailored to individual patient.

Abbreviations: NRT = nicotine replacement therapy

Figure 2: **Assessment of Patients with Nicotine Dependence**

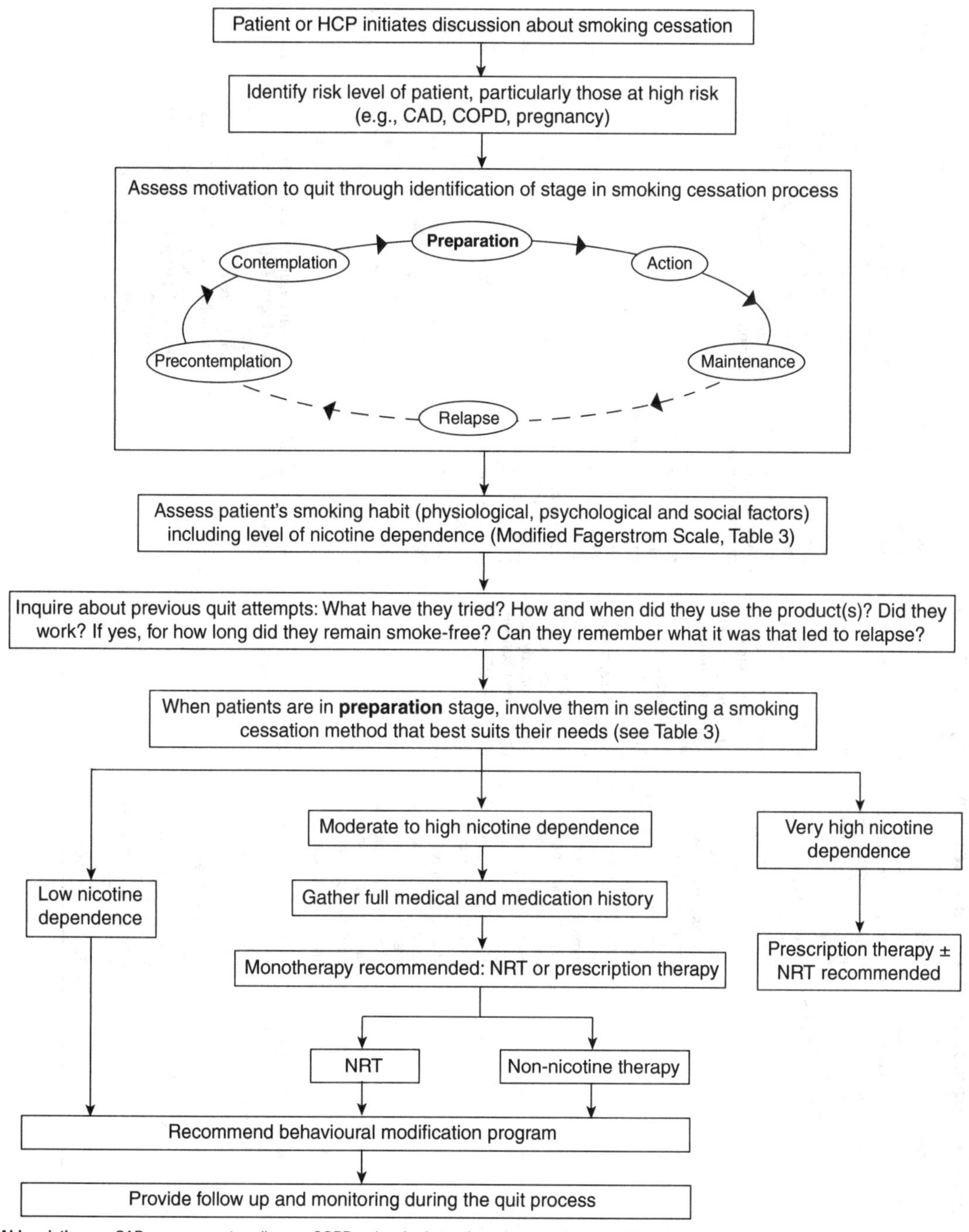

Abbreviations: CAD = coronary artery disease; COPD = chronic obstructive pulmonary disease; HCP = healthcare professional; NRT = nicotine replacement therapy

Table 8: Nicotine Replacement Therapy for Smoking Cessation

Class	Drug	Dosage	Adverse Effects	Contraindications	Comments	Cost[a]
Nicotine replacement, immediate-release	*nicotine gum/chewing pieces (nicotine polacrilex)* Nicorette Gum, Thrive Gum, generics	Initial strength: Nicorette: 2 mg if Fagerström score is ≤6, 4 mg if ≥7 (see Table 3). Thrive: 4 mg if ≥25 cigarettes/day, 2 mg if <25 cigarettes/day Initial dose: 10–12 pieces per day po; may increase to 20 pieces per day if needed Place 1 piece of gum in the mouth. Bite down once or twice then park it between the teeth and gums for about 1 min. Repeat when the desire to smoke arises or once the 'tingling' sensation stops, up to once per min for up to 30 min, then discard piece At weekly intervals, reduce by 1 piece/day over 3 months, as withdrawal symptoms allow. Continue for maximum of 6 months Peak: 20–30 min	Jaw, mouth or throat soreness. CNS: depression, anxiety, irritability, insomnia; dizziness, weakness, headache. Gastrointestinal: changes in taste perception, hiccoughs dyspepsia, nausea, vomiting. Cardiovascular: hypertension, palpitations, tachycardia, chest pain. Skin: erythema, itching, rash, urticaria. Respiratory: dyspnea, cough, hoarseness, sneezing, wheezing.	Life-threatening arrhythmia; severe angina pectoris; history of recent stroke; temporomandibular joint disease; within 2 wk following myocardial infarction. Relative contraindications: pregnancy, smoking while using this medication (nicotine toxicity), breastfeeding, age <18 y. Caution in hyperthyroidism, pheochromocytoma, insulin-dependent diabetes, active peptic ulcer, uncontrolled hypertension.	Caution patients not to chew like regular gum (increased side effects). Avoid use of acidic beverages and foods (coffee, fruit juices, soft drinks, alcohol) while chewing and 15 min before as this decreases absorption. Favourable dosing flexibility compared with patch.	$
	nicotine lozenges (nicotine bitartrate dihydrate) Thrive Lozenges	Initial strength: 1 mg if <20 cigarettes per day, 2 mg if ≥20 cigarettes per day Dosing frequency: see nicotine polacrilex lozenges; maximum 15/day po for 2 mg strength, 25/day po for 1 mg strength Peak: 20–60 min	See nicotine gum/ chewing pieces.	See nicotine gum/ chewing pieces.	Caution patients not to swallow or chew lozenges (increased side effects). Avoid acidic beverages and foods (e.g., coffee, fruit juices, soft drinks, alcohol) during and 15 min prior to using the lozenge as this decreases absorption. Favourable dosing flexibility compared with patch.	$$

Class	Drug	Dosage	Adverse Effects	Contraindications	Comments	Cost[a]
	nicotine lozenges (nicotine polacrilex) Nicorette Lozenge	Use initial strength of 2 mg if first cigarette of the day >30 min after waking, 4 mg if ≤30 min Weeks 1–6: Dissolve 1 lozenge in the mouth Q1–2H PRN for withdrawal symptoms (maximum 15 lozenges/day) Weeks 7–9: Use 1 lozenge Q2–4H PRN po Weeks 10–12: Use 1 lozenge Q4–8H PRN po Discontinue when the dose has been reduced to 1–2 lozenges/day Use beyond 6 months is not generally recommended Lozenges should be allowed to slowly dissolve and moved from one side of the mouth to the other periodically Peak: 20–60 min	See nicotine gum/chewing pieces.	See nicotine gum/chewing pieces.	See nicotine lozenges.	$$
	nicotine inhaler Nicorette Inhaler	Initial therapy: Use at least 6 cartridges/day (maximum 12 per day) for the first 3–6 wk. Begin to taper slowly over the next 6–12 wk. Discontinue once usage is down to 1–2 times per day (after 3 months ideally). Use may be continued with tapering dosage up to 6 months. Use for >6 months not recommended	Mainly mild local irritation, cough, throat irritation, pharyngitis, stomatitis, rhinitis. Headache, dyspepsia, nausea may also be present. Side effects are usually transient and decrease with continued use.	See nicotine gum/chewing pieces.	Each 10 mg cartridge delivers 4 mg of nicotine (of which about 2 mg is systemically absorbed); approximately equivalent to 20 min of puffing. Nicotine vapour is absorbed through the buccal lining of the mouth, not from the lungs. Colder ambient temperatures decrease absorption rate. Cartridge can be used for up to 24 h once punctured.	$$

(cont'd)

Table 8: **Nicotine Replacement Therapy for Smoking Cessation** *(cont'd)*

Class	Drug	Dosage	Adverse Effects	Contraindications	Comments	Cost[a]
		Inhalers should be puffed similarly to a cigarette (~5–10 min at a time) Peak: 15 min				
	nicotine mouthspray Nicorette QuickMist	Use 1 or 2 sprays every 30–60 min po Maximum dose: 2 sprays/episode, 4 sprays/h, 64 sprays/day Spray must be primed with first use or after 2 days of not using Peak: 16 min	Altered sense of taste, headache, hiccoughs, nausea and vomiting, dyspepsia, oral soft tissue pain, stomatitis, salivary hypersecretion, burning lips, dry mouth.	Life-threatening arrhythmia; severe angina pectoris; history of recent stroke; temporomandibular joint disease; within 2 wk following myocardial infarction. Relative contraindications: pregnancy, smoking while using this medication (nicotine toxicity), breastfeeding, age <18 y. Caution in hyperthyroidism, pheochromocytoma, insulin-dependent diabetes, active peptic ulcer, GI disease, uncontrolled hypertension, hepatic or renal impairment.	Each spray delivers 1 mg of nicotine. Mouthspray absorbed through buccal mucosa. Avoid acidic beverages and foods (coffee, fruit juices, soft drinks, alcohol) during use and 15 min before use as this may decrease absorption.	$$

Class	Drug	Dosage	Adverse Effects	Contraindications	Comments	Cost[a]
Nicotine replacement, sustained-release	*nicotine transdermal patch* Habitrol, Nicoderm, generics	Apply patch to nonhairy, clean, dry skin site on upper arm or hip; use a different site each day; avoid using the same site more than once weekly Apply upon waking and wear 16–24 h per day, depending on product General dosing instructions involve 6 wk of use of highest strength (21 mg for Nicoderm or Habitrol, 15 mg for Nicorette) followed by 2 wk at the intermediate strength then 2 wk at the lowest strength Consult individual product monographs for details Peak: 2–6 h	Local skin reactions: erythema, pruritus, edema, blisters, rash, burning sensation. CNS: headache, dizziness, paresthesias, insomnia, abnormal dreams, depression, somnolence, anxiety, emotional lability. Cardiovascular: palpitations, chest pain, blood pressure changes, tachycardia. Gastrointestinal: abdominal pain, dyspepsia, nausea, diarrhea, constipation, dry mouth, nausea and vomiting, flatulence, stomatitis. Respiratory: cough, pharyngitis, rhinitis, dyspnea, sinusitis. Other: myalgia, arthralgia, dysmenorrhea, toothache, sweating, taste perversion.	Life-threatening arrhythmia; severe angina pectoris; history of recent stroke; temporomandibular joint disease; within 2 wk following myocardial infarction; generalized skin disorders (severe eczema or psoriasis); hypersensitivity to topical adhesives or nicotine. Relative contraindications: pregnancy, smoking while using this medication (nicotine toxicity), breastfeeding, age <18 y; mild atopic or eczematous dermatitis. Caution in hyperthyroidism, pheochromocytoma, insulin-dependent diabetes, active peptic ulcer, uncontrolled hypertension.	Assess patient in first 2 wk to ensure smoking has been discontinued. Wearing patch during strenuous exercise may increase absorption and adverse effects. Used patches should be folded so that medicated sides are facing inward and discarded safely out of reach of children or pets. Manufacturers do not recommend cutting patches as this may damage the delivery device. Patients who experience insomnia from the 24-hour patch may benefit from removing the patch at night and using an immediate-release product first thing in the morning, then applying a new patch.	$$$

[a] Cost of 100 pieces of gum or lozenges, 42 cartridges, 150 sprays or 28 patches; includes drug cost only.

Legend: $ < $25 $$ $25–50 $$$ $50–75

Table 9: **Non-nicotine Therapy for Smoking Cessation**

Class	Drug	Dosage	Adverse Effects	Drug Interactions	Comments	Cost[a]
Alpha$_2$-adrenergic Receptor Agonists	*clonidine* Catapres, generics	0.1 mg BID po starting up to 3 days before or on the quit date. Titrate up by 0.1 mg/day po once per week as tolerated to a maximum of 0.4 mg/day. Duration of therapy ranges from 3–10 wk	Common: sedation, dizziness, hypotension, dry mouth. Less common: anxiety, irritability, memory problems.	Avoid concurrent use with tricyclic antidepressants. Additive effects with other CNS depressants such as ethanol. Additive hypotensive effect when combined with antihypertensive drugs.	Monitor blood pressure and heart rate during treatment initiation. Taper gradually to avoid rebound hypertension when stopping treatment.	$
Antidepressants	*bupropion* Zyban	150 mg daily po × 3 days then 150 mg BID po × 7–12 wk Begin 1–2 wk before the selected quit date	Usual: insomnia, dry mouth, dizziness, restlessness, difficulty concentrating. Unusual: hypersensitivity reactions, increased risk of seizures at higher dosages; agitation-type reactions involving mood/behavioural changes.	Inhibits CYP2D6; may decrease clearance of atomoxetine, duloxetine, fluoxetine, fluvoxamine, paroxetine, risperidone, sertraline, venlafaxine; may decrease effectiveness of codeine and tamoxifen. Do not use with MAO inhibitors (possible mania, excitation, hyperpyrexia). May be safely combined with NRT (monitor for treatment-emergent hypertension).	Not recommended in patients with conditions predisposing to seizures, history of seizures, current eating disorder or severe hepatic impairment. Least expensive of oral medications. Officially indicated for smoking cessation.	$$
	nortriptyline Aventyl	25 mg/day po titrated to 75–100 mg/day po Quit day is usually set between 1 and 4 wk; medication is continued for 12 wk	Common: dry mouth, blurred vision, constipation, dizziness, sedation. Less common: confusion, arrhythmias, urinary retention.	Do not use with MAO inhibitors (may cause mania, excitation, hyperpyrexia). Inducers of CYP2D6 or CYP3A4 such as carbamazepine, phenytoin or rifampin may decrease effect. Inhibitors of CYP2D6 or CYP3A4 such as clarithromycin, erythromycin, grapefruit juice, fluoxetine or paroxetine may increase effect and toxicity.	Not recommended in patients with conditions predisposing to seizures, history of seizures, current eating disorder or severe hepatic impairment. Least expensive of oral medications officially indicated for smoking cessation. Caution in patients with cardiovascular disease or arrhythmias. Consider measuring serum levels to reach therapeutic dose (based on efficacy data for depression).	$$

Class	Drug	Dosage	Adverse Effects	Drug Interactions	Comments	Cost[a]
Nicotine Receptor Partial Agonists	*varenicline* (kidney symbol) Champix	0.5 mg daily po for 3 days then BID for 4 days then 0.5–1 mg BID po for 12 wk. Patient should quit smoking 1–2 wk after starting varenicline. If patient is still smoking 4 wk after starting, reassess therapy; can be continued for an additional 12 wk if patient has benefited. If 1 mg BID not tolerated, can reduce to 0.5 mg BID. No tapering necessary when discontinuing	Nausea (30%); may be mitigated by taking on a full stomach, increasing water intake or reducing dose. May cause insomnia; take second daily dose at suppertime. Neuropsychiatric side effects such as suicidal/homicidal ideation have been reported; monitor closely for changes in mood/behaviour. Close monitoring by healthcare practitioner for those with pre-existing psychiatric disorders.	Combination with nicotine replacement therapy may increase risk of adverse effects.	Does not induce cytochrome P450 enzymes; excreted renally unchanged. Efficacy is dose related.	$$$$

[a] Cost of 30-day supply; includes drug cost only.

(Kidney symbol) Dosage adjustment may be required in renal impairment.

Legend: $ < $25 $$ $25–50 $$$ $50–75 $$$$ $75–100

Resource Tips

Canadian Lung Association. Available from: www.lung.ca. Note: World "No Tobacco Day" is May 31st each year. Partner with your local Lung Association for more resources (such as pamphlets and handouts) to assist you with a display or clinic day venue.

Health Canada. Quit4Life. Available from: www.quit4life.com.

Motivational Interviewing Network of Trainers (MINT). Available from: www.motivationalinterviewing.org.

Physicians for a Smoke-Free Canada. Available from: www.smoke-free.ca.

Suggested Readings

Centre for Addiction and Mental Health. Canadian Action Network for the Advancement, Dissemination and Adoption of Practice-informed Tobacco Treatment. *Canadian smoking cessation clinical practice guideline*. Toronto: CAN-ADAPTT; 2011. Available from: www.nicotinedependenceclinic.com/English/CANADAPTT/Guideline/Introduction.aspx.

The Lung Association. *Making quit happen: Canada's challenges to smoking cessation*. 2009. Available from: www.lung.ca/news/advocacy-tools/our-publications.

Mallin R. Smoking cessation: integration of behavioral and drug therapies. *Am Fam Phys* 2002;65:1107-14.

Marcano Belisario JS, Bruggeling MN, Gunn LH et al. Interventions for recruiting smokers into cessation programmes. *Cochrane Database Syst Rev* 2012;12:CD009187.

Selby P. Smoking cessation. In: Jovaisas B, ed. *Compendium of therapeutic choices*. 7th ed. Ottawa: Canadian Pharmacists Association; 2014. p. 172-88.

References

1. *Tobacco, nicotine and addiction: a committee report*. Prepared at the Request of The Royal Society of Canada for the Health Protection Branch, Health and Welfare Canada. Ottawa: The Society; 1989.
2. Brunton LL, Lazo JS, Parker KL, eds. *Goodman & Gilman's pharmacological basis of therapeutics*. 11th ed. New York: McGraw-Hill Medical; 2006.
3. American Psychiatric Association. DSM-5 Task Force. *Diagnostic and statistical manual of mental disorders: DSM-5*. 5th ed. Washington: American Psychiatric Publishing; 2013.
4. Gossel TA. The physiological and pharmacological effects of nicotine. *U.S. health professional supplement*. 1992 February.
5. Gourlay SG, McNeil JJ. Antismoking products. *Med J Aust* 1990;153:699-707.
6. Health Canada. *Canadian Tobacco Use Monitoring Survey (CTUMS) 2012*. Available from: www.hc-sc.gc.ca/hc-ps/tobac-tabac/research-recherche/stat/ctums-esutc_2012-eng.php. Accessed June 18, 2015.
7. Fiore MC, Jaen CR, Baker TB et al. *Treating tobacco use and dependence: 2008 update*. Rockville: U.S. Department of Health and Human Services; 2008.
8. Pollin W. The role of the addictive process as a key step in causation of all tobacco-related diseases. *JAMA* 1984;252:2874.
9. The Lung Association. *Making quit happen: Canada's challenges to smoking cessation*. 2009. Available from: www.lung.ca/news/advocacy-tools/our-publications. Accessed July 10, 2015.
10. Henningfield JE, Kozlowski LT, Benowitz NL. A proposal to develop meaningful labeling for cigarettes. *JAMA* 1994;272:312-4.
11. DiFranza JR, Lew RA. Effect of maternal cigarette smoking on pregnancy complications and sudden infant death syndrome. *J Fam Pract* 1995;385-94.
12. Taylor G, McNeill A, Girling A et al. Change in mental health after smoking cessation: systematic review and meta-analysis. *BMJ* 2014;348:g1151.
13. Health Canada. *On the road to quitting program*. Available from: www.hc-sc.gc.ca/hc-ps/tobac-tabac/quit-cesser/now-maintenant/road-voie/index-eng.php. Accessed February 16, 2010.
14. Pirie K, Peto R, Reeves GK et al. The 21st century hazards of smoking and benefits of stopping: a prospective study of one million women in UK. *Lancet* 2013;381:133-41.
15. Sakata R, McGale P, Grant EJ et al. Impact of smoking on mortality and life expectancy in Japanese smokers: a prospective cohort study. *BMJ* 2012;324:e7093.
16. Jha P, Ramasundarahettige C, Landsman V et al. 21st-century hazards of smoking and benefits of cessation in the United States. *N Engl J Med* 2013;368:341-50.
17. International Agency for Research on Cancer; World Health Organization. IARC Monographs on the Evaluation of Carcinogenic Risks to Humans; 83. *Tobacco smoke and involuntary smoking*. Switzerland: WHO; 2004. Available from: monographs.iarc.fr/ENG/Monographs/vol83/index.php. Accessed March 3, 2010.
18. Feldman HA, Johannes CB, Derby CA et al. Erectile dysfunction and coronary risk factors: prospective results from the Massachusetts male aging study. *Prev Med* 2000;30:328-38.

19. McGill HC. The cardiovascular pathology of smoking. *Am Heart J* 1988;115:250-7.
20. Silverstein P. Smoking and wound healing. *Am J Med* 1992;93:22S-24S.
21. Canadian Association of Occupational Therapists, Canadian Association of Social Workers, Canadian Dental Association et al. Tobacco: the role of health professionals in smoking cessation. *Can Pharm J* 2001;134:34-5.
22. Facchini FS, Hollenbeck CB, Jeppesen J. Insulin resistance and cigarette smoking. *Lancet* 1992;339:1128-30.
23. Hollenbach KA, Barrett-Connor E, Edelstein SL et al. Cigarette smoking and bone mineral density in older men and women. *Am J Public Health* 1993;83:1265-70.
24. Ill PO, Alexandre C. [Tobacco as risk factor of osteoporosis, myth or reality?] *Rev Rhum Ed Fr* 1993;60:280-6. [French].
25. Law MR, Hackshaw AK. A meta-analysis of cigarette smoking, bone mineral density and risk of hip fracture: recognition of a major effect. *BMJ* 1997;315:841-6.
26. Farley TM, Meirik O, Chang CL et al. Combined oral contraceptives, smoking, and cardiovascular risk. *J Epidemiol Community Health*1998;52:775-85.
27. Health Canada. *Smoking and oral cancer.* 2011. Available from: www.hc-sc.gc.ca/hc-ps/tobac-tabac/legislation/label-etiquette/oral-bouche-eng.php. Accessed June 18, 2015.
28. Delpisheh A, Brabin L, Brabin BJ. Pregnancy, smoking and birth outcomes. *Womens Health (Lond Engl)* 2006;2:389-403.
29. Southall DP, Samuels MP. Reducing risks in the sudden infant death syndrome. *BMJ* 1992;304:265-6.
30. Doherty SP, Grabowski J, Hoffman C et al. Early life insult from cigarette smoke may be predictive of chronic diseases later in life. *Biomarkers* 2009;14;97-101.
31. U.S. Department of Health and Human Services. *The health consequences of smoking: the changing cigarette: a report of the Surgeon General.* Washington: Public Health Service, Office of the Surgeon General; 1981. Available from: profiles.nlm.nih.gov/NN/B/B/S/N/_/nnbbsn.pdf. Accessed June 18, 2015.
32. McCusker K. Mechanisms of respiratory tissue injury from cigarette smoking. *Am J Med* 1992;93:18S-21S.
33. Stead LF, Buitrago D, Preciado N et al. Physician advice for smoking cessation. *Cochrane Database Syst Rev* 2013;5:CD000165.
34. Godenick MT. Review of available smoking cessation methods, 1989. *Md Med J* 1989;38:277-9.
35. Godenick MT. Review of available smoking cessation methods, 1989: Part II. *Md Med J* 1989;38:377-80.
36. Prochaska JO, Velicer WF, Rossi JS et al. Stages of change and decisional balance for 12 problem behaviors. *Health Psychol* 1994;13:39-46.
37. Lindson-Hawley N, Aveyard P, Hughes JR. Reduction versus abrupt cessation in smokers who want to quit. *Cochrane Database Syst Rev* 2012;11:CD008033.
38. Cornuz J, Willi C. Nonpharmacological smoking cessation interventions in clinical practice. *Eur Respir Rev* 2008;17:187-91. Available from: err.ersjournals.com/content/17/110/187.full.pdf.
39. Lindson-Hawley N, Thompson TP, Begh R. Motivational interviewing for smoking cessation. *Cochrane Database Syst Rev* 2015;3:CD006936.
40. West R, McNeill A, Raw M. Smoking cessation guidelines for health professionals: an update. Health Education Authority.*Thorax* 2000;55:987-99.
41. Stead LF, Lancaster T. Combined pharmacotherapy and behavioural interventions for smoking cessation. *Cochrane Database Syst Rev* 2012;10:CD008286.
42. Chen YF, Madan J, Welton N et al. Effectiveness and cost-effectiveness of computer and other electronic aids for smoking cessation: a systematic review and network meta-analysis. *Health Technol Assess* 2012;16:1-205.
43. Whittaker R, McRobbie H, Bullen C et al. Mobile phone-based interventions for smoking cessation. *Cochrane Database Syst Rev* 2012;11:CD006611.
44. Civljak M, Stead LF, Hartmann-Boyce J et al. Internet-based interventions for smoking cessation. *Cochrane Database Syst Rev* 2013;7:CD007078.
45. Stead LF, Lancaster T. Group behaviour therapy programmes for smoking cessation. *Cochrane Database Syst Rev* 2005;(2):CD001007.
46. Prokhorov AV, Hudmon KS, Marani S et al. Engaging physicians and pharmacists in providing smoking cessation counseling. *Arch Intern Med* 2010;170:1640-46.
47. Schwartz JL. *Review and evaluation of smoking cessation methods: the United States and Canada 1978-1985.* Washington: Division of Cancer Prevention and Control, National Cancer Institute; 1987. p. 2940.
48. White AR, Rampes H, Liu JP et al. Acupuncture and related interventions for smoking cessation. *Cochrane Database Syst Rev* 2014;1:CD000009.
49. Schwartz JL. Methods for smoking cessation. *Clin Chest Med* 1991;12:737-53.
50. Centers for Disease Control (CDC). Illnesses possibly associated with smoking clove cigarettes. *MMWR Morb Mortal Wkly Rep* 1985;34:297-9.
51. Addiction Research Foundation. *Information alert: tobacco-less cigarettes*. October 1993.
52. Healthy Canadians. *Health Canada advises Canadians not to use electronic cigarettes*. Available from: healthycanadians.gc.ca/recall-alert-rappel-avis/hc-sc/2009/13373a-eng.php.
53. U.S. Food and Drug Administration (FDA). *Summary of results: laboratory analysis of electronic cigarettes conducted by FDA*. Available from: www.fda.gov/newsevents/publichealthfocus/ucm173146.htm.
54. Healthy Canadians. *Nicotine addiction*. Available from: www.healthycanadians.gc.ca/health-sante/tobacco-tabac/addiction-dependance-eng.php.
55. McRobbie H, Bullen C, Hartmann-Boyce J, Hajek P. Electronic cigarettes for smoking cessation and reduction. *Cochrane Database Syst Rev* 2014;12:CD010216.
56. Kalkhoran S, Glantz SA. E-cigarettes and smoking cessation in real-world and clinical settings: a systematic review and meta-analysis. Lancet Respir Med. 2016;4(2):116-28.
57. Halpern SD, French B, Small DS et al. Randomized trial of four financial-incentive programs for smoking cessation. *N Engl J Med* 2015;372:2108-17.
58. Troxel AB, Volpp KG. Effectiveness of financial incentives for longer-term smoking cessation: evidence of absence or absence of evidence? *Am J Health Promot* 2012;26:204-7.
59. Reda AA, Kotz D, Evers SM, Van schayck CP. Healthcare financing systems for increasing the use of tobacco dependence treatment. *Cochrane Database Syst Rev* 2012;6:CD004305.

60. Pederson LL, Scrimgeour WG, Lefcoe NM. Comparison of hypnosis plus counseling, counseling alone, and hypnosis alone in a community service smoking withdrawal program. *J Consult Clin Psychol* 1975;43:920.
61. Baker TB, Piper ME, Stein JH et al. Effects of Nicotine Patch vs Varenicline vs Combination Nicotine Replacement Therapy on Smoking Cessation at 26 Weeks: A Randomized Clinical Trial. JAMA 2016;315(4):371-9.
62. Cahill K, Stevens S, Perera R et al. Pharmacological interventions for smoking cessation: an overview and network meta-analysis. *Cochrane Database Syst Rev* 2013;5:CD009329.
63. Smith SS, McCarthy DE, Japuntich SJ et al. Comparative effectiveness of 5 smoking cessation pharmacotherapies in primary care clinics. *Arch Intern Med* 2009;169:2148-55.
64. Stead LF, Perera R, Bullen C et al. Nicotine replacement therapy for smoking cessation. *Cochrane Database Syst Rev* 2012;11:CD000146.
65. Nicotine replacement therapy for smoking cessation or reduction: a review of the clinical evidence. Ottawa: Canadian Agency for Drugs and Technologies in Health; 2014 Jan. *CADTH Rapid Response Reports*.
66. Gourlay S. The pros and cons of transdermal nicotine therapy. *Med J Aust* 1994;160:152-9.
67. Dale LC, Hurt RD, Offord KP et al. High-dose nicotine patch therapy. Percentage of replacement and smoking cessation. *JAMA* 1995;274:1353-8.
68. Dale LC, Hurt RD, Hays JT. Drug therapy to aid in smoking cessation. Tips on maximizing patients' chances for success. *Postgrad Med* 1998;104:75-8, 83-4.
69. Hughes JR, Stead LF, Hartmann-Boyce J, et al. Antidepressants for smoking cessation. *Cochrane Database Syst Rev* 2014;1:CD000031.
70. Zyban [product monograph]. In: Jovaisas B, ed. *Compendium of pharmaceuticals and specialties: Canada's trusted drug reference*. Ottawa: Canadian Pharmacists Association; 2016. p. 3842-6.
71. Ebbert JO, Hughes JR, West RJ et al. Effect of varenicline on smoking cessation through smoking reduction: a randomized clinical trial. *JAMA* 2015;313:687-94.
72. Rigotti NA, Pipe AL, Benowitz NL et al. Efficacy and safety of varenicline for smoking cessation in patients with cardiovascular disease: a randomized trial. *Circulation* 2010;121:221-9.
73. Singh S, Loke YK, Spangler JG et al. Risk of serious adverse cardiovascular events associated with varenicline: a systemic review and meta-analysis. *CMAJ* 2011;183:1359-66.
74. Healthy Canadians. *Health Canada reviewing stop-smoking drug Champix (varenicline tartrate) and potential risk of heart problems in patients with heart disease*. 2011. Available from: www.healthycanadians.gc.ca/recall-alert-rappel-avis/hc-sc/2011/13619a-eng.php. Accessed June 18, 2015.
75. Healthy Canadians. *Champix: updated safety information for the smoking-cessation drug*. 2012. Available from: healthycanadians.gc.ca/recall-alert-rappel-avis/hc-sc/2012/13633a-eng.php. Accessed June 26, 2015.
76. Prochaska JJ, Hilton JF. Risk of cardiovascular serious adverse events associated with varenicline use for tobacco cessation: systematic review and meta-analysis. *BMJ* 2012;344:e2856.
77. Svanstrom HS, Pasternak B, Hviid A. Use of varenicline for smoking cessation and risk of serious cardiovascular events: nationwide cohort study. *BMJ* 2012;324:e7176.
78. Mills EJ, Thorlund K, Eapen S et al. Cardiovascular events associated with smoking cessation pharmacotherapies: a network meta-analysis. *Circulation* 2014;129:28-41.
79. Gibbons RD, Mann JJ. Varenicline, smoking cessation, and neuropsychiatric adverse events. *Am J Psychiatry* 2013;170:1460-7.
80. Thomas KH, Martin RM, Knipe DW et al.. Risk of neuropsychiatric adverse events associated with varenicline: systematic review and meta-analysis. *BMJ* 2015;350:h1109.
81. Molero Y, Lichtenstein P, Zetterqvist J et al. Varenicline and risk of psychiatric conditions, suicidal behaviour, criminal offending, and transport accidents and offences: population based cohort study. *BMJ* 2015;350:h2388.
82. Healthy Canadians. *Champix (varenicline tartrate)—changes to the Canadian product monograph—for health professionals*. Available from: www.healthycanadians.gc.ca/recall-alert-rappel-avis/hc-sc/2010/14595a-eng.php. Accessed June 18, 2015.
83. Champix [product monograph]. In: Jovaisas B, ed. *Compendium of pharmaceuticals and specialties: Canada's trusted drug reference*. Ottawa: Canadian Pharmacists Association; 2016. p. 718-23.
84. Gourlay SG, Stead LF, Benowitz NL. Clonidine for smoking cessation. *Cochrane Database Sys Rev* 2004;(3):CD000058.
85. William M. Effectiveness of clonidine in smoking cessation. *Can J Hosp Pharm* 1992;45:77-8.
86. Walker N, Howe C, Glover M et al. Cytisine versus nicotine for smoking cessation. *N Engl J Med* 2014;371:2353-62.
87. Ramon JM, Morchon S, Baena A et al. Combining varenicline and nicotine patches: a randomized controlled trial study in smoking cessation. *BMC Med* 2014;12:172.
88. Koegelenberg CF, Noor F, Bateman ED et al. Efficacy of varenicline combined with nicotine replacement therapy vs varenicline alone for smoking cessation: a randomized clinical trial. *JAMA* 2014;312:155-61.
89. Rose JE, Behm FM. Combination treatment with varenicline and bupropion in an adaptive smoking cessation paradigm. *Am J Psychiatry* 2014;171:1199-205.
90. Jorenby DE, Leischow SJ, Nides MA et al. A controlled trial of sustained-release bupropion, a nicotine patch, or both for smoking cessation. *N Engl J Med* 1999;340:685-91.
91. Stapleton J, West R, Hajek P et al. Randomized trial of nicotine replacement therapy (NRT), bupropion and NRT plus bupropion for smoking cessation: effectiveness in clinical practice. *Addiction* 2013;108:2193-201.
92. Evins AE, Cather C, Culhane MA et al. A 12-week double-blind, placebo-controlled study of bupropion sr added to high-dose dual nicotine replacement therapy for smoking cessation or reduction in schizophrenia. *J Clin Psychopharmacol* 007;27:380-6.
93. Lumley J, Chamberlain C, Dowswell T et al. Interventions for promoting smoking cessation during pregnancy. *Cochrane Database Syst Rev* 2009;(3):CD001055.
94. Chamberlain C, O'Mara-Eves A, Oliver S et al. Psychosocial interventions for supporting women to stop smoking in pregnancy. *Cochrane Database Syst Rev* 2013;10:CD001055.
95. Coleman T, Chamberlain C, Davey MA et al. Pharmacological interventions for promoting smoking cessation during pregnancy. *Cochrane Database Syst Rev* 2015;12CD010078.
96. Benowitz N, Dempsey D. Pharmacotherapy for smoking cessation during pregnancy. *Nicotine Tob Res* 2004;6:S189-202.
97. Berlin I, Grangé G, Jacob N et al. Nicotine patches in pregnant smokers: randomised, placebo controlled, multicentre trial of efficacy. *BMJ* 2014;348:g1622.

98. Cooper S, Lewis S, Thornton JG et al. The SNAP trial: a randomised placebo-controlled trial of nicotine replacement therapy in pregnancy—clinical effectiveness and safety until 2 years after delivery, with economic evaluation. *Health Technol Assess* 2014;18:1-128.
99. Joseph AM, Norman SM, Ferry LH et al. The safety of transdermal nicotine as an aid to smoking cessation in patients with cardiac disease. *N Engl J Med* 1996;335:1792-8.
100. Wennberg P, Eliasson M, Hallmans G et al. The risk of myocardial infarction and sudden cardiac death amongst snuff users with or without a previous history of smoking. *J Intern Med* 2007;262:360-7.
101. Benowitz NL. Pharmacology of nicotine: addiction, smoking-induced disease, and therapeutics. *Annu Rev Pharmacol Toxicol* 2009;49:57-71.
102. Fletcher C, Peto R. The natural history of chronic airflow obstruction. *Br Med J* 1977;1:1645-8.
103. Mons U, Müezzinler A, Gellert C et al. Impact of smoking and smoking cessation on cardiovascular events and mortality among older adults: meta-analysis of individual participant data from prospective cohort studies of the CHANCES consortium. *BMJ* 2015;350:h1551.
104. Cawkwell PB, Blaum C, Sherman SE. Pharmacological smoking cessation therapies in older adults: a review of the evidence. *Drugs Aging* 2015; 32:443-51.
105. Patnode CD, O'Connor E, Whitlock EP et al. Primary care-relevant interventions for tobacco use prevention and cessation in children and adolescents: a systematic evidence review for the U.S. Preventative Services Task Force. *Ann Intern Med* 2013;158:253-60.
106. Johnston V, Liberato S, Thomas D. Incentives for prevention smoking in children and adolescents. *Cochrane Database Syst Rev* 2012;10:CD008645.
107. Arefalk G, Hambraeus K, Lind L et al. Discontinuation of smokeless tobacco and mortality risk after myocardial infarction. *Circulation* 2014;130:325-32.
108. Ebbert JO, Elrashidi MY, Stead LF. Interventions for smokeless tobacco use cessation. *Cochrane Database Syst Rev* 2015;10:CD004306.
109. Ebbert JO, Fagerström K. Pharmacological interventions for the treatment of smokeless tobacco use. *CNS Drugs* 2012;26:1-10.
110. QUIT (Quit Using and Inhaling Tobacco) Smoking Cessation Program, Canadian Pharmacists Association, Ottawa, 2015.
111. Kroon LA. Drug interactions with smoking. *Am J Health Syst Pharm* 2007;64:1917-21.
112. Fankhauser MP. Drug interactions with tobacco smoke: implications for patient care. *Curr Psychiatr* 2013;12:12-6. Available from: www.currentpsychiatry.com.
113. Lucas C, Martin J. Smoking and drug interactions. *Aust Prescr* 2013;36:102-4. Available from: www.australianprescriber.com/magazine/36/3/102/4.
114. O'Hara P, Connett JE, Lee WW et al. Early and late weight gain following smoking cessation in the Lung Health Study. *Am J Epidemiol* 1998;148:821-30.
115. Aubin HJ, Farley A, Lycett D et al. Weight gain in smokers after quitting cigarettes: meta-analysis. *BMJ* 2012;345:e4439.

Quitting Smoking—What You Need to Know

Congratulations on deciding to quit smoking! Whether this is your first time quitting, or you have tried to quit before, follow these tips to be successful.

- Set a quit date. It should be within the next 2 weeks. Avoid a time when you will be under stress.
- Think about why you want to quit and all the good things that you expect as a result of quitting.
- If you have tried to quit before, you have probably learned some valuable tips of what *not* to do this time. Think about what was most difficult last time and why you stopped trying. Think about the things you need to avoid or change this time.
- Decide what kind of support will be most helpful over the next 6 months to a year. For example, you can join a smoking cessation group or plan to meet regularly with a healthcare provider (such as a pharmacist, nurse or doctor).
- Tell your family and friends that you are quitting. Ask them to help you to stick to your plan. If they smoke, ask them to respect your decision to quit and to not smoke in front of you. Think of things you can do to avoid smoking while with them.
- Choose someone you know who does not smoke and ask them to help you to quit.
- Make a diary for a few days to keep track of when and why you smoke.
- Think of ways to avoid situations when you usually smoke.
- Think of things you can do instead of smoking (for example, chewing gum, sipping water, playing cards or calling a friend).
- It is possible that you might gain weight while quitting. You can avoid this by eating healthy foods and increasing daily activity. Keep healthy snacks around for times when you get the urge to nibble.
- Keep busy with healthy activities like walking or an exercise program. Starting a new activity will help to break old habits connected with smoking.
- If you are taking medication to help you to quit, follow the instructions carefully. Be sure to ask your pharmacist any medication-related questions.
- If you are using nicotine replacement therapy, you should either not smoke at all or reduce smoking as much as possible, to avoid side effects such as nausea or headaches.
- Smoking (and quitting) can affect your metabolism. After you quit, reduce your caffeine intake to prevent side effects, and talk to your pharmacist or other healthcare provider about other medicines you may be taking, in case the dose needs to be adjusted.
- For some people, cutting down on the number of cigarettes smoked is an important first step in quitting. Many people may find this more manageable. If you decide to reduce your smoking, cut down the amount you smoke each month until you feel you can try quitting for good.

Chapter 7
Fever

Yvonne M. Shevchuk, BSP, PharmD, FCSHP

Fever is a regulated elevation in core body temperature that is generally considered to be caused by infection; however, noninfectious causes include inflammatory diseases, neoplasms and immunologically mediated conditions such as some drug fevers.[1,2] The definition of fever varies; anything above the normal range for body temperature can be defined as fever.[1,2] Fever in children is most often defined as rectal temperature >38°C if the child is appropriately dressed and resting.[3] In adults and children, an individual's body temperature varies with the time of day (normal circadian variation); it is lowest at approximately 6 a.m. and highest between 4 and 6 p.m.[1] The mean amplitude of variability is 0.5°C. Oral temperatures >37.2°C in early morning or ≥37.8°C any time during the day may also be used to define fever.[1,4] Outside the neonatal period, children generally have a higher temperature than adults; however, this is poorly documented.[5,6] Basal core temperatures decrease toward the adult range by 1 year of age and continue to decline until puberty. The degree of response to antipyretics does not distinguish serious bacterial infections from viral infections.[3]

Mild elevations in body temperature occur with exercise, ovulation, pregnancy, excessive clothing (overbundling of infants), ingestion of hot foods or liquids and chewing gum or tobacco.[1]

Rectal temperatures are approximately 0.6°C higher and axillary temperatures approximately 0.5–1°C lower than oral temperatures.[3] A high fever is usually defined as a temperature >40.5°C. Fever is a regulated physiologic response and temperatures >41°C are rare.[2,7]

Pathophysiology

The thermoregulatory centre in the anterior hypothalamus normally controls core temperature within a narrow range by balancing heat production by muscle and liver tissues with heat dissipation from skin and lungs. With fever, the thermoregulatory set-point is elevated.[1,2] Endothelial cells of the organum vasculosum laminae terminalis, a network of enlarged capillaries surrounding the hypothalamus, release arachidonic acid metabolites when exposed to pyrogens in the circulation. Prostaglandin E_2, released by the hypothalamus, is thought to be the major substance producing an elevation of the thermoregulatory set-point. Initially, with an elevated set-point, there is vasoconstriction of peripheral blood vessels to conserve heat, shivering to increase heat production, and behavioural changes such as seeking warmer environments and clothing. When the set-point is reduced through administration of antipyretics or disappearance of pyrogens, the reverse occurs—vasodilation and sweating to dissipate heat, as well as behavioural changes such as removal of clothing.[2]

Sources of pyrogens (substances that cause fever) are both exogenous and endogenous.[1,2] The most common exogenous sources are microorganisms and their products or toxins (e.g., lipopolysaccharide endotoxin of gram-negative bacteria). Exogenous pyrogens induce formation and release of endogenous pyrogens. Endogenous pyrogens or pyrogenic cytokines are polypeptides produced by host cell macrophages, monocytes and other cells. The most common are interleukin 1α and 1β (IL 1α and 1β), tumor necrosis factor alpha (TNF α), IL-6, ciliary neurotropic factor (CNF) and interferon gamma (IFN γ).

Goals of Therapy

- Provide patient comfort

- Reduce parental anxiety
- Reduce metabolic demand caused by fever in patients with cardiovascular or pulmonary disease
- Prevent or alleviate fever-associated mental dysfunction in the elderly (common practice but evidence is unclear)

Patient Assessment

Figure 1 presents an algorithm for the assessment of patients with fever.

Fever is a symptom or sign of illness, not a disease, and the reason for fever should be determined.[3] Most commonly it is due to infection, often viral. Children <6 months of age with a fever should be assessed by an appropriate healthcare practitioner.[8] Fever persisting longer than 3 days in those >6 months, recurrent fever, or high fever (>40.5°C) should be evaluated by an appropriate healthcare practitioner.

Once fever is established, the body initiates processes to permit homeostasis. Peripheral vasodilation causes the skin to feel hot. Sweating may occur. Malaise and fatigue may be seen at higher temperatures. Headache, backache, myalgia, arthralgia, somnolence, chills and rigors may also be associated with fever.

Drug-induced fever is a symptom of hypersensitivity but can occur with other symptoms such as myalgia, chills and headache. Table 1 lists several medications associated with drug-induced fever.[9,10,11]

Fever differs from hyperthermia, which is an increase in core temperature without an increase in hypothalamic set-point. If hyperthermia is suspected, refer the patient to an appropriate healthcare practitioner; antipyretics are not useful (see Chapter 9: Heat-related Disorders).

Table 1: **Selected Drugs Associated with Fever[9,10,11]**

allopurinol	digoxin	methyldopa
amphotericin B	diltiazem	metoclopramide
antacids	doxepin	mycophenolate
antibacterials/antibiotics (e.g., cephalosporins, penicillins, SMX/TMP)	epinephrine	nifedipine
anticholinergics	folic acid	NSAID (e.g., ibuprofen, naproxen)
antihistamines	furosemide	oral contraceptives
antineoplastics (e.g., cisplatin, hydroxyurea)	griseofulvin	phenytoin
antipsychotics	heparin	procainamide
atropine	hydralazine	propylthiouracil
azathioprine	hydrochlorothiazide	quinidine
barbiturates	H_2-receptor antagonists (e.g., cimetidine)	quinine
carbamazepine	insulin	rifampin
clofibrate	interferon	salicylates
corticosteroids	iodides	sulfasalazine
cyclosporine	iron dextran	tacrolimus
	isoniazid	triamterene
	MAOI	vitamins

Abbreviations: MAOI = monoamine oxidase inhibitor; NSAID = nonsteroidal anti-inflammatory drug; SMX/TMP = sulfamethoxazole/trimethoprim

Measurement of Body Temperature

For comparative features of nonprescription products, consult the *Compendium of Products for Minor Ailments*—Home Testing Products: Thermometers.

There are a number of methods of measuring temperature in an ambulatory setting—oral, rectal, axillary, tympanic membrane, temporal artery and transcutaneous (see Table 2).[8] Oral, rectal and axillary temperatures may be taken with an electronic thermometer with a digital display (digital probe). Standard mercury-in-glass thermometers are no longer recommended due to potential toxicity if they break,[8] environmental concerns and problems with proper use including long equilibration times, difficulty in reading them properly and inability to reset the thermometer. Electronic thermometers are safer and easier to use because they are faster and easier to read and avoid the environmental concerns of mercury. Generally, equilibration times require 30–60 seconds, while up to 10 minutes are required for standard glass thermometers.

It is difficult to make clear recommendations on the ideal method of measuring temperature since many of the studies are small or have methodologic flaws. In addition, most studies are conducted in emergency departments or inpatient settings. Few studies are conducted in patients' homes which may be the most relevant to self-care. Recommendations from Caring for Kids remain the most reliable source of information. See Suggested Readings.

Normal, route-specific temperature ranges and preferred routes based on age are listed in Table 3 and Table 4.

Table 2: **Methods of Measuring Body Temperature**

Method	Description	Instructions For Use
Rectal[8]	Considered the most accurate and the standard against which other routes of temperature measurement are compared.[1,7,12] This route is preferred for newborns, for children less than 4–5 y when an axillary temperature is not sufficient, and when the oral route is not suitable due to mouth breathing. May be less acceptable to toddlers. It is contraindicated in premature infants,[1] the immunocompromised[7] and in the presence of rectal anomalies, recent anorectal surgery or severe hemorrhoids. A rare complication is perforation of the rectum. This route may also transmit infections.[7]	Children: ▪ Place the infant on his back with knees bent or lay infant or young child face down across parent's lap or in fetal position on flat surface. ▪ Lubricate anus and thermometer with petroleum jelly (pea-size quantity). ▪ With one hand gently insert thermometer 2–3 cm into rectum. ▪ Hold buttocks closed against thermometer with other hand. ▪ Leave thermometer in place until it beeps and temperature is displayed.
Oral[8]	This route can be used in children over 5 y and adults;[7] younger children may bite the thermometer or have difficulty keeping it in the closed mouth. This may also be a problem for individuals who have difficulty understanding instructions, e.g., the mentally impaired or elderly with dementia.[1] Avoid the oral route when nasal breathing is difficult (e.g., due to viral upper respiratory tract infection); mouth breathing will cause spuriously low temperatures. Beverages, either hot or cold, and smoking should be avoided for at least 10 min prior to taking an oral temperature.[1,7]	▪ Place thermometer on either side of mouth (between gum and cheek) or under the tongue. ▪ Hold in place with lips or fingers (not the teeth). ▪ Breathe through nose with mouth closed. ▪ Leave thermometer in place until it beeps and temperature is displayed.
Axilla[8]	Axillary (armpit) temperatures have many disadvantages.[7] They take a longer time to measure and are affected by a number of factors including hypotension, cutaneous vasodilation and prior cooling of the patient. Axillary temperature may be a poor alternative to rectal temperatures in children aged 3 months to 6 y.[13,14] Although axillary temperatures are generally considered to be approximately 0.5°C lower than oral temperatures, reliable data are not available to correlate axillary with oral	▪ Place thermometer in apex of axilla. ▪ Hold elbow against chest to stabilize the thermometer. ▪ Leave thermometer in place until it beeps and temperature is displayed.

(cont'd)

Table 2: **Methods of Measuring Body Temperature** *(cont'd)*

Method	Description	Instructions For Use
	or rectal temperatures. The advantages of axillary temperatures are that this route is very accessible, safe and less frightening to children than rectal temperatures.[7] The reading should be confirmed via another route if the axillary temperature is >37.2°C.	
Ear[15]	A tympanic thermometer (TT) measures infrared emissions from the tympanic membrane.[1,16] The tympanic membrane and the hypothalamus share the same blood supply. TT may better reflect core temperature measurements.[1] The temperature is then converted by the thermometer to reflect oral or rectal temperatures, which may lead to some inaccuracy in the temperature reading. Proper placement in the ear canal is important.[6] Improper placement can result in a lower reading that reflects the outer ear canal wall temperature.[6] There may be a poor correlation between typmanic and rectal temperatures and TT may not be sensitive enough to screen for fever in pediatric patients.[17,18,19] Performance was good in adults, including the elderly.[20] The Canadian Paediatric Society does not recommend TT for children <2 y.[8] Advantages of TT include simplicity, speed and patient acceptance.[7] Less than 2 seconds is needed to obtain a reading. Other advantages include lack of external influences such as hot beverage ingestion, and no mucous membrane contact, therefore minimal risk of disease transmission.[7] Acute otitis media and nonobstructive cerumen do not appear to affect the accuracy of TT.[16] A disadvantage is high cost.	▪ Follow specific manufacturers' directions as they may vary. ▪ Apply a clean probe tip. ▪ Gently tug on ear, pulling it back. This helps to straighten the ear canal so an accurate reading can be obtained. ▪ Gently insert the thermometer into the ear until the ear canal is fully sealed off. ▪ Squeeze and hold down the button for 1 second (or until the device beeps). ▪ Remove from the ear and read temperature.
Transcutaneous	"Fever strips" contain encapsulated thermophototropic esters of cholesterol (called liquid crystals) that change colour in response to temperature changes. They are easier to read and require less time than a standard thermometer, but are less reliable because skin temperature is not a reliable indicator of core temperature.[1,6,7,8,21,22] When studied in emergency departments, fever strips were poor predictors of fever.[22,23] Accuracy is affected by ambient temperature such as cold hands holding the strip or nearby heat sources such as a lamp. A truly febrile child may register as afebrile, possibly delaying medical attention.	Based on poor performance in studies, use cannot be recommended for children or adults.
Temporal artery (forehead)[24]	Like the TT, the temporal artery (TA) thermometer uses infrared technology to measure the temperature using a heat balance method.[25] Infrared sensors compute a temporal artery temperature by rapid, repeated measures to synthesize skin surface and ambient temperature. It is similar to the TT in that it is very quick (3 seconds) and avoids any mucous membrane contact.[25] It may be prone to less error than the TT[26] but is not considered as accurate as rectal temperatures in children.[26,27,28] A clinically significant difference of 0.5°C was found between the oral and TA route in 49% of patients.[29] A geriatric study (age >75) determined that diagnostic accuracy for infection was lower for temporal artery thermometry compared with rectal or tympanic measurement.[30]	▪ Follow specific manufacturers' directions as they may vary. ▪ Remove dirt, hair or sweat from forehead area. ▪ Turn unit on. ▪ Press button a second time. ▪ Place thermometer probe gently and flush onto the area approximately 1.25 cm above the centre of the eyebrow. ▪ Sweep the skin from above eyebrow to temple until you hear a beep. ▪ Read the temperature display.

Table 3: **Normal Pediatric Temperature Ranges Associated with Measurement Technique**

Measurement Technique	Normal Temperature Range
Rectum	36.6–38°C (97.9–100.4°F)
Mouth	35.5–37.5°C (95.9–99.5°F)
Armpit	34.7–37.3°C (94.5–99.1°F)
Ear	35.8–38°C (96.4–100.4°F)

Source: Canadian Paediatric Society, 2015. *Fever and temperature taking*. For more information, visit www.caringforkids.cps.ca.

Table 4: **Recommendations for Temperature Measuring Techniques**

Age	Recommended Technique	
Birth to 2 y	First choice:	Rectum (for an exact reading)
	Second choice:	Armpit (to check for fever)
	Not recommended:	Tympanic membrane thermometers
Between 2 and 5 y	First choice:	Rectum
	Second choice:	Ear, armpit
Older than 5 y	First choice:	Mouth
	Second choice:	Ear, armpit

Source: Canadian Paediatric Society, 2015. *Fever and temperature taking*. For more information, visit www.caringforkids.cps.ca.

Nonpharmacologic Therapy

Nonpharmacologic interventions include removal of excess clothing and bedding, increased fluid intake to replace increased insensible water loss during fever, maintenance of ambient temperatures around 20–21°C, and avoidance of physical exertion.[8]

Sponging increases evaporation and promotes heat loss. Tepid water sponging may help reduce body temperature; however, it does not reset the thermoregulatory set-point.[31] Therefore, the body actually works harder to maintain the elevated temperature by shivering, which results in increased oxygen consumption. Sponging often causes significant patient discomfort.[32] Studies show no additional benefit from sponging after antipyretic administration.[33,34,35] If used, administer antipyretics 30 minutes before sponging to reduce thermoregulatory set-point.

If tepid sponging is performed, use water only. Though rarely, isopropyl alcohol sponging has resulted in hypoglycemia, intoxication and coma as a result of absorption through the skin or inhalation of fumes, and is not recommended.[32,36]

Pharmacologic Therapy

For comparative ingredients of nonprescription products, consult the *Compendium of Products for Minor Ailments*—Analgesic Products: Internal Analgesics and Antipyretics.

There are many arguments against treating a fever:[1,2,37,38,39]

- Fever is an important defence mechanism; it enhances the immune response.
- Use of antipyretics may impair the use of temperature as an important clinical tool for monitoring the progress of an infection or response to antibiotics.
- Fever is usually self-limiting, and though sometimes distressing, the consequences of fever (mild dehydration, discomfort, febrile delirium or febrile seizures) are usually not harmful.

Therefore, the decision to use antipyretics must be individualized. The goal should be reduction of fever rather than "normal" body temperature. Assessment of the patient should not depend solely on the elevation of temperature (see Figure 1).

Acetaminophen, ASA, ibuprofen and naproxen sodium are all currently indicated to reduce fever. These drugs reduce body temperature in febrile patients by decreasing prostaglandin synthesis in the brain and reducing the thermoregulatory set-point.[1,37] They do not lower normal body temperature. Short-term treatment with these drugs is associated with few side effects. Intermittent administration of antipyretics may result in drug-induced fluctuations in temperature and concomitant shivering which may make the individual feel worse. Use at regular intervals may reduce patient discomfort and the risk of increased metabolic demand caused by shivering.

Acetaminophen is a relatively safe and effective antipyretic with few contraindications, and can be used in any age group.[40,41] Many years of clinical experience is also an advantage. Using a loading dose of acetaminophen 30 mg/kg in children 4 months to 9 years of age resulted in a more rapid and sustained response and a greater reduction in temperature compared with 15 mg/kg.[42] Although used in some emergency departments, the safety of this practice has not been evaluated and the dose is an initial dose only; subsequent doses should be 10–15 mg/kg. Do *not* recommend a loading dose to parents. Acetaminophen overdose resulting in hepatotoxicity remains a concern. In response to this concern, Health Canada has developed labelling standards which includes warnings regarding hepatotoxicity and maximum package sizes for pediatric products and is reviewing the option of decreasing the maximum recommended daily dose.[43,44] It is the preferred agent in those with renal dysfunction or risk factors for GI bleeding.

Standard dosing is provided in Table 5.

Ibuprofen is an alternative to acetaminophen when there are no contraindications to its use. There is less experience with ibuprofen and it is more expensive, but with short-term use in children there appears to be no difference in adverse event rates compared with acetaminophen.[45,46,47,48] However, renal failure in children has been reported, particularly when the child is dehydrated; therefore, avoid in children with diarrhea and vomiting.[8,49] In one study, time without fever in the first 4 hours after administration was greater and time to fever clearance was shorter with ibuprofen compared with acetaminophen.[50] A meta-analysis showed that ibuprofen (5–10 mg/kg) as compared with acetaminophen (10–15 mg/kg) was a better antipyretic producing greater temperature reductions at 2, 4 and 6 hours after dosing.[51] Ibuprofen may also have a longer duration of action[51] than acetaminophen and is less toxic in overdose.[52,53]

ASA should be avoided in children younger than 18 years who have a viral illness because of its association with Reye's syndrome in influenza and varicella. Reye's syndrome consists of acute encephalopathy with cerebral edema, fatty infiltration of the liver and metabolic derangements such as hypoglycemia. It occurs in otherwise healthy children. Since the cause of fever is unknown initially in many circumstances, avoid ASA in children.[54,55,56]

Naproxen sodium is the most recent nonprescription NSAID available for fever. It has a longer half-life with a corresponding less frequent administration schedule. There are no data on the use of naproxen sodium for treatment of fever in children.

Alternating Antipyretics

In the past, alternating acetaminophen with ASA was recommended for management of fever unresponsive to a single agent. This practice has been abandoned due to an association with Reye's syndrome. Recommendations to alternate acetaminophen with ibuprofen have emerged.[57,58] Alternating or combining acetaminophen and ibuprofen may result in a greater period of time without fever but the clinical significance is uncertain.[50,59,60,61] The goal of treating a febrile child should be to reduce discomfort rather than to normalize the temperature. It is important to note that no difference was found in patient discomfort in the only 2 trials to assess it.[50,60,62] Safety and superior effectiveness of the combination has not been proven.[63,64] In fact, the practice of combining or alternating antipyretics may not be as safe as previously thought. A review of FDA's AERS database concluded that concomitant use of ibuprofen and acetaminophen in children may be associated with an increased risk of acute kidney injury.[65]

Parents and caregivers often find the recommendation to combine antipyretics confusing and it may result in increased dosing errors.[66,67] In addition, it may serve to reinforce fever phobia. Both caregivers and healthcare practitioners should be educated to avoid combination therapy with acetaminophen and ibuprofen.[68]

Table 5 outlines dosing, side effects, contraindications and precautions for ASA, acetaminophen, ibuprofen and naproxen sodium.

Fever in Specific Patient Groups

Children

Young children have an immature thermoregulatory system. In the first 2 months of life, infants may have minimal or no fever during an infectious illness. Since neonates and infants are less able to mount a febrile response, a fever is more likely to indicate a major illness. Evaluation based on symptoms and physical examination is more challenging, and it is more difficult to accurately predict serious bacterial infection than in older children. After 3 months of age, the degree of fever more closely approximates that seen in older children.[69]

Fever is common in children and is frequently due to bacterial or viral infection. Because children have had less exposure to infectious agents than adults, they are more susceptible upon initial contact. Reactions to vaccinations may also be a cause of fever. Compared with adults, children are more sensitive to ambient temperature (due to a greater body surface area for heat exchange) and at higher risk of dehydration.[69]

In children ages 3 months to 5 years, seizures occur with 2–5% of febrile episodes.[70] Although simple febrile seizures are rarely associated with neurologic damage or permanent seizure disorders, they concern and frighten parents. For this reason, antipyretics are often recommended for children in this age group, particularly those with previous febrile seizures or neurologic problems. Using antipyretics at the first sign of fever does not prevent recurrent febrile seizures even though this practice is frequently recommended.[70,71,72,73]

Patients with Cardiovascular or Pulmonary Disorders

Increased metabolic demands which occur during the chill phase (increased metabolic rate, norepinephrine-mediated peripheral vasoconstriction, increased arterial blood pressure) may aggravate comorbid disease states in patients with heart failure or coronary, pulmonary or cerebral insufficiency. Fever may result in deterioration in cognitive function and delirium.[1]

The Elderly

Older individuals exhibit less intense fevers in response to infection compared with younger individuals.[74] They also become hypothermic more often when infected and suffer greater morbidity and mortality from infections.[74] Fever in individuals older than 60 years is less likely to be a benign febrile illness than in younger individuals;[75] therefore, careful assessment of fever in the elderly is important. The elderly are more likely to experience the cardiovascular and pulmonary conditions described above. **Acetaminophen** is safer in older individuals with risk factors predisposing to GI and renal toxicity of **NSAID**.

Pregnancy

Studies in humans suggest that exposure to fever and other heat sources during the first trimester of pregnancy is associated with increased risk of neural tube defects and multiple congenital abnormalities.[76,77] Although one study indicated a possible benefit of antipyretic therapy,[78] others have not[79] and a recent meta-analysis suggests additional research is required.[80]

Acetaminophen crosses the placenta and is relatively safe for short-term use in pregnancy when therapeutic doses are used.

Use of **ASA** and **NSAID** can result in a number of problems during pregnancy, including cardiac issues. They should be avoided in the first and third trimesters of pregnancy. Low-dose ASA is considered compatible with pregnancy.[81] Since these drugs inhibit prostaglandin synthesis, they may interfere with labour and cause premature closure of the ductus arteriosus resulting in persistent pulmonary hypertension in the infant. Platelet aggregation is inhibited in the newborn if ASA is ingested by the mother within 7 days of delivery and salicylates displace bilirubin from protein binding sites. Increased bleeding has been reported in both mothers and infants if ASA is ingested close to the time of delivery.[52] See Appendix V: Pregnancy and Breastfeeding: Self-care Therapy for Common Conditions.

Both acetaminophen and ibuprofen are considered safe to take while breastfeeding.[81]

Fever Phobia

The term "fever phobia" describes unrealistic concerns and misconceptions of parents and healthcare practitioners regarding fever in children.[82,83,84,85,86,87,88] Healthcare practitioners should undertake educational interventions to ensure appropriate management of fever and rational use of antipyretics.

Optimizing Dosing and Administration

Review the following points with all parents when recommending an antipyretic preparation:

- Ensure parents/caregivers understand that fever is rarely harmful and does not have to be treated
- Explain that comfort is the goal and not achievement of an arbitrary "normal" temperature
- Assist parents in calculating the correct mg/kg dose of the drug and ensure they know the maximum number of doses that can be administered in a 24-hour period
  - In a study of 100 caregivers given a mock dosing scenario that required caregivers to determine and measure a correct dose of acetaminophen for their child, only 40% stated an appropriate dose for their child[89]
  - Of 118 children given an antipyretic at home and subsequently brought to the emergency department, only 47% had been given a proper dose.[90] Underdosing may be a cause of

unnecessary emergency department visits.[91] This also leads to added stress for both the parent and sick child[92]

- Ensure the parent has and will use an appropriate measuring device
  - In the mock dosing study reported above, only 67% of caregivers accurately measured the amount they intended to give. Forty-three percent measured out a correct amount of acetaminophen; however, 30% of these did so by accident by inaccurately measuring an improper dose[89]
  - Consider demonstrating the correct use of the dosing device. Ask the caregiver to repeat instructions back to you. It may be helpful to mark the dosing device with the correct dose[93]
- Ask what form of product they have at home and calculate the appropriate volume of liquid or number of tablets for the child. Explain the differences in concentration between drops and syrup and that tablets come in different strengths for children[93]
  - Multiple miscalculated overdoses of acetaminophen given by parents represent an important cause of acetaminophen toxicity[94,95,96]
  - Use of incorrect measuring devices, differences in medication concentrations (e.g., pediatric drops vs. suspensions), use of adult formulations for pediatric patients and unrecognized acetaminophen content in multiple-ingredient cough and cold products contribute to this problem[95]
- Ask about other preparations, particularly cough and cold products, they may be coadministering and ensure they are aware of the antipyretic content of these products. The coadministration of these products should be carefully monitored to ensure the cumulative dose is within the recommended range.

Monitoring of Therapy

Recommendations for frequent monitoring of temperature likely contribute to parental concern and fever phobia. The temperature should be taken if the patient feels warm or looks ill, to determine the initial temperature. Subsequently, temperatures need not be taken more than 2–4 times daily unless the patient has recently received chemotherapy. If the fever persists for 24 hours without an apparent cause, or for more than 3 days, medical attention should be sought. The degree of illness and not the temperature should guide therapy and referral.

Monitor:

- All patients given antipyretics for development of rash or other allergic reactions
- Patients with pre-existing comorbid illness for edema and decreased urine output
- For other common side effects, such as GI intolerance and tinnitus (see Table 5)
- To ensure appropriate doses, products and measuring devices are being used, and the patient is not receiving excessive amounts of antipyretics through use of cough and cold or analgesic products
- To ensure the patient is not receiving interacting medications (see Table 5). Recommend avoiding alcohol.

Figure 1: **Assessment of Patients with Fever**[1,3,6,8]

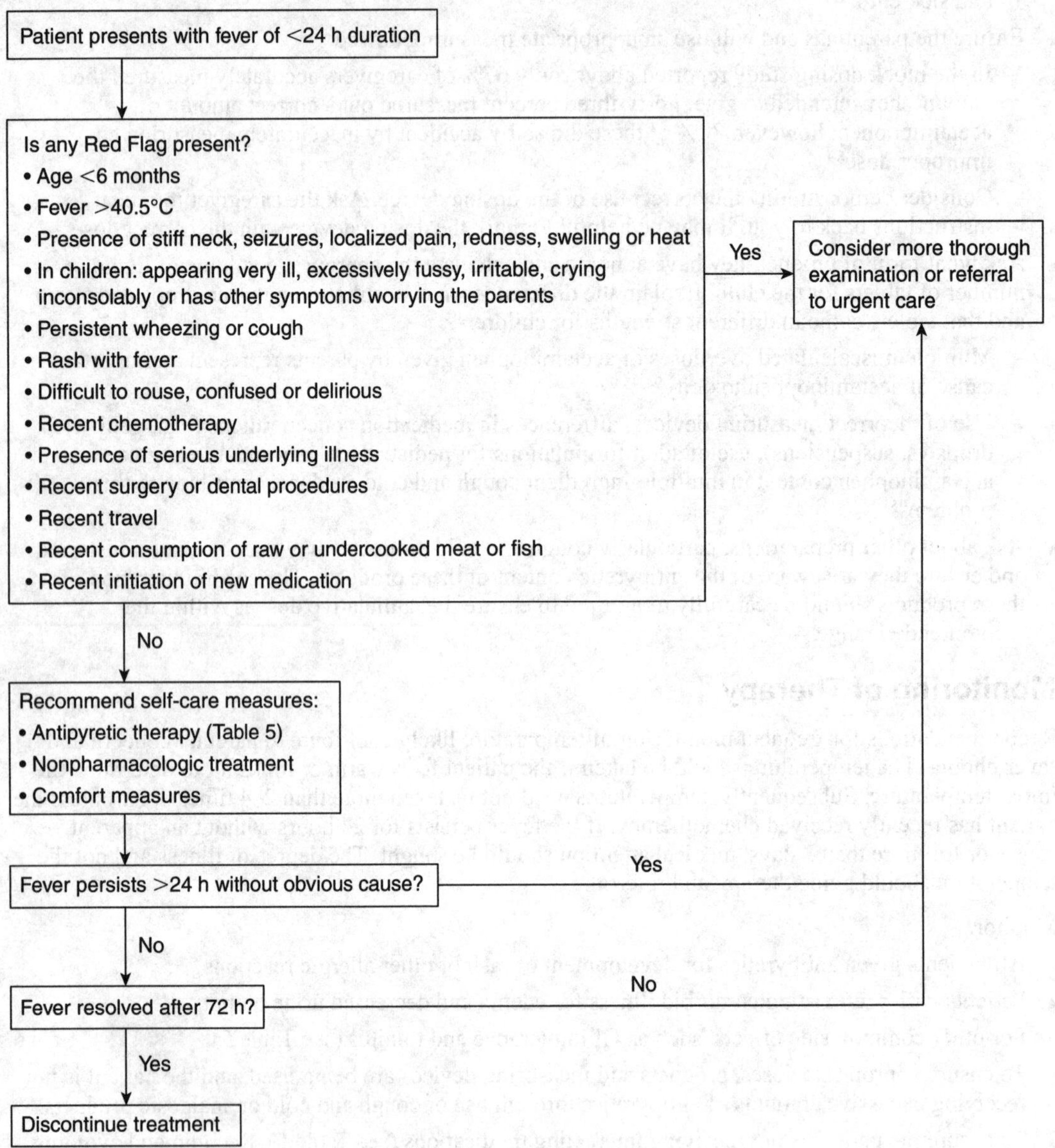
Patient presents with fever of <24 h duration
Is any Red Flag present?
• Age <6 months
• Fever >40.5°C
• Presence of stiff neck, seizures, localized pain, redness, swelling or heat
• In children: appearing very ill, excessively fussy, irritable, crying inconsolably or has other symptoms worrying the parents
• Persistent wheezing or cough
• Rash with fever
• Difficult to rouse, confused or delirious
• Recent chemotherapy
• Presence of serious underlying illness
• Recent surgery or dental procedures
• Recent travel
• Recent consumption of raw or undercooked meat or fish
• Recent initiation of new medication
Yes
Consider more thorough examination or referral to urgent care
No
Recommend self-care measures:
• Antipyretic therapy (Table 5)
• Nonpharmacologic treatment
• Comfort measures
Fever persists >24 h without obvious cause?
Yes
No
Fever resolved after 72 h?
No
Yes
Discontinue treatment

Table 5: **Drug Therapy for Fever**

Class	Drug	Dosage	Adverse Effects	Drug Interactions	Comments	Cost[a]
NSAID	*ibuprofen* Advil, Advil Children/Pediatric, Advil Junior Strength, Advil Liqui-Gels, Motrin, Motrin (Children's), Motrin IB, Motrin Liquid Gels, generics	Adults: 200–400 mg Q4-6H po PRN (maximum for self-care 1200 mg/day; supervised maximum 2400 mg/day) Children >6 months: 5–10 mg/kg Q6–8H po PRN for symptom management; maximum 40 mg/kg/day Children <6 months: 5 mg/kg Q8H Do not exceed adult dose	Uncommon with infrequent use and recommended dose. GI intolerance and bleeding, allergic reactions, tinnitus, visual disturbances, nephropathy. Sodium and water retention. Dehydration enhances risk of renal toxicity. Platelet dysfunction can result in increased bleeding risk.	Alcohol and corticosteroids: Increased risk of GI pain/ulceration. Antagonism of hypotensive effects of ACEI, diuretics, beta-blockers. Anticoagulants: increased risk of bleeding. Increased risk of bleeding with SSRIs. Increased levels of cyclosporine and risk of nephrotoxicity. Increased levels of lithium, methotrexate.[b] Reduction of antiplatelet effects of ASA.[97]	Renal dysfunction: No adjustment required; however, should be avoided in renal dysfunction due to effects of prostaglandin inhibition on renal function. Limited data exist for the use of ibuprofen in children <2 months. Do not give if dehydration is present; ensure adequate intake of fluids. NSAIDs have been associated with an increased risk of severe skin and soft tissue infections in children with chicken pox and to a lesser extent adults with shingles.[98] Some nonprescription products contain ibuprofen in combination with other drugs. Advise patients and caregivers to check labels carefully to avoid inadvertent administration of excessive doses.	$
	naproxen sodium Aleve, Anaprox, Maxidol, generics	Adults: 220 mg Q8–12H po PRN; maximum 440 mg/day Children: Not recommended under 12 y	See ibuprofen.	See ibuprofen.	See ibuprofen.	$

(cont'd)

Table 5: **Drug Therapy for Fever** *(cont'd)*

Class	Drug	Dosage	Adverse Effects	Drug Interactions	Comments	Cost[a]
Para-aminophenol Derivatives	*acetaminophen* Atasol Preparations, Tempra, Tylenol, generics	Adults: 325–650 mg Q4-6H po/pr PRN (maximum 4000 mg/day) Children: 10–15 mg/kg/dose Q4–6H po as needed for symptom management; maximum 75 mg/kg/day; do not exceed adult dose	Uncommon with infrequent use and recommended dose. Hypersensitivity, agranulocytosis and anemia (rare). Chronic use and overdose associated with hepatotoxicity, nephropathy. Potential for toxicity enhanced if concurrent dehydration, prolonged fasting, diabetes mellitus, obesity, concomitant viral infection or family history of hepatotoxic reaction.	Alcohol: Increased risk of hepatotoxicity. Isoniazid: Increased risk of hepatotoxicity. Enzyme inducers (e.g., barbiturates, carbamazepine, isoniazid, phenytoin) decrease acetaminophen levels. Acetaminophen has been reported to increase INR in warfarin-treated patients.[99] Check INR if acetaminophen ≥2 g/day is used for ≥3 consecutive days. Adjust warfarin dosage as required.	Use with caution in patients with liver dysfunction or active liver disease. Rectal administration results in erratic absorption and should be used under healthcare practitioner supervision. Available as oral drops, tablets, chewable tablets, suppositories and suspension. Acetaminophen may be associated with exacerbation of wheezing in febrile children.[100] Many nonprescription products contain acetaminophen in combination with other drugs. Advise parents and caregivers to check labels carefully to avoid inadvertent administration of excessive doses.	$

Class	Drug	Dosage	Adverse Effects	Drug Interactions	Comments	Cost[a]
Salicylates	*ASA* Aspirin, Coated Aspirin, generics	Adults: 325–650 mg Q4H po; maximum 4000 mg/day Children: Avoid use with fever under 18 y	GI upset. Avoid in patients with renal failure, peptic ulcer disease, heart failure and ASA-sensitive asthma.	Alcohol and corticosteroids: Increased risk of GI pain/ulceration. Anticoagulants: Increased risk of bleeding. Increased levels of methotrexate.[b] ASA may decrease therapeutic effect of uricosuric agents (probenecid, sulfinpyrazone) Increased risk of GI bleeding with SSRIs. Antihypertensives (diuretics, beta-blockers, ACEI, alpha-blockers): Possible reduction in antihypertensive effect; may require additional antihypertensive therapy.	Avoid if ClCr <10 mL/min. Enteric-coated products will have delayed onset of action.	$

[a] Cost per day; includes drug cost only.

[b] More likely to occur with antineoplastic doses of methotrexate.

Abbreviations: ACEI = angiotensin converting enzyme inhibitor; GI = gastrointestinal; NSAID = nonsteroidal anti-inflammatory drug

Legend: $ <$1

Suggested Readings

American Academy of Pediatrics. Committee on Drugs. Acetaminophen toxicity in children. *Pediatrics* 2001;108:1020-4.

Aronoff DM, Neilson EG. Antipyretics: mechanisms of action and clinical use in fever suppression. *Am J Med* 2001;111:304-15.

Canadian Paediatric Society. Caring for Kids. *Fever and temperature taking*. Available from: www.caringforkids.cps.ca/handouts/fever_and_temperature_taking.

Crocetti M, Moghbeli N, Serwint J. Fever phobia revisited: have parental misconceptions about fever changed in 20 years? *Pediatrics* 2001;107:1241-6.

Fields E, Chard J, Murphy MS et al. Assessment and initial management of feverish illness in children younger than 5 years: summary of updated NICE guidance. *BMJ* 2013;346:f2866.

Plaisance KI. Toxicities of drugs used in the management of fever. *Clin Infect Dis* 2000;31:S219-23.

Section on Clinical Pharmacology and Therapeutics; Committee on Drugs, Sullivan JE et al. Fever and antipyretic use in children. *Pediatrics* 2011;127:580-7.

Simon HK, Weinkle DA. Over-the-counter medications. Do parents give what they intend to give? *Arch Pediatr Adolesc Med* 1997;151:654-6.

Steering Committee on Quality Improvement and Management, Subcommittee on Febrile Seizures. Febrile seizures: clinical practice guideline for the long-term management of the child with simple febrile seizures. *Pediatrics* 2008;121:1281-6.

References

1. Mackowiak PA. Temperature regulation and the pathogenesis of fever. In: Mandell GL, Bennett JE, Dolin R, eds. *Mandell, Douglas, and Bennett's principles and practice of infectious diseases*. 7th ed. Philadelphia: Churchill Livingstone/Elsevier; 2010. p. 765-78.
2. Mackowiak P. Concepts of fever. *Arch Intern Med* 1998;158:1870-81.
3. Alpern ER, Henretig FM. Fever. In: Fleisher GR, Ludwig S, Henretig FM, eds. *Textbook of pediatric emergency medicine*. 5th ed. Philadelphia: Lippincott Williams & Wilkins; 2006. p. 295-306.
4. Mackowiak PA, Wasserman SS, Levine MM. A critical appraisal of 98.6 degrees F, the upper limit of the normal body temperature, and other legacies of Carl Reinhold August Wunderlich. *JAMA* 1992;268:1578-80.
5. Mackowiak PA, Bartlett JG, Borden EC et al. Concepts of fever: recent advances and lingering dogma. *Clin Infect Dis* 1997;25:119-38.
6. Bonadio WA. Defining fever and other aspects of body temperature in infants and children. *Pediatr Ann* 1993;22:467-8, 470-3.
7. El-Radhi AS, Barry W. Thermometry in paediatric practice. *Arch Dis Child* 2006;91:351-6.
8. Canadian Paediatric Society. Caring for Kids. *Fever and temperature taking*. Available from: www.caringforkids.cps.ca/handouts/fever_and_temperature_taking. Accessed November 6, 2015.
9. Mackowiak PA, LeMaistre CF. Drug fever: a critical appraisal of conventional concepts. An analysis of 51 episodes in two Dallas hospitals and 97 episodes reported in the English literature. *Ann Intern Med* 1987;106:728-33.
10. Patel RA, Gallagher JC. Drug fever. *Pharmacotherapy* 2010;30:57-69.
11. Sylvia LM. eChapter 22. Allergic and pseudoallergic drug reactions. In: DiPiro JT, Talbert RL, Yee GC et al., eds. *Pharmacotherapy: a pathophysiologic approach*. 9th ed. New York: McGraw-Hill; 2014. Available from: accesspharmacy.mhmedical.com. Accessed November 6, 2015.
12. Varney SM, Manthey DE, Culpepper VE et al. A comparison of oral, tympanic, and rectal temperature measurement in the elderly. *J Emerg Med* 2002;22:153-7.
13. Zengeya ST, Blumenthal I. Modern electronic and chemical thermometers used in the axilla are inaccurate. *Eur J Pediatr* 1996;155:1005-8.
14. Craig JV, Lancaster GA, Williamson PR et al. Temperature measured at the axilla compared with rectum in children and young people: systematic review. *BMJ* 2000;320:1174-8.
15. Vicks. Ear thermometer package insert.
16. Terndrup TE. An appraisal of temperature assessment by infrared emission detection tympanic thermometry. *Ann Emerg Med* 1992;21:1483-92.
17. Hooker EA. Use of tympanic thermometers to screen for fever in patients in a pediatric emergency department. *South Med J* 1993;86:855-8.
18. Selfridge J, Shea SS. The accuracy of the tympanic membrane thermometer in detecting fever in infants aged 3 months and younger in the emergency department setting. *J Emerg Nurs* 1993;19:127-30.
19. Dodd SR, Lancaster GA, Craig JV et al. In a systematic review, infrared ear thermometry for fever diagnosis in children finds poor sensitivity. *J Clin Epidemiol* 2006;59:354-7.
20. Onur OE, Guneysel O, Akoglu H et al. Oral, axillary, and tympanic temperature measurements in older and younger adults with or without fever. *Eur J Emerg Med* 2008;15:334-7.
21. Reisinger KS, Kao J, Grant DM. Inaccuracy of the Clinitemp skin thermometer. *Pediatrics* 1979;64:4-6.
22. Scholefield JH, Gerber MA, Dwyer P. Liquid crystal forehead temperature strips. A clinical appraisal. *Am J Dis Child* 1982;136:198-201.
23. Lewit EM, Marshall CL, Salzer JE. An evaluation of a plastic strip thermometer. *JAMA* 1982;247:321-5.
24. Vicks. Forehead thermometer package insert.
25. Titus MO, Hulsey T, Heckman J et al. Temporal artery thermometry utilization in pediatric emergency care. *Clin Pediatr (Phila)* 2009;48:190-3.

26. Greenes DS, Fleisher GR. Accuracy of a noninvasive temporal artery thermometer for use in infants. *Arch Pediatr Adolesc Med* 2001;155:376-81.
27. Hebbar K, Fortenberry JD, Rogers K et al. Comparison of temporal artery thermometer to standard temperature measurements in pediatric intensive care unit patients. *Pediatr Crit Care Med* 2005;6:557-61.
28. Schuh S, Komar L, Stephens D et al. Comparison of the temporal artery and rectal thermometry in children in the emergency department. *Pediatr Emerg Care* 2004;20:736-41.
29. Bodkin RP, Acquisto NM, Zwart JM et al. Differences in noninvasive thermometer measurements in the adult emergency department. *Am J Emerg Med* 2014;32:987-9.
30. Singler K, Bertsch T, Heppner HJ et al. Diagnostic accuracy of three different methods of temperature measurement in acutely ill geriatric patients. *Age Ageing* 2013;42:740-6.
31. Steele RW, Tanaka PT, Lara RP et al. Evaluation of sponging and of oral antipyretic therapy to reduce fever. *J Pediatr* 1970;77:824-9.
32. Axelrod P. External cooling in the management of fever. *Clin Infect Dis* 2000;31:S224-9.
33. Newman J. Evaluation of sponging to reduce body temperature in febrile children. *Can Med Assoc J* 1985;132:641-2.
34. Purssell E. Physical treatment of fever. *Arch Dis Child* 2000;82:238-9.
35. Thomas S, Vijaykumar C, Naik R et al. Comparative effectiveness of tepid sponging and antipyretic drug versus only antipyretic drug in the management of fever among children: a randomized controlled trial. *Indian Pediatr* 2009;46:133-6.
36. Garrison RF. Acute poisoning from use of isopropyl alcohol in tepid sponging. *JAMA* 1953;152:317-8.
37. Aronoff DM, Neilson EG. Antipyretics: mechanisms of action and clinical use in fever suppression. *Am J Med* 2001;111:304-15.
38. Styrt B, Sugarman B. Antipyresis and fever. *Arch Intern Med* 1990;150:1589-97.
39. El-Radhi AS. Why is the evidence not affecting the practice of fever management? *Arch Dis Child* 2008;93:918-20.
40. Eccles R. Efficacy and safety of over-the-counter analgesics in the treatment of common cold and flu. *J Clin Pharm Ther* 2006;31:309-19.
41. Goldman RD, Ko K, Linett JL et al. Antipyretic efficacy and safety of ibuprofen and acetaminophen in children. *Ann Pharmacother* 2004;38:146-50.
42. Treluyer JM, Tonnelier S, d'Athis P et al. Antipyretic efficacy of an initial 30-mg/kg loading dose of acetaminophen versus a 15-mg/kg maintenance dose. *Pediatrics* 2000;108:E73.
43. Health Canada. *Guidance document—acetaminophen labelling standard.* Available from: www.hc-sc.gc.ca/dhp-mps/prodpharma/applic-demande/guide-ld/label_stand_guide_ld-2015-eng.php. Accessed November 5, 2015.
44. Healthy Canadians. *Health Canada taking new action to improve acetaminophen safety, reminds Canadians about safe use.* 2015. Available from: healthycanadians.gc.ca/recall-alert-rappel-avis/hc-sc/2015/54178a-eng.php. Accessed November 10, 2015.
45. Lesko SM, Mitchell AA. Renal function after short-term ibuprofen use in infants and children. *Pediatrics* 1997;100:954-7.
46. Lesko SM, Mitchell AA. The safety of acetaminophen and ibuprofen among children younger than two years old. *Pediatrics* 1999;104:e39.
47. Lesko SM, Mitchell AA. An assessment of the safety of pediatric ibuprofen. A practitioner-based randomized clinical trial. *JAMA* 1995;273:929-33.
48. Southey ER, Soares-Weiser K, Kleijnen J. Systematic review and meta-analysis of the clinical safety and tolerability of ibuprofen compared with paracetamol in paediatric pain and fever. *Curr Med Res Opin* 2009;25:2207-22.
49. Moghal NE, Hegde S, Eastham KM. Ibuprofen and acute renal failure in a toddler. *Arch Dis Child* 2004;89:276-7.
50. Hay AD, Costelloe C, Redmond NM et al. Paracetamol plus ibuprofen for the treatment of fever in children (PITCH): randomised controlled trial. *BMJ* 2008;337:a1302.
51. Perrott DA, Piira T, Goodenough B et al. Efficacy and safety of acetaminophen vs ibuprofen for treating children's pain or fever: a meta-analysis. *Arch Pediatr Adolesc Med* 2004;158:521-6.
52. Hersh EV, Moore PA, Ross GL. Over-the-counter analgesics and antipyretics: a critical assessment. *Clin Ther* 2000;22:500-48.
53. Seifert SA, Bronstein AC, McGuire T. Massive ibuprofen ingestion with survival. *J Toxicol Clin Toxicol* 2000;38:55-7.
54. Aspirin and Reye syndrome. Committee on Infectious Diseases. *Pediatrics* 1982;69:810-2.
55. Starko KM, Ray CG, Dominguez LB et al. Reye's syndrome and salicylate use. *Pediatrics* 1980;66:859-64.
56. Waldman RJ, Hall WN, McGee H et al. Aspirin as a risk factor in Reye's syndrome. *JAMA* 1982;247:3089-94.
57. Mayoral CE, Marino RV, Rosenfeld W et al. Alternating antipyretics: is this an alternative? *Pediatrics* 2000;105:1009-12.
58. Wright AD, Liebelt EL. Alternating antipyretics for fever reduction in children: an unfounded practice passed down to parents from pediatricians. *Clin Pediatr (Phila)* 2007;46:146-50.
59. Erlewyn-Lajeunesse MD, Coppens K, Hunt LP et al. Randomised controlled trial of combined paracetamol and ibuprofen for fever. *Arch Dis Child* 2006;91:414-6.
60. Wong T, Stang AS, Ganshorn H et al. Combined and alternating paracetamol and ibuprofen therapy for febrile children. *Cochrane Database Syst Rev* 2013;10:CD009572.
61. Kramer LC, Richards PA, Thompson AM et al. Alternating antipyretics: antipyretic efficacy of acetaminophen versus acetaminophen alternated with ibuprofen in children. *Clin Pediatr (Phila)* 2008;47:907-11.
62. Sarrell EM, Wielunsky E, Cohen HA. Antipyretic treatment in young children with fever: acetaminophen, ibuprofen, or both alternating in a randomized, double-blind study. *Arch Pediatr Adolesc Med* 2006;160:197-202.
63. Schmitt BD. Concerns over alternating acetaminophen and ibuprofen for fever. *Arch Pediatr Adolesc Med* 2006;160:757.
64. Allen GM, Ivers N, Shevchuk Y. Treatment of pediatric fever: are acetaminophen and ibuprofen equivalent? *Can Fam Physician* 2010;56:773.
65. Yue Z, Jiang P, Sun H et al. Association between an excess risk of acute kidney injury and concomitant use of ibuprofen and acetaminophen in children, retrospective analysis of a spontaneous reporting system. *Eur J Clin Pharmacol* 2014;70:479-82.
66. Mofenson HC, McFee R, Caraccio T et al. Combined antipyretic therapy: another potential source of chronic acetaminophen toxicity. *J Pediatr* 1998;133:712-4.
67. Saphyakhajon P, Greene G. Alternating acetaminophen and ibuprofen in children may cause parental confusion and is dangerous. *Arch Pediatr Adolesc Med* 2006;160:757.
68. Purssell E. Systematic review of studies comparing combined treatment with paracetamol and ibuprofen, with either drug alone. *Arch Dis Child* 2011;96:1175-9.
69. McCarthy PL. Fever in infants and children. In: Mackowiak PA, ed. *Fever: basic mechanisms and management.* 2nd ed. Philadelphia: Lippincott-Raven; 1997. p. 351-62.
70. Steering Committee on Quality Improvement and Management, Subcommittee on Febrile Seizures. Febrile seizures: clinical practice guideline for the long-term management of the child with simple febrile seizures. *Pediatrics* 2008;121:1281-6.

71. van Stuijvenberg M, Derksen-Lubsen G, Steyerberg EW et al. Randomized controlled trial of ibuprofen syrup administered during febrile illnesses to prevent febrile seizure recurrences. *Pediatrics* 1998;102:E51.
72. Camfield PR, Camfield CS, Shapiro SH et al. The first febrile seizure–antipyretic instruction plus either phenobarbital or placebo to prevent recurrence. *J Pediatr* 1980;97:16-21.
73. Offringa M, Newton R. Prophylactic drug management for febrile seizures in children. *Cochrane Database Syst Rev* 2012;4:CD003031.
74. Bender B, Scarpace PJ. Fever in the elderly. In: Mackowiak PA, ed. *Fever: basic mechanisms and management.* 2nd ed. Philadelphia: Lippincott-Raven; 1997. p. 363-73.
75. Keating HJ, Klimek JJ, Levine DS et al. Effect of aging on the clinical significance of fever in ambulatory adult patients. *J Am Geriatr Soc* 1984;32:282-7.
76. Milunsky A, Ulcickas M, Rothman KJ et al. Maternal heat exposure and neural tube defects. *JAMA* 1992;268:882-5.
77. Edwards MJ. Review: hyperthermia and fever during pregnancy. *Birth Defects Res A Clin Mol Teratol* 2006;76:507-16.
78. Czeizel AE, Puho EH, Acs N et al. High fever-related maternal diseases as possible causes of multiple congenital abnormalities: a population-based case-control study. *Birth Defects Res A Clin Mol Teratol* 2007;79:544-51.
79. Li Z, Ren A, Liu J et al. Maternal flu or fever, medication use, and neural tube defects: a population-based case-control study in northern China. *Birth Defects Res A Clin Mol Teratol* 2007;79:295-300.
80. Dreier JW, Andersen A, Berg-Beckhoff G. Systematic review and meta-analyses: fever in pregnancy and health impacts in the offspring. *Pediatrics* 2014;133:e674-88.
81. Briggs GG, Freeman RK. *Drugs in pregnancy and lactation: a reference guide to fetal and neonatal risk.* 10th ed. Philadelphia: Wolters Kluwer Health; 2015.
82. Crocetti M, Moghbeli N, Serwint J. Fever phobia revisited: have parental misconceptions about fever changed in 20 years? *Pediatrics* 2001;107:1241-6.
83. Schmitt BD. Fever phobia: misconceptions of parents about fevers. *Am J Dis Child* 1980;134:176-81.
84. May A, Bauchner H. Fever phobia: the pediatrician's contribution. *Pediatrics* 1992;90:851-4.
85. Karwowska A, Nijssen-Jordan C, Johnson D et al. Parental and health care provider understanding of childhood fever: a Canadian perspective. *CJEM* 2002;394-400.
86. Walsh A, Edwards H, Fraser J. Parents' childhood fever management: community survey and instrument development. *J Adv Nurs* 2008;63:376-88.
87. Enarson MC, Ali S, Vanderneer B et al. Beliefs and expectations of Canadian parents who bring febrile children for medical care. *Pediatrics* 2012;130:e905-12.
88. Wallenstein MB, Schroeder AR, Hole MK et al. Fever literacy and fever phobia. *Clin Pediatr (Phila)* 2012;52:254-9.
89. Simon HK, Weinkle DA. Over-the-counter medications. Do parents give what they intend to give? *Arch Pediatr Adolesc Med* 1997;151:654-6.
90. McErlean MA, Bartfield JM, Kennedy DA et al. Home antipyretic use in children brought to the emergency department *Pediatr Emerg Care* 2001;17:249-51.
91. Goldman RD, Scolnik D. Underdosing of acetaminophen by parents and emergency department utilization. *Pediatr Emerg Care* 2004;20:89-93.
92. Li SF, Lacher B, Crain EF. Acetaminophen and ibuprofen dosing by parents. *Pediat Emerg Care* 2000;16:394-7.
93. Chiappini E, Principi N, Longhi R et al. Management of fever in children: summary of the Italian Pediatric Society guidelines. *Clin Ther* 2009;31:1826-43.
94. Rivera-Penera T, Gugig R, Davis J et al. Outcome of acetaminophen overdose in pediatric patients and factors contributing to hepatotoxicity. *J Pediatr* 1997;130:300-4.
95. Heubi JE, Bien JP. Acetaminophen use in children: more is not better. *J Pediatr* 1997;130:175-7.
96. Heubi JE, Barbacci MB, Zimmerman HJ. Therapeutic misadventures with acetaminophen: hepatotoxicity after multiple doses in children. *J Pediatr* 1998;132:22-7.
97. Antman EM, Bennett JS, Daugherty A et al. Use of nonsteroidal anti-inflammatory drugs: an update for clinicians: a scientific statement from the American Heart Association. *Circulation* 2007;115:1634-42.
98. Mikaeloff Y, Kezouh A, Suissa S. Nonsteroidal anti-inflammatory drug use and the risk of severe skin and soft tissue complications in patients with varicella or zoster disease. *Br J Clin Pharmacol* 2008;65:203-9.
99. Lopes RD, Horowitz JD, Garcia DA et al. Warfarin and acetaminophen interaction: a summary of the evidence and biologic plausibility. *Blood* 2011;118:6269-73.
100. Kanabar D, Dale S, Rawat M. A review of ibuprofen and acetaminophen use in febrile children and the occurrence of asthma-related symptoms. *Clin Ther* 2007;29:2716-23.

Fever—What You Need to Know

Hints to help you manage a fever:

- Treat the person, not the fever. By itself, fever is rarely dangerous. It is not always necessary to use drugs to lower a fever.
- **Do not** wake a sleeping child to give drugs for fever.
- **Do not** use fever medication for more than 3 days without consulting a healthcare provider.
- Use acetaminophen or ibuprofen for fever in children and adolescents. **Do not** use ASA—it can cause Reye's syndrome, a serious disorder.
- Use one drug only. **Do not** alternate acetaminophen and ibuprofen.
- Read the labels carefully. Make sure you use the right form of medicine for your child (liquid or pills). Determine the dosage based on your child's weight. Use the proper measuring device to be sure the amount is accurate. Ask your pharmacist or other healthcare provider for help.
- Check other medications, especially medications for cough and cold, to see if they contain acetaminophen, ibuprofen or ASA. Be sure you are not giving your child too much of these medicines.
- Keep all medications out of reach of children.
- Encourage the person with fever to drink lots of fluids.
- Keep the person cool by removing excess clothing and bedding.

When should you contact a healthcare provider?

- Contact a healthcare provider for:
  - fever over 40.5°C
  - children less than 6 months old who have fever
  - a child who appears very ill, has a stiff neck, has a seizure, is confused or delirious, or is crying without stopping
  - fever that lasts longer than 3 days
- Contact a healthcare provider if the person with a fever has recently had chemotherapy.

Chapter 8
Headache

Irene Worthington, BScPhm

This chapter focuses on 3 of the most common headache disorders: tension-type headache and migraine (primary headache disorders), and medication-overuse headache (secondary headache disorder). A full list of headache disorders and their classification is published by the International Headache Society (IHS).[1]

Pathophysiology

Tension-type Headache

Tension-type headache (TTH) is the most common type of headache. It is diagnosed mainly by the presence of a headache lasting 30 minutes to 7 days that has at least 2 of the following criteria: bilateral location, a pressing/tightening quality, mild or moderate intensity, not aggravated by routine physical activity, and an absence of features found in other types of headache (e.g., migraine). Although mental stress and tension are frequently thought to precipitate TTH, the exact pathophysiology is unknown. Both peripheral (myofascial tissues) and central mechanisms are thought to contribute to pain in TTH.[2] Since there are significant overlapping features, some headache experts believe that TTH is a variant of migraine; however, epidemiologic studies have concluded that migraine and TTH are different disorders that coexist in many patients.[1] TTH can be episodic or chronic (headache on ≥15 days per month). The lifetime prevalence of TTH is around 80%, and about 3% for chronic TTH. TTH appears to be more prevalent in women, and declines with age in both women and men.[2]

Migraine

Migraine is a common, underdiagnosed, often incapacitating neurovascular disorder characterized by recurrent attacks of headache pain (generally moderate to severe), autonomic nervous system dysfunction, and neurologic symptoms in some patients.[3] The IHS describes the diagnostic features of migraine subtypes.[1] The 2 most common are migraine with aura and migraine without aura. The specific cause of migraine is unknown but genetic factors are likely involved. It has been proposed that specific triggers can provoke CNS dysfunction in susceptible individuals, leading to dilation of intracranial and extracerebral blood vessels and activation of the trigeminal sensory nerves (resulting in release of vasoactive peptides such as calcitonin gene-related peptide), with subsequent relaying of pain signals to the brain. Migraine attacks may be episodic or chronic (≥15 days per month). Approximately 15% of patients experience migraine attacks preceded or accompanied by transient focal neurologic symptoms (usually visual), referred to as an aura. Aura is thought to be caused by neuronal dysfunction, not ischemia or vasoconstriction as previously believed. Aura can also occur without a subsequent headache. In North America and Western Europe, the 1-year prevalence of migraine is 11% overall: 15–18% among women and 6% among men. Attacks may last from 4–72 hours.[3,4] Status migrainosus is a debilitating migraine attack that lasts more than 72 hours.

Medication-overuse Headache

Medication-overuse headache (MOH) is an under-recognized condition that may occur in patients who suffer from migraines (primarily) or tension-type headaches. Recognition and treatment of MOH may lead to long-term improvement in headache relief and quality of life for many patients. Frequent use of analgesics or other acute migraine medications for ≥3 months can lead to MOH (headache present on ≥15 days per month) in patients with migraine/tension-type headaches. MOH can occur in association with simple analgesics (e.g., acetaminophen, ASA) or, less commonly, with NSAIDs. It is more common with combination products containing barbiturates, caffeine and/or opioids. Overuse of ergotamine or triptans and withdrawal from substances such as caffeine, opioids and estrogen have also been implicated.[1,5]

Goals of Therapy

- Identify potentially serious causes of headache and refer patient for diagnosis/treatment. Patients with sudden, severe headache should go to an emergency room
- Relieve pain and associated symptoms (e.g., nausea/vomiting) so that patient can return to normal functioning
- Prevent recurrence of migraine headache
- Prevent medication-overuse headache

Patient Assessment

The IHS has established criteria for the diagnosis of various headache disorders.[1] There are no diagnostic tests for primary headache disorders (e.g., tension-type headache, migraine, cluster headache). Diagnosis is based on symptoms, after ruling out any serious underlying disorders.[6,7,8,9,10,11] Secondary headache disorders are those associated with organic causes (e.g., trauma, meningitis, space-occupying lesion). Some medical procedures are associated with headache (e.g., lumbar puncture, rhinoscopy).

Patients with occasional tension-type headache do not require further assessment unless the headaches become chronic (≥15 days/month). Patients with features of migraine require assessment, diagnosis and appropriate treatment. Patients with any unusual headache require further assessment; if the headache is very severe, with a sudden onset, refer immediately to an emergency room (see Red Flags for Serious Headache).

A stepwise approach to headache assessment and treatment is provided in Figure 1.

Common Signs and Symptoms

Table 1 outlines the clinical features of tension-type and migraine headache.

Table 1: **Clinical Features of Tension-type Headache and Migraine**

Clinical Feature	Tension-type Headache	Migraine
Quality of headache	Pressing/tightening (nonpulsating)	Throbbing/pulsating (at least part of the time)
Severity	Mild to moderate	Usually moderate to severe, although can be mild
Location	Bilateral	Usually unilateral (can be bilateral, especially in children)
Frequency	Episodic (<15 days/month) or chronic (≥15 days/month)	Episodic (<15 days/month) or chronic (≥15 days/month)
Duration	30 min to 7 days	4–72 h
Aggravated by physical activity	No	Yes
Associated symptoms	No nausea/vomiting (anorexia may occur) Photophobia or phonophobia but not both	At least one of the following: 1. nausea and/or vomiting 2. photophobia and phonophobia May occur with or without aura (usually visual)

Differential Diagnosis

In addition to the primary headache disorders listed in Table 1, other possible etiologies of headache include:[1,6,7,8,12]

- Primary headache types such as benign cough headache, benign exertional headache, cluster headache and other trigeminal autonomic cephalgias, hemicrania continua, cold-stimulus headache, primary stabbing headache and new daily persistent headache
- Infections such as meningitis and encephalitis
- Temporal arteritis (an important cause of headache in those over 50 years of age; associated with systemic symptoms and elevated erythrocyte sedimentation rate; if left untreated, often leads to permanent blindness)
- Cerebral ischemia (stroke); cervicogenic headache (originating from the neck); glaucoma; headache following stroke or transient ischemic attack (TIA); space-occupying lesions (e.g., brain tumour); subarachnoid hemorrhage or intracerebral hemorrhages; subdural hematoma; systemic/CNS vasculitides (e.g., systemic lupus erythematosus); and others
- Note: "sinus" headaches occur only in the presence of a sinus infection (fever, purulent nasal discharge)[12]
- Medications (see Table 2)

Drugs Associated with Headache

Table 2 lists drugs that commonly cause headache as a side effect.

Table 2: **Drugs Associated with Headache**[7,13,14,15]

Drugs associated with intracranial hypertension[a]	
Antibiotics	minocycline, sulfamethoxazole/trimethoprim, tetracycline
Corticosteroids	
Other	cimetidine, isotretinoin, tamoxifen
Drugs with headache as a side effect[a]	
ACEIs	e.g., captopril
Antihypertensives, miscellaneous	hydralazine, methyldopa
Beta-blockers	e.g., atenolol, propranolol (also used for migraine prophylaxis)
Calcium channel blockers	nifedipine
H_2 antagonists	e.g., cimetidine, ranitidine
Nitrates	e.g., nitroglycerin
NSAIDs	diclofenac, indomethacin (also used to treat certain types of headache)
Oral contraceptives and HRT (in some patients predisposed to migraine)	
SSRIs	citalopram, escitalopram, fluoxetine, fluvoxamine, paroxetine, sertraline
Other	caffeine (especially caffeine withdrawal), cyclosporine, danazol, latanoprost ophthalmic drops,[16] metronidazole

[a] Most common drug-related causes (not exhaustive).

Abbreviations: ACEI = angiotensin-converting enzyme inhibitor; HRT = hormone replacement therapy; NSAID = nonsteroidal anti-inflammatory drug; SSRI = selective serotonin reuptake inhibitor

Red Flags for Serious Headache

- Severe/abrupt onset ("worst headache ever")
- Onset in middle age or older (>40 years)
- Neurologic signs: stiff neck, focal signs, reduced consciousness
- Systemic signs: appears ill, fever, nausea/vomiting (not explained by migraine or systemic illness)
- Significant change in pattern of headaches: increased frequency and/or progressive severity
- Nocturnal occurrence or on awakening in the morning; if patient consistently has headache on awakening or is awakened by a headache, brain tumour is a possible cause; however, migraines sometimes occur on awakening
- Onset with exercise or sexual activity (may be benign or serious)

Nonpharmacologic Therapy

Patient education is important in the management of headache. Provide patients with an explanation of their headache disorder and use printed materials to reinforce verbal information. Reassure them (in some cases, once the diagnosis has been confirmed) that they do not have a serious underlying cause for headaches (e.g., brain tumour). Establish realistic goals and expectations of treatment; explain benefits and limitations of various treatment options in collaboration with the patient's healthcare team. Patients may also benefit from referral to self-help groups.[11,14]

Acute/Symptomatic Treatment

During a migraine attack, simple measures such as resting in a dark, quiet room and applying a cold cloth/ice pack to the head are helpful, although not evidence-based. Sleep often alleviates migraine headaches.

Prevention

Migraine and other headaches are often triggered by 1 or more factors. Triggers vary among individual patients. Advise patients to identify and avoid the triggers associated with their migraines. Lifestyle changes such as maintaining regular sleeping and eating schedules, reducing stress and limiting caffeine intake may reduce the frequency of headaches, particularly migraine. A sudden decrease in caffeine consumption may lead to a withdrawal headache; caffeine may help alleviate headache in some migraine sufferers. Ask patients to maintain a headache diary (available from www.headachenetwork.ca or www.migrainecanada.org), that includes food ingested within 24 hours prior to an attack, to identify dietary migraine triggers.[14] If feasible, discontinue drugs implicated in triggering a headache (see Table 2) on a trial basis. Common migraine triggers are listed in Table 3.

Biobehavioural measures such as biofeedback, relaxation therapy, cognitive behavioural therapy and acupuncture may help to prevent migraine in some individuals.[14] While aerobic exercise (e.g., 40 minutes 3 times weekly) may trigger a headache for some patients, in others it may reduce headache frequency and provide an option for patients who cannot or choose not to take prophylactic medication.[17]

Controversial measures include chiropractic and other physical therapies, transcutaneous electrical stimulation, hypnosis, occipital or supraorbital nerve blockade and homeopathic remedies.[14,18]

Pharmacologic Therapy

For comparative ingredients of nonprescription products, consult the *Compendium of Products for Minor Ailments*—Analgesic Products: Internal Analgesics and Antipyretics; Herbal and Natural Health Products: Single Entity; Vitamin and Mineral Products: Single Entity.

Table 3: **Migraine Triggers**[9,14]

Types of Triggers[a]	Examples
Chemical	Benzene, insecticides, perfumes or other strong odours.
Drugs	See Table 2.
Environmental	Weather changes (barometric pressure changes), bright/flickering lights, loud noise, strong odours (e.g., perfume), cigarette smoke, travel across time zones.
Foods and beverages that contain nitrites, monosodium glutamate (MSG), aspartame or neurotransmitter precursors (e.g., tyramine, tyrosine, phenylalanine)	Aged cheeses, cured meats (e.g., hot dogs, bacon), chocolate, alcoholic beverages (especially red wine), caffeine-containing beverages. Missed or delayed meals can also trigger migraine.
Hormonal	Menstruation, pregnancy (especially in first trimester), perimenopause.
Other	Sleep-wake cycle alterations, stress/anxiety (or let-down from stress), intense activity/physical exertion, sexual activity.

[a] Most common triggers are listed (not an exhaustive list).

Symptomatic Treatment

See Table 4 for information on drug therapy for acute headache.

Tension-type Headaches

Analgesics

Mild tension-type headache may not require treatment. Appropriate doses of simple analgesics (e.g., **acetaminophen**, **ASA**) or NSAIDs (e.g., **ibuprofen**, **naproxen sodium**) will often alleviate tension-type headaches.[2,11]

Migraine Headaches

The goal of acute drug therapy for migraine headaches is to alleviate pain within 2 hours of treatment.[10] Several agents may be tried before finding the most effective therapy. Patients may need ≥1 medication depending on the migraine severity. Moderate to severe migraine attacks often require the use of triptans with or without simple analgesics, and possibly antiemetics.[10] Consider prophylactic therapy if migraine attacks have a significant impact on quality of life despite appropriate use of acute medications or if frequency of attacks and reliance on acute medications puts patients at risk of MOH[30] (see Preventive Therapy).

Analgesics

Mild to moderate migraine attacks may respond to adequate doses of simple analgesics (e.g., **acetaminophen**, **ASA**) or NSAIDs (e.g., **ibuprofen**, **naproxen sodium**).[2,11,26,31]

There is a lack of evidence of efficacy for codeine (8 mg) in combination with ASA or acetaminophen (plus caffeine) in the treatment of migraine. It may be considered if other options are ineffective or contraindicated. Recommended dosage is 1–2 tablets Q4H PRN in adults and 1–2 tablets up to QID in adolescents. Side effects associated with codeine include constipation, sedation, dependence and tolerance. Codeine has been associated with an increased incidence of congenital anomalies including cleft palate and inguinal hernias.[21] To avoid MOH, these combination products should be used <10 days/month. Overuse of caffeine can lead to withdrawal headache. Use codeine with caution in a breastfeeding mother: choose the lowest effective dose and limit treatment to less than 3–4 days.[32] For more information on opioid use in this population, consult the *Compendium of Pharmaceuticals and Specialties*: Drug Use during Breastfeeding.

Unfortunately many migraine sufferers do not achieve adequate pain relief by relying exclusively on simple analgesics.[33,34,35,36,37,38] Furthermore, most published trials of nonprescription agents in migraine have systematically excluded patients with more severe attacks.

Triptans

Triptans or $5\text{-HT}_{1B/1D}$ receptor agonists (e.g., **almotriptan**, **eletriptan**, **frovatriptan**, **naratriptan**, **rizatriptan**, **sumatriptan** and **zolmitriptan**) are considered to be the most efficacious agents for acute migraine treatment.[39,40] They alleviate headache pain and migraine-associated symptoms (nausea/vomiting, photophobia/phonophobia). In randomized controlled trials, all triptans have demonstrated efficacy in the treatment of acute migraine; however, individuals may differ in their response to a particular triptan. The triptans are available in various formulations: subcutaneous injection (sumatriptan), oral tablets (all), orally disintegrating tablets (rizatriptan, zolmitriptan) and intranasal (sumatriptan, zolmitriptan).[41] If oral agents are not effective or cannot be used due to nausea/vomiting, consider an intranasal formulation or the triptan showing the greatest efficacy—subcutaneous sumatriptan.[10]

The combination of an NSAID (e.g., naproxen sodium) and a triptan (e.g., sumatriptan) has better efficacy compared with either agent alone, and reduces headache recurrence.[42,43]

Ergotamine Derivatives

Nasal or injectable **dihydroergotamine** (DHE) has been shown to be effective for migraine.[10,44] Oral ergot preparations (e.g., ergotamine tartrate; no longer available in Canada) have limited efficacy and excessive side effects.[10,45]

Other Agents

In the emergency room, various parenteral agents may be used for treatment of severe migraine. Adjunctive antiemetics (e.g., **metoclopramide**), **chlorpromazine**, **prochlorperazine**, **ketorolac**, **dexamethasone** or opioids (not considered first-line therapy) may be given with other agents such as DHE.[10]

Butalbital (in combination with ASA, caffeine and/or codeine) is sometimes used in the management of acute migraine, but has a very limited role due to the potential for dependence, abuse, medication-overuse headache and the possibility of a withdrawal syndrome following discontinuation of high doses.[10]

Adjunctive drugs for the management of nausea/vomiting associated with migraine include **dimenhydrinate** (though there is a lack of evidence), **domperidone**, **metoclopramide** or **prochlorperazine**.[10]

For further discussion of pharmacologic therapy for migraine, consult the *Compendium of Therapeutic Choices*: Headache in Adults; Headache in Children.

Medication-overuse Headache

Treatment of medication-overuse headache (MOH) involves discontinuation of the drug(s) that are implicated, relief of withdrawal symptoms, use of migraine-specific medications (adhering to recommended limits in frequency of use) to treat recurrent headaches, and initiation of prophylactic therapy (e.g., **divalproex sodium**, **propranolol**, **topiramate**, **tricyclic antidepressants**). The causative agents are usually stopped abruptly or sometimes tapered, while titrating prophylactic therapy. Advise patients not to discontinue high doses of butalbital-containing analgesics abruptly, since seizures may occur on withdrawal. Ideally, refer these patients to a neurologist/headache specialist. Primary care healthcare practitioners can play a key role in preventing and managing MOH. Monitor the patient's use of prescription and nonprescription medications, counsel on appropriate use of antimigraine medications and provide support to patients who are withdrawing from medications.[46,47,48,49,50,51]

Preventive Therapy

Tension-type Headache

Most strategies to prevent tension-type headache are nonpharmacologic (see Nonpharmacologic Therapy). For disabling and/or chronic tension-type headache, pharmacologic prophylaxis may be considered (e.g., **amitriptyline, mirtazapine, nortriptyline, venlafaxine**).[52]

Migraine

Prophylactic therapy is usually administered daily to reduce the frequency and severity of attacks in patients with migraine. Guidelines for migraine prophylaxis are available from the Canadian Headache Society.[30]

Prophylactic migraine therapy is appropriate in the following circumstances:[10,11,30]

- Migraine attacks (any number) that significantly impair normal activity or quality of life despite appropriate use of acute therapies
- Optimal acute therapies have failed, are contraindicated or have produced serious side effects
- Frequent attacks that result in the potential overuse of acute therapies and may lead to medication-overuse headache.

Prophylaxis is considered successful if headache frequency, or number of days with headache, is reduced by ≥50%. Typically only 1 preventive agent is used at a time; however, neurologists may prescribe combinations of agents in resistant cases. Start medications at a low dose and titrate to the most effective tolerated dose. A trial period of at least 2 months is needed to assess the efficacy of most prophylactic medications. If effective, prophylactic agents may be continued for 6–12 months, then tapered gradually (to assess ongoing need and prevent rebound headaches). Prophylactic therapy may be required for prolonged periods in some patients. Consider the patient's concurrent medical conditions (e.g., hypertension, depression or obesity) and/or drug contraindications (e.g., beta-blockers are contraindicated in patients with asthma) when selecting a prophylactic agent. Advise patients to keep a headache diary (available from www.headachenetwork.ca or www.migrainecanada.org) to monitor their response to therapy.[30]

Preventive Agents

Medications used for migraine prophylaxis include beta-blockers without intrinsic sympathomimetic activity (e.g., **propranolol, nadolol, metoprolol**), tricyclic antidepressants (e.g., **amitriptyline, nortriptyline**), calcium channel blockers (e.g., **flunarizine, verapamil**), serotonin (5-HT_2) receptor antagonists (e.g., **pizotifen**), **valproic acid/divalproex sodium, topiramate, candesartan, lisinopril, gabapentin** and NSAIDs (e.g., **naproxen sodium** 550 mg twice daily for 1 week per month for menstrual migraine prophylaxis).[10,11,30,52]

For more information on preventive therapy, consult the *Compendium of Therapeutic Choices*: Headache in Adults; Headache in Children.

Natural Health Products

See Table 5 for information on natural health products used for migraine headache prophylaxis.

Butterbur (*Petasites hybridus* extract) 75 mg, and not 50 mg, was significantly more effective than placebo in a controlled trial that randomized patients with migraine (n=245) to butterbur 50 mg, 75 mg or placebo twice daily.[54] Sixty-eight percent of patients receiving butterbur 75 mg BID achieved ≥50% reduction in attack frequency after 4 months compared with 49% for the placebo arm. Butterbur was well tolerated; the most frequently reported adverse events included mild GI events, primarily burping. There have been rare reports of hepatotoxicity.[53] Caution patients to avoid consuming any part of the *Petasites* plant other than specific commercially prepared products that have had plant carcinogens and hepatotoxic alkaloids removed.

Coenzyme Q10 (300 mg/day) was well tolerated and superior to placebo in a small, randomized, controlled trial of migraine prophylaxis in 42 patients.[56] Better studies are needed to determine the efficacy of coenzyme Q10 in migraine prophylaxis.

The potential role of **magnesium** deficiency in the pathogenesis of migraine has been investigated. Prophylactic oral magnesium supplementation was effective in 2 double-blind studies. The lack of response in a third study is thought to be due to the poor absorption of magnesium preparation used.[57,58,59] In 1 study that demonstrated the efficacy of magnesium, patients received magnesium 600 mg (24 mmol) daily in the form of trimagnesium dicitrate (not available in Canada; an alternative may be magnesium citrate).[57] More definitive, large-scale studies are needed to assess the role of magnesium in migraine prevention.

Riboflavin (vitamin B_2) 400 mg daily for 3 months was compared with placebo for migraine prophylaxis in a randomized, double-blind trial with 55 patients.[60] Approximately 50% of patients taking riboflavin had ≥50% reduction in frequency of attacks compared with 15% in the placebo arm. The exact mechanism of action is not known but may be related to its effects on mitochondrial energy metabolism. It is thought that mitochondrial dysfunction, resulting in impaired oxygen metabolism, may play a role in migraine pathogenesis. Only minor adverse effects (1 case each of diarrhea and polyuria) were reported in the riboflavin group. Riboflavin can also cause insignificant yellow discoloration of the urine.[60] In a randomized, double-blind study of 48 children with migraine, a high placebo response rate suggested that riboflavin 200 mg daily is not effective in preventing migraine in children.[61] Further large-scale and comparative studies are needed to determine the efficacy of riboflavin in migraine prophylaxis.

Although **feverfew** (*Tanacetum parthenium*) has been used for migraine prophylaxis, evidence for its efficacy is conflicting and it appears to be no better than placebo. Therefore, it is no longer recommended for migraine prophylaxis in the Canadian guidelines.[30] Furthermore, discontinuation of feverfew can result in post-feverfew syndrome, characterized by severe headache, insomnia, nervousness and joint pain.[55]

Medication-overuse Headache

To prevent the development of MOH when treating primary headache disorders such as migraine or tension-type headache, use simple analgesics (e.g., acetaminophen, ASA) <15 days per month and combination analgesics or opioids <10 days per month. Frequent use (≥10 days per month) of ergot or triptan medications can also result in MOH. Headache associated with overuse of analgesics tends to resemble a tension-type headache (migraine headaches can also be superimposed) whereas triptan overuse manifests as increased migraine frequency.[46,47,48,49,50,51]

Monitoring of Therapy

Acute/Symptomatic Therapy

Ideally, medications should relieve headaches (no pain or mild pain) and associated nausea/vomiting and photophobia/phonophobia within about 2 hours.[10] Advise patients to report any significant adverse effects to their healthcare practitioner (see Table 4 for side effects and drug interactions of nonprescription medications).

Preventive Therapy

Continue prophylactic medications for migraine for at least 2 months to determine efficacy. A ≥50% reduction in the frequency of migraine attacks is considered a good response. Advise patients to record exercise, food intake, medication use and migraine attacks in a headache diary,[4] and to report any medication adverse effects to their healthcare practitioner (see Table 5 for side effects of natural health products for migraine prophylaxis).

Figure 1: Assessment and Management of Patients with Headache

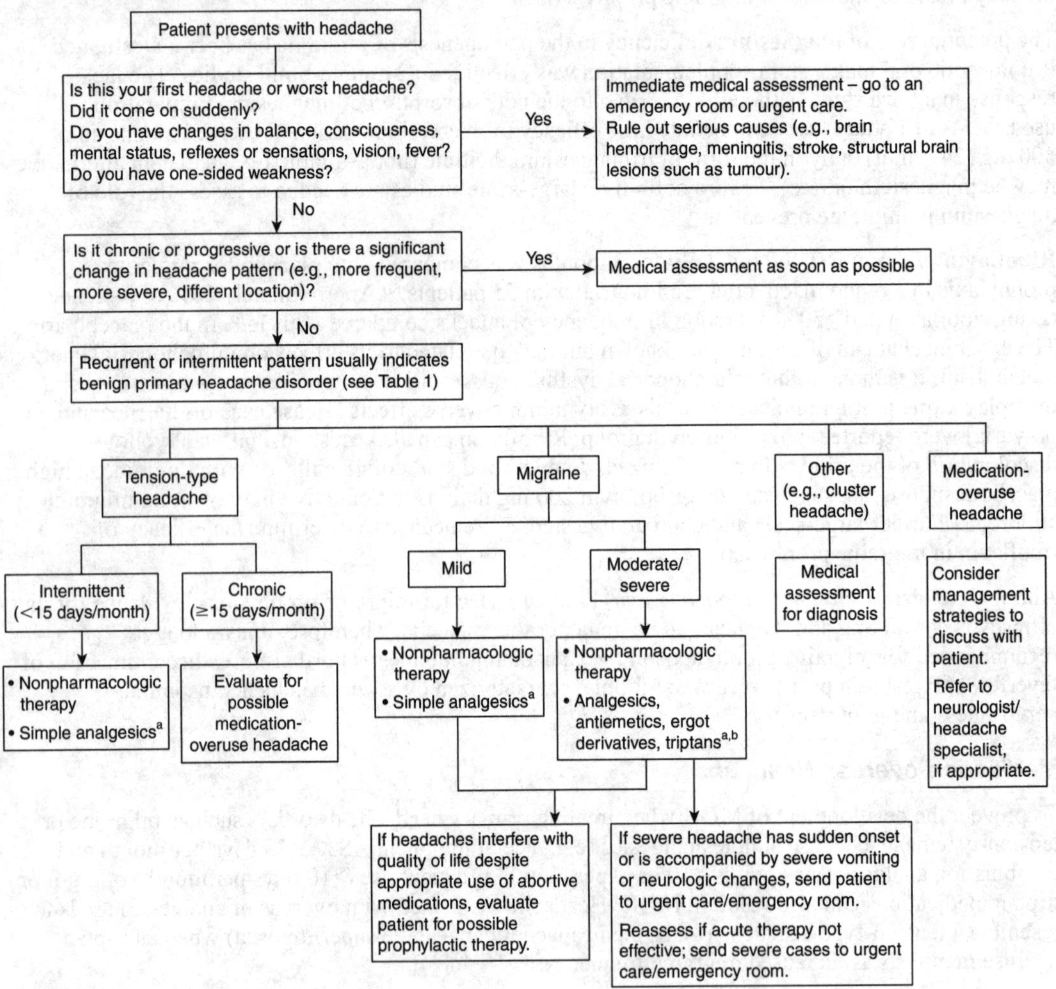

[a] Limit use of simple analgesics (e.g., acetaminophen, NSAIDs) to <15 days/month and combination analgesics (e.g., acetaminophen with codeine) to <10 days/month.
[b] Limit use of ergot and triptan products to <10 days/month.

Table 4: **Drug Therapy for Treatment of Mild Tension-type and Migraine Headaches**

Class	Drug	Dosage	Adverse Effects	Drug Interactions	Comments	Cost[a]
NSAIDs	*ASA* Aspirin, Coated Aspirin, generics	**Adult:** 975–1000 mg po[b] **Pediatric (≥12 y):** 500–650 mg single dose	GI upset—usually the only more common adverse effect when single doses are used to treat acute headache. With continuous or frequent NSAID use: Cardiovascular: MI, stroke, heart failure, fluid retention, hypertension. CNS: Dizziness, drowsiness, headache, tinnitus, confusion (especially in the elderly); CNS effects may be dose related and respond to decreased dosage. GI: Dyspepsia, epigastric pain, nausea/vomiting, diarrhea, gastric and duodenal ulcers, GI bleeding. Nephrotoxicity may occur; avoid NSAIDs in patients with severe renal impairment (ClCr <30 mL/min). Minor or serious skin rashes, pruritus.	Increased risk of bleeding with anticoagulants (e.g., warfarin) or antiplatelet drugs (e.g., clopidogrel). May decrease effect of antihypertensives. May decrease renal clearance of lithium; monitor lithium levels when NSAID added. Increased risk of GI bleeding when used with SSRIs.	Use <15 days/month to avoid MOH. Good evidence for efficacy in migraine (975–1000 mg).[19] A meta-analysis of 3 trials concluded that effervescent ASA 1000 mg was as effective as sumatriptan 50 mg for acute migraine.[20] Because of the possible risk of Reye's syndrome, ASA should not be used in the presence of viral illness or fever in children. Enteric-coated preparations will result in a delayed onset of action. Pregnancy: Relatively safe in intermittent doses during first and second trimesters; avoid use in third trimester (may be associated with prolonged gestation and labour, premature narrowing of ductus arteriosus, persistent pulmonary hypertension of the newborn).[21]	$
	ibuprofen Advil, Advil Children/ Pediatric, Advil Junior Strength, Advil Liquid Gels, Motrin, Motrin (Children's), Motrin IB, Motrin Liquid Gels, generics	**Adult:** 400 mg po[b] **Pediatric:** Children ≥6 months: 5–10 mg/kg Q6–8H po PRN for symptom management; maximum 40 mg/kg/day; do not exceed adult dose	See ASA.	See ASA.	Use <15 days/month to avoid MOH. Good evidence for efficacy in migraine.[22] A meta-analysis concluded that ibuprofen at doses of 200 mg or 400 mg is effective in rendering migraine sufferers pain-free at 2 h; however, photophobia and phonophobia improved only with the 400 mg dose.[23] Pregnancy: See ASA.	$

(cont'd)

Table 4: Drug Therapy for Treatment of Mild Tension-type and Migraine Headaches *(cont'd)*

Class	Drug	Dosage	Adverse Effects	Drug Interactions	Comments	Cost[a]
	naproxen Naprosyn, Pediapharm Naproxen Suspension, generics	Adult: 500 mg po[b]	See ASA.	See ASA.	Use <15 days/month to avoid MOH. In studies showing efficacy in migraine, prescribed doses of 500–825 mg were used.[24] Pregnancy: See ASA.	$
	naproxen sodium Aleve, Anaprox, generics	Adult: 550 mg po[b] Recommended self-care dose: 220 mg Q12H po	See ASA.	See ASA.	See naproxen.	$
Simple Analgesics	*acetaminophen* Atasol Preparations, Tempra, Tylenol, Tylenol Children's, generics	**Adult:** 1000 mg po[b] (do not exceed 4 g/day) **Pediatric:** 10–15 mg/kg Q4–6H po PRN for symptom management; maximum 75 mg/kg/day; do not exceed adult dose	Potential liver (and rarely kidney) dysfunction with chronic use of high doses or with acute overdose.	Acetaminophen has been reported to increase INR in warfarin-treated patients.[25] Check INR if acetaminophen ≥2 g/day is used for ≥3 consecutive days. Adjust warfarin dosage as required.	Limit use to <15 days/month to avoid MOH. Effective in childhood migraine.[26] In adults, it is considered to be less effective than ASA or NSAIDs for migraine.[10] 1 g dose shown to be effective for migraine in adults, although patients with severe migraine were excluded.[27,28] Pregnancy: Relatively safe during all trimesters; considered to be analgesic of first choice during pregnancy.[21,29]	$

[a] Cost per dose; includes drug cost only.

[b] In acute migraine, only single doses have been studied in randomized controlled trials.

Abbreviations: MOH = medication-overuse headache; NSAID = nonsteroidal anti-inflammatory drug

Legend: $ <$1

Table 5: **Natural Health Products for Prevention of Migraine Headaches**

Class	Drug	Dosage	Adverse Effects	Drug Interactions	Comments	Cost[a]
Natural Health Products	*butterbur*	**Adult:** 75 mg BID po **Pediatric:** No recommendations; some evidence for safe use in children 6–17 y for up to 4 months	Generally well tolerated; mild gastrointestinal events (mainly burping). Rare reports of hepatotoxicity.[53]	No significant interactions.	Good evidence for efficacy in adults.[54] Derived from *Petasites hybridus* root extract; product should be standardized to contain a minimum of 15% petasins (e.g., Petadolex—Weber & Weber, GmbH & Co, Germany). Caution patients against consuming any part of *Petasites* plant in any form other than commercially prepared products, in which plant carcinogens and hepatotoxic alkaloids have been removed. Preparations containing hepatotoxic alkaloid might be teratogenic and hepatotoxic. Safety has not been established in pregnancy, breastfeeding, or children <6 years.[55]	$$$
	coenzyme Q10	**Adult:** 300 mg/day po in 3 divided doses **Pediatric:** No recommendations; some evidence of efficacy in children who have low levels of coenzyme Q10	Generally well tolerated; GI effects (<1%; minimized by giving in divided doses 2 or 3 times daily).	May have additive blood pressure lowering effects when used with antihypertensive agents. May reduce anticoagulant effects of warfarin. Monitor patient's INR closely. May lower efficacy of chemotherapeutic agents (e.g., doxorubicin; preliminary evidence).	One small trial showed efficacy in adults.[56] May take up to 3 months for significant benefit. Insufficient data regarding use in pregnancy.	$$

(cont'd)

Table 5: **Natural Health Products for Prevention of Migraine Headaches** *(cont'd)*

Class	Drug	Dosage	Adverse Effects	Drug Interactions	Comments	Cost[a]
Minerals	*magnesium*	**Adult:** 300 mg (elemental magnesium) BID po **Pediatric:** No recommendations; some evidence of efficacy in children	Generally well tolerated; diarrhea, GI upset.	May decrease absorption of bisphosphonates (e.g., alendronate, risedronate), tetracyclines or quinolone antibiotics (e.g., ciprofloxacin, levofloxacin, moxifloxacin); separate administration by at least 2 h.	Conflicting evidence for efficacy.[57,58,59] Some magnesium salts are poorly absorbed; suggest citrate salt. Considered reasonably safe to use in pregnancy.	$
Vitamins	*riboflavin*	**Adult:** 400 mg/day po **Pediatric:** Insufficient evidence	Generally well tolerated; yellow discoloration of urine (benign).	No significant interactions.	One small trial in adults showed efficacy.[60] Lack of efficacy in pediatric migraine prophylaxis.[61] Use in pregnancy: safety of high-dose therapy not shown to be safe but not considered teratogenic.	$

[a] Cost per month; includes drug cost only.

Legend: $ <$10 $$ $10–20 $$$ $20–30

Resource Tips

Canada. Canadian Headache Society. Available from: www.migrainecanada.org.

Canada. Headache Network Canada. Available from: www.headachenetwork.ca (bilingual—English and French).

Ontario. Help for Headaches. Available from: www.headache-help.org.

U.S. American Committee for Headache Education, American Headache Society. Available from: www.achenet.org.

Suggested Readings

Becker WJ, Findlay T Moga C et al. Guideline for primary care management of headache in adults. *Can Fam Physician* 2015;61:670-9.

Evers S, Marziniak M. Clinical features, pathophysiology, and treatment of medication-overuse headache. *Lancet Neurol* 2010;9:391-401.

Purdy RA. Headache in adults. In: Jovaisas B, ed. *Compendium of therapeutic choices: CTC 7*. 7th ed. Ottawa: Canadian Pharmacists Association; 2014. p. 211-28.

Worthington I. Migraine headache: management strategies and optimizing therapy for acute attacks. *Pharm Pract* 2014;1:23-9.

Worthington I. Migraine prophylaxis: drug selection and treatment strategies for individual patients. *Pharm Pract* 2012;28:28-34.

References

1. Headache Classification Committee of the International Headache Society (IHS). The International Classification of Headache Disorders, 3rd edition (beta version). *Cephalalgia* 2013;33:629-808.
2. Fumal A, Schoenen J. Tension-type headache: current research and clinical management. *Lancet Neurol* 2008;7:70-83.
3. Goadsby PJ, Lipton RB, Ferrari MD. Migraine–current understanding and treatment. *N Engl J Med* 2002;346:257-70.
4. Silberstein SD. Migraine. *Lancet* 2004;363:381-91.
5. Saper JR, Da Silva AN. Medication overuse headache: history, features, prevention and management strategies. *CNS Drugs* 2013;27:867-77.
6. Dodick D. Headache as a symptom of ominous disease. What are the warning signals? *Postgrad Med* 1997;101:46-50, 55-6, 62-4.
7. Clinch CR. Evaluation of acute headaches in adults. *Am Fam Physician* 2001;63:685-92.
8. Campbell JK, Sakai F. Diagnosis and differential diagnosis. In: Olesen J, Tfelt-Hansen P, Welch KM, eds. *The headaches*. 2nd ed. Philadelphia: Lippincott William & Wilkins; 2000. p. 359-63.
9. Worthington I. Migraine headache: management strategies and optimizing therapy for acute attacks. *Pharm Pract* 2014;1:23-9.
10. Worthington I, Pringsheim T, Gawel MJ et al. Canadian Headache Society Guideline: acute drug therapy for migraine headache. *Can J Neurol Sci* 2013;40:S1-S80.
11. Purdy RA. Headache in adults. In: Jovaisas B, ed. *Compendium of therapeutic choices: CTC 7*. 7th ed. Ottawa: Canadian Pharmacists Association; 2014. p. 211-28.
12. Cady RK, Dodick DW, Levine HL et al. Sinus headache: a neurology, otolaryngology, allergy, and primary care consensus on diagnosis and treatment. *Mayo Clin Proc* 2005;80:908-16.
13. Silberstein SD. Drug-induced headache. *Neurol Clin* 1998;16:107-23.
14. Pryse-Phillips WE, Dodick DW, Edmeads JG et al. Guidelines for the nonpharmacologic management of migraine in clinical practice. Canadian Headache Society. *CMAJ* 1998;159:47-54.
15. Askmark H, Lundberg PO, Olsson S. Drug-related headache. *Headache* 1989;29:441-4.
16. Weston BC. Migraine headache associated with latanoprost. *Arch Ophthalmol* 2001;119:300-1.
17. Varkey E, Cider A, Carlsson J et al. Exercise as migraine prophylaxis: a randomized study using relaxation and topiramate as controls. *Cephalgia* 2011;31:1428-38.
18. Li Y, Liang F, Yang X et al. Acupuncture for treating acute attacks of migraine: a randomized controlled trial. *Headache* 2009;49:805-16.
19. Kirthi V, Derry S, Moore RA et al. Aspirin with or without an antiemetic for acute migraine headaches in adults. *Cochrane Database Syst Rev* 2010;(4):CD008041.
20. Lampl C, Voelker M, Diener HC. Efficacy and safety of 1,000 mg effervescent aspirin: individual patient data meta-analysis of three trials in migraine headache and migraine accompanying symptoms. *J Neurol* 2007;254:705-12.
21. Briggs GG, Freeman RK, Yaffe SJ. *Drugs in pregnancy and lactation: a reference guide to fetal and neonatal risk*. 10th ed. Philadelphia: Wolters Kluwer; 2015.
22. Rabbie R, Derry S, Moore RA et al. Ibuprofen with or without an antiemetic for acute migraine headaches in adults. *Cochrane Database Syst Rev* 2010;(11):CD008039.
23. Suthisisang C, Poolsup N, Kittikulsuth W et al. Efficacy of low-dose ibuprofen in acute migraine treatment: systematic review and meta-analysis. *Ann Pharmacother* 2007;41:1782-91.
24. Suthisisang C, Poolsup N, Suksomboon N et al. Meta-analysis of the efficacy and safety of naproxen sodium in the acute treatment of migraine. *Headache* 2010;50:808-18.

25. Lopes RD, Horowitz JD, Garcia DA et al. Warfarin and acetaminophen interaction: a summary of the evidence and biologic plausibility. *Blood* 2011;118:6269-73.
26. Whiting S. Headache in children. In: Jovaisas B, ed. *Compendium of therapeutic choices: CTC 7*. 7th ed. Ottawa: Canadian Pharmacists Association; 2014. p. 229-39.
27. Lipton RB, Baggish JS, Stewart WF et al. Efficacy and safety of acetaminophen in the treatment of migraine: results of a randomized, double-blind, placebo-controlled, population-based study. *Arch Intern Med* 2000;160:3486-92.
28. Derry S, Moore RA, McQuay HJ. Paracetamol (acetaminophen) with or without an antiemetic for acute migraine headaches in adults. *Cochrane Database Syst Rev* 2010;(11):CD:008040.
29. Menon R, Bushnell CD. Headache and pregnancy. *Neurologist* 2008;14:108-19.
30. Pringsheim T, Davenport W, Mackie G et al. Canadian Headache Society guideline for migraine prophylaxis. *Can J Neurol Sci* 2012;39:S1-59.
31. Worthington I. Pediatric migraine. *Pharm Pract* 1999;15:48-57.
32. Sachs HC, Committee On Drugs. The transfer of drugs and therapeutics into human breast milk: an update on selected topics. *Pediatrics* 2013;132:e796-809.
33. Wenzel RG, Sarvis CA, Krause ML. Over-the-counter drugs for acute migraine attacks: literature review and recommendations. *Pharmacotherapy* 2003;23:494-505.
34. Rapoport AM. Emerging nonspecific migraine therapies: targets and unmet needs. *Headache* 1999;39:S27-34.
35. Sheftell FD. Role and impact of over-the-counter medications in the management of headache. *Neurol Clin* 1997;15:187-98.
36. Lipton RB, Stewart WF, Goadsby PJ. Headache-related disability in the management of migraine. *Neurology* 2001;56:S1-3.
37. Edmeads J, Findlay H, Tugwell P et al. Impact of migraine and tension-type headache on life-style, consulting behaviour, and medication use: a Canadian population survey. *Can J Neurol Sci* 1993;20:131-7.
38. Lipton RB, Stewart WF. Acute migraine therapy: do doctors understand what patients with migraine want from therapy? *Headache* 1999;39:S20-266.
39. Gawel MJ, Worthington I, Maggisano A. A systematic review of the use of triptans in acute migraine. *Can J Neurol Sci* 2001;28:30-41.
40. Ferrari MD, Roon KI, Lipton RB et al. Oral triptans (serotonin 5-HT(1B/1D) agonists) in acute migraine treatment: a meta-analysis of 53 trials. *Lancet* 2001;358:1668-75.
41. Worthington I. Delivery systems for acute migraine medications. *Can Fam Physician* 2001;47:322-9.
42. Brandes JL, Kudrow D, Stark SR et al. Sumatriptan-naproxen for acute treatment of migraine: a randomized trial. *JAMA* 2007;297:1443-54.
43. Smith TR, Sunshine A, Stark SR et al. Sumatriptan and naproxen sodium for the acute treatment of migraine. *Headache* 2005;45:983-91.
44. Saper JR, Silberstein S. Pharmacology of dihydroergotamine and evidence for efficacy and safety in migraine. *Headache* 2006;46:S171-81.
45. Tfelt-Hansen P, Saxena PR, Dahlof C et al. Ergotamine in the acute treatment of migraine: a review and European consensus. *Brain* 2000;123:9-18.
46. Bigal ME, Lipton RB. Excessive acute migraine medication use and migraine progression. *Neurology* 2008;71:1821-8.
47. Saper JR, Da Silva AN. Medication overuse headache: history, features, prevention and management strategies. *CNS Drugs* 2013;27:867-77.
48. Turner CJ, Pryse-Phillips W. Pilot study to improve health outcomes for medication-induced headache sufferers. *Can J Clin Pharmacol* 1999;6:113-7.
49. Tepper SJ, Tepper DE. Breaking the cycle of medication overuse headache. *Cleve Clin J Med* 2010;77:236-42.
50. Dodick D. Freitag F. Evidence-based understanding of medication-overuse headache: clinical implications. *Headache* 2006;46:S202-11.
51. Grazzi L, Andrasik F. Medication-overuse headache: description, treatment, and relapse prevention. *Curr Pain Headache Rep* 2006;10:71-7.
52. Becker WJ, Findlay T Moga C et al. Guideline for primary care management of headache in adults. *Can Fam Physician* 2015;61:670-9.
53. Medicines and Healthcare Products Regulatory Agency. *Consumers are advised not to take unlicensed Butterbur (Petasites hybridus) herbal remedies*. London: MHRA; 2012. Available from: webarchive.nationalarchives.gov.uk/20141205150130/http://www.mhra.gov.uk/Safetyinformation/Generalsafetyinformationandadvice/Herbalmedicines/Herbalsafetyupdates/Allherbalsafetyupdates/CON140849.
54. Lipton RB, Gobel H, Einhaupl KM et al. Petasites hybridus root (butterbur) is an effective preventive treatment for migraine. *Neurology* 2004;63:2240-4.
55. D'Andrea G, Cevoli S, Cologno D. Herbal therapy in migraine. *Neurol Sci* 2014;35:135-40.
56. Sandor PS, Di Clemente MD, Coppola G et al. Efficacy of coenzyme Q10 in migraine prophylaxis: a randomized controlled trial *Neurology* 2005;64:713-5.
57. Mauskop A, Altura BM. Magnesium for migraine: rationale for use and therapeutic potential. *CNS Drugs* 1998;9:185-90.
58. Peikert A, Wilimzig C, Kohne-Volland R. Prophylaxis of migraine with oral magnesium: results from a prospective, multi-centre, placebo-controlled and double-blind randomized study. *Cephalalgia* 1996;16:257-63.
59. Pfaffenrath V, Wessely P, Meyer C et al. Magnesium in the prophylaxis of migraine–a double-blind, placebo-controlled study. *Cephalalgia* 1996;16:436-40.
60. Schoenen J, Jacquy J, Lenaerts M. Effectiveness of high-dose riboflavin in migraine prophylaxis. A randomized controlled trial. *Neurology* 1998;50:466-70.
61. MacLennan SC, Wade FM, Forrest KM et al. High-dose riboflavin for migraine prophylaxis in children: a double-blind, randomized, placebo-controlled trial. *J Child Neurol* 2008;23:1300-4.

Headache—What You Need to Know

Headache is very common. Some headaches will go away after a short time without treatment, or with a nonprescription pain reliever. Other headaches (migraines) may be more severe and you may need to have treatment prescribed by a healthcare practitioner. Most headaches are not caused by serious health problems.

What should you do about headaches?

Tension-type headaches

- The most common type of headache is called a "tension-type headache". This kind of headache may be caused by many things, not only tension. You may get a tension-type headache if you have a cold or the flu.
- The pain is usually mild to moderate. It may be on both sides of the head or across the forehead. It often feels like there is tightness or pressure in your head and sometimes in the shoulders and back of the neck.
- The pain usually goes away on its own. Pain relievers such as ASA, acetaminophen, ibuprofen or naproxen sodium might help. If you have this kind of headache often (more than 15 times in 1 month), seek medical advice.

Migraine headaches

- Migraine headaches are fairly common. Migraine headaches are more common in women than in men. Migraines tend to run in families. Both children and adults can get migraines.
- Migraine headaches usually occur on 1 side of the head. Some people, especially children, feel pain on both sides of the head.
- The pain is usually moderate to severe and throbbing. Physical activity tends to make the pain worse.
- A person may have other symptoms in addition to the pain. For example:
  - nausea or vomiting, or both
  - sensitivity to light and sound
  - a visual sensation that sometimes occurs just before the headache. This is called an aura and may appear as flashes or bursts of light, zig-zag lines, dark spots surrounded by light.

What triggers migraine headaches?

Many things can trigger a migraine headache. Triggers are different for each person. Keep a diary about your headaches to help you figure out what causes them. Some common triggers are:

- Food (such as aged cheeses, cured meats, chocolate, red wine)
- Caffeine (from coffee, tea, some carbonated or energy drinks, etc.—having too much or suddenly reducing the amount you normally have)
- Hormones (in women—at the time of your monthly menstrual period or during menopause)
- Chemicals (such as MSG in foods)
- Environment (changes in weather, bright lights, loud noises, strong odours, cigarette smoke)
- Other factors (such as anxiety/stress, too much or too little sleep, not eating regularly)

How can you treat a migraine?

Prevention

- Avoid foods and other things that may trigger a migraine.
- Some people find that biofeedback, relaxation, acupuncture and cognitive behavioural therapy help to prevent migraine headaches.

Mild Migraine Headaches

- Many patients get relief by lying down in a dark, quiet room and applying a cold cloth or ice pack to the head. Falling asleep often provides relief as well.
- Pain relievers such as ASA, acetaminophen, ibuprofen or naproxen sodium might help.
- It is important not to use pain relievers more than 15 days per month, or products containing codeine or caffeine more than 10 days per month. If you use them more often, you may begin to get more frequent or daily headaches called "medication-overuse headache".
- Seek medical advice if you have headaches every day or almost every day. You may be asked to stop taking pain relievers for a while. If your headaches are severe, you will usually be prescribed other medication.

Moderate or Severe Migraine Headache

- Seek medical advice. You may need a prescription medication.
- It is important not to use migraine therapy such as triptans and ergot medication more than 10 days per month.
- You may need medication to treat nausea. Dimenhydrinate (Gravol) may help to reduce nausea. You may also need prescription medication such as domperidone or metoclopramide to treat nausea or vomiting.
- Go to an emergency room if you have a very severe headache and/or severe vomiting that starts suddenly. Consider going to an urgent care facility if your migraine isn't relieved by medication.
- You may be prescribed medication that you take every day to prevent migraines that happen often, that are severe, or that last a long time.
- Certain vitamins or herbal remedies may help to prevent migraines. Talk to a healthcare practitioner before taking any medication to prevent migraines.

Other Headaches

There are many other less common types of headache. Seek medical advice to find out what is causing your headache. Many people who think they have "sinus" headaches are actually suffering from migraine or another type of headache. Sinus headaches only occur if a sinus infection is present.

Severe, New or Unusual Headaches

Some headaches may be the first sign of a more serious health problem. **Go to the emergency room or an urgent care facility if:**

- You suddenly have a severe headache that is worse than any you have had before.
- You have symptoms such as fever, stiff neck, drowsiness, confusion, seizures or a general feeling of weakness, as well as a headache.

Seek medical advice as soon as possible if:

- You experience a new or unusual type of headache.

- There is a change in your usual headache pattern—for example, headaches that happen more often or become severe.
- You start to have headaches in middle age or later (age 40 or over).

For more information on migraine headaches, visit these websites:

Canadian Headache Society. Available from: www.migrainecanada.org

Headache Network Canada. Available from: www.headachenetwork.ca.

American Headache Society. Available from: www.achenet.org.

Chapter 9
Heat-related Disorders

Dorothy Tscheng, BScPhm, CGP

Heat-related illnesses and mortality are preventable.[1] There is a wide spectrum of heat-related disorders, ranging from mild heat edema or heat rash to potentially fatal heat stroke. With timely treatment, the mortality rate for heat stroke is around 10%, but when treatment is delayed, death can occur in up to 80% of cases.[2] The incidence of these disorders increases with higher temperature and humidity, e.g., during an extended heat wave. A study of hospital admissions during heat waves found that older adults had a 2.5-fold increase in risk of being hospitalized for heat stroke compared with non-heat wave periods.[3] Deaths due to heat-related disorders are under-reported as cardiovascular and respiratory illnesses also increase during heat waves and may not be attributed directly to the heat.[4] Because increases in atmospheric greenhouse gas levels are leading to more frequent and intense heat events, the incidence of heat stress disorders is likely to increase.[5] Healthcare practitioners need to be aware of the consequences of these environmental conditions and to actively promote preventive measures.

Pathophysiology

The body's thermoregulatory centre (the hypothalamus) is responsible for the maintenance of core body temperature (approximately 37°C).[2,6] The body acquires heat through different sources or processes including shivering, thyrotoxicosis, physical activity and high ambient temperatures. Heat illness results from an imbalance of heat generated within and absorbed by the body and its ability to dissipate excessive heat.[1,2,6] Because heat dissipation occurs primarily through the skin, preventing or correcting a heat imbalance requires normal skin condition as well as sufficient cardiac output and blood volume to maintain adequate blood flow to the skin.[2,7]

The body eliminates heat by 4 different mechanisms:[2,6]

- Evaporation of moisture from the skin or respiratory tract results in loss of heat. In low humidity conditions, evaporation is an effective mechanism of heat dissipation. This mechanism becomes more important at higher ambient temperatures when evaporation of perspiration is key
- Radiation is the transfer of heat through electromagnetic waves. It accounts for about 65% of heat loss when ambient temperature is lower than body temperature. At higher ambient temperatures, heat gain can result
- Conduction is the transfer of heat through physical contact with a cooler object. At higher temperatures, conduction is the least effective of the 4 mechanisms
- Convection is the transfer of heat to the air and vapour. Both air flow and vasodilation contribute to heat loss by convection.

A reduction in the efficacy of any of the above mechanisms can increase the risk of developing a heat-related illness. As ambient temperature and humidity increase, heat dissipation becomes less efficient. If not treated in time, excessive body temperature initiates a series of processes that leads to the collapse of the cardiovascular system, multiorgan failure and potentially death.[2]

There are 2 types of heat stroke: classic and exertional. Hallmark symptoms for both include an elevated body temperature of over 40°C (measured rectally as this is the most reliable method to determine body temperature compared with oral or tympanic methods) and changes in mental status.

Older individuals with predisposing health risks who are exposed to poor environmental conditions usually present with classic heat stroke. These patients differ from exertional heat stroke sufferers in that they typically present with hot, dry skin and the increase in core body temperature is relatively less pronounced.[1,2] This type of heat stroke can develop over several days.[1]

Exertional heat stroke, as its name depicts, usually occurs in younger, healthy individuals who have participated in strenuous physical activity. Competitive athletes and military personnel are population groups that typically develop this form of heat stroke, distinguished by the presence of sweat and a more marked increase in core body temperature.[1,2] Symptoms can occur rapidly, often within a few hours of the activity.[1]

Risk Factors

Several population groups are at risk of developing heat-related disorders:[1,2,7,8]

- Infants and young children
- Older adults
- Outdoor labourers (e.g., firefighters, military personnel)
- Competitive athletes
- Individuals in poor socioeconomic situations

Table 1 outlines risk factors for development of heat-related illness.[1,2,3,5,9,10,11,12]

Children are thought to be at increased risk of heat-related illnesses due to physiologic and anatomical differences (e.g., reduced sweating due to a greater surface area to body mass ratio, immature thermoregulatory system) and a reduced thirst response to dehydration as compared with healthy adults.[2,7,8] However, some recent information suggests that these differences are not as significant, especially in older children. Infants and preschool children are still considered an at-risk group partly due to the dependence of young children on others to ensure they stay hydrated and are removed from risky environments.[7] Regardless of the reason, caregivers need to be mindful of the potential risks when exposing this population to hot and humid environments.

Older adults are predisposed to heat illnesses because of comorbid illnesses (including cardiovascular limitations), multiple medications and poor thermoregulatory response.[2,3,8] Social and behavioural factors such as home containment (not leaving the home on a daily basis), social isolation, bed confinement and an inability to provide self-care put this population at particular risk, especially in more dependent older adults.[3,8,9]

In addition to heat-related disorders, cardiovascular and respiratory deterioration have long been identified as consequences of heat waves. An association has been found between heat exposure and higher hospital admission rates in older adults for fluid-related disorders, renal failure, urinary tract infections and septicemia.[3] The risk of these additional health consequences increased as the period and intensity of the heat wave increased and remained elevated for up to 5 days after the heat wave.

Medication-related Causes

Medications listed in Table 2 can predispose patients to heat-related disorders through various mechanisms that include:[1,6,7,9,10,13,14,15]

- Inhibition of sweat excretion (anticholinergic effects and hypovolemic causes)
- Vasoconstriction of cutaneous vessels
- Disruption of hypothalamic thermoregulation
- Increase in heat production
- Increased fluid loss through diarrhea or vomiting leading to dehydration

Table 1: Common Risk Factors for Developing Heat-related Illnesses

Demographic/Medical Factors	Behavioural/Environmental Factors
Age (young children, elderly) Alcoholism Bed confinement Cardiovascular disorders Dehydration Dermatologic diseases such as scleroderma, miliaria Fever Homelessness Hyperthyroidism Lower socioeconomic environment Obesity Peripheral vascular disease Psychiatric disorders Pulmonary disorders Use of medications listed in Table 2	Lack of acclimatization Lack of air conditioning or ventilation Lack of breaks during exercise Living in urban areas with greater number of paved surfaces and buildings Poor physical condition Social isolation Strenuous activity in hot, humid conditions Unable to perform self-care Use of heavy clothing or equipment

Table 2: Medications that can Predispose to Heat-related Illnesses

Mechanism	Drug/Class[a]
Disruption of hypothalamic regulation	antipsychotics amphetamines (including MDMA/"ecstasy")
Increased heat production	excessive thyroid medication sympathomimetics
Reduction of sweat excretion (either by direct effects on the skin/sweat glands or through reduced blood flow to the skin)	alcohol anticholinergics antihistamines antiparkinsonian (anticholinergic) agents antipsychotics (anticholinergic) belladonna alkaloids beta-blockers calcium channel blockers cholinesterase inhibitors creatine[b] diuretics laxatives lithium topiramate tricyclic antidepressants
Vasoconstriction of cutaneous vessels	alpha-agonists monoamine oxidase inhibitors sympathomimetics (including ephedrine, cocaine, amphetamines, diet products containing ma huang)

[a] In addition, any medication or substance (e.g., tranquilizers, cocaine) that can alter a person's behaviour, including the perception of their environment or need for proper hydration, may increase the risk of heat-related illnesses in the right conditions.[10]

[b] Evidence has been contradictory; however, use of creatine ≤28 days or when exercising ≤60 min does not appear to influence hydration status or temperature regulation.[16] It is not clear whether creatine use >28 days or with exercise >60 min affects thermoregulation.

Goals of Therapy

Prevention of any heat-related disorder is the foremost goal. However, once an individual has experienced symptoms, the goals of therapy are:

- Reduce mortality
- Prevent long-term consequences
- Normalize body temperature
- Reduce and eliminate symptoms

Patient Assessment

Information about the assessment of patients with a suspected heat-related disorder can also be found in Figure 1.[1,2,17]

Symptoms of various heat-related problems present differently depending on the degree or stage of the illness. Patients' complaints range from edema in the feet to more serious concerns of confusion or coma. The spectrum of disorders is described (from mildest to most severe) in Table 3.[1,2,13,18,19,20]

If any acute neurologic symptoms (altered mental status, confusion or hallucinations, seizures) are present, the person must be taken to the hospital immediately, preferably in an air-conditioned vehicle, to be assessed and treated. In addition to heat stroke, differential diagnosis includes meningitis, neuroleptic malignant syndrome, hyperthyroidism, encephalopathy, tetanus, delirium and overdose of various substances including cocaine and salicylates.[2]

Other hyperthermia syndromes include neuroleptic malignant syndrome (NMS) and malignant hyperthermia (MH); however, the underlying causes are drug related rather than heat related. Both NMS and MH present with hyperthermia and muscle rigidity but have different etiologies; NMS is induced by antipsychotics and MH by inhaled anesthetics or succinylcholine (post-surgery) in susceptible individuals.

For further discussion of management of NMS and MH, consult the *Compendium of Therapeutic Choices:* Thermoregulatory Disorders in Adults.

Prevention

Prevention of heat-related illnesses is the primary goal. The first step in prevention is the identification of individuals at risk and keeping a careful watch over them during heat waves. Healthcare practitioners can offer proactive education and tips for these population groups, and when possible could check on identified at-risk patients during heat waves.[8]

If possible, remove these individuals to an air-conditioned location and encourage them to participate in social activities. Both have been shown to lower the risk of heat-related deaths during heat waves. Fluid intake should be increased, without waiting for the appearance of thirst.[21] Other potentially helpful measures include taking extra showers or baths.[11]

Environment Canada's Humidex tables help predict environmental situations where the risk of heat stroke is increased and vigilant monitoring of at-risk individuals is indicated. The Humidex tables can be found at www.ec.gc.ca/meteo-weather/.

Health Canada has a toolkit intended for use by public health and emergency management officials to warn Canadian residents about impending heat events. Healthcare practitioners may find many aspects of the toolkit useful in developing a communication plan for their own patients and reinforcing the public health message. The toolkit can be found at www.hc-sc.gc.ca/ewh-semt/pubs/climat/heat-chaleur/index-eng.php.

Table 3: **Spectrum of Heat-related Disorders: Symptoms and Therapy**

Type of Illness	Features/Symptoms	Therapy
Heat rash	"Prickly heat" that appears as a group of small blisters or rash Due to irritation from excessive sweating Usually located on the neck, upper chest, under the breasts, in the groin area or in elbow creases	Retreat to a cooler and less humid environment Keep the area dry
Heat edema	Edema in the extremities from transient vasodilation of vessels, sodium and water retention and with prolonged standing More frequent during the summer months	Elevate feet or hands No specific treatment Prevention with acclimatization
Heat cramps	Thought to be due to water and sodium depletion Cramps in muscles of the arms, legs and stomach are most common Warning sign of heat exhaustion Common in athletes	Stop activity and rest in a cool, shaded area Rehydrate with an oral rehydration solution containing glucose and sodium (see Chapter 42: Sports Nutrition, Table 3) Lightly stretch or massage affected muscles Avoid heavy activity for a few hours See healthcare practitioner if no improvement in 1 h or if symptoms worsen
Heat syncope	Dizziness Fainting episode	Stop activity and rest in a cool, shaded area Patients often recover quickly after falling to the ground (secondary to fainting) Slowly get up from a sitting or laying position
Heat exhaustion	Weakness Nausea and/or vomiting Tachycardia, hypotension Fatigue Dizziness Headache Slightly elevated core body temperature (up to 40°C) Fainting Reversible, but can lead to heat stroke if untreated	Stop activity and rest in a cool, shaded area Rehydrate with oral rehydration solution Recovery is usually quick, within 2–3 h
Heat stroke	**Medical emergency**—can result in death Similar to heat exhaustion with the added feature, in most cases, of neurologic symptoms such as: – altered mental status – hallucinations – seizures – confusion – coma – ataxia Other symptoms include hot, dry skin Core body temperature above 40°C Leads to hepatic and renal failure, CNS injury, coagulopathy and cardiovascular collapse	**Call 911**—take patient to **emergency room** as soon as possible In the interim: – stop activity immediately and rest in an air-conditioned environment (or if not possible, a cool, shaded area) – remove excessive clothing – rehydrate – ensure good air circulation around patient – cool the body (on the way to the hospital) with ice water towels or packs to the groin, neck, axillae and head

If outdoor activities cannot be avoided during periods of high temperature and humidity, the following strategies are recommended to help reduce the risk of heat-related disorders:

- Ensure proper hydration before the activity and drink cool fluids (approximately 500 mL to 1 L) during each hour of heavy exercise.[18,19] Oral rehydration solutions or sport drinks are useful as they contain sodium and glucose that are lost during exercise. Thirst should not be relied upon as a reminder to drink.[2] It is important to remind people of salt and sugar content and to avoid use of sports drinks in those patients with diabetes, hypertension, heart failure, renal failure or fluid restrictions
- Stay out of the sun if possible. Take 10- to 20-minute breaks per hour of activity, either in the shade or in an air-conditioned environment[19,22]
- Avoid strenuous outdoor activities during peak sun hours (10 a.m. to 3 p.m.)
- Wear light-coloured, lightweight clothing, including a wide-brimmed hat[18]
- Acclimatize to the environment. Gradual exposure to ambient conditions can prevent heat-related illnesses. The average adult should start at about 50% of expected activity in the environment, increasing gradually to 80% over the next few days. However, the recommendation for inexperienced workers is to start at 20% of expected activity and increase it by 20% daily. Up to 10–14 days of exposure is required for full acclimatization in a hot environment.[6,20,22] There is no consensus on how to acclimatize children.[22]

Figure 2 provides a step-wise approach to aiding patients in the prevention of heat-related disorders.

Nonpharmacologic Therapy

It is imperative to address heat stroke immediately as delaying treatment results in poorer patient outcomes.[2] After seeking medical attention, the first priority is to move the patient to a shaded or preferably air-conditioned environment and to cool the patient using external methods such as cool compresses applied to the groin, neck, axillae and head. Increase air flow around the patient and promote evaporation by removal of unnecessary clothing, use of fans and misting with moderate temperature water.[1,2] Cold water immersion has been shown to reduce morbidity and mortality in exertional heat stroke.[1] However, in the elderly and those with comorbidities and in situations where cold water immersion is not available, other cooling methods as described above should be used. Internal cooling methods, such as cold water irrigation to the stomach or rectum, are used in hospital as necessary.[1]

Other types of heat-related illnesses are not considered emergent and can be addressed appropriately depending on severity. Table 3 outlines treatment options for various heat-related disorders.

Pharmacologic Therapy

Medications, such as antipyretics, do not help reduce the body's internal temperature and should not be used. Although not the mainstay of therapy, medications can be helpful in treating some of the complications of heat stroke. **Benzodiazepines** such as diazepam are used to treat seizures and control shivering. **Barbiturates** have also been used for seizures, if benzodiazepines are not effective. **Mannitol** is used to promote osmotic diuresis and prevent or treat renal failure in patients with rhabdomyolysis.[2] **Dantrolene** is a muscle relaxant that has been evaluated for the treatment of heat stroke, but has not proven to be effective. **Dobutamine** is the drug of choice for circulatory support.[2,23]

Monitoring of Therapy

Monitoring by friends and family of individuals at risk of developing heat-related disorders is a critical preventive strategy. Healthcare practitioners can play an important role by ensuring patients and caregivers are able to recognize symptoms that require intervention or medical attention.

For those involved in outdoor activities, proper hydration (see Prevention) is important as thirst is an unreliable sign of body fluid loss. Aim for maintaining light yellow urine.

The extent of recommended monitoring of patients who have suffered a heat-related illness depends on the severity of the illness. Patients with heat exhaustion should avoid further heat exposure for 24–48 hours after even a mild injury.[1,20] Heat stroke patients require more intensive monitoring after hospital discharge to manage potential complications, such as chronic renal failure and other organ damage.

Figure 1: **Assessment of Patients with Heat-related Disorders**

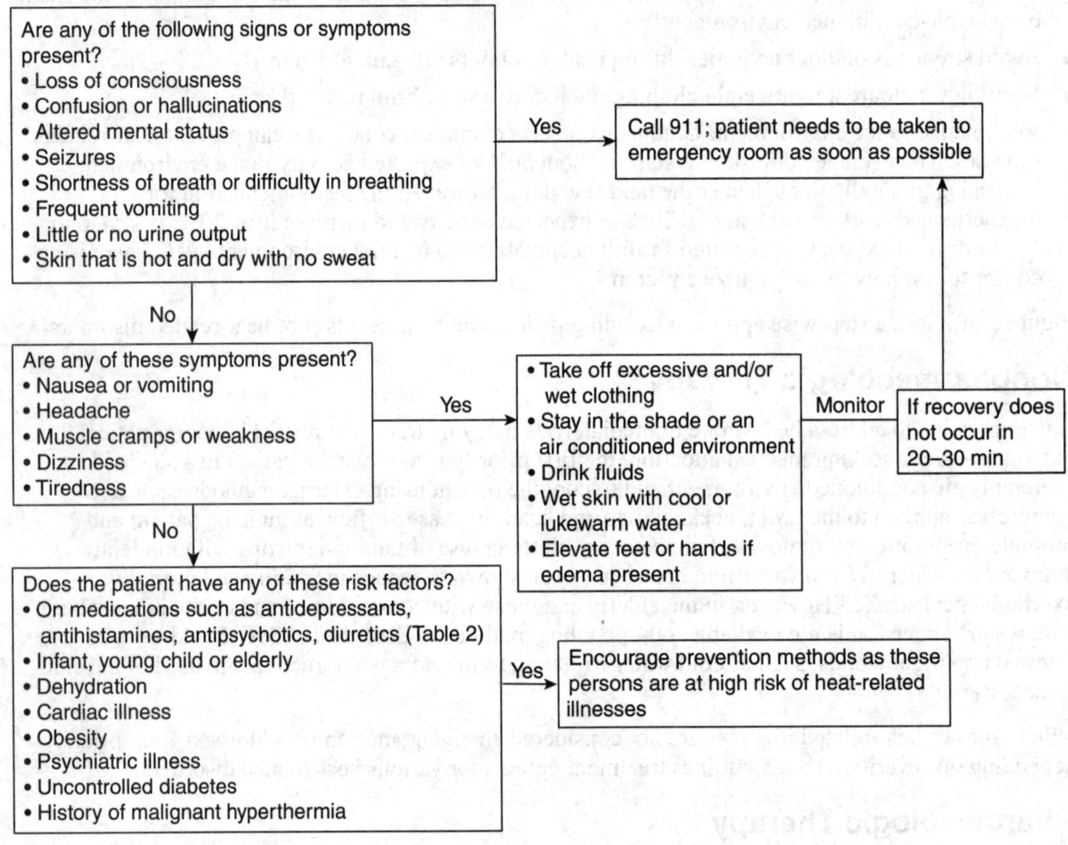

Figure 2: **Approach to Implementing Preventive Strategies for Heat-related Disorders**

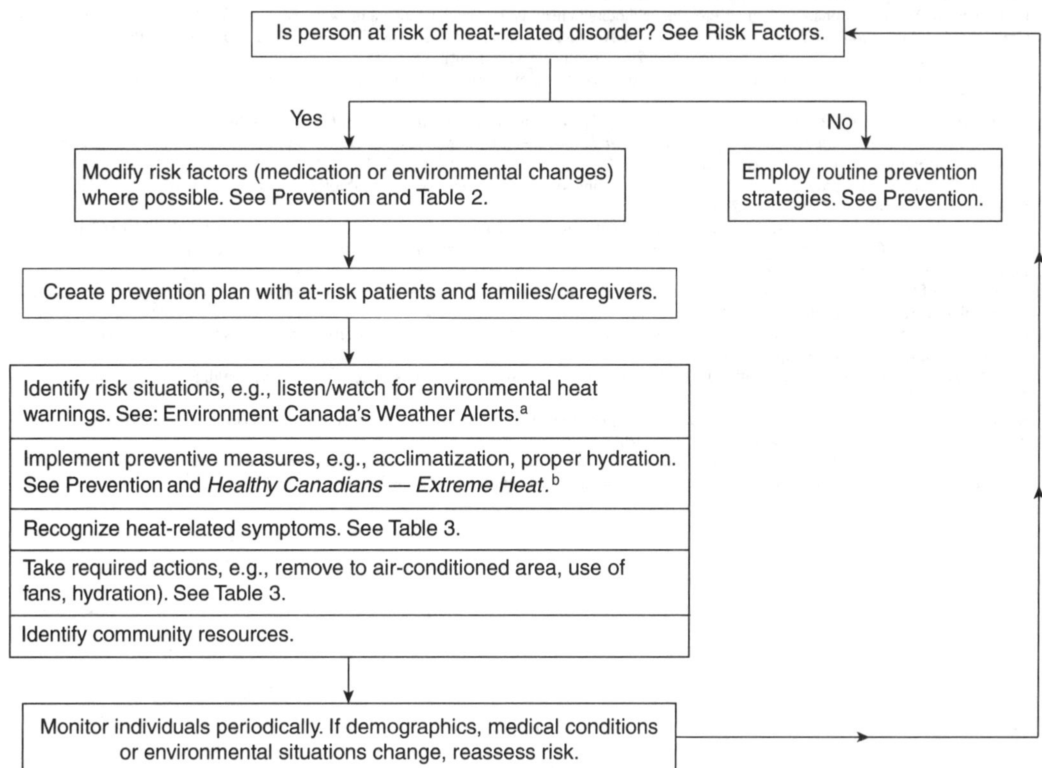

[a] See Environment Canada's Weather Alerts, available at www.weather.gc.ca/mainmenu/alert_menu_e.html

[b] See Healthy Canadians: Extreme heat – heat waves, available at www.healthycanadians.gc.ca/healthy-living-vie-saine/environment-environnement/sun-soleil/heat-extreme-chaleur-eng.php

Suggested Readings

Becker JA, Stewart LK. Heat-related illness. *Am Fam Physician* 2011;83:1325-30.

Health Canada. *Acute care during extreme heat. Recommendations and information for health care workers*. Available from: http://www.hc-sc.gc.ca/ewh-semt/pubs/climat/actue_care-soins_actifs/index-eng.php.

Kenny GP, Yardley J, Brown C et al. Heat stress in older individuals and patients with common chronic diseases. *CMAJ* 2010;182:1053-60.

Tscheng D. Heat-stroke and medications. *Can Pharm J* 2000;133:30-2.

References

1. Becker JA, Stewart LK. Heat-related illness. *Am Fam Physician* 2011;83:1325-30.
2. Medscape by WebMD. Helman RS, Habal R. *Heatstroke*. Updated May 1, 2015. Available from: emedicine.medscape.com. Accessed June 2, 2015. Registration required.
3. Bobb JF, Obermeyer Z, Wang Y et al. Cause-specific risk of hospital admission related to extreme heat in older adults. *JAMA* 2014;312:2659-67.
4. Patz JA, Frumkin H, Holloway T et al. Climate change: challenges and opportunities for global health. *JAMA* 2014;312:1565-80.
5. Public Health Agency of Canada. *Climate change and public health factsheets*. Modified August 11, 2015. Available from: phac-aspc.gc.ca/hp-ps/eph-esp/fs-fi-a-eng.php. Accessed 10 March 2016.
6. Moreau TP, Deeter M. Heatstroke–predictable, preventable, treatable. *JAAPA* 2005;18:30-5.
7. Xu Z, Etzel RA, Su H et al. Impact of ambient temperature on children's health: a systematic review. *Environ Res* 2012;117:120-31.
8. Groot E, Abelsohn A, Moore K. Practical strategies for prevention and treatment of heat-induced illnesses. *Can Fam Physician* 2014;60:729-30.

9. Tscheng D. Heat-stroke and medications. *Can Pharm J* 2000;133:30-2.
10. Martinez M, Devenport L, Saussy J et al. Drug-associated heat stroke. *South Med J* 2002;95:799-802.
11. Bouchama A, Dehbi M, Mohamed G et al. Prognostic factors in heat wave related deaths: a meta-analysis. *Arch Intern Med* 2007;167:2170-6.
12. Crowley RA; Health and Public Policy Committee of the American College of Physicians. Climate Change and Health: A Position Paper of the American College of Physicians. *Ann Intern Med* 2016. [Epub ahead of print].
13. Bailes JE, Cantu RC, Day AL. The neurosurgeon in sport: awareness of the risks of heatstroke and dietary supplements. *Neurosurgery* 2002;51:283-6.
14. de Carolis P, Magnifico F, Pierangeli G et al. Transient hypohidrosis induced by topiramate. *Epilepsia* 2003;44:974-6.
15. Health Canada. *Acute care during extreme heat. Recommendations and information for health care workers*. Available from: http://www.hc-sc.gc.ca/ewh-semt/pubs/climat/actue_care-soins_actifs/index-eng.php. Accessed April 22, 2016.
16. Lopez RM, Casa DJ, McDermott BP et al. Does creatine supplementation hinder exercise heat tolerance or hydration status? A systematic review with meta-analyses. *J Athl Train* 2009;44:215-23.
17. Kenny GP, Yardley J, Brown C et al. Heat stress in older individuals and patients with common chronic diseases. *CMAJ* 2010;182:1053-60.
18. Centers for Disease Control and Prevention. *Frequently asked questions (FAQ) about extreme heat*. Available from: emergency.cdc.gov/disasters/extremeheat/faq.asp. Accessed April 22, 2016.
19. Government of Canada. *Extreme heat—heat waves*. Available from: www.healthycanadians.gc.ca/health-sante/environment-environnement/sun-soleil/heat-extreme-chaleur-eng.php. Accessed April 22, 2016.
20. American College of Sports Medicine, Armstrong LE, Casa DJ et al. American College of Sports Medicine position stand. Exertional heat illness during training and competition. *Med Sci Sports Exerc* 2007;39:556-72.
21. Hajat S, O'Connor M, Kosatsky T. Health effects of hot weather: from awareness of risk factors to effective health protection. *Lancet* 2010;375:856-63.
22. Larsen T, Kumar S, Grimmer K et al. A systematic review of guidelines for the prevention of heat illness in community-based sports participants and officials. *J Sci Med Sport* 2007;10:11-26.
23. McNamara R, Ryan D, McCarthy G. Towards evidence based emergency medicine: best BETs from the Manchester Royal Infirmary. Bet 4: in patients with classic heat stroke does adding treatment with dantrolene improve outcome? *Emerg Med J* 2008;25:441-2.

Heat-related Illness—What You Need to Know

What is a heat-related illness?

- Your body has ways to keep itself cool when the weather is hot or if you are exercising. When your body has difficulty keeping cool, you may develop a heat-related illness such as heat cramps or something more serious such as heat stroke.
- Awareness is the key to preventing heat-related illness before it happens.

What are the warning signs of a heat-related illness?

The different forms of heat-related illnesses present differently. The 2 most important illnesses to be aware of are heat exhaustion and heat stroke. Heat exhaustion can lead to heat stroke if not treated and **heat stroke is a medical emergency**.

The symptoms for heat exhaustion include (but are not limited to):

- Headache
- Nausea, vomiting or both
- Muscle weakness or cramps
- Dizziness
- Sweating

The symptoms for heat stroke include (but are not limited to):

- Red, hot dry skin (for classic heat stroke)
- High core body temperature (greater than 40°C)
- Nausea
- Confusion
- Unconsciousness

What are some factors that increase the risk of heat-related illness?

- Age (young children, elderly)
- Certain chronic diseases (e.g., alcoholism, heart, kidney, lung, psychiatric or thyroid disease, obesity)
- Dehydration
- Medications (e.g., antidepressants, antihistamines, antipsychotics, diuretics, drugs for overactive bladder or Parkinson's disease)—talk to your pharmacist about your own medications
- Activity in hot, humid conditions
- Lack of breaks during exercise
- Lack of air-conditioning or ventilation
- Living in cities and surrounding suburbs where there is a lot of concrete and pavement.

How can you prevent heat-related illness?

- If possible, avoid heavy outdoor activities when the sun is hottest (between 10 a.m. and 3 p.m.).
- Try to stay in the shade. If you have to stay in direct sun, wear loose-fitting, light-coloured clothing.
- Take several breaks from your activity.

- Drink plenty of fluids before, during and after any outdoor activity. Limit the amount of coffee, tea, cola and alcoholic beverages you drink.

What should you do if you do not feel well?

- Rest in the shade or in an air-conditioned building if possible.
- Take off as much clothing as possible.
- Drink water or oral rehydration fluids.
- Wet yourself with cool water.
- Get medical attention or call 911 if you are not urinating (peeing) or sweating, if you vomit several times, or if you start to feel confused.

What should you do if you are at risk of a heat-related illness?

- Let your family and friends know what symptoms to watch for. They can help you in case you develop symptoms and can make sure you get the help you need.
- Wear a Medic-Alert identification bracelet or something similar.

Chapter 10
Tinnitus

Yvonne M. Shevchuk, BSP, PharmD, FCSHP

Pathophysiology

Although tinnitus can occur at any age, it is less common in children and most common in the elderly. Hearing loss is the most important risk factor for development of tinnitus.[1] Objective tinnitus is caused by a sound produced within the head due to either vascular (e.g., arteriovenous malformations, carotid stenosis, valvular heart disease, states of high cardiac output and other conditions causing turbulent blood flow), mechanical (e.g., palatal myoclonus, patulous eustachian tube) or spontaneous (spontaneous otoacoustic emissions) causes.[2] Subjective tinnitus, which is more common, is the perception of sound or noise without any external stimulation. Causes include otologic (e.g., noise-induced hearing loss, presbycusis, impacted cerumen, Meniere's disease), neurologic (e.g., head injury, multiple sclerosis), infectious (e.g., otitis media, sequelae of meningitis), drug-related (e.g., adverse effect of loop diuretics, salicylates, aminoglycosides) and other (e.g., temporomandibular-joint dysfunction) factors.[2]

Tinnitus can be described as buzzing, hissing, cricket-like sounds, ringing, whistling, humming or a combination of these.[2,3] It can also occur as continuous, intermittent or pulsatile tinnitus.[3] Tinnitus can have a major impact on the quality of a patient's life with symptoms such as frustration, annoyance, insomnia, anxiety, depression, irritation and difficulty concentrating, in addition to the "ringing in the ears".[3]

The pathophysiology is incompletely understood; however, central mechanisms are involved. A distributed tinnitus brain network, including sensory auditory areas and cortical regions involved in perceptual, emotional mnemonic, attentional and salience functions, has been hypothesized.[3]

Goals of Therapy

- Treat the underlying medical condition if possible
- Correct hearing loss if correctable
- Reduce or eliminate tinnitus, although this is not usually possible
- Improve the patient's quality of life

Patient Assessment

Assess potential drug-related causes of tinnitus and address any potential drug causes.[4,5] Review the patient's drug history, both current and past, for potentially ototoxic drugs (see Table 1 and Chapter 17: Assessment of Patients with Hearing Loss, Ear Pain and Ear Drainage, Table 2). Reassess the need for any ototoxic drug found; removal of the offending agent may resolve tinnitus.[2] All patients with tinnitus lasting >24 hours should be assessed by an appropriate healthcare practitioner. The severity of tinnitus and the impact on quality of life should be assessed. The Tinnitus Handicap Inventory (THI) and the Tinnitus Reaction Questionnaire (TRQ) are two commonly used instruments. See Resource Tips for patient resources.

Table 1: **Drugs Reported to Cause Tinnitus**[a,4,5]

almotriptan	doxycycline	nortriptyline
amiloride/hydrochlorothiazide	eletriptan	NSAIDs
aminoglycosides	enalapril	quinine
amitriptyline	frovatriptan	risedronate
ASA	gabapentin	sulfamethoxazole/trimethoprim
atorvastatin	galantamine	sulfasalazine
buprenorphine	imipramine	timolol
bupropion	irbesartan	trazodone
chlorpheniramine	linezolid	trimipramine
ciprofloxacin	loop diuretics	valsartan
citalopram	mefloquine	varenicline
clomipramine	norfloxacin	venlafaxine

[a] List is not comprehensive. See Suggested Readings.

Nonpharmacologic Therapy

- Avoid loud noises. Use noise protectors if loud noise cannot be avoided.
- Avoid caffeinated beverages and stimulants and stop smoking (significant reduction in tinnitus may be noted with caffeine and nicotine avoidance).
- Use masking techniques or devices (an external noise is used to cover the tinnitus).[2]
- Use hearing aids and cochlear implants in patients with hearing loss.[2]
- Try stress management and biofeedback.
- Try tinnitus retraining therapy (multidisciplinary program to habituate patients to the sounds of tinnitus) combined with cognitive behavior therapy.[2,6]
- Acupuncture has not been shown to be of benefit.[2]

Pharmacologic Therapy

Many drugs have been studied in the management of tinnitus, including alprazolam, baclofen, gabapentin, SSRIs, tricyclic antidepressants, zinc and others, and none have been shown to be effective.[7,8,9] **Ginkgo biloba** has been studied in the management of tinnitus and is commonly used;[10,11] however, evidence of efficacy is lacking.[12,13] Adverse effects of ginkgo biloba include mild GI complaints, headache, dizziness, palpitations and allergic skin reactions. It is also associated with bleeding and seizures. The risk of bleeding may increase when ginkgo biloba is combined with warfarin or antiplatelet drugs. Advise patients to avoid this combination.

A number of other **natural health products** (e.g., bupleurum, feverfew, cordyceps, glossy privet, goldenseal, ground ivy, lycium, melatonin, poria mushroom), **vitamin A** and **zinc** are also purported to be useful for tinnitus, but no evidence is available to confirm or refute any potential benefit.[12]

For treatment of tinnitus and other aspects of Meniere's disease, see Chapter 11: Vertigo and Dizziness.

Monitoring of Therapy

Most trials indicate that drugs will have little benefit. If a drug trial is elected despite this, determine a stopping time with the patient if there is no improvement in the tinnitus. There is no evidence to guide how long the drug should be tried; clinical trials ran from 6–14 weeks.[9,13]

Advice for the Patient

Advise patients on:

- Nonpharmacologic therapy
- Realistic expectations of drug therapy
- Possible side effects and their management

Resource Tips

American Speech-Language-Hearing Association. *Tinnitus*. Available from www.asha.org/public/hearing/Tinnitus/.

Canadian Academy of Audiology. *Tinnitus*. Available from canadianaudiology.ca/for-the-public/tinnitus.

National Institute on Deafness and Other Communication Disorders. *Tinnitus*. Available from www.nidcd.nih.gov/health/hearing/pages/tinnitus.aspx.

Suggested Readings

Cianfrone G, Pentangelo D, Cianfrone F et al. Pharmacological drugs inducing ototoxicity, vestibular symptoms and tinnitus: a reasoned and updated guide. *Eur Rev Med Pharmacol Sci* 2011;15:601-36.

Lockwood AH. Tinnitus. *Neurol Clin* 2005;23:893-900.

Seligmann H, Podoshin L, Ben-David J et al. Drug-induced tinnitus and other hearing disorders. *Drug Saf* 1996;14:198-212.

Tunkel DE, Bauer CA, Sun GH et al. Clinical practice guideline: tinnitus. *Otolaryngol Head Neck Surg* 2014;151:S1-S40.

References

1. Lockwood AH. Tinnitus. *Neurol Clin* 2005;23:893-900.
2. Lockwood AH, Salvi RJ, Burkard RF. Tinnitus. *N Engl J Med* 2002;347:904-10.
3. Langguth B, Elgoyhen A. Current pharmacological treatments for tinnitus. *Expert Opin Pharmacother* 2012;13;2495-509.
4. Cianfrone G, Pentangelo D, Cianfrone F et al. Pharmacological drugs inducing ototoxicity, vestibular symptoms and tinnitus: a reasoned and updated guide. *Eur Rev Med Pharmacol Sci* 2011;15:601-36.
5. Miell M. Can tricyclic antidepressants cause tinnitus? Available from: www.evidence.nhs.uk.
6. Cima RF, Maes IH, Joore MA et al. Specialised treatment based on cognitive behaviour therapy versus usual care for tinnitus: a randomised controlled trial. *Lancet* 2012;379:1951-9.
7. Tunkel DE, Bauer CA, Sun GH et al. Clinical practice guideline: tinnitus.*Otolaryngol Head Neck Surg* 2014;151:S1-S40.
8. Pichora-Fuller MK, Santaguida P, Hammill A et al. Evaluation and treatment of tinnitus: comparative effectiveness. *AHRQ Comparative Effectiveness Reviews* 2013. Report No.:13-EHC110-EF.
9. Baldo P, Doree C, Molin P et al. Antidepressants for patients with tinnitus. *Cochrane Database Syst Rev* 2012;9:CD003853.
10. Holgers KM, Axelsson A, Pringle I. Ginkgo biloba extract for the treatment of tinnitus. *Audiology* 1994;33:85-92.
11. Drew S, Davies E. Effectiveness of Ginkgo biloba in treating tinnitus: double blind, placebo controlled trial. *BMJ* 2001;322:73.
12. Natural Medicines Comprehensive Database. Jellin JM, ed. Stockton: Therapeutic Research Faculty. Available from: naturaldatabase.therapeuticresearch.com. Keyword search: tinnitus. Accessed February 2013. Subscription required.
13. Hilton M, Stuart E. Ginkgo biloba for tinnitus. *Cochrane Database Syst Rev* 2004;2:CD003852.

Tinnitus—What You Need to Know

What is tinnitus?

Tinnitus is the sensation of hearing an abnormal sound in the ears. It may be a ringing, clicking, buzzing, hissing or whistling sound.

What causes tinnitus?

Tinnitus may be caused by a number of things, including medications and exposure to loud noises. If you take medications, check with your pharmacist or other health care professional to see if they may be connected to the problem. Use ear protection if you must be exposed to loud noises.

When should you see a healthcare provider?

See a healthcare provider if your tinnitus lasts longer than 24 hours.

What is the treatment for tinnitus?

- You may be able to manage your tinnitus by avoiding smoking, caffeine and stimulants.
- Ask your doctor, pharmacist or audiologist for information about these methods:
  - using noise to mask tinnitus
  - using a hearing aid or cochlear implants
  - stress management or biofeedback
  - tinnitus retraining therapy
- If your healthcare provider recommends medication, be sure to ask about possible side effects.
- **Do not** take ginkgo biloba for tinnitus if you are on warfarin or drugs that affect blood clotting (such as ASA or clopidogrel).

Chapter 11
Vertigo and Dizziness

Yvonne M. Shevchuk, BSP, PharmD, FCSHP

Pathophysiology

Dizziness refers to a variety of sensations such as lightheadedness, fainting, spinning and giddiness.[1] Vertigo is one type of dizziness defined as a sensation of motion where there is none, or an exaggerated sense of motion in response to a given bodily movement.[2] It is the cardinal symptom of vestibular disease resulting from lesions or disturbances in the inner ear, eighth cranial nerve or vestibular nuclei and their pathways in the brain stem and cerebellum. Vertigo is usually accompanied by varying degrees of nausea and vomiting as well as pallor and perspiration. It may be acute, chronic or recurrent. Specific conditions that produce vertigo are listed in Table 1.

Dizziness has a number of causes unrelated to ear conditions, including cardiovascular conditions (e.g., arrhythmias, hypertension), metabolic or endocrine conditions (e.g., anemia, diabetes), psychiatric conditions, and neurologic conditions (e.g., migraine, head injury).[3]

Table 1: **Specific Conditions that Produce Vertigo**

Type	Description	Treatment[a]
Benign paroxysmal positional vertigo (BPPV)	Most common type of vertigo (20–42% of all cases).[4,5] Probable causes such as viral neuritis (see Vestibular neuritis), surgery, infection, vasculitis and trauma, identified in approximately 50% of cases.[6] Presence of debris or small crystals of calcium carbonate (canaliths) in semicircular canals.[4] Recurrent bouts of vertigo (brief) resulting from changes in head position.[6] Hearing loss and tinnitus not usually present. Symptoms may disappear in a few weeks but may recur.	Physical manipulation of the head (e.g., Epley manoeuvre)[5,7,8] much more useful than drug therapy.[4] Epley manoeuvre is a specific sequence of head position changes, performed by an appropriately trained healthcare practitioner, that moves particles into the posterior semicircular canal toward the utricle.[7] The Epley manoeuvre has been found to be more effective than several other repositioning manoeuvres.[9] Routine use of antihistamines and benzodiazepines not recommended. Vestibular suppressants (Table 3) may be used for short-term management of severe nausea and vomiting.[4,5] Vestibular rehabilitation (physical therapy program to improve balance, eye-hand coordination and habituate the patient to feelings of dizziness) may be offered as initial or adjunctive therapy.[5]
Meniere's disease	Second most common cause of vertigo of otologic origin.[4] Associated with distention of the endolymphatic compartment of the inner ear. Fluctuating hearing, roaring tinnitus, aural fullness and vertigo.[6] Vertigo has acute onset and persists from 30 min to several hours.	**Vestibular suppressants** (Table 3) with or without antiemetics to treat acute attacks.[4] **Prophylaxis** ▪ Dietary salt restriction (1–2 g/day), avoidance of caffeine and smoking.[4] ▪ **Diuretics**, e.g., hydrochlorothiazide/triamterene (avoid loop diuretics) often recommended but little evidence for benefit.[10] ▪ **Betahistine** is commonly used but has been shown to be no more effective than placebo.[11,12]

(cont'd)

Table 1: **Specific Conditions that Produce Vertigo** *(cont'd)*

Type	Description	Treatment[a]
		▪ Avoid **vestibular suppressants** for prophylaxis as they may impair vestibular compensation.[4] ▪ Conflicting results have been reported for positive pressure therapy (Meniett device).[13,14] Minor surgery is required to place ventilation tubes in the tympanic membrane.
Vestibular neuritis	Self-limiting, preceded by a nonspecific viral infection.[4,6] Due to viral infection of the vestibular portion of the eighth cranial nerve.[4] Sudden onset vertigo, nausea, ataxia and nystagmus.[4,6] Generally no hearing impairment; referred to as labyrinthitis if hearing impairment present.[4] Symptoms constant for 2–3 days.[4]	Reassurance and explanation; prognosis is excellent. Avoid movement as this exacerbates symptoms and use **vestibular suppressants** and **antiemetics** for 2–3 days after which symptoms have usually significantly decreased.[4] Use as few medications as possible and encourage as much activity as tolerated so compensation is not delayed.[4,6] **Methylprednisolone** may have a role in vestibular recovery.[15] BPPV may occur in up to 15% of patients with vestibular neuritis.
Central vertigo	Less than 5% of cases.[4] Often caused by vascular disorders, e.g., stroke, transient ischemic attack, migraine.[4]	Treat underlying cause.[4]

[a] See Table 3 for description of pharmacologic agents.

Drug-induced causes of dizziness are listed in Table 2. Ototoxic drugs may also produce vertigo (see Chapter 17: Assessment of Patients with Hearing Loss, Ear Pain and Ear Drainage, Table 2).

Goals of Therapy

- Reduce or eliminate symptoms of vertigo[4]
- Reduce or eliminate nausea and anxiety[4]
- Avoid compromising the process of vestibular compensation (allowing the brain to find a new sensory equilibrium despite the vestibular lesion) by appropriate use of medications[4]

Patient Assessment

Always seek potential drug-induced causes of vertigo and dizziness. Medication was reported to be the cause of vertigo/dizziness in 0.8% of patients under age 45 and 2.5% of patients over age 45.[18] All patients with vertigo should be assessed by an appropriate healthcare practitioner. If the vertigo is accompanied by numbness, tingling or weakness in any part of the body, visual disturbances, confusion or difficulty speaking, this is an emergency. Call 911 as the patient may be experiencing a transient ischemic attack or stroke.

Nonpharmacologic Therapy

Nonpharmacologic therapy depends on the cause of the vertigo; see Table 1.

Table 2: **Medications That May Cause Dizziness**[a,16,17]

Dizziness reported in ≥10% of patients		
carbamazepine	pergolide	sertraline
carvedilol	pregabalin	tenofovir
clomipramine	quetiapine	tramadol
emtricitabine/tenofovir	rivastigmine	tretinoin
indinavir		
Dizziness reported in 1–10% of patients		
acebutolol	infliximab	quinapril
almotriptan	leflunomide	rabeprazole
alprazolam	letrozole	ritonavir
aripiprazole	levetiracetam	rizatriptan
bisoprolol	levonorgestrel	ropinirole
botulinum toxin A	lisinopril	rosiglitazone
buprenorphine	lorazepam	rosuvastatin
bupropion	losartan	selegiline
cabergoline	mefloquine	sildenafil
cilazapril	metformin	sotalol
citalopram	methadone	stavudine
dantrolene	metoprolol	sulindac
desipramine	mirtazapine	sumatriptan
diuretics	naltrexone	tacrolimus
donepezil	olanzapine	tamsulosin
doxazosin	olmesartan	telmisartan
eletriptan	oseltamivir	terazosin
emtricitabine	oxcarbazepine	topiramate
enfuvirtide	parathyroid hormone	trimipramine
escitalopram	paroxetine	vardenafil
famotidine	perindopril	venlafaxine
fluconazole	pindolol	verapamil
fluoxetine	pioglitazone	voriconazole
fluvoxamine	pramipexole	zolmitriptan
fosamprenavir		
galantamine		

[a] List is not comprehensive. See Suggested Readings.

Pharmacologic Therapy

For comparative ingredients of nonprescription products, consult the *Compendium of Products for Minor Ailments*—Gastrointestinal Products: Antiemetics.

Drug therapy for vertigo is symptomatic; in the majority of cases the mechanism of the vertigo is unknown and specific therapy can therefore not be determined. Unless a specific cause of vertigo is known (e.g., Meniere's disease), the choice of pharmacologic agent for treatment depends on the adverse effect profile of the drug, presence of contraindications and cost. Most drugs used in vertigo down-regulate vestibular excitability (vestibular suppressants).[4] Table 3 describes drugs used to treat vertigo. Many drugs have been used for vertigo, including **benzodiazepines**,[4] and **flunarizine**.[4,11,19] Few drugs have been properly evaluated for the treatment of vertigo. Benzodiazepines in particular have significant disadvantages and little evidence of benefit. They should be avoided unless use is warranted by comorbidities such as anxiety.

Betahistine was studied in patients with Meniere's disease. No difference was found between placebo and either dose of betahistine (48 mg daily or 144 mg daily) in terms of frequency or severity of symptoms.[12] This confirms the findings of a previous Cochrane review that questioned the usefulness of betahistine in patients with Meniere's disease.[20]

Although these drugs may reduce vertigo, they also reduce vestibular function in the normal ear, which is a disadvantage. Vestibular suppressants reduce or slow down vestibular compensation and prevent the CNS from receiving the necessary feedback to facilitate compensation.[4] For this reason, vestibular suppressants are not intended for long-term use. In most cases the duration of treatment should be a week or less.

For seniors in particular, reassessment of effectiveness of medications that may cause dizziness or reduce CNS feedback is important. When conducting medication assessments, consider the ongoing need for medications that can affect balance.[21,22]

Monitoring of Therapy

Vertigo is often self-limiting. Evaluate the need for continued use of daily medication, at least initially. Determine the severity, duration and frequency of the vertigo. Monitor the patient for relief of vertigo and associated symptoms such as nausea, vomiting and anxiety. If no improvement of vertigo is noted, discontinue drug therapy. Monitor patients for adverse effects such as drowsiness and anticholinergic effects.

Advice for the Patient

Advise patients who receive drug therapy regarding:

- Expected duration of treatment
- Management of side effects (Table 3)
- Instructions not to combine drug therapy with alcohol.

Table 3: Drug Therapy for Vertigo

Class	Drug	Dosage	Adverse Effects	Drug Interactions	Comments	Cost[a]
Antiemetics	*promethazine* Histantil	25 mg Q6–8H po for nausea	Drowsiness, anticholinergic effects (dry mouth, mydriasis, blurred vision, constipation, urinary retention, confusion). Extrapyramidal reactions.	Metoclopramide: Increased risk of extrapyramidal symptoms. Additive sedation with alcohol or other sedating medications. May increase absorption of digoxin.	Avoid combining with CNS depressants. Contraindicated in angle closure glaucoma, prostatic hyperplasia and urinary retention.	$
Antivertigo Agents	*betahistine* Serc, generics	24–48 mg divided in 2–3 doses daily po	Vomiting, GI pain, abdominal distention and bloating can be reduced by taking with a meal or by reducing the dose. Drowsiness, confusion.	Antihistamines may antagonize effects of betahistine. Monitor patients using $beta_2$-agonists. Betahistine may counteract clinical effect of bronchodilators. MAOIs may inhibit metabolism. Dosage reduction may be required.	Warnings about use in patients with ulcer or hyperacidity may be unfounded. Based on one small study conducted in healthy individuals, no increase in gastric acid was found.[23] Research has shown no benefit in Meniere's disease.[12]	$
Calcium Channel Blockers	*flunarizine* generics	Initial: 5 mg QHS po; increase to 10 mg QHS po after 1–2 wk	Weight gain, extrapyramidal effects, drowsiness, depression.	Additive sedation with other CNS depressants, such as alcohol, benzodiazepines, opioids.	Many patients have side effects. Contraindicated in hypotension, heart failure and arrhythmia. Avoid in severe constipation. Do not use in depressed patients or those with extrapyramidal disorders.	$$
Vestibular Suppressants/ Antiemetics	*dimenhydrinate* Gravol, generics	25–50 mg Q6H po or 100 mg Q8H pr	Drowsiness, anticholinergic effects (dry mouth, mydriasis, blurred vision, constipation, urinary retention, confusion).	Additive sedation with alcohol or other sedating medications. May increase absorption of digoxin.	Avoid combining with CNS depressants. Contraindicated in angle closure glaucoma, prostatic hyperplasia and urinary retention.	$
	scopolamine Transderm-V	Transdermal patch (1.5 mg delivers 1 mg over 3 days) 1 patch Q72H	See dimenhydrinate. Local reactions, allergies.	Additive sedation with alcohol or other sedating medications.	See dimenhydrinate.	$$$/patch

[a] Cost per day; includes drug cost only.

Legend: $ <$1 $$ $1–2 $$$ $2–5

Suggested Readings

Ponka D, Kirlew M. Top 10 differential diagnoses in family medicine: Vertigo and dizziness. *Can Fam Physician* 2007;53:1959.

Post RE, Dickerson LM. Dizziness: a diagnostic approach. *Am Fam Physician* 2010;82:361-8, 369.

Sloane PD, Coeytaux RR, Beck RS et al. Dizziness: state of the science. *Ann Intern Med* 2001;134:823-32.

Swartz R, Longwell P. Treatment of vertigo. *Am Fam Physician* 2005;71:1115-22.

References

1. Walker MF, Daroff RB. Dizziness and vertigo. In: Fauci AS et al., eds. *Harrison's principles of internal medicine*. 19th ed. New York: McGraw-Hill; 2015. Available from: accessmedicine.mhmedical.com/content.aspx?bookid=1130&Sectionid=79724668. Accessed August 30, 2015. Subscription required.
2. Swartz R, Longwell P. Treatment of vertigo. *Am Fam Physician* 2005;71:1115-22.
3. Kerber KA. Vertigo and dizziness in the emergency department. *Emerg Med Clin North Am* 2009;27:39-50.
4. Hain TC, Uddin M. Pharmacologic treatment of vertigo. *CNS Drugs* 2003;17:85-100.
5. Bhattacharyya N, Baugh RF, Orvidas L et al. Clinical practice guideline: benign paroxysmal positional vertigo. *Otolaryngol Head Neck Surg* 2008;139:S47-81.
6. Hanley K, O'Dowd, Considine N. A systematic review of vertigo in primary care. *Br J Gen Pract* 2001;51:666-71.
7. Froehling DA, Bowen JM, Mohr DN et al. The canalith repositioning procedure for the treatment of benign paroxysmal positional vertigo: a randomized controlled trial. *Mayo Clin Proc* 2000;75:695-700.
8. Fife TD, Iverson DJ, Lempert T et al. Practice parameter: therapies for benign paroxysmal positional vertigo (an evidence-based review): report of the Quality Standards Subcommittee of the American Academy of Neurology. *Neurology* 2008;70:2067-74.
9. Hilton MP, Pinder DK. The Epley (canalith repositioning) manoeuvre for benign paroxysmal positional vertigo. *Cochrane Database Syst Rev* 2014;12:CD003162.
10. Burgess A, Kundu S. Diuretics for Meniere's disease or syndrome. *Cochrane Database Syst Rev* 2006;3:CD003599.
11. James AL, Burton MJ. Betahistine for Meniere's disease or syndrome. *Cochrane Database Syst Rev* 2001;1:CD001873.
12. Adrion C, Fischer CS, Wagner J, et al. Efficacy and safety of betahistine treatment in patients with Meniere's disease: primary results of a long term, multicentre, double blind, randomised, placebo controlled, dose defining trial (BEMED trial). BMJ 2016;352:h6816.
13. van Sonsbeek S, Pullens B, van Benthem PP. Positive pressure therapy for Ménière's disease or syndrome. *Cochrane Database Syst Rev* 2015;3:CD008419.
14. Ahsan SF, Standring R, Wang Y. Systematic review and meta-analysis of Meniett therapy for Meniere's disease. *Laryngoscope* 2015;125:203-8.
15. Strupp M, Zingler VC, Arbusow V et al. Methyprednisolone, valacyclovir, or the combination for vestibular neuritis. *N Engl J Med* 2004;351:354-61.
16. Sloane PD, Coeytaux RR, Beck RS et al. Dizziness: state of the science. *Ann Intern Med* 2001;134:823-32.
17. Cianfrone G, Pentangelo D, Cianfrone F et al. Pharmacological drugs inducing ototoxicity, vestibular symptoms and tinnitus: a reasoned and updated guide. *Eur Rev Med Pharmacol Sci* 2011;15:601-36.
18. Ponka D, Kirlew M. Top 10 differential diagnoses in family medicine: Vertigo and dizziness. *Can Fam Physician* 2007;53:1959.
19. Haid T. Evaluation of flunarizine in patients with Meniere's disease. Subjective and vestibular findings. *Acta Otolaryngol Suppl* 1988;460:149-53.
20. Della Pepa C, Guidetti M, Eandi M. Betahistine in the treatment of vertiginous syndromes: a meta-analysis. *Acta Otorhinolaryngol Ital* 2006;26:208-15.
21. Public Health Agency of Canada. *Seniors' falls in Canada: second report*. Ottawa: Public Health Agency of Canada; 2014.
22. Al-Aama T. Falls in the elderly: spectrum and prevention. *Can Fam Physician* 2011;57:771-6.
23. Cochran KM, Allan JG, Russell RI. A study of the effect of betahistine on gastric acid secretion in man. *Curr Med Res Opin* 1974;2:63-6.

Vertigo—What You Need to Know

What is vertigo?

Vertigo is a kind of dizziness where it feels like you or your surroundings are moving or spinning. It often makes people feel sick to their stomach.

What causes vertigo?

Vertigo can be caused by many things, including viral infections and inner ear problems. Sometimes it goes away on its own. Other times the body learns to ignore the feeling. **Anyone with vertigo should see a healthcare provider to find out what is causing it.**

What is the treatment for vertigo?

A healthcare provider may try a series of positions called the Epley manoeuvre to see if it helps relieve your vertigo.

Medication can be used to treat vertigo and the upset stomach it causes. However, medications will not fix the problem. They may even keep your body from learning to ignore the vertigo.

If you suffer from attacks of vertigo, avoid activities that may be dangerous (such as climbing ladders, driving and operating machinery).

Important information about medications used to treat vertigo:

- Medications used to treat vertigo may cause:
  - drowsiness or blurred vision—use caution driving and operating dangerous machinery
  - dry mouth—sugarless candy or gum may help relieve dryness
  - constipation—drink plenty of water and eat high-fibre foods
- Don't combine these medications with alcohol or other drugs that might make you drowsy or less alert.
- Talk to your pharmacist or other healthcare provider if the side effects are unusual or really bother you.

Chapter 12
Assessment of Patients with Eye Conditions

Anne M. Friesen, BSc(Pharm), MSc

Figure 1: Assessment of Patients with Eye Conditions

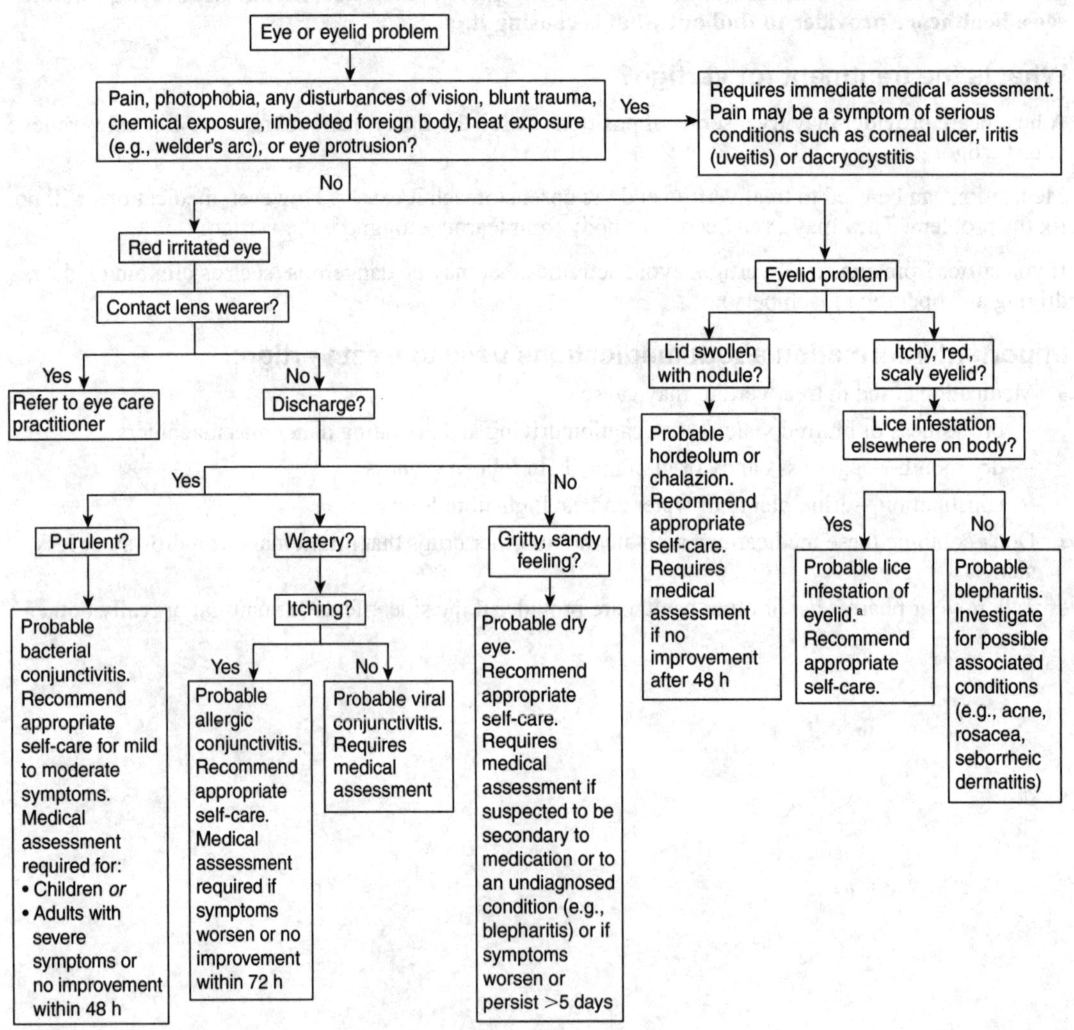

[a] See Chapter 69: Parasitic Skin Infections: Lice and Scabies.

Chapter 13
Conjunctivitis

Anne M. Friesen, BSc(Pharm), MSc

Pathophysiology

The conjunctiva is a thin, translucent, relatively elastic tissue layer that lines the inside of the eyelids (palpebral portion) and the anterior aspect of the globe (bulbar portion); see Chapter 16: Eyelid Conditions: Hordeolum, Chalazion and Blepharitis, Figure 1. As the outermost layer of the exterior surface of the globe, the conjunctiva is exposed to many microorganisms and other environmental factors. The combined action of the tears and eyelids protect the conjunctiva by trapping and diluting debris and organisms, then flushing the tears into the nasolacrimal duct.[1,2]

Common causes of conjunctivitis are listed in Table 1.

Table 1: **Causes of Conjunctivitis[2,3,4,5]**

Bacterial	Neonates: *Chlamydia trachomatis*, *Staphylococcus aureus*, *Haemophilus influenzae*, *Streptococcus pneumoniae*, *Neisseria gonorrhoeae*, *Neisseria meningitidis*
	Children: *H. influenzae*, *S. pneumoniae*, *S. aureus*
	Adults: *S. aureus*, coagulase-negative Staphylococcus organisms, *H. influenzae*, *S. pneumoniae*, *N. gonorrhoeae*, *N. meningitidis*
Viral	Adenovirus Herpes simplex virus
Immunologic	Immediate hypersensitivity reactions: hay fever, vernal keratoconjunctivitis, atopic keratoconjunctivitis, giant papillary conjunctivitis
	Autoimmune disease: keratoconjunctivitis sicca with Sjögren's syndrome, ocular cicatricial pemphigoid
	Delayed hypersensitivity reactions
Chemical or irritative	Iatrogenic: miotics, idoxuridine, preservatives, contact lens solutions
	Occupational: acids, alkalies, smoke, wind, UV light
	Irritative: superior limbic keratoconjunctivitis
Associated with dermatologic condition	Ocular rosacea Psoriasis Stevens-Johnson syndrome (erythema multiforme major)
Associated with systemic disease	Thyroid disease Kawasaki disease
Lacrimal system infections	Canaliculitis Dacryocystitis

Conjunctivitis is a general term that refers to any inflammatory condition of the membrane that lines the inside of the eyelids and covers the exposed surface of the sclera. The inflammation can be hyperacute, acute or chronic in presentation and may be caused by infection or many other factors (see Table 1). Conjunctivitis is the most common cause of red eye worldwide.[2,3] This chapter addresses bacterial (hyperacute, acute and chronic), viral and allergic conjunctivitis.

Goals of Therapy

- Relieve symptoms
- Prevent complications (preserve eyesight)
- Prevent recurrence
- Cure or control infection, where present
- Prevent transmission of infection to others

Patient Assessment

An algorithm for the assessment of eye conditions is presented in Chapter 12: Assessment of Patients with Eye Conditions.

Typically, patients present with some degree of redness in the conjunctiva, as well as some type of discharge. Other descriptions of symptoms include a scratching or burning sensation, a foreign body sensation, a feeling of fullness around the eyes, itching and mild photophobia. Often the eyes are crusty or sticky after sleeping, particularly with bacterial conjunctivitis.

Signs and symptoms of the most common types of conjunctivitis are listed in Table 2.

Table 2: **Signs and Symptoms of Conjunctivitis**

Clinical Findings	Viral	Bacterial	Allergic
Itching	Minimal	Minimal	Severe
Redness	Generalized	Generalized	Generalized
Discharge	Profuse, serous	Moderate, mucopurulent or purulent	Moderate, serous or mucoid

Acute Bacterial Conjunctivitis

Approximately 60% of suspected and documented cases of bacterial conjunctivitis are self-limiting and resolve without treatment in 1–2 weeks.[6] However, antibiotic treatment can reduce the duration of the disease and may decrease the risk of more serious corneal complications, recurrences, and person-to-person spread.[2,3,5,7,8,9,10] The most common causative organism is *S. aureus*, but *S. pneumoniae* and *H. influenzae* are also common, especially in children.[1,5,11,12,13]

Nonpharmacologic Therapy

- The patient, family and other care providers should be careful to prevent contamination by avoiding direct hand-to-eye contact, and should employ proper hand-washing techniques to avoid transmitting the infection (see Chapter 16: Eyelid Conditions: Hordeolum, Chalazion and Blepharitis, Infections of the Eyelids or Conjunctiva—What you Need to Know).
- If eyelids are stuck together in the morning, soak with a warm compress and open carefully.

- The conjunctival sac can be irrigated with sterile saline or a commercial eye wash product as necessary to remove conjunctival secretions.
- Because of an increased risk of developing serious infections, advise contact lens wearers with conjunctivitis to stop using their lenses and seek medical advice.[6]
- Patients who use eye drops, e.g., for glaucoma or dry eye, should replace the eye drop bottles in case the bottles have been inadvertently contaminated.

Pharmacologic Therapy

For comparative ingredients of nonprescription products, consult the *Compendium of Products for Minor Ailments*—Ophthalmic Products: Anti-infectives.

For mild cases of bacterial conjunctivitis in adults, **polymyxin B/gramicidin** eye drops can be instilled in the affected eye(s) 4–6 times a day for 7–10 days. Generally, continue treatment for 2 days after symptoms have resolved.[1,2,3,5,7,12,14,15]

Polymyxin B-based combinations are not reliably bactericidal.[15] If there is no improvement within 48 hours of starting treatment, refer the patient to a physician or eye care practitioner; all children with conjunctivitis should be referred to a physician.

When the infection is moderate to severe, or if polymyxin-based products have been ineffective, the use of standard empiric treatment with broad spectrum antibacterial drops is warranted (e.g., **trimethoprim/polymyxin B**, ophthalmic ointments containing **erythromycin** or **bacitracin**).[5,7,12,14] Adults and adolescents generally prefer ophthalmic drops. Ointments may be better tolerated by young children, who may not be bothered by ointment-induced blurred vision and may find drop administration irritating.

Tobramycin provides good gram-negative coverage and relatively poor gram-positive coverage with systemic use but is sufficiently effective in the topical treatment of conjunctivitis. Toxicity to the corneal epithelium can occur, especially with prolonged use. Reserve fluoroquinolone antibiotics (**ciprofloxacin**, **gatifloxacin**, **moxifloxacin**, **ofloxacin**) for serious infections such as bacterial keratitis.[1,2,3,5,7,12,14]

For more information on antibacterial therapy for conjunctivitis, consult the *Compendium of Therapeutic Choices:* Red Eye.

Hyperacute Bacterial Conjunctivitis

This infection is most commonly seen in neonates or sexually active young people (15–24 years old).[2,3,5,7,11,14] It is a severe, sight-threatening ocular infection caused by *N. gonorrhoeae* or *N. meningitidis*. It is characterized by a copious, yellow-green purulent discharge, redness, irritation and tenderness to palpation. Symptoms are rapidly progressive, leading to severe corneal damage, perforation and loss of vision if there is any delay in treatment. In adults, the organism is usually transmitted from the genitalia to the hands and then to the eyes. In infants, transmission of the organism occurs during vaginal delivery, and they typically develop bilateral discharge 3–5 days after birth. As a preventive measure, ophthalmic antibiotic ointments have been routinely applied to infants immediately after delivery. However, the Canadian Pediatric Society currently recommends abolishing the mandatory application of antibiotic ophthalmic ointment to newborns.[16] Instead, they recommend screening all pregnant women for gonorrhea and chlamydia, and subsequently treating infants with effective antibiotics if the mother had untreated infection at time of delivery.

Nonpharmacologic Therapy

Immediate medical assessment is required. After treatment has been initiated, the same adjunctive nonpharmacologic measures as used for acute bacterial conjunctivitis can be implemented.[2,5,14]

Pharmacologic Therapy

Medical assessment is imperative.

Treatment consists of immediate Gram staining of specimens, followed by systemic and ophthalmic antibacterials and saline irrigation. In adults, **ceftriaxone** 1–2 g im is the therapy of choice.

For more information on therapy for hyperacute bacterial conjunctivitis, consult the *Compendium of Therapeutic Choices:* Red Eye.

Chronic Bacterial Conjunctivitis

Chronic bacterial conjunctivitis is defined as a condition that lasts 4 weeks or longer. It is often associated with blepharitis, and is sometimes found in conjunction with facial seborrhea, acne rosacea, nasolacrimal duct obstruction or chronic dacryocystitis. *S. aureus* and *Moraxella lacunata* are most commonly involved, the latter occurring in clusters in women who share contaminated makeup.[4,14]

Nonpharmacologic Therapy

Treatment is similar to the treatment of blepharitis. See Chapter 16: Eyelid Conditions: Hordeolum, Chalazion and Blepharitis. Eyelid hygiene and warm compresses are important as a daily routine. Contaminated facial care products and makeup should be discarded.[2,3,14]

Pharmacologic Therapy

Chronic bacterial conjunctivitis has a protracted course with periods of exacerbation and appropriate treatment should be carefully managed by an appropriate healthcare practitioner.

Topical antibacterials are used during periods of exacerbation. Patients whose chronic conjunctivitis is associated with meibomian gland dysfunction or severe acne rosacea may benefit from oral agents such as **doxycycline** or **erythromycin**. Topical **metronidazole** therapy for acne rosacea may also ameliorate associated conjunctivitis.

For further discussion of antibacterial prescription therapy for chronic conjunctivitis, consult the *Compendium of Therapeutic Choices:* Red Eye.

Viral Conjunctivitis

Patients with viral conjunctivitis usually present with an acutely red eye, watery discharge, conjunctival swelling, foreign body sensation and mild photophobia. There may be tenderness around the preauricular node. Occasionally, patients may have subconjunctival hemorrhage.[3,17] Both eyes may be affected at the same time, or the second eye may become infected a few days after the first. If this happens, the infection is usually more severe in the first eye.

The most common causative organism is adenovirus. Viral infections are highly contagious and can be spread through respiratory tract-to-eye, finger-to-eye, or instrument-to-eye (physician's office) contact, and via contaminated swimming pools. Some patients have an associated respiratory tract infection.[2,3,11,14,17] The incubation period ranges from 2–14 days and the infection can last from 2–4 weeks.[11] It is contagious for 2 weeks after the second eye becomes involved.[5]

Herpes simplex virus (HSV) and *herpes zoster* can also cause viral conjunctivitis. The risk of progressive keratitis is higher with these types of infection.

Nonpharmacologic Therapy

All patients with suspected viral conjunctivitis require medical assessment to determine the cause.

Treatment of adenovirus conjunctivitis is supportive. Cold compresses may increase patient comfort.[18] Instruct patients to avoid direct contact with other persons for at least 14 days after the onset of symptoms or until the eyes are no longer red and weeping.[17] Children should be kept out of school until there is no ocular discharge (approximately 1 week).[3,19]

Pharmacologic Therapy

Ocular lubricants may be useful in improving patient comfort.[18] **Ophthalmic decongestants** or **antihistamines** may help with severe itching, but are generally not indicated.

Antiviral agents are usually not indicated in adenovirus infection, although **cidofovir** (available only through Health Canada's Special Access Programme) has been used successfully.[18] Corticosteroid eye drops may prolong the course of the disease by allowing viral proliferation and should only be used under the direction of an ophthalmologist.[18]

Treatment of HSV usually consists of topical (**trifluridine**) or oral antiviral agents (**acyclovir**, **famciclovir**, **valacyclovir**), while only oral agents are used for herpes zoster infection.[2,3,14,18]

For further discussion of pharmacologic therapy for HSV or herpes zoster, consult the *Compendium of Therapeutic Choices:* Red Eye.

Allergic Conjunctivitis

Allergic conjunctivitis encompasses a group of ocular surface diseases that vary in severity, but are typically associated with Type I hypersensitivity reactions.[20] Seasonal allergic conjunctivitis (SAC) and perennial allergic conjunctivitis (PAC) comprise approximately 95% of allergic conjunctivitis cases. Vernal keratoconjunctivitis (VKC), atopic keratoconjunctivitis (AKC) and giant papillary conjunctivitis (GPC) are rare but more serious conditions which require assessment and management by an ophthalmologist.

In SAC, also known as hay fever, patients experience ocular itching, tearing, redness and mild eyelid swelling.[2,3,4] Although ragweed is the most common airborne cause of allergic rhinitis, grass pollen is considered the most common cause of ocular symptoms.[21,22] Dry eye can also be a factor in SAC—reduced tear volume leads to decreased capacity to dilute and wash away allergens.

PAC exhibits the same symptoms as SAC, but reactions are triggered by environmental allergens commonly found in the home (e.g., dust mites, mold spores, animal dander). Patients suffer throughout the year, but may have seasonal exacerbations in addition to chronic symptoms.[23]

Although other ocular conditions (e.g., blepharitis, dry eye) present similarly, the hallmark symptom of SAC is ocular itching, while patients with PAC have red eyes as their primary symptom.[20] For further information on allergic conjunctivitis in relation to allergic rhinitis, see Chapter 22: Allergic Rhinitis.

Nonpharmacologic Therapy

Allergen avoidance is an important first step in the treatment of allergic conjunctivitis.[24,25] In SAC, minimize exposure to grassy fields, trees and flowers and keep windows closed to prevent pollens from entering the home. Wash hands after being outdoors and avoid touching/rubbing the eyes while outdoors. Wraparound eyeglasses are an effective means to protect the eyes from pollens and reduce symptoms of SAC.[26]

In PAC, allergen avoidance may be more problematic as it could involve the family pet.[23] However, dust mite control measures, proper ventilation of home and office environments, air filtration systems, and awareness of allergen prevalence (pollen and mold counts) can all help to ease symptoms. Washing the hair prior to going to bed can also help reduce allergen exposure.

Cold compresses over the eyes offer considerable symptom relief, especially ocular pruritus.[25]

Pharmacologic Therapy

For comparative ingredients of nonprescription products, consult the *Compendium of Products for Minor Ailments*—Ophthalmic Products: Anti-allergy Agents, Antihistamines and Decongestants; Ocular Lubricants.

Ocular lubricants help to wash out allergens and may act as a barrier to pollens.[25] Benzalkonium chloride (a preservative in some lubricants) may irritate eyes, especially if used ≥4 times per day; avoid when possible. Saline or commercial eyewashes can help wash out allergens and reduce eyelid swelling, chemosis (conjunctival edema) and hyperemia (redness due to increased blood flow). These are both first-line treatment options; refrigeration may improve their soothing effect.

Ophthalmic **decongestants** (e.g., **naphazoline, oxymetazoline, phenylephrine, tetrahydrozoline**) decrease eye redness and eyelid edema through vasoconstriction. They may cause rebound ocular congestion with prolonged use (time frame not clearly defined, but probably with use >10 days).[27] If rebound congestion occurs, it is likely to be mild and harmless.[27] Ophthalmic decongestants are second-line treatment options for mild-moderate SAC; they are not indicated for prolonged use in PAC. Because they are vasoconstrictors, they are contraindicated in patients with narrow angle (angle-closure) glaucoma.

Oral H_1 **antihistamines** may relieve itching associated with SAC, but do not decrease redness.[24] Ophthalmic antihistamines are available in combination with decongestants (e.g., **pheniramine** in combination with decongestants listed above), and are preferred over systemic antihistamines because they act faster and are less drying.[25,28] **Emedastine** is a topical histamine H_1 antagonist with a rapid onset of action. It is more effective than antihistamine/vasoconstrictor combinations or oral antihistamines in relieving itchy, watery eyes;[27] however it is not available as a self-care option.

Mast cell stabilizers prevent degranulation of mast cells and are useful in both SAC and PAC as they treat the late phase of the allergic response.[20] Regular use during allergy season will prevent redness, itching and eyelid edema. Mast cell stabilizers may take up to 10 days for maximum effect; they must be started before allergy season to prevent symptoms. **Nedocromil, lodoxamide** and **sodium cromoglycate** are mast cell stabilizing agents that alleviate the signs and symptoms of mild to moderate allergic conjunctivitis.[2,22,24,28,29]

Agents that have both antihistaminic and mast cell stabilizing properties (e.g., **olopatadine, ketotifen**) will relieve itching quickly while providing long-term activity against ocular irritation by allergens.[20]

Nonsteroidal anti-inflammatory eye drops such as **ketorolac** can decrease the amount of ocular itching and conjunctival redness in allergic conjunctivitis.[2,22,24] These agents may cause stinging upon instillation; limit to short-term use to avoid serious corneal effects, such as keratitis, ulceration, or even corneal perforation. Patients at increased risk of corneal effects include those with dry eye syndrome and those recovering from recent surgery.

Once the immediate problem of allergic symptoms is addressed, question the patient about possible dry eye symptoms. Patients with moderate to severe allergic conjunctivitis, or those who do not respond to self-care measures within 72 hours, require further medical assessment. Severe cases of

SAC may require the use of topical corticosteroids or other immunomodulatory agents under the care of an ophthalmologist.[2,22,24]

For further discussion of pharmacologic therapy for allergic conjunctivitis, consult the *Compendium of Therapeutic Choices:* Red Eye.

Monitoring of Therapy

Table 3 provides a monitoring plan that should be individualized for the patient and the condition.

Table 3: **Monitoring of Therapy for Conjunctivitis**[1,2,3,17]

Eye Condition	Monitoring	Goals/Endpoint of Therapy	Actions
Bacterial conjunctivitis[5,14]	Patient: Daily Healthcare practitioner: Within 2 days of initiating drug therapy	Resolution of infection. A decrease in signs and symptoms should occur within 48 h.	Adults: Requires consultation for further therapy if worsening or no improvement within 48 h. Children: Requires consultation for further therapy. Do not recommend self-treatment.
Chronic bacterial conjunctivitis[5,14]	Patient: Daily Healthcare practitioner: Each visit	Control of infection. Reduce the risk of long-term complications.	Encourage lid hygiene regimen (see Chapter 16: Eyelid Conditions: Hordeolum, Chalazion and Blepharitis). Remind patient to cleanse only the margin of the eyelid and not to scratch the eyeball or conjunctiva. Requires consultation for further therapy if recurrence or acute exacerbation occurs.
Viral conjunctivitis (adenovirus)[14]	Patient/family: Daily Healthcare practitioner: Within 1 wk of initiating treatment	Ease symptoms while infection resolves. Prevent transmission to others.	Requires medical assessment to rule out other viral causes. If decongestant or lubricant drops cause irritation, discontinue use or suggest a preservative-free product.
Seasonal allergic conjunctivitis[21,30]	Patient: Daily Healthcare practitioner: Within 3 days of initiating drug therapy	Ease patient discomfort. Stop allergic/inflammatory process. Prevent recurrence in future seasons.	If decongestant or lubricant drops cause irritation, discontinue use or suggest a preservative-free product. Requires consultation for further therapy if no improvement within 3 days, or if symptoms persist despite treatment. Requires consultation for further therapy if symptoms are severe.

Suggested Readings

American Academy of Ophthalmology. *Conjunctivitis PPP-2013*. Available from: www.aao.org/preferred-practice-pattern/conjunctivitis-ppp–2013.

Merck manual: professional version. *Overview of conjunctival and scleral disorders*. Available from: www.merckmanuals.com/professional/eye-disorders/conjunctival-and-scleral-disorders/overview-of-conjunctival-and-scleral-disorders.

Narayana S, McGee S. Bedside diagnosis of the 'red eye': a systematic review. *Am J Med* 2015;128:1220-4.

Sheikh A, Hurwitz B, van Schayck CP et al. Antibiotics versus placebo for acute bacterial conjunctivitis. *Cochrane Database Syst Rev* 2012;9:CD001211.

References

1. Baum J. Infections of the eye. *Clin Infect Dis* 1995;21:479-86.
2. Garcia-Ferrer FJ, Schwab IR, Shetlar DJ. Conjunctiva. In: Riordan-Eva P, Whitcher J, eds. *Vaughan & Asbury's general ophthalmology*. 17th ed. New York: Lange Medical Books/McGraw-Hill Medical; 2008.
3. Morrow GL, Abbott RL. Conjunctivitis. *Am Fam Physician* 1998;57:735-46.

4. Kanski JJ. *Clinical ophthalmology: a systematic approach.* 4th ed. Boston: Butterworth-Heinemann; 1999.
5. Tarabishy AB, Jeng BH. Bacterial conjunctivitis: a review for internists. *Cleve Clin J Med* 2008;75:507-12.
6. Amir AA, Barney NP. Conjunctivitis: a systematic review of diagnosis and treatment. *JAMA* 2013;310:1721-9.
7. Hovding G. Acute bacterial conjunctivitis. *Acta Ophthalmol* 2008;86:5-17.
8. Sheikh A, Hurwitz B, van Schayck CP et al. Antibiotics versus placebo for acute bacterial conjunctivitis. *Cochrane Database Syst Rev* 2012;9:CD001211.
9. Hutnik C, Mohammed-Shahi MH. Bacterial conjunctivitis. *Clin Ophthalmol* 2010;4:1451-7.
10. Epling J. Bacterial conjunctivitis. *Clin Evid (Online)* 2012;pii:0704.
11. Jackson WB. Differentiating conjunctivitis of diverse origins. *Surv Ophthalmol* 1993;38:91-104.
12. Weiss A, Brinser JH, Nazar-Stewart V. Acute conjunctivitis in childhood. *J Pediatr* 1993;122:10-4.
13. Golde KT, Gardiner MF. Bacterial conjunctivitis in children: a current review of pathogens and treatment. *Int Ophthalmol Clin* 2011;51:85-92.
14. Thielen TL, Castle SS, Terry JE. Anterior ocular infections: an overview of pathophysiology and treatment. *Ann Pharmacother* 2000;34:235-46.
15. Karpecki P, Paterno MR, Comstock TL. Limitations of current antibiotics for the treatment of bacterial conjunctivitis. *Optom Vis Sci* 2010;87:908-19.
16. Moore DL, MacDonald NE; Canadian Paediatric Society, Infectious Diseases and Immunization Committee. Preventing ophthalmia neonatorum. *Paediatr Child Health* 2015;20:93-6.
17. Galor A, Jeng BH. Red eye for the internist: when to treat, when to refer. *Cleve Clin J Med* 2008;75:137-44.
18. Skevaki CL, Galani IE, Pararas MV et al. Treatment of viral conjunctivitis with antiviral drugs. *Drugs* 2011;71:331-47.
19. LaMattina K, Thompson L. Pediatric conjunctivitis. *Dis Mon* 2014;60:231-8.
20. O'Brien TP. Allergic conjunctivitis: an update on diagnosis and management. *Curr Opin Allergy Clin Immunol* 2013;13:543-9.
21. Bielory L. Allergic and immunologic disorders of the eye. Part II: ocular allergy. *J Allergy Clin Immunol* 2000;106:1019-32.
22. Bielory L, Friedlaender MH. Allergic conjunctivitis. *Immunol Allergy Clin North Am* 2008;28:43-58.
23. Bielory L, Meltzer EO, Nichols KK et al. An algorithm for the management of allergic conjunctivitis. *Allergy Asthma Proc* 2013;34:408-20.
24. Bielory L. Ocular allergy treatment. *Immunol Allergy Clin North Am* 2008;28:189-224.
25. Bilkhu PS, Wolffsohn JS, Naroo SA. A review of non-pharmacological and pharmacological management of seasonal and perennial allergic conjunctivitis. *Cont Lens Anterior Eye* 2012;35:9-16.
26. Comert S, Karakaya G, Kalyoncu AF. Wraparound eyeglasses improve symptoms and quality of life in patients with seasonal allergic rhinoconjunctivitis. *Int Forum Allergy Rhinol* 2016 Feb 25. [Epub ahead of print].
27. Friedlaender MH. Ocular allergy. *Curr Opin Allergy Clin Immunol* 2011;11:477-82.
28. Bielory L. Ocular allergy. *Mt Sinai J Med* 2011;78:740-58.
29. Castillo M, Scott NW, Mustafa MS et al. Topical antihistamines and mast cell stabilisers for treating seasonal and perennial allergic conjunctivitis. *Cochrane Database Syst Rev* 2015;6:CD009566.
30. Hingorani M, Lightman S. Therapeutic options in ocular allergic disease. *Drugs* 1995;50:208-21.

Chapter 14
Contact Lens Care

David S. Wing, BSP, MS
Ken Gellatly, OD

Contact lenses can correct refractive errors associated with hyperopia (farsightedness), myopia (nearsightedness), astigmatism (related to shape of eye or cornea), presbyopia (age-related decline in acuity of near objects) and aphakia (reduced near and far vision related to absence of lens). Contact lenses are foreign bodies that sit on a tear cushion and do not actually make contact with the eye as implied by their name. As tears constantly bathe the cornea and supply oxygen, contact lenses act as physical barriers, leading to progressive hypoxia and edema. Development of clinical symptoms depends on lens materials, design and fit; the duration of wear and the adherence to the care regimen.

Contact lenses offer many advantages over eyeglasses:[1,2]

- An entire field of view in focus
- Natural appearance
- No fogging from temperature changes, perspiration or weather
- No annoying reflections and peripheral obstructions.

Types of Contact Lenses

The 2 major types of contact lenses are soft and rigid gas-permeable (RGP). Soft lenses are worn by over 90% of Canadian contact lens users, thus the chapter will focus on their maintenance and care.[3] Table 1 compares some of the important features of RGP and soft lenses.

Rigid Gas-permeable Lenses

RGP lenses, also known as hard lenses, retain the optical qualities and durability of PMMA (polymethyl methacrylate, the original, but now obsolete, hard lens) but have increased oxygen permeability and comfort.[4] RGP lenses have a sufficiently high oxygen permeability to prevent clinically observable corneal edema with normal wear. Hence, they offer better long-term visual acuity and, in general, result in fewer complications than either PMMA or soft lenses. Although RGP lenses have replaced the original PMMA lenses as the standard of care for hard lenses, their use is decreasing and accounts for only 10% of contact lenses.[5]

Soft Lenses

Soft lenses, or hydrogels, are made of a flexible polymeric material, usually hydroxyethyl methacrylate (HEMA), that has a high capacity for water absorption.[6,7] Most soft lenses currently available are silicone hydrogels, also made of HEMA, with the addition of silicone. Silicone hydrogels are the new standard in soft contact lenses and have replaced old (conventional) hydrogels.[8] Silicone hydrogels contain a much better polymer with increased oxygen permeability compared with conventional hydrogels, which has enabled longer wear times, and dramatically decreased incidence of hypoxia and corneal edema.[9] Silicone hydrogels also adsorb less protein;[10] when used with nonpreserved care solutions, they may be the safest choice[11] although a study found no decrease in the risk of microbial keratitis.[12]

The main advantage of soft lenses over RGP lenses is increased comfort. This is due to their flexibility (which increases with increasing water content), soft thin edges and hydrophilic nature. The vast majority of contact lens users wear soft lenses. Unfortunately, these lenses have an open matrix in which tear film lipoproteins, ophthalmic preparations, environmental pollutants, chemical vapors, oil and dust from fingers, cosmetics and some contact lens solution preservatives concentrate, all of which can lead to ocular irritation. Soft lens materials also tend to develop lens deposits (accumulation of proteins and lipids), a risk factor for the development of microbial keratitis, more rapidly than RGP lens materials.

Combination RGP/Soft Lenses

In combination lenses, an RGP centre is fused to a heme skirt to provide the great optics of RGP with the comfort of HEMA. The combination is indicated for keratoconus and other corneal dystrophies. Soft lens solutions are used with these combination lenses.

Table 1: **Comparative Features of Rigid Gas-permeable and Soft Contact Lenses**

Characteristics	Soft Lenses	RGP Lenses
Composition	Silicone hydrogel	PMMA/silicone, fluorosilicone acrylate
Water content	29–85% (hydrophilic); silicone hydrogels are made of hydrophobic material but have a hydrophilic surface treatment	≤2% (hydrophobic)
Life expectancy of lens	1 day to 1 year	5 years (unless lost earlier)
Solution requirements	Only soft lens solutions	Only RGP solutions
Visual acuity	Good	Excellent
Initial cost	Similar	Similar
Maintenance cost	More	Less
Gas permeability	Less	More
Initial comfort	Most comfortable	Intermediate
Adaptability (days until new lenses feel comfortable)	<1	5–10
Long-term comfort	Most comfortable	Intermediate
Daily wear time (hours)	>12	>12
Extended wear (days)	≤7 (hydrogels) ≤30 (silicone hydrogels)	≤7
Strength	Fragile	Strong
Accumulation of deposits from tear film	Most susceptible	Least susceptible
Effect of humidity	Easily affected	Minimally affected
Risk of microbial contamination	Greatest	Slight

Abbreviations: PMMA = polymethyl methacrylate; RGP = rigid gas-permeable

Wear Schedules

Lenses are worn according to various replacement schedules: conventional (1 year or more), planned replacement (lenses replaced every 2 weeks, every month or every 3 months) or daily (brand new soft lenses inserted every day). The vast majority of contact lens users follow a planned replacement schedule; a decreasing number of people follow a conventional schedule while an increasing number use daily disposables.[3,8,13,14]

Adherence problems related to conventional schedules (e.g., inadequate cleaning, disinfection and rinsing, reuse of old solutions, poor hygiene, using lenses for a longer time than recommended), lead to the development of planned replacement programs (PRPs).

Advantages of PRPs include:

- More frequent insertion of a new, sterile lens
- Lower cost because of reduced need for solutions (multipurpose solutions can replace single-purpose solutions)
- Improved vision (from more frequent replacement)
- Improved comfort (deposits are reduced, which increases lens wettability and reduces dryness)
- Improved adherence (from increased monitoring)
- More convenience (multipurpose solutions can be used, in association with increased monitoring)
- Fewer complaint-related office visits (reduction in giant papillary conjunctivitis, acute red eye and infective or inflammatory keratitis)
- Fewer problems associated with lost lenses (wearer has immediate access to a new set of lenses) or damaged lenses (wearer has no need to keep an old spare pair of lenses on hand).

In addition to supplied lenses, a disposable system that includes solutions and storage cases that are replaced at regular intervals may decrease the risk of ocular infections.

Daily disposables are sterile soft lenses that are opened fresh each day, worn for the day, and then disposed of in the evening. These lenses require no regular solutions for daily care and offer advantages for wearers who may have adherence problems with one of the other wear schedules.[15] Reuse of lenses increases the risk of contamination.[16]

Extended wear is defined as continuous use of a contact lens for 24 hours or more. The lenses are usually soft; however, RGP lenses are increasingly being used in extended-wear schedules. Early uncontrolled trials suggested that the rate of serious complications was not excessive and many wearers adopted extended-wear schedules. However, extended wear of contact lenses was eventually implicated in promoting microbial keratitis.[17,18] The most likely causes are increased protein accumulation, decreased flushing of bacteria during sleep and decreased immunologic activity during sleep. The prevalence of extended wear has decreased, likely due to increased risk of infection.[19]

Goals of Contact Lens Care

- Optimize vision
- Promote lens longevity and comfort
- Minimize complications such as eye irritation and infection

Patient Assessment

Use the following questions and answers to identify potential problems and aid in appropriate and timely referral to eye care professionals.

What type of contact lenses are you wearing?

The lens type (RGP or soft) determines the care regimen. Solutions for a specific lens type from the same manufacturer can likely be interchanged. Advise patients to consult their eye care professional for confirmation.

Do you have any of the following symptoms:

- Pain when inserting or wearing the lenses or after wearing them?
- Burning that causes excessive tearing?
- Inability to keep your eyes open?
- Severe or persistent haze, fog or halos while wearing the lenses?
- Redness, irritation or itching?
- Poor vision?

These symptoms may be due to poor lens fit, damaged lenses, improper handling, microbial conjunctivitis, solution or lens intolerance, ocular or systemic disease or improper lens care. Painful lid swelling and photophobia may be due to over wear. Advise patients to discontinue lens wear and consult their eye care professional if any of these symptoms occur.[20]

How long have you worn lenses?

Most contact lens wearers experience mild discomfort during the first few days while the eyes adapt. Since it may not be obvious at first which problems are significant, advise wearers to contact their eye care professional.

What medications are you taking?

Advise patients to consult an eye care professional before using any ophthalmic preparation with their lenses in place. Almost any ophthalmic product that is not specifically designed for use with contact lenses will cause temporary discomfort.

Numerous systemic medications can alter eye dynamics sufficiently to warrant therapeutic intervention. Sedatives (including alcohol), hypnotics, antihistamines and muscle relaxants can affect the eyelid, producing incomplete blinking or a decreased rate of blinking. Antihistamines, anticholinergics, tricyclic antidepressants and diuretics can decrease tear volume, leading to significant discomfort. See Table 2 and Table 3.

What products do you use for the care of your lenses?

Eye care professionals recommend specific products for lenses. When purchasing these products, patients may need guidance to select or substitute appropriately. Refer the wearer to an eye care professional if there is any confusion or uncertainty regarding the correct solution to use. See also Prevention of Complications.

Describe how you use your lens care products.

To ensure wearers adhere to prescribed care, ask them to describe their care regimen (Figure 1). Nonadherence is the greatest threat to eye comfort and lens life. Inadequate cleaning and disinfection cause about 50% of all problems associated with contact lenses.

Table 2: **Interactions between Contact Lenses and Systemic Drugs[21,22,23,24,25]**

Drug	Effect on Lenses
Oral contraceptives[26]	Lens intolerance due to exacerbation of dry eye
Antihistamines[27,28] Hypnotics Sedatives	Decrease in blink rate (blinking is required to maintain hydration in soft lens wearers and helps supply oxygen to the cornea in RGP lens wearers)
Muscle relaxants	Incomplete blinking
Anticholinergics Antihistamines Tricyclic antidepressants[29,30]	Decreased tear volume (leading to irritation and deposits in soft lens wearers, and corneal drying in RGP lens wearers)
Isotretinoin[31]	Itching and decreased wear time in soft lens wearers
ASA[32]	Ocular irritation and redness in soft lens wearers
Nitrofurantoin Phenazopyridine Rifampin[33,34] Sulfasalazine[35] Tetracycline	Discoloration of soft lenses

Abbreviations: RGP = rigid gas-permeable

Table 3: **Interactions between Soft Contact Lenses and Ophthalmic Products[22,25,36,37]**

Ophthalmic Agent	Effect on Soft Lenses
Phenylephrine Tetrahydrozoline	Dark discoloration of lens with repeated use
Benzalkonium chloride (preservative)	Can concentrate in soft lenses and cause ocular toxicity
Fluorescein[38] Rose bengal (diagnostic ophthalmic dyes)	Can concentrate in soft lenses and cause staining

What measures do you take before reinsertion after the lens has been dropped?

Unfortunately, wearers often pick up and promptly reinsert the lens along with whatever it has collected when removed from the eye. The proper technique is to reclean RGP lenses with soaking/wetting solution; rinse soft lenses with an appropriate rinsing solution (normal saline or multipurpose solution) before reinserting.

Prevention of Complications

Proper care of contact lenses is crucial in maintaining optimal eye health. The ideal contact lens care system would be economical, easy to use, free of side effects and would maintain all types of contact lenses in a clean and sterile state. Improved contact lens technology (e.g., daily disposables, improvements in oxygen permeability, multipurpose solutions) have brought the standard of practice closer to the ideal.[39,40] Figure 1 outlines the steps required to maintain soft contact lenses.

Nonadherence with proper lens care is the greatest threat to eye health and lens life, and affects as many as 50–99% of contact lens wearers.[41] Common forms of nonadherence include inadequate cleaning or rinsing, and economizing by using old solutions and old cases. Solution contamination (e.g., topping up old contaminated solution containers rather than replacing them), inadequate lens disinfection, manipulation of the lens in the eye and poor hygiene increase the exposure of the eye to pathogens, that can lead to microbial keratitis and corneal ulcers.[42,43,44,45,46,47,48,49] Adherence may be improved by explaining its benefits along with consequences of nonadherence.[50] New methods of improving adherence are required as education alone may be insufficient.[51]

Products for Contact Lenses

Contact Lens Solutions

For comparative ingredients of lens care products, consult the *Compendium of Products for Minor Ailments*—Contact Lens Products: Contact Lens Solutions for Soft and Rigid Gas-Permeable Lenses, Rigid Gas-Permeable Contact Lens Cleaning Systems, Soft Contact Lens Cleaning Chemical Systems, Soft Contact Lens Hydrogen Peroxide Cleaning Systems.

General Principles

When contact lenses are purchased, the wearer usually receives a contact lens case and a multipurpose solution, with or without various other solutions (e.g., rinsing, wetting). Once the sample is finished, wearers tend to replace their solutions with the same brand if the solutions have been well tolerated. If not tolerated, the eye care professional will recommend a different set of solutions on a trial basis. This trial-and-error scenario is repeated until the eye care professional considers the effect of the solutions on the corneal epithelium, as viewed by a biomicroscope, is considered acceptable. Unless otherwise instructed by their eye care professional, advise wearers to always use solutions from a single manufacturer. Each manufacturer formulates all components of its care regimen to be compatible with each other. The effect of substituting even one solution from a different manufacturer is not predictable, even if it has the same active ingredients in the same concentration. In addition, all solutions that are recommended by an eye care professional will have been found to be compatible with the wearer.

Although the majority of contact lens wearers use a multipurpose solution, single-purpose solutions are still discussed for educational purposes.

Multipurpose Solutions

In the past, eye care professionals may have recommended as many as 5 single products to use as part of a contact lens care regimen. To increase convenience, many products combine 2 or more functions in a single multipurpose solution.[52,53] The increase in use of multipurpose solutions has paralleled the increase in use of silicone hydrogels; accordingly, the majority of contact lens users employ a multipurpose solution for the maintenance of their lenses.[54] Although some researchers suggest that cleaning is compromised with the use of multipurpose solutions, clinical evaluations of multipurpose products for both soft and RGP lenses have shown they improve adherence and exhibit acceptable cleaning efficacy, leading to their wide acceptance. Some multipurpose solutions have been shown to disinfect at a rate faster than their recommended time.[55]

Initial positive results with no-rub formulations[56,57] were countered by other studies with varying results and led to more cautious recommendations.[58,59] Since then, many studies[60,61,62,63,64,65] and a literature review[66] have all recommended the reinstitution of rubbing as more effective than not rubbing.

Two separate outbreaks (*Acanthamoeba* and *Fusarium*) of keratitis were traced to multipurpose solutions.[67,68] There has also been an increase in corneal staining and low-grade infiltrates, 2 measures of solution-related toxicity. Low-impact lens/multipurpose solution combinations, daily disposable lenses or hydrogen peroxide disinfection are recommended to minimize the risk of these complications. It has been suggested that RGP lenses should be rinsed with saline before insertion and artificial tears be used for rewetting.[69]

Although the majority of contact lens wearers use a multipurpose solution, single-purpose solutions are still discussed for educational purposes.

Cleaning Solutions

Cleaning optimizes visual acuity, comfort, eye health and lens life and is the most important step in the proper care of all contact lenses.[70] Debris from numerous sources collects on the lens from the moment of insertion. The risk of complications such as blurred vision, ocular discomfort, local allergic reactions, ocular infection or blindness increases as the interval between cleanings lengthens. Most contact lens wearers use a multipurpose solution for cleaning their lenses. If they choose to use single-purpose solutions, there are two main types of cleaning solutions: surfactants (to remove loose debris) and protein cleaners (to remove embedded protein). The global acceptance of disposable soft lenses has made protein cleaning almost obsolete for soft lenses; for RGP lenses, enzyme cleaning is optional and is generally redundant when surfactants are properly used.

Since many contact lens contaminants are not water soluble, rinsing without cleaning is inadequate.[71] Proper cleaning and rinsing can remove more than 99.9% of the contaminants prior to disinfection.[70] Surfactants emulsify and suspend organisms and other debris, thereby reducing contamination and facilitating disinfection (the presence of debris can inactivate disinfectants).

Daily surfactant cleaning is similar for soft and RGP lenses. Surfactants for soft lenses contain preservatives that do not concentrate in the lens (e.g., polyquaternium-1). Immediately after lens removal, a few drops of surfactant are applied to each lens surface. The lenses are cleaned in the palm of the hand using the index finger in a circular motion for 30–60 seconds. An alternative method involves vigorous friction rubbing between the thumb and forefinger for 30–60 seconds. The surfactant is then thoroughly rinsed off with a rinsing solution (normal saline or multipurpose solution) before disinfection. A surfactant cleaner is used before an enzyme cleaner; the surfactant acts on the lipids that may hide protein deposits, making the enzyme cleaner more effective. Surfactants must be thoroughly rinsed off the lens and hands to minimize the risk of chemical keratoconjunctivitis, stinging, allergic reactions, conjunctival hyperemia and eyelid edema.[71]

Unorthodox cleaners include toothpaste, baking soda, laundry detergent, hair shampoo and skin cleaners.[72] These nonsterile products can damage lenses and are not recommended.

Disinfecting Solutions

A disinfectant actively kills microorganisms on lenses, while a preservative maintains the sterility of a solution.[73] Some compounds can be used for both purposes. Most disinfecting solutions for soft lenses contain disinfectants and preservatives. Some also contain surfactants but in a lower concentration than in cleaning solutions, so disinfecting still requires a separate step.

Most contact lens wearers use a multipurpose solution for disinfection. If they choose to use single-purpose solutions, there are 2 basic forms of chemical disinfection solutions for soft lenses: oxidizing agents (hydrogen peroxide) and disinfecting agents (e.g., polyquaternium-1, polyaminopropyl-biguanide and alkyltriethanolammonium chloride). Benzalkonium chloride (BAC) and chlorobutanol are used in solutions for RGP lenses only; these chemicals would be adsorbed by the HEMA polymer in soft lenses and cause ocular tissue damage when they are subsequently released.[73]

Chemical disinfection of soft lenses is similar to the soaking process for RGP lenses, as the lenses are soaked or stored overnight in a chemical disinfecting solution.[74] All soft lenses can be chemically disinfected with the appropriate solution. After disinfection, soft lenses must be thoroughly rinsed with at least 25 mL of rinsing solution (usually normal saline or a multipurpose solution) before lenses are inserted into the eye. With RGP lenses, saline or the disinfecting solution itself is used for rinsing. Water (e.g., tap, bottled, distilled) is not recommended for any lens because of potential accumulation of minerals in the lens and possible microbial contamination.[74,75]

Hydrogen peroxide was one of the more popular chemical disinfectants for soft lenses, but use fell to less than 10% of chemical disinfection systems due to the advent of more convenient multipurpose solutions.[76,77] However, when used properly, hydrogen peroxide is the most effective chemical disinfectant and produces the mildest ocular response when properly neutralized. Oxidizing agents like hydrogen peroxide are inherently unstable and, in the presence of organic debris, form free radicals that attach to debris and disperse it.[78] Their effervescence is a secondary means of removing debris from the lens matrix. Following disinfection, hydrogen peroxide is neutralized by a platinum catalyst, sodium pyruvate, catalase or thiosulfite. Hydrogen peroxide does not affect the tints of contact lenses, although hydrogen peroxide first aid products may cause tints to fade. Hydrogen peroxide first aid products are not designed for ophthalmic use and may contain impurities, stabilizers and other additives that irritate ocular tissue.[79,80]

Commercially available hydrogen peroxide products come with a specially designed lens case that contains a built-in neutralizing disc, in which the lenses must be soaked for 4–6 hours after disinfection, depending on the product. If the lenses are not soaked for the entire recommended duration, or not neutralized all together, patients are at risk of placing unneutralized hydrogen peroxide into their eyes, which is highly irritating. Patients are commonly unaware that hydrogen peroxide solutions differ from multipurpose solutions, and often experience eye irritation if not counseled appropriately.[81] Advise patients that hydrogen peroxide containers have red tips, which serve as a reminder that the solution is *not* safe to put directly into the eyes. Also, contact lenses must be free of multipurpose solution before placing them in hydrogen peroxide; otherwise the solution will foam and overflow the lens case. To avoid this, rinse the lenses thoroughly with the hydrogen peroxide solution before soaking them.

Wetting and Rewetting Solutions

Accessory solutions provide wetting/rewetting, lubrication and cushioning functions in various combinations.[82] Wetting/rewetting agents are artificial tears preserved with chemicals that are compatible with soft lenses. Lubrication and cushioning actions are imparted by viscosity agents, large colloidal molecules (e.g., hydroxypropylcellulose, sodium hyaluronate) that increase resistance to flow, holding the tears in the eyes and reducing the drying-out effect of solutions. They produce a cushioning and lubricant effect between the lens and eyelid and between the lens and cornea. Unlike wetting solutions without added viscosity agents, lubricants do not enhance the flow of tears over the cornea. Wearers of silicone hydrogels who are suffering from dryness benefit from lubricants but comforting effects seldom last longer than 1–2 hours, even with increasing viscosity.[83]

Solutions in this class have all 3 properties to varying degrees. Since the clinical significance of these differences is unknown, their uses are interchangeable.

Unit-dose or multidose saline is available in preserved or unpreserved formulations.[84] Preserved saline minimizes the risk of contamination during repeated use. Unpreserved unit-dose saline eliminates potential sensitivity reactions to preservatives. However, microbial contamination can occur if the solution stands for longer than 1 hour or if it is used improperly.

Soft Lenses

Soft lenses tend to dry out throughout the day, especially in a dry or polluted environment, leading to dry eye symptoms in up to 75% of soft lens wearers.[85] Additional risk factors for dry eye include the use of diuretics or hormones (e.g., oral contraceptives), lack of adequate tearing (e.g., due to age), certain conditions (e.g., rheumatoid arthritis and to a lesser extent hypertension), air conditioning and low humidity. Dry eye is usually not associated with adherence factors.[86] Rewetting solutions can be used to relieve dryness, but limit use to 1 drop every 4–5 hours. More frequent use can result in red, irritated eyes and a foreign body sensation. No one product is consistently superior to any other, although unpreserved solutions are generally recommended because they minimize the potential for allergic reactions. Lubricants have not been found to be significantly superior to saline.[85] Artificial tears that are not specifically formulated for contact lenses should not be used for rewetting soft lenses because most contain preservatives (e.g., BAC) that can accumulate in the lens matrix.

RGP Lenses

RGP lenses require wetting to reduce the foreign body sensation upon insertion.[87] The mucin layer of the tear film contains highly hydrated polysaccharides that wet the lens. However, this deposition can take up to 15 minutes to develop, during which time the wearer experiences discomfort. A wetting and cushioning solution minimizes the transitional discomfort until the eyes adjust. The solution is applied to the concave side of the lens immediately before insertion. Wetting agents reduce surface tension between tears and the contact lens or between tears and the cornea, allowing tears to spread evenly. Although natural saliva has excellent wetting properties, it contains many potential pathogens and should never be used as a wetting agent.

Lens Cases

Store contact lenses in their cases, completely covered by disinfecting or multipurpose solution.[88] If lenses dry out, their shape can temporarily change, rendering them useless until they can regain their original shape. Maintain storage cases with the same vigilance as lenses, since a dirty case will nullify the previous steps taken in the care of contact lenses. Even in asymptomatic contact lens wearers, the potential risk of fungal keratitis remains.[89] About 40% of bacterial eye infections among contact lens wearers can be attributed to carrying cases. Lens case care was the only area of improvement in an adherence study.[90] Routinely (at least monthly) boil storage cases in water for 10 minutes. Allow the lens case to cool for 30–45 minutes before lenses are placed in it. If a case can not be boiled at least once a month, it should be replaced. Even when cleaned properly on a regular basis, replace a lens case every 3 months. Fortunately, lens case replacement is being incorporated into PRPs. Replace the soaking solution daily. Flush the case of old solution and air-dry it before adding new solution.[91] Digital rubbing, rinsing with multipurpose solution, tissue wiping and air drying face down will reduce contamination further.[92,93] Effective education can improve lens case hygiene.[94]

Monitoring of Therapy

Care can be optimized when contact lens wearers are made aware of the many systemic and ophthalmic medications that can affect contact lenses by altering eye shape, affecting the blink reflex, altering tear volume and composition, concentrating in the lens or discoloring the lens (Table 2 and Table 3). Inform the wearer that drug-lens interactions are possible and can negatively affect the success of contact lens wear. Advise all wearers to maintain a current list of their medications and share it with their eye care professional.

Figure 1: **Steps for Proper Care of Soft Contact Lenses[a,b]**

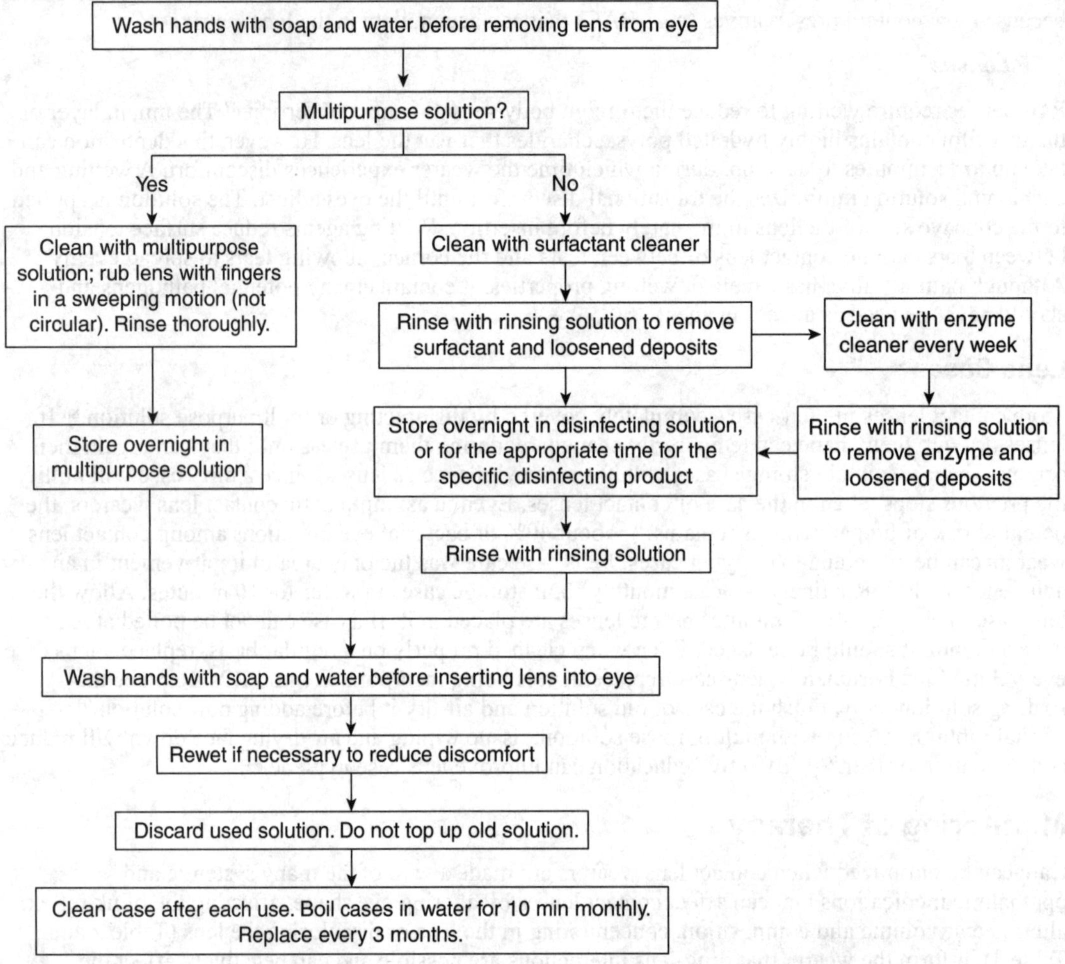

[a] There may be variations to these regimens (e.g., an enzyme cleaner may not be required in a planned replacement program).
[b] With multipurpose solutions, 2 or more functions (usually cleaning and disinfecting, but may include rinsing and storing) are combined in 1 formulation.

Resource Tips

American Optometric Association. Available from: www.aoa.org.

British Contact Lens Association. Available from: www.bcla.org.uk.

Canadian Association of Optometrists. Available from: www.opto.ca.

Contact Lens Association of Ophthalmologists. Available from: www.clao.org.

Suggested Readings

Donshik PC, Ehlers WH, Anderson LD et al. Strategies to better engage, educate, and empower patient compliance and safe lens wear: compliance: what we know, what we do not know, and what we need to know. *Eye Contact Lens* 2007;33:430-3.

Foulks GN. Prolonging contact lens wear and making contact lens wear safer. *Am J Ophthalmol* 2006;141:369-73.

Suchecki JK, Donshik P, Ehlers WH. Contact lens complications. *Ophthalmol Clin North Am* 2003;16:471-84.

Szczotka-Flynn LB, Pearlman E, Ghannoum M. Microbial contamination of contact lenses, lens care solutions and their accessories: a literature review. *Eye Contact Lens* 2010;36:116-29.

U.S. Food and Drug Administration. FDA Executive Summary prepared for the May 13, 2014 Meeting of the Ophthalmic Devices Panel of the Medical Devices Advisory Committee. *Contact lens and care product guidance documents*. Available from: www.fda.gov/downloads/AdvisoryCommittees/CommitteesMeetingMaterials/MedicalDevices/MedicalDevicesAdvisoryCommittee/OphthalmicDevicesPanel/UCM395577.pdf.

U.S. Food and Drug Administration. Hampton D. *Contact lens safety*. Available from: www.fda.gov/downloads/AdvisoryCommittees/CommitteesMeetingMaterials/MedicalDevices/MedicalDevicesAdvisoryCommittee/OphthalmicDevicesPanel/UCM397603.pdf.

Woods CA, Jones DA, Jones LW et al. A seven year survey of the contact lens prescribing habits of Canadian optometrists. *Optom Vis Sci* 2007;84:505-10.

References

1. Alberta Association of Optometrists. *Contact lenses*. Available from: www.optometrists.ab.ca/contact-lenses. Accessed March 22, 2016.
2. Contact Lens Manufacturers Association. *Wouldn't you rather wear contacts than glasses?* Available from: www.contactlenses.org/clsglasses.htm. Accessed March 22, 2016.
3. Woods CA, Jones DA, Jones LW et al. A seven year survey of the contact lens prescribing habits of Canadian optometrists. *Optom Vis Sci* 2007;84:505-10.
4. Contact lenses now. *Drug Ther Bull* 1988;26:39-40.
5. Efron N, Morgan PB, Woods CA et al. International survey of rigid contact lens fitting. *Optom Vis Sci* 2013;90:113-8.
6. Lum VJ, Lyle WM. Chemical components of contact lens solutions. *Can J Optom* 1981;43:136-51.
7. Mandell RB. *Contact lens practice*. 3rd ed. Springfield: Thomas; 1981. p. 495-518.
8. Efron N, Nichols JJ, Woods CA et al. Trends in US contact lens prescribing 2002 to 2014. *Optom Vis Sci* 2015;92:758-67.
9. Sweeney DF. Have silicone hydrogel lenses eliminated hypoxia? *Eye Contact Lens* 2013;39:53-60.
10. Santos L, Rodrigues D, Lira M et al. The influence of surface treatment on hydrophobicity, protein adsorption and microbial colonisation of silicone hydrogel contact lenses. *Cont Lens Anterior Eye* 2007;30:183-8.
11. Robertson DM, Petroll WM, Jester JV et al. The role of contact lens type, oxygen transmission, and care-related solutions in mediating epithelial homeostasis and pseudomonas binding to corneal cells: an overview. *Eye Contact Lens* 2007;33:394-8.
12. Dart JK, Radford CF, Minassian D et al. Risk factors for microbial keratitis with contemporary contact lenses: a case-control study. *Ophthalmology* 2008;115:1647-54.
13. Lane I. Daily disposable: putting them into practice. *Rev Optom* 1995;132:66-8.
14. Gellatly KW. Disposable contact lenses: a clinical performance review. *Can J Optom* 1993;55:166-73.
15. Nason RJ, Boshnick EL, Cannon WM et al. Multisite comparison of contact lens modalities. Daily disposable wear vs. conventional daily wear in successful contact lens wearers. *J Am Optom Assoc* 1994;65:774-80.
16. Boost M, Poon KC, Cho P. Contamination risk of reusing daily disposable contact lenses. *Optom Vis Sci* 2011;88:1409-13.
17. Schein OD, Glynn RJ, Poggio EC et al. The relative risk of ulcerative keratitis among users of daily-wear and extended-wear soft contact lenses. A case-control study. Microbial Keratitis Study Group. *N Engl J Med* 1989;321:773-8, 824-6.
18. Lee SY, Kim YH, Johnson D et al. Contact lens complications in an urgent-care population: the University of California, Los Angeles, contact lens study. *Eye Contact Lens* 2012;38:49-52.
19. Efron N, Morgan PB, Woods CA et al. International survey of contact lens prescribing for extended wear. *Optom Vis Sci* 2012;89:122-9.
20. Suchecki JK, Donshik P, Ehlers WH. Contact lens complications. *Ophthalmol Clin North Am* 2003;16:471-84.
21. Aucamp A. Drug excretion in human tears and its meaning for contact lens wearers. *South Afr Optom* 1980;39:128-36.
22. Chang FW. The possible adverse effects of over-the-counter medications on the contact lens wearer. *J Am Optom Assoc* 1977;48:319-23.
23. Fraunfelder FT. *Drug-induced ocular side effects and drug interactions*. 2nd ed. Philadelphia: Lea & Febiger; 1982.
24. Miller D. Systemic medications. *Int Ophthalmol Clin* 1981;21:177-83.
25. Garston M. When meds disrupt contact lens wear. *Rev Optom* 1993:49-50.
26. Chen SP, Massaro-Giordano G, Pistilli M et al. Tear osmolarity and dry eye symptoms in women using oral contraception and contact lenses. *Cornea* 2013;32:423-8.
27. Farber AS. Ocular side effects of antihistamine-decongestant combinations. *Am J Ophthalmol* 1982;94:565.
28. Koffler BH, Lemp MA. The effect of an antihistamine (chlorpheniramine maleate) on tear production in humans. *Ann Ophthalmol* 1980;12:217-9.
29. Litovitz GL. Amitriptyline and contact lenses. *J Clin Psychiatry* 1984;45:188.
30. Troiano G. Amitriptyline and contact lenses. *J Clin Psychiatry* 1985;46:199.
31. Simmerman JS. Contact lens fitting after Accutane treatment. *Rev Optom* 1985;122:102.
32. Valentic JP, Leopold IH, Dea FJ. Excretion of salicylic acid into tears following oral administration of aspirin. *Ophthalmology* 1980;87:815-20.
33. Lyons RW. Orange contact lenses from rifampin. *N Engl J Med* 1979;300:372-3.
34. Harris J, Jenkins P. Discoloration of soft contact lenses by rifampicin. *Lancet* 1985;2:1133.

35. Riley SA, Flegg PJ, Mandal BK. Contact lens staining due to sulphasalazine. *Lancet* 1986;1:972.
36. Krezanoski JZ. Topical medications. *Int Ophthalmol Clin* 1981;21:173-6.
37. Lemp MA, Hamill JR. Factors affecting tear film breakup in normal eyes. *Arch Ophthalmol* 1973;89:103-5.
38. Hardman Lea SJ, Loades J, Rubinstein MP. The interaction between hydrogel lenses and sodium fluorescein. Theoretical and practical considerations. *Acta Ophthalmol (Copenh)* 1989;67:441-6.
39. Nichols KK, Mitchell GL, Simon KM et al. Corneal staining in hydrogel lens wearers. *Optom Vis Sci* 2002;79:20-30.
40. Foulks GN. Prolonging contact lens wear and making contact lens wear safer. *Am J Ophthalmol* 2006;141:369-73.
41. Donshik PC, Ehlers WH, Anderson LD et al. Strategies to better engage, educate, and empower patient compliance and safe lens wear: compliance: what we know, what we do not know, and what we need to know. *Eye Contact Lens* 2007;33:430-3.
42. Levy B. Infectious keratitis: what have we learned? *Eye Contact Lens* 2007;33:418-20.
43. Willcox MD. New strategies to prevent Pseudomonas keratitis. *Eye Contact Lens* 2007;33:401-3.
44. Kuzman T, Kutija MB, Masnec S et al. Compliance among soft contact lens wearers. *Coll Antropol* 2014;38:1217-21.
45. Dumbleton KA, Spafford MM, Sivak A et al. Exploring compliance: a mixed-methods study of contact lens wearer perspectives. *Optom Vis Sci* 2013;90:898-908.
46. Wilcox MD. Solutions for care of silicone hydrogel lenses. *Eye Contact Lens* 2013;39:24-8.
47. Stapleton F, Edwards K, Keay L et al. Risk factors for moderate and severe microbial keratitis in daily wear contact lens wearers. *Ophthalmology* 2012:119:1516-21.
48. Fraser MN, Wong Q, Shah L et al. Characteristics of an Acanthamoeba keratitis outbreak in British Columbia between 2003 and 2007. *Ophthalmology* 2012;119:1120-5.
49. Robertson DM, Cavanagh HD. Non-compliance with contact lens wear and care practices: a comparative analysis. *Optom Vis Sci* 2011;88:1402-8.
50. McMonnies CW. Improving contact lens compliance by explaining the benefits of compliant procedures. *Cont Lens Anterior Eye* 2011;34:249-52.
51. Bui TH, Cavanagh HD, Robertson DM. Patient compliance during contact lens wear: perceptions, awareness and behavior. *Eye Contact Lens* 2010;36:334-9.
52. Mulford MB, Houlsby RD, Langston JB et al. Rigid lens care revisited. *Contact Lens Forum* 1980:33-43.
53. Roth HW, Roth-Wittig M. Multipurpose solutions for soft lens maintenance. *Int Contact Lens Clin* 1980;7:92-5.
54. Papas EB, Carnt N, Willcox MD et al. Complications associated with care product use during silicone daily wear of hydrogel contact lens. *Eye Contact Lens* 2007;33:392-3.
55. Scheuer C, Zhao F, Erb T et al. Multipurpose solutions and rates of biocidal efficacy. *Eye Contact Lens* 2009;35:88-91.
56. Guillon M, Maissa C. Clinical acceptance of two multipurpose solutions: MPS containing HPMC versus citrate-based MPS without rubbing. *CLAO J* 2002;28:186-91.
57. Borazjani RN, Kilvington S. Effect of a multipurpose contact lens solution on the survival and binding of Acanthamoeba species on contact lenses examined with a no-rub regimen. *Eye Contact Lens* 2005;31:39-45.
58. Stiegemeier MJ, Cedrone R, Evans D et al. Clinical performance of "no rub" multi-purpose solutions. *Cont Lens Anterior Eye* 2004;27:65-74.
59. Mok KH, Cheung RW, Wong BK et al. Effectiveness of no-rub contact lens cleaning on protein removal: a pilot study. *Optom Vis Sci* 2004;81:468-70.
60. Nichols JJ. Deposition rates and lens care influence on galyfilcon A silicone hydrogel lenses. *Optom Vis Sci* 2006;83:751-7.
61. Zhang S, Ahearn DG, Stulting RD et al. Differences among strains of the Fusarium oxysporum-F. solani complexes in their penetration of hydrogel contact lenses and subsequent susceptibility to multipurpose contact lens disinfection solutions. *Cornea* 2007;26:1249-54.
62. Ahearn DG, Zhang S, Stulting RD et al. Fusarium keratitis and contact lens wear: facts and speculations. *Med Mycol* 2008;46:397-410.
63. Cho P, Cheng SY, Chan WY et al. Soft contact lens cleaning: rub or no-rub? *Ophthalmic Physiol Opt* 2009;29:49-57.
64. Kilvington S, Lonnen J. A comparison of regimen methods for the removal and inactivation of bacteria, fungi and Acanthamoeba from two types of silicone hydrogel lenses. *Cont Lens Anterior Eye* 2009;32:73-7.
65. Zhu H, Bandara MB, Vijay AK et al. Importance of rub and rinse in use of multipurpose contact lens solution. *Optom Vis Sci* 2011;88:967-72.
66. Butcko V, McMahon TT, Joslin CE et al. Microbial keratitis and the role of rub and rinsing. *Eye Contact Lens* 2007;33:421-3.
67. Patel A, Hammersmith K. Contact lens-related microbial keratitis: recent outbreaks. *Curr Opin Ophthalmol* 2008;19:302-6.
68. Tu EY, Joslin CE. Recent outbreaks of atypical contact lens-related keratitis: what have we learned? *Am J Ophthalmol* 2010;150:602-8.
69. Choy CK, Cho P, Boost MV. Cytotoxicity of rigid gas-permeable lens care solutions. *Clin Exp Optom* 2013;96:467-71.
70. Sibley MJ, Shih KL, Hu JC. The microbiological benefit of cleaning and rinsing contact lenses. *Int Contact Lens Clin* 1985;12:235-42.
71. Sibley MJ. Cleaning solutions for contact lenses. *Int Contact Lens Clin* 1982;9:291-4.
72. Diefenbach CB, Seibert CK, Davis LJ. Analysis of two "home remedy" contact lens cleaners. *J Am Optom Assoc* 1988;59:518-21.
73. Ernst RR. Sterilization by heat. In: Block SS, ed. *Disinfection, sterilization and preservation.* 2nd ed. Philadelphia: Lea & Febiger; 1977. p. 481-521.
74. Sibley MJ. Disinfection solutions. *Int Ophthalmol Clin* 1981;21:237-47.
75. Penland RL, Wilhelmus KR. Microbiologic analysis of bottled water: is it safe with contact lenses? *Ophthalmology* 1999;106:1500-3.
76. Holden B. A report card on hydrogen peroxide for contact lens disinfection. *CLAO J* 1990;16:S61-4.
77. Johnson & Johnson Vision Care. *2000 survey data.* Markham: Johnson & Johnson Vision Care.
78. Gasset AR, Ramer RM, Katzin D. Hydrogen peroxide sterilization of hydrophilic contact lenses. *Arch Ophthalmol* 1975;93:412-5.
79. Gordon KD. The effect of oxidative disinfecting systems on tinted hydrogel lenses. *Can J Optom* 1989;51:175-6.
80. Anonymous. Contact lens questions and answers. Generic peroxide. *Rev Optom* 1986;123:77.
81. Health Canada. Product confusion alert. Risk of eye injury with improper use of hydrogen peroxide-based contact lens solution. *Health Product InfoWatch* 2016 February. Available from: www.hc-sc.gc.ca/dhp-mps/medeff/bulletin/hpiw-ivps_2016-02-eng.php. Accessed April 6, 2016.
82. Weissman BA, Tari LA. A solution for the dry eye. *Contact Lens Forum* 1982:5-7.
83. Ozkan J, Papas E. Lubricant effects on low Dk and silicone hydrogel lens comfort. *Optom Vis Sci* 2008;85:773-7.
84. Harris MG, Higa CK, Lacey LL et al. The pH of aerosol saline solution. *Optom Vis Sci* 1990;67:84-8.
85. Efron N, Golding TR, Brennan NA. The effect of soft lens lubricants on symptoms and lens dehydration. *CLAO J* 1991;17:114-9.
86. Ramamoorthy P, Nichols JJ. Compliance factors associated with contact lens-related dry eye. *Eye Contact Lens* 2014;40:17-22.
87. Mauger TF, Hill RM. Solutions that soothe. *Contact Lens Forum* 1982:75-7.

88. Simmons PA, Edrington TB, Hsieh L et al. Bacterial contamination rate of soft contact lens cases. *Int Contact Lens Clin* 1991;18:188-91.
89. Mela EK, Anastassiou ED, Gartaganis SP et al. Fungal isolation from disinfection solutions of contact lens storage cases among asymptomatic users. *Eye Contact Lens* 2015;41:87-90.
90. Yung AM, Boost MV, Cho P et al. The effect of a compliance enhancement strategy (self-review) on the level of lens care compliance and contamination of contact lenses and lens case accessories. *Clin Exp Optom* 2007;90:190-202.
91. Larragoiti ND, Diamos ME, Simmons PA et al. A comparative study of techniques for decreasing contact lens storage contamination. *J Am Optom Assoc* 1994;65:161-3.
92. Wu YT, Teng YJ, Nicholas M et al. Impact of lens case hygiene guidelines on contact lens case contamination. *Optom Vis Sci* 2011;88:E1180-7.
93. Wu YT, Zhu H, Willcox M et al. The effectiveness of various cleaning regimens and current guidelines in contact lens case biofilm removal. *Invest Ophthalmol Vis Sci* 2011;52:5287-92.
94. Tilia D, Lazon de la Jara P, Zhu H et al. The effect of compliance on contact lens case contamination. *Optom Vis Sci* 2014;91:262-71.

Contact Lenses and Cosmetics—What You Need to Know

People who wear contact lenses must be very careful when using cosmetics and other products. Some products (such as mascara or sprays) can irritate the eyes if they get on or under the lenses. To avoid eye problems, choose products carefully and use them safely.

How to use cosmetics safely:

- Before handling your lenses, wash your hands and fingers well with soap and water to remove any product that could irritate your eyes (examples—perfume, cologne, lotion, suntan oil, nail polish and remover).
- **Do not** apply cosmetics if your eyes are swollen, red or infected.
- Apply cosmetics, nail polish, hand creams and perfumes **after** inserting lenses.
- Remove lenses **before** removing makeup.
- Apply eye makeup lightly and remove it daily.
- Use oil-free and fragrance-free eye makeup.
- Use a good quality "water-resistant" mascara that does not flake off. Avoid "waterproof" mascara, which likely contains oils.
- Choose cream eye shadow instead of powder.
- Make sure anyone giving you advice on cosmetics knows that you wear contact lenses.
- Never use another person's eye makeup. It may contain bacteria that are dangerous to your eyes.
- Remove your lenses before using hair dye, bleach, perm lotion or medicated shampoo.
- Protect your eyes and your lenses when using spray products (such as deodorant or hair spray). Close your eyes when you spray, then walk away from the area. Use pump sprays if possible. If spray particles get on your lenses, you may have to replace them.
- If you have to remove your lenses temporarily while wearing makeup, you can avoid smearing your makeup by tilting your head to one side after putting your lenses back in. This makes the tears run to the side.

Chapter 15

Dry Eye

Anne M. Friesen, BSc(Pharm), MSc

Pathophysiology

Anatomy/Physiology

The lacrimal functional unit is composed of the lacrimal glands, the ocular surface (cornea and conjunctiva), meibomian glands, eyelids and the sensory and motor nerves that connect them. This unit controls the production of the tear film and responds to environmental, endocrine and cortical influences in order to maintain the tear film, the transparency of the cornea and the quality of the image projected onto the retina.

The tear film is composed of 3 layers:

- The mucous layer is the layer closest to the eye and contains multiple mucins, produced by goblet cells in the conjunctiva. It stabilizes the tear film by interacting with epithelial layers in the cornea and conjunctiva and the aqueous layer. It also removes waste materials such as mucous threads and fibrils.
- The aqueous layer is the thickest part of the tear film and is produced by the lacrimal glands. It contains inorganic salts, glucose, urea, trace elements, antibacterial proteins (including lactoferrin and lysozyme), vitamins (particularly vitamin A) and growth factors. This layer hydrates the mucous layer, supplies oxygen and electrolytes to the ocular surface and provides antibacterial defense and wound healing.
- The lipid layer is primarily secreted by the meibomian glands and is the outermost layer of the tear film. It is responsible for slowing tear evaporation, enhancing tear film spreading and providing a smooth optical surface.

Although this is the classic view of the tear film, it is probably better described as a hydrated, mucin gel, where the mucin concentration is highest at the epithelial cell surface (the eye) and lowest as it comes in contact with the air.[1,2]

Dry Eye Disease

The International Dry Eye Workshop (2007) defined dry eye disease (DED) as "a multifactorial disease of the tears and ocular surface that results in symptoms of discomfort, visual disturbance, and tear film instability with potential damage to the ocular surface. It is accompanied by increased osmolarity of the tear film and inflammation of the ocular surface".[3]

DED has 2 major classifications: aqueous tear-deficient dry eye (Table 1) and evaporative dry eye (Table 2). However, there can be considerable overlap between these classes and DED may involve multiple mechanisms.[1,3,4,5,7] For example, contact lens wearers may experience decreased corneal sensitivity with reflex sensory block, leading to aqueous deficiency. These patients may also blink less, which can result in increased tear evaporation. There may also be incomplete lid closure during blinking, leading to further evaporation of the tear film. If the patient is also taking a medication with anticholinergic side effects, tear secretion may be decreased even further.[8]

Regardless of the mechanism(s) for the development of DED, the impact on a patient's quality of life can be significant. Severe DED may result in ocular surface erosions, epithelial damage and, rarely, ocular surface keratinization, ulceration, perforation, scarring and markedly reduced vision.[1,3,5,9,10]

Aging is a risk factor for the development of DED.[3,4,5,11] Also, DED occurs more often in females; however, this may be more related to the finding that androgen deficiency promotes meibomian gland dysfunction (MGD), leading to evaporative DED.

Occupational risk factors include prolonged visual attention to a task (e.g., looking through a microscope, working at a computer) resulting in a reduced blink rate.[3,4] Tasks that require an upward gaze (e.g., playing billiards) can expose more of the ocular surface, resulting in greater tear film evaporation. Likewise, patients with a naturally wider palpebral aperture expose more of the ocular surface to evaporation.

Environmental factors that lead to DED include low humidity, high temperature, wind or high air velocity and air pollution (e.g., tobacco smoke).[1,3,4,12] A diet low in omega-3 fatty acids or vitamin A may also contribute to DED.

Systemic medications may play an important role in the development or progression of DED (see Prevention).[3,4,5,8,13,14]

Diagnosis of DED can prove difficult as symptoms do not necessarily reflect the severity of the disease.[1,3,4] Patients who are highly symptomatic may not have clinical evidence of DED, while some patients who already have damage to the ocular surface may not complain of symptoms. This lack of concordance between signs and symptoms makes it difficult for investigators to meet primary efficacy endpoints in DED trials.

Goals of Therapy

- Ease patient discomfort and minimize symptoms
- Prevent or delay complications
- Educate patients about their condition and encourage adherence, especially in those with long-term disease

Table 1: **Classification of Aqueous Tear-deficient Dry Eye**

Non-Sjögren[1,3,4,5]	**Lacrimal gland deficiency**	**Primary:** Age-related, congenital alacrima, familial dysautonomia
		Secondary: Lacrimal gland infiltration, e.g., in sarcoidosis, lymphoma, AIDS, graft-versus-host disease; lacrimal gland ablation; lacrimal gland denervation
	Lacrimal duct obstruction	Trachoma, cicatricial pemphigoid, mucous membrane pemphigoid, erythema multiforme, chemical and thermal burns
	Reflex hyposecretion	**Sensory block:** Secondary to factors that decrease corneal sensation including corneal surgery (e.g., LASIK, PRK), contact lens wear, diabetes mellitus, ophthalmic infection (e.g., herpes simplex keratitis, herpes zoster ophthalmicus), neurotrophic keratitis
		Motor block: Secondary to damage to the VII cranial nerve; neuromatosis; systemic medication use
Sjögren[6]	**Primary**	Autoimmune disease affecting exocrine glands
	Secondary	Associated with other autoimmune diseases, e.g., rheumatoid arthritis, systemic lupus erythematosus

Table 2: **Classification of Evaporative Dry Eye**[1,3,4,5]

Intrinsic	**Meibomian gland dysfunction**: Associated with dermatoses such as acne rosacea, seborrheic dermatitis and atopic dermatitis
	Medications: Isotretinoin therapy
	Disorders of lid aperture: Exophthalmos (hyperthyroidism; eyelid deformity; poor lid apposition)
	Low blink rate: Parkinson's disease
Extrinsic	**Decreased blink rate**: Tends to occur during activities such as reading, watching television, computer work
	Ocular surface abnormalities: Vitamin A deficiency; exposure to eye drops containing benzalkonium chloride or anesthetic agents
	Contact lens wear
	Allergic conjunctivitis

Patient Assessment

An algorithm for the assessment of eye conditions is presented in Chapter 12: Assessment of Patients with Eye Conditions.

Patients with DED may complain of a foreign body sensation in the eye.[3,4,5] Words like "sandy" or "scratchy" are used to convey this symptom. Eyes often feel like they are burning, itchy or tired. Other symptoms include photophobia, blurred vision, redness, discomfort and difficulty in moving the lids.

Although most patients state that their eyes feel dry, some will report increased tearing, especially when exposed to wind or when concentrating on tasks such as reading or computer work.[3,4,5] This is a reflex tearing that does little to increase comfort.

Unlike blepharitis and conjunctivitis, dry eye symptoms tend to worsen over the course of the day.[3,4]

Prevention

Many systemic medications have the potential to cause DED, including amiodarone, antiandrogenic agents, anticholinergics or medications with anticholinergic side effects, beta-blockers, diuretics, interferon, isotretinoin and postmenopausal hormone replacement therapy.[3,15,16] Natural health products have also been known to cause DED; niacin, echinacea, kava kava, and herbal products that contain anticholinergic alkaloids have all been associated with DED.[17] Frequent use of eye drops, particularly those containing benzalkonium chloride as a preservative, may contribute to DED by further damaging the ocular surface.[18,19,20] Advise patients of this potential effect and provide treatment options in case it occurs.

Contact lens wearers need to pay careful attention to proper cleaning and wear of their lenses (see Chapter 14: Contact Lens Care). It is common to blink less frequently during activities requiring concentration such as reading, computer work and video games; remind patients to blink more often during these activities. Encourage patients with chronic blepharitis to maintain lid hygiene. Ask patients with autoimmune or dermatologic diseases (e.g., Sjögren syndrome, rheumatoid arthritis, systemic lupus erythematosus, acne rosacea) about any symptoms of dry eye. Because of the severity of DED that has been associated with these diseases, referral to an eye care practitioner may be suggested to optimize therapy and prevent complications.

Nonpharmacologic Therapy

Nonpharmacologic therapy of DED may involve environmental changes.[6,9,13,21] Encourage patients to avoid smoking and smoky rooms since tobacco smoke is a common cause of eye irritation. Humidifiers, especially in winter, can improve conditions for dry eye sufferers. Moisture chamber spectacles, or ski or swim goggles, can be worn to increase humidity in the eye area as well as decrease the evaporation of tears. A moistened gauze placed inside the goggles helps maintain a moist environment. A cool, moist washcloth placed over closed eyelids may provide short-term relief.

In severe or chronic DED, tear duct (punctal) occlusion may be used to prevent drainage of existing tears via the nasolacrimal ducts. Punctal plugs, inserted by an eye care practitioner trained in this technique, are used to assess whether a patient will benefit from this treatment.[3,15,21,22,23] It is possible to dislodge the plugs, especially if patients rub their eyelids. Therefore, nasolacrimal occlusion for eye drop instillation is not recommended or required in patients with punctal plugs. Permanent occlusion can be achieved through heat or electrocautery but can also occur spontaneously following insertion of punctal plugs, and can persist even after the plugs are lost.[24]

Pharmacologic Therapy

For comparative ingredients of nonprescription products, consult the *Compendium of Products for Minor Ailments*—Ophthalmic Products: Ocular Lubricants.

Pharmacologic therapy generally begins with administration of **artificial tears** that contain a volume-enhancing agent to supplement tear production or an **ocular lubricant** that contains a contact-enhancing agent to help retain existing tears.[3,21] Artificial tear drops have demonstrated efficacy for relieving symptoms of DED in several clinical trials.[25]

Although there are a number of solutions available, it is difficult to identify the solution of choice in DED. Clinical trials do not provide definitive conclusions because of the difficulty in meeting primary efficacy endpoints. Much of the information relating to pharmacologic treatments is proprietary, and large, head-to-head clinical trials are lacking.[25] Until more evidence is available, choosing the best therapy is achieved through a trial and error approach.[2,3,15,16,21,23,26,27] This can be frustrating, both for the patient and for the healthcare practitioner. A 1- to 2-week trial of eye drops is needed to determine the subjective efficacy of the product (patient comfort, improvement in symptoms).

Consider the following factors in choosing a tear replacement product:

- Electrolyte composition:[3,15,16,21,23] Potassium and bicarbonate are the most critical electrolytes. Potassium is important in maintaining corneal thickness, while bicarbonate appears to aid the recovery of epithelial barrier function in a cornea that has already been damaged. It may also be important in maintaining the mucous layer of the tear film
- Crystalloid osmolarity (the concentration of small dissolved particles, such as ions):[3,15,16,21,23] Patients with DED have a higher tear film osmolarity than the normal population. This results in biochemical changes to the cornea and a pro-inflammatory state. Hypo-osmotic tears were developed to counteract this increased osmolarity
- Colloidal osmolality (the concentration of macromolecules or compatible solutes):[3,15,16,21,23] Also known as oncotic pressure, this relates to water transport across the ocular surface epithelium. An artificial tear product with a high colloidal osmolality could protect against epithelial damage from hyperosmolar tears by stabilizing the volume of corneal epithelial cells. Compatible solutes (e.g., glycerin) are taken up by cells, increasing intracellular osmolarity so that the cells do not have to increase their internal electrolyte concentration to achieve the same goal
- Viscosity agents:[3,7,15,16,18,23] Artificial tear products with higher viscosity increase tear retention time and help protect the ocular surface. However, they are merely a palliative treatment. These agents include substituted cellulose ethers such as **carboxymethyl cellulose** and **hypromellose**

(hydroxypropylmethylcellulose), **polyvinyl alcohol**, **polyethylene glycol**, **glycol 400** and **propylene glycol**. **Hydroxypropyl-guar** (HP-guar) appears to form a bioadhesive gel when exposed to the eye, protecting the eye by mimicking the mucous layer of the tear film. **Castor oil** or **mineral oil** may be used in ocular lubricants to decrease tear evaporation by restoring the lipid layer of the tear film. **Sodium hyaluronate** is a polysaccharide polymer that acts as a viscoelastic solution at physiologic pH, with a viscosity 500 000 times that of saline. Ophthalmic solutions in concentrations of 0.1–0.5% have been successful in treating symptoms of dry eye. **Carbomer** resins are synthetic high molecular weight polymers of acrylic acid cross-linked to a polyalkyl polyether. Although carbomer 940 resembles an ointment, it causes less blurred vision than petrolatum-based ophthalmic ointments

- Cytotoxic additives:[3,15,16,21,23] **Ethylenediaminetetraacetic acid** (EDTA), an additive in some eye drops, can damage corneal epithelial cells. **Lanolin** is an additive in some ophthalmic ointments but can cause ocular irritation especially in patients who are sensitive to wool
- Preservatives:[3,28,29,30]
  - Advise patients with mild dry eye who require more than 4 applications per day for long periods of time to use a preservative-free product to prevent toxicity. The detergent preservative **benzalkonium chloride** is the most frequently used preservative in eye drops. However, it is known to be toxic to the corneal epithelium. Advise patients with moderate to severe DED to avoid benzalkonium chloride whenever possible[3,4,15,18]
  - Oxidative preservatives, such as **polyquaternium-1** (Polyquad), **sodium chlorite** (Purite) or **sodium perborate** are safer alternatives to benzalkonium chloride. The latter 2 preservatives are termed "vanishing" preservatives: sodium chlorite degrades to chloride ions and water after instillation, while sodium perborate converts to water and oxygen after making contact with the tear film. However, these preservatives may not always disappear completely in patients with moderate to severe DED because of decreased tear volume
  - Ophthalmic ointments do not support bacterial growth and generally do not require preservatives. **Petrolatum**-containing ophthalmic ointments have a longer retention time in the eye than drops but can cause unacceptable blurred vision. This limits their application to bedtime use for most patients.

A long-acting artificial tear containing **hyprolose** (hydroxypropylcellulose) is available as an insert to be placed in the conjunctival sac daily or twice daily, depending on dry eye severity. It dissolves over several hours, allowing long-term ocular lubrication. Blurred vision is common for the first few hours, but it is preservative-free. Manual dexterity and education are required for proper insertion. Ophthalmic anti-inflammatories such as **cyclosporine** and **loteprednol** are used in the management of patients who are not responsive to ocular lubricants and artificial tears.[31]

Autologous serum eye drops have been used to treat DED.[32,33] They contain biologically active substances required to maintain the tear film, which are believed to be a better substitute than artificial tears. Concerns about autologous serum eye drops include the risk of microbial growth in the protein-rich product and the risks associated with periodic patient blood draws. The optimal concentration and diluent are also unknown. A Cochrane review reported insufficient evidence to prove the safety and efficacy of autologous serum eye drops for the treatment of DED; high-quality randomized control trials are required.[34]

Other treatments that have been investigated for severe dry eye include topical **acetylcysteine**[9,18,21] (removes excessive mucus), topical **methylprednisolone**,[35] topical **estradiol**[36] and periorbital intramuscular injections of **botulinum toxin**.[37]

For more detailed information regarding ophthalmic products used in the management of dry eye disease, consult the *Compendium of Therapeutic Choices*: Red Eye.

Patients with meibomian gland dysfunction associated–DED may benefit from **omega-3 fatty acid**–rich foods or supplementation.[38,39] Omega-3 fatty acids are thought to have anti-inflammatory properties which may reduce the inflammatory component of DED.[40,41,42] Preliminary evidence suggests that even **omega-6 fatty acids**, which are considered pro-inflammatory, show some benefit in decreasing the symptoms of DED.[40] Randomized controlled trials have demonstrated that supplementation with omega-3 fatty acids increases tear break-up time (TBUT) and significantly improves dry eye symptoms.[43,44] Encourage patients to consume higher amounts of food rich in omega-3 fatty acids (herring, mackerel, salmon, sardines, tuna, canola oil, chia, and pumpkin and sunflower seeds). **Flaxseed** and **flaxseed oil** are other sources of omega-3 fatty acids.[40,45]

Oral **pilocarpine** is indicated for the treatment of dry eye associated with Sjögren syndrome.[46]

Monitoring of Therapy

Patients with intermittent symptoms of dry eye can be treated effectively with 1 or more of the numerous ocular lubricants available. The patient should be assessed if symptoms do not resolve within 3–5 days or if they worsen.

Signs of preservative toxicity include stinging upon instillation and conjunctival inflammation.[3,4,15,18] If these symptoms are present, the patient may need a product with a different preservative, a preservative-free product or referral for assessment.

Periodic assessment of eye drop and ointment instillation technique will help patients make best use of the agents (see Chapter 16: Eyelid Conditions: Hordeolum, Chalazion and Blepharitis, Proper Use of Eye Drops, Proper Use of Eye Ointments—What You Need to Know). Devices such as the Auto-Drop and Auto-Squeeze (Owen Mumford, www.owenmumford.com) are usually available through local wholesalers and can be offered to patients to aid in ocular medication administration.

Resource Tips

eMedicine from WebMD. Foster CS, Yuksel E. *Dry eye syndrome*. Available from: emedicine.medscape.com. Registration required.

Suggested Readings

Bron AJ, Tomlinson A, Foulks GN et al. Rethinking dry eye disease: a perspective on clinical implications. *Ocul Surf* 2014;12:S1-31.

Pucker AD, Ng SM, Nichols JJ. Over the counter (OTC) artifical tear drops for dry eye syndrome. *Cochrane Database Syst Rev* 2016;2:CD009729.

Tear Film and Ocular Surface Society (TFOS). *Introduction to the 2007 report of the International Dry Eye Workshop*. Available from: www.tearfilm.org/dewsreport.

References

1. Lemp MA. Advances in understanding and managing dry eye disease. *Am J Ophthalmol* 2008;146:350-6.
2. Tavares FdeP, Fernandes RS, Bernandes TF et al. Dry eye disease. *Semin Ophthalmol* 2010;25:84-93.
3. 2007 report of the International Dry Eye Workshop (DEWS). *Ocul Surf* 2007;5:65-204.
4. Perry HD. Dry eye disease: pathophysiology, classification, and diagnosis. *Am J Manag Care* 2008;14:S79-87.
5. eMedicine from WebMD. Foster CS, Yuksel E. *Dry eye syndrome*. Available from: emedicine.medscape.com. Registration required.
6. Friedlaender MH. Ocular manifestations of Sjögren's Syndrome: keratoconjunctivitis sicca. *Rheum Dis Clin North Am* 1992;18:591-608.
7. Semes L. Diagnosis and primary care management of tear film deficiencies. *Optom Clin* 1995;4:87-104.
8. Jaanus SD, Bartlett JD, Hiett JA. Ocular effects of systemic drugs. In: Bartlett JD, Jaanus SD, eds. *Clinical ocular pharmacology*. 3rd ed. Boston: Butterworth-Heinemann; 1995. p. 957-1006.
9. Sullivan JH, Crawford JB, Witcher JP. Lids, lacrimal apparatus, and tears. In: Vaughan D, Asbury T, Riordan-Eva P, eds. *General ophthalmology*. 15th ed. Stamford: Appleton & Lange; 1999. p. 74-91.
10. Pflugfelder SC. Advances in the diagnosis and management of keratoconjunctivitis sicca. *Curr Opin Ophthalmol* 1998;9:50-3.
11. Shimazaki J, Goto E, Ono M et al. Meibomian gland dysfunction in patients with Sjögren syndrome. *Ophthalmology* 1998;105:1485-8.

12. Gaby AR. Nutritional therapies for ocular disorders: part three. *Altern Med Rev* 2008;13:191-204.
13. Asbell PA, Torres MA. Therapeutic dilemmas in external ocular diseases. *Drugs* 1991;42:606-15.
14. Fraunfelder FT. *Drug-induced ocular side effects*. 4th ed. Baltimore: Williams & Wilkins; 1996.
15. Lemp MA. Management of dry eye disease. *Am J Manag Care* 2008;14:S88-101.
16. Foulks GN. Treatment of dry eye disease by the non-ophthalmologist. *Rheum Dis Clin North Am* 2008;34:987-1000.
17. Askeroglu U, Alleyne B, Guyuron B. Pharmaceutical and herbal products that may contribute to dry eyes. *Plast Reconstr Surg* 2013;131:159-67.
18. Jaanus SD. Lubricants and other preparations for ocular surface disease. In: Bartlett JD, Jaanus SD, eds. *Clinical ocular pharmacology*. 3rd ed. Boston: Butterworth-Heinemann; 1995. p. 355-67.
19. Baudouin C, Pisella PJ, Fillacier K et al. Ocular surface inflammatory changes induced by topical antiglaucoma drugs: human and animal studies. *Ophthalmology* 1999;106:556-63.
20. Semes LP, Clompus RJ. Diseases of the lacrimal system. In: Bartlett JD, Jaanus SD, eds. *Clinical ocular pharmacology*. 3rd ed. Boston: Butterworth-Heinemann; 1995. p. 601-30.
21. Fechner PU, Teichmann KD. *Ocular therapeutics: pharmacology and clinical application*. Thorofare: SLACK; 1998.
22. Cohen EJ. Punctal occlusion. *Arch Ophthalmol* 1999;117:389-90.
23. Latkany R. Dry eyes: etiology and management. *Curr Opin Ophthalmol* 2008;19:287-91.
24. Karcioglu ZA, Fleming JC. Long-term retention rates and complications of silicone punctal plugs in dry eye. *Am J Ophthalmol* 2008;145:586.
25. Pucker AD, Ng SM, Nichols JJ. Over the counter (OTC) artifical tear drops for dry eye syndrome. *Cochrane Database Syst Rev* 2016;2:CD009729.
26. Fiscella, RG. Understanding dry eye disease: a managed care perspective. *Am J Manag Care* 2011;17:S432-9.
27. Shields SR. Managing eye disease in primary care. Part 2. How to recognize and treat common eye problems. *Postgrad Med* 2000;108:83-6, 91-6.
28. Gobbels M, Spitznas M. Corneal epithelial permeability of dry eyes before and after treatment with artificial tears. *Ophthalmology*1992;99:873-8.
29. Lopez Bernal D, Ubels JL. Quantitative evaluation of the corneal epithelial barrier: effect of artificial tears and preservatives. *Curr Eye Res* 1991;10:645-56.
30. Lopez Bernal D, Ubels JL. Artificial tear composition and promotion of recovery of the damaged corneal epithelium. *Cornea* 1993;12:115-20.
31. Pavesio CE, Decory HH. Treatment of ocular inflammatory conditions with loteprednol etabonate. *Br J Ophthalmol* 2008;92:455-9.
32. Hussain M, Shtein RM, Sugar A et al. Long-term use of autologous serum 50% eye drops for the treatment of dry eye disease. *Cornea* 2014;33:1245-51.
33. Celebi AR, Ulusoy C, Mirza GE. The efficacy of autologous serum eye drops for severe dry eye syndrome: a randomized double-blind crossover study. *Graefes Arch Clin Exp Ophthalmol* 2014;252:619-26.
34. Pan Q, Angelina A, Zambrano A et al. Autologous serum eye drops for dry eye. *Cochrane Database System Rev* 2013;8:CD009327.
35. Marsh P, Pflugfelder SC. Topical nonpreserved methylprednisolone therapy for keratoconjunctivitis sicca in Sjögren syndrome. *Ophthalmology* 1999;106:811-6.
36. Sator MO, Joura EA, Golaszewski T et al. Treatment of menopausal keratoconjunctivitis sicca with topical oestradiol. *Br J Obstet Gynaecol* 1998;105:100-2.
37. Spiera H, Asbell PA, Simpson DM. Botulinum toxin increases tearing in patients with Sjögren's syndrome: a preliminary report. *J Rheumatol* 1997;24:1842-3.
38. Pinna A, Piccinini P, Carta F. Effect of oral linoleic and gamma-linolenic acid on meibomian gland dysfunction. *Cornea* 2007;26:260-4.
39. Macsai MS. The role of omega-3 dietary supplementation in blepharitis and meibomian gland dysfunction (an AOS thesis). *Trans Am Ophthalmol Soc* 2008;106:336-56.
40. Rand AL, Asbell PA. Nutritional supplements for dry eye syndrome. *Curr Opin Ophthalmol* 2011;22:279-82.
41. Dogru M, Tsubota K. Pharmacotherapy of dry eye. *Expert Opin Pharmcother* 2011;12:325-34.
42. Al Mahmood AM, Al-Swailem SA. Essential fatty acids in the treatment of dry eye syndrome. A myth or reality? *Saudi J Ophthalmol* 2014;23:195-7.
43. Bhargava R, Kumar P, Kumar M et al. A randomized controlled trial of omega-3 fatty acids in dry eye syndrome. *Int J Ophthalmol* 2013;6:811-6.
44. Bhargava R, Kumar P, Phogat H et al. Oral omega-3 fatty acids treatment in computer vision syndrome related dry eye. *Cont Lens Anterior Eye* 2015;38:206-10.
45. Lewin GA, Schachter HM, Yuen D et al. Effects of omega-3 fatty acids on child and maternal health. *Evid Rep Technol Assess (Summ)* 2005;118:1-11.
46. Vivino FB, Al-Hashimi I, Khan Z et al. Pilocarpine tablets for the treatment of dry mouth and dry eye symptoms in patients with Sjögren syndrome: a randomized, placebo-controlled, fixed-dose, multicenter trial. P92-01 Study Group. *Arch Intern Med* 1999;159:174-81.

Chapter 16

Eyelid Conditions: Hordeolum, Chalazion and Blepharitis

Anne M. Friesen, BSc(Pharm), MSc

Eye Anatomy

Eyelids and lashes protect the globe (eyeball) from foreign bodies and injuries and help maintain a wet corneal surface. The eyelid is a complex structure of skin, muscle and fibrous tissue. The skin of the eyelid is among the thinnest anywhere on the body, which allows for the mobility of the eyelids. Underneath the skin lies loose, areolar tissue that is capable of significant edema and swelling. The next layer is the orbicularis muscle, responsible for closing the eyelids and innervated by the seventh cranial nerve.[1,2]

Posteriorly in the eyelid is the tarsus, a dense fibrous connective tissue plate that supports the lid margins and forms the skeleton of the eyelid (Figure 1). Modified sebaceous glands, known as meibomian glands, are contained within the tarsal plates and secrete the lipid layer of the tear film. There are 20–30 glands in the upper lid and 10–20 in the lower lid.[1,2,3]

The glands of Zeis and Moll lie in the anterior section of the eyelid. Zeis's glands are modified sebaceous glands that are associated with the lash follicles. Moll's glands are modified sweat glands whose ducts open either into a lash follicle or directly onto the anterior lid margin between the lashes (Figure 2).[4]

Figure 1: **Anatomy of the Eyelids and Anterior Eye**

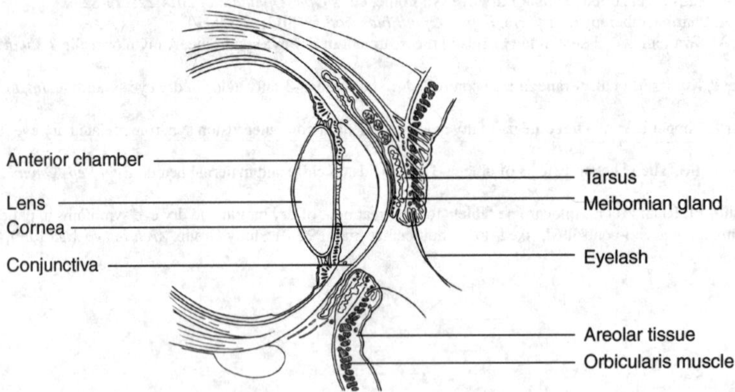

Figure 2: **Cross-section of Upper Eyelid**

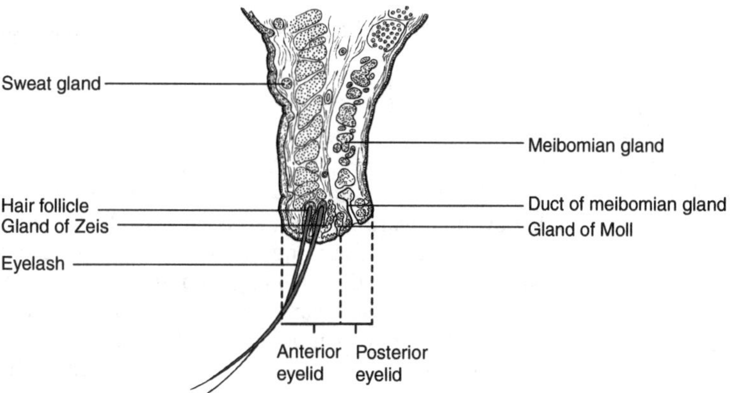

Hordeolum

Pathophysiology

A hordeolum (stye) is an infection of the sebaceous glands of the eyelids. It is the most common eyelid infection in ophthalmology.[3,5,6,7] When the glands of Zeis are involved, the infection is smaller, more superficial and referred to as an external hordeolum. In this type of infection the lesion always points toward the skin. An internal hordeolum is marked by a larger swelling that usually involves the meibomian glands, and the lesion can point either to the skin or to the conjunctival surface. As compared with the external stye, the internal hordeolum generally has a more prolonged course because it rarely drains spontaneously. Microbiologic cultures are seldom required for either type of hordeolum since the most common infecting organism is *Staphylococcus aureus*.

Goals of Therapy

- Resolve infection
- Prevent recurrence
- Prevent transmission to other eye or to household contacts

Patient Assessment

Patients with hordeolum present with unilateral, localized lid swelling, tenderness and erythema. The amount of discomfort increases with the degree of lid swelling. Hordeola are often associated with blepharitis and have a tendency to recur.[2,5]

An algorithm for the assessment of eye conditions is presented in Chapter 12: Assessment of Patients with Eye Conditions.

Prevention

A common sense approach to avoid infecting the fellow eye or transmitting the infection to other persons in the household includes the following instructions for the patient:

- Avoid touching the eyes and wash the hands after any contact with the infected eye.
- Change compresses and towels after each use.

- Take care not to allow the tip of eye drop bottles or ophthalmic ointments to touch the eye or eyelashes.

Conscientious attention to treating symptoms of blepharitis may help to decrease the incidence of recurrent hordeola.

Nonpharmacologic Therapy

External hordeola usually drain spontaneously within 48 hours, but warm compresses applied for 10–15 minutes 3 or 4 times a day may hasten resolution.[2,3,8] Following the application of warm compresses, gently massaging the eyelid toward the lid margin can also be helpful. Warm tap water is sufficient to use in compresses. There is a risk of burning the skin when using the microwave to heat warm compresses.[9] One study showed that a hard-boiled egg, kept in the shell, retained heat longer than a warm compress.[10] The authors suggest that a hard-boiled egg wrapped in a handkerchief or compress is a convenient and cost-effective way to apply heat to the eyelid. The same egg can be reboiled prior to each application. Caution patients against applying pressure on the warm compress or hard-boiled egg, as corneal deformation can occur resulting in blurred vision (usually transient following short-term use).[11,12] If patients find it difficult to control the amount of pressure using the hard-boiled egg, they may try bending forward and holding the wrapped egg close to the eye without touching it.[11] Patients should seek medical advice if they have external hordeola that do not spontaneously drain within 48 hours. In these situations incision and drainage may be required.[2,3,8,13]

Acute internal hordeola generally resolve within 1–2 weeks and can be treated with warm compresses for 5–10 minutes several times a day. Patients should seek medical advice if they have internal hordeola that do not resolve spontaneously in 1 week.[13,14]

Pharmacologic Therapy

Self-medication with nonprescription ophthalmic antibacterials is not necessary and is not recommended.[15]

If incision and drainage are required, an ophthalmic antibacterial ointment such as **bacitracin** or **erythromycin**, applied to the conjunctival sac several times a day, may help prevent further infection.[2,3,8] The presence of cellulitis is an indication for the use of systemic antibacterials.

For further discussion of pharmacologic therapy for bacterial eye infections, consult the *Compendium of Therapeutic Choices*: Red Eye.

Chalazion

Pathophysiology

A chalazion is an idiopathic, sterile, chronic inflammation of a meibomian gland. Blockage of the meibomian gland orifices results in stagnation of sebaceous secretions.[2,8,16] A lesion develops over a period of weeks and is characterized by painless, localized swelling. Most chalazia point toward the conjunctival surface, causing conjunctival redness and swelling.

Chalazia are more common in people with blepharitis, acne rosacea or seborrheic dermatitis. Other risk factors for chalazion include smoking, gastritis and irritable bowel syndrome.[17] These patients are also at greater risk of developing multiple or recurrent chalazia. Patients with recurrent or persistent chalazion require evaluation for more serious conditions such as meibomian gland carcinoma.

Goals of Therapy

- Resolve lesion
- Prevent recurrence

Patient Assessment

The initial symptoms of chalazion (mild inflammation and tenderness) may resemble hordeolum, but without the acute inflammatory signs.[1,2,16] Chalazia may be distinguished from hordeola by the lack of pain.[18] Large chalazia may press on the eyeball and cause astigmatism or visual distortion. An algorithm for the assessment of eye conditions is presented in Chapter 12: Assessment of Patients with Eye Conditions.

Prevention

Encourage patients who have recurrent chalazia associated with blepharitis to maintain good lid hygiene (see Blepharitis, Nonpharmacologic Therapy). Advise patients with dermatologic conditions such as acne rosacea and seborrheic dermatitis to adhere to treatment of these conditions. Encourage and support smoking cessation.

Nonpharmacologic Therapy

Initial treatment for chalazion is similar to that for hordeolum, especially for small lesions.[16,19,20] Warm compresses, applied several times a day, are used to soften sebaceous secretions that may be blocking meibomian gland orifices. Approximately 25–50% of lesions resolve with this treatment. Following the application of warm compresses, gently massaging the eyelid toward the lid margin may also be helpful.

Further assessment is required if the lesion does not begin to resolve within a few days of initiating warm compress treatment. Immediate referral to an appropriate healthcare practitioner is required for patients experiencing eye pain or impaired vision.

Pharmacologic Therapy

Self-medication with nonprescription ophthalmic antibacterials is not necessary and is not recommended for chalazia.[1,16,18]

Larger chalazia may require surgical excision, **intralesional steroid injections**, or both.[16,19,20] These procedures should be performed by an ophthalmologist. When excision is required, the ophthalmologist makes a vertical incision on the conjunctival surface, followed by careful curettement of the gelatinous material. Topical antibacterials or corticosteroid drops may be prescribed after surgery to prevent infection and decrease inflammation. The presence of cellulitis is an indication for the use of systemic antibacterials. For further information on ophthalmic therapy, consult the *Compendium of Therapeutic Choices*: Red Eye.

Blepharitis

Pathophysiology

Blepharitis is a chronic condition, with periods of exacerbation, that usually affects the eyelids bilaterally.[6,7] Although the different types can be defined as anterior and posterior, blepharitis often occurs as a mixed condition in patients, making it difficult to accurately diagnose and treat. It is often associated with chronic dermatologic conditions such as acne rosacea and seborrheic dermatitis,[21] as well as pterygia, ulcerative colitis, irritable bowel syndrome, anxiety and gastritis.[22] These conditions must also be treated, for optimal control of blepharitis.

Long-term complications of this chronic disorder include physical damage to the eyelids and the cornea.[6,7] Inflammation of the cornea can result in scarring, loss of surface smoothness and loss of visual acuity. If the inflammation is severe, corneal perforation may occur.

Anterior Blepharitis

Staphylococcal blepharitis is usually caused by *S. aureus* or *S. epidermidis*.[6,7] Patients present with inflammation and erythema along the anterior margin of the eyelid. The lid margins are scaly, with crusts and tiny ulcerations around the lashes. In chronic inflammatory staphylococcal blepharitis, loss of eyelashes (madarosis) may occur. Complications of staphylococcal blepharitis include recurrent hordeola or chalazia, epithelial keratitis of the lower third of the cornea and marginal corneal infiltrates.

Seborrheic blepharitis (nonulcerative) presents with less inflammation and redness along the anterior border of the eyelid and the scales are more oily or greasy than in staphylococcal blepharitis.[6,7] Seborrheic blepharitis is often associated with seborrheic dermatitis affecting other parts of the body.

Although 2 types of anterior blepharitis have been identified, it is more common for patients to present with a mix of staphylococcal and seborrheic types.[6,7] Patients with either form of anterior blepharitis are also predisposed to developing conjunctivitis.

Posterior Blepharitis

Meibomian gland dysfunction can lead to inflammation of the posterior aspect of the eyelid (closer to the eyeball).[2,6,7] This is a bilateral, chronic condition that sometimes coexists with anterior blepharitis.

Meibomian seborrhea is characterized by excessive glandular secretions.[2,6,7] Symptoms can include photophobia, burning sensation, an excessively oily or foamy tear film and froth on the lid margin. Although they may be difficult to detect, small oil globules may be sitting at the meibomian gland orifices on the lid margin. There are usually few signs of inflammation.

Meibomianitis is characterized by inflammation and obstruction of the meibomian glands.[2,6,7] Signs include diffuse or localized inflammation of the posterior lid margin. In chronic cases the meibomian gland orifices become obstructed and the posterior lid margin may become thick, rounded and notched. When pressure is applied over the glands, a soft cheesy substance is expressed. In very severe cases the glands are completely blocked so no secretions can be expressed.

Goals of Therapy

- Reduce inflammation and discomfort associated with blepharitis
- Reduce the risk of recurrence of severe symptoms
- Reduce the risk of complications such as conjunctivitis and keratitis

Patient Assessment

Generally, symptoms of blepharitis include irritation, burning and itching of the lid margins. There may also be a foreign-body sensation in the eye.[7,23,24] Patients may complain of a sandy or gritty sensation in the eyes that is worse upon awakening since, during sleep, the inflamed eyelids lie against the cornea, tear secretion decreases, and inflammatory mediators have several hours to act on the surface of the eye. See also Pathophysiology, anterior and posterior blepharitis.

An algorithm for the assessment of eye symptoms is presented in Chapter 12: Assessment of Patients with Eye Conditions.

Prevention

Blepharitis is almost always a chronic condition that frustrates patients, physicians and eye care practitioners. Inadequate instruction and nonadherence with lid hygiene are the most common reasons for treatment failure.[8] Encourage patients to maintain a long-term lid hygiene program as this helps prevent exacerbations and long-term complications. Treatment of dermatologic disorders elsewhere in the body, such as seborrheic dermatitis, is important in achieving long-term control of blepharitis.[5,15,23]

Nonpharmacologic Therapy

For comparative ingredients of nonprescription products, consult the *Compendium of Products for Minor Ailments*—Ophthalmic Products: Cleansers and Washes.

Treatment for all types of blepharitis consists of regular and long-term eyelid margin hygiene:[6,23,24,25]

1. Warm compresses, applied to closed eyelids for 5–10 minutes, help to melt solidified material in the glands
2. Gentle cleansing of the lid margin follows. Instruct the patient to gently scrub only the lid margin, not the conjunctiva or outer lid area, using warm water with a facecloth, a commercial **eyelid scrub** (e.g., Lid-Care), or a cotton swab dipped in a solution of baby shampoo diluted with warm water
3. Mechanical expression, performed by an ophthalmologist, may be necessary to decrease the amount of irritating lipids within the glands. The patient may be instructed to perform firm massage of the lid margins after applying warm compresses, to enhance secretion from the meibomian glands. One hand holds the eyelid taut at the outer corner, while the index finger of the other hand presses along the lid from the inner corner out. Alternatively, the patient may simply apply direct pressure to the lid if that is more comfortable.

Lid hygiene may be required once or twice daily, immediately after initial diagnosis or during periods of exacerbation, but may be reduced to twice a week once control has been achieved.[6,23,25] This decision should be made by the treating healthcare practitioner. Very few patients will be able to completely discontinue a lid hygiene regimen.

If blepharitis persists despite treating with standard therapy, consider assessing whether the patient used a lid hygiene product containing cocoamidopropyl betaine (CAPB). CAPB is a surfactant present in many cosmetic and self-care products, including baby shampoo and eyelid scrub products, that is known to cause contact dermatitis and eyelid dermatitis.[26] Recalcitrant blepharitis has been associated with the use of products containing CAPB.

Pharmacologic Therapy

For comparative ingredients of nonprescription products, consult the *Compendium of Products for Minor Ailments*—Herbal and Natural Health Products: Single Entity.

Advise patients to use topical nonprescription antibacterials for blepharitis only with medical advice. **Omega-3 fatty acids** (e.g., flaxseed oil supplements), which have anti-inflammatory properties and may enhance lubrication, may be useful in patients with tear deficiencies.[21]

Treatment of anterior blepharitis may include topical antistaphylococcal antibiotics, used after eyelid cleansing.[23,24] Antibacterial ointments, applied on the lid margins, are preferred to drops because of increased contact time between the drug and tissues. Ointments that cover gram-positive organisms, such as **bacitracin** and **erythromycin**, are applied 1–4 times per day for 1–2 weeks. If effective, treatment can be reduced to once daily at bedtime for a further 4–8 weeks. Continue treatment for a month after all signs of inflammation have subsided.

Short-term treatment with **topical corticosteroids** or **corticosteroid/antibacterial** combinations may be necessary during exacerbations, or for severe inflammation and complications.[23,24] For further information on ophthalmic therapy, consult the *Compendium of Therapeutic Choices*: Red Eye.

In posterior blepharitis, patients may require systemic antibacterial therapy for several weeks or even months, in addition to lid hygiene.[23,24] Tetracyclines (**Tetracycline, doxycycline** or **minocycline**) are usually the drugs of choice. **Erythromycin** is an alternative when tetracyclines are contraindicated (e.g., allergy or during pregnancy). **Azithromycin** can be used as pulse therapy for the treatment of meibomian gland dysfunction because of its long half-life.[27,28] More information on antimicrobial therapy for blepharitis can be found in Table 2.

Monitoring of Therapy

Table 1 provides a monitoring plan, which should be individualized.[3,5,8,15,23]

Table 1: Monitoring of Therapy for Eyelid Conditions

Eye Condition	Monitoring	Goals/Endpoint of Therapy	Actions
Hordeolum	Patient: Daily Healthcare practitioner: After 48 h	Spontaneous drainage within 48 h.	Requires assessment for further therapy if drainage does not occur within 48 h, if pain worsens or if there are signs of infection.
Chalazion	Patient: Daily Healthcare practitioner: After 2–3 days	Improvement should begin within a few days. Complete resolution can take weeks to months.	Requires assessment for further therapy if the lesion is large and/or painful or if spontaneous drainage does not occur. For patients with blepharitis, encourage regular lid hygiene[a] to prevent chalazion recurrence.
Blepharitis	Patient: Daily during exacerbation. Less often when controlled Healthcare practitioner: Each visit in chronic disease. Within 1 wk if patient requires anti-infective therapy	Control inflammation and discomfort. Reduce the risk of severe, long-term complications.	Encourage adherence with lid hygiene regimen.[a] Ensure that patients cleanse only the margin of the eyelid and do not scratch the eyeball or conjunctiva. Requires assessment for further therapy if new onset of blepharitis is suspected. For exacerbations, assessment required for anti-infective or other therapy.

[a] See Blepharitis, Nonpharmacologic Therapy.

Table 2: **Antimicrobials Used in the Treatment of Blepharitis**[21,27,28]

Class	Drug	Dosage	Adverse Effects	Drug Interactions	Comments	Cost[a]
Tetracycline	*doxycycline* generics	100 mg daily	GI effects, yeast overgrowth, photosensitivity, acute renal failure.	Products containing aluminum, calcium, magnesium or iron may impair the absorption of oral tetracyclines. Separate doses by 2 h. May also interact with warfarin, retinoids, digoxin, antiepileptics, penicillin.	Not for use in pregnancy.	$
	minocycline generics	50–100 mg daily	See doxycycline. Also dizziness, vertigo, abnormal cutaneous pigmentation.	See doxycycline.	See doxycycline.	$
	tetracycline (kidney symbol) generics	250 mg QID	See doxycycline.	See doxycycline.	See doxycycline. Dose may be tapered to 250–500 mg daily. Take on an empty stomach, 1 h before or 2 h after food or milk ingestion.	$
Macrolide	*erythromycin* Eryc, generics	250 mg QID	GI effects: Nausea, vomiting, epigastric distress, diarrhea. QT_c interval prolongation.	Avoid use with highest risk QT_c-prolonging agents, amiodarone, fluconazole, lovastatin, pimozide, simvastatin. Moderate CYP3A4 inhibitor, concurrent use with CYP3A4 substrates may result in increased effects of the substrate.	May be used cautiously in pregnancy.	$
	azithromycin Zithromax, generics	1 g weekly or 500 mg daily for 3 days, repeated weekly	See erythromycin. GI effects not as common as with erythromycin.	See erythromycin. Not expected to inhibit CYP3A4.	See erythromycin.	$$$/week

[a] Cost per day unless otherwise specified; includes drug cost only.

(kidney symbol) Dosage adjustment may be required in renal impairment.

Legend: $ <$1 $$ $1–5 $$$ $5–10

Resource Tips

Mayo Clinic. *Blepharitis*. Available from: www.mayoclinic.org/diseases-conditions/blepharitis/basics/definition/con-20024605.

National Eye Institute. *Facts about blepharitis*. Available from: nei.nih.gov/health/blepharitis/blepharitis.

WedMD. *Styes and chalazia—topic overview*. Available from: www.webmd.com/eye-health/tc/styes-and-chalazia-topic-overview.

Suggested Readings

American Academy of Ophthalmology. *Blepharitis PPP-2013*. Available from: www.aao.org/preferred-practice-pattern/blepharitis-ppp–2013.

Carlisle RT, Digiovanni J. Differential diagnosis of the swollen red eyelid. *Am Fam Physician* 2015;92:106-12.

Gupta A, Stacey S, Amissah-Arthur KN. Eyelid lumps and lesions. *BMJ* 2014;348:g3029.

Merck manual: professional version. *Chalazion and hordeolum (stye)*. Available from: www.merckmanuals.com/professional/eye-disorders/eyelid-and-lacrimal-disorders/chalazion-and-hordeolum-%28stye%29.

Vagefi MR, Sullivan JH, Corrêa ZM et al. Lids & lacrimal apparatus. In: Riordan-Eva P, Cunningham ET, eds. *Vaughan & Asbury's general ophthalmology*. 18th ed. New York: McGraw-Hill Medical; 2011.

References

1. Rubin S, Hallagan L. Lids, lacrimals, and lashes. *Emerg Med Clin North Am* 1995;13:631-48.
2. Sullivan JH, Shetlar DJ, Whitcher JP. Lids, lacrimal apparatus, & tears. In: Riordan-Eva P, Whitcher J, eds. *Vaughan & Asbury's general ophthalmology*. 17th ed. New York: Lange Medical Books/McGraw-Hill Medical; 2008.
3. Lederman C, Miller M. Hordeola and chalazia. *Pediatr Rev* 1999;20:283-4.
4. Kanski JJ. *Clinical ophthalmology: a systematic approach*. 4th ed. Oxford: Butterworth-Heinemann; 1999.
5. Shields SR. Managing eye disease in primary care. Part 2. How to recognize and treat common eye problems. *Postgrad Med* 2000;108:83-6, 91-6.
6. Raskin EM, Speaker MG, Laibson PR. Blepharitis. *Infect Dis Clin North Am* 1992;6:777-87.
7. Thielen TL, Castle SS, Terry JE. Anterior ocular infections: an overview of pathophysiology and treatment. *Ann Pharmacother* 2000;34:235-46.
8. Mueller JB, McStay CM. Ocular infection and inflammation. *Emerg Med Clin North Am* 2008;26:57-72.
9. Jones YJ, Georgesuc D, McCann JD et al. Microwave warm compress burns. *Ophthal Plast Reconstr Surg* 2010;26:219.
10. Freedman HL, Preston KL. Heat retention in varieties of warm compresses: a comparison between warm soaks, hard-boiled eggs and the re-heater. *Ophthalmic Surg* 1989;20:846-8.
11. McMonnies CW, Korb DR, Blackie CA. The role of heat in rubbing and massage-related corneal deformation. *Cont Lens Anterior Eye* 2012;35:148-54.
12. Lam AK, Lam CH. Effect of warm compress therapy from hard-boiled eggs on corneal shape. *Cornea* 2007;26:163-7.
13. Deibel JP, Cowling K. Ocular inflammation and infection. *Emerg Med Clin N Am* 2013;31:387-97.
14. Lindsley K, Nichols JJ, Dickersin K. Interventions for acute internal hordeolum. *Cochrane Database Syst Rev* 2013;(4):CD007742.
15. Baum J. Infections of the eye. *Clin Infect Dis* 1995;21:479-86.
16. Gilchrist H, Lee G. Management of chalazia in general practice. *Aust Fam Physician* 2009;38:311-4.
17. Nemet AY, Vinker S, Kaiserman I. Associated morbidity of chalazion. *Cornea* 2011;30:1376-81.
18. Arbabi EM, Kelly RJ, Carrim ZI. Chalazion. *BMJ* 2012;341:c4044.
19. Cottrell DG, Bosanquet RC, Fawcett IM. Chalazions: the frequency of spontaneous resolution. *Br Med J (Clin Res Ed)* 1983;287:1595.
20. Smythe D, Hurwitz JJ, Tayfour F. The management of chalazion: a survey of Ontario ophthalmologists. *Can J Ophthalmol* 1990;25:252-5.
21. Bernardes TF, Bonfioli AA. Blepharitis. *Semin Ophthalmol* 2010;25:79-83.
22. Nemet AY, Vinker S, Kaiserman I. Associated morbidity of blepharitis. *Ophthalmology* 2011;118:1062-8.
23. Jackson WB. Blepharitis: current strategies for diagnosis and management. *Can J Ophthalmol* 2008;43:170-9.
24. Medscape from WebMD. Lowery RS. *Adult blepharitis*. Available from: emedicine.medscape.com. Accessed April 7, 2016. Registration required.
25. Morrow GL, Abbott RL. Conjunctivitis. *Am Fam Physician* 1998;57:735-46.
26. Welling JD, Mauger TF, Schoenfield LR et al. Chronic eyelid dermatitis secondary to cocamidopropyl betaine allergy in a patient using baby shampoo eyelid scrubs. *JAMA Ophthalmol* 2014;132:357-9.
27. Greene JB, Jeng BH, Fintelmann RE et al. Oral azithromycin for the treatment of meibomitis. *JAMA Ophthalmol* 2014;132:121-2.
28. Igami TZ, Hozchuh R, Osaki TH et al. Oral azithromycin for treatment of posterior blepharitis. *Cornea* 2011;30:1145-9.

Safe Use of Eye Products—What You Need to Know

General information about eye products (drops, ointments):

- Eye products are only for external use.
- Follow the directions carefully.
- Keep eye products out of the reach of children.
- Never share your eye products with another person.
- Close containers tightly after use.
- Store eye products in a cool, dark place. Some products have to be stored in the refrigerator. Ask your pharmacist how to store the products.
- Discard the product:
  - if it changes colour or appearance
  - if it was opened more than 1 month ago
  - immediately after use if it is a single-dose package without preservatives. **Do not** use the leftover product later.

Hints for using eye products:

- If you have difficulty using your eye product, ask a family member or friend to help you. You can also ask your pharmacist about devices that might help.
- Wash hands well with soap and water before and after using the product.
- **Do not** allow the tip of the container to touch the eyes, eyelids, eyelashes, fingers or counter surface. Contact with any surface can contaminate the product.
- Be sure to put the cap of the container on a clean tissue when you use the product to avoid contamination of the cap. Replace the cap as soon as possible.
- Some products may blur your vision for a short time. **Do not** drive or perform hazardous tasks until you can see clearly again.

How to deal with problems:

- Discontinue using the medication and see your eye care professional if:
  - you have pain in your eye
  - your eyes become sensitive to light
  - your vision changes in any way
  - the eye irritation and redness continues
  - the condition lasts longer than 48 hours after you stop using the medication
  - the condition does not improve after 48 hours of treatment with anti-infectives or 72 hours of treatment with other agents
  - the condition gets worse

Proper Use of Eye Drops—What You Need to Know

Hints to help you use eye drops safely:

- Wash hands well with soap and warm water before using eye drops.
- If the medication is a suspension, shake the bottle before using it. Ask your pharmacist if you're not sure.
- Remove the bottle cap carefully. Lay the cap on its side on a clean, dry tissue. Do not touch the rim of the bottle or the inside of the cap. You may contaminate them.
- Tilt your head back or lie down.
- Keep both eyes open. Gently pull the lower eyelid of the affected eye down to form a pouch.
- Hold the bottle almost horizontally. Bring it up to your eye from the side. This reduces the risk of accidentally hitting your eye with the tip of the bottle.
- Hold the tip about 2.5 cm (1 inch) away from the eyelid. Do not touch the lid or lashes with the tip of the bottle.
- Look upwards by moving your eyes only (keep your head tilted back). Looking up moves the centre of the eyeball away from where the drop is going. It will keep your eye from blinking hard when the drop goes in.
- Put one drop into the pouch of the lower eyelid. Continue to hold your head back so the drop can fall as deeply as possible into the pouch.
- Look down for several seconds and then slowly release the lower lid. Looking down allows the medication to reach the centre of the eye. This is especially important for infections of the cornea.
- Gently close the eyes. Do not squeeze the eyes shut—you may force the medication out. Keep eyes closed for at least 30 seconds—longer is better (up to 5 minutes). This will keep the medication in contact with the eye for as long as possible.
- You can press gently on the side of the bridge of the nose with your thumb and index finger to help keep the medication from going down the tear duct. If you have recently had eye surgery or have had punctal plugs inserted, ask your eye doctor whether it is safe to apply pressure to the bridge of your nose.
- Before opening the affected eye, use a clean tissue to blot away excess medication. *Do not* rub the eye. Try not to blink.
- *Do not* rinse the tip of the eye drop bottle. Replace the bottle cap.
- Wash hands well with soap and warm water.
- If more than one drop of the same medication is prescribed, wait 3–5 minutes between drops. This ensures the first drop is not flushed away and the second drop is not diluted by the first.
- If you are using more than 1 medication, wait 5–10 minutes before applying another medication.
- If you have problems with balance or dizziness, lie down or sit down in a very stable position before using your drops. This will reduce your risk of falling.
- If you have tremors (shaking) or arthritis, ask your pharmacist or eye care professional about devices to help you use eye drops.
- Eye drop bottles usually contain a preservative to prevent the medication from being contaminated. However, the bottle can become contaminated over time, especially if the bottle tip has come into contact with the eye or the eyelashes. It's a good idea to throw out any bottles that have been open for a month or more.

Figure 1: **Eye Drop Instillation**

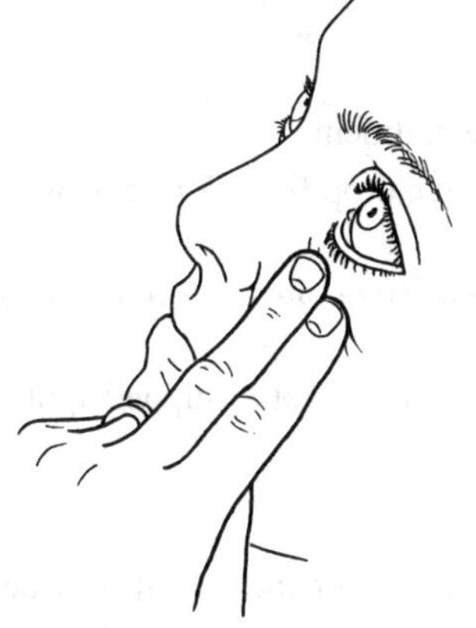

Step 1
Gently pull down on the lower eyelid to form a pouch.

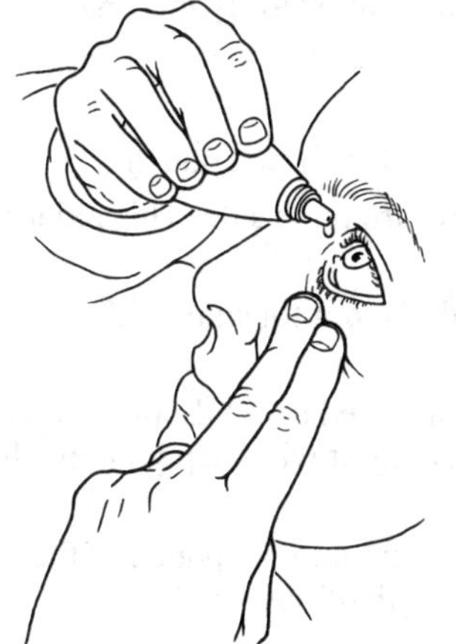

Step 2
Hold bottle horizontally, approach the eye from the side. Hold tip at least 2.5 cm away from the eyelid.

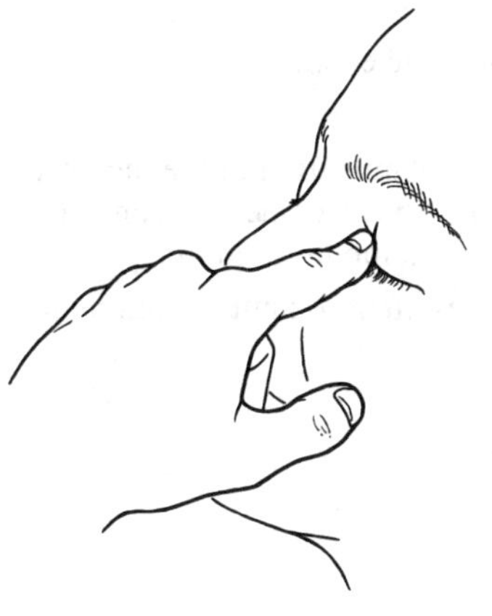

Step 3
Keep eye closed for at least 30 seconds (up to 5 minutes). Apply gentle pressure to the side of the bridge of the nose. If you had eye surgery recently or have had punctal plugs inserted, ask the doctor if it is safe to apply pressure.

Proper Use of Eye Ointments—What You Need to Know

General instructions:

- Wash hands well with soap and water before using an eye ointment.
- If you have to use both an ointment and eye drop, use the eye drop first. Wait at least 5 minutes before using the ointment.
- If you have to use different types of ointments, wait at least 10 minutes before using the second one.
- If you have to apply the ointment to the outer eyelids, use a sterile cotton-tipped applicator to apply the ointment.

How to apply eye ointment:

- Hold the tube in your hand for a few minutes to warm the ointment and help it flow better. Remove the container cap. Lay it on its side on a clean, dry tissue.
- When you open the tube for the first time, squeeze out and throw away the first 0.25 cm (0.1 inch) of ointment as it may be too dry.
- Tilt your head back or lie down.
- Keep your eyes open. Gently pull down on the lower eyelid to form a pouch.
- Hold the tube almost horizontally. Bring it up to your eye from the side. This reduces the risk of accidentally hitting your eye with the tip of the tube.
- Hold the tip about 2.5 cm (1 inch) away from the eyelid. **Do not** touch the lids or lashes with the tip of the tube.
- Look upwards by moving your eyes only (keep your head tilted back). Looking up moves the centre of the eyeball away from where the ointment is going. It will keep your eye from blinking hard when the ointment goes in.
- Place 0.6–1.25 cm (one-quarter to one-half inch) of ointment into the pouch of the lower eyelid. It is not necessary to place the ointment along the entire length of the pouch.
- Gently close the eye for 1–2 minutes and roll the eyeball in all directions.
- Replace the container cap.
- Use a clean tissue to remove excess ointment from around the eyelid.
- Wash hands thoroughly.
- Eye ointments usually contain a preservative to prevent contamination of the medication. However, they can become contaminated over time, especially if the tip has come into contact with the eye or the eyelashes. Throw out any tubes that have been open for a month or more.
- **Remember:** Your vision may be blurred for a few minutes after you put the ointment in. **Do not** drive or operate machinery until you can see clearly.

Figure 1: **Eye Ointment Instillation**

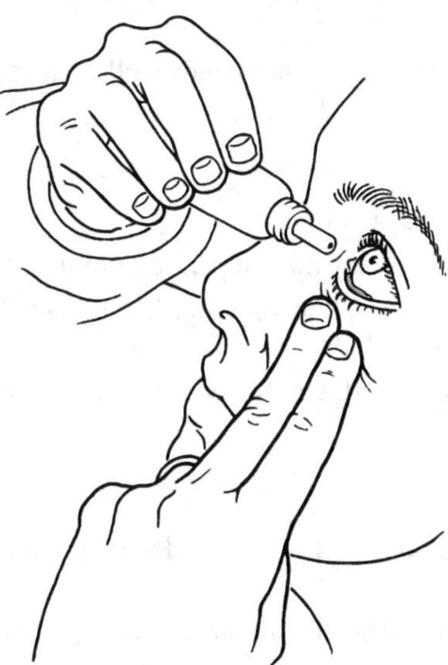

Eye Drops for Children—What You Need to Know

Before you put drops in a child's eyes, wash your hands well with soap and water. It is also important to get the child in a good position.

Positioning:

- Have the child lie down and close the eyes.
- For infants and small children who may not cooperate, try this alternative method:
  - sit on the floor and have the child sit on your lap, facing you. Their legs should be open over yours. Your legs may be spread slightly.
  - while supporting the back and head, gently lower the child backwards until the child is lying along your legs.

Holding the child's head:

You may use several methods to hold the child's head, depending on how much control you want. You may need another person to help.

- With the child lying down, hold the head with one hand. Use your other hand to put drops in the eye on the side you are holding.
- If the child resists, you may gently clamp the head between your legs and wedge the child's feet against your body under your arms.

Putting the drops into the eyes (instillation):

- Wash your hands well with soap and water before you begin.
- If the medication is a suspension, shake the bottle before using it. Ask the pharmacist if you are not sure.
- Hold the container horizontally as you bring it up to the eye. Rest your hand on the child's cheek to prevent injury to the eye if the child moves suddenly.

Open-eye method:

If the child is able to cooperate you can use this method:

- Tilt the child's head back or have the child lie down.
- Gently pull the lower eyelid of the affected eye down to form a pouch.
- Hold the tip of the bottle about 2.5 cm (1 inch) away from the eyelid. **Do not** touch the lid or the lashes with the tip of the bottle.
- Have the child look upward, moving only the eyes. This will help to keep the child from blinking when the drop goes in.
- Put the recommended dose into the pouch of the lower eyelid. Keep the child's head back so the medicine can get deeply into the pouch.
- Have the child look down, moving only the eyes. Looking down allows the medication to reach the centre of the eye.
- Allow the child to close the eyes gently for about 30 seconds. Tell the child not to squeeze the eyes shut tightly. Squeezing may force the medication out.
- Before the child opens the eye, use a clean tissue to blot any excess medication. **Do not** allow the child to rub the eye. Ask the child to try not to blink.

Alternative methods:

These methods work better for younger children or children that are resisting the medication. They are also useful for adults with a strong blink reflex.

1. Place the drop on the eyelid in the inner corner of the eye, then have the child open the eye so the drop falls in by gravity.
2. Pull the lower lid down and instil the drop through the lashes. Avoid touching the bottle to the lashes.

Remember: If the medication is important, it is better to get some drops or ointment on the lids and lashes (with the eye closed) where it could seep onto the surface of the eye, than not to use the drops or ointment at all.

Infections of the Eyes or Eyelids—What You Need to Know

When should you seek more medical advice?

See your eye care professional if:

- you have pain or severe redness in your eyes
- your vision is altered—you can't see as well as usual
- you have had this problem before
- you have a disease (such as diabetes) along with your eye problem
- you have used a nonprescription treatment for 48 hours or more but the condition has not improved
- the condition gets worse with treatment
- without treatment, the condition has lasted longer than 48 hours

Hints to help you manage an infection of the eye or eyelids:

- Use separate facecloths, towels, pillows and sheets from other family members to prevent the infection from spreading. Use a clean facecloth and towel each time you clean your eye.
- Wash your hands with soap and water before and after touching your eyes.
- It is important to clean the eye area before applying any medication. This is particularly true when there is a sticky discharge or an eyelid infection. Clean the lids well with soap and water.
- If you need to use a device to put in your eye drops, wash it with soap and warm water after each use.
- **Do not** use an eye patch unless your eye care professional recommends it.
- Avoid using mascara and other cosmetics while your eye is infected. Cosmetics may need to be discarded as they may contain bacteria that can reinfect your eye later on.

Chapter 17

Assessment of Patients with Hearing Loss, Ear Pain and Ear Drainage

Yvonne M. Shevchuk, BSP, PharmD, FCSHP

Signs and Symptoms

Ear symptoms may occur in many conditions. Table 1 describes signs and symptoms associated with various otic conditions and Figure 1 provides an algorithm for patient assessment. Signs and symptoms commonly associated with ear disease include ear pain, ear drainage, tinnitus, vertigo, dizziness and hearing loss. Assessment should include determining the patient's age, location and characteristics of the pain, and the presence or absence of pruritus, hearing loss, discharge from the ear, or any aggravating factors associated with the symptoms.

Table 1: **Signs and Symptoms Associated with Various Ear Conditions**

Condition	Pain	Pruritus	Discharge	Hearing Loss	Comments
Acute bacterial otitis externa	Yes (acute onset)	Sometimes	Frequent	Sometimes	Associated with excessive moisture, trauma to EAC, attempts to scratch or remove wax from EAC. Pain with chewing, movement of auricle.
Barotrauma	Yes	No	Yes if TM ruptures	Yes	Associated with air travel (descent) and diving. Tinnitus and vertigo may also be present.
Eczematous otitis externa	Sometimes	Yes	Sometimes (crusting, oozing)	Sometimes	Characteristic features of underlying dermatologic condition may be present (e.g., psoriatic plaques; erythema and scaling with atopic dermatitis). May become secondarily infected.
Foreign body	Yes	Sometimes	If becomes infected	Yes	Fullness and pressure in the ear.
Impacted earwax	Rarely unless infected	Frequent	Rarely unless infected	Yes (gradual)	May be described as fullness or pressure.
Otitis media	Yes (abrupt onset)	No	Yes if TM ruptures	Sometimes	Primarily in children. Pain relieved with rupture of TM. Commonly preceded by viral URTI.
Ruptured tympanic membrane	Yes (sudden, sharp)	No	Yes	Yes (abrupt)	May be associated with acute otitis media, barotrauma and other conditions.

Abbreviations: EAC = external auditory canal; TM = tympanic membrane; URTI = upper respiratory tract infection

Ear Pain (Otalgia)

Otalgia is usually associated with inflammation of the external or middle ear, but pain may be referred to the ear from other sites such as the teeth, temporomandibular joint, pharynx or sinuses.[1,2,3] If pain lasts more than 2–3 days, refer the patient for medical evaluation.

Ear Drainage (Otorrhea)

Otorrhea may be caused by a simple scratch in the ear or by serious medical conditions. Otorrhea is often a sign of otitis externa, otitis media with perforation of the tympanic membrane or drainage from the middle ear from tympanostomy tubes.[3,4] Bloody drainage can occur with several conditions, including trauma, neoplasm and foreign bodies. Clear drainage may be from the middle ear or a cerebrospinal fluid leak. Drainage resulting from mild otitis externa (e.g., eczematous) may be self-treated; however, unless this is specifically identified as the cause, the patient should be referred for assessment and treatment.

Tinnitus, Vertigo and Dizziness

These symptoms are discussed in detail in Chapter 10: Tinnitus and in Chapter 11: Vertigo and Dizziness.

Hearing Loss

Hearing loss is classified as either conductive or sensorineural.[5,6,7] Conductive hearing loss occurs when sound is prevented from gaining access to the inner ear, and may result from diseases of the external or middle ear. Examples include otitis externa, impacted earwax, upper respiratory tract infections, otitis media, foreign objects or water trapped in the ear and tumors. Rupture of the tympanic membrane due to acute otitis media or trauma also produces hearing loss. Sensorineural hearing loss involves the inner ear or cochlea, the auditory nerve or a central nerve lesion. These conditions are not managed by self-care. Unless hearing loss is identified as due to impacted earwax or an upper respiratory tract infection, all patients with hearing loss should be referred to an appropriate healthcare practitioner for assessment.

Drug-induced Ototoxicity

Hearing loss, tinnitus and vertigo may be drug-induced. It is important to review a patient's medication profile to ensure that symptoms are not due to drug-induced ototoxicity. Many drugs have been associated with ototoxicity, sometimes only as a single case report.[8] Drugs more commonly associated with ototoxicity are found in Table 2. This is not an exhaustive list; a more comprehensive list can be found in Cianfrone et al (see Suggested Readings).

Miscellaneous Conditions Affecting the Ear

Conditions affecting the auricle such as dermatitis (Chapter 55: Atopic, Contact, and Stasis Dermatitis), infections (Chapter 56: Bacterial Skin Infections: Impetigo, Furuncles and Carbuncles, Chapter 65: Fungal Skin Infections), burns (Chapter 57: Burns), frostbite (Chapter 63: Frostbite) and lacerations (Chapter 68: Minor Cuts and Wounds), are amenable to self-treatment if not severe. More detailed assessment by an appropriate healthcare provider is required if these are not easily distinguishable by history and appearance.

Figure 1: Assessment of Patients with Ear Complaints[1,5,6,7,2,3]

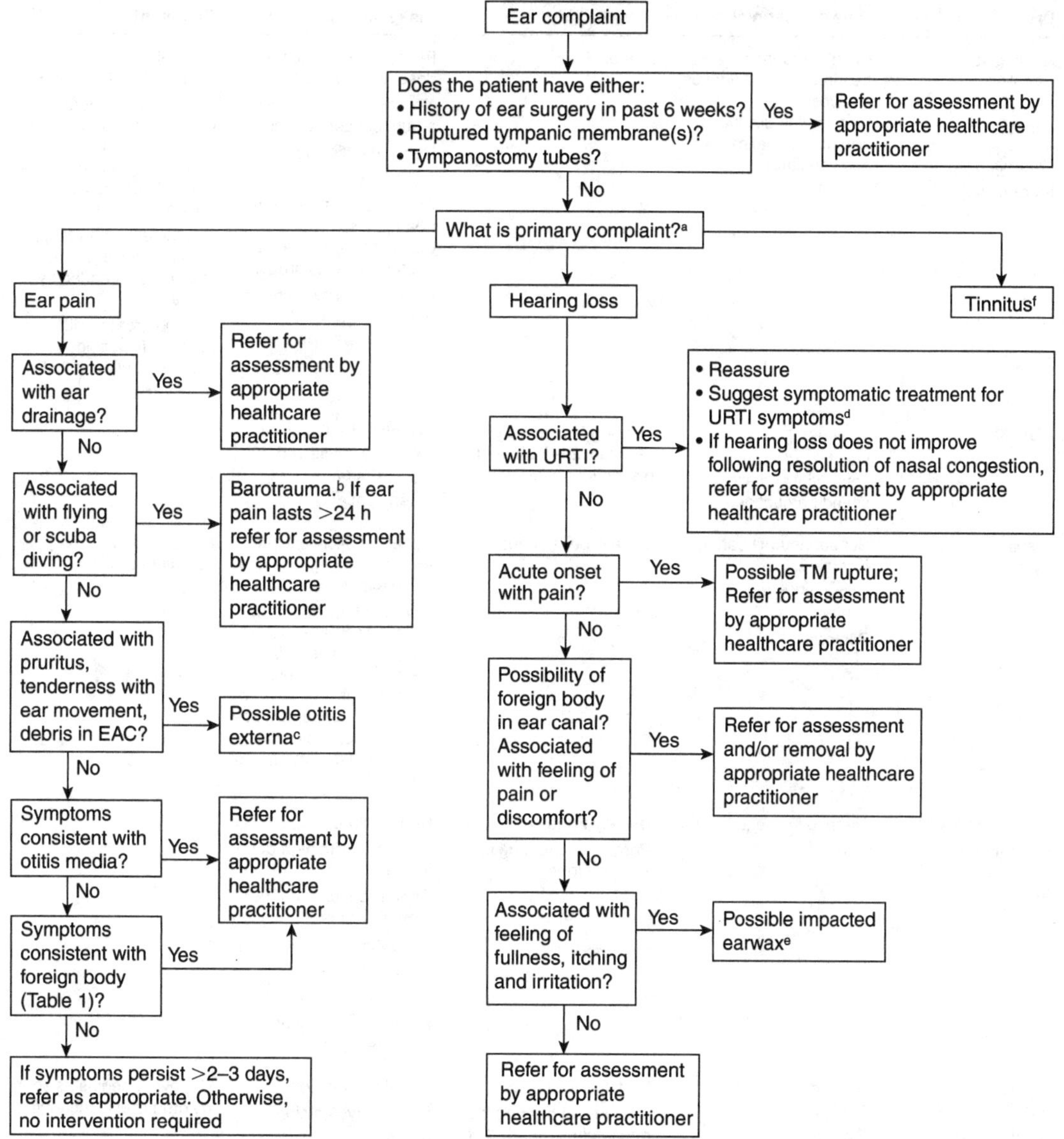

[a] Ear conditions often present as a constellation of symptoms (Table 1). The predominant symptom often varies between individuals. For this reason, more than one path of this algorithm may apply to a particular case.
[b] See Chapter 18: Complications Affecting the Ear: Ear Piercing, Foreign Bodies and Barotrauma.
[c] See Chapter 20: Otitis Media and Otitis Externa.
[d] See Chapter 24: Viral Rhinitis, Influenza, Rhinosinusitis and Pharyngitis.
[e] See Chapter 19: Impacted Earwax.
[f] See Chapter 10: Tinnitus.

Abbreviations: EAC = external auditory canal; TM = tympanic membrane; URTI = upper respiratory tract infection

Table 2: **Drugs Associated with Ototoxicity**

Drug	Type of Hearing Loss	Reversibility	Risk Factors	Comments
Aminoglycosides[9,10,11,12] (amikacin, gentamicin, neomycin, streptomycin, tobramycin)	Cochlear (sensorineural hearing loss and tinnitus) and vestibular (unrelenting dizziness with occasional nausea and vomiting).	Irreversible	Possibly related to total dose administered. Not correlated well with serum concentrations. Renal insufficiency. Age >60 y. Previous sensorineural hearing loss, noise exposure, concurrent use of other ototoxic drugs. Duration of treatment >10 days.	Discontinuation at first sign may limit damage. Audiology monitoring recommended by some as initial hearing loss may be higher frequency and not noticed by patient. Vestibular testing (e.g., dynamic illegible E or DIE) recommended by some. Risk no greater with once-daily dosing compared with multiple daily doses.
ASA[13,14]	Tinnitus. Decreased acoustic sensitivity and altered sound perception.	Hearing loss usually recovers 24–72 h after discontinuation.	Correlated with serum salicylate levels and higher doses. Elderly patients.	
Cisplatin[15]	Sensorineural hearing loss. Some patients exhibit tinnitus. Bilateral.	Usually permanent.	Renal insufficiency, pre-existing hearing loss and noise exposure. Increased risk with renal insufficiency, high serum drug levels, age >60 y, previous sensorineural hearing loss, noise exposure, concurrent use of other ototoxic drugs, duration of treatment >10 days.	Dose-related, cumulative.
Loop diuretics[13,16,17] (bumetanide, ethacrynic acid, furosemide)	Hearing loss and tinnitus.	Usually transient. Permanent hearing loss also reported.	Renal failure. Generally with high-dose iv use. Concurrent use of ototoxic drugs. Hypoalbuminemia. Liver disease. Heart failure. Furosemide infusion rates >4 mg/min.	
Macrolides[18,19,20,21,22] (azithromycin, clarithromycin, erythromycin)	Sensorineural with tinnitus. Bilateral.	Usually reversible. Irreversible hearing loss and tinnitus reported at low doses as well.	Renal dysfunction. Hepatic dysfunction. Female sex. Erythromycin dose >4 g/day.	Recovery begins as soon as drug is discontinued.
Phosphodiesterase type 5 inhibitors[23] (sildenafil, tadalafil, vardenafil)	Sudden hearing loss sometimes accompanied by tinnitus and dizziness.	Usually unilateral. Reversible in one-third of cases.	Unknown.	

(cont'd)

Table 2: **Drugs Associated with Ototoxicity** *(cont'd)*

Drug	Type of Hearing Loss	Reversibility	Risk Factors	Comments
Quinine[13,14]	High frequency sensorineural hearing loss. Vestibular toxicity also seen.	Reversible. Bilateral.	Initiation of high-dose therapy or chronic lower dose therapy.	Cinchonism: headache, nausea, vertigo, tinnitus, deafness, blindness and dysphoria.
Tetracyclines (doxycycline,[24] minocycline[25,26])	Vestibular symptoms such as lightheadedness, loss of balance, dizziness and tinnitus.	Generally self-limiting.	More common in women.	Occurs at usual oral doses and usually disappears within 2 days.

Suggested Readings

Cianfrone G, Pentangelo D, Cianfrone E et al. Pharmacological drugs inducing ototoxicity, vestibular symptoms and tinnitus: a reasoned and updated guide. *Eur Rev Med Pharmacol Sci* 2011;15:601-36.

Ely JW, Hansen MR, Clark EC. Diagnosis of ear pain. *Am Fam Physician* 2008;77:621-8.

References

1. Stallard TC. Emergency disorders of the ear, nose, sinuses, oropharynx & mouth. In: Stone C, Humphries RL, eds. *Current diagnosis & treatment emergency medicine*. 7th ed. New York: McGraw-Hill; 2011. Available from: accessmedicine.mhmedical.com. Accessed August 30, 2015.
2. Shah RK, Blevins NH. Otalgia. *Otolaryngol Clin North Am* 2003;36:1137-51.
3. Ely JW, Hansen MR, Clark EC. Diagnosis of ear pain. *Am Fam Physician* 2008;77:621-8.
4. Pankhania M. Otorrhoea. *BMJ* 2011;342:d2299.
5. Lustig LR, Schindler JS. Ear, nose and throat disorders. In: Papadakis MA, McPhee SJ, Rabow MW, eds. *Current medical diagnosis & treatment 2015*. New York: McGraw Hill. Available from: accessmedicine.mhmedical.com. Accessed August 30, 2015. Subscription required.
6. Friedman NR, Scholes MA, Yoon PJ. Ear, nose, and throat. In: Hay WW, Levin MJ, Deterding RR et al., eds. *Current diagnosis and treatment: pediatrics*. 22nd ed. New York: McGraw Hill; 2013. Available from: accessmedicine.mhmedical.com. Accessed August 30, 2015. Subscription required.
7. Lalwani AK. Disorders of hearing. In: Kasper D, Fauci A, Hauser S et al., eds. *Harrison's principles of internal medicine*. 19th ed. New York: McGraw-Hill; 2015. Available from: accessmedicine.mhmedical.com. Accessed August 30, 2015. Subscription required.
8. Seligmann H, Podoshin L, Ben-David J et al. Drug-induced tinnitus and other hearing disorders. *Drug Saf* 1996;14:198-212.
9. Rizzi MD, Hirose K. Aminoglycoside ototoxicity. *Curr Opin Otolaryngol Head Neck Surg* 2007;15:352-7.
10. Ariano RE, Zelenitsky SA, Kassum DA. Aminoglycoside-induced vestibular injury: maintaining a sense of balance. *Ann Pharmacother* 2008;42:1282-9.
11. Barza M, Ioannidis JP, Cappelleri JC et al. Single or multiple daily doses of aminoglycosides: a meta-analysis. *BMJ* 1996;312:338-45.
12. Palmay L, Walker SA, Walker SE et al. Symptom reporting compared with audiometry for the detection of cochleotoxicity in patients on long-term aminoglycoside therapy. *Ann Pharmacother* 2011;45:590-5.
13. Yorgason JG, Fayad JN, Kalinec F. Understanding drug ototoxicity: molecular insights for prevention and clinical management. *Expert Opin Drug Saf* 2006;5:383-99.
14. Jung TT, Rhee CK, Lee CS et al. Ototoxicity of salicylate, nonsteroidal antiinflammatory drugs, and quinine. *Otolaryngol Clin North Am* 1993;26:791-810.
15. Rybak LP. Mechanisms of cisplatin ototoxicity and progress in otoprotection. *Curr Opin Otolaryngol Head Neck Surg* 2007;15:364-9.
16. Ikeda K, Oshima T, Hidaka H et al. Molecular and clinical implications of loop diuretic ototoxicity. *Hear Res* 1997;107:1-8.
17. Baldwin KA, Budzinski CE, Shapiro CJ. Acute sensorineural hearing loss: furosemide ototoxicity revisited. *Hosp Pharm* 2008;43:982-7,1007.
18. Principi N, Esposito S. Comparative tolerability of erythromycin and newer macrolide antibacterials in paediatric patients. *Drug Saf* 1999;20:25-41.
19. Whitener CJ, Parker JE, Lapp NL. Erythromycin ototoxicity: a call to heighten recognition. *South Med J* 1991;84:1214-6.
20. Ress BD, Gross EM. Irreversible sensorineural hearing loss as a result of azithromycin ototoxicity. A case report. *Ann Otol Rhinol Laryngol* 2000;109:435-7.
21. Hajiioannou JK, Florou V, Kousoulis P, et al. Clarithromycin induced reversible sensorineural hearing loss. B-ENT. 2011;7(2):127-30.
22. Coulston J, Balaratnam N. Irreversible sensorineural hearing loss due to clarithromycin. Postgrad Med J. 2005 Jan;81(951):58-9.
23. Maddox PT, Saunders J, Chandrasekhar SS. Sudden hearing loss from PDE-5 inhibitors: a possible cellular stress etiology. *Laryngoscope* 2009;119:1586-9.
24. Segelnick SL, Weinberg MA. Doxycycline-induced dizziness in dental patient. Case report. *N Y State Dent J* 2010;76:28-32.
25. Jacobson JA, Daniel B. Vestibular reactions associated with minocycline. *Antimicrob Agents Chemother* 1975;8:453-6.
26. Fanning WL, Gump DW, Sofferman RA. Side effects of minocycline: a double-blind study. *Antimicrob Agents Chemother* 1977;11:712-7.

Chapter 18
Complications Affecting the Ear: Ear Piercing, Foreign Bodies and Barotrauma

Yvonne M. Shevchuk, BSP, PharmD, FCSHP

Complications of Ear Piercing

Ear piercing complications are common (up to 35% of patients) and most frequently include infection and allergic reactions to metals.[1,2] Mild redness, swelling and crusting is part of the normal course of healing post-piercing. Healing typically takes 6–8 weeks or longer depending on what part of the ear is pierced. To prevent infection, the piercing site should be washed twice daily with soap and water. Alcohol is no longer recommended because of excessive drying. If a mild bacterial infection develops secondary to piercing, it can be managed with local therapy (cleansing, warm compresses and topical antibiotics) without removing the earring. If the inflammation or swelling is significant, the earring may need to be removed in which case a ring can be made from a nylon suture material or a 20-gauge Teflon catheter with silicone tubing (available from surgical supply manufacturer) and inserted into the hole to keep it open.[1] High ear piercings can produce infections of the cartilage which are much more serious.[1,2,3] These patients require further assessment and management. Allergic dermatitis is managed by avoidance of the inciting compound (nickel or gold) and may include short-term use of a mild to moderate topical corticosteroid, such as **hydrocortisone** 0.5% or 1% or **clobetasone butyrate** 0.05%. See Ear Piercing—What You Need to Know for recommendations to reduce the risk of ear piercing complications and information on caring for the ears after piercing.

For comparative ingredients of nonprescription products, consult the *Compendium of Products for Minor Ailments*—Skin Care Products: Dermatitis and Dry Skin.

Foreign Bodies

Foreign bodies in the ear canal occur more frequently in children than adults.[4,5] Often the patient (or witness in the case of a child) will give a history of a foreign object entering the ear. Patients experience pain, which may be dull or severe, a feeling of fullness or pressure in the ear and loss of hearing. Foreign objects should always be removed by a healthcare practitioner. If patients attempt to remove objects by syringing, especially if they are organic (e.g., beans, peas, insects), the object may swell when moistened and occlude the canal. If the objects are sharp they may scratch the canal or perforate the tympanic membrane. Cotton-tipped applicators may push the foreign object further into the canal. Insects are particularly annoying because of their movement. Provided the tympanic membrane is not perforated, insects may be drowned at home by using a dropper to fill the ear canal with mineral oil, olive oil or baby oil before removal by the healthcare practitioner.

Barotrauma

Otic barotrauma, also referred to as aerotitis media, occurs when an individual cannot equalize the pressure gradient between the middle ear and the atmosphere.[6,7,8] This occurs during air travel (descent) and underwater diving (descent). The eustachian tube closes, causing a painful pressure change in the middle ear and extravasation of fluid and blood into the middle ear space. Tympanic membrane perforation may result. The symptoms are a sensation of ear blockage followed by ear pain, tinnitus, vertigo and transient conductive hearing loss. With diving, tympanic membrane rupture may result in severe vertigo due to cold water entering the middle ear. This may become life threatening due to disorientation.[9] The condition may last 2 or 3 days and usually resolves spontaneously. More severe injury can occur with deep sea dives. Occasionally, surgery may be required. Treatment includes **analgesics** for pain, **oral**[10] or **topical decongestants**[6] to encourage opening of the eustachian tube and attempts to auto-inflate using the Valsalva manoeuvre (forced expiration keeping the mouth tightly closed and the nostrils pinched) or the Toynbee manoeuvre (holding the nose and swallowing hard with the mouth closed). The Valsalva manoeuvre may cause syncope or cardiac arrhythmia and should not be recommended to patients with cardiac disease.

The Divers Alert Network (DAN) has guidelines for flying after recreational diving. They suggest waiting 12 hours after a single recreational dive. For multiple dives in one day or multiple dives over multiple days, DAN suggests waiting at least 18 hours before flying. For dives requiring decompression stops, a wait time of at least 18 hours is recommended although DAN states there is little evidence to support this recommendation.[11] More information on recreational diving can be found on the DAN website at www.diversalertnetwork.org.

If symptoms of barotrauma do not subside in 24 hours, or if bloody fluid drains from the ear indicating a ruptured tympanic membrane, refer the patient for further assessment and management.

As mentioned above, poor functioning of the eustachian tube can result in failure of pressure equilibration during descent while flying or diving. This may be due to congenital and anatomic conditions, but upper respiratory tract infections, eustachian tube edema resulting from allergies, chronic middle ear disease and nasal chamber edema during pregnancy also produce eustachian tube dysfunction. Flying or diving should be postponed in these individuals if possible; in some cases diving may be contraindicated (e.g., if the tympanic membrane is perforated).[12] The eustachian tube also does not function normally while an individual is asleep.

Beginning early in the descent while flying, individuals should swallow, yawn and auto-inflate frequently. They should ensure they are awakened prior to descent. Children can be given gum to chew or candy to suck; small children can be breastfed or given a bottle during descent to reduce discomfort. When diving, various techniques are used during descent, such as the Valsalva manoeuvre, yawning, swallowing or moving the jaw from side to side.[9]

Nasal sprays and oral decongestants are often recommended to prevent barotrauma. In adults, **pseudoephedrine** 120 mg sustained-release formulation taken 30 minutes before flying has been shown to reduce pain, blockage and hearing loss in individuals with a history of ear discomfort,[13,14] but oxymetazoline nasal spray is not better than placebo.[13] Efficacy has not been demonstrated in children ≤6 years and Health Canada advises against their use in this age group;[15] therefore, decongestants should not be used in this population.[16] The most appropriate recommendation is for 60 mg (regular-release) or 120 mg (sustained-release) of oral pseudoephedrine in adults. Administration 30 minutes prior to takeoff is appropriate for short flights under 4 hours. Because it is the descent that causes problems, on long international flights, pseudoephedrine should be taken 30–60 minutes prior to the anticipated arrival time. Drowsiness was the only adverse effect reported in clinical trials specific to barotrauma.[14] Data on insomnia were not presented. The product selected should have sufficient duration of action to match the length of the flight.

Pseudoephedrine 60 mg taken 30 minutes before diving decreased the incidence and severity of middle ear barotrauma in first-time divers.[17] For contraindications and precautions, see Table 1.

For comparative ingredients of nonprescription products, consult the *Compendium of Products for Minor Ailments*—Analgesic Products: Internal Analgesic and Antipyretics; Cough, Cold and Allergy Products.

Table 1: Drugs Used in the Management and Prevention of Barotrauma

Class	Drug	Dosage	Adverse Effects	Drug Interactions	Comments	Cost[a]
Decongestants, oral	*pseudoephedrine* ❥ Eltor 120, Sudafed Decongestant 12 Hour, generics	Adults and children ≥12 y: 60 mg Q4–6H po Sustained-release: 120 mg Q12H po Maximum: 240 mg per day Children 6–11 y: 30 mg Q4–6H po Maximum: 120 mg per day	Mild CNS stimulation (nervousness, excitability, restlessness, dizziness, weakness, insomnia). Peripheral vasoconstriction. Tachycardia or palpitation may occur. Blood pressure may be increased in hypertensive patients. May adversely affect blood sugar control in diabetics.	Beta-blockers: Antihypertensive effects may be reduced. MAOIs and ergot derivatives may enhance the hypertensive effect of pseudoephedrine. Concurrent use and use within 14 days of discontinuation of MAOIs is contraindicated.	Caution in patients with heart disease, high blood pressure, hyperthyroidism, diabetes, angle-closure glaucoma or prostatic enlargement. Onset of action 30 min.	$$

[a] Cost of 12 tablets; includes drug cost only.

❥ Dosage adjustment may be required in renal impairment.

Legend: $ < $3 $$ $3–6

Suggested Readings

Csortan E, Jones J, Haan M et al. Efficacy of pseudoephedrine for the prevention of barotrauma during air travel. *Ann Emerg Med* 1994;23:1324-7.

Holbrook J, Minocha J, Laumann A. Body piercing: complications and prevention of health risks. *Am J Clin Dermatol* 2012;13:1-17.

Meltzer DI. Complications of body piercing. *Am Fam Physician* 2005;72:2029-34.

Newbegin C, Ell S. Ear barotrauma after flying and diving. *Practitioner* 2000;244:96-9, 101-2, 105.

References

1. Meltzer DI. Complications of body piercing. *Am Fam Physician* 2005;72:2029-34.
2. Holbrook J, Minocha J, Laumann A. Body piercing: complications and prevention of health risks. *Am J Clin Dermatol* 2012;13:1-17.
3. Manca DP, Levy M, Tariq K. Case report: infected ear cartilage piercing. *Can Fam Physician* 2006;52:974-5.
4. Ely JW, Hansen MR, Clark EC. Diagnosis of ear pain. *Am Fam Physician* 2008;77:621-8.
5. Friedman NR, Scholes MA, Yoon PJ. Ear, nose, and throat. In: Hay WW, Levin MJ, Sondheimer JM et al. *Current pediatric diagnosis and treatment*. 22nd ed. New York: McGraw-Hill; 2013. Available from: accessmedicine.mhmedical.com. Accessed August 31, 2015. Subscription required.
6. DeGorordo A, Vallejo-Manzur F, Chanin K et al. Diving emergencies. *Resuscitation* 2003;59:171-80.
7. Wright T. Middle-ear pain and trauma during air travel. *BMJ Clin Evid* 2015;pii:0501.
8. Lynch JH, Deaton TG. Barotrauma with extreme pressures in sport: from scuba to skydiving. *Curr Sports Med Rep* 2014;13:107-12.
9. Hamilton-Farrell M, Bhattacharyya A. Barotrauma. *Injury* 2004;35:359-70.
10. Mirza S, Richardson H. Otic barotrauma from air travel. *J Laryngol Otol* 2005;119:366-70.
11. Sheffield, P, Vann R; Divers Alert Network. *Flying after recreational diving: workshop proceedings, May 2, 2002*. Durham: DAN; 2004. Available from: www.diversalertnetwork.org/files/FADWkshpBook_web.pdf.
12. McMullin A. Scuba diving: what you and your patients need to know. *Cleve Clin J Med* 2006;73:711-2, 714, 716.
13. Jones JS, Sheffield W, White LJ et al. A double-blind comparison between oral pseudoephedrine and topical oxymetazoline in the prevention of barotrauma during air travel. *Am J Emerg Med* 1998;16:262-4.
14. Csortan E, Jones J, Haan M et al. Efficacy of pseudoephedrine for the prevention of barotrauma during air travel. *Ann Emerg Med* 1994;23:1324-7.
15. Government of Canada. *Concerns about children's medication*. Date modified: 2015-03-26. Available from: www.healthycanadians.gc.ca.
16. Buchanan BJ, Hoagland J, Fischer PR. Pseudoephedrine and air travel-associated ear pain in children. *Arch Pediatr Adolesc Med* 1999;153:466-8.
17. Brown M, Jones J, Krohmer J. Pseudoephedrine for the prevention of barotitis media: a controlled clinical trial in underwater divers. *Ann Emerg Med* 1992;21:849-52.

Ear Piercing—What You Need to Know

Recommendations to reduce the risk of ear piercing problems:

- Ear piercing should be done only by individuals who have proper training. All piercing equipment must be sterile. There is a higher rate of infection and other problems for people who pierce their ears at home.
- Do not pierce the ears of children under 5 years of age. The earrings may get caught during play and injure the child's ears. Also it is more difficult to keep a child's piercings cleaned properly.
- Do not have your ears pierced if you have any of the following health problems: valvular heart disease, diabetes, glomerulonephritis or a history of rheumatic fever. The risk of infection is higher and more serious for these individuals.
- Do not have your ears pierced if you have had problems with scarring in the past, such as thick, raised scars (keloid formation).
- Avoid using earrings that contain nickel or gold in newly pierced ears. This will help to reduce the risk of an allergic skin reaction (dermatitis).
- Be sure that the studs are made in a single piece from surgical grade stainless steel.
- Before the ears are pierced: Clean the earlobes with alcohol or chlorhexidine soap. Allow the lobes to dry completely.

Care of the ears following piercing:

- Wash the piercing twice daily with soap and water for the first 6 weeks. Be sure to get between the stud and skin on the front, and between the earring back and skin on the back of the lobe.
- Examine the ears carefully after they are pierced. Watch for redness, swelling or rash. Feel the lobes for small lumps (which could be cysts or nodules). See a doctor right away if you have any of these problems.
- Do not turn or twist the earrings except when cleaning; this increases the risk of infection. Leave studs in place for 6 weeks.
- When you wash your hair, make sure you rinse all shampoo from the ear area. Avoid using hair spray and perfume until the lobes are well healed.
- When the earlobes are completely healed (at least 6 weeks), you can take out the studs. Wet the earlobes with water and soap to make it easier to remove the studs.
- Once earlobes are healed, wash daily with soap and water, just as you would wash your face.
- Always wash earrings with soap and water before you put them in your earlobes.

Ear Conditions

Chapter 19

Impacted Earwax

Yvonne M. Shevchuk, BSP, PharmD, FCSHP

Pathophysiology

The skin lining the lateral two-thirds of the external auditory canal (EAC) contains hair follicles, ceruminous glands (producing cerumen) and sebaceous glands (producing sebum).[1,2,3] Earwax is composed of secretions from these glands mixed with exfoliated squamous epithelium, sweat and foreign substances such as dirt, hairspray and shampoo. Earwax, rather than cerumen, is the more correct term to use although the two are often used interchangeably.[4] Earwax lubricates and protects the ear; it is water repellent, preventing maceration of the EAC, and is bacteriostatic. It is normally secreted in small amounts and moves out of the ear through the action of cilia, talking and chewing. Factors that disrupt the normal migration of earwax to the outer EAC increase the risk of impaction (see Table 1).

Accumulation of earwax may:[1,3,5,6]

- Prevent visualization of the tympanic membrane (required when attempting to diagnose middle ear conditions)
- Cause impaction of wax
- Produce hearing loss
- Produce ear discomfort (sensation of fullness in the ear, or pruritis), ear pain, vertigo or tinnitus
- Produce chronic cough
- Contribute to infection by impairing the natural cleansing mechanism of the ear.

Table 1: **Risk Factors for Earwax Impaction**

Bony growths in the canal (osteophyte or osteoma)
Hearing aids and ear plug–type hearing protectors
History of previous impaction
Numerous ear canal hairs
Older age: ceruminous glands atrophy, creating drier cerumen that is more difficult to expel from the ear
Use of cotton-tipped applicators

Goals of Therapy

- Relieve symptoms
- Allow visualization of tympanic membrane
- Avoid damage to the EAC
- Prevent infection
- Prevent recurrence

Patient Assessment

Figure 1 illustrates the assessment pathway for a patient with suspected earwax impaction. Ideally, earwax impaction is diagnosed by direct visualization with an otoscope.

Question the patient regarding the common symptoms of earwax impaction (sensation of fullness in the ear, hearing loss and discomfort) and modifiable risk factors for impaction. There is often a history of attempted removal of wax with cotton-tipped swabs or other foreign objects, which have actually pushed the wax further into the ear and exacerbated symptoms. If there is discharge from the ear (pus or blood), coexisting otitis externa or injury of the EAC may be present (see Chapter 20: Otitis Media and Otitis Externa).

Referral for assessment and further treatment should be considered if:[1]

- the ear has been injured
- the tympanic membrane is perforated
- there is a history of recent ear surgery
- the patient has tympanostomy tubes
- the patient has chronic otitis media
- there is drainage from the ear, hearing loss, tinnitus or dizziness
- the patient is a child
- the patient has congenital or anatomical abnormalities.

Prevention

The ear is usually self-cleaning. The external opening can be cleaned using a washcloth over the index finger. Discourage attempts at removing earwax with cotton-tipped applicators, hair pins, matches, fingernails and other objects. This may cause damage to the EAC and push wax farther into the canal, causing impaction.

Instillation of **olive oil**, **light mineral oil**, **hydrogen peroxide**, **glycerin** or **sodium bicarbonate** are sometimes recommended in individuals prone to earwax impaction as preventive therapy although there is no evidence to support this effect. When used, a few drops of the agent is instilled into the ear or ears daily to twice weekly.

Nonpharmacologic Therapy

Since the ear is generally self-cleaning, products or techniques to aid in earwax removal should be recommended only when required (for example, when there is a need to see the tympanic membrane) or for symptomatic relief. Discourage use by the patient to simply "keep the ears clean."

A common method used to remove earwax is syringing the ear with water at body temperature, with or without prior instillation of eardrops to soften the wax. Self-irrigation with bulb syringes can reduce the demand for ear irrigation by healthcare practitioners and has been shown to be safe.[7,8] Suggest assistance from a caregiver as it may be difficult to perform the procedure on oneself. See Impacted Earwax—What You Need to Know for steps outlining proper syringing technique.

Syringing is contraindicated if the tympanic membrane is perforated or has been perforated in the past, infection is present, tympanostomy tubes are present, there is a history of ear surgery, the patient is a young child who is uncooperative, or the affected ear is the patient's only hearing ear.[1,9]

Complications of syringing include failure to remove wax, pain or discomfort, vertigo, otitis media or otitis externa, damage to the EAC and perforation of the tympanic membrane.[1,5,9,10,11] Major complications occur in approximately 1 in 1000 ears.[11]

Wax can also be manually removed with a curette, forceps or suction by a healthcare practitioner with the appropriate training.[1,3]

Pharmacologic Therapy

A number of agents are purported to enhance removal of wax from the ear (see Table 2). These products are instilled for the required period of time, after which the wax is allowed to be expelled naturally or the ear syringed to remove the softened wax. Few studies exist to provide evidence of their effectiveness. Studies comparing the effectiveness of various agents with each other or with syringing are of poor quality, making it difficult to recommend one method over another.

Water-based ceruminolytics (see Table 2) and **carbamide peroxide** expand and loosen or dissolve wax plugs while oil-based products simply lubricate the EAC and wax plug.[3,4,12] In vitro data suggest oil-based products (olive oil and urea hydrogen peroxide 5% in glycerol) are not effective in disintegrating cerumen.[13]

No earwax-softening agent has been demonstrated to be superior to others. **Water** or **saline** appears to be as effective as **sodium bicarbonate**,[14] **chlorbutol**,[14] **docusate sodium**,[14,15] or **carbamide peroxide**[12,16] to facilitate clearing earwax with or without syringing.[5] Instillation of any of these agents into the ear canal for 15 minutes followed by syringing is as effective as using oil in the canal for 3 nights followed by syringing.[5,12,17] Instillation of oil is still commonly recommended by healthcare practitioners; however, use of an non-oil-based earwax-softening agent followed by syringing is often more convenient for the patient and offers more immediate relief of symptoms.

Commercially prepared otic products are available in a dropper bottle. If household products such as olive oil are chosen, the patient should purchase a dropper and instil the substance in a manner similar to other ear drops. "Home remedies" such as dilutions of hydrogen peroxide or solutions of sodium bicarbonate should be freshly prepared and used immediately (see Table 2).

For comparative ingredients of nonprescription products, consult the *Compendium of Products For Minor Ailments*—Otic Products.

Ceruminolytics should not be used if the tympanic membrane is not intact or if tympanostomy tubes are present.

Ear candling is a procedure that has been claimed to remove earwax by creating a vacuum or negative pressure within the ear canal. Studies have disproven the claims and have shown it may cause serious injury.[18,19] Risks associated with ear candling include burns, occlusion from candle wax, temporary loss of hearing, punctured eardrum and fire. Health Canada has received several reports of ear injury from ear candling.[19] The sale of ear candles in Canada is illegal. Discourage the use of ear candles.

Monitoring of Therapy

Relief of symptoms (ear fullness, hearing loss, ear discomfort) should occur as soon as the wax is expelled. Initially, hearing loss or fullness may be exacerbated due to swelling of the wax within the canal. If irritation of the canal occurs, use of the product should be discontinued. This is generally sufficient; however if the irritation is severe or otitis externa develops, appropriate treatment may be required. The healthcare practitioner should follow up with the patient after the third or fourth day of use to determine whether symptom relief has occurred. Relief may occur more gradually (5–7 days) with oil-based products without syringing; follow up after 5–7 days. If relief does not occur, further assessment and treatment may be required.

Figure 1: Assessment of Patients with Impacted Earwax Symptoms[1]

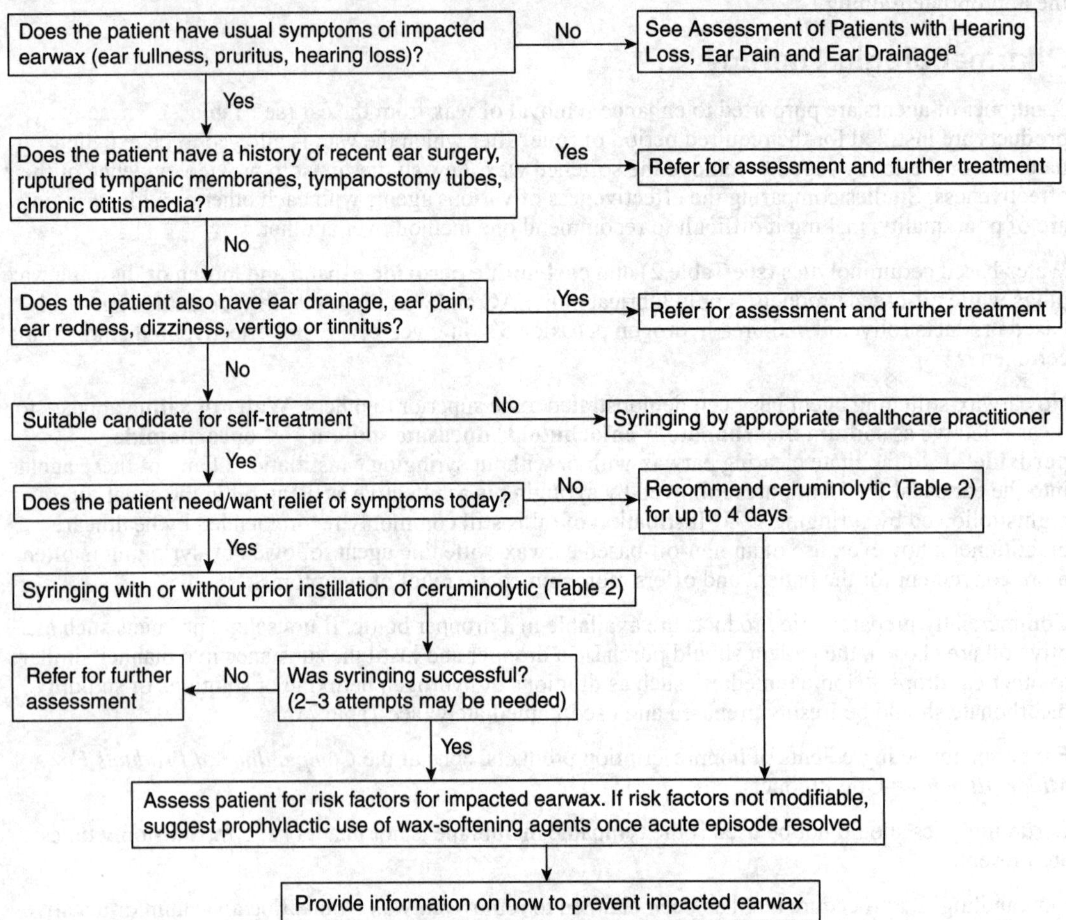

[a] See Figure 1 in Chapter 17: Assessment of Patients with Hearing Loss, Ear Pain and Ear Drainage.

Table 2: Agents to Remove Excessive or Impacted Earwax

Class	Drug	Dosage[a]	Comments	Cost[b]
Softening Agents, Oil-based	*olive oil, mineral oil (light), almond oil*	4–6 drops in the ear canal BID for up to 4 days *or* 3 drops in the affected ear QHS for 3–4 nights	Intended to soften earwax prior to syringing, or wax may be allowed to be expelled naturally. In vitro data suggest oils are ineffective for disintegrating earwax.[13] Generally not irritating. Effects are delayed (unless used just prior to syringing). Hearing loss and fullness may initially be exacerbated due to swelling of wax. These agents may be instilled periodically (daily or 2–3 times weekly) for prevention of impaction.	$
Softening Agents, Water-based	*water, saline, sodium bicarbonate (10–15%), hydrogen peroxide 3%*	Fill ear canal for 15–30 min prior to syringing	In vitro data suggest water-based products are more effective than oil-based products.[13] May use a few drops of sodium bicarbonate or hydrogen peroxide 2–3 times weekly to prevent impaction.	$
	chlorbutol 5% Cerumol	Use 5–10 drops for 10–15 min	The commercially available chlorbutol product contains oil of terbinth (turpentine oil), paradichlorobenzene and peanut oil. Turpentine is a rubefacient and counterirritant used topically to provide analgesia. It can cause skin irritation. Paradichlorobenzene gives the characteristic smell to moth balls and is used to repel insects. Their inclusion in a product used to remove earwax is questionable. Arachis oil may induce allergic reactions and patients allergic to peanuts should not use this product. Health Canada has received a report of anaphylaxis in a peanut-allergic child with use of the commercial product.[20]	$$
	docusate sodium 10 mg/mL generics	1 mL in the affected ear for 10–15 min followed by syringing	No commercial otic preparation available; use oral solution.	$$
Softening Agents, Non-water, non-oil-based	*carbamide peroxide 6.5%* Murine Ear Drops, Murine Ear Wax System	5–10 drops in affected ear; leave in ear several minutes; any wax remaining can be removed by gently flushing the ear with warm water. Use BID for up to 4 days		$$

[a] For instructions on proper instillation of eardrops, see Eardrops—What You Need to Know in Chapter 20: Otitis Media and Otitis Externa

[b] Cost of smallest available pack size.

Legend: $ < $4 $$ $4–8

Suggested Readings

Aung T, Mulley GP. Removal of ear wax *BMJ* 2002;325:27.

McCarter DF, Courtney AU, Pollart SM. Cerumen impaction. *Am Fam Physician* 2007;75:1523-8.

Roland PS, Smith TL, Schwartz SR et al. Clinical practice guideline: cerumen impaction. *Otolaryngol Head Neck Surg* 2008;139:S1-S21.

References

1. Roland PS, Smith TL, Schwartz SR et al. Clinical practice guideline: cerumen impaction. *Otolaryngol Head Neck Surg* 2008;139:S1-S21.
2. Arnett A. Pain-earache. In: Fleisher GR, Ludwig S, Henretig FM, eds. *Textbook of pediatric emergency medicine*. 5th ed. Philadelphia: Lippincott Williams & Wilkins; 2006. p. 505-10.
3. McCarter DF, Courtney AU, Pollart SM. Cerumen impaction. *Am Fam Physician* 2007;75:1523-8.
4. Hawke M. Update on cerumen and ceruminolytics. *Ear Nose Throat J* 2002;81:23-4.
5. Browning GG. Ear wax. *Clin Evid (Online)* 2008;pii:0504.
6. Raman R. Impacted ear wax–a cause for unexplained cough? *Arch Otolaryngol Head Neck Surg* 1986;112:679.
7. Coppin R, Wicke D, Little P. Randomized trial of bulb syringes for earwax: impact on health service utilization. *Ann Fam Med* 2011;9:110-4.
8. Rogers N, Stevermer JJ. PURLs: Ear wax removal: help patients help themselves. *J Fam Pract* 2011;60:671-3.
9. Aung T, Mulley GP. Removal of ear wax *BMJ* 2002;325:27.
10. Sharp JF, Wilson JA, Ross L et al. Ear wax removal: a survey of current practice. *BMJ* 1990;301:1251-3.
11. Bird S. The potential pitfalls of ear syringing. Minimising the risks. *Aust Fam Physician* 2003;32:150-1.
12. Hand C, Harvey I. The effectiveness of topical preparations for the treatment of earwax: a systematic review. *Br J Gen Pract* 2004;54:862-7.
13. Saxby C, Williams R, Hickey S. Finding the most effective cerumenolytic. *J Laryngol Otol* 2013;127:1067-70.
14. Burton MJ, Doree C. Ear drops for the removal of ear wax. *Cochrane Database Syst Rev* 2009;(1):CD004326.
15. Whatley VN, Dodds CL, Paul RI. Randomized clinical trial of docusate, triethanolamine polypeptide, and irrigation in cerumen removal in children. *Arch Pediatr Adolesc Med* 2003;157:1177-80.
16. Roland PS, Eaton DA, Gross RD et al. Randomized, placebo-controlled evaluation of Cerumenex and Murine earwax removal products. *Arch Otolaryngol Head Neck Surg* 2004;130:1175-7.
17. Eekhof JA, de Bock GH, Le Cessie S et al. A quasi-randomised controlled trial of water as a quick softening agent of persistent earwax in general practice. *Br J Gen Pract* 2001;51:635-7.
18. Seely DR, Quigley SM, Langman AW. Ear candles–efficacy and safety. *Laryngoscope* 1996;106:1226-9.
19. Government of Canada. *Ear candling*. Available from: healthycanadians.gc.ca/drugs-products-medicaments-produits/buying-using-achat-utilisation/medical-procedures-medicales/ear-oreille-eng.php. Accessed February 13, 2013.
20. Health Canada. Case presentation: Cerumol and anaphylaxis. *Canadian Adverse Reaction Newsletter* 2013;23:5. Available from: www.hc-sc.gc.ca/dhp-mps/alt_formats/pdf/medeff/bulletin/carn-bcei_v23n1-eng.pdf. Accessed February 26, 2013.

Impacted Earwax—What You Need to Know

General information about caring for your ears:

- Ears generally clean themselves. It is not usually necessary to remove wax.
- If you put any object into the ear canal (in particular cotton-tipped swabs), you may push wax further in. This can cause a wax buildup that blocks the ear (impaction). It may result in discomfort and hearing loss.
- If earwax becomes impacted, you may need to use something to soften the wax so it will come out. You can use:
  - 4–6 drops of olive oil, almond oil or light mineral oil;

  or
  - a commercial eardrop. Follow the directions on the package.
- For some products, such as olive oil, almond oil, light mineral oil or carbamide peroxide, you may have to put drops in your ear twice a day for several days before the wax softens enough to come out on its own.
- Some products (such as those containing chlorbutol) should remain in the ear for no more than 15 minutes before you syringe them out.
- Water or saline work as well as commercial products when used prior to syringing.
- If you buy a commercial product, make sure you know how to use it safely before you leave the pharmacy. Ask your pharmacist for advice.
- Stop using any product that irritates your ears.
- You may have heard or read about the use of ear candling to clean the ear canal. Ear candling is dangerous and does not work. It can lead to injury of the ear and burns to the ears or face.
- If you have repeated problems with earwax, you may be able to prevent the problem by using 4–6 drops of olive oil, vegetable oil, light mineral oil, hydrogen peroxide or sodium bicarbonate 15% solution in your ears 2–3 times a week.

See a healthcare provider if:

- You have any of the symptoms of a burst eardrum. Symptoms of a burst eardrum include:
  - bleeding or discharge from the ear
  - dizziness
  - pain in the ear
  - ringing in the ears
  - hearing loss
- You have:
  - a rash in your ear
  - a history of ear surgery
  - tubes in your ears
  - ear infection
  - received radiation treatment to the area
  - sharp foreign objects in the ear canal

Your ears should not be syringed in these cases.

How to syringe the ears:

- **Never attempt to flush out the ear canal if there is any possibility the eardrum has burst (see above) or ear tubes are present. If you think you have a burst eardrum, see a healthcare provider.**
- It is difficult to syringe your ears by yourself—get someone to help you.
- Fill the ear syringe with warm water (body temperature).
- Hold a basin just below the ear to catch the water coming out of the ear. Lay a towel over the shoulder.
- For adults, straighten the ear canal by gently pulling the ear up and back. For a child, pull the ear down and back.
- Insert the ear syringe just into the opening of the ear canal. Do not put it in further—you could damage the ear.
- Using the syringe, direct a stream of water along the upper surface of the ear canal so that the returning flow pushes the earwax out from behind. Squeeze the syringe gently. Don't force the water into the ear.

Chapter 20

Otitis Media and Otitis Externa

Yvonne M. Shevchuk, BSP, PharmD, FCSHP

Otitis Media

Pathophysiology

Acute otitis media (AOM) is an infection of the middle ear cavity and is one of the most common bacterial infections in childhood.[1] Seventy-five percent of children experience at least 1 episode prior to entering school.[2] To diagnose AOM, 3 criteria need to be met: 1) signs and symptoms of middle ear inflammation 2) the presence of middle ear effusion and 3) acute onset (often abrupt) of signs and symptoms of middle ear inflammation and effusion.[1] Symptoms include acute ear pain (often unilateral and developing over a few hours), fever and reduced hearing.[1] Tugging or pulling on the ears is often described, but this is a very nonspecific sign.[1] Children too young to complain of pain or pressure in the ears may display irritability, excessive fussiness, poor feeding and disrupted sleep patterns. Acute otitis media is more common in the winter months. A recent history of viral upper respiratory tract infection is often present.[2] The microorganisms most commonly associated with AOM are *Streptococcus pneumoniae*, *Haemophilus influenzae* and *Moraxella catarrhalis*.[1,2]

AOM has a high spontaneous recovery rate; 80% of children experience spontaneous symptomatic relief with placebo or no drug therapy.[3,4] For this reason, the concept of "watchful waiting" is advocated after appropriate healthcare practitioner assessment and diagnosis of AOM. Rather than immediate initiation of antibiotic therapy, appropriately selected children are managed with analgesic therapy for the first 24–48 hours. This includes children >6 months of age with no craniofacial abnormalities who have uncomplicated AOM (normal host, no otorrhea, no history of chronic or recurrent AOM) without severe pain or systemic illness, and whose caregivers are able to recognize severe illness, take the child for immediate assessment, and provide access to follow-up care.[1,2]

Goals of Therapy

- Relieve symptoms of fever, pain and irritability
- Eliminate bacteria from the middle ear
- Ensure appropriate therapy to reduce the risk of resistant pathogens and drug-related adverse effects such as antibiotic-associated diarrhea
- Prevent complications, e.g., mastoiditis, intracranial infection, facial paralysis

Nonpharmacologic Therapy

Comfort measures, such as warmed oils, warm or cold compresses and heating pads have been used by parents and caregivers for years, although there are no studies evaluating their effectiveness. If tried, heat therapy should be used cautiously and with close supervision in children, to avoid burns. A young child should never sleep with a hot water bottle or heating pad. Question the caregiver about whether there has been any drainage from the ear prior to recommending any topical therapy. Warmed oil should not be used if there is a chance of perforation or any suspicion of drainage. Warming of drops or oil should be done by rolling the bottle between the palms; other methods such as placing the bottle in a glass of warm water or using the microwave oven should be avoided as serious burns have been reported.

Pharmacologic Therapy

For more information on management of acute otitis media, consult the *Compendium of Therapeutic Choices*: Acute Otitis Media in Childhood.

- If **antibiotics** are used, systemic therapy is required; topical agents are not used in AOM.
- Adequate analgesia with usual doses of **acetaminophen** or **ibuprofen** is important (see Chapter 7: Fever, Table 5).
- **Topical analgesics** may provide short-term analgesia in children with AOM, but should not replace oral analgesics.[5,6] Topical analgesics may cause local hypersensitivity reactions.
- Decongestants and antihistamines, which were recommended in the past, do not speed the resolution of effusion and can have significant adverse effects in children and therefore should not be used.[7,8]

For a more complete discussion of acute otitis media, see Suggested Readings.

Otitis Externa

Pathophysiology

Otitis externa is defined as inflammation of the external auditory canal (EAC) and may also involve the pinna or tympanic membrane (TM). Otitis externa is often due to infection.[9,10,11,12] The EAC is warm, dark and prone to becoming moist. This provides an excellent environment for bacteria or fungi to proliferate, particularly if the EAC is traumatized. Otitis externa can be categorized as acute diffuse, acute localized, chronic, eczematous or necrotizing.[12] The main focus of this chapter is acute diffuse otitis externa.

Acute Diffuse Otitis Externa

Predisposing factors for acute diffuse otitis externa include:[9,10,11,13]

- Too little cerumen—cerumen provides antibacterial action by physically protecting the canal and maintaining a low pH
- Too much cerumen, which can lead to occlusion and maceration
- Moisture (swimming, bathing, water sports, perspiration, increased humidity)—macerates underlying skin and raises pH
- Trauma to EAC (caused by fingernails, cotton-tipped swabs, other foreign objects, overzealous wax removal)—abrasion and laceration allowing inoculation of organisms
- Chronic dermatologic disorders
- Hearing aids
- Narrow, hairy ear canal.

The most common etiology of acute otitis externa is bacterial infection. Fungal overgrowth occurs rarely, and primarily in patients who have received prior antibiotic therapy. The 2 most common microorganisms causing acute otitis externa are *Pseudomonas aeruginosa* (20–60%) and *Staphylococcus aureus* (10–70%).[10,11]

Bacterial otitis externa produces ear pain or discomfort (otalgia), otorrhea, pruritus and tenderness, especially on manipulation of the ear.[10,11] These symptoms may be more intense than those seen with fungal otitis externa. Cellulitis of the pinna and regional lymphadenopathy may be present.[10] Fungal otitis externa may be asymptomatic or may produce pruritus and fullness in the ear. It classically occurs after prolonged treatment of bacterial otitis externa with antibiotics which alter the bacterial flora of the EAC. The EAC may contain black, grey, bluish green, yellow or white fungal elements and debris.

Acute Localized Otitis Externa (Furunculosis)

This is an acute localized "boil" (infected hair follicle) in the ear canal usually due to *S. aureus*. It produces localized pain, itching, edema, erythema and possibly a fluctuance or abscess. The pain subsides when the boil comes to a head and bursts. Topical mupirocin or fusidic acid can be used for mild cases.[14] Incision and drainage may be required for some patients. Patients appearing to need incision and drainage should be seen by a healthcare practitioner with appropriate training. In more severe cases, systemic antibiotics active against *S. aureus* should be considered.[10]

Chronic Otitis Externa

Chronic otitis externa is characterized as a thickening of the EAC skin secondary to low-grade infection and inflammation. There is usually unrelenting pruritus, mild discomfort and dry, flaky skin in the EAC with lack of cerumen. This is often due to nonbacterial causes including allergic contact dermatitis.[9]

Eczematous Otitis Externa

Eczematous otitis externa may be due to a variety of skin conditions, including atopic, seborrheic or contact dermatitis, psoriasis, lupus erythematosus, neurodermatitis and infantile eczema. Lesions typically occur elsewhere on the body, especially the head and neck, as well as the auricle and EAC. Appearance may range from mild erythema and scaling with atopic dermatitis to the typical adherent scales of psoriasis (see Chapter 55: Atopic, Contact, and Stasis Dermatitis; Chapter 58: Dandruff and Seborrheic Dermatitis; and Chapter 71: Psoriasis for a more complete description of the lesions). The most common symptom is pruritus, although erythema, edema, crusting and oozing may be present. The lesions may become secondarily infected with bacteria or fungi. Treatment is primarily management of the underlying condition.[15]

Necrotizing (Malignant) Otitis Externa

This is an infection that extends to the mastoid or temporal bone and is usually seen in immunocompromised patients or those with diabetes. Urgent referral and systemic antimicrobial therapy are required.[10,11]

This chapter focuses on the management of acute diffuse otitis externa.

Goals of Therapy

- Eliminate pathogenic microorganisms
- Control pain
- Restore the canal to normal health so it resists infection—return to normal acidic pH and adequate cerumen

Patient Assessment

Acute otitis externa is characterized by otalgia (70% of cases), itching (60%) or fullness (22%) with or without hearing loss (32%) and discharge in or coming from the ear (otorrhea).[10,16] Incidence peaks in children age 7–12 years and declines after the age of 50.[16] It is unilateral in 90% of cases.[16] The discomfort can range from pruritus to severe pain. The pain is often worse with motion of the ear (pushing the tragus or pulling the pinna),[10] including movement caused by chewing.[11] Determining the type of otitis externa (infectious vs. noninfectious) can be assisted by the description of the signs and symptoms above and the presence of contributing factors (e.g., history of swimming or trauma to the EAC), or the presence of dermatologic conditions on areas of the body other than the EAC.

The drug must be delivered to the infected tissue if topical therapy is to be successful.[10,16] Cleansing must be done by a healthcare practitioner with appropriate training. Therefore, if there is significant edema or debris in the EAC, the patient may need to be referred so that aural toilet can be performed or for a wick to be placed.[10] In mild cases, a topical product may be initiated without cleansing; recommendations for pain management are important.

Nonpharmacologic Therapy

Adequate cleansing of the ear canal with removal of debris may be required frequently so that topical therapy can be effective.[9,10] If the canal is not patent, ear wicks may be inserted by a healthcare practitioner to reduce edema and swelling and provide a mechanism for drug delivery to the canal.[10,11] These may remain in place for 2–5 days.

Pharmacologic Therapy

For comparative ingredients of nonprescription products, consult the *Compendium of Products for Minor Ailments*—Analgesic Products: Internal Analgesics and Antipyretics; Otic Products.

Topical treatment is the mainstay of therapy, although in more severe cases, when infection has spread beyond the EAC, when otitis media coexists, or if the patient has a condition such as diabetes or immunodeficiency, systemic antibiotics may be required.[10] In uncomplicated cases, systemic therapy does not improve outcomes compared with topical therapy and increases the risk of adverse effects and antibiotic resistance and time to clinical cure.[17] Topical therapy options include **acidifying agents, antibiotics** alone or **antibiotic/corticosteroid** combinations (see Table 1). Comparative trials show similar outcomes among approaches; therefore, the choice is determined by healthcare practitioner and patient preference, the side effect profile of the agents and cost.[10,11,12,18,19] One trial demonstrated that corticosteroid drops (with either **acetic acid** or antibiotic) are more effective than acetic acid alone and recommended that acetic acid alone not be used in adult patients.[20] In patients whose symptoms last longer than a week, acetic acid may be less effective than an antibiotic/corticosteroid combination; efficacy at 1 week is similar.[18] Advantages and disadvantages of the various products are outlined in Table 1.

Antibiotic drops are available as both otic and ophthalmic preparations. Both nonprescription and prescription products are available. Otic products are more acidic than ophthalmic preparations and may cause burning on instillation. If a patient cannot tolerate otic preparations, ophthalmic preparations may be more comfortable.[21] Preparations for treatment of otitis externa may contain corticosteroids, which reduce inflammation and edema and may resolve symptoms more quickly; however, this has not been shown in all studies and corticosteroids may occasionally be topical sensitizers.[18]

One particular concern with topical therapy of acute otitis externa is the potential ototoxicity of **aminoglycosides**.[22] This is a documented adverse effect of systemically administered aminoglycosides. If the tympanic membrane is intact, the risk with topical administration is extremely small. Risk factors for ototoxicity include ruptured tympanic membrane, use of the product for more than 1 week and continued use after otorrhea has subsided. Topical **fluoroquinolones** have not been associated with ototoxicity.

Enough liquid to fill the canal (3–4 drops) should be instilled 3–4 times daily (most products except fluoroquinolones). Symptoms will last for approximately 6 days after treatment begins; however, improvement in symptoms should occur within 48–72 hours.[10] Patients should be treated for 1 week. If symptoms are not completely gone, therapy can be continued until symptoms resolve plus a few days beyond (up to 2 weeks).[18] In 65–90% of patients, clinical resolution occurs in 7–10 days.[10] For information on correct instillation of eardrops, see Eardrops—What You Need to Know.

Fungal otitis externa often responds to cleansing and acidification alone, although topical antifungal agents (**clioquinol**, **clotrimazole**, **tolnaftate**) may also be used.[16] Some preparations may need to be compounded.

Otitis externa can be very painful. Usual doses of **acetaminophen**, **ibuprofen** or **naproxen sodium** can be used for analgesia (**ASA** can be used in adults).[10,11] Although some otic preparations contain topical anesthetics, the efficacy of these agents has not been determined in acute otitis externa, and topical hypersensitivity reactions can occur.[10] If topical anesthetic agents are used in addition to other topical therapy, this will dilute the acidifier or antibiotic present in the canal. Avoid their use in otitis externa. Systemic analgesia is the preferred recommendation.

Eczematous Otitis Externa

Eczematous otitis externa is managed by treating the underlying dermatologic disease (e.g., seborrhea, psoriasis, acne).[9,15] Contact dermatitis commonly occurs on or in the ears, and grooming products (e.g., shampoos, hair sprays and hair dyes) are common allergens.[10] Hearing aids and earplugs may also cause dermatitis of the EAC. Neomycin is one of the topical medications that most commonly causes allergic contact dermatitis.[10] Patients sensitive to neomycin may also react to tobramycin. Other agents commonly placed in the ear that are reported to cause contact dermatitis include benzalkonium chloride, benzocaine and propylene glycol.[23]

Management includes avoiding the offending agent, applying **acetic acid** solution to dry oozing lesions and re-acidify the canal, or symptomatic therapy with a **topical corticosteroid**.

Prevention of Recurrence

Provide information on how to prevent a recurrence to individuals who develop acute otitis externa:

- After swimming or bathing, dry the external canal with a blow dryer on low setting or by instillation of acidifying or alcohol drops.[10,11,16]
- Avoid overzealous cleansing and scratching (trauma) of the ear canal.[10]
- Avoid cotton-tipped swabs.[11,16,24]
- Avoid water sports for at least 7–10 days during treatment.[10]
- Ear plugs and bathing caps may be used to keep the ears dry; however, there is little evidence to guide recommendations.[10] Frequent use of ear plugs may also act as a local irritant and promote infection.

Monitoring of Therapy

Symptoms should be significantly reduced by day 3 of therapy,[10,11] and for most patients symptoms should have completely resolved in a week. Occasionally up to 14 days of treatment is needed.[18] Follow up with the patient in 3–5 days to ensure symptoms are improving and at the end of treatment to ensure resolution. If symptoms worsen or do not resolve, consider the following: the patient may be reacting to the medication (contact dermatitis); a superinfection may have developed; the diagnosis may be incorrect; improper or infrequent use of eardrops; inadequate penetration of topical agents due to debris or narrowing of the canal; immunosuppression or malignant otitis externa; or the organism is not susceptible to the topical agent selected.[9,10] Assessment for further treatment will be required.

Advice for the Patient

Advise patients on:

- Prevention of recurrences
- Methods of pain control
- Correct use of eardrops
- Possible side effects of treatment and their management (see Table 1)
- When to see a healthcare practitioner.

Table 1: Drugs for Otitis Externa

Class	Drug	Indications	Adverse Effects	Comments	Cost[a]
Acidifying Agents	*acetic acid 2%*	Prevention and treatment of mild AOE	Can be irritating to inflamed canal. Possibly ototoxic.	Broad-spectrum antibacterial.[25] Restores acidity to canal. Lower cost than antibiotics. No commercial product available. May be prepared by diluting white vinegar with equal parts isopropyl alcohol or water.[10]	$
Antibiotics	*ciprofloxacin* Ciloxan, generics	Treatment of AOE	Well tolerated. Not associated with ototoxicity.	Active against many gram-negative organisms including *P. aeruginosa* and some gram-positive (*S. aureus*). Twice-daily dosing. Topical quinolones provide similar clinical cure rates as other topical antibiotics.[19] Ophthalmic solutions can be used in the ears.	$
	gramicidin/polymyxin B Optimyxin Ear Drops, Polysporin Eye/Ear Drops	Treatment of AOE	Potentially ototoxic.	Gramicidin—active against gram-positive organisms. Polymyxin B—active against gram-negative organisms.	$$
	moxifloxacin Vigamox	Treatment of AOE	See ciprofloxacin.	See ciprofloxacin. Ophthalmic solutions can be used in the ears.	$$
	ofloxacin Ocuflox, generics	Treatment of AOE	See ciprofloxacin.	See ciprofloxacin. Ophthalmic solutions can be used in the ears.	$
	tobramycin Tobrex, generics	Treatment of AOE	Potentially ototoxic, particularly with perforated tympanic membrane, tympanostomy tubes or use >1 wk.	Aminoglycosides active against gram-negative organisms (e.g., *Pseudomonas*) and *S. aureus*. Ophthalmic solutions can be used in the ears.	$
Corticosteroids	*dexamethasone* Maxidex	Dermatologic causes of AOE	May cause hypersensitivity reactions.	Anti-inflammatory properties reduce swelling and edema. If bacterial etiology combine with acidifier or antibiotic. Ophthalmic solutions can be used in the ears.	$

(cont'd)

Table 1: **Drugs for Otitis Externa** *(cont'd)*

Class	Drug	Indications	Adverse Effects	Comments	Cost[a]
Antibiotic/ Corticosteroid Combinations	*ciprofloxacin/ dexamethasone* Ciprodex	Treatment of AOE	See ciprofloxacin. See dexamethasone.	See ciprofloxacin. See dexamethasone.	$$$
	clioquinol/flumethasone pivalate Locacorten Vioform Eardrops	Treatment of AOE	Negligible gram-negative activity. Bacteriostatic. See dexamethasone.	Clioquinol active against fungi and gram-positive bacteria. See dexamethasone.	$$
	framycetin/gramicidin/ dexamethasone Sofracort	Treatment of AOE	See tobramycin. See dexamethasone.	Framycetin active against gram-negative organisms (but not *Pseudomonas*) and *S. aureus.* Gramicidin—active against gram-positive organisms. See dexamethasone.	$$
Miscellaneous	*antipyrine/benzocaine* Auralgan	Topical analgesia	Benzocaine may produce topical hypersensitivity reactions. Antipyrine—mild anesthetic; can cause burning and itching. May mask symptoms of worsening AOE.	Do not use with ruptured tympanic membrane. Oral analgesics preferred.	$
	isopropyl alcohol 95% glycerin 5% Auro-Dri Ear Water	Prevention of AOE	Painful when used in acute otitis externa.	Useful drying agent.	$

[a] Cost of smallest available pack size; includes drug cost only.

Abbreviations: AOE = acute otitis externa

Legend: $ < $10 $$ $10–20 $$$ $20–30

Suggested Readings

Otitis Externa

Hui CP; Canadian Paediatric Society, Infectious Diseases and Immunization Committee. Acute otitis externa. *Paediatr Child Health* 2013;18:96-101.

Rosenfeld RM, Schwartz SR, Cannon CR et al. Clinical practice guideline: acute otitis externa. *Otolaryngol Head Neck Surg* 2014;150:S1-S24.

Schaefer P, Baugh RF. Acute otitis externa: an update. *Am Fam Physician* 2012;86:1055-61.

Otitis Media

Le Saux N, Robinson J. Management of acute otitis media in children six months of age and older. *Paediatr Child Health* 2016;21(1):39–44.

Lieberthal AS, Carroll AE, Chonmaitree T et al. Diagnosis and management of acute otitis media. *Pediatrics* 2013:131:e964-99.

Vergison A, Dagan R, Arguedas A et al. Otitis media and its consequences: beyond the earache. *Lancet Infect Dis* 2010;10:195-203.

References

1. Lieberthal AS, Carroll AE, Chonmaitree T et al. Diagnosis and management of acute otitis media. *Pediatrics* 2013;131:e964-99.
2. Le Saux N, Robinson J. Management of acute otitis media in children six months of age and older. *Paediatr Child Health* 2016;21(1):39–44.
3. Rosenfeld RM, Vertrees JE, Carr J et al. Clinical efficacy of antimicrobial drugs for acute otitis media: metaanalysis of 5400 children from thirty-three randomized trials. *J Pediatr* 1994;124:355-67.
4. Venekamp RP, Sanders SL, Glasziou PP et al. Antibiotics for acute otitis media in children. *Cochrane Database of Syst Rev* 2015;1:CD000219.
5. Carley SD. Best evidence topic reports. Towards evidence based emergency medicine: Best BETs from the Manchester Royal Infirmary. *Emerg Med J* 2008;25:103.
6. Foxlee R, Johansson A, Wejfalk J et al. Topical analgesia for acute otitis media. *Cochrane Database Syst Rev* 2006;3:CD005657.
7. Mandel EM, Rockette HE, Bluestone CD et al. Efficacy of amoxicillin with and without decongestant-antihistamine for otitis media with effusion in children. Results of a double-blind, randomized trial. *N Engl J Med* 1987;316:432-7.
8. Cantekin EI, Mandel EM, Bluestone CD et al. Lack of efficacy of a decongestant-antihistamine combination for otitis media with effusion ("secretory" otitis media) in children. Results of a double-blind, randomized trial. *N Engl J Med* 1983;308:297-301.
9. Schaefer P, Baugh RF. Acute otitis externa: an update. *Am Fam Physician* 2012;86:1055-61.
10. Rosenfeld RM, Schwartz SR, Cannon CR et al. Clinical practice guideline: acute otitis externa. *Otolaryngol Head Neck Surg* 2014;150:S1-S24.
11. Hui CP; Canadian Paediatric Society, Infectious Diseases and Immunization Committee. Acute otitis externa. *Paediatr Child Health* 2013;18:96-101.
12. Hajioff D, Mackeith S. Otitis externa. *Clin Evid (Online)* 2008;pii:0510.
13. Klein JO. Otitis externa, otitis media and mastoiditis. In: Mandell GL, Bennett JE, Dolin R, eds. *Mandell, Douglas and Bennett's principles and practice of infectious diseases*. 7th ed. Philadelphia: Churchill Livingston/Elsevier; 2010. p. 831-8.
14. Blondel-Hill E, Fryters S. Bugs & Drugs app. Edmonton (AB): Alberta Health Services; 2015.
15. Shea CR. Dermatologic diseases of the external auditory canal. *Otolaryngol Clin North Am* 1996;29:783-94.
16. Osguthorpe JD, Nielsen DR. Otitis externa: review and clinical update. *Am Fam Physician* 2006:74:1510-6.
17. Pabla L, Jindal M, Latif K. The management of otitis externa in UK general practice. *Eur Arch Otorhinolaryngol* 2012;269:753-6.
18. Kaushik V, Malik T, Saeed SR. Interventions for acute otitis externa. *Cochrane Database Syst Rev* 2010;1:CD004740.
19. Rosenfeld RM, Singer M, Wasserman JM et al. Systematic review of topical antimicrobial therapy for acute otitis externa. *Otolaryngol Head Neck Surg* 2006;134:S24-48.
20. van Balen FA, Smit WM, Zuithoff NP et al. Clinical efficacy of three common treatments in acute otitis externa in primary care: randomised controlled trial. *BMJ* 2003;327:1201-5.
21. Ong YK, Chee G. Infections of the external ear. *Ann Acad Med Singapore* 2005;34:330-4.
22. Haynes DS, Rutka J, Hawke M et al. Ototoxicity of ototopical drops–an update. *Otolaryngol Clin North Am* 2007;40:669-83.
23. Fraki JE, Kalimo K, Tuohimaa P et al. Contact allergy to various components of topical preparations for treatment of external otitis. *Acta Otolaryngol* 1985;100:414-8.
24. Nussinovitch M, Rimon A, Volovitz B et al. Cotton-tipped applicators as a leading cause of otitis externa. *Int J Pediatr Otorhinolaryngol* 2004;68:433-5.
25. Thorp MA, Kruger J, Oliver S et al. The antibacterial activity of acetic acid and Burow's solution as topical otological preparations. *J Laryngol Otol* 1998;112:925-8.

Acute Otitis Externa (Swimmer's Ear)—What You Need to Know

What is acute otitis externa?

Acute otitis externa, or "swimmer's ear," is an infection of the ear canal. The symptoms are itching or pain in the ear and liquid draining from it. The ear may become plugged. Your hearing may be affected.

What causes acute otitis externa?

The skin in your ears may become infected because of:

- Too much water in the ear (from bathing, swimming or water sports)
- Removing the natural earwax that protects the ear canal
- Skin conditions in the ear canal (such as eczema)
- Using cotton-tipped swabs, fingernails or other sharp objects in the ear canal
- Wax buildup due to hearing aids or other ear devices

What is the treatment for acute otitis externa?

- The usual treatment is prescription eardrops. A healthcare provider may have to clean the ear canal for the drops to work.
- Most drops need to be used 3 or 4 times a day.
- Use the drops until 3 days after all symptoms are gone.
- Symptoms are usually much better in 3 days and should be gone in 10 days.
- While you are using eardrops:
  - Keep your ears as dry as possible. Take a bath instead of a shower. Avoid swimming and water sports until the treatment is done.
  - Don't poke your fingers or other objects into your ears.

What can you do to prevent acute otitis externa?

- Keep the ear canal as dry as possible:
  - Dry ears with a towel after swimming or bathing. Use a blow dryer set on low to dry the ear canal. You can also use diluted vinegar or alcohol drops in the ear.
  - Try using a bathing cap or ear plugs when swimming. If this makes it worse, stop using.
- **Do not** clean earwax out of your ears:
  - Earwax protects against infection. The ears generally clean themselves. If you have pain in your ears from earwax, see your healthcare provider.
- **Do not** put anything in the ear canal except eardrops. Fingernails, cotton-tipped swabs and other objects irritate and damage the skin. If the skin is damaged you are more likely to get an infection.

Eardrops—What You Need to Know

Hints to help you use eardrops safely:

If possible, get someone to put the drops in your ear for you.

- Warm the eardrops to body temperature by holding the bottle in your hands for a few minutes. **Do not** heat the drops in hot water or the microwave because this could cause pain and dizziness or serious burns.
- Always wash your hands with soap and water before administering the eardrops.
- The eardrops must be kept clean. Do not let the dropper touch the ear or anything else that could have germs on it and let germs get into your eardrops.
- Shake the bottle before using if there is a "Shake Well" label on the bottle. Lie on your side so that the ear you are treating is facing up.
- The ear canal must be straight so that the eardrops can reach the affected tissue. The direction that you pull the top of the ear depends on the person's age.
  - **For adults and children over 3 years**, gently pull the top of the ear **up and back**.
  - **For children under 3 years**, gently pull the top of the ear **down and back**
- Hold the dropper above the ear. Place the prescribed number of drops into the ear. Do not put the dropper into the ear canal. It could injure the ear.
- Stay in the same position for 3–5 minutes after using the drops. This will allow the eardrops to run down into the ear canal.
- A gentle to-and-fro movement of the ear will sometimes help in getting the drops to their intended destination. You can also press with an in/out movement on the small piece of cartilage in front of the ear.
- Dry the earlobe if there are any eardrops on it.
- If you have had a wick placed in your ear, do not remove it. It may fall out on its own as the swelling and infection in the ear improves.

If you have to put drops in both ears:

Wait about 5–10 minutes before putting drops in the second ear. You want to be sure that the medicine stays in the ear canal of the first ear long enough to reach the eardrum before you tilt your head to put drops in the other ear.

These instructions may be changed by your healthcare provider depending on your medical condition or the type of medicine in the eardrops.

Chapter 21

Acute Cough

Daniel J.G. Thirion, BPharm, MSc, PharmD, FCSHP

Pathophysiology

Cough is a common symptom of many respiratory diseases and is a normal physiological response aimed at protecting the respiratory tract. It is a voluntarily induced or involuntarily activated reflex arc that can be triggered by a wide range of chemical and mechanical stimuli. First, receptors in the head, neck and chest are stimulated. This information is then transmitted to the cough centre in the medulla via the afferent limb of the vagus nerve, resulting in increased neural activity in the efferent pathway to both the respiratory musculature and airway.[1] Cough is present in many respiratory diseases. To help guide clinical assessment, it can be useful to classify cough according to duration within the following 3 categories: acute (lasting <3 weeks), subacute (lasting 3–8 weeks) and chronic (lasting >8 weeks).[2]

Viral infections of the upper respiratory tract are the most common causes of acute cough and can lead to a "post-infectious" cough.[2] Cough due to viral infections appears to arise from stimulation of the cough reflex in the upper respiratory tract caused by postnasal drip (referred to as upper airway cough syndrome—formerly postnasal drip syndrome), clearing of the throat or both.[3] Other frequent causes include acute bacterial sinusitis, chronic bronchitis, allergic rhinitis, and rhinitis due to environmental irritants. See Table 1. *Bordetella pertussis* or *Bordetella parapertussis* infection may be suspected in those with persistent cough.[4]

Table 1: **Causes of Cough**[5]

Common Causes of Cough	Less Common Causes of Cough
Asthma	Bronchiectasis
Chronic bronchitis	Cystic fibrosis
Drugs, e.g., ACE inhibitors, beta-blockers, ASA or NSAIDs in sensitive individuals	Interstitial lung disease
Environmental/occupational irritants, e.g., air pollution, cigarette smoke, asbestos	Lung cancer
Foreign body	Other lung diseases
Gastroesophageal reflux disease	Psychogenic cough
Heart failure	Unexplained cough (idiopathic)
Pulmonary embolism	Zenker's diverticulum (esophageal pouch)
Upper airway cough syndrome (sinusitis, allergic rhinitis, postinfectious)	
Upper/lower respiratory tract infection (viral or bacterial)	

Goals of Therapy

- Alleviate symptoms
- Diagnose and treat the underlying cause when possible
- Prevent complications

Patient Assessment

An assessment algorithm for patients presenting with cough is presented in Figure 1.

Nonpharmacologic Therapy

Although evidence is lacking, hydration with oral liquids and humidification of room air may be beneficial. Room humidifiers used as preventive measures should be well cleaned to avoid aerosolizing mould.

Mechanical methods such as postural drainage and chest percussion can improve airway clearance for conditions such as increased production of secretions or dysfunctional clearance of secretions.[6]

Avoid exposure to inhaled irritants such as smoke, dust, pollutants and allergens.

Pharmacologic Therapy

For comparative ingredients of nonprescription products, consult the *Compendium of Products for Minor Ailments*—Cough, Cold and Allergy Products.

Treatment of underlying conditions contributing to cough is paramount. For example, in gastroesophageal reflux disease, treatment of the reflux itself can alleviate associated cough. Smokers presenting with cough are prime candidates for discussing smoking cessation strategies.[7]

A specific treatment is not always possible. For example, there is no cure for the viral infection that causes the common cold. Despite a lack of evidence to support their use, nonspecific treatments such as nonprescription antitussives and protussives (expectorants) are frequently used in these cases depending on the presence/absence of mucus (sputum) production.

The efficacy of drugs used in the treatment of cough has been evaluated in numerous studies including many systematic reviews.[8,9,10] They show a lack of evidence for the effectiveness of nonprescription products in terms of reducing the frequency or severity of cough in children or adults. Some studies have shown benefit; however, the positive results in these studies were often of questionable clinical relevance.[11,12,13] Overall, there is little evidence for or against the effectiveness of nonprescription cough medicines. When counselling patients on selecting products, also consider the placebo effect, which can be significant.[14]

Nonprescription agents used in the management of cough are described in Table 3.

Antihistamines

First-generation antihistamines may have a small effect on cough caused by upper respiratory tract infections.[8,9,10,15] Their anticholinergic properties may reduce postnasal drip, which is one of the mechanisms responsible for cough in the common cold. The effect is modest and side effects such as drowsiness, dry mouth and confusion may outweigh potential benefit.

Second-generation antihistamines lack significant anticholinergic effects and therefore are not effective for this indication.[15]

For dosage of antihistamines, see Chapter 22: Allergic Rhinitis, Table 5.

Antitussives

The available nonprescription antitussives act centrally to suppress cough.[15] The exact mechanism is unknown; however, the brainstem is thought to be the main region where antitussive agents act to inhibit motor control of cough.

Dextromethorphan and **codeine** are commonly used to treat cough related to upper respiratory tract infections although there is little evidence for efficacy.[8,9,10] Some studies have shown that they are no more effective than placebo, while others demonstrated a modest benefit.[15,16,17] The reason for this discrepancy may be related to the limited efficacy of dextromethorphan in inhibiting cough, requiring larger numbers of subjects to demonstrate a significant effect.[15] Consequently, the American College of Chest Physicians (ACCP) 2006 guideline on the management of cough does not recommend centrally acting cough suppressants for cough secondary to upper respiratory tract infections.[18] On the other hand, codeine and dextromethorphan are effective for cough due to COPD, suppressing cough counts by 40–60%, and may be used for short-term relief.[15]

Antitussives are not recommended when a cough performs a useful function. If used by a patient with a productive cough, more mucus is retained.[19]

Expectorants

The protussive agents act peripherally. **Guaifenesin** is purported to enhance cough effectiveness by promoting the clearance of airway secretions.[15] The efficacy and safety of **guaiacol** and **ammonium chloride** have not been established. Expectorants are reported to reduce sputum viscosity permitting more effective removal of secretions from the respiratory tract.[2] As with antitussives, there is a lack of evidence to support the efficacy of expectorants. They do not thin sputum or increase sputum volume, even at doses higher than recommended.[19] Good hydration with oral liquids and inhalation of humidified air is perhaps the best protussive or "expectorant" measure.

Other Agents

Limited evidence suggests **honey** may be an effective cough suppressant in children.[20,21] A Cochrane review concluded that honey administered before sleep may be moderately better than no treatment or diphenhydramine, and no different from dextromethorphan, for reducing cough severity and improving sleep quality.[20] Honey has demulcent, antioxidant and antibacterial effects. It is proposed that the demulcent effect may act to decrease cough. Because of the risk of botulism, give pasteurized honey only, to immunocompetent children over the age of 1 year.

Zinc lozenges have been used to alleviate cough due to the common cold. Studies evaluating the efficacy of zinc in common cold symptoms have yielded conflicting results, and 2 meta-analyses have concluded there is insufficient evidence to recommend zinc preparations.[15] Therefore, the ACCP guidelines do not recommend zinc preparations for acute cough due to the common cold. In addition, zinc can be associated with unpleasant taste, mouth irritation and nausea.

Anesthetics such as **benzocaine**, **phenol** or **menthol** may reduce the sensitivity of peripheral nociceptors. They have been used as antitussives, but evidence for efficacy is poor.

Prescription Therapy

Bronchodilators such as **salbutamol** or **formoterol** are recommended only for cough due to obstructive lung disease such as asthma or COPD.[18,22,23] Following a respiratory infection, patients sometimes develop a cough for which corticosteroids could be beneficial. The potential benefit of inhaled corticosteroids requires confirmation through further studies before making recommendations for their routine use.

Cough in Special Populations

Children

For comparative ingredients of nonprescription products, consult the *Compendium of Products for Minor Ailments*—Baby Care Products: Cough and Cold.

In 2008, Health Canada required manufacturers to relabel nonprescription cough and cold medicines with certain active ingredients to indicate that they should not be used in children under 6 years.[24] **Dextromethorphan**, **guaifenesin** and **first-generation antihistamines** contained in cough and cold products are included in the list of active ingredients in the Health Canada advisory. See Chapter 24: Viral Rhinitis, Influenza, Rhinosinusitis and Pharyngitis, Table 3.

Although cough and cold medicines have been used by children for many years, little evidence supports their effectiveness in this population.[10,17,25] In addition, reports of misuse, overdose and very rare serious side effects have raised concerns about the use of these medicines in children under 6 years.[26] Rare but serious potential side effects include seizures, increased heart rate, decreased level of consciousness, abnormal heart rhythms and hallucinations.[24,25]

In children ≥6 years, **dextromethorphan** can be used to treat nonproductive cough, though evidence of efficacy in children is absent. Codeine should not be used in children <12 years.[27]

Pregnancy and Breastfeeding

See Appendix V: Pregnancy and Breastfeeding: Self-care Therapy for Common Conditions.

Monitoring of Therapy

Table 2 contains information on monitoring therapy.

Table 2: **Monitoring of Therapy for Cough**

Symptoms	Monitoring	Endpoint of Therapy	Actions if Endpoint Not Met
Cough	Patient: Daily Healthcare practitioner: Next visit or by telephone 2–3 days later	Patient able to perform daily activities. Patient able to sleep.	Optimize nonpharmacologic measures. Change treatment.
Drowsiness (antitussive)	Patient: Daily Healthcare practitioner: Next visit or by telephone when checking for efficacy	No drowsiness.	Change medication schedule (bedtime only) or change treatment.

Advice for the Patient

Advise patients regarding:

- Nonpharmacologic therapy
- Proper use of medication
- Expected results and management of side effects
- When to contact a physician

Figure 1: **Assessment of Patients with Cough**

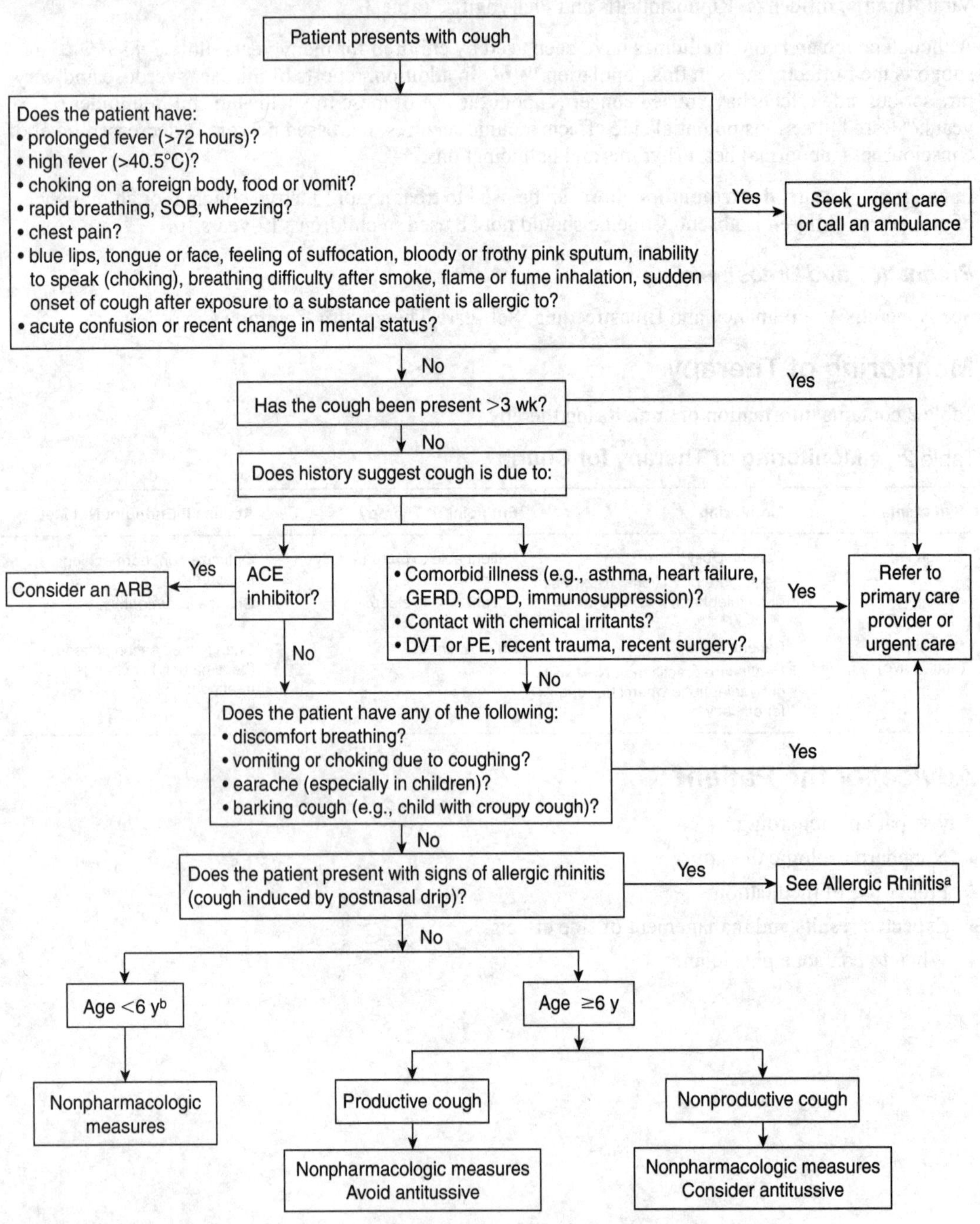

[a] See Chapter 22: Allergic Rhinitis.

[b] Cough and cold medicines are not recommended in children under 6 years of age (see Cough in Special Populations, Children).

Abbreviations: ACE = angiotensin converting enzyme; ARB = angiotensin receptor blocker; COPD = chronic obstructive pulmonary disease; DVT = deep vein thrombosis; GERD = gastroesophageal reflux disease; PE = pulmonary embolus; SOB = shortness of breath

Table 3: Nonprescription Medications for Cough

Class	Drug	Dosage[a]	Adverse Effects	Drug Interactions	Comments	Cost[b]
Antitussives	*codeine* Combination products: CoActifed, Dimetane Expectorant-C, Dimetapp-C, Robitussin AC, generics	Adults: 10–20 mg Q4–6H po Maximum: 120 mg/day Children ≥12 y: Give adult dose Health Canada recommends against use of codeine in children <12 y For combination products, consult label for additional ingredients. Follow directions on label.	Drowsiness, sedation, nausea, vomiting, constipation.	CNS depressants, including alcohol, enhance CNS side effects. MAOIs: Risk of serotonin syndrome. CYP2D6 inhibitors, e.g., fluoxetine, paroxetine, may inhibit conversion of codeine to its active metabolite and reduce clinical effect.	Causes less sedation than hydrocodone. Metabolized to morphine. Children are more sensitive to adverse effects of codeine. Potential for addiction. Nonprescription codeine products always contain other ingredients.	$$
	dextromethorphan Balminil DM, Benylin DM; Combination products: Robitussin DM, others	Adults and Children ≥12 y: 10–20 mg Q4H po *or* 30 mg Q6–8H po Maximum: 120 mg/day Children: 6–11 y: 5–10 mg Q4H po *or* 15 mg Q6–8H po Maximum: 60 mg/day For combination products, consult label for additional ingredients. Follow directions on label.	Generally well tolerated. Occasional dizziness, drowsiness and nausea.	Modulators of serotonin: Risk of serotonin syndrome, e.g., linezolid, MAOIs (including moclobemide), sibutramine, SSRIs. CYP2D6 inhibitors, e.g., fluoxetine, paroxetine, may inhibit DM metabolism resulting in increased DM levels and potential for adverse effects.	Causes less sedation than codeine and other opioids. DM has been abused for its euphoric effects.	$$

(cont'd)

Table 3: Nonprescription Medications for Cough *(cont'd)*

Class	Drug	Dosage[a]	Adverse Effects	Drug Interactions	Comments	Cost[b]
Expectorants	*guaifenesin* Robitussin Mucus & Phlegm, generics	Adults and Children ≥12 y: 200–400 mg Q4H po Maximum: 2.4 g/day Children ≥6 y: 12 mg/kg/day in divided doses Q4H po Maximum: 1.2 g/day For combination products, consult label for additional ingredients. Follow directions on label.	Side effects are rare. Dizziness, drowsiness, headache, nausea and vomiting have been reported at high doses.	No known interactions.		$$

[a] Cough and cold medicines are not recommended for use in children <6 years (see Cough in Special Populations, Children).

[b] Cost of 100 mL, unless otherwise specified; includes drug cost only

Dosage adjustment may be required in renal impairment.

Legend: $ <$2 $$ $2–5

Suggested Readings

Bolser DC. Cough suppressant and pharmacologic protussive therapy: ACCP evidence-based clinical practice guidelines. *Chest* 2006;129:238S-49S.

Morice AH, McGarvey L, Pavord I et al. Recommendations for the management of cough in adults. *Thorax* 2006;61:i1-24.

Smith SM, Schroeder K, Fahey T. Over-the-counter (OTC) medications for acute cough in children and adults in ambulatory settings. *Cochrane Database Syst Rev* 2014;11:CD001831.

References

1. Canning BJ, Chang AB, Bolser DC et al. Anatomy and neurophysiology of cough: CHEST Guideline and Expert Panel report. *Chest* 2014;146:1633-48.
2. Dicpinigaitis PV. Cough: an unmet clinical need. *Br J Pharmacol* 2011;163:116-24.
3. Pratter MR. Cough and the common cold: ACCP evidence-based clinical practice guidelines. *Chest* 2006;129:72S-4S.
4. Braman SS. Postinfectious cough: ACCP evidence-based clinical practice guidelines. *Chest* 2006;129:138S-46S.
5. Pratter MR, Brightling CE, Loulet LP et al. An empiric integrative approach to the management of cough: ACCP evidence-based clinical practice guidelines. *Chest* 2006;129:222S-31S.
6. Strickland SL. Year in review 2014: airway clearance. *Respir Care* 2015;60:603-5.
7. Morice AH, McGarvey L, Pavord I et al. Recommendations for the management of cough in adults. *Thorax* 2006;61:i1-24.
8. Irwin RS, Madison JM. The diagnosis and treatment of cough. *N Engl J Med* 2000;343:1715-21.
9. Schroeder K, Fahey T. Systematic review of randomised controlled trials of over the counter cough medicines for acute cough in adults. *BMJ* 2002;324:329-31.
10. Smith SM, Schroeder K, Fahey T. Over-the-counter (OTC) medications for acute cough in children and adults in ambulatory settings. *Cochrane Database Syst Rev* 2014;11:CD001831.
11. Parvez L, Vaidya M, Sakhardande A et al. Evaluation of antitussive agents in man. *Pulm Pharmacol* 1996;9:299-308.
12. Curley FJ, Irwin RS, Pratter MR et al. Cough and the common cold. *Am Rev Respir Dis* 1988;138:305-11.
13. Thackray P. A double-blind, crossover controlled evaluation of a syrup for the night-time relief of the symptoms of the common cold, containing paracetamol, dextromethorphan hydrobromide, doxylamine succinate and ephedrine sulphate. *J Int Med Res* 1978;6:161-5.
14. Paul IM, Beiler JS, Vallati JR et al. Placebo effect in the treatment of acute cough in infants and toddlers: a randomized clinical trial. *JAMA Pediatr* 2014;168:1107-13.
15. Bolser DC. Cough suppressant and pharmacologic protussive therapy: ACCP evidence-based clinical practice guidelines. *Chest* 2006;129:238S-49S.
16. Freestone C, Eccles R. Assessment of the antitussive efficacy of codeine in cough associated with common cold. *J Pharm Pharmacol* 1997;49:1045-9.
17. Taylor JA, Norvack AH, Almquist JR et al. Efficacy of cough suppressants in children. *J Pediatr* 1993;122:799-802.
18. Irwin RS, Baumann MH, Bolser DC et al. Diagnosis and management of cough executive summary: ACCP evidence-based clinical practice guidelines. *Chest* 2006;129:1S-23S.
19. Irwin RS, Curley FJ, Bennett FM. Appropriate use of antitussives and protussives. A practical review. *Drugs* 1993;46:80-91.
20. Oduwole O, Meremikwu MM, Oyo-Ita A et al. Honey for acute cough in children. Cochrane Database Syst Rev 2014;12:CD007094.
21. Cohen HA, Rozen J, Kristal H et al. Effect of honey on nocturnal cough and sleep quality: a double-blind, randomized, placebo-controlled study. *Pediatrics* 2012;130:465-71.
22. El-Gohary M, Hay AD, Coventry P et al. Corticosteroids for acute and subacute cough following respiratory tract infection: a systematic review. *Fam Pract* 2013;30:492-500.
23. Becker LA, Hom J, Villasis-Keever M et al. Beta$_2$-agonists for acute cough or a clinical diagnosis of acute bronchitis. *Cochrane Database Syst Rev.* 2015;9:CD001726.
24. Government of Canada. Healthy Canadians. *Health Canada releases decision on the labelling of cough and cold products for children.* Available from: www.healthycanadians.gc.ca/recall-alert-rappel-avis/hc-sc/2008/13267a-eng.php. Accessed November 12, 2009.
25. Use of codeine- and dextromethorphan-containing cough remedies in children. American Academy of Pediatrics. Committee on Drugs. *Pediatrics* 1997;99:918-20.
26. Peterson RG, Cran B, Knoppert D et al. *Scientific Advisory Panel on nonprescription pediatric cough and cold medications (SAP-NPCCM).* Ottawa: Health Canada; March 20, 2008.
27. Government of Canada. Healthy Canadians. *Health Canada's review recommends codeine only be used in patients aged 12 and over.* Available from: healthycanadians.gc.ca/recall-alert-rappel-avis/hc-sc/2013/33915a-eng.php?_ga=1.94474908.1833075375.1359051823. Accessed April 22, 2014.

Cough—What You Need to Know

What causes cough?

There are many possible reasons for a cough. The most common cause is a viral infection, such as the common cold or the flu. In this case, it will go away by itself in a couple of weeks. Other causes include:

- Worsening asthma
- Allergies
- Environmental irritants (air pollution, cigarette smoke)
- Side effect of certain drugs
- Other infections such as bronchitis or pneumonia

When to see a healthcare provider:

- You've had a cough longer than 3 weeks
- You have difficulty breathing or chest pain
- You are coughing up bloody or coloured mucous
- You have a fever >40.5ºC or any fever lasting longer than 3 days
- Your child is <3 months old and has a cough
- Your child is between 3 and 6 months old and has a cough and fever >38.5ºC
- You have a medical condition such as asthma, chronic obstructive pulmonary disease (COPD) or heart failure

Treatment for cough

There is not a lot of proof that cough medicines work well. Some medicines may help control a cough (cough suppressants) while others help clear chest phlegm (expectorants). Cough suppressants should not be used if you have a cough with mucous. Talk to your pharmacist about which medicine may be right for you.

Cough in children

- Cough medicines are not recommended for children <6 years old
- You can try a teaspoon of pasteurized honey before going to bed
- **Do not** give honey to children less than 1 year old or if you have an immune condition, because of the risk of botulism
- Brush teeth after giving or taking honey.

Chapter 22
Allergic Rhinitis

Jennifer Kendrick, BScPharm, ACPR, PharmD

Pathophysiology

Allergic rhinitis affects 10–30% of the population, and the prevalence is increasing.[1,2,3] It is estimated that more than 500 million people worldwide are affected.[3] The prevalence of allergic rhinitis is thought to be highest in school-age children; 80% of people with allergic rhinitis are diagnosed before 20 years of age.[1,4] Allergic rhinitis is associated with a genetic predisposition; children have a 30% chance of developing allergic rhinitis if one parent is affected and a 50% chance if both are affected.[5,6]

Allergic rhinitis is characterized by inflammation of the nasal mucosa following inhalation of an allergen.[1,4,6,7] The allergic reaction is mediated by antigen-antibody responses and takes place in 3 phases. The first phase, sensitization, occurs on first contact with the allergen. IgE is produced and binds to receptors on the surface of mast cells and basophils. The second and third phases occur on re-exposure to an allergen in a sensitized individual. The second phase, immediate reaction, occurs within minutes of re-exposure and lasts up to 30–90 minutes. In this phase the allergen binds to allergen-specific IgE and the mast cells release preformed mediators, histamine and tumor necrosis factor alpha (TNF-α), and newly generated mediators, leukotrienes LTC4, LTD4, LTE4, prostaglandin D2 and kinins. The third phase, late reaction, occurs 4–8 hours after exposure. It is characterized by migration of inflammatory cells, eosinophils, monocytes, macrophages and basophils.

Allergic rhinitis was previously classified as seasonal or perennial; however, this classification was determined to be inadequate for a number of reasons. For example, outdoor pollens and moulds may be perennial in some regions and symptoms of perennial allergy may not be present year-round. The Allergic Rhinitis and its Impact on Asthma (ARIA) guideline proposed the classifications of intermittent allergic rhinitis (IAR) and persistent allergic rhinitis (PAR) in 2008.[3] IAR is defined as symptoms of allergic rhinitis occurring <4 days/week or for <4 weeks at a time. PAR is defined as symptoms of allergic rhinitis occurring ≥4 days/week and for ≥4 weeks at a time. Allergic rhinitis is further classified based on severity. In mild allergic rhinitis, symptoms are present but not troublesome and there is no impairment in daily activities, school or work and no sleep disturbance. In moderate/severe allergic rhinitis, one or more is present: troublesome symptoms, impairment in daily activities, school or work, or sleep disturbance.[3,7] The ARIA classification has been validated in both adults and children.

Rhinitis may also be nonallergic. Conditions associated with nonallergic rhinitis are listed in Table 1. Drugs associated with rhinitis are listed in Table 2.

Goals of Therapy

- Prevent symptoms by avoiding exposure to allergen(s)
- Alleviate signs and symptoms produced by the allergic response
- Improve quality of life

Table 1: **Possible Nonallergic Causes of Acute and Chronic Rhinitis**[3,4,6,7]

- Drug-induced (see Table 2)
- Hormones
  - pregnancy, menstruation, hypothyroidism
- Infection
  - viral, bacterial, fungal, other
- Nonallergic rhinitis with eosinophilia syndrome (NARES)
- Other
  - emotions, e.g., stress, sexual arousal
  - vasomotor rhinitis, e.g., exercise, cold air
  - anatomic abnormalities, e.g., nasal septal deviation, enlarged adenoids and tonsils, nasal tumors, choanal atresia[a]
  - food and alcohol
  - nasal polyps
  - atrophy
  - foreign body

[a] A congenital defect where the posterior nares do not communicate with the nasopharynx.

Table 2: **Drugs Associated with Rhinitis**[6,8]

- ACE inhibitors
- ASA and other NSAIDs
- Cocaine
- Diuretics, e.g., amiloride, hydrochlorothiazide
- Gabapentin
- Hydralazine
- Oral contraceptives
- Phosphodiesterase-5 inhibitors, e.g., sildenafil
- Psychotropics, e.g., chlorpromazine, risperidone
- Sympatholytics, e.g., clonidine, doxazosin, methyldopa, phentolamine, prazosin
- Topical decongestants (prolonged use)

Patient Assessment

The sensitization phase of allergic rhinitis is asymptomatic. Symptoms of the second or immediate phase include sneezing, nasal and palatal pruritus, congestion and clear rhinorrhea.[9] Symptoms of the delayed phase are similar but nasal congestion predominates.[4] Patients may also have itchy, red, watery eyes (allergic conjunctivitis), itchy throat, ear fullness and popping, and a feeling of pressure over the cheeks and forehead.[4] Facial signs of allergic rhinitis are illustrated in Figure 1. The allergic salute is a sign more commonly seen in children, where the patient wipes the nose with the palm of the hand in an upward motion.

Some patients present primarily with symptoms of sneezing and rhinorrhea, whereas others are mostly bothered by nasal blockage and have little or no itching or sneezing.[6] Eye symptoms are more commonly associated with outdoor allergens.[3,7]

Allergic rhinitis can have a significant impact on a patient's quality of life. Patients may have headache, difficulty concentrating, fatigue or sleep disturbance.[6] Malaise or fatigue may be presenting complaints in children.[9] Complications of allergic rhinitis include sinusitis, otitis media, asthma, and sleep apnea. In children, there may be dental overbite and a high-arched palate due to chronic mouth breathing.[3,6]

An assessment plan for patients suffering from allergic rhinitis is illustrated in Figure 2. During the assessment, also identify precipitating factors/allergens and assess occupational exposure and response to previous therapy.

Figure 1: **Facial Signs of Allergic Rhinitis**

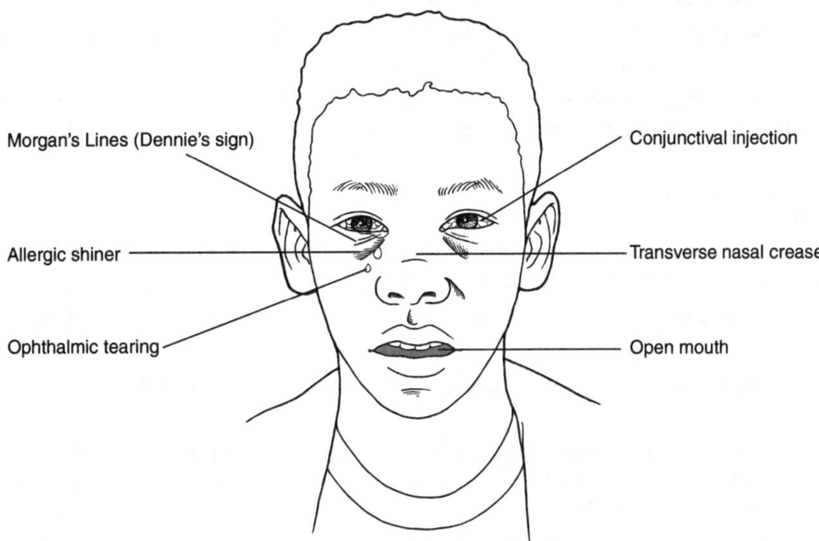

Morgan's Lines or Dennie's sign or folds are extra creases at the lower eyelids due to edema. Allergic shiners describe discoloured infraorbital areas due to venous stasis resulting from nasal swelling. The transverse nasal crease is a crease seen at the junction of the bulbous portion of the nose and the nosebridge and is caused by recurrent nose rubbing (allergic salute). Conjunctival injection refers to conjunctival redness fading toward the edges.

Consider the need for prescription therapy or referral for allergy testing if the patient has already tried appropriate nonprescription therapy for 2 weeks without an adequate response, or if the allergen responsible for symptoms cannot be readily identified.[3] Also refer patients for further assessment if they have signs or symptoms that are unilateral or are not usually associated with allergic rhinitis (e.g., fever, pain, loss of smell or taste, recurrent epistaxis, purulent nasal or ocular secretions, postnasal drip with or without rhinorrhea) or symptoms suggesting complications such as asthma.[3]

Prevention

Prevention is the first step in the management of allergic rhinitis. Although consensus is that improvement in symptoms should occur with allergen avoidance, little evidence supports individual measures.[3] While some measures such as washing pets, impermeable covers for bedding, and air filtration have been shown to reduce the allergen level, a corresponding reduction in allergic symptoms has not been shown.[9] The benefits of environmental control may take weeks or months to fully manifest. Avoidance measures for common allergens are presented below.[1,3,6,7]

Pollen

- Keep windows and doors closed when at home or in the car.
- If using air conditioning, keep the unit on recirculate or the indoor cycle, if the choice is available.
- Do not use window or attic fans.
- Monitor weather reports on pollen counts, if available. Decrease outdoor exposure during periods of high pollen counts. Pollen counts tend to be highest on sunny, windy days.
- Do not dry clothing outdoors.
- Shower or bathe and wash hair after outdoor activity to remove pollen from hair and skin and prevent contamination of bedding.

Outdoor Moulds

- Remain in a closed environment as much as possible.
- If using air conditioning, keep the unit on the indoor cycle, if the choice is available; note, however, that units can be heavily contaminated with mould.
- Use of face masks for activities such as raking leaves or working with compost or dry soil may have limited value because air seeps around the edges of the mask and the mask does not protect the eyes.

Indoor Moulds

- Use fungicide on sinks, shower stalls, nonrefrigerated vegetable storage areas and garbage pails. A solution of equal parts household bleach and water effectively kills mould.
- Avoid console humidifiers and cool mist vaporizers; if these must be used, keep them scrupulously clean.
- If the home is built over a crawl space, install a plastic vapor barrier over exposed soil and keep foundation vents open.
- If the basement is damp or tends to flood, avoid carpeting or furnishing the basement. Use a dehumidifier at all times and empty the extracted water from the air frequently; remove any standing water as soon as possible.
- Remove houseplants, which are a common source of mould. Alternatively, keep soil surface dry and clean of debris to reduce mould.

House Dust Mites

- Avoid carpeting the bedroom and main living areas.
- Plastic, leather or wood furniture is best.
- Some **acaricides** (e.g., benzyl benzoate, tannic acid) appear to reduce the mite population if used regularly. However, their clinical effect is not established and they are not routinely recommended.[3]
- If possible, clean while the allergic individual is not at home.
- Mite-sensitive persons should avoid vacuuming or making beds. Those who must do their own cleaning should wear a facemask during cleaning and for 10–15 minutes afterward.
- Use a vacuum cleaner with an efficient double filtration system.
- Keep indoor humidity between 40% and 45%.
- Minimize use of humidifiers as excess humidity promotes mite growth.
- Encase all mattresses, box springs and pillows in the allergic individual's bedroom in zippered, allergen-proof casings.
- Consider replacing old mattresses.
- Wash bedding in hot (>55°C) water at least every 2 weeks. Cooler water temperatures will not kill dust mites, nor will detergents.
- Avoid stuffed toys that cannot be washed. Alternatively, put stuffed toys or pillows in a hot dryer or in plastic bags and freeze every 2 weeks to kill dust mites.
- Do not store items under the bed.
- Use window shades instead of venetian blinds.
- Evidence suggests the best strategy is a combination of the above interventions.[10]

Animal Allergens

- Permanent removal of pets from the home is the best way to control animal allergens. This should be followed by thorough cleaning of the house, including washing carpets. "Trial" removal of pets is not helpful; it can take 20 weeks or longer for cat allergen levels to drop to levels comparable to homes without cats.
- If the family is unable to remove the animal from the home then:
  - remove carpets and replace with hard flooring
  - keep the animal away from the allergic individual's bedroom and other living areas where the allergic individual spends time
  - a high-efficiency particulate air (HEPA) filter or electrostatic air purifier may be helpful
  - washing cats weekly and dogs once or twice weekly may help but evidence to support this approach is lacking
  - eliminate litter boxes if possible; otherwise place them in an area unconnected to the air supply for the rest of the house.

Occupational Allergens

- For individuals affected by occupational rhinitis, recommend minimizing or eliminating exposure.
- Common causes of occupational rhinitis include animal or vegetable proteins (e.g., mouse, rat, wheat, grains, latex), enzymes, pharmaceuticals (e.g., antibiotics) and chemicals (e.g., resins).

Nonpharmacologic Therapy

Intranasal saline spray and irrigation has been shown to reduce nasal symptoms and the need for pharmacologic therapy in children and nonpregnant adults.[11] The effect of intranasal saline irrigation in pregnant women is less clear.[12] Isotonic saline is preferred to hypertonic saline, as it improves mucociliary clearance; however, the optimal dose, frequency and delivery have not been established.[11]

Tobacco smoke can aggravate symptoms and should be avoided by all patients with allergic rhinitis.[3] Other irritants that should be avoided include insect sprays, air pollution and fresh tar or paint.[3]

Pharmacologic Therapy

When avoidance of allergens is ineffective or impractical, consider pharmacologic options. If it is possible to predict the onset of symptoms (e.g., intermittent exposure), prophylactic medication should be started before exposure.

For comparative ingredients of nonprescription products, consult the *Compendium of Products for Minor Ailments*—Cough, Cold and Allergy Products.

Table 3 summarizes the pharmacologic activity of different therapies for the treatment of allergic rhinitis.

Medications for treatment of allergic rhinitis are described in Table 5 and Table 6.

Several guidelines for the treatment of allergic rhinitis are available and each provides similar treatment recommendations.[3,6,7,9] For mild symptoms, **second-generation antihistamines** are the drugs of choice, although they produce only a modest improvement in nasal congestion. **First-generation antihistamines** are no longer recommended first-line due to their adverse effect profile.[6] For moderate to severe allergic rhinitis, regularly administered **intranasal corticosteroids** are recommended as first-line therapy.[14]

Table 3: **Comparative Symptom Relief of Allergic Rhinitis Therapies**[7,13]

Medication	Rhinorrhea	Congestion	Sneezing	Nasal Itch	Eye Symptoms[a]
Oral antihistamines	+	+/-	+	+	+/-
Intranasal mast cell stabilizers	+/-	+/-	+/-	+/-	-
Decongestants (oral and topical)	-	+	-	-	-
Intranasal corticosteroids	++	++	++	++	+/-
Leukotriene receptor antagonists	+	+	+/-	+/-	+/-
Intranasal anticholinergics	++	-	-	-	-
Intranasal antihistamines	++	++	++	++	+/-

[a] See Chapter 13: Conjunctivitis.

Abbreviations: (+/-) = modest or variable effect

Antihistamines

Introduced in the 1940s, antihistamines were the first medications used for the treatment of allergic rhinitis. They act as competitive antagonists for the histamine-1 (H_1) receptor found on the surface of target cells in the nose, lung, conjunctiva and skin.[15] They also act as a reverse agonist, meaning that they change the three-dimensional configuration of the receptor, decreasing its affinity for histamine and down-regulating histamine-driven symptoms.[15] Antihistamines decrease nasal itching, sneezing, rhinorrhea, conjunctival itching and lacrimation but generally do not relieve nasal congestion. **Desloratadine, fexofenadine** and **cetirizine** have modest effects on nasal congestion.[16] Antihistamines are first-line treatment in mild cases of allergic rhinitis.[3,6,9]

Antihistamines are divided into 2 major classes: first- and second-generation. All are similarly effective; however, adverse effect profiles and pharmacology differ.[15,17,18,19,20,21]

First-generation antihistamines have a rapid onset but relatively short duration of action due to their short half-life.[22,23] They are poorly selective for the H_1 receptor and also exert effects on cholinergic receptors. The anticholinergic effect manifests as dry mouth and nasal passages, difficulty voiding urine, constipation and tachycardia. They are also highly lipophilic and therefore cross the blood-brain barrier and interact with central H_1 receptors. This results in CNS effects such as sedation and psychomotor and cognitive impairment. In children, paradoxical excitation may occur.[24] Performance impairment has been documented using various measures (e.g., reaction time, visual-motor coordination, arithmetical exercises and memory, learning and driving tests) although more recent data suggest that the magnitude of these effects has been overstated.[25,26] CNS depression and impairment can be independent of any subjective complaints by the patient.[27] First-generation antihistamines also impair learning and academic performance in children.[27] Workers taking first-generation antihistamines have lower work performance and are more likely to be involved in workplace accidents. Daytime performance effects are noted even when the antihistamine is taken only at bedtime.[6,27]

First-generation antihistamines can decrease rhinorrhea, but mucus secretion may be thickened and can be more bothersome for some patients.[15]

The first-generation antihistamines should be used with caution in patients with narrow-angle glaucoma, stenosing peptic ulcer, pyloroduodenal obstruction, symptomatic prostatic hypertrophy or bladder-neck obstruction, cardiovascular disease and chronic lung disease.

Second-generation antihistamines are more selective for H_1 receptors and less lipophilic. Consequently, they do not have significant anticholinergic adverse effects and do not cross the blood-brain barrier.[20] Use of **cetirizine** in standard doses is associated with more sedation compared with placebo, but less than first-generation antihistamines.[6] Administration of standard doses of **loratadine** and **desloratadine** results in an incidence of sedation equivalent to placebo; however, drowsiness has been reported at higher than recommended doses, or rarely in susceptible individuals at recommended doses.[6] **Fexofenadine** appears to be nonsedating, even at increased doses. Due to their improved adverse effect profile, especially with regard to sedation and psychomotor performance, second-generation antihistamines represent a better choice than first-generation agents for the treatment of allergic rhinitis.[6,14] Clinical trials comparing various second-generation antihistamines demonstrate similar reduction of symptoms.[2,19,21,28] They are less effective than intranasal corticosteroids for most symptoms of allergic rhinitis.[6] Two meta-analyses demonstrated intranasal corticosteroids were more effective than antihistamines for relieving congestion and sneezing; for ocular symptoms, no difference was found.[29,30]

The intranasal antihistamine **levocabastine** is effective for sneezing, nasal pruritus and rhinorrhea. It has a rapid onset of action (<15 minutes), but must be used 2–4 times daily.[22] The intranasal antihistamine **azelastine** (available only in combination with fluticasone in Canada) is clinically similar to oral second-generation antihistamines for the relief of nasal symptoms.[30]

Antihistamines are more effective when taken before allergen exposure. The best results are obtained with chronic dosing compared with intermittent dosing; therefore, patients should take the antihistamine for as long as they are in contact with the allergen.[14] If one antihistamine is not effective, switching to another antihistamine may be beneficial.[31]

Mast Cell Stabilizers

Sodium cromoglycate (also called cromolyn sodium) modestly reduces itching, sneezing and rhinorrhea but is not effective for nasal congestion.[3] Treatment should begin before exposure to the allergen and continue for the entire allergen season.[22] If treatment begins after allergen exposure, relief may be delayed up to 4 weeks. Sodium cromoglycate is less effective than corticosteroids for allergic rhinitis and has not been adequately compared with leukotriene receptor antagonists and antihistamines.[6,30]

Decongestants

Decongestants are available in oral and topical formulations. Oral decongestants generally have a weaker effect on nasal obstruction than the topical formulations.[22] When given orally, decongestants can cause systemic adverse effects (see Table 5). Most available agents do not cause blood pressure elevations in normotensive persons unless the recommended dose is significantly exceeded.[32] Elevation of blood pressure may occur at standard doses in hypertensive patients.[33]

Systemic absorption from topical formulations is low, resulting in mainly local adverse effects (see Table 6). Rhinitis medicamentosa (rebound vasodilation) can occur if topical decongestants are used for more than 3–5 days.[34] In one study, 49% of patients reported using an intranasal decongestant daily for at least one year, even though 80% reported having received education about limiting the duration of use. Intranasal decongestant overuse was less common in patients who were using intranasal corticosteroid or oral antihistamine.[35] Overuse can lead to nasal congestion when the topical agent is stopped, and to permanent overgrowth of nasal tissue with chronic overuse. This condition is more likely to occur with shorter-acting agents (**phenylephrine**) than with longer-acting agents (**oxymetazoline** and **xylometazoline**). Many solutions to this problem have been proposed, including slow tapering of the decongestant, adding or switching to intranasal corticosteroids, or abrupt discontinuation of the topical decongestant. Abrupt cessation is effective but may be uncomfortable for the patient as nasal congestion may persist for several days or weeks.[34]

Corticosteroids

Intranasal corticosteroids are more effective against the nasal symptoms of allergic rhinitis than oral and intranasal antihistamines, nasal cromoglycate and leukotriene receptor antagonists.[29,30] Intranasal corticosteroids are the drugs of choice for moderate to severe or persistent allergic rhinitis, and for mild allergic rhinitis that does not respond to antihistamines.[3,6,9] Some intranasal corticosteroids (**mometasone furoate** and **fluticasone furoate**) have a modest benefit on allergic conjunctivitis symptoms.[6,10,36,37,38] A meta-analysis suggests that intranasal corticosteroids as a class are effective for ocular symptoms of allergic rhinitis; however the magnitude of effect has not been quantified.[39] Onset of action of intranasal corticosteroids is within 6–8 hours of first dose, although maximum effect may take a few weeks. Short courses of oral corticosteroids may be required for severe cases of allergic rhinitis that is unresponsive to other treatment.[6] Patients may prefer intranasal corticosteroids in aerosol form compared with spray form; therefore, switching to another intranasal corticosteroid formulation may be recommended if patient tolerability is affecting therapy.[40] Regular use of intranasal steroids is more effective than intermittent use.[14]

Leukotriene Receptor Antagonists (LTRA)

Montelukast is superior to placebo but less effective than intranasal corticosteroids for nasal symptoms of allergic rhinitis.[30] Montelukast is similar in efficacy to loratadine, but patient response is more variable than with antihistamines.[30] There may be additive effects when it is used concomitantly with antihistamines. Montelukast is more effective than oral antihistamines and comparable to intranasal corticosteroids for reduction of asthma symptoms and use of rescue asthma medication.[30] As a result, montelukast may be a reasonable option for allergic rhinitis coexisting with asthma.[6,7,9] Otherwise, montelukast is not recommended as first-line therapy for allergic rhinitis.[9]

Immunotherapy

According to clinical practice guidelines, allergen immunotherapy should be considered for patients who continue to have moderate to severe symptoms despite treatment or those who require systemic corticosteroids.[2,9] Immunotherapy may be indicated when the exposure to allergens is significant and unavoidable (e.g., grass pollen), and when the symptom complex is severe enough to warrant the time, expense and small risk of anaphylaxis.[6] Allergen immunotherapy is the only treatment that can modify the natural history of allergic rhinitis and potentially induce long-term disease remission after cessation of treatment. It may also prevent the development of new allergies and reduce the risk of development of asthma in children. Therefore, allergen immunotherapy may be considered even in milder cases of allergic rhinitis. Immunotherapy is administered by subcutaneous injection, although sublingual immunotherapy seems to be somewhat effective as well.[6,41,42]

Anticholinergics

Intranasal **ipratropium bromide** is effective for rhinorrhea secondary to allergic rhinitis but not for other symptoms.[22]

Combination Therapies

Combination therapy is recommended by some guidelines when patients have inadequate response to monotherapy.[9] Some combinations have been shown to be more effective than monotherapy while others have not.

First- and Second-generation Antihistamines

Some experts suggest a second-generation antihistamine during the day and a first-generation antihistamine at bedtime to promote sleep. Evidence to support this practice is lacking and next-day sedation is possible.[2] If sleep is disturbed due to allergies, symptom relief itself can be expected to improve sleep.

Antihistamine plus Decongestant

Because antihistamines may have only a modest effect on nasal congestion, antihistamines and decongestants are often combined. Some patients may respond to this combination when corticosteroids have failed or when either medication alone does not provide adequate relief of nasal symptoms.[2,30]

Antihistamine plus Corticosteroid

Intranasal corticosteroids are often combined with oral antihistamines to treat severe or resistant cases of allergic rhinitis.[6] This strategy seems logical because the 2 drugs have different mechanisms of action. Evidence is insufficient to support the combination of intranasal corticosteroids and oral antihistamines, as it has not been consistently shown to be superior to either medication alone.[2,30] However, intranasal corticosteroid in combination with intranasal antihistamine (fluticasone/azelastine) is more effective for the nasal symptoms of allergic rhinitis than either medication alone.[30]

Antihistamine or Intranasal Corticosteroid plus LTRA

An additive effect has been shown when LTRAs and either oral antihistamines or intranasal corticosteroids are used concomitantly.[30] The efficacy of oral antihistamines in combination with a LTRA is less than that of intranasal corticosteroids alone.[6] However, antihistamine-LTRA combination therapy may provide an alternative for patients who are unresponsive or nonadherent to intranasal corticosteroid therapy.

Special Populations

Children

The guidelines for treatment of allergic rhinitis in children are similar to those for adults.[6] Healthcare practitioners must ensure they select the correct dosage, ensure proper administration and minimize adverse effects.[3,7,24] Most **second-generation antihistamines** are now available in pediatric formulations for children >6 months and are generally preferred over first-generation agents due to improved adverse effect profiles. Table 5 and Table 6 provide dosage guidelines and age limits for oral and intranasal agents. **Intranasal corticosteroids** are also effective and are considered safe in children >2 years of age, depending on the formulation.[24] Intranasal **budesonide** and **mometasone furoate** have not shown growth suppression with prolonged use at recommended doses.[6,43,44] Intranasal **beclomethasone dipropionate**, **fluticasone propionate** and **triamcinolone acetonide** have been shown to reduce growth velocity by 0.2–0.9 cm per year within the first year of treatment.[45,46,47] Longer term studies have not been conducted. If intranasal corticosteroids are used, use the lowest possible dose, monitor growth and use other therapies (e.g., antihistamines) to minimize the dose of corticosteroid required for symptom control.[6] **Decongestants** are not recommended for use in children under 6 years.[48,49] In those children, intranasal saline drops or spray may be used to clear nasal passages before eating or sleeping.

Pregnancy

Intranasal cromoglycate and **intranasal corticosteroids** are both considered safe during pregnancy although **beclomethasone**, **budesonide** and **fluticasone propionate** have accumulated more safety data than other intranasal corticosteroids.[6] Neither **first-** nor **second-generation antihistamines** have been associated with teratogenic effects in pregnancy.[50,51] First-generation antihistamines were previously favoured because of substantially greater experience; however, safety data for **cetirizine** and **loratadine** now indicate these are acceptable options. **Chlorpheniramine** has a good safety record in pregnancy. Although **diphenhydramine** has good safety data and is still recommended and frequently used in pregnancy, there have been isolated reports of cleft palate.[51] Sedation and impaired performance may limit the use of first-generation antihistamines. **Oral decongestants** should be avoided in the first trimester.[51] A **topical decongestant** may be used; at usual doses, they do not present a risk to the fetus. **Immunotherapy** generally should not be started during pregnancy. Courses of immunotherapy started prior to conception may be continued if beneficial and not causing systemic reactions; doses should not be increased during pregnancy.[52] See Appendix V: Pregnancy and Breastfeeding: Self-care Therapy for Common Conditions.

Breastfeeding

Recommendations for breastfeeding are similar to those during pregnancy. Both **first-** and **second-generation antihistamines** are considered safe while breastfeeding.[53] First-generation antihistamines may in theory diminish milk production via their anticholinergic effect; however, this has not been reported in practice. Infant somnolence should be monitored when a first-generation antihistamine or cetirizine is used.

The systemic absorption of **topical decongestants** is low and transfer into breast milk is unknown. Consequently, these agents are expected to be reasonably safe during breastfeeding.

The American Academy of Pediatrics considers **pseudoephedrine** to be compatible with breastfeeding.[51] Information on the use of other oral decongestants during breastfeeding is limited.

Information on the use of topical **sodium cromoglycate** during breastfeeding is not available, although the manufacturer recommends caution.

Monitoring of Therapy

Table 4 provides a monitoring plan framework that should be individualized.

Table 4: **Monitoring of Therapy for Allergic Rhinitis**

Symptoms	Monitoring	Endpoint of Therapy	Actions
Allergic symptoms (sneezing, runny nose, itchy and watery eyes, congestion, rhinorrhea)	Patients: Daily Healthcare practitioner: Next visit or by telephone 1 wk later	Patient able to perform daily activities. Patient able to sleep.	If nonprescription therapy is ineffective after 1 wk, optimize allergen avoidance and medication dose (if applicable). If symptoms not controlled after a further wk of therapy, consider another agent. Refer as necessary.[3]
Drowsiness (antihistamine)	Patient: Daily Healthcare practitioner: Next visit or by telephone when checking for efficacy	Patient not drowsy during the day.	Switch to a less sedating antihistamine. If using cetirizine, could give dose at bedtime.
Insomnia (oral decongestant)	Patient: Daily Healthcare practitioner: 1 wk	No insomnia.	Change medication schedule so last dose taken 4–6 h before bedtime or discontinue medication.
Elevated blood pressure in hypertensive patients (oral decongestant)	Patient: Daily Healthcare practitioner: Monitor blood pressure of hypertensive patients twice in the first wk	No elevation in blood pressure above baseline.	Stop decongestant if blood pressure elevated above baseline.

Advice for the Patient

Advise all patients about allergen avoidance. In addition, patients who require drug therapy should receive counselling regarding proper use of the medication, expected results and management of adverse effects (see Table 4).

Figure 2: **Assessment and Initial Treatment of Patients with Allergic Rhinitis**[3,4,6,7]

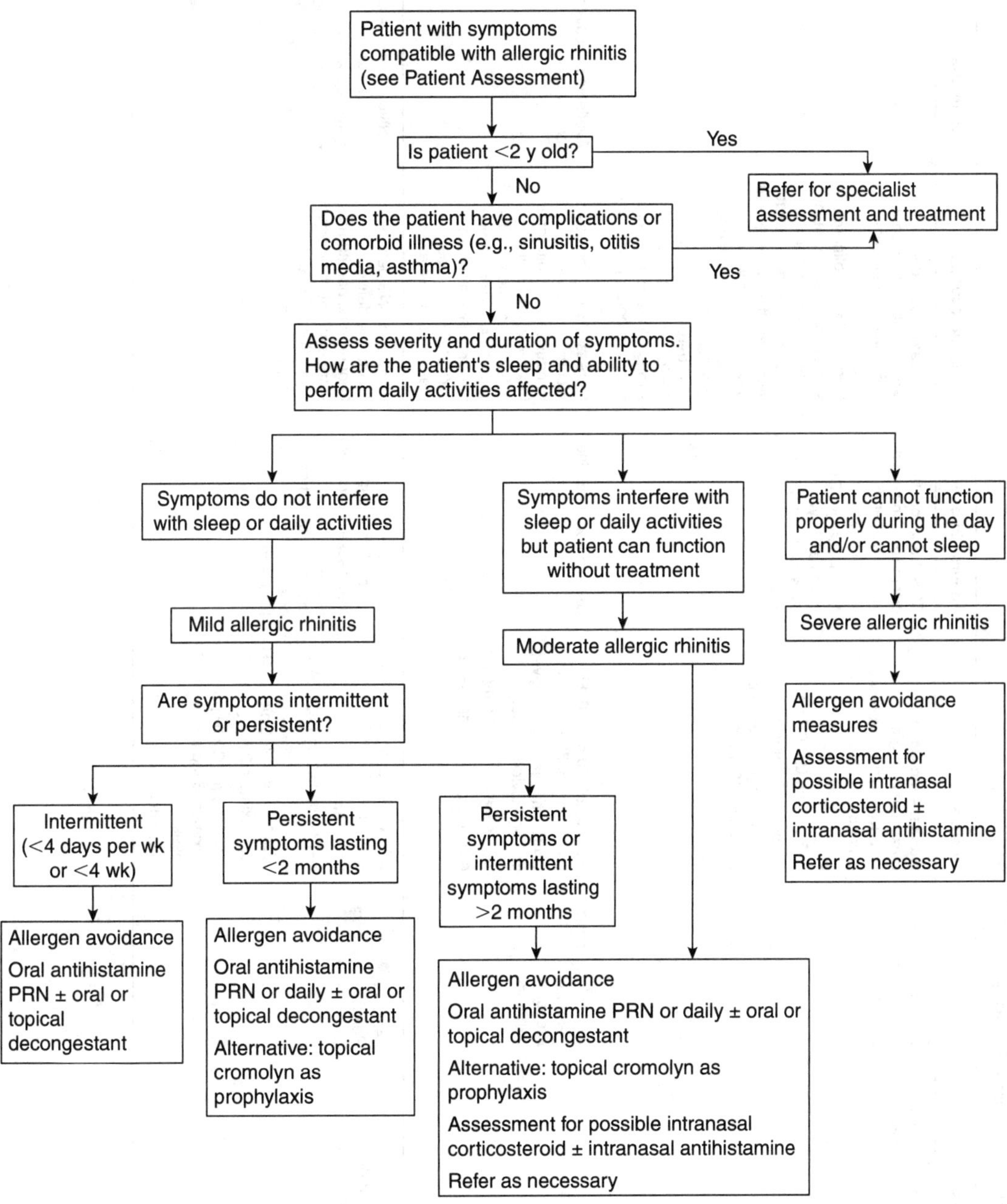

Table 5: Oral Agents for Allergic Rhinitis

Class	Drug	Dosage	Adverse Effects	Drug Interactions	Comments	Cost[a]
Antihistamines, First-generation	*chlorpheniramine* Chlor-Tripolon, generics	**Adults**: 4 mg Q4–6H po; maximum 24 mg/day **Children**: 0.35 mg/kg/day divided Q4–6H po *or* 2–5 y: 1 mg Q4–6H po; maximum 6 mg/day 6–11 y: 2 mg Q4–6H po; maximum 12 mg/day	CNS: Sedation, fatigue, dizziness, impairment of cognition and performance. Anticholinergic: Dry mouth and eyes, constipation, urinary retention.	Increased CNS depression when combined: Alcohol, sedatives, tranquilizers, barbiturates. Increased anticholinergic side effects when combined with: TCAs, scopolamine. Increase chlorpheniramine levels resulting in increased adverse effects when combined with moderate CYP2D6 inhibitors, e.g., amiodarone, celecoxib. Avoid combination with strong CYP2D6 inhibitors, e.g., bupropion, paroxetine.		$
	diphenhydramine Benadryl Preparations, generics	**Adults**: 25–50 mg Q6–8H po; maximum 300 mg/day **Children**: 5 mg/kg/day given in 3 or 4 divided doses po 2–5 y: Maximum 37.5 mg/day 6–11 y: Maximum150 mg/day	See chlorpheniramine.	Increased CNS depression: Alcohol, sedatives, tranquilizers, barbiturates. Increased anticholinergic side effects when combined with: TCAs, scopolamine. May increase levels of CYP2D6 substrates, e.g., metoprolol, venlafaxine.	Available in pediatric liquid formulation.	$
Antihistamines, Second-generation	*cetirizine* Reactine, generics	**Adults**: 5–10 mg Q24H po; maximum 20 mg Q24H po **Children**: 6–12 months: 2.5 mg Q24H po 12–23 months: 2.5 mg Q24H po; maximum 2.5 mg Q12H 2–5 y: 2.5 mg Q24H po; maximum 5 mg/day in 1 or 2 doses ≥6 y: Adult dosage	Minimal to no anticholinergic effects. May cause drowsiness in some individuals especially at higher doses. Headache.	Increased CNS depression: Alcohol, sedatives, tranquilizers, barbiturates. Increased anticholinergic side effects: TCAs, scopolamine.	Active metabolite of hydroxyzine. Available in pediatric 5 mg rapid-dissolve tablet. Available as 5 mg/5 mL syrup.	$

Class	Drug	Dosage	Adverse Effects	Drug Interactions	Comments	Cost[a]
	desloratadine Aerius, generics	**Adults**: 5 mg Q24H po **Children**: 6–11 months: 1 mg Q24H po 1–5 y: 1.25 mg Q24H po 6–11 y: 2.5 mg Q24H po	Minimal to no anticholinergic effects. Headache.	P-gp inhibitors (e.g., erythromycin, ketoconazole) may increase loratadine levels while P-gp inducers (e.g., carbamazepine, dexamethasone) may decrease loratadine levels; clinical effect probably minimal.	Active metabolite of loratadine. Available in pediatric liquid formulation.	$
	fexofenadine Allegra	**Adults**: 60 mg Q12H po Sustained-release: 120 mg Q24H po **Children**: 2–11 y: 30 mg Q12H po	See desloratadine.	Decreased fexofenadine level: Aluminum- and magnesium-containing antacids. Ingestion of fruit juices such as apple, grapefruit or orange may decrease bioavailability.	Active metabolite of terfenadine. Only 5% of a dose is metabolized.	$
	loratadine Claritin, Claritin Liquid Capsules, generics	**Adults**: 10 mg Q24H po **Children**: 2–5 y: 5 mg Q24H po ≥5 y: 10 mg Q24H po	See desloratadine.	QT_c prolongation reported with concomitant use of loratadine and amiodarone. Caution is advised. P-gp inhibitors (e.g., erythromycin, ketoconazole) may increase loratadine levels while P-gp inducers (e.g., carbamazepine, dexamethasone) may decrease loratadine levels; clinical effect probably minimal.	Available in pediatric liquid formulation and rapid-dissolve tablets.	$

(cont'd)

Table 5: **Oral Agents for Allergic Rhinitis** *(cont'd)*

Class	Drug	Dosage	Adverse Effects	Drug Interactions	Comments	Cost[a]
Decongestants	*pseudoephedrine* Eltor 120, Sudafed, generics	**Adults**: 60 mg Q4–6H po; maximum 240 mg/day Sustained-release: 120 mg Q12H po; maximum 240 mg/day **Children**: 6–11 y: 30 mg Q4–6H po; maximum 120 mg/day ≥12 y: adult dose	Mild CNS stimulation (nervousness, excitability, restlessness, dizziness, weakness, insomnia). Peripheral vasoconstriction. Tachycardia or palpitation may occur. Blood pressure may be increased in hypertensive subjects. May adversely affect blood sugar control in diabetics.	Beta-blockers: Antihypertensive effects may be reduced. Contraindicated with MAOIs and ergot derivatives. Avoid use with phenothiazines and selective serotonin reuptake inhibitors.	Caution in patients with heart disease, high blood pressure, hyperthyroidism, diabetes, angle closure glaucoma and prostatic enlargement. Concurrent use with or use within 2 weeks of MAOIs may cause hypertensive crisis.	$$
Antihistamine, Second-generation/ Decongestant Combinations	*cetirizine/ pseudoephedrine* Reactine Complete	**Adults**: 1 tab (5 mg/120 mg) Q12H po **Children**: ≥12 y: Give adult dose	See cetirizine. See pseudoephedrine.	See cetirizine. See pseudoephedrine.	See cetirizine. See pseudoephedrine.	$$
	desloratadine/ pseudoephedrine Aerius Dual Action 12 Hour	**Adults**: 1 tab (2.5 mg/120 mg) Q12H po **Children**: ≥12 y: Give adult dose	See desloratadine. See pseudoephedrine.	See desloratadine. See pseudoephedrine.	See desloratadine. See pseudoephedrine.	$$
	fexofenadine/ pseudoephedrine Allegra-D	**Adults**: 1 tab (60 mg/ 120 mg) Q12H po **Children**: ≥12 y: Give adult dose	See desloratadine. See pseudoephedrine.	See fexofenadine. See pseudoephedrine.	See fexofenadine. See pseudoephedrine.	$$
	loratadine/ pseudoephedrine Claritin Allergy + Sinus, Claritin Allergy + Sinus Extra Strength	**Adults**: 1 tab (5 mg/120 mg) Q12H po *or* 1 tab (10 mg/240 mg) Q24H po **Children**: ≥12 y: Give adult dose	See desloratadine. See pseudoephedrine.	See loratadine. See pseudoephedrine.	See loratadine. See pseudoephedrine.	$$

Class	Drug	Dosage	Adverse Effects	Drug Interactions	Comments	Cost[a]
Leukotriene Receptor Antagonists	*montelukast* Singulair, Montelukast, other generics	**Adults and children ≥15 y**: 10 mg QHS **Children**: 6–14 y: 5 mg QHS 2–5 y: 4 mg QHS	Headache, abdominal pain, flu-like symptoms.	Strong CYP2C9 and 3A4 inducers (e.g., carbamazepine, phenobarbital, phenytoin, rifampin) may decrease montelukast levels whereas, strong CYP2C9 inhibitors (e.g., sulfadiazine) may increase montelukast levels; clinical significance is uncertain; however, monitor for reduced efficacy or adverse effects.	Strong CYP2C9 and 3A4 inducers (e.g., carbamazepine, phenobarbital, phenytoin, rifampin) may decrease montelukast levels whereas, strong CYP2C9 inhibitors (e.g., fluconazole) may increase montelukast levels; clinical significance is uncertain; however, monitor for reduced efficacy or adverse effects	$$

[a] Cost of 10-day supply; includes drug cost only

Dosage adjustment may be required in renal impairment.

Abbreviations: CNS = central nervous system; MAOI = monoamine oxidase inhibitor; SR = sustained-release

Legend: $ < $10 $$ $10–20

Table 6: **Intranasal Agents for Allergic Rhinitis**

Class	Drug	Dosage	Adverse Effects	Comments	Cost[a]
Antihistamines	*levocabastine* Livostin Nasal Spray	**Adults and Children (≥12–65 y):** 2 sprays (50 µg/spray) per nostril BID; may increase to 2 sprays TID–QID	Nasal irritation.	Shake well before use. Initial priming required. Discontinue if no improvement seen within 3 days.	$$$
Antihistamine/ Corticosteroid Combinations	*azelastine/fluticasone* Dymista	**Adults and children ≥12 y**: 1 spray (137 µg/50 µg) in each nostril BID	Burning or stinging, nosebleeds. Dysgeusia may occur if patient tilts head back too far during administration.	Avoid use with ritonavir due to potential for systemic corticosteroid effects. Rarely causes drowsiness.	$100
Corticosteroids	*beclomethasone* generics	**Adults and children ≥6 y**: 2 sprays (50 µg/spray) in each nostril BID Adults: Maximum 12 sprays/day Children: Maximum 8 sprays/day Use lowest effective dose for maintenance therapy	Burning or stinging, nosebleed. May cause mild growth suppression with prolonged use.[45,46,47]	Use at regular intervals. Slow onset (7–14 days for maximal effect). Drug may fail to reach the site of action if excessive nasal mucus secretion or edema of the nasal mucosa is present. May use a vasoconstrictor (intranasal decongestant) 2–3 days prior to the suspension. Aim spray up towards turbinates and away from septum. Liquid forms may be more effective than metered-dose inhalers.	$$

Class	Drug	Dosage	Adverse Effects	Comments	Cost[a]
	budesonide Rhinocort Aqua, Rhinocort Turbuhaler	**Nasal suspension**: **Adults and children ≥6 y (64 µg/metered dose)**: Initial dose 2 sprays in each nostril daily *or* 1 spray in each nostril BID; may decrease maintenance dose to 1 spray in each nostril daily **Nasal powder**: **Adults and children ≥6 y (100 µg/dose)**: Initial dose 2 applications in each nostril in the morning *or* 1 application in each nostril BID; may decrease maintenance dose to 1 spray in each nostril daily Maximum 400 µg/day	See beclomethasone.	See beclomethasone. For the nasal suspension, initial priming needed. Re-prime if not used ≥4 days.	$$-$$$
	ciclesonide Omnaris	**Adults and children ≥12 y**: 2 sprays (50 µg/spray) in each nostril daily; maximum 200 µg/day	Burning or stinging, nosebleeds.	See beclomethasone. Initial priming needed.	$$$
	flunisolide generics	**Adults**: 2 sprays (25 µg/metered spray) in each nostril BID, may increase to TID if needed; maximum 300 µg/day **Children 6–14 y**: 1 spray in each nostril TID; maximum 150 µg/day	See ciclesonide.	See beclomethasone.	$$
	fluticasone propionate Flonase, generics	**Adults and children ≥12 y**: 2 sprays (50 µg/spray) in each nostril daily, may increase to BID in severe situations; maximum 400 µg/day **Children 4–11 y**: 1–2 sprays in each nostril daily; maximum 200 µg/day	See beclomethasone.	See beclomethasone.	$$$

(cont'd)

Table 6: **Intranasal Agents for Allergic Rhinitis** *(cont'd)*

Class	Drug	Dosage	Adverse Effects	Comments	Cost[a]
	fluticasone furoate Avamys	**Adults and children ≥12 y**: 2 sprays (27.5 µg/spray) in each nostril once daily; maximum 110 µg/day **Children ≥2 y to <12 y**: 1 spray in each nostril once daily, may increase to 2 sprays in each nostril once daily if needed. Decrease to 1 spray in each nostril daily for maintenance; maximum 110 µg/day	See ciclesonide.	See beclomethasone. Initial priming needed. Re-prime if not used ≥30 days or if cap left off for ≥5 days.	$$$
	mometasone Nasonex	**Adults and children ≥12 y**: 2 sprays (50 µg/spray) in each nostril daily, may decrease to 1 spray in each nostril daily for maintenance; may increase to BID in severe situations **Children 3–11 y**: 1 spray in each nostril daily	See ciclesonide.	See beclomethasone.	$$$
	triamcinolone Nasacort AQ	**Adults and children ≥12 y**: 2 sprays (55 µg/spray) in each nostril once daily, may decrease to 1 spray in each nostril once daily **Children 4–11 y**: 1 spray (55 µg/spray) in each nostril once daily, may increase to 2 sprays in each nostril once daily if needed. Decrease to 1 spray in each nostril daily for maintenance; maximum 110 µg/day	See ciclesonide.	See beclomethasone.	$$$

Class	Drug	Dosage	Adverse Effects	Comments	Cost[a]
Decongestants	*oxymetazoline* Claritin Allergy Decongestant, Dristan Long Lasting Nasal Mist, Dristan Long Lasting Mentholated Nasal Spray	**Adults and children ≥6 y**: 0.05% solution 2–3 drops or sprays/nostril Q12H	Burning, stinging, sneezing, dryness of the nasal mucosa. Bradycardia, tachycardia, hypotension and hypertension have been reported.	Onset of action: 5–10 min. Long duration of action lasting up to 12 h. Do not use longer than 3–5 days.	$
	phenylephrine Dristan Nasal Mist	**Adults and children ≥6 y**: 0.25% or 0.5% solution 2–3 drops or sprays/nostril Q4H	See oxymetazoline.	See oxymetazoline.	$
	xylometazoline Otrivin, Balminil Nasal Decongestant	**Adults and children ≥6 y**: 0.05% or 0.1% solution 2–3 drops or 1–2 sprays/nostril Q8-10H	See oxymetazoline.	See oxymetazoline.	$
Mast Cell Stabilizers	*sodium cromoglycate* Rhinaris CS Anti-allergic	**Adults and children >2 y**: 1 spray/nostril 3–6 times daily	Local: Sneezing, nasal stinging or irritation, bad taste in the mouth, epistaxis.	Less effective than other agents. Onset of action delayed up to 4 wk.	$$

[a] Cost of 1 unit (spray pump); includes drug cost only.

Legend: $ < $10 $$ $10–20 $$-$$$ $10–30 $$$ $20–30

Suggested Readings

Brozek JL, Bousquet J, Baena-Cagnani CE et al. Allergic Rhinitis and its Impact on Asthma (ARIA) guidelines: 2010 revision. *J Allergy Clin Immunol* 2010;126:466-76.

Seidman MD, Gurgel RK, Lin SY et al. Clinical practice guideline: Allergic rhinitis. *Otolaryngol Head Neck Surg* 2015;152:S1-43.

Wallace DV, Dykewicz MS, Bernstein DI et al. The diagnosis and management of rhinitis: an updated practice parameter. *J Allergy Clin Immunol* 2008;122:S1-84.

Wheatley LM, Togias A. Clinical practice. Allergic rhinitis. *N Engl J Med* 2015;372:456-63.

References

1. Mucci T, Govindaraj S, Tversky J. Allergic rhinitis. *Mt Sinai J Med* 2011;78:634-44.
2. Plaut M, Valentine MD. Clinical practice. Allergic rhinitis. *N Engl J Med* 2005;353:1934-44.
3. Brozek JL, Bousquet J, Baena-Cagnani CE et al. Allergic Rhinitis and its Impact on Asthma (ARIA) guidelines: 2010 revision. *J Allergy Clin Immunol* 2010;126:466-76.
4. Greiner A, Hellings PW, Rotiroti G et al. Allergic rhinitis. *Lancet* 2011;378:2112-22.
5. Kay AB. Allergy and allergic diseases. First of two parts. *N Engl J Med* 2001;344:30-7.
6. Wallace DV, Dykewicz MS, Bernstein DI et al. The diagnosis and management of rhinitis: an updated practice parameter. *J Allergy Clin Immunol* 2008;122:S1-84.
7. Scadding GK, Durham SR, Mirakian R et al. BSACI guidelines for the management of allergic and non-allergic rhinitis. *Clin Exp Allergy* 2008;38:19-42.
8. Varghese M, Glaum MC, Lockey RF. Drug-induced rhinitis. *Clin Exp Allergy* 2010;40:381-4.
9. Seidman MD, Gurgel RK, Lin SY et al. Clinical practice guideline: Allergic rhinitis. *Otolaryngol Head Neck Surg* 2015;152:S1-43.
10. Nurmatov U, van Schayck CP, Hurwitz B et al. House dust mite avoidance measures for perennial allergic rhinitis: an updated Cochrane systematic review. *Allergy* 2012;67:158-65.
11. Hermelingmeier KE, Weber RK, Hellmich M et al. Nasal irrigation as an adjunctive treatment in allergic rhinitis: a systematic review and meta-analysis. *Am J Rhinol Allergy* 2012;26:e119-25.
12. Garavello W, Somigliana E, Acaia B et al. Nasal lavage in pregnant women with seasonal allergic rhinitis: a randomized study. *Int Arch Allergy Immunol* 2010;151:137-41.
13. Wilson AM, O'Byrne PM, Parameswaran K. Leukotriene receptor antagonists for allergic rhinitis: a systematic review and meta-analysis. *Am J Med* 2004;116:338-44.
14. Laekeman G, Simoens S, Buffels J et al. Continuous versus on-demand pharmacotherapy of allergic rhinitis: evidence and practice. *Respir Med* 2010;104:615-25.
15. Krouse JH. Allergic rhinitis–current pharmacotherapy. *Otolaryngol Clin North Am* 2008;41:347-58.
16. Bachert C. A review of the efficacy of desloratadine, fexofenadine, and levocetirizine in the treatment of nasal congestion in patients with allergic rhinitis. *Clin Ther* 2009;31:921-44.
17. Lehman JM, Blaiss MS. Selecting the optimal oral antihistamine for patients with allergic rhinitis. *Drugs* 2006;66:2309-19.
18. Simons FE. Advances in H_1-antihistamines *N Engl J Med* 2004;351:2203-17.
19. Slater JW, Zechnich AD, Haxby DG. Second-generation antihistamines: a comparative review. *Drugs* 1999;57:31-47.
20. Horak F, Stubner UP. Comparative tolerability of second generation antihistamines. *Drug Saf* 1999;20:385-401.
21. Simons FE. H_1-receptor antagonists. Comparative tolerability and safety. *Drug Saf* 1994;10:350-80.
22. Melvin TA, Patel AA. Pharmacotherapy for allergic rhinitis. *Otolaryngol Clin North Am* 2011;44:727-39.
23. Sur DK, Scandale S. Treatment of allergic rhinitis. *Am Fam Physician* 2010;81:1440-6.
24. Turner PJ, Kemp AS. Allergic rhinitis in children. *J Paediatr Child Health* 2012;48:302-10.
25. Bender BG, Berning S, Dudden R et al. Sedation and performance impairment of diphenhydramine and second-generation antihistamines: a meta-analysis. *J Allergy Clin Immunol* 2003;111:770-6.
26. Weiler JM, Bloomfield JR, Woodworth GG et al. Effects of fexofenadine, diphenhydramine and alcohol on driving performance. A randomized, placebo-controlled trial in the Iowa driving simulator. *Ann Intern Med* 2000;132:354-63.
27. Church MK, Maurer M, Simons FE et al. Risk of first-generation H(1)-antihistamines: a GA(2)LEN position paper. *Allergy* 2010;65:459-66.
28. Walsh GM, Annunziato L, Frossard N et al. New insights into the second generation antihistamines. *Drugs* 2001;61:207-36.
29. Weiner JM, Abramson MJ, Puy RM. Intranasal corticosteroids versus oral H_1 receptor antagonists in allergic rhinitis: systematic review of randomised controlled trials. *BMJ* 1998;317:1624-9.
30. Glacy J, Putnam K, Godfrey S et al. *Treatments for seasonal allergic rhinitis*. Rockville: Agency for Healthcare Research and Quality; 2013. (Comparative Effectiveness Reviews, No. 120.) Available from: www.ncbi.nlm.nih.gov/books/NBK153714.
31. Golightly LK, Greos LS. Second-generation antihistamines: actions and efficacy in the management of allergic disorders. *Drugs* 2005;65:341-84.
32. Johnson DA, Hricik JG. The pharmacology of alpha-adrenergic decongestants. *Pharmacotherapy* 1993;13:110S-15S.
33. Chua SS, Benrimoj SI, Gordon RD et al. A controlled clinical trial on the cardiovascular effects of single doses of pseudoephedrine in hypertensive patients. *Br J Clin Pharmacol* 1989;28:369-72.
34. Graf P. Rhinitis medicamentosa: aspects of pathophysiology and treatment. *Allergy* 1997;52:28-34.
35. Mehuys E, Gevaert P, Brusselle G et al. Self-medication in persistent rhinitis: overuse of decongestants in half of the patients. *J Allergy Clin Immunol Pract* 2014;2:313-9.
36. Ratner P, Van Bavel JV, Mohar D et al. Efficacy of daily intranasal fluticasone propionate on ocular symptoms associated with seasonal allergic rhinitis. *Ann Allergy Asthma Immunol* 2015;114:141-7.
37. van Drunen C, Meltzer EO, Bachert C et al. Nasal allergies and beyond: a clinical review of the pharmacology, efficacy, and safety of mometasone furoate. *Allergy* 2005;60:5-19.

38. Kaiser HB, Naclerio RM, Given J et al. Fluticasone furoate nasal spray: a single treatment option for the symptoms of seasonal allergic rhinitis. *J Allergy Clin Immunol* 2007;119:1430-7.
39. Hong J, Bielory B, Rosenberg JL. Efficacy of intranasal corticosteroids for the ocular symptoms of allergic rhinitis: a systematic review. *Allergy Asthma Proc* 2011;32:22-35.
40. Berger WE, Prenner B, Turner R et al. A patient preference and satisfaction study of ciclesonide nasal aerosol and mometasone furoate aqueous nasal spray in patients with perennial allergic rhinitis. *Allergy Asthma Proc* 2013;34:542-50.
41. Kowalski ML. Systemic and specific treatment for a global disease: allergen immunotherapy revisited. *Allergy* 2006;61:791-5.
42. Jacobsen L, Niggemann B, Dreborg S et al. Specific immunotherapy has long term preventive effect of seasonal and perennial asthma: 10-year follow-up on the PAT study. *Allergy* 2007;62:943-8.
43. Allen DB. Systemic effects of intranasal steroids: an endocrinologist's perspective. *J Allergy Clin Immunol* 2000;106:S179-90.
44. Skoner DP, Gentile DA, Doyle WJ. Effect on growth of long-term treatment with intranasal triamcinolone acetonide aqueous in children with allergic rhinitis. *Ann Allergy Asthma Immunol* 2008;101:431-6.
45. Skoner DP, Rachelefsky GS, Meltzer EO et al. Detection of growth suppression in children during treatment with intranasal beclomethasone dipropionate. *Pediatrics* 2000;105:E23.
46. Lee LA, Sterling R, Maspero J et al. Growth velocity reduced with once-daily fluticasone furoate nasal spray in prepubescent children with perennial allergic rhinitits. *J Allergy Clin Immunol Pract* 2014;2:421-7.
47. Skoner DP, Berger WE, Gawchik SM et al. Intranasal triamcinolone and growth velocity. *Pediatrics* 2015;135:e348-56.
48. Healthy Canadians. *Health Canada releases decision on the labelling of cough and cold products for children*. Available from: www.healthycanadians.gc.ca/recall-alert-rappel-avis/hc-sc/2008/13267a-eng.php. Accessed November 30, 2009.
49. Peterson RG, Cran B, Knoppert D et al. Scientific Advisory Panel on Nonprescription Paediatric Cough and Cold Medications (SAP-NPCCM). *Record of proceedings*. Ottawa: Health Canada; March 20, 2008.
50. Mazzotta P, Loebstein R, Koren G. Treating allergic rhinitis in pregnancy. Safety considerations. *Drug Saf* 1999;20:361-75.
51. Briggs GG, Freeman RK. *Drugs in pregnancy and lactation: a reference guide to fetal and neonatal risk*. 10th ed. Baltimore: Lippincott Williams & Wilkins; 2015.
52. Oykhman P, Kim HL, Ellis AK. Allergen immunotherapy in pregnancy. *Allergy Asthma Clin Immunol* 2015;11:31.
53. Hale TW. *Medications and mothers' milk: a manual of lactational pharmacology*. 15th ed. Amarillo: Hale Publishing; 2012.

Allergic Rhinitis—What You Need to Know

Allergic rhinitis is a condition caused by allergens in the air. Allergens are things that cause allergies. Some of the symptoms of allergic rhinitis are sneezing, coughing, runny nose, and itchy or watery eyes. The most important thing you can do to feel better is to avoid the things that cause your allergies. Also avoid exposure to cigarette smoke and strong smells. If you do not know what causes your allergies, see your doctor.

Helpful Hints for People Who Have Allergies

If you are allergic to pollen:

- Keep the windows and doors of your house closed.
- If you need to use air conditioning, set the unit to the indoor cycle.
- Do not use window or attic fans.
- Check the weather report to find out about the pollen count. The pollen count tells you what kind of pollen is in the air and how much. Avoid spending time outdoors when the pollen count is high. The pollen count is highest on sunny, windy days and in the morning.
- Do not dry your clothing outdoors.
- Shower or take a bath and wash your hair after outdoor activity. This will remove pollen from your hair and skin. You want to avoid getting pollen into your bedding.

If you are allergic to outdoor moulds:

- Stay indoors as much as possible.
- If you need to use air conditioning, set the unit to the indoor cycle. Have your air conditioner cleaned regularly. Air conditioners can be heavily contaminated with mould.
- Use a facemask if you rake leaves or work with compost or dry soil.

If you are allergic to indoor moulds:

- Kill mould with a solution of equal parts household bleach and water. Wash sinks, shower stalls, nonrefrigerated vegetable storage areas and garbage pails with this solution.
- Avoid using a humidifier or cool mist vaporizer. Moulds grow easily where it is damp. If you must use a humidifier or vaporizer, clean it often with a solution of equal parts bleach and water.
- If your home is built over a crawl space, install a plastic vapor barrier over exposed soil and keep the foundation vents open.
- If your basement is damp or tends to flood, do not put carpet or furniture there. For a damp basement, run a dehumidifier at all times. Empty water from the machine often and clean it regularly. For a flooded basement, drain the water as quickly as possible.
- Fix any leaky faucets or pipes promptly.
- Do not keep houseplants.

If you are allergic to dust mites:

- Do not put carpet in your bedroom or main living areas.
- Plastic, leather or wood furniture is best.
- If possible, have someone else clean the house while you are not at home.
- If you must do your own cleaning, wear a facemask while you clean and for 10–15 minutes afterward.

- Use a vacuum cleaner with an efficient double-filtration system.
- Keep indoor humidity between 40% and 45%. You can buy a hygrometer to measure the humidity in your house at a hardware store or home centre.
- Avoid using a humidifier or cool mist vaporizer.
- Use zippered, allergen-proof casings on all mattresses, box springs and pillows.
- Consider replacing old mattresses.
- Wash your bedding in hot (>55°C) water at least every 2 weeks. Cooler water will not kill dust mites.
- Do not keep stuffed toys that cannot be washed.
- Do not store items under your bed.
- Use window shades instead of venetian blinds.

If you are allergic to a pet:

- The best choice is to find another home for the animal. It can take several months before the allergen levels return to normal.
- If you are not able to give up your pet, then:
  - You may find it helps to install a HEPA or electrostatic air purifier in your home.
  - Keep animals out of your bedroom at all times.
  - Keep animals out of rooms that have carpets.
  - Try to keep animals off furniture.
  - Washing cats weekly and dogs twice weekly may help, though this has not been proven.
  - Get rid of litter boxes if possible. If not, put them in an area that is not connected to the air supply for the rest of your home.
  - If the animal lives in a cage, keep it in a room without carpet, far away from your bedroom.

Medication to Help with Allergy Symptoms

You may want to try medication if:

- You don't feel better even when you avoid the things that cause your allergies.
- Your allergies are interfering with your sleep or your daily activities.

Your pharmacist can help you pick the best medication for you and show you how to use it. See Table 1. You can choose between pills or a nasal spray.

Table 1: **How to Use a Nasal Spray or Drops**

Nasal Spray (Adults only)
1. Gently blow your nose. 2. Gently shake bottle and remove cap or lid. 3. With your head upright but not tilted backward, press your finger against one side of your nose to close the nostril. Spray the medication into the open nostril, with the tip directed away from the middle of the nose and back towards the nasal cavity. Squeeze the bottle quickly and breathe in slowly through the nose. 4. Remove tip of nasal spray from your nostril and breathe out through your mouth. 5. Do the same thing on the other side. 6. Blow your nose in 3–5 minutes.

(cont'd)

Table 1: How to Use a Nasal Spray or Drops *(cont'd)*

7. Rinse the tip of the spray bottle with hot water, but try not to get water in the bottle. Replace lid.
8. Do not use more nose spray than the recommended amount.

Nose Drops (Adult or child)

1. Gently blow your nose.
2. Lie on your back on a bed with your head hanging slightly over the side.
3. Gently shake bottle. Fill the dropper with the recommended amount of medication. Put the dropper just inside one nostril (about 0.8 cm or one-third inch). If possible, don't let the dropper touch the skin.
4. Apply the recommended number of drops. Apply the medication to the other nostril in the same way.
5. Stay in the same position for about 5 minutes. Tilt head from side to side.
6. Blow the nose 3–5 minutes later.
7. You can also take nose drops by tilting your head back (instead of lying down). Use the recommended number of drops for each nostril. Then bend over at the waist and hold that position for a few seconds before coming up straight again.
8. Rinse the dropper with hot water and return it to the bottle.
9. Do not use nose drops more than is recommended on the package.

Chapter 23

Assessment of Patients with Upper Respiratory Tract Symptoms

Daniel J.G. Thirion, BPharm, MSc, PharmD, FCSHP

Upper respiratory tract infection is a nonspecific term used to describe a spectrum of acute infections that may involve the nose, sinuses, pharynx, larynx and trachea. These infections are common in adults and children and may be caused by a virus, by bacteria or (less frequently) by fungi. Most viral infections are self-limited, resolve spontaneously and are managed symptomatically. Some patients are at risk of complications of viral infections including influenza (see Table 1) and respiratory syncytial virus and may require specific antiviral treatment. Bacterial infections or complications should be medically evaluated to determine the need for antibiotic therapy and further specific intervention.

Viral and bacterial infections can be difficult to differentiate. Signs and symptoms, along with a medical history, can help determine the next steps of care (see Figure 1). Investigation for possible bacterial infection is indicated in the presence of fever lasting more than 72 hours, high fever, chills, severe sudden throat pain, prolonged congestion (>7 days), difficulty breathing, earache (especially in children) or double sickening (worsening after a few days of initial improvement). The patient should be assessed for the presence of complications, intensity of care required and the need for antibiotics.

Patients suffering from the common cold usually first complain of discomfort of the throat (dryness, scratchiness), followed by nasal congestion and rhinorrhea. Nasal discharge is clear and watery at the beginning and becomes mucopurulent as the infection progresses. Cough may be present and may persist for 1–2 weeks. Usually dry at the beginning, the cough often becomes productive.

Compared with the common cold, the onset of throat pain in pharyngitis is more rapid and the pain is more severe. Prolonged nasal congestion and purulent drainage are consistent with possible sinusitis; especially if accompanied by fever, headache and facial pain.

Cough is present in most upper respiratory tract infections, such as the common cold and influenza, but may be caused by many other conditions, many of which require diagnosis by an appropriate healthcare practitioner (see Chapter 21: Acute Cough, Table 1). Cough persisting longer than 3 weeks should be assessed more thoroughly.

Table 1: **Persons at High Risk of Complications or Hospitalization Due to Influenza**[1]

- Adults and children with chronic conditions, such as cardiac or pulmonary disorders, diabetes mellitus or other metabolic disease, cancer, immunodeficiency or immunosuppression, renal disease, anemia or hemoglobinopathy, morbid obesity (BMI ≥40)
- Any resident of a nursing home or other chronic care facility, regardless of age
- Persons 65 years of age and older
- Conditions that compromise the management of respiratory secretions and are associated with an increased risk of aspiration
- Children and adolescents with conditions treated for long periods with acetylsalicylic acid
- Healthy children under 5 years of age
- Pregnant women
- Aboriginal persons

See Table 2 for a comparison of common upper respiratory tract ailments. For more detailed information, see Chapter 24: Viral Rhinitis, Influenza, Rhinosinusitis and Pharyngitis. Symptoms suggestive of croup, epiglottitis or otitis media (see Table 3) require further assessment for a tailored workup and treatment.

Allergic rhinitis can resemble the common cold but does not have an infectious etiology. Allergic rhinitis is characterized by sneezing and rhinorrhea which may progress to nasal congestion. Eye symptoms, such as conjunctivitis and lacrimation may also be present. See Chapter 13: Conjunctivitis and Chapter 22: Allergic Rhinitis.

Table 2: **Differential Diagnosis of Upper Respiratory Tract Conditions**

Symptom/Cause	Common Cold[2,3,4,5,6,7,8]	Allergic Rhinitis[9,10,11]	Influenza[6,7,8]	Sinusitis[6,7,8,12,13]	Pharyngitis[6,7,8,14]
Nasal discharge and congestion	Clear at the beginning, then can become mucopurulent Nasal congestion is common	Abundant; aqueous and clear Nasal congestion may be present	Clear at the beginning, then mucopurulent Nasal congestion is rare	Persistent, purulent rhinorrhea Coloured (yellow, green)	Rare
Fever	Rare, mild	No	Yes (38–40°C) Sudden onset	Possible	Yes
Sore throat	Common Mild (dry, scratchy, sore)	Rarely	Sometimes	No	Severe, sudden onset
Cough	Mild to moderate Dry at the beginning; often becomes productive as the cold progresses	Possible via post-nasal drip	Common Nonproductive	Possible via postnasal drip	Rare
Headache	Rare, via sinus congestion	Via sinus congestion	Yes	Common, via sinus congestion	
General aches and pain	Rare, mild	Earaches, especially in children	Common (myalgia)	Rare	Possible
Other	Sneezing in the first couple of days	Pruritus (palate, nose, eyes) Sneezing, lacrimation	Fatigue, weakness, chills	Facial tenderness; jaw and tooth pain	
Duration	Usually 5–7 days but 25% last 14 days	As long as exposed to the allergen	10 days	Days to weeks	3 days
Etiology	Viral	Noninfectious	Viral	Viral, bacterial, fungal (rare)	Viral (most common), bacterial

Table 3: **Croup, Epiglottitis and Otitis Media in Children**

Condition	Croup[6,15,16]	Epiglottitis[6,16]	Otitis Media[6,17]
Possible signs and symptoms	Barking, seal-like cough, usually nonproductive Gradually worsening inspiratory stridor Dyspnea Fever Hoarseness	Sore throat and difficulty swallowing Fever, chills Stridor Use of accessory muscles and positioning for breathing (laboured, sitting upright, and leaning slightly forward) Hoarseness Drooling Cyanosis	Fever, especially one beginning several days after the start of a cold Earache or child tugging at or fingering ear Irritability and/or lethargy Purulent drainage from ear
Other characteristics	Fluctuating course with rapid improvements and declines; symptoms often worse at night Prodrome (2–5 days) consisting of mild fever, rhinorrhea, malaise, sore throat and cough For more information, consult the *Compendium of Therapeutic Choices*: Croup.	Rapidly progressive, usually absence of cough	For more information, consult the *Compendium of Therapeutic Choices*: Acute Otitis Media in Childhood.

Figure 1: Assessment of Patients with Upper Respiratory Tract Symptoms[2,3,4,5,6,7,8,9,10,11,12,13,14]

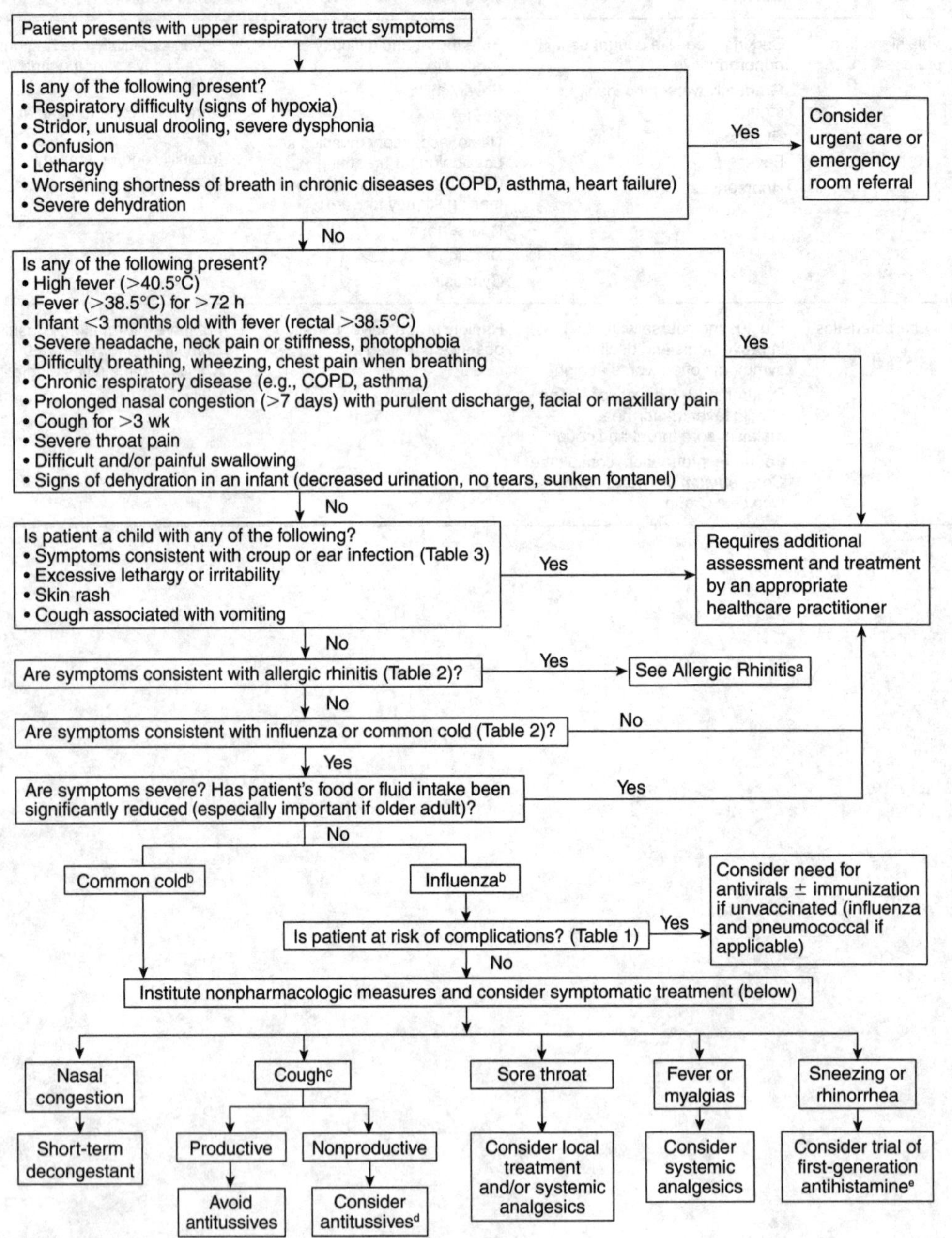

[a] See Chapter 22: Allergic Rhinitis.
[b] See Chapter 24: Viral Rhinitis, Influenza, Rhinosinusitis and Pharyngitis.
[c] See Chapter 21: Acute Cough.
[d] Antitussives are not recommended in children <6 years. See Chapter 21: Acute Cough.
[e] First-generation antihistamines are not recommended in children <6 years. See Chapter 24: Viral Rhinitis, Influenza, Rhinosinusitis and Pharyngitis.

Suggested Readings

Allan GM, Arroll B. Prevention and treatment of the common cold: making sense of the evidence. *CMAJ* 2014;186:190-9.

Committee on Infectious Diseases, American Academy of Pediatrics. Principles of appropriate use for upper respiratory tract infections. In: Pickering LK, ed. *Red Book: 2012 report of the Committee on Infectious Diseases*. 29th ed. Elk Grove Village: American Academy of Pediatrics; 2012. p. 802-5.

Small P, Kim H. Allergic rhinitis. *Allergy Asthma Clin Immunol* 2011;7:S3.

References

1. National Advisory Committee on Immunization (NACI). An Advisory Committee Statement (ACS). *Canadian Immunization Guide chapter on influenza and statement on seasonal influenza vaccine for 2015-2016*. Ottawa (ON): PHAC; 2015. Available from: www.phac-aspc.gc.ca/naci-ccni/flu-2015-grippe-eng.php. Accessed November 20, 2015.
2. Heikkinen T, Jarvinen A. The common cold. *Lancet* 2003;361:51-9.
3. Pratter MR. Cough and the common cold: ACCP evidence-based clinical practice guidelines. *Chest* 2006;129:72S-74S.
4. Canadian Paediatric Society. Caring for Kids. *Colds in children*. Available from: www.caringforkids.cps.ca/handouts/colds_in_children. Accessed November 20, 2015.
5. Irwin RS, Madison JM. The diagnosis and treatment of cough. *N Engl J Med* 2000;343:1715-21.
6. Committee on Infectious Diseases, American Academy of Pediatrics. Principles of appropriate use for upper respiratory tract infections. In: Pickering LK, ed. *Red Book: 2012 report of the Committee on Infectious Diseases*. 29th ed. Elk Grove Village: American Academy of Pediatrics; 2012. p. 802-5.
7. Frei C, Frei B. Upper respiratory tract infections. In: DiPiro JT et al., eds. *Pharmacotherapy: a pathophysiologic approach*. 9th ed. New York: McGraw-Hill Medical; 2014. p. 1717-29.
8. Nahata MC, O'Mara NB, Benavides S. Viral infections. In: Koda-Kimble MA, Young LL, eds. *Applied therapeutics: the clinical use of drugs*. 9th ed. Philadelphia: Lippincott Williams & Wilkins; 2009. p. 72-1-72-20.
9. May JR, Smith PH. Allergic rhinitis. In: DiPiro JT et al., eds. *Pharmacotherapy: a pathophysiologic approach*. 9th ed. New York: McGraw-Hill Medical; 2014. p. 1541-53.
10. Plaut M, Valentine MD. Clinical practice. Allergic rhinitis. *N Engl J Med* 2005;353:1934-44.
11. Small P, Kim H. Allergic rhinitis. *Allergy Asthma Clin Immunol* 2011;7:S3.
12. Desrosiers M, Evans GA, Keith PK et al. Canadian clinical practice guidelines for acute and chronic rhinosinusitis. *Allergy Asthma Clin Immunol* 2011;7:2.
13. Worrall G. Acute sinusitis. *Can Fam Physician* 2011;57:565-7.
14. Worrall G. Acute sore throat. *Can Fam Physician* 2011;57:791-4.
15. Worrall G. Croup. *Can Fam Physician* 2008;54:573-4.
16. Sobol SE, Zapata S. Epiglottitis and croup. *Otolaryngol Clin North Am* 2008;41:551-66.
17. Canadian Paediatric Society. Management of acute otitis media. *Paediatr Child Health* 2009;14:457-64.

Chapter 24

Viral Rhinitis, Influenza, Rhinosinusitis and Pharyngitis

Daniel J.G. Thirion, BPharm, MSc, PharmD, FCSHP

Upper respiratory tract infections (URTIs) are a group of diseases of the upper airway caused by many different viruses or bacteria. Each infection shares some common symptoms, involving, to variable degrees, sneezing, nasal congestion and discharge (rhinorrhea), sore throat, cough, low grade fever, headache and malaise. This chapter describes each infection and their symptomatic management.

Pathophysiology

Viral Rhinitis (Common Cold)

The common cold is a viral infection caused by more than 200 different viruses. Among these, rhinoviruses (30–50%) are the most common in all age groups. More than 100 serotypes of rhinovirus have been identified. Coronaviruses are also frequently involved, accounting for 10–20% of infections. Other common viruses are respiratory syncytial virus (RSV), adenovirus, parainfluenza and enterovirus.[1,2,3]

The common cold is one of the most common infectious diseases of humankind. Preschool children average 6 episodes annually and adults 2–3.[2] Daycare attendance is an important risk factor for children.[1] It is estimated that 40% of time lost from work and 30% of absences from school are due to the common cold.[1,4,5] It can occur at any time of year but is less common during the summer months. Rhinoviruses are more prevalent during fall and spring, and coronaviruses during mid-winter and early spring.[1]

The transmission of viruses that cause upper respiratory tract infection can occur by any of the following 3 mechanisms:[1]

- hand contact with secretions that contain the virus, either directly from an infected person or indirectly from environmental surfaces
- small-particle aerosols lingering in the air
- direct hit by large-particle aerosols from an infected person.

All 3 mechanisms are possible for each virus but the primary routes of transmission may differ between them. Hand-to-hand contact appears to be the major transmission route for rhinovirus infection.

Contact between the virus and nasal mucosa appears to be important for initiation of the infection. The increase in vascular permeability, glandular secretion and vasodilatation that follows are responsible for the symptoms.[1,3] The detailed mechanisms by which viral infection causes such changes in the nasal mucosa are still incompletely understood.[1] The host's humoral and cellular immune responses seem to play pivotal roles. Cholinergic stimulation leads to increased mucous gland secretion and sneezing. No increase in histamine concentration is noted.[1] Viral replication peaks in 48 hours but viral shedding can continue for up to 3 weeks.[1]

The common cold is characterized by a sore throat usually resolving within a few days, followed by nasal congestion, rhinorrhea, sneezing and cough. Nasal discharge can sometimes be purulent and mistaken for bacterial sinus infection.[4] Fever is infrequent in adults but common in children.[5] Symptoms peak around 2–4 days and begin to resolve by day 7. For a small proportion of patients, symptoms such as cough can still be present after 3 weeks.

The common cold is usually a self-limiting illness confined to the upper respiratory tract.[1] It can sometimes predispose individuals to bacterial complications, such as otitis media (especially in children via dysfunction of the eustachian tube[6]), bacterial rhinosinusitis and pneumonia. It may also cause exacerbations of asthma.[1]

Influenza

Influenza in humans is caused by influenza A and/or B virus. Influenza A viruses are categorized into subtypes on the basis of 2 surface antigens, hemagglutinin and neuraminidase. Influenza B viruses are separated into 2 distinct genetic lineages but are not categorized into subtypes.[7] Immunity to 1 subtype does not confer protection against another subtype, and mutations occur often.[8] Although influenza A is more common and tends to cause more severe illness, it is impossible to differentiate clinically between influenza A and B.[9,10]

Influenza is normally seen between November and April in the northern hemisphere. Debate exists as to how influenza virus is transmitted: airborne, droplet, contact or a combination of these.[11] The incubation period for influenza virus averages 2 days.[7] Viral replication occurs in the superficial epithelium of the airway tract. Symptoms, usually having an abrupt onset, are related to the presence of the virus in the airway or to the host immune response. Initial symptoms tend to be systemic in nature, with respiratory symptoms becoming prominent as systemic symptoms subside.[12] Common systemic symptoms include fever, myalgia, headache, malaise and chills. Respiratory symptoms include sore throat, nonproductive cough and rhinitis.[12] The infectivity period starts before the onset of symptoms and usually lasts 5–7 days, but shedding of the virus may continue for 7 days or longer after the start of symptomatic illness, especially in children and immunocompromised patients.[13] Complications of influenza include pneumonia and even death. Influenza may worsen chronic obstructive pulmonary disease, asthma and pulmonary conditions of patients with cystic fibrosis. In 2011, influenza and pneumonia together were responsible for 5767 deaths and ranked 8th among leading causes of death in Canada.[14] Persons at high risk of experiencing complications due to influenza are described in Chapter 23: Assessment of Patients with Upper Respiratory Tract Symptoms, Table 1.

Rhinosinusitis

Acute rhinosinusitis is characterized by inflammation of the nasal cavity and paranasal sinuses in response to infection, that lasts less than 4 weeks.[15,16] Symptoms include nasal congestion and obstruction, purulent nasal discharge, maxillary tooth discomfort and facial pain or pressure, hyposmia or anosmia, cough, headache, fever and malaise.[17]

Rhinosinusitis is often preceded by a viral upper respiratory tract infection. Viral and bacterial infections, as well as allergic rhinitis, affect mucociliary transport thereby disrupting evacuation of microorganisms. Although it is often preceded by a viral upper respiratory tract infection, only 0.5–2% of episodes of viral rhinosinusitis are complicated by acute bacterial infection.[18] The most common viruses are rhinovirus, influenza virus and parainfluenza virus. *Streptococcus pneumoniae* or *Haemophilus influenzae* cause 70% of bacterial rhinosinusitis.[16] *Moraxella catarrhalis* is also a common pathogen in children.[19,20] Other events that introduce microorganisms into the sinuses (such as dental extraction) or anatomical abnormality may also be precipitants.

Complications of acute rhinosinusitis include periorbital and orbital cellulitis, orbital abscess, blindness and cavernous sinus thrombosis.[20] Complications of chronic rhinosinusitis can include mucoceles (airless, expanded sinuses) and nasal polyps.[20]

Rhinosinusitis is considered chronic if symptoms persist more than 3 months. Risk factors for developing chronic rhinosinusitis include: anatomical abnormalities (e.g., deviation of the nasal septum, septal spurs, hypertrophic turbinates, nasal polyps); conditions that affect the normal function of the mucociliary sinus epithelium (e.g., cystic fibrosis); and conditions that affect the normal immune defenses of the upper respiratory tract. Sixty percent of chronic rhinosinusitis is caused by *H. influenzae*. Other responsible organisms are *Staphylococcus aureus*, alpha-hemolytic streptococci, *Bacteroides* species, *Veillonella* species, *Corynebacterium* species, *Pseudomonas aeruginosa* (patients with nasal polyps or cystic fibrosis) and fungi (diabetic or immunocompromised patients).[15,16]

Pharyngitis

Acute pharyngitis is an inflammatory syndrome of the pharynx. Many bacterial and viral organisms are capable of inducing pharyngitis, but the majority (90%) are viral.[21] Pharyngitis may be present in Epstein-Barr infection, influenza, the common cold, measles, varicella, allergic rhinitis and rhinosinusitis, or may be due to exposure to irritating substances or environmental pollutants, ingestion of caustic substances or direct trauma to the pharynx. Among bacterial causes, group A beta-hemolytic streptococcus (GABHS) is by far the most commonly implicated (15–30% of cases in children aged 5–15 years and 5–10% in adults).[22] Pharyngitis due to GABHS is usually seen during the winter and early spring. Suppurative complications (peritonsillar or retropharyngeal abscess, cervical lymphadenitis, mastoiditis and rhinosinusitis), rheumatic fever and post-streptococcal glomerulonephritis may occur secondary to bacterial pharyngitis.[22] Rheumatic fever is prevented by treatment of GABHS within 9 days of onset of the infection.[22]

Goals of Therapy

- Alleviate symptoms
- Eradicate infection or shorten the duration of infection
- Prevent complications of the infection

Patient Assessment

Determine symptoms, duration and risk factors for serious disease. See Figure 1 in Chapter 23: Assessment of Patients with Upper Respiratory Tract Symptoms for an assessment algorithm plus Table 2 in Chapter 23: Assessment of Patients with Upper Respiratory Tract Symptoms which summarizes differentiating characteristics of upper respiratory tract disorders.

Viral Rhinitis

Viral rhinitis is a self-limiting disease that rarely causes complications. Currently, no therapy is available to change the course of disease. Management is targeted at alleviating symptoms rather than treating the infection.

Influenza

Typical symptoms include fever/chills, myalgia, headache, nonproductive cough and fatigue. GI symptoms (e.g., nausea, vomiting, diarrhea) are generally uncommon in adults but more common in children. GI symptoms may occur in up to 30% of cases depending on the infecting strain.[23,24] Persons at risk of complications (see Chapter 23: Assessment of Patients with Upper Respiratory Tract Symptoms, Table 1) require immediate assessment of the need for antiviral therapy.[24]

Rhinosinusitis

Most cases of rhinosinusitis are viral and are self-limiting. Differentiating bacterial from viral rhinosinusitis is a challenge because the clinical features of the 2 etiologies are similar.[18] A change in the colour of the nasal discharge is not a specific sign of bacterial infection since mucopurulent nasal secretions may also occur a few days after onset of a viral infection.[18] Bacterial rhinosinusitis is suggested when sinus symptoms do not improve within 10 days or worsen after 5–7 days, and by the presence of nasal obstruction or purulence plus one or both of facial pain/pressure/fullness or hyposmia/anosmia.[15,18] These patients should be assessed for antibiotic therapy. Other symptoms (e.g., headache, dental pain, cough, halitosis) may be present but are not used for the diagnosis of acute bacterial rhinosinusitis.

Pharyngitis

A sore throat is common to many URTIs and usually does not require specific treatment. Symptoms suggestive of GABHS include sore throat with a sudden onset, fever and headache. Nasal congestion, conjunctivitis and cough are not generally suggestive of bacterial pharyngitis.[25] After eliminating other causes of sore throat, a modified Centor score can be used to help determine the likelihood of GABHS and therefore the need for antibiotic treatment.[26,27] The score is determined using the criteria listed in Table 1. If the cumulative score is ≥2 points, refer the patient for culture and possibly antibiotics. The score is not a diagnostic tool and should not be relied upon as such. As many as 25–30% of all GABHS-positive culture results in adults with pharyngitis occur in those with a modified Centor score of less than 2.[26] Conversely, up to 50% of patients with a score of ≥4 may have a GABHS-negative throat culture result and not need antibiotic treatment.

If a patient with a sore throat also presents with painful dysphagia, they should be assessed for the presence of epiglottitis.

Table 1: **Modified Centor Score**[27]

Criteria	Points
Temperature >38°C	1
Absence of cough	1
Swollen, tender anterior cervical nodes	1
Tonsillar swelling or exudate	1
Age	
3–14 years	1
15–44 years	0
≥45 years	−1

Adapted with permission from McIsaac WJ, White D, Tannenbaum D, Low DE. A clinical score to reduce unnecessary antibiotic use in patients with sore throat. *CMAJ* 1998;158:75-83. Copyright © 1998 Canadian Medical Association.

Prevention

Upper respiratory tract viruses are transmitted by direct contact (hand-to-hand), aerosol particles or contact with settled droplets. Routine handwashing is recommended to prevent transmission of infection.[1,28] One should also try not to touch the face and eyes. Proper handwashing technique is described in Common Cold and Influenza—What You Need to Know at the conclusion of this chapter. Alcohol-based hand sanitizers are widely used in healthcare settings or in situations when water is not available but may be of limited value for preventing spread of respiratory infections.[29,30] Handwashing remains the first and most important step for cleaning hands, especially if they are visibly soiled. Hand sanitizers are to be used as a supplement to regular, effective handwashing, when water is not readily available, and when hands are not visibly soiled.

Sneeze and cough etiquette is another method traditionally advised for the prevention of URTIs. This involves coughing or sneezing into an arm, sleeve or tissue. If a tissue is used, it should be promptly thrown away and the hands washed.[31]

Prevention of Influenza

Annual **influenza vaccination** is the most effective way to prevent influenza and its complications. Health Canada has approved trivalent and quadrivalent vaccines, most of which are inactivated, but one live attenuated quadrivalent vaccine is available. Refer to current statement from the National Advisory Committee on Immunization (NACI) for details regarding yearly vaccine availability.[32] The vaccines are modified each year according to the viruses expected to circulate in the population that season. The efficacy of the vaccine depends on the degree of antigenic match between the vaccine virus and the circulating virus. Influenza vaccine can provide moderate protection against influenza, but protection is greatly reduced or absent in some seasons.[33] Healthy school-age children and adults respond well to vaccination, whereas preschool children, the elderly and the immunocompromised respond less well.[32,34,35] The live-attenuated influenza vaccine provides improved efficacy compared with inactivated vaccines in children ≤6 years but should be avoided in certain populations (those <2 years or >59 years of age, pregnant women, those with immunodeficiencies, severe asthma or egg allergy, or children receiving ASA therapy).[32] With a good antigenic match, influenza vaccination prevents influenza in 56–91% of healthy children and adults. Protection is lower in elderly and immunocompromised patients.[32] Vaccination also reduces rates of illness, numbers of physician visits and sick days in healthy, working adults. Protection is generally achieved approximately 2 weeks after vaccine administration, and usually lasts less than 1 year.

Vaccination is encouraged for all appropriate candidates but is particularly important for those at high risk of complications due to influenza (Chapter 23: Assessment of Patients with Upper Respiratory Tract Symptoms, Table 1). It is also recommended for people capable of transmitting influenza to those at high risk, such as healthcare workers and household contacts (including children) of people at high risk who either cannot receive the vaccine or may respond inadequately to it (e.g., elderly, immunocompromised, infants <6 months), those providing regular care to children <5 years of age, or persons who provide essential community services.[32,36]

The optimal time for vaccination is mid-October to mid-November. However, if this time frame is missed, vaccination should be performed at any opportunity that becomes available prior to the end of the flu season, typically the end of April in Canada.[32] The inactivated vaccine is safe in all stages of pregnancy and during breastfeeding.[32]

Antiviral chemoprophylaxis is no longer recommended other than in select circumstances, such as control of outbreaks in long-term care facilities that house large numbers of patients at high risk of influenza complications.[24] In other circumstances, the preferred approach is early treatment of infected persons because of the potential risk of oseltamivir resistance emerging during postexposure prophylaxis (see Table 2).

Nonpharmacologic Therapy

For the common cold, influenza, pharyngitis and rhinosinusitis, nonpharmacologic treatment consists of bed rest, good hydration and increased humidity (>50%).

Pharmacologic Therapy

Irritated nasal tissue may be soothed with commercial **nasal saline** solutions. Nasal saline can improve symptoms and decrease medication use in rhinosinusitis.[37] **Petrolatum** may be applied to a raw nose to increase patient comfort.

Table 2: **Recommendations for Chemoprophylaxis vs. Early Therapy for Influenza**[24]

In general, early treatment of symptomatic illness is recommended in preference to postexposure prophylaxis after contact with infectious individuals.

In exposed, susceptible, profoundly immunosuppressed individuals at very high risk of complications, presumptive treatment should be initiated prior to the onset of symptomatic illness.

Prophylaxis, combined with treatment for ill persons, is indicated to control outbreaks in nursing homes and other long-term care facilities where large numbers of patients are at high risk of acquiring infections due to their housing arrangements and influenza complications.

Neither early treatment nor prophylaxis should be prescribed:

- for groups of healthy individuals based on possible exposure in the community
- if the close contact did not occur during the infectious period of the person with suspected or confirmed influenza
- If >4 days have elapsed since the last infectious contact.

Acetaminophen and **NSAID** are used in upper respiratory conditions to reduce associated headaches, pain and fever. Usual analgesic/antipyretic doses are used. They do not alter viral shedding or antibody response.[38,39] **ASA** should not be used in children and adolescents with viral illnesses due to its association with Reye's syndrome.

For comparative ingredients of nonprescription products, consult the *Compendium of Products for Minor Ailments*—Analgesic Products: Internal Analgesics and Antipyretics; Cough, Cold and Allergy Products.

Viral Rhinitis

Symptomatic treatment remains the mainstay of managing the common cold, because there is no effective antiviral cure and few effective preventive measures. The literature on the common cold is extensive, but inconsistent in its rigour. These limitations restrict the ability to make confident and specific recommendations about treatments.

Agents used to treat symptoms of viral rhinitis include **decongestants** (topical and oral) alone or in combination with **antihistamines**. For treatment of an accompanying cough see Chapter 21: Acute Cough.

Decongestants

Decongestants are sympathomimetic agents that can relieve nasal congestion associated with the common cold, influenza and rhinosinusitis. They are available in oral and topical formulations.

Several systematic reviews including studies that evaluated systemic and topical decongestants, in single or repeat doses, have evaluated the efficacy of decongestants.[40,41,42] Single doses of nasal decongestants are moderately effective in relieving nasal congestion due to the common cold in adults. The multiple dosing studies are conflicting; some show benefit while others do not. Given these results, the use of topical or oral decongestants for a few days is reasonable and consistent with standard practice.[2]

There is no published evidence that decongestants are effective in children under 12 years of age.[40,43]

Decongestants used in the symptomatic management of upper respiratory tract infections are described in Table 5. Side effects differ between oral and topical formulations. Oral decongestants are generally not recommended in patients with hypertension. While most decongestants cause blood pressure elevations in normotensive persons only at doses that significantly exceed the recommended range, elevation of blood pressure may occur at standard doses in hypertensive patients.[44,45]

Rhinitis medicamentosa refers to rebound vasodilation that occurs after prolonged regular use (3–5 days) of topical decongestants and results in nasal congestion when the topical agent is discontinued. This condition is more likely to arise with shorter-acting agents (**phenylephrine**) than with longer-acting agents (**oxymetazoline**, **xylometazoline**). Many treatments for this problem have been proposed, including a slow reduction in use of the decongestant, a switch to inhaled corticosteroid or an abrupt discontinuation of the topical decongestant. Abrupt cessation is effective but is difficult because the patient will be congested for several days or weeks.[46]

Antihistamines

The efficacy of antihistamines in the management of the common cold is marginal at best because histamine is not involved in the pathology of this infection. Due to their anticholinergic properties, first-generation antihistamines may be minimally helpful in managing rhinorrhea associated with the common cold.[47,48] Antihistamines reduce overall symptoms compared with placebo for the first two days of a cold but have no additional benefit beyond the first two days.[49] There is concern that by making mucus thicker, antihistamines may make secretions more difficult to expel, leading to increased congestion of the nose and/or chest. This is also a concern if used to treat rhinosinusitis.[50] The adverse effect profile of the first-generation antihistamines must also be considered as they generally outweigh the benefit.[51]

First-generation antihistamines may reduce cough associated with the common cold (see Chapter 21: Acute Cough).[52,53] Second-generation antihistamines have no effect on symptoms of the common cold. Antihistamines are not recommended for treatment of cough in children younger than 6 years old.

Menthol

Menthol has long been used for the treatment of congestion and cough associated with the common cold. Menthol may increase the perception of nasal breathing; however, objective measurements of nasal flow do not indicate improvement.[54]

Influenza

Symptomatic treatment is the usual management approach for influenza. **Acetaminophen** or **NSAID** can help with the fever, aches and pain associated with influenza. **ASA** should not be used in children and adolescents due to its association with Reye's syndrome. Antivirals can be of benefit if started rapidly after the onset of symptoms and should be considered for patients at high risk of complications (Chapter 23: Assessment of Patients with Upper Respiratory Tract Symptoms, Table 1). See Chapter 7: Fever, for information and dosing of medications used for fever and pain.

Neuraminidase Inhibitors

Oseltamivir and **zanamivir** inhibit neuraminidase, an enzyme essential for the replication of influenza (see Table 6). The neuraminidase inhibitors have fewer side effects than amantadine and are effective against both influenza A and B. They prevent symptoms and shorten the duration of illness by about 1 day if taken within 48 hours of the onset of symptoms.[55,56,57,58,59,60] Evidence for or against their benefit in preventing complications of seasonal influenza in otherwise healthy adults is lacking.[61] Oseltamivir may reduce mortality in high-risk populations.[62] Resistance is rare among currently circulating strains but may eventually emerge, especially if antivirals are misused.[63]

Amantadine

Amantadine is not used for treatment or prevention of influenza due to almost complete resistance of circulating viruses.[24]

Rhinosinusitis

The majority of cases of acute rhinosinusitis will resolve on their own.[18] Symptomatic treatment such as **saline nasal irrigation**, **decongestants** (systemic and topical) and **analgesics** may be used to alleviate the symptoms. There have been few rigorous studies of the effect of nonprescription treatments on the symptoms of rhinosinusitis; available evidence suggests that the effect of these treatments is minimal.[19] In severe cases, **nasal corticosteroids** may be used.[64] If secondary bacterial infection occurs, **antibiotics** are required.

Pharyngitis

The pain associated with pharyngitis may be eased with systemic (e.g., **acetaminophen**, **ibuprofen**) or local analgesics (e.g., **benzocaine**, **diclonine hydrochloride**, **phenol**). Local analgesics (anesthetics) are available as lozenges, sprays and gargles and provide short-term relief (30–45 minutes). Methemoglobinemia is an uncommon but serious adverse effect that has been reported with the use of benzocaine applied to the oral mucosa.[65] Some lozenges contain antiseptics (e.g., **cetylpyridinium**, **dequalinium**); however, there is no evidence of benefit particularly since most cases of pharyngitis are viral. Nonmedicated lozenges may reduce the discomfort of a sore throat by their demulcent effect on the throat and their ability to increase salivation. Topical treatments should not be recommended if severe pain upon swallowing and dysphagia is present. Abrupt closure/spasm of the epiglottis leading to death has been reported with their use in the presence of epiglottitis.[66]

The objectives of **antibiotic** treatment for group A streptococcal infections are mainly to prevent suppurative complications and rheumatic fever, and to decrease contagiousness.

Nonprescription agents used in the management of upper respiratory tract infections are described in Table 5.

For comparative ingredients of nonprescription products, consult the *Compendium of Products for Minor Ailments*—Analgesic Products: Internal Analgesics and Antipyretics; Cough, Cold and Allergy Products.

Use of Combination Products

Selection of a combination product over a single-ingredient product is preferred for practical reasons from a patient's perspective. Antihistamine-decongestant and antihistamine-decongestant-analgesic combinations appear to have an impact on common cold symptoms.[67] However, combination products complicate dose tailoring of specific ingredients. Increasing the dose for a desired selected effect may lead to toxic effects of another ingredient. It is also less flexible when trying to adapt choice of specific ingredients to the continuously changing symptomatic picture over the course of an upper respiratory tract infection.

Natural Health Products

Echinacea

Echinacea is hypothesized to stimulate the immune system and is widely used to prevent and treat the common cold and other respiratory infections.[68] Three species of echinacea are available: *Echinacea angustifolia*, *Echinacea purpurea* and *Echinacea pallida*. *E. purpurea* is the most frequently studied, but *E. angustifolia* is most commonly used in North America. Numerous studies have evaluated the efficacy and safety of echinacea for this indication. Though it appears to be safe, evidence regarding its efficacy is inconclusive.[69,70] Several rigorously designed studies and meta-analyses have failed to demonstrate a beneficial effect in prevention or treatment of upper respiratory tract infections.

The dose that has been used is 1 g 3 times daily. Treatment begins at the first sign of symptoms and continues at least 10–14 days.[68] Echinacea is generally well tolerated. Adverse effects are uncommon but have included allergy, nausea and dizziness, tingling of the tongue and excessive salivation. Allergic cross-sensitivity can occur with members of the Asteraceae/Compositae family (e.g., ragweed); echinacea should be used with caution in atopic individuals.[71] It is contraindicated in immunosuppressed patients, including those with HIV and autoimmune diseases or those taking immunosuppressant medication. Safety in pregnancy or during breastfeeding has not been established.

Garlic

Garlic demonstrates some antiviral and antibacterial activity possibly related to allicin, a compound that is produced when garlic is chopped up. Allicin has been evaluated for prevention and treatment of the common cold in several trials.[72] However, given the poor quality of these trials, evidence is insufficient to provide any recommendations on use of garlic.

North American Ginseng

A popular natural remedy for the prevention and treatment of the common cold is North American ginseng (*Panax quinquefolius*). A systematic review found insufficient evidence that ginseng reduces the incidence or severity of the common cold.[73] However, ginseng reduced the duration of the common cold by about 6 days if used daily for up to 4 months. The main side effect was GI upset. There was great heterogeneity among a small number of trials in this systematic review. In addition, results may be applicable only to healthy adults. The authors found no trials that evaluated ginseng for the treatment of the common cold.

Vitamin C (Ascorbic Acid)

It is a popular belief that large doses of vitamin C can treat or prevent the common cold but there is no reliable evidence to support this belief. Treatment with vitamin C at doses of ≥200 mg/day does not have an impact on the duration or severity of the common cold in the general population.[74] In addition, daily use of vitamin C (1 g/day) does not reduce the incidence of the common cold in the general population but may be of benefit in preventing colds in persons engaged in extreme physical exercise and/or exposed to significant stress due to extreme cold temperatures.[74]

Prolonged intake of more than 1 g per day of vitamin C may cause oxaluria, uricosuria, renal stones or diarrhea. Abrupt discontinuation of prolonged intake of >1 g per day may lead to rebound scurvy.

Zinc

Zinc (gluconate or acetate) lozenges have been purported to decrease the duration and severity of the common cold. In vitro, zinc has the capacity to inhibit viral replication.[75] However, evidence for its efficacy in vivo is inconsistent and inconclusive.[75,76,77,78,79,80] Meta-analyses also provide conflicting results.[81,82] Explanations for the divergent results include widely varying dosages, inadequate blinding and bioavailability issues.

If zinc is used, the lozenge should contain at least 13.3 mg of elemental zinc, similar to lozenges studied, and should be free of agents that chelate zinc and inhibit its absorption, such as citric acid and tartaric acid.[75] Treatment should begin within 48 hours of symptom onset. The dose is 1 lozenge every 2 hours while awake for the duration of the cold. Common side effects are bad taste, mouth irritation, nausea and diarrhea. Side effects and the frequency of dosing often lead to discontinuation of therapy. Because of its potential to cause mouth irritation and gastric erosions, zinc should be avoided in cases of aphthous or peptic ulcers. Zinc may decrease absorption of tetracyclines or quinolones; avoid concomitant therapy. The use of intranasal zinc has been associated with long-term or permanent loss of smell and is not recommended.[80]

For comparative ingredients of nonprescription products, consult the *Compendium of Products for Minor Ailments*—Herbal and Natural Health Products: Single Entity; Vitamin and Mineral Products: Single Entity.

Considerations in Special Populations

Children

Acetaminophen or **ibuprofen** may be used for relief of aches and pains or fever >38.5°C. Avoid **ASA** due to its association with Reye's syndrome. See Chapter 7: Fever for more information on the management of fever.

Nonprescription cough and cold remedies should be avoided in children under 6 years of age.[43,83] In December 2008, Health Canada required manufacturers to relabel nonprescription cough and cold medicines with certain active ingredients to indicate that they should not be used in children under 6 years.[83] Active ingredients affected by Health Canada's decision on cough and cold products for children include **antihistamines**, **antitussives**, **expectorants** and **decongestants** that are given orally for treatment of the common cold (see Table 3). Medications given by a route of administration other than oral or for another indication (e.g., antihistamine for allergic rhinitis) are not included in the Health Canada advisory. Although cough and cold medicines have been used by children for many years, little evidence supports their effectiveness in this group.[40,49,84] In addition, reports of misuse, overdose and, on rare occasions, serious side effects have raised concerns about the use of these medicines in children younger than 6 years. The rare but serious potential side effects include convulsions, increased heart rate, decreased level of consciousness, abnormal heart rhythms and hallucinations.

Table 3: **Medications Not to Be Used for Cough and Cold in Children <6 Years[83]**

Therapeutic Categories	Active Ingredients
Antihistamines in cough and cold medicines	brompheniramine maleate chlorpheniramine maleate clemastine hydrogen fumarate dexbrompheniramine maleate diphenhydramine hydrochloride diphenylpyraline hydrochloride doxylamine succinate pheniramine maleate phenyltoloxamine citrate promethazine hydrochloride pyrilamine maleate triprolidine hydrochloride
Antitussives	dextromethorphan dextromethorphan hydrobromide diphenhydramine hydrochloride
Expectorants	guaifenesin
Decongestants	ephedrine hydrochloride/sulfate phenylephrine hydrochloride/sulfate pseudoephedrine hydrochloride/sulfate

Therapeutic strategies for use in children include:

- Prop the child upright to sleep in the daytime (e.g., in a car seat) to help prevent nasal congestion.
- Use **saline drops** and a nasal aspirator to suction mucus from the nasal passages. This is especially important if children have difficulty feeding.
- Use a humidifier to keep the oropharynx moist (avoid steam vaporizers, which can cause burns if the child tips it over). It is important to clean the humidifier regularly to prevent mould growth.
- Ensure the child drinks plenty of clear fluids (e.g., water, diluted nonsweetened fruit juice or clear soups) to prevent dehydration and keep the throat moist.

Parents can consult Health Canada or the Canadian Paediatric Society websites for more information.

Pregnancy and Breastfeeding

See Appendix V: Pregnancy and Breastfeeding: Self-care Therapy for Common Conditions.

Monitoring of Therapy

Table 4 contains information on monitoring therapy.

Table 4: **Monitoring of Therapy for the Common Cold, Influenza, Rhinosinusitis and Pharyngitis**

Symptoms	Monitoring	Endpoint of Therapy	Actions
Common cold symptoms (congestion, rhinorrhea, cough, sore throat)	Patient: Daily Healthcare practitioner: Next visit or by telephone 2–3 days later	Patient able to perform daily activities. Patient able to sleep.	Optimize nonpharmacologic measures. Change treatment if not effective.
Insomnia (oral decongestant)	Patient: Daily Healthcare practitioner: 1 wk	No insomnia.	Change medication schedule (daytime use only) or discontinue medication.
High blood pressure (oral decongestant in hypertensive patients only)	Patient or healthcare practitioner: Monitor blood pressure 2 times in the first week	No elevation in blood pressure above baseline.	Stop decongestant if blood pressure elevated above baseline. Recommend trial of topical decongestant.
Drowsiness (antihistamine)	Patient: Daily Healthcare practitioner: Next visit or by telephone when checking for efficacy	No drowsiness.	Change medication schedule (bedtime only) or discontinue treatment.
Drowsiness (antitussive)	Patient: Daily Healthcare practitioner: Next visit or by telephone when checking for efficacy	No drowsiness.	Change medication schedule (bedtime only) or treatment.

Advice for the Patient

Advise patients regarding:

- Nonpharmacologic therapy
- Proper use of medication
- Expected results and management of side effects
- Lack of efficacy of antibiotics against viral infections and potential to contribute to antimicrobial resistance with misuse/overuse
- When to contact a healthcare provider.

Table 5: Decongestant Medications for Upper Respiratory Tract Infections

Class	Drug	Dosage	Adverse Effects	Drug Interactions	Comments	Cost[a]
Decongestants, oral	*pseudoephedrine* Eltor 120, Sudafed Decongestant 12 hour, generics. Combination products: Advil Cold and Sinus Plus, Benylin, Robitussin, Sinutab Sinus and Allergy, Tylenol Children's, others	Adults and children ≥12 y: 60 mg Q4–6H po SR: 120 mg Q12H po Maximum: 240 mg per day Children 6–11 y: 30 mg Q4–6H po Maximum: 120 mg per day For combination products, consult label for additional ingredients. Follow directions on label.	Mild CNS stimulation (nervousness, excitability, restlessness, dizziness, weakness, insomnia). Peripheral vasoconstriction. Tachycardia or palpitation may occur. Blood pressure may be increased in hypertensive patients. May adversely affect blood sugar control in diabetics.	Beta-blockers: Antihypertensive effects may be reduced. MAOI and ergot derivatives may enhance the hypertensive effect of pseudoephedrine. Concurrent use and use within 14 days of discontinuation of MAOI is contraindicated.	Caution in patients with heart disease, high blood pressure, hyperthyroidism, diabetes, angle-closure glaucoma or prostatic enlargement. Onset of action 30 min.	$$
	phenylephrine Combination products: Dimetapp, generics	Consult individual product labels Dose based on phenylephrine content: Adults: 10 mg Q4H; maximum 60 mg/24h po Children 6–11 y: 5 mg Q4H; maximum 30 mg/24h po	Decongestant: See pseudoephedrine. Antihistamine: Drowsiness, fatigue, anticholinergic effects such as dry eyes, dry mouth and urinary retention. Paradoxical stimulatory effects may occur in children and the elderly.	Decongestant: MAOI: Avoid combination. Risk persists for 2 wk following discontinuation of nonselective MAOI (e.g., phenelzine). Risk of severely elevated blood pressure when combined with ergot derivatives (e.g., bromocriptine, cabergoline, ergotamine). Antagonizes effects of alpha$_1$-blockers (e.g., alfuzosin, doxazosin, prazosin, silodosin, tamsulosin, terazosin). Antihistamine: Additive effects with other anticholinergic drugs and CNS depressants.	Caution in patients with heart disease, high blood pressure, hyperthyroidism, diabetes, angle-closure glaucoma or prostatic enlargement. Onset of action 30 min.	$$

(cont'd)

Table 5: **Decongestant Medications for Upper Respiratory Tract Infections** *(cont'd)*

Class	Drug	Dosage	Adverse Effects	Drug Interactions	Comments	Cost[a]
Decongestants, topical	*oxymetazoline* Claritin Allergy Decongestant, Dristan Long Lasting Nasal Mist, Drixoral, generics	Adults and children ≥12 y: 0.05% solution: 2–3 drops or sprays/nostril Q12H Maximum duration: 3–5 days	Local burning and stinging, sneezing, dryness of the nasal mucosa. Rhinitis medicamentosa when used for more than 3–5 days. Bradycardia, tachycardia, hypertension and hypotension have been reported.	MAOI: Avoid combination. Risk persists for 2 wk following discontinuation of nonselective MAOI (e.g., phenelzine).	Onset of action: 5–10 min. Long duration of action lasting up to 12 h. Concurrent therapy with MAOI may cause hypertensive crisis.	$
	phenylephrine Dristan Nasal Mist, Soframycin Nasal Spray	Adults and children ≥12 y: 0.25% or 0.5% solution: 2–3 drops or sprays/nostril Q4H Maximum duration: 3–5 days	See oxymetazoline.	See oxymetazoline.	Onset of action: 5–10 min. Short duration of action lasting up to 4 h. Concurrent therapy with MAOI may cause hypertensive crisis.	$$
	xylometazoline Balminil Nasal Decongestant, Otrivin, generics	Adults and children ≥12 y: 0.05% or 0.1% solution: 2–3 drops or sprays/nostril Q8–10H Maximum duration: 3–5 days	See oxymetazoline.	See oxymetazoline.	See oxymetazoline.	$

[a] Cost of 1 unit (spray pump, drops) or 100 mL of liquid or 12 tablets; includes drug cost only.

Dosage adjustment may be required in renal impairment.

Legend: $ < $3 $$ $3–6

Table 6: **Neuraminidase inhibitors**

Class	Drug	Dosage	Adverse Effects	Drug Interactions	Comments	Cost[a]
Antivirals, neuraminidase inhibitors[85]	*oseltamivir* (renal symbol) Tamiflu	**Treatment**:[24,86,87] Adults: 75 mg BID po × 5 days Children: ≥1 y and ≤15 kg: 30 mg BID po × 5 days >15–23 kg: 45 mg BID po × 5 days >23–40 kg: 60 mg BID po × 5 days >40 kg: 75 mg BID po × 5 days **Prophylaxis**:[86,87] Adults and children ≥13 y: 75 mg once daily po Children: ≥1 y and ≤15 kg: 30 mg once daily po >15–23 kg: 45 mg once daily po >23–40 kg: 60 mg once daily po >40 kg: 75 mg once daily po Duration of prophylaxis is variable; used for the duration of the outbreak	Nausea, vomiting.	Avoid administration 48 h prior to and for 2 wk after influenza vaccine.	Take with food. Safety in pregnancy not established but currently recommended as first-line agent in pregnant women. For dose adjustments, consult the *Compendium of Therapeutic Choices*: Influenza.	$$
	zanamivir Relenza	Treatment for ≥7 y: 10 mg (2 inhalations) BID × 5 days Prophylaxis for ≥7 y: 10 mg (2 inhalations) daily × 10 days	Nausea, vomiting.	Avoid administration 48 h prior to and for 2 wk after influenza vaccine.	Safety in pregnancy not established.	$$

[a] Cost of a course of treatment; includes drug cost only.

(renal symbol) Dosage adjustment may be required in renal impairment.

Legend: $ < $25 $$ $25–50

Suggested Readings

Desrosiers M, Evans GA, Keith PK et al. Canadian clinical practice guidelines for acute and chronic rhinosinusitis. *Allergy Asthma Clin Immunol* 2011;7:2.

Fashner J, Ericson K, Werner S. Treamtent of the common cold in children and adults. *Am Fam Physician* 2012;86:153-9.

Heikkinen T, Jarvinen A. The common cold. *Lancet* 2003;361:51-9.

National Advisory Committee on Immunization (NACI). An Advisory Committee Statement (ACS). *Canadian Immunization Guide Chapter on Influenza and Statement on seasonal influenza vaccine for 2016-2017*. Ottawa (ON): PHAC; 2016. Available from: www.phac-aspc.gc.ca/naci-ccni/flu-2016-grippe-eng.php.

Smith MB, Feldman W. Over-the-counter cold medications. A critical review of clinical trials between 1950 and 1991. *JAMA* 1993;269:2258-63.

References

1. Heikkinen T, Jarvinen A. The common cold. *Lancet* 2003;361:51-9.
2. Allan GM, Arroll B. Prevention and treatment of the common cold: making sense of the evidence. *CMAJ* 2014;186:190-9.
3. Fashner J, Ericson K, Werner S. Treamtent of the common cold in children and adults. *Am Fam Physician* 2012;86:153-9.
4. Keast DH, Marshall JN, Stewart MA et al. Why do patients seek family physicians' services for cold symptoms? *Can Fam Physician* 1999;45:335-40.
5. Putto A, Ruuskanen O, Meurman O. Fever in respiratory virus infections. *Am J Dis Child* 1986;140:1159-63.
6. Heikkinen T. The role of respiratory viruses in otitis media. *Vaccine* 2000;19:S51-5.
7. Williams JM. 2009 update in prevention, evaluation, and outpatient treatment of influenza. *Curr Med Res Opin* 2009;25:817-28.
8. Cate TR. Clinical manifestations and consequences of influenza. *Am J Med* 1987;82:15-9.
9. Prevention and treatment of influenza A and B. *Therapeutics Letter* 2000;38:1-2. Available from: www.ti.ubc.ca/PDF/38.PDF. Accessed April 28, 2010.
10. Nahata MC, O'Mara NB, Benavides S. Viral infections. In: Alldredge BK, et al. eds. *Koda Kimble & Young's Applied therapeutics: the clinical use of drugs*. 10th ed. Philadelphia: Lippincott, Williams & Wilkins; 2012. p. 1772-90.
11. Brankston G, Gitterman L, Hirji Z et al. Transmission of influenza A in human beings. *Lancet Infect Dis* 2007;7:257-65.
12. Dolin R, Cohen YZ. Chapter 224: Influenza. In: Kasper DL et al., eds. *Harrison's principles of internal medicine*. 19th ed. New York: McGraw-Hill; 2012.
13. Leekha S, Zitterkopf NL, Espy MJ et al. Duration of influenza A virus shedding in hospitalized patients and implications for infection control. *Infect Control Hosp Epidemiol* 2007;28:1071-6.
14. Statistics Canada. *Leading causes of death, total population, by age group and sex, Canada*. 2011. Catalogue no. 82-625-X. Available from: www.statcan.gc.ca/pub/82-625-x/2014001/article/11896-eng.htm. Accessed April 2, 2015.
15. Desrosiers M, Evans GA, Keith PK et al. Canadian practice guidelines for acute and chronic rhinosinusitis. *Allergy Asthma Clin Immunol* 2011;7:2.
16. Evans KL. Recognition and management of sinusitis. *Drugs* 1998;56:59-71.
17. Rosenfeld RM, Piccirillo JF, Chandrasekhar SS et al. Clinical practice guideline (update):adult sinusitis. *Otolaryngol Head Neck Surg* 2015;152:S1-39.
18. Chow AW, Benninger MS, Brook I et al. IDSA clinical practice guideline for acute bacterial rhinosinusitis in children and adults. *Clin Infect Dis* 2012;54:e72-112.
19. Piccirillo JF. Clinical practice. Acute bacterial sinusitis. *N Engl J Med* 2004;351:902-10.
20. American Academy of Pediatrics. Principles of appropriate use for upper respiratory tract infections. In: Pickering LK, ed. *Red Book: report of the Committee on Infectious Diseases*. 28th ed. Elk Grove Village: American Academy of Pediatrics; 2009. p. 740-2.
21. Bisno AL. Acute pharyngitis. *N Engl J Med* 2001;344:205-11.
22. American Academy of Pediatrics. Group A streptococcal infections. In: Pickering LK, ed. *Red Book: report of the Committee on Infectious Diseases*. 28th ed. Elk Grove Village: American Academy of Pediatrics; 2009. p. 616-28.
23. Writing Committee of the WHO Consultation on Clinical Aspects of Pandemic (H1N1) 2009 Influenza et al. Clinical aspects of pandemic influenza A (H1N1) virus infection. *N Engl J Med* 2010;362:1708-19.
24. Aoki FY, Allen UD, Stiver HG et al. The use of antiviral drugs for influenza: a foundation document for practitioners. *Can J Infect Dis Med Microbiol* 2013;24:1C-15C. Available from: www.ammi.ca/guidelines. Accessed November 24, 2014.
25. Shulman ST, Bisno AL, Clegg HW. Clinical practice guideline for the diagnosis and management of group A streptococcal pharyngitis: 2012 update by the Infectious Diseases Society of America. *Clin Infect Dis* 2012;55:1279-82.
26. McIsaac WJ, Kellner JD, Aufricht P et al. Empirical validation of guidelines for the management of pharyngitis in children and adults. *JAMA* 2004;291:1587-95.
27. McIsaac WJ, White D, Tannenbaum D et al. A clinical score to reduce unnecessary antibiotic use in patients with sore throat. *CMAJ* 1998;158:75-83.
28. Jefferson T, Del Mar CB, Dooley L et al. Physical interventions to interrupt or reduce the spread of respiratory viruses. *Cochrane Database Syst Rev* 2011;(7):CD006207.
29. Aiello AE, Coulborn RM, Perez V et al. Effect of hand hygiene on infectious disease risk in the community setting: a meta-analysis. *Am J Public Health* 2008;98:1372-81.
30. Wong VW, Cowling BJ, Aiello AE. Hand hygiene and risk of influenza virus infections in the community: a systematic review and meta-analysis. *Epidemiol Infect* 2014;142:922-32.

31. Public Health Agency of Canada. *Flu prevention checklist*. Available from: publications.gc.ca/site/eng/341997/publication.html.
32. National Advisory Committee on Immunization (NACI). An Advisory Committee Statement (ACS). *Canadian Immunization Guide Chapter on Influenza and Statement on seasonal influenza vaccine for 2016-2017*. Ottawa (ON): PHAC; 2016. Available from: www.phac-aspc.gc.ca/naci-ccni/flu-2016-grippe-eng.php. Accessed May 20, 2016.
33. Osterholm MT, Kelley NS, Sommer A et al. Efficacy and effectiveness of influenza vaccines: a systematic review and meta-analysis. *Lancet Infect Dis* 2012;12:36-44.
34. Ahmed F, Singleton JA, Franks AL. Clinical practice. Influenza vaccination for healthy young adults. *N Engl J Med* 2001;345:1543-7.
35. Langley JM, Faughnan ME. Prevention of influenza in the general population: recommendation statement from the Canadian Task Force on Preventive Health Care. *CMAJ* 2004;171:1169-70.
36. American Academy of Pediatrics Committee on Infectious Diseases. Recommendations for prevention and control of influenza in children, 2011-2012. *Pediatrics* 2011;128:813-25.
37. Achilles N, Mösges R. Nasal saline irrigations for the symptoms of acute and chronic rhinosinusitis. *Curr Allergy Asthma Rep* 2013;13:229-35.
38. Sperber SJ, Hendley JO, Hayden FG et al. Effects of naproxen on experimental rhinovirus colds. A randomized, double-blind, controlled trial. *Ann Intern Med* 1992;117:37-41.
39. Kim SY, Chang YJ, Cho HM et al. Non-steroidal anti-inflammatory drugs for the common cold. *Cochrane Database Syst Rev* 2013;6:CD006362.
40. Taverner D, Latte J. Nasal decongestants for the common cold. *Cochrane Database Syst Rev* 2007;1:CD001953.
41. Del Mar C, Glasziou P. Upper respiratory tract infection. *Clin Evid* 2003;10:1747-56.
42. Kollar C, Schneider H, Waksman J, et al. Meta-analysis of the efficacy of a single dose of phenylephrine 10 mg compared with placebo in adults with acute nasal congestion due to the common cold. *Clin Ther* 2007;29:1057-70.
43. Peterson RG, Cran B, Knoppert D et al. Scientific Advisory Panel on Nonprescription Paediatric Cough and Cold Medications (SAP-NPCCM). *Record of proceedings*. Ottawa: Health Canada; March 20, 2008.
44. Chua SS, Benrimoj SI, Gordon RD et al. A controlled clinical trial on the cardiovascular effects of single doses of pseudoephedrine in hypertensive patients. *Br J Clin Pharmacol* 1989;28:369-72.
45. Johnson DA, Hricik JG. The pharmacology of alpha-adrenergic decongestants. *Pharmacotherapy* 1993;13:110S-5S.
46. Graf P. Rhinitis medicamentosa: aspects of pathophysiology and treatment. *Allergy* 1997;52:28-34.
47. Hendeles L. Efficacy and safety of antihistamines and expectorants in nonprescription cough and cold preparations. *Pharmacotherapy* 1993;13:154-8.
48. Howard JC, Kantner TR, Lilienfield LS et al. Effectiveness of antihistamines in the symptomatic management of the common cold. *JAMA* 1979;242:2414-7.
49. De Sutter AI, Saraswat A, van Driel ML. Antihistamines for the common cold. *Cochrane Database Syst Rev*. 2015;11:CD009345.
50. Stafford CT. The clinician's view of sinusitis. *Otolaryngol Head Neck Surg* 1990;103:870-4.
51. Sutter AI, Lemiengre M, Campbell H et al. Antihistamines for the common cold. *Cochrane Database Syst Rev* 2003;3:CD001267.
52. Pratter MR. Cough and the common cold: ACCP evidence-based clinical practice guidelines. *Chest* 2006;129:72S-74S.
53. Bolser DC. Older-generation antihistamines and cough due to upper airway cough syndrome (UACS): efficacy and mechanism. *Lung* 2008;186:S74-7.
54. Kenia P, Houghton T, Beardsmore C. Does inhaling menthol affect nasal patency or cough? *Pediatr Pulmonol* 2008;43:532-7.
55. Hayden FG, Osterhaus A, Treanor JJ et al. Efficacy and safety of the neuraminidase inhibitor zanamivir in the treatment of influenza virus infections. GG167 Influenza Study Group. *N Engl J Med* 1997;337:874-80.
56. Aoki FY, Macleod MD, Paggiaro P et al. Early administration of oral oseltamivir increases the benefits of influenza treatment. *J Antimicrob Chemother* 2003;51:123-9.
57. Randomised trial of efficacy and safety of inhaled zanamivir in treatment of influenza A and B virus infections. The MIST (Management of Influenza in the Southern Hemisphere Trialists) Study Group. *Lancet* 1998;352:1877-81.
58. Nicholson KG, Aoki FY, Osterhaus AD et al. Efficacy and safety of oseltamivir in treatment of acute influenza: a randomised controlled trial. Neuraminidase Inhibitor Flu Treatment Investigator Group. *Lancet* 2000;355:1845-50.
59. Heneghan CJ, Onakpoya I, Thompson M et al. Zanamivir for influenza in adults and children: systematic review of clinical study reports and summary of regulatory comments. *BMJ* 2014;348:g2547.
60. Dobson J, Whitley RJ, Pocock S et al. Oseltamivir treatment for influenza in adults: a meta-analysis of randomized controlled trials. *Lancet* 2015;385:1729-37.
61. Jefferson T, Jones MA, Doshi P et al. Neuraminidase inhibitors for preventing and treating influenza in healthy adults and children. *Cochrane Database Syst Rev* 2014;4:CD008965.
62. Hsu J, Santesso N, Mustafa R et al. Antivirals for treatment of influenza: a systematic review and meta-analysis of observational studies. *Ann Intern Med* 2012;156:512-24.
63. Moscona A. Oseltamivir resistance—disabling our influenza defenses. *N Engl J Med* 2005;353:2633-6.
64. Zalmanovici A, Trestioreanu A, Yaphe J. Intranasal steroids for acute sinusitis. *Cochrane Database Syst Rev* 2013;12:CD005149.
65. Health Canada. *Notice to hospitals—Health Canada issued important safety information on benzocaine sprays*. November 23, 2006. Available from: www.healthycanadians.gc.ca/recall-alert-rappel-avis/hc-sc/2006/14393a-eng.php.
66. Additional warning(s) for products indicated for relief of sore throat. *Fed Regist* 1991;56:48339-40.
67. De Sutter AIM, van Driel ML, Kumar AA et al. Oral antihistamine-decongestant-analgesic combinations for the common cold. *Cochrane Database Syst Rev* 2012;2:CD004976.
68. Giles JT, Palat CT, Chien SH et al. Evaluation of echinacea for treatment of the common cold. *Pharmacotherapy* 2000;20:690-7.
69. Grimm W, Muller HH. A randomized controlled trial of the effects of fluid extract of Echinacea purpurea on the incidence and severity of colds and respiratory infections. *Am J Med* 1999;106:138-43.
70. Karsch-Völk M, Barrett B, Kiefer D et al. Echinacea for preventing and treating the common cold. *Cochrane Database Syst Rev* 2014;2:CD000530.
71. Mullins RJ, Heddle R. Adverse reactions associated with echinacea: the Australian experience. *Ann Allergy Asthma Immunol* 2002;88:42-51.
72. Lissiman E, Bhasale AL, Cohen M. Garlic for the common cold. *Cochrane Database Syst Rev* 2014;11:CD006206.
73. Seida JK, Durec T, Kuhle S. North American (Panax quinquefolius) and Asian Ginseng (Panax ginseng) preparations for prevention of the common cold in healthy adults: a systematic review. *Evid Based Complement Alternat Med* 2011;2011:282151.

74. Hemila H, Chalker E. Vitamin C for preventing and treating the common cold. *Cochrane Database Syst Rev* 2013;1:CD000980.
75. Marshall S. Zinc gluconate and the common cold. Review of randomized controlled trials. *Can Fam Physician* 1998;44:1037-42.
76. Mossad SB, Macknin ML, Medendorp SV et al. Zinc gluconate lozenges for treating the common cold. A randomized, double-blind, placebo-controlled study. *Ann Intern Med* 1996;125:81-8.
77. Garland ML, Hagmeyer KO. The role of zinc lozenges in the treatment of the common cold. *Ann Pharmacother* 1998;32:63-9.
78. Macknin ML, Piedmonte M, Calendine C et al. Zinc gluconate lozenges for treating the common cold in children: a randomized controlled trial. *JAMA* 1998;279:1962-7.
79. Turner RB, Cetnarowski WE. Effect of treatment with zinc gluconate or zinc acetate on experimental and natural colds. *Clin Infect Dis* 2000;31:1202-8.
80. Caruso TJ, Prober CG, Gwaltney JM. Treatment of naturally acquired common colds with zinc: a structured review. *Clin Infect Dis* 2007;45:569-74.
81. Jackson JL, Peterson C, Lesho E. A meta-analysis of zinc salts lozenges and the common cold. *Arch Intern Med* 1997;157:2373-6.
82. Science M, Johnstone J, Roth DE et al. Zinc for the treatment of the common cold: a systematic review and meta-analysis of randomized controlled trials. *CMAJ* 2012;184:E551-61.
83. Health Canada. *Health Canada releases decision on the labelling of cough and cold products for children*. Available from: www.healthycanadians.gc.ca/recall-alert-rappel-avis/hc-sc/2008/13267a-eng.php. Accessed December 4, 2014.
84. Smith MB, Feldman W. Over-the-counter cold medications. A critical review of clinical trials between 1950 and 1991. *JAMA* 1993;269:2258-63.
85. Stiver HG, Evans GA, Aoki FY et al. Guidance on the use of antiviral drugs for influenza in acute care facilities in Canada, 2014-2015. *Can J Infect Dis Med Microbiol* 2015;26:e5-8.
86. Oo C, Barrett J, Hill G et al. Pharmacokinetics and dosage recommendations for an oseltamivir oral suspension for the treatment of influenza in children. *Paediatr Drugs* 2001;3:229-36.
87. Oo C, Hill G, Dorr A et al. Pharmacokinetics of anti-influenza prodrug oseltamivir in children aged 1-5 years. *Eur J Clin Pharmacol* 2003;59:411-5.

Common Cold and Influenza—What You Need to Know

The common cold and influenza (the flu) are viral infections. They usually go away in 7–10 days. Antibiotics for bacterial infections will not help you get better from a cold or flu.

Hints to help you feel better if you have a cold or the flu:

- Drink lots of fluids and get plenty of rest.
- You can try a cool-mist humidifier. Be sure to clean it regularly to prevent bacteria or mould growth.
- Soothe your irritated nose with a saline nose spray. Use saline drops in young children.

Medications for colds and the flu

Many medications for cold and flu symptoms are available without a prescription. Ask your pharmacist if medication can help you or not.

- Check with your doctor or pharmacist before giving cough or cold products to children. Cough, cold or flu products should not be used in children less than 6 years old.
- Use acetaminophen or ibuprofen if you have a fever, aches or pains. **Do not** give ASA (such as Aspirin) to a child or teenager who has a cold or the flu.
- **Do not** give medicine labelled for older children or adults to young children.
- **Do not** use more than 1 cough and cold product at a time. Many products contain the same ingredients.
- Measure the right dose with a measuring device. **Do not** use a regular spoon.

See a healthcare provider if any of these things happen:

- You have trouble breathing
- You make strange sounds when you breathe
- Your throat is very sore
- You have a lung disease such as asthma, emphysema or chronic bronchitis
- You have a fever for more than 24 hours
- Your cold or flu lasts for more than 7–10 days

Take a child to a healthcare provider if any of these things happen:

- They seem to have an earache
- They have a high fever (temperature above 39°C or 102°F)
- They seem very sleepy most of the time
- They seem very cranky or fussy most of the time
- They have rapid breathing or trouble breathing
- They have a cough that lasts more than 10 days
- They have a skin rash
- They seem to be dehydrated (dry mouth, no urine output over 6 hours, crying without tears)

How can you prevent colds and flu?

There is no sure way to prevent colds and flu. A yearly flu shot will help to cut your chance of getting the flu. You can also help protect yourself by washing your hands often. Clean hands help to prevent colds and flu from spreading.

Always wash your hands:

- Before cooking or eating
- Before feeding a baby or child
- Before giving someone medication
- After wiping your nose

Follow these steps for proper hand-washing:

1. Wet your hands under running water.
2. Using soap, scrub your hands for 20 seconds (the time it takes to sing *Twinkle Twinkle Little Star*).
3. Rinse your hands under running water for 10 seconds.
4. Dry your hands with a clean towel.

Chapter 25

Diabetes Care

Lori MacCallum, BScPhm, PharmD, CDE

CPhA acknowledges the contribution of Maryann Hopkins as a previous author of this chapter.

It is estimated that more than 2 million Canadians have known diabetes plus an estimated 400 000 are unaware they have diabetes, and these numbers are continuing to rise. By 2018–2019, the number diagnosed with diabetes is expected to reach 3.7 million.[1] Diabetes is the leading cause of adult-onset blindness, kidney disease, and nontraumatic lower limb amputations. In addition, people with diabetes have a much higher risk of cardiovascular disease, the leading cause of death in this population.[2] People with diabetes have higher mortality rates and decreased quality of life, primarily due to the complications of the disease. There are tremendous fiscal implications. It is estimated that diabetes costs the Canadian healthcare system $12.2 billion annually, mainly due to the costs of diabetic complications.[3]

Pathophysiology

Type 1 diabetes is primarily the result of the destruction of pancreatic β-cells. It includes those cases due to an autoimmune process and those for which the etiology of β-cell destruction is unknown. It is thought to be multifactorial (a genetic predisposition combined with environmental factors), but the exact cause remains unknown. Type 1 diabetes can be diagnosed at any age but most commonly presents between 5 and 7 years of age or around puberty, and insulin replacement is needed for survival. Type 1 diabetes that develops in adults may be difficult to distinguish from type 2 diabetes.[4]

β-cell failure and insulin resistance in muscle and liver are the primary defects in type 2 diabetes. Insulin resistance in the liver leads to an overproduction of glucose in the fasting state and impaired suppression following a meal. Insulin resistance in the muscle leads to impaired uptake of glucose following a meal, leading to postprandial hyperglycemia. There are also abnormalities of the fat cell (increased lipolysis leading to increased free fatty acids which impairs insulin secretion), gastrointestinal tract (deficiency or resistance to the incretin gut hormones), α-cells of the pancreas (increased secretion of glucagon which increases production of glucose by the liver), kidney (increased glucose reabsorption) and brain (insulin resistance). All of these lead to the development of glucose intolerance, and have been described by DeFronzo as the Ominous Octet.[5] Heredity plays a major role in the development of insulin resistance. This genetic predisposition to insulin resistance, combined with obesity and decreased physical activity, both insulin resistant states, puts major stress on the β-cells to maintain normal glucose. Initially, β-cells compensate for insulin resistance with increased insulin production. Eventually the β-cells fail, first leading to a rise in postprandial glucose and then fasting plasma glucose, and eventually type 2 diabetes.[5]

Individuals with prediabetes have higher than normal blood glucose values but not high enough to meet the diagnosis of diabetes. Prediabetes includes impaired fasting glucose, impaired glucose tolerance or an HbA_{1c} of 6–6.4%. Individuals with prediabetes are at risk of developing type 2 diabetes although not all will progress. Once patients have impaired glucose tolerance, they already have insulin resistance and may have lost up to 80% of their β-cell function.[5] These patients should be carefully monitored and screened for the development of diabetes as well as an assessment of cardiovascular risk factors as they are at higher risk of cardiovascular disease, particularly those with impaired glucose tolerance.

Diabetes in pregnancy includes pregestational diabetes (type 1 and type 2) or gestational diabetes. Pregestational diabetes is diabetes that was present before pregnancy. Gestational diabetes refers to diabetes diagnosed during pregnancy. Those with gestational diabetes are at high risk of developing type 2 diabetes in subsequent years and should be screened between 6 weeks and 6 months postpartum to detect prediabetes and diabetes.[6]

For more information on gestational diabetes, consult the *Compendium of Therapeutic Choices*: Diabetes Mellitus.

Diabetes may also be caused by other endocrine diseases (e.g., Cushing's disease, acromegaly), other genetic defects, infections or toxins, or may be associated with drug therapy (Table 1). Patients with known risk factors for diabetes (see Table 2) should be screened.

Table 1: **Examples of Drugs Known to Raise Blood Glucose**[7,8,9,10]

Alpha-interferon	HMG CoA-reductase inhibitors
Antipsychotics, second-generation	Nicotinic acid
Beta-adrenergic agonists	Pentamidine
Beta-blockers	Phenytoin
Calcineurin inhibitors	Protease inhibitors
Diazoxide	Thiazide diuretics
Gatifloxacin	Thyroid hormone
Glucocorticoids	

Table 2: **Known Risk Factors for Type 2 Diabetes**[11]

- Member of a high-risk population e.g., Aboriginal, African, Asian, South Asian or Hispanic descent
- Acanthosis nigricans
- Age ≥40 y
- First-degree relative with type 2 diabetes
- Giving birth to a macrosomic infant
- History of prediabetes (impaired fasting glucose, impaired glucose tolerance or HbA_{1c} 6–6.4%)
- History of gestational diabetes
- Presence of vascular risk factors: abdominal obesity, HDL cholesterol <1 mmol/L in males or <1.3 in females, hypertension, triglycerides ≥1.7 mmol/L, overweight
- Presence of associated diseases: bipolar disorder, depression, HIV infection, obstructive sleep apnea, polycystic ovary syndrome, schizophrenia
- Presence of end-organ damage associated with diabetes:
  - microvascular: nephropathy, retinopathy, neuropathy
  - macrovascular: coronary, cerebrovascular or peripheral artery disease
- Use of drugs associated with increased risk of diabetes e.g., glucocorticoids, protease inhibitors, second-generation antipsychotics

Goals of Therapy

- Adopt a healthy lifestyle
- Prevent microvascular and macrovascular complications
- Establish a regular follow-up schedule based on established recommendations
- Avoid blood glucose values outside of established targets
- Recognize, prevent and treat hypoglycemia

Patient Assessment

Though many people with type 2 diabetes are asymptomatic, signs and symptoms may be present (Table 3). The diagnosis of diabetes is dependent upon laboratory testing following specific diagnostic criteria.

Table 3: **Possible Signs and Symptoms of Diabetes**

▪ Blurred vision	▪ Frequent urination
▪ Cuts and bruises that are slow to heal	▪ Tingling or numbness in hands or feet
▪ Extreme fatigue	▪ Unusual thirst
▪ Frequent or recurring infections	▪ Weight change (gain or loss)

Diagnostic Criteria for Diabetes

The diagnosis of diabetes requires blood glucose or HbA_{1c} results obtained in the laboratory. Capillary blood glucose readings suggesting the presence of diabetes should be confirmed with plasma glucose (PG) levels:[12]

- Fasting plasma glucose (FPG; no caloric intake for at least 8 hours) ≥7 mmol/L, *or*
- An HbA_{1c} ≥6.5% using a standardized, validated assay in the absence of factors that affect the accuracy of the test (not for suspected type 1 diabetes, children, adolescents or pregnancy), *or*
- A plasma glucose level 2 hours after a 75 g glucose load ≥11.1 mmol/L, *or*
- Random plasma glucose ≥11.1 mmol/L

HbA_{1c} may be misleading in people with hemoglobinopathy, iron deficiency, hemolytic anemia or severe renal or hepatic disease.[13] In addition, African Americans, Aboriginals, Hispanics and Asians have HbA_{1c} values that are 0.4% higher than those of Caucasians at similar levels of glycemia.[14,15] HbA_{1c} is also affected by age, rising by up to 0.1% per decade of life. More studies are required in these populations to determine whether age or ethnic-specific thresholds are required.[16,17]

In the absence of symptomatic hyperglycemia, if a single laboratory test result is in the diabetes range, a confirmatory laboratory test (e.g., FPG, HbA_{1c}) must be done on another day. It is preferable that the same test be repeated for confirmation, but a random PG in the diabetes range in an asymptomatic individual should be confirmed with an alternative test. In the case of symptomatic hyperglycemia, the diagnosis has been made and a confirmatory test is not required before treatment is initiated. In individuals in whom type 1 diabetes is likely (younger or lean or symptomatic hyperglycemia, especially with ketonuria or ketonemia), confirmatory testing should not delay initiation of insulin, to avoid rapid deterioration. If results of 2 different tests are available and both are above the diagnostic cutpoints, the diagnosis of diabetes is confirmed. When the results of more than 1 test are available and the results are discordant, the test whose result is above the diagnostic cutpoint should be repeated and the diagnosis made on the basis of the repeat test.[12]

Optimal glycemic control is critical to both the management of diabetes and prevention of complications. Both the Diabetes Control and Complications Trial (DCCT), a prospective randomized control trial in type 1 diabetes, and the United Kingdom Prospective Diabetes Study (UKPDS), which was conducted in patients with newly diagnosed type 2 diabetes, demonstrated a reduction in microvascular complications with tighter glycemic control.[18,19] In the UKPDS there was a 25% relative risk reduction in microvascular complications.[19] The DCCT showed a relative risk reduction of 76% in incident retinopathy, a 54% reduction in progression of retinopathy, a 54% reduction in nephropathy and a 60% reduction in clinical neuropathy.[20,21] Ten-year observational follow up of the UKPDS participants demonstrated that despite a loss of glycemic control, the reduction in microvascular complications persisted, MI was reduced by 15% and death from any cause by 13% in the intensively treated group.[22] Follow-up of the DCCT showed that intensive treatment reduced the risk of any cardiovascular event by 42% and the risk of nonfatal MI, stroke, or death from cardiovascular disease by 57%.[23]

Glycemic targets should be individualized based on age, duration of diabetes, risk of severe hypoglycemia, presence of cardiovascular disease and life expectancy (Table 4).[24] Both the fasting and postprandial blood glucose contribute to the HbA_{1c} value and correlate with the risk of complications. For most individuals with diabetes, the target should be an $HbA_{1c} \leq 7\%$ to reduce the risk of microvascular complications and if implemented early in the course of the disease, may also reduce the risk of macrovascular complications. To achieve target HbA_{1c} levels, individuals should aim for a preprandial or fasting plasma glucose of 4–7 mmol/L and a 2-hour postprandial glucose of 5–10 mmol/L. If an $HbA_{1c} \leq 7\%$ cannot be achieved with a postprandial glucose target of 5–10 mmol/L, lower the target to 5–8 mmol/L.[24]

Table 4: **Targets for Adults with Type 1 or Type 2 Diabetes**[24]

Target Value	Patient Group
$HbA_{1c} \leq 6.5\%$	Some patients with type 2 diabetes, to further lower risk of nephropathy and retinopathy balanced against the increased risk of hypoglycemia
$HbA_{1c} \leq 7\%$	Most patients with type 1 or type 2 diabetes
HbA_{1c} 7.1–8.5%	Patients with: limited life expectancy, high-level functional dependency, extensive coronary artery disease at high risk of ischemic events, multiple comorbidities, recurrent severe hypoglycemia, hypoglycemia unawareness, long-standing diabetes where lower HbA_{1c} cannot be achieved despite effective doses of multiple medications

Age alone is not an indicator for more or less stringent targets. In the frail elderly, prevention of hypoglycemia is the priority as the risk of hypoglycemia increases markedly with age. While avoiding symptomatic hyperglycemia, glycemic targets are an $HbA_{1c} \leq 8.5\%$ and fasting or preprandial glucose of 5–12 mmol/L.[25]

Nonpharmacologic Therapy

Intensive lifestyle interventions in people with type 2 diabetes can produce improvements in weight management, fitness, glycemic control and cardiovascular risk factors. The Look AHEAD trial was a large (n=5145) randomized control trial that examined whether intensive lifestyle intervention for weight loss would decrease cardiovascular morbidity and mortality in overweight or obese individuals with type 2 diabetes. Although the intervention arm did achieve greater weight loss, greater reduction in HbA_{1c} and greater initial improvements in fitness and cardiovascular risk factors (with the exception of LDL), there was no difference between the lifestyle intervention and the control arm in the primary composite endpoint of cardiovascular morbidity and mortality after a median follow up of 9.6 years.[26] However, because of the many other benefits of adopting a healthy lifestyle including weight loss, lifestyle intervention remains the mainstay of diabetes care.

The recommendation for people with diabetes is a minimum of 150 minutes per week of moderate- to vigorous-intensity exercise. This should be spread over at least 3 days of the week with no more than 2 consecutive days without exercise. This should be combined with at least 2 sessions per week (3 sessions preferable) of resistance exercise (i.e., exercise bands or weights).[27] Patients are encouraged to follow Canada's Food Guide to Healthy Eating. A nutritionally balanced, calorie-reduced diet is further recommended in overweight or obese patients to achieve a 5–10% weight loss.[28] Finally, it is important to determine the smoking status of all patients and to encourage patients who currently smoke to begin the process of quitting by providing resources, support and medication if indicated.

Pharmacologic Therapy

Antihyperglycemic medications target different pathophysiologic abnormalities associated with type 2 diabetes, including insulin resistance, decreased insulin secretion, excessive glucose output by the liver and increased glucose reabsorption by the kidneys. To achieve recommended glycemic targets, combinations of different agents may be used.

The **sulfonylureas** and **meglitinides** are insulin secretagogues, and stimulate endogenous insulin release from the β-cells of the pancreas. **Metformin** acts primarily by improving insulin action in the liver (reduces glucose production) and enhances insulin activity in muscle and fat cells. The thiazolidinediones (**pioglitazone**, **rosiglitazone**) decrease insulin resistance in peripheral tissues and the liver. **Acarbose** is an alpha-glucosidase inhibitor that slows the breakdown of certain sugars and starches in the gut, thus slowing glucose absorption. Dipeptidyl peptidase-4 inhibitors (**alogliptin**, **linagliptin**, **saxagliptin**, **sitagliptin**) prevent the breakdown of the gut hormones, GLP-1 and GIP, thereby increasing the release of insulin from β-cells and suppressing the release of glucagon from α-cells. Glucagon-like peptide agonists (**dulaglutide**, **exenatide**, **liraglutide**) also increase insulin release and suppress glucagon. Sodium glucose co-transporter 2 (SGLT2) inhibitors (**canaglifozin**, **dapaglifozin**, **empagliflozin**) act on the kidney and lower glucose by increasing urinary glucose excretion.

For more information on pharmacologic therapy for diabetes, consult the *Compendium of Therapeutic Choices*: Diabetes Mellitus.

Insulin

For comparative ingredients of nonprescription products, consult the *Compendium of Products for Minor Ailments*—Diabetes Products: Insulin Products.

To achieve normal blood glucose levels, those with type 1 diabetes require exogenous insulin. Those with type 2 diabetes may also require insulin therapy in certain circumstances: at diagnosis in those with symptomatic hyperglycemia and metabolic decompensation, if blood glucose targets are not being reached with lifestyle changes or other antihyperglycemics, temporarily during illness, pregnancy or stress, or for a medical procedure or surgery.

The insulin dose, type of insulin required and the time of day the insulin needs to be administered depend on individual circumstances. Table 5 describes some common insulin regimens used in the management of diabetes.

Various insulin products are available in Canada; their characteristics are listed in Table 6.

Insulin Storage

Unopened insulin vials and cartridges should be stored in the refrigerator (2–8°C). Once in use, insulin may be stored at room temperature. Insulin stored at room temperature causes less irritation and burning when administered. Insulin should not be frozen or exposed to extreme heat (>30°C) for prolonged periods as this will affect its action. Caps should be kept on insulin pens to protect insulin from light, and insulin should not be stored in direct sunlight. Once insulin is opened, it may be used for up to 28 days when stored at room temperature, with the exception of insulin detemir, which may be used for up to 42 days.[31]

Insulin Absorption[31]

Insulin is absorbed most rapidly and consistently from the abdomen. Moderate absorption rates occur at the upper arm and the lateral side of the thigh. The slowest rate of absorption occurs from the buttock. Massaging the injection site immediately before or after the injection increases the absorption rate. Increased temperature of the injection site (e.g., from a hot bath, sauna, or exercise) may increase the absorption rate.

Lipohypertrophy can develop from repeated use of the same injection site. Lesions vary in size and may be detected visually or by palpation. Injecting into a lipohypertrophic site can result in a decrease and variable rate of insulin absorption. Instruct patients not to inject into a lipohypertrophic area. Injection sites should be inspected by a healthcare practitioner routinely to monitor for the development of lipohypertrophy. To prevent lipohypertrophy and to ensure consistent absorption of insulin, injection sites should be rotated within an anatomical area and a new needle should be used for each injection. When changing from a lipohypertropic injection site to a healthy site, patients may need to reduce their insulin dose. Blood glucose should be monitored more frequently.

Table 5: **Common Insulin Regimens**[29,30]

Regimen	Advantages	Disadvantages
Basal insulin once daily One injection daily (usually at bedtime). Analogues may be given at bedtime or in the morning. Can continue oral agents	▪ Convenient ▪ Causes less weight gain and hypoglycemia ▪ Easy method for starting patients on insulin	▪ Lack of mealtime control
Premixed insulin twice daily One injection of premixed insulin before breakfast and one injection before supper. Continue metformin. Insulin secretagogues are often stopped to avoid hypoglycemia	▪ Convenient—only 2 injections per day	▪ Less flexibility in dosing as insulin is premixed (must adhere to schedule) ▪ Lack of flexibility in activity levels, meal sizes and times ▪ Requires a bedtime snack to avoid nocturnal hypoglycemia ▪ Requires a consistent and predictable lifestyle with regard to meals and activity
Basal plus bolus Bolus insulin with each meal and basal insulin at bedtime. Continue metformin. Insulin secretagogues are stopped to avoid hypoglycemia	▪ Flexibility for mealtimes ▪ Useful for those with shift work or unpredictable lifestyle	▪ Requires frequent blood glucose monitoring ▪ More complex ▪ Inconvenience of multiple injections
Insulin pumps	▪ Better glycemic control ▪ Less severe hypoglycemia ▪ Greater flexibility	▪ Extensive training ▪ Rapid blood glucose deterioration if insulin delivery fails (remind patients to have insulin for manual injection as backup)

Best Practice Recommendations for Insulin Administration[31]

- Provide proper education and ensure regular assessment of injection sites and techniques.
- Rotation of injection sites within all zones of an anatomical area is essential to avoid lipohypertrophy.
- Healthcare practitioners should know how to inspect and palpate injection sites and prevent lipohypertrophy.
- Shorter pen needles (4 mm, 5 mm and 6 mm) are suitable for all people with diabetes, regardless of BMI; 6 mm needles are recommended for syringe use.
- The abdomen is the preferred injection area for consistency of absorption.
- Splitting of large insulin doses to reduce the volume of injection should be based on individual need.

- Glycemic variability and poor glycemic control may be related to injection techniques.
- For cloudy insulin (e.g., NPH), the vial or cartridge should be rolled gently 10 times and then tipped (not shaken) 10 times. The vial or cartridge should be inspected visually to ensure the suspension has a consistent milky white appearance.
- The lateral sides of the abdomen are the preferred injection sites for pregnant women.

Table 6: **Characteristics of Insulin and Analogues**[29,30]

Class	Type	Onset (h)[a]	Peak (h)[a]	Duration (h)[a]
Rapid-acting insulin analogues	aspart	10–15 min	1–1.5	3–5
	glulisine	10–15 min	1–1.5	3–5
	lispro	10–15 min	1–2	3.5–4.75
Short-acting insulin	human insulin regular, Toronto	0.5	2–3	6.5
	pork insulin	0.5	2–4	5–7
Intermediate-acting insulin	human NPH	1–3	5–8	up to 18
	pork NPH	1–3	6–12	24–28
Long-acting insulin analogues	glargine	1.5	No peak	up to 24
	glargine U300	6	No peak	30
	detemir	1.5	No peak	16–24

[a] Onset, peak and duration may vary depending on product and patient characteristics.

Natural Health Products

A Canadian study found that 78% of people with diabetes reported taking a natural health product.[32] It is important for healthcare practitioners to ask patients about their use of natural health products, assess for drug interactions and adverse events, and provide information on risks and benefits. Although some natural health products have been shown to lower HbA_{1c} in people with type 2 diabetes, the 2013 CDA Clinical Practice Guidelines do not recommend their use at this time and further research is needed.[33]

Microvascular Complications (Retinopathy, Nephropathy, Neuropathy)

Retinopathy

Diabetic retinopathy is the most common cause of new-onset blindness in the working age population. Data showed a prevalence rate of 23% in people with type 1 diabetes, 14% in people with type 2 diabetes on insulin therapy, and 3% in people receiving oral antihyperglycemic therapies.[34] Risk factors for the development or progression of diabetic retinopathy are longer duration of diabetes, elevated HbA_{1c}, increased blood pressure, dyslipidemia, low hemoglobin, pregnancy (in type 1 diabetes), proteinuria and severe retinopathy itself.[35,36] Because laser therapy can reduce the risk of blindness, it is imperative that patients with diabetes be screened regularly for diabetic retinopathy to allow early diagnosis and treatment. Landmark trials demonstrated that glycemic control ($HbA_{1c} \leq 7\%$) reduced the development and progression of retinopathy in patients with type 1 (DCCT[18]) and type 2 diabetes (UKPDS[19]). Blood pressure control is also an important risk factor and the UKPDS trial demonstrated that tighter blood pressure control reduced the progression of retinopathy.[37] The target blood pressure for people with diabetes is less than 130/80 mm Hg.[38,39]

Recommendations[34]

- Screen/evaluate for retinopathy annually beginning 5 years after the onset of diabetes in all patients with type 1 diabetes (at or after age 15).
- Screen for retinopathy in all patients at the time of diagnosis of type 2 diabetes. Follow up every 1–2 years unless severity dictates more frequent evaluation that is tailored to the severity of the retinopathy.
- Evaluate women with diabetes prior to pregnancy (when possible), in the first trimester, throughout the pregnancy as needed and within the first year postpartum.
- To prevent the onset and delay the progression of diabetic retinopathy, people with diabetes should be treated to achieve optimal control of blood glucose and blood pressure. Fenofibrate, in addition to statin therapy, may be used in patients with type 2 diabetes to slow the progression of retinopathy.[40]
- Changes in vision should be reported to a physician or optometrist.
- Note: Individuals who start intensive diabetes management or pump therapy should have their eyes checked pre- and post-intervention as there is a risk of worsening retinopathy (short-term) due to intensification of diabetes therapy.

Nephropathy

Diabetes is the leading cause of kidney disease in Canada and kidney disease can decrease both life expectancy and quality of life.[41,42] People with diabetes can develop various forms of kidney disease including diabetic nephropathy, ischemic damage and other renal diseases; up to half of patients with diabetes will demonstrate signs of kidney damage over their lifetime.[43,44,45] Diabetic nephropathy involves the development or worsening of proteinuria. Patients with diabetes should be screened for chronic kidney disease (CKD) by screening for albuminuria with a random urinary albumin-to-creatinine ratio (ACR) and by assessing renal function with eGFR. Because all patients with CKD are considered at high risk for cardiovascular disease, cardiovascular risk factors should also be assessed and optimized.

Optimal glycemic and blood pressure control have been shown to reduce the risk of development and progression of diabetic nephropathy.[19,46] The use of renin-angiotensin-aldosterone system (RAAS) blockers (ACE inhibitors and ARBs) has been shown to reduce the risk of development[47,48] and progression[49,50] of diabetic nephropathy, independent of blood pressure lowering in those with diabetes and hypertension.

Recommendations[51]

- Screen with a random ACR and a serum creatinine converted to an eGFR in postpubertal individuals with type 1 diabetes annually, beginning 5 years after diagnosis. Those with type 2 diabetes should be similarly screened at diagnosis and then annually. Recent fever, major exercise, urinary tract infection, menstruation, decompensated heart failure or acute severe elevation of blood pressure or blood glucose can elevate the ACR. Screening for albuminuria should be delayed until these conditions are resolved.
- Maintain optimal blood glucose to prevent or delay the progression of diabetic nephropathy.
- Maintain optimal blood pressure control to prevent or delay the progression of diabetic nephropathy.
- The use of an ACE inhibitor or ARB can delay the progression of diabetic nephropathy.
- Advise women of child-bearing potential about the importance of avoiding pregnancy if taking an ACE inhibitor or an ARB because of the risk of congenital malformations.

- Reduce or eliminate all modifiable risk factors for heart disease, e.g., smoking, excessive alcohol intake, obesity, high cholesterol and blood pressure, physical inactivity.
- All patients with diabetes, but especially those with CKD, should be aware of the "sick day" medication list (see Table 7). They should be instructed to hold these medications if they become ill and are unable to maintain adequate fluid intake due to vomiting and/or diarrhea, because their kidney function may worsen. Patients should be instructed to monitor blood glucose more frequently and adjust their doses of insulin or other antihyperglycemic agents as necessary.
- Regularly assess medications in patients with CKD to determine whether their renal function warrants dosage adjustment or discontinuation of renally eliminated medications.

Table 7: **Sick-day Medication List**[52]

Letter	Drug/Class	Reason for Caution with Inadequate Fluid Intake
S	**S**ulfonylureas	Renal clearance may be reduced, leading to increased risk of adverse effects
A	**A**CE inhibitors	May impair renal function
D	**D**iuretics, direct renin inhibitors	May impair renal function
M	**M**etformin	Renal clearance may be reduced leading to increased risk of adverse effects
A	**A**ngiotensin receptor blockers	May impair renal function
N	**N**onsteroidal anti-inflammatory drugs	May impair renal function
S	**S**GLT2 inhibitors	May impair renal function

Neuropathy

Detectable sensorimotor polyneuropathy will develop within 10 years of the onset of diabetes in 40–50% of individuals.[53] Diabetic neuropathy can lead to foot ulceration and eventual amputation, and continues to be the leading cause of lower extremity amputation. Optimal glycemic control has been shown to prevent or reduce the progression of diabetic neuropathy and is the only disease-modifying treatment available. Patients often experience neuropathic pain and anticonvulsants and antidepressants are recommended for symptomatic relief. However, they do not affect the progression of the complication. Opioids are also used for symptomatic relief but are considered a less favorable option because of risks such as dependence, tolerance and diversion.[54]

Recommendations[54]

- Screen for peripheral neuropathy by assessing loss of sensitivity to the 10-g monofilament or to vibration at the dorsum of the great toe, when type 2 diabetes is diagnosed and annually thereafter. In those with type 1 diabetes, screening should begin 5 years after diagnosis in postpubertal individuals and annually thereafter.
- Optimal glycemic control is recommended for reducing onset and progression of neuropathy.
- Antidepressants (amitriptyline, duloxetine and venlafaxine) and anticonvulsants (gabapentin, pregabalin and valproate) may be used alone or in combination for symptomatic relief of peripheral neuropathic pain.
- Counsel all patients on the importance of foot care, to reduce the risk of ulceration and amputation resulting from reduced foot sensitivity.

Cardiovascular Health and Hypertension in Patients with Diabetes

People with diabetes are at increased risk of cardiovascular disease, presenting as coronary heart disease, stroke and peripheral vascular disease. People with diabetes have a cardiovascular age 10–15 years higher than their chronological age.[55] All patients with diabetes, regardless of age, require education on implementing a healthy lifestyle (maintaining a healthy body weight, physical activity and smoking cessation) as a way to reduce cardiovascular risk. The need for pharmacologic therapy for vascular protection, including statins, ACE inhibitors/ARBs and acetylsalicylic acid, depends on the individual risk of the patient.

Recommendations

To promote optimal cardiovascular health, the treatment of all patients with diabetes should include:[56]

- Optimal blood glucose control
- Blood pressure less than 130/80 mm Hg
- Optimal lipid control
- Healthy body weight
- Regular physical activity
- Smoking cessation
- Healthy diet

The use of pharmacologic therapy for vascular protection is based on the patient's cardiovascular risk. The CDA 2013 Clinical Practice Guidelines have established the following criteria:[56]

- Statin therapy is recommended if:
  - Age ≥40 years, *or* irrespective of age in the following situations:
    - macrovascular disease
    - microvascular disease
    - diabetes present for >15 years and age >30 years
    - presence of other risk factors (male, smoker, family history of premature CVD, ECG abnormalities, ACR >2 mg/mmol)
- ACE inhibitor or ARB is recommended if:
  - Age ≥55 years, *or* irrespective of age in the following situations:
    - macrovascular disease
    - microvascular disease

Low-dose **ASA** (81–325 mg) once daily may be used for secondary prevention in those who already have established CVD. **Clopidogrel** 75 mg once daily may be used in those unable to tolerate ASA. ASA should not be routinely used for primary prevention in people with diabetes. In people with diabetes, ASA has shown little or no benefit in the reduction of CAD events and stroke in primary prevention and there is an increased risk of GI hemorrhage.[56]

Pneumonia and Influenza Vaccinations

Patients with diabetes are at high risk of morbidity and mortality from influenza and pneumococcal disease. They should receive the **influenza vaccine** yearly. They should also receive a one-time **pneumococcal vaccine**. For those >65 years, revaccination is recommended if the first vaccination was given >5 years ago and before the age of 65.[57]

Alcohol Consumption

Alcohol may be incorporated into a diabetes meal plan, provided there are no other contraindications. Alcohol consumption may mask symptoms of hypoglycemia, reduce hepatic glucose production and increase ketones. However, when used in moderation it can be safe and even beneficial from a cardiovascular perspective. Alcohol consumption should be limited to ≤2 standard drinks per day and <10 drinks per week in nonpregnant, nonlactating females with diabetes and ≤3 standard drinks per day and <15 drinks per week in men. One standard drink is defined as 10 g of alcohol which will be contained in 341 mL of 5% alcohol beer, 43 mL of 40% alcohol spirits or 142 mL of 12 % alcohol wine.[28]

- Increased physical activity and reduced or no food intake can increase the risk of hypoglycemia with alcohol ingestion. In those with type 1 diabetes, moderate consumption of alcohol with or a few hours after the evening meal can result in hypoglycemia the following morning or up to 24 hours later.[28]
- Those using insulin or insulin secretagogues (e.g., **meglitanides**, **sulfonylureas**) should be informed of the risk of delayed hypoglycemia resulting from alcohol consumption with or after the previous evening meal and advised of measures to prevent hypoglycemia including: consuming alcohol with food, eating a carbohydrate-containing snack before bed, adjusting insulin and monitoring blood glucose.
- Inform patients who use **metformin** that consuming alcohol within the suggested limits is unlikely to be problematic, but that acute or chronic ingestion of larger quantities of alcohol can contribute to the development of lactic acidosis.
- Alcohol contains 29 kJ or 7 cal/g, and can therefore contribute to weight gain. Alcohol-containing medications are unlikely to contribute to poor blood glucose management or weight gain when used in moderation.

Safe Use of Nonprescription Medications

It is important for individuals with diabetes to seek medical attention for more severe health problems before they become problematic. However, many minor conditions may be safely treated with the same nonprescription choices used by the general public.

Instruct patients with diabetes to use low-sugar/sugar-free products, as many liquid pharmaceuticals may contain significant amounts of sugar. Also, the frequency of glucose monitoring needs to be increased during illness to avoid loss of glucose control. Patients should have a sick-day management plan.

Occasional use of nonprescription **analgesics** has little or no effect on blood sugar. However, **NSAIDs** can adversely affect blood pressure. Regular use of NSAIDs can also exacerbate renal impairment. Therefore, refer patients with diabetes who require regular analgesia to their healthcare practitioner. Topical **capsaicin** may be used for painful symptoms of diabetic neuropathy, but short-term burning and itching may limit its use. Patients with peripheral neuropathic pain should be encouraged to optimize their blood glucose levels in order to prevent progression of neuropathy.

Oral **decongestants** should be avoided in those with diabetes and hypertension. Another reason for cautious use in patients with diabetes is the vasoconstriction caused by these agents, which can be more significant in those with vascular complications such as poor circulation. Topical decongestants are less likely to raise blood pressure than oral decongestants but should be avoided or used with caution in patients with diabetes.

Patients experiencing heartburn, indigestion or reflux can be treated with nonprescription **H_2-receptor antagonists** or with low-sugar/sugar-free **antacids**. However, diabetes management may be complicated if significant gastroparesis is present. Encourage patients to discuss use of these nonprescription medications with the healthcare practitioner treating their diabetes.

Constipation or diarrhea can be treated with the usual nonprescription remedies (see Chapter 29: Constipation and Chapter 30: Diarrhea). However, repeated constipation or diarrhea may signal gastroparesis that requires further assessment.

Patients may travel to other countries where medication accessibility is different from Canada. Advise patients to seek advice from a healthcare practitioner if they are choosing foreign nonprescription products.

Dental Care

Periodontitis is a chronic inflammatory disease characterized by destruction of the supporting structures of the teeth. Epidemiological studies have shown that people with diabetes have a threefold higher prevalence of periodontitis than those without diabetes.[58] There is some evidence of improvement in glycemic control after treating periodontal disease but additional large, well-conducted studies are required.[59] People with diabetes should be educated on the importance of good oral and periodontal health through regular dental visits, brushing and flossing (see Chapter 86: Oral Hygiene, Dental Plaque and Caries). Smoking is a major risk factor and assistance with smoking cessation is recommended.

Skin Care

Hyperglycemia, poor circulation due to vascular abnormalities and peripheral neuropathy contribute to impaired host defenses against infection. Nerve damage from diabetic neuropathy may also decrease sweating, especially in the hands and feet, which normally helps to keep the skin moist. Patients with diabetes are at increased risk of skin infections and delayed healing. Careful skin care is important, to prevent serious skin problems. See Chapter 62: Dry Skin and Chapter 68: Minor Cuts and Wounds for discussion of these topics.

Foot Care

Foot problems are a major cause of morbidity and mortality, and individuals with diabetes are more prone to developing serious foot problems than the general population. People with diabetes, peripheral neuropathy and peripheral arterial disease are predisposed to foot ulceration and infection, and this can lead to lower extremity amputation. Other risk factors include previous ulceration or amputation, structural deformity, limited joint mobility, microvascular complications, high HbA_{1c} and onychomycosis.[60,61,62] Prevention of ulceration and infection is critical and patients need to be educated on the importance of daily foot examinations.[63] Foot ulcers require early treatment using an interprofessional approach that addresses glycemic control, infection, offloading of high-pressure areas, assessment of lower extremity vascular status and wound care (see Foot Care for People with Diabetes—What You Need to Know).

Managing Hypoglycemia

Hypoglycemia is defined as the development of autonomic or neuroglycopenic symptoms (see Table 8) that respond to the administration of carbohydrate, and a plasma glucose <4 mmol/L. Drug-induced hypoglycemia is a complication of diabetes management and may limit the ability to achieve glycemic targets. It is important that individuals receiving insulin or insulin secretagogues (sulfonylureas and meglitinides) understand how to prevent, recognize and treat hypoglycemia. Severe hypoglycemia can lead to confusion, seizure, coma and death.

Table 8: **Symptoms of Hypoglycemia**

Neurogenic (autonomic)	Neuroglycopenic
Trembling	Difficulty concentrating
Palpitations	Confusion
Sweating	Weakness
Anxiety	Drowsiness/dizziness
Hunger	Vision changes
Nausea	Headache

To prevent hypoglycemia:

- Review medication/insulin timing in relation to meals
- Ensure each meal contains a source of carbohydrates
- Snacks may be required before exercise
- Review appropriate blood glucose monitoring including technique, frequency and interpretation of results
- Have the patient consume foods containing carbohydrates, if alcohol is consumed.

Some medications that may contribute to hypoglycemia are listed in Table 9.

Table 9: **Examples of Drugs Known to Contribute to Hypoglycemia[9,64]**

Alcohol	Pentamidine
Beta-blockers	Quinine/Quinidine
Gatifloxacin	Tramadol

Patients taking an alpha-glucosidase inhibitor (**acarbose**) must use glucose/dextrose tablets (or if unavailable, milk or honey) to treat hypoglycemia.[65]

See also Low Blood Sugar (Hypoglycemia)—What You Need to Know.

Prevention of Diabetes

Type 1 Diabetes

Therapies to prevent the onset of type 1 diabetes are considered experimental and range from primary prevention studies (in individuals with a genetic risk for type 1 diabetes but without pancreatic islet autoantibodies) to secondary prevention (in individuals with multiple pancreatic islet autoantibodies but without overt hyperglycemia).[4]

Type 2 Diabetes

Lifestyle intervention in individuals with prediabetes has been shown to reduce the progression to type 2 diabetes by as much as 58% through comprehensive programs that support dietary modification and moderate physical activity (brisk walking) that results in a 5% weight loss.[66,67,68] Long-term follow up of individuals enrolled in these studies demonstrated sustained benefit up to 10–20 years.[69,70] Pharmacologic therapy, including **metformin**, **acarbose** and **thiazolidinediones**, has also been shown to reduce the progression from prediabetes to type 2 diabetes.[66,71,72] However, in the Diabetes Prevention Trial, the benefit of lifestyle intervention in preventing progression to diabetes was greater than with metformin.[66] The CDA 2013 Clinical Practice Guidelines recommend that a structured program of lifestyle intervention that includes moderate weight loss and regular physical activity be implemented in those with impaired glucose tolerance or impaired fasting glucose to decrease the risk of progression to type 2 diabetes. Those with prediabetes, particularly impaired glucose tolerance, are also considered at higher risk of cardiovascular disease and therefore should be assessed for cardiovascular risk factors as well.[73]

Resource Tips

Patients can find useful information from the Canadian Diabetes Association. Available from: www.diabetes.ca.

Suggested Readings

American Diabetes Association. Available from: www.diabetes.org.

American Diabetes Association. Standards of medical care in diabetes—2015. *Diabetes Care* 2015;38:S1-93.

Beaser RS, ed. *Joslin's diabetes deskbook: a guide for primary care providers*. 3rd ed. Philadelphia: Wolters Kluwer Health/Lippincott Williams & Wilkins; 2014.

Canadian Diabetes Association. Current guidelines for management of diabetes. Available from: www.diabetes.ca.

Canadian Diabetes Association Clinical Practice Guidelines Expert Committee. Canadian Diabetes Association 2013 Clinical Practice Guidelines for the Prevention and Management of Diabetes in Canada. *Can J Diabetes* 2013;37:S1-S212.

MacCallum L. *Guidebook for pharmacists on diabetes management: helping patients reach treatment goals*. 1st ed. Toronto: Banting & Best Diabetes Centre, University of Toronto; 2014.

References

1. Public Health Agency of Canada. *Diabetes in Canada: Facts and figures from a public health perspective*. 2011. Available from: www.phac-aspc.gc.ca. Accessed August 28, 2015.
2. Kannel WB, McGee DL. Diabetes and cardiovascular disease. The Framingham study. *JAMA* 1979;241:2035-8.
3. Canadian Diabetes Association. *An economic tsunami: the cost of diabetes in Canada* . 2009. Available from: www.diabetes.ca. Accessed August 28, 2015.
4. Atkinson M, Eisenbarth GS, Michels AW. Type 1 diabetes. *Lancet* 2014;383:69-82.
5. DeFronzo RA. Banting Lecture. From the triumvirate to the ominous octet: a new paradigm for the treatment of type 2 diabetes mellitus. *Diabetes* 2009;58:773-95.
6. Canadian Diabetes Association Clinical Practice Guidelines Expert Committee, Thompson D, Berger H et al. Diabetes and pregnancy. *Can J Diabetes* 2013;37:S168-83.
7. Canadian Diabetes Association Clinical Practice Guidelines Expert Committee. Appendix 1. Etiologic classification of diabetes mellitus. *Can J Diabetes* 2013;37:S197.
8. Park-Wyllie LY, Juurlink DN, Kopp A et al. Outpatient gatifloxacin therapy and dysglycemia in older adults. *N Engl J Med* 2006;354:1352-61.
9. Luna B, Feringlos MN. Drug-induced hyperglycemia. *JAMA* 2001;286:1945-8.
10. Abdur R, Setter SM, Vue MH. Drug-induced glucose alterations part 2: drug-induced hyperglycemia *Diabetes Spectr* 2011;24:234-8.
11. Canadian Diabetes Association Clinical Practice Guidelines Expert Committee, Ekoé JM, Punthakee Z et al. Screening for type 1 and 2 diabetes. *Can J Diabetes* 2013;37:S12-5.
12. Canadian Diabetes Association Clinical Practice Guidelines Expert Committee, Goldenberg R, Punthakee Z. Definition, classification, and diagnosis of diabetes, prediabetes and metabolic syndrome. *Can J Diabetes* 2013;37:S8-11.
13. Gallagher EJ, Le Roith D, Bloomgarden Z. Review of hemoglobin A(1c) in the management of diabetes. *J Diabetes* 2009;1:9-17.
14. Herman WH, MA Y, Uwaifo G et al. Differences in A1C by race and ethnicity among patients with impaired glucose tolerance in the Diabetes Prevention Program. *Diabetes Care* 2007;30:2453-7.
15. Ziemer DC, Kolm P, Weinstraub WS et al. Glucose-independent, black-white differences in hemoglobin A1C levels. *Ann Intern Med* 2010;152:770-7.
16. Davidson MB, Schriger DL. Effect of age and race/ethnicity on HbA1C levels in people without known diabetes mellitus: implications for the diagnosis of diabetes. *Diabetes Res Lin Pract* 2010;87:415-21.
17. Pani LN, Korenda L, Meigs JB et al. Effect of aging on A1C levels in persons without diabetes: evidence from the Framingham Offspring Study and the National Health and Nutrition Examination Survey 2001-2004. *Diabetes Care* 2008;31:1991-6.
18. The effect of intensive treatment of diabetes on the development and progression of long-term complications in insulin-dependent diabetes mellitus. The Diabetes Control and Complications Trial Research Group. *N Engl J Med* 1993;329:977-86.
19. Intensive blood-glucose control with sulphonylureas or insulin compared with conventional treatment and risk of complications in patients with type 2 diabetes (UKPDS 33). UK Prospective Diabetes Study (UKPDS) Group. *Lancet* 1998;352:837-53.

20. The Writing Team for the Diabetes Control and Complications Trial/Epidemiology of Diabetes Intervention and Complications Research Group. Effects of intensive therapy on the microvascular complications of type 1 diabetes. *JAMA* 2002;287:2563-9.
21. Martin CL, Albers J, Herman WH et al. Neuropathy among the diabetes control and complications trial cohort 8 years after trial completion. *Diabetes Care* 2006;29:340-4.
22. Holman RR, Sanjoy PK, Bethel MA et al. 10-year follow-up of intensive glucose control in type 2 diabetes. *N Engl J Med* 2008;359:1577-89.
23. Nathan DM, Clearly PA, Backlund JY et al. Intensive diabetes treatment and cardiovascular disease in patients with type 1 diabetes. *N Engl J Med* 2005;353:2643-53.
24. Canadian Diabetes Association Clinical Practice Guidelines Expert Committee, Imran SA, Rabasa-Lhoret R et al. Targets for glycemic control. *Can J Diabetes* 2013;37:S31-4.
25. Canadian Diabetes Association Clinical Practice Guidelines Expert Committee, Meneilly GS, Knip A et al. Diabetes in the elderly. *Can J Diabetes* 2013;37:S184-90.
26. The Look AHEAD Research Group, Wing RR, Bolin P et al. Cardiovascular effects of intensive lifestyle intervention in type 2 diabetes. *N Engl J Med* 2013;369:145-54.
27. Canadian Diabetes Association Clinical Practice Guidelines Expert Committee, Sigal RJ, Armstrong MJ et al. Physical activity and diabetes. *Can J Diabetes* 2013;37:S40-4.
28. Canadian Diabetes Association Clinical Practice Guidelines Expert Committee, Dworatzek PD, Arcudi K et al. Nutrition therapy. *Can J Diabetes* 2013;37:S45-55.
29. MacCallum L. *Guidebook for pharmacists on diabetes management: helping patients reach treatment goals*. 1st ed. Toronto: Banting & Best Diabetes Centre, University of Toronto; 2014.
30. Canadian Diabetes Association Clinical Practice Guidelines Expert Committee, McGibbon A, Richardson C et al. Pharmacotherapy in type 1 diabetes. *Can J Diabetes* 2013;37:S56-60.
31. FIT Forum for Injection Technique Canada. *Recommendations for best practice in injection technique*. 2012; Available from: www.fit4diabetes.com/canada-english/fit-recommendations/. Accessed August 25, 2015.
32. Ryan EA, Pick ME, Marceau C. Use of alternative medicines in diabetes mellitus. *Diabet Med* 2001;18:242-5.
33. Canadian Diabetes Association Clinical Practice Guidelines Expert Committee, Nahas R, Goguen J. Natural health products. *Can J Diabetes* 2013;37:S97-9.
34. Canadian Diabetes Association Clinical Practice Guidelines Expert Committee, Boyd R, Advani A et al. Retinopathy. *Can J Diabetes* 2013;37:S137-41.
35. Klein R, Klein BE, Moss SE et al. The Wisconsin Epidemiologic Study Of Diabetic Retinopathy. IX. Four-year incidence and progression of diabetic retinopathy when age at diagnosis is less than 30 years. *Arch Ophthalmol* 1989;107:237-43.
36. Klein R, Klein BE, Moss SE et al. The Wisconsin epidemiologic study of diabetic retinopathy. II. Prevalence and risk of diabetic retinopathy when age at diagnosis is less than 30 years. *Arch Ophthalmol* 1984;102:520-6.
37. Tight blood pressure control and risk of macrovascular and microvascular complications in type 2 diabetes: UKPDS 38. UK Prospective Diabetes Study Group. *BMJ* 1998;317:703-13.
38. Daskalopoulou SS, Rabi DM, Zamke KB et al. The 2015 Canadian hypertension education program recommendations for blood pressure measurement, diagnosis, assessment of risk, prevention, and treatment of hypertension. *Can J Cardiol* 2015;31:549-68.
39. Gilbert RE, Rabi D, LaRochelle P et al. Treatment of Hypertension. *Can J Diabetes* 2013;37:S117-8.
40. Keech AC, Mitchell P, Summanen PA et al. Effect of fenofibrate on the need for laser treatment for diabetic retinopathy (FIELD study): a randomised controlled trial. *Lancet* 2007;370:1687-97.
41. Fortin CM, Williams B, Ivis F et al. *Treatment of end-stage organ failure in Canada, 2000 to 2009*. Ottawa: Canadian Institute for Health Information; 2011.
42. Foley RN, Parfrey PS, Sarnak MJ. Clinical epidemiology of cardiovascular disease in chronic renal disease. *Am J Kidney Dis* 1998;32:S112-9.
43. Warram JH, Gearin G, Laffel L et al. Effect of duration of type I diabetes on the prevalence of stages of diabetic nephropathy defined by urinary albumin/creatinine ratio. *J Am Soc Nephrol* 1996;7:930-7.
44. Reenders K, de Nobel E, van den Hoogen HJ et al. Diabetes and its long-term complications in general practice: a survey in a well-defined population. *Fam Pract* 1993;10:169-72.
45. Weir MR. Albuminuria predicting outcome in diabetes: incidence of microalbuminuria in Asia-Pacific Rim. *Kidney Int* 2004;66:S38-9.
46. Maki DD, Ma JZ, Louis JZ et al. Long-term effects of antihypertensive agents on proteinuria and renal function. *Arch Intern Med* 1995;155:1073-1080.
47. Effects of ramipril on cardiovascular and microvascular outcomes in people with diabetes mellitus: results of the HOPE study and MICRO-HOPE substudy. Heart Outcomes Prevention Evaluation Study Investigators. *Lancet* 2000;355:253-9.
48. Ruggenenti P, Fassi A, Ilieva AP et al. Preventing microalbuminuria in type 2 diabetes. *N Engl J Med* 2004;351:1941-51.
49. Lewis EJ, Hunsicker LG, Clarke WR et al. Renoprotective effect of the angiotensin-receptor antagonist irbesartan in patients with nephropathy due to type 2 diabetes. *N Engl J Med* 2001;345:851-0.
50. Brenner BM, Cooper ME, de Zeeum D et al. Effects of losartan on renal and cardiovascular outcomes in patients with type 2 diabetes and nephropathy. *N Engl J Med* 2001;345:861-9.
51. Canadian Diabetes Association Clinical Practice Guidelines Expert Committee, McFarlane P, Gilbert RE et al. Chronic kidney disease in diabetes. *Can J Diabetes* 2013;37:S129-36.
52. Canadian Diabetes Association Clinical Practice Guidelines Expert Committee. Appendix 7. Sick day medication list. *Can J Diabetes* 2013;37:S209.
53. Dyck PJ, Kratz KM, Karnes JL et al. The prevalence by staged severity of various types of diabetic neuropathy, retinopathy, and nephropathy in a population-based cohort: the Rochester Diabetic Neuropathy Study. *Neurology* 1993;43:817-24.
54. Canadian Diabetes Association Clinical Practice Guidelines Expert Committee, Bril V, Perkins B et al. Neuropathy. *Can J Diabetes* 2013;37:S142-4.
55. Booth GL, Kapral MK, Fung K et al. Relation between age and cardiovascular disease in men and women with diabetes compared with non-diabetic people: a population-based retrospective cohort study. *Lancet* 2006;368:29-36.
56. Canadian Diabetes Association Clinical Practice Guidelines Expert Committee, Stone JA, Fitchett D et al. Vascular protection in people with diabetes. *Can J Diabetes* 2013;37:S100-4.
57. Canadian Diabetes Association Clinical Practice Guidelines Expert Committee, Husein N, Woo V. Influenza and pneumococcal immunization. *Can J Diabetes* 2013;37:S93.

58. Preshaw PM, Alba AL, Herrera D et al. Periodontitis and diabetes: a two-way relationship. *Diabetologia* 2012;55:21-31.
59. Simpson TC, Weldon JC, Worthington HV et al. Treatment of periodontal disease for glycaemic control in people with diabetes. *Cochrane Database Syst Rev* 2015;11:CD004714. [Epub ahead of print].
60. Boyko EJ, Ahroni JH, Stensel V et al. A prospective study of risk factors for diabetic foot ulcer. The Seattle Diabetic Foot Study. *Diabetes Care* 1999;22:1036-42.
61. Fernando DJ, Masson EA, Veves A. Relationship of limited joint mobility to abnormal foot pressures and diabetic foot ulceration. *Diabetes Care* 1991;14:8-11.
62. Boyko EJ, Ahroni JH, Cohen V et al. . Prediction of diabetic foot ulcer occurrence using commonly available clinical information: the Seattle Diabetic Foot Study. *Diabetes Care* 2006;29:1202-7.
63. Canadian Diabetes Association Clinical Practice Guidelines Expert Committee. Appendix 9. Diabetes and foot care: a patient's checklist. *Can J Diabetes* 2013;37:S211.
64. Murad MH, Coto-Yglesias F, Wang AT et al. Clinical review: drug-induced hypoglycemia: a systematic review. *J Clin Endocrinol Metab* 2009;94:741-5.
65. Canadian Diabetes Association Clinical Practice Guidelines Expert Committee, Clayton D, Woo V et al. Hypoglycemia. *Can J Diabetes* 2013;37:S69-71.
66. Knowler WC, Barrett-Conner E, Fowler SE et al. Reduction in the incidence of Type 2 diabetes with lifestyle intervention or metformin. *N Engl J Med* 2002;346:393-403.
67. Tuomilehto J, Lindstrom J, Eriksson JG et al. Prevention of type 2 diabetes mellitus by changes in lifestyle among subjects with impaired glucose tolerance. *N Engl J Med* 2001;344:1343-50.
68. Pan XR, Li GW, Hu YH et al. Effects of diet and exercise in preventing NIDDM in people with impaired glucose tolerance. The Da Qing IGT and Diabetes Study. *Diabetes Care* 1997;20:537-44.
69. Diabetes Prevention Program Research Group, Knowler WC, Flower SE et al. 10-year follow-up of diabetes incidence and weight loss in the Diabetes Prevention Program Outcomes Study. *Lancet* 2009;374:1677-86.
70. Li G, Zhang P, Wang J et al. The long-term effect of lifestyle interventions to prevent diabetes in the China Da Qing Diabetes Prevention Study: a 20-year follow-up study. *Lancet* 2008;371:1783-9.
71. DREAM (Diabetes REduction Assessment with ramipril and rosiglitazone Medication) Trial Investigators, Gerstein HC, Yusuf SJ et al. Effect of rosiglitazone on the frequency of diabetes in patients with impaired glucose tolerance or impaired fasting glucose: a randomised controlled trial. *Lancet* 2006;368:1096-105.
72. Chiasson JL, Josse RG, Gomis R et al. Acarbose treatment and the risk of cardiovascular disease and hypertension in patients with impaired glucose tolerance: the STOP-NIDDM trial. *JAMA* 2003;290:486-94.
73. Canadian Diabetes Association Clinical Practice Guidelines Expert Committee, Ransom T, Goldenberg R et al. Reducing the risk of developing diabetes. *Can J Diabetes* 2013;37:S16-9.

Self-care for People with Diabetes—What You Need to Know

Suggestions to help you manage your diabetes:

- Follow a healthy, well-balanced meal plan. Ask to see a dietitian to establish a plan.
- Establish a regular exercise routine that a healthcare provider thinks is safe for you. Wear proper footwear and inspect your feet after exercising. Exercise in a cool environment. When weather is hot, exercise outdoors earlier or later in the day if possible. Postpone exercise if you are finding it unusually difficult to control your blood sugar levels.
- Aim to reach a healthy weight and stay there. Ask to see a dietitian.
- Get advice on how to take care of your feet. See: Foot Care for People with Diabetes—What You Need to Know.
- See a healthcare provider if you have difficulty sensing heat or cold or if you feel tingling in your hands or feet.
- Keep blood pressure and cholesterol levels at the target you and your healthcare provider have established.
- Keep blood sugar levels and HbA_{1c} in your target range (follow your meal plan and activity plan, and take the medications you have been prescribed).
- **Do not** smoke. Smoking increases the rate of illness and death for people with diabetes.
- Have a flu shot each fall; have the pneumonia vaccine once, and repeated once if your healthcare provider determines you need a second vaccination.
- Have regular checkups with your healthcare provider, dentist and eye specialist.
- Learn about diabetes through a diabetes education program.
- Ask your healthcare provider about medications that can help prevent damage to your heart and kidneys.
- Become a knowledgeable health care consumer. Ask questions and get a second opinion if you have any concerns.
- Wear a MedicAlert bracelet or other diabetes identification at all times.

Low Blood Sugar (Hypoglycemia)—What You Need to Know

What is hypoglycemia?

Hypoglycemia occurs when a person's blood sugar level is too low. It can be a serious condition for people who have diabetes. If you are taking certain medications you are at risk of hypoglycemia. Ask your healthcare provider if you are taking one of these medications. Make sure you understand how to prevent, detect and properly manage hypoglycemia.

What are the signs of hypoglycemia?

Early signs of hypoglycemia include sweating, hunger, nausea, shakiness, heart palpitations (heavy, fast heartbeats), anxiety, feeling irritable, mood or behaviour changes, numb lips or tongue and headache.

Tips to manage hypoglycemia:

- Always carry a source of fast sugar (such as glucose tablets) and a snack (such as 6 crackers and cheese or peanut butter).
- At the first sign(s) of low blood sugar, check your blood glucose value and if less than 4 mmol/L eat one of the following fast sugar (carbohydrate) sources right away:
  - 15 grams glucose (glucose tablets)
  - 6 Life Savers candies (chewed)
  - 15 mL or 3 packets of sugar dissolved in water, or 15 mL (3 teaspoonfuls) of honey
  - 3/4 cup (6 oz; 180 mL) juice or regular soft drink
- Wait 15 minutes and then retest your blood glucose. If your blood glucose is still less than 4 mmol/L, take one of the items listed above again. Eat your next meal at the regular time. If your next mealtime is more than 1 hour away, eat a snack with 15 grams carbohydrate and one source of protein to prevent the return of hypoglycemia.
- If the hypoglycemia is severe (you need help from another person) eat 20 grams of carbohydrate (for example glucose tablets or 4 packets of sugar). Wait 15 minutes and then retest your blood glucose. If your blood glucose is still less than 4 mmol/L take 15 grams of carbohydrate.
- If you are having hypoglycemia and are unconscious or not able to swallow, caregivers or support persons should get medical attention for you as soon as possible. Your diabetes healthcare team should also be told about the event.
- If you are taking the medication acarbose (Prandase/Glucobay) and have hypoglycemia, you must take a commercially available source of glucose such as glucose tablets, milk or honey. Acarbose prevents other sugars from being quickly absorbed.
- For those at risk of severe hypoglycemia, support persons should be taught how to administer glucagon by injection.
- It is important not to overtreat hypoglycemia. This can lead to high blood glucose and weight gain.
- Avoid driving immediately following hypoglycemia. Be aware of provincial driving regulations regarding hypoglycemia.

Foot Care for People with Diabetes—What You Need to Know

People who have diabetes must take good care of their feet. Although not all people with diabetes suffer from circulation or nerve defects in their feet, everyone with diabetes should know about foot care and should watch for changes in the condition of their feet. Here are some tips to help you keep your feet in good condition:

1. **Inspect**
   - Check your feet every day. Look for scratches, cracks between the toes, blisters, corns and other sores. Watch for swelling and changes in the temperature or colour of your feet and legs. If you cannot see all parts of your feet, use a mirror. Another person can also help you inspect your feet.
   - Your doctor should check your feet at each appointment. Other healthcare providers involved in managing your diabetes (e.g., an endocrinologist) may also check your feet during your appointments.
2. **Bathe**
   - Wash your feet daily with warm (not hot) soapy water. Check the water temperature with your elbow. Your hands and feet may not be able to tell you how hot the water is.
   - Do not soak your feet. Dry your feet well, especially between the toes.
   - Do not scrub with abrasive cloths or loofas.
3. **Moisturize**
   - Apply moisturizer to the tops and bottoms of your feet. Do not apply lotion, cream or oil between the toes. You can use a small amount of foot powder on your feet. Avoid putting it in your shoes or in between toes as it may cake and rub against the foot.
4. **Trim**
   - Cut your toenails straight across. Have a professional cut your nails, especially if you have vision problems, if the nails are thick or if you have poor circulation or nerve defects in your feet.
   - Do not treat your own corns, calluses or warts with over-the-counter medications as they may damage your skin. See a professional trained in foot care if you have corns or calluses.
   - Do not treat your own ingrown toenails or slivers.
5. **Shoes and Socks**
   - Always wear shoes and breathable, clean, soft socks or nylons. Do not wear socks that have been mended, have holes or seams that may irritate your feet or that are too tight. Change your socks every day.
   - Select shoes that fit well, preferably made of breathable material (e.g., leather). Avoid sandals, plastic shoes, pointed toes and high heels.
   - Check the inside of your shoes for sharp objects or rough spots before you wear them.
   - Protect your feet at the beach. Sand, shells and rocks can damage your feet. Wear protective shoes.
6. **Avoid Extreme Cold and Heat (including the sun)**
   - Do not use heating pads, electric blankets or hot water bottles and do not warm your feet by a fireplace.
   - Wear warm boots in the winter to help you avoid frostbite.

7. **Circulation**
    - Avoid anything that puts pressure on your feet and legs (such as tight socks or stockings, garters, elastics or knee highs). They may reduce circulation to the legs and feet.
    - Avoid smoking.
    - Maintain a healthy body weight.
    - Do not sit for long periods of time.
8. **Injuries/Infections**
    - See your healthcare provider as soon as possible if you injure your feet or legs or you see changes in their condition. If you need treatment, it should be started as soon as possible.
    - Treat athlete's foot at the first sign of infection.
9. **Exercise**
    - Ask your healthcare provider to recommend safe exercises to improve circulation.
    - Do your exercises every day.
10. **Control**
    - Follow your healthcare provider's advice to control your blood glucose, cholesterol and blood pressure.

Chapter 26
Diabetes Care Devices

Ronald Silver, BSc, BScPharm

Diabetes Management

Technology has empowered patients with diabetes by giving them the tools to be more responsible for their health management on a daily basis. The primary goals of therapy are to maintain health and avoid acute and long-term complications. Diabetes care depends upon the daily commitment of those with diabetes to self-management practices, with support from their healthcare practitioners. Effective diabetes self-management improves HbA_{1c} values and restores blood glucose (BG) levels to near-normal range.[1] This reduces the frequency of microvascular complications in patients with type 1 or type 2 diabetes, as well as macrovascular risk in individuals with type 1 diabetes and some with type 2 diabetes.[1,2,3,4]

Blood Glucose Levels

Optimal BG levels are associated with a low risk of complications (Table 1). However, in some cases these levels may be impossible to attain because of severe side effects (e.g., hypoglycemia),[3] diminished quality of life, or cost.

Table 1: **Recommended Targets for Glycemic Control**[4]

	HbA_{1c} (%)	FPG or Preprandial PG (mmol/L)	2-hour Postprandial PG (mmol/L)
Type 1 and type 2 diabetes	≤7[a]	4–7	5–10 (5–8 if HbA_{1c} targets not being met)

[a] Higher or lower target values may be appropriate in specific individuals as discussed in the text.

Abbreviations: FPG = fasting plasma glucose; HbA_{1c} = glycated hemoglobin; PG = plasma glucose

Fasting BG >5.6 mmol/L is associated with an increased risk of cardiovascular disease; however, postprandial hyperglycemia appears to be a better predictor, with values >7.8 mmol/L associated with an increase in all-cause mortality, and values >10 mmol/L with both microvascular complications and risk of MI.[4] Blood glucose levels correlate well with HbA_{1c} levels. When HbA_{1c} values are high, the major influence is the fasting BG. When HbA_{1c} levels approach 7%, postprandial plasma glucose becomes more significant.[4]

Glycemic targets should be individualized based on the age, duration of diabetes, risk of severe hypoglycemia, presence or absence of cardiovascular disease, and life expectancy.[4] More intensive control with an HbA_{1c} <6.5% may be beneficial if it can be achieved without a significant increase in hypoglycemia, and may be appropriate in patients with a shorter duration of diabetes, no evidence of significant cardiovascular disease, and a longer life expectancy.[4] An HbA_{1c} target of <8.5% may be considered in patients with a limited life expectancy, a higher level of functional dependency, a history of severe hypoglycemia, or advanced comorbidities.[4]

Blood Glucose Monitoring

For comparative features of nonprescription products, consult the *Compendium of Products for Minor Ailments*—Diabetes Products: Blood Glucose Meters.

Blood glucose monitoring can help inform adjustments in diabetes medications, particularly with insulin treatment. If used appropriately it may help empower patients with diabetes to engage in self-care behaviours such as diet selection, exercise and foot care.[5]

All available blood glucose meters test a capillary blood sample, which is whole blood. Meanwhile, laboratories use venous plasma glucose as the benchmark (plasma is whole blood without the red blood cells). Blood glucose meters are adjusted to give results which correlate with lab test results. At BG levels >4.2 mmol/L, a difference of <20% is considered acceptable.[6] Experts recommend comparing laboratory and meter results at least annually, or when meter results do not appear to match HbA_{1c} or other indicators.

Frequency of Testing

Healthcare practitioners care can assist patients in determining the frequency and timing of their blood glucose measurements since the quality of evidence to support testing is variable.[7] Factors to consider are the potential benefits of monitoring vs. cost and pain associated with the procedure.[8]

Patients with type 1 diabetes should test at least 3 times daily; this has been associated with a 1% reduction of HbA_{1c} levels.[6] Testing can be done on a twice-daily basis: before breakfast and after supper one day, and after lunch and at bedtime the next day. Patients with type 2 diabetes using insulin more than once a day should also test 3 times daily.[6] Patients using multiple insulin injections or insulin pump therapy should be testing 3 times daily or more.[9]

Patients with type 2 diabetes on oral medication should test periodically, testing once or twice weekly to ensure that glycemic targets are being met between HbA_{1c} tests. Tests should reflect pre-meal, after-meal and bedtime levels. The Canadian Diabetes Association has a tool available on its website to help patients determine how often to test, along with a recommended pattern of testing.[10] Testing in these patients has demonstrated a reduction in HbA_{1c} levels of 0.2–0.6%.[6] Testing may also be used to achieve postprandial glucose targets.[9] Additional testing (more than twice daily) may be suggested for patients with pharmacotherapy changes, those starting a drug that may cause hyperglycemia, or those with an acute illness.[10]

Daily blood glucose testing is not recommended for pre-diabetes and for patients diagnosed with diabetes who are being treated only by diet and lifestyle if they are meeting their glycemic targets.[10]

Testing

Advise patients to track their results in a journal log, or use meters with memory and graphing options so they can share this information with their physician and other healthcare practitioners. For optimal self-monitoring of blood glucose, the patient is educated on the use of a meter, interprets the results and modifies treatment based on current blood glucose levels according to individual guidelines provided by healthcare practitioners.[9]

Encourage patients to adhere to storage directions for test strips, keeping them in their original containers at room temperature or cooler. Expired and mishandled test strips can lead to errors in testing. Once a vial of test strips is open, the strips keep longest in a refrigerator (35–50 days), but deteriorate quickly in direct light and humidity (3–14 days).[11]

Lancing Devices

The first step in blood glucose monitoring is obtaining a blood sample. A capillary blood sample is collected by puncturing the skin with a lancet, which is a small needle of varying gauge or size. When the lancing device is triggered, the needle is projected into the skin and then retracts.

Since patients with diabetes are more susceptible to infection, the area must be well cleansed. Washing hands with soap and water is acceptable. When travelling, patients can use alcohol swabs instead. Most lancets are designed to be used 2–4 times.

Most lancing devices have a depth adjustment. The majority of models are pen-shaped and accept a variety of lancets. However, some lancets can be used only by a specific lancing device. For example, Softclix devices accept only Softclix lancets.

To use a lancet device, apply the device to the skin, exert gentle pressure and press the trigger. Site rotation is also important. Frequent users will rotate between fingers; occasionally, right-handed users might prefer lancing the left hand and vice versa. The target area is the side of the finger beside the fingernail.

Health Canada recommends against the use of multi-patient lancing devices due to the risk of disease transmission, even if a new lancet is used for every patient. Only auto-disabling lancet devices should be used in multi-patient settings.

Alternate Site Testing

Meters are available that allow the use of blood samples from sites other than the fingertip, such as the forearm, palm of the hand or thigh. During periods of rapid change in BG levels (e.g., after meals, after exercise and during periods of hypoglycemia), fingertip testing is the most accurate.[6] Blood samples taken from the palm near the base of the thumb provide a closer correlation to fingertip samples than the forearm or thigh.

Blood Glucose Meters

There are many meters available, and healthcare practitioners can assist patients in choosing an appropriate device by considering the following factors:

- The amount of blood required for the sample
- The calibration method: for some models it is as simple as putting in a test strip; others require pushing a button or inserting a code for calibration
- The size of the test strips: patients with poor dexterity may prefer larger strips
- The screen size and display size are important to visually impaired patients
- The ability to provide an audible readout is important for those who are blind
- The battery type and battery life
- The ability to link to a computer for in-depth reports
- The ability to add comments, such as meals and levels of activity, and access built-in graphs
- The ability to communicate with insulin pumps.

Testing with a Blood Glucose Meter

Healthcare practitioners assisting patients with blood glucose meters must have a thorough knowledge of available products. Demonstrations and detailed owner's manuals are available. As well, a quick reference guide is available with each meter for rapid consultation. Canadian blood glucose meters are set to measure glucose in mmol/L and this cannot be changed by the user. To avoid confusion, patients should be made aware that information designed to the American standard will use units of mg/dL.

Troubleshooting Blood Glucose Meters

Although newer meters are easier to use, patients may still experience difficulties. Many meters provide directions or error codes that patients or healthcare practitioners can verify in the owner's manual or discuss with the manufacturer's technical support team.

Most problems are due to:

- Errors in user technique
- Improper meter calibration. It is important that the meter's calibration number corresponds with the calibration number on the strip container
- Outdated or poorly stored strips. Check manufacturer's specifications regarding temperature, light and humidity
- Inadequacy of blood samples, e.g., size, traces of alcohol used to clean puncture site
- Change in patient's situation (e.g., illness, stress, pregnancy), which can produce unexpected but accurate results
- Changes in medications (including adding or discontinuing nonprescription drugs).

Diabetes Management Software

With the appropriate interface, data can be downloaded from a blood glucose meter to a computer. The software will enable the patient to see the information in different formats, such as patient profiles, logbooks, means, variations, deviations from pre-set goals, charts, standard day and insulin doses. This information can also be printed. The software may be available through the manufacturer, or it may be possible to download the file from the manufacturer's website. Cables to link meters to computers are available from the manufacturer. Pharmacists may wish to set up their own computer so they are able to download patients' data and provide interpretive counselling.

Blood glucose values can also be transferred directly to some smart phone apps. In addition to recording blood glucose data, these apps may include food databases and allow the tracking of diet, exercise routines and medications.[12] Selecting which app to use should be done carefully since they are not regulated, privacy is not guaranteed and the units of measure in the app may not be compatible with Canadian standards.

Urine Glucose Monitoring

For comparative features of nonprescription products, consult the *Compendium of Products for Minor Ailments*—Diabetes Products: Urine Glucose and Ketone Test Kits.

Urinary glucose measurement is not ideal, as it does not reflect current blood glucose levels and will not detect hypoglycemia. However, there may be select circumstances under which urine glucose monitoring may be used, such as when blood glucose monitoring is not available, too costly or too painful.

Ketone Monitoring

For comparative features of nonprescription products, consult the *Compendium of Products for Minor Ailments*—Diabetes Products: Urine Glucose and Ketone Test Kits.

When insulin levels fall too low, the body shifts from carbohydrate to fat metabolism. Ketones are a by-product of this process. Ketones are normally excreted by the kidneys, but under these circumstances, elimination is not rapid enough and ketones accumulate in the bloodstream, causing the blood to become acidic. The levels of blood glucose continue to rise, causing diabetic ketoacidosis

(DKA), which is accompanied by the following symptoms: thirst, dry mouth, frequent urination, nausea and vomiting, blurred vision, abdominal pain and fruity-smelling breath.

Ketone testing is recommended for those with type 1 diabetes during periods of acute illness accompanied by elevated BG, when preprandial BG levels are >14 mmol/L, or when symptoms of DKA are present. If all of these conditions are present in individuals with type 2 diabetes, ketone testing should also be considered.[6]

During DKA, there is a shift in the equilibrium that is usually present among ketone bodies, favouring the formation of betahydroxybutyric acid. Blood assays of this acid have been associated with an earlier detection of DKA than urine testing for acetoacetate or acetone levels.[6] Ketones can be detected in urine using test strips such as Ketostix; to test for ketones in blood, ketone-measuring test strips are used with a blood glucose meter such as Precision Xtra.

Continuous Glucose Monitoring Systems

Continuous glucose monitoring (CGM) systems have been shown to improve HbA_{1c} levels and reduce the duration of hypoglycemia, hyperglycemia and nocturnal hypoglycemia in patients treated with insulin.[6] CGM, used in conjunction with intensive insulin regimens, can be a useful tool to lower HbA_{1c} in selected adults (>25 years) with type 1 diabetes.[13] CGM may also be helpful in children.[6] CGM may be a supplemental tool to BG monitoring in those patients with hypoglycemia unawareness and/or with frequent hypoglycemic episodes.

CGM systems measure glucose levels in interstitial fluids. These levels relate well with BG values, although there may be significant differences due to lag time, particularly when BG levels are rapidly changing (such as a few hours after eating). BG tests are still required during these times, for the purpose of calibrating the CGM system device and for making decisions regarding medication changes.[14]

The glucose sensor is a tiny electrode inserted subcutaneously that continuously records glucose levels. The sensor is worn for up to 3 days before it is discarded and replaced. Glucose readings are transmitted to a meter or insulin pump where the readings are displayed. Trend reports and charts can be viewed after the data are downloaded to a computer. Using a CGM system chart is like watching a movie—anyone can follow the storyline and anticipate what is going to occur next. CGM systems allow patients and their healthcare practitioners to discover how diet, exercise, medication and lifestyle affect their glucose levels. CGM system devices that display real-time readings allow patients to see how fast, and in what direction, their glucose levels are changing, allowing them to intervene earlier to reduce the frequency and severity of high and low blood sugar episodes.[14,15]

Insulin Administration Devices

For comparative features of nonprescription products, consult the *Compendium of Products for Minor Ailments*—Diabetes Products: Insulin Products.

When insulin is administered by injection it is important that patients receive appropriate training in the device they are using. Consensus guidelines on good injection technique contain tips for optimal insulin administration.[16]

Insulin pens look like large fountain pens. Instead of retrieving the insulin from vials, the pen either comes prefilled with insulin, or uses insulin cartridges. Insulin pens are more convenient and easier to use than insulin syringes. For the visually impaired, the audible clicks are a useful guide for selecting the correct number of units to administer.

Once an insulin cartridge is installed into a refillable pen it can be stored between 2–30°C for up to 28 days. Unused cartridges can be refrigerated and kept until their expiry date. Disposable pens should be refrigerated until opened, then kept at room temperature (below 30°C) for up to 28–42 days depending on the insulin brand. Ensure that patients understand the particular technique associated with the use of the pen. Advise patients to keep a few syringes at home in case of pen malfunction.

There are a number of major companies in the pen/cartridge market and patients must be aware that cartridges are not interchangeable.

Needles vary in length and diameter. Needle length ranges from 4–12.7 mm. The diameter will vary from 28–33 gauge, with higher numbers indicating a smaller diameter. Thinner and shorter needles cause less resistance in skin penetration and usually less discomfort for the patient, and are therefore preferred. Some patients, such as those who are obese, may find longer needles provide better penetration to the subcutaneous tissue and reduce insulin leakage from the injection site. Waiting 3–5 seconds before taking a needle out of the skin after injection will help prevent insulin leakage. If 5 seconds is not sufficient, this interval should be prolonged. Reusing needles diminishes the point sharpness and removes the silicon coating. This may lead to micro-traumas which are linked to nodule formation; manufacturers recommend single use only.

Syringes can be used for the administration of insulin but their use has declined significantly with the introduction of insulin pens. Various sizes and measurement increments are available. The 100-unit size has 2-unit increments for measuring larger doses, while the 50- and 30-unit syringes have 1-unit increments. The choice of syringes should be based on the total amount of insulin to be administered, keeping in mind that smaller-volume syringes will offer a more accurate measurement. Occasionally, patients require syringes to be prefilled with measured insulin doses. Follow appropriate procedures for preparation and storage to maintain insulin stability.[17]

Insulin Pumps

An insulin pump is a battery-operated device that is designed to be worn 24 hours a day. A small plunger pushes insulin out of a reservoir or cartridge through tubing to a cannula that has been inserted in the patient's subcutaneous tissue.

It can be easier to match insulin requirements with lifestyle (allowing for more flexibility with meals and activity) using an insulin pump rather than multiple daily doses of insulin. Insulin pumps provide a constant supply of insulin to the patient, adjustable to the time of day, with the option of providing extra insulin for meals and snacks.

Advantages of pump therapy:[14]

- Can be used for type 1 diabetes (most common use) or type 2 diabetes
- May provide more consistent blood glucose control than daily and multiple daily injections
- More convenient than multiple daily injections and allows the patient more flexibility in the timing and size of meals
- Less variation in the rate of insulin absorption (3% vs. 25%) due to fewer injection sites
- May result in lower HbA_{1c} values without increasing the risk of hypoglycemia.

Disadvantages of pump therapy:[14]

- An insulin pump can cost between $6000 and $8000, and pump supplies can cost about $250/month. Many provinces have programs to offset some of these costs
- Malfunctions may occur, resulting in ketoacidosis within a few hours due to a disruption in insulin delivery
- Patients need to change their infusion sites every 2–3 days; other considerations include the requirement for regular skin care and wearing a pump 24 hours a day

- Patients must be trained by an experienced diabetes educator and be comfortable with the device operation.

Pump Features

Insulin pumps are programmed to provide a basal rate of insulin, which can vary for each patient and at different times of the day. More insulin is usually required at night for those who experience the dawn phenomenon.

Patients can adjust the pump to provide a bolus amount of insulin according to what and when they are eating. The insulin pump helps to calculate the dose required based on the number of grams of carbohydrates eaten, but this can be overridden depending on planned activities or other factors. Patients must learn the skill of carbohydrate counting. Some meters have a database of favourite foods, which can make the calculations easier and faster. The pump can also be programmed to provide the bolus all at once for a regular meal, or over a period of time (e.g., 1–2 hours) when a patient wishes to nibble.[14]

Insulin pumps can be linked to a blood glucose meter through wireless technology, and adjustments to insulin delivery can be made and monitored. The CGM device communicates with the insulin pump every 5 minutes, showing the direction and rate of change in glucose levels. The advantage of this is to foresee problems regarding hypo- or hyperglycemia before they arise. The disadvantage of CGM is that the sensors must be calibrated 2–3 times daily with a blood glucose meter when blood glucose values are stable. Also, the sensors are expensive and need to be replaced every 3 days.[14]

The insulin pump may be worn around the abdominal area, or at various other sites including the leg. The pump contains a reservoir to hold fast-acting insulin. Insulin is withdrawn from a vial and moved to the reservoir with a needle-attached adapter. The reservoir typically holds 170–300 units of insulin. The pump can be programmed to set basal rates and bolus settings, along with connectivity to a glucose meter and/or computer for reporting activity.

An infusion set consists of tubing with either a needle or a cannula to deliver insulin from the pump to the body. Infusion sets are available with 2 lengths of tubing, ranging from 24 inches (60 cm) to 43 inches (110 cm). These lengths allow users to wear their pumps in a variety of locations. The tubing needs to be replaced every 3 days. For sc administration, patients have a choice between steel needles (which must be changed every 1–2 days) or soft Teflon cannula sets (which can be used for 2–3 days). These are available in 2 or 3 lengths and are designed to be inserted either at a 90-degree angle or at a 30- to 45-degree angle. An autoinjector is available to assist insertions. The 90-degree insertion provides better penetration for obese patients. Shorter needles can be used (an advantage for those with needle phobias) but they are more prone to kinking, which may inhibit insulin flow.[14]

Pharmacists can assist patients who are using pumps by having consumable supplies available. These include infusion sets, reservoirs, transparent dressings, batteries and adhesive removers.

For information on available insulin pumps, consult the Canadian Diabetes Association website (see Resource Tips).

Miscellaneous Supplies

Plastic syringe cases allow for the transportation of pre-filled syringes without accidentally applying pressure to the plunger. They are available for 1 or 7 syringes. This tool is excellent for healthcare practitioners who pre-fill and deliver insulin to patients with special needs.

Travel kits organize all diabetes needs in one place. Most travel kits contain ice packs, useful for patients travelling to areas of extreme temperature.

Sharps containers (which are tamper-proof) should be used to dispose of used syringes, needles and lancets. The containers should be taken to a needle disposal site for safe destruction. There are also manual and electric needle cutters which retain the exposed needle in a compartment, which when full can be safely destroyed.

Logbooks can be used by patients to record their blood glucose results, diet and activity level.

Specialized socks provide extra cushioning and warmth while wicking perspiration away from the feet. They also have loose elastics and no rough seams, so as not to impair circulation or irritate the feet. The long-term benefit of using these in foot care has not been established.

Callus and blister protectors are also useful for individuals with diabetes, to prevent damage to the skin on the feet.

Dextrose gels or tablets are a useful means to treat hypoglycemia by providing an exact amount of sugar in a convenient format. Tablets are recommended over gels because they are faster-acting.

Glucagon is a hormone that counteracts the action of insulin. Glucagon stimulates the release of glucose from the liver into the bloodstream, thereby easing the symptoms of low blood glucose. Glucagon kits contain a preloaded syringe, and are mainly for use by family or friends in treating a severe insulin reaction in patients unable to take sugar by mouth. Seek medical attention for patients not recovering after a few minutes.

Filling new and refill prescriptions for diabetes medications is a convenient opportunity to ask patients if they are using and/or require diabetes supplies:[9]

- Alcohol swabs
- Blood glucose strips
- Glucagon
- Glucose tablets
- Lancets
- Needles/syringes
- Needle disposal containers
- Pump supplies
- Urine ketone strips
- Other aids

Resource Tips

American Diabetes Association. Available from: www.diabetes.org.

Canadian Diabetes Association. Available from: www.diabetes.ca.

Diabetes in Control. News and information for medical professionals. Available from: www.diabetesincontrol.com.

FIT Forum for Injection Technique Canada. *Recommendations for best practice in injection technique.* Available from: www.bd.com/resource.aspx?IDX=25063.

Insulin Pumpers. Provides information and support for adults and children with diabetes and their families interested in insulin pump therapy. Available from: www.insulin-pumpers.org.

Mayo Clinic. *Health Information*. Available from: www.mayoclinic.com.

Mendosa D. On-line diabetes resources. *Part 14: Blood glucose meters*. Available from: www.mendosa.com/meters.htm.

Public Health Agency of Canada. *Diabetes*. Available from: www.phac-aspc.gc.ca/cd-mc/diabetes-diabete/index-eng.php.

References

1. Jones H, Berard LD, MacNeill G et al. Canadian Diabetes Association 2013 Clinical Practice Guidelines for the Prevention and Management of Diabetes in Canada: Self-management education. *Can J Diabetes* 2013;37:S26-30. Available from: guidelines.diabetes.ca/Browse/Chapter7.
2. Holman RR, Paul SK, Bethel MA et al. 10-year follow-up of intensive glucose control in type 2 diabetes. *N Engl J Med* 2008;359:1577-89.
3. The effect of intensive treatment of diabetes on the development and progression of long-term complications in insulin-dependent diabetes mellitus. The Diabetes Control and Complications Trial Research Group. *N Engl J Med* 1993;329:977-86.
4. Imran SA, Rabasa-Lhoret R, Ross S. Canadian Diabetes Association 2013 Clinical Practice Guidelines for the Prevention and Management of Diabetes in Canada: Targets for glycemic control. *Can J Diabetes* 2013;37:S31-4. Available from: guidelines.diabetes.ca/Browse/Chapter8.
5. Tidy C. *Self-monitoring in diabetes mellitus*. Available from: patient.info/doctor/self-monitoring-in-diabetes-mellitus.
6. Berard LD, Blumer I, Houlden R et al. Canadian Diabetes Association 2013 Clinical Practice Guidelines for the Prevention and Management of Diabetes in Canada: Monitoring glycemic control. *Can J Diabetes* 2013;37:S35-9. Available from: guidelines.diabetes.ca/Browse/Chapter9.
7. Ahuja TK, Bai A, Belanger D et al. Systematic review of use of blood glucose test strips for the management of diabetes mellitus. Ottawa: Canadian Optimal Medication Prescribing and Utilization Service (COMPUS), Canadian Agency for Drugs and Technologies in Health (CADTH). *COMPUS Optimal Therapy Report* 2009;3:1-157.
8. Goldstein DE, Little RR. Monitoring glycemia in diabetes. Short-term assessment. *Endocrinol Metab Clin North Am* 1997;26:475-86.
9. American Diabetes Association. Standards of medical care in diabetes–2012. *Diabetes Care* 2012;35:S11-63.
10. Canadian Diabetes Association 2013 Clinical Practice Guidelines for the Prevention and Management of Diabetes in Canada: Self-monitoring of blood glucose tool (SMBG) recommendation tool for healthcare providers. *Can J Diabetes* 2013;37:S202-3. Available from: guidelines.diabetes.ca/bloodglucoselowering/smbgtoolpwd.
11. Bamberg R, Schulman K, MacKenzie M et al. Effect of adverse storage conditions on performance of glucometer test strips. *Clin Lab Sci,* 2005;18:203-9.
12. El-Gayar O, Timsina P, Nawar N et al. Mobile applications for diabetes self-management: status and potential. *J Diabetes Sci Technol* 2013;7:247-62.
13. Canadian Diabetes Association Clinical Practice Guidelines Expert Committee. Monitoring glycemic control. *Can J Diabetes* 2008;32:S32-3.
14. Montopoli T. Pump it up, a pharmacist's guide to insulin pump therapy. *Pharmacy Practice* 2009 April/May:D6-D9.
15. Medtronic MiniMed. *Distinctions between standard glucose meters and glucose sensors*. 2006.
16. FIT Forum for Injection Technique Canada. *Recommendations for best practice in injection technique*. Available from: www.bd.com/resource.aspx?IDX=25063.
17. Manitoba Pharmaceutical Association. *Guidelines for the pre-filling of insulin syringes*. Available from: napra.ca/Content_Files/Files/Manitoba/PreFilling-of-Insulin-Syringes.pdf.

Chapter 27
Lifestyle Management and Disease Prevention

L. Maria Gutschi, BScPharm, PharmD

Using the knowledge, skills and ability of health professionals, including pharmacists, to improve lifestyle management is becoming increasingly important. Many drugs are used to treat diseases for which disease prevention strategies and lifestyle management are also recommended. Healthcare practitioners may have frequent contact with patients who could potentially benefit from lifestyle modification, so knowledge of these issues helps in providing patients with information, guidance and counselling to prevent disease.

Risk Factors for Mortality in Canada

Developments in public health as well as increased affluence have changed the causes of death in Western countries such as Canada. Infectious diseases are no longer the major causes of death; the leading causes of death in 2011[1] were primarily chronic conditions, specifically:

- cancer (29.9%)
- cardiovascular diseases (19.7%) and stroke (5.5%)
- chronic respiratory diseases (4.6%)
- diabetes (3%)
- Alzheimer's disease (2.6%)

Acute conditions that were the leading causes of death include:

- influenza and pneumonia (2.4%)
- accidental death and suicide (5.9%)

Genetic and environmental factors play a role in the risks of chronic diseases; however, much of the variation in the incidence of chronic conditions may be due to modifiable causes. An analysis of the "actual causes of death" (from external, nongenetic causes), found that many chronic conditions are often rooted in lifestyle, dietary and metabolic risk factors,[2] in particular:

- high blood glucose or LDL cholesterol
- high blood pressure
- overweight or obesity
- physical inactivity
- poor diet practices
- tobacco use

In addition, alcohol use is an important risk factor for road traffic and other injuries, violence, cancers and hemorrhagic stroke.[2] Both excess and insufficient sun exposure are risk factors for preventable disease that is often associated with lifestyle behaviours.[3]

Since a small number of preventable behaviours and exposures may explain a large proportion of all deaths,[2] interventions to increase smoking cessation, avoid excess alcohol, control high blood pressure, improve diet and increase physical activity are high priorities in health care.

Obesity

Obesity has reached epidemic proportions in Canada as well as globally; over 2 billion adults worldwide are considered overweight.[4] Epidemic rates of obesity are found in both developed and developing countries and it is a chronic condition with serious social and psychological dimensions, affecting Canadians of all age and socioeconomic groups. Current surveys reveal that approximately 62% of the Canadian population is overweight and 25.4% are obese.[5] The obesity rate in children has also risen significantly; the prevalence of obesity in children aged 6–17 years is 8.6% using International Obesity Task Force (IOTF) definitions. This is important since complications, both physical and psychological, and comorbidities of obesity may begin during childhood. Being overweight or obese increases the risk of chronic disease and health conditions such as hypertension, dyslipidemia, insulin resistance, type 2 diabetes, coronary heart disease, stroke, gallbladder and liver disease, osteoarthritis and sleep apnea.[5,6] Less well known is that obesity is associated with cancers such as colon cancer and those that are hormonally related, particularly prostate, endometrial and breast cancers.[4,5,7] Furthermore, obesity is an independent risk factor for all-cause mortality.[5,7,8]

Obesity is defined by the WHO as a body mass index (BMI) >30 measured as kg/(height in m)^2. A BMI of 40–45 kg/m^2 is associated with a reduced median survival of 8–10 years, comparable to the effects of smoking.[9] However, the use of BMI to assess obesity does not apply to people over 65 or to conditioned athletes.[10] Further discussion of obesity and treatment options can be found in Chapter 43: Weight Management.

Visceral adiposity may be a better indicator of increased risk for cardiovascular disease and all-cause mortality.[11] Patients at high risk have a waist measurement of >40 inches (102 cm) for males and >35 inches (88 cm) for females.[5,7] Waist circumference cut-offs for South Asian, Chinese and Japanese ethnic groups are lower.

Physical Inactivity

Seventy-five percent of adults are not active enough to meet Canada's physical activity recommendations, a figure much lower than estimated using self-reported surveys.[12] In addition, a large proportion of children are considered sedentary.

Evidence supporting a physically active lifestyle to improve health is robust. Regular exercise benefits health by increasing longevity and reducing morbidity and mortality due to coronary heart disease (CHD), stroke, hypertension, obesity, diabetes and osteoporosis.[12,13,14] Exercise also may help with depression[15] and improves mental outlook in patients with chronic illness.[16] Exercise reduces the risk of colon, prostate and breast cancer.[8,13,14] Exercise is beneficial even if the participant is older,[17] in persons with disabilities and significantly protects against cognitive decline.[18] Being fit in midlife is associated with significantly decreased risk of developing a chronic illness in later life.[19] Furthermore, the reduction in CHD risk provided by moderate exercise compares favourably with interventions for smoking, hypertension and high cholesterol levels. If an inactive person becomes active at age 50, life gain is estimated to be 1.3–3.7 years while those who quit smoking at age 50 are expected to gain 2.3-2.5 years.[14] Most importantly, the least fit individuals obtain the most benefit.[14] Exercise has been called the miracle drug,[20] since regular physical activity prevents disease and promotes health. Improved physical fitness levels should be a priority for Canadians of all ages.

Alcohol

The regular intake of alcohol is associated with both benefits and risks.[21] Most studies have shown alcohol consumption demonstrates a J-shaped curve: a lower risk of death in people who are light to moderate drinkers compared with lifetime abstainers and heavy drinkers.[22] Low to moderate doses of alcohol are beneficial for reducing the risk of CHD,[21,22] stroke,[23] and diabetes[24] compared with no alcohol use. Based on observational trials, health benefits from alcohol consumption are seen only from middle age and onward and total caloric intake may increase with alcohol consumption without a commensurate increase in nutritional benefit.[22] Cardiovascular benefits can be obtained from as little as one standard drink (13.6 g alcohol or 45 mL spirits, 150 mL table wine, 360 mL beer) every 2 days.

Alcohol consumption is associated in a dose-dependent manner with cancers of the mouth, pharynx, larynx, esophagus and liver.[22] Alcohol consumption in persons who smoke increases the rates of these cancers more than the independent effect of either smoking or drinking alone.[25] Doses greater than 50 g/day or 4 standard drinks were significantly associated with the risk of developing cancer at various sites. Cardiovascular protection due to alcohol is lost at doses greater than 72 g/day (5 standard drinks/day). Women are at increased risk of harms from both chronic and acute ingestion of alcohol for a given consumption level.[22] Differences in women's physiology (lower body weight, less volume of distribution and smaller livers) may be responsible for this.

Risk of injury from motor and nonmotor vehicle accidents rises with increasing ingestion of alcohol.[22] Sporadic drinking of 5 or more drinks in a single day leads to worse long-term health outcomes than the same amount spread evenly over several days.[22] Alcohol use during pregnancy is associated with fetal alcohol spectrum disorder (FASD).[26]

Smoking

Smoking is the greatest known cause of avoidable morbidity and mortality and contributes directly or indirectly to 17% of all deaths in Canada.[27]

Second-hand smoke is associated with an increased risk of respiratory and heart disease with regular exposure and is estimated to be responsible for the death of 831 Canadians in 2002.[27] Although overall smoking rates in the decade prior to 2012 have decreased to 16% in people aged 15 years and older, this represents a hard-to-reach group.[27] Consumption of other tobacco products such as cigarillos has increased, especially among youth.[28]

A recommendation from a healthcare practitioner is one of the most important ways of influencing a patient to consider quitting.[29,30,31] Since it is estimated that most smokers start smoking as teenagers,[27] strategies to prevent smoking are as important as getting patients to quit.

Influenza and Pneumonia

Influenza and pneumonia cause significant morbidity and mortality in patients with chronic medical conditions, particularly in the elderly (see Chapter 24: Viral Rhinitis, Influenza, Rhinosinusitis and Pharyngitis).[32,33,34] Vaccination is the most effective method for preventing or attenuating influenza, yet only 35.8% of adults aged 18–64 years with a chronic medical condition received the influenza vaccine in 2008 in Canada.[33] Vaccination rates of non-institutionalized seniors are greater at 66.5% but these rates fall short of the national target of 80%.[33] Emerging research suggests influenza vaccination may provide indirect protection to others in the household or community.[35]

Invasive pneumococcal disease is a serious illness, which affects the very young, the elderly and individuals with immunosuppression or other chronic conditions.[36] Vaccination with **pneumococcal conjugate vaccine** is recommended for patients undergoing stem cell transplantation, patients with HIV and immunocompromised adults (e.g., asplenia, long-term immunosuppressive therapy, solid organ transplantation).[37] Use of the conjugate pneumococcal vaccine in infants appears to confer secondary protection in the elderly as a decline in invasive pneumococcal disease has been reported in this population.[38]

The **pneumococcal polysaccharide vaccine** is recommended for adults who required medical care for asthma within the last 12 months,[39] all immunocompetent adults 65 years of age and older, those <65 years of age in long-term care facilities, persons with alcoholism, smokers, persons who are homeless and individuals who use illicit drugs.[36]

Sun Exposure and Vitamin D

Skin cancer is the most frequently diagnosed cancer in Canada and the rate of diagnosis is increasing.[40] The Canadian Cancer Society recommends reduced exposure to the sun, particularly between 11 a.m. and 4 p.m. when the sun's rays are the strongest. Intermittent, intense sun exposure during childhood or adolescence, along with a history of sunburn, shows the strongest association with risk of melanoma.

A sunscreen with a sun protection factor (SPF) 15 or higher and SPF 30 for persons who work outdoors or will be outside for most of the day is recommended. Protection from ultraviolet radiation with hats, sunglasses and clothing that covers most of the skin should be used[40] (see Chapter 72: Prevention and Treatment of Sun-induced Skin Damage).

Most Canadians, including children and adolescents, may have insufficient vitamin D levels.[41,42] Persons with little sun exposure such as the elderly, individuals with dark skin and exclusively breastfed babies may be deficient in vitamin D. Sufficient vitamin D intake through diet alone is impractical and skin exposure to ultraviolet light may be poor due to Canada's northern latitudes and modern indoor lifestyle. Excessive exposure is associated with skin cancer. Therefore, oral supplementation may be required.

The effects of vitamin D on bone health (lowering risk of fracture) and improved muscle strength (lowering risk of falling) are well established.[43] In addition, epidemiologic evidence of vitamin D deficiency has been associated with a variety of nonmusculoskeletal diseases including cancer (particularly colon and breast), cardiovascular disease, infectious diseases, depression, dementia and other conditions.[44] However, prospective trials with vitamin D supplements using primary end points of other health risks, overall cancer rates, cardiovascular disease or mortality are lacking.[3] The Institute of Medicine (IOM) concluded there was insufficient high quality evidence to support supplementation above that required for bone health.[45] Further controlled and randomized trials are required to determine whether low vitamin D intake and stores is a marker of illness and which Canadians have insufficient vitamin D levels and require supplementation.

Goals of Disease Prevention

- Prevent or decrease risk of disease occurrence and minimize the need for future drug therapy
- Lower risk of developing some cancers (e.g., breast, colon, prostate, oral, esophageal)
- Lower risk of developing cardiovascular disease, diabetes, influenza and pneumonia
- Prevent fetal alcohol spectrum disorder
- Lower risk of cognitive decline

Patient Assessment

Gather information on lifestyle behaviours to quantify and document:

- tobacco use status (never used, ex-user, current tobacco use)
- diet and dietary patterns (fruit and vegetable intake, fibre intake, caloric intake)
- physical activity (types, quantity, frequency and duration)
- alcohol intake (e.g., number of standard drinks/day, occurrence of large amounts at one sitting)
- influenza vaccination (e.g., never, sporadically, yearly) and pneumococcal vaccine if indicated
- sun exposure habits

A risk assessment tool to determine the impact of lifestyle behaviours associated with increased longevity has been proposed by the Project Big Life. This self-assessment tool provides patients with information regarding their highest risk behaviour and allows persons to determine the amount of increased longevity if these behaviours were modified.

In addition to waist circumference cut-offs, the waist to height ratio (WHtR) is an easy-to-use tool for self-assessment of obesity-related health risks (Figure 1). Although not well known, the WHtR can be used in both children and adolescents[46] and as a screening tool for cardiometabolic risk in both Asian and non-Asian populations.[47]

Figure 1: Ashwell Shape Chart

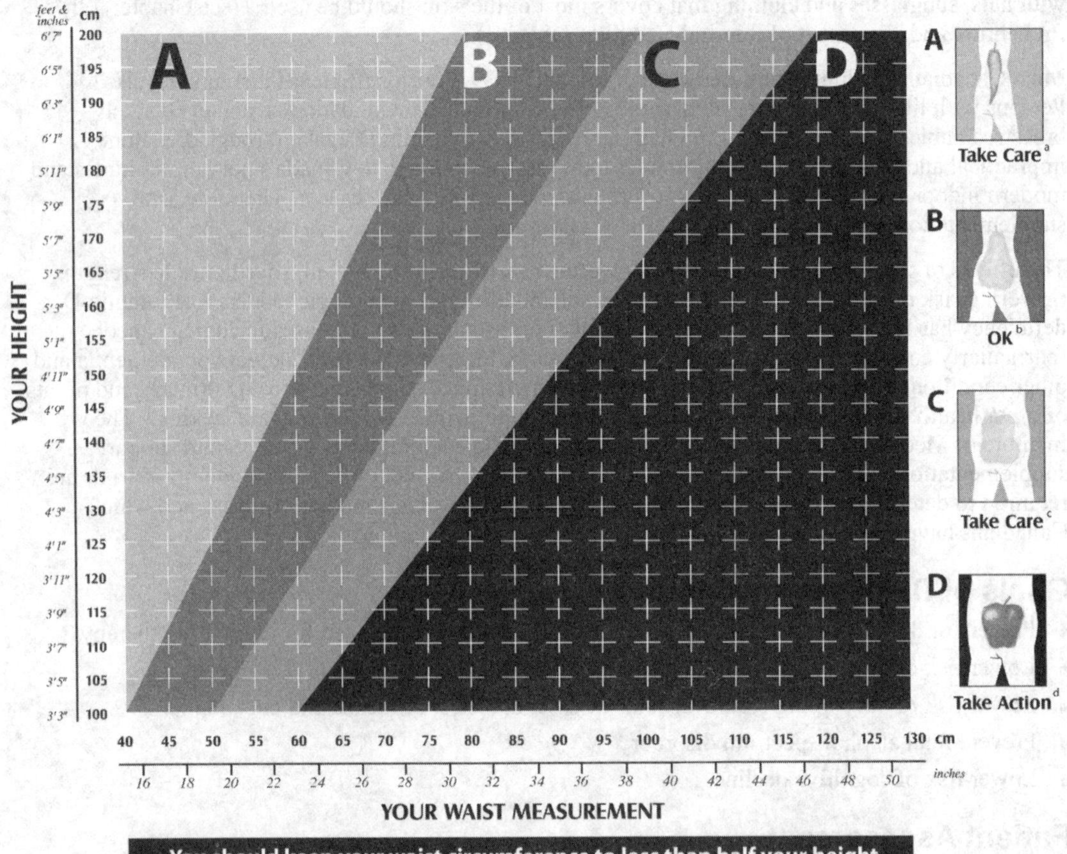

a If your shape is in this 'chili' region, you should **Take Care**. You will not need to decrease your waistline.
b If your shape is in this 'pear' region, you have a healthy **OK** shape.
c If your shape falls in this 'pearapple' region (particularly the upper end), you should **Take Care**. Adults over 18 years should consider action, children over 5 years should take action. Make sure you don't increase your waistline any more.
d If your shape falls into this 'apple' region, your health is probably at risk. Find out what you can do to **Take Action**.

Adapted from *The Ashwell Shape Chart: Are you an apple or a pear?* Available from: www.ashwell.uk.com with permission from Ashwell Associates.

Who Can Benefit from Health Promotion and Disease Prevention?

Surveys from the Behavioral Risk Factor Surveillance System show that only 5.1% of people without cardiovascular disease and 7.2% of people with coronary heart disease adhere to the public health promotion recommendations for physical activity, fruit and vegetable intake and smoking abstinence.[48] As a result, most patients will likely benefit from lifestyle modification and disease prevention behaviours. Examples of how patient presentation may suggest possible lifestyle interventions are shown in Table 1. Techniques for presenting lifestyle change to patients are discussed later in the chapter.

Table 1: **Patient Presentation and Possible Lifestyle Intervention**

Patient Presentation	Lifestyle Intervention	Resource Tip
Chronic headache	Regular physical activity	Chapter 8: Headache, exerciseismedicine.ca
Chronic insomnia	Regular physical activity	Chapter 5: Insomnia, exerciseismedicine.ca
Cough/cold	Smoking cessation, flu vaccination	Chapter 6: Smoking Cessation
Dyspepsia	Weight loss and exercise	Chapter 43: Weight Management, exerciseismedicine.ca
Mild low back pain	Regular physical activity	Chapter 45: Low Back Pain, exerciseismedicine.ca
Osteoarthritis	Diet and exercise, and potentially weight loss	Chapter 46: Osteoarthritis, exerciseismedicine.ca
Osteoporosis	Regular physical activity	Chapter 47: Osteoporosis, exerciseismedicine.ca

Strategies to Improve Lifestyle Management and Disease Prevention

The following strategies are addressed in Table 2.

Weight Control

A multimodal approach including dietary therapy, physical activity and behavioural therapy is essential for weight control.[5,61] To initiate weight loss a caloric deficit is the goal, while during weight maintenance, caloric intake of food needs to be equivalent to daily energy expenditure. A caloric deficit of 500 kcal/day should result in a weight loss of 0.5–1 kg per week. Professional help may be required; continuous monitoring and support are necessary and are provided by some commercial weight loss programs.[62] Further discussion of options for weight control can be found in Chapter 43: Weight Management.

Unfortunately, dietary interventions for obesity have shown little longterm efficacy, and initial weight loss of 5–10% is often reversed in 3–5 years regardless of the type of diet utilized.[63] However, weight losses of 3–4 kg on average are obtained in dietary interventions after 2 years;[54] this is often a clinically relevant effect. Emphasize eating whole foods such as fruits, vegetables, whole grains and reducing intake of processed, sugar-sweetened beverages[56] and foods high in fat and salt. Both low-fat and low-carbohydrate diets can produce significant weight loss; recommend a diet the patient can adhere to.[58]

Table 2: Disease Prevention and Health Promotion for Adults

Disease Prevention Strategy	Recommendations	Expected Benefits	Onset of Benefit	Cautions	Comments
Physical activity[49,50,51]	At least 2.5 h/wk of moderate to vigorous aerobic activity in bursts of 10 min or more: ▪ Moderate activity: Brisk walking (6 km/h), skating, bike riding. Person can talk but cannot sing ▪ Vigorous activity: Running, basketball, soccer, cross-country skiing. Person cannot speak in full sentences without taking a breath ▪ 45–60 min of intentional physical activity is preferable. Resistance or strength training twice weekly: ▪ push-ups, sit-ups, lifting weights, climbing stairs, digging in the garden ▪ bone strengthening (walking, running, yoga, dance). Children and adolescents should engage in at least 60 min per day of moderate to vigorous physical activity at least 5 times weekly. Limit or avoid prolonged sitting.	Reduction in all mortality causes Reduced risk of development of disease and type 2 DM, HTN, CHD Reduced risk of stroke Reduced risk of obesity Reduced risk of breast and colon cancer Improved mental outlook Reduced stress Improved balance and energy Improved sleep Beneficial in some chronic musculoskeletal disorders Prevents cognitive decline Slows progression of osteoporosis Weight control	3–4 wk for lipid values 4–6 wk for mental outlook and mild depression 10 y for all-cause mortality Benefits lost if exercise not continued; cannot be "stored up"	Patients should self-assess exercise risks based on their health conditions using the PAR-Q+[52] (see Resource Tips).	Emphasize the harms of sedentary behaviours. Discourage vigorous exercise in otherwise sedentary adults. Suggest gardening, walking, using stairs instead of an elevator, cleaning house and recreational activities. Walking suggested for most, as costs are low and no training required. Indoor walking or treadmills are options if weather poor. Encourage use of pedometer. 10-min sessions accumulated throughout the day is as effective as a single 30-min session. Additional health benefits seen with moderate to vigorous activity for >150 min/wk. Total energy expenditure is most important.
Nutrition[53,54,55,56,57]	Diet high in fruits, vegetables (6–10 servings), fibre, whole grains, rich in omega-3 fatty acids and protein sources that are low in trans-fat, saturated fat and cholesterol. Sodium intake of ≤1500 mg/day (approximately 1 tsp of table salt) is also recommended. Caloric intake matched to energy expenditure. Mediterranean diet associated with increased longevity, independent of weight.[58,59] Limit sugar sweetened beverages.	Reduced risk of cancers (colon, esophageal) Reduced risk of developing CHD Reduced risk of developing type 2 DM Reduced risk of stroke	3–4 wk for lipid values 1–5 y for CHD, DM, stroke	Clinical nutritionist or other professional with specialized nutritional expertise for patients with DM, dyslipidemia and CHD, morbid obesity. Patients with unstable medical or mental illnesses should be temporarily excluded from weight loss programs.	Healthy nutrition, exercise and weight control is key. Weight loss indicated if BMI >30 and comorbidity (DM, HTN, sleep apnea) or abdominal obesity as measured by waist circumference. Self assessment of health risks may be accomplished using the Ashwell Shape Chart (Figure 1). Encourage daily breakfast, weekly weighing and limiting fast food intake.

Disease Prevention Strategy	Recommendations	Expected Benefits	Onset of Benefit	Cautions	Comments
	Increase intake of vegetables. Other foods high in polyphenols (e.g., green/black tea, cocoa/dark chocolate) may be beneficial. Moderate coffee consumption (3–4 cups/day) not associated with health risks and may be beneficial. Caution in the elderly, persons with hypertension and children.			Unintentional weight loss should be referred to a physician. Evidence for weight loss in those >60 y without obesity-related factors is lacking. Weight stability is important.	
Tobacco cessation	Abstinence	Reduced risk of cancer, including breast cancer Reduced risk of CVD including stroke Reduced risk of osteoporosis Reduced risk of lung diseases	6 months for improvement in respiratory symptoms 3 y for risk reduction of CVD 10-y abstinence results in risk reduction of cancer to similar to that of nonsmokers	None	Address concern for increase in weight as absolute risk of smoking is greater than absolute risk of obesity. Discuss benefits and risks of smoking cessation drugs.
Alcohol[22,25,26]	Low to moderate alcohol consumption.[a] Abstinence if pregnant. Abstinence while driving a motor vehicle or boat.	Reduced risk of CVD achieved with consumption of approximately 1 drink every other day	5–10 y for benefit of CVD in patients >45 y Younger patients unlikely to benefit	Consumption outside low-risk guidelines associated with: ▪ Increased risk of cancer (esophageal, liver, mouth, pharynx, larynx) ▪ Increased risk of hypertension ▪ impaired social functioning. Consult appropriate healthcare practitioner if problem drinking identified.	Alcohol can potentiate post-prandial triglyceridemia; excessive alcohol intake combined with high carbohydrate intake can induce hypertriglyceridemia.

(cont'd)

Table 2: **Disease Prevention and Health Promotion for Adults** *(cont'd)*

Disease Prevention Strategy	Recommendations	Expected Benefits	Onset of Benefit	Cautions	Comments
Influenza/ pneumonia[36]	Influenza vaccination for: ▪ >65 y of age ▪ adults <65 y at high risk of influenza-related complications, their household contacts, healthcare workers, and all those wishing to be protected against influenza ▪ immunosuppression ▪ HIV Pneumococcal vaccination: ▪ adults ≥65 y ▪ adults <65 at increased risk of pneumococcal disease, i.e., those with asplenia, sickle cell disease, cirrhosis, alcoholism.	Reduced mortality due to influenza or pneumonia Reduced risk of hospitalization due to these diseases in patients >65 y	2 wk; influenza vaccination required yearly 2- to 3-wk onset for >10 y protection with pneumococcal vaccination	Contraindications to vaccination: ▪ egg allergy for influenza vaccination ▪ previous pneumococcal vaccination Address concerns regarding common vaccination myths.	Pneumococcal vaccination usually given only once.
Sun exposure and vitamin D supplementa-tion[42,43,44]	1000 IU of cholecalciferol (vitamin D_3) for adults during the fall and winter months.[60] Children and infants should receive 400 IU/day with sensible skin exposure. Patients with inadequate skin exposure due to religious or cultural dress, dark skin or lifestyle, malabsorption syndromes, obesity, chronic kidney disease are at higher risk.	Improved bone health and muscle strength Decreased risk of fracture Potential reduced mortality from cancer Potential reduced risk of respiratory diseases	3–5 y for cancer risk 1 y or longer for fracture risk reduction and bone health 3–4 wk for correction of insufficiency	Avoid excessive sun exposure, particularly sunburns. Vitamin D likely safe at total intake of ≤2000 IU/day. Patients with chronic granulomatous disorders (TB, sarcoidosis, some lymphomas) should be referred for assessment by appropriate healthcare practitioner. Doses >50 000 IU per day are associated with hypercalcemia and hyperphosphatemia.	Vitamin D toxicity does not occur with sun exposure but risk of skin cancer increased with exposure. Sensible skin exposure of 5–30 min, depending on skin type, of arms and legs at half minimal erythemal dose[b] can provide 400 IU of vitamin D. Exposure to 1 minimal erythemal dose in a swimsuit during the hours of 10:00 a.m. to 3:00 p.m. can provide the equivalent of 10 000 IU of vitamin D.

[a] Defined as ≤9 standard drinks per week for females or ≤14 standard drinks per week for males.
[b] Defined as amount of sunlight exposed before skin turns slightly red.

Abbreviations BMI = body mass index; CHD = coronary heart disease; CVD = cardiovascular disease; CSF = cerebrospinal fluid; DM = diabetes mellitus; HTN = hypertension; HIV = human immunodeficiency virus; MI = myocardial infarction; PAR-Q = physical activity readiness questionnaire; SBP = systolic blood pressure; TB = tuberculosis

Nutrition for Disease Prevention

Principles for nutrition include:

- eating a balanced proportion of food from different food groups
- eating a wide variety of foods from each food group
- eating in moderation

Canada's Food Guide recommends that carbohydrates comprise 45–55%, protein 10–35% and fat 20–35% of calories in the diet. The diet should be low in saturated fat, sugar and salt. Vegetables, fruits and grains are emphasized.[64]

The Mediterranean diet pyramid has been shown to improve mortality and morbidity in the secondary prevention of coronary artery disease, even if no weight loss occurs.[58,65] This diet is high in legumes, minimally processed whole grain products, fruits, vegetables, nuts and fish, and low in red and processed meat and dairy products. Olive oil is the major source of lipids. For prevention of disease, higher adherence to all aspects of the Mediterranean diet is associated with a lower risk of mortality, cardiovascular disease or mortality, cancer incidence or mortality and neurodegenerative diseases.[59] Nut consumption was associated with reduced CV risk as part of the Mediterranean diet[59] and has not been associated with weight gain if used as a replacement to other foods.[66]

The Dietary Approaches to Stop Hypertension (DASH) diet is a proven dietary pattern to treat hypertension. High fiber foods, vegetables, fruits and low-fat dairy products are emphasized while sodium, sweets, red meats and sugar-sweetened beverages are discouraged.[67]

The American Cancer Society also recommends a diet high in fruits and vegetables, a healthy weight and physical activity to reduce cancer risk.[8]

Green tea and cocoa contain polyphenolic flavanoids; green tea consumption in particular is associated with decreased CV and stroke risk.[57]

Physical Activity

Promote regular moderate physical activity to virtually all patients. Populations who may particularly benefit are cancer survivors, the elderly and those with chronic medical conditions. To identify potential risks, individualized exercise recommendations must be preceded by patients completing the revised PAR-Q+ which stratifies patients into low, intermediate (moderate) and high-risk categories.

For general or low risk patients the questions are:[52]

- Has your doctor ever said that you have a heart condition or high blood pressure?
- Do you feel pain in your chest at rest, during your activities of daily living, or when you do physical activity?
- Do you lose your balance because of dizziness, or have you lost consciousness in the last 12 months? (Please answer no if your dizziness was associated with over-breathing, including during vigorous exercise).
- Have you been diagnosed with another chronic medical condition? (other than heart disease or high blood pressure).
- Are you currently taking prescribed medications for a chronic medical condition?
- Do you have a bone or joint problem that could be made worse by a change in your physical activity? (Please answer no if you had a joint problem in the past but it does not limit your current ability to be physically active).
- Has your doctor ever said that you should only do medically supervised physical activity?

Patients who have answered no to all of the questions are cleared for physical activity and can exercise at moderate intensities with minimum supervision. If any of these questions are answered in the positive, the patient should be referred to the electronic Physical Activity Readiness Medical Examination (ePARmed-X+) available from eparmedx.com/. This online assessment tool further stratifies patients into intermediate or high risk and provides specific recommendations for physical activity and need for professional guidance and/or medical supervision. Most patients with relative contraindications can still exercise, but at lower levels of intensity; the risk of an adverse event related to exercise is very low even in those living with a chronic condition.[52] Patients should be clearly told to stop exercising and seek medical attention if they develop chest pain, light-headedness, or palpitations.

Moderate to vigorous aerobic activity is recommended in adults, including older adults, in order to achieve health benefits.[51] Moderate physical activity such as brisk walking (defined as 5–6 km/h or 3–4 mph), cycling, yoga or noncompetitive swimming is sufficient to reduce the risk of cardiovascular mortality and confers many other benefits, but more activity produces more benefits.[13,14,51] Resistance training or muscle-strengthening exercises are also recommended at least twice weekly for maintaining muscle mass and bone health and older adults should perform physical activity to maintain balance and prevent falls.[51] Combining aerobic activities of differing types and intensities, such as housekeeping, leisure and recreational activities is appropriate. It is important to know that a large volume of physical activity is required for weight loss if there is no concomitant caloric deficit. For weight maintenance, however, regular moderate amounts of intentional physical activity are required.

Success should be evaluated according to improvements in chronic disease factors or symptoms and by adopting healthy lifestyle habits, not by weight loss alone.[13,14] Despite little or no weight loss, increased exercise decreases visceral adiposity[68] and decreases mortality.[13,14,19,51] More physical activity provides greater health benefits but even 15 minutes/day may increase longevity compared to inactivity.[49] Exercise is also beneficial for maintaining flexibility and decreasing health risks in those who are sedentary or have significant limitations in their ability to exercise.[13] However, activity of moderate intensity and duration is required to achieve specific health outcomes such as reduction in the risk of type 2 diabetes.

Children are also encouraged to participate in moderate to intensite physical activity every day and to minimize sedentary behaviours such as screen time and time spent in sedentary transport.[51]

Pedometers provide an accurate, objective measure of walking and other ambulatory activity (see Table 3); for an average person 2000 steps is the equivalent of a 1.6-km (1-mile) walk. Pedometer-measured activity has shown Canadian adults average approximately 9000 steps/day,[12] which is considered a somewhat active lifestyle. Although the use of pedometers can increase physical activity over baseline and they are used to set and keep goals, current evidence suggests that pedometer use results in only modest increase in walking behaviours and weight loss.[69] However, this may be sufficient to limit weight re-gain.

Table 3: Pedometer-measured Activity[8,50]

Number of Steps per Day	Lifestyle Category
<5000	Sedentary
5000–7499	Low active (typical of daily activity excluding sports/exercise)
7500–9999	Somewhat active
≥10 000	Active

Primary care providers are using prescriptions for exercise, using validated tools. These tools may be accessed at exerciseismedicine.ca and are safe for healthy adults and those with stable chronic conditions. The tool includes the frequency, intensity, type and time format for exercise, and can include a referral to an exercise specialist. The addition of very accurate piezoelectrical pedometers to an exercise prescription can be useful, especially for those who ambulate at slower speeds like the elderly.[70] The Piezo Step Rx Series pedometer is classified as a medical device and maybe included as an insurable benefit. Pharmacists can initiate or support exercise prescriptions in their patients, display signage and provide appropriate pedometers to support these initiatives.

Vitamin D Supplementation

The optimal dietary requirement for vitamin D in healthy adults is currently evolving. Vitamin D is naturally present in very few foods, mainly fatty fish and egg yolks. The major sources of vitamin D in Canada are fortified foods such as cow's milk, soy beverages and calcium-fortified orange juice.[64] Endogenous vitamin D is produced in the skin with exposure to ultraviolet light but virtually none is produced during the winter months in Canada. To improve bone health, the recommended Dietary Reference Intakes (DRIs) for vitamin D are 600 IU (15 µg) for men and women aged 1–70 years and 800 IU (20 µg) for people older than 70 years.[71] Although more data are required to define optimal blood and intake levels, based on emerging data the Canadian Cancer Society recommends supplementation with 1000 IU of vitamin D (cholecalciferol) daily during the fall and winter to reduce the risk of breast, colon and prostate cancer.[60] In Canada, exclusively breastfed infants <1 year of age should receive 400 IU of vitamin D per day. Without adequate sun exposure, children and adults may require approximately 800–1000 IU per day.[71] Skin exposure of arms and legs for 5–30 minutes between 10 a.m. and 3 p.m. twice weekly is sufficient for vitamin D synthesis. However, because of the risks of ultraviolet radiation, a balanced diet, supplementation and limited skin exposure are the preferred methods of obtaining vitamin D. See Appendix VI: Nutritional Supplements for more information.

Immunization

Encourage pneumococcal vaccination in those at high risk. Refer to the Canadian Guidelines for Immunization by the National Advisory Committee on Immunization (NACI)[36] for further recommendations on pneumococcal vaccinations for infants and children. Review whether the patient is a candidate for other recommended vaccines such as tetanus.

Tobacco Cessation

Ask for the smoking status of patients and document this in the patient's profile. Recommend and initiate smoking cessation programs as appropriate (see Chapter 6: Smoking Cessation). Recommend stopping other tobacco products.

Alcohol

Encourage low-risk drinking for patients who drink alcohol, and in particular those who are receiving drugs known to have potentiating effects with alcohol. Patients who abstain from alcohol should not be encouraged to start drinking for its cardiovascular benefits, as there are other options and they may have a reason for abstinence. Inform all pregnant women of the risks of alcohol consumption and FASD. Emphasize abstinence in this population.[21] Consult the Society of Obstetricians and Gynaecologists of Canada website for more information.

Approaches to Health Behaviour Change

A high degree of awareness exists among the Canadian population regarding strategies for disease prevention and lifestyle modifications, and patients are very interested in preventive care.[72,73]

However, long-term improvements in dietary changes and physical activity levels have been hard to achieve[5,14,54] although smoking rates have fallen over the last decade.[27]

Effective approaches to improve lifestyle among patients are not yet established despite evidence of specific targets for physical activity, smoking and dietary behaviours known to improve longevity and decrease morbidity.[74] According to several behavioural and social theories, health promotion interventions that include interpersonal, intrapersonal, organizational and environmental factors may be more effective than those that focus solely on individuals.[74,75]

Population-based

Public health agencies, workplace integration, recreation, planning and regional, national and international partnerships have been suggested to increase physical activity levels at the population level.[75] This approach was successful in decreasing smoking rates.

Population-based strategies include media and educational campaigns, labeling and consumer information, economic incentives, school and workplace approaches, local environmental changes and direct restrictions and mandates.[75] Decision prompts encouraging the use of stairs versus elevators are one example of a successful public strategy.[76]

Individual-based

Strategies to assist clinicians in lifestyle management in the ambulatory setting have been proposed in 3 broad categories:[77]

- appropriate ways to discuss lifestyle changes including body weight
- multidisciplinary collaboration
- information technology strategies.

Approaching the Patient

Discussions with patients should always include the medical consequences of unhealthy lifestyle behaviours and should be delivered in a respectful and nonjudgemental manner. Emphasizing the harms of inactivity for example, instead of the benefits, has been suggested as a strategy to increase physical activity.[78]

Brief, effective interventions are often successful.[79,80,81] A new diagnosis of a chronic disease with a new prescription for drug therapy or other important life events can be a catalyst, increasing the likelihood that patients themselves identify the need for a lifestyle change.[81]

The model used for brief advice regarding smoking cessation has been adapted for health behaviours, including advice on lifestyle:[77]

- Ask (Do you perform physical activity regularly? Have you been told you have weight-related diseases?)
- Assess readiness for change (Are you interested in increasing physical activity?)
- Advise (Provide specific detailed information with an end point and time frame. Define small achievable goals)
- Assist (Identify barriers, personalize lifestyle changes, provide information and goal setting)
- Follow up (Include plans for self-monitoring, reinforcement and follow up).

Validated practical tools to assess diet and lifestyle that are quick to use may provide an efficient and accurate assessment of eating and physical activity behaviours.[82,83]

Multidisciplinary Collaboration/Multi-component Program

Programs to deliver lifestyle interventions usually consist of a weight loss goal of >5% of body weight, an increase in physical activity to at least 150 minutes/week, and a psychosocial intervention. A portion-controlled diet during the initial phase, then behavioural techniques, diet modification, physical activity and social support are the usual components of a lifestyle intervention. These programs do improve weight loss but effects wane over time.[84] Since intense lifestyle interventions require significant human resources, ongoing intervention and support are usually required, as is true with all chronic diseases.

Internet and Other Technologies

Since lifestyle interventions are a large component of primary care, technologies that can affect human resource and time constraints have generated much interest.

Most Internet-based lifestyle interventions include:[77]

- education about diet, physical activity, weight loss and maintenance
- self-monitoring
- individual goal setting
- motivation enhancement through online or electronically by a counsellor
- peer social support.

Internet behavioural weight loss programs with email counselling, or on-line support have been found to be effective in weight loss programs.[85] Mobile or digital health interventions have been used to improve CVD outcomes[86] including hypertension, increase smoking cessation rates,[87] and to improve physical activity and dietary recommendations.[88]

Online lifestyle interventions generally work as well as face-to-face interventions,[85] even in those older than 50 years.[89] However, long-term effects, potential risks and possible limitations to these approaches require further study.

Monitoring the Patient for Lifestyle Changes

Self-monitoring is important for lifestyle change as it is for any chronic condition.Table 4 provides a framework that requires individualization. Provide reinforcement with written or technology based plans and logs for self-monitoring, as this has been found to be useful especially for nutrition and exercise recommendations.[13]

Table 4: **Monitoring of Disease Prevention and Health Promotion**

Lifestyle Change	Monitoring	Endpoint	Actions
Weight loss and nutrition	Patient: Weight weekly while on diet, monitor fit of clothing, increased mobility, reduced drug requirements Healthcare practitioner: After 3–6 months	Decrease in 5–10% of body weight over 6 months.	If ineffective, consider referral to a formal weight management program and/or dietitian. If effective, moderately vigorous exercise recommended to prevent weight regain.
Exercise	Patient: Daily using activity logs/electronic methods and pedometers, increased stamina, flexibility and energy	2.5 h/wk moderate intensity: walking at 6 km/h or 4 mph pace spread out into sessions of 10 min or more. Muscle strengthening exercise twice	Start with 10 min per day, slowly increasing by 10 min, every 8–10 wk in elderly or sedentary patients.

(cont'd)

Table 4: **Monitoring of Disease Prevention and Health Promotion** *(cont'd)*

Lifestyle Change	Monitoring	Endpoint	Actions
	Healthcare practitioner: After 8–12 wk	weekly such as climbing stairs, lifting weights or yoga.	If walking, set goals, using a pedometer, of an increase of 2000–3000 steps a day over baseline; aim for 8000–10 000 steps per day if no functional limitations, lower amounts in the elderly or very sedentary. If ineffective, refer to other community resources.
Smoking	See Chapter 6: Smoking Cessation		
Alcohol	Patient: Weekly intake Healthcare practitioner: after 3–6 months	Alcohol intake within low-risk guidelines.	If ineffective, counsel to stage of change (see Chapter 2: Facilitating Behaviour Change). If problem drinking (impaired social functioning), refer for further assessment and treatment.
Sun exposure and vitamin D supplementation	Patient: Daily intake; limit exposure to sun during peak hours in summer Healthcare practitioner: after 3–6 months	No sunburn or excessive exposure.	Supplementation with vitamin D during winter months is suggested for patients >50 y.
Influenza/pneumococcal vaccines	Patient: In the fall for influenza via pharmacy or clinic, at any time for pneumococcal Healthcare practitioner: In the fall for influenza, at any time for pneumococcal	Yearly immunization with influenza, once for pneumococcal vaccine.	If ineffective, record in patient profile for recommendation the following year. Assess and address reasons for nonvaccination, counsel to stage of change.

Resource Tips

Smart Phone Applications:

Fitbit. Available from: www.fitbit.com/product/mobile/iphone.

Lose It. Available from: www.loseit.com.

MyFitnessPal. Available from: www.myfitnesspal.com/mobile.

SparkPeople. Available from: www.sparkpeople.com/mobile-apps.asp.

Web Sites:

Exercise is Medicine Canada. Available from: exerciseismedicine.ca

Mediterranean Diet Pyramid. Available from: oldwayspt.org/sites/default/files/images/Med_pyramid_flyer.jpg.

Pace Canada. Health provider's guide to counseling for healthy active living. Available from: www.idocc.ca/Guideline/References/23_PACE_Guide_for_Healthy_Active_Living.pdf.

PAR-Q+ and eParmed-X+ Online. Available from: eparmedx.com.

Physical Activity Line. Available from: www.physicalactivityline.com.

Project Big Life. Health calculators. Life expectancy. Available from: www.projectbiglife.ca/life/.

Simple Lifestyle Indicator Questionnaire and its scoring scheme. Available from: www.cfp.ca/content/54/1/76/F1.expansion.html

Suggested Reading

Canadian Society for Exercise Physiology. *Canadian physical activity and sedentary behaviour guidelines handbook.* . Available from: csep.ca/CMFiles/Guidelines/CSEP_Guidelines_Handbook.pdf.

Health Canada. *Eating well with Canada's food guide.* Available from: www.hc-sc.gc.ca/fn-an/food-guide-aliment/index-eng.php.

Lenz TL. *Lifestyle modifications in pharmacotherapy.* Philadelphia: Wolters Kluwer/Lippincott Williams & Wilkins; 2008.

References

1. Statistics Canada. *The 10 leading causes of death, 2011.* Available from: www.statcan.gc.ca/pub/82-625-x/2014001/article/11896-eng.htm. Accessed April 21, 2015.
2. Danaie G, Ding EL, Mozaffarian D et al. The preventable causes of death in the United States: comparative risk assessment of dietary lifestyle, and metabolic risk factors. *PLoS Med* 2009;6:e1000058.
3. Goodwin PJ. Vitamin D in cancer patients: above all, do no harm. *J Clin Oncol* 2009;27:2117-9.
4. World Health Organization. *Obesity and overweight. Fact sheet no. 311.* Geneva: WHO; 2015. Available from: www.who.int/mediacentre/factsheets/fs311/en/. Accessed June 4, 2015.
5. Public Health Agency of Canada. *Obesity in Canada.* Available from: www.phac-aspc.gc.ca/hp-ps/hl-mvs/oic-oac/intro-eng.php. Accessed April 21, 2015.
6. Roberts KC, Shields M, de Groh M et al. *Overweight and obesity in children and adolescents: results from the 2009 to 2011 Canadian Health Measures Survey.* Available from: www.statcan.gc.ca/pub/82-003-x/2012003/article/11706-eng.htm. Accessed June 19, 2015.
7. Lau DC, Douketis JD, Morrison KM et al. 2006 Canadian clinical practice guidelines on the management and prevention of obesity in adults and children [summary]. *CMAJ* 2007;176:S1-13.
8. Kushi LH, Doyle C, McCullough M et al. American Cancer Society Guidelines on nutrition and physical activity for cancer prevention: reducing the risk of cancer with healthy food choices and physical activity. *CA Cancer J Clin* 2012;62:30-67.
9. Prospective Studies Collaboration et al. Body-mass index and cause-specific mortality in 900 000 adults: collaborative analyses of 57 prospective studies. *Lancet* 2009;373:1083-96.
10. Douketis JD. Body weight classification. *CMAJ* 2005;172:1274-5.
11. Staiano AE, Reeder BA, Elliott S et al. Body mass index versus waist circumference as predictors of mortality in Canadian adults. *Int J Obes* 2012;36:1450-4.
12. Statistics Canada. *Directly measured physical activity of adults, 2012 and 2013.* Available from: www.statcan.gc.ca/pub/82-625-x/2015001/article/14135-eng.htm. Accessed April 27, 2015.
13. Warburton DE, Charlesworth S, Ivey A et al. A systematic review of the evidence for Canada's Physical Activity Guidelines for Adults. *Int J Behav Nutr Phys Act* 2010;7:39.
14. Lee IM, Shiroma EJ, Lobelo F et al. Effect of physical inactivity on major non-communicable disease worldwide: an analysis of burden of disease and life expectancy. *Lancet* 2012;380:219-29.
15. Rimer J, Dwan K, Lawlor DA et al. Exercise for depression. *Cochrane Database Syst Rev* 2012;7:CD004366.
16. Herring MP, Puetz TW, O'Connor PJ et al. Effect of exercise training on depressive symptoms among patients with a chronic illness: a systematic review and meta-analysis of randomized controlled trials. *Arch Intern Med* 2012;172:101-11.
17. Chou CH, Hwang CL, Wu YT. Effect of exercise on physical function, daily living activities, and quality of life in the frail older adults: a meta-analysis. *Arch Phys Med Rehab* 2012;93:237-44.
18. Sofi F, Valecchi D, Bacci D et al. Physical activity and risk of cognitive decline: a meta-analysis of prospective studies. *J Intern Med* 2011;269:107-17.
19. Willis BL, Gao A, Leonard D et al. Midlife fitness and the development of chronic conditions in later life. *Arch Intern Med* 2012;172:1333-40.
20. Pimlott N. The miracle drug. *Can Fam Physician* 2010;56:407, 409.
21. Bondy SJ, Rehm J, Ashley MJ et al. Low-risk drinking guidelines: the scientific evidence. *Can J Public Health* 1999;90:264-70.
22. Butt P, Beirness D, Gliksman L et al. *Alcohol and health in Canada: a summary of evidence and guidelines for low-risk drinking.* Ottawa: Canadian Centre on Substance Abuse. Available from: www.ccsa.ca/Resource%20Library/2011-Summary-of-Evidence-and-Guidelines-for-Low-Risk%20Drinking-en.pdf. Accessed April 27, 2015.
23. Berger K, Ajani UA, Kase CS et al. Light-to-moderate alcohol consumption and the risk of stroke among U.S. male physicians. *N Engl J Med* 1999;341:1557-64.
24. Howard AA, Amsten JH, Gourevitch MN. Effect of alcohol consumption in diabetes mellitus: a systematic review. *Ann Intern Med* 2004;140:211-9.
25. Bagnardi V, Blangiardo M, La Vecchia C et al. Alcohol consumption and the risk of cancer: a meta-analysis. *Alcohol Res Health* 2001;25:263-70.
26. Cook JL, Green CR, Lilley CM et al. Fetal alcohol spectrum disorder: a guideline for diagnosis across the lifespan. *CMAJ* 2016;188(3):191-7.
27. Health Canada. *Canadian Tobacco Use Monitoring Survey (CTUMS), 2012.* Available from: www.hc-sc.gc.ca/hc-ps/tobac-tabac/research-recherche/stat/ctums-esutc_2012-eng.php. Accessed April 25, 2015.
28. Physicians for a Smoke-Free Canada. *Cigarillo smoking in Canada: a review of results from CTUMS, Wave 1-2007.* Ottawa: Physicians for a Smoke-Free Canada; 2008. Available from: www.smoke-free.ca/pdf_1/cigarillos-2008.pdf. Accessed November 26, 2009.
29. Stead LF, Bergson G, Lancaster T. Physician advice for smoking cessation. *Cochrane Database Syst Rev* 2008;(2):CD00165.

30. U.S. Preventive Services Task Force. Counseling and interventions to prevent tobacco use and tobacco-caused disease in adults and pregnant women: U.S. Preventive Services Task Force reaffirmation recommendation statement. *Ann Intern Med* 2009;150:551-5.
31. ASHP therapeutic position statement on smoking cessation. American Society of Health-System Pharmacists. *Am J Health Syst Pharm* 1999;56:460-6.
32. Christenson B, Lundbergh P, Hedlund J et al. Effects of a large-scale intervention with influenza and 23-valent pneumococcal vaccines in adults aged 65 years or older: a prospective study. *Lancet* 2001;357:1008-11.
33. National Advisory Committee on Immunization (NACI). Statement on influenza vaccination for the 2012-2013 season. *Can Commun Dis Rep* 2012;38(ACS-4). Available from: www.phac-aspc.gc.ca/publicat/ccdr-rmtc/12vol38/acs-dcc-4/index-eng.php. Accessed October 9, 2012.
34. Treanor JD. Influenza-the goal of control. *N Engl J Med* 2007;357:1439-41.
35. Loeb M, Russell ML, Moss L et al. Effect of influenza vaccination of children on infection rates in Hutterite communities: a randomized trial. *JAMA* 2010;303:943-50.
36. Part 4. Active vaccines. Pneumococcal vaccine. In: *Canadian immunization guide*. Evergreen ed. Public Health Agency of Canada. National Advisory Committee on Immunization (NACI). Available from: www.phac-aspc.gc.ca/publicat/cig-gci/p04-pneu-eng.php. Accessed April 25, 2015.
37. National Advisory Committee on Immunization (NACI). An Advisory Committee Statement (ACS). Statement on the use of pneumococcal vaccine-13 valent in adults (Pneu-C-13). *Can Commun Dis Rep* 2013;39(ACS-5):1-52. Available from: www.phac-aspc.gc.ca/publicat/ccdr-rmtc/13vol39/acs-dcc-5/index-eng.php. Accessed April 25, 2015.
38. Whitney CG, Farley MM, Hadler J et al. Decline in invasive pneumococcal disease after the introduction of protein-polysaccharide conjugate vaccine. *N Engl J Med* 2003;348:1737-46.
39. National Advisory Committee on Immunization (NACI). An Advisory Committee Statement (ACS). *Update on the use of pneumococcal vaccines: addition of asthma as a high-risk condition*. Available from: www.phac-aspc.gc.ca/naci-ccni/acs-dcc/2014/pvaa-vaaa_0414-eng.php. Accessed April 27, 2015.
40. Canadian Cancer Society. *Canadian Cancer Statistics 2014. Special topic: skin cancers*. Available from: www.cancer.ca/~/media/cancer.ca/CW/cancer%20information/cancer%20101/Canadian%20cancer%20statistics/Canadian-Cancer-Statistics-2014-EN.pdf. Accessed April 27, 2015.
41. Statistics Canada. *Vitamin D levels of Canadians, 2012-2013*. Available from: www.statcan.gc.ca/pub/82-625-x/2014001/article/14125-eng.htm. Accessed April 27, 2015.
42. Schwalfenberg G. Not enough vitamin D: health consequences for Canadians. *Can Fam Physician* 2007;53:841-54.
43. Holick MF. Vitamin D deficiency. *N Engl J Med* 2007;357:266-81.
44. Haines ST, Park SK. Vitamin D supplementation: what's known, what to do, and what's needed. *Pharmacotherapy* 2012;32:354-82.
45. Ross AC, Manson JE, Abrams SA et al. The 2011 report on dietary reference intakes for calcium and vitamin D from the Institute of Medicine: what clinicians need to know. *J Clin Endocrinol Metab* 2011;96:53-8.
46. Freedman DS, Kahn HS, Mei Z et al. Relation of body mass index and waist-to-height ratio to cardiovascular disease risk factors in children and adolescents: the Bogalusa Heart Study. *Am J Clin Nutr* 2007;86:33-40.
47. Savva, SC, Lamnisos D, Kafatos AG. Predicting cardiometabolic risk: waist-to-height ratio or BMI. A meta-analysis. *Diabetes Metab Syndr Obes* 2013;6:403-19.
48. Miller RR, Sales AE, Kopjar B et al. Adherence to heart-healthy behaviors in a sample of the U.S. population. *Prev Chronic Dis* 2005;2:A18.
49. Wen CP, Wai JP, Tsai MK et al. Minimum amount of physical activity for reduced mortality and extended life expectancy: a prospective cohort study. *Lancet* 2011;378:1244-53.
50. Tudor-Locke C, Bassett DR. How many steps/day are enough? Preliminary pedometer indices for public health. *Sports Med* 2004;34:1-8.
51. Canadian Society for Exercise Physiology. *Canadian physical activity guidelines and Canadian sedentary behaviour guidelines*. Available from: www.csep.ca/guidelines. Accessed October 5, 2012.
52. Warburton DE, Jamnik VK, Bredin SS et al. The Physical Activity Readiness Questionnaire (PAR-Q+) and electronic Physical Activity Readiness Medical Examination (ePARmed-X+). *Health & Fitness Journal of Canada* 2011;4:3-23. Available from: www.healthandfitnessjournalofcanada.com/index.php/html/article/viewFile/103/66. Accessed October 5, 2012.
53. Bosomworth NJ. The downside of weight loss: realistic intervention in body-weight trajectory. *Can Fam Physician* 2012;58:517-23.
54. Katan MB. Weight-loss diets for the prevention and treatment of obesity. *N Engl J Med* 2009;360:923-5.
55. Hopper I, Billah B, Skiba M et al. Prevention of diabetes and reduction in major cardiovascular events in studies of subjects with prediabetes: meta-analysis of randomised controlled clinical trials. *Eur J Cardiovasc Prev Rehabil* 2011;18:813-23.
56. Malik VS, Popkin B, Bray GA et al. Sugar-sweetened beverages and risk of metabolic syndrome and type 2 diabetes: a meta-analysis. *Diabetes Care* 2010;33:2477-83.
57. Eilat-Adar S, Sinai T, Yosefy C et al. Nutritional recommendations for cardiovascular disease prevention. *Nutrients* 2013; 5(9): 3646-3683.
58. de Lorgeril M, Renaud S, Mamelle N et al. Mediterranean alpha-linolenic acid-rich diet in secondary prevention of coronary heart disease. *Lancet* 1994;343:1454-9.
59. Estruch R, Ros E, Salas-Salvado J et al. Primary prevention of cardiovascular disease with a Mediterranean diet. *N Engl J Med* 2013;368:1279-90.
60. Canadian Cancer Society. *Vitamin D*. Available from: www.cancer.ca/en/prevention-and-screening/live-well/vitamin-d/?region=on. Accessed November 12, 2015.
61. Kumanyika SK, Obarzanek E, Stettler N et al. Population-based prevention of obesity: the need for comprehensive promotion of healthful eating, physical activity, and energy balance: a scientific statement from the American Heart Association Council on Epidemiology and Prevention, Interdisciplinary Committee for Prevention (formerly the expert panel on population and prevention science). *Circulation* 2008;118:428-64.
62. Gudzune KA, Doshi RS, Mehta AK et al. Efficacy of commercial weight-loss programs: an updated systematic review. *Ann Intern Med* 2015;162:501-12.
63. Sacks FM, Bray GA, Carey VJ et al. Comparison of weight-loss diets with different compositions of fat, protein, and carbohydrates. *N Engl J Med* 2009;360:859-73.
64. Health Canada. *Eating well with Canada's food guide*. Available from: www.hc-sc.gc.ca/fn-an/food-guide-aliment/index-eng.php. Accessed October 9, 2012.
65. Willet WC, Sacks F, Trichopoulou A et al. Mediterranean diet pyramid: a cultural model for healthy eating. *Am J Clin Nutr* 1995;61:1402S-6S.

66. Jackson CL, Hu FB. Long-term associations of nut consumption with body weight and obesity. *Am J Clin Nutr* 2014;100:408S-11S.
67. Appel LJ, Moore TJ, Obarzanek E et al. A clinical trial of the effects of dietary patterns on blood pressure. *N Eng J Med* 1997;366:1117-24.
68. Irwin ML, Yasui Y, Ulrich CM et al. Effect of exercise on total and intra-abdominal body fat in postmenopausal women: a randomized controlled trial. *JAMA* 2003;289:323-30.
69. Khangura S, Grimshaw J, Moher D. *KTA evidence summary: pedometer-based interventions to reduce risk for and manage chronic disease*. Ottawa Hospital Research Institute; September 2010. Available from: www.ohri.ca/kta/docs/KTA-Pedometers-Evidence-Summary.pdf. Accessed October 9, 2012.
70. Melanson EL, Knoll JR, Bell ML et al. Commercially available pedometers: considerations for accurate step counting. *Prev Med* 2004;39:361-8.
71. Health Canada. *Vitamin D and calcium: updated Dietary Reference Intakes*. Available from: www.hc-sc.gc.ca/fn-an/nutrition/vitamin/vita-d-eng.php. Accessed September 24, 2015.
72. Cogswell B, Eggert MS. People want doctors to give more preventative care. A qualitative study of healthcare consumers. *Arch Fam Med* 1993;2:611-9.
73. Flocke SA, Clark A, Schlessman K et al. Exercise, diet, and weight loss advice in the family medicine outpatient setting. *Fam Med* 2005;37:415-21.
74. Mozaffarian D, Afshin A, Benowitz NL et al. Population approaches to improve diet, physical activity, and smoking habits: a scientific statement from the American Heart Association. *Circulation* 2012;126:1514-63.
75. Heath GW, Parra DC, Sarmiento OL et al. Evidenced-based intervention in physical activity: lessons from around the world. *Lancet* 2012;380:272-81.
76. Soler RE, Leeks KD, Buchanan LR et al. Point-of-decision prompts to increase stair use. A systematic review update. *Am J Prev Med* 2010;38:S292-300.
77. Rao G, Burke LE, Spring BJ et al. New and emerging weight management strategies for busy ambulatory settings: a scientific statement from the American Heart Association endorsed by the Society of Behavioral Medicine. *Circulation* 2011;124:1182-203.
78. Wen CP, Wu X. Stressing harms of physical inactivity to promote exercise. *Lancet* 2012;380:192-3.
79. Christian JG, Bessesen DH, Byers TE et al. Clinic-based support to help overweight patients with type 2 diabetes increase physical activity and lose weight. *Arch Intern Med* 2008;168:141-6.
80. Petrella RJ, Lattanzio CN. Does counseling help patients get active? Systematic review of the literature. *Can Fam Physician* 2002;48;72-80.
81. Keenan PS. Smoking and weight change after new health diagnoses in older adults. *Arch Intern Med* 2009;169:237-42.
82. Paxton AE, Strycker LA, Toobert DJ et al. Starting the conversation performance of a brief dietary assessment and intervention tool for health professionals. *Am J Prev Med* 2011;40:67-71.
83. Greenwood JL, Nurtaugh MA, Omura EM et al. Creating a clinical screening questionnaire for eating behaviors associated with overweight and obesity. *J Am Board Fam Med* 2008;21:539-48.
84. Dansinger ML, Tatsioni A, Wong JB et al. Meta-analysis: the effect of dietary counseling for weight loss. *Ann Intern Med* 2007;147:41-50.
85. Wieland LS, Falzon L, Sciamanna CN et al. Interactive computer-based interventions for weight loss or weight maintenance in overweight or obese people. *Cochrane Database Syst Rev* 2012;8:CD007675.
86. Widmer RJ, Collins NM, Collins CS et al. Digital health interventions for the prevention of cardiovascular disease: a systematic review and meta-analysis. *Mayo Clin Proc* 2015;90:469-80.
87. Spohr SA, Nandy R, Gandhiraj D et al. Efficacy of SMS text message interventions for smoking cessation: a meta-analysis. *J Subst Abuse Treat* 2015;56:1-10.
88. Liu F, Kong X, Cao J et al. Mobile phone intervention and weight loss among overweight and obese adults: a meta-analysis of randomized controlled trials. *Am J Epidemiol* 2015;181:337-48.
89. Aalbers T, Baars MA, Rikkert MG. Characteristics of effective Internet-mediated interventions to change lifestyle in people aged 50 and older: a systematic review. *Ageing Res Rev* 2011;10:487-97.

Healthy Active Living—What You Need to Know

Be active:

- Take part in moderate to vigorous activity, such as brisk walking, for at least 2.5 hours per week. You can do your activities in three 10-minute sessions spaced out during the day.
- More exercise is better.
- Add stair climbing or lifting weights to your regimen at least twice weekly.
- Use an activity record and pedometers to keep track of what you do every day—see Table 1 for an example.

Consult *Tips to Get Active* available from www.phac-aspc.gc.ca/hp-ps/hl-mvs/pa-ap/04paap-eng.php.

Eat sensibly:

- Weigh yourself regularly.
- Eat breakfast every day and limit fast food meals.
- Eat 5 to 10 servings a day of fruit and vegetables.
- Increase fibre by eating oatmeal, barley, brown rice, whole wheat and dried beans, peas and lentils.
- Cut down on fat in cooking and reduce the amount you add to food (e.g., butter on bread).
- Limit red and processed meats—choose poultry or fish instead.
- Avoid high-fat and sugary desserts, sweetened beverages, snack foods and processed foods.
- Cut down on calories and have smaller portions if you have been told to lose weight.
- Use a food record to keep track of what you eat—see Table 2 for an example.

Consult *Canada's Food Guide* available from www.hc-sc.gc.ca/fn-an/food-guide-aliment/index-eng.php.

Stop smoking:

- If you don't smoke, don't start.
- Talk to your doctor or pharmacist about how to quit. There are many choices to help you.

If you drink alcohol, drink moderately:

- Do not drink and drive a motor vehicle or a boat.
- Do not drink if you are pregnant.
- Moderate drinking means:
  - No more than 2 standard drinks a day for men
  - No more than 1 standard drink a day for women
  - A standard drink is: 1.5 oz (45 mL) hard liquor or spirits, *or* 5 oz (150 mL) wine, *or* 12 oz (360 mL) beer.

Protect yourself from the flu and pneumonia:

- Get the flu shot every year.
- Get vaccinated against pneumococcal pneumonia if you are at high risk.
- Discuss vaccination with your doctor or pharmacist or contact the public health unit.

- For more information on flu shots and vaccination visit healthycanadians.gc.ca/diseases-conditions-maladies-affections/disease-maladie/flu-grippe/index-eng.php/.

Could you benefit from Vitamin D supplements?

- All adults >51 years of age
- Little sun exposure, poor dietary intake of vitamin D, obesity
- Consider taking at least 1000 IU/day of vitamin D_3 (cholecalciferol) in the fall and winter months

Table 1: **Example of a Physical Activity Log**

Week #		Endurance	Strength	Flexibility	Total Minutes	Total Steps
	Mon					
	Tues					
	Wed					
	Thurs					
	Fri					
	Sat					
	Sun					
	Weekly Totals					
Place a ✓ (checkmark) in the appropriate box for every 10 minutes of activity. If you are using a pedometer, record the daily total in the Total Steps column.						

Table 2: **Example of a Food Record Log**

Date	Food Description	Serving Size	Time	Hunger Level
Breakfast				
Snack				
Lunch				
Snack				
Dinner				
Snack				

Chapter 28

Assessment of Patients with Abdominal Pain

Peter Thomson, BSc(Pharm), PharmD

Abdominal pain is a nonspecific symptom arising from a variety of sources both within and external to the GI tract. Virtually everyone experiences abdominal symptoms on an intermittent basis, which can have an impact on both personal and societal resources (e.g., dyspepsia alone can account for 5% of family physician visits[1]). Fortunately, the vast majority of symptoms are benign in nature.

Pathophysiology

Excluding an acute abdomen, sites within the GI tract that contribute to the majority of GI complaints include the esophagus (e.g., GERD), stomach (e.g., peptic ulcer disease), liver (e.g., hepatitis), gallbladder (e.g., cholelithiasis), pancreas (e.g., pancreatitis) and intestines (e.g., abdominal hernia, cancer of the colon, constipation, diverticulitis, inflammatory bowel disease, lactose intolerance).

Irritable bowel syndrome (IBS) and functional dyspepsia (FD) are common functional disorders of the GI tract; these are prevalent in both the adult and pediatric populations. Formal classification of functional GI disorder subtypes can be found in the ROME III criteria.[2]

Although not a requirement, pain and abdominal discomfort due to IBS are more often localized below the umbilicus in combination with alteration in the frequency of bowel movements and/or consistency of the stool, whereas symptoms of dyspepsia usually arise from the epigastrium and include heartburn, reflux, pain (or discomfort) and nausea. IBS and FD are not likely to increase the risk of pathologic GI disorders yet they may significantly impair quality of life and increase utilization of healthcare resources. Together they can account for roughly half of all referrals to outpatient gastroenterology clinics.[3]

There are a number of evidence-based guidelines for the assessment and management of dyspepsia in adults.[1,4,5,6] In general, the goal is to ensure that those with serious GI pathology seek prompt investigation and treatment and to minimize overuse of diagnostic investigations unlikely to provide useful information.[5,7,8]

Patient Assessment

Indications of Serious GI Pathology

Individuals presenting with common symptoms associated with serious GI pathology should seek timely medical attention. In a study of over 150 patients who developed gastric or esophageal cancer under the age of 55 years, over 97% had at least 1 the following serious signs and symptoms: dysphagia, weight loss (>3 kg over 6 months), persistent vomiting, bleeding, anemia, hematemesis or melena.[9] Additional "red flags" include: age >50 years (especially if new onset dyspepsia or recent change in symptoms), jaundice, cancer history (strong family history) and multiple treatment failures. Fever and chills can represent an infectious source of abdominal pain requiring medical assessment (see Figure 1).

Figure 1: **Assessment of Patients with Chronic Abdominal Pain**

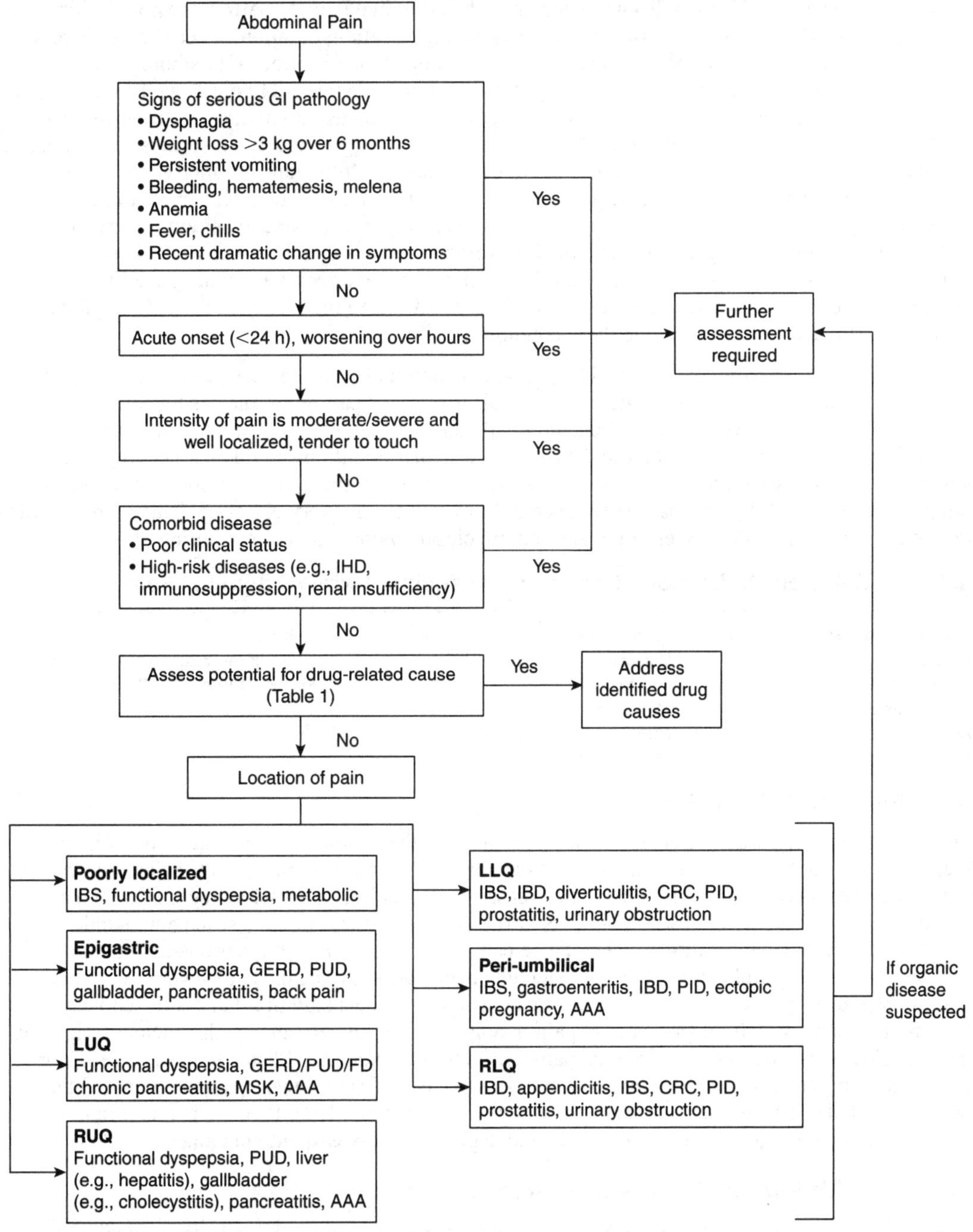

Abbreviations: AAA = abdominal aortic aneurysm; CRC = colorectal cancer; FD = functional dyspepsia; IBD = inflammatory bowel disease; IBS = irritable bowel syndrome; IHD = ischemic heart disease; LLQ = left lower quadrant; LUQ = left upper quadrant; MSK = musculoskeletal; PID = pelvic inflammatory disease; RLQ = right lower quadrant; RUQ = right upper quadrant

Assessment of Patient Acuity

Obtain a detailed medical history from the person with abdominal pain, to narrow the possibilities to a few key potential diagnoses. Key assessment issues include location, duration, severity and triggers of pain, comorbid medical conditions and medication use. If no signs of serious GI pathology are apparent, undertake a systematic assessment of abdominal pain. Acute (<24 hours), well-localized, moderate or severe pain worsening over hours and tender to touch usually indicates a need for medical attention. Triggers of pain such as medications and foods may suggest specific disorders such as peptic ulcer disease (PUD), GERD, lactase deficiency or celiac disease. Intolerance to foods can also give rise to abdominal pain. Spicy foods, citrus fruits and foods with a high fat content are examples. Postprandial pain is often associated with overindulgence. High fat intake and certain foods can produce indigestion and trigger symptoms of IBS. Review timing of pain with meals and current medications (including herbals and vitamins). Evaluate alcohol and recreational drug use (if appropriate). Certain disease states such as renal failure and heart failure may cause abdominal pain. Frequently, pain is diffuse in nature in these conditions.

Medications are commonly associated with epigastric abdominal pain (Table 1) and the presence of medication-induced dyspepsia is not necessarily indicative of GI pathology such as bleeding. Comorbid diseases can produce or mimic abdominal pain and may warrant further assessment (e.g., ischemic heart disease, psychiatric disorders). Particular attention should be given to patients using immunosuppressive medications such as systemic corticosteroids, in whom the symptoms of clinically important GI disease may be attenuated. Extremes in age (very elderly, infants <1 month old) are often at risk of rapid decompensation and require closer evaluation and monitoring.[10]

Table 1: **Selected Medications Commonly Associated with Abdominal Pain**

Amiodarone (especially loading dose)	Antiretrovirals	Opioids
Antibiotics	Dabigatran	Sildenafil (especially in the treatment of pulmonary hypertension)
Antiepileptic drugs	Iron salts	SSRIs
Antineoplastics	Metformin	Sulfasalazine
Antipsychotics	NSAIDs, ASA and other antiplatelet agents	

Location of Abdominal Pain

Pain is often, but not always, localized to different areas of the abdomen. Localization often helps determine the most likely causes of the pain. It may also assist in assessing when to refer a patient for medical care. Pain commonly arises from the epigastric, periumbilical or pelvic regions as well as from the right, left, upper and lower quadrants. More common causes of epigastric pain include GERD, PUD, FD and pancreatitis (the latter also causes back pain). Right upper quadrant pain often involves the liver or gallbladder but can also include pancreatitis. Acute onset of severe right upper quadrant pain usually requires medical assessment, as this may be a sign of biliary colic, cholecystitis or biliary obstruction. Left upper quadrant pain may involve the spleen but can also include epigastric and musculoskeletal sources of abdominal pain. Periumbilical pain may be due to gastroenteritis or inflammatory bowel disease (IBD) in addition to IBS. Causes of right lower quadrant pain include appendicitis, IBD, IBS and pelvic organs. Small bowel obstruction, IBD, IBS and pelvic inflammatory disease (or ectopic pregnancy) can appear as either right or left lower quadrant pain.[10]

Caveats to Abdominal Pain Assessment

In many cases, the cause of abdominal pain varies with patient age as well as comorbid medical conditions. There is a considerable overlap in symptoms among many of the common disorders that cause abdominal pain. For example, over 80% of patients with IBS will also exhibit symptoms of dyspepsia.[11] Moderate to intense pain is not a characteristic feature of dyspepsia. In biliary tract disease and pancreatitis, the pain is usually acute and more intense in nature.[11]

Recurrent periumbilical abdominal pain occurs in various intensities in approximately 10% of school-aged children. Nausea and vomiting may also occur but weight loss is uncommon. In over 90% of cases there is no organic cause. Stress (e.g., school) may be a component. Drug therapy is generally not recommended.[12]

Suggested Readings

Gans SL, Pols MA, Stoker J et al. Guideline for the diagnostic pathway in patients with acute abdominal pain. *Dig Surg* 2015;32:23-31.

Marsicano E, Vuong GM, Prather CM. Gastrointestinal causes of abdominal pain. *Obstet Gynecol Clin North Am* 2014;41:465-89.

References

1. National Institute for Health and Care Excellence (NICE). *Gastro-oesophageal reflux disease and dyspepsia in adults: investigation and management.* NICE guidelines [CG184]; November 2014. Available from: www.nice.org.uk/guidance/cg184. Accessed February 25, 2016.
2. Rome Foundation. *Appendix A: Rome III diagnostic criteria for functional gastrointestinal disorders.* Available from: www.romecriteria.org/assets/pdf/19_RomeIII_apA_885-898.pdf. Accessed February 25, 2016.
3. Jones J, Boorman J, Cann P et al. British Society of Gastroenterology guidelines for the management of the irritable bowel syndrome. *Gut* 2000;47:ii1-19.
4. Talley NJ; American Gastroenterological Association. American Gastroenterological Association medical position statement: evaluation of dyspepsia. *Gastroenterology* 2005;192:1753-5.
5. Veldhuyzen van Zanten SJ, Flook N, Chiba N et al. An evidence-based approach to the management of uninvestigated dyspepsia in the era of Helicobacter pylori. Canadian Dyspepsia Working Group. *CMAJ* 2000;162:S3-23.
6. Mason JM, Delaney B, Moayyedi P et al. Managing dyspepsia without alarm signs in primary care: new national guidance for England and Wales. *Aliment Pharmacol Ther* 2005;21:1135-43.
7. Suzuki H, Nishizawa R, Hibi T. Therapeutic strategies for functional dyspepsia and the introduction of the Rome III classification. *J Gastroenterol* 2006;41:513-23.
8. Veldhuyzen van Zanten SJ, Bradette M, Chiba N et al. Evidence-based recommendations for short- and long-term management of uninvestigated dyspepsia in primary care: an update of the Canadian Dyspepsia Working Group (CanDys) clinical management tool. *Can J Gastroenterol* 2005;19:285-303.
9. Gillen D, McColl KE. Does concern about missing malignancy justify endoscopy in uncomplicated dyspepsia in patients aged less than 55? *Am J Gastroenterol* 1999;94:75-9.
10. Millham FH. Acute abdominal pain. In: Feldman M, Friedman LS, Brandt LJ, eds. *Sleisenger and Fordtran's gastrointestinal and liver disease: pathophysiology, diagnosis, management.* 10th ed. Philadelphia: Saunders/Elsevier; 2016. p 161-74.
11. Tack J. Dyspepsia. In: Feldman M, Friedman LS, Brandt LJ, eds. *Sleisenger and Fordtran's gastrointestinal and liver disease: pathophysiology, diagnosis, management.* 10th ed. Philadelphia: Saunders/Elsevier; 2016. p. 183-96.
12. Hay WW. Recurrent abdominal pain. In: Hay WW, Hayward AR, Levin MJ et al., eds. *Current pediatric diagnosis and treatment.* 14th ed. Old Tappan: Appleton & Lange; 1999. p. 550-2.

Chapter 29
Constipation

Jane Bowles-Jordan, BScPhm, CDE

Pathophysiology

Constipation is generally defined as defecation fewer than 3 times per week accompanied by other symptoms including hard stools, feeling of incomplete evacuation, excessive straining, a sense of rectal blockage and abdominal discomfort, bloating and distention.[1] Some patients incorrectly believe that a daily bowel movement is necessary and that anything less means they are constipated. In fact, the average number of bowel movements for adults and children 3 years of age or older in the Western world varies from 3 daily to 1 every 3 days.[2,3]

Constipation can be a symptom secondary to a drug or disease (see Table 1).[4,5,6,7] Chronic constipation that does not have drug, anatomic or physiologic causes is termed functional or chronic idiopathic constipation and is defined by the ROME III criteria (see Table 2).[4,8]

If left untreated, chronic constipation may lead to serious complications such as bowel perforation, obstruction, fecal impaction, peritoneal infection, anal fissures, hemorrhoids, megacolon, pelvic organ prolapse in women and volvulus.[9,10,11]

Risk factors for chronic or acute constipation include:[12,13,14,15]

- Female gender
- Non-white
- Living in rural, northern or mountainous areas in North America[13]
- Age over 65 years
- Fewer years of formal education
- Low caloric intake
- Greater number of medications used
- Lower socioeconomic status
- Physical and sexual abuse
- Sedentary lifestyle
- Travelling
- Toilet training (in children)
- Ignoring the urge to defecate (habituates the rectum to the stimulus of the fecal mass).

Table 1: Medications and Conditions Associated with Chronic Constipation

Medications

5-HT3 receptor antagonists
ondansetron
Anticholinergics
Antidepressants
bupropion
mirtazapine
monoamine oxidase inhibitors
trazodone
tricyclic antidepressants
venlafaxine
Antidiarrheal agents
diphenoxylate
loperamide

Antiepileptics
gabapentin
phenytoin
pregabalin
Antihistamines
diphenhydramine
hydroxyzine
Antihypertensives
clonidine
nifedipine
verapamil

Antinauseants
dimenhydrinate
prochlorperazine
promethazine
scopolamine
Antiparkinsonian agents
amantadine
benztropine
bromocriptine
levodopa
pramipexole
ropinirole
Antipsychotics

Antispasmodics
dicyclomine
Cation-containing agents
aluminum
barium
bismuth
calcium
iron
Diuretics
NSAIDs
Opioids
Resins
cholestyramine
sodium polystyrene sulfonate
Vinca alkaloids

Conditions

Anatomic obstructions
Diverticulosis
Post surgical abnormalities
Stricture
Cancer
Chemotherapy-induced dehydration
Direct intestinal radiation
Hormonal changes
Hypercalcemia
Tumor compression of large intestine
Tumor interference with colonic innervations
Dementia

Endocrine/metabolic disorders
Chronic renal failure/uremia
Cystic fibrosis
Diabetes
Hyper/hypocalcemia
Hyperparathyroidism
Hypokalemia
Hypomagnesemia
Hypothyroidism
Panhypopituitarism
Porphyria
Uremia

GI motor disorders
Hirschsprung's disease
Irritable bowel syndrome
Megarectum and megacolon
Pelvic floor dysfunction
Rectoceles
Neurogenic disorders
Autonomic neuropathy
Intestinal pseudo-obstruction
Multiple sclerosis
Parkinson's disease
Spinal cord injury
Stroke
Systemic sclerosis

Older age
Pain
Secondary to anal fissures, hemorrhoids
Pregnancy
Psychiatric disorders
Abuse, anxiety, brain injury, depression, eating disorders

Table 2: ROME III Diagnostic Criteria for Chronic Functional Constipation[8]

The following must be present for at least 3 months with an onset of at least 6 months prior to diagnosis:

1. Loose stool rarely present without use of laxatives, *and*
2. Insufficient criteria to classify as irritable bowel syndrome, *and*
3. At least 2 of the following criteria:
   - Straining[a]
   - Lumpy or hard stools[a]
   - Sensation of incomplete evacuation[a]
   - Sensation of anorectal obstruction/blockage[a]
   - Manual manoeuvres to facilitate defecation (e.g., digital evacuation, support of the pelvic floor)[a]
   - Fewer than 3 defecations per week

[a] Must be present in at least a quarter of the defecations.

Goals of Therapy

- Treat or correct the secondary cause of constipation
- Return frequency of stool to previous normal or at minimum ≥3 defecations per week
- Eliminate symptoms of straining, incomplete emptying, bloating, pain and obstruction
- Improve stool consistency
- Improve quality of life
- Avoid complications of constipation
- Use laxatives appropriately

Patient Assessment

Assessment of patients with constipation is necessary to delineate root causes (Figure 2).[16,17] The Bristol Stool Scale is a valuable medical communication aid designed to assist patients in describing bowel patterns in a way that is more useful for diagnosis and evaluation of treatment (Figure 1).

Diagnostic colon motility tests (e.g., colonic transit studies, colon motility, colonic barostat testing) are usually reserved for patients with chronic idiopathic constipation who are unresponsive to regular laxative therapy.[6,8]

Figure 1: **Bristol Stool Chart**[a]

Stool form	Appearance	Type
Separate hard lumps like nuts, (hard to pass). Result of slow transit.	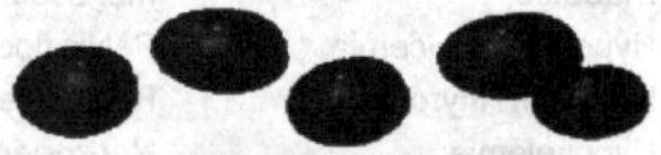	1
Sausage-shaped but lumpy.		2
Like a sausage but cracks on its surface.	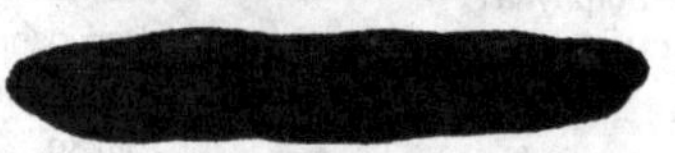	3
Like a sausage or snake—smooth and soft.		4
Soft blobs with clear cut edges (easy to pass).	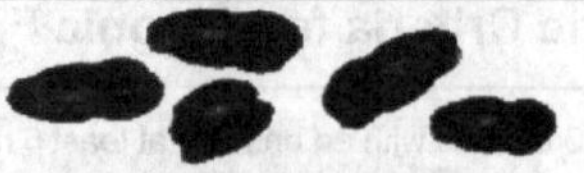	5
Fluffy pieces with ragged edges, a mushy stool.		6
Watery, no solid pieces. Result of very fast transit.		7

[a] Types 1–2 indicate constipation, types 3–4 represent ideal stool consistencies as they are easier to pass and types 5–7 may indicate diarrhea and urgency.

Reproduced with permission from Thompson WG, Heaton KW. *Fast facts: irritable bowel syndrome*. 2nd ed. Oxford (GB): Health Press Limited; 2003.

Signs and symptoms of constipation include:

- infrequent defecation
- abdominal distention
- nausea
- vomiting
- anorexia
- early satiety
- stools that are small, hard and/or difficult to evacuate
- incomplete rectal emptying
- rectal bleeding due to fissures or hemorrhoids
- weight loss (in chronic constipation).

Fecal impaction is the inability to pass a hard collection of stool. Symptoms of impaction include rectal discomfort, anorexia, nausea, vomiting, abdominal pain, urinary frequency and both fecal and urinary overflow incontinence. Physically or mentally incapacitated persons and the elderly are at particular risk of impaction, as are those who require long-term use of medications associated with constipation (Table 1).

In the initial patient assessment, review prescription and nonprescription medications to rule out drug-induced causes (Table 1). This review must also include natural health products since their overuse could cause gut dysfunction and paradoxical constipation.[17]

Examine diet, exercise and relevant social or psychological problems. Patients often have self-medicated prior to asking for assistance. Address the patient's most bothersome symptoms and inquire about past laxative use and failed therapies, to help maximize adherence and reduce possible side effects.[2]

Further assessment is required if constipation is accompanied by the following red flags:

- children <2 years old
- constipation for more than 2 weeks (or no bowel movement for more than 7 days) despite use of laxatives, particularly in the elderly and in those with chronic medical conditions such as diabetes or Parkinson's disease
- blood or mucus in stool or rectal bleeding, fever
- symptoms suggestive of anemia such as fatigue or lethargy
- family history of colon cancer (particularly if patient is >50 years old)
- persistent abdominal pain
- vomiting
- severe pain upon defecation
- unremitting nocturnal symptoms
- diarrhea alternating with constipation (could signify irritable bowel syndrome)
- recent abdominal surgery
- eating disorders such as bulimia nervosa
- moderate to extreme thirst
- unexplained weight loss of greater than 5%
- chronic illness associated with constipation (Table 1)
- rectal or abdominal mass.

After a thorough assessment, if the above red flag symptoms are absent and further investigation not required, then nonpharmacologic and pharmacologic therapy can be recommended for mild-moderate acute cases.

Prevention

The following strategies may be used to prevent constipation:[18]

- High-fibre diet (should be complemented with a minimum fluid consumption of 1500 mL daily)
- Regular, private toilet routine
- Heed the urge to defecate
- Use of a prophylactic laxative if using constipating medication or in presence of diseases associated with constipation
- Moderate daily physical activity may be helpful in mild constipation, particularly in the elderly. Vigorous exercise does not affect bowel habits in healthy subjects[19]
- Increasing the amount of fluid intake has been controversial unless patient usually drinks very little or is dehydrated.[9]

Daily fibre intake of at least 25 g for adult females and 38 g for adult males younger than 50 years is currently recommended for increased laxation and softening of stool.[20] Few adults consume this level; 10 g per day of total dietary fibre is often sufficient as a daily minimum goal. Stool weight increases and fecal transit time usually decreases with adequate fibre supplementation but pain or stool frequency usually do not improve.[9] Soluble fibre (e.g., psyllium) may improve symptoms of straining and pain and may increase the number of bowel movements in patients with chronic idiopathic constipation. Data for insoluble fibre (e.g., dark leafy vegetables, rye bread, wheat bran, whole grains) are conflicting.[21] Patients with confirmed slow-transit constipation or pelvic floor dyssynergia respond poorly to a high fibre diet. Table 3 lists the fibre content of some common foods.

Table 3: **Dietary Fibre in Selected Raw Foods**[22]

Food Source	≥5 g fibre/100 g	2–5 g fibre/100 g	<2 g fibre/100 g
Vegetables	Artichoke heart Beans, pinto Beans, red kidney Chickpeas Lentils Peas, green	Asparagus Beets Broccoli Brussels sprouts Cabbage Carrots Cauliflower Eggplant Garlic Kale Parsnips Potato with skin Snow peas Spinach Sweet corn	Celery Cucumber Iceberg lettuce Mushrooms Onions Pepper, green Radish Rhubarb Tomato Turnip Winter squash Zucchini
Fruits	Avocado Blackberries Plums Prunes	Apples with skin Apricots Banana Blueberries	Cantaloupe Grapefruit Grapes Honeydew melons

(cont'd)

Table 3: **Dietary Fibre in Selected Raw Foods**[22] *(cont'd)*

Food Source	≥5 g fibre/100 g	2–5 g fibre/100 g	<2 g fibre/100 g
	Raspberries	Cherries, sweet Figs Kiwi Orange, navel Pears Raisins, seedless Strawberries	Mango Papaya Peaches Pineapple Watermelons
Cereals	All Bran Bran Buds Bran Flakes Cheerios Fiber1 Just Right Life Mini Wheats Multigrain Cheerios Oat Bran Puffed Wheat Raisin Bran Shredded Wheat Weetabix	Captain Crunch Corn Flakes Special K	Rice Krispies
Breads	Pita bread, whole wheat Pumpernickel bread Rye bread Whole-wheat bread	Bagel, oat bran Bagel, plain English muffin Kaiser roll Muffin, oat bran Nutrigrain waffle Pita bread, white Taco shell	
Nuts	Almonds Brazil nuts Hazelnut Macadamia Peanuts Pistachio Walnuts		
Miscellaneous	Popcorn		Brown rice White rice Wild rice

Nonpharmacologic Therapy

Adults

- Increase calories in low calorie diets: This helps improve colonic transit.[9]
- Have a regular bowel regimen: Patients should attempt to have a bowel movement at the same time each day especially after breakfast since colonic activity is highest at that time. Encourage patients to heed the urge to defecate and discourage them from spending prolonged periods of time at the

toilet. Placing a footstool in front of the toilet helps elevate the thighs, thus placing the pelvis in the optimum position for defecation.[2,5]

- Consume a high-fibre diet: The target is 25–38 g of fibre daily or 10–20 g/1000 cal.[20,23] Table 3 lists the fibre content of some common foods. Patients with poor dentition can eat foods that are easy to chew such as bran muffins, bran cereal, fibre biscuits, applesauce and baked beans. Fibre-enriched formulations of nutritional supplement drinks are available for those patients unable to prepare meals, or as snacks between meals. Two to 6 tablespoonsful (30–90 mL) of wheat bran daily taken with a 250 mL glass of water or juice can be used to supplement dietary fibre. Gas production from soluble fibre metabolism may limit acceptance.
- Eat more fruits: Apples, pears and prunes contain the natural laxative sorbitol.
- Exercise: Because inactivity is associated with constipation, exercise has been advocated as a treatment option. Though not clearly shown to be effective, it is still worth recommending for many preventive health reasons.
- Weight loss: Weight loss is suggested for the treatment of chronic constipation in overweight patients. Like exercise, benefit has not been proven but is still worth recommending. The goal is to reach a weight compatible with a body mass index (BMI) of 18.5–24.9 (see Chapter 43: Weight Management).
- Biofeedback and relaxation: Biofeedback and relaxation training has been used in the treatment of constipation caused by pelvic floor dysfunction. This trains patients to relax their pelvic floor muscles and to coordinate relaxation and pushing during defecation.[12] Further well-designed trials are necessary to confirm effectiveness.

Children

- Aim for a daily dietary fibre level ≥10 g for children 3–7 years old and ≥15 g for children 8–14 years.[24]
- In infants, juices that contain sorbitol (e.g., prune, apple and pear) can increase the frequency of bowel movements and water content of stools. Barley malt extract (2–10 mL in 250 mL milk or juice) or corn syrup can be used as stool softeners.[25]
- Children with functional constipation should be encouraged to attempt defecation 5–15 minutes after each meal until they have a bowel movement that day.[3,25,26]
- Biofeedback may be beneficial for the treatment of a small subgroup of children with intractable constipation.[27]

Pharmacologic Therapy

For further discussion of pharmacologic therapy for constipation, consult the *Compendium of Therapeutic Choices*: Constipation in Adults.

For comparative ingredients of nonprescription products, consult the *Compendium of Products for Minor Ailments*—Gastrointestinal Products: Colon Electrolyte Lavage, Laxatives.

Constipation should not be managed through medications in the presence of an obstruction or ileus.[28]

There are 4 basic groups of laxatives: bulk forming, emollient, osmotic and stimulant (see Table 6).[29,30,31,32] Other drug classes include μ-opioid receptor antagonists (e.g., **methylnaltrexone**, **naloxegol**), prokinetic agents (e.g., **domperidone**, **erythromycin**, **prucalopride**) and guanylate cyclase C-agonists (e.g., **linaclotide**).

Detailed discussions regarding acute and chronic constipation as well as constipation in special populations can be found under Acute Constipation, Chronic Constipation and Constipation in Special Populations.

Bulk-forming Laxatives

Bulk-forming laxatives increase stool volume and are considered the safest agents suitable for long-term use.[8] Their fermentation in the colon leads to gas formation, increased osmotic load, water retention and wall stress which stimulate motility.[8,33] Each dose of a bulk-forming laxative should be administered with at least 250 mL of water or juice to prevent fecal impaction and/or esophageal obstruction.[8] Do not use if patient is dehydrated or fluid restricted. **Psyllium** improves stool frequency and consistency and **bran** reduces the use of laxatives in the elderly. Although there is insufficient evidence regarding the efficacy of **calcium polycarbophil** and **methylcellulose** in the management of constipation, these agents are still recommended if patients cannot use or tolerate other bulk-forming laxatives.[8,21] Fibre shows consistent beneficial effect for relieving overall symptoms and bleeding in the treatment of symptomatic hemorrhoids.[8]

Emollients/Stool Softeners

Stool softeners (e.g., **docusate sodium** or **docusate calcium**) act as surfactants to soften the stool by allowing the mixing of aqueous and fatty substances.[10] Although stool softeners have minimal if any effect on improving symptoms of chronic constipation and supporting evidence for their effectiveness is lacking, these agents may be useful for some patients who cannot tolerate more potent laxatives or when constipation is mild.[34]

Heavy mineral oil is not generally recommended due to risk of lipid aspiration and binding of fat-soluble medications. Studies in pediatric patients have shown it is superior to senna-based laxatives for frequency and stool consistency and inferior to osmotic agents which have fewer risks.[3,25,35]

Osmotic Laxatives

This class contains poorly absorbed ions or molecules that create an osmotic gradient and retain water within the intestinal lumen; the increased pressure on the lumen wall induces gastric motility.[7,36,37] **Polyethylene glycol (PEG)** and **lactulose** are examples of osmotic laxatives.[7,36,37]

PEG is a safe, effective and well-tolerated agent and causes less flatulence and bloating in adults compared with other osmotic laxatives.[38] PEG is superior to lactulose in outcomes of stool frequency per week, stool form and consistency, relief of abdominal pain and need for additional products.[39,40] PEG is considered more palatable than lactulose. Daily use of PEG (up to 6 months) is safe and effective[41] and may facilitate the discontinuation of other laxatives. As many as 40% of patients, however, could experience diarrhea with PEG or lactulose. Lower doses help prevent bloating, cramping, flatulence and electrolyte abnormalities. PEG may also be effective in the management of opioid-induced constipation.[42]

Glycerin suppositories act osmotically and have a quicker onset of action (approximately 15–30 minutes). They are less effective if the stool is dry and hard. Glycerin suppositories should be moistened with lukewarm water before insertion and retained as long as possible.

There is some evidence that **milk of magnesia** can be used for chronic constipation in patients with normal renal function.[43] Limitations include frequent diarrhea, multiple electrolyte abnormalities (e.g., hypermagnesemia, hyperphosphatemia, hypercalcemia, hyponatremia, hypokalemia) and hypovolemia.[44] These side effects may occur even in the absence of pre-existing renal failure. They should be administered with sufficient water to prevent dehydration.[43] **Oral sodium phosphate** products should *not* be used as purgatives since they may cause serious electrolyte, kidney, cardiovascular and neurologic problems, but they are still considered safe and effective for laxative use. **Magnesium citrate** is generally reserved for bowel cleansing.

Osmotic laxatives alone or in combination with stimulants are most commonly used as cathartics before surgery or intestinal procedures.

Stimulant Laxatives

This group of laxatives (e.g., **bisacodyl**, **senna**, **sodium picosulfate**) increase colonic peristalsis by producing rhythmic muscle contractions in the intestines and may be recommended if osmotic laxatives fail or are not tolerated.[43,45] All 3 medications are prodrugs. Senna is activated in the large bowel whereas bisacodyl and sodium picosulfate are activated in the alkaline medium of the small intestine.[46] Limiting their use helps minimize melanosis coli, abdominal discomfort, electrolyte imbalances, allergic reactions and hepatotoxicity.

Stimulant laxatives are likely safe in the treatment of chronic constipation.[43] Some evidence supports the short-term (4 weeks) efficacy and safety of **bisacodyl**[47] and **sodium picosulfate**[48] in chronic constipation.[49] Continuous daily usage may cause hyponatremia, hypokalemia and dehydration. Stimulant laxatives are usually administered at bedtime due to 6–12 hour delay in onset and are the laxatives of choice for opioid-induced constipation.

Castor oil use as a laxative is no longer recommended and is contraindicated in pregnancy and the elderly. It produces abdominal cramping and pain and stimulates uterine contractions during pregnancy and can be aspirated by the elderly.

Enemas

There is only anecdotal evidence for the value of enemas in the management of chronic constipation. However, many clinicians and patients find them useful and effective for the treatment of acute constipation and as a means of preparing or cleansing the distal colon for endoscopic or surgical procedures. Enemas generally have faster onset than suppositories and produce cleansing within an hour of administration. They are, however, less "socially" accepted by North Americans for chronic constipation and are mainly used for bowel cleansing prior to intestinal procedures. Caution is warranted when using enemas in the elderly since they are associated with increased mortality.[50]

Instructions for Administering an Enema

The patient should:

- Lubricate the enema nozzle if it is not pre-lubricated
- Lie on left side with knees bent
- Insert the enema nozzle into the rectum, with the nozzle pointing towards the navel
- Gently squeeze the container until the dose is expelled; if discomfort is felt at this point, the flow is probably too fast
- Retain the solution until definite abdominal cramping is felt.

Probiotics

Evidence is insufficient to support the use of probiotics in the treatment of chronic idiopathic constipation. There has been no direct comparison of different probiotic regimens in the management of constipation and the most beneficial strains, doses, dosing frequency and duration remain unclear.[51,52,53]

Natural Health Products

Only a few small randomized controlled trials and little other evidence supports the efficacy and/or safety of the following herbal treatments: aloes, bitter orange, buckthorn, dandelion, elderberry, hemp seed, lavender, licorice, rhubarb and soy. Yellow dock is an effective laxative but its safety has not been definitively established.[54,55]

Homeopathic Therapy

No clinical trials could be found investigating the use of homeopathy in constipation. Some commonly used remedies include alumina, byronia, calcarea carbonica, conium, lycopodium, natrum muriaticum, nux vomica, sepia and silicea.[54,55]

Long-term Use of Laxatives

Most patients suffering from constipation will self-medicate. They may overuse laxatives and anti-diarrheals resulting in a pendulum effect between constipation and diarrhea. This type of abuse is present in about 4% of laxative users.[2] Long-term use of stimulant laxatives has traditionally been discouraged based on tests linking long-term use to damage of the enteric nervous system in the mesenteric plexus and smooth muscles of the colon. However, the results of these tests have not been confirmed by newer technologic methods. Many experts now believe that the risks of long-term stimulant laxative use have been overemphasized, and that they are safe for daily use.[56] However, due to the increased cost and side effects such as cramping, reserve stimulants for third-line therapy when previous treatment has failed.

Melanosis coli is a melanotic hyperpigmentation of the colonic mucosa that occurs after long-term use of the anthraquinones. It is benign and reverses 3–12 months after discontinuation of the laxative.[16]

Other side effects of laxative overuse include various electrolyte abnormalities; hypermagnesemia, hypernatremia and hyperphosphatemia can occur due to accumulation of absorbed ions derived from the laxative.[44] Hypernatremia can also arise when large volumes of osmotic laxatives cause substantial water loss from the GI tract. Hypokalemia may result as the body tries to regain fluid losses by activating the renin-aldosterone system.[6]

Acute Constipation

Acute and chronic constipation require different management. Acute constipation is a term without a clear definition and its optimal management has not been well studied. Prevalence of acute constipation is not known, as the definition varies; however, it is more common than chronic constipation as defined by the ROME III criteria.[8]

Therapy is often based on the patient's level of discomfort. In general, it is best to clear out hard stool in the distal bowel before using a bulk agent or an aggressive oral regimen.[57] A reasonable approach is to use an agent with a relatively quick onset of action, e.g., **glycerin** or **bisacodyl** suppositories.[5] As well, saline laxatives are used to treat acute constipation if there is no indication of bowel obstruction, heart failure or renal impairment.[5]

If constipation is not relieved within 48 hours, add an agent with a quicker onset of action such as an enema. If fecal impaction is present, it must be relieved before maintenance treatment can begin. Disimpaction may be initiated manually, and then a tap water, phosphate, saline or mineral oil enema (with or without a local anesthetic lubricant) can be inserted daily for up to 3 days. Avoid soapsuds enemas because of an irritant effect on the colonic mucosa that may result in proctitis or colitis.[16] If the stool blockage is higher up in the colon than can be reached with enemas and the patient has no sign of bowel obstruction, use **polyethylene glycol** orally to disimpact the patient (2 litres for 1–2 days or 1 litre for 3 days).[58] Patients should not self-disimpact unless trained to do so. Avoid bulk-forming laxatives if impacted.

Chronic Constipation

Chronic constipation may cause atonic bowels and dependency on laxatives to stimulate motility. Slowly weaning the patient from a stimulant laxative to an osmotic laxative may improve long-term control particularly if the patient experiences permanent loss of smooth muscle contractility. Stimulant laxatives may be necessary in patients with slow motility secondary to diabetes or use of opioid medications. In most cases, the laxative should be tapered down to the lowest effective dose in order to minimize side effects.

Chronic constipation is treated in a stepwise approach (Table 4).[59]

Table 4: **Management of Chronic Constipation**

Step I	Unless a modifiable cause is identified, chronic constipation is initially managed by patient education, lifestyle modification and dietary changes, including fibre supplementation (bran) and/or bulk-forming laxatives. Fibre intake should be increased gradually every 7–10 days. Saline laxatives, glycerin suppository and/or enemas may be used as rescue treatment if no bowel movement has occurred for 2 consecutive days.
Step II	After a 4- to 6-wk trial, if the problem persists, second-line agents such as an osmotic or saline laxative may be added.
Step III	Third-line agents such as emollients and stimulants should be limited to short-term use after other agents have failed. This is due to the high incidence of side effects from these classes.

Constipation in Special Populations

Pediatrics

The overwhelming majority of children with chronic constipation suffer from functional constipation, involving a cycle of pain on defecation, fecal retention and chronic rectal distention.[25] Chronic constipation is estimated to occur in 1–5% of children. A third of these children have chronic constipation beyond puberty.[25] Management of constipation specific to the treatment of infants and children is presented below.

Infants

- The use of enemas is not recommended in infants.[3,25,35]
- Rectal disimpaction of infants can be achieved with pediatric **glycerin** suppositories.[3]
- **Barley malt extract**, **corn syrup**, **lactulose** or **sorbitol** can be used as stool softeners.[25]
- Heavy mineral oil and stimulant laxatives are not recommended for infants.[35]
- Constipation may be linked to milk intolerance in some children. A time limited trial of a cow's milk–free diet may be useful to rule out this as a cause.

Children ≥1 Year

Increased consumption of dietary fibre may improve stool frequency and consistency in children with constipation but does not reduce the need of laxatives.[60] Aim for a daily dietary fibre intake ≥10 g for children 3–7 years and ≥15 g for children 8–14 years.[24] There are no trials assessing the effectiveness of bulk-forming laxatives (e.g., psyllium) in children. **PEG**,[61] **lactulose** or **sorbitol** are considered first-line agents for the treatment of constipation whereas **magnesium hydroxide** and **heavy mineral oil** are second-line.[25,26] PEG may be superior to lactulose and magnesium hydroxide in this population.[61] Side effects include flatulence, abdominal pain, nausea, diarrhea and headache. Of the different polyethylene glycols, the PEG 3350 is better tolerated and accepted by children than the PEG with electrolytes.[62] Young children are at increased risk of lipoid pneumonia due to aspiration of mineral oil.[26] No evidence supports the use of stool softeners. **Senna** and **bisacodyl** can be used as rescue medication when other agents have failed.[25]

Disimpaction with enemas is recommended after diagnosis of impaction via rectal examination or, in some cases, abdominal radiography; higher doses of oral PEG 3350 1–1.5 g/kg/day may also be effective but may take up to 5 days of treatment.[36] Biofeedback therapy can be an effective short-term treatment of intractable constipation.[27]

Pregnancy and Breastfeeding

Constipation affects up to 25–30% of women in late pregnancy and up to 3 months postpartum.[63,64] It is thought to be secondary to elevated progesterone levels causing muscle relaxation in the intestine. It may also be due to the use of calcium and iron supplements and the gravid uterus pushing on the colon.[65] Dietary **bran or wheat fibre** is preferred as initial treatment of constipation during pregnancy to increase the frequency of defecation and soften stools.[66] **Docusate** has traditionally been added if fibre supplementation has failed during pregnancy but there is little evidence to support this practice. Heavy mineral oil is not absorbed systemically but may impede vitamin or mineral absorption. If stools remain hard, consider adding or switching to **lactulose** or **PEG**. **Stimulant laxatives** are more effective than dietary or medicinal fibre therapy but cause more side effects of diarrhea and abdominal pain; they are reserved for short-term use when other agents have failed.[66] Use stimulant and osmotic laxatives short term to prevent possible dehydration and electrolyte disturbances.[67] Occasional use of **glycerin** or **bisacodyl** suppositories is also an option. One study found no association between senna and higher risk of congenital abnormalities in pregnant women.[68]

Elderly

Treatment of the older adult is often complicated by comorbidities, cognitive impairment and polypharmacy.[59] There is a paucity of evidence-based recommendations in the management of constipation in the elderly.[69] Management should be tailored to each individual's needs and expectations regardless of age or place of residence.

Functional abilities related to mobility, following instructions, communicating needs, eating, drinking and cognitive status must be assessed.[14]

Fluid intake should target 1500–2000 mL daily unless fluid restrictions are imposed as in those with heart failure. Low fluid consumption with bulk forming laxatives can exacerbate constipation. Dietary **fibre** should be targeted at 25–30 g daily which may allow discontinuation of laxatives and may increase the senior's well-being.[69] Exercise may be performed to patient's capacity; pelvic tilt, trunk rotation and leg lifts are recommended for bedridden patients.[70] Medication review should rule out polypharmacy and drug-induced constipation.[18]

Renal impairment must be determined prior to using laxatives. The use of **saline laxatives** is contraindicated in renal and heart failure. Limitations for use include possible multiple electrolyte abnormalities such as hypermagnesemia, hyperphosphatemia, hypocalcemia and hypokalemia.[71] When used, oral saline laxatives (e.g., **sodium phosphate**) should be administered with sufficient water to prevent dehydration. **Magnesium citrate** is generally reserved for bowel cleansing and should be used with caution in renal impairment. **PEG** is safe and effective for use in seniors suffering from acute or chronic constipation.[41] Stimulant laxatives (e.g., **senna**, **bisacodyl**) may cause severe cramping and electrolyte losses when used long term.

Encourage institutions to establish an interdisciplinary team approach to prevent and manage constipation.[18]

Palliative Care and Cancer Patients

Constipation is prevalent in 50% of cancer patients and rises to 78% in the palliative patient due to the use of high-dose opioids.[45] Decreased GI motility, tumour compression of the large intestine or interference with colonic neural innervation is the usual mechanism involved (Table 1).[72]

The best therapy to manage constipation in this population is uncertain. Traditionally, **stimulant laxatives** have been the mainstay of therapy with rescue enemas or bisacodyl suppositories used when required for a period not exceeding 3 days. Higher doses of stimulant laxatives may be necessary in palliative patients (e.g., senna 34.4 mg TID, bisacodyl 20 mg TID or sodium picosulfate 30 mg at bedtime). Laxative dose may be increased every 24–48 hours until response or a ceiling dose is reached. It is best to maximize doses of stimulant laxative prior to adding an osmotic agent. **Lactulose** and **PEG** are alternatives but may cause nausea.[37] Impaction should be ruled out if the patient has not passed a stool in more than 3 days.[45]

There is significant evidence supporting the use of μ-opioid receptor antagonists (e.g., **methylnaltrexone**, **naloxegol**) in treatment of opioid-induced constipation. These agents are considered second-line if traditional laxatives fail.

Avoid bulk-forming agents since they may cause impaction.[45] Stool softeners are unlikely to have any benefit in this population. In neutropenic or thrombocytopenic patients, avoid rectal manipulation to prevent infection or bleeding; give oral laxatives and cathartics only.

Monitoring of Therapy

Table 5 provides a monitoring plan framework that should be individualized.

The use of a daily bowel log may be helpful in patients with chronic constipation, including children. A sample log is included in Constipation—What You Need to Know.

Table 5: Monitoring of Therapy for Constipation

Symptoms	Monitoring	Endpoint of Therapy	Actions
Inability to have bowel movement	Acute constipation: Patient: Daily Healthcare practitioner: After 1–3 days of therapy, depending upon the agent chosen	Full bowel movement.	Add agent with a relatively quick onset of action (e.g., glycerin suppository). If other laxative not effective, or if patient has not had a bowel movement in 7 days, reassess.
	Chronic constipation: As above plus: Patient: Keep daily bowel log (see Daily Bowel Log sample table below) Healthcare practitioner: Check with patient weekly for 4 wk	Chronic constipation: As above, plus patient should have established regular bowel patterns after 1 month.	Chronic constipation: If patient has not established regular patterns after 1 month, reassess treatment plan.
Bloating, cramping	Acute constipation: Patient: Daily Healthcare practitioner: Day 3	Bloating and cramping should be relieved shortly after full bowel movement occurs.	If full bowel movement has occurred but bloating and cramping are not relieved, reassess.

Advice for the Patient

All patients should receive advice regarding:

- Normal variation in frequency of bowel movements
- Nonpharmacologic methods of treating and preventing constipation
- Development of an individualized bowel routine
- Evaluation of the signs and symptoms and when they should contact a healthcare practitioner.

In addition, all patients who require drug therapy should receive advice regarding:

- The expected onset of action of the laxative and what to do if constipation is not relieved (long-term constipation may require weeks to months of therapy for bowel habits to adjust)
- Usual side effects of the medication.

Figure 2: **Assessment and Treatment of Patients with Constipation**

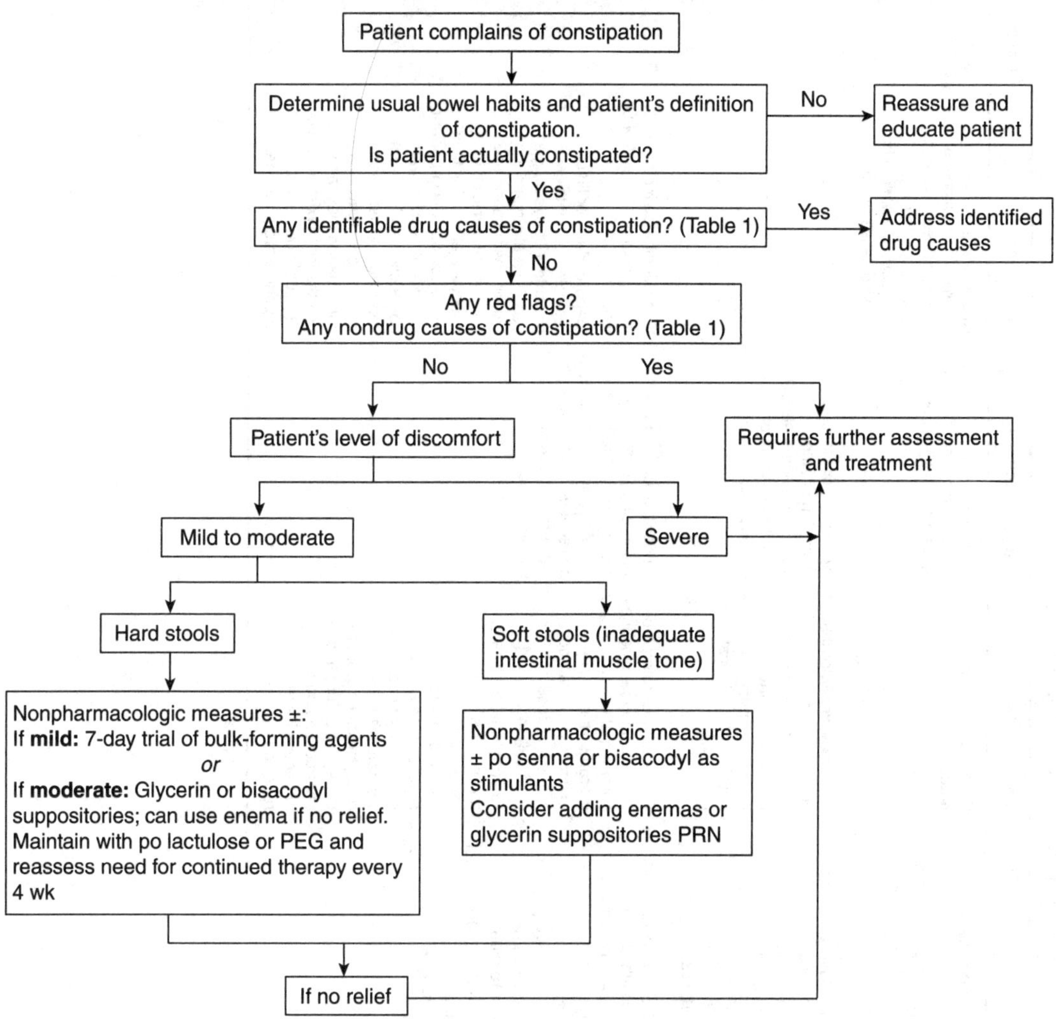

Table 6: Pharmacologic Treatment and Prevention of Constipation

Class	Drug	Dosage	Adverse Effects	Drug Interactions	Comments	Cost[a]
Bulk-forming Agents	*bran*	**>12 y:** 1–7 g/dose daily to BID po; maximum 14 g/day **6–12 y:** 1–3.5 g/dose daily to BID po; maximum 7 g/day **Onset:** 3–5 days	Diarrhea, bloating, flatulence.	May interfere with absorption of iron, calcium and fat-soluble vitamins.	Reduces total cholesterol and risk of colon cancer. Can be added to yogurt, cereals, soups or applesauce. If patient has celiac disease use rice bran.	$
	polycarbophil calcium Prodiem Tablets	**>12 y:** 1 g daily to QID po; maximum 4 g/day **6–12 y:** 0.5 g daily to QID po; maximum 2 g/day **2–5 y:** 0.5 g daily to BID po; maximum 1 g/day **Onset:** 12–72 h	Generally well-tolerated, some flatulence, bloating. Other adverse reactions reported include esophageal obstruction and fecal impaction.	If possible, do not take within 2 h of other medication or the effect of the other medication may be reduced.		$
	psyllium Metamucil Preparations, generics	**>12 y:** 2.5–7.5 g/dose daily to TID po with 250 mL of water or juice; maximum 30 g/day **6–12 y:** 2.5–3.75 g/dose 1–3 times daily po with 250 mL of water or juice; maximum 15 g/day **<6 y:** Safety and efficacy not established **Onset:** 12–72 h	Generally well tolerated; some flatulence, bloating common at start of therapy. This can be minimized by starting with a low dose and gradually increasing. Anaphylaxis, asthma and other allergic reactions have been reported. Allergic reactions may occur in up to 18% of healthcare workers with occupational exposure to psyllium. Esophageal obstruction and fecal impaction have been reported.	If possible, do not take within 2 h of other medication or the effect of the other medication may be reduced. May cause calcium and iron malabsorption.	Contraindicated if partial mechanical obstruction of GI tract. Inappropriate for fluid-restricted patients or patients with dysphagia, esophageal strictures or partial obstructions of GI tract. Administration of adequate amount of fluid with each dose is important to prevent esophageal obstruction and/or fecal impaction. When used to treat chronic functional constipation may take 2–3 months for maximum effect. Psyllium powder and capsules are gluten-free.	$

Class	Drug	Dosage	Adverse Effects	Drug Interactions	Comments	Cost[a]
Enemas	*mineral oil retention enema* Fleet Enema Mineral Oil	**>12 y:** 120 mL as a single dose pr **2–12 y:** 60 mL as a single dose pr **<2 y:** Not recommended **Onset:** 5–15 min	Incontinence. Risk of mechanical trauma to rectal wall.	No known drug interactions.	Softens and lubricates stool.	$$$
	phosphate enema Fleet Enema, generics	**>12 y:** 120 mL as a single dose pr **2–12 y:** 60 mL as a single dose pr Under a physician's supervision doses of 6 mL/kg (up to 135 mL) have been used **<2 y:** Avoid **Onset:** 5–15 min	Abdominal distension, vomiting. Hyperphosphatemia and hypocalcemia have occurred; most common in patients with renal dysfunction or when enema is retained too long.	No known drug interactions.	Avoid in patients with potential for prolonged retention (e.g., paralytic ileus, congenital megacolon) and those with cardiac disease, renal dysfunction or pre-existing electrolyte abnormalities. Risk of mechanical trauma to rectal wall.	$$
	tap water enema	**Adults:** 500 mL pr **<2 y:** Not recommended **Onset:** 5–15 min	Water intoxication and dilutional hyponatremia have occurred in children, the elderly and patients with megacolon. Risk of mechanical trauma to rectal wall.	No known drug interactions.	Evacuation induced by distended colon; mechanical lavage. May be uncomfortable for patient. Use warm, but not hot, tap water.	$

(cont'd)

Table 6: **Pharmacologic Treatment and Prevention of Constipation** *(cont'd)*

Class	Drug	Dosage	Adverse Effects	Drug Interactions	Comments	Cost[a]
Lubricants	*mineral oil* Lansoyl, others	**>12 y:** 15–45 mL HS po while sitting up **6–12 y:** 5–15 mL HS po while sitting up **1–5 y:** 1–3 mL/kg HS po while sitting up; maximum 15 mL HS **<1 y:** Not recommended **Onset:** 6–8 h	Lipoid pneumonia if aspirated. Theoretical interference with fat-soluble drug and vitamin absorption. Foreign body reaction, dehydration. Seepage from rectum may cause perianal pruritus.	May reduce absorption of vitamins A, D, E and K. May increase anticoagulant effect due to decreased absorption of vitamin K. Do not use with docusate, which increases absorption of mineral oil.	Not generally recommended. Lubricates contents of GI tract for the relief of occasional constipation. Can be mixed with fruit juice or carbonated beverage. Not recommended for periods >1 wk. Light mineral oil should not be used internally. Young children and elderly may be at higher risk of aspiration. Due to aspiration risk, not recommended for those who are bedridden or have swallowing difficulties, gastric retention or GERD. Crosses placenta. Has caused hemorrhagic disease of the newborn; not recommended for prolonged periods in pregnancy. Minimally absorbed but not metabolized; accumulates in tissues with repeated use. Light mineral oil should not be used internally. Young children and elderly may be at higher risk of aspiration. Due to aspiration risk, not recommended for those who are bedridden or have swallowing difficulties, gastric retention or GERD. Crosses placenta.	$

Class	Drug	Dosage	Adverse Effects	Drug Interactions	Comments	Cost[a]
Osmotic Agents	*glycerin* Glycerin Suppositories, generics	**Adults:** 2.6 g suppository pr daily or BID PRN. Insert high into rectum and retain for 15 min if possible **Children:** 1.44 g suppository pr daily or BID PRN. Insert high into rectum and retain for 15 min if possible **Onset:** 15–30 min	Rectal irritation.	No known drug interactions.	May dissolve in hands if not inserted soon after unwrapping.	$
	lactulose generics	**>12 y:** 15–30 mL daily or BID po **6–12 y:** 10 mL BID po **1–5 y:** 5 mL BID po **Onset:** 24–48 h	Flatulence and abdominal cramps are common, especially at the beginning of therapy. Nausea is more common with higher doses. Diarrhea is a sign of overdosage.	Slower absorption of medication from the intestine due to acidification. Ideally, do not take within 2 h of other medication.	Many patients find sweet taste intolerable. Avoid in patients who require a galactose-free diet. 667 mg lactulose = 147 mg galactose, <80 mg lactose. Not absorbed systemically. Can be used by patients with diabetes.	$
	magnesium citrate Citro-Mag, generics	**Adults:** 75–150 mL once daily po as laxative. 300 mL once po as cathartic Drink 250 mL water before and after each dose **Children (maintenance):** **>12 y:** 150–300 mL once daily po **6–12 y:** 50–100 mL once daily po **<6 y:** 1–3 mL/kg once daily po Do not exceed adult dose **Onset:** 0.5–3 h	Risk of hypermagnesemia increased with overdose, in infants and those with renal impairment.	May reduce bioavailability of digoxin and the tetracyclines.	Caution with dehydration. Not recommended with cardiac or renal disease. Chill solution before administration for greater palatability. Often used as a cathartic prior to surgery or GI procedures.	$$$

(cont'd)

Table 6: **Pharmacologic Treatment and Prevention of Constipation** *(cont'd)*

Class	Drug	Dosage	Adverse Effects	Drug Interactions	Comments	Cost[a]
	magnesium hydroxide Milk of Magnesia, generics	**Adults:** 15–30 mL daily or BID po **Children:** 80–240 mg/kg daily po Do not exceed adult dose **Onset:** 0.5–3 h	Risk of hypermagnesemia increased with overdose and in infants and those with renal impairment. Hypokalemia may also occur with prolonged use or overdose. Dehydration, abdominal cramps, incontinence.	No known drug interactions.	Caution with dehydration. Not recommended with cardiac or renal disease.	$
	polyethylene glycol Lax-A-Day, Pegalax, RestoraLAX	**Adults:** 17 g (1 heaping tablespoonful) in 250 mL of liquid once daily po **Children 2–18 y:** 0.4–0.8 g/kg/day po in 240 mL liquid (not to exceed adult dose) **Onset:** 48–96 h	Transient diarrhea, flatulence, nausea, retching, abdominal bloating, cramping, anal irritation. Pulmonary edema may occur if powder is aspirated. Mallory-Weiss tears have occurred.	Slower absorption of medication from the intestine due to acidification. Ideally, do not take within 2 h of other medication.	Available with or without electrolytes (both formulations are equally effective in the treatment of constipation). Causes retention of water in GI lumen. Not fermented into hydrogen or methane by the GI microbiota and has no effect on the absorption or secretion of glucose or electrolytes. Do not use if bowel obstruction. Space 2 h from other medication. Avoid high doses in the elderly due to increased risk of diarrhea.	$
	sodium phosphate generics	All doses of concentrated solution are diluted in 125 mL water and followed by 250 mL water **≥13 y:** 20 mL of concentrated solution (with water as above) once daily po **10–12 y:** 10 mL of concentrated solution (with water as above) once daily po	Hypocalcemia, hypokalemia and hypernatremia have also been reported. Caution with renal or cardiac disease.	ACE inhibitors, angiotensin receptor blockers, diuretics and NSAIDs may enhance the nephrotoxic effect of sodium phosphate.	Considered to be safe as laxative but unsafe if used as purgative due to association with electrolyte disturbances and kidney injury. Best taken on an empty stomach upon rising, 30 min before a meal, or at bedtime. Not recommended for pregnant or nursing women. Not recommended for sodium-restricted patients or for chronic use.	$$$

Class	Drug	Dosage	Adverse Effects	Drug Interactions	Comments	Cost[a]
		6–9 y: 5 mL of concentrated solution (with water as above) once daily po **Onset:** 0.5–3 h Each 5 mL of concentrated solution contains 2.4 g monobasic sodium phosphate monohydrate and 0.9 g dibasic sodium phosphate heptahydrate				
	sorbitol 70% solution	**Adults:** 15–30 mL daily or BID po Rectal enema 120 mL pr as 25–30% solution **Children:** 1–3 mL/kg in divided doses po (not to exceed adult dose) Rectal enema 30–60 mL pr as 25–50% solution **Onset:** po: 24–48 h pr: 5–15 min	Flatulence, abdominal cramps, nausea, diarrhea.	No known drug interactions.	Cost-effective alternative to lactulose. Caution in severe cardiopulmonary or renal impairment.	$

(cont'd)

Table 6: **Pharmacologic Treatment and Prevention of Constipation** *(cont'd)*

Class	Drug	Dosage	Adverse Effects	Drug Interactions	Comments	Cost[a]
Stimulants	*bisacodyl* Dulcolax, Carters Little Pills, generics	**>12 y:** 5–10 mg HS po or 10 mg suppository pr **6–12 y:** 5 mg HS po or 5 mg suppository pr **Onset:** po: 6–12 h pr: 0.5–1 h	Abdominal pain, cramps, diarrhea, hypokalemia. Incontinence. Rectal administration may cause rectal irritation or burning.	Should not be taken with milk, antacids or proton pump inhibitors because these products increase the pH of the upper GI tract causing the premature disintegration of the enteric coating in the stomach before the product reaches the colon.	Appears in breast milk. Tablets should not be crushed, broken or chewed.	$
	cascara sagrada	**Adults:** 2–5 mL or 0.3–1 g HS po Not for use in children **Onset:** 6–12 h	Abdominal discomfort, diarrhea, hypokalemia, allergic reactions.	No known drug interactions.	Avoid in pregnancy. Aromatic formulation contains 0.2% alcohol. Excreted into breast milk. May discolour urine red to pink or brown to black.	$
	senna Senokot Preparations, others	**>12 y:** 10–15 mL (1.7 mg/mL) or 2–4 tablets (8.6 mg/tablet) HS po; maximum 15 mL or 4 tablets BID po **Pregnancy and children** **6–12 y:** 5–10 mL or 1–2 tablets HS po; maximum 10 mL or 2 tablets BID po **2–5 y:** 3–5 mL once daily po; maximum 5 mL BID po **Onset:** 6–12 h	Abdominal pain, diarrhea, hypokalemia, dehydration, allergic reactions and, rarely, proctitis and idiosyncratic hepatitis, melanosis coli.	No known drug interactions.	Excreted into breast milk. May discolour urine red to pink or brown to black. Not first-line in pregnancy.	$

Class	Drug	Dosage	Adverse Effects	Drug Interactions	Comments	Cost[a]
Stool Softeners	*docusate calcium* generics	**Adults:** 240 mg daily or BID po **Onset:** 12–72 h	Usually well tolerated. Mild, transient nausea or GI cramps may occur. Occasional rash.	Absorption of mineral oil may be increased.	Evidence weak regarding efficacy of stool softeners.	$
	docusate sodium generics	**>12 y:** 100 mg BID po **6–12 y:** 40–150 mg once daily or divided BID po **3–5 y:** 20–60 mg once daily or divided BID po **<3 y:** 10–40 mg once daily or divided BID po **Onset:** 12–72 h	See docusate calcium.	See docusate calcium.	Available as capsules or liquid.	$

a Cost per day; includes drug cost only.

Dosage adjustment may be required in renal impairment.

Legend: $ <$1 $$ $1–3 $$$ $3–6

Suggested Readings

American Gastroenterological Association, Bharucha AE, Dorn SD et al. American Gastroenterological Association medical position statement on constipation. *Gastroenterology* 2013;144:211-7.

Basilisco G, Coletta M. Chronic constipation: a critical review. *Dig Liver Dis* 2013;45:886-93.

Gandell D, Straus SE, Bundookwala M et al. Treatment of constipation in older people. *CMAJ* 2013;185:663-70.

Paré P, Fedorak RN. Systematic review of stimulant and nonstimulant laxatives for the treatment of functional constipation. *Can J Gastroenterol Hepatol* 2014;28:549-57.

Shah BJ, Rughwani N, Rose S. In the clinic. Constipation. *Ann Intern Med* 2015;162:ITC1.

References

1. American Gastroenterological Association, Bharucha AE, Dorn SD et al. American Gastroenterological Association medical position statement on constipation. *Gastroenterology* 2013;144:211-7.
2. Bharucha AE, Pemberton JH, Locke GR. American Gastroenterological Association technical review on constipation. *Gastroenterology* 2013;144:218-38.
3. Levy J, Volpert D. Know thy laxatives: a parent's guide to the successful management of chronic functional constipation in infants and children. *Digestive Health Matters* Summer 2004.
4. Chang JY, Locke GR McNally MA et al. Impact of functional gastrointestinal disorders on survival in the community. *Am J Gastroenterol* 2010;105:822-32.
5. Wong PW, Kadakia S. How to deal with chronic constipation. A stepwise method of establishing and treating the source of the problem. *Postgrad Med* 1999;106:199-200, 203-4, 207-10.
6. Medscape. *Chronic constipation: understanding issues in gut physiology and implications for therapy.* Available from: www.medscape.org/viewprogram/17096. Registration required.
7. Johanson JF. Review of the treatment options for chronic constipation. *MedGenMed* 2007:9:25.
8. Longstreth GF, Thompson WG, Chey WD et al. Functional bowel disorders. *Gastroenterology* 2006;130:1480-91.
9. Thompson WG. Constipation: a physiological approach. *Can J Gastroenterol* 2000;14:155D-162D.
10. Borum ML. Constipation: evaluation and management. *Prim Care* 2001;28:577-90.
11. Leung L, Riutta T, Kotecha J et al. Chronic constipation: an evidence-based review. *J Am Board Fam Med* 2011;24:436-51.
12. Locke GR, Pemberton JH, Phillips SF. American Gastroenterological Association medical position statement: guidelines on constipation. *Gastroenterology* 2000;119:1761-6.
13. Higgins PD, Johanson JF. Epidemiology of constipation in North America: a systematic review. *Am J Gastroenterol* 2004;99:750-9.
14. Towers AL, Burgio KL, Locher JL et al. Constipation in the elderly: influence of dietary, psychological and physiological factors. *J Am Geriatr Soc* 1994;42:701-6.
15. Wexner SD, Duthie GS, eds. *Constipation: etiology, evaluation, and management*. 2nd ed. London: Springer; 2006.
16. Longe RL, DiPiro JT. Diarrhea and constipation. In: DiPiro JT, Talbert RL, Yee GC et al., eds. *Pharmacotherapy: a pathophysiologic approach*. 4th ed. Stamford: Appleton &Lange; 1999. p. 599-613.
17. Prather CM, Ortiz-Camacho CP. Evaluation and treatment of constipation and fecal impaction in adults. *Mayo Clin Proc* 1998;73:881-7.
18. Registered Nurses' Association of Ontario (RNAO). *Prevention of constipation in the older adult population.* Toronto: RNAO; 2005. Available from: rnao.ca/bpg/guidelines/prevention-constipation-older-adult-population. Accessed February 17, 2016.
19. Dukas L, Willett WC, Giovannucci EL. Association between physical activity, fiber intake, and other lifestyle variables and constipation in a study of women. *Am J Gastroenterol* 2003;98:1790-6.
20. Position of the American Dietetic Association: health implications of dietary fiber. *J Am Diet Assoc* 1997;97:1157-9.
21. Suares NC, Ford AC. Systematic review: the effects of fibre in the management of chronic idiopathic constipation. *Aliment Pharmacol Ther* 2011;33:895-901.
22. USDA National Nutrient Database for Standard Reference. Beltsville: U.S. Department of Agriculture. Available from: ndb.nal.usda.gov. Accessed February 17, 2016.
23. Muller-Lissner SA. Effect of wheat bran on stool weight and gastrointestinal transit time: a meta analysis. *Br Med J (Clin Res Ed)* 1988;296:615-7.
24. Chao HC, Lai MW, Kong MS et al. Cutoff volume of dietary fiber to ameliorate constipation in children. *J Pediatr* 2008;153:45-9.
25. Baker SS, Liptak GS, Colletti RB et al. Constipation in infants and children: evaluation and treatment. A medical position statement of the North American Society for Pediatric Gastroenterology and Nutrition. *J Ped Gastroenterol Nutr* 1999;29:612-26.
26. Youssef NN, Di Lorenzo C. Childhood constipation: evaluation and treatment. *J Clin Gastroenterol* 2001;33:199-205.
27. van Kuyk EM, Wissink-Essink M, Brugman-Boezeman AT et al. Multidisciplinary behavioral treatment of defecation problems: a controlled study in children with anorectal malformations. *J Pediatr Surg* 2001;36:1350-6.
28. Shah BJ, Rughwani N, Rose S. In the clinic. Constipation. *Ann Intern Med* 2015;162:ITC1.
29. Pare P, Bridges R, Champion MC et al. Recommendations on chronic constipation (including constipation associated with irritable bowel syndrome) treatment. *Can J Gastroenterol* 2007;21:3B-22B.
30. Nurko S, Youssef NN, Sabri M et al. PEG3350 in the treatment of childhood constipation: a multicenter, double-blinded, placebo-controlled trial. *J Pediatr* 2008;153:254-61, 261.e1.
31. Seinelä L, Sairanen U, Laine T et al. Comparison of polyethylene glycol with and without electrolytes in the treatment of constipation in elderly institutionalized patients: a randomized, double-blind, parallel-group study. *Drugs Aging* 2009;26:703-13.
32. Rowan-Legg A, Canadian Paediatric Society. Managing functional constipation in children. *Paediatr Child Health* 2011;16(10):661-70.
33. Johanson JF, Kralstein J. Chronic constipation: a survey of the patient perspective. *Aliment Pharmacol Ther* 2007;25:599-608.

34. Treatments for constipation: a review of systematic reviews. Ottawa: CADTH; 2014. *CADTH Rapid Response Reports*.
35. Constipation Guideline Committee of the North American Society for Pediatric Gastroenterology, Hepatology and Nutrition. Evaluation and treatment of constipation in infants and children: recommendations of the North American Society for Pediatric Gastroenterology, Hepatology and Nutrition. *J Pediatr Gastroenterol Nutr* 2006;43:e1-13.
36. PendoPharm. *Lax-A-Day product monograph and utilization in the pediatric population*. April 30, 2009.
37. van der Spoel JI, Oudemans-van Straaten HM, Kuiper MA et al. Laxation of critically ill patients with lactulose or polyethylene glycol: a two-center randomized, double-blind, placebo-controlled trial. *Crit Care Med* 2007;35:2726-31.
38. Belsey JD, Geraint M, Dixon TA. Systematic review and meta analysis: polyethylene glycol in adults with non-organic constipation. *Int J Clin Pract* 2010;64:944-55.
39. Lee-Robichaud H, Thomas K, Morgan J et al. Lactulose versus polyethylene glycol for chronic constipation. *Cochrane Database Syst Rev* 2010;(7):CD007570.
40. Zurad EG, Johanson JF. Over-the-counter laxative polyethylene glycol 3350: an evidence-based appraisal. *Curr Med Res Opin* 2011;27:1439-52.
41. Dipalma JA, Cleveland MV, McGowan J et al. A randomized, multicenter, placebo-controlled trial of polyethylene glycol laxative for chronic treatment of chronic constipation. *Am J Gastroenterol* 2007;102:1436-41.
42. Wirz S, Nadstawek J, Elsen C et al. Laxative management in ambulatory cancer patients on opioid therapy: a prospective, open-label investigation of polyethylene glycol, sodium picosulphate and lactulose. *Eur J Cancer Care (Engl)* 2012;21:131-40.
43. Petticrew M. Effectiveness of laxatives in adults. *Eff Health Care* 2001;7:1-12.
44. Corbi G, Acanfora D, Iannuzzi GL et al. Hypermagnesemia predicts mortality in elderly with congestive heart disease: relationship with laxative and antacid use. *Rejuvenation Res* 2008;11:129-38.
45. Miles CL, Fellowes D, Goodman ML et al. Laxatives for the management of constipation in palliative care patients. *Cochrane Database Syst Rev* 2006;(4):CD003448.
46. Twycross R, Sykes N, Mihalyo M et al. Stimulant laxatives and opioid-induced constipation. *J Pain Symptom Manage*. 2012;43:306-13.
47. Kamm MA, Mueller-Lissner S, Wald A et al. Oral bisacodyl is effective and well-tolerated in patients with chronic constipation. *Clin Gastroenterol Hepatol* 2011;9:577-83.
48. Mueller-Lissner S, Kamm MA, Wald A et al. Multicenter, 4-week, double-blind, randomized, placebo-controlled trial of sodium picosulfate in patients with chronic constipation. *Am J Gastroenterol* 2010;105:897-903.
49. Kienzle-Horn S, Vix JM, Schuijt C et al. Comparison of bisacodyl and sodium picosulphate in the treatment of chronic constipation. *Curr Med Res Opin* 2007;23:691-9.
50. Niv G, Grinberg T, Dickman R et al. Perforation and mortality after cleansing enema for acute constipation are not rare but are preventable. *Int J Gen Med* 2013;6:323-8.
51. Dimidi E, Christodoulides S, Fragkos KC et al. The effect of probiotics on functional constipation in adults: a systematic review and meta-analysis of randomized controlled trials. *Am J Clin Nutr* 2014;100:1075-84.
52. Chmielewska A, Szajewska H. Systematic review of randomised controlled trials: probiotics for functional constipation. *World J Gastroenterol* 2010;16:69-75.
53. Ford AC, Quigley EM, Lacy BE et al. Efficacy of prebiotics, probiotics, and synbiotics in irritable bowel syndrome and chronic idiopathic constipation: systematic review and meta-analysis. *Am J Gastroenterol* 2014;109:1547-61.
54. Ernst E, Pittler MH, Wider B, eds. *The desktop guide to complementary and alternative medicine: an evidenced-based approach*. New York: Mosby; 2001.
55. Boon H, Smith M. *Health care professional training program in complementary medicine*. Botanica Consulting Inc; 1998. p. 126-33.
56. Muller-Lissner SA, Kamm MA, Scarpignato C et al. Myths and misconceptions about chronic constipation. *Am J Gastroenterol* 2005;100:232-42.
57. Kienzle-Horn S, Vix JM, Schuijt C et al. Efficacy and safety of bisacodyl in the acute treatment of constipation: a double-blind, randomized, placebo-controlled study. *Aliment Pharmacol Ther* 2006;23:1479-88.
58. Candy D, Belsey J. Macrogol (polyethylene glycol) laxatives in children with functional constipation and faecal impaction: a systematic review. *Arch Dis Child* 2009;94:156-60.
59. Ginsberg DA, Phillips SE, Wallace J et al Evaluating and managing constipation in the elderly. *Urol Nurs* 2007;27:191-200, 212.
60. Weber TK, Toporovski MS, Tahan S et al. Dietary fiber mixture in pediatric patients with controlled chronic constipation. *J Pediatr Gastroenterol Nutr* 2014;58:297-302.
61. Gordon M, Naidoo K, Akobeng AK et al. Osmotic and stimulant laxatives for the management of childhood constipation. *Cochrane Database Syst Rev* 2012;7:CD009118.
62. Savino F, Viola S, Erasmo M et al. Efficacy and tolerability of peg-only laxative on faecal impaction and chronic constipation in children. A controlled double blind randomized study vs a standard peg-electrolyte laxative. *BMC Pediatr* 2012;12:178.
63. Cullen G, O'Donoghue D. Constipation and pregnancy. *Best Pract Res Clin Gastroenterol* 2007;21:807-18.
64. Bradley CS, Kennedy CM, Turcea AM et al. Constipation in pregnancy: prevalence, symptoms, and risk factors. *Obstet Gynecol* 2007;110:1351-7.
65. Smith J, Taddio A, Koren G. Drugs of choice for pregnant women. In: Koren G, ed. *Maternal-fetal toxicology: a clinician's guide*. 2nd ed. New York: Dekker; 1994.
66. Jewell DJ, Young G. Interventions for treating constipation in pregnancy. *Cochrane Database Syst Rev* 2001;(2):CD001142.
67. Trottier M, Erebara A, Bozzo P. Treating constipation during pregnancy. *Can Fam Physician* 2012;58:836-8.
68. Acs N, Banhidy F, Puho EH et al. Senna treatment in pregnant women and congenital abnormalities in their offspring–a population-based case-control study. *Reprod Toxicol* 2009;28:100-4.
69. Gallagher P, O'Mahony D. Constipation in old age. *Best Pract Res Clin Gastroenterol* 2009;23:875-87.
70. Minaker K, Harai D. Constipation in the elderly. *Hospital Practice* 1995:67-76.
71. Beloosesky Y, Grinblat J, Weiss A et al. Electrolyte disorders following oral sodium phosphate administration for bowel cleansing in elderly patients. *Arch Intern Med* 2003;163:803-8.
72. Droney J, Ross J, Gretton S et al. Constipation in cancer patients on morphine. *Support Care Cancer* 2008;16:453-9.

Constipation—What You Need to Know

What is constipation?

Constipation means difficulty having a bowel movement.

What is a normal bowel movement?

A normal bowel movement is different for each person. Some people have them 3 times a day while others have them only 3 times a week. A normal bowel movement should be soft, hold its shape and be easy to pass (no straining).

Causes of Constipation

Constipation can be caused by many things, including prescription and nonprescription medications. If you take medication, check with your healthcare provider to see if it could be making you constipated. Constipation is often due to simple factors such as not going to the bathroom when you have the urge.

Tips to Prevent Constipation:

- Drink at least 6–8 glasses (8 ounces or 250 mL each) of water daily.
- Eat a balanced diet that is high in fibre and includes fruit, vegetables and bran. Foods high in fibre include 100% bran cereal, beans, peas, raspberries and broccoli.
- Exercise regularly.
- Try to have a bowel movement at the same time each day. For many people the best time is shortly after breakfast.
- Go to the bathroom when you have the urge; waiting will cause problems. Do not rush; take time to pass the entire stool.

Using Laxatives

The most natural way to regulate your bowels is by eating a healthy diet and following the tips shown above. Sometimes, however, you may need a laxative. The safest laxative for most people is a bulk-forming laxative such as psyllium. It should work within 3 days. If this is too long to wait, other laxatives are available that work more quickly, such as suppositories. Do not use laxatives for more than a week unless your healthcare provider tells you to do this. Talk to your healthcare provider about which laxative is best for you.

When to See Your Healthcare Provider?

If you are constipated *and*:

- You have not had a bowel movement for 7 days, *or*
- You are extremely uncomfortable because you are constipated, *or*
- You have pain in your rectum (back passage) or rectal bleeding, *or*
- You have a fever, your belly hurts or you feel like throwing up, *or*
- Your bowel movements are thin as a pencil, *or*
- You have a problem with your bowels that lasts longer than 2 weeks or keeps coming back.

If you are often constipated, you may find it helpful to keep track of your bowel movements for a few days. You can use a Daily Bowel Log like the one shown below. Try making changes in your diet and the amount of fluid you drink to see if that helps your constipation.

Table 1: **Daily Bowel Log**

Date	Number of bowel movements and consistency of each (for example hard, soft, loose)	Straining (yes/no)	Complete movement (yes/no)	Fibre and fluid intake (number of glasses juice/ water and servings of fibre)	Methods used to treat constipation

Chapter 30
Diarrhea

Antonietta Forrester, BScPhm

Diarrhea is the unusually frequent excretion of watery stools. It is associated with loss of electrolytes and loss of fecal matter at a rate of >200 g/24 hours.[1] A more practical working definition is ≥3 loose or watery stools per day or a definite decrease in consistency and increase in frequency based on an individual baseline.[2] Decreased fluid absorption or increased fluid secretion can lead to dehydration, which can ultimately lead to death, particularly in children and the elderly. This chapter has 2 parts, (1) Acute and Chronic Diarrhea and (2) Travellers' Diarrhea which could have an acute or chronic course.

Acute and Chronic Diarrhea

Although temporal definitions vary, diarrhea can be classified as acute (<14 days in duration) or chronic (>14 days in duration or repeated episodes of diarrhea lasting <14 days each).

Diarrhea is believed to be underreported.[3] The incidence of acute diarrhea in industrialized countries is approximately 0.5–2 episodes per person yearly and considerably higher in developing and underdeveloped countries.[4] In older children, adolescents and adults, diarrhea accounts for about 2.8 billion episodes annually worldwide.[5] Diarrhea is common in the pediatric population; statistics indicate that children <5 years experience 1.3–2.7 episodes of diarrhea yearly.[6] Eighteen percent of all deaths in children under the age of 5 years are attributed to diarrhea and 78% of those deaths occur in African and South East Asian regions. In this age group, diarrhea is the second leading cause of death following pneumonia.[7] As a result, the integrated Global Action Plan for the Prevention and Control of Pneumonia and Diarrhea hopes to reduce death from diarrhea in children under 5 years to <1 in 1000 by 2025.[8]

Aside from dehydration, complications of diarrhea include electrolyte imbalances, hypotension, vascular collapse, metabolic acidosis, hypokalemia, hypomagnesemia, hemorrhoids and rectal prolapse. Diarrhea often results in a decreased ability to perform daily activities.

Pathophysiology

Chronic diarrhea is often indicative of a functional bowel disorder such as irritable bowel syndrome. Intestinal diseases with underlying inflammation (e.g., inflammatory bowel disease) are also prevalent. Food intolerances and sensitivities, ischemic colitis, microscopic colitis, GI infections, radiation or chemotherapy and maldigestion or malabsorption of fat or carbohydrates (celiac disease, lactose intolerance) can also be responsible for chronic diarrhea. Foods that contain large amounts of sorbitol or mannitol can cause osmotic diarrhea.[9]

The most common causes of acute diarrhea are bacterial and viral infections and food toxins. Acute childhood diarrheal pathogens are transmitted by close contact and in particular the oral-fecal route.

Childcare settings are a common place for acquiring infectious diarrhea. Infectious viral agents include:[9]

- Rotavirus—responsible for causing severe diarrhea in infants and children, and the most common cause of gastroenteritis among children worldwide.[10]
- Norwalk-like virus—responsible for a milder form of diarrhea affecting older children and adults
- Adenovirus
- Calicivirus

Drugs are also a common cause of diarrhea (Table 1). In particular, broad-spectrum antibiotics such as penicillins, cephalosporins and erythromycins are implicated in altering the bacterial flora of the gut, resulting in diarrhea. This usually occurs 2–3 days after starting the antibiotic and resolves when the antibiotic is discontinued. An uncommon but potentially serious result of antibiotics use is *Clostridium difficile*-associated diarrhea. The agents most often implicated as causes of *C. difficile*-associated diarrhea are clindamycin, ampicillin and the cephalosporins,[13] although any antimicrobial agent can cause it, including those used to treat it. The condition can occur in anyone who has received an antibiotic within the previous 3 months and is characterized by significant loss of fluid, fever and abdominal pain.

Table 1: **Drugs Associated with Diarrhea**[1,11,12]

Acetylcholinesterase inhibitors	Cholinergics	Orlistat
Alcohol	Dopamine antagonists	Potassium supplements
Antacids—magnesium salts	Histamine H_2-receptor antagonists	Prostaglandins
Antibiotics	HIV medications	Proton pump inhibitors
Anticoagulants	Immunosuppressants	Quinidine
Antidiabetics	Lactose-containing pharmaceuticals (in lactose intolerant patients)	SSRIs
Antihypertensives	Laxatives	Sulfasalazine
Antimetabolites	Lithium	Theophylline
Cardiovascular drugs	NSAIDs	Ticlopidine
Chemotherapeutic agents		

Other causes of diarrhea include: nervousness or anxiety, gastrointestinal or pancreatic tumors, diabetes mellitus, opiate withdrawal, rapid increase of fibre in the diet, enteral nutritional supplements, deficiencies of specific nutrients such as vitamin A and zinc,[14] excesses of specific nutrients such as vitamin C and magnesium,[1,9] certain metals, organic toxins and plant products (e.g., arsenic, insecticides, mushroom toxins, caffeine).[15]

Goals of Therapy

- Determine the specific etiology where possible and treat appropriately
- Decrease the symptoms and re-establish normal stools
- Avoid and treat complications such as dehydration
- Identify red flags (see Table 2) and cases requiring further diagnostic testing

Patient Assessment

For those with noninfectious diarrhea, conducting a thorough patient history may be helpful in elucidating the underlying cause. This can include travel and animal exposure history, sources of water (e.g., well water), recent food consumption, history of past diarrheal episodes and recent antibiotic use.

Aside from frequent loose stools, symptoms of infectious diarrhea may include nausea, vomiting, abdominal pain, headache, fever, chills and malaise. Presence of "red flags" (Table 2) requires further detailed patient assessment. Table 3 presents symptoms of dehydration in children and adults. Figure 1 depicts decreased skin turgor.

Question patients with repeated episodes of diarrhea about any relationship between symptoms and consumption of dairy or grain products to rule out lactose or gluten intolerance (see Chapter 41: Special Diets).

Table 2: Red Flags Associated with Diarrhea

Red Flags
Blood or abnormal mucus in stool
Extensive abdominal cramping or pain
Fever >38.5°C
Frail elderly
Immunocompromised (e.g., HIV infection, immunosuppressants)
Persistent or chronic diarrhea
Persistent vomiting for >4 h
Pregnancy
Presence of chronic medical conditions (e.g., diabetes, heart failure, kidney dysfunction)
Recent use of antibiotics particularly those associated with *C. difficile* colitis (e.g., clindamycin, ampicillin, cephalosporins)
Severe diarrhea (>6 unformed stools per day for >48 h)
Signs or symptoms of debilitating dehydration (Table 3 and Figure 1)
Weight loss due to diarrhea
Worsening diarrhea
Young age (<2 y)

Table 3: Signs and Symptoms of Dehydration in Children and Adults[16,17]

Children	Adults
Dry mouth, tongue and skin	Increased thirst
Few or no tears when crying	Decreased urination
Decreased urination (less than 4 wet diapers in 24 h)	Feeling weak or lightheaded
Sunken eyes, cheeks or abdomen	Dry mouth/tongue
Greyish skin	
Sunken soft spot (fontanel) in infants	
Decreased skin turgor (Figure 1)	
Irritability or listlessness	

Figure 1: Decreased Skin Turgor

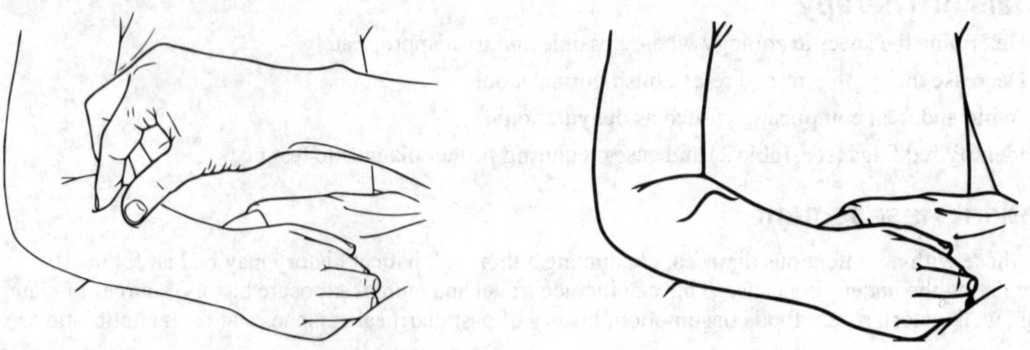

When pinched and released, the skin flattens slowly

An assessment and management plan for patients suffering from diarrhea not related to travel is illustrated in Figure 2.

Prevention

Nonpharmacologic Preventive Measures

- Encourage handwashing after going to the toilet or changing a diaper and before preparing and eating food. Transmission of GI infections in the childcare setting is reduced significantly if infection control procedures are followed. High compliance with handwashing decreases episodes of diarrhea by 66%.[18]
- Avoid lactose-containing products if lactose intolerance is suspected or diagnosed.
- Avoid gluten-containing products if celiac disease is diagnosed.
- Encourage maintenance of a diet diary to uncover food intolerances or sensitivities and consider an elimination diet to see if improvement of symptoms occurs.
- Prevent food poisoning:[19]
  - Avoid milk and fruit juices that are unpasteurized
  - Cook foods thoroughly, especially red meat, poultry and eggs
  - Eat foods soon after they have been cooked so that pathogens do not have time to grow
  - Rinse foods that are not cooked before they are eaten (fresh fruits and vegetables) under running water
  - Keep hot foods hot (60°C) and cold foods cold (4°C)
  - When preparing raw meats and poultry, keep them separated from cooked food, fresh fruits and vegetables
  - Use separate cutting boards for raw meats and vegetables
  - Reheat foods completely when serving leftovers
  - Wash hands with hot, soapy water before and after preparing food
  - Use mild solution of hot water and soap to clean counters, cutting boards and utensils
  - Protect food from insects and animals.

Pharmacologic Preventive Measures

Two vaccines are available to protect against rotavirus infection (Table 10).[20,21,22]

Probiotics are live microorganisms (bacteria and yeast) that exert a beneficial effect by improving the balance of the host's intestinal flora.[23,24]

There are few well-designed clinical trials of the use of probiotics to prevent or treat diarrhea. However, in children, *Lactobacillus rhamnosus* strain GG (e.g., Culturelle) may reduce the duration of diarrhea due to rotavirus[24] and decrease the incidence of antibiotic-associated diarrhea.[25,26]

Saccharomyces boulardii (e.g., Florastor) has been effective for prevention of antibiotic-associated diarrhea in adults and children as well as prevention of recurrence of *C. difficile* diarrhea in adults.[27] This effectiveness does not extend to elderly, hospitalized patients.[28,29,30] It is generally well tolerated; however, it can cause fungaemia particularly in immunocompromised patients.[27,31,32,33,34,35]

The combination of *Lactobacillus bulgaricus*, *Streptococcus thermophilus* and *Lactobacillus casei Defensis* (DanActive) may be helpful in reducing severity of acute diarrhea in infants and young children.[36,37,38] It may also prevent antibiotic-associated diarrhea caused by *C. difficile* in hospitalized adults.[36,37,38]

Administering a daily dose of fermented milk combining *L. acidophilus* CL1285 and *L. casei* (e.g., Bio-K) is another effective option for preventing antibiotic- and *C. difficile*-associated diarrhea.[39,40] Daily administration of Lactobacillus reuteri DSM 17938 (e.g., Bio-Gaia) or Lactobacillus plantarum 299v (e.g., Metagenics Ultra Flora Intensive Care; TuZen) were also shown to be effective in preventing antibiotic-associated diarrhea.[41,42] Enteral administration of Lactobacillus plantarum 299v was also shown to decrease colonization by *C. difficile* in critically ill patients.[43]

Most probiotics appear relatively safe.[44] There have been isolated reports of serious adverse effects, including a case report of liver abscess due to *L. rhamnosus* in a 74-year-old diabetic with Mirizzi syndrome.[45] Probiotics should be used cautiously in patients who are immunosuppressed or have a badly damaged GI tract.[23]

Dairy products and many commercially available probiotics may contain organisms that, unlike *L. rhamnosus* strain GG, have not been shown to survive in the human GI tract.[23] Yogurt and kefir, in particular, have not been shown to prevent antibiotic-associated diarrhea.[46,47] Product standardization can also be a problem. Despite this heterogeneity, the overall evidence suggests a protective effect of probiotics in preventing antibiotic-associated diarrhea.[48] Products may contain microorganisms not listed on the label or contain quantities of microorganisms other than that listed.[49] As a result, the health benefits of one strain cannot be extrapolated to probiotics in general particularly those of unknown strain composition.

Nonpharmacologic Therapy

For comparative ingredients of nonprescription products, consult the *Compendium of Products for Minor Ailments*—Oral Rehydration Products.

Rehydration and maintaining electrolyte balance are the cornerstones of therapy for diarrhea.[50] **Oral rehydration therapy** (ORT) can treat the majority of patients with diarrhea as well as prevent most diarrhea-related complications.[6] Oral rehydration solution (ORS) utilizes the sodium/glucose-coupled absorption mechanism in the small intestine.[51] ORS is composed of sodium and glucose in the concentration and osmolarity of the luminal fluid. It is recommended by the World Health Organization (WHO) and should be used early, particularly when treating children and the elderly. Diarrhea is the second leading cause of child deaths with 1.9 million children dying yearly mainly from dehydration.[52] The WHO along with UNICEF currently advocate the use of a new ORS formulation which has a decreased osmolarity of 245 mOsm/L compared with an osmolarity of 311 mOsm/L in the previous formulation. This new formulation was recommended in 2002 and has decreased concentrations of glucose and sodium chloride. Studies have shown that a reduced-osmolarity solution decreases stool output by 20%, reduces vomiting by 30% and decreases the need for intravenous therapy by about 30%.[53,54] The WHO formula for ORS is presented in Table 4 as are those of the commercially available Gastrolyte, Pedialyte and Hydralyte.[55,56,57] It should be noted that liquid Hydralyte can be stored in the refrigerator for 30 days once opened compared with 24 and 48 hours for Gastrolyte and Pedialyte respectively. The use of fruit juices, pop or tea with sugar is unsuitable due to the high carbohydrate concentration of these drinks. Homemade ORS can also be used although this is discouraged because mixing errors often occur. Examples of homemade ORS recipes are described in Table 5.

ORT is contraindicated in the following instances:[60]

- Protracted vomiting despite small frequent feedings
- Worsening diarrhea and an inability to keep up with losses
- Stupor or coma
- Intestinal ileus.

Rapid refeeding with age-appropriate foods should immediately follow rehydration.[50] Withholding food for bowel rest, formula dilution and systematic elimination of lactose are no longer standard recommendations.

Table 4: Composition of Oral Rehydration Solution Preparations

Component	WHO	Gastrolyte	Pedialyte	Hydralyte
Sodium (mmol/L)	75	60	45	45
Potassium (mmol/L)	20	20	20	20
Chloride (mmol/L)	65	60	35	45
Bicarbonate (mmol/L)	30	10		
Citrate (mmol/L)	10		10	
Glucose (mmol/L)	75			81 (as monohydrate)
Dextrose (g/L)		17.8	25	

Table 5: Recipes for Homemade Oral Rehydration Solution[58,59]

	Ingredients	Amount
Recipe #1	Fruit juice	240 mL (1 cup)
	Honey (pasteurized)	2.5 mL (one-half teaspoonful)
	Salt	0.5 mL (one-eighth teaspoonful)
	Baking soda	1 mL (one-quarter teaspoonful)
Recipe #2[a]	Purified water	1 L (4 cups)
	Salt	5 mL (1 teaspoonful)
	Sugar	30 mL (2 tablespoonfuls)

[a] Amount of sugar in original reference is reduced from 40 mL to 30 mL, to match the current WHO recommendations.

Children

In most cases, diarrhea in children is self-limiting and non-life-threatening. However, this population can be more susceptible to the adverse consequences of dehydration and should be monitored closely.

The treatment of childhood diarrhea focuses on correcting dehydration with ORT. Although oral rehydration solutions are readily available, effective, safe and economical, they are often underutilized.[50] Underutilization may be due to the inconvenience of ORT administration and a preference for intravenous versus oral rehydration.

Breastfeeding should be continued during episodes of diarrhea[50] and ORS should be offered. If a child is not being breastfed, age appropriate foods should be given as well as ORS as described in Table 6. ORT should start as soon as diarrhea begins and continue until diarrhea is less frequent.

Even if a child refuses ORS by the cup or bottle, the solution is to be given by a medicine dropper or small teaspoon. If vomiting occurs, ORS should be continued with a spoon, giving 15 mL every 10–15 minutes until vomiting stops, then resuming with the regular amount (Table 6). If vomiting does not stop after 4–6 hours, the child should undergo further assessment.

Table 6: **Administration of Oral Rehydration Solution to Non-breastfed Infants**[16]

Age of Child	Amount of Oral Rehydration Solution to Give
0–6 months	30–90 mL every hour
6–24 months	90–125 mL every hour
>2 y	125–250 mL every hour

Early refeeding should begin within 6 hours of beginning ORS. For infants who are formula-fed, start with small, frequent feedings of the child's usual formula. If the diarrhea persists for 2 days, switch to a soy-based or lactose-free formula as lactose intolerance may be suspected.[60]

For older children, early refeeding with age-appropriate, previously tolerated foods is recommended.[50,60] After 24–48 hours, the child's normal diet can resume. It may take 7–10 days for stools to become completely formed. Restricting a child to a complex carbohydrate diet (e.g., BRATT diet: bananas, rice, applesauce, tea and toast) is inappropriate.[61]

For dehydrating, persistent diarrhea the use of hypo-osmolar ORS (e.g., the new WHO ORS, Gastrolyte, Pedialyte, Hydralyte) is beneficial and superior to the older iso-osmolar WHO ORS (see Table 4).[62] Hypo-osmolar ORS results in a shorter period of diarrhea, less stool output and less need for maintenance therapy.

Pharmacologic Therapy

Antidiarrheal medications are indicated for relief of debilitating symptoms that accompany diarrheal illness. Select agents useful in the management of diarrhea are described in Table 11.

For further discussion of pharmacologic therapy for diarrhea, consult the *Compendium of Therapeutic Choices*: Diarrhea.

For comparative ingredients of nonprescription products, consult the *Compendium of Products for Minor Ailments*—Gastrointestinal Products: Antidiarrheals.

The World Health Organization and UNICEF now recommend supplementation with **zinc** 20 mg daily for 10–14 days for infants >6 months and 10 mg per day for infants <6 months of age. Zinc supplementation decreases both the severity and the duration of acute or persistent diarrhea in children.[52,63,64] Supplementing with a combination of micronutrients and vitamins is not superior to zinc alone.[65] The addition of zinc and prebiotics to ORS limits the duration of diarrhea in children.[66]

Other pharmacologic therapies for diarrhea include:

- **Cholestyramine:** useful in treatment of bile acid-induced diarrhea[1]
- **Fidaxomicin**, **metronidazole** and **oral vancomycin**: useful in treating diarrhea due to *C. difficile* [67,68]
- **Codeine:** doses necessary for antidiarrheal effect may not be safely attainable with nonprescription products and may result in acetaminophen toxicity
- **Clonidine:** effective against diarrhea associated with opioid withdrawal and diabetic autonomic neuropathy[1]
- **Diphenoxylate with atropine:** less effective than loperamide[69]
- **Octreotide:** useful in diarrhea due to chemotherapy, short bowel syndrome, neuroendocrine tumors, AIDS-associated diarrhea and other chronic diarrhea not responding to standard treatment.[70,71]

Natural Health Products

Natural health products that have been used for the treatment of diarrhea include German chamomile, carob, marshmallow, slippery elm, bayberry, blackberry leaf, raspberry leaf, bilberry, agrimony, quercetin and berberine.[72] None have been found to be effective.

Pregnancy

Acute diarrhea in pregnancy is mainly due to viral or bacterial causes and is usually self-limiting. Maintenance of fluid intake is important. **Bulking agents** may be of use and systemic agents such as **loperamide** should be reserved for severe cases when the risk of dehydration outweighs the risk of the drug used.[73]

Elderly

The elderly are particularly susceptible to dehydration due to diarrhea. Nursing homes are similar to childcare settings where pathogens are spread by the oral-fecal route. Prompt rehydration is essential to avoid damage to vital organs.

Monitoring of Therapy

Table 7 provides a monitoring plan framework that should be individualized.

Table 7: **Monitoring of Therapy for Diarrhea**

Symptoms	Monitoring	Endpoint	Actions
Loose, watery stools	Patient: Regularly as long as symptoms persist. Healthcare practitioner: Ask for symptom report; call patient within 48 h to see if symptoms have resolved.	Resolution of symptoms. Return to usual bowel evacuation pattern.	Antidiarrheal medications may be necessary within first 2 days to alleviate symptoms. If symptoms persist beyond 48 h, seek medical attention.
Signs and symptoms of dehydration (Table 3)	Patient: Continually.	No signs of dehydration.	If signs of dehydration (Table 3 and Figure 1) occur despite oral rehydration therapy, reassess.
Fever or blood in stools	Patient: Regularly as long as symptoms persist.	No fever; no blood in stools.	Reassess if this occurs.

Travellers' Diarrhea

Travellers' diarrhea (TD) is known by many colloquial names including Montezuma's revenge, GI trots, Turkey trots, turista and Delhi belly. It is defined by 3 or more loose, unformed stools per day along with at least 1 symptom of enteric infection such as fever, abdominal cramps, nausea, fecal urgency or dysentery.[74] TD is a generally self-limiting illness which usually resolves within 3–4 days even without treatment. However, infants, the elderly, patients with severe chronic diseases (e.g., chronic renal failure, heart failure, insulin-dependent diabetes mellitus, inflammatory bowel disease) and immunocompromised hosts may experience significant complications. It is estimated that TD could affect up to 50% of persons travelling from industrialized countries to developing countries like Latin America, Asia and Africa.[75] In many cases symptoms develop during the first week of travel and more than 90% of cases occur within the first 2 weeks of travel.[76] An episode of TD does not protect against future attacks and more than 1 episode could be experienced in a single trip.[77,78]

Pathophysiology

TD is associated with food or water that is contaminated by bacteria, viruses or parasites (Table 8). However, up to 50% of TD cases may have no identifiable cause.[79] The microorganisms are primarily spread by the fecal-oral route and vary depending on the geographical area visited as well as the time of year (more in summer months and rainy seasons.) Low-risk areas include Canada, the United States, Australia, New Zealand, Japan, and Northern and Western Europe. Intermediate-risk areas include Southern Europe, South Africa, Israel, Russia and some Caribbean Islands (e.g., Haiti and Dominican Republic). High-risk areas include large areas of Asia, Africa and Latin America.[76,80,81] Factors associated with an increased likelihood of acquiring TD include travel from an industrialized country to a developing tropical or semitropical region, contraction of TD on a previous trip, low-budget or adventure travel, adventurous eating habits, daily use of proton pump inhibitors and a relative lack of gut immunity seen in younger individuals.[58,80,82]

Table 8: **Common Causes of Travellers' Diarrhea**

Bacterial (up to 80% of cases)	Viral (5–25% of cases)	Parasitic (up to 10% of cases)
Aeromonas spp.—common in Thailand	Norwalk virus	*Cryptosporidium* spp.—common in Russia
Campylobacter jejuni—common in Mexico, Thailand, Morocco (dry winter)	Rotavirus	*Cyclospora cayetanensis*—common in Guatemala, Haiti, Nepal and Peru
Enterotoxigenic *Escherichia coli* (ETEC)—common in Latin America, Africa	Astrovirus	*Cystoisospora belli*
Plesiomonas spp.	Enteric adenoviruses	*Dientamoeba fragilis*
Salmonella spp.		*Entamoeba histolytica*
Shigella spp.		*Giardia lamblia*—common in Nepal and Russia
Vibrio cholerae—common in Bali, Ecuador, India and Indonesia		
Yersinia spp.		

Goals of Therapy

- Assess/reduce the risk of experiencing TD at the travel destination
- Assess patient's existing medical conditions that may contribute to experiencing TD
- Educate travellers about food hygiene and safe drinking water to reduce the risk of TD
- Educate travellers about effective treatment regimens in case they experience symptoms
- Educate travellers about when to be evaluated by a healthcare practitioner
- Minimize suffering/interruption of vacation or business plans and associated costs
- Prevent complications such as dehydration
- Reduce symptoms in the period immediately following travel

Patient Assessment

Assess travellers to determine their risk of experiencing TD before travel. This assessment allows patients at increased risk to seek appropriate medications before travelling.

Risk factors for developing TD or its complications include:

- Children or young adults (particularly those with adventurous eating habits)
- Destination has poor standards of hygiene, accommodation or sanitation amenities (e.g., Africa, most of Asia, Central and South America and Middle East)
- Elderly or frail
- Immunocompromised

- Inflammatory bowel disease
- Reduced stomach acidity
- Diabetes
- Travelling to remote areas with few or no medical amenities.

The assessment and management of TD is illustrated in Figure 3. Any red flags would require further detailed assessment (Table 2).[83]

Prevention

The incidence of TD can be minimized by choosing appropriate foods and avoiding those associated with the illness (Table 9).

Table 9: **Food and Travellers' Diarrhea**

Safe Foods/Beverages	Unsafe Foods/Beverages
Beer or wine	Buffet food at room temperature
Boiled or bottled water	Cold salads
Carbonated beverages (with no ice cubes)	Condiments in open bottles
Cooked vegetables	Custards, mousses, mayonnaise, hollandaise sauce
Dry food (e.g., bread)	Food from street vendors
Hot beverages (e.g., tea, coffee)	Fresh soft cheese
Pasteurized milk (if properly stored)	Ice cubes/chips
Peeled fruit (preferably done by self)	Large reef fish from the Caribbean and South Pacific (e.g., snapper, barracuda, grouper, jack, moray eel)
Piping hot food	Leafy and/or raw vegetables
Thoroughly and recently cooked meats and fish	Leftovers
	Raspberries/strawberries/watermelon
	Shellfish
	Uncooked, cold sauces
	Undercooked hamburger/meat/fish
	Unpeeled fruit

Other measures that travellers should follow include:

- Follow the adage "Boil it, cook it, peel it or forget it"
- Use purified water or water from the hot tap to brush teeth
- Wash hands frequently while travelling, particularly before handling or consuming food (if soap and water are unavailable, consider using commercially available waterless hand sanitizing agents)[58]
- Avoid drinking the water while swimming
- Avoid drinking local water
- Drink bottled beverages in their original containers and ensure the cap is sealed
- Bismuth subsalicylate is 60–65% effective as a prophylactic agent[58] (Table 12) and may be used to prevent TD.

Consider antibiotic prophylaxis only in selected cases:

- People who cannot tolerate even a brief illness (e.g., elite athletes, business or political travellers)
- People at high risk of TD due to achlorhydria, gastrectomy or history of repeated episodes of severe TD
- Those who are immunosuppressed

- Those with chronic illness at increased risk of experiencing complications due to TD.

Routine antibiotic prophylaxis is not recommended for a number of reasons which include antibiotic resistance, photosensitivity reactions, severe allergic reactions (e.g., Stevens-Johnson syndrome), *C. difficile*-associated diarrhea and candidal vaginitis.[77]

A number of studies have shown the effectiveness of **probiotics** such as *Lactobacillus GG* (e.g., Culturelle) and *Saccharomyces boulardii* (e.g., Florastor) to prevent TD. These regimens typically involve starting the probiotic 2–3 days before travel and continuing until the end of travel or until 2 days after returning from travel. While routine recommendations are not yet advised, studies continue to show promise. However, these data should not be extrapolated to all strains of probiotics since variation can be present.[87,88]

Methods for purifying untreated water are discussed in Appendix III: Information for the Traveller.

Nonpharmacologic Therapy

For comparative ingredients of nonprescription products, consult the *Compendium of Products for Minor Ailments*—Oral Rehydration Products.

Travellers are advised to maintain and possibly increase their fluid intake during bouts of diarrhea, though dehydration is not a major concern. Health Canada suggests that children and the elderly use ORS, while healthy adults maintain hydration with canned juices, purified water, carbonated soft drinks or clear salty soups to maintain light-coloured urine and relieve thirst.[58] Dairy products, alcohol, caffeine, prune juice, orange juice and apple juice should be avoided.

Pharmacologic Therapy

Select agents for the prevention of TD are described in Table 12. Table 13 lists some medications used in the treatment of TD. For further discussion of pharmacologic therapy for travellers' diarrhea, consult the *Compendium of Therapeutic Choices*: Travellers' Diarrhea.

For comparative ingredients of nonprescription products, consult the *Compendium of Products for Minor Ailments*—Gastrointestinal Products: Antidiarrheals.

Antibiotics useful in treating TD include the **fluoroquinolones (ciprofloxacin**, **levofloxacin**, **norfloxacin** or **ofloxacin**) and **azithromycin**.[88] Azithromycin is particularly useful in pregnant patients or children since fluoroquinolones are contraindicated in these populations. Azithromycin may be preferred over the fluoroquinolones where ciprofloxacin-resistant Campylobacter is a growing concern (e.g., Asia).[88]

Sulfamethoxazole/trimethoprim and doxycycline are of limited use due to widespread resistance.[58] Prior to departure, travellers should have antibiotics on hand for use in case of diarrhea while travelling in order to reduce duration and severity of the illness.[89]

Goldenseal (*Hydrastis canadensis*) has been used to treat TD. The primary active constituent is thought to be berberine. There are insufficient human data to support the efficacy of goldenseal or berberine in the treatment of infectious diarrhea. The dose of **berberine sulfate** used in clinical studies was 400 mg per day given in 1–4 divided doses. The adult dose of dried herb is 0.5–1 g, 3 times daily. Safety in children or during breastfeeding has not been established. Goldenseal is contraindicated during pregnancy. The use of goldenseal extracts as outlined appears safe. However, administration of high doses of berberine may result in serious adverse effects (e.g., hypertension, seizures, respiratory failure).[90,91]

Monitoring of Therapy

Patients can monitor their condition based on the frequency and severity of symptoms. They can expect a fairly brief illness if they take medication and in some cases even without medication.[58] Monitoring includes reduction of loose, watery stools to ≤1 per day within 2–3 days.[58,83] Medical attention should be sought if the patient develops signs of dehydration, or if a child <2 years develops bloody stools, a rectal temperature >38.5°C or persistent vomiting.[58,83] If symptoms persist longer than 14 days without pharmacologic treatment or longer than 2 days despite optimum pharmacologic treatment a healthcare practitioner should be consulted.

Figure 2: **Assessment and Management of Patients with Diarrhea Not Related to Travel**[9,16]

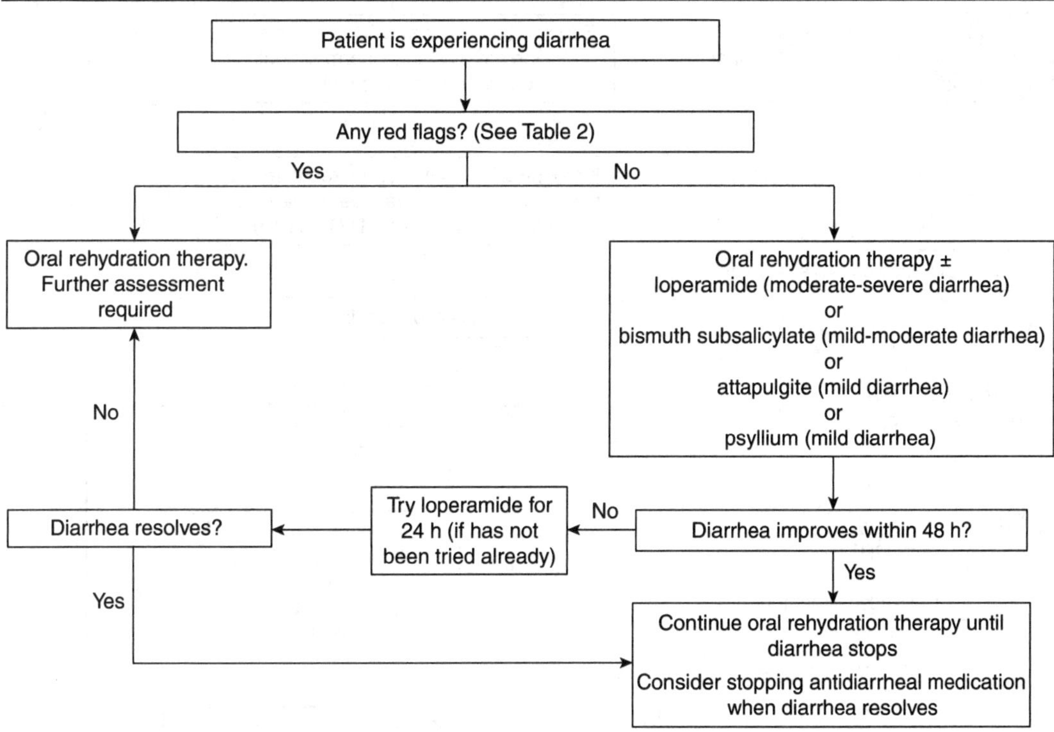

Figure 3: **Assessment and Self-management of Travellers' Diarrhea**[58,83]

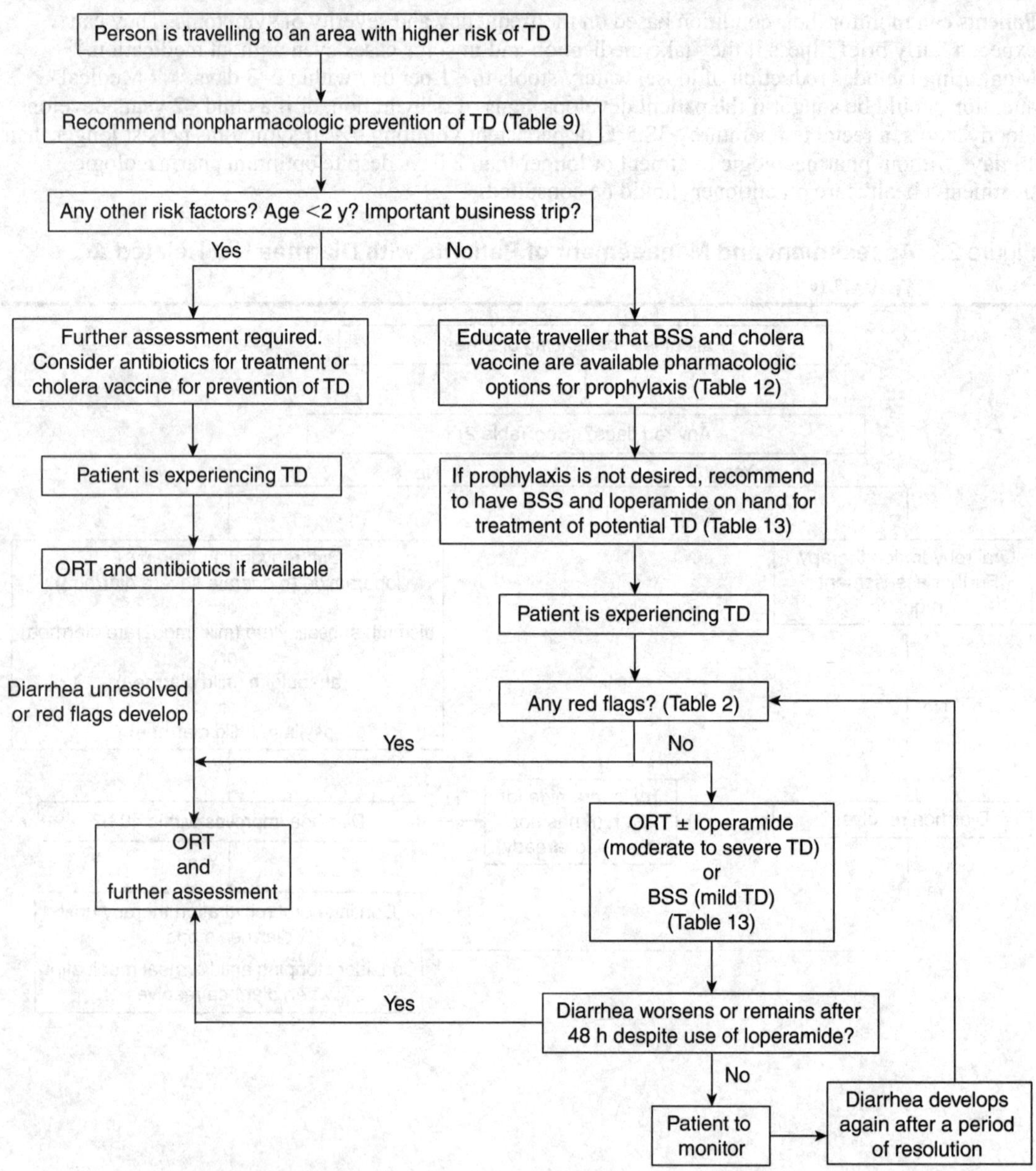

Abbreviations: BSS = bismuth subsalicylate; ORT = oral rehydration therapy; TD = travellers' diarrhea

Table 10: Vaccines for Rotavirus Prevention

Class	Drug	Dosage	Adverse Effects	Drug Interactions	Comments	Cost[a]
Vaccines	*rotavirus pentavalent, live oral vaccine* RotaTeq	3 total doses First dose usually given between 6 and 12 weeks of age; subsequent doses should have 4–10 wk between them. Can be given with other routine immunizations	Mild fever (20%), diarrhea (24.1%), vomiting (15.2%), otitis media (14.5%), bronchospasm (1.1%).	Immunosuppressive therapies (e.g., anti-TNF-α agents) passed from the mother to the fetus may remain in the newborn's blood for up to 6 months postdelivery; avoid administering any live vaccines to the newborn until at least 6 months of age.	Contains 5 rotavirus strains responsible for about 95% of rotavirus disease in Canada. 85–98% effective against severe rotavirus disease. Can decrease hospitalizations by up to 96%.	$60
	rotavirus monovalent, live oral vaccine Rotarix	2 total doses First dose usually given after 6 weeks of age; subsequent dose given at least 4 wk later but no later than 24 weeks of age. Can be given with other routine immunizations	Rarely intussusception (type of bowel blockage).	See rotavirus pentavalent.	85–98% effective against severe rotavirus disease.	$90

[a] Cost per dose; includes drug cost only.

Table 11: **Nonprescription Drug Therapy for Diarrhea**[a]

Class	Drug	Dosage	Adverse Effects	Drug Interactions	Comments	Cost[b]
Adsorbent Agents	*attapulgite* Kaopectate	**>12 y:** 1200–1500 mg po initially, then 1200–1500 mg after each BM Maximum: 8400 mg/day **6–12 y:** 600–750 mg po initially, then 600–750 mg after each BM Maximum: 4200 mg per day **3–5 y:** 300 mg po initially, then 300 mg after each BM Maximum: 2100 mg per day	Well tolerated.	No known drug interactions.	May be useful for treatment of mild to moderate acute diarrhea.	$
Antimotility Agents	*loperamide* Imodium, generics	**>12 y:** 4 mg po initially, then 2 mg after each loose BM Maximum: 16 mg per day **9–12 y:** 2 mg TID po for 1 day then 0.1 mg/kg/dose after each loose BM (not to exceed 2 mg/dose) **6–8 y:** 2 mg BID po for 1 day then 0.1 mg/kg/dose after each loose BM (not to exceed 2 mg/dose) **2–5 y:** 1 mg TID po for 1 day then 0.1 mg/kg/dose after each loose BM (not to exceed 1 mg/dose)	Abdominal cramps or discomfort, drowsiness, dizziness, dry mouth, skin rash.	Concomitant administration of loperamide with quinidine or ritonavir may increase loperamide's plasma levels.	Do not use in children <3 y or in those who are malnourished, moderately or severely dehydrated or systemically ill or in those with bloody diarrhea. Use with caution in children <12 y. Discontinue if symptoms persist longer than 48 h. Opiate-like CNS effects have been observed in children <3 y. Monitor patients with hepatic dysfunction for signs of CNS toxicity.	$
Antisecretory Agents	*bismuth subsalicylate* Pepto-Bismol, generics	**>14 y:** 524 mg every 30–60 min PRN po (maximum 4.2 g/day) **10–14 y:** 262 mg every 30–60 min PRN po (maximum 2.1 g/day) **5–9 y:** 131 mg every 30–60 min PRN po (maximum 1 g/day) **2–4 y:** 88 mg every 30–60 min PRN po (maximum 0.7 g/day)	Black tongue and stools, tinnitus.	Avoid in patients taking anticoagulants, methotrexate, probenecid, salicylates.	Used to treat chronic idiopathic diarrhea with a reduction in stool weight and frequency. Bismuth subsalicylate is available as a 17.6 mg/mL liquid or 262 mg tablets.	$

Class	Drug	Dosage	Adverse Effects	Drug Interactions	Comments	Cost[b]
Hydrophilic Bulking Agents	*psyllium* Metamucil Preparations, generics	**Adults:** up to 40 g/day po in 2–4 divided doses **Children >6 y:** 5 g up to 2–4 times daily po	Cramping, flatulence.	Concomitant administration may interfere with the absorption of carbamazepine and lithium.	Separate administration of other medications by 2 h. Contraindicated in patients with dysphagia. Allergic reactions have occurred. Esophageal obstruction has occurred when insufficient liquid was administered with the dose.	$

[a] For more information on pharmacologic therapy for diarrhea, consult the *Compendium of Therapeutic Choices*: Diarrhea.

[b] Cost per day; includes drug cost only.

Legend: $ <$1

Table 12: **Drug Therapy for Prevention of Travellers' Diarrhea**[a]

Class	Drug	Dosage	Adverse Effects	Drug Interactions	Comments	Cost[b]
Antisecretory Agents	*bismuth subsalicylate* Pepto-Bismol, generics	**>14 y:** 524 mg QID po **10–14 y:** 262 mg QID po **5–9 y:** 131 mg QID po **2–4 y:** 88 mg QID po Start 1 day before travel and continue until 2 days after leaving destination	Black tongue/stool, tinnitus.	Avoid in patients taking anticoagulants, methotrexate, probenecid, salicylates. Can interfere with absorption of doxycycline (which may be used for malaria prevention).	Avoid in patients with history of ASA allergy, renal insufficiency and gout. Limit prophylaxis to 3 wk. Not for children <2 y. Can decrease incidence of travellers' diarrhea from 40% to 14%.	$
Vaccines	*cholera vaccine, inactivated oral* Dukoral	**>2 y:** 2 doses po First dose at least 2 wk before departure Second dose 1 wk after the first dose and at least 1 wk before departure If more than 6 wk elapse between the first and second dose, the primary immunization should be restarted	No significant or common adverse effects.	Separate administration of encapsulated oral typhoid vaccine by at least 8 h. Oral administration of other vaccines and medicinal products should be avoided 1 h before and 1 h after vaccination.	About 43% short-term protection against diarrhea caused by enterotoxigenic *E. coli*.[84,85] A booster dose is required every 3 months if the risk is ongoing. Food should be avoided 1 h before and after administration. Not recommended for routine use since it may not be effective for prevention of TD;[86] can be considered when risk is high.	$40/dose

[a] For more information on pharmacologic prevention of travellers' diarrhea, consult the *Compendium of Therapeutic Choices*: Travellers' Diarrhea.

[b] Cost per day unless otherwise specified; includes drug cost only.

Legend: $ <$1

Table 13: Drug Therapy for Treatment of Travellers' Diarrhea[a]

Class	Drug	Dosage	Adverse Effects	Drug Interactions	Comments	Cost[b]
Antimotility Agents	*loperamide* Imodium, generics	Prevention: Not recommended Treatment: **>12 y:** 4 mg stat then 2 mg after each loose BM po Maximum: 16 mg per day **9–12 y:** 2 mg TID po for 1 day then 0.1 mg/kg/dose after each loose BM (not to exceed 2 mg/dose) **6–8 y:** 2 mg BID po for 1 day then 0.1 mg/kg/dose after each loose BM (not to exceed 2 mg/dose) **2–5 y:** 1 mg TID po for 1 day then 0.1 mg/kg/dose after each loose BM (not to exceed 1 mg/dose)	Abdominal cramps or discomfort, drowsiness, dizziness, dry mouth, skin rash.	Concomitant administration of loperamide with quinidine or ritonavir may increase loperamide's plasma levels.	Do not use in children <3 y or in those who are malnourished, moderately or severely dehydrated or systemically ill or in those with bloody diarrhea. Use with caution in children <12 y. Discontinue if symptoms persist longer than 48 h. Opiate-like CNS effects have been observed in children <3 y. Monitor patients with hepatic dysfunction for signs of CNS toxicity.	$
Antisecretory Agents	*bismuth subsalicylate* Pepto-Bismol, generics	2 × 262 mg tablets or equivalent suspension every 30 min × 8 doses	Black tongue and stools, tinnitus.	Avoid in patients taking anticoagulants, methotrexate, probenecid, salicylates.	Bismuth subsalicylate is also available as a 17.6 mg/mL suspension. Bismuth subsalicylate is also available as 17.5 mg/mL, 35.2 mg/mL and 35 mg/mL.	$

[a] For more information on pharmacologic therapy for travellers' diarrhea, consult the *Compendium of Therapeutic Choices*: Travellers' Diarrhea.

[b] Cost per day; includes drug cost only.

Legend: $ <$1

Suggested Readings

Diarrhea

Guarino A, Dupont C, Gorelov AV et al. The management of acute diarrhea in children in developed and developing areas: from evidence base to clinical practice. *Expert Opin Pharmacother* 2012;13:17-26.

Hempel S, Newberry SJ, Maher AR et al. Probiotics for the prevention and treatment of antibiotic-associated diarrhea: a systematic review and meta-analysis. *JAMA* 2012;307:1959-69.

McClarren RL, Lynch B, Nyayapati N. Acute infectious diarrhea. *Prim Care* 2011;38:539-64.

Parashar UD, Gibson CJ, Bresse JS et al. Rotavirus and severe childhood diarrhea. *Emerg Infect Dis* 2006;12:304-6.

Pilotto A, Franceschi M, Vitale D et al. The prevalence of diarrhea and its association with drug use in elderly outpatients: a multicenter study. *Am J Gastroenterol* 2008;103:2816-23.

Venugopal AA, Johnson S. Current state of Clostridium difficile treatment options. *Clin Infect Dis* 2012;55:S71-6.

Travellers' Diarrhea

Kollaritsch H, Paulke-Korinek M, Wiedermann U. Traveler's diarrhea. *Infect Dis Clin North Am* 2012;26:691-706.

Paredes-Paredes M, Flores-Figueroa J, Dupont HL. Advances in the treatment of travelers' diarrhea. *Curr Gastroenterol Rep* 2011;13:402-7.

Shah N, DuPont HL, Ramsey DJ. Global etiology of travelers' diarrhea: systematic review from 1973 to the present. *Am J Trop Med Hyg* 2009;80:609-14.

Singh E, Redfield D. Prophylaxis for travelers' diarrhea. *Curr Gastroenterol Rep* 2009;11:297-300.

References

1. Deepak P, Ehrenpreis ED. Diarrhea. *Dis Mon* 2011;57:490-510.
2. Wanke C. *Epidemiology and causes of acute diarrhea in resource rich countries*. Available from: www.uptodate.com. Accessed May 4, 2015. Subscription required.
3. Sandler RS, Stewart WF, Liberman JN et al. Abdominal pain, bloating and diarrhea in the United States: prevalence and impact. *Dig Dis Sci* 2000;45:1166-71.
4. Manatsathit, S, Dupont HL, Farthing M et al. Guideline for the management of acute diarrhea in adults. *J Gastroenterol Hepatol* 2002;17:S54-71.
5. Lamberti L, Fischer Walker CL et al. Systematic review of diarrhea duration and severity in children and adults in low-middle income countries. *BMC Public Health* 2012;12:276.
6. Ladinsky M, Duggan A, Santosham M et al. The World Health Organization oral rehydration solution in US pediatric practice: a randomized trial to evaluate parent satisfaction. *Arch Pediatr Adolesc Med* 2000;154:700-5.
7. World Gastroenterology Organisation Global Guidelines. *Acute diarrhea in adults and children: a global perspective*. February 2012 p. 3. Available from: www.worldgastroenterology.org/guidelines/global-guidelines/acute-diarrhea/acute-diarrhea-english. Accessed May 4, 2015.
8. World Health Organization. *Ending preventable deaths from pneumonia and diarrhea by 2025*. Available from: www.who.int/maternal_child_adolescent/news_events/news/2013/gappd_launch/en. Accessed May 4, 2015.
9. Grimwood K, Forbes DA. Acute and persistent diarrhea. *Pediatr Clin North Am* 2009;56:1343-61.
10. Dennehy PH. Rotavirus infection: an update on management and prevention. *Adv Pediatr* 2012;59:47-74.
11. Thomas RE, Wyer M. Nausea, vomiting, diarrhea and constipation. In: Herfindal ET, Gourley DR, Hart LL, eds. *Clinical pharmacy and therapeutics*. 4th ed. Baltimore: Williams & Wilkins; 1998. p. 306-7.
12. U.S. National Library of Medicine. MedlinePlus. Eisner T. *Drug-induced diarrhea*. Updated November 2, 2014. Available from: www.nlm.nih.gov/medlineplus/ency/article/000293.htm. Accessed May 4, 2015.
13. Owens RC, Donskey CJ, Gaynes RP et al. Antimicrobial-associated risk factors for Clostridium difficile infection. *Clin Infect Dis* 2008;46:S19-31.
14. Mehta DI, Blecker U. Chronic diarrhea in infancy and childhood. *J La State Med Soc* 1998;150:419-29.
15. Bowen R. *Pathophysiology of diarrhea*. Updated July 27, 2006. Available from: www.vivo.colostate.edu/hbooks/pathphys/digestion/smallgut/diarrhea.html. Accessed May 4, 2015.
16. Canadian Paediatric Society. Caring for Kids. *Dehydration and diarrhea in children: prevention and treatment*. Updated June 2013. Available from: www.caringforkids.cps.ca/handouts/dehydration_and_diarrhea. Accessed February 8, 2016.
17. Thomas DR, Cote TR, Lawhorne L et al. Understanding clinical dehydration and its treatment. *J Am Med Dir Assoc* 2008;9:292-301.
18. Roberts L, Jorm L, Patel M et al. Effect of infection control measures on the frequency of diarrheal episodes in child care: a randomized, controlled trial. *Pediatrics* 2000;105:743-6.
19. Canadian Paediatric Society. Caring for Kids. *Food safety at home*. Updated October 2014. Available from: www.caringforkids.cps.ca/handouts/food_safety_at_home. Accessed February 8, 2016.
20. Kollaritsch H, Wiedermann U. [Examples for vaccines against diarrheal diseases—rotavirus and traveller's diarrhea]. *Wien Med Wochenschr* 2007;157:102-6. [German].

21. CPS online. Ottawa: Canadian Pharmacists Association; 2015. *Rotarix* [product monograph]. Available from: www.e-therapeutics.ca. Subscription required.
22. CPS online. Ottawa: Canadian Pharmacists Association; 2013. *RotaTeq* [product monograph]. Available from: www.e-therapeutics.ca. Subscription required.
23. Elmer GW. Probiotics: "living drugs". *Am J Health Syst Pharm* 2001;58:1101-9.
24. Alvarez-Olmos MI, Oberhelman RA. Probiotic agents and infectious diseases: a modern perspective on a traditional therapy. *Clin Infect Dis* 2001;32:1567-76.
25. Johnston BC, Supina AL, Ospina M et al. Probiotics for the prevention of pediatric antibiotic-associated diarrhea. *Cochrane Database Syst Rev* 2007;(2):CD004827.
26. Vanderhoof JA, Whitney DB, Antonson DL et al. Lactobacillus GG in the prevention of antibiotic-associated diarrhea in children. *J Pediatr* 1999;135:564-8.
27. Pillai A, Nelson R. Probiotics for treatment of Clostridium difficile-associated colitis in adults. *Cochrane Database Syst Rev* 2008;(1):CD004611.
28. Pozzoni P, Riva A, Bellatorre AG et al. Sacchromyces boulardii for the prevention of antibiotic associated diarrhea in adult hospitalized patients: a single-center, randomized, double-blind, placebo-controlled trial. *Am J Gastroenterology* 2012;107:922-31.
29. Allen SJ, Wareham K, Wang D et al. Lactobacilli and bifidobacteria in the prevention of antibiotic-associated diarrhea and Clostridium difficile diarrhea in older inpatients (PLACIDE): a randomized, double-blind, placebo-controlled, multicenter trial. *Lancet* 2013;382:1249-57.
30. Allen SJ, Wareham K, Wang D et al. A high-dose preparation of lactobacilli and bifidobacteria in the prevention of antibiotic-associated and Clostridium difficile diarrhea in older people admitted to hospital: a multicenter, randomized , double-blind, placebo, controlled, parallel arm trial (PLACIDE). *Health Technol Assess* 2013;17:1-140.
31. Guarino A, LoVecchio A, Canani RB. Probiotics as prevention and treatment for diarrhea. *Curr Opin Gastroenterol* 2009;25:18-23.
32. Szajewska H, Skorka A, Dylag M. Meta-analysis: Saccharomyces boulardii for treating acute diarrhoea in children. *Aliment Pharmacol Ther* 2007;25:257-64.
33. Guslandi M. Are probiotics effective for treating Clostridium difficile disease and antibiotic-associated diarrhea? *Nat Clin Pract Gastroenterol Hepatol* 2006;3:606-7.
34. McFarland LV, Surawicz CM, Greenberg RN et al. A randomized placebo-controlled trial of Saccharomyces boulardii in combination with standard antibiotics for Clostridium difficile disease. *JAMA* 1994;271:1913-8.
35. Feizizadeh S, Salehi-Abargouei A, Akbari V. Efficacy and safety of Sacchromyces boulardii for acute diarrhea. *Pediatrics* 2014;134:e176-91.
36. Pedone CA, Bernabeu AO, Postaire ER et al. The effect of supplementation with milk fermented by Lactobacillus casei (strain DN-114 001) on acute diarrhoea in children attending day care centres. *Int J Clin Pract* 1999;53:179-84.
37. Pedone CA, Arnaud CC, Postaire ER et al. Multicentric study of the effect of milk fermented by Lactobacillus casei on the incidence of diarrhoea. *Int J Clin Pract* 2000;54:568-71.
38. Hickson M, D'Souza AL, Muthu N et al. Use of probiotic Lactobacillus preparation to prevent diarrhoea associated with antibiotics: randomised double blind placebo controlled trial. *BMJ* 2007;335:80.
39. Beausoleil M, Fortier N, Guenette S et al. Effect of a fermented milk combining Lactobacillus acidophilus CL1285 and Lactobacillus casei in the prevention of antibiotic-associated diarrhea: a randomized, double-blind, placebo-controlled trial. *Can J Gastroenterol* 2007;21:732-6.
40. Gao XW, Mubasher M, Fang CY et al. Dose-response efficacy of a proprietary probiotic formula of Lactobacillus acidophilus CL1285 and Lactobacillus casei LBC 80R for antibiotic associated diarrhea and Clostridium difficile-associated diarrhea prophylaxis in adult patients. *Am J Gastroenterol* 2010;105:1636-41.
41. Gutierrez-Castrellon P, Lopez-Velazquez G, Diaz-Garcia L et al. Diarrhea in preschool children and Lactobacillus reuteri: a randomized controlled trial. *Pediatrics* 2014;133:e904-9.
42. Lonnermark E, Friman V, Lappas G et al. Intake of Lactobacillus plantarum reduces certain gastrointestinal symptoms during treatment with antibiotics. *J Clin Gastroenterol* 2010;44:106-12.
43. Klarin B, Wullt M, Palmquist I et al. Lactobacillus plantarum 299v reduces colonization of Clostridium difficile in critically ill patients treated with antibiotics. *Acta Anaesthesiol Scand* 2008;52:1096-102.
44. Allen SJ, Martinez EG, Gregorio GV et al. Probiotics for treating acute infectious diarrhea. *Cochrane Database Syst Rev* 2010;(11):CD003048.
45. Chan JF, Lau SK, Woo PC et al. Lactobacillus rhamnosus hepatic abscess associated with Mirizzi syndrome: a case report and review of the literature. *Diagn Microbiol Infect Dis* 2010;66:94-7.
46. Conway S, Hart A, Clark A et al. Does eating yogurt prevent antibiotic-associated diarrhoea? A placebo-controlled randomised controlled trial in general practice. *Br J Gen Pract* 2007;57:953-9.
47. Merenstein DJ, Foster J, D'Amico F. A randomized clinical trial measuring the influence of kefir on antibiotic-associated diarrhea: the measuring the influence of Kefir (MILK) Study. *Arch Pediatr Adolesc Med* 2009;163:750-4.
48. Johnston BC, Goldenberg JZ, Vandvik PO et al. Probiotics for the prevention of pediatric antibiotic-associated diarrhea. *Cochrane Database Syst Rev* 2011;(11):CD004827.
49. Hamilton-Miller JM, Shah S, Smith CT. "Probiotic" remedies are not what they seem. *BMJ* 1996;312:55-6.
50. Guarino A, Dupont C, Gorelov AV et al. The management of acute diarrhea in children in developed and developing areas: from evidence base to clinical practice. *Expert Opin Pharmacother* 2012;13:17-26.
51. Institute of Medicine; Marriott BM, ed. *Fluid replacement and heat stress*. Washington: National Academies Press; 1994. Available from: www.nap.edu/openbook.php?record_id=9071&page=13. Accessed February 8, 2016.
52. World Health Organization. *Improved formula for oral rehydration salts to save children's lives*. Available from: www.who.int/mediacentre/news/releases/2006/pr14/en/index.html. Accessed February 8, 2016.
53. World Health Organization. *New formula for oral rehydration salts will save millions of lives*. Available from: www.who.int/mediacentre/news/releases/release35/en/index.html. Accessed February 8, 2016.
54. Hartling L, Bellemare S, Wiebe N et al. Oral versus intravenous rehydration for treating dehydration due to gastroenteritis in children. *Cochrane Database Syst Rev* 2006;(3):CD004390.
55. World Health Organization. *Oral rehydration salts: production of the new ORS*. Available from: whqlibdoc.who.int/hq/2006/WHO_FCH_CAH_06.1.pdf. Accessed February 8, 2016.

56. RxMed: comprehensive resource for physicians, drug and illness information. *Gastrolyte*. Available from: www.rxmed.com/b.main/b2.pharmaceutical/b2.1.monographs/CPS-%20Monographs/CPS-%20(General%20Monographs-%20G)/GASTROLYTE.html. Accessed February 8, 2016.
57. RxMed: comprehensive resource for physicians, drug and illness information. *Pedialyte, Pedialyte freezer pops*. Available from: www.rxmed.com/b.main/b2.pharmaceutical/b2.1.monographs/CPS-%20Monographs/CPS-%20(General%20Monographs-%20P)/PEDIALYTE.html. Accessed February 8, 2016.
58. Committee to Advise on Tropical Medicine and Travel (CATMAT). An Advisory Committee Statement (ACS). *Statement on travellers' diarrhea*. Ottawa: Public Health Agency of Canada; 2015. Available from: www.phac-aspc.gc.ca/tmp-pmv/catmat-ccmtmv/assets/pdfs/diarrhea-diarrhee-eng.pdf.
59. World Health Organization. *WHO position paper on oral rehydration salts to reduce mortality from cholera*. Available from: www.who.int/cholera/technical/ORSRecommendationsForUseAtHomeDec2008.pdf. Accessed February 8, 2016.
60. Canadian Paediatric Society. Nutrition Committee. *Oral rehydration therapy and early refeeding in the management of childhood gastroenteritis*. Available from: www.cps.ca/en/documents/position/oral-rehydration-therapy. Accessed February 8, 2016.
61. Pieścik-Lech M, Shamir R, Guarino A et al. Review article: the management of acute gastroenteritis in children. *Aliment Pharmacol Ther* 2013;37:289-303.
62. Dutta P, Mitra U, Dutta S et al. Hypo-osmolar oral rehydration salts solution in dehydrating persistent diarrhoea in children: double-blind, randomized, controlled clinical trial. *Acta Paediatr* 2000;89:411-6.
63. Lazzerini M, Ronfani L. Oral zinc for treating diarrhoea in children. *Cochrane Database Syst Rev* 2008;(3):CD005436.
64. Lukacik M, Thomas RL, Aranda JV. A meta-analysis of the effects of oral zinc in the treatment of acute and persistent diarrhea. *Pediatrics* 2008;121:326-36.
65. Dutta P, Mitra U, Dutta S et al. Zinc, vitamin A and micronutrient supplementation in children with diarrhea: a randomized controlled clinical trial of combination therapy vs monotherapy. *J Pediatr* 2011;159:633-7.
66. Passariello A, Terrin G, De Marco G et al. Efficacy of a new hypotonic oral rehydration solution containing zinc and prebiotics in the treatment of childhood acute diarrhea: a randomized controlled trial. *J Pediatr* 2011;158:288-92.
67. Cohen SH, Gerding DN, Johnson S et al. Clinical practice guidelines for Clostridium difficile infection in adults: 2010 update by the society for healthcare epidemiology of America (SHEA) and the infectious diseases society of America (IDSA). *Infect Control Hosp Epidemiol* 2010;31:431-55.
68. Bassetti M, Villa G, Pecori D et al. Epidemiology, diagnosis and treatment of Clostridium difficile infection. *Expert Rev Anti Infect Ther* 2012;10:1405-23.
69. Kollaritsch H, Paulke-Korinek M, Wiedermann U. Traveler's diarrhea. *Infect Dis Clin North Am* 2012;26:691-706.
70. Szilagyi A, Shrier I. Systematic review: the use of somatostatin or octreotide in refractory diarrhoea. *Aliment Pharmacol Ther* 2001;15:1889-97.
71. Cascinu S. Management of diarrhea induced by tumors or cancer therapy. *Curr Opin Oncol* 1995;7:325-9.
72. University of Maryland Medical Centre. Ehrlich S. *Diarrhea*. Reviewed on June 6, 2014. Available from: umm.edu/health/medical/altmed/condition/diarrhea. Accessed February 8, 2016.
73. Einarson A, Mastroiacovo P, Arnon J et al. Prospective, controlled, multicentre study of loperamide in pregnancy. *Can J Gastroenterol* 2000;14:185-7.
74. Itokasu GS, Bearden DT, Danzinger LH. Infectious diarrhea. In: Koda-Kimble MA, Young LL, eds. *Applied therapeutics: the clinical use of drugs*. 10th ed. Philadelphia: Wolters Kluwer/Lippincott Williams & Wilkins; 2013.
75. Leung AK, Robson WL, Davies HD. Traveler's diarrhea. *Adv Ther* 2006;23:519-27.
76. Diemert DJ. Prevention and self-treatment of traveler's diarrhea. *Clin Microbiol Rev* 2006;19:583-94.
77. Connor BA. Travelers' diarrhea. In: Centers for Disease Control and Prevention. *Travelers' health: Yellow book 2010*. Available from: wwwnc.cdc.gov/travel/yellowbook/2010/chapter-2/travelers-diarrhea.aspx. Accessed February 8, 2016.
78. Health Protection Agency. *Travellers' diarrhoea*. Available from: www.hpa.org.uk/HPA/Topics/InfectiousDiseases/InfectionsAZ/1191942149569/. Accessed February 8, 2016.
79. Spira AM. Assessment of travellers who return home ill. *Lancet* 2003;361:1459-69.
80. de la Cabada Bauche J, Dupont HL. New developments in traveler's diarrhea. *Gastroenterol Hepatol (N Y)* 2011;7:88-95.
81. Government of Canada. *Travellers' diarrhea*. Modified March 2, 2015. Available from: travel.gc.ca/travelling/health-safety/diseases/diarrhea. Accessed February 8, 2016.
82. DuPont HL. Travellers' diarrhoea: contemporary approaches to therapy and prevention. *Drugs* 2006;66:303-14.
83. An Advisory Committee Statement (ACS). Committee to Advise on Tropical Medicine and Travel (CATMAT). Persistent Diarrhea in the returned traveller. *Can Commun Dis Rep* 1998;24:1-8.
84. Jelinek T, Kollaritsch H. Vaccination with Dukoral against travelers' diarrhea (ETEC) and cholera. *Expert Rev Vaccines* 2008;7:561-7.
85. Lopez-Gigosos R, Garcia-Fortea P, Calvo MJ et al. Effectiveness and economic analysis of the whole cell/recombinant B subunit (WC/rbs) inactivated oral cholera vaccine in the prevention of traveller's diarrhoea. *BMC Infect Dis* 2009;9:65.
86. Nickonchuk T, Lindblad AJ, Kolber MR. Oral cholera vaccine for traveler's diarrhea prophylaxis. *Can Fam Physician* 2014;60:451.
87. McFarland LV. Meta-analysis of probiotics for the prevention of traveler's diarrhea. *Travel Med Infect Dis* 2007;5:97-105.
88. DuPont HL. Travelers' diarrhea: antimicrobial therapy and chemoprevention. *Nat Clin Pract Gastroenterol Hepatol* 2005;2:191-8.
89. De Bruyn G, Hahn S, Borwick A. Antibiotic treatment for travellers' diarrhoea. *Cochrane Database Syst Rev* 2000;(3):CD002242.
90. Ernst E, Pittler MH, Wider B, eds. *The desktop guide to complementary and alternative medicine: an evidence-based approach*. New York: Mosby Elsevier; 2001.
91. Smith M. Golden seal. In: Chandler F, ed. *Herbs: everyday reference for health professionals*. Ottawa: Canadian Pharmacists Association/Canadian Medical Association; 2000. p. 139-41.

Diarrhea—What You Need to Know

What is diarrhea?

Diarrhea refers to loose and watery bowel movements. Almost everyone has diarrhea at some time in their life. It is especially common in children, who may have diarrhea 2 or 3 times a year.

What causes diarrhea?

Diarrhea is usually caused by an infection or food poisoning. It may also be caused by stress, anxiety, diseases, medications or difficulty digesting some foods.

What can you do to prevent diarrhea from infections or food poisoning?

- Wash your hands after going to the toilet or changing a diaper.
- Always wash your hands before eating or preparing food.
- **Do not** drink milk or fruit juices that have not been pasteurized (check the label).
- Cook foods thoroughly, especially red meat, poultry (chicken and turkey) and eggs.
- Eat food soon after it is cooked so that germs do not have time to grow.
- Rinse fresh fruits and vegetables under running water before you eat them.
- Keep hot foods hot (60°C) and cold foods cold (4°C).
- Keep raw meat and poultry away from other foods, especially when you are preparing food.
- Use separate cutting boards for raw meats and other foods.
- If serving leftovers, make sure they are reheated all the way through.
- Use soap and water to clean counters, cutting boards and utensils.

How do you treat diarrhea?

- Make sure you get enough fluids
- Dehydration can be a serious problem for children, older people and people with chronic medical conditions. Ask your pharmacist about using an oral rehydration solution (a special mixture of water and salts) for these people
- Talk to your pharmacist about medications used to treat diarrhea.

When should you see your healthcare provider?

See a healthcare provider if you have *any* of these symptoms:

- a high fever (over 38.5°C or 101°F)
- a bowel movement that has blood in it or looks black
- diarrhea that lasts longer than 2 days
- severe pain in your belly
- more than 6 bowel movements in 1 day
- vomiting
- signs of dehydration (very thirsty, weak or lightheaded, dry mouth or tongue, not urinating as often as usual).

Take children with diarrhea to the doctor if:

- They are less than 6 months old, *or*
- They have vomiting that lasts longer than 4–6 hours, *or*
- They show any of these signs of dehydration:
  - dry mouth or tongue
  - no tears when they cry
  - less than 4 wet diapers in 24 hours
  - their eyes or soft spot are sunken
  - they are irritable or have low energy.

Travellers' Diarrhea—What You Need to Know

Travellers to developing countries in Latin America, Asia and Africa may develop diarrhea during their trip. It is almost always caused by contaminated food or water. It usually gets better on its own in a few days without causing serious problems.

Hints to prevent diarrhea while travelling:

- Pack a thermometer and medicine to treat diarrhea. Talk to your pharmacist about what medicine is right for you.
- Before you travel, talk to your healthcare provider about antibiotics. Many people bring antibiotics with them in case they get seriously ill. A few people need to take medication to prevent diarrhea from happening at all.
- Be careful when you eat and drink. Remember the saying, "Boil it, cook it, peel it or forget it"
- Only **eat** or **drink** things that are not likely to make you sick. These are:
  - piping hot foods
  - fruit you peel yourself
  - cooked vegetables
  - carbonated beverages (with no ice cubes)
  - boiled or bottled water
  - pasteurized milk (properly stored)
- **Avoid** foods that will likely make you sick. These include:
  - buffet foods at room temperature
  - fresh soft cheese
  - food from street vendors
  - cold salads
  - raw vegetables
  - uncooked/cold sauces
  - unpeeled fruit
  - raspberries, strawberries, watermelon
  - ice cubes
  - undercooked meat or fish
  - shellfish
  - large reef fish such as snapper, barracuda, grouper, jack and Moray eel
  - custard, mousse, mayonnaise and hollandaise sauce
- Wash your hands, especially before you eat.
- Avoid swallowing water while swimming.
- **Do not** drink local water.
- Drink bottled beverages from their original containers. Make sure the cap is properly sealed.
- Talk to your healthcare provider about what to do if you have diarrhea while you are away.

Chapter 31
Dyspepsia and GERD

Co Q. D. Pham, BSc, BA, BScPharm, ACPR, PharmD

Dyspepsia is defined as a chronic or recurrent epigastric (upper abdomen) pain or burning, postprandial fullness or early satiety with no evidence of structural disease to explain the symptoms.[1] Other symptoms may also include bloating, nausea or vomiting.[1] In contrast, the predominant symptom in gastroesophageal reflux disease (GERD) is troublesome or frequent acid regurgitation or heartburn (a burning feeling in the stomach or lower chest rising up to the neck).[2] GERD is also associated with epigastric pain, nausea, dysphagia (difficulty swallowing) and odynophagia (pain with swallowing).[2] Extraesophageal or atypical manifestations of GERD are also possible and include cough, sore throat, chest pain, hoarseness, shortness of breath and wheezing.[2,3,4,5,6,7,8,9] It is important to recognize that there is considerable symptom overlap between dyspepsia and GERD, and it may be difficult to differentiate between them in a patient who has not been investigated.[3]

Although the incidence of dyspepsia is poorly documented, the prevalence rate in western countries approximates 25%; if heartburn symptoms are also considered then the prevalence rate increases to 40%.[1,4] GERD has a prevalence of approximately 40%, and up to half of the sufferers may show erosive esophagitis upon endoscopic investigation.[3,5,10] GERD with a normal esophagus at endoscopy is referred to as nonerosive reflux disease (NERD) or as endoscopy-negative reflux disease (ENRD). Dyspepsia and GERD remain costly chronic conditions where a significant proportion of patients self-manage without seeking medical attention.[5,11]

Pathophysiology

Dyspepsia

Dyspepsia can be caused by identifiable abnormalities such as chronic peptic ulcer disease (PUD), GERD and gastric or esophageal cancer (Table 1).[1,3,4] Dyspepsia is referred to as functional, idiopathic or nonulcer dyspepsia (NUD) when no identifiable structural or biochemical abnormalities are found (Table 1). The pathophysiology of functional dyspepsia is considered an overlap of psychosocial factors, upper GI motor abnormalities (delayed gastric emptying, impaired gastric accommodation to meals) and altered organ sensory function (gastric or duodenal hypersensitivity to mechanical distention or nerve-related mechano-sensory dysfunction).[1,3,4] In general, the symptoms of dyspepsia are minor and infrequent, although with a relapsing course.[1,3,4]

Table 1: **Causes of Dyspepsia**

Structural abnormalities/identifiable causes (40%):
Peptic ulcer disease (15–25%)
Reflux esophagitis (5–15%)
Gastric or esophageal cancer (<2%)
Other diseases: e.g., cholecystitis, pancreatitis, celiac disease, Crohn's disease, sarcoidosis, hypothyroidism, hypercalcemia, hepatoma, intestinal angina, renal failure, diabetic gastroparesis

(cont'd)

Table 1: **Causes of Dyspepsia** *(cont'd)*

Food intolerance: e.g., lactase deficiency
Medications: e.g., acarbose, amiodarone, antibiotics (e.g., erythromycin), bisphosphonates, digitalis, iron supplements, NSAIDs, potassium supplements, theophylline
Natural health products: e.g., garlic, feverfew, chaste tree berry, white willow
Infections: e.g., cytomegalovirus, *Giardia lamblia*, *Strongyloides stercoralis*
No identifiable structural abnormalities or causes (60%)
Functional or idiopathic (nonulcer) dyspepsia

Gastroesophageal Reflux Disease (GERD)

The pathogenesis of GERD is multifactorial and includes:

- Defective lower esophageal sphincter (LES); in the normal state, the LES prevents reflux of gastric contents into the esophagus
- Hiatal hernia
- Impaired esophageal peristalsis
- Delayed gastric emptying
- Excessive gastric acid production
- Bile reflux.

The pathophysiology of GERD is multifactorial and determining the primary etiology can be challenging. The abnormalities that contribute to GERD can result from various components in the system, including the esophagus, LES and the stomach. Poor esophageal motility may decrease the clearance of acidic material. A dysfunctional LES valve can permit reflux of gastric content. As well, delayed gastric emptying can increase both the volume and pressure in the stomach, overwhelming the LES valve and leading to GERD. A hiatal hernia (herniation of the stomach above the diaphragm) can also be viewed as part of the GERD continuum, presenting in patients with severe erosive esophagitis. Therefore, therapy should consider the components that may be deficient, to apply effective treatment.[12,13]

GERD symptoms may be exacerbated when a patient bends over, lies down, smokes, is obese, eats certain foods (fatty meals) or takes certain medications (Table 2).[4,5,6] GERD may also result in structural damage to the esophagus, and the resulting esophagitis can lead to complications such as ulcers, erosions, hemorrhage, strictures, Barrett's esophagus and esophageal adenocarcinoma. Barrett's esophagus involves the replacement of the normal esophageal squamous epithelium with columnar intestinal-like epithelium. Studies estimate the annual incidence of esophageal adenocarcinoma among patients with Barrett's esophagus to be 0.1–2.9%.[14,15] Severity of GERD symptoms is not always related to the severity of structural esophageal damage. In healthy individuals a certain amount of normal acid-reflux does occur. However, with further refluxate exposure, the esophagus becomes more vulnerable to damage.[7,8,9]

Table 2: **GERD: Triggers or Exacerbating Factors**

Disease states	Asthma (possibly) Sjögren's syndrome
Drugs (reduce lower esophageal sphincter pressure)	Alpha-blockers Anticholinergics Benzodiazepines Beta-blockers Calcium channel blockers Nicotine Nitrates Opioids Theophylline
Lifestyle	Obesity Smoking[a] Diet ▪ fatty foods delay gastric emptying ▪ chocolate,[a] coffee[a] and alcohol[a] may reduce LES tone ▪ carbonated drinks may cause gastric distention and increased transient lower esophageal sphincter relaxations
Other Factors	Age >65 y Hiatus hernia Pregnancy Stress and anxiety

[a] Association with GERD is weak but some patients may experience worsening symptoms.

Goals of Therapy

- Reduce or eliminate symptoms
- Reduce or prevent recurrence of symptoms (frequency or duration)
- Induce healing of any damaged mucosa
- Prevent complications such as Barrett's esophagus or esophageal adenocarcinoma
- Educate patients to recognize worsening symptoms of GERD

Patient Assessment

For uninvestigated dyspepsia, patient assessment should start with a review of alarm features (Table 3), symptoms and history. Patients would require prompt investigation and assessment if alarm features are present or if age is >50 years with new onset or worsening of symptom severity or frequency (Figure 1).

In patients with GERD, a similar initial assessment should review the presence of alarm features (Table 3) and symptoms (Figure 1).[5,6] If GERD is not evaluated and treated in a timely manner, complications may arise. These complications include esophageal inflammation, ulcers, hemorrhage, strictures and cancer as well as anemia, aspiration pneumonia, gingivitis, halitosis and tooth decay.

Table 3: **Assessment of Dyspepsia and GERD: Alarm Symptoms[1,5]**

Further evaluation is required immediately if the patient experiences any of the following symptoms:

Symptom	Description
Chest pain	Resembling cardiac pain
Choking	Sensation of acid refluxed into the windpipe causing shortness of breath, coughing or hoarseness
Dysphagia	Difficulty swallowing
GI bleeding	Vomiting blood or having tarry or black bowel movements
Odynophagia	Pain upon swallowing
Unintentional weight loss	
Vomiting	

Nonpharmacologic Therapy

Evidence for lifestyle modifications has been inconclusive. Still many patients derive symptomatic benefit from inexpensive and usually simple measures. Some recommendations are provided in Table 4 and Table 5. These likely have their greatest impact in patients with mild symptoms.[1,16,17]

Table 4: **Preventive and Nonpharmacologic Treatments for Dyspepsia[1,17]**

Lifestyle modifications	Avoid foods that precipitate events Avoid lying down right after meals Achieve ideal body weight Quit smoking Reduce alcohol intake Reduce caffeine intake Smaller, more frequent meals
Psychological	Reassure patients regarding the benign nature of functional dyspepsia Stress reduction

Table 5: **Lifestyle Modifications in the Treatment of GERD[5,18,19]**

Avoid exercising or bending on a full stomach	Avoid tight-fitting clothes around the waist
Avoid foods that delay gastric emptying or increase acid exposure: chocolate, onions, carminatives (spearmint, peppermint), high-fat meals	Elevate head of bed about 10 cm
Avoid large meals	Avoid excessive alcohol consumption
Limit use of drugs that may cause or worsen dyspepsia (e.g., antibiotics, bisphosphonates, corticosteroids, iron, metformin, NSAIDs, opioids, potassium salts)	Stop smoking if a smoker
Avoid lying down following meals, or eating before bedtime	Achieve ideal body weight if obese

Pharmacologic Therapy

For comparative ingredients of nonprescription products, consult the *Compendium of Products for Minor Ailments*—Gastrointestinal Products: Antacid, Antiflatulent and Antireflux.

For further discussion of pharmacologic therapy for GERD, consult the *Compendium of Therapeutic Choices*: Gastroesophageal Reflux Disease.

In the absence of alarm features the initial management of mild or intermittent GERD should consist of diet and lifestyle modifications. Consider **alginates, antacids** or **histamine type 2 receptor antagonists** (H_2RAs) for mild and infrequent GERD symptoms (Figure 1). H_2RAs decrease the frequency of nighttime awakenings for GERD. Overall, symptom relief appears similar to antacids but the duration of effect is longer.[23] All H_2RAs appear to have similar efficacy. H_2RAs may become less effective with time and may not suppress meal-related acid secretion as well as proton pump inhibitors (PPIs).

PPIs decrease stomach acid production. Studies have demonstrated that PPIs decrease the overall days of symptoms of GERD and dyspepsia, as well as nighttime symptoms.[8] Patients with moderate to severe or frequent symptoms of GERD occurring >2 times per week can be treated with PPIs. **Prokinetic agents** or H_2RAs may also be useful. Antacids or sodium alginate can be used for breakthrough symptom control in these patients.[3,17]

Patients with dyspepsia should be followed up for *H. pylori* test-and-treat strategy (Figure 1).[1] The test-and-treat strategy works on the principle that 1) some patients with dyspepsia not yet investigated with an endoscope will test positive for *H. pylori* infection, 2) patients who are *H. pylori* positive are more likely to have definite ulcers and 3) treatment of *H. pylori* in patients with ulcers is likely to lead to remission of dyspeptic symptoms.

Patients who have ongoing symptoms despite a test-and-treat strategy and a trial of PPIs likely have functional dyspepsia. The majority of trials have demonstrated that most of the available pharmacologic agents for functional dyspepsia are of no proven benefit. The natural history of functional dyspepsia is such that the majority of patients improve without therapy.[1] Despite this, almost all patients with functional dyspepsia who seek medical help will be prescribed a drug. However, only a minority of patients require continuous chronic therapy with medications (PPIs, prokinetic agents, H_2RAs) and a significant portion will have difficulty achieving complete symptom relief.[1,3] Step-up therapy (starting with antacids) has similar efficacy to step-down therapy (starting with PPIs) but treatment cost may be lower for the former.[16]

Patients with minor or intermittent dyspeptic/GERD symptoms may use an antacid, sodium alginate or H_2RAs for symptomatic therapy (Table 6).

Antacids

Little evidence supports the efficacy of antacids in functional dyspepsia despite their widespread use.[20] In GERD, relief of heartburn occurs in approximately 20% of patients and the esophagus is protected from gastric contents for roughly 1.5 hours.[21] Antacids do provide therapeutic benefits in PUD but their inconvenience (frequent dosing, volume) and taste of suspensions makes other acid suppression therapy more attractive. Four basic types of antacids are available: sodium bicarbonate, and salts of aluminum, calcium and magnesium. The order of acid-neutralizing potency is aluminum hydroxide (least potent), followed by magnesium hydroxide, sodium bicarbonate and calcium carbonate (most potent). Some products contain a combination of salts, especially aluminum and magnesium. The rationale for the aluminum-magnesium combination is to offset the tendency of the respective agents to cause constipation and diarrhea. Table 6 provides an overview of the different products and precautions with each agent.

Dosing equivalency amongst antacids is based upon their ability to neutralize a molar amount of acid, which is called the acid neutralizing capacity (ANC). Doses of 10–40 mEq ANC are commonly recommended for functional dyspepsia in adults. GERD usually requires doses ranging from 80–160 mEq ANC. ANCs are dependent on the formulation and quantity of each antacid. Doses are therefore individual to each preparation. Because ANCs are not provided in Canadian labelling information or product monographs, antacid doses are often based on manufacturers' recommendations. The most common dose is 10–20 mL or 2–4 tablets after meals and at bedtime, as needed. Doses used in GERD are higher, e.g., 30 mL 1 hour after meals and at bedtime.

Antacids are available in a variety of formulations. If the patient can tolerate the taste, suspensions are preferred over solid dosage forms since suspensions have a greater ANC (owing to their smaller particle size).[22] Some tablet formulations overcome this by incorporating more active ingredient per dose. Other factors to consider in product selection include concomitant clinical conditions and cost. Sodium content is important in salt-sensitive patients. Fortunately most products have a low sodium content.

Although antacids appear to be of limited to no benefit in NUD,[23,24] adequate doses (based on ANC of agent) can raise the gastric pH sufficiently to prevent pepsin activation. Pepsin is an enzyme that begins the digestion of proteins in the stomach, and contributes to the stomach acid that regurgitates into the esophagus.[18] Antacids maintain an increased stomach pH only while they are in the stomach, so the duration of effect is dependent on the gastric emptying time. After a large meal, the duration of effect may be 1–3 hours. On an empty stomach it may be less than 1 hour.[18] If the dose of antacid neutralizes 90% of stomach acid the pH rises only one full point, e.g., pH 1.3–2.3.[22] Despite the lack of evidence, many clinicians feel that antacids may resolve some dyspeptic symptoms (e.g., heartburn) related to the presence of acid in the stomach.[22] The LES pressure may also increase with the use of antacids, likely due to increased gastric pH.[18] Placebo-controlled trials provide limited data to support the role of antacids.[18]

Sodium bicarbonate is suitable only for occasional use because of its high sodium content. It should be avoided in hypertension, heart failure, renal dysfunction, edema, cirrhosis, pregnancy and other situations where excess sodium intake may be harmful. Adverse effects include flatulence, belching and abdominal distention. Sodium bicarbonate can also cause metabolic alkalosis, which may become significant in patients with renal dysfunction or with high doses or prolonged use.

Calcium carbonate is generally the preferred agent in patients with compromised renal function as these patients often have hypocalcemia and hyperphosphatemia. Patients with compromised renal function are predisposed to developing the milk-alkali syndrome. This rare syndrome refers to the development of hypercalcemia, metabolic alkalosis and renal insufficiency with oral intake of more than 2–2.5 g/day of elemental calcium with absorbable alkali. This can result from ingesting calcium as an antacid (e.g., calcium carbonate) or from the combination of other antacids with calcium from another source such as milk. Symptoms include nausea, vomiting, weakness and altered mental status. Chronic ingestion of calcium carbonate may cause hypophosphatemia in predisposed patients; e.g., those with poor dietary intake of phosphates, such as malnourished alcoholics. Characteristic features of hypophosphatemia include muscle weakness, tiredness and, in its most severe form, breathing difficulties and heart failure.

Magnesium-based antacids should be avoided in renal failure and limited in the elderly due to the risk of hypermagnesemia. Signs of magnesium toxicity include nausea and vomiting, flushing, drowsiness and muscle weakness.

Alginic acid acts by physical means and tends to form a layer on top of the gastric contents. The rationale for its action is to be preferentially refluxed into the esophagus over other gastric contents, thereby decreasing esophageal exposure to acid and bile. Evidence of this agent's ability to prevent or reverse esophageal injury is lacking. In short-term trials, the combination of alginic acid with an antacid has not produced a therapeutic advantage over antacid alone.[25]

Pregnancy and Breastfeeding

See Chapter 82: Prenatal and Postpartum Care and Appendix V: Pregnancy and Breastfeeding: Self-care Therapy for Common Conditions.

Monitoring of Therapy

Further investigation is required for patients with symptoms that persist for >2 weeks, in those with worsening symptoms, when symptoms are incompletely relieved by antacids, H_2RAs and PPIs, and when symptoms recur a number of times per year. Due to the variability of GERD and dyspeptic symptomologies, clinical judgment is required in conducting follow-up care. This should be based on the individual patient's symptoms and response to treatments. Follow up on days 2 and 7 of therapy would be reasonable to ensure that the medication is effective and that the patient is experiencing no adverse side effects. Patients should monitor their symptoms and response to treatments on regular basis, and keep track of factors that may exacerbate their symptoms.

Advice for the Patient

Advise patients on:

- Nonpharmacologic interventions
- Expected side effects and their management
- Seeing a healthcare practitioner if the condition lasts >2 weeks or if alarm features appear.

Figure 1: Assessment and Management of Patients with Dyspepsia and GERD[1]

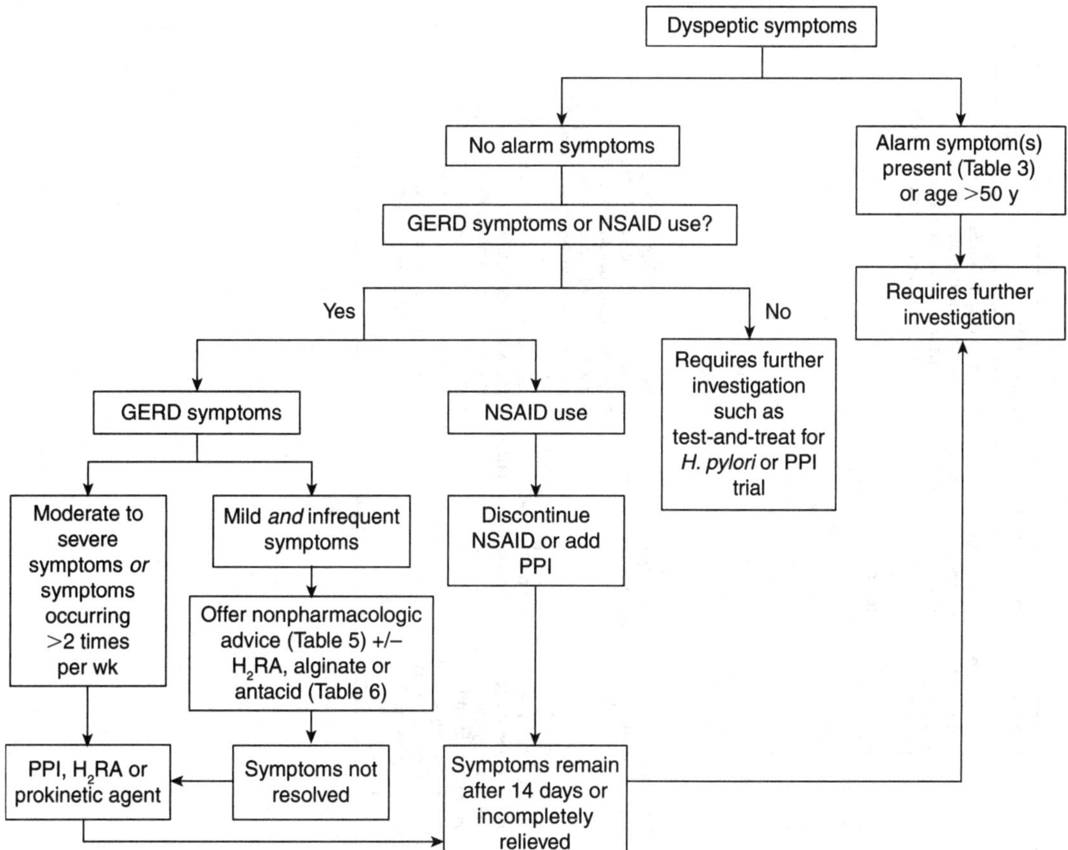

Abbreviations: GERD = gastroesophageal reflux disease; H_2RA = histamine type 2 receptor antagonist; PPI = proton pump inhibitor

Table 6: **Drug Therapy for GERD and Dyspepsia[a]**

Class	Drug	Dosage	Adverse Effects	Drug Interactions	Comments	Cost[b]
Antacids	*alginic acid/antacid combinations* Gaviscon, generics	Alginates (sodium salt)/aluminum hydroxide liquid: **Adults:** 10–20 mL PC and HS PRN po, followed by a glass of water Alginic acid/ magnesium carbonate tablets: **Adults:** 2–4 tablets (chewed) PC and HS PRN, followed by a glass of water	Constipation common with liquid formulation. Hypophosphatemia has occurred with prolonged use or high doses. Long-term use in endstage renal disease can cause dementia and osteomalacia.	All antacids are expected to decrease the absorption of fluoroquinolone and tetracycline antibiotics, digoxin, iron and isoniazid. They may also decrease serum concentrations of ASA but only when large doses of ASA are used.	Available in combination with aluminum, magnesium and calcium antacids. Aluminum-containing antacids should not be used in infants.	$
	aluminum hydroxide Alugel, Amphogel, others	**Adults:** 500–1800 mg, 2–6 times daily po, between meals and HS PRN	See alginic acid/ antacid combinations.	See alginic acid/ antacid combinations.	Avoid use in patients prone to constipation or bowel obstruction. Avoid long-term use in those with renal disease. Aluminum-containing antacids should not be used in infants.	$$
	aluminum hydroxide/ magnesium hydroxide combinations Diovol, others	**Adults:** 30 mL 1 h PC and HS PRN po	Diarrhea. Long-term use in end-stage renal disease may cause osteomalacia and dementia. May cause hypermagnesemia in those with renal dysfunction.	See alginic acid/ antacid combinations.	Avoid high doses or prolonged use in those with renal dysfunction. Constipating effect of aluminum is meant to offset the diarrhea-producing action of magnesium, but in most patients diarrhea predominates. Aluminum-containing antacids should not be used in infants.	$$

Class	Drug	Dosage	Adverse Effects	Drug Interactions	Comments	Cost[b]
	calcium carbonate Tums, others	**Adults:** 500–1500 mg per day in divided doses PRN po	Constipation, belching, flatulence. In high doses can cause milk-alkali syndrome or hypercalcemia.	See alginic acid/ antacid combinations.	Stimulates gastrin release, thereby increasing acid production. Up to 10% systemic absorption. Calcium carbonate 500 mg = elemental calcium 200 mg.	$
	magnesium salts Milk of Magnesia, generics	**Adults and children >12 y:** 650–1300 mg per day, in 4 divided doses PRN po	Diarrhea common. May cause hypermagnesemia in those with renal dysfunction. Renal stones have been reported with the trisilicate salt.	See alginic acid/ antacid combinations.	Available as hydroxide, carbonate and trisilicate salts. Avoid use in renal failure.	$
H_2-receptor Antagonists	*famotidine* (kidney symbol) Pepcid AC, Pepcid AC Maximum Strength, generics	**Adults and children >12 y:** 10–20 mg BID PRN po Maximum: 40 mg per day For prevention of acid-related symptoms associated with the consumption of food and/or beverage, take 10–15 min AC	Headache and dizziness.	Concurrent administration of antacid of medium to high potency (75 mEq) is not recommended. Do not take antacids within 0.5–1 h of H_2-receptor antagonist ingestion. May decrease bioavailability of ketoconazole.	Patients should be investigated further if symptoms get worse or continue after 2 wk of treatment.	$$$
	ranitidine (kidney symbol) Zantac, Zantac Maximun Strength Non-Prescription, Ranitidine, other generics	**Adults and children >16 y:** 75–150 mg BID PRN po Maximum: 300 mg per day For prevention of acid-related symptoms associated with the consumption of food and/or beverage, take 30–60 min AC	Headache, nausea, vomiting and diarrhea.	See famotidine.	See famotidine.	$$$

[a] For more information on pharmacologic therapy for GERD, consult the *Compendium of Therapeutic Choices*: Gastroesophageal Reflux Disease.

[b] Cost of 30-day supply, includes drug cost only.

(kidney symbol) Dosage adjustment may be required in renal impairment.

Legend: $ <$5 $$ $5–10 $$$ $10–15

Suggested Readings

Armstrong D, Marshall JK, Chiba N et al. Canadian Consensus Conference on the management of gastroesophageal reflux disease in adults–update 2004. *Can J Gastroenterol* 2005;19:15-35.

Kahrilas PJ. Clinical practice. Gastroesophageal reflux disease. *N Engl J Med* 2008;359:1700-7.

Lacy BE, Talley NJ, Locke GR et al. Review article: current treatment options and management of functional dyspepsia. *Aliment Pharmacol Ther* 2012;36:3-15.

Vakil N, van Zanten SV, Kahrilas P et al. The Montreal definition and classification of gastroesophageal reflux disease: a global evidence-based consensus. *Am J Gastroenterol* 2006;101:1900-20.

References

1. Talley NJ, Ford AC. Functional dyspepsia. *N Engl J Med* 2015;373:1853-63.
2. Vakil N, van Zanten SV, Kahrilas P et al. The Montreal definition and classification of gastroesophageal reflux disease: a global evidence-based consensus. *Am J Gastroenterol* 2006;101:1900-20.
3. Thomson AB, Barkun AN, Armstrong D et al. The prevalence of clinically significant endoscopic findings in primary care patients with uninvestigated dyspepsia: the Canadian Adult Dyspepsia Empiric Treatment-Prompt Endoscopy (CADET-PE) study. *Aliment Pharmacol Ther* 2003;17:1481-91.
4. El-Serag HB, Talley NJ. Systematic review: the prevalence and clinical course of functional dyspepsia. *Aliment Pharmacol Ther* 2004;19:643-54.
5. Kahrilas PJ, Shaheen NJ, Vaezi MF et al. American Gastroenterological Association Institute technical review on the management of gastroesophageal reflux disease. *Gastroenterology* 2008;135:1392-413.
6. Storr M, Meining A, Allescher HD. Pathophysiology and pharmacological treatment of gastroesophageal reflux disease. *Dig Dis* 2000;18:93-102.
7. Orlando RC. The pathogenesis of gastroesophageal reflux disease: the relationship between epithelial defense, dysmotility, and acid exposure. *Am J Gastroenterol* 1997;92:3S-5S.
8. Kahrilas PJ. Clinical practice. Gastroesophageal reflux disease. *N Engl J Med* 2008;359:1700-7.
9. Spechler SJ. GERD and its complications. *Mt Sinai J Med* 2000;67:106-11.
10. Devault KR. Review article: the role of acid suppression in patients with non-erosive reflux disease or functional heartburn. *Aliment Pharmacol Ther* 2006;23:33-9.
11. Piessevaux H, De Winter B, Louis E et al. Dyspeptic symptoms in the general population: a factor and cluster analysis of symptom groupings. *Neurogastroenterol Motil* 2009;21:378-88.
12. de Vries DR, van Herwaarden MA, Smout AJ et al. Gastroesophageal pressure gradients in gastroesophageal reflux disease: relations with hiatal hernia, body mass index, and esophageal acid exposure. *Am J Gastroenterol* 2008;103:1349-54.
13. Pandolfino JE, Shi G, Trueworthy B et al. Esophagogastric junction opening during relaxation distinguishes nonhernia reflux patients, hernia patients and normal subjects. *Gastroenterology* 2003;125:1018-24.
14. Shaheen NJ, Crosby MA, Bozymski EM et al. Is there publication bias in the reporting of cancer risk in Barrett's esophagus? *Gastroenterology* 2000;119:333-8.
15. Hvid-Jensen F, Pedersen L, Drewes AM et al. Incidence of adenocarcinoma among patients with Barrett's esophagus. *N Engl J Med* 2011;365:1375-83.
16. van Marrewijk CJ, Mujakovic S, Fransen GA et al. Effect and cost-effectiveness of step-up versus step-down treatment with antacids, H2-receptor antagonists, and proton pump inhibitors in patients with new onset dyspepsia (DIAMOND study): a primary-care-based randomised controlled trial. *Lancet* 2009;373:215-25.
17. Veldhuyzen van Zanten SJ, Flook N, Chiba N et al. An evidence-based approach to the management of uninvestigated dyspepsia in the era of Helicobacter pylori. Canadian Dyspepsia Working Group. *CMAJ* 2000;162:S3-23.
18. Kitchen LI, Castell DO. Rationale and efficacy of conservative therapy for gastroesophageal reflux disease. *Arch Intern Med* 1991;151:448-54.
19. Bazaldua OV, Schneider FD. Evaluation and management of dyspepsia. *Am Fam Physician* 1999;60:1773-84.
20. Maton PN, Burton ME. Antacids revisited: a review of their clinical pharmacology and recommended therapeutic use. *Drugs* 1999;57:855-70.
21. DeVault KR. Overview of medical therapy for gastroesophageal reflux disease. *Gastroenterol Clin North Am* 1999;28:831-45.
22. McEvoy GK, American Society of Health-System Pharmacists. *AHFS drug information 2010*. Bethesda: American Society of Health-System Pharmacists; 2010.
23. Fisher RS, Parkman HP. Management of nonulcer dyspepsia. *N Engl J Med* 1998;339:1376-81.
24. Holtmann G, Talley NJ. Functional dyspepsia. Current treatment recommendations. *Drugs* 1993;45:918-30.
25. Lanza FL, Sibley CM. Role of antacids in the management of disorders of the upper gastrointestinal tract. Review of clinical experience 1975-1985. *Am J Gastroenterol* 1987;82:1223-41.

Dyspepsia—What You Need to Know

What is dyspepsia?

Dyspepsia refers to mild stomach upsets such as heartburn. Almost everyone experiences some kind of stomach upset from time to time. Some people have it more frequently. Dyspepsia is generally not associated with an increased risk of serious diseases such as cancer.

What can you do to relieve stomach upsets?

- Ask your healthcare provider about medication to relieve stomach upsets.
- Read the instructions on the package carefully to find out how much to take and how often.
- For liquid antacids, shake well. Take before or after meals.

When should you see your healthcare provider?

See your healthcare provider if you have frequent heartburn or stomach upsets or if the symptoms last more than 2 weeks. Your symptoms should not require more than 2 weeks of continuous medication every 6 months. See your healthcare provider if the symptoms do not go away after treatment.

See a healthcare provider **right away** if you have any of the following symptoms:

- Severe abdominal pain
- Pain that stays in the same spot on the side of your abdomen
- Unexplained weight loss of more than 3 kg in the past 6 months
- New feelings of shortness of breath or chronic tiredness
- Difficult or painful swallowing
- Persistent vomiting
- Coughing up blood
- Blood in the stool or black stools that look like tar.

Chapter 32
Gastrointestinal Gas

Co Q. D. Pham, BSc, BA, BScPharm, ACPR, Pharm D

Intestinal gas represents a normal and common biological process in healthy adults. Excess gas in the digestive tract can be found in the esophagus, stomach, small intestine and large intestine. These gases are removed via flatulence or eructation.[1,2] Common terms used to refer to gastrointestinal (GI) gas or its expulsion to the outside world include abdominal gas, gas, intestinal gas, flatus, farting, passing wind, bloating, belching, burping, abdominal pain, cramping, abdominal distention and abdominal discomfort.

Pathophysiology

The passage of gas is a normal daily process.[1] The gut typically contains <200 mL of gas, while daily gas expulsion averages 500–700 mL.[2,3] The main complaints about intestinal gas include excessive eructation, distention (bloating) and excessive flatus (Table 1).[1,2,4] There is poor correlation between the volume of gas in the digestive tract and actual symptoms.[5]

Eructation: Eructation (belching) results from swallowed air into the GI tract (aerophagia) or the ingestion of carbonated beverages. Aerophagia is a normal process occurring while people eat and drink. However, many individuals will swallow air unconsciously while smoking, when anxious or when trying to induce belching. Other causes of aerophagia include excessive salivation, respiratory disorders, not chewing food thoroughly, GI disorders (dyspepsia, acid-reflux), some medications, gum chewing, ill-fitted dental apparatus and sensations of nausea. Eructation may also be a sign of more serious underlying GI disorders such as peptic ulcer disease, gastroparesis or gastroesophageal reflux disease (GERD).[6,7,8] Normally, most of the air swallowed is eructated to prevent excess accumulation of gas in the GI tract.[2,6,8]

Abdominal Discomfort: Abdominal discomfort (bloating, cramping or pain) is often attributed to excess intestinal gas, although evidence does not always link it to these complaints. Abdominal discomfort may present in isolation or may occur as a result of underlying GI disorders: functional GI disorders (e.g., irritable bowel syndrome, dyspepsia), inflammatory bowel disease (e.g., Crohn's disease, ulcerative colitis), GERD, altered GI motility or colon cancer. Other conditions such as eating disorders (e.g., bulimia, anorexia) may also be associated with symptoms of abdominal discomfort. Some individuals have hypersensitive intestinal tracts, where minor changes in gas volume may result in abdominal discomfort. Thus, the causes of abdominal discomfort vary and should be assessed thoroughly.[2,4]

Abdominal pain deserves a careful note, because the region of pain may be confused in many cases with other medical conditions. Right-sided colonic pain may resemble gallstones or appendicitis, and left-sided colonic pain may be misdiagnosed in heart disease. Severe abdominal pain should be investigated promptly (see alarm symptoms in Patient Assessment).[4,6]

Flatulence: Gas is always present in the GI tract. The average person passes gas 10–25 times daily. The elderly may pass gas more frequently, but this is not well defined. Although there is considerable variability in the frequency and quantity of flatulence, passing gas more than 25 times a day may be considered excessive. Flatus results from the normal metabolic by-products of nonabsorbable foods digested and fermented by intestinal bacteria. Very little is due to aerophagia. The small intestine is unable to digest and absorb certain carbohydrates (e.g., fibre and nonabsorbable carbohydrates such as raffinose, stachyose and verbascose) found in foods. As a result the undigested food passes to the large intestine, where normal bacterial flora break down the food. The primary components of flatus are 5 gases: nitrogen, hydrogen, carbon dioxide, methane and oxygen. The odour of flatus stems from trace gases: skatoles, indoles and sulfur compounds. The frequency and quantity of flatus are related to an individual's diet and intestinal flora.[1,2,4]

Common dietary sources of intestinal gas include lactose, fibre and other nonabsorbable carbohydrates. A deficiency of lactase in the GI tract permits lactose to reach the colon where it is metabolized into fatty acids and 2 gases: hydrogen and carbon dioxide.[1,2] Lactase deficiency can be congenital or secondarily acquired. The acquired disorder is more commonly seen in older children and adults, and may be due to celiac disease, infectious gastroenteritis or giardiasis. Congenital causes of lactase deficiency are due to a mutation in the gene that is responsible for producing lactase (absent from birth) and are more prevalent in Asians than Caucasians.

Table 1: **Causes of Gastrointestinal Gas**

Symptoms	Causes
Eructation (belching)	Aerophagia (air swallowing): eating quickly, excessive salivation, gum chewing, mal-fitted dental apparatus, nausea, respiratory disorders, smoking
	Consumption of carbonated beverages
Abdominal discomfort (bloating, cramping, pain)	Aerophagia
	Cancer
	Eating disorders (anorexia, binge eating, bulimia, compulsive eating)
	GI disorders: functional GI disorders (irritable bowel syndrome, dyspepsia), inflammatory bowel disease (Crohn's disease, ulcerative colitis), GI motility disorders
Flatus	Celiac disease/tropical sprue
	Dietary consumption: beans, complex carbohydrates, dairy, vegetables
	Disaccharidase deficiency
	Pancreatic insufficiency

Goals of Therapy

- Educate patients about the normal aspects of GI gas
- Relieve symptoms (belching, pain, bloating, flatulence)
- Educate patients regarding preventive measures

Patient Assessment

The symptoms of gas are variable and subjective.[2,3,4,6] An important first step is to review the patient history. Patients with eructation should have a history of aerophagia, whereas flatus or abdominal discomfort may be associated with timing, quantity and type of foods consumed, bowel habits or other underlying medical conditions. The history should also elicit any relevant medical conditions (respiratory disorders, GI disorders such as celiac disease, lactose intolerance or gastroparesis).

Patients with recurrent symptoms of abdominal fullness, distention or bloating relieved by defecation may have features of underlying irritable bowel syndrome (see Chapter 35: Irritable Bowel Syndrome). Weight loss associated with GI gas may suggest a malabsorption syndrome.

Be vigilant for alarm symptoms in the history, which may include weight loss, blood in stool or vomit, moderate to severe abdominal pain or swelling, sudden changes in bowel habits, nausea or vomiting, or fever and chills. Investigate patients promptly if they present with any alarm symptoms.[4]

In general, testing for GI gas is not required. However, in some severe cases testing for carbohydrate intolerance, bacterial overgrowth, bacterial cultures or endoscopic examinations may be warranted. Figure 1 outlines a general approach to assessing patients with GI gas.

Nonpharmacologic Therapy

The majority of patients have symptoms that do not require any treatment, but many may seek advice in selecting treatments for more excessive or intolerable symptoms. Typically, changes in diet and lifestyle allow for quick corrections in the symptoms of gas.[4]

Eructation: Recognize the history and activities of aerophagia. Some patients gulp air with each belch. This is often associated with multiple small belches over seconds. Educating the patient to stop gulping air with each belch or instructing a forced cessation of belching should relieve this.[3] Adjusting poorly fitting dental apparatus or decreasing excess salivation by reducing gum chewing, cigar chomping or cigarette smoking can help improve eructation. Also, reducing ingestion of gas-producing or gas-releasing substances (e.g., carbonated beverages, sodium bicarbonate) may be helpful. Encourage patients to eat meals slowly to decrease the likelihood of gulping air when swallowing.[2,6,7] Abdominal breathing exercises may also be considered.[8]

GI Discomfort: The feeling of bloating with the desire to belch can simply be due to overeating. Very large meals ingested in the late evening may induce symptoms; eating less and earlier in the day may reduce them. Abdominal cramping may arise from a number of dietary and pharmaceutical sources, such as osmotic laxatives.[2,4]

Flatulence: Eating smaller more frequent meals throughout the day may help decrease symptoms. A proper exercise program may also help improve and maintain the function of the GI system and reduce gas production.[1,2,4]

Dietary therapy with foods low in fermentable oligo-, di-, and mono-saccharides and polyols (FODMAPs) may be an option in the management of patients with functional gut symptoms.[9] FODMAPs include fructans, fructose, galacto-oligosaccharides, lactose, mannitol and sorbitol. Foods rich in FODMAPs include apples, artichokes, cauliflower, garlic, honey, legumes, mango, milk, mushrooms, onions, pears, rye, stone fruits, sugar-free mints/gums, watermelon and wheat.[10,11]

Pharmacologic Therapy

For comparative ingredients of nonprescription products, consult the *Compendium of Products for Minor Ailments*—Gastrointestinal Products: Antacid, Antiflatulent and Antireflux; Nutrition Products: Lactose Digestants.

Evidence-based pharmacotherapy for GI gas is limited and no consensus guidelines for the management of this condition exist. Currently there is no evidence-based therapy for aerophagia; the proper approach and treatment for eructation is unclear. It is important to identify the underlying causes of eructation and correct them whenever possible. Otherwise, further medical evaluation for GI disorders such as GERD should be considered.

Information on selected nonprescription therapies for GI gas can be found in Table 2.

Activated charcoal tablets have not demonstrated efficacy in reducing symptoms of intestinal gas and should not be recommended.[4,12] External charcoal devices for reducing odour can be effective in binding sulfur gases.[13] These devices exist as pads, cushions or briefs and may be useful depending on patient preference.

Alpha-D-galactosidase is effective in reducing symptoms of flatus and abdominal discomfort associated with the consumption of nonabsorbable carbohydrates.[14] Enzyme products should not be put on hot foods (too hot to eat or during cooking) as heat renders the enzyme inactive. Instruct patients to place the liquid enzyme on the first spoonful of food.

The use of **antibiotics** in the general treatment of gas is not required. However, if bacterial overgrowth is suspected, antibiotics may be required.[15]

Baclofen is a muscle relaxant that has been studied in the reduction of eructation. It may reduce reflux, air swallowing and belching.[16] More research is needed to confirm these findings. Baclofen has CNS side-effects that may limit longer term use in eructation.

Bismuth subsalicylate is capable of binding a considerable amount of sulfide gas. Therefore, it may be very effective in the short-term relief of intestinal gas. However, to avoid salicylate toxicity, do not recommend bismuth for long-term use (>3–4 weeks) or at high doses (>150 mg/kg).[17,18]

Lactase supplementation taken with or prior to ingestion of lactose products can prevent flatulence in patients with lactase deficiency. The amount of supplementation required is dependent on the amount of lactose ingested. Dairy products with lactose should still be consumed in moderation as large doses of lactose will not be completely broken down by the lactase supplement. Patients with suspected lactose malabsorption require further investigation for proper diagnosis.

Laxatives may have an important role in reducing symptoms of intestinal gas, notably those associated with constipation (see Chapter 29: Constipation).

Probiotics are live microorganisms that confer a health benefit. Although not all commonly used probiotics have been adequately studied in randomized-controlled trials, some data have demonstrated a reduction in both short- and long-term symptoms of abdominal distention, bloating, and gas. Commercially available products are not always consistent in the quantity and type of bacterial species combined.[19,20,21,22,23]

Simethicone acts by preventing bubbling of liquids in the stomach and does not appear to be absorbed from the GI tract. However, data do not show a clear benefit in the reduction of symptoms from intestinal gas. Despite this fact, it is generally used for treatment of flatulence and abdominal bloating. Simethicone in combination with loperamide may be effective in reducing abdominal bloating and flatus associated with acute diarrhea.[24]

Information on selected nonprescription therapies for GI gas can be found in Table 2. Other specific pharmacotherapy options might be indicated if there is underlying pathology affecting GI motility, functional GI disorders (irritable bowel disease, inflammatory bowel disease) or infection.

Natural Health Products

Peppermint probably acts by reducing lower esophageal sphincter pressure, theoretically making it easier to pass gas from the stomach into the esophagus.[25] This pressure reduction potentially increases the likelihood of GERD.

Garlic and **ginger** are other alternative products promoted for treatment of intestinal gas. However, there is insufficient evidence to recommend their use.

Monitoring of Therapy

Investigate patients further if they experience alarm symptoms or if their symptoms persist for more than 1–2 weeks despite pharmacotherapy.

Exclusion diets (e.g., diets free of lactose or nonabsorbable carbohydrates) should be monitored for effective resolution of symptoms. If symptoms persist, both diet and other sources of the triggers (e.g., lactose in medications and herbals) should be more rigorously evaluated.

Functional GI conditions presenting with symptoms of abdominal distention (bloating), pain and flatus may be chronic or intermittent and may only be partially managed with pharmacotherapy. It is important to be positive and reassure patients with functional GI disorders that these symptoms are not detrimental to their health.

Figure 1: **Assessment of Patients with Gastrointestinal Gas**

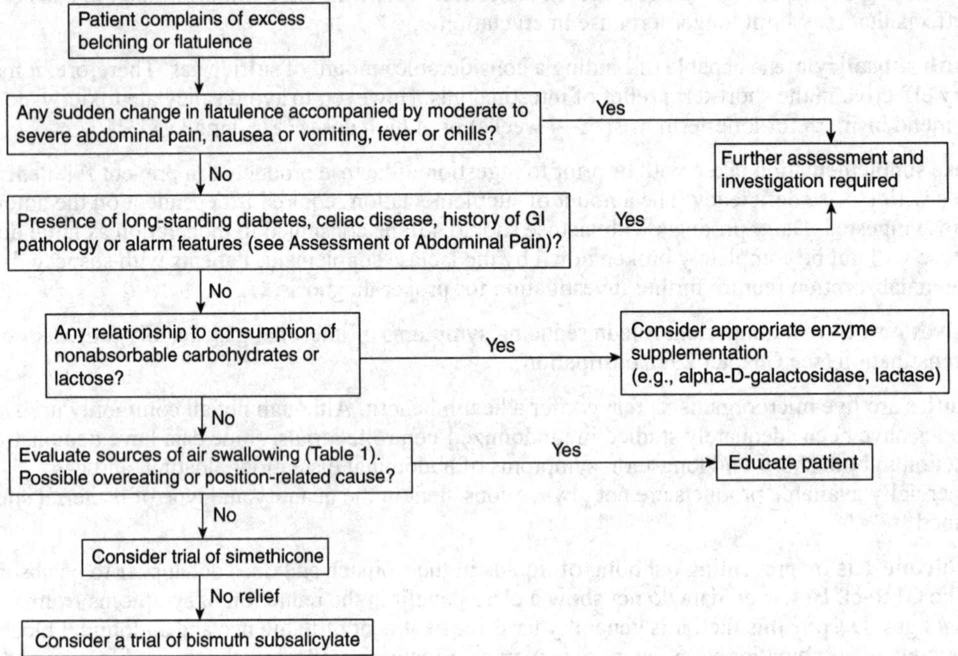
Patient complains of excess belching or flatulence
Any sudden change in flatulence accompanied by moderate to severe abdominal pain, nausea or vomiting, fever or chills?
Yes
Further assessment and investigation required
No
Presence of long-standing diabetes, celiac disease, history of GI pathology or alarm features (see Assessment of Abdominal Pain)?
Yes
No
Any relationship to consumption of nonabsorbable carbohydrates or lactose?
Yes
Consider appropriate enzyme supplementation (e.g., alpha-D-galactosidase, lactase)
No
Evaluate sources of air swallowing (Table 1). Possible overeating or position-related cause?
Yes
Educate patient
No
Consider trial of simethicone
No relief
Consider a trial of bismuth subsalicylate

Table 2: Drug Therapy for Intestinal Gas and Cramps

Class	Drug	Dosage	Adverse Effects	Cost[a]
Adsorbents	*bismuth subsalicylate* Pepto-Bismol, generics	524 mg QID po (maximum 8 doses/day)	Constipation, diarrhea, nausea, tongue discolouration, grayish-black stool, vomiting	$
Antiflatulents	*simethicone* Ovol, Gas X, others	80–160 mg per meal po	None reported	$
Enzymes	*alpha-D-galactosidase* Beano	150–450 GalU po with the first bite of food (300–1200 GalU/day)	Rare allergic reactions (rash, pruritus)	$

[a] Cost per day; includes drug cost only.

Legend: $ <$1

Suggested Readings

Bailey J, Carter NJ, Neher JO. FPIN's Clinical Inquiries: Effective management of flatulence. *Am Fam Physician* 2009;79:1098-100.

Kessing BF, Bredenoord AJ, Smout AJ. The pathophysiology, diagnosis and treatment of excessive belching symptoms. *Am J Gastroenterol* 2014;109:1196-203.

Lacy BE, Gabbard SL, Crowell MD. Pathophysiology, evaluation, and treatment of bloating: hope, hype, or hot air? *Gastroenterol Hepatol (N Y)* 2011;7:729-39.

References

1. Serra J, Azpiroz F, Malagelada JR. Intestinal gas dynamics and tolerance in humans. *Gastroenterology* 1998;115:542-50.
2. Azpiroz F. Intestinal gas dynamics: mechanisms and clinical relevance. *Gut* 2005;54:893-5.
3. Bharucha AE. Gas-related complaints. In: *The Merck manual of diagnosis and therapy.* Rahway: Merck Sharp and Dohme; 2007.
4. Bailey J, Carter NJ, Neher JO. FPIN's Clinical Inquiries: Effective management of flatulence. *Am Fam Physician* 2009;79:1098-100.
5. Morken MH, Berstad AE, Nysaeter G et al. Intestinal gas in plain abdominal radiographs does not correlate with symptoms after lactulose challenge. *Eur J Gastroenterol Hepatol* 2007;19:589-93.
6. Bredenoord AJ, Smout AJ. Physiologic and pathologic belching. *Clin Gastroenterol Hepatol* 2007;5:772-5.
7. Lin M, Triadafilopoulos G. Belching: dyspepsia or gastroesophageal reflux disease? *Am J Gastroenterol* 2003;98:2139-45.
8. Kessing BF, Bredenoord AJ, Smout AJ. The pathophysiology, diagnosis and treatment of excessive belching symptoms. *Am J Gastroenterol* 2014;109:1196-203.
9. Gibson PR, Shepherd SJ. Evidence-based dietary management of functional gastrointestinal symptoms: The FODMAP approach. *J Gastroenterol Hepatol* 2010;25:252-8.
10. Barrett JS, Gibson PR. Fermentable oligosaccharides, disaccharides, monosaccharides and polyols (FODMAPs) and nonallergic food intolerance: FODMAPs or food chemicals? *Therap Adv Gastroenterol* 2012;5:261-8.
11. Azpiroz F, Hernandez C, Guyonnet D et al. Effect of a low-flatulogenic diet in patients with flatulence and functional digestive symptoms. *Neurogastroenterol Motil* 2014;26:779-85.
12. Suarez FL, Furne J, Springfield J et al. Failure of activated charcoal to reduce the release of gases produced by the colonic flora. *Am J Gastroenterol* 1999;94:208-12.
13. Ohge H, Furne JK, Springfield J et al. Effectiveness of devices purported to reduce flatus odor. *Am J Gastroenterol* 2005;100:397-400.
14. Di Stefano M, Miceli E, Gotti S et al. The effect of oral alpha-galactosidase on intestinal gas production and gas-related symptoms. *Dig Dis Sci* 2007;52:78-83.
15. Sharara AI, Aoun E, Abdul-Baki H et al. A randomized double-blind placebo-controlled trial of rifaximin in patients with abdominal bloating and flatulence. *Am J Gastroenterol* 2006;101:326-33.
16. Blondeau K, Boecxstaens V, Rommel N et al. Baclofen improves symptoms and reduces postprandial flow events in patients with rumination and supragastric belching. *Clin Gastroenterol Hepatol* 2012;10:379-84.
17. Suarez FL, Furne JK, Springfield J et al. Bismuth subsalicylate markedly decreases hydrogen sulfide release in the human colon. *Gastroenterology* 1998;114:923-9.
18. Chyka PA, Erdman AR, Christianson G et al. Salicylate poisoning: an evidence-based consensus guideline for out-of-hospital management. *Clin Toxicol (Phila)* 2007;45:95-131.
19. Kim HJ, Vazquez Roque MI, Camilleri M et al. A randomized controlled trial of a probiotic combination VSL#3 and placebo in irritable bowel syndrome with bloating. *Neurogastroenterol Motil* 2005;17:687-96.
20. Bittner AC, Croffut RM, Stranahan MC et al. Prescript-assist probiotic-prebiotic treatment for irritable bowel syndrome: an open-label, partially controlled, 1-year extension of a previously published controlled clinical trial. *Clin Ther* 2007;29:1153-60.
21. Di Stefano M, Miceli E, Armellini E et al. Probiotics and functional abdominal bloating. *J Clin Gastroenterol* 2004;38:S102-3.
22. Kajander K, Hatakka K, Poussa T et al. A probiotic mixture alleviates symptoms in irritable bowel syndrome patients: a controlled 6-month intervention. *Aliment Pharmacol Ther* 2005;22:387-94.
23. Lacy BE, Gabbard SL, Crowell MD. Pathophysiology, evaluation, and treatment of bloating: hope, hype, or hot air? *Gastroenterol Hepatol (N Y)* 2011;7:729-39.
24. Hanauer SB, DuPont HL, Cooper KM et al. Randomized, double-blind, placebo-controlled clinical trial of loperamide plus simethicone versus loperamide alone and simethicone alone in the treatment of acute diarrhea with gas-related abdominal discomfort. *Curr Med Res Opin* 2007;23:1033-43.
25. Suarez FL, Springfield J, Levitt MD. Identification of gases responsible for the odour of human flatus and evaluation of a device purported to reduce this odour. *Gut* 1998;43:100-4.

Gastrointestinal Gas—What You Need to Know

What causes GI gas symptoms?

Excess eructation (belching) is often caused by swallowing air or eating things that release gas. If you have gas in your abdomen, it can cause cramps. Here are some hints to help prevent gas and reduce belching:

- **Do not** chew gum, chomp on cigars or smoke cigarettes.
- **Do not** drink carbonated beverages such as colas.
- Eat your meals slowly.

If you often feel abdominal discomfort (bloating or pain), avoid eating large meals, especially late in the day.

If your gas and abdominal discomfort seem to be related to certain foods, consider changing your diet or avoiding foods that cause these symptoms. Alternatively, there may be a medication that could help you.

When should you see a healthcare provider?

See a healthcare provider if:

- Your symptoms last for more than 1–2 weeks.
- Your symptoms are very painful and come on suddenly.
- You lose weight without trying.
- Your stools (bowel movements) contain blood or dramatically change in colour (for example, pale whitish or black, tar-like stools).
- You develop fever or chills.
- Your stomach or intestines feel unwell.

What can you do?

It may help to change what you eat—you may need to avoid some foods or modify your diet. Exercise can improve and maintain the stomach and intestinal function. Check with a healthcare provider before you make changes to your diet and exercise routines.

Chapter 33
Hemorrhoids

Joyce Chan, BScPhm, MSc, PharmD

CPhA acknowledges the contribution of Patricia Carruthers-Czyzewski as a previous author of this chapter.

Pathophysiology

Hemorrhoids are a normal anatomic feature of the anal canal and contribute to continence. Commonly referred to as cushions, they consist of connective tissue, an arteriovenous plexus and suspensory smooth muscle. The existence of hemorrhoidal cushions alone does not constitute disease. Once symptoms appear (typically bleeding, itch, protrusion or pain) due to swelling and/or prolapse, then hemorrhoids are diseased.[1]

Hemorrhoids can be classified as internal, external or mixed hemorrhoids (Figure 1). Internal hemorrhoids originate above the dentate/pectinate/anorectal line and may be further classified into 4 stages (see below). Internal hemorrhoids should not cause pain unless complications develop, since this area has no nerve fibres. External hemorrhoids originate below the dentate line and can cause pain, since this area is well innervated by pain fibres. The term "mixed hemorrhoids" is used when internal and external hemorrhoids coexist.[2,3]

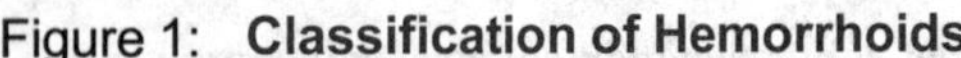
Figure 1: **Classification of Hemorrhoids**

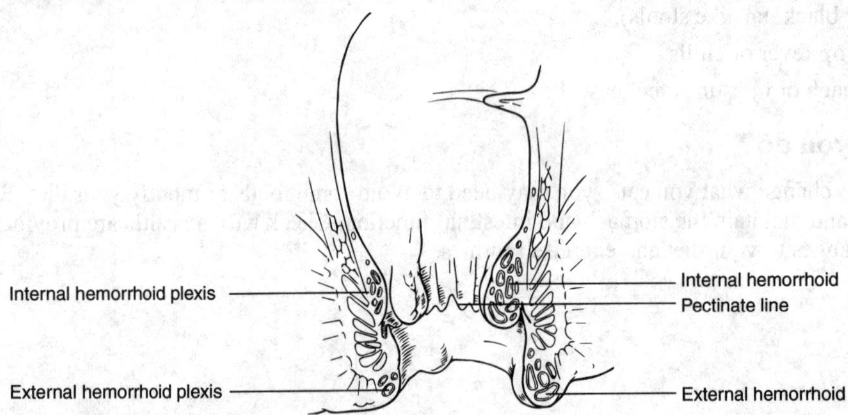

Internal hemorrhoids can be classified symptomatically according to their degree of formation. First-degree hemorrhoids swell in the anal cushion due to straining and are usually painless. During the second stage, a small part of the anal mucosa or cushion may protrude at the anus during defecation. After the bowel movement, the hemorrhoid spontaneously returns to its normal position. Third-degree hemorrhoids remain in the prolapsed position after defecation, but may be re-placed manually within the anus. Fourth-degree hemorrhoids cannot be re-placed after a bowel movement, and thus create a permanent bulge at the anus. This condition is quite painful, and it is usually at this stage that individuals should consult their physician. Fourth-degree hemorrhoids are at risk of thrombosis and gangrene.[4]

Hemorrhoids are common. Fifty-eight to 86% of individuals will have symptomatic hemorrhoids at some point in their lives.[5,6] A US survey showed a prevalence of 4.4% in the general population. Hemorrhoids occur equally in both sexes, peaking between the ages of 45 and 65, and declining thereafter.[7] The incidence of hemorrhoids may be overestimated. Some studies have indicated that when patients complain of hemorrhoids, only 50% actually have simple hemorrhoids; other problems include thrombosed hemorrhoids in approximately 18.5% of patients with anal complaints, fissures in 8% and miscellaneous problems in 23%.[8]

Many factors may be associated with the development of hemorrhoids: constipation, diarrhea, pregnancy, advancing age and possibly type of work and physical exertion.[8,9,10] When the individual tries to pass small, firm stools, the intrarectal pressure rises, blocking the venous return from the anal canal and leading to more straining. The shearing action of the fecal mass passing over the area causes a loosening of the underlying connective tissue. Diarrhea, either acute or chronic, can also cause hemorrhoids due to futile and protracted straining. Heredity is not an important factor. The only connection between heredity and hemorrhoids is the similarity of diet and personal habits in members of the same family.[9]

Pregnancy is believed to precipitate the onset of hemorrhoids in susceptible women. The woman who experiences hemorrhoids in the last few months of pregnancy may have become symptomatic due to increased abdominal pressure, allowing already existing hemorrhoids to present themselves. Other possibilities are that during pregnancy there may be a softening of the elastic tissue that supports anal cushions or that the woman may be more constipated. In many cases, these hemorrhoids resolve after parturition.[11]

Other possible causes of hemorrhoids include increased abdominal pressure due to heavy lifting and prolonged standing or sitting. Prolonged periods of time on the toilet and chronic straining can increase the risk of hemorrhoids; in this position, the perineum is relaxed and the anal cushions are unsupported.[9] Evidence of any of these risk factors as primary causes of hemorrhoids is nonexistent. Rather, it is probable that each can worsen asymptomatic hemorrhoids that are already present.[9]

Hemorrhoids are found primarily in populations consuming a diet high in white flour, sugar and fibre-depleted carbohydrate foods. However, there is no association between fibre intake and the prevalence of hemorrhoids. There is no evidence that spicy foods worsen the irritation and pruritus of hemorrhoids.[12]

Goals of Therapy

- Relieve symptoms
- Prevent complications
- Promote good bowel habits and anal hygiene

Patient Assessment

For some patients, the first symptom is a painful mass at the anus lasting several days to weeks (thrombosed hemorrhoid), sometimes accompanied by the sudden relief of pain following rupture of the skin overlying the thrombus and bleeding. Other symptoms include itching, swelling and burning. Swelling is probably the main cause of pruritus. Fecal soiling of underwear often occurs. Prolapse often coincides with the beginning of a troublesome amount of discharge as a result of increased mucus production. The degree of discomfort experienced by the patient is dependent on the type of hemorrhoids and their severity. Internal hemorrhoids lack nerves and are painless. When hemorrhoids bleed, the blood is usually bright red and seen on the outer part of stools after defecation. The patient does not usually bleed at other times.

Healthcare practitioners should base the diagnosis of hemorrhoids on the patient's history and results of a physical exam. If bleeding exists, its source would often require confirmation by endoscopy.[13] Since many patients delay seeking help for hemorrhoids until symptoms have become unbearable, referral to a qualified healthcare practitioner is often required.[13]

Prevention

The most important preventive measure is to avoid constipation (see Chapter 29: Constipation). Advise patients not to remain on the toilet more than 1–2 minutes and to avoid straining.

Nonpharmacologic Therapy

Fibre supplementation may help improve constipation, pruritus due to fecal soilage and bleeding.[14] The benefit of fibre for irritation and pruritus is less well established than for bleeding.[14] Adding fibre to the diet is usually adequate to relieve symptoms of hemorrhoids in individuals with first- and second-degree hemorrhoids. When recommending fibre supplementation suggest starting at a low dose and slowly increasing (up to a total of 20–30 g per day) to minimize problems with bloating and abdominal discomfort.[13] Patients should also ensure adequate fluid intake with fibre supplementation.

If these general measures do not relieve hemorrhoidal symptoms, recommend the use of a Sitz bath 3–4 times daily. Sitz baths help relieve irritation and pruritus. Their effectiveness may in part be related to relaxation of the internal anal sphincter.[15] A Sitz bath consists of a tub of warm water (about 46°C) in which the individual sits for 15 minutes at a time. Plastic Sitz baths may be fitted over the toilet seat rim for greater convenience.

Any prolapsed hemorrhoids must be replaced using a moistened tissue. After each bowel movement, the anorectal area should be cleaned with mild soap and water and gently wiped with a wet toilet tissue.

Nonsurgical therapies (e.g., rubber-banding or infrared coagulation) are widely used although there have been no placebo-controlled trials to establish their efficacy.[16] In-office rubber band ligation may result in a lower need for repeated treatment compared with injection sclerotherapy and infrared coagulation in the management of first- to third-degree hemorrhoids.[17] Surgical hemorrhoidectomy is the most effective treatment but is associated with the highest complication rates and most postoperative disability. It is recommended in only a minority of patients (e.g., for treatment failures, for third- and fourth-degree hemorrhoids and for acute thrombosed hemorrhoids).[18] More than 80% of people respond to medical treatment, rubber-banding placed endoscopically or infrared coagulation; these methods cause less discomfort and entail less time off work compared with hemorrhoidectomy.[2,3]

Pharmacologic Therapy

For comparative ingredients of nonprescription products, consult the *Compendium of Products for Minor Ailments*—Gastrointestinal Products: Hemorrhoids.

Pharmacologic treatments are directed towards relief of symptoms; none are curative. A variety of hemorrhoidal products are available (see Table 1). There is no good evidence that commercially available hemorrhoidal products reduce bleeding or prolapse.[10] However, they can provide short-term relief of pain, burning, itch, discomfort and irritation while swelling subsides and healing occurs. Many commercially available hemorrhoidal products are formulated in a lubricating or emollient base with combinations of 2 or more active ingredients, including anti-inflammatory agents, astringents, local anesthetics, protectants and vasoconstrictors.

Local anesthetics are included in some topical hemorrhoidal preparations to relieve pain. If used for less than 7 days, local anesthetics are relatively safe and may relieve pain. Longer duration of use increases the risk of contact dermatitis. Good evidence of their efficacy is lacking.[10] Penetration of intact skin by local anesthetics is generally poor, but with excessive application to the rectal mucosa, absorption can occur.[10] Adverse effects associated with systemic use of local anesthetics include CNS effects (restlessness, excitement, nervousness, paresthesias, dizziness, tinnitus, blurred vision, nausea and vomiting, muscle twitching and tremors, convulsions) and cardiovascular effects (hypotension, bradycardia).[10] Products containing local anesthetics should be used only in the perianal region or the lower anal canal to reduce systemic absorption.

Hydrocortisone is used for temporary relief of anal itch and as an anti-inflammatory agent in the treatment of hemorrhoids.[19] The maximum recommended duration of treatment is 1 week, but up to 14 days may be appropriate if significant improvement is occurring.[20] Hydrocortisone 1% is available in various combinations with zinc sulfate and/or local anesthetics. Ointments are recommended for external hemorrhoids. For internal hemorrhoids, the ointment (applied manually using a finger cot) is preferred to using rectal tubes or suppositories.[20]

Astringents cause coagulation (clumping) of proteins in the cells of the perianal skin or the lining of the anal canal. This action promotes dryness of the skin, which in turn helps relieve burning, itching and pain. These are effective for mild symptoms but if there is significant itching and discharge, a preparation that includes **hydrocortisone** can be recommended.

Protectants prevent irritation of the perianal area by forming a physical barrier on the skin. This barrier reduces irritation, itch, pain and burning by preventing contact of the irritated skin with liquid or stool from the rectum. Their lubricating effect further protects the skin from irritation. For example, when included in hemorrhoidal products, petrolatum allows the stool to pass through the rectum more easily and freely, potentially minimizing further tissue damage.

Hemorrhoidal preparations are available in a variety of dosage forms (e.g., creams, ointments, suppositories and cleaning pads). Ultimately, the choice of delivery form lies with the consumer. Many people prefer suppositories, but these products may not be effective because they tend to slip into the rectum and melt, thus bypassing the anal canal where the medication is needed. To prevent a suppository from slipping into the rectum, advise patients to avoid inserting it too far up, and to lie down for a few minutes on their side after insertion. In general, creams and ointments are preferable to suppositories. They are easy to apply and usually contain the same or similar ingredients.

Hemorrhoidal products for external use should be applied sparingly and not inserted into the rectum. Before any hemorrhoidal product is applied, the anorectal area should be washed with mild soap and warm water, rinsed thoroughly and dried gently by patting or blotting with toilet tissue or a soft cloth.

Hemorrhoidal products are not recommended for children under the age of 12 years, unless the child has been examined.[21]

Oral analgesics such as **acetaminophen** may provide relief of mild discomfort or pain. Opioids should not be recommended as they may cause constipation and worsen the hemorrhoids. Management of constipation also decreases discomfort during defecation.

Natural Health Products

Phlebotonic agents such as the bioflavonoids **diosmin** and **hesperidin** have demonstrated efficacy in the treatment of hemorrhoids.[6,22] Though the precise mechanism is not known, phlebotonics are associated with strengthening of vessel walls and increased venous tone. These preparations are considered safe. Another therapy that is described as helping to reduce hemorrhoids is **topical bovine cartilage**; the 5% cream relieves itching and the 2% suppository works as a stool softener.[23]

Horse chestnut has also been used for symptomatic relief of hemorrhoids. The active ingredients in horse chestnut appear to be saponins, of which aescin is considered the most important. **Aescin** appears to reduce swelling and inflammation.[24] Adverse effects include pruritus, nausea, stomach complaints, bleeding, nephropathy and allergic reactions. There is little evidence to support the topical use of horse chestnut for hemorrhoids. Horse chestnut and aescin are contraindicated during pregnancy and breastfeeding or in patients who have bleeding disorders. In addition, it may interact with ASA and other antithrombotics leading to an increased bleeding risk.[23,25]

Pregnancy

At present, there are no reproductive safety data available for any of the compounds commonly used for hemorrhoids. Hemorrhoids in pregnancy should be treated by increasing fibre content in the diet, administering stool softeners, increasing liquid intake, and training in toilet habits.[11] Correcting constipation and taking Sitz baths are usually helpful in reducing the discomfort from hemorrhoids. External medications are preferred over those inserted into the rectum because the drugs can be well absorbed from the rectal mucosa. Products containing local anesthetics and corticosteroids, in the recommended dosages, can be used during pregnancy with medical supervision.[26] Systemic absorption after excessive use of a topical corticosteroid has been associated with intrauterine growth retardation.[26,27]

Monitoring of Therapy

Assess relief of symptoms such as itching, pain or burning. Check with the patient in 1 week. If there is no relief within 7 days, if symptoms worsen, or if bleeding, protrusion or seepage occur, reassess and consider referral to specialist care as symptoms associated with rectal cancer, anal fissure, anal abscess, anal fistula, perianal hematoma and other diseases may be similar to those produced by hemorrhoids.[28]

Advice for the Patient

Advise patients regarding:

- Nonpharmacologic therapy, such as increasing fibre in diet
- Management of constipation, if applicable (see Chapter 29: Constipation)
- Proper use and side effects of chosen medication
- When to see a healthcare practitioner.

Table 1: Drug Therapy for Hemorrhoids

Class	Drug	Dosage	Adverse Effects	Comments	Cost[a]
Anesthetics, Local	*dibucaine* Proctosedyl, generics	0.5–1% ointment/cream; 5 mg suppository Use each morning and evening and after each bowel movement	Allergic reactions, locally and systemically; local reactions (burning and itching).	Amide type Common ingredient in hemorrhoidal products. Also referred to as cinchocaine.	$$
	pramoxine Anusol Plus, Anugesic HC, generics	1% ointment; 20 mg suppository Use each morning and evening and after each bowel movement	Allergic reactions, locally and systemically; local reactions (burning and itching).	Exhibits less cross-sensitivity because it does not have the usual amide or ester structure. Lower incidence of sensitization. Generally used in combination with hydrocortisone and/or zinc.	$
Anti-infectives	*framycetin* Proctosedyl, generics	1% ointment; suppositories Use every morning and evening and after each bowel movement PRN	Local irritation, itching, sensistivity.	Used to reduce superimposed bacterial infection to alleviate edema, inflammation and pruritus.	$$
Anti-inflammatory Agents	*hydrocortisone acetate* Anusol HC, Anugesic HC, Proctosedyl , generics	0.5% and 1% ointment; 5–10 mg suppositories Use every morning and evening and after each bowel movement PRN	Mucosal atrophy (more common with prolonged use).	Should not be used for longer than 7 days, but up to 14 days may be appropriate if significant improvement is occurring.	$$
Astringents	*hamamelis* Preparation H-PE Gel	50% gel; available as pads or wipes Use up to 6 times daily after each bowel movement PRN	No significant adverse effects.	Generally used in combination with phenylephrine.	$$
	zinc sulfate Anusol, Anusol Plus, Anusol HC, Anugesic HC, generics	0.5% ointment/cream; 10 mg suppository Use up to 6 times daily after each bowel movement PRN	No significant adverse effects.	Common ingredient in hemorrhoidal products.	$
Protectants	*glycerin*	10% ointment Apply up to QID	No significant adverse effects.		$
	petrolatum	Apply up to QID	No significant adverse effects.		$

(cont'd)

Table 1: **Drug Therapy for Hemorrhoids** *(cont'd)*

Class	Drug	Dosage	Adverse Effects	Comments	Cost[a]
Vasoconstrictors	*phenylephrine* Preparation H-PE Gel	0.25% gel Apply every morning and evening and after each bowel movement PRN	Possible systemic absorption if applied to abraded skin (increased blood pressure, CNS disturbances, cardiac arrhythmia, aggravation of symptoms of hyperthyroidism).	Onset of action ranges from a few seconds to 1 min. Duration of action is 2–3 h. Theoretically may interact with MAOIs, including RIMAs (increased systemic adverse effects of vasoconstrictor) but no published reports. Caution if heart disease, hypertension, thyroid disease, diabetes, prostatic hypertrophy.	$$
Yeast Derivatives	*yeast* Preparation H	1% ointment/cream; 22 mg suppository Use every morning and evening and after each bowel movement PRN to improve wound healing	No significant adverse effects.	Insufficient evidence to confirm efficacy.	$$

[a] Cost of smallest available pack size; includes drug cost only.

Abbreviations: CNS = central nervous system; MAOI = monoamine oxidase inhibitor; RIMA = reversible inhibitor of monoamine oxidase type A

Legend: $ <$5 $$ $5–10

Suggested Readings

Lohsiriwat V. Hemorrhoids: from basic pathophysiology to clinical management. *World J Gastroenterol* 2012;18:2009-17.

Ross NP, Hildebrand DR, Tiernan JP et al. Haemorrhoids: 21st-century management. *Colorectal Dis* 2012;14:917-9.

Wald A, Bharucha AE, Cosman BC et al. ACG clinical guideline: management of benign anorectal disorders. *Am J Gastroenterol* 2014;109:1141-57.

References

1. Haas PA. The prevalence of confusion in the definition of hemorrhoids. *Dis Colon Rectum* 1992;35:290-1.
2. Pfenninger JL, Zainea GG. Common anorectal conditions: Part I. Symptoms and complaints. *Am Fam Physician* 2001;63:2391-8.
3. Pfenninger JL, Zainea GG. Common anorectal conditions: Part II. Lesions. *Am Fam Physician* 2001;64:77-88.
4. Brisinda G. How to treat haemorrhoids. Prevention is best; haemorrhoidectomy needs skilled operators. *BMJ* 2000;321:582-3.
5. Hulme-Moir M, Bartolo DC. Hemorrhoids. *Gastroenterol Clin North Am* 2001;30:183-97.
6. MacKay D. Hemorrhoids and varicose veins: a review of treatment options. *Altern Med Rev* 2001;6:126-40.
7. Johanson JF, Sonnenberg A. The prevalence of hemorrhoids and chronic constipation. An epidemiological study. *Gastroenterology* 1990;98:380-6.
8. Mazier WP. Hemorrhoids, fissures and pruritus ani. *Surg Clin North Am* 1994;74:1277-92.
9. Johannsson HO, Graf W, Pahlman L. Bowel habits in hemorrhoid patients and normal subjects. *Am J Gastroenterol* 2005;100:401-6.
10. Madoff RD, Fleshman JW; Clinical Practice Committee, American Gastroenterological Association. American Gastroenterological Association technical review on the diagnosis and treatment of hemorrhoids. *Gastroenterology* 2004;126:1463-73.
11. Staroselsky A, Nava-Ocampo AA, Vohra S et al. Hemorrhoids in pregnancy. *Can Family Physician* 2008;54:189-90.
12. Altomare DF, Rinaldi M, La Torre F et al. Red hot chili pepper and hemorrhoids: the explosion of a myth: results of a prospective, randomized, placebo-controlled, crossover trial. *Dis Colon Rectum* 2006;49:1018-23.
13. Wald A, Bharucha AE, Cosman BC et al. ACG clinical guideline: management of benign anorectal disorders. *Am J Gastroenterol* 2014;109 (8):1141-57.
14. Alonso-Coello P, Guyatt G, Heels-Ansdell D et al. Laxatives for the treatment of hemorrhoids. *Cochrane Database Syst Rev* 2005; (4):CD004649.
15. Shafik A. Role of warm-water bath in the anorectal conditions. The "thermosphincteric reflex". *J Clin Gastroenterol* 1993;16:304-8.
16. Johanson JF. Nonsurgical treatment of hemorrhoids. *J Gastrointest Surg* 2002;6:290-4.
17. MacRae HM, McLeod RS. Comparison of hemorrhoidal treatment modalities. A meta-analysis. *Dis Colon Rectum* 1995;38:687-94.
18. Clinical Practice Committee, American Gastroenterological Association. American Gastroenterological Association medical position statement: Diagnosis and treatment of hemorrhoids. *Gastroenterology* 2004;126:1461-2.
19. American Society of Health-System Pharmacists. *AHFS drug information*. Bethesda: Board of the American Society of Health-System Pharmacists; 2015.
20. Univeristy of Saskatchewan. medSask. *Hemorrhoids: guidelines for prescribing rectal hydrocortisone combination products*. Available from: medsask.usask.ca/professional/guidelines/hemorrhoids.php. Accessed February 16, 2016.
21. Health Canada. *Anorectal drug products. Labelling standard*. Available from: www.hc-sc.gc.ca/dhp-mps/prodpharma/applic-demande/guide-ld/label-etiquet-pharm/anorecta-eng.php. Accessed February 16, 2016.
22. Perera N, Liolitsa D, Iype S et al. Phlebotonics for haemorrhoids. *Cochrane Database Syst Rev* 2012;8:CD004322.
23. Natural Medicines Comprehensive Database. Jellin JM, ed. Stockton: Therapeutic Research Faculty. Available from: naturaldatabase.therapeuticresearch.com. Subscription required.
24. Sirtori CR. Aescin: pharmacology, pharmacokinetics and therapeutic profile. *Pharmacol Res* 2001;44:183-93.
25. Ernst E, ed. *The desktop guide to complementary and alternative medicine*. London: Harcourt Publishers; 2001.
26. Zip C. A practical guide to dermatological drug use in pregnancy. *Skin Therapy Lett* 2006;11:1-4.
27. Ward KE, O"Brien BM. Pregnancy and lactation: therapeutic considerations. In: DiPiro JT, Talbert RL, Yee GC et al., eds. *Pharmacotherapy: a pathophysiologic approach*. 9th ed. New York: McGraw-Hill Education; 2014. p. 1253.
28. Kaidar-Person O, Person B, Wexner SD. Hemorrhoidal disease: a comprehensive review. *J Am Coll Surg* 2007;204:102-17.

Hemorrhoids—What You Need to Know

What are hemorrhoids?

Hemorrhoids are displaced anal cushions (pads). Hemorrhoids may be internal or external or both. Internal hemorrhoids usually do not hurt but they can bleed. External hemorrhoids, however, do hurt.

What causes hemorrhoids?

Hemorrhoids are a common problem. They may be brought on by many things, including:

- Constipation or diarrhea
- Pregnancy
- Heavy lifting
- Standing or sitting for long periods of time

What are the symptoms of hemorrhoids?

Hemorrhoids can cause itching, burning and irritation around the anus. They can also bleed when you have a bowel movement.

What can you do to help prevent hemorrhoids?

- Avoid constipation by drinking lots of fluid and eating a healthy diet that is high in fibre.
- Do not sit on the toilet for long periods of time.
- Do not strain to have a bowel movement.

When should you see your healthcare provider?

See your healthcare provider if any of the following things happen:

- The hemorrhoid does not go back in place after a bowel movement
- You have bleeding from your rectum (back passage)
- The problem lasts longer than 7 days
- Stool or mucus leaks from your rectum between bowel movements

What is the treatment for hemorrhoids?

Medications may help to control the symptoms of hemorrhoids, but do not fix the problem. Talk to your healthcare provider for advice on which product may be best for you.

Chapter 34
Infant Colic

Shelita Dattani, BSc(Pharm), PharmD

Colic is reported in approximately 10–20% of healthy infants.[1,2] The most accepted definition of colic is the Wessel "rule of three", which defines colic as unexplained paroxysmal bouts of fussing and crying that last more than 3 hours a day, for more than 3 days a week, and for greater than 3 weeks.[1,3,4,5]

The term colic is imprecise and frequently overused. Although crying is an integral component of colic, a behavioural definition includes increased motor activity and altered patterns of sleeping and eating.[1,5,6] It is often associated with clenched fists, reddening of the face, drawing up of the legs, abdominal distention and flatus.[1] Occasionally, excessive regurgitation and vomiting can occur.[1,5,7,8]

Pathophysiology

Infantile colic is a diagnosis of exclusion and is considered when an otherwise thriving infant presents with crying that is often inconsolable and when other causes such as infections, trauma, metabolic disorders, foreign bodies, gastrointestinal, central nervous system or cardiovascular issues are ruled out. It usually starts around the second week of life and is most common in infants aged 4–6 weeks. It gradually improves, becomes uncommon at 3–4 months of age and beyond, and is not associated with any long-term consequences.[9] A normal diurnal variation has been noted, with crying more often in the late afternoon or evening.[5,10,11] Males and females are affected with equal frequency.[1,3,10] Limited data suggest that colic may be more likely in babies whose mothers smoke.[12] Colic occurs in both breastfed and formula-fed babies. There is no evidence of a genetic predisposition to colic.[1,10,11]

Although the exact etiology of colic is unknown, proposed causes include organic, behavioural and psychological components (Table 1).[13] A combination of these factors may be implicated in any given infant. Some experts feel that colic may be best viewed as a clinical manifestation of normal emotional development, in which an infant has diminished capacity to regulate crying duration.[6,8,9] Parents will become frustrated if they try to pinpoint the exact cause of the baby's colic.

Table 1: **Proposed Causes of Infant Colic[14]**

Proposed Cause	Possible Rationale
Organic	Carbohydrate intolerance, intestinal gas, motility disorder, gastroesophageal reflux, immature central and autonomic nervous system, milk or food allergy, altered intestinal microflora.
Behavioural	Improper feeding or feeding technique, smoking in the home.
Psychological	Difficulties with parent-child interaction.

Goals of Therapy

- Decrease frequency or duration of crying episodes to less than 3 hours per day, less than 3 days per week[6,8,10]
- Infant eating well and thriving
- Less or minimal fussiness after eating

- Avoid dehydration of infant
- Infant is able to fall asleep
- Minimize adverse effects of recommended therapies
- Minimize parental stress and frustration and help strengthen coping skills

Patient Assessment

An assessment algorithm for infants with colic is illustrated in Figure 3. A complete history and physical examination should be performed to rule out any organic causes of crying or underlying medical conditions.

Nonpharmacologic Therapy

Nonpharmacologic therapy is the mainstay of treatment of colic. Since the cause of colic is unknown, there are as many nonpharmacologic treatments as there are proposed etiologies. Furthermore, there is a lack of evidence to support the efficacy of these interventions.[1,6,11] Take a holistic approach when advising parents of treatment strategies, and provide information on community support to give parents the opportunity to share and consult with other parents. Parents should be reassured that any given strategy may or may not work and that flexibility is essential to success.

Physical Methods

Methods that have been attempted include gentle pressure to the abdomen, carrying, rocking, swaddling, skin-to-skin contact, use of infant carriers or massage. There are several forms of massage, including whole-body massage and belly massage (infant facing downward in one hand; parent starts from the navel and massages abdomen in clockwise motion).[15] Figure 1 illustrates how to hold the baby and Figure 2 illustrates the correct method of belly massage.

Figure 1: **How to Hold the Baby**

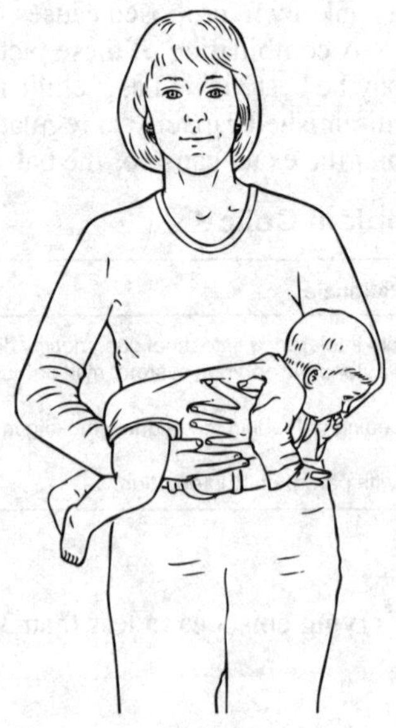

Figure 2: **How to Massage the Baby**

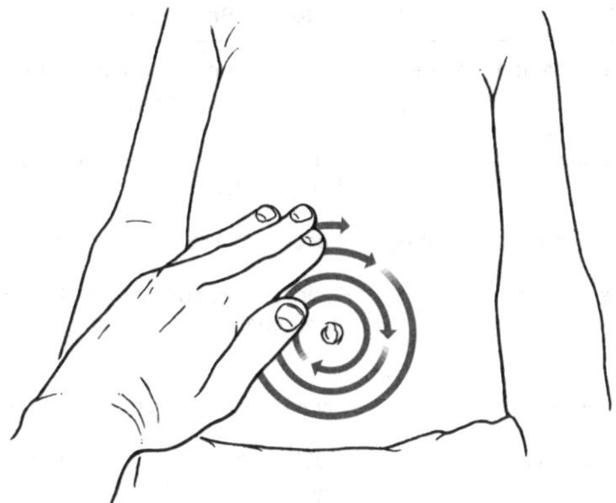

Babies who demonstrate possible gastric distress by pulling their legs up and arching their backs may derive some relief if their legs are gently pushed back and forth, in an alternating or "bicycle" motion. Repetitive motion relaxes infants and physical contact from the parent or caregiver may have a calming effect.[1,6]

Warm baths may relieve gastrointestinal spasm. Heating pads should not be used due to the risk of burning the infant. Evidence for the efficacy of chiropractic spinal manipulation is inconclusive—parents should be discouraged from trying this approach.[7]

Behavioural Management

Table 2 lists some common causes of crying and provides some basic management strategies. Crying is one of the few ways a baby can communicate, and the parental response reassures the infant that someone is listening. The strategies below can be attempted in any order. If the baby continues to cry, parents should move on to another strategy and not persist with any one measure.[6]

A colic diary that documents crying and fussing spells can assist parents and healthcare practitioners in creating a management strategy by helping to establish some patterns in the infant's day. Parents can log their behaviours, look for patterns and then try to modify these behaviours to see if the situation improves. A routine schedule for feeding, holding, playtime and general care can be developed once patterns are established. At the very least, keeping a diary gives a parent a better sense of control and a clearer perspective of a frustrating situation.[1,16]

It is imperative that the caregiver has sufficient rest breaks when symptoms can no longer be tolerated. Parental tension will make everyone's distress worse.

Even though colic is usually self-limiting for the infant, it can take some time to repair the parent-infant attachment relationship. If families continue to have difficulty coping with their usual sources of support and despite reassurance by their healthcare practitioner, they may be referred to a mental health professional (e.g., counsellors, psychologists).[1,6]

Environmental Manipulation

Although white noise has anecdotally been comforting to some infants, evidence of the efficacy of strategies using vibration or sound comes from uncontrolled studies and is inconclusive.[17]

Additionally, available evidence suggests that increased carrying, car rides or car-ride simulators and baby swings are not effective in the management of colic symptoms.[1,7,8,17]

Table 2: **Behavioural Management Strategies for Parents of Crying Babies**[1,5,6]

Problem	Symptoms	Potential Strategies
Hunger	Crying between feedings. Inadequate weight gain	Hunger periods often do not follow a regular pattern. Increase feeding frequency as needed.
Poor feeding	Refusing bottle or breast	Poor feeding may be indicative of a serious health problem and may lead to dehydration. Consult with a healthcare practitioner.
Overheated	Crying when tightly swaddled or layered	Loosen covers, reduce clothing, reduce room temperature.
Need for attention or physical contact	Crying or fussiness when left alone	Hold, rock or cuddle baby. Do not worry about spoiling the infant or contributing to a bad habit.
Insomnia	Crying, inability to sleep at bedtime	Avoid excessive stimulation or arousal before bedtime.
Tiredness	Crying or fussiness when handled	Put the baby down in a dark, quiet room. Unless crying excessively, babies can be left alone for short intervals to see if they will fall asleep on their own. Babies who are crying loudly should be picked up and held or rocked quietly until they fall asleep.
Lack of stimulation	Crying or fussiness when left alone	Play with the baby, provide a visual or auditory distraction or place baby in an infant seat or swing where there is a lot of activity, e.g., kitchen.
Ear infection	Crying or irritability; infant may be fingering or pulling on ear. Infant may not be sleeping or eating well. May be accompanied by or preceded by a cold. Occasionally, fluid may be draining out of the ear canal. Fever may be present	Requires further assessment and possibly treatment, particularly if temperature >38°C and <3 months of age (even if other symptoms of ear infection are absent).
Teething	Crying, excessive salivation, inflamed gums. Typically begins after 5 months of age	Rub the baby's gums with a clean finger or offer a rubber teething ring. Refrain from using teething biscuits.

If parents try a series of calming techniques without using any one consistently for at least a day, the infant may get overstimulated, which can make the colicky situation worse. Other parents give up trying and withdraw from their infants, which can lead to spiralling parent and infant stress.[1,6]

Dietary Manipulation

The majority of the dietary manipulations recommended below require specialized follow up.

Breastfeeding

Breastfeeding should be continued since the incidence of colic in breastfed and bottle-fed infants is similar, and weaning a colicky infant to formula can result in symptoms worsening.[1,8]

Limited data suggest that prolonged emptying of 1 breast at each feed (vs. equal drainage of both breasts at each feed) is associated with a lower incidence of colic.[18]

The link between food allergies and infant colic in children without other symptoms of atopy is controversial.[19] However, if there is suspicion of food allergies in a colicky baby, healthcare practitioners may advise that bottle-fed babies receive extensively hydrolyzed cow's proteins. If the baby is breastfeeding, the mother could be advised to eliminate certain foods from her diet (e.g., cow's milk protein and dairy products, soy, wheat, eggs, peanuts, tree nuts and fish for 1–2 weeks; recommend that the mother takes calcium supplementation if milk and its products are eliminated from her diet).[1,5,19,20,21]

Foods noted to aggravate colic in breastfed infants include cabbage, broccoli, caffeine, citrus fruit and chocolate. Limited data suggest that eliminating these foods from the mother's diet for a period of time may help with colicky symptoms.[1,19] Removing too many foods, however, may have an adverse effect on the mother's nutrition and generate additional stress. Consider referral to a dietitian before significant modifications occur.[1,5]

Formula Feeding

Substituting traditional formulas with hypoallergenic (casein hydrolysate, whey hydrolysate) formula may reduce duration of crying but may be associated with an increased cost to families and may be less palatable than traditional infant formulas.[5,17,19,22] Hypoallergenic formulas should be reserved for infants with confirmed allergies to cow's milk protein.[7] The use of soy protein-based formulas in the treatment of colic is not supported by adequate data.[11,22]

Evidence for the use of lactose-reduced formula or lactase enzyme supplementation is not sufficient to draw conclusions about efficacy of these treatments for colic.[6,10,19,22] The addition of fibre to formula is not effective.[8,10,19]

If formula changes are made, they should not be pursued if symptoms do not improve after 1 week.[6,8] Frequent formula changes are not recommended.[6,8]

Feeding Techniques

The following simple techniques can be helpful in feeding a colicky bottle-fed infant:

- To prevent regurgitation and promote the exit of swallowed air, infants should be held in a vertical position during feeding, with the head higher than the feet[1,6]
- It is important to use the correct bottle and nipple size for the infant's age. Curved bottles allow the infant to be fed while sitting up, and bottles with a collapsible bag may decrease air swallowing. Changing the nipple of the bottle to one with a smaller hole or anticolic design may prevent frequent colic attacks. The effects of these measures have not been formally studied[1]
- Infants should be burped in an upright position, with the baby held over the shoulder or in a gentle chin grasp. Burping should be encouraged after every 30–60 mL of formula ingested or after every 5–10 minutes of breastfeeding.[1,6]

Pharmacologic Therapy

For comparative ingredients of nonprescription products, consult the *Compendium of Products for Minor Ailments*—Baby Care Products: Gastrointestinal.

Over the years, different medications have been recommended for the management of colic. The efficacy of pharmacologic agents in the treatment of colic is difficult to assess due to the highly subjective nature of the problem, undetermined etiology, poorly designed trials, conflicting results and high placebo effect noted in clinical trials.[9,17,19] Furthermore, the age of the patient group and fear of possible harm to the infant makes it difficult to conduct research aimed at developing more effective medications. Before pharmacologic agents are tried, ensure that nonpharmacologic measures have been used to their fullest potential. Table 4 describes various pharmacologic therapies for colic.

If pharmacologic therapy is attempted:

- Start with the lowest dose and increase incrementally only when necessary based on symptoms
- Use only intermittent dosing when necessary based on symptoms
- NOTE: most of the pharmacologic agents available provide questionable benefit and are not routinely recommended in the treatment of colic

- Treatment with probiotics requires more study before being widely adopted. Unlike other agents used in the treatment of colic, probiotics would require at least 2–4 weeks of continuous treatment at appropriate doses to show effect.

Natural Health Products and Probiotic Remedies

Preparations containing fennel oil or the probiotic *Lactobacillus reuteri* appear to be effective in reducing crying times in colicky infants.[26,27] No clinically meaningful adverse effects have been reported but long-term safety has not been established.

Monitoring of Therapy

Table 3 provides a framework for a monitoring plan that should be individualized for each patient.

Table 3: Monitoring of Therapy for Infant Colic[16]

Symptoms	Monitoring	Endpoint of Therapy	Actions
Excessive crying	Parent: Daily—log behaviour in a colic diary to assess patterns Document associated symptoms Healthcare practitioner: After 3 days or at next visit. Review diary with parent	Decrease in frequency or duration of crying episodes to less than 3 h per day, less than 3 days per week.	If current treatment strategy is not effective, try another strategy based on patterns noted in diary. If still ineffective after 3 days, further investigation would be required to rule out organic etiology for crying. If crying is associated with poor feeding, fever, vomiting, dehydration or significant change in stool or urination pattern, or if infant cries for ≥3 h without stopping, an immediate and thorough assessment would be required.
Parental anxiety	Parent: Daily Healthcare practitioner: After 3 days or at next visit	Decrease in parental anxiety and frustration. Improved parental coping skills.	Reassure parents and re-emphasize coping strategies. Remind them to take "time out" rest periods away from the infant. If they continue to seem frustrated or overwhelmed, refer to an appropriate healthcare practitioner for counselling.
Infant agitated or unable to fall asleep	Parent: Daily—log behaviour in diary and document associated symptoms Healthcare practitioner: After 3 days or at next visit. Review diary with parent	Infant able to fall asleep. Infant calm before bedtime or naptime.	Healthcare practitioner should perform a complete history and physical examination. If serious issues are ruled out, environmental manipulation or other soothing techniques can be tried.
Refusal to eat or excessive fussiness after eating	Parent: Daily—log behaviour in diary and indicate whether related to other symptoms such as gas, fever, constipation. If signs of dehydration are noted (e.g., tearless crying, reduced urination to <4 diapers/day, sunken eyes, dry skin and mouth, sunken fontanelle), the child should be assessed by a healthcare practitioner immediately Healthcare practitioner: Look for signs of dehydration and monitor infant's body weight as required. Infants <2–3 months of age may require hospital admissions to rule out sepsis	Less or minimal fussiness after eating. No weight loss or signs of dehydration.	A thorough physical assessment for weight loss or signs of dehydration is required. Suggest that caregiver discuss with an appropriate healthcare practitioner alterations in maternal diet or formula to rule out allergenic component to colic.

Advice for the Caregiver

Advise caregivers of colicky babies regarding:

- When to seek medical advice (Table 3)
- Nonpharmacologic management strategies

- Proper use of any drug therapy chosen
- Expected results of any drug therapy and management of adverse effects.

Figure 3: **Assessment of Infants with Suspected Colic**

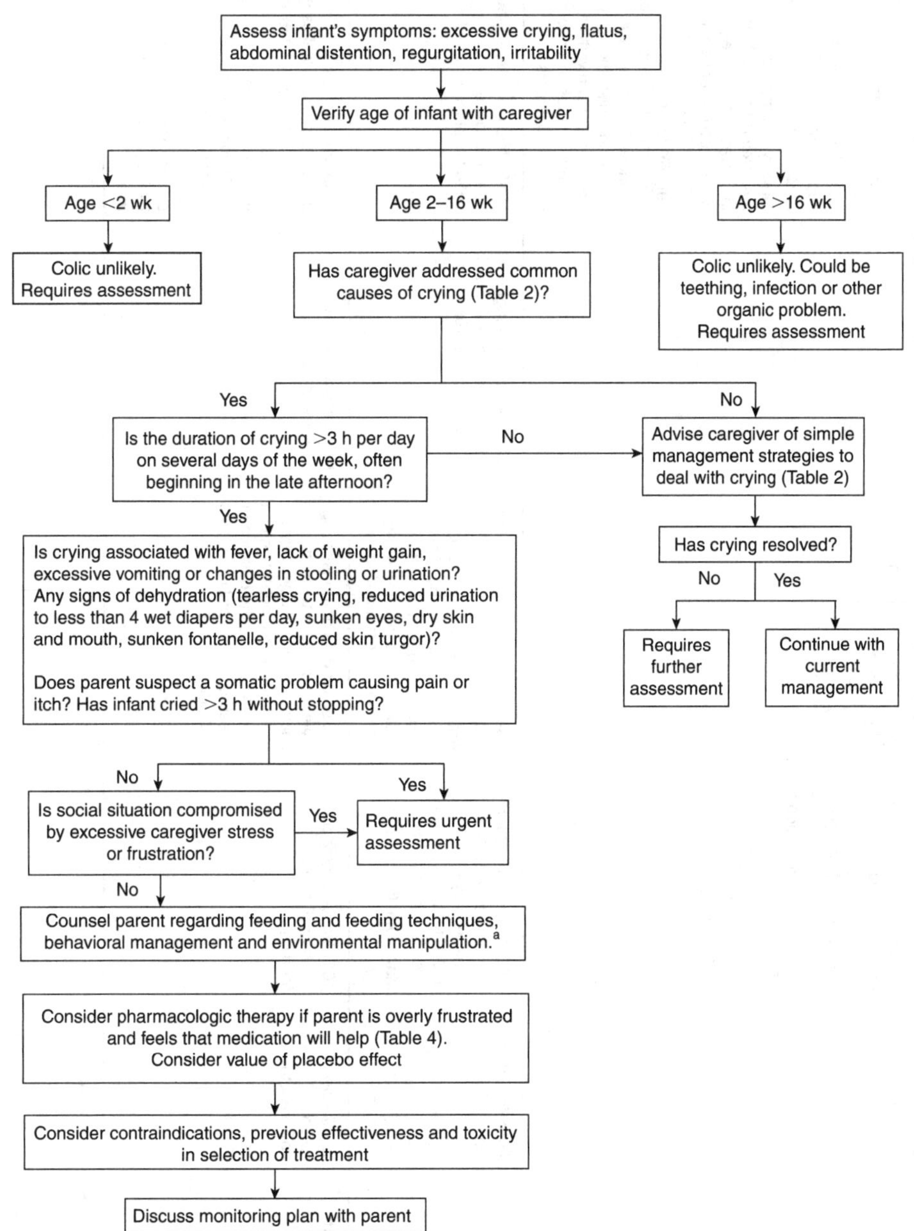
Assess infant's symptoms: excessive crying, flatus, abdominal distention, regurgitation, irritability
Verify age of infant with caregiver
Age <2 wk
Age 2–16 wk
Age >16 wk
Colic unlikely. Requires assessment
Has caregiver addressed common causes of crying (Table 2)?
Colic unlikely. Could be teething, infection or other organic problem. Requires assessment
Yes
No
Is the duration of crying >3 h per day on several days of the week, often beginning in the late afternoon?
No
Advise caregiver of simple management strategies to deal with crying (Table 2)
Yes
Has crying resolved?
No
Yes
Requires further assessment
Continue with current management
Is crying associated with fever, lack of weight gain, excessive vomiting or changes in stooling or urination? Any signs of dehydration (tearless crying, reduced urination to less than 4 wet diapers per day, sunken eyes, dry skin and mouth, sunken fontanelle, reduced skin turgor)?
Does parent suspect a somatic problem causing pain or itch? Has infant cried >3 h without stopping?
No
Yes
Is social situation compromised by excessive caregiver stress or frustration?
Yes
Requires urgent assessment
No
Counsel parent regarding feeding and feeding techniques, behavioral management and environmental manipulation.[a]
Consider pharmacologic therapy if parent is overly frustrated and feels that medication will help (Table 4). Consider value of placebo effect
Consider contraindications, previous effectiveness and toxicity in selection of treatment
Discuss monitoring plan with parent

[a] Recommend that caregiver maintain a colic diary for 48–72 hours that documents crying and fussing spells and associated symptoms. Parents should also log sleeping, feeding, playtime and bowel movements in this diary.

Table 4: **Pharmacologic Therapy for Infant Colic**

Class	Agents	Dosage	Mechanism of Action	Adverse Effects	Comments	Cost
Carbohydrates	*sucrose*	Dissolve 5 g of sucrose (table or granulated sugar) in 40 mL water (12% solution) and give 2 mL to infant via dropper. Increase concentration to 25–50% if necessary (7.5–15 g sucrose in 30 mL water, respectively)	Proposed analgesic effect in infants. Short-acting response; lasts <30 min.	None reported.	Limited data show 63% of infants respond with decrease in symptoms but short duration of action of sucrose may limit its practical use.[23] More well-controlled research is needed before this treatment can be widely recommended. If solution is not administered right away, store in refrigerator and inspect for changes in appearance before administration. Do not substitute with honey because of risk of botulism in infants.	$
Carminatives	*simethicone* Infacol, Ovol, generics	0.25–0.5 mL (10–20 mg) with or after each feeding as necessary May be added to formula or given directly from dropper Maximum: 6 mL per 24 h	Based on the possible etiology of gas in colic. Antiflatulent; alters surface tension of mucus and allows entrapped gas bubbles to coalesce and be more easily released by the mouth or anus.	No clinically meaningful adverse effects due to lack of systemic absorption.	Ineffective but safe.[22] May be useful because of potential placebo effect.	$
Probiotic Agents	*Lactobacillus reuteri* BioGaia, others	10^8 colony-forming units per day 30 min after feeding	Based on data demonstrating lower counts of intestinal Lactobacilli in colicky infants. Probiotic supplementation can favourably alter the balance of intestinal Lactobacilli in infants with colic.	No clinically meaningful adverse effects.	Data demonstrate meaningful and significant reduction in crying times as early as 7 days of treatment.[13,14,24,25] Additional studies are needed to determine whether other probiotic strains may be beneficial. Refrigerate when not in use.	$

[a] Cost of 1 dose; includes drug cost only.

Legend: $ <$2

Resource Tips

Parents can call their regional health department's parent-child information line or their local children's hospital hotline for more information on community support for parents of colicky babies. The Internet can be an extensive source of information but is also inundated with endorsements or advertisements for products that have not been proven effective or safe in the treatment of colic. Parents should be cautioned about this and encouraged to look for legitimate websites such as the site maintained by the Canadian Paediatric Society.[8]

Internet-based Information on Colicky Infants:

Canadian Paediatric Society. Available from: www.cps.ca.

Keyword search: colic.

WebMD. Available from: www.webmd.com.

Keyword search: colic.

Suggested Readings

Canadian Paediatric Society. *Infantile colic: is there a role for dietary interventions?* Available from: www.cps.ca/documents/position/infantile-colic-dietary-interventions.

Cohen-Silver J, Ratnapalan S. Management of infantile colic: a review. *Clin Pediatr (Phila)* 2009;48:14-7.

Dobson D, Lucassen PL, Miller JJ et al. Manipulative therapies for infantile colic. *Cochrane Database Syst Rev* 2012;12:CD004796.

Gupta SK. Update on infantile colic and management options. *Curr Opin Investig Drugs* 2007;8:921-6.

Kheir AE. Infantile colic, facts and fiction. *Ital J Pediatr* 2012;38:34.

References

1. Berkowitz CD. Management of the colicky infant. *Compr Ther* 1997;23:277-80.
2. Sferra TJ, Heitlinger LA. Gastrointestinal gas formation and infantile colic. *Pediatr Clin North Am* 1996;43:489-510.
3. Reust CE, Blake RL. Diagnostic workup before diagnosing colic. *Arch Fam Med* 2000;9:282-3.
4. Wessel MA, Cobb JC, Jackson EB et al. Paroxysmal fussing in infancy, sometimes called colic. *Pediatrics* 1954;14:421-35.
5. Gupta SK. Update on infantile colic and management options. *Curr Opin Investig Drugs* 2007;8:921-6.
6. Balon AJ. Management of infantile colic. *Am Fam Physician* 1997:55:235-42, 245-6.
7. Cohen-Silver J, Ratnapalan S. Management of infantile colic: a review. *Clin Pediatr (Phila)* 2009;48:14-7.
8. Roberts DM, Ostapchuk M, O'Brien JG. Infantile colic. *Am Fam Physician* 2004;70:735-40.
9. Kanabar D. Infantile colic. *J Fam Health Care* 2004;14:1-2.
10. Clemons RM. Issues in newborn care. *Prim Care* 2000;27:251-67.
11. Savino F. Focus on infantile colic. *Acta Paediatr* 2007;96:1259-64.
12. Reijneveld SA, Lanting CI, Crone MR et al. Exposure to tobacco smoke and infant crying. *Acta Paediatr* 2005;94:217-21.
13. Savino F, Cordisco L, Tarasco V et al. Lactobacillus reuteri DSM 17938 in infantile colic: a randomized, double-blind, placebo-controlled trial. *Pediatrics* 2010;126:e526-33.
14. Szajewska H, Gyrczuk E, Horvath A. Lactobacillus reuteri DSM 17938 for the management of infantile colic in breastfed infants: a randomized, double-blind, placebo-controlled trial. *J Pediatr* 2013;162:257-62.
15. Larsen JH. Infants' colic and belly massage. *Practitioner* 1990;234:396-7.
16. *Personal communication*. Barry Lester, PhD, Director of Infant Development Center, Professor in Departments of Psychiatry and Pediatrics, Brown University.
17. Lucassen PL, Assendelft WJ, Gubbels JW et al. Effectiveness of treatments for infantile colic: systematic review. *BMJ* 1998;316:1563-9.
18. Evans K, Evans R, Simmer K. Effect of the method of breast feeding on breast engorgement, mastitis and infantile colic. *Acta Paediatr* 1995;84:849-52.
19. Nocerino R, Pezzella V, Cosenza L et al. The controversial role of food allergy in infantile colic: evidence and clinical management. *Nutrients* 2015;7:2015-25..
20. Lucassen PL, Assendelft WJ, Gubbels JW et al. Infantile colic: crying time reduction with a whey hydrolysate: a double-blind, randomized, placebo-controlled trial. *Pediatrics* 2000;106:1349-54.
21. Hill DJ, Roy N, Heine RG et al. Effect of a low-allergen maternal diet on colic among breastfed infants: a randomized, controlled trial. *Pediatrics* 2005;116:e709-15.
22. Wade S, Kilgour T. Extracts from "Clinical Evidence". Infantile colic. *BMJ* 2001;323:437-40.
23. Markestad T. Use of sucrose as a treatment for infant colic. *Arch Dis Child* 1997;76:356-7.

24. Savino F, Pelle E, Palumeri E et al. Lactobacillus reuteri (American Type Culture Collection Strain 55730) versus simethicone in the treatment of infantile colic: a prospective randomized study. *Pediatrics* 2007;119:e124-30.
25. Savino F, Cordisco L, Tarasco V et al. Lactobacillus reuteri DSM 17938 in infantile colic: a randomized, double-blind, placebo-controlled trial. *Pediatrics* 2010;126:e526-33.
26. Harb T, Matsuyama M et al. Infant colic—what works: a systematic review of interventions for breastfed infants. *J Pediatr Gastroenterol Nutr* 2015 Dec 10. [Epub ahead of print].
27. Xu M, Wang J, Wang N et al. The efficacy and safety of the probiotic Bacterium Lactobacillus reuteri DSM 17938 for infantile colic: a meta-analysis of randomized controlled trials. *PLoS One* 2015;10:e0141445.

Infant Colic—What You Need to Know

Many babies have colic. It usually goes away by the time the baby is 3–4 months old. Babies that have colic cry more than other babies—sometimes a lot more. That can be hard on the parents. Don't feel guilty that your baby has colic. It's not your fault.

What causes colic?

No one is sure what causes colic. Colic does not mean that your baby is sick or that there is anything wrong with your baby. Colic is not caused by the way the baby is handled or treated. It does not mean that your baby is mad at you, rejecting you or manipulating you. Don't take your baby's colic personally.

How does a baby with colic act?

Babies that have colic may draw their legs in towards their bodies. They may clench their fists. It may seem like they are in pain. Sometimes, they stretch out their arms and legs and go stiff, then draw in again. They may turn bright red from crying. Babies with colic often get fussy at the end of the day but colic can happen at any time.

What can you do to manage colic?

- **Never** shake your baby.
- Keep a diary of your baby's fussy periods for 2 or 3 days to see if there is a pattern. If you know when the baby is fussy, it can help you feel more in control of the situation. It can also help you and your doctor decide how to deal with it (see Table 1).
- You can try many different things to soothe your baby, such as:
  - holding your baby in a different position
  - giving your baby a warm bath
  - rocking him/her in a cradle or rocking chair
  - playing music
  - walking the baby in a stroller
  - taking the baby for a ride in the car

  Remember that what works on one day may not work on the next day. Try to be flexible.
- Having a colicky baby can be very stressful. You may feel overwhelmed, especially if you are not getting much sleep. Don't be afraid to take time for yourself and don't feel guilty about it. Ask your spouse, a grandparent or a babysitter to watch the baby while you have a rest break.

When should you see your healthcare provider?

See your healthcare provider if:

- Your baby:
  - does not drink enough milk
  - develops a fever
  - is vomiting or spitting up a lot of milk
  - is having difficulty breathing

  - has any change in the number of wet or dirty diapers
  - cries for 3 hours without stopping
  - cries without tears
- You have tried for more than 3 days to find a way to soothe your baby but nothing seems to work.
- You are so stressed you are worried you might hurt your baby.

What about nonprescription medication for colic?

If you are thinking of using nonprescription medication to treat your baby's colic:

- Be aware that there is little proof that these medications work. Talk to your healthcare provider before trying any medication.
- Do not use the medication for more than a few days. Use it only when your baby has symptoms of colic. If the medication does not help to relieve the colic symptoms, stop using it.
- Make sure that you give your baby the right amount of medicine. Read the label carefully to find out how much to give.
- Use a calibrated dropper or an oral syringe to give your baby liquid medication. A dropper or syringe makes it easier to measure the amount of medication accurately. Do not use a spoon—the amount will not be accurate. Read the label carefully to make sure that you are giving the right dose.
- If you use a calibrated dropper: Hold the dropper up at eye level to measure the liquid. Give it to your baby quickly to avoid dripping any liquid.
- If you use an oral syringe: Measure the liquid, then hold the syringe with the tip pointing up. Tap air bubbles toward the end. Push the plunger gently to force air out. Check that you have the right amount of medication in the syringe. Give small amounts of medicine slowly to avoid choking. Let the baby swallow all of the medicine before giving more.
- Clean droppers and syringes with soap and water and store the parts in a clean, dry place.
- Be sure to close medication bottles tightly. Keep all medicine out of the reach of children.

Table 1: **Sample Colic Diary for Parents**

Hour	Crying ("C" for crying or "F" for fussy)—note how long the crying spell goes on and how hard the baby is crying	Other symptoms (for example, gas or arching back)	Comments (for example, hungry, tired)—make a note in this column of when the baby is sleeping, feeding, crying, playing or having a bowel movement	Measures you use to soothe your baby (for example, holding, car ride, change in feeding technique)
6:00 AM				
7:00 AM				
8:00 AM				
9:00 AM				
10:00 AM				
11:00 AM				
12:00 PM				
1:00 PM				
2:00 PM				
3:00 PM				
4:00 PM				
5:00 PM				
6:00 PM				
7:00 PM				
8:00 PM				
9:00 PM				
10:00 PM				
11:00 PM				
12:00 AM				
1:00 AM				
2:00 AM				
3:00 AM				
4:00 AM				
5:00 AM				

Chapter 35
Irritable Bowel Syndrome

Lynette Kosar, BSP, MSc (Pharm)

Irritable bowel syndrome (IBS), also referred to as spastic colon or irritable colon, is a common functional bowel disorder with no identifiable structural or biochemical abnormalities. Generalizations about IBS are difficult as patient presentation varies. The condition encompasses abdominal pain or discomfort with altered bowel habits.[1,2] Other symptoms that characterize the disorder include abdominal bloating, cramping and/or passage of mucus in the stool. IBS can be divided into 3 subtypes: constipation-predominate (IBS-C), diarrhea-predominate (IBS-D), and mixed (IBS-M), a combination of both diarrhea and constipation.[1] Symptoms cycle through phases of exacerbations and remissions, and subtypes may change over time. Patients will often seek medical care when they are concerned their symptoms may represent a life-threatening disorder.

Canada has one of the highest rates of IBS in the world with approximately 5 million Canadians living with this condition.[3] Women are 1.5–2 times more likely to be diagnosed with IBS than men, and it is more common in lower socioeconomic groups and those younger than 50 years.[1,4] Patients often endure a significantly impaired quality of life, an impact similar to that of diabetes, renal disease or hypertension. Mental health may be negatively affected and clinicians should be vigilant for signs of depression. IBS patients use >50% more healthcare resources than those without IBS.[1]

Pathophysiology

A variety of pathophysiologic changes occur in patients with IBS. These include altered neurologic function and sensitivity to stimuli, altered GI motility and abnormal psychosocial features.

Nociceptive stimuli in the GI tract provide input to pain centres that are augmented by psychosocial factors leading to the patient's sensation and interpretation of pain.[5] Patients with IBS are often found to have increased sensitivity to distension in the rectum, ileum and esophagus.[6,7] Pain may be associated with altered motility in the small intestine. An altered balance of neurotransmitters in the GI tract may also be involved. Emotional stress is known to cause changes in GI motility in both the small and large intestine.[5]

Within IBS referral clinics, reports of psychological features can be high, with over half of patients meeting the clinical criteria for depression.[8] In addition, anxiety and somatization (the tendency to overinterpret physiological symptoms) disorders also appear more frequently in patients with IBS. Abuse (physical, sexual) may be reported in one-third of subjects. In patients with IBS who do not seek physician assessment, it is not certain whether these psychological features are present.

Between 60% and 70% of patients with IBS believe certain foods trigger their symptoms.[1] The prevalence of lactose intolerance in the IBS population is estimated to be 38% compared with 26% in the general population.[1] The odds of having celiac disease are 5 times higher in patients with IBS compared with the general population.[1,9]

After an acute illness with a GI pathogen (e.g., *Campylobacter*, *Shigella*, *Salmonella*), some previously healthy individuals may develop persistent IBS symptoms. Likely less than one-third of IBS can be related to an infectious precipitant.[10]

Goals of Therapy

- Improve quality of life by minimizing (or eliminating, if possible) diarrhea, constipation, abdominal pain, bloating, or intestinal spasms
- Treat any existing psychiatric disorders
- Reassure and educate patient regarding the benign nature of IBS

Patient Assessment

IBS is diagnosed when the patient has experienced recurrent abdominal pain or discomfort at least 3 days per month in the past 3 months with symptom onset at least 6 months prior to the diagnosis, and is associated with at least 2 of the following:

- improvement with defecation
- onset associated with a change in frequency of stool
- onset associated with a change in form (appearance) of stool.

The accuracy of IBS diagnosis is further strengthened by the absence of alarm signs and symptoms (e.g., rectal bleeding, iron deficiency anemia, fever, weight loss, onset of symptoms in patients >50 years old, family history of colorectal cancer, nocturnal symptoms, recent progressive symptoms). Patients with alarm features, mental health impacted by IBS symptoms or IBS-D or IBS-M subtypes should undergo further diagnostic evaluation.

When assessing GI symptoms, consider their duration, severity and course. Recurrent symptoms over months to years are suggestive of a functional GI disorder such as IBS. Symptoms of recent onset or becoming steadily more severe, especially over a short time period, are suggestive of an organic GI disorder. Patients with symptoms of IBS should initially undergo a basic diagnostic workup to confirm the diagnosis of IBS and to rule out organic GI disorders such as infections, when applicable. Patients with IBS-D or IBS-M should be tested for celiac disease.

The Bristol Stool Scale can help patients communicate their stool consistency to healthcare practitioners, especially when the patient is hesitant to discuss his/her bowel patterns in a public setting (e.g., community pharmacy). The Bristol Stool Scale distinguishes diarrhea from constipation, and is useful for monitoring response to therapy (see Figure 1).[11]

Acute flares of IBS may be altered by removing triggers and dealing with psychological issues. Perform a careful medication history on all patients. Medications and natural health products can be potential sources of GI adverse effects. Constipation, for example, could be caused by opioids, minerals (iron, calcium, aluminum), anticholinergic agents, loperamide and the calcium channel blockers verapamil and diltiazem. Diarrhea, on the other hand, could be caused by antibiotics, magnesium and laxatives. NSAIDs may cause either constipation or diarrhea.

Important complications of IBS are the loss of productivity and consumption of healthcare resources related to the disorder. Many patients see a number of different healthcare practitioners. Unrealistic expectations can arise, especially with regard to drug therapy. The patient's goals can be unrealistic; goal planning with the patient and other healthcare providers is an important part of the treatment plan. Prevention of IBS is difficult to achieve on a consistent basis.

Figure 1: **Bristol Stool Chart**[a]

Stool form	Appearance	Type
Separate hard lumps like nuts, (hard to pass). Result of slow transit.	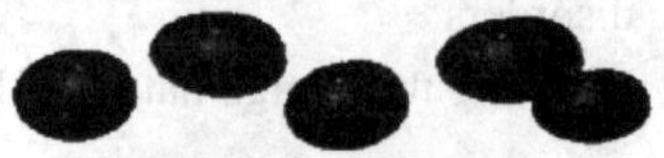	1
Sausage-shaped but lumpy.		2
Like a sausage but cracks on its surface.		3
Like a sausage or snake—smooth and soft.		4
Soft blobs with clear cut edges (easy to pass).	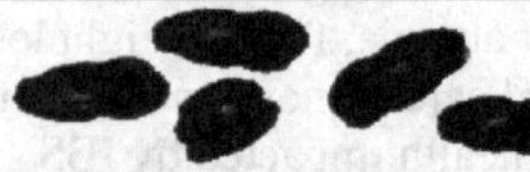	5
Fluffy pieces with ragged edges, a mushy stool.	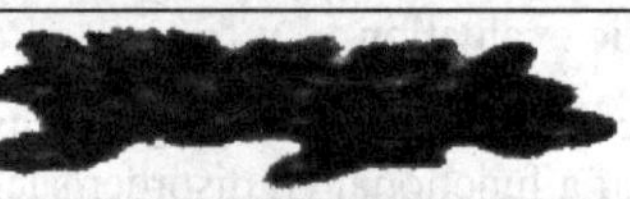	6
Watery, no solid pieces. Result of very fast transit.		7

[a] Types 1–2 indicate constipation, types 3–4 represent ideal stool consistencies as they are easier to pass and types 5–7 may indicate diarrhea and urgency.

Reproduced with permission from Thompson WG, Heaton KW. *Fast facts: irritable bowel syndrome*. 2nd ed. Oxford (GB): Health Press Limited; 2003.

Nonpharmacologic Therapy

Patient symptoms should guide the therapeutic plans (e.g., pain, bloating, gas, diarrhea, constipation). A key component of the therapeutic plan is patient reassurance. The likelihood of a serious organic GI disease such as cancer is likely no different in IBS than the general population.[1] In general, therapies are likely to offer only limited relief over the long term. Counselling patients on the high likelihood for recurrence is important.

Nondrug therapies for IBS include establishing a nonjudgmental therapeutic relationship with the patient, exercise,[12] stress management[13] and counselling for psychological issues.[14] Consider lactose intolerance; consumption of dairy products may be decreased, at least on a trial basis. Patients with IBS-D or IBS-M may benefit from serologic testing for celiac sprue.

Avoidance of lifestyle triggers such as excessive caffeine or fruit intake is a usual component of the treatment plan. Gluten-free and low-FODMAP (fermentable oligosaccharides, disaccharides, monosaccharides and polyols) diets may improve IBS symptoms; however, there is insufficient evidence to recommend food allergy testing or exclusion diets.[2] If patients insist on dietary restrictions, instruct them to keep a food diary and monitor to avoid nutritional deficiencies. The diary is particularly helpful in determining whether lactose is a trigger. This may be accomplished with guidance from a dietitian.

Foods that are most often reported to contribute to IBS symptoms include:

- dairy products
- cereals (e.g., wheat, oats and corn)
- citrus fruit
- potatoes
- caffeinated drinks
- fat
- alcohol
- simple sugar alternatives (e.g., fructose, lactose, sorbitol)
- an excess or insufficient intake of dietary fibre.

Pharmacologic Therapy

For further discussion of pharmacologic therapy for IBS, consult the *Compendium of Therapeutic Choices*: Irritable Bowel Syndrome.

For comparative ingredients of nonprescription products, consult the *Compendium of Products for Minor Ailments*—Gastrointestinal Products: Antidiarrheals, Laxatives.

Selected agents used in the management of IBS are described in Table 1.

In general, drug therapies for IBS are only marginally more effective than placebo over the long term. Short-term benefits over a few weeks may be dramatic as there is a high placebo response (about 50%) to therapy in IBS.[15] To date, only psychological and dietary treatments have been found to provide sustained benefits.[6] With any therapy, 4 weeks is generally considered the minimum duration needed to determine efficacy.

Constipation

If lifestyle modifications (diet, exercise, increased fluids) fail, patients suffering from constipation can try fibre supplementation.[16,17] **Soluble fibre** (e.g., **psyllium**, **calcium polycarbophil**) is more effective than placebo in relieving constipation and global IBS symptoms.[2] Insoluble fibre (e.g., wheat or corn bran) is no different from placebo and may actually worsen abdominal pain or bloating.[16]

Laxatives (e.g., **bisacodyl**, **lactulose**, **magnesium salts**, **polyethylene glycol**, **senna**) may be tried if fibre supplementation is unsuccessful.[17] Stimulant laxatives may cause abdominal cramps and lactulose may result in bloating.

Diarrhea

Loperamide is helpful in the management of diarrhea due to IBS (by decreasing stool frequency and urgency). Some patients may experience nighttime abdominal pain when using loperamide.[18] Fibre supplementation has been studied for IBS-related diarrhea, but there is insufficient evidence to recommend its use.[19]

Abdominal Pain

Antidepressants

Expert recommendations are conflicting regarding the use and effectiveness of tricyclic antidepressants (TCAs) and SSRIs in the management of IBS.[2,20,21] **SSRIs** may improve global assessment and **TCAs** may improve abdominal pain and symptom score in all IBS subtypes.[22] Comorbid depression does not predict response. Since TCAs exhibit anticholinergic properties and tend to increase GI transit time,[23] they may be most appropriate for use in patients with IBS-D. Conversely, SSRIs may decrease GI transit time and may be a more suitable choice in patients with IBS-C.[23,24]

St. John's wort is ineffective in the treatment of IBS.[25]

Antispasmodics

Low-quality evidence suggests that antispasmodics may provide short-term relief from abdominal pain and may improve global assessment and symptom score.[16] Available antispasmodics include **dicyclomine**, **hyoscine**, **peppermint oil**, **pinaverium** and **trimebutine**.[16,22] If recommending peppermint oil, ensure the formulation has a Natural Product Number to reduce the risk of exposure to contaminated or inappropriately labelled products. Monitor IBS-C patients for worsening of constipation as this is a potential side effect of these agents. For acute attacks, recommend dosing on as-needed basis. In patients suffering from postprandial symptoms, scheduling an antispasmodic before meals may be warranted.

Bloating and Gas

Bloating and gas associated with IBS are usually managed with dietary changes (limitation of fibre intake and avoidance of gas-producing vegetables). Treating constipation, if present, may alleviate bloating and gas. Fibre supplementation should be used cautiously as it may worsen gas and bloating symptoms. Weak evidence suggests that **fluoxetine** may help relieve constipation, abdominal pain and bloating in patients with IBS-C suffering from abdominal pain.[24]

Other Therapies

Probiotics have been investigated in the management of IBS symptoms. In general, probiotics may improve IBS symptoms, disease severity score and quality of life but the magnitude of benefit and the most effective species and strain are uncertain.[26,27,28,29,30] Lactobacilli alone offers little if any improvements in IBS symptoms.[1] *Bifidobacteria* shows promise; however, additional evidence is required. Combinations of probiotics may be more effective than single entities.[1]

There are insufficient data to support the use of other alternative therapies in IBS.[1] Acupuncture provides no benefit when compared with sham acupuncture in IBS patients.[31]

Monitoring of Therapy

Monitor diets as they often become more restrictive over time since many patients with IBS associate their symptoms with particular foods. Ensure that patients who withhold dairy products maintain supplemental intake of calcium and vitamin D. Advise patients of the alarm features of serious GI pathology (see Patient Assessment).

Symptoms often recur or present differently over the course of time. In more difficult cases, patient dissatisfaction with care increases. A long-term care plan is important as patients frequently seek new alternative sources of heath care to deal with persisting or recurrent symptoms. Good communication with other healthcare practitioners is especially important in this difficult-to-manage group of patients with functional GI disorders.

Most therapeutic trials should be at least 1 month in length. Antidepressants often require 6 weeks or more to assess their effectiveness. More than 1 antidepressant is often tried as there is interpatient variability in response to individual agents.

Table 1: **Pharmacologic Therapy for Irritable Bowel Syndrome**[a]

Class	Drug	Dosage	Adverse Effects	Drug Interactions	Comments	Cost[b]
Antispasmodics	*dicyclomine* Bentylol, generics	10–20 mg TID–QID PRN or scheduled before meals	Dry mouth, drowsiness, constipation, confusion, blurred vision.	Contraindicated in patients taking aclidinium, glucagon and glycopyrrolate.	Used to relieve abdominal pain. Avoid in patients with tachyarrythmias, angle-closure glaucoma, urinary retention, hyperthyroidism. The elderly are more susceptible to adverse effects. Has been used in doses of up to 40 mg QID.	$
	peppermint oil	0.2–0.4 mL in enteric-coated capsules TID po taken between meals	Heartburn, nausea, vomiting, flushing, headache, diarrhea, anal burning. May be hepatotoxic in high doses.	May increase cyclosporine serum levels. Contraindicated in patients taking pimozide.	Used to relieve abdominal pain. Enteric-coated capsules reduce risk of heartburn. Separate administration of antacids, H_2-antagonists and proton pump inhibitors by 2 h.	$
Antidiarrheals	*loperamide* Imodium, generics	2–4 mg up to QID	Abdominal cramps, drowsiness, dry mouth, nausea and vomiting, skin rash.	No significant drug interactions.	Used to relieve diarrhea. Individual dose varies; can cause constipation. Highest dose in IBS trials was 12 mg/day. No significant drug interactions.	$
Bulk-forming Laxatives	*polycarbophil calcium* Prodiem Tablets	1000 mg daily po Gradually titrate to QID as tolerated; drink 240 mL of fluid with each dose	Abdominal pain/ bloating, epigastric fullness, flatulence.	May impair absorption of oral bisphosphonates, fluoroquinolones, tetracylcines and thyroid hormones.	May cause less gas or bloating than psyllium.	$
	psyllium Metamucil Preparations, generics	3.4 g BID po with meals Gradually titrate to 12–20 g/day as tolerated; drink 240 mL of fluid with each dose	Abdominal pain/ bloating, flatulence, cramps. Risk of intestinal impaction/ obstruction if inadequate fluid intake.	No significant drug interactions.	If palatability an issue, try another formulation or mix in beverage to mask taste.	$

(cont'd)

Table 1: **Pharmacologic Therapy for Irritable Bowel Syndrome[a]** *(cont'd)*

Class	Drug	Dosage	Adverse Effects	Drug Interactions	Comments	Cost[b]
Osmotic Laxatives	*lactulose* generics	15–60 mL per day in 1 or 2 divided doses	Flatulence, abdominal cramps, diarrhea. May cause bloating. Nausea more common with higher doses.	No significant drug interactions.	Used to relieve constipation. Palatability may be an issue (very sweet); may mix in beverage. No significant drug interactions.	$
	magnesium hydroxide Milk of Magnesia, generics	15–30 mL daily or BID po	Diarrhea. Risk of hypermagnesemia increased in patients with renal dysfunction.	Contraindicated in patients taking misoprostol, polystyrene sulfonate, quinine. Oral magnesium salts may decrease bioavailability of allopurinol, bisphosphonates, cefuroxime, chloroquine, corticosteroids, dabigatran, fluoroquinolones, fosinopril, iron salts, itraconazole, ketoconazole, levothyroxine, mycophenolate, sotalol and tetracyclines. Magnesium salts may decrease effectiveness of bisacodyl, mesalamine and methenamine.	Used to relieve constipation. Avoid in patients with renal dysfunction. Do not recommend maximum dose for more than 2 weeks unless monitored by an appropriate healthcare practitioner.	$
	polyethylene glycol Lax-A-Day, Pegalax, RestoraLAX	17 g daily po	Nausea, abdominal bloating, cramping, flatulence, diarrhea, urticaria.	No significant drug interactions.	Used to relieve constipation. May require 2–4 days of therapy to produce a bowel movement. Treatment duration should be limited to 1 wk unless monitored by an appropriate healthcare practitioner.	$

[a] For more information on pharmacologic therapy for IBS, consult the *Compendium of Therapeutic Choices*: Irritable Bowel Syndrome.

[b] Cost per day; includes drug cost only.

Dosage adjustment may be required in renal impairment.

Legend: $ <$1

Suggested Readings

Chang L, Lembo A, Sultan S. American Gastroenterological Association Institute Technical Review on the pharmacological management of irritable bowel syndrome. *Gastroenterology* 2014;147:1149-72.e2.

Ford AC, Moayyedi P, Lacy BE et al. American College of Gastroenterology monograph on the management of irritable bowel syndrome and chronic idiopathic constipation. *Am J Gastroenterol* 2014;109:S2-26.

Kosar L, Schuster B, Regier L et al. Irritable bowel syndrome–drugs for symptom management. *RxFiles drug comparison charts*. 10th ed. Saskatoon: Saskatoon Health Region; 2014. p. 66.

References

1. Brandt LJ, Chey WD, Foxx-Orenstein AE et al. An evidence-based position statement on the management of irritable bowel syndrome. *Am J Gastroenterol* 2009;104:S1-35.
2. Ford AC, Moayyedi P, Lacy BE et al. American College of Gastroenterology monograph on the management of irritable bowel syndrome and chronic idiopathic constipation. *Am J Gastroenterol* 2014;109:S2-26.
3. Canadian Digestive Health Foundation. *Digestive disorders*. Available from: www.cdhf.ca/en/statistics#Irritable Bowel Syndrome. Accessed February 16, 2016.
4. Chey WD, Kurlander J, Eswaran S. Irritable bowel syndrome: a clinical review. *JAMA* 2015;313:949-58.
5. Drossman DA. Diagnosing and treating patients with refractory functional gastrointestinal disorders. *Ann Intern Med* 1995;123:688-97.
6. Jones J, Boorman J, Cann P et al. British Society of Gastroenterology guidelines for the management of the irritable bowel syndrome. *Gut* 2000;47:ii1-19.
7. Horwitz BJ, Fisher RS. The irritable bowel syndrome. *N Engl J Med* 2001;344:1846-50.
8. Clouse RE. Antidepressants for functional gastrointestinal syndromes. *Dig Dis Sci* 1994;39:2352-63.
9. Wong BS, Camilleri M, Carlson P et al. Increased bile acid biosynthesis is associated with irritable bowel syndrome with diarrhea. *Clin Gastroenterol Hepatol* 2012;10:1009-15.e3.
10. Camilleri M. Management of the irritable bowel syndrome. *Gastroenterology* 2001;120:652-68.
11. Wilkins T, Pepitone C, Alex B et al. Diagnosis and management of IBS in adults. *Am Fam Physician* 2012;86:419-26.
12. Johannesson E, Simrén M, Strid H et al. Physical activity improves symptoms in irritable bowel syndrome: a randomized controlled trial. *Am J Gastroenterol* 2011;106:915-22.
13. Fjorback LO, Arendt M, Ornbøl E et al. Mindfulness therapy for somatization disorder and functional somatic syndromes: randomized trial with one-year follow-up. *J Psychosom Res* 2013;74:31-40.
14. Labus J, Gupta A, Gill HK et al. Randomised clinical trial: symptoms of the irritable bowel syndrome are improved by a psycho-education group intervention. *Aliment Pharmacol Ther* 2013;37:304-15.
15. Patel SM, Stason WB, Legedza A et al. The placebo effect in irritable bowel syndrome trials: a meta-analysis. *Neurogastroenterol Motil* 2005;17:332-40.
16. Ford AC, Talley NJ, Spiegel BM et al. Effect of fibre, antispasmodics and peppermint oil in the treatment of irritable bowel syndrome: a systematic review and meta-analysis. *BMJ* 2008;337:a2313.
17. Drugs for irritable bowel syndrome. *Treat Guidel Med Lett* 2006;4:11-6.
18. Efskind PS, Bernklev T, Vatn MH. A double-blind placebo-controlled trial with loperamide in irritable bowel syndrome. *Scand J Gastroenterol* 1996;31:463-8.
19. Chouinard LE. The role of psyllium fibre supplementation in treating irritable bowel syndrome. *Can J Diet Pract Res* 2011;72:e107-14.
20. Weinberg DS, Smalley W, Heidelbaugh JJ et al. American Gastroenterological Association Institute Guideline on the pharmacological management of irritable bowel syndrome. *Gastroenterology* 2014;147:1146-8.
21. National Institute for Health and Care Excellence (NICE). *Irritable bowel syndrome in adults: diagnosis and management*. NICE guidelines [CG61]; Modified February 2015. Available from: /www.nice.org.uk/guidance/cg61. Accessed February 16, 2016.
22. Ruepert L, Quartero AO, de Wit NJ et al. Bulking agents, antispasmodics and antidepressants for the treatment of irritable bowel syndrome. *Cochrane Database Syst Rev* 2011;(8):CD003460.
23. Gorard DA, Libby GW, Farthing MJ. Influence of antidepressants on whole gut and orocaecal transit times in health and irritable bowel syndrome. *Aliment Pharmacol Ther* 1994;8:159-66.
24. Vahedi H, Merat S, Rashidioon A et al. The effect of fluoxetine in patients with pain and constipation-predominant irritable bowel syndrome: a double-blind randomized-controlled study. *Aliment Pharmacol Ther* 2005;22:381-5.
25. Saito YA, Rey E, Almazar-Elder AE et al. A randomized, double-blind, placebo-controlled trial of St John's wort for treating irritable bowel syndrome. *Am J Gastroenterol* 2010;105:170-7.
26. Williams EA, Stimpson J, Wang D et al. Clinical trial: a multistrain probiotic preparation significantly reduces symptoms of irritable bowel syndrome in a double-blind placebo-controlled study. *Aliment Pharmacol Ther* 2009;29:97-103.
27. Brenner DM, Moeller MJ, Chey WD et al. The utility of probiotics in the treatment of irritable bowel syndrome: a systematic review. *Am J Gastroenterol* 2009;104:1033-49.
28. Ritchie ML, Romanuk TN. A meta-analysis of probiotic efficacy for gastrointestinal diseases. *PLoS One* 2012;7:e34938.
29. Kruis W, Chrubasik S, Boehm S et al. A double-blind placebo-controlled trial to study therapeutic effects of probiotic Escherichia coli Nissle 1917 in subgroups of patients with irritable bowel syndrome. *Int J Colorectal Dis* 2012;27:467-74.
30. Whelan K. Probiotics and prebiotics in the management of irritable bowel syndrome: a review of recent clinical trials and systematic reviews. *Curr Opin Clin Nutr Metab Care* 2011;14:581-7.
31. Manheimer E, Cheng K, Wieland LS et al. Acupuncture for treatment of irritable bowel syndrome. *Cochrane Database Syst Rev* 2012;5:CD005111.

Irritable Bowel Syndrome—What You Need to Know

What is irritable bowel syndrome (IBS)?

Irritable bowel syndrome (IBS) is a chronic disorder with symptoms such as diarrhea and/or constipation, stomach pain, bloating and cramps. It tends to come back but it is not predictable. The triggers vary for different people. IBS does not mean that you have a higher risk for serious gastrointestinal diseases such as stomach cancer.

What can you do to manage IBS?

It is unlikely that any therapy will completely get rid of IBS symptoms. However, you can learn to manage it.

- Keep track of your bowel movements if they are irregular. Try to identify things that may be triggers for you (such as certain foods).
- Avoid caffeine and sugarless gum or candies.
- Avoid eating too much fruit.
- Stress can make IBS worse. Try to reduce stress through relaxation, hobbies or vacation time.
- You may be able to reduce symptoms of IBS by changing your lifestyle. Talk to your doctor or other healthcare provider.

When should you see a healthcare provider?

See your healthcare provider if any of these things happen:

- Your bowel movements (stools) contain blood.
- Your bowel movements change colour significantly (for example, pale whitish or black, tar-like stools).
- You are losing weight without trying to.
- You have lost more than 3 kg (about 6 or 7 pounds) over 6 months.
- Your symptoms are very severe.
- Your symptoms last for more than 3 days in a row.

Chapter 36
Nausea and Vomiting

Christine Hughes, BScPharm, PharmD

Pathophysiology

Nausea is the unpleasant sensation of the imminent need to vomit and may or may not lead to vomiting. Vomiting is the forceful expulsion of gastric contents with contraction of the abdominal and chest wall musculature.[1] Retching or "dry heaves" is the same physiologic process as vomiting but without expulsion of gastric contents.

Nausea and vomiting can be associated with disorders of the gastrointestinal, endocrine or central nervous systems or may be due to infections, medications, toxins or aberrant metabolic processes.[1] Some causes of nausea and vomiting are listed in Table 1.[2] This chapter addresses the most commonly encountered causes of nausea and vomiting. Syndromes that have a high incidence of nausea and vomiting, such as migraine headaches, are addressed in other chapters (see Chapter 8: Headache).

The pathophysiology of nausea and vomiting is complicated by the involvement of numerous neurotransmitters and nerve systems arising from different organs and activated by a variety of stimuli (Figure 1).[3,4] Because of this, it is often difficult to determine which stimulus is most responsible for a patient's symptoms and to design a therapeutic plan.

Complications of prolonged or severe nausea and vomiting include esophageal rupture, Mallory-Weiss tears, dehydration, hypokalemia, hypomagnesemia, hypo- or hypernatremia, metabolic alkalosis, malnutrition and dental caries.

Table 1: **Selected Causes of Nausea and Vomiting**

CNS	**Gastrointestinal**
Head trauma	Appendicitis
Increased intracranial pressure	Cholecystitis/cholangitis
Migraine[a]	Gastric outlet obstruction
Vestibular disorders (including motion sickness)[a]	Gastroparesis
Endocrine/Metabolic	Hepatitis (acute)
Diabetic ketoacidosis	Intestinal obstruction
Pregnancy[a]	Nonulcer dyspepsia[a]
Renal disease (uremia)	Pancreatitis
Infectious	Peptic ulcer disease
Acute otitis media	**Miscellaneous**
Gastroenteritis[a]	Postoperative nausea and vomiting[a]
Pyelonephritis	Noxious odours[a]
	Medication/toxin-induced[a]

[a] Common causes of nausea and vomiting.

Figure 1: **Pathways Involved in Nausea and Vomiting**

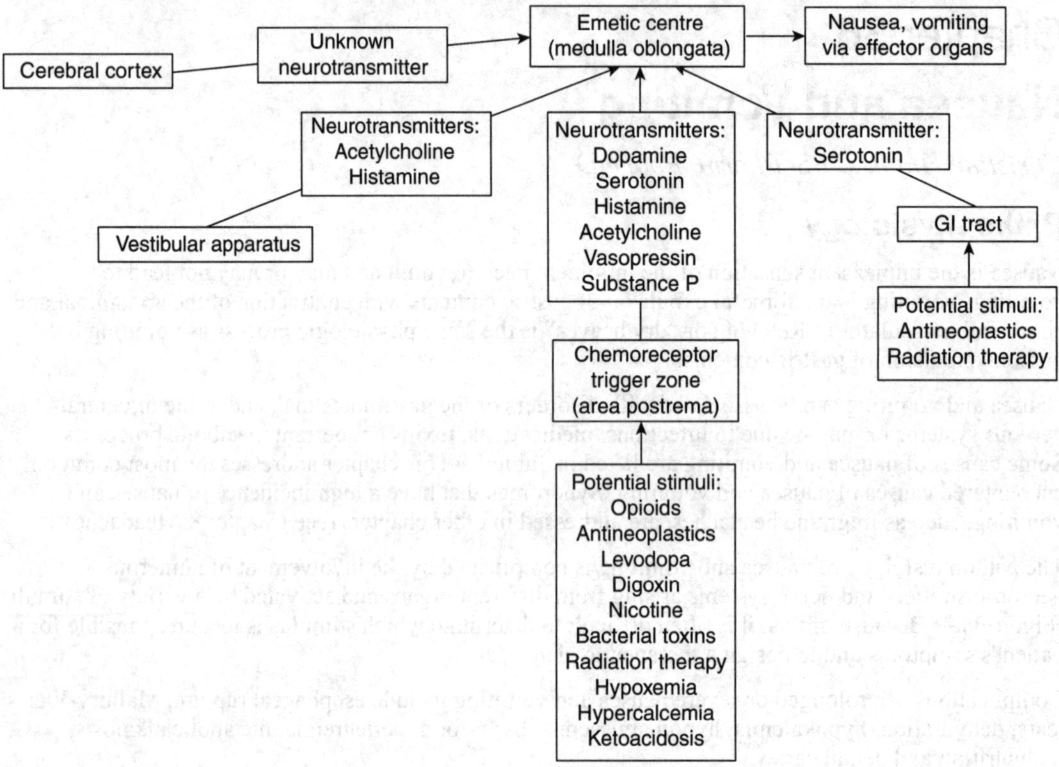

Motion Sickness

Motion sickness refers to the normal physiologic response to unusual perception of motion.[5] It can be precipitated by abrupt changes in movement, such as during bumpy rides, turbulent flights and rough seas, and is also referred to as airsickness, seasickness or carsickness. The development of motion sickness depends on a number of factors including the characteristics of the stimulus (frequency, intensity, direction and duration) as well as individual susceptibilities including age and gender.[5,6,7] Women are more prone to developing motion sickness than men. Susceptibility to motion sickness is highest between the ages of 3 and 12 years, and gradually decreases thereafter. Children under the age of 2 years are typically immune to motion sickness. Motion sickness begins with a feeling of "stomach awareness," followed by nausea, increasing malaise, pallor and sweating. As symptoms worsen, patients may also experience increased salivation, a feeling of body warmth, dizziness and vomiting or retching.[5,6,7] The severity of symptoms varies with the intensity of the stimulus and the susceptibility of the individual.

Theories of the cause of motion sickness centre around a mismatch between the motion one expects to occur (either through visual cues or previous experiences) and the actual motion sensed by the vestibular apparatus in the ear.[5,7] The vertical component of the motion is believed to be most important in causing motion sickness, and the movement must be repetitive, relatively slow, and prolonged.[5] This may explain why ship travel, characterized by low-frequency continuous heaving, is such a potent cause of motion sickness while travelling in a speedboat is not.

Neurotransmitters thought to be most responsible for motion sickness include histamine and acetylcholine. Drugs used for treatment are aimed at modulating receptors for these chemicals.

Postchemotherapy Nausea and Vomiting (PCNV)

Nausea and vomiting associated with chemotherapy are divided into 3 types: acute, delayed and anticipatory. Whether acute or delayed nausea and vomiting is experienced depends most strongly on the actual chemotherapy drug(s) administered and their dosage and infusion rate.[4,8,9,10]

Acute PCNV:

- Starts within a few hours after chemotherapy administration and usually does not persist beyond 24 hours
- Occurs in >90% of patients receiving highly emetogenic chemotherapy regimens (e.g., cisplatin, cyclophosphamide)[9,10]
- Patient-related risk factors include younger age, female sex, past history of low alcohol intake, poor control of symptoms in prior cycles and history of motion sickness or nausea in pregnancy[9,10]
- The neurotransmitter most responsible is serotonin (5-HT_3 receptors) while type 2 dopamine and neurokinin-1 receptors also play a role[9,10]
- Chemotherapy and radiation therapy cause enterochromaffin cells lining the GI tract to release serotonin in large amounts, activating 5-HT_3 receptors in the GI tract, which stimulate the vomiting centre in the medulla oblongata (Figure 1).[9,10]

Delayed PCNV:

- Begins at least 24 hours after administration of chemotherapy and may last up to 6 or 7 days[9]
- Cisplatin and cyclophosphamide are the most commonly used drugs that cause acute as well as delayed nausea and vomiting, often with a nausea and vomiting–free period in between. With cisplatin, the incidence of delayed nausea and/or vomiting may be as high as 80%[4,9,10]
- Serotonin is less important in delayed nausea and vomiting, while substance P-dependent mechanisms appear to play a significant role.[11]

Anticipatory vomiting:

- Is a conditioned or learned response to previously poorly managed nausea and vomiting in chemotherapy patients
- Occurs in approximately 25% of patients by the fourth course of chemotherapy[12]
- Occurs before, during or immediately after chemotherapy administration but before acute nausea and vomiting would be expected to occur.

Nausea and Vomiting of Pregnancy (NVP)

Also known as "morning sickness," nausea and vomiting of pregnancy occurs in 70–80% of pregnancies.[13] These symptoms are normal in pregnancy. While the underlying pathophysiology is not well understood, a combination of processes is likely involved including genetic, endocrine, environmental, gastrointestinal and psychosocial factors.[13,14] Other theories suggest evolutionary adaptation where NVP serves to protect mother and fetus from ingestion of foods that might potentially be dangerous.[15] Meat, fish, poultry and eggs (all of which carry the risk of infectious diseases) produce the most aversion in North America. Morning sickness is less common in societies that do not eat such foods.[15] Experiencing NVP is associated with better pregnancy outcomes, including a lower risk of miscarriages and preterm deliveries.[13,16,17]

Virtually all women who develop NVP have some symptoms by 9 weeks' gestation, and more than half have symptoms by 6 weeks.[18] For the vast majority of women, the symptoms subside by 16 weeks; however, approximately 10% of women have NVP that persists beyond 20 weeks' gestation. Nausea and vomiting may occur at any time of day and be constant throughout the day.

Hyperemesis gravidarum is a serious condition occurring in up to 2% of pregnant women.[18] It is characterized by intractable vomiting, beginning in the first trimester and possibly continuing throughout the pregnancy. Vomiting may lead to dehydration, electrolyte disturbances, nutritional deficiency and weight loss. This condition can threaten the survival of the fetus and the mother, and requires early identification and treatment. Such symptoms must also prompt investigation for specific diseases such as urinary tract infections, diabetic ketoacidosis, thyrotoxicosis and hepatitis.[18] Hyperemesis gravidarum is typically diagnosed when other possible causes of nausea and vomiting have been ruled out.

Postoperative Nausea and Vomiting (PONV)

Postoperative nausea and vomiting, defined as nausea and/or vomiting occurring within 24 hours following surgery, occurs in up to 70–80% of patients at high risk (e.g., female sex, nonsmoker, history of PONV or motion sickness, use of nitrous oxide, use of intraoperative and postoperative opioids, high doses of neostigmine, longer duration of surgery).[19,20] Nausea and/or vomiting may be present in the recovery room immediately following surgery or may begin several hours later. The cause of PONV is thought to be multifactorial, with individual, surgical and anesthetic risk factors. Four primary risk factors are well recognized: female sex, nonsmokers, history of PONV/motion sickness and opioid use.[19] In one study, the incidence of PONV in the presence of none, 1, 2, 3 and all 4 risk factors was 10%, 20%, 40%, 60% and 80%, respectively.[21] Longer duration of surgery and the type of surgery also influence the incidence of PONV. Intra-abdominal surgery, ophthalmic surgery (particularly strabismus), gynecologic surgery and ear-nose-throat surgery are associated with higher rates of PONV.[1,19] Furthermore, even if the absolute risk of PONV is low with a particular surgery, aggressive prevention of nausea and vomiting might be preferred if the effects of PONV have a high likelihood of causing undesirable surgical complications as seen in some cosmetic procedures with tight suture lines. In terms of anesthesia, nitrous oxide has been associated with an increased risk of PONV, and volatile anesthetics are strongly associated with nausea and vomiting in the early postoperative period (within 0–2 hours). Besides the obvious unpleasantness for the patient, PONV can sometimes result in overnight hospital stays when day surgery was planned, interfere with pain management efforts, lead to wound dehiscence if vomiting or retching occurs following abdominal procedures, or result in fluid and electrolyte imbalances.

Almost all of the known mechanisms for nausea and vomiting (dopaminergic, serotonergic, cholinergic, histaminergic, cortical) may be active to varying degrees in patients who experience PONV.[1,19,22]

Medication-induced Nausea and Vomiting

Almost all medications are capable of producing nausea and, to a lesser degree, vomiting. Some of the most commonly used and/or emetogenic nonchemotherapy drugs are listed in Table 2.

The mechanisms by which some drugs cause nausea and vomiting are unknown but likely involve extensions of their pharmacologic action. Drugs that cause vomiting by acting on the area postrema include dopaminergic agonists (e.g., levodopa), nicotine, digoxin and opioid analgesics. Agents such as NSAIDs and erythromycin activate peripheral afferent pathways, most likely vagal, which then stimulate the brainstem nuclei to coordinate the act of vomiting. This chapter specifically addresses opioid analgesics.

Opioid-induced nausea and vomiting:[1,23,24]

- Approximately 25–30% of patients started on opioids experience nausea

- Nausea and vomiting are most common during the first few days of therapy and tolerance develops rapidly thereafter
- There is little evidence of differences between opioids in their propensity to cause nausea and vomiting. Rather, the increase in the dose of opioid raises the risk of nausea and vomiting
- Opioids may cause nausea and vomiting by stimulating afferent input into the vomiting centre, via the vestibular apparatus, the cerebral cortex or the chemoreceptor trigger zone.

Table 2: **Commonly Used Drugs that Frequently Cause Nausea and/or Vomiting**

Antibiotics:	**Antidiabetics:**
Antituberculous agents	Metformin
Erythromycin	Sulfonylureas
Sulfonamides	**Cardiovascular:**
Tetracycline	Amiodarone
Anticonvulsants:	Beta-blockers
Carbamazepine	Calcium channel blockers
Phenobarbital	Digoxin
Phenytoin	Procainamide
Valproic acid	**Others:**
Anti-inflammatories:	Acyclovir
ASA	Levodopa
Auranofin	Nicotine
Colchicine	Opioids
NSAIDs	Oral contraceptives
	Theophylline

Goals of Therapy

- Eliminate nausea and vomiting
- If not possible, then reduce severity, frequency and duration as much as possible
- Prevent complications of nausea and vomiting
- Prevent recurrence of nausea and vomiting
- Decrease time off work and lifestyle disruptions caused by nausea and vomiting
- Reduce or prevent side effects of medications used to treat nausea and vomiting

Patient Assessment

Figure 4 presents an approach to patient assessment for nausea and vomiting.[25] Table 3 presents symptoms of dehydration.[26,27] Figure 2 depicts decreased skin turgor.

Nonpharmacologic Therapy

General nonpharmacologic measures for managing nausea and vomiting include eating small meals, avoiding spicy foods and noxious odours and reducing physical activity. If pain and nausea coexist, successful treatment of the pain often reduces the nausea.

Maintaining fluid intake helps prevent dehydration and electrolyte disturbances. The amount of fluid required depends on the amount lost through vomiting and/or diarrhea. Normally, 2.5 L of fluid intake is required to maintain water balance.[26] In patients who are vomiting several times daily, 3–5 L of water per day may be needed. For mild dehydration, drinking adequate amounts of water may be all that is required. To treat moderate to severe dehydration, it is necessary to replace electrolytes (especially sodium and potassium). Oral rehydration solutions with appropriate amounts of electrolytes are recommended under these circumstances.[27]

Table 3: **Symptoms of Dehydration in Children and Adults**

Children	Adults
Dry mouth, tongue and skin	Increased thirst
Few or no tears when crying	Decreased urination
Decreased urination (less than 4 wet diapers in 24 h)	Feeling weak or light-headed
Sunken eyes	Dry mouth/tongue
Greyish skin	
Sunken soft spot (fontanel) in infants	
Decreased skin turgor (Figure 2)	

Figure 2: **Decreased Skin Turgor**

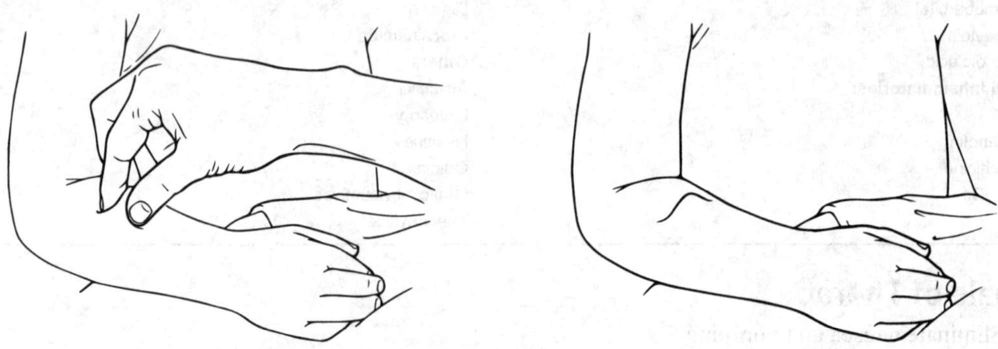

When pinched and released, the skin flattens slowly.

Motion Sickness

To prevent motion sickness, counsel patients to:

- Avoid eating a large meal within 3 hours of travel
- Avoid dairy products and foods high in protein, calories or sodium before travel
- Avoid alcohol, smoking and disagreeable odours
- Avoid visual stimuli that commonly precipitate motion sickness, such as reading and watching videos during travel
- While travelling, focus on a stable external object or the horizon
- While on a boat, stay in a central location least susceptible to motion
- While in a vehicle, sit in a front seat with a clear forward view, and, if possible, drive the vehicle rather than be a passenger
- Increase ventilation and exposure to cool fresh air
- Minimize head movement by pressing head into headrest.

Acupressure wristbands (Sea-Bands) have not been shown to be beneficial for preventing motion sickness.[28,29] In a controlled study of experimental motion sickness, neither acupressure nor acustimulation were of benefit.[30]

Postchemotherapy Nausea and Vomiting (PCNV)

Although potent antiemetic medications are usually required in patients receiving highly emetogenic chemotherapy, hypnosis reduces anticipatory nausea and reduces the amount of antiemetic medication required in both children and adults.[31,32]

Other behavioural manoeuvres aimed at producing relaxation, diverting attention and enhancing feelings of control may be effective, particularly for anticipatory nausea and vomiting.

Nausea and Vomiting of Pregnancy (NVP)

Although not well studied, the following measures may be recommended to reduce NVP:

- Eat small, bland, frequent meals and avoid fatty, fried or spicy foods[13,14]
- Eat at times of the day when nausea is less severe[18,33]
- Eat before getting out of bed in the morning to help early morning nausea
- Try cold food if the smell of hot food is bothersome
- Avoid cooking if possible
- Drink small amounts of fluid regularly between meals.

Prenatal vitamins may worsen nausea, primarily due to the iron content as well as large size of tablets. In the first trimester, women can take folic acid alone or a multivitamin that does not contain iron.[34]

In patients with frequent vomiting, maintenance of fluid and electrolyte status orally or intravenously is essential.

Acupuncture and P6 acupressure have been the subject of numerous trials for NVP. P6 is also known as Nei Guan ("inner guard") and is the sixth point along the pericardial meridian. P6 is anatomically located about 5 cm proximal to the distal crease of the wrist, between the tendons of palmaris longus and flexor carpi radialis of either forearm (Figure 3). The point can be stimulated with the tip of a finger, with or without moderate-pressure massaging. There is no consensus regarding how long or how often to apply the pressure, but some practitioners recommend 5 minutes of pressure every 4 hours.[33] Patients may be taught to do this themselves. Wearing Sea-Bands continuously is an alternative, but some studies (in motion sickness) have shown less efficacy than manual pressure because the Sea-Bands tend to slip out of position. Some patients find them too conspicuous. Studies evaluating the effectiveness of acupuncture or acupressure at P6 have shown equivocal results.[35,36,37] While acupressure has not been clearly shown to be better than dietary or lifestyle advice or "dummy" acupressure, the manual application of acupressure is harmless and without cost.

Reassure patients that most mild to moderate forms of nausea and vomiting are normal, not harmful to the fetus and usually subside as the pregnancy progresses.

Postoperative Nausea and Vomiting (PONV)

General measures that may be useful in preventing PONV include avoiding significant intake of food for 48 hours postoperatively, slow and gradual increase in physical activity postoperatively, avoiding noxious odours and stimuli and maintaining adequate hydration. Smooth transportation of the patient from the postanesthetic recovery room to the ward is also important. Comfort measures such as cool cloths and sucking on ice chips may be beneficial.

Low quality evidence suggests that P6 acupressure may be as effective as antiemetics in preventing and treating PONV.[38,39,40,41]

Figure 3: **P6 Acupressure Point**

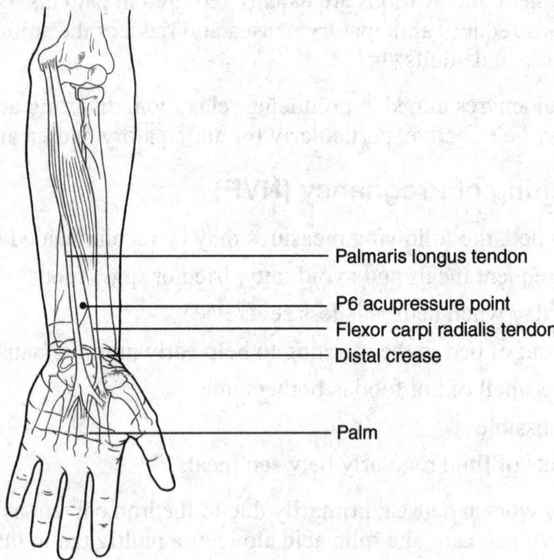

Pharmacologic Therapy

For comparative ingredients of nonprescription products, consult the *Compendium of Products for Minor Ailments*—Gastrointestinal Products: Antiemetics; Vitamin and Mineral Products: Single Entity.

Selected agents used in the management of nausea and vomiting are described in Table 5.[42,43,44] For further discussion of pharmacologic therapy for nausea and vomiting, consult the *Compendium of Therapeutic Choices*: Nausea in Adults.

For treatment of nausea and vomiting associated with viral gastroenteritis there is no evidence that one antiemetic is superior to another. The initial choice should be made on the basis of previous response, available routes of administration, cost, adverse effects and patient preference. These criteria often result in **dimenhydrinate** being tried first.

If symptoms are worsened by movement, it may be surmised that acetylcholine is a significant contributor and anticholinergic agents such as dimenhydrinate may be tried first. If symptoms are associated with a feeling of fullness in the stomach, a prokinetic agent such as **metoclopramide** or **domperidone** may be a logical starting point. Caution is warranted with these agents since domperidone is associated with a small increased risk of serious ventricular arrhythmias or sudden cardiac death and metoclopramide is associated with extrapyramidal symptoms (even in children) and tardive dyskinesia (involuntary movements of the tongue, face, mouth or jaw). If patients fail to respond to these initial measures, selection of other antiemetics is based on adverse effects, available routes of administration, patient preference and cost. Consider trying agents with different mechanisms of action if combinations of antiemetics are to be used.

Motion Sickness

Since acetylcholine and histamine are thought to be the most important neurotransmitters causing motion sickness, it follows that anticholinergic and antihistaminergic drugs are fairly effective in controlling it. Prevention is more effective than treatment in established nausea and vomiting.

- For short duration of exposure, **dimenhydrinate** is effective for most patients. **Diphenhydramine** is an alternative. Because motion sickness induces gut stasis, it is important to take oral medications at least 60 minutes in advance[6,7]
- **Scopolamine** transdermal patch applied at least 4 hours before exposure is effective and superior to placebo, and has the advantage of a longer duration of action[45]
- **Promethazine** has a longer duration of action as compared to dimenhydrinate and may be an alternative in patients with refractory nausea or when dimenhydrinate is ineffective
- If alertness is required, transdermal scopolamine or oral promethazine have been combined with dextroamphetamine or ephedrine.[45,46] These combinations have been used in extreme situations (e.g., by airline pilots) after the patient has become thoroughly accustomed to their CNS effects, as these may be unpredictable[47]
- The most appropriate agent for children older than 2 years is dimenhydrinate given 1 hour before exposure, then every 6 hours as needed. Diphenhydramine may also be used as an alternative and may help children sleep better while travelling. Some children experience paradoxical excitability with these agents, so a test dose should be administered well before travelling
- Controlled clinical trials have not consistently demonstrated the benefit of **ginger root** for motion sickness,[48,49,50] although it is widely promoted for its antinausea effects.

Since dimenhydrinate is recommended by Canada's Motherisk program for augmenting **doxylamine/pyridoxine** (Diclectin) therapy in pregnancy[34] and it is considered generally safe in pregnancy, it can be considered for intermittent therapy of motion sickness in pregnant patients. Promethazine may also be used.[34]

Postchemotherapy Nausea and Vomiting (PCNV)

Effective agents are available for the treatment and prevention of PCNV (e.g., 5-HT_3 receptor antagonists, neurokinin-1 antagonists, dexamethasone). For further discussion of pharmacologic therapy for postchemotherapy nausea and vomiting, consult the *Compendium of Therapeutic Choices*: Chemotherapy-induced Nausea and Vomiting.

Nausea and Vomiting of Pregnancy (NVP)

When nonpharmacologic methods fail to control nausea and vomiting, medication can play a role in relieving symptoms and preventing weight loss, dehydration and hospitalization. In patients with hyperemesis gravidarum, the combination of intravenous fluids and antiemetic drugs is often necessary. For further discussion of pharmacologic therapy for nausea and vomiting of pregnancy, consult the *Compendium of Therapeutic Choices*: Nausea in Adults.

Treatment of nausea and vomiting of pregnancy:

- Diclectin, containing 10 mg each of **pyridoxine** (vitamin B_6) and **doxylamine**, is the drug of choice for NVP in Canada[34,35,51]
- Pyridoxine alone may safely reduce NVP and may be used in place of Diclectin in women who prefer a "natural" remedy or in whom doxylamine is not tolerated[14,35]
- **Dimenhydrinate** is both safe and effective for NVP. Typically, this agent is second-line therapy after Diclectin has been tried. Other agents that appear to be safe in pregnancy and can be used in women who do not respond to Diclectin or dimenhydrinate include **chlorpromazine**, **prochlorperazine**, **promethazine**, **metoclopramide** and **ondansetron**[14,34,35]
- Evidence suggests that **ginger** is effective in reducing NVP in divided doses of 500–1500 mg/day.[35,52,53] In a systematic review of randomized controlled trials, 4 of the 6 trials showed ginger was superior to placebo, and in the other 2 trials it was as effective as vitamin B_6.[52] Safety concerns have been raised regarding the presence of natural cytotoxic chemicals in ginger.

However, based on available data there appear to be no significant adverse effects on pregnancy outcomes if the daily dose is limited to 1 g.

Postoperative Nausea and Vomiting (PONV)

Treatment of postoperative nausea and vomiting:

- The most effective strategy to manage PONV is to reduce risk factors when appropriate.[19,22,23] Whenever possible, regional anesthesia should be used in place of general anesthesia, intravenous propofol should be used in place of nitrous oxide and volatile inhaled anesthetics, and nonopioid analgesics (e.g., NSAIDs) should be used in place of opioids. Prophylaxis of PONV should be reserved for patients who are at moderate to high risk (≥2 risk factors or a history of PONV)
- Appropriate preventive therapies include 5-HT_3 receptor antagonists, dexamethasone, droperidol and, to a lesser extent, prochlorperazine. In a meta-analysis of 18 trials, **dimenhydrinate** was found to be an effective antiemetic for prophylaxis of PONV when compared with placebo.[54] Transdermal **scopolamine** also may be effective,[55] but should be applied the evening before surgery or 4 hours before the end of anesthetic action. Limitations of transdermal scopolamine include its slow onset of action and adverse effect profile. Because numerous neurotransmitters are involved in the pathogenesis of PONV, combination therapy is more effective than monotherapy.[19] Drugs with different mechanisms of action may be used when necessary. Combination therapy with 5-HT_3 receptor antagonists and droperidol or dexamethasone is equally efficacious[56,57]
- Treatment of established PONV has not been thoroughly studied, but available evidence and experience support the use of the following agents as needed postoperatively: **5-HT_3 receptor antagonists**, **promethazine**, **prochlorperazine**, **droperidol** and **dexamethasone**. When prophylaxis with one drug has failed, a repeat dose of this drug should not be initiated as rescue therapy and a drug from a different class of antiemetics should be used[19,58]
- Although data are limited, treatments such as **peppermint oil** or **isopropyl alcohol** aromatherapy have reduced PONV.[59,60]

Opioid-induced Nausea and Vomiting

Therapeutic options for opioid-induced nausea and vomiting include:

- Alter the administration schedule so that nausea does not interfere with meals
- Reduce the dose of the opioid as low as possible or avoid large increases in the opioid dose since this may lead to comparatively large increases in the opioid's serum concentrations, which may in turn induce or worsen nausea and vomiting
- If pain is not controlled, attempt an increase in dosage since nausea is sometimes caused by pain
- Consider switching to another opioid at 75% of the equivalent daily dose. No solid evidence for differences between opioids exists in terms of emetogenicity, but patient responses are highly variable[24]
- Addition of an antiemetic drug is often helpful, although the possibility of additive CNS side effects must be carefully weighed. Appropriate antiemetic agents include metoclopramide, diphenhydramine, dimenhydrinate, prochlorperazine, promethazine, haloperidol and the 5-HT_3 receptor antagonists[23,24]
- When managing refractory opioid-induced nausea and vomiting, instead of replacing one antiemetic agent with another, adding additional therapies with different mechanisms of action may result in a synergistic effect
- Tolerance to nausea and vomiting frequently develops in patients receiving opioids for chronic pain. However, changes to the opioid drug therapy regimen should be made as part of a team approach, closely involving the patient's other healthcare practitioners.

Monitoring of Therapy

Efficacy

For all of the conditions discussed in this chapter, monitoring therapy involves paying close attention to the patient's description of the nausea response, changes in frequency of vomiting and vigilant monitoring for emergence of serious complications such as weight loss, dehydration, changes in mental status (which may signal electrolyte disturbances) and blood loss from any source. Assess adherence to nonpharmacologic measures when response to therapy is suboptimal (see Table 4).

Safety

Table 5 shows the most common adverse effects encountered with the antiemetic agents discussed. If a patient experiences an intolerable adverse effect, consider dosage reduction, switching to another agent or relying on nondrug measures alone. Reassess patient if PONV persists beyond 48 hours postoperatively. The most common cause of nausea and vomiting >48 hours postoperatively is opioid analgesics.

Table 4: **Monitoring of Therapy for Nausea and Vomiting**

Symptoms	Monitoring	Endpoint of Therapy	Actions
Pregnancy-associated nausea	Patient: Continuously Healthcare practitioner: Day 3	Minimal/no nausea.	Diclectin might be helpful if dimenhydrinate or pyridoxine do not provide adequate relief after 3 days of therapy.
Pregnancy-associated vomiting	Patient: Continuously Healthcare practitioner: Day 3	Vomiting does not interfere with daily activities and does not result in other morbidity (dehydration, weight loss, electrolyte disturbances).	Diclectin might be helpful if dimenhydrinate or pyridoxine do not provide adequate relief after 3 days of therapy.
Motion sickness	Patient: Whenever exposed to stimulus Healthcare practitioner: After next visit	Minimal/no nausea. No vomiting.	Depending on the drug being used, increase dosage or switch to another agent; ensure dose given approximately 60 min before stimulus.
Postoperative nausea and vomiting	Patient: Continuously for 72 h after surgery Healthcare practitioner: For 72 h after surgery	Minimal or no nausea, no vomiting during 48 h postoperative period.	If dimenhydrinate ineffective, other agents may be tried.
Opioid-induced nausea and vomiting	Patient: Continuously Healthcare practitioner: Daily or as often as is practical	Minimal or no nausea. No vomiting.	If dimenhydrinate ineffective, alternative agents may be tried and/or opioid dosage may be adjusted.
Symptoms of dehydration (Table 3)	Patient: Continuously Healthcare practitioner: Daily or as often as is practical	No symptoms of dehydration.	If symptoms of dehydration occur, further evaluation would be required immediately.

Advice for the Patient

Advise all patients with nausea and vomiting regarding:

- When medical attention should be sought (warning signs include symptoms of dehydration such as dizziness and sunken eyes, severe abdominal pain, blood in vomitus, repeated vomiting and inability to keep liquids down for >8 hours)
- Nonpharmacologic measures to improve nausea and vomiting, tailored to the specific cause in their case
- Possible adverse effects of drug therapy, especially sedation, which may preclude performing activities requiring mental alertness such as driving or operating dangerous machinery
- The risk of combining antiemetic medications with alcohol
- The importance of handwashing after handling the scopolamine patch, as severe eye irritation or mydriasis can occur if the eyes are touched.

Figure 4: **Assessment of Patients with Nausea and Vomiting**

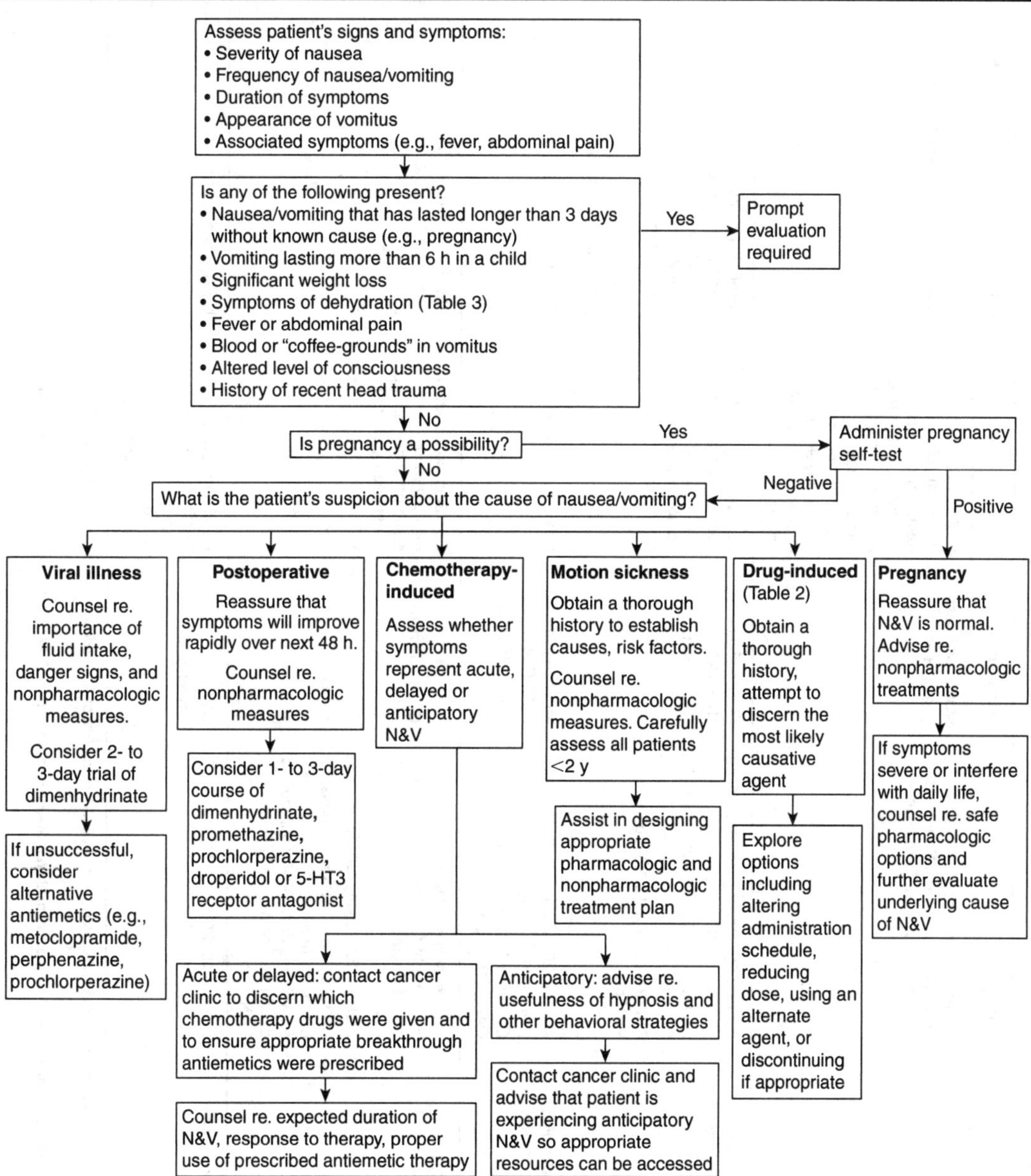
Assess patient's signs and symptoms:
• Severity of nausea
• Frequency of nausea/vomiting
• Duration of symptoms
• Appearance of vomitus
• Associated symptoms (e.g., fever, abdominal pain)
Is any of the following present?
• Nausea/vomiting that has lasted longer than 3 days without known cause (e.g., pregnancy)
• Vomiting lasting more than 6 h in a child
• Significant weight loss
• Symptoms of dehydration (Table 3)
• Fever or abdominal pain
• Blood or "coffee-grounds" in vomitus
• Altered level of consciousness
• History of recent head trauma
Yes
Prompt evaluation required
No
Is pregnancy a possibility?
Yes
Administer pregnancy self-test
No
Negative
What is the patient's suspicion about the cause of nausea/vomiting?
Positive
Viral illness
Counsel re. importance of fluid intake, danger signs, and nonpharmacologic measures.
Consider 2- to 3-day trial of dimenhydrinate
If unsuccessful, consider alternative antiemetics (e.g., metoclopramide, perphenazine, prochlorperazine)
Postoperative
Reassure that symptoms will improve rapidly over next 48 h.
Counsel re. nonpharmacologic measures
Consider 1- to 3-day course of dimenhydrinate, promethazine, prochlorperazine, droperidol or 5-HT3 receptor antagonist
Chemotherapy-induced
Assess whether symptoms represent acute, delayed or anticipatory N&V
Acute or delayed: contact cancer clinic to discern which chemotherapy drugs were given and to ensure appropriate breakthrough antiemetics were prescribed
Counsel re. expected duration of N&V, response to therapy, proper use of prescribed antiemetic therapy
Anticipatory: advise re. usefulness of hypnosis and other behavioral strategies
Contact cancer clinic and advise that patient is experiencing anticipatory N&V so appropriate resources can be accessed
Motion sickness
Obtain a thorough history to establish causes, risk factors.
Counsel re. nonpharmacologic measures. Carefully assess all patients <2 y
Assist in designing appropriate pharmacologic and nonpharmacologic treatment plan
Drug-induced (Table 2)
Obtain a thorough history, attempt to discern the most likely causative agent
Explore options including altering administration schedule, reducing dose, using an alternate agent, or discontinuing if appropriate
Pregnancy
Reassure that N&V is normal. Advise re. nonpharmacologic treatments
If symptoms severe or interfere with daily life, counsel re. safe pharmacologic options and further evaluate underlying cause of N&V

Abbreviations: N&V = nausea and vomiting

Table 5: **Nonprescription Pharmacologic Therapies for Nausea and Vomiting**[a]

Class	Drug	Dosage	Uses/Onset	Adverse Effects	Drug Interactions	Cost[b]
Anticholinergics	*scopolamine* Transderm-V	**Adults:** 1 patch applied to skin every 72 h if required. Should not be used in children. Caution in elderly.	Motion sickness Onset: 4 h	Sedation, constipation, dry mouth, blurred vision, rash, allergic contact dermatitis, eye irritation if hands touch eyes after handling patch. Disorientation, delirium. The elderly are at increased risk of CNS effects.	Sedatives, anticholinergics (additive effects).	$$
Antihistamines	*dimenhydrinate* Gravol Preparations, generics	**Adults:** 50–100 mg Q4-6H PRN po (maximum 400 mg/day) **Children 6–12 y:** 25–50 mg Q6–8H PRN po **Children 2–5 y:** 15–25 mg Q6–8H PRN po	Motion sickness, NVP, PONV Onset: 30 min	Sedation, dry mouth, constipation, urinary retention, blurred vision, paradoxical excitation in children.	Alcohol and any other medication that causes drowsiness may enhance sedative effects of the antihistamine, increase confusion, ataxia and paradoxical excitation.	$
	diphenhydramine Benadryl, generics	**Adults:** 25–50 mg Q4–6H PRN po (maximum 200 mg/day) **Children 6–12 y:** 12.5–25 mg Q4–6H PRN po	Motion sickness, NVP, PONV Onset: 30 min	See dimenhydrinate.	See dimenhydrinate.	$
Phenothiazines	*promethazine* Histantil	**Adults:** Motion sickness: 25 mg BID po with first dose 30–60 min before departure and repeat dose in 8–12 h PRN PONV: 12.5–25 mg Q4–6H PRN po **Children ≥2 y:** Motion sickness: 0.5 mg/kg (maximum 25 mg/dose) po with first dose 30–60 min before departure and repeat 12 h later PRN	All types Onset: 30 min	Sedation, somnolence, extrapyramidal symptoms, dry mouth, constipation, blurred vision.	Alcohol and other CNS depressants (additive effects).	$
Vitamins	*pyridoxine (vitamin B6)*	**Adults:** 10–25 mg po TID	NVP Onset: 1–2 h	Abdominal pain, headache, loss of appetite, paresthesia, photosensitivity, skin irritation, somnolence.	No significant drug interactions.	$

[a] For more information on pharmacologic management of nausea and vomiting, consult the *Compendium of Therapeutic Choices*: Nausea in Adults.

[b] Cost per day; includes drug cost only.

Abbreviations: NVP = nausea and vomiting of pregnancy; PCNV = postchemotherapy nausea and vomiting; PONV = postoperative nausea and vomiting

Legend: $ <$1 $$ $1–2

Resource Tips

Motherisk web site: www.motherisk.org.

Motherisk Morning Sickness Helpline: 1-800-436-8477.

Suggested Readings

Einarson A, Maltepe C, Boskovic R et al. Treatment of nausea and vomiting in pregnancy: an updated algorithm. *Can Fam Physician* 2007;53:2109-11.

Gan TJ, Diemunsch P, Habib AS et al. Consensus guidelines for the management of postoperative nausea and vomiting. *Anesth Analg* 2014;118:85-113.

Jordan K, Gralla R, Jahn F, Molassiotis A. International antiemetic guidelines on chemotherapy induced nausea and vomiting (CINV): content and implementation in daily routine practice. *Eur J Pharmacol* 2014;722:197-202.

Murdin L, Golding J, Bronstein A. Managing motion sickness. *BMJ* 2011;343:d7430.

Swegle JM, Logemann C. Management of common opioid-induced adverse effects. *Am Fam Physician* 2006;74:1347-54.

References

1. Quigley EM, Hasler WL, Parkman HP. AGA technical review on nausea and vomiting. *Gastroenterology* 2001;120:263-86.
2. Scorza K, Williams A, Phillips JD et al. Evaluation of nausea and vomiting. *Am Fam Physician* 2007;76:76-84.
3. Hasler WL. Nausea, vomiting, and indigestion. In: Kasper D, Fauci A, Hauser S et al., eds. *Harrison's principles of internal medicine*. 19th ed. New York: McGraw-Hill; 2015.
4. Hesketh PJ. Chemotherapy-induced nausea and vomiting. *N Engl J Med* 2008;358:2482-94.
5. Shupak A, Gordon CR. Motion sickness: advances in pathogenesis, prediction, prevention, and treatment. *Aviat Space Environ Med* 2006;77:1213-23.
6. Murdin L, Golding J, Bronstein A. Managing motion sickness. *BMJ* 2011;343:d7430.
7. Golding JF. Motion sickness susceptibility. *Auton Neurosci* 2006;129:67-76.
8. Jordan K, Gralla R, Jahn F, Molassiotis A. International antiemetic guidelines on chemotherapy induced nausea and vomiting (CINV): content and implementation in daily routine practice. *Eur J Pharmacol* 2014;722:197-202.
9. Lohr L. Chemotherapy-induced nausea and vomiting. *Cancer J* 2008;14:85-93.
10. Jordan K, Sippel C, Schmoll HJ. Guidelines for antiemetic treatment of chemotherapy-induced nausea and vomiting: past, present, and future recommendations. *Oncologist* 2007;12:1143-50.
11. Hesketh PJ. Understanding the pathobiology of chemotherapy-induced nausea and vomiting. Providing a basis for therapeutic progress. *Oncology (Williston Park)* 2004;18:9-14.
12. Roscoe JA, Morrow GR, Aapro MS et al. Anticipatory nausea and vomiting. *Support Care Cancer* 2011;19:1533-8.
13. Lee NM, Saha S. Nausea and vomiting of pregnancy. *Gastroenterol Clin North Am* 2011;40:309-34.
14. Jarvis S, Nelson-Piercy C. Management of nausea and vomiting in pregnancy. *BMJ* 2011;342:d3606.
15. Flaxman SM, Sherman PW. Morning sickness: a mechanism for protecting mother and embryo. *Q Rev Biol* 2000;75:113-48.
16. Furneaux EC, Langley-Evans AJ, Langley-Evans SC. Nausea and vomiting of pregnancy: endocrine basis and contribution to pregnancy outcome. *Obstet Gynecol Surv* 2001;56:775-82.
17. Koren G, Madjunkova S, Maltepe C. The protective effects of nausea and vomiting of pregnancy against adverse fetal outcome—a systematic review. *Reprod Toxicol* 2014;47:77-80.
18. Goodwin TM. Hyperemesis gravidarum. *Obstet Gynecol Clin North Am* 2008;35:401-17.
19. Le TP, Gan TJ. Update on the management of postoperative nausea and vomiting and postdischarge nausea and vomiting in ambulatory surgery. *Anesthesiol Clin* 2010;28:225-49.
20. McCracken G, Houston P, Lefebvre G et al. Guideline for the management of postoperative nausea and vomiting. *J Obstet Gynaecol Can* 2008;30:600-7, 608-16.
21. Apfel CC, Laara E, Koivuranta M et al. A simplified risk score for predicting postoperative nausea and vomiting: conclusions from cross-validations between two centers. *Anesthesiology* 1999;91:693-700.
22. Horn CC, Wallisch WJ, Homanics GE et al. Pathophysiological and neurochemical mechanisms of postoperative nausea and vomiting. *Eur J Pharmacol* 2014;722:55-66.
23. Harris JD. Management of expected and unexpected opioid-related side effects. *Clin J Pain* 2008;24:S8-S13.
24. Smith HS, Smith JM, Seidner P. Opioid-induced nausea and vomiting. *Ann Palliat Med* 2012;1:121-9.
25. Metz A, Hebbard G. Nausea and vomiting in adults—a diagnostic approach. *Aust Fam Physician* 2007;36:688-92.
26. Scales K, Pilsworth J. The importance of fluid balance in clinical practice. *Nurs Stand* 2008;22:50-7.
27. Allen K. The vomiting child—what to do and when to consult. *Aust Fam Physician* 2007;36:684-7.
28. Bruce DG, Golding JF, Hockenhull N et al. Acupressure and motion sickness. *Aviat Space Environ Med* 1990;61:361-5.
29. Warwick-Evans LA, Masters IJ, Redstone SB. A double-blind placebo controlled evaluation of acupressure in the treatment of motion sickness. *Aviat Space Environ Med* 1991;62:776-8.
30. Miller KE, Muth ER. Efficacy of acupressure and acustimulation bands for the prevention of motion sickness. *Aviat Space Environ Med* 2004;75:227-34.

31. Marchioro G, Azzarello G, Viviani F et al. Hypnosis in the treatment of anticipatory nausea and vomiting in patients receiving cancer chemotherapy. *Oncology* 2000;59:100-4.
32. Mundy EA, DuHamel KN, Montgomery GH. The efficacy of behavioral interventions for cancer treatment-related side effects. *Semin Clin Neuropsychiatry* 2003;8:253-75.
33. Sheehan P. Hyperemesis gravidarum—assessment and management. *Aust Fam Physician* 2007;36:698-701.
34. Einarson A, Maltepe C, Boskovic R et al. Treatment of nausea and vomiting in pregnancy: an updated algorithm. *Can Fam Physician* 2007;53:2109-11.
35. Matthews A, Haas DM, O'Mathúna DP et al. Interventions for nausea and vomiting in early pregnancy. *Cochrane Database Syst Rev* 2015;9:CD007575.
36. Heazell A, Thorneycroft J, Walton V et al. Acupressure for the in-patient treatment of nausea and vomiting in early pregnancy: a randomized control trial. *Am J Obstet Gynecol* 2006;194:815-20.
37. Jamigorn M, Phupong V. Acupressure and vitamin B6 to relieve nausea and vomiting in pregnancy: a randomized study. *Arch Gynecol Obstet* 2007;276:245-9.
38. Doran K, Halm MA. Integrating acupressure to alleviate postoperative nausea and vomiting. *Am J Crit Care* 2010;19:553-6.
39. Cheong KB, Zhang JP, Huang Y et al. The effectiveness of acupuncture in prevention and treatment of postoperative nausea and vomiting—a systematic review and meta-analysis. *PLoS One* 2013;8:e82474.
40. Lee A, Done ML. The use of nonpharmacologic techniques to prevent postoperative nausea and vomiting: a meta-analysis. *Anesth Analg* 1999;88:1362-9.
41. White PF, Issioui T, Hu J et al. Comparative efficacy of acustimulation (ReliefBand) versus ondansetron (Zofran) in combination with droperidol for preventing nausea and vomiting. *Anesthesiology* 2002;97:1075-81.
42. Flake ZA, Scalley RD, Bailey AG. Practical selection of antiemetics. *Am Fam Physician* 2004;69:1169-74.
43. Chepyala P, Olden KW. Nausea and vomiting. *Curr Treat Options Gastroenterol* 2008;11:135-44.
44. CPS online. Ottawa: Canadian Pharmacists Association; 2016. Available from: www.e-therapeutics.ca. Accessed February 2, 2016. Subscription required.
45. Spinks A, Wasiak J. Scopolamine (hyoscine) for preventing and treating motion sickness. *Cochrane Database Syst Rev* 2011;6:CD002851.
46. Zajonc TP, Roland PS. Vertigo and motion sickness. Part II: Pharmacologic treatment. *Ear Nose Throat J* 2006;85:25-35.
47. Gillingham KK, Previc FH. Spatial orientation in flight. In: DeHart RL, ed. *Fundamentals of aerospace medicine*. 2nd ed. Baltimore: Williams & Wilkins; 1996. p. 309-97.
48. Stewart JJ, Wood MJ, Wood CD et al. Effects of ginger on motion sickness susceptibility and gastric function. *Pharmacology* 1991;42:111-20.
49. Lien HC, Sun WM, Chen YH et al. Effects of ginger on motion sickness and gastric slow-wave dysrhythmias induced by circular vection. *Am J Physiol Gastrointest Liver Physiol* 2003;284:G481-9.
50. Grøntved A, Brask T, Kambskard J et al. Ginger root against seasickness. A controlled trial on the open sea. *Acta Otolaryngol* 1988;105:45-9.
51. Koren G, Clark S, Hankins GD et al. Effectiveness of delayed-release doxylamine and pyridoxine for nausea and vomiting of pregnancy: a randomized placebo controlled trial. *Am J Obstet Gynecol* 2010;203:571.e1-7.
52. Borrelli F, Capasso R, Aviello G et al. Effectiveness and safety of ginger in the treatment of pregnancy-induced nausea and vomiting. *Obstet Gynecol* 2005;105:849-56.
53. Boone SA, Shields KM. Treating pregnancy-related nausea and vomiting with ginger. *Ann Pharmacother* 2005;39:1710-3.
54. Kranke P, Morin AM, Roewer N et al. Dimenhydrinate for prophylaxis of postoperative nausea and vomiting: a meta-analysis of randomized controlled trials. *Acta Anaesthesiol Scand* 2002;46:238-44.
55. Apfel CC, Zhang K, George E et al. Transdermal scopolamine for the prevention of postoperative nausea and vomiting: a systematic review and meta-analysis. *Clin Therap* 2010;32:1987-2002.
56. Sanchez-Ledesma MJ, Lopez-Olaondo L, Pueyo FJ et al. A comparison of three antiemetic combinations for the prevention of postoperative nausea and vomiting. *Anesth Analg* 2002;95:1590-5.
57. Habib AS, El-Moalem HE, Gan TJ. The efficacy of the 5-HT3 receptor antagonists combined with droperidol for PONV prophylaxis is similar to their combination with dexamethasone. A meta-analysis of randomized controlled trials. *Can J Anaesth* 2004;51:311-9.
58. Wilhelm SM, Dehoorne-Smith ML, Kale-Pradhan PB. Prevention of postoperative nausea and vomiting. *Ann Pharmacother* 2007;41:68-78.
59. Pellegrini J, DeLoge J, Bennett J et al. Comparison of inhalation of isopropyl alcohol vs promethazine in the treatment of postoperative nausea and vomiting (PONV) in patients identified as at high risk for developing PONV. *AANA J* 2009;77:293-9.
60. Mamaril ME, Windle PE, Burkard JF. Prevention and management of postoperative nausea and vomiting: a look at complementary techniques. *J Perianesth Nurs* 2006;21:404-10.

Motion Sickness—What You Need to Know

Hints to help you manage motion sickness:

- **Before you travel:**
  - Avoid eating a large meal within 3 hours of travel.
  - Avoid dairy products and foods high in salt, calories or protein (such as meat or nuts).
- **While you are travelling:**
  - Try to get cool fresh air by opening air vents or using air conditioning.
  - Avoid alcohol, smoking and disagreeable odours.
  - Avoid reading and watching videos.
  - Focus on the horizon or an object that does not move outside the car, plane or boat.
  - Try pressing your head into the headrest.
  - On a boat, try to stay in the middle.
  - In a vehicle (such as a car or truck), sit in the front seat with a clear forward view.
  - If possible, drive the vehicle rather than be a passenger.
- **Natural health products:**
  Some people find that natural health products help them. However, there is no proof that they work. Try the suggestions above before trying natural health products, such as:
  - Eat or drink any of the following: apricot juice, carrot juice, unroasted pumpkin or squash seeds, parsley, peppermint tea.
  - Try ginger root. This comes as candied ginger, powder, capsules and tea.
  - Try SeaBands acupressure wristbands.

How to take antinausea medication:

Your healthcare provider may recommend medication for motion sickness. Here are some things you should know about these medications:

- **Do not** take antinausea medication with alcohol.
- Most antinausea medications can cause drowsiness. **Do not** drive a car or operate dangerous machinery while you are taking these medications. They are as dangerous as alcohol when driving.
- If you need to be alert, talk to your healthcare provider about taking a medication that does not cause much drowsiness.
- Antinausea medications can cause the following side effects: dizziness, shakiness, anxiety, blurred vision and constipation. Ask your healthcare provider if your medication will cause side effects.
- When children take antinausea medications, they sometimes get very excitable instead of drowsy. Be sure to test the medication on the child before you travel.

Morning Sickness—What You Need to Know

Nausea and vomiting are **completely normal** during the first 12 weeks of a pregnancy (12 weeks after your last period). Morning sickness can happen at any time of the day, not just in the morning. **Remember:** Morning sickness usually gets better as your pregnancy progresses!

Suggestions to help you manage nausea or vomiting:

- Avoid smells that make you feel nauseated.
- Eat crackers or dry toast before you get out of bed in the morning.
- Eat any food that looks and smells appealing to you. You may find that bland foods will bother you less.
- Avoid foods that are fatty, fried or spicy.
- Eat 5 or 6 small meals each day instead of eating 3 large meals; eating large meals or having an empty stomach can worsen nausea.
- Drink small amounts of fluid regularly between meals.
- Avoid lying down right after eating.
- Take your prenatal vitamins or iron supplements after meals, never on an empty stomach.
- Iron supplements or prenatal vitamins which contain higher amounts of iron can contribute to nausea and vomiting. You may stop these supplements for a while and continue to take folic acid alone or a multivitamin that does not contain iron.
- Heartburn, gas and constipation can make nausea worse. Talk to your healthcare provider about ways to manage these problems.
- Products that contain ginger may help to settle your stomach. Talk to your healthcare provider about safe use of ginger products.
- Avoid warm places and dress in layers so you can remove some clothing if feeling too warm. Being too hot can make you feel sick.
- Try to get lots of rest and reduce your stress.
- Try eating at times of the day when nausea is less severe.
- Talk to your healthcare provider about trying acupressure.

Are there safe medications for nausea and vomiting?

Several medications have been proven safe to treat nausea during pregnancy. They do not increase the risk of birth defects. If you find your nausea or vomiting is not reduced by any of the suggestions above, talk to your healthcare providers. They can tell you about safe and effective medications for nausea.

When should you see your healthcare provider?

Pregnant women who have severe vomiting require special treatment to prevent dehydration. See your healthcare provider right away if you have any of the following symptoms:

- Your vomiting does not respond to any type of treatment.
- You are losing weight, or not gaining weight as you should be.
- Diarrhea.
- Fever or body temperature above 39°C.
- You vomit any amount of blood or the vomit contains what looks like coffee grounds.

- You cannot keep fluids down and you feel very thirsty or faint when you get up from lying down. This may mean you are dehydrated.

For more information:

- Call the University of Toronto's Motherisk program toll-free helpline at **1-800-436-8477**. They can answer your questions or concerns about nausea and vomiting in pregnancy. They also have an excellent website with information about morning sickness and many other issues. Go to www.motherisk.org.
- You can learn more about healthy eating during pregnancy from your local public health department or at www.healthyalberta.com/HEALPregnancy-Sept2012.pdf.

Chapter 37
Ostomy Care

Marie Berry, BScPharm, BA, LLB

Types of Ostomies

An ostomy is an artificial opening made surgically in the body. The opening itself is called a stoma, derived from the Greek word *stoma*, meaning mouth. A colostomy involves the colon, an ileostomy the ileum or small intestine and a urostomy the urinary tract. Ostomies may be permanent or temporary, and the type of ostomy used depends upon the condition being treated.

Half a million North Americans have ostomies and over 90 000 ostomy operations are performed each year in the United States and Canada.[1] No particular age or ethnic group has more ostomies, but in general more women than men have ostomies. Birth defects account for the majority of ostomies in children.

The older the adult the more likely the ostomy surgery will be a colostomy because of cancer or obstruction related to disease. Ileostomies are more common in young women, especially those resulting from inflammatory bowel disease.

Ileostomy

To construct an ileostomy, the entire colon and possibly part of the ileum are removed or bypassed. Usually the ileum end is brought to the skin surface.

For some persons, instead of an ileostomy the surgeon creates a continent fecal diversion, such as an ileoanal reservoir ("S" or "J" pouch). In this procedure, a permanent external ostomy bag is not needed. The entire colon and rectum are removed and the ileum is refashioned into an internal pouch with the end of the ileum joined to the anal canal. The internal pouch serves as a reservoir which is able to store waste material that then can be eliminated in the normal way.

Crohn's disease and ulcerative colitis are the most common reasons for an ileostomy. An ileostomy may also be required because of trauma, cancer, familial polyp disease or necrotizing enterocolitis.

Colostomy

To construct a colostomy, part of the colon is removed and the GI tract ends with a portion of the colon. The different types of colostomy are illustrated in Figure 1. A colostomy may be required due to obstruction of the colon or rectum, genetic malformation, trauma, radiation colitis, loss of anal muscle control, diverticulitis, or cancer of the colon or rectum. Colorectal cancer is the most common indication for this procedure.

Temporary ileostomies and colostomies are sometimes performed to allow a diseased or surgically repaired bowel to heal, and once the bowel has healed it is reversed.

Colostomies and ileostomies show a characteristic output or effluent, as described in Table 1.

Table 1: **Description of Output from Different Colostomies and Ileostomies**

Ileostomy	Initially the output is liquid. With time, as the ileum becomes more absorptive, the output becomes semi-soft. The output is continuous and contains enzymes that may cause skin irritation but is less odourous than output from a colostomy. An appliance must be worn at all times.
Ascending colostomy (uncommon)	The output is liquid or semi-solid, malodourous and irritating. An appliance must be worn at all times.
Transverse colostomy (commonly used for temporary colostomies)	The output is semi-solid, malodourous and irritating; an appliance must be worn at all times.
Descending and sigmoid colostomies (more common)	Output is pasty. Irrigation may be an option and an appliance may not be needed.

Urostomies

Urostomies (urinary diversions) are most common in infants and the elderly. They are performed to correct bladder loss or dysfunction resulting from genetic malformation, cancer or neurogenic bladder. These allow the elimination of urine through an opening in the abdominal wall. Because urine always remains liquid and is discharged continuously, urostomy surgery usually requires an appliance. There are many types of urostomies (see Figure 2):

- Ileal and colonic conduits (more common): The colon or (more commonly) ileum is used to fashion the conduit into which the ureters are implanted. Mucus shreds may be seen in urine because the bowel has been used. Urine output from the stoma is continuous and an appliance is required at all times.
- Ureterostomy (uncommon): The ureters are brought to the skin surface; with time the ureters tend to narrow.
- Nephrostomy: A tube is placed into the renal pelvis of kidney to divert urine from the kidneys. It may be temporary in the case of reversible ureteral obstruction.
- Cystotomy: A suprapubic cystostomy is a surgically created passage from the abdominal wall directly into the urinary bladder. A catheter tube is then inserted into the bladder to continuously drain urine.
- Continent urinary diversion: A pouch is created using the small or large bowel and is emptied by intermittently inserting a catheter in the stoma. Some examples are the Kock, Indiana, Florida or Miami pouches. In the Mitrofanoff procedure, the appendix is used to create the conduit and a stoma is constructed that can be intermittently catheterized. A passage is created with a reservoir valve to channel from the urinary bladder to the abdominal skin. No external collection pouch is required.
- Orthotopic neobladder, i.e., Studer pouch, is a new or neobladder constructed from intestine to replace a diseased or dysfunctional urinary bladder. The detubularized bowel segment is surgically attached to the urethra. No stoma is present and it is possible to void normally through the urethra but some persons may require urethral catheterization.

Patient Assessment

A healthy stoma is shiny, moist and either dark pink or red (see Healthy Stoma in Photo Section). It has no pain sensation because it does not contain nerve fibres. The stoma size in adults usually ranges from 2–5 cm depending upon the portion of the bowel or urinary tract used. After surgery, it shrinks gradually over several months to its permanent size.

A careful history and inspection of the ostomy site can help determine whether the patient is experiencing a problem. See Common Problems section for more information.

Figure 1: **Types of Colostomies**

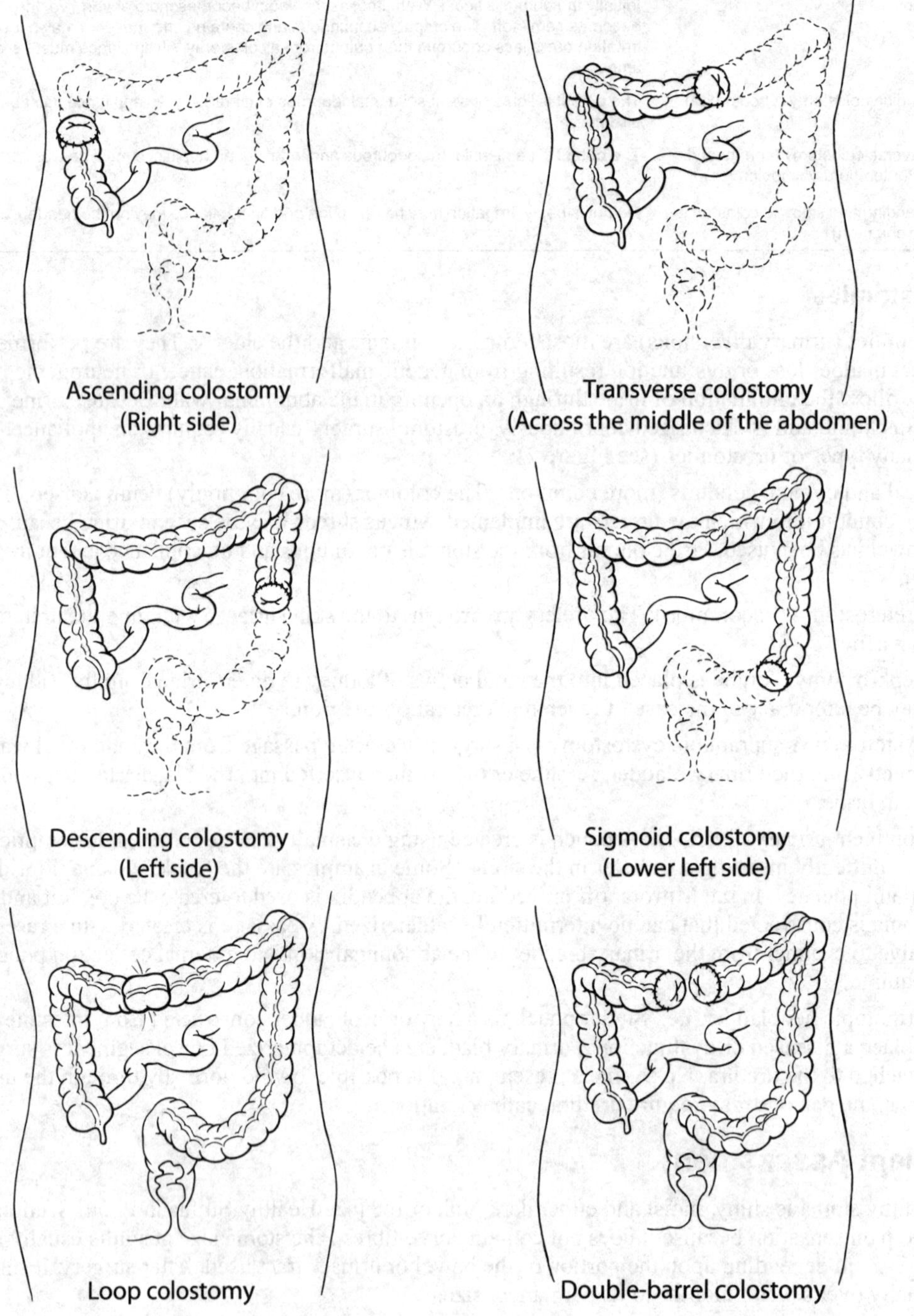

Figure 2: **Types of Urostomies**

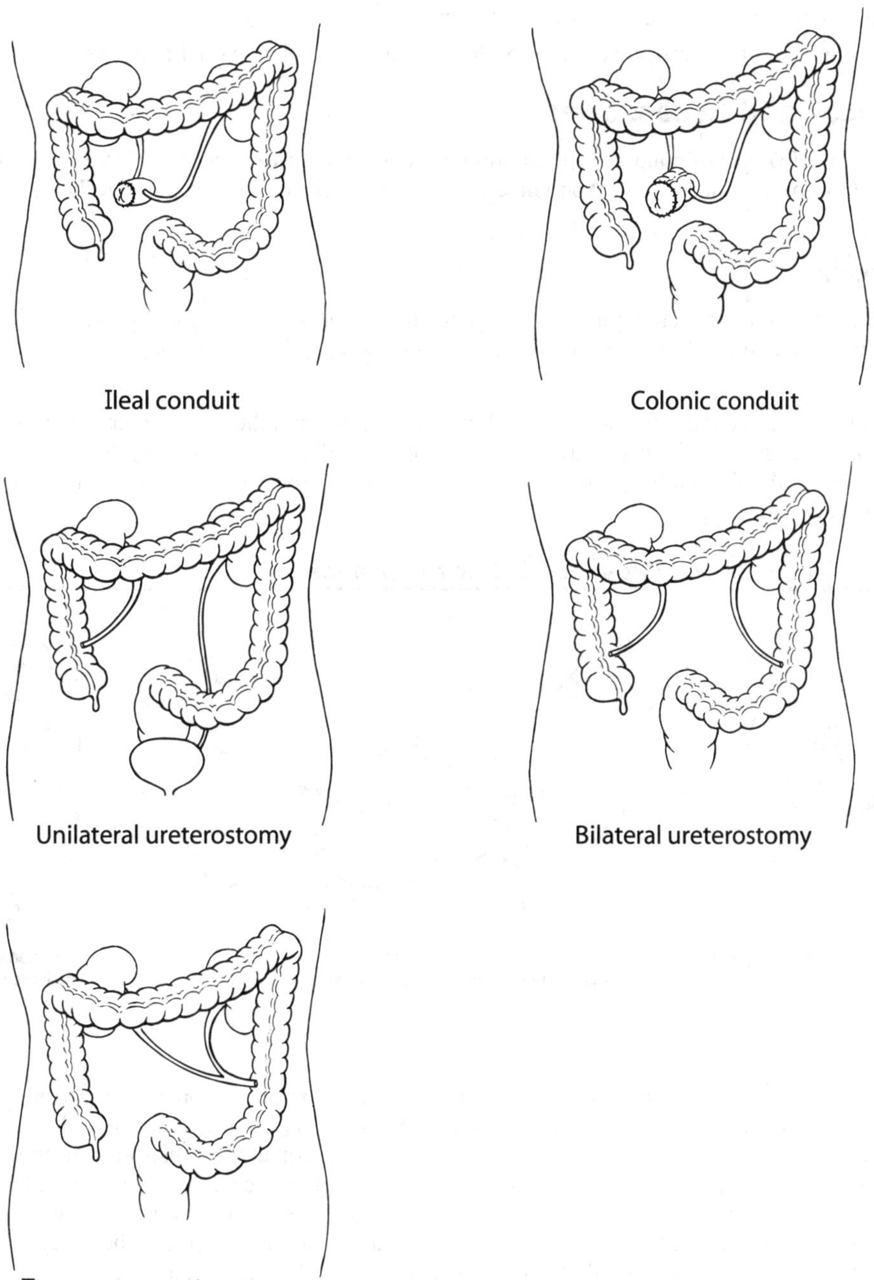

Goals of Ostomy Care

- Contain output or effluent
- Prevent common problems such as skin irritation
- Minimize impact of ostomy on activities of daily living and optimize quality of life

Appliances and Accessories

For comparative features of nonprescription products, consult the *Compendium of Products for Minor Ailments*—Ostomy Products: Adult Appliances; Pediatric Appliances; Protectants, Adhesives and Cleansers.

Appliances

An appliance is used to collect output from the stoma but not all stomas require appliances. The ideal ostomy appliance permits effective containment with no leakage, does not damage skin and is odour-free.

An ostomy appliance includes the pouch, which collects output, and the skin barrier with a flange (plastic ring on the skin barrier that attaches to the pouch) or adhesive coupling system. The skin barrier attaches to the skin on the person's abdomen (Figure 3). Appliances are available in both pediatric and adult sizes.

Figure 3: **Placement of a Two-piece Ostomy Appliance**

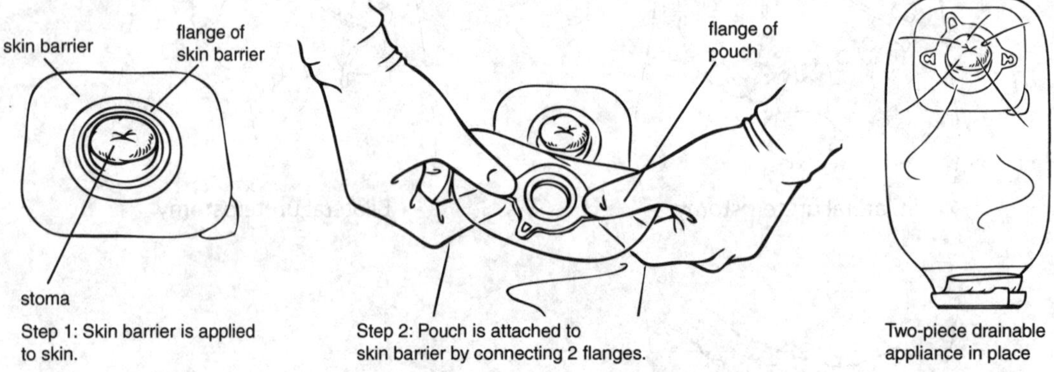

Step 1: Skin barrier is applied to skin.

Step 2: Pouch is attached to skin barrier by connecting 2 flanges.

Two-piece drainable appliance in place

Pouch

Pouches (see Figure 4) are available in different lengths and capacities to contain the varying amounts of output. Pouches may be open-ended (drainable) or close-ended (not drainable). Whether a drainable or non-drainable pouch is selected depends upon the site of the stoma, the consistency of the output and whether the task or cost of emptying and cleaning the pouch is acceptable to the individual. Open-ended appliances afford frequent emptying and are more often used for ileostomies and when a colostomy is not regulated. It is usually recommended that pouches are emptied when they are half to a third full. If a drainable pouch is used, the drainage end needs to be kept clean.

Pouches are selected based on the individual's choice and their ability to care for the ostomy. Pouches come in various lengths, can be clear or opaque and some may have a fabric backing for comfort or discretion. Most pouches are odour proof and some have an embedded charcoal filter to minimize odour while allowing gas to escape.[2]

Flange

The flange is the plastic ring on the skin barrier that attaches to the pouch. The selection of the flange size depends upon the size of the stoma. Skin barriers with flanges are also available in different sizes, shapes (e.g., round, oval) and convexities, and in rigid or flexible formats to accommodate different body contours and stoma sizes, shapes and locations.

One-piece vs. Two-piece Appliances

Appliances are available as both one- and two-piece units (Figure 4).

One-piece appliances combine a pouch/skin barrier and attach directly to the skin. Closed-ended appliances are discarded after one use while open-ended versions can be emptied and reused until the skin barrier requires changing. Two-piece appliances consist of a skin barrier with a flange, which is attached directly to the skin and separate pouches. The benefits of using a two-piece appliance include: pouch can be cleaned for reuse, and less frequent removal/replacement which can irritate the skin. While this ability to interchange appliance components exists within a manufacturer's line of products, it does not usually extend between various manufacturers. Of note, two-piece appliances can be difficult to use if a person has diminished manual dexterity or eyesight.

Figure 4: **Ostomy Appliances**

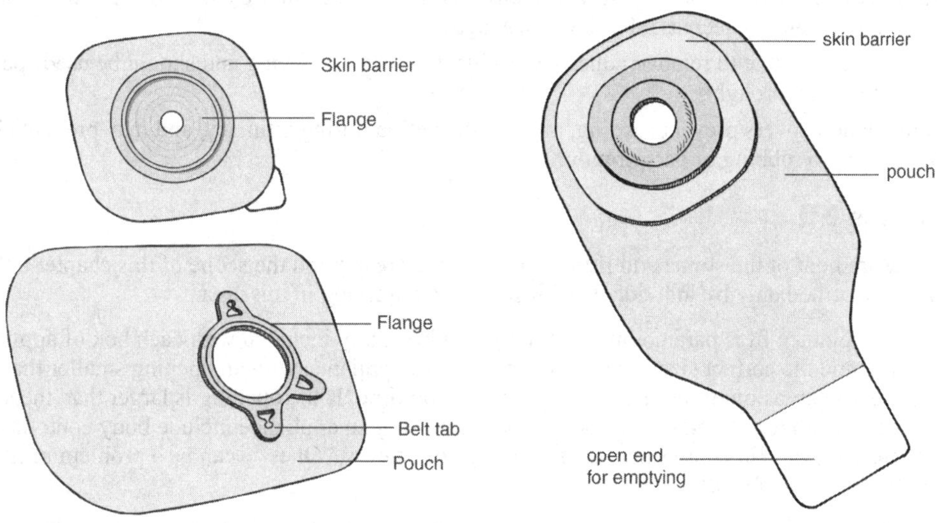

Two-piece closed appliance.

One-piece drainable appliance.

Accessories

Skin Barriers

Skin barriers help keep the skin surrounding a stoma intact, protecting it and keeping it dry. Skin barrier wafers are usually composed of pectin, gelatin and cellulose. The skin barrier wafer can be flat, convex, rigid or flexible to accommodate different body contours and stoma sizes, shapes and locations. Stomas that drain urine or loose/liquid stool require special barriers commonly labelled for "extended wear". Flanges are incorporated in skin barrier wafers and are an essential component of the ostomy appliance. If the person has a confirmed allergy to any of the components of the product it would be best to test the skin barrier before using it. Applying the product to an inconspicuous area of skin for 48 hours is usually sufficient to determine whether there is any reaction.

Skin barrier powders are formulated of pectin, gelatin and cellulose and used to absorb moisture from the skin. Skin barrier pastes are also formulated of pectin, gelatin and cellulose and contain alcohol and preservatives. They are used like caulking, to improve the seal between the skin barrier wafer and the skin on the abdomen. Skin barrier paste is also available in strip format that is alcohol-free.

Adhesives

Although no longer in common use, adhesives are applied either as cement, which must be allowed to dry before the appliance is attached, or as a pad. Some adhesives include skin barriers in their formulations. Some ostomy pouches have adhesive integrated into the flange and/or skin barrier, making application simple.

Adhesives are the most common cause of allergies. A patch test should be performed prior to use as described in Skin Barriers.

Other Accessories

- Sometimes adhesive tape is used to secure an appliance. If so, it should be hypoallergenic.
- Belts are often used by urostomy patients to reduce the strain on the skin barrier wafer from the weight of the urine in the pouch. However, any ostomy patient can use a belt to assist with improved wear and to decrease the risk of leakage.
- Solvents are available to remove adhesive residue, but they are drying and should be used sparingly and washed off thoroughly.
- Ostomy pouch covers prevent rustling, provide discretion during intimacy, and may prevent skin irritation due to rubbing or perspiration.

Appliance Fit

Note: Measurement of the stoma and fitting an appliance are beyond the scope of this chapter and should be performed only by individuals with specialized training in this area.

The correct appliance fit is paramount. A fitting guide is usually included with each box of appliances to help determine the correct size based on the stoma. An appliance with an opening smaller than the stoma may cause abrasion of the stoma and poor wearing time. If the opening is larger than the stoma, skin excoriation can result. Other considerations in choosing an appliance include body contour, stoma location, presence of skin creases and scars, and type of ostomy.[3] Obesity can be a problem in fitting and maintaining an appliance.

The type of appliance may change postsurgically as the stoma heals, and as body contour changes due to weight changes, aging, pregnancy or concurrent medical conditions.

Changing the Appliance

Routine emptying of the pouch is required, usually when it is about one-third full. This would help prevent the weight of the pouch from compromising the seal on the skin.

The directions for changing the appliance vary somewhat from model to model and the directions accompanying the particular pouch should be consulted. However, some general principles do apply:

- Hands should be washed before beginning.
- The appliance should be carefully peeled off to avoid damaging the skin.

- The stoma and peristomal skin should be gently washed with warm water and soap, then thoroughly dried.
- Soap must be completely washed off.
- Alcohol should not be used to clean the peristomal skin.
- All adhesive areas should be in contact with skin.
- All skin folds should be smoothed out.
- Once applied, the appliance should be pressed gently into place.

Irrigation

For some persons with colostomies, irrigation is sometimes an alternative to wearing an appliance. It is less expensive and affords some control of fecal outflow. In irrigation, squirting water through the stoma into the intestine stimulates peristalsis which forces waste out. It is usually performed in the bathroom with an irrigation bag, which is much like an enema bag.

In addition to an irrigation bag, irrigation systems include an irrigation sleeve, skin barrier and stoma cone. The stoma cone is used with its pointed end inserted into the stoma to act like tubing, but to prevent bowel perforation, which could accompany the use of tubing alone. The irrigation sleeve, attached to the skin barrier, carries the waste material to the toilet.

When not being irrigated, a stoma cap or even a pad is all that is required to cover the stoma. Irrigation is performed regularly, the interval ranging from every one to four days. A convenient time may be after the largest meal of the day, because of the peristalsis stimulated by the meal.

Common Problems

Common problems usually involve the stoma or peristomal skin. The actual incidence of skin problems is difficult to determine; however, peristomal skin problems seem to occur frequently involving anywhere from 18–55% of persons living with an ostomy.[4,5] Functional, psychological and social factors may contribute to ostomy problems. Poor manual dexterity, visual problems, clothing incompatibilities and dietary issues can lead to appliance leakage and odour. Other concerns, such as depression, anxiety, sexual or body image concerns, lack of education about the stoma and inability to return to work, can exacerbate any problem.

Peristomal Skin Problems

Allergies

Skin barrier adhesives and pastes are the most common cause of allergies, and allergic contact dermatitis is the most common manifestation (itching, burning or stinging, redness and areas of moist, denuded skin).[6] A switch to another adhesive or appliance may be necessary. A skin barrier may help, but it needs to extend beyond the damaged area. The majority of modern appliances are latex-free, reducing the risk of a latex allergy.

Infections

Infections can occur under the skin barrier and/or flange. These may be bacterial or fungal; culture and sensitivity testing may be needed to identify the pathogen responsible and ensure appropriate treatment. Proper maintenance is important in preventing infections.

Ostomy sites are susceptible to fungal infections with *Candida* species because they provide a warm, moist environment conducive to fungal growth. The primary symptom of *Candida* infection is itching, accompanied by a red rash with satellite lesions.[7] With an unchecked infection, skin excoriation and additional skin irritation can occur. Use of broad spectrum antibiotics can contribute to *Candida* infections by changing the normal flora; thus, knowing a patient's medication history is important.

Nystatin powder may be used to treat *Candida* infections. The appliance is applied directly over the powder, with any excess powder brushed off. Another antifungal option is the silver based **Arglaes** powder. Usually antifungal powder is continued for 1 week after the *Candida* infection clears. Treatment may be extended further if the individual is also undergoing treatment with antibiotics. Greasy topical products should be avoided since they may interfere with the adherence of skin barriers.

Refer any person living with an ostomy to an appropriate healthcare practitioner (e.g., wound ostomy and continence nurse, enterostomal therapy nurse, physician) if experiencing symptoms of infection, fever, chills, foul odour or purulent output from the stoma.

Skin Damage

The most common peristomal skin problem is sore skin, usually the result of frequent removal of the appliance. The skin around the stoma becomes damaged—red, swollen, burning, itchy. Skin damage may be also related to mechanical irritation caused by a poor-fitting appliance, a stoma that is difficult to access or clothing that is too tight.

Skin Excoriation

Skin excoriation or irritant dermatitis is abrasion of the skin by digestive enzymes, which may result in bleeding, painful skin (see Peristomal Skin Excoriation in Photo Section). The most common cause is an appliance that is too big for the stoma and allows leakage. Delayed replacement or maintenance may also result in waste material containing digestive enzymes coming into contact with skin. Choosing the proper size of appliance, routine maintenance of the appliance, and use of a skin barrier will avoid the problem.

Folliculitis

Folliculitis is an inflammation of hair follicles around the stoma and is characterised by redness at the base of hair follicles. Aggressive removal of an appliance may also pull hair from follicles, resulting in inflammation and infection. Shaving the area surrounding the stoma will prevent folliculitis. An electric razor is preferred because it will leave the skin intact. Clipping the hair is an alternative if shaving with an electric razor does cause skin damage.

Leakage

Ill-fitting or badly applied appliances result in leakage around the seal. Proper fit and maintenance of the appliance are the solution to this issue.

Bleeding

Bleeding of the stoma is usually due to aggressive cleaning. Proper cleaning technique is required—gentle yet thorough. If bleeding persists, it may be an indication that the original disease has recurred, or that a new condition is developing. Referral to an appropriate healthcare professional is necessary.

Odour

Diet is the most common source of odour. Identifying what food is causing the odour and changing the diet usually solves the problem (Table 2). Pouches usually have an odour barrier and thus are considered odour-free, provided they are changed regularly, emptied as needed, cleaned properly, are without flaws or pinholes and are reliably sealed. Emptying a pouch is often accompanied by odour.

Table 2: **Foods with Implications for Ostomy Patients**[8]

Bulk-forming foods	Celery, coconut, coleslaw, foods with seeds or kernels (e.g., corn), dried fruits, nuts, meats in casings, popcorn, whole grains, whole vegetables, wild rice
Gas-forming foods	Beer, broccoli, brussels sprouts, cabbage, carbonated drinks, cauliflower, corn, cucumbers, dairy products, dried beans, mushrooms, onions, peas, radishes, spinach, string beans or chewing gum with an open mouth
Diarrhea-causing foods	Broccoli, beer (other alcoholic beverages are not common offenders), green beans, highly seasoned food, raw fruit, spinach
Odour-forming foods	Asparagus, beans, broccoli, cabbage, eggs, fish, garlic, onions, peas, some spices, turnips

Deodorants are available to help control odour. These are placed into the pouch after each emptying. Oral **deodorants**, such as **activated charcoal**, **chlorophyllin copper complex** and **bismuth subgallate**, act on the digestive system to eliminate odours from digested foods.

Gas

Foods that caused gas prior to surgery usually cause gas after surgery. Travel in pressurized aircraft cabins can cause distention of an appliance. Careful dietary choices and relaxation techniques to reduce stress due to travel can reduce this distention. Some appliances have charcoal filters—the gas is released and the charcoal absorbs odours.

Strategies for decreasing gas include:

- Using an antacid
- Eating yogurt[7]
- Eating slowly and chewing food well (with a closed mouth)
- Avoiding drinking from a straw
- Avoiding chewing gum
- Limiting intake of gas-producing foods, especially prior to social occasions (Table 2).

Crystalline Phosphate Deposits

Crystalline phosphate deposits may build up on urostomies, making the stoma fragile and cutting into the mucosa. These deposits are the major cause of blood in a urostomy pouch. To dissolve the crystals, vinegar mixed with one-third to two-thirds water can be dabbed on the stoma when the appliance is cleaned. Acidifying the urine by consuming foods such as cranberry juice or even ascorbic acid will reduce the formation of these deposits. An ammonia odour may be the first sign of this problem and some individuals monitor the urine pH with urine dip sticks.

Fluid and Electrolyte Depletion

Persons living with an ileostomy lack normal reserve capacity for absorption of water, sodium and potassium, and should be advised to take extra fluid and electrolytes after exercise and in hot weather. Specialized fluid and electrolyte replacement drinks used by athletes are ideal but beverages with high sugar content should be avoided because they can precipitate diarrhea. Some individuals need routine potassium supplementation and particular attention should be paid to plasma potassium levels if a diuretic is used.

To avoid dehydration, fluid intake must be sufficient. This is especially important during illness and for infants. Signs and symptoms of dehydration and common electrolyte abnormalities are summarized in Table 3 and Table 4.

Table 3: **Symptoms of Dehydration in Children and Adults[9,10]**

Children	Adults
Dry mouth, tongue and skin	Increased thirst
Few or no tears when crying	Decreased urination
Decreased urination (less than 4 wet diapers in 24 h)	Feeling weak or light-headed
Sunken eyes	Dry mouth/tongue
Grayish skin	
Sunken soft spot (fontanel) in infants	
Decreased skin turgor	

Table 4: **Symptoms of Hyponatremia and Hypokalemia[11,12]**

Hyponatremia	Hypokalemia
Nausea, malaise, headache, lethargy, confusion, obtundation	Muscle weakness, fatigue, shortness of breath, decreased sensation in arms and legs, abdominal bloating (secondary to paralytic ileus)

Constipation

Individuals with colostomies are prone to constipation; fluid, fibre and exercise are recommended to avoid this problem. The causes of constipation are diverse, but it is often related to medications or diet (see Chapter 29: Constipation). Laxatives should be used only on the advice of an individual's healthcare practitioner.

Diarrhea

Persons with ostomies who are experiencing diarrhea may be at increased risk of fluid and/or electrolyte imbalances (Table 3 and Table 4). Fluid intake should be increased; oral rehydration solutions may be used to replenish electrolytes. Foods like bananas, potatoes, pasta, applesauce, yogurt, cheese and creamy peanut butter can help thicken the stoma output. Refer ostomy patients with diarrhea to an appropriate healthcare practitioner for further assessment.

Urinary Tract Infections

Individuals with urostomies have an increased risk of urinary tract infections which may require further assessment and treatment. They should be aware of the symptoms of these infections: chills, fever, bloody or cloudy urine, foul-smelling urine, back pain in the kidney area, abdominal pain.

Structural Problems

Fistula Formation, Prolapse and Retraction

Fistula formation appears as leakage around the base of the stoma, causing skin erosion. All fistula formation should be investigated as it may indicate an underlying disease or condition (e.g., inflammatory bowel disease, cancer, abscess formation, trauma, foreign body retention). The underlying problem should be addressed and sometimes surgical refashioning of the stoma is required.

Inward retraction of the stoma or outward prolapse of the stoma and/or bowel may occur. Either may be due to the way the stoma was originally fashioned or to major changes in the individual's weight. Anything that increases abdominal pressure (e.g., coughing, pregnancy) increases the risk of prolapse.

If the bowel is prolapsed, strangulation can occur. A prolapse should be reduced, and sometimes surgery is required.

Retraction may be controlled by the use of a convex appliance, but as with a prolapse, surgery may be needed.[13]

Stenosis

Stenosis is a narrowing of the stoma, usually caused by formation of scar tissue due to the surgical construction, ischemia, active bowel disease or dermatitis. Dilation and/or surgery may be required for correction.

Diet

Unless there are medical contraindications, individuals can eat a normal, varied diet, making their own adjustments to omit foods that change the consistency of the feces or cause odour or gas (Table 2).[14] A food diary may aid in determining foods that are well tolerated and those that cause problems. Fluid intake is important, especially for individuals with an ileostomy or urostomy. Eight to 10 glasses of fluid each day is recommended. The foods most often cited as causing odour, gas or frequent watery discharge are brans, fish, onions, carbonated beverages and beer.

People with an ileostomy will notice that high-fibre foods remain undigested. Sometimes this undigested food can cause a blockage or obstruction of the stoma. These foods should be introduced into the diet one at a time. Eating them in small quantities, chewing well and drinking fluids with them will help avoid problems. Symptoms of obstruction (e.g., no output from stoma, cramping, abdominal pain, vomiting, stoma swelling and watery, foul-smelling waste material) should be investigated further by an appropriate healthcare practitioner.

Medication Use

With an ostomy, GI transit times for medications are altered, which may in turn affect the medication's pharmacokinetics. Extended-release formulations may be unsuitable, and some medications are implicated in specific complications seen with ostomies, e.g., broad-spectrum antibiotics increase the risk of diarrhea and fungal infections. Table 5 summarizes some medication concerns.

Lifestyle Considerations

Persons living with an ostomy can be assured that they can wear their usual clothing and that if the pouch is changed and emptied as necessary it will not be visible. Women can continue to wear control-top panty hose, but an elastic girdle may need to be adapted with an opening to prevent pressure on the stoma and pouch.

Having an ostomy does not necessarily interfere with exercise, sports, occupational work or sexual activity. However, because of the potential for injury to the stoma, avoiding very heavy lifting and extremely rough contact sports is recommended. Specialized stomal caps and pouches are available for wear when swimming. A smaller sized pouch or even emptying the regular sized pouch, along with bathing suits of patterned fabric or boxer trunks for men, may help an ostomy patient feel more comfortable on the beach.[15]

Bathing and showering is possible with or without the appliance in place. Soap and water will not injure a stoma, but bath oils and soaps may leave a greasy film that can prevent the appliance from adhering. If a long soak in the bathtub is contemplated and the stoma will be below the water line, a cap can be used to prevent water from seeping into the stoma and the bowel. A person with a urinary stoma who wishes to attach a night drainage system to their appliance will require a free-standing holder or one that slides between the box spring and mattress.

Table 5: **Medication Concerns for Persons with Ostomies**

Drugs that may affect ostomy function	
Antacids	Aluminum-containing antacids can cause constipation in persons with colostomies; calcium-containing antacids can cause calcium stone formation in persons with urostomies and ileostomies; magnesium-containing antacids can cause diarrhea in persons with ileostomies
Antibiotics	Broad-spectrum antibiotics may alter the normal flora of the intestinal tract resulting in diarrhea or fungal infections of the skin surrounding the stoma. For persons with urostomies, the use of sulfa-containing antibiotics can lead to crystallization in the urine when high concentrations are obtained or when the urine is acidic. Persons with a urostomy that use urinary acidifiers to prevent urinary tract infection or encrustations are at high risk of sulfa crystal development in the kidneys or ureters. Persons with urostomies often stop taking urinary acidifiers while being treated with sulfa-containing antibiotics
Antidiarrheals	May cause constipation and possible obstruction in persons with colostomies
Antimotility drugs	May cause constipation in persons with colostomies and in some with ileostomies
Corticosteroids	Immunosuppressants can delay healing and increase risk of infections
Diuretics	May cause excess fluid loss and dehydration; with ileostomies monitor fluid balance and electrolytes
Laxatives	May result in perforations of colostomies; stool softeners are preferred; enemas should not be used with colostomies or ileostomies; avoid laxatives. Laxatives are also to be avoided in persons with ileostomies because of the high risk of dehydration and electrolyte imbalance
Opioids	May cause constipation
Salt substitutes	May cause hyponatremia in persons with ileostomies
Stool softeners	May cause diarrhea in persons with ileostomies
Sulfa drugs	Crystallization in the kidney may be more prominent if the individual is having difficulty with fluid and electrolyte balance; more common with urostomies. Good fluid intake is required
Drugs that may be ineffective because they are poorly absorbed	
Vitamins A, D, E, K, B_{12}	Variable absorption can occur with extensive resection of the ileum[5]
Oral contraceptives	May not be adequately absorbed in some persons with ileostomies
Digoxin	Variable bioavailability depending on length of bowel
Warfarin	Hypoprothrombinemia has occurred in some persons with short bowel syndrome
Drug formulations that may be problematic	
Enteric-coated or timed-release formulations	Enteric-coated formulations that require the alkaline environment of the small intestine to dissolve may pass through the intestinal tract intact. They are often ineffective in persons with ileostomies and only partially effective for persons with a colostomy. Checking in the pouch for undissolved tablets will identify the problem; alternatives include chewable tablets and liquids. Avoid timed-release preparations, especially with an ileostomy
Drugs that discolour the feces	Examples: Iron (black), bismuth (greenish black), amitriptyline (blue or green), phenothiazines (pink-red), vitamin B_{12} (yellow), salicylates (pink to red or black), senna (yellow), aluminum-containing antacids (whitish or speckled)

Hot weather or physical activity can cause sweating between the appliance and skin which can be uncomfortable and may lead to skin problems. Some antiperspirants may be used on the skin; however, check with the individual's nurse or physician. An adhesive change or the use of a breathable skin barrier are other options. With education, persons living with an ostomy will continue to enjoy their previous quality of life.

Ensure that persons with ostomies know about:

- The surgical technique, resulting stoma position/characteristics and type of output or effluent
- The postoperative care with an emphasis on stoma and skin care
- What is considered normal and when to contact a healthcare practitioner

- Appliance fit, techniques and options
- The amount of time an appliance should be worn—scheduling changes may help prevent problems
- The available cleansers and deodorants
- Recognizing and treating common skin problems
- What to do if abdominal changes occur, e.g., weight changes, pregnancy.

Travelling with an Ostomy

It is usually recommended to travel with more supplies than needed and to empty the pouch immediately before boarding an airplane. Supplies should be protected from the extremes of hot and cold temperature. For example, ostomy supplies should not be left in the glove compartment of a very hot car. The changes in temperature, diet and activities that occur during travelling usually decrease the usual wear times for appliances. Compliance with vehicle seat belt legislation is essential. However, placement of a seat belt across the appliance or directly on the stoma may cause pressure or friction. To prevent potential injury place a soft foam padding or a small pillow between the stoma location and the seat belt. When travelling by airplane, persons with ostomies should carry their ostomy supplies in their carry-on luggage and ensure they have sufficient supplies.

It is recommended to carry a physician's letter stating that ostomy supplies are required and mentioning that a private area may be necessary for a search. Currently, for security reasons, most airports prohibit scissors in carry-on luggage. Scissors, if required, will need to be packed in checked luggage.

Resource Tips

Canadian Association for Enterostomal Therapy. 66 Leopolds Drive, Ottawa, Ontario K1V 7E3. Telephone: 1-888-739-5072. Available from: www.caet.ca.

Canadian Cancer Society. National Office, 55 St. Clair Avenue West, Suite 300, Toronto, Ontario, M4V 2Y7. Telephone: 416-961-7223. Available from: www.cancer.ca.

Crohn's and Colitis Canada. 600-60 St. Clair Avenue East, Toronto, Ontario, M4T 1N5. Telephone: 1-800-387-1479. E-mail: support@crohnsandcolitis.ca. Available from: www.crohnsandcolitis.ca.

International Ostomy Association. P.O. Box 512, Northfield, Minnesota, 55057. Telephone: 1-800-826-0826. Available from: www.ostomyinternational.org.

Ostomy Canada Society. 5800 Ambler Drive, Suite 210, Mississauga, Ontario, L4W 4J4. Telephone: 1-888-969-9698. Available from: www.ostomycanada.ca.

Wound, Ostomy and Continence Nurses Society. 1120 Rt. 73, Suite 200, Mount Laurel, New Jersey, 08054. Available from: www.wocn.org (more suitable for health care professionals).

Suggested Readings

Basic ostomy skin care: a guide for patients and healthcare providers. Mount Laurel: WOCN; 2006.

Dorman C. Ostomy basics. *RN* 2009;72:22-7.

Floruta CV. Dietary choices of people with ostomies. *J Wound Ostomy Continence Nurs* 2001;28:28-31.

Hampton BG, Bryant RA. *Ostomies and continent diversions: nursing management*. St Louis: Mosby Year Book; 1992.

Patient Education Series. *Managing your ostomy*. Libertyville: Hollister Inc.; 2003.

A professional's guide for counselling ostomy patients. Princeton: ConvaTec; 1998.

Zanni GR, Wick JY. Ostomy care and the consultant pharmacist. *Consult Pharm* 2006;21:262-4, 267-70, 272-4.

References

1. Wound, Ostomy and Continence Nurses Society. Available from: www.wocn.org. Accessed August 31, 2009.
2. Mitchel JV. A clinical pathway for ostomy care in the home: process and development. *J Wound Ostomy Continence Nurs* 1998;25:200-5.
3. Rozen BL. The value of a well-placed stoma. *Cancer Pract* 1997;5:347-52.
4. Colwell JC, Goldberg M, Carmel J. The state of the standard diversion. *J Wound Ostomy Continence Nurs* 2001;28:6-17.
5. Rarliff CR, Donovan AM. Frequency of peristomal complications. *Ostomy Wound Manage* 2001;47:26-9.
6. ConvaTec Inc. *Maintaining healthy peristomal skin*. Available from: www.convatec.com/ostomy/living-with-an-ostomy/skin-care-tips/maintaining-healthy-peristomal-skin. Accessed February 2, 2016.
7. Bradley M, Pupiales M. Essential elements of ostomy care. *Am J Nurs* 1997;97:38-45.
8. Chicago Dietetic Association; South Suburban Dietetic Association; Dietitians of Canada. *Manual of clinical dietetics*. 6th ed. Chicago: American Dietetic Association; 2000.
9. Canadian Paediatric Society. Caring for Kids. *Dehydration and diarrhea in children: prevention and treatment*. Available from: www.caringforkids.cps.ca/handouts/dehydration_and_diarrhea. Accessed October 25, 2010.
10. JAMA patient page. Preventing dehydration from diarrhea. *JAMA* 2001;285:362.
11. Singer GG, Brenner BM. Fluid and electrolyte disturbances. In: Fauci AS, Braunwald E, Isselbacher KJ et al., eds. *Harrison's principles of internal medicine*. 14th ed. New York: McGraw-Hill; 1998. p. 265-77.
12. Schultz NJ, Slaker RA. Electrolyte homeostasis. In: DiPiro JT, Talbert RL, Yee GC et al., eds. *Pharmacotherapy: a pathophysiologic approach*. 4th ed. Stamford: Appleton & Lange; 1999. p. 890-917.
13. Metcalf C. Stoma care: empowering patients through teaching skills. *Br J Nurs* 1999;8:593-600.
14. Wood S. Nutrition and stoma patients. *Nurs Times* 1998;94:65.
15. Aron S, Carrareto R, Prazeres SM et al. Self-perceptions about having an ostomy: a postoperative analysis. *Ostomy Wound Manage* 1999;45:46-50, 52-4, 56.

Chapter 38
Perianal Symptom Assessment

Joyce Chan, BScPhm, MSc, PharmD

CPhA acknowledges the contribution of Patricia Carruthers-Czyzewski as a previous author of this chapter.

Assessment Algorithm

Figure 1: **Assessment of Patients with Perianal Symptoms**

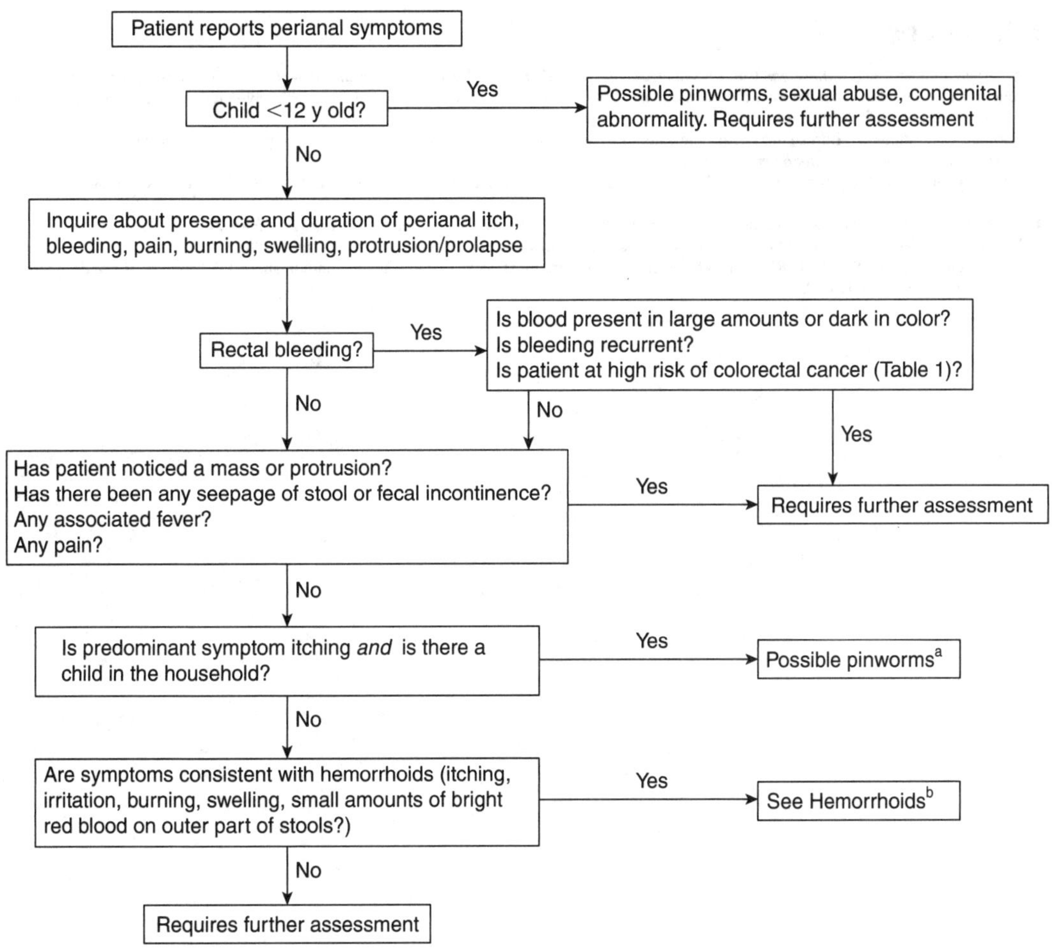

a See Chapter 39: Pinworms.
b See Chapter 33: Hemorrhoids.

Patients may erroneously attribute any perianal symptom to hemorrhoids. In fact, these symptoms may be due to a number of conditions, ranging in severity from poor hygiene to colorectal cancer (Table 1).[1] An assessment plan for patients reporting perianal symptoms is illustrated in Figure 1.[2,3,4,5,6] All too often, patients seeking relief with nonprescription agents have delayed consulting a healthcare practitioner until the symptoms have become unbearable and the condition has advanced to the point where medical referral is necessary.

Table 1: **Risk Factors for Colorectal Cancer**[1]

- Age >50 y
- History of colorectal cancer or adenomatous polyposis
- Family history of familial adenomatous polyposis or hereditary nonpolyposis colon cancer (Lynch syndrome)
- Inflammatory bowel disease
- Strong family history (either cancer or polyps in a first-degree relative <60 y or 2 first-degree relatives of any age)

References

1. American Cancer Society. *American Cancer Society recommendations for colorectal cancer early detection*. Available from: www.cancer.org/cancer/colonandrectumcancer/moreinformation/colonandrectumcancerearlydetection/colorectal-cancer-early-detection-acs-recommendations. Accessed February 18, 2016.
2. Turnbull GK, Vanner SJ, Burnstein M et al. The colon. In: Thomson AB, Shaffer EA, eds. *First principles of gastroenterology: the basis of disease and an approach to management*. 5th ed. Toronto: Janssen-Ortho; 2005.
3. Zuber TJ. Diseases of the rectum and anus. In: Taylor RB, ed. *Family medicine: principles and practice*. 6th ed. New York: Springer; 2003. p. 776-83.
4. Pfenniger JL, Zainea GG. Common anorectal conditions: Part I. Symptoms and complaints. *Am Fam Physician* 2001;63:2391-8.
5. Pfenniger JL, Zainea GG. Common anorectal conditions: Part II. Lesions. *Am Fam Physician* 2001;64:77-88.
6. Schubert MC, Sridhar S, Schade RR et al. What every gastroenterologist needs to know about common anorectal disorders. *World J Gastroenterol* 2009;15:3201-9.

Chapter 39

Pinworms

Joyce Chan, BScPhm, MSc, PharmD

CPhA acknowledges the contribution of Patricia Carruthers-Czyzewski as a previous author of this chapter.

Pathophysiology

Enterobiasis is an intestinal infection caused by the nematode *Enterobius vermicularis* (commonly referred to as pinworm, seatworm, roundworm or threadworm).[1] Although the adult worms resemble white cotton threads about 1 cm in length, the name threadworm is best reserved for *Strongyloides stercoralis*.

Humans are the only natural host of *E. vermicularis*. Cats and dogs have been shown to hold eggs on their fur, probably as a result of dust contamination (e.g., shaking bedclothes in their presence) but there is no evidence they can act as carriers of the infection.[2,3]

Transmission of *E. vermicularis* follows ingestion of mature eggs. The larvae mature in the gut in approximately 1–2 months. The eggs are not released into the gut contents but the mature female migrates to the anus at night and lays its eggs on the perianal or perineal skin. The eggs become infective within 6 hours and are transferred from the perianal region to night clothes, bedding, dust and air. The most common mode of transmission is on hands and under fingernails, either through scratching or handling infected clothes and linen.[4,5,6] Eggs can remain infective for up to 20 days.[5]

Pinworms are particularly common in young children 5–10 years of age and uncommon in children younger than 2 years. An estimated one-third of Canadian children will be infested during their childhood. It is the most common intestinal parasite seen in the primary care setting, regardless of race, socioeconomic or cultural circumstances.[4,7]

Enterobiasis is more prevalent in temperate and cold climates because of less frequent bathing and infrequent changing of underclothing.[3] It is facilitated by factors such as overcrowding in schools and family groupings as well as inadequate personal and community hygiene. The infestation is more common in homosexual men, institutionalized patients, residents of native reserves, travellers to areas of high incidence such as India and Iran, families with school-aged children and primary caregivers of infected children.[2]

Despite the high prevalence of pinworms, it is a rather innocuous parasite. The usual consequences of infection include loss of sleep, discomfort due to anal itching and embarrassment due to the social connotations of having "worms." Often an entire family is affected. Only rarely have infections been associated with significant pathology, including appendicitis, chronic salpingitis and ulcerative lesions of the small and large intestine.[4]

Goals of Therapy

- Relieve symptoms such as itchiness
- Eliminate the infection
- Promote good hygiene
- Prevent transmission
- Prevent complications

- Prevent reinfection

Patient Assessment

Though many infections are asymptomatic, enterobiasis is often associated with perianal or perineal itching.[4] The itching is worse at night, when the females lay eggs that are attached to the perianal area by a sticky substance that causes pruritus. The itching may contribute to insomnia and restlessness.

Scratching may cause skin irritation. If severe scratching occurs, the skin may break down and allow development of a secondary bacterial infection, eczematous dermatitis or bleeding.[8] If the worm migrates to the genital area in females, vulvovaginitis, vaginal discharge and irritation may be seen.[9] Enuresis has also been attributed to pinworms.[3] Although symptoms may alert the parent or patient to a potential problem, studies have shown no difference in the incidence of "classic" symptoms between infected and noninfected children.[4] This reinforces the need for actual viewing of the pinworm or its ova for definite diagnosis (see Diagnosis of Pinworm).

Conditions such as diaper dermatitis, constipation, psoriasis of the anogenital region, and perianal eczema may mimic symptoms of pinworms and should be considered in patients presenting with perianal itching.

An uncomplicated pinworm infection does not usually cause abdominal pain, severe diarrhea, bloody bowel movements, dysuria, fever or extreme poor appetite. If the patient has any of these signs or symptoms, or if neurotic excoriation (self-inflicted lesions produced by repetitive scratching) or sexual abuse is suspected, further assessment and medical attention are required.[8]

Refer all those with suspected pinworm infestation to a physician so the diagnosis can be confirmed. This is especially important in pregnant women, children under 12 and those with renal or hepatic impairment.

Diagnosis of Pinworm

Pinworm diagnosis is contingent on visual identification of either the ova or the worm itself.[1,4,7] The 3 most common diagnostic methods are:

- Inspection of the perianal area:[1] parents may observe the worms during ovipositing by putting the child to bed without underpants and using a flashlight to examine the anus after the child has been sleeping for 1 hour. Worms obtained by the parents should be placed in alcohol or vinegar and brought to the clinic for confirmation of the diagnosis.
- Scotch-tape test (cellulose-tape slide test):[1] this test is performed at home in the morning before defecation or washing. A piece of transparent adhesive tape is pressed on the perianal skin, then stuck to a slide to be examined under a microscope. Diagnosis is confirmed by identification of pinworm ova. The test may have to be repeated several times. A single examination will confirm the diagnosis in 50%, 3 exams in 90% and 5 exams in 99% of cases.
- Microscopic analysis of subungual samples:[6] ova may be found under the fingernails of infected patients since anal itching is a common symptom of pinworm infection.

Prevention

Prevention is difficult. However, proper hygiene is helpful and includes careful handwashing after going to the toilet, after scratching the perianal area and before and after eating or preparing food.[2]

Nonpharmacologic Therapy

As with prevention, proper hygiene is an important component of nonpharmacologic management of pinworm infestations. If ingestion of eggs can be avoided, the infection is usually self-limiting. In practice, however, this is difficult to achieve and pharmacologic therapy is usually necessary for eradication.

Nonpharmacologic measures should always be used as adjunctive therapy in combination with any drug treatment. These include:

- Showering each morning
- Regular cleaning of bedding (every 3–7 days for 3 weeks)[8]
- Washing night clothes, underwear and hand towels daily for 2 weeks[8]
- Changing night clothes and sheets frequently and at the start of each treatment course
- Handwashing and fingernail cleaning, especially prior to meals and after using the bathroom or scratching the perianal area
- Keeping fingernails short and clean[8]
- During the week following treatment, all family members should wear cotton underpants that have been washed in hot soapy water. These should be worn day and night and changed twice daily
- Cleansing of the floors of sleeping quarters as thoroughly as possible with household cleaner and water or by airing and vacuuming around beds, curtains and other articles in the bedroom where the highest concentrations of eggs are likely to occur
- Frequent washing of the toilet seat
- Avoiding shaking linens or clothing prior to washing
- Discouraging thumb sucking.

Cleaning or vacuuming the entire house or washing the sheets every day is probably not effective in preventing reinfection.

Pharmacologic Therapy

For comparative ingredients of nonprescription products, consult the *Compendium of Products for Minor Ailments*—Anthelmintic Products.

A confirmed diagnosis by an appropriate healthcare practitioner is recommended before pharmacologic treatment is initiated to minimize unnecessary exposure to potential adverse effects of the anthelmintics. Pinworm infections respond readily to drug therapy but reinfection is common.[7] Treatment failure is usually due to reinfection.

Treatment with the anthelmintics **mebendazole** or **pyrantel pamoate** results in a high cure rate with minimal side effects (see Table 2).[5] Since these anthelmintics do not reliably kill pinworm eggs it is prudent to retreat 2 weeks later.[2,8,10] Since reinfection occurs easily, prevention (e.g., handwashing) should always be discussed at the time of treatment. Since pinworms can be passed from one person to another, some experts suggest treating all close contacts of a person with pinworms even if they are asymptomatic. Treating contacts can help prevent reinfection and the spread of pinworms. This is especially important in households where more than one member is infected or where repeated, symptomatic infections occur. However, medical treatment may not be always appropriate for infants or pregnant or breastfeeding women (see Pregnancy and Breastfeeding). The use of laxatives to facilitate removal of pinworms after anthelmintic therapy is not necessary.

To relieve the intense itching that often accompanies pinworm infection, a soothing ointment or cream (e.g., a **zinc oxide** preparation) can be recommended.

Pregnancy and Breastfeeding

If possible, asymptomatic pregnant women should be treated after delivery since there are no harmful effects to mother or fetus from the pinworm infection. When a pregnant woman is symptomatic and natural cure by scrupulous attention to personal hygiene is unlikely, treatment with **mebendazole** or **pyrantel pamoate** may be used after the first trimester (preferably in the third trimester) on a case-by-case basis.[2,11,12,13,14,15]

Mebendazole and pyrantel pamoate are considered compatible with breastfeeding.[16,17]

Monitoring of Therapy

Table 1 provides a monitoring plan framework, which should be individualized.

Table 1: **Monitoring of Therapy for Pinworms**

Symptoms	Monitoring	Endpoint of Therapy	Actions
Perianal itching	Parent/patient: Daily Healthcare practitioner: Day 7	Resolution of itching	If itching has not resolved within 7–14 days of starting medication, repeat treatment. If itching has not resolved within 7 days of beginning second course, or if signs of bacterial superinfection occur, refer to an appropriate healthcare practitioner for further assessment.
Adverse effects: nausea, vomiting, diarrhea, abdominal cramps	Parent/patient: Daily Healthcare practitioner: Day 1 after treatment	Minimal GI effects	If adverse GI effects interfere with functioning or persist more than 3 days after treatment ends, consult with an appropriate healthcare practitioner.
Adverse effects: dizziness, drowsiness	Parent/patient: Daily Healthcare practitioner: Day 1 after treatment	Minimal drowsiness or dizziness	Caution patient not to drive or use hazardous machinery until effect of drug is known. If symptoms interfere with function or persist more than 24 h after treatment, consult with an appropriate healthcare practitioner.

Advice for the Patient

Advise patient regarding:

- Proper use of the drug and need for any repeat doses
- The need to treat infected family members or close household contacts at the same time (unless there is a contraindication)
- Adjunctive nonpharmacologic measures and proper hygiene
- Expected results of drug therapy and management of side effects
- The mostly innocuous nature of a pinworm infection
- Visiting a healthcare practitioner if symptoms recur.

Table 2: Pharmacologic Therapy for Pinworm Infection

Class	Drug	Dosage	Adverse Effects	Drug Interactions	Comments	Cost[a]
Anthelmintics	*mebendazole* Vermox	**Adults and children ≥2 y**: 100 mg single dose po; repeat in 2 wk	Abdominal pain, anemia, diarrhea, dizziness, drowsiness, eosinophilia, flatulence, headache, hematuria, itching, neutropenia, vomiting.	Mebendazole may raise risk of Stevens-Johnson syndrome or toxic epidermal necrolysis when coadministered with metronidazole; avoid combination. Mebendazole plasma levels may be decreased by carbamazepine or phenytoin and increased by cimetidine.	No special procedures such as fasting or bowel evacuation are required when treating with mebendazole.	$12
	pyrantel pamoate Combantrin, generics	**Adults and children >1 y**: 11 mg/kg (base) single dose po; repeat in 2 wk **Maximum:** 1 g (base)	Anorexia, nausea, vomiting, abdominal cramps, diarrhea, headache, dizziness, drowsiness; transient elevation of aspartate aminotransferase has been reported.	Pyrantel pamoate and piperazine have antagonistic effects; avoid combination.	11 mg/kg base equals 31.9 mg/kg pyrantel pamoate. Liquid form (50 mg/mL base) should be shaken well before use. Tablets available as 125 mg pyrantel base. Avoid in the first trimester of pregnancy. Caution in hepatic impairment.	$14

[a] Cost of 2 doses based on 70 kg body weight; includes drug cost only.

Suggested Readings

eMedicineHealth by WebMD. Mersch J. *Pinworms*. Available from: www.emedicinehealth.com. Registration required.

Kucik CJ, Martin GL, Sortor BV. Common intestinal parasites. *Am Fam Physician* 2004;69:1161-8.

References

1. Health Canada. Drugs and Health Products. *Anthelmintics: labelling standard.* Available from: www.hc-sc.gc.ca/dhp-mps/prodpharma/applic-demande/guide-ld/label-etiquet-pharm/anthelmi-eng.php. Accessed May 3, 2016.
2. Cook GC. Enterobius vermicularis infection. *Gut* 1994;35:1159-62.
3. Russell LJ. The pinworm, Enterobius vermicularis. *Prim Care* 1991;18:13-24.
4. Maguire JH. Intestinal nematodes (roundworms). In: Mandell GL, Bennett JE, Dolin R et al., eds. *Mandell, Douglas and Bennett's principles and practice of infectious diseases*. 7th ed. Philadelphia: Elsevier Churchill Livingstone; 2009. p. 3577-86.
5. Grencis RK, Cooper ES. Enterobius, trichuris, capillaria, and hookworm including ancylostoma caninum. *Gastroenterol Clin North Am* 1996;25:579-97.
6. Centers for Disease Control and Prevention. *Parasites—Enterobiasis (also known as pinworm infection)*. Available from: www.cdc.gov/parasites/pinworm/. Accessed April 1, 2016.
7. Juckett G. Common intestinal helminths. *Am Fam Physician* 1995;52:2039-48, 2051-2.
8. eMedicineHealth by WebMD. Mersch J. *Pinworms*. Available from: www.emedicinehealth.com. Registration required.
9. Centers for Disease Control and Prevention. Laboratory Identification of Public Health Concern. Division of Parasitic Diseases (DPDx). *Parasites and health: enterobiasis*. Available from: www.dpd.cdc.gov/dpdx/HTML/Enterobiasis.htm. Accessed May 3, 2016.
10. Drugs for parasitic infections. *Med Lett Drugs Ther* 2007;(Suppl):1-15.
11. Tietze PE, Jones JE. Parasites during pregnancy. *Prim Care* 1991;18:75-99.
12. Van Riper G. Pyrantel pamoate for pinworm infestation. *Am Pharm* 1993;NS33:43-5.
13. Leach FN. Treatment of threadworm infestation during pregnancy. *Arch Dis Child* 1990;65:399-400.
14. de Silva NR, Sirisena JL, Gunaskera DP et al. Effect of mebendazole therapy during pregnancy on birth outcome. *Lancet* 1999;353:1145-9.
15. Diav-Citrin O, Shechtman S, Arnon J et al. Pregnancy outcome after gestational exposure to mebendazole: a prospective controlled cohort study. *Am J Obstet Gynecol* 2003;188:282-5.
16. World Health Organization. *Breastfeeding and maternal medication: recommendations for drugs in the eleventh WHO model list of essential drugs*. Available from: apps.who.int/iris/bitstream/10665/62435/1/55732.pdf.
17. Centers for Disease Control and Prevention. *Parasites—Enterobiasis (also known as pinworm infection): resources for health professionals.* Available from: www.cdc.gov/parasites/pinworm/health_professionals/.

Pinworms—What You Need to Know

Pinworms are an infection of the intestine caused by a tiny worm. The infection is very common, especially in children. Pinworms do not usually cause serious problems.

How do you get pinworms?

Pinworms spread easily from one person to another. If one person in a family has pinworms, there is a good chance that everyone in the family will have them. You may become infected with pinworms if you get pinworm eggs on your hands and transfer them to your mouth or food.

You cannot see pinworm eggs because they are very small. The eggs can live on sheets, clothing, toys, bathroom walls or toilets. They also live on an infected person's hands.

What are the signs of pinworms?

A person with pinworms may have a very itchy bottom (anus) or belly pain. They may have trouble sleeping or be irritable. Many people with pinworms show no signs at all.

How do you treat pinworms?

See your doctor if you think that you or someone you live with may have pinworms. Do not use any medicine until you have an accurate diagnosis.

If you need medicine, it is important to take the right amount and to follow the directions exactly. Talk to the pharmacist to make sure you understand the directions. Most people need to take a second dose of the medicine after about 2 weeks to be sure the infection is gone.

How can you prevent pinworms from coming back?

- Everyone in the house should keep their nails cut short.
- Everyone should wash their hands and scrub their nails after using the toilet and before eating or preparing meals.
- Wash underwear and sleepwear in hot water every day for 2 weeks to destroy the eggs.
- Wear pajamas or pants at night to prevent yourself from scratching while you are asleep.
- To stop the spread of eggs, do not shake sleepwear, sheets or blankets before washing them. Fold them up and wash them right away (in hot water).
- Do not use disinfectants to kill the eggs. They do not work.

Chapter 40
Infant Nutrition

Joan Brennan-Donnan, BASc, RD

CPhA acknowledges the contribution of Sandra Bjelajac Mejia as a previous author of this chapter.

Breastfeeding

Exclusive breastfeeding of infants (defined by the World Health Organization as only breast milk—no solids and no other liquids, not even water, with the exception of drops or syrups consisting of vitamins, mineral supplements or medicines) is considered the gold standard for feeding infants for the first 6 months of life.[1,2,3,4] However, the consensus is that breastfeeding continues to benefit the nutritional, emotional and immunologic health of the child until up to 2 years of age.[1,2]

Statistics Canada reported that a majority (90%) of mothers in Canada attempt to breastfeed their babies.[5] This is higher than the rate of breastfeeding in the United States (77%), but lower than the rates in both Norway and Australia (95% and 92% respectively).[6] However, only 27% of Canadian mothers breastfeed exclusively for at least 6 months.[5] With breastfeeding initiation rates low in some provinces and duration rates below ideal levels across Canada, healthcare practitioners have a role to play in promotion of this important preventive health measure.

Peer support groups provide information, practical assistance and emotional support for breastfeeding mothers using a mother-to-mother approach. These include local La Leche League Canada groups or breastfeeding classes. Many hospitals offer women breastfeeding support and/or a breastfeeding clinic. Healthcare professionals can augment this support by ensuring that therapeutic or other interventions, if possible, allow a mother to maintain the breastfeeding relationship with her baby.[7] Problems encountered by women that may compromise continuation of breastfeeding should be addressed by breastfeeding experts, who may be public health nurses, dietitians, the mother's physician, La Leche League Canada leaders or International Board Certified Lactation Consultants (IBCLCs).

Benefits of Breastfeeding

Human milk feeding has acknowledged short-term and long-term benefits including improvement in health (specifically GI function, host defense and neurodevelopment) as well as social, psychological and economic advantages.[3,7,8] All alternative feeding products are measured against the known benefits of human milk with regard to growth and development. Research shows that human milk feeding reduces the incidence and in many cases the severity of a number of illnesses, such as asthma, atopic dermatitis, childhood leukemia, type 1 and type 2 diabetes, necrotizing enterocolitis, nonspecific gastroenteritis, otitis media, severe lower respiratory tract infections and sudden infant death syndrome.[9] Preterm infants fed human milk show improved developmental outcomes when compared with formula-fed infants.[10,11,12] Although the evidence is not as compelling as for preterm infant data, studies have shown improved neurodevelopmental outcomes in full-term breastfed infants.[13] Further research is needed to clarify any potential effect on cardiovascular disease, infant mortality, obesity[14,15,16,17] and childhood cancers.[9,18]

For mothers, breastfeeding contributes to a number of health benefits.[9] These include decreased postpartum bleeding and more rapid return to pre-pregnancy uterine size,[19] reduced risk of type 2 diabetes, reduced risk of postpartum depression and a decreased risk of some cancers (breast and ovarian).[9,20] The relationship between breastfeeding and improved bone health[21] and more rapid return to pre-pregnancy weight[22] requires further study.[9]

Contraindications to Breastfeeding

Contraindications to breastfeeding in the mother are few and occur rarely. Breastfeeding might be contraindicated when the mother:[3,23]

- is HIV antibody–positive
- is acutely infected with H1N1 influenza (may resume once afebrile)
- has cancer and is undergoing chemotherapy (or tamoxifen treatment for breast cancer[24])
- has untreated, active tuberculosis (a mother being treated for active tuberculosis can breastfeed if she is considered noninfectious, i.e., has been treated for at least 2 weeks)
- has untreated brucellosis[25]
- has active herpes simplex virus outbreak on her breast
- has human T-cell lymphotropic virus (HTLV) type I or II
- is taking a drug not compatible with breastfeeding.

Breastfeeding is also contraindicated when the baby has galactosemia, an inborn error of metabolism where the ability to break down galactose is absent and the baby cannot tolerate breast milk.

Establishing Breastfeeding

Breastfed babies nurse for both food and comfort. Direct skin-to-skin contact between mother and baby soon after birth can help to establish breastfeeding.[26] Pacifiers and artificial nipples may be detrimental to establishing breastfeeding, and should be avoided if possible.[1] Mothers should be encouraged to breastfeed every 2–3 hours (8–12 feedings in a 24-hour period) during the first weeks postpartum. Educate mothers about the signs of hunger, satiety and a good latch and letdown. Breastfed babies may seem to be more wakeful and to feed more frequently, because the components in human milk are easily and readily digested. Colostrum, the yellowish milk produced in the first day or two is high in nutrients and immunoglobulins. Because this substance is present in small amounts, the baby is stimulated to nurse frequently, which establishes an appropriate milk supply. On day 3 or 4 postpartum the milk comes in as the colostrum changes to mature milk. Milk supply then increases to the individualized quantity required by the baby or babies in the case of twins or triplets. Removal of milk, through breastfeeding or expressing, acts to increase production of milk.

Infants who do not readily arouse for feeding should be wakened to feed if more than 4 hours have elapsed since the start of the last feeding. Signs of adequate intake include 3–5 wet diapers daily by day 3–5, and 4–6 wet diapers daily by day 5–7. After breastfeeding is established, the number of feedings usually declines to 6–8 every 24 hours.[3]

Once the mother's milk supply comes in, a well-hydrated, healthy baby will have 3–5 wet diapers and pale, odourless urine. Brick-coloured crystals in the baby's diaper indicate the infant is not receiving appropriate amounts of fluid and necessitates referral, especially if the child is under 6 weeks of age. Once the baby's first stool, called meconium, has passed in the first several days, the breastfed baby will have 2–5 loose, unformed yellow/green/tan bowel movements per day. After 6 weeks of age the number of bowel movements and wet diapers may become less frequent. Healthy breastfed infants require no extra water, even in hot weather, as long as breastfeeding is readily available to the infant.

At ages 3 weeks, 6 weeks and 3 months, it is normal for babies to nurse more frequently for a few days to increase milk supply to meet their growing needs. By reviewing the signs of adequate milk supply (above), healthcare professionals can help a mother differentiate a growth spurt from a change in milk supply.

Some mothers may not produce enough milk to maintain their baby's needs. A breastfeeding expert should assess the problem and initiate counseling, relaxation techniques or mechanical expression. If nonpharmacologic therapy is unsuccessful, treatment with **domperidone** 30 mg/day is an option. By blocking D_2 and D_3 dopamine receptors in the pituitary gland, domperidone increases prolactin levels and breast milk production. Potential QT prolongation, ventricular arrhythmias and sudden cardiac death have been reported when doses of domperidone >30 mg/day are used in patients at risk of sudden cardiac death.[27] Prior to initiation, screen mothers for comorbid medical conditions, the use of QT-prolonging medications and drugs that may interact with domperidone. Regularly monitor for efficacy and adverse reactions.[27]

Fenugreek is a commonly recommended natural health product to increase breast milk supply, although evidence of its efficacy is minimal.[28] The standard dose of fenugreek capsules is 580–610 mg 3–4 times daily. Fenugreek seeds (one-quarter teaspoonful) may also be steeped in 8 oz (250 mL) of water for 10 minutes to produce a tea, of which the standard dose is 1 cup 3 times daily.

Products that Support Breastfeeding

For comparative features of nonprescription products, consult the *Compendium of Products for Minor Ailments*—Breastfeeding Products: Collection Accessories, Nipple Accessories, Pumps.

Breast Pumps

A breast pump (Figure 1) may be used to express and store milk when breastfeeding is not possible. With practice, hand expression is learned. Many types of electric or manual breast pumps are available; funnels (flanges) are available in various sizes as one size will not suit all mothers.

Figure 1: **Breast Pump**

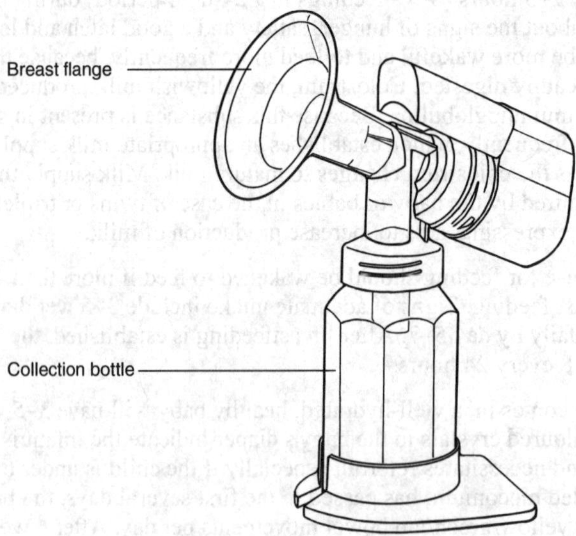

Several companies offer a range of electric breast pumps for purchase or rent. Advise mothers to speak with their local hospital's breastfeeding support clinic for information. Electric breast pumps are most effective and are recommended when a mother is separated from a hospitalized baby, when the mother must remove milk quickly and efficiently, or when the baby is unable to nurse (when the mother's breasts are engorged). Most electric pumps have adapter kits that allow mothers to pump both breasts at the same time. This increases stimulation, which in turn increases her milk supply and facilitates removal of milk. The kits can often be turned into manual cylinder or handle-squeeze pumps with the purchase of adapter parts.

Usually a good quality, manual (hand-operated) pump will suffice for the occasional feed when breastfeeding is not possible. Bicycle horn–type pumps are not recommended as lack of control on suction may bruise the breast, and milk can collect in and contaminate the bulb.

Report any instances of breast pumps causing damage or injuring a mother during use to Health Canada's Medical Device Problem Reporting program. Information may be found at www.hc-sc.gc.ca/dhp-mps/compli-conform/prob-report-rapport/md_prob_rep-rap_incident_im-eng.php.

Breast Pads

Reusable, washable, cotton breast pads are recommended, as disposable pads with plastic or occlusive liners promote dampness and increase the risk of a yeast (*Candida*) infection on the breast. Breast pads should be changed with each feeding. Mothers should not use cut-up disposable baby diapers, as the water-retaining beads in the diapers can be harmful to the baby if accidentally ingested. Once breastfeeding is established, after 6–8 weeks, leaking is not usually a problem.

Nipple Shields

Silicone nipple shields are worn over sore or abraded nipples while the baby nurses, to overcome latch problems or to help infants with physical challenges or impaired suck mechanisms. Over time, the use of a nipple shield may lower a mother's milk supply and should be used only on the recommendation of a breastfeeding expert.

Breast Shells

Breast shells are firm, plastic, cup-shaped devices that can be worn inside the bra between feeds to provide air flow during healing of an abraded nipple, or to shape the nipple between feeds for easier latch of the baby. Wearing the shells inside the bra for several hours per day for 6–12 weeks before delivery may draw out flat or inverted nipples. An estimated 10% of women have nipples that retract rather than protrude when the areola is compressed. However, proper latch of the baby after birth may overcome this problem.[29] Breast shells are not to be used to collect milk or in place of breast pads. Constant pressure on the ducts interferes with natural control mechanisms for leaking.

Mother Care

While breastfeeding, a mother should drink to satisfy her thirst and eat according to *Canada's Food Guide*, which also recommends supplementation with a multivitamin that includes folic acid.[30] For information regarding galactogogues, see Establishing Breastfeeding.

Nipple Trauma

Nipple trauma is a cutaneous lesion in the area of the nipple and areola manifesting as fissures, ulceration, erythema, edema, blisters, pain or bruising. Nipple trauma is common among newly breastfeeding mothers with an incidence ranging from 29–76%.[31] The most common cause of nipple trauma is improper latch of the baby to the breast. Proper latch is attachment that causes no overt pain and maximizes transfer of milk to baby. Advise a mother with nipple pain to contact a breastfeeding expert to check the baby's position on the breast. **Lanolin**, alone or with breast shells, and breast milk expressed and applied before and after each feeding have demonstrated efficacy in reducing nipple trauma.[31] Applying **olive oil** before suckling was effective for sore nipples in a preliminary study.[32] Irrespective of which treatment is used (including no treatment), most nipple pain subsides to low levels at 7–10 days postpartum (see Establishing Successful Latch in Photo Section).[33]

Thrush (due to the yeast-like fungus *Candida albicans*) is another common cause of nipple and breast pain, usually occurring later in the course of breastfeeding. Burning or stabbing pain as well as red, shiny skin on the nipple and areola are characteristic signs. Prior treatment with antibiotics predisposes mothers to yeast infections on the breast. If the mother is diagnosed with thrush on the breast, it is important that both the mother and baby are treated. The mother may use a **topical antifungal** cream, e.g., **nystatin** or **clotrimazole** (see Chapter 65: Fungal Skin Infections). The baby may be prescribed an **oral antifungal** medication such as **nystatin**. Mothers should practise good hygiene to prevent infecting or reinfecting the baby, or developing a vaginal yeast infection.

Any product applied to the breast or nipple area should be wiped off by the mother before she nurses her baby.

Sore Breasts

A common cause of pain and swelling of the breasts during the establishment of breastfeeding is engorgement, typically caused by the arrival of new milk.[34] Mild engorgement is normal and reassures the mother that an adequate milk supply exists. However, if the engorgement is severely symptomatic and painful, it should be treated. Nonpharmacologic options include applying gentle pressure to the areola to move the swelling upward into the breast; this helps with the infant's latch. If this does not enable the infant to latch, manual expression should be tried. **Acetaminophen** and **ibuprofen** are also safe treatment options for the management of breast engorgement.

Mastitis is a painful inflammatory condition of the breast usually resulting from a plugged duct or a breast infection. A plugged duct occurs when a milk duct does not drain properly and becomes inflamed, causing soreness, redness and sometimes a lump. Fever and flu-like symptoms may be present as a result of the inflammation, but may also indicate the presence of an infection. When a plugged duct is not resolved within 24 hours by increased breastfeeding on the affected side, locally applied heat, massage and rest, and an infection ensues, an antibiotic must be prescribed.[35] Most antibiotics are safe to use during breastfeeding. Mothers with recurrent mastitis should be referred to a breastfeeding expert.

Principles of Drug and Natural Health Product Use during Breastfeeding

A mother may continue to breastfeed her baby while on medication depending on whether the benefit to the mother outweighs the risk of the baby's exposure to the medication. Most drugs are excreted to some extent in breast milk; however, drugs considered compatible with breastfeeding far outnumber those that are not.[36,37,38,39]

The texts *Drugs in Pregnancy and Lactation* (Briggs and Freeman)[40] and *Medications and Mothers' Milk* (Hale and Rowe)[41] are comprehensive sources of information on drugs and breastfeeding. Knowledge about safety of medications transferred from mother's milk to baby is evolving. For a selection of reliable and authoritative web-based resources see Table 1.

Table 1: **Online Sources of Information about Compatibility of Drugs and Natural Health Products with Breastfeeding**

Database	Web Address (URL)
Drug Use during Breastfeeding	www.myrxtx.ca (formerly www.e-therapeutics.ca) Requires subscription
LactMed—Drugs and Lactation Database housed within the TOXNET web site	www.toxnet.nlm.nih.gov/cgi-bin/sis/htmlgen?LACT Free of charge
Motherisk—provides evidence-based information and guidance about the safety or risk to the developing fetus or infant arising from maternal exposure to drugs, chemicals, diseases, radiation and environmental agents	www.motherisk.org Free of charge

For more information on pharmacotherapies during breastfeeding, see Chapter 82: Prenatal and Postpartum Care and Appendix V: Pregnancy and Breastfeeding: Self-care Therapy for Common Conditions.

Infant Formula

For comparative ingredients of nonprescription products, consult the *Compendium of Products for Minor Ailments*—Nutrition Products: Infant Formulas.

In both Canada and the United States, regulatory bodies are responsible for ensuring the safety and nutritional adequacy of infant formulas. In Canada, this responsibility lies with Health Canada under provision of the Canadian Food and Drug Regulations.

If the mother chooses not to breastfeed exclusively, commercial iron-fortified infant formulas are an acceptable alternative until 9–12 months of age.

Most infant formulas are available as powder concentrate, liquid concentrate and/or ready-to-use varieties. Not all products are available in all forms. Powdered formulas tend to be more appealing as they are less expensive than both liquid concentrate and ready-to-use forms. They are more portable than the liquid options and the unreconstituted powder does not require refrigeration. Powder formulas are a convenient option if a mother wishes to supplement breastfeeding.

Once the can is opened, powdered formula can be used for up to 1 month as long as it is stored in a cool, dry place. It is usually reconstituted with 1 scoop (provided with each product) of powder to 60 mL of boiled or commercially prepared, sterilized water. Cold tap water should be boiled for at least 2–5 minutes.[42] If the formula will be fed immediately after preparation, it is safe to mix with cooled water that was previously boiled. However, if the formula is prepared in advance, it should be prepared with boiled water that is still very hot.[1] Once formula made from powder has been reconstituted, it should be covered, refrigerated and used within 24 hours. Once a feeding has been started, the formula should be used within 2 hours or discarded.

Concerns have been raised regarding powdered infant formula and its relationship to a number of diseases including necrotizing enterocolitis and meningitis.[43,44,45] *Enterobacter sakazakii* outbreaks in infants have been linked to powdered infant formula and the equipment used to prepare it. As a result, regulatory bodies have issued warnings about the use of powdered infant formula, especially in immunocompromised infants as well as those born prematurely. It is important to emphasize that proper hygiene, preparation, use and storage of powdered infant formula minimizes the risks of acquiring *E. sakazakii*. Bottles, nipples, caps and any other mixing equipment should be boiled for at least 2 minutes, and allowed to air dry and cool.

Liquid concentrate formulas are sterile and require reconstitution with boiled or commercially prepared, sterilized water in a 1:1 ratio. Once a can of liquid concentrate is opened, it must be refrigerated and used within 48 hours. Once mixed with water, the reconstituted formula must be used within 24 hours.

Ready-to-use infant formula is sterile and does not require mixing or the availability of a clean water supply. Although convenient for the occasional bottle, it is expensive for daily routine feeding.

Infant formulas can be used as a sole source of nutrition or as a supplement to human milk feeding. In general, commercial infant formulas contain 0.67 kcal/mL with 40–45% of calories from carbohydrate, 8–12% of calories from protein and approximately 45–50% of calories from fat. Both micro- and macronutrient content differ slightly between products but all are designed to mimic human milk as closely as possible.

Cow's Milk–Based Formulas

Cow's milk–based formulas are the most commonly used substitution or supplement to breast milk.

The protein content of these formulas is higher than that of breast milk and can vary in the proportion of the common protein components, whey and casein. Most formula manufacturers try to have the ratio of whey to casein resemble that of human milk as much as possible. When acidified, whey proteins remain in solution whereas casein proteins precipitate into curds. Whey-based formulas may accelerate gastric emptying faster than casein-predominant formulas and may be associated with fewer episodes of emesis or gastroesophageal reflux.[46] The carbohydrate source of standard cow's milk–based formula is either lactose, the carbohydrate found in human milk, or a combination of lactose and maltodextrin. Maltodextrins are easily digestible polysaccharides produced from the hydrolysis of starch.

Standard term formulas (for healthy term infants) usually contain a combination of vegetable oils, including palm, coconut, soy, sunflower and safflower oils. Approximately 50% of the energy contained in a standard term formula is derived from fat. Although these formulas do contain the essential fatty acids linoleic acid and alpha-linolenic acid, the fat blends used in commercially available formulas are different from those found in human milk. Arachidonic acid (ARA) and docosahexaenoic acid (DHA) have been added to some infant formulas as a few studies suggest that they may improve short-term visual and cognitive function, although the body of evidence is inconclusive.[7,47] Other variations of cow's milk–based formulas include products with lower iron or with probiotics.

Lactose-free Cow's Milk–Based Formulas

As the name suggests, in these formulas the milk sugar lactose is replaced with either corn syrup solids or maltodextrin and sucrose. The protein source remains as cow's milk-based protein. Parents may purchase a lactose-free formula if they suspect that symptoms of gassiness or fussiness in infancy are related to the lactose content of the formula. Some parents may select this feeding after a bout of infant diarrhea where there may be a temporary, secondary disaccharidase deficiency. Lactose-free formulas may contain residual amounts of lactose and galactose, which makes them an inappropriate formula choice for infants with galactosemia.[1] For infants with this condition, see Soy Protein Isolate–Based Formulas.

Lactose has an important role in mineral absorption and nonpathogenic bacterial colonization of the GI tract. Therefore, a decision to switch to a lactose-free formula should be made with careful consideration of the risks and benefits.

Soy Protein Isolate–Based Formulas

Soy-based formulas are free of cow's milk protein and lactose. They are iron-fortified and are designed to meet the nutritional needs of term-born infants. The protein fraction of these formulas is composed of soy protein isolate. Starch, corn syrup solids, corn maltodextrin and sucrose form the carbohydrate fraction. The fat blend is the same as the cow's milk–based product of that particular brand. Minerals are added in greater concentration than in cow's milk–based formula as mineral bioavailability is reduced by the presence of phytates in the soy protein isolate.

Soy protein formulas are recommended for term infants with galactosemia or congenital lactase deficiency. They can be used as a supplement to breastfeeding for infants of mothers who follow a vegetarian diet or for infants whose mothers wish to feed them nonanimal protein-based formula. They are not recommended for infants with cow's milk protein–induced enteropathy or enterocolitis as 30–60% will also be sensitive to soy. However, infants who have an immunoglobulin E–associated reaction to cow's milk protein may tolerate soy formulas.[48]

Soy formulas contain soy isoflavones, which are phytoestrogens that had been linked to reduced reproductive function. However, an expert panel did not support this link conclusively.[49]

The cost of soy protein formulas is comparable to that of milk-based formulas.

Hydrolyzed Protein Formulas

Hydrolyzed formulas available in Canada can be either partially or extensively hydrolyzed. The 2 types cannot be used interchangeably.

Partially hydrolyzed whey formula contains lactose and is less expensive and more palatable than extensively hydrolyzed protein–containing formula. Partially hydrolyzed formulas are used commonly as a substitute for or supplement to breast milk. The perceived benefits of a partially hydrolyzed whey formula, such as fewer spitting-up episodes and softer stools, are likely related to the β-lactoglobulin (which remains soluble in the stomach) moving faster to the upper jejunum.[50] These benefits may be more pronounced in children with underlying gastroesophaeal reflux disease.

Extensively hydrolyzed protein-containing formulas contain casein proteins that have been heat-treated and enzymatically hydrolyzed into peptide chains and free amino acids. They are recommended for infants with intolerance to intact cow's milk protein and soy protein.[51] They contain either long-chain triglycerides or a mixture of both long-chain and medium-chain triglycerides. The advantages of medium-chain triglycerides (MCT) in these formulas are their ability to bypass the lymphatic system and their requirement for less pancreatic enzymes and bile salts for digestion and absorption. Extensively hydrolyzed formulations benefit infants with malabsorptive diseases such as short bowel syndrome, liver disease, cystic fibrosis and intractable diarrhea.[7] Infants with cholestasis and lymphangiectasia also benefit from extensively hydrolyzed formulations, especially those containing a higher percentage of medium-chain triglycerides. Extensively hydrolyzed protein-containing formulas are lactose-free, and the carbohydrate is usually corn syrup solids, cornstarch and occasionally sucrose. These formulas are more expensive and less palatable than milk-based formulas.

Infants who cannot exclusively breastfeed and are at high risk of allergy and atopic disease, should be given extensively hydrolyzed protein formula, which may delay or prevent occurrence.[1,51,52]

Amino Acid–Based Formulas

Amino acid-based formulas, also known as "elemental" formulas, contain 100% free amino acids. They are designed for infants with severe milk protein hypersensitivity and are also used for infants with malabsorption-associated diseases who have persistent symptoms when receiving a partially hydrolyzed formula. These formulas are lactose-free and usually contain a combination of long-chain and medium-chain triglycerides. Amino acid–based formulas are more expensive than hydrolyzed formulas and are equally unpalatable.

Pre-thickened Formulas

Commercially available pre-thickened formulas for the treatment of regurgitation and vomiting offer advantages over standard formulas thickened with cornstarch or rice cereal. When standard formulas are thickened with infant cereal or cornstarch, nutrients and fluids are displaced; this practice is not recommended. The nutrient composition of pre-thickened formulas more closely resembles that of standard formula. Although symptoms of regurgitation and vomiting have been reduced in infants fed commercially prepared pre-thickened formula,[53] these formulas may not be as effective for reducing reflux symptoms.[54]

Follow-up Formulas

Follow-up formulas are designed for infants between 6 and 24 months who are consuming some complementary foods. They are usually less expensive than starter formulas and contain higher amounts of protein, vitamins and minerals. Although there does not appear to be superior health benefits to using a follow-up formula compared with a starter formula, they may deter parents from the early introduction of unmodified cow's milk.

Formulas for Premature Infants

These formulas are designed to meet the accelerated growth needs of infants born prematurely. They are available in sterile, ready-to-use form and are available only in a hospital setting. These formulations are available as standard and higher energy (0.67 kcal/mL and 0.8 kcal/mL). The protein, vitamins and minerals are also present in higher amounts than term formula in order to support third trimester growth. Premature formulas contain fat blends of 40–50% MCT to improve digestion and absorption in immature GI tracts. The fatty acids DHA and ARA have been added to all premature formulas in North America based on research suggesting that there are visual, cognitive and other developmental advantages to supplementing premature formulas.[55,56] Because of the immaturity of the GI tract and lower amount of lactase enzyme, glucose polymers replace some of the lactose in the carbohydrate portion of these formulas.

Postdischarge Formulas for Preterm Infants

The unique nutritional needs of preterm infants do not end when they reach term age. Many preterm infants remain undergrown compared with their term-born counterparts. Postdischarge formulas for preterm infants are designed to provide the additional energy, protein and other nutrients necessary for catch-up growth. Preterm infants fed a postdischarge formula up to 9 months post-term have higher weights and lengths compared with preterm infants fed standard-term formula.[57] However, little evidence supports using these formulas beyond 9 months post-term. At standard dilution, these formulas provide 0.74 kcal/mL.

Other Considerations

Alternative Milks and Beverages

Unmodified cow's milk (whole/3.25%, 2%, 1% or skim) and evaporated cow's milk are not recommended during the first 9–12 months of life. Once introduced, only whole cow's milk should be used until the age of 2 years.[58] Cow's milk contains much higher protein content than human milk and limited amounts of the essential fatty acids linoleic and alpha-linolenic acid. In addition, the renal solute load is higher than that of human milk due to significantly higher mineral and protein concentrations. This puts a greater stress on the kidneys especially if the infant has any illness that will increase insensible water loss. Unmodified cow's milk is also associated with increased blood loss through the GI tract. This blood loss, in addition to the low concentration and bioavailability of iron in unmodified cow's milk, may predispose the infant to iron deficiency anemia.[7] For more information regarding iron supplementation, see Vitamins and Minerals.

Pasteurized and unpasteurized goat milk, soy beverages, rice beverages or other vegetarian beverages are not considered complete nutritional alternatives to breast milk or commercial infant formula.

Water and juice are not necessary for breastfed infants during the first 6 months of life and may displace nutrient-rich human milk and introduce contaminants and potential allergens. Infants older than 6 months should be offered water if they are thirsty. Sweetened beverages are not encouraged; if consumed, they should be limited to 125–175 mL per day.[58] Carbonated beverages are not recommended for infants because they contain few nutrients and may contain caffeine and excess sugar, exposing infants to an unnecessary stimulant and predisposing them to dental caries. As well, carbonated beverages may interfere with the intake of more nutrient-rich foods. Sports drinks are not recommended for infants because of their high sugar content and lack of other nutrients. There is a lack of evidence to support the safe use of herbal teas and drinks in infants and therefore they are not recommended.[1]

Complementary Foods for Babies Older than 6 Months

Exclusive breastfeeding or an iron-enriched commercial term formula is sufficient to support growth and development during the first 6 months of life.[3] The introduction of complementary foods before 6 months of age provides no advantage to energy intake, rate of growth or the duration of sleep during the night, and may displace the intake of human milk or result in less milk production in the mother. Usually around 6 months of age, when an infant has good head and neck control and shows signs of readiness such as an interest in food when others are eating, iron-rich foods can be introduced gradually.

In Canada, the most common "first food" is iron-fortified infant cereal. However, other iron-containing foods (e.g., meats, eggs, tofu and legumes) can be introduced first at this stage and will vary depending on family and culture.[1] Once iron-rich foods are introduced, there is no specific order in which to introduce the infant to fruits, vegetables and dairy products.[58] Initially, foods are introduced in a pureed consistency, but as the child becomes more mature and confident with new foods, different safe textures should be progressively introduced until the child is eating a varied diet by the age of 1 year (Table 2).

Delaying common food allergens (egg, fish, peanut, wheat, soy) beyond 4–6 months is not recommended for prevention of food allergy; it may even increase the risk of developing such allergies, even in high-risk infants with a family history.[58,59] Once a potential allergen has been introduced, it should be regularly fed to the infant several times per week.[59] Parents should avoid introducing more than one common allergen per day, and should separate the introduction of different allergens by at least 2 days.[58] For more information regarding food allergy in infants, see Food Allergy.

Consider the safety of infants when offering complementary foods. While finger foods are encouraged to promote self-feeding, they should have a low choking risk (e.g., soft fruits and vegetables, grated cheese, ground meat and toast).[58] Avoid hard, small, round and sticky solid foods, raw and undercooked meats and eggs, and unpasteurized dairy products and juices. Also avoid honey in children under 1 year due to risk of botulism. Infant consumption of rice products, including infant cereals and toddler snacks, has been associated with arsenic exposure that exceeds standard recommendations.[60] Although the health implications of increased arsenic exposure are unknown, strategies to limit infants' exposure may be appropriate; these include feeding with other iron-rich foods, and supplementing the diet with a variety of grains.

Table 2: **Infant Feeding Guide**

Age of Infant	Breast Milk or Iron-fortified Formula	Iron-fortified Infant Cereal and Other Grain Products	Vegetables and Fruit	Meat and Alternatives	Milk Products
Birth–6 months	Breast milk feeding on demand every 2–3 h (8–12 feedings every 24 h) Exclusively and partially breastfed infants should receive vitamin D 400 IU/day, not to exceed 1000 IU/day Formula feeding on demand every 3–4 h (6–8 feedings every 24 h) Exclusive breastfeeding or iron-fortified infant formula is sufficient to achieve optimal growth, development and health until 6 months of age	None	None	None	Breast milk or iron-fortified formula only
6–9 months Introduce meat, meat alternatives and iron-fortified cereals as first complementary foods Transition from runny purees to thick or finely mashed soft foods	Breast milk feeding on demand Exclusively and partially breastfed infants should receive vitamin D 400 IU/day, not to exceed 1000 IU/day Formula feeding on demand, usually 3–5 feedings every 24 h Ensure introduction of solids does not interfere with adequate volume of breast milk or formula being consumed	Introduce iron-containing single food, e.g., iron-fortified infant cereal Begin with 5–10 mL increasing to 30–60 mL BID Introduce other grain products as developmentally appropriate, e.g., dry toast, unsalted crackers, rice and pasta	Offer pureed cooked vegetables and/or fruit after iron-fortified cereal and/or meat introduced, 120–200 mL total per day Offer ripe mashed fruit such as banana, mango, peach, avocado	Introduce iron-fortified single food, e.g., meat, meat alternative, egg or cereal. Iron from meat sources is better absorbed than iron from non-meat sources Offer more variety of meat and meat alternatives, e.g., pureed fish, chicken, tofu, mashed beans and legumes, 15–50 mL daily	Offer plain yogurt, cottage cheese, grated hard cheese, 15–30 mL daily Breast milk or iron-fortified formula only
9–12 months Transition from thick or finely mashed foods to minced or diced finger and table foods; encourage self-feeding	Breast milk feeding on demand Exclusively and partially breastfed infants should receive vitamin D 400 IU/day, not to exceed 1000 IU/day Formula feeding on demand, usually 3–4 feedings every 24 h Transition from breast/bottle to some cup feeding	Offer bread, rice and pasta, 120–150 mL daily Choose whole grain options	Offer mashed or diced cooked vegetables, 100–150 mL daily; soft ripe peeled, seeded, diced fresh or canned fruits packed in water or juice, 100–150 mL per day	Offer minced, diced, cooked meat, fish, chicken, tofu, beans, legumes, egg, 50–60 mL daily	Pasteurized whole cow's milk may be introduced Continue with yogurt, cottage cheese, grated hard cheese, 30–60 mL daily

Vitamins and Minerals

For comparative ingredients of nonprescription products, consult the *Compendium of Products for Minor Ailments*—Vitamin and Mineral Products: Single Entity.

Human milk contains small amounts of **vitamin D**, but not enough to prevent rickets. With decreased sun exposure, either through the use of sunscreen or coverage of the skin with hats and clothing, the usual mechanism of vitamin D production is hindered. Dark-skinned infants born to dark-skinned mothers and infants living in northern climates are at greater risk of vitamin D deficiency.[61] All fully and partially breastfed babies require a vitamin D supplement of 400 IU/day, not to exceed 1000 IU/day.[62,63] Vitamin D supplementation should continue until 1 year of age. Exclusively formula-fed babies do not require additional vitamin D.[1] If direct infant supplementation is not possible, an alternative would be for the breastfeeding mother to take 6400 IU/day to adequately supply the infant with the appropriate amount of vitamin D.[64]

According to the Canadian Dental Association (CDA), **fluoride** supplements are not recommended before the eruption of the first permanent tooth.[65] Fluoride supplements may be appropriate in communities that do not have access to fluoride in any other form, such as toothpaste. The CDA Position on Fluorides in Caries Prevention states "When, on an individual basis, the benefit of supplemental fluoride outweighs the risk of dental fluorosis, practitioners may elect to use these supplements at appropriate dosages in younger children. In doing so, the total daily fluoride intake from all sources should not exceed 0.05–0.07 mg fluoride/kg body weight, to minimize risk of dental fluorosis."

Healthy, full-term, breastfed infants do not need extra **iron** until 6 months of age, at which time the iron in complementary foods provides appropriate intake.[1,66,67] Healthy, full-term infants who are not breastfed will receive adequate iron through iron-fortified infant formula. Infants at risk of iron deficiency include those with a low birth weight, premature infants, those born to iron-deficient mothers, and infants older than 6 months who drink breast milk or an excessive amount of cow's milk without an adequate supply of iron-rich foods.[1] Symptoms of iron deficiency include pallor, irritability, poor appetite and delayed growth and development. If iron-deficiency is suspected, the infant should be screened and given supplementation accordingly.

Infant Colic

For comparative ingredients of nonprescription products, consult the *Compendium of Products for Minor Ailments*—Baby Care Products: Gastrointestinal.

Infant colic is defined as periods of fussiness or crying without apparent cause or failure to thrive.[1] Possible causes include immaturity of gut function, altered visceral perception, or, rarely, cow's milk allergy. Although foods the mother eats may appear in her milk, colic in the baby is seldom the result of the mother's diet. Therefore, feeding changes (e.g., interrupting breastfeeding, supplementing with formula, restricting the diet of the breastfeeding mother) are not an effective means to manage infant colic.

Breastfed babies may be fussy for a number of other reasons, such as hunger, the need to be near the mother, an oversupply of breast milk or an overactive milk ejection reflex. Oversupply or overactive ejection reflex occur when the mother has a generous milk supply and the baby gets an overabundance of foremilk (higher in lactose) that overwhelms the intestinal lactase. Consider this condition if a thriving infant presents with excessive crying, gas and explosive, loose, watery stools. A breastfeeding expert can provide management techniques. This is not an indication for use of lactose-free infant formula.

For more information regarding infant colic, see Chapter 34: Infant Colic.

Gastroesophageal Reflux in Healthy Infants

Gastroesophageal reflux (GER) in healthy infants is a normal physiologic occurrence. Most GER episodes cause few symptoms and infants gain weight and grow out of their symptoms, without the need for treatment. However, a subset of infants with gastroesophageal reflux disease (GERD) requires more aggressive treatment, often as a combination of nonpharmacologic and pharmacologic therapies. Rarely are the symptoms of reflux so severe that breastfeeding should be discontinued.[68] However, if regurgitation and vomiting persist for more than 1 month in formula-fed infants, the switch to an extensively hydrolyzed formula or an amino acid–based formula may be warranted.[68]

Constipation

Stool patterns in childhood vary, ranging from several times per day to once every 3–4 days.[1] True constipation during infancy is rare. When introducing complementary foods such as rice cereal, stool patterns may change temporarily. Careful attention should be paid to fluid intake to reduce the incidence of hard, painful bowel movements. For infants older than 6 months, the use of prune juice and the addition of whole grain cereal, cooked legumes, fruits and vegetables into the diet may be helpful. There are no dietary fibre recommendations for children under 2 years. Recommendations do exist for children over 2 years[69] but are not based on evidence of disease prevention.[1] For more information, see Chapter 29: Constipation.

Food Allergy

Food allergy is an adverse reaction that develops after an offending food or ingredient is eaten. A true food allergy is an immunologically mediated adverse reaction which is different from a "food intolerance" (a reaction not mediated by the immune system).[70] Milk, egg and peanut are the most common food allergies in infancy followed by soy, nuts and wheat. Many food allergies resolve spontaneously with age but peanut, tree nuts and seafood allergies are less likely to do so. In the majority of children, allergies to milk, egg, soy and wheat resolve by school age.

The most effective way to manage food allergy is avoidance of the offending food.[70] In exclusively breastfed infants, elimination of the offending protein from the mother's diet is no longer considered a first-line measure to reduce the likelihood of sensitization, except if the allergen is peanut.[51] If allergy is suspected a mother may continue to breastfeed unless the symptoms are bothersome to her or the baby, e.g., skin rash, runny nose, diarrhea. If allergies persist, the recommended treatment is to use a formula containing hydrolyzed proteins. In infants who continue to be symptomatic, an elemental amino acid-based formula is the only alternative.[71] For more information on these types of formulas see Hydrolyzed Protein Formulas and Amino Acid–Based Formulas. For more information regarding the introduction of solid foods and food allergy prevention, see Complementary Foods for Babies Older than 6 Months.

Resource Tips

Canadian Lactation Consultant Association. Available from: www.clca-accl.ca

Friedman J, Saunders N. *Canada's baby care book: a complete guide from birth to 12 months old.* Toronto: The Hospital for Sick Children; 2007.

International Lactation Consultant Association search tool to find an International Board Certified Lactation Consultant (IBCLC) from: www.ilca.org/why-ibclc/falc.

Koren G. *The complete guide to everyday risks in pregnancy and breastfeeding: answers to all your questions about medications, morning sickness, herbs, diseases, chemical exposures and more.* Toronto: The Hospital for Sick Children; 2004.

La Leche League Canada. Available from: www.lllc.ca.

La Leche League International. Center for Breastfeeding Information. Available from: www.llli.org/cbi/CBI.html.

Saunders N, Friedman J, eds. *Caring for kids: the complete Canadian health guide for children.* Toronto: The Hospital for Sick Children; 2006.

Suggested Readings

Kalnins D, Stone D, Touw J. *Better breastfeeding: a mother's guide to feeding and nutrition.* Toronto: The Hospital for Sick Children; 2007.

Kramer MS, Kakuma R. Optimal duration of exclusive breastfeeding. *Cochrane Database Syst Rev* 2012;8:CD003517.

Nutrition for healthy term infants: recommendations from birth to six months—a joint statement of Health Canada, Canadian Paediatric Society, Dietitians of Canada, and Breastfeeding Committee for Canada. Ottawa: Minister of Public Works and Government Services; 2012. Available from: www.hc-sc.gc.ca/fn-an/nutrition/infant-nourisson/recom/index-eng.php.

Nutrition for healthy term infants: recommendations from six to 24 months—a joint statement of Health Canada, Canadian Paediatric Society, Dietitians of Canada, and Breastfeeding Committee for Canada. Ottawa: Minister of Public Works and Government Services; 2014. Available from: www.hc-sc.gc.ca/fn-an/nutrition/infant-nourisson/recom/recom-6-24-months-6-24-mois-eng.php.

Section on Breastfeeding. Breastfeeding and the use of human milk. *Pediatrics* 2012;129:e827-41.

References

1. *Nutrition for healthy term infant: recommendations from birth to six months—a joint statement of Health Canada, Canadian Paediatric Society, Dietitians of Canada, and Breastfeeding Committee for Canada.* Ottawa: Minister of Public Works and Government Services; 2012. Available from: www.hc-sc.gc.ca/fn-an/nutrition/infant-nourisson/recom/index-eng.php. Accessed October 26, 2015.
2. World Health Organization. *Global strategy for infant and young child feeding.* Geneva: WHO; 2003. Available from: www.who.int/nutrition/publications/gs_infant_feeding_text_eng.pdf. Accessed October 26, 2015.
3. American Academy of Pediatrics. Breastfeeding and the use of human milk. *Pediatrics* 2012;129:e827.
4. Kramer MS, Kakuma R. Optimal duration of exclusive breastfeeding. *Cochrane Database Syst Rev* 2012;8:CD003517.
5. Statistics Canada. *Health trends.* Statistics Canada catalogue no. 82-213-XWE. Ottawa; 2014. Released June 12, 2014.
6. Statistics Canada. Gionet L. Breastfeeding trends in Canada. *Health at a Glance.* Statistics Canada catalogue no. 82-624-X. Ottawa; 2013.
7. American Academy of Pediatrics. Formula feeding for term infants. In: Kleinman RE, ed. *Pediatric nutrition handbook.* 5th ed. Washington: American Academy of Pediatrics; 2004. p. 87-97.
8. American Academy of Pediatrics. Breastfeeding. In: Kleinman RE, ed. *Pediatric nutrition handbook.* 5th ed. Washington: American Academy of Pediatrics; 2004. p. 55-86.
9. Ip S, Chung M, Raman G et al. Breastfeeding and maternal and infant health outcomes in developed countries. *Evid Rep Technol Assess (Full Rep)* 2007;153:1-186.
10. Schanler RJ, Shulman RJ, Lau C. Feeding strategies for premature infants: beneficial outcomes of feeding fortified human milk versus preterm formula. *Pediatrics* 1999;103:1150-7.
11. Schanler RJ. The use of human milk for premature infants. *Pediatr Clin North Am* 2001;48:207-19.
12. Lucas A, Morley R, Cole TJ. Randomised trial of early diet in preterm babies and later intelligence quotient. *BMJ* 1998;317:1481-7.
13. Jain A, Concato J, Leventhal JM. How good is the evidence linking breastfeeding and intelligence? *Pediatrics* 2002;109:1044-53.
14. Arenz S, Ruckerl R, Koletzko B et al. Breast-feeding and childhood obesity–a systematic review. *Int J Obes Relat Metab Disord* 2004;28:1247-56.
15. Grummer-Strawn LM, Mei Z. Does breastfeeding protect against pediatric overweight? Analysis of longitudinal data from the Centers for Disease Control and Prevention Pediatric Nutrition Surveillance System. *Pediatrics* 2004;113:e81-6.
16. Kramer MS, Fombonne E, Igumnov S et al. Effects of prolonged and exclusive breastfeeding on child behavior and maternal adjustment: evidence from a large, randomized trial. *Pediatrics* 2008;121:e345-40.
17. Martin RM, Patel R, Kramer MS et al. Effects of promoting longer-term and exclusive breastfeeding on adiposity and insulin-like growth factor-I at age 11.5 years: a randomized trial. *JAMA* 2013;309:1005-13.
18. Bener A, Denic S, Galadari S. Longer breast-feeding and protection against childhood leukemia and lymphomas. *Eur J Cancer* 2001;37:234-8.
19. Chua S, Arulkumaran S, Lim I et al. Influence of breastfeeding and nipple stimulation on postpartum uterine activity. *Br J Obstet Gynaecol* 1994;101:804-5.
20. Collaborative Group on Hormonal Factors in Breast Cancer. Breast cancer and breastfeeding: collaborative reanalysis of individual data from 47 epidemiological studies in 30 countries including 50302 women with breast cancer and 96973 women without the disease. *Lancet* 2002;360:187-95.
21. Paton LM, Alexander JL, Nowson CA et al. Pregnancy and lactation have no long-term deleterious effect on measures of bone mineral in healthy women: a twin study. *Am J Clin Nutr* 2003;77:707-14.

22. Dewey KG, Heinig MJ, Nommsen LA. Maternal weight-loss patterns during prolonged lactation. *Am J Clin Nutr* 1993;58:162-6.
23. American Academy of Pediatrics. Recommendations for the care of children in special circumstances. In: Pickering LK, ed. *Red Book: report of the Committee on Infectious Diseases*. 28th ed. Elk Grove Village: American Academy of Pediatrics; 2009. p. 118-24.
24. Helewa M, Levesque P, Provencher D et al. Breast cancer, pregnancy and breastfeeding. *J Obstet Gynaecol Can* 2002;24:164-80.
25. Arroyo CI, Lopez RMJ, Sapina AM et al. Probable transmission of brucellosis by breast milk. *J Trop Pediatr* 2006;52:380-1.
26. Moore ER, Anderson GC, Bergman N et al. Early skin-to-skin contact for mothers and their healthy newborn infants. *Cochrane Database Syst Rev* 2012;5:CD003519.
27. Flanders D, Lowe A, Kramer M et al. *A consensus statement on the use of domperidone to support lactation*. International Lactation Consultation Association. Available from: http://kindercarepediatrics.ca/wp-content/uploads/Domperidone-Consensus-Statement-Final-May-11-2012.pdf. Accessed April 13, 2016.
28. Academy of Breastfeeding Medicine Protocol Committee. ABM clinical protocol #9: use of galactogogues in initiating or augmenting the rate of maternal milk secretion (first revision January 2011). *Breastfeed Med* 2011;6:41-9.
29. Alexander JM, Grant AM, Campbell MJ. Randomised controlled trial of breast shells and Hoffman's exercises for inverted and non-protractile nipples. *BMJ* 1992;304:1030-2.
30. Health Canada. *Eating well with Canada's food guide*. Available from: www.hc-sc.gc.ca/fn-an/food-guide-aliment/index-eng.php. Accessed October 26, 2015.
31. Vieira F, Bachion MM, Mota DD et al. A systematic review of the interventions for nipple trauma in breastfeeding mothers. *J Nurs Scholarsh* 2013;45:116-25.
32. Gungor AN, Oguz S, Vurur G et al. Comparison of olive oil and lanolin in the prevention of sore nipples in nursing mothers. *Breastfeed Med* 2013;8:334-5.
33. Dennis CL, Jackson K, Watson J. Interventions for treating painful nipples among breastfeeding women. *Cochrane Database Syst Rev* 2014;12:CD007366.
34. The Academy of Breastfeeding Medicine Protocol Committee. ABM clinical protocol #20: engorgement. *Breastfeed Med* 2009;4:111-113.
35. Jahanfar S, Ng CJ, Teng CL. Antibiotics for mastitis in breastfeeding women. *Cochrane Database Syst Rev* 2013;2:CD005458.
36. Brochet MS, Ito S. Drug use during breastfeeding. In: CPS online. Ottawa: Canadian Pharmacists Association; 2015. Available from: www.e-therapeutics.ca. Accessed October 26, 2015. Subscription required.
37. American Academy of Pediatrics Committee on Drugs. The transfer of drugs and other chemicals into human milk. *Pediatrics* 2001;108:776-89.
38. Moretti ME, Lee A, Ito S. Which drugs are contraindicated during breastfeeding? *Motherisk Update* 2000 Sept. Available from: www.motherisk.org.
39. Ito S. Drug therapy for breast-feeding women. *N Engl J Med* 2000;343:118-26.
40. Briggs GG, Freeman RK. *Drugs in pregnancy and lactation: a reference guide to fetal and neonatal risk*. 10th ed. Philadelphia: Wolters Kluwer Health; Lippincott Williams & Wilkins; 2015.
41. Hale TW, Rowe HE. *Medications and mothers' milk: a manual of lactational pharmacology*. 16th ed. Plano: Hale Publishing; 2014.
42. O'Connor DL, Brennan J, Dello S et al. Use of nonsterile nutritionals for neonates in-hospital and after hospital discharge: control measures currently instituted at one tertiary care institution. In: Farber JM, Forsythe SJ, eds. *Enterobacter sakazakii*. Washington: ASM Press; 2008. p. 187-220.
43. Farber JM, Forsythe SJ, eds. *Enterobacter sakazakii and Salmonella in powdered infant formula: meeting report, MRA Series 10*. Washington: ASM Press; 2008. Available from: www.who.int/foodsafety/publications/micro/mra10/en/index.html. Accessed October 26, 2015.
44. U.S. Food and Drug Administration. *Health professionals letter on Enterobacter sakazakii infections associated with use of powdered (dry) infant formulas in neonatal intensive care units*. 2002. Available from: www.fda.gov/food/recallsoutbreaksemergencies/safetyalertsadvisories/ucm111299.htm. Accessed April 14, 2016.
45. World Health Organization. *Safe preparation, storage and handling of powdered infant formula: guidelines*. 2007. Available from: www.who.int/foodsafety/publications/micro/pif_guidelines.pdf. Accessed October 26, 2015.
46. Staelens S, Van den Driessche M, Barclay D et al. Gastric emptying in healthy newborns fed an intact protein formula, a partially and an extensively hydrolysed formula. *Clin Nutr* 2008;27:264-8.
47. Koletzko B, Baker S, Cleghorn G et al. Global standard for the composition of infant formula: recommendations of an ESPGHAN coordinated international expert group. *J Pediatr Gastroenterol Nutr* 2005;41:584-99.
48. Bhatia J, Greer F; American Academy of Pediatrics Committee on Nutrition. Use of soy protein-based formulas in infant feeding. *Pediatrics* 2008;121;1062-8.
49. Rozman KK, Bhatia J, Calafat AM et al. NTP-CERHR expert panel on the reproductive and developmental toxicity of soy formula. *Birth Defects Res B Dev Reprod Toxicol* 2006;77:280-397.
50. Meyer R, Foong RX, Thapar N et al. Systematic review of the impact of feed protein type and degree of hydrolysis on gastric emptying in children. *BMC Gastroenterol* 2015;15:137.
51. Greer FR, Sicherer SH, Burks AW et al. Effects of early nutritional interventions on the development of atopic disease in infants and children: the role of maternal dietary restriction, breastfeeding, timing of introduction of complementary foods, and hydrolyzed formulas. *Pediatrics* 2008;121:183-91.
52. Osborn DA, Sinn J. Formulas containing hydrolysed protein for prevention of allergy and food intolerance in infants. *Cochrane Database Syst Rev* 2006;4:CD003664.
53. Vanderhoof JA, Moran JR, Harris CL et al. Efficacy of a pre-thickened infant formula: a multicenter, double-blind, randomized, placebo-controlled parallel group trial in 104 infants with symptomatic gastroesophageal reflux. *Clin Pediatr (Phila)* 2003;42:483-95.
54. Penna FJ, Norton RC, Carvalho AS et al. [Comparison between pre-thickened and home-thickened formulas in gastroesophageal reflux treatment]. *J Pediatr (Rio J)* 2003;79:49-54. [Portuguese].
55. American Academy of Pediatrics. Nutritional needs of the preterm infant. In: Kleinman RE, ed. *Pediatric nutrition handbook*. 5th ed. Washington: American Academy of Pediatrics; 2004. p. 23-54.
56. O'Connor DL, Hall R, Adamkin D et al. Growth and development in preterm infants fed long-chain polyunsaturated fatty acids: a prospective, randomized control trial. *Pediatrics* 2001;108:359-71.
57. Lucas A, Fewtrell MS, Morley R et al. Randomized trial of nutrient-enriched formula versus standard formula for postdischarge preterm infants. *Pediatrics* 2001;108:703-11.

58. *Nutrition for healthy term infants: recommendations from six to 24 months—a joint statement of Health Canada, Canadian Paediatric Society, Dietitians of Canada, and Breastfeeding Committee for Canada*. Ottawa: Minister of Public Works and Government Services; 2012. Available from: www.hc-sc.gc.ca/fn-an/nutrition/infant-nourisson/recom/index-eng.php.

59. Chan ES, Cummings C, Atkinson A et al. Dietary exposures and allergy prevention in high-risk infants: a joint position statement of the Canadian Society of Allergy and Clinical Immunology and the Canadian Paediatric Society. *Allergy Asthma Clin Immunol* 2014;10:45.

60. Karagas MR, Punshon T, Sayarath V et al. Association of rice and rice-product consumption with arsenic exposure early in life. *JAMA Pediatr* 2016 Apr 25. [Epub ahead of print].

61. Bodnar LM, Simhan HN, Powers RW et al. High prevalence of vitamin D insufficiency in black and white pregnant women residing in the northern United States and their neonates. *J Nutr* 2007;137:447-52.

62. Vitamin D supplementation: recommendations for Canadian mothers and infants. *Pediatr Child Health* 2007;12:583-98.

63. Wagner CL, Greer FR; American Academy of Pediatrics Section on Breastfeeding et al. Prevention of rickets and vitamin D deficiency in infants, children, and adolescents. *Pediatrics* 2008;122:1142-52.

64. Hollis BW, Wagner CL, Howard CR et al. Maternal versus infant vitamin D supplementation during lactation: a randomized controlled trial. *Pediatrics* 2015;135(4):625-34.

65. Canadian Dental Association. *CDA Position on use of fluorides in caries prevention*. Available from: www.cda-adc.ca/_files/position_statements/fluoride.pdf. Accessed October 26, 2015.

66. Oddy WH, Sly PD, de Klerk NH et al. Breast feeding and respiratory morbidity in infancy: a birth cohort study. *Arch Dis Child* 2003;88:224-8.

67. Marild S, Hansson S, Jodal U et al. Protective effect of breastfeeding against urinary tract infection. *Acta Paediatr* 2004;93:164-8.

68. Vandenplas Y, Rudolph CD, Di Lorenzo C et al. Pediatric gastroesophageal reflux clinical practice guidelines: joint recommendations of the North American Society for Pediatric Gastroenterology, Hepatology, and Nutrition (NASPGHAN) and the European Society for Pediatric Gastroenterology, Hepatology, and Nutrition (ESPGHAN). *J Pediatr Gastroenterol Nutr* 2009;49:498-547.

69. Williams CL. Importance of dietary fiber in childhood. *J Am Diet Assoc* 1995;95:1140-6, 1149.

70. Sampson HA. The evaluation and management of food allergy in atopic dermatitis. *Clin Dermatol* 2003;21:183-92.

71. Vanderhoof JA, Young RJ. Allergic disorders of the gastrointestinal tract. *Curr Opin Clin Nutr Metab Care* 2001;4:553-6.

Feeding Your Baby—What You Need to Know

How to Clean Equipment, Nipples and Soothers

First step—sterilize:

- Before you use any equipment that will be in contact with the milk or the baby's mouth, you must sterilize it. Sterilizing kills any germs on the equipment. You should sterilize the following things:
  - breast pump and breast pump kit
  - infant feeding bottles, nipples and soothers
- To sterilize: Place the equipment in a pot of boiling water for 2–5 minutes. All parts should be covered by the water.

Regular cleaning:

- Clean equipment by washing in hot soapy water and rinsing with hot water. Let it air-dry—do not dry it with a dish towel. You can also wash equipment in a dishwasher with a heat dry cycle.
- *Do not* squeeze liquid dish soap into breast pump parts, bottles or nipples. Soap may remain in the equipment and spoil the milk.

Special cases:

- For infants who are ill or in the hospital, you may need to sterilize more often. Check with your nurse, doctor or hospital.
- For babies with oral thrush (yeast) infection, sterilize bottles, nipples and soothers regularly. Replace worn nipples and soothers as yeast may collect in tiny cracks and re-infect the baby.

How to Use a Breast Pump—General Instructions

- Read the instructions that came with the pump.
- Wash your hands before you start.
- Moisten the funnel (flange) of the breast pump with milk or water before beginning to pump. Centre the funnel on the breast.
- A gentle rhythmic pattern of pumping works best. Set pumps at the lowest setting to start.
- If you are using a hand piston pump, hold the piston underneath to prevent strain on your wrists.
- If you are using an electric pump, turn pump setting to low. Turn pump off before removing from breast.
- If pumping is uncomfortable or does not seem to be working, make sure you have the funnel placed correctly. If you are still having trouble after several tries, contact a breastfeeding expert for advice. You may need a different kind of pump.
- You can also learn how to express milk from your breasts by hand.
- You can call the La Leche League Canada for information about breastfeeding and help with any problems. They will give you the name of a person near you. Call 1-800-665-4324.

Hints for Collecting Milk:

- If you are separated from your baby:
  - apply warm moist cloths to the breast
  - massage gently with your hands to help begin the flow of milk (called let-down)
  - pump 7–8 times a day, about 15 minutes each time. Switch sides twice during each pumping session

- it is not necessary to switch if you are using a double pump. Pump 10–15 minutes each time.
- If you are collecting milk for occasional feedings:
  - pump after the baby has breastfed (morning may work best)
  - don't worry if you only get a few drops the first time. It may take several days of regular pumping or expressing by hand for your milk supply to increase
  - plan ahead. You may have to collect milk for several days to make sure you have enough stored. Follow the instructions below for storing breast milk
  - reduce the amount of pumping for several days before you will be away from the baby. This will help reduce your milk supply and help prevent leakage.

Storing Breast Milk

- Breast milk may be kept at room temperature (19–22°C) for up to 2 hours.
- Refrigerated breast milk (0–4°C) may be kept up to 48 hours.
- **Do not** keep breast milk that is left in a bottle after feeding the baby.
- Breast milk that is collected away from home should be stored in a fridge or cooler. To take the milk home, pack it between frozen cool packs in a small, insulated lunch bag or picnic cooler.

Freezing Breast Milk

- Freeze breast milk in quantities of 60–100 mL. Write the date on each container when you freeze it.
- Cooled fresh milk may be added to frozen milk.
- Store frozen milk in hard plastic or glass containers, or plastic bags specially designed to store breast milk. Disposable bottle liners and freezer bags are not recommended for freezing milk. Fat from the milk, which your baby needs, may cling to these bags.
- Length of time you can store frozen milk safely:
  - freezer inside a fridge—2 weeks
  - self-contained (separate) freezer unit of a fridge—3–4 months
  - deep freezer at a constant temperature of minus 19°C—at least 6 months.

Using Frozen Breast Milk

- Thaw frozen milk by running it under warm water. Shake or swirl the container to mix.
- Do not thaw frozen breast milk in a microwave. High temperatures can reduce the quality of the milk. A microwave can also cause hot spots in the milk that could burn the baby.
- Previously frozen milk that has thawed can be kept in the refrigerator for 24 hours.
- Do not refreeze thawed milk.

Tips on Bottle-feeding a Breastfed Baby

- Be sure to choose a bisphenol A-free bottle.
- Feed before the baby becomes very hungry and upset. A calm breastfed baby is more likely to take a bottle.
- Have someone other than the mother bottle-feed the baby.
- Always hold the baby while feeding. Holding helps the baby feel more comfortable.
- Use a different feeding position than the one used for breastfeeding.
- Use a nipple with a small hole (1 drop per second or less). Breastfed babies have a strong suck. The milk may come out too fast from a nipple with a large hole. If baby refuses 1 type of nipple, try another.

- Do not put the baby to bed with a bottle. The baby may choke on the milk. Using a bottle as a pacifier can cause the baby's teeth to decay (called infant caries).
- Use a small cup, a tiny spoon or an eyedropper to feed a breastfed baby who refuses to use an artificial nipple.

How to Mix and Use Infant Formula

- Only use water that is safe for drinking.
- Use water from the cold water tap. Hot water may contain lead and other metals. If the water is softened, hot water will contain a lot of salt. Do not use carbonated or mineral waters.
- Bring the water to a rolling boil and boil it for 2 minutes. Boiled water should *always* be used for infants under 4 months. Boiled water should be used for older babies if there is any chance that the water is not safe for drinking.
- You can store boiled water in a sterilized, tightly closed container for 2–3 days in the refrigerator. It can be kept at room temperature for 24 hours.
- If you use canned formula (ready-to-use or concentrate), pour boiling water over the top of the can before opening.
- Mix liquid concentrate with the same amount of cooled boiled water (equal parts).
- Use only the measuring spoon provided with cans of powdered concentrate. Do not use a spoon from a different brand. Mix powder concentrate with the manufacturer's recommended amount of cooled boiled water.
- Use prepared formula that is at room temperature within 1 hour.
- Store prepared formula in the refrigerator. Use it within 24 hours.
- Refrigerate opened cans of ready-to-use or concentrated formula. Use within 24–48 hours.
- Use cans of powdered concentrate within 30 days of opening. Once mixed with water, refrigerate and use within 24 hours.
- To feed baby, warm prepared infant formula in a pan of hot water or use a commercial warmer. Heating a bottle in the microwave can be dangerous. It can cause hot spots that will burn the baby. Shake the bottle well and always test the temperature before feeding.

Nutrition

Chapter 41
Special Diets

Shirley Heschuk, BScPharm, MSc

Some patients require diets that are either restricted or enhanced in certain nutrients for health reasons.[1] An appropriate assessment is necessary to determine whether a special diet would benefit a specific patient.

Sodium-restricted Diet

The purpose of a sodium-restricted diet is to prevent accumulation of fluid and/or promote a net loss of excess body water. The diet is indicated in:

- Essential hypertension: Blood pressure reduction is correlated with a moderately reduced sodium intake.[2,3] To decrease blood pressure, the Canadian Hypertension Education Program recommends reducing sodium intake toward 2 g (5 g of salt or 87 mmol of sodium) per day[4] (see also Diets for Cardiovascular Diseases, Diet for Hypertension)
- Heart failure: Sodium restriction is the primary diet therapy in treating heart failure. A sodium intake of ≤2–3 g/day is recommended for all patients with symptomatic heart failure with a further reduction to ≤1–2 g/day for patients with more advanced heart failure or fluid retention[5]
- Renal disease: Sodium intake should be modified to facilitate blood pressure control, to maintain normal hydration status and to help prevent heart failure and pulmonary edema. Fluid status and appropriateness of sodium intake can be monitored through measuring blood pressure, interdialytic weight gains, signs of edema and thirst. In people with chronic kidney disease (CKD), sodium reduction lowered blood pressure considerably and reduced proteinuria consistently.[6] However, long-term studies are required to determine the effect on mortality and progression to end-stage kidney disease.[6] Generally, the recommended intake of sodium is 2–3 g per day (87–130 mmol)[1]
- Liver disease: In patients with liver disease, fluid and electrolyte status must be monitored and sodium restriction may be required.

Although sodium reduction is recommended, an aggressive sodium limit of ≤1.5 g/day has not demonstrated a mortality benefit and may even increase risk of adverse health effects in some populations.[7]

Choose fresh or frozen food and reduce intake of high-sodium processed food, beverages and condiments, e.g., fast foods, smoked and/or salted meats, canned or prepackaged foods, snack foods, salad dressings. Limit use of salt in cooking and at the table: use salt substitutes (KCl) or other seasoning such as herbs, spices, seasoning blends (e.g., Mrs. Dash), lemon juice and garlic during food preparation. Most salt substitutes contain less than 1 mmol of sodium per teaspoon but large amounts of potassium (30–50 mmol per teaspoon). Patients with renal disease should not use salt substitutes, as ingestion of additional potassium could result in hyperkalemia. Note: 2.4 g elemental sodium = 6 g NaCl = 1 teaspoon of table salt.

Advise patients to read the Nutrition Facts table on food packages for sodium content. Sources of sodium include sodium chloride (table salt), celery salt, garlic salt or onion salt, sea salt, baking soda, baking powder, brine for pickling, soy sauce, substances with Na (abbreviation for sodium), monosodium glutamate (Accent or MSG), sodium benzoate, sodium citrate, sodium nitrate, disodium phosphate and sodium gluconate.

Health Canada allows the following sodium-related label claims on food products:

- Sodium-free/salt-free = <5 mg sodium per serving
- Very low sodium = ≤35 mg sodium per serving
- Low sodium = ≤140 mg sodium per serving
- Reduced sodium/less sodium = at least 25% less than the regular product

Potassium-modified Diets

The purpose of both high-potassium and low-potassium diets is to maintain normal potassium levels (3.5–5 mmol/L) in hypo- and hyperkalemic patients.

High-potassium diets may be indicated during use of certain medications such as potassium-wasting thiazide-type diuretics or antibiotics (e.g., gentamicin). Evidence suggests that a diet with increased potassium may reduce blood pressure and risk of stroke[8] and is associated with lower risk of death and cardiovascular events.[9]

Low-potassium diets may be indicated in patients with impaired renal function or those taking medications that increase potassium levels, such as potassium supplements, potassium-sparing diuretics and ACE inhibitors. To decrease dietary potassium intake, restrict fruits and vegetables high in potassium content, such as potatoes, bananas, melons, juices (orange, prune, tomato), spinach, fresh meat, milk and salt substitutes containing potassium chloride (KCl). Patients who follow a very low potassium diet may become deficient in calcium, iron, vitamin C, folate and B vitamins.

Fat-restricted Diet

Fat-restricted diets prevent symptoms of intolerance (diarrhea, flatulence, abdominal pain) due to high intakes of dietary fat, and control nutrient losses caused by malabsorption disorders. Fat-restricted diets are not intended for weight reduction (see Weight ManagementChapter 43: Weight Management) or for lowering serum lipids (see Diets for Cardiovascular Diseases, Diet for Dyslipidemia).

Fat-restricted diets may be used in the treatment of diseases of the hepatobiliary tract (gall bladder disease, chronic cholecystitis), pancreas (chronic pancreatitis), intestinal mucosa (GERD, Crohn's disease, small bowel resection) and lymphatic system (intestinal lymphangiectasia).

Those with malabsorption syndromes may be deficient in fat-soluble vitamins and other micronutrients; supplement with vitamins A, D, E and K. Water-miscible forms of the fat-soluble vitamins are available.

In severe fat restriction, patients may need to supplement protein.

Fibre-modified Diets

Fibre is a substance found in plants that cannot be hydrolyzed by the digestive system. It is classified as soluble or insoluble based on physiochemical properties. Soluble fibre occurs as pectins (e.g., bananas, apples), mucilage (e.g., psyllium) and gum (e.g., oatmeal, legumes). Insoluble fibre includes cellulose (e.g., wheat bran, apples), hemicellulose (e.g., whole wheat) and lignin (e.g., potatoes). For a table of fibre content of common foods, see Chapter 29: Constipation.

A fibre-restricted diet reduces the frequency and volume of fecal output while prolonging intestinal transit time and prevents blockage of stenosed gastrointestinal tract. A fibre-restricted diet is indicated in diverticulitis, stenosis of the intestine and acute inflammatory bowel disease (ulcerative colitis, Crohn's disease) to limit the pain and frequency of stools and to prevent obstruction when the lumen of the colon is narrowed or stenosed.[10]

Patients can reduce indigestible carbohydrate intake by limiting amounts of well-cooked or canned vegetables and canned, cooked or very ripe fruit products, replacing whole-grain breads and cereals with refined products and avoiding nuts, seeds and legumes.

High-fibre diets increase fecal bulk and promote regularity, normalize serum lipid levels and blunt postprandial blood glucose response.

High-fibre diets are indicated in:

- Inflammatory bowel disease: When the disease is in remission or under control, a high-fibre diet (as tolerated) is recommended to stimulate peristalsis and improve the tone of the muscular wall of the GI tract, especially the colon[10]
- Irritable bowel syndrome (IBS): Research has shown that soluble fibre, but not bran, is effective in treating IBS[11]
- Colon cancer: A systematic review of dietary fibre intake and the incidence of colorectal cancer concluded a high intake of dietary fibre, cereal fibre and whole grains in particular, was associated with a reduced risk of colon cancer[12]
- Hypercholesterolemia: Small but significant decreases in total and LDL cholesterol are seen with various soluble fibres[13,14]
- Diabetes: Soluble fibre has a small effect on inhibiting blood glucose absorption from the small intestine[15]
- Cardiovascular disease: Increased fibre intake is associated with a lower risk of coronary heart disease and cardiovascular disease[16]
- All-cause mortality: For each 10 g/day increase in fibre intake, a 10% reduction in risk of death has been shown.[17] Increasing fibre in patients who survived MI is significantly associated with lower all-cause and cardiovascular mortality.[18]

Fibre content should be increased gradually to minimize abdominal distress, bloating, flatulence, cramps and diarrhea, and adequate amounts of noncaffeinated fluid (2 L/day) should be consumed.

Iron-rich Diet

The purpose of an iron-rich diet is to promote adequate intake, especially for individuals with increased iron requirements. It is used to prevent and/or treat low iron stores and iron deficiency anemia:

- For individuals who are at risk for suboptimal iron intake, such as young children and older adults
- For individuals with increased iron requirements, such as pregnant women, premenopausal women, endurance athletes or those consuming a vegetarian or vegan diet.

Iron-rich diets include foods high in iron as well as foods that enhance iron absorption. There are 2 types of iron in the diet:

- heme iron, found in meats, fish and poultry, is highly bioavailable (15–35%). Sources include liver (pork, beef and chicken), venison, beef, clams, oysters, mussels and shrimp
- nonheme iron, found in vegetables, is less bioavailable (2–20%). Sources include cooked beans, lentils, chickpeas and soybeans, pumpkin seeds, tofu, tempeh, blackstrap molasses, enriched breakfast cereals and enriched pasta.

Iron absorption can be increased by consuming iron-absorbing enhancers together with iron-rich foods and by not eating the iron-rich foods together with foods that inhibit absorption (Table 1). Cooking with iron skillets, steel woks and stainless steel cookware (to a lesser extent) may add extra iron to the food.

Table 1: **Foods that Affect Iron Absorption**

Iron Absorption Enhancers	Iron Absorption Inhibitors[a]
Meats, fish, poultry	Calcium (milk, yogurt, cheese, sardines)
Vitamin C–containing fruits (oranges, orange juice, cantaloupe, strawberries, grapefruit) and vegetables (broccoli, brussel sprouts, tomatoes, tomato juice, potatoes, red and green peppers)	Eggs
	Oxalates (spinach, chard, beet greens, rhubarb, sweet potatoes)
	Phytates (whole grains, bran)
	Tannins and polyphenols (red wine, coffee, tea)

[a] Bind to iron and prevent absorption.

Gluten-restricted Diet

Gluten is a protein contained in wheat, rye, triticale (a cross between wheat and rye) and barley (see Table 2). In patients with gluten sensitivity, ingestion causes damage to the mucosa of the small intestine, leading to a variety of GI symptoms (cramps, bloating, diarrhea) and nutritional deficiencies.

Table 2: **Selected Gluten-containing Food Ingredients and Substitutions[a]**

Ingredients to Avoid (contain gluten)	Gluten-free Substitutes	
Barley	Amaranth	Potato
Beer, ale[b]	Arrowroot	Quinoa
Buckwheat (kasha)[c]	Beans	Rice
Graham	Corn	Sago
Rye	Distilled alcoholic beverages[b]	Sorghum
Seminola	Flax seed	Soy
Triticale	Millet	Tapioca
Vinegar (malt)	Nut	Vinegar
Wheat (spelt, durum, kamut, semolina, farina)	Oat[d]	(cider or wine)

[a] Includes ingredient and products made from it (e.g., flours); not an exhaustive list.
[b] Beer and ale are generally made from barley and contain prolamines, a subfraction of gluten. Alcohol made from fermented grains (e.g., vodka, whiskeys) is distilled, removing the prolamines; these products are allowed unless otherwise contraindicated.
[c] Although buckwheat itself does not contain gluten, some celiac patients cannot tolerate it; also, commercial buckwheat products (e.g., some buckwheat flours, pancake mixes, pasta) may be mixed with or contain wheat flour.
[d] Pure and uncontaminated oats are safe in limited amounts: 50–70 g/day (one-half to three-quarters cup dry rolled oats) for adults and 20–25 g/day (one-quarter cup dry rolled oats) for children with celiac disease.[19]

Patients with celiac disease and those who cannot tolerate gluten must follow a restricted diet to eliminate virtually all gluten intake. Patients must avoid all gluten products; any product entering the digestive system must be gluten-free. It is important to carefully review ingredient lists on food and drug labels to determine whether gluten-containing ingredients are present. Canadian regulations permit fortification of gluten-free flours to match the enrichment requirements of white flour for B vitamins, folic acid and iron, but there is no requirement to do so; additional sources of these nutrients may be required. For gluten content of specific pharmaceutical products, the manufacturer should be contacted.

Screening tests for celiac disease include either or both of the following blood tests: IgA human tissue transglutaminase (TTG) or IgA endomysial antibody (EMA). If the symptoms suggest celiac disease and the TTG and/or EMA are negative, the physician should consider upper endoscopy and intestinal biopsy.

Lactose-restricted Diet

For comparative ingredients of nonprescription products, consult the *Compendium of Products for Minor Ailments*—Nutrition Products: Lactose Digestants.

Lactose is a disaccharide sugar (glucose and galactose) found in dairy products and is digested by the enzyme lactase. A deficiency of lactase results in lactose intolerance which manifests as intestinal symptoms (bloating, flatulence, cramping, nausea and diarrhea). The purpose of a lactose-restricted diet is to reduce lactose intake in intolerant patients to a level that will prevent or reduce these symptoms while providing adequate nutrient intake.

The 3 main types of lactase deficiency are:

- Primary: The most prevalent type; presents with a late onset. It usually occurs with increasing age and individuals exhibit tolerance to various levels of lactose
- Secondary: Transient in nature and develops secondary to illness or disease involving mucosal injury
- Congenital: Extremely rare and requires a lifelong lactose-free or very-low-lactose diet.

Lactose-intolerant individuals vary in their ability to digest lactose and the amount of lactase in their systems. Total lactose avoidance is usually not necessary except in galactosemia. True lactase deficiency can be clinically diagnosed with a breath hydrogen test, which measures hydrogen produced by colonic bacteria in the presence of unabsorbed sugars.

Enzymatic **lactase** products break down lactose into digestible sugars—glucose and galactose. They are available in various forms: tablets, chewable tablets and drops.

Lactase-treated food products (e.g., milk, cheeses) and yogurts contain negligible amounts of lactose. Lactose-intolerant individuals may meet their calcium and vitamin D requirements from other food sources, but supplementation may be required depending upon their dietary intake and age. For more information on calcium and vitamin D, see Chapter 47: Osteoporosis.

Note: It is important to read ingredient lists on food and drug labels, as many fillers contain lactose. For lactose content of specific pharmaceutical products, contact the manufacturer.

Phenylalanine-restricted Diet

Phenylalanine is an amino acid found in protein which is metabolized to tyrosine by the enzyme phenylalanine hydroxylase. The absence of this enzyme is the result of a rare genetic disorder called phenylketonuria (PKU). In patients with PKU, phenylalanine can build up in the blood and brain to toxic levels and affect brain development and function. PKU is detected by a simple blood test which is part of the newborn screening panel in Canada and the United States and it is treated by strictly following a diet that is extremely low in phenylalanine, particularly during the years of growth and development.

Phenylalanine is present in significant amounts in high protein foods such as dairy products, meat, fish, chicken, eggs, beans and nuts. The artificial sweetener aspartame also contains phenylalanine and should be avoided. Special diets devoid of phenylalanine but containing protein, vitamins, minerals and energy (calories) can be used for life. Foods allowed include: fruit, vegetables, juices, low-protein breads and pastas. A consult with a dietician is highly recommended.

It is important for patients' progress to be monitored through food diaries, monthly blood tests and regular follow-up care.

Purine-restricted Diet

Purines include the nucleotides adenine and guanine. They are found in virtually all food, but are more concentrated in some (see Table 3). Purines are metabolized to uric acid, so a purine-restricted diet decreases blood and urine uric acid levels. A purine-restricted diet is beneficial to patients with hyperuricemia, gouty arthritis and urinary uric acid lithiasis (in conjunction with medication).

In a 12-year study of men with no gout at baseline, moderate intake of purine-rich vegetables (peas, beans, mushrooms, cauliflower, spinach) and total protein intake were not associated with increased risk of gout. Higher meat and seafood consumption increased the risk of gout, whereas consumption of low-fat dairy products reduced the risk.[20]

Patients with gout should consume meat, seafood and alcoholic beverages in moderation, meet protein needs with purine-rich vegetables rather than animal products and use low-fat dairy products. Monounsaturated fats and complex carbohydrates are preferred and portion sizes and the content of noncomplex carbohydrates should be monitored to prevent the development of insulin resistance.[21] For more information regarding dietary recommendations in gout, see Table 3.

Several studies have shown that obese patients are at an increased risk of developing gout.[22,23,24] Weight reduction diets that are high in fat and purine-rich foods such as meat and seafood (e.g., Atkins Diet) can induce ketosis and hyperuricemia. Research is required to determine the most effective weight loss diet for people with gout.

Table 3: **General Dietary Measures for Patients with Gout**

Avoid	Limit	Encourage
Organ meats high in purine content (e.g., sweetbreads, liver, kidney)	Serving sizes of: beef, lamb, pork, seafood with high purine content (e.g., sardines, shellfish)	Low-fat or nonfat dairy products
High-fructose corn syrup–sweetened sodas, other beverages or food	Servings of naturally sweet fruit juices, table sugar, sweetened beverages and desserts, table salt (including sauces and gravies)	Vegetables
Alcohol overuse (>2 servings/day for males and >1 serving/day for females)	Alcohol (particularly beer but also wine and spirits)	—

Adapted with permission from Khanna D, Fitzgerald JD, Khanna P et al. 2012 American College of Rheumatology guidelines for management of gout. Part 1: systematic nonpharmacologic and pharmacologic therapeutic approaches to hyperuricemia. *Arthritis Care and Research* 64:(10);1431-46.

Tyramine-controlled Diet

Tyramine is an indirect sympathomimetic amine found naturally in some foods and created when food is cured, aged, fermented or spoiled. It is metabolized by the monoamine oxidase enzyme and prolongs the action of adrenergic transmitters also metabolized by this enzyme. Tyramine also stimulates transmitter release from adrenergic terminals which can lead to an adrenergic crisis (sudden increase in blood pressure and tachycardia), particularly in the presence of monoamine oxidize inhibitors (MAOIs) such as phenelzine or tranylcypromine.

A tyramine-controlled diet aims to minimize consumption of foods containing tyramine. Patients taking MAOIs follow this diet to prevent hypertensive crisis and other adverse reactions associated with ingesting MAOIs in combination with tyramine.

Patients limiting their intake of tyramine-containing foods should avoid aged, mature cheeses, dry fermented sausages (salami), smoked or pickled fish, nonfresh meat or poultry, leftovers containing meat, fish, or poultry, red wine, and overripe, spoiled, moldy or fermented fruit or vegetables. Cottage cheese and processed cheese are allowed. Cooking food does not reduce the amount of tyramine it contains.

High-calorie, High-protein Diet

High-calorie, high-protein diets provide energy and nutrients in excess of usual requirements to prevent malnutrition, promote weight gain, meet the need for increased nutrients and optimize an individual's ability to respond to medical treatment. This type of diet is indicated for patients with poor intake, e.g., cancer, HIV/AIDS, chronic GI problems, burns, wounds, trauma, renal dialysis, failure to thrive, preparation for planned surgery.

Calorie-dense and protein-dense foods are suggested, e.g., whole milk, peanut butter, nuts, seeds, beef, chicken, fish, pork and eggs.

Modified Consistency Diets

Table 4 compares modified consistency diets and Table 5 provides a detailed list of foods permitted on a clear liquid diet.

Table 4: **Comparison of Modified Consistency Diets**[1]

Consistency	Purpose	Indications	Description
Clear liquid diet	Supply fluid, electrolytes and energy in a form that requires minimal digestion and stimulation of the GI tract.	For short-term use or transition: ▪ In preparation for bowel surgery or prior to colonoscopic examination ▪ After a period of intravenous feeding (as a transition diet) ▪ In acute GI disturbances (such as gastroenteritis or pancreatitis).	Provides adequate water, 500–1000 kcal as simple sugar and some electrolytes. It is fibre-free and requires minimal digestion or intestinal motility. Because of the low calorie and minimal protein content, it is used only for short periods. For detailed list of foods permitted on a clear liquid diet, see Table 5.
Full liquid diet	Provide food in a liquid form for patients who are unable to chew, swallow or tolerate solid foods. The diet can be designed to provide adequate calories and protein.	For patients: ▪ Following oral or facial surgery. ▪ With esophageal abnormalities, e.g., strictures, anatomical irregularities. ▪ In preparation for some diagnostic procedures. ▪ Who have been on clear liquid diets for a long time (to advance the diet).	Fluids and foods are liquefied using a blender or food processor. The appropriate thickness and temperature will depend on patient condition and tolerance. Dairy products, soups, eggs and soft cereals are used to supplement clear liquids. Commercial oral supplements (e.g., Boost, Ensure) can be used. Use of broth, gravy, vegetable juices, cream soups, cheese and tomato sauces, milk and fruit juices, rather than water, is recommended to increase nutritional value, colour and flavour. Liquefied foods should be used immediately, but can be refrigerated up to 48 h or frozen to prevent growth of harmful bacteria. Vitamins and minerals may have to be supplemented.
Soft diet	Provide texture-modified foods that require minimal chewing.	▪ To assist in progression from full liquid diets to regular diets in postoperative patients. ▪ After head and neck surgery. ▪ In patients with esophageal strictures. ▪ In patients whose dentition is too poor to handle a general diet. ▪ In other patients who have difficulty chewing or swallowing.	Food modified in texture to promote ease of mastication, e.g., chopped, ground, mashed and pureed foods. A food processor is recommended as blenders tend to liquefy foods. Individual patient assessment is important to determine the appropriate consistency of food provided. The patient's acceptance and tolerance of the diet also dictate the extent of texture modification. The soft diet can be designed to meet all nutritional requirements. Most raw fruits and vegetables are excluded, as are any foods containing seeds, nuts and dried fruits. However, soft ripened fruits, e.g., peaches, pears and bananas can be mashed to an appropriate consistency. Vegetables, e.g., broccoli, peas, carrots and yams can be cooked and mashed. The diet can be modified to comply with medical nutrition therapy for specific conditions.

Table 5: **Clear Liquid Diet**

Type of Food	Allowed	Not Allowed
Beverages	Clear fruit juices, e.g., apple, grape, cranberry Low-pulp or pulp-free juices, e.g., orange, lemonade, grapefruit	All others including nectars, milk, fruit juices with pulp, cocoa, prune juice, tomato and vegetable juices
Soups	Bouillon, consommé or clear broth	All others
Sweets/desserts	Clear fruit-flavoured or unflavoured gelatin Fruit ice made from clear fruit juice Plain hard candy, sugar, honey, sugar substitutes, frozen pops	All others and any not tolerated or contraindicated by medical condition
Miscellaneous	Commercially prepared low-residue, lactose-free nutritional supplements Herbs, mild seasonings, salt and flavour extracts	Regular formulations of nutritional supplements Pepper and spices, all others

Meal Replacements and Oral Supplements

For comparative ingredients of nonprescription products, consult the *Compendium of Products for Minor Ailments*—Nutrition Products: Adult Nutrition Products.

While some meal replacement products are nutritionally complete (e.g., Ensure), others require at least 1 regular meal daily to meet nutrient requirements (e.g., Boost, Carnation Instant Breakfast).

Oral supplements: Formulated liquid diets are nutritionally complete for oral or feeding-tube use. Some are modified for specific disease states. A multitude of nutritionally complete formulated liquid diets are available for oral use (e.g., Isocal) or tube feeding (e.g., Jevity). Elemental liquid formulas (e.g., Vital HN) are useful for patients with difficulties in digestion and absorption as they are readily absorbed. More specialized formulated liquid diets have been designed to fulfill the nutrition requirements of patients suffering from certain diseases (e.g., Pulmocare for COPD, Oxepa for ventilated patients).

Diets for Cardiovascular Diseases

For other general principles of healthy living for disease risk reduction, see Chapter 27: Lifestyle Management and Disease Prevention. For a summary of the effects of dietary interventions on surrogate markers of cardiovascular disease, see Table 6.

Diet for Hypertension

Dietary modifications can help to prevent or control primary (essential) and secondary hypertension, alone or in conjunction with antihypertensive drug therapy.

Reductions in dietary sodium intake can reduce blood pressure.[32,33,34,35,36] However, long-term effect on cardiovascular events and mortality is unclear (see also Sodium-restricted Diet).[37] About 50–60% of the population is "sodium sensitive", with blood pressure that responds to alterations in dietary sodium intake.[38] Sodium-sensitive persons are predisposed to hypertension because of inherited susceptibility and can benefit most from sodium-restricted diets. African Americans, older adults and persons with hypertension or diabetes are more sensitive to changes in sodium chloride.[39]

Table 6: **Effect of Dietary Interventions on Metabolic Parameters**

Dietary Interventions	Advantages	Disadvantages
High-carbohydrate (low-glycemic index)	Decreases HbA_{1c}, CRP, hypoglycemia, need for diabetes medications	Non known
High-fibre	Decreases HbA_{1c}, TC, LDL-C, need for diabetes medications	Decreases HDL-C GI side effects
Low-carbohydrate	Decreases TG	Decreases micronutrients Increases renal load
High-protein	Decreases HbA_{1c}, BP, TG	Decreases micronutrients Increases renal load
High–omega-3 fatty acids	Decreases TG	Mercury exposure, environmental impact
Vegetarian	Decreases HbA_{1c}, LDL-C, BMI, TC, BP[25] Increases HDL-C	Decreases vitamin B_{12}
Mediterranean	Decreases HbA_{1c}, BP, CRP, TC, TG, major CV events, diabetes[26], metabolic syndrome[27], mortality[28,29] Increases HDL-C	None known
DASH	Decreases HbA_{1c}, weight, BP, CRP, LDL-C Increases HDL-C	None known
Portfolio	Decreases LDL[30,31]	

Abbreviations: BMI = body mass index; BP = blood pressure; CV = cardiovascular; CRP = C-reactive protein; HbA_{1c} = glycosylated hemoglobin; HLD-C = high-density lipoprotein cholesterol; LDL-C = low-density lipoprotein cholesterol; TG = triglycerides; TC = total cholesterol

The Canadian Hypertension Education Program (CHEP) recommendations advise reducing sodium intake toward 2000 mg (5 g of salt or 87 mmol of sodium) per day to decrease blood pressure.[4] CHEP also recommends consuming a diet that emphasizes fruits, vegetables, low-fat dairy products, dietary and soluble fibre, whole grains and protein from plant sources that is low in saturated fat and cholesterol.

The Institute of Medicine (IOM) does not recommend an aggressive sodium limit in hypertension; their systematic review indicates that ≤1.5 g/day of sodium does not confer a mortality benefit and may even increase risk of adverse health effects in some patient populations.[7] The IOM does recommend a moderate reduction in sodium with a limit of ≤2.3 g/day.

The US National Institutes of Health's DASH diet (Dietary Approaches to Stop Hypertension) and *Canada's Food Guide* are 2 examples of recommendations for healthy eating encouraged by the Heart and Stroke Foundation of Canada. The DASH diet is promoted to control hypertension; it limits sodium intake, encourages consumption of nuts, whole grains, fish, poultry, fruits and vegetables, and suggests lower consumption of red meats, sweets and sugar.[40] It is also rich in calcium, magnesium, potassium, protein and fibre. DASH and *Canada's Food Guide* are similar; *Canada's Food Guide* has a greater range in the number of servings, whereas DASH recommends a higher level of vegetable and fruit intake.

Diet for Dyslipidemia

Dyslipidemia refers to high blood levels of low-density lipoprotein cholesterol (LDL-C), triglycerides (TGs) or both, or low blood levels of high-density lipoprotein cholesterol (HDL-C), all of which contribute to the development of atherosclerosis. Causes may be primary (genetic) or secondary, which includes excessive dietary intake of saturated fat, cholesterol and trans fat. A modified diet can improve the lipoprotein and lipid levels of individuals with dyslipidemia and can help prevent and/or slow the progression of coronary heart disease (CHD).

Lowering total cholesterol and LDL-C decreases risk for fatal and nonfatal coronary events.[41] The *2012 Update of the Canadian Cardiovascular Society Guidelines for the Diagnosis and Treatment of Dyslipidemia for the Prevention of Cardiovascular Disease in the Adult* has established target lipid values based on degree of risk of CHD.

The guidelines recommend the following dietary measures to help achieve these target values:[42]

- moderate energy (caloric) intake to achieve and maintain a healthy body weight
- emphasize a diet rich in vegetables, fruit, whole-grain cereals, and polyunsaturated and monosaturated oils, such as omega-3 fatty acids, particularly from fish
- avoid trans fats; limit saturated fats to <7% and total fats to <30% of daily total energy intake
- increase daily fibre intake to >30 g
- limit cholesterol intake to 200 mg daily for individuals with dyslipidemia or at increased risk of cardiovascular disease
- increase consumption of cholesterol-lowering foods such as phytosterols, soluble fibre, soy and nuts
- follow any of the following diets: Mediterranean[43] (see also Chapter 43: Weight Management), DASH (see also Diets for Cardiovascular Diseases, Diet for Hypertension), or Portfolio (emphasizing cholesterol lowering foods such as soluble fibre, soy protein, plant sterols and nuts).[30,31] See Resource Tips.

Trans fats are formed from the partial hydrogenation of vegetable oils, which turns the oils into solids. Trans fats have been shown to raise LDL-C levels and decrease HDL-C levels. These fats are often listed as 'partially hydrogenated oil' on food labels and are often found in vegetable oil shortening, hard margarines, commercially prepared baked goods, potato and corn chips, crackers, microwave popcorn and deep-fried foods. The Heart and Stroke Foundation of Canada states that trans fats are at least 5 times more harmful than saturated fats and has appealed to Health Canada to introduce regulations to severely limit the trans fat content of foods.[44,45]

Cholesterol is primarily produced by the liver, but dietary cholesterol found in animal foods may contribute to elevated blood cholesterol levels. Foods that have high levels of dietary cholesterol include egg yolks and organ meats, but all animal products contribute to the cholesterol level of the diet. Every ounce of beef, lamb, pork, poultry and fish contains approximately 25 mg of dietary cholesterol and 1 cup of milk contains 4–33 mg, depending on the fat content. Restricting dietary cholesterol intake can achieve a 1–3% reduction in LDL-C.[46]

Saturated fats are the strongest contributor to elevated LDL-C levels. They are found primarily in animal foods (beef, chicken, pork, whole-fat dairy products, eggs and lard) and in some plant-based foods (coconut, palm and palm kernel oils and cocoa butter). Restricting saturated fat intake can achieve a 5–10% reduction in LDL-C.[46,47] A large, prospective cohort study found that replacing 5% of energy intake from saturated fats with equivalent energy intake from polyunsaturated fats, monounsaturated fats or carbohydrates from whole grains was associated with a 25%, 15%, and 9% lower risk of CHD, respectively. However, carbohydrates from refined starches or added sugars (e.g., sugar sweetened beverages or foods) have been positively associated with a risk of CHD and should not be used to replaced saturated fat.[48,49]

Unsaturated fats include monounsaturated and polyunsaturated fats.[47]

- **Monounsaturated fats (MUFAs)** include omega-7 (palmitoleic) and omega-9 (oleic).

- They have been shown to improve blood cholesterol levels and are found in avocados, nuts, and vegetable oils (canola, olive, peanut, safflower, sesame and sunflower oil).

- **Polyunsaturated fats (PUFAs)** include both omega-3 and omega-6 fatty acids.
  - **Omega-3 fatty acids** can lower triglycerides and help prevent clotting of blood. They are found in cold-water fish (mackerel, herring, sardines, salmon and trout), canola and soybean oils, nuts (walnuts, pecans, pine nuts) and seeds (flaxseed, sunflower seed).
  - **Omega-6 fatty acids** lower LDL-C. They are found in vegetable oils (soybean, safflower, sunflower, corn oil), non-hydrogenated margarine, nuts (almonds, pecans, brazil nuts) and seeds (sunflower).

Health Canada requires food products to state fat content (saturated fats, unsaturated fats, cholesterol and trans fats) on the labels. Some guidelines to permitted food claims include:[50]

- Fat-free: <0.5 g fat per serving of stated size
- Low-fat: ≤3 g fat per serving of stated size
- Reduced fat: modified to contain at least 25% less fat than a similar reference food
- Light in fat: modified to contain at least 25% less fat than a similar reference food.

Beware of potentially misleading labels, such as:

- "cholesterol-free" as only animal products contain cholesterol
- "partially hydrogenated fat" as trans fats are formed in the processing
- "low-fat" as fat may be replaced with refined carbohydrates (sugars) and the resulting product may be higher in calories.

Diet for Diabetes

Diet control is the first step in the treatment of diabetes. Proper diet can help control blood sugar levels. In many cases of type 2 diabetes, proper diet, along with exercise, can control the disease without the need for oral medications.

An appropriate diet helps achieve and maintain optimal blood glucose and lipid levels through appropriate food choices. It is recommended for individuals diagnosed with type 1 diabetes, type 2 diabetes, gestational diabetes, impaired fasting glucose and impaired glucose tolerance.

Meal planning is crucial. A typical meal plan includes breakfast, lunch, dinner and a night time snack. Some people also need to plan other between-meal snacks. Being consistent in a diet is the most important part of meal planning. It is advisable to eat the same number of calories, the same amounts of food and the same types of food at the same times each day. Regular scheduling of meals helps to avoid sharp ups and downs in blood sugar. Individuals using insulin therapy should adjust their insulin based on the carbohydrate content of their meals. This involves carbohydrate counting where dietary fibre is subtracted from the total carbohydrates.

Dietitians with expertise in diabetes management can help individualize nutrition recommendations and also provide information on carbohydrate counting and timing of insulin.

The Canadian Diabetes Association's 2013 Clinical Practice Guidelines for the Prevention and Management of Diabetes in Canada makes the following nutrition therapy recommendations:[51]

1. People with diabetes should receive nutrition counselling by a registered dietitian to lower HbA_{1c} levels and to reduce hospitalization rates.
2. Nutrition education is effective when delivered in either a small group or a one-on-one setting. Group education should incorporate adult education principles, such as hands-on activities, problem solving, role playing and group discussions.

3. Individuals with diabetes should be encouraged to follow *Canada's Food Guide* to meet their nutritional needs.
4. In overweight or obese people with diabetes, a nutritionally balanced, calorie-reduced diet should be followed to achieve and maintain a lower, healthier body weight.
5. In adults with diabetes, the macronutrient distribution as a percentage of total energy can range from 45–60% carbohydrate, 15–20% protein and 20–35% fat to allow for individualization of nutrition therapy based on preferences and treatment goals.
6. Adults with diabetes should consume no more than 7% of total daily energy from saturated fats and should limit intake of trans fats to a minimum.
7. Added sucrose or added fructose can be substituted for other carbohydrates as part of mixed meals up to a maximum of 10% of total daily energy intake, provided adequate control of blood glucose and lipids is maintained.
8. People with type 2 diabetes should maintain regularity in timing and spacing of meals to optimize glycemic control.
9. Dietary advice may emphasize choosing carbohydrate food sources with a low glycemic index to help optimize glycemic control.
10. Alternative dietary patterns may be used in people with type 2 diabetes to improve glycemic control:
    a. Mediterranean-style dietary pattern
    b. Vegan or vegetarian dietary pattern
    c. Incorporation of dietary pulses (e.g. beans, peas, chick peas, lentils)
    d. Dietary Approaches to Stop Hypertension (DASH) dietary pattern.
11. An intensive lifestyle intervention program combining dietary modification and increased physical activity may be used to achieve weight loss and improvements in glycemic control and cardiovascular risk factors.
12. People with type 1 diabetes should be taught how to match insulin to carbohydrate quantity and quality or should maintain consistency in carbohydrate quantity and quality.
13. People using insulin or insulin secretagogues should be informed of the risk of delayed hypoglycemia resulting from alcohol consumed with or after the previous evening's meal and should be advised on preventive actions such as carbohydrate intake and/or insulin dosage adjustments and increased blood glucose monitoring.

Resource Tips

Canadian Diabetes Association. Available from: www.diabetes.ca.

Health Canada. *Eating well with Canada's food guide*. Available from: www.hc-sc.gc.ca/fn-an/food-guide-aliment/index-eng.php.

DASH Diet (hypertension)

National Institutes of Health. National Heart, Lung, and Blood Institute. *Your guide to lowering your blood pressure with DASH*. Available from: www.nhlbi.nih.gov/files/docs/public/heart/new_dash.pdf.

Gluten Intolerance

Canadian Celiac Association. Available from: www.celiac.ca.

Gluten Intolerance Group. Available from: www.gluten.net.

Mediterranean Diet

Mayo Clinic. *Mediterranean diet: a heart-healthy eating plan.* Available from: www.mayoclinic.org/healthy-lifestyle/nutrition-and-healthy-eating/in-depth/mediterranean-diet/art-20047801.

Portfolio Diet

Harvard Health Publications. Harvard Medical School. *What foods are included in the portfolio diet?* Available from: www.health.harvard.edu/diet-and-weight-loss/what-foods-are-included-in-the-portfolio-diet.

Suggested Readings

Adopting healthful lifestyle habits to lower LDL cholesterol and reduce CHD risk; and diet Appendices A, B and C. In: National Institutes of Health. National Heart Lung and Blood Institute. *Third report of the National Cholesterol Education Program (NCEP) Expert Panel on detection, evaluation, and treatment of high blood cholesterol in adults (Adult Treatment Panel III): final report.* Available from: www.nhlbi.nih.gov/sites/www.nhlbi.nih.gov/files/Circulation-2002-ATP-III-Final-Report-PDF-3143.pdf.

Anderson TJ, Gregoire J, Hegele RA et al. 2012 update of the Canadian Cardiovascular Society guidelines for the diagnosis and treatment of dyslipidemia for the prevention of cardiovascular disease in the adult. *Can J Cardiol* 2013;29:151-67.

Canadian Diabetes Association Clinical Practice Guidelines Expert Committee. Canadian Diabetes Association 2013 Clinical Practice Guidelines for the Prevention and Management of Diabetes in Canada. *Can J Diabetes* 2013;37:S1-S212. Available from: guidelines.diabetes.ca/fullguidelines.

Khanna D, Fitzgerald JD, Khanna PP et al. 2012 American College of Rheumatology guidelines for management of gout. Part 1: systematic nonpharmacologic and pharmacologic therapeutic approaches to hyperuricemia. *Arthritis Care Res (Hoboken)* 2012;64:1431-46.

References

1. Chicago Dietetic Association; South Suburban Dietetic Association (Ill.); Dietitians of Canada. *Manual of clinical dietetics*. 6th ed. Chicago: American Dietetic Association; 2000.
2. Cutler JA, Follmann D, Allender PS. Randomized trials of sodium reduction: an overview. *Am J Clin Nutr* 1997;65:643S-651S.
3. Midgley JP, Matthew AG, Greenwood CM et al. Effect of reduced dietary sodium on blood pressure: a meta-analysis of randomized controlled trials. *JAMA* 1996;275:1590-7.
4. Daskalopoulou SS, Rabi DM, Zarnke KB et al. The 2015 Canadian Hypertension Education Program recommendations for blood pressure measurement, diagnosis, assessment of risk, prevention, and treatment of hypertension. *Can J Cardiol* 2015;31:549-68.
5. Arnold JM, Liu P, Demers Cet al. Canadian Cardiovascular Society consensus conference recommendations on heart failure 2006: diagnosis and management. *Can J Cardiol* 2006;22:23-45.
6. McMahon EJ, Campbell KL, Bauer JD et al. Altered dietary salt intake for people with chronic kidney disease. *Cochrane Database Syst Rev* 2015;2:CD010070.
7. Institute of Medicine of the National Academies. Strom BL, Yaktine AL, Oria M, eds. *Sodium intake in populations: assessment of evidence (2013)*. Washington: National Academies Press; 2013.
8. Aburto NJ, Hanson S, Gutierrez H et al. Effect of increased potassium intake on cardiovascular risk factors and disease: systematic review and meta-analyses. *BMJ* 2013;346:f1378.
9. O'Donnell M, Mente A, Rangarajan S et al. Urinary sodium and potassium excretion, mortality, and cardiovascular events. *N Engl J Med* 2014;371:612-23.
10. O'Sullivan MA, O'Morain CA. Nutritional therapy in Crohn's disease. *Inflamm Bowel Dis* 1998;4:45-53.
11. Moayyedi P, Quigley EM, Lacy BE et al. The effect of fiber supplementation on irritable bowel syndrome: a systematic review and meta-analysis. *Am J Gastroenterol* 2014;109:1367-74.
12. Aune D, Chan DS, Lau R et al. Dietary fibre, whole grains, and risk of colorectal cancer: systematic review and dose-response meta-analysis of prospective studies. *BMJ* 2011;343:d6617.
13. Gorman MA, Bowman C. Position of the American Dietetic Association: health implications of dietary fiber. *J Am Diet Assoc* 1993;93:1446-7.
14. Brown L, Rosner B, Willett WW et al. Cholesterol-lowering effects of dietary fiber: a meta-analysis. *Am J Clin Nutr* 1999;69:30-42.
15. Frans MJ, Horton ES, Bantle JP et al. Nutrition principles for the management of diabetes and related complications. *Diabetes Care* 1994;17:490-518.
16. Threapleton DE, Greenwood DC, Evans CE et al. Dietary fibre intake and risk of cardiovascular disease: a systematic review and meta-analysis. *BMJ* 2013;347:f6879.
17. Yang Y, Zhao LG, Wu QJ et al. Association between dietary fiber and lower risk of all-cause mortality: a meta-analysis of cohort studies. *Am J Epidemiol* 2015;181:83-91.

18. Li S, Flint A, Pai JK et al. Dietary fiber intake and mortality among survivors of myocardial infarction: a prospective cohort study. *BMJ* 2014;348:g2659.
19. Rashid M, Butzner D, Burrows V et al. Consumption of pure oats by individuals with celiac disease: a position statement by the Canadian Celiac Association. *Can J Gastroenterol* 2007;21:649-51.
20. Choi HK, Atkinson K, Karlson EW et al. Purine-rich foods, dairy and protein intake, and the risk of gout in men. *N Engl J Med* 2004;350:1093-103.
21. Lee SJ, Terkeltaub RA, Kavanaugh A. Recent developments in diet and gout. *Curr Opin Rheumatol* 2006;18:193-8.
22. Campion EW, Glynn RJ, DeLabry LO. Asymptomatic hyperuricemia. Risks and consequences in the Normative Aging Study. *Am J Med* 1987;82:421-6.
23. Roubenoff R. Gout and hyperuricemia. *Rheum Dis Clin North Am* 1990;16:539-50.
24. Choi HK, Curhan G. Adiposity, hypertension, diuretic use and risk of incident gout in women: the Nurses Health Study. *Arthritis Rheum* 2005;52:S733.
25. YokoyamaY, Nishimura K, Barnard ND et al. Vegetarian diets and blood pressure: a meta-analysis. *JAMA Intern Med* 2014;174:577-87.
26. Salas-Salvado J, Bullo M, Estruch R et al. Prevention of diabetes with Mediterranean diets: a subgroup analysis of a randomized trial. *Ann Intern Med* 2014;160:1-10.
27. Babio N, Toledo E, Estruch R et al. Mediterranean diets and metabolic syndrome status in the PREDIMED randomized trial. *CMAJ* 2014;186:E649-57.
28. Guasch-Ferré M, Bulló M, Martínez-González MÁ et al. Frequency of nut consumption and mortality risk in the PREDIMED nutrition intervention trial. *BMC Med* 2013;11:164.
29. Guasch-Ferré M, Hu FB, Martínez-González MA et al. Olive oil intake and risk of cardiovascular disease and mortality in the PREDIMED Study. *BMC Med* 2014;12:78.
30. Jenkins DJ, Kendall CW, Marchie A et al. Effects of a dietary portfolio of cholesterol-lowering foods vs lovastatin on serum lipids and C-reactive protein. *JAMA* 2003;290:502-10.
31. Jenkins DJ, Jones PJ, Lamarche B et al. Effect of a dietary portfolio of cholesterol-lowering foods given at 2 levels of intensity of dietary advice on serum lipids in hyperlipidemia: a randomized controlled trial. *JAMA* 2011;306:831-9.
32. He FJ, MacGregor GA. Effect of longer-term modest salt reduction on blood pressure. *Cochrane Database Syst Rev* 2004;3:CD004937.
33. Joffres MR, Campbell NR, Manns B et al. Estimate of the benefits of a population-based reduction in dietary sodium additives on hypertension and its related care costs in Canada. *Can J Cardiol* 2007;23:437-43.
34. Penz ED, Joffres MR, Campbell NR. Reducing dietary sodium and decreases in cardiovascular disease in Canada. *Can J Cardiol* 2008;24:497-1.
35. He FJ, Li J, Macgregor GA. Effect of longer-term modest salt reduction on blood pressure. *Cochrane Database Syst Rev* 2013;4:CD004937,
36. Aburto NJ, Ziolkovska A, Hooper L et al. Effect of lower sodium intake on health: systematic review and meta-analyses. *BMJ* 2013;346:f1326.
37. Adler AJ, Taylor F, Martin N et al. Reduced dietary salt for the prevention of cardiovascular disease. *Cochrane Database Syst Rev* 2014;12:CD009217.
38. Williams GH, Hollenberg NK. Sodium-sensitive essential hypertension: emerging insights into an old entity. *J Am Coll Nutr* 1989;8:490-4.
39. Weinberger MH. Salt sensitivity of blood pressure in humans. *Hypertension* 1996;27:481-90.
40. National Institutes of Health. National Heart, Lung, and Blood Institute. *Your guide to lowering your blood pressure with DASH*. Available from: www.nhlbi.nih.gov/health/public/heart/hbp/dash/new_dash.pdf. Accessed April 21, 2016.
41. Scandinavian Simvastatin Survival Study Group. Randomised trial of cholesterol lowering in 4444 patients with coronary heart disease: the Scandinavian Simvastatin Survival Study (4S). *Lancet* 1994;344:1383-9.
42. Anderson TJ, Gregoire J, Hegele RA et al. 2012 update of the Canadian Cardiovascular Society guidelines for the diagnosis and treatment of dyslipidemia for the prevention of cardiovascular disease in the adult. *Can J Cardiol* 2013;29:151-67.
43. Estruch R, Rose E, Salas-Salvado J et al. Primary prevention of cardiovascular disease with a Mediterranean diet. *N Engl J Med* 2013;368 (14):1279-90.
44. Dietitians of Canada. *Trans fats*. Available from: www.dietitians.ca/Dietitians-Views/Food-Regulation-and-Labelling/Trans-Fats.aspx. Accessed April 21, 2016.
45. Heart and Stroke Foundation of Canada. Position Statement. *Trans fatty acids ('trans fat') and heart disease and stroke*. Available from: www.heartandstroke.com/site/c.ikIQLcMWJtE/b.3799313/k.C112/Position_Statements__Trans_fatty_acids_position_statement.htm. Accessed April 21, 2016.
46. Denke, MA. Dietary prescriptions to control dyslipidemias. *Circulation* 2002;105(2):132-5.
47. Health Canada. Fats: the good the bad and the ugly. *It's Your Health* 2012 April. Available from: publications.gc.ca/collections/collection_2012/sc-hc/H13-7-118-2012-eng.pdf. Accessed April 21, 2016.
48. Li Y, Hruby A, Bernstein AM et al. Saturated fats compared with unsaturated fats and sources of carbohydrates in relation to risk of coronary heart disease: a prospective cohort study. *J Am Coll Cardiol* 2015;66:1538-48.
49. Malik VS, Hu FB. Fructose and cardiometabolic health: what the evidence from sugar-sweetened beverages tells us. *J Am Coll Cardiol* 2015;66:1615-24.
50. Canadian Food Inspection Agency. Specific Nutrient Content Claim Requirements. *Fat claims*. Available from: inspection.gc.ca/food/labelling/food-labelling-for-industry/nutrient-content/specific-claim-requirements/eng/1389907770176/1389907817577?chap=4. Accessed April 21, 2016.
51. Canadian Diabetes Association Clinical Practice Guidelines Expert Committee. Canadian Diabetes Association 2013 Clinical Practice Guidelines for the Prevention and Management of Diabetes in Canada. *Can J Diabetes* 2013;37:S1-S212.

Chapter 42
Sports Nutrition

Shirley Heschuk, BScPharm, MSc

This chapter discusses the macronutrient, micronutrient and hydration requirements of athletes, as well as nutritional supplements used as ergogenic aids (performance enhancers).

Macronutrients

Nutrition and Athletic Performance, the 2016 joint position statement of the Academy of Nutrition and Dietetics, Dietitians of Canada and the American College of Sports Medicine, provides guidelines for energy, nutrient and fluid intakes for active adults and competitive athletes.[1] The position statement expresses macronutrient (carbohydrate and protein) recommendations based on body weight to allow amounts to be scaled to the range in body sizes of athletes (Table 1).

Table 1: **Macronutrient Goals for Athletes[1]**

Nutrient	Recommended Daily Intake
Carbohydrate	3–10 g/kg body weight Up to 12 g/kg body weight for extreme and prolonged activities
Protein	1.2–2 g/kg body weight
Fat	Individualize based upon training level and body composition goals. 20–35% total energy intake from fat is common in athletes. *Canada's Food Guide*[2] recommends consuming 30–45 mL (2–3 tbsp) of unsaturated fat and limiting total energy to <10% saturated fat.

For optimal performance, energy consumed must be sufficient to match energy expended. The energy intake required depends on the basal metabolic rate (BMR), the energy expended in physical activity and the thermic effect of food (energy required to digest, absorb, transport, metabolize and store food). Adequate energy needs to be consumed during periods of high-intensity and/or long-duration training to maintain body weight and health and to maximize training effects. Loss of muscle mass, menstrual dysfunction, increased risk of fatigue, injury and illness and a prolonged recovery process may occur if energy intakes are low.

Competitive athletes need an adequate energy intake for athletic performance, to maintain or increase lean body mass and to repair tissue. They must consume enough calories to meet this energy demand. Some athletes require >5000 calories per day.[3] In addition, timing of nutrient intake and nutritional support should be individualized to the athlete and his/her particular sport. It is best to consult a sports dietitian listed with the Coaching Association of Canada (CAC) for specific meal plans for athletes (see Resource Tips).

Carbohydrate

Carbohydrate-rich diets can help maximize muscle and liver glycogen stores before exercise and promote faster recovery of stores after exercise. Complex carbohydrates (e.g., starch, dextrin) are preferred because they are digested slowly compared with simple sugars and supply a sustained release of energy. They also provide fibre, iron (if enriched) and many of the B vitamins necessary for energy metabolism. A summary of guidelines for carbohydrate intake by athletes can be found in Table 2.

Table 2: Guidelines for Carbohydrate Intake by Athletes

Situation	Carbohydrate Targets	Comments on Type and Timing of Carbohydrate Intake
Daily needs for fuel and recovery		
1. The following targets are intended to provide high carbohydrate availability (to meet the carbohydrate needs of muscle and CNS) for different exercise loads for scenarios where it is important to exercise with high quality and/or at high intensity. These general recommendations should be fine-tuned with individual consideration of total energy needs, specific training needs, and feedback from training performance. 2. On other occasions, when exercise quality or intensity is less important, it may be less crucial to achieve these carbohydrate targets or to arrange carbohydrate intake over the day to optimize availability for specific sessions. In these cases, carbohydrate intake may be chosen to suit energy goals, food preferences or food availability. 3. In some scenarios, when the focus is on enhancing the training stimulus or adaptive response, low carbohydrate availability may be deliberately achieved by reducing total carbohydrate intake, or by manipulating carbohydrate intake related to training sessions (e.g., training in a fasted state or undertaking a second session of exercise without adequate opportunity for refuelling after the first session).		
Light: Low intensity or skill-based activities	3–5 g/kg body weight per day	Timing of intake of carbohydrate over the day may be manipulated to promote high carbohydrate availability for a specific session by consuming carbohydrate before or during the session, or during recovery from a previous session. Otherwise, as long as total fuel needs are provided, the pattern of intake may simply be guided by convenience and individual choice. Athletes should choose nutrient-rich carbohydrate sources to allow overall nutrient needs to be met.
Moderate: Moderate exercise program (e.g., 1 h/day)	5–7 g/kg body weight per day	
High: Endurance program (e.g., 1–3 h/day moderate- to high-intensity exercise)	6–10 g/kg body weight per day	
Very high: Extreme commitment (e.g., >4–5 h/day moderate- to high-intensity exercise)	8–12 g/kg body weight per day	
Acute fueling strategies[a]		
General fueling up: Preparation for events involving <90 min exercise	7–12 g/kg body weight per 24 h as for daily fuel needs	Athletes may choose carbohydrate-rich sources that are low in fiber/residue and easily consumed to ensure that fuel targets are met, and to meet goals for gut comfort or lighter "racing weight".
Carbohydrate loading: Preparation for events involving >90 min of sustained/ intermittent exercise	10–12 g/kg body weight per 24 h × 36–48 h	
Speedy refueling: <8 h recovery between 2 fuel-demanding sessions	1–1.2 g/kg body weight per h for first 4 h then resume daily fuel needs	There may be benefit in consuming small, regular snacks. Carbohydrate-rich foods and drinks may help to ensure that fuel targets are met.
Pre-event fueling: Before exercise >60 min duration	1–4 g/kg body weight consumed 1–4 h before exercise	Timing, amount and type of carbohydrate foods and drinks should be chosen to suit the practical needs of the event and individual preferences/experiences. Choices high in fat/protein/fiber may need to be avoided to reduce risk of GI issues during the event. Low-glycemic-index choices may provide a more sustained source of fuel for situations where carbohydrate cannot be consumed during exercise.
During brief exercise: <45 min	Not needed	
During sustained high-intensity exercise: 45–75 min	Small amounts, including mouth rinse	A range of drinks and sports products can provide easily consumed carbohydrate. The frequent contact of carbohydrate with the mouth and oral cavity can stimulate parts of the brain and CNS to enhance perceptions of well-being and increase self-chosen work outputs.

(cont'd)

Table 2: **Guidelines for Carbohydrate Intake by Athletes** *(cont'd)*

During endurance exercise, including "stop and start" sports: 1–2.5 h	30–60 g/h	Carbohydrate intake provides a source of fuel for the muscles to supplement endogenous stores. Opportunities to consume foods and drinks vary according to the rules and nature of each sport. A range of everyday dietary choices and specialized sports products ranging in form from liquid to solid may be useful. The athlete should practice to find a refuelling plan that suits his or her individual goals, including hydration needs and gut comfort.
During ultra-endurance exercise: >2.5–3 h	Up to 90 g/h	As per endurance exercise. Higher intakes of carbohydrate are associated with better performance. Products providing multiple transportable carbohydrates (glucose/fructose mixtures) achieve high rates of oxidation of carbohydrate consumed during exercise.

[a] These guidelines promote high carbohydrate availability to promote optimal performance during competition or key training sessions.

Adapted from Burke LM, Hawley JA, Wong SH et al. Carbohydrates for training and competition. *J Sports Sci* 2011;29:S17–27. With permission of Taylor & Francis Ltd, www.tandfonline.com.

Carbohydrate loading is recommended for athletes who compete in events that last 90 minutes or longer, such as marathons, triathlons and cross-country skiing. The athlete consumes 60–70% of calories from carbohydrate, while simultaneously decreasing the intensity and duration of exercise prior to competition.[3] The type of carbohydrate consumed is less important than the amount ingested.[4] Athletes who follow this regimen for up to a week before competition can significantly increase the glycogen content of exercised muscles; this elevation can persist for 5 days with limited physical exercise and taking in 60% of calories from carbohydrate.[4,5] This strategy has been shown to enhance performance, presumably by delaying fatigue.[4] The type and duration of dietary manipulation and the exercise/training activities varies and is flexible enough to personalize the athlete's pre-event preparation.[4]

Carbohydrate loading in women has not been well studied. Research has shown that up to 93% of total energy as carbohydrate is required, and this could disrupt daily energy requirements.[6] The menstrual cycle may play a role as there is a greater capacity for storage of glycogen during the luteal phase than during the follicular phase.[7]

The downside of carbohydrate loading is that for every 1 g of glycogen stored in muscle tissue, the body also stores 2.7 g of water. This causes weight gain and a feeling of sluggishness.[3]

Fat

Fat is a necessary component of a healthy diet; it provides energy, helps maintain cell membranes and aids absorption of fat-soluble vitamins. Fat intake should comprise 20–35% of total energy intake. Intake of fat by athletes should be in accordance with public health guidelines and should be individualized based on training level and body composition goals.[1] *Canada's Food Guide* recommends consuming 30–45 mL (2–3 tbsp) of unsaturated fat daily and limiting total daily energy to <10% saturated fat.[2] Extreme fat restriction limits food choices and sources of protein, fat-soluble vitamins (A, D, E and K), iron, zinc and essential fatty acids. Reducing fat intake to less than 15% of total calories (e.g., weight restriction to lose weight for an event) compromises fat stores and therefore endurance performance.[8] Athletes requiring a high caloric intake (>5000 calories per day) are recommended to consume ≤35% of calories from fat.[3,9] A high-fat diet is associated with impairment in exercise capacity[10] and an increased risk of cardiovascular disease.[11] For more information on dietary fat, see Chapter 41: Special Diets.

Protein

For adults >18 years of age, *Canada's Food Guide* recommends protein intake of 10–35% of total calories or an intake of 0.8 g protein/kg body weight per day for the sedentary person. For athletes, *Nutrition and Athletic Performance* recommends protein intake from 1.2–2 g/kg body weight per day to support metabolic adaptation, repair, remodeling and protein turnover.[1] Intensive training for short periods, reduction of energy intake or sudden inactivity (e.g., as result of injury) may require even higher protein intake.[12,13]

Athletes do not usually have difficulty consuming enough protein unless they are on a restricted diet. Meeting this increased amount of protein does not require the use of protein or amino acid supplements. The best way is to consume foods that contain high-quality protein, including low-fat dairy products, soy products (e.g., tofu, tempeh), legumes, nuts, seeds, lean meats and fish. Intact, high-quality sources of protein such as whey, casein or soy have been shown to be effective for maintenance, repair and synthesis of skeletal muscle protein in response to training.[14] When inconvenient to consume such protein sources, more portable protein sources (bars, drinks, powders) offer a practical alternative. The content should be closely scrutinized for quality. A dose of 20–25 g of high-quality protein appears to maximally stimulate protein synthesis; above this point protein synthesis is not additionally stimulated, but increases in amino acid oxidation and urea synthesis may result.[15] Protein consumption as soon as possible after exercise promotes recovery and possibly enhances the rate of adaptation of muscle to improve function.[12]

Contrary to what many athletes believe, excess dietary protein does not have an anabolic effect and any excess will be oxidized for energy production or stored as fat. In adult athletes, increased training rather than excess protein intake builds muscle. There are few side effects from daily protein intakes under 2 g/kg in healthy people.

Some concerns regarding high protein intake include:

- Diets high in protein are often high in fat
- Excessive protein intake enhances diuresis, thus increasing the risk of dehydration as the body attempts to excrete excess nitrogen
- Acceleration of the progression of pre-existing renal disease[16]
- Increased urinary calcium excretion, resulting in adverse effects on bone (osteoporosis).[17]

Amino Acids

High intake of single amino acids may impair absorption of other amino acids. The safety and quality of amino acid supplements are questionable. They are expensive and their efficacy has not been established.[18,19,20] Amino acids are commonly taken by athletes as growth hormone-releasing agents.[21] Arginine, lysine and ornithine used in high doses may cause transient increases in human growth hormone levels, but their effect is not sustained enough to increase muscle mass or decrease body fat.[22] Large doses may cause diarrhea and nausea while inhibiting the absorption of other amino acids. Supplementation with protein or amino acids has not been shown to positively impact athletic performance.[23,24,25,26]

Micronutrients

For comparative ingredients of nonprescription products, consult the *Compendium of Products for Minor Ailments*—Vitamin and Mineral Products: Liquid Combinations, Single Entity, Solid Combinations.

Restriction of energy intake, severe weight-loss practices, elimination of one or more food groups from the diet or consumption of high- or low-carbohydrate diets of low micronutrient density can increase the risk of micronutrient deficiencies. Athletes should consume the Recommended Dietary Allowance (RDA)[27] of all micronutrients.

B vitamins are essential for energy metabolism and are adequately supplied if sufficient calories and plenty of complex carbohydrates, fruits and vegetables are part of an athlete's diet. Those following a gluten-free diet may have difficulty meeting their vitamin B requirements as many gluten-free products are not fortified. Vegans and some vegetarians require a vitamin B_{12} supplement.

Calcium helps to protect against stress fractures and, coupled with exercise, delays the onset of osteoporosis (for more information, see Chapter 47: Osteoporosis). The RDA of elemental calcium is 1300 mg for children and adolescents 9–18 y, 1000 mg for adults 19–50 y, 1000 mg for men 51–70 y, 1200 mg for women 51–70 y and 1200 mg for all adults >70 y. The RDA should ideally be met from food sources rather than supplements. Some good dietary sources of calcium include dairy products, fortified dairy alternatives (nut, rice or soy-based products), fortified orange juice, tofu, dried figs, cooked beans, collards and broccoli.

Vitamin D is required for adequate calcium absorption and regulation of serum calcium and phosphorus levels. It also regulates the development and homeostasis of the nervous system and skeletal muscle. While the current RDA for persons 1–70 years of age is 600 IU/day, growing evidence shows that this level might be too low.[28,29] Those who live in northern climates or train primarily indoors year-round are at risk of vitamin D deficiency, especially if they do not consume foods fortified with vitamin D.

The female athlete triad includes the three interrelated conditions of amenorrhea, disordered eating and low bone mineral density. For more information, see Resource Tips. Female athletes with inadequate diets and/or amenorrhea or menstrual disturbances are at higher risk of early osteoporosis, and may have higher calcium and vitamin D requirements.[30]

The International Olympic Committee (IOC) recommends 1500 mg/day of calcium and 1500–2000 IU/day of vitamin D to optimize bone health in athletes with low energy intake or menstrual dysfunction.[31]

Magnesium plays a role in regulating metabolism, including energy utilization and work performance. Engaging in intensive exercise may decrease tissue magnesium levels, partly due to magnesium losses in perspiration. Persons with a low magnesium status exhibit reduced physiological strain during exercise when their magnesium intake is increased.[32] According to several studies, magnesium supplementation produces benefits such as improved aerobic performance, greater strength and fewer exercise-induced muscle injuries.[33,34] In another clinical trial, magnesium supplementation did not improve exercise performance.[35] Supplementation or increased dietary intake of magnesium has a beneficial effect on exercise performance in magnesium-deficient individuals but has questionable effects in individuals with adequate magnesium status.[36] Counsel athletes on good food sources of magnesium (e.g., halibut, cashews, artichoke, peanut butter, pinto beans, banana, potato, broccoli).

Iron is needed to carry oxygen to active muscle cells. Female athletes are at higher risk of iron deficiency (depletion) as a result of menstrual losses. Iron depletion is more common in endurance athletes, regular blood donors and in those who consume a vegetarian or vegan diet (see Micronutrient Requirements of the Vegetarian/Vegan Athlete). Lack of iron leads to fatigue; however, mild iron deficiency has little effect on performance.[37] Any concern about iron deficiency should be discussed with a healthcare practitioner.

Strenuous exercise can lower the body's reserve of other trace minerals such as **copper** (essential for red blood cell synthesis) and **zinc** (important in many enzymes related to energy production). This may cause marginal deficiencies, but does not necessarily require supplementation. High-dose supplements of iron, copper or zinc can interfere with the normal absorption of these and other minerals, such that an excess of one can cause a deficiency in another.[9]

Antioxidants: Vitamin C, vitamin E, beta-carotene and **selenium** help protect the body's cells from free-radical damage. Exercise produces free radicals which are capable of damaging muscle fibres; however, the body synthesizes a variety of endogenous antioxidants to counteract this effect. Also, physical training may enhance the antioxidant defense system to offset the reactive oxygen species generated during exercise.[38] Exogenous antioxidants (i.e., dietary antioxidants) interact with endogenous antioxidants to protect against radical-mediated cellular damage. Antioxidant supplementation in sports is controversial. Vitamin C and vitamin E supplementation was shown to hamper cellular adaptations in exercised muscles and therefore caution is advised when considering supplementation.[39] A review of the impact of antioxidant supplementation on performance found that acute dietary intake of antioxidants is likely to be beneficial on sport performance but chronic intake has a harmful effect.[40] Until research confirms that the use of antioxidant supplementation is safe and effective, the recommendation for physically active individuals is to ingest a diet rich in antioxidants. Nutrient-rich foods include: fruits, vegetables, nuts, whole grains and legumes.

A sports dietitian listed with the CAC can suggest a training diet to meet an athlete's needs for vitamins and minerals through food, which is preferable to taking supplements; if the diet is nutritionally complete, using supplements has not been shown to enhance performance.[41]

Micronutrient Requirements of the Vegetarian/Vegan Athlete

Vegetarian or vegan athletes may, with a well-planned diet, meet all of their micronutrient (vitamin and mineral) needs. Nutrients that may be of concern are presented in Table 3.[3,9,42]

Table 3: **Micronutrient Needs of the Vegetarian/Vegan Athlete**

Micronutrient	Comment	Plant Sources
Calcium	May need fortified foods and supplements to meet calcium needs.	Calcium-fortified beverages (soy milk, orange juice), firm tofu, cooked beans, greens (kale, broccoli, bok choy), almonds, figs, oranges.
Iron	Vegetarians should consume 1.8 times the iron of non-vegetarians since the nonheme iron in plant sources has lower bioavailability than heme iron from animal sources.	Legumes, enriched cereals/breads, dark green leafy vegetables, nuts, dried fruit, blackstrap molasses, tofu. Spinach and beets have a high iron content but they contain phytates, which bind the iron and prevent absorption. Absorption of iron from plant foods can be increased if eaten together with a vitamin C source, e.g., citrus fruits, tomatoes, strawberries, red peppers (see Chapter 41: Special Diets). Cooking, sprouting and fermenting vegetables will release iron from phytates.
Riboflavin	Important for the release of energy from food.	Bean sprouts, green peas, seaweed, nutritional yeast, almonds, mushrooms, cooked soybeans, fortified soy beverages.
Vitamin B_{12}	Found only in animal products or fortified plant products.	Fortified soy beverages, fortified breakfast cereal, nutritional yeast; if fortified foods are not eaten, 5–10 µg daily as a supplement.
Vitamin D	Levels may be low if vitamin D–fortified foods are not consumed (in addition to other risk factors for deficiency).	Vitamin D–fortified soy beverages, fortified rice beverages, fortified margarine.
Zinc	Better absorbed from animal sources than plant sources.	Whole grains, seeds: soaking, sprouting and grinding removes the phytates and improves absorption.

Hydration

Exercise generates body heat, which is lost through evaporation of fluid (sweat) from the skin. Some elite athletes lose as much as 1–2 L of fluid per hour and dehydration can occur quickly without fluid replacement.[3,9]

Common signs of dehydration include:

- thirst
- dizziness
- tiredness
- nausea
- chills
- headache
- muscle cramps.

Adequate fluid intake before, during and after exercise is necessary to prevent dehydration, which can decrease exercise performance and increase risk of potentially life-threatening heat injury such as heat stroke. Athletes are encouraged to consume a fluid volume of 5–10 mL/kg body weight in the 2–4 hours before exercise (until urine is pale yellow in colour), sufficient fluid to replace sweat losses during exercise and sufficient fluid to restore any deficit after exercise. Hydration strategies must be customized as sweat rates vary during exercise from 0.3–2.4 L/h depending on exercise duration and intensity, climate, altitude and the athlete's level of fitness. Acute changes in body weight reflect change in body water and allow athletes to track their hydration status. Pre- and post-exercise body weight measurements aid in estimation of fluid loss; a loss of 1 kg body weight correlates to 1 L sweat loss. While the sensation of thirst is a good indication of the need for fluid, it is not a sign of dehydration. Older athletes should be advised there is an age-related decrease in thirst sensation.[1]

Water can replace fluid lost in sweat but may not be adequate for rehydration because it does not contain energy or electrolytes. Sodium helps to retain ingested fluids and should be included in fluid replacement during and after exercise when large sweat losses occur.[1]

Sports drinks provide energy (from glucose, glucose polymers, sucrose) and electrolytes. Beverages containing 6–8% glucose or sucrose are absorbed as rapidly as water and provide energy needed for prolonged exercise.[43] Electrolytes replace lost sodium, chloride and potassium, and enhance the palatability of the beverage. Sodium and chloride help ensure an adequate intake of fluid and stimulate greater rehydration or thirst after exercise.

Dietitians of Canada suggests that sports drinks contain:[44]

- Carbohydrates: 30–60 g/L from different sources such as glucose, sucrose, fructose and/or maltodextrin
- Sodium: 460–690 mg/L (or at least 70 mg/250 mL)
- Potassium: 78–195 mg/L

Fruit juices and soft drinks are concentrated sources of carbohydrate (>10% carbohydrate concentration), which may deter fluid replacement and cause GI discomfort.[43] A homemade sports drink can be made by diluting unsweetened fruit juice with water and adding iodized table salt, e.g., 500 mL unsweetened orange juice, 500 mL water and 1–2 mL (one-quarter to one-half teaspoonful) iodized table salt (one-quarter teaspoonful table salt = 500 mg Na+);[45] the resulting 1 L mixture contains 54 g (5.4%) carbohydrate.

Most people exercising for <1 hour should drink water only. Sports drinks may be appropriate when participating for <1 hour in intense sports, when doing endurance sports (>1 hour) or when exercising in hot weather.[3,9,43,45,46]

Hyperhydration

Excessive drinking of water during exercise can cause hyponatremia (blood sodium <135 mmol/L).

Signs of hyponatremia include:

- weight/fluid gain
- mental confusion
- general weakness.

Hyponatremia can lead to seizures, coma and even death. Recreational athletes have been identified as being at risk of over-hydration and hyponatremia as their work output and sweat rates are lower, and their belief in the need to drink and opportunities to drink are often greater, compared with competitive athletes.[1] To prevent over-hydrating during an event, recreational athletes are encouraged to drink only enough water to quench thirst.

Nutritional Supplements as Ergogenic Aids

Most sports nutritional supplements are marketed as ergogenic aids and lack rigorous clinical trials to evaluate efficacy. They are unnecessary when athletes select the right variety of foods to meet their energy needs.

The safety of some of these products may be questionable, largely due to possible contamination with extraneous substances. These substances may be dangerous, prohibited during sports competitions or illegal, e.g., androstenedione, dehydroepiandrosterone (DHEA) and other anabolic androgenic steroids, *Tribulus terrestris*, ephedra, strychnine or human growth hormone. Ingestion of prohibited substances may jeopardize the athlete's eligibility to compete (see Chapter 44: Drug Use and Abuse in Sports).

Vitamins, minerals and amino acids have been added to many food products and have been regulated as Natural Health Products (NHPs). Health Canada is in the process of moving these products to the food regulatory framework to resolve confusion while maintaining safety. Examples of these products include energy drinks, waters and juices with added vitamins and minerals, and yogurts and bars with specific health claims. Maximum allowable levels of vitamins, minerals and amino acids are defined. Since December 2013, caffeinated drinks that contain 200–400 ppm (mg/L) of caffeine from all sources and are prepackaged, ready-to-consume and predominately water-based have been classified as food products (formerly NHPs). "Energy shots" containing ≤90 mL liquid and intended as a single dose are classified as NHPs. A list of permitted and prohibited ingredients and monographs for NHPs can be found on Health Canada's website (see Resource Tips).

Liquid supplements and sports bars that contain carbohydrate, protein and fat provide an easy way to increase energy intake. Athletes should read labels in order to incorporate these into their daily diet. Sports drinks can contribute needed fluids and carbohydrates before, during and after exercise. Some of these products may contain other components promoted as ergogenic (e.g., chromium, amino acids, ginseng) which make them more expensive.

Supplements with Evidence to Support Claims

Table 4 summarizes sports food and supplements that have evidence to support the claimed benefits. For more information on sports supplements, see Chapter 44: Drug Use and Abuse in Sports.

Table 4: Supplements with Evidence-based Uses in Sports Nutrition

Category	Examples	Uses	Concerns
Sports food[47]	sports drinks sports bars sports confectionery sports gels electrolyte supplements protein supplements liquid meal supplements	Practical choice to meet sports nutrition goals especially when access to food, opportunities to consume nutrients, or GI concerns make it difficult to consume traditional food and beverages	More expensive than whole foods May be used unnecessarily or in inappropriate protocols
Medical supplements[47]	iron supplements calcium supplements vitamin D supplements multivitamin/mineral omega-3 fatty acids	Prevention or treatment of nutrient deficiency under the supervision of appropriate medical/ nutrition expert	May be self-prescribed unnecessarily without appropriate supervision or monitoring
Specific Performance Supplements	**Ergogenic Effects**	**Physiological Effects/ Mechanism of Ergogenic Effect**	**Concerns Regarding Use[a]**
Creatine[48]	Improves performance of repeated bouts of high-intensity exercise with short recovery periods ▪ Direct effect on competition performance ▪ Enhanced capacity for training	Increases creatine and phosphocreatine concentrations May also have other effects such as enhancement of glycogen storage and direct effect on muscle protein synthesis	Associated with acute weight gain (0.6–1 kg), which may be problematic in weight-sensitive sports May cause GI discomfort Some products may not contain appropriate amounts or forms of creatine
Caffeine[48,49,50]	Reduces perception of fatigue Allows exercise to be sustained at optimal intensity/output for longer	Adenosine antagonist with effects on many body targets, including CNS Promotes Ca^{2+} release from sarcoplasmic reticulum	Causes side effects (e.g., tremor, anxiety, increased heart rate) when consumed in high doses Toxic when consumed in very large doses Rules of National Collegiate Athletic Association competition prohibit the intake of large doses that produce urinary caffeine levels exceeding 15 µg/mL Some products do not disclose caffeine dose or may contain other stimulants
Sodium bicarbonate[51]	Improves performance of events that would otherwise be limited by acid-base disturbances associated with high rates of anaerobic glycolysis ▪ High-intensity events of 1–7 min ▪ Repeated high-intensity sprints ▪ Capacity for high-intensity "sprint" during endurance exercise	When taken as an acute dose pre-exercise, increases extracellular buffering capacity	May cause GI side effects that cause performance impairment rather than benefit

(cont'd)

Table 4: **Supplements with Evidence-based Uses in Sports Nutrition** *(cont'd)*

Beta-alanine[52]	Improves performance of events that would otherwise be limited by acid-base disturbances associated with high rates of anaerobic glycolysis ▪ Mostly targeted at high-intensity exercise lasting 60–240 s ▪ May enhance training capacity	When taken in a chronic protocol, achieves increase in muscle carnosine (intracellular buffer)	Some products with rapid absorption may cause paresthesia (i.e., tingling sensation)
Nitrate[53]	Improves exercise tolerance and economy Improves performance in endurance exercise at least in nonelite athletes	Increases plasma nitrite concentrations to increase production of nitric oxide with various vascular and metabolic effects that reduces O_2 cost of exercise	Consumption in concentrated food sources (eg, beetroot juice) may cause gut discomfort and discoloration of urine Efficacy seems less clear cut in high-caliber athletes

[a] Athletes should be assisted to undertake a cost-to-benefit analysis[47] before using any sports food and supplements with consideration of potential nutritional, physiological, and psychological benefits for their specific event weighed against potential disadvantages. Specific protocols of use should be tailored to the individual scenario (see references for further information) and specific products should be chosen with consideration of the risk of contamination with unsafe or illegal chemicals.

Adapted with permission from Position of the Academy of Nutrition and Dietetics, Dietitians of Canada, and the American College of Sports Medicine: Nutrition and athletic performance. *Can J Diet Pract Res* 2016;77:54. Available from Dietitians of Canada at www.dietitians.ca/sports.

Resource Tips

Coaching Association of Canada. *Find a dietitian*. Available from: www.coach.ca/find-a-dietitian-p140496.

Coaching Association of Canada. *Sport nutrition*. Available from: www.coach.ca/sport-nutrition-tips-s13426.

Dietitians of Canada. *Nutrition A-Z (alphabetical listing of materials)*. Available from: www.dietitians.ca/Your-Health/Nutrition-A-Z.aspx.

Female Athlete Triad Coalition. An International Consortium. Available from: www.femaleathletetriad.org/.

Health Canada. *Natural and non-prescription health products*. Available from: www.hc-sc.gc.ca/dhp-mps/prodnatur/index-eng.php.

National Institutes of Health. Office of Dietary Supplements. *Dietary supplement fact sheets*. Available from: ods.od.nih.gov/factsheets/list-all/.

Sportscience: a peer-reviewed journal and site for sport research. Available from: www.sportsci.org.

World Anti-Doping Agency. Available from: www.wada-ama.org.

Suggested Readings

Rodriguez NR, DiMarco NM, Langley S et al. Position of the American Dietetic Association, Dietitians of Canada, and the American College of Sports Medicine: Nutrition and athletic performance. *J Am Diet Assoc* 2009;109:509-27.

Rosenbloom CA, Coleman EJ, eds. *Sports nutrition: a practice manual for professionals*. 5th ed. Chicago: Academy of Nutrition and Dietetics; 2012.

Sarubin A. *The health professional's guide to popular dietary supplements*. 3rd ed. Chicago: American Dietetic Association; 2007.

Thomas DT, Erdman KA, Burke LM. Position of the Academy of Nutrition and Dietetics, Dietitians of Canada, and the American College of Sports Medicine: Nutrition and athletic performance. *J Acad Nutr Diet* 2016;116:501-28.

References

1. Thomas DT, Erdman KA, Burke LM. Position of the Academy of Nutrition and Dietetics, Dietitians of Canada, and the American College of Sports Medicine: Nutrition and athletic performance. *J Acad Nutr Diet* 2016;116:501-28.
2. Health Canada. *Eating well with Canada's food guide*. Available from: www.hc-sc.gc.ca/fn-an/food-guide-aliment/index-eng.php. Accessed April 26, 2016.
3. Turner RE, Ross D. Sports nutrition. In: Insel PM, ed. *Nutrition*. Sudbury: Jones and Barlett; 2001. p. 480-521.
4. Sedlock DA. The latest on carbohydrate loading: a practical approach. *Curr Sports Med Rep* 2008;7:209-13.
5. Arnall DA, Nelson AG, Quigley J et al. Supercompensated glycogen loads persist 5 days in resting trained cyclists. *Eur J Appl Physiol* 2007;99:251-6.
6. Tarnopolsky MA, Atkinson SA, Phillips SM et al. Carbohydrate loading and metabolism during exercise in men and women. *J Appl Physiol* 1995;78:1360-8.
7. McLay RT, Thomson CD, Williams SM et al. Carbohydrate loading and female endurance athletes: effect of menstrual-cycle phase. *Int J Sport Nutr Exerc Metab* 2007;17:189-205.
8. Horvath PJ, Eagen CK, Fisher NM et al. The effects of varying dietary fat on performance and metabolism in trained male and female runners. *J Am Coll Nutr* 2000;19:52-60.
9. Rodriguez NR, DiMarco NM, Langley S et al. Position of the American Dietetic Association, Dietitians of Canada, and the American College of Sports Medicine: Nutrition and athletic performance. *J Am Diet Assoc* 2009;109:509-27.
10. Hawley JA, Brouns F, Jeukendrup A. Strategies to enhance fat utilization during exercise. *Sports Med* 1998;25:241-57.
11. Sarna S, Kaprio J. Life expectancy of former elite athletes. *Sports Med* 1994;17:149-51.
12. Phillips SM, Van Loon LJ. Dietary protein for athletes: from requirements to optimum adaptation. *J Sports Sci* 2011;29:S29-38.
13. Wall BT, Morton JP, van Loon LJ. Strategies to maintain skeletal muscle mass in the injured athlete: nutritional considerations and exercise mimetics. *Eur J Sport Sci* 2015;15:53-62.
14. Tipton KD, Elliott TA, Cree MG et al. Stimulation of net muscle protein synthesis by whey protein ingestion before and after exercise. *Am J Physiol Endocrinol Metab* 2007;292:E71-6.
15. Phillips SM, Moore DR, Tang JE. A critical examination of dietary protein requirements, benefits, and excesses in athletes. *Int J Sport Nutr Exerc Metab* 2007;17:S58-76.
16. Brenner BM, Meyer TW, Hostetter TH. Dietary protein intake and the progressive nature of kidney disease: the role of hemodynamically mediated glomerular injury in the pathogenesis of progressive glomerular sclerosis in aging, renal ablation, and intrinsic renal disease. *N Engl J Med* 1982;307:652-9.
17. Barzel US, Massey LK. Excess dietary protein can adversely affect bone. *J Nutr* 1998;128:1051-3.
18. Slavin JL, Lanners G, Engstrom MA. Amino acid supplements: beneficial or risky? *Phys Sportsmed* 1988;16:221-4.
19. Otten JJ, Hellwig JP, Meyers LD, eds. *DRI, Dietary reference intakes: the essential guide to nutrient requirements*. Washington: National Academies Press; 2006.
20. Di Luigi L. Supplements and the endocrine system in athletes. *Clin Sports Med* 2008;27:131-51.
21. Chromiak JA, Antonio J. Use of amino acids as growth hormone-releasing agents by athletes. *Nutrition* 2002;18:657-61.
22. Suminski RR, Robertson RJ, Gross FL et al. Acute effect of amino acid ingestion and resistance exercise on plasma growth hormone concentration in young men. *Int J Sport Nutr* 1997;7:48-60.
23. Ivy JL, Res PT, Sprague RC et al. Effect of a carbohydrate-protein supplement on endurance performance during exercise of varying intensity. *Int J Sport Nutr Exerc Metab* 2003;13:382-95.
24. van Essen M, Gibala MJ. Failure of protein to improve time trial performance when added to a sports drink. *Med Sci Sports Exerc* 2006;38:1476-83.
25. Abel T, Knechtle B, Perret C et al. Influence of chronic supplementation of arginine aspartate in endurance athletes on performance and substrate metabolism–a randomized, double-blind, placebo-controlled study. *Int J Sports Med* 2005;26:344-9.
26. Sutton EE, Coill MR, Deuster PA. Ingestion of tyrosine: effects on endurance, muscle strength, and anaerobic performance. *Int J Sport Nutr Exerc Metab* 2005;15:173-85.
27. Health Canada. *Dietary reference intakes tables*. Available from: www.hc-sc.gc.ca/fn-an/nutrition/reference/table/index-eng.php. Accessed April 26, 2016.
28. Holick MF. Vitamin D deficiency. *N Engl J Med* 2007;357:266-81.
29. Hanley DA, Cranney A, Jones G et al. Vitamin D in adult health and disease: a review and guideline statement from Osteoporosis Canada (summary). *CMAJ* 2010;182:1315-9.
30. Rauh MJ, Nichols JF, Barrack MT. Relationship among injury and disordered eating, menstrual dysfunction, and low bone mineral density in high school athletes: a prospective study. *J Athl Train* 2010;45:243-52.
31. Mountjoy M, Sundgot-Borgen J, Burke L et al. The IOC consensus statement: beyond the Female Athlete Triad–Relative Energy Deficiency in Sport (RED-S). *Br J Sports Med* 2014;48:491-7.
32. Lukaski HC, Nielsen FH. Dietary magnesium depletion affects metabolic responses during submaximal exercise in postmenopausal women. *J Nutr* 2002;132:930-5.
33. Golf SW, Bender S, Gruttner J. On the significance of magnesium in extreme physical stress. *Cardiosvasc Drugs Ther* 1998;12:197-202.
34. Brilla LR, Haley TF. Effect of magnesium supplementation on strength training in humans. *J Am Coll Nutr* 1992;11:326-9.
35. Weller E, Bachert P, Meinch HM et al. Lack of effect of oral Mg-supplementation on Mg in serum, blood cells, and calf muscle. *Med Sci Sports Exerc* 1998;30:1584-91.
36. Nielsen FH, Lukaski HC. Update on the relationship between magnesium and exercise. *Magnes Res* 2006;19:180-9.
37. Zhu YI, Haas JD. Iron depletion without anemia and physical performance in young women. *Am J Clin Nutr* 1997;66:334-1.
38. Tauler P, Aguillo A, Gimeno I et al. Response of blood cell antioxidant enzyme defences to antioxidant diet supplementation and to intense exercise. *Eur J Nutr* 2006;45:187-95.
39. Paulsen G, Cumming KT, Holden G et al. Vitamin C and E supplementation hampers cellular adaptation to endurance training in humans: a double-blind, randomised, controlled trial. *J Physiol* 2014;592:1887-901.
40. Braakhuis AJ, and Hopkins WG. Impact of dietary antioxidants on sport performance: a review. *Sports Med* 2015;45:939–55.
41. Lukaski HC. Vitamin and mineral status: effects on physical performance. *Nutrition* 2004;20:632-44.
42. Coaching Association of Canada. Sport Nutrition Advisory Committee (SNAC). *Vegetarian ways of eating: finding the nutrients*. Available from: coach.ca/vegetarian-ways-of-eating-finding-the-nutrients-p154670. Accessed April 26, 2016.

43. Marriage B, Schnurr H, Carter-Erdman KA et al. *Sports nutrition: resource manual*. 2nd ed. Edmonton: Sport Medicine Council of Alberta; 1999.
44. Dietitians of Canada. *Sports nutrition (adult). Sports hydration*. Available from: www.dietitians.ca/Your-Health/Nutrition-A-Z/Sports-Nutrition-%28Adult%29/Sports-Hydration.aspx. Accessed April 26, 2016.
45. Coaching Association of Canada. Sport Nutrition Advisory Committee. *Fluids and foods during training/competition*. Available from: coach.ca/fluids-and-foods-during-training-competition-p154683. Accessed April 26, 2016.
46. von Duvillard SP, Arciero PJ, Tietjen-Smith T et al. Sports drinks, exercise training, and competition. *Curr Sports Med Rep* 2008;7:202-8.
47. Burke LM, Cato L. Supplements and sports foods. In: Burke LM, Deakin V, eds. *Clinical sports nutrition*. 5th ed. North Ryde: McGraw- Hill; 2015. p. 493-591.
48. Tarnopolsky MA. Caffeine and creatine use in sport. *Ann Nutr Metab* 2010;57:1-8.
49. Astorino TA, Roberson DW. Efficacy of acute caffeine ingestion for short-term high-intensity exercise performance: a systematic review. *J Strength Cond Res* 2010;24:257-65.
50. Burke L, Desbrow B, Spriet L. *Caffeine for sports performance*. Champagne: Human Kinetics; 2013.
51. Carr AJ, Hopkins WG, Gore CJ. Effects of acute alkalosis and acidosis on performance: a meta-analysis. *Sports Med* 2011;41:801-14.
52. Quesnele JJ, Laframboise MA, Wong JJ et al. The effects of beta-alanine supplementation on performance: a systematic review of the literature. *Int J Sport Nutr Exerc Metab* 2014;24:14-27.
53. Jones AM. Influence of dietary nitrate on the physiological determinants of exercise performance: a critical review. *Appl Physiol Nutr Metab* 2014;39:1019-28.

Nutrition for Athletes—What You Need to Know

Athletes can improve their health and athletic performance by eating well. A good diet is important whether you play recreational or competitive sports. Here's what you need to know about eating well for sports.

- **A high-carbohydrate diet enables your body to store energy.**
  - Recreational athletes should get 45–65% of their energy from carbohydrates.
  - Endurance (competitive) athletes should get 60–70% of their energy from carbohydrates.
  - To increase your carbohydrate intake, eat more whole-grain products, vegetables and fruit.
- **Keep your fat intake low and avoid saturated fats.** You should get 20–35% of your energy from fats, but less than 10% from saturated fats. To reduce saturated fat:
  - Reduce intake of animal products
  - Choose lower-fat dairy products (skim milk, 1% milk, cheese with less than 20% milk fat, yogurt with less than 2% milk fat)
  - Choose lean cuts of meat (lean ground beef, sirloin and flank steaks)
  - Bake or broil foods, rather than frying.
- **Your body needs protein to keep your muscles strong and to produce antibodies to fight infection. However, you do not need a large amount of protein.** The amount varies with your body size and your level of activity. People who are not active or only occasionally participate in physical activity (e.g., recreational sports) should consume 0.8 g of protein for every kilogram of body weight per day. Athletes who train regularly require 1.2–2 g of protein for every kilogram of body weight per day, depending upon the intensity of their training. Daily protein requirements can easily be met if protein makes up 10–35% of the diet.
- **You do not need vitamin and mineral supplements if you eat the right variety of foods every day.**
- **It is important to be well hydrated during sports.** Follow these guidelines to get the right amount of fluid:
  - During exercise, drink enough to replace water lost through sweat
  - Drinking after the activity to satisfy thirst is also important to replace lost fluids
  - For exercise lasting less than 1 hour, water is best
  - For exercise lasting over 1 hour, for intense exercise lasting less than 1 hour or if exercising in hot weather, use diluted glucose and electrolyte solutions (sports drinks with 6–8% carbohydrate).

Chapter 43
Weight Management

Shirley Heschuk, BSc Pharm, MSc

Overweight/Obesity

Overweight/obesity is a chronic condition characterized by an accumulation of body fat in adipose tissue resulting from excessive caloric intake and inadequate caloric loss. Various methods are used for objective measurement of overweight/obesity. The body mass index (BMI) is the most commonly used clinical measurement and is calculated by dividing the person's weight in kilograms by the person's height in metres squared (kg/m^2). See Resource Tips for suggested sources of BMI calculators.

The internationally recognized cut-off BMI values for adults are shown in Table 1.[1,2]

The lower end of the BMI ranges is for the small-framed person with less muscle and the higher end of the range is for a large-framed person or one who carries more muscle. BMI measurements are useful for ages 20–65.[3] The definitions do not apply to infants, children, adolescents, pregnant or breastfeeding women, or adults over 65 years of age.[4]

For infants, children and adolescents ages 2–19 years, Canadian dietitians adapted World Health Organization (WHO) growth charts to assess obesity.[5] The weight-for-length or BMI-for-age percentile determines the cut-offs for obesity (see Table 2). More cautious cut-offs are recommended for younger children (birth to 2 years) to avoid the risk of putting young children on diets.

In the elderly (>65 years), the ideal BMI may be in a higher range, as research has shown that overweight and obese BMI does not appear to confer increased risk of mortality,[6] and underweight BMI can pose a greater threat than being overweight or obese.[7,8] More research is needed to determine optimal BMI in the elderly.

Table 1: **Definition of Adult Overweight and Obesity**

Parameter	Underweight	Normal Weight	Overweight	Obesity		
				Mild or Class I	Moderate or Class II	Severe or Class III
BMI (kg/m^2)	<18.5	18.5–24.9	25–29.9	30–34.9	35–39.9	≥40

Table 2: **Definition of Pediatric Overweight and Obesity**

	Category (cut-off percentile)			
Age Group	**Risk of Overweight**	**Overweight**	**Obesity**	**Severe Obesity**
Birth to 2 y[a]	>85th	>97th	>99.9th	Not applicable
2–5 y[b]	>85th	>97th	>99.9th	Not available
5–19 y[b]	Not available	>85th	>97th	>99.9th

[a] Weight-for-length
[b] BMI-for-age

Physically active people who regularly perform muscle-resistance exercise may have an overweight or obese BMI even though they have normal or even low body fat content. BMI measurement does not provide information about the distribution of body fat. Central body fat distribution, or abdominal fatness, can be determined indirectly by measuring waist circumference.

To measure waist circumference:[9]

- Patient should be in the standing position
- Place measuring tape horizontally around waist at the level of the iliac crest (top of the hip bones)
- Measurement is made at the end of a normal expiration.

Cut-off values have been proposed for healthy waist circumference. Measurements higher than these show an increased prevalence of comorbidities. These values can vary with gender, age and ethnicity (Table 3).

Waist circumference has been incorporated with the measurement of BMI to determine obesity-related health risk and morbidity (Table 4).

Table 3: **Ethnicity-specific Values for Waist Circumference as a Measure of Central Obesity[10]**

Country or Ethnic Group	Waist Circumference (cm)	
	Men	Women
North American (NCEP-ATP III)	>102	>88
Caucasian	≥94	≥80
South Asian, Chinese, Japanese	≥90	≥80
South and Central American	Use South Asian values until more specific data are available	
Sub-Saharan African	Use Caucasian values until more specific data are available	
Eastern Mediterranean and Middle East (Arab)	Use Caucasian values until more specific data are available	

Abbreviations: NCEP-ATP III = National Cholesterol Education Program—Adult Treatment Panel III

Adapted with the permission from International Diabetes Federation. *The IDF consensus worldwide definition of the metabolic syndrome.* Available from: www.idf.org/webdata/docs/MetS_def_update2006.pdf.

Prevalence

The rates of overweight and obesity in Canada classified by age group and gender are presented in Table 5.[11,12]

The prevalence of overweight and obesity has increased in Canada over the last several years in both adults and children. Obesity rates have tripled, from 6.1% to 18.3%, between 1985 and 2011, with a disproportionate increase within obesity classes II and III (correlating with a BMI ≥35). If the current trend continues, it is predicted that 21% of the Canadian adult population will be obese by 2019.[13]

Data from the Canadian health surveys administered between 2001 and 2011 show significant provincial variations in the prevalence and rate of change of adult obesity levels over time. Compared with the national average of 18.3% obese adults in 2011, rates were lower in Quebec and British Columbia, similar in Ontario and Alberta, and higher in the remaining 6 provinces. The Atlantic provinces reported the highest levels of obesity in the country and Newfoundland and Labrador showed a much higher rate of increase (73.3%) compared with other provinces. It is predicted that half of Canadian provinces will have more overweight or obese adults than normal weight adults by 2019.[13]

Table 4: **Classification of Overweight and Obesity by Body Mass Index (BMI), Waist Circumference and Associated Disease Risk[1]**

Weight Category	BMI (kg/m²)	Obesity Class	Disease Risk[a]	
			Waist Circumference: Men ≤40 in (≤102 cm) Women ≤35 in (≤88 cm)	Waist Circumference: Men >40 in (>102 cm) Women >35 in (>88 cm)
Underweight	<18.5			
Normal[b]	18.5–24.9		Least	Increased
Overweight	25–29.9		Increased	High
Obesity	30–34.9	I	High	Very high
	35–39.9	II	Very high	Very high
Extreme obesity	≥40	III	Extremely high	Extremely high

[a] Disease risk of increased waist circumference (increased abdominal fat) added to disease risk of BMI for type 2 diabetes, hypertension and cardiovascular disease. Indicates relative risk; relative to risk at normal weight and waist circumference.
[b] Increased waist circumference can also be a marker for increased risk, even in persons of normal weight.
Adapted with permission from National Institutes of Health. Clinical guidelines on the identification, evaluation, and treatment of overweight and obesity in adults—the evidence report. *Obes Res* 1998;6(Suppl 2):51-209S.

The prevalence of obesity, in both men and women, increases with age. Prevalence is also affected by socioeconomic status, education level and ethnic or cultural differences. Poverty and lower educational attainment are associated with higher than average rates of obesity.[14] In Canada, those at highest risk of overweight and obesity are Canada's aboriginal peoples, followed by individuals of Latin American and African ancestry.[15]

Level of physical activity is inversely related to development of obesity. Obesity is more prevalent in persons with sedentary lifestyles or a disability that restricts activity.[16]

Table 5: **Rates of Overweight and Obesity in Canada by Age and Gender**

Weight Category	Age 5–11 y		Age 12–17 y		Age 18–79 y	
	Females	Males	Females	Males	Females	Males
Overweight	19%	14%	18%	23%	28%	43%
Obese	9%	8%	12%	21%	26%	27%

Health Risks of Obesity

- Cardiovascular:
  - Obesity is a major modifiable cardiovascular disease risk factor.[17] It is associated with an increase in hypertension, heart failure, dyslipidemia, atrial fibrillation, stroke, arrhythmias and venous disease.[18] Obesity is associated with premature acute MI[19] and causes a 3.3-fold increase in cardiovascular disease in American women with a BMI >29 compared with a BMI <21[1,20]
  - Incidence of hypertension is 3 times higher in obese patients. In the Framingham study, hypertension developed 10 times more often in persons who were overweight by 20% or more than in those of normal weight[21]
  - A 14-year follow up of Framingham Heart Study participants showed that every 1 kg/m² increase in BMI increased the risk of heart failure 5% in men and 7% in women[18]
  - Obesity is associated with low high-density lipoprotein cholesterol (HDL-C), high triglycerides and high low-density lipoprotein cholesterol (LDL-C). In the Framingham study, every 10%

increase in relative weight was associated with an increase in plasma cholesterol of 0.3 mmol/L[21,22]

- Varicose veins, venous stasis and pulmonary embolism are more common in obese patients.

- Cancer: A population-based cohort study of 5.24 million United Kingdom adults found that BMI was associated with 17 of 22 cancers investigated.[23] A linear association was found with leukemia and cancers of the uterus, gallbladder, kidney, cervix and thyroid for each 5 kg/m^2 increase in BMI. A positive association was also observed in several cancer types (e.g., liver, colon, ovarian and postmenopausal breast cancers). Similarly, a systematic review and meta-analysis assessed the association between BMI and incidence of cancer by cancer site, gender and ethnic group.[24] A 5 kg/m^2 increase in BMI in men was strongly associated with esophageal adenocarcinoma, thyroid, colon and renal cancers. In women, a strong association between increased BMI and endometrial, gallbladder, esophageal adenocarcinoma and renal cancers was observed. Associations were similar in North American, European, Australian and Asia-Pacific populations, but there was stronger association in Asia-Pacific populations between increased BMI and pre- and postmenopausal breast cancers.[24]
- Endocrine and metabolic:
  - Mildly obese persons have a twofold risk, moderately obese a fivefold risk, and severely obese a tenfold risk of developing type 2 diabetes.[25] Seventy-five percent of Canadians with type 2 diabetes are overweight or obese[26]
  - The enlarged fat cell is less sensitive to the antilipolytic and lipogenic actions of insulin
  - Obese patients have a slightly higher risk of hypothalamic, pituitary, thyroid, adrenal, ovarian and pancreatic syndromes as well as irregular menses, reduction of fertility and toxemia.
- Gastrointestinal:
  - Gallstones occur 3–4 times more often in obese than nonobese persons
  - Gastroesophageal reflux disease (GERD): Overweight and obese patients have a high prevalence of GERD symptoms (37%). A prospective intervention trial showed that a structured weight-loss program reduced and resolved GERD symptoms in 81% and 65% of subjects, respectively.[27]
- Gout: The Canadian Health Survey found that the percentage of men with uric acid levels >416 μmol/L increased from 7% to 31% as the BMI increased from 21 to 31. Women were not affected until they reached a BMI >31, when the percentage prevalence was 7%.[28] Among participants (age ≥20 years) of the US National Health and Nutrition Examination Surveys in 1988–1994 and 2007–2010, a 1-unit higher BMI was associated with a 5% greater prevalence of gout.[29]
- Infection: Obesity increases the risk of nosocomial infections,[30] surgical site infections, periodontitis and skin infections.[31] Fungal and yeast infections are more common in the obese population.
- Liver: Obesity is a main risk factor for NAFLD (nonalcoholic fatty liver disease) and NASH (non-alcoholic steatohepatitis). A prospective study confirmed NAFLD in 63% and NASH in 26% of obese patients undergoing gastric bypass.[32]
- Mortality: Incidence of mortality in subjects with a BMI >26 is 1.67 times higher than those with a BMI <22.5.[1,33] However, in adults ≥65 y of age the risk of mortality increased with a BMI <23 and being overweight was not found to be associated with an increase in mortality.[8]
- Osteoarthritis: Obesity is associated with increased risk of both development and progression of osteoarthritis of the knee.[34,35]
- Pregnancy: Obesity may complicate pregnancy and negatively affect pregnancy outcomes. Obese women have an increased risk of Cesarean delivery and post-Cesarean wound complications, gestational diabetes, gestational hypertension, preeclampsia, preterm delivery and postpartum anemia.[36,37,38] Additionally, neonates born to obese mothers are at higher risk of negative outcomes

(e.g., bacterial sepsis, hypoglycemia or respiratory distress syndrome).[39,40] Studies looking at neonates through childhood and into adult life have also found that maternal pre-pregnancy obesity has a negative impact on several outcomes (e.g., hypertension, childhood obesity and infertility).[39]

- Psychological: Poor self-image and impaired social relationships, depression and anxiety are all worsened by obesity.
- Respiratory: Obstruction by local accumulation of fat leads to hypoventilation and hypoxia, resulting in sleep apnea. Obstructive sleep apnea (OSA) can lead to cardiac arrhythmias, nocturnal hypoxia, heart failure and pulmonary hypertension.[1] OSA is very common in bariatric surgery patients (71%) with a higher prevalence in males (90%) than females (60%).[41]
- Other: Stretch marks (striae) are more common in the obese population.

Economic Burden of Obesity

The combined annual economic burden of overweight and obesity in Canada was estimated at $19 billion in 2012, with $7.5 billion attributed to overweight and $11.5 billion to obesity. This comprises both direct costs to the healthcare system (hospital care, pharmaceuticals, physician care and institutional care) and indirect costs to productivity (the value of economic output lost as a result of premature death and short- and long-term disability) and the total is expected to increase as the population grows. A 1% relative reduction in the incidence of overweight and obesity could have substantial positive economic impact over time.[42]

Pathophysiology

Obesity is a chronic disease developed from interactive influences of numerous factors: organic, hereditary (genetic), physiologic, metabolic (set-point theory), medications, psychological and environmental.

An identifiable organic cause can only be found in a small percentage of people. Weight gain in excess of 1 kg per day invariably implies fluid retention and is frequently a sign of a cardiovascular, renal or hepatic disorder. Other causes may be endocrinopathies such as insulinoma, Cushing's disease or thyroid dysfunction.

Although obesity is associated with several genetic syndromes (e.g., Prader-Willi, Bardet-Biedl and Cohen),[43] in the absence of a genetic syndrome the role of heredity is not easily assessed as environmental factors pertaining to food intake greatly confound this issue. If both parents are of normal weight, the incidence of having an obese child is approximately 9%. If one parent is obese, the rate increases to 50% and if both parents are obese, the rate is 80%.[44]

Adipose tissue grows through an increase in both size and number of cells. Fat infants have a higher chance of being obese in adulthood than do lean infants but obesity is not inevitable for those in the high percentiles of weight for height, age and gender in the early years.[45] Childhood obesity accounts for only a minority of cases of obesity in adults.[46,47]

Many physiologic factors may affect obesity, such as neurotransmitters, neuropeptides and hormones. The hypothalamus receives input from peripheral satiety sites, leptin (a hormone produced by fat cells to signal satiety), ghrelin (a hormone produced from the stomach to increase appetite) and the indoleamine neurotransmitter system in the brain, all of which are thought to play a role in obesity.

Sleep deprivation may be associated with overweight and obese status, as demonstrated in several studies.[48] Reduced sleep decreases the secretion of leptin and increases the secretion of ghrelin, resulting in increased hunger and appetite.[49] Individuals who are awake longer are more exposed to food stimuli, leading to a greater propensity to overeat.[50]

Concerning metabolic influences, the set-point theory proposes that the body has an internal control mechanism, a set-point, probably located in the hypothalamus, which drives the body to maintain a particular level of body fat. Exercise can lower the particular setting, whereas dieting has no effect. Each time we manage to reduce our fat level below our "natural" set-point, the body makes internal adjustments to resist this change and conserve or replenish body fat, making it difficult to lose weight. There is little evidence to support adaptive metabolic changes as an explanation for the tendency of weight-reduced persons to regain weight.[51]

Weight gain is also a common side effect of certain medications (see Table 6).[52,53,54]

Psychiatric disorders may be associated with obesity.[55] Depression and obesity may contribute to each other in a cyclical manner; more study is warranted to determine the mechanism of this relationship.[56] Integrating treatment for psychiatric disorders with weight loss measures may be beneficial.[55]

Environmental factors such as social and cultural background, an increase in sedentary behavior, and economic forces (food prices, agricultural subsidies, wages, availability of low-cost, high-energy-dense foods, portion sizes) have caused waist girth and weight to rise dramatically in modernized societies.[57]

Table 6: **Medications Associated with Weight Gain**

Class	Drugs	Mechanism	Typical Weight Gain	Possible Alternatives
Antidepressants	tricyclic antidepressants (e.g., amitriptyline) mirtazapine	Unclear; may attenuate serotonin-mediated signal transduction, can produce a reduction in BMR.	Appears to be related to the particular drug and the dose and duration of therapy, e.g., amitriptyline (1.8 kg), mirtazapine (1.5 kg). Continued weight gain can be predicted to occur with continued treatment, but at a slower rate than the initial 3 months of therapy.	bupropion fluoxetine sertraline
	monoamine oxidase inhibitors	Unclear; increases hunger and craving for sweets.	Less profound than with TCAs.	
Antiepileptic drugs	valproic acid	Unclear; enhances GABA functions which stimulate carbohydrate intake and reduce BMR.	15–20 kg over variable lengths of treatment.	Topiramate lamotrigine
	carbamazepine	Water retention; mechanism unclear. Possible antidiuretic hormone involvement. Possible norepinephrine or serotonin effect.	Up to 15 kg during a 3-month treatment course.	
Antihyperglyce-mic agents	insulin	Elimination of glycosuria results in increase in fat mass.	Up to 8 kg during an intensive 3-month course of therapy.	acarbose metformin DPP-4 inhibitors GLP-1 receptor agonists SGLT2 inhibitors
	meglitinides, sulfonylureas, thiazolidinediones	Unclear	Up to 5 kg during 3–12 months of treatment.	

(cont'd)

Table 6: **Medications Associated with Weight Gain** *(cont'd)*

Class	Drugs	Mechanism	Typical Weight Gain	Possible Alternatives
Antimanic agents	lithium	Produces polydipsia, causes sodium and water retention, inhibits synthesis of thyroid hormone, blocks dopamine receptors inducing feeding, increases GABA functions (see above).	10 kg or more in 6–10 y; up to 28 kg has been reported.	
Antineoplastic agents	tamoxifen	Unclear	Average 2.5–6 kg, up to 10 kg or more.	
Antipsychotic agents	first-generation antipsychotics	Blocks dopamine D_2 and serotonin receptors to cause increased appetite.	Clozapine: average 12 kg over 16 wk of therapy.	aripiprazole ziprasidone
	second-generation (atypical) antipsychotics		Loxapine: 9 kg in 36 wk.	
Corticosteroids	e.g., dexamethasone, prednisone	Stimulates food intake, causes hyperinsulinemia which promotes fat deposition.	Prednisone; average of 2 kg during a 6-month daily course of therapy.	
Hormones	estrogen, progesterone, testosterone or other anabolic/androgenic steroids	Unclear; possible increased appetite or body fat.	Variable	For contraception: barrier methods or copper IUD
Migraine prophylaxis agents	flunarizine	Possible increased appetite; dopamine effect.	4 kg at dose of 10 mg per day for 60 days of treatment.	
	pizotifen	Unclear; possible serotonin effect.	2–10.5 kg in 8 wk of treatment.	

Abbreviations: BMR = basal metabolic rate; GABA = gamma-aminobutyric acid; TCA = tricyclic antidepressant; IUD = intrauterine device

Goals of Therapy

- Refocus from weight change alone, which is aimed at appearance, to weight management, achieving the best weight possible in the context of overall health
- Reduce body weight or at least prevent further gain—for initial weight loss, a realistic goal of 10% weight reduction should be set (approximately 1 kg weight loss per week over 6 months)
- Abate the complications associated with obesity
- Achieve and maintain a healthy weight range (BMI between 18.5 and 24.9) long term

Patient Assessment

The Canadian Task Force on Preventive Health Care strongly recommends primary care providers measure weight and height to calculate BMI and measure waist circumference to assess obesity-related health risks at all appropriate visits, to identify underweight, overweight and obese patients.[2] If this is done on a regular basis, early intervention can address any unwanted change in BMI and health risk factors.

The 5As intervention, which was developed for smoking cessation, has been modified by the College of Family Physicians of Canada for use in obesity management. The 5As (ask, assess, advise, agree and assist) comprises a manageable, evidence-based, behavioural intervention strategy that has the potential to improve the success of weight management within primary care (see Table 7).[58]

Approaches to use in the treatment of obesity include nutrition therapy, physical activity, cognitive behavioural therapy, pharmacotherapy and surgery.[1] An assessment tool for stepwise management of the overweight or obese adult is presented in Figure 1.

Table 7: **The 5As of Obesity Management and Counselling[58]**

A	Definition	Rationale	Counseling
Ask	Ask permission to discuss weight; be nonjudgmental; explore readiness for change	Weight is a sensitive issue; avoid verbal cues that imply judgment; indication of readiness might predict outcomes	**Ask permission to discuss weight:** "May I talk to you about your weight?" "Are you concerned about the effects of your weight on your health or quality of life?" "Would it be alright if we discussed your weight?" Be sure to affirm that you hear what the patient says **Explore readiness to change:** "Are you ready to work on your weight? Would it be okay if I helped?" "How important is it for you to work on your weight?" "How confident are you that you can take action on your goal?"
Assess	Assess BMI, WC, obesity stage; explore drivers and complications of excess weight	BMI alone should never serve as an indicator for obesity interventions; obesity is a complex and heterogeneous disorder with multiple causes; drivers and complications of obesity will vary among individuals	Assess health status, BMI, WC, waist-hip ratio, root causes of weight gain, and effects of weight on psychosocial functioning Use the Edmonton Obesity Staging System[59,60]
Advise	Advise on health risks of obesity, benefits of modest weight loss, the need for a long-term strategy, and treatment options	Health risks of excess weight can vary; avoidance of weight gain or modest weight loss can have health benefits; considerations of treatment options should account for risks	**Advise about the risks of obesity; explain the benefits of modest weight loss and the need for long-term strategies** "Now that we have a better understanding of your situation, can we explore and come up with a plan of action to improve things?" **Explore all treatment options**
Agree	Agree on realistic weightloss expectations and targets, behavioural changes using the SMART framework,[61] and specific details of the treatment options	Most patients and many physicians have unrealistic expectations; interventions should focus on changing behaviour; providers should seek patients' "buy-in" to proposed treatment	The agree step is about respectful negotiation to achieve "best weight" focused on SMART goals and health outcomes Any treatment plan should use effective behaviour modification principles such as goal setting and behaviour shaping
Assist	Assist in identifying and addressing barriers; provide resources and assist in identifying and consulting with appropriate providers; arrange regular follow up	Most patients have substantial barriers to weight management; patients are confused and cannot distinguish credible and noncredible sources of information; follow up is an essential principle of chronic disease management	Address facilitators (motivation, support) and barriers (social, medical, emotional and economic) that make weight management challenging The clinician's role is to identify, educate, recommend and support Arrange follow up to keep the conversation going

Abbreviations: BMI = body mass index; SMART = specific, measurable, achievable, rewarding, timely; WC = waist circumference

Adapted with permission from Vallis M, Piccinini-Vallis H, Sharma AM et al. Clinical review: modified 5 As: minimal intervention for obesity counseling in primary care. *Can Fam Physician* 2013;59:27-31.

Nonpharmacologic Therapy

Diet Therapy

Calorie Restriction

There is strong evidence that low-calorie diets consisting of approximately 1000–1200 kcal per day can reduce body weight by an average of 8% over 3–12 months.[62] If caloric intake is reduced by 500 kcal per day, it will result in weight loss of approximately 0.5 kg per week. The diet must be nutritionally adequate (diets under 1100 kcal per day may not contain adequate amounts of vitamins and minerals; supplementation may be recommended). Eating less than 1000 kcal per day long term is not recommended as compliance is difficult. It may cause a reduction in resting metabolic rate, promoting weight regain upon cessation of energy restriction.[25]

Reduced-calorie diets result in clinically meaningful weight loss regardless of whether they emphasize protein, fat or carbohydrates.[63,64] Even in overweight or obese children and adolescents, the dietary macronutrient distribution of a reduced-energy diet is not important, as improved weight status can be achieved regardless.[65] Since weight loss among diets is similar, the best option is to recommend any diet that a patient will adhere to.

See Table 8 for a comparison of macronutrient and calorie content of various diets.

Diet Types

Very-low-calorie Diets

Very-low-calorie diets are usually liquid diets that supply about 400–800 kcal per day and produce rapid weight loss while minimizing the protein losses of starvation.[73] They are recommended only for obese patients (BMI ≥30) and must only be administered under close medical supervision. When rapid weight loss (achieved with very-low-calorie diet) was compared with slower weight loss (achieved with low-energy diets), there was no significant difference with respect to weight loss at the end of long-term follow up.[74] Evidence from randomized trials shows a greater initial weight loss may result in improved sustained weight maintenance.[75] Examples include the Cambridge, Optifast, Dr. Bernstein's and hCG (human chorionic gonadotropin) diets.

Table 8: **Nutrient Content of *Canada's Food Guide* Compared with Other Diets**

Diet	Kilocalories/ Day	Total Fat (%)	Saturated Fat (%)	Protein (%)	CHO (%)	Fibre (g)
Canada's Food Guide	1800	30	10	15	55	30
Typical American Diet[66]	2200	35	16	15	50	9
Weight Watchers[66]	1462	25	6	20	56	26
Dr. Atkins (New Diet Revolution)[66,67,68]	1800	60[a]	18	30[b]	10	10
The Zone[69]	1000	30	8	30[b]	40	10
Carbohydrate Addict's	1476	54[a]	24	23[b]	24	8
Sugar Busters[70]	1521	28	7	33[b]	39	25
Dr. Ornish[66,71]	1273	9	2	15	81[c]	38
Mediterranean Diet[72]	2000	37	9	15	43	31

[a] High-fat diet.
[b] High-protein diet.
[c] High-carbohydrate diet.

Abbreviations: CHO = carbohydrate

High-protein, Low-carbohydrate Diets

High-protein, low-carbohydrate diets are based on the idea that by limiting the amount of carbohydrate, the body is forced to burn stored fat. There is no scientific evidence for this and high-protein diets may increase bone calcium loss.[66] These diets can also trigger ketosis, which could lead to dehydration, gout, orthostatic hypotension and electrolyte imbalance, and possibly result in kidney and liver damage.[25] Weight loss induced by high-protein, low-carbohydrate diets is largely attributable to loss of water, glycogen and lean tissue. Adverse effects include headache, bad breath and constipation.

At 3 and 6 months, there is greater weight loss than with low-fat diets but the difference is no longer significant after 1 year. Low-carbohydrate diets are associated with unfavourable changes in total cholesterol and LDL-C but favourable changes in TG (triglycerides) and HDL-C. The long-term benefit is not known as diets high in protein are generally higher in fat, and therefore effects on heart disease, colorectal conditions and cancer are yet to be determined. A systematic review could not recommend use for or against a low-carbohydrate diet.[76] Examples include the Montignac Diet, the Carbohydrate Addict's Lifespan Program, Dr. Atkins New Diet Revolution and Protein Power.[67,68]

Low-fat Diets

Low-fat diets produce significant weight loss for up to 3 years. A 2012 review concluded that low-fat and energy-reduced diets are comparable in terms of weight loss. Low-fat diets are most successful in maintaining weight loss. A diet high in vegetables, fruits, complex carbohydrates (whole grains and legumes) and low-fat dairy is a moderate-fat, low-calorie diet that prevents weight gain and results in weight loss and weight maintenance. Fewer patients drop out from a low-fat diet than a low-carbohydrate diet, suggesting that energy from carbohydrate is more satiating than from fat.[77,78] Weight Watchers is an example of this type of diet.

High-fibre, Low-glycemic-index Diets

These diets promote weight loss through consumption of large amounts of fibre. Increasing dietary fibre may facilitate weight loss.[79] Both soluble fibre (e.g., pectins, gums, psyllium, oat bran) and insoluble fibre (e.g., cellulose, lignins) promote satiety by delaying gastric emptying and causing a feeling of fullness.[80] Insoluble fibre adds bulk and increases water in the stool, which speeds the passage of food through the intestinal tract, allowing less time for absorption of nutrients.[81] Examples include Dr. Ornish's Eat More, Weigh Less and Dr. Bob Arnot's Revolutionary Weight Control Program.

Glycemic index is a term used to compare the blood glucose response to ingestion of 50 g of available carbohydrate from a test food with that of a reference food (either glucose or white bread). When foods with a higher glycemic index are eaten, they produce more of an insulin spike than foods with a lower glycemic index. This may be followed by reactive hypoglycemia and eventually insulin resistance. An index greater than 50 denotes a high-index food. Examples are: white bread (73), baked potato (85), corn flakes (85), bananas (52). Low-glycemic-index foods (<50) include: All-Bran (42), apples (38), lentils (29), carrots (47).[82]

Glycemic load may be more important than glycemic index.[83] Glycemic load takes into account the amount of carbohydrate in the food portion. For example, watermelon has a high glycemic index (72); however, since only 5% of watermelon is carbohydrate it actually has a low glycemic load (3.6). A glycemic load of less than 10 is considered low.

A systematic review on the effects of high-glycemic-index and low-glycemic-index foods on appetite and energy balance did not show a difference.[84] When a high-glycemic-load diet was compared with a low-glycemic-load diet, the long-term weight loss was similar.[85] Use of glycemic index is not endorsed by the American Diabetic Association. However, consumption of lower-glycemic-index foods (whole grains) is encouraged. Examples of low-glycemic-index diets for weight management include the GI Diet; Good Carbs, Bad Carbs; and the South Beach Diet.

Mediterranean Diet

While there are variations in the definition of a Mediterranean diet, it is generally characterized by high intake of extra virgin (cold pressed) olive oil and plant foods (vegetables including leafy greens, fruits, cereals, nuts and pulses/legumes), moderate intake of fish, poultry, dairy and red wine, and low intake of red meat, eggs and sweets.[72] Adherence to a Mediterranean-type diet has been associated with longer survival, reduced risk of cardiovascular or cancer mortality and reduced risk of neurodegenerative disease.[86] Compared with low-carbohydrate diets, the Mediterranean diet showed similar effect on weight and more favorable effect on glycemic control.[87] A subgroup analysis of the PREDIMED trial that looked at the potential health benefits of a Mediterranean diet supplemented with either extra-virgin olive oil or nuts compared with a control diet (advice on a low-fat diet) showed that a Mediterranean diet supplemented with extra-virgin olive oil reduced diabetes risk among persons with high cardiovascular risk.[88] Similarly, a Mediterranean diet enriched with extra-virgin olive oil or nuts resulted in a decrease in diastolic blood pressure compared with the control diet[89] and was more likely to cause reversion of the metabolic syndrome.[90]

Food-specific Diets

These diets make the unfounded claim that some foods have special properties that can cause weight loss. Eventually boredom sets in and one stops eating the allowed food, or at least enough of the allowed food to maintain weight. Examples include the Blood Type Diet, GenoType Diet, Dukan Diet, Paleo Diet, Abs Diet and Wheat Belly Diet.

The Blood Type Diet and GenoType Diet advise tailoring diet and lifestyle to correspond to blood type or genetic make up; e.g., those with blood type A are advised to follow a vegetarian diet.[91] The Dukan Diet is a high-protein diet in which one eats specific food in phases, e.g., in the first phase, one consumes only high protein for a week; in the second phase, vegetables are allowed.[92] The Paleo Diet suggests eating only natural foods that our ancestors have hunted, fished and gathered (no processed food, modern grains or dairy) and eating until full.[93] The Abs Diet promotes building muscle to increase the metabolism of fat. It limits the diet to 12 "power foods" including nuts, fruits, beans, low-fat dairy, whole-grain bread, eggs, turkey and whey protein.[94] Strength training and cardiovascular and abdominal exercises are essential. The Wheat Belly Diet suggests that consuming genetically modified wheat is the cause of being overweight and calls for the elimination of all wheat products.[95]

Fasting

Fasting to cleanse the body and jump-start weight loss has traditionally been used. But fasting deprives the body of nutrients and results in low energy, weakness and light-headedness. Any weight loss is water and muscle, not fat, and weight will be regained when eating is started again. It does not clear toxins from the body; rather, ketones can build up when carbohydrates are not available for energy.[25]

Canadian Guidelines for Diet Therapy

The 2006 Canadian guidelines on the management and prevention of obesity recommend that a nutritionally balanced diet (designed to reduce energy intake) be combined with other supportive interventions. They suggest a **high-protein** or a **low-fat** diet (within acceptable macronutrient distribution ranges indicated in the Dietary Reference Intakes—see Table 9) as a reasonable short-term (6–12 months) treatment option for obese adults as part of their weight-loss program.[1]

Table 9: **Dietary Reference Intakes for Macronutrients**[a]

Age Group (males and females)[b]	Total Carbohydrate (% Energy)	Total Protein (% Energy)	Total Fat (% Energy)	Omega-6 Polyunsaturated Fatty Acids (linoleic acid) (% Energy)	Omega-3 Polyunsaturated Fatty Acids (α-linolenic acid) (% Energy[c])
1–3 y	45–65	5–20	30–40	5–10	0.6–1.2
4–18 y	45–65	10–30	25–35	5–10	0.6–1.2
≥19 y	45–65	10–35	20–35	5–10	0.6–1.2

[a] These are reference values for normal, apparently healthy individuals eating a typical mixed North American diet. An individual may have physiological, health or lifestyle characteristics that may require tailoring of specific nutrient values.
[b] Includes pregnant and breastfeeding women.
[c] Up to 10% of the allowed macronutrient dietary reference can be consumed as eicosapentaenoic acid (EPA) and/or docosahexaenoic acid (DHA).

 Dietary Reference Intake Tables. Health Canada, 2006. Reproduced with permission from the Minister of Health, 2016. Available from: www.hc-sc.gc.ca/fn-an/nutrition/reference/table/ref_macronutr_tbl-eng.php.

For successful weight loss, consume a diet that is:

- Energy-reduced (500 kcal less per day)
- High-protein (within dietary reference value: 10–35%), emphasizing lean protein
- Low-fat (within dietary reference values: 20–35%); decrease saturated fat (<10%), emphasize mono- and poly-unsaturated fats
- Low-glycemic-index (carbohydrate within dietary reference values: 45–65%)
- High-fibre (30 g/day), whole grains.

Other Lifestyle Therapies

Physical Activity/Exercise

Physical activity plus diet produces more weight loss than either diet or physical activity alone.[1] The Canadian Society for Exercise Physiology and Health Canada established an overall goal for individual Canadians to accumulate at least 60 minutes of physical activity every day (in periods of at least 10 minutes each) to stay healthy or to improve health.[25] Exercise reduces obesity and related glucose tolerance and while aerobic exercise (e.g., walking, running) is the most effective for burning fat, it was found that similar reductions in abdominal obesity occur with fixed amounts of exercise, whether of high or low intensity.[96] While walking is safe for most ambulatory people, the Physical Activity Readiness Questionnaire for Everyone (PAR-Q+) can be used to determine whether medical evaluation is required before becoming more physically active (see Resource Tips).

Behavioural Modification

The goal of behavioural modification is to reduce, change or eradicate lifestyle habits that have caused or contributed to weight gain. Through maintenance of a diary, patients become aware of what and how much they eat as a background for changing that behaviour. The aim is to break learned associations between environmental cues and food intake. Strategies include self-monitoring, eating "mindfully" (slower meals, with increased attention to the food and greater awareness of hunger and satiety cues), physical activity, stress management, stimulus control, problem solving, contingency management, cognitive restructuring and social support.[97,98,99]

Interventions that incorporate these strategies produce gradual and moderate weight loss.[100] With systematic manipulation of all factors associated with eating and exercise patterns, there is evidence that with an average length of 18 weeks of treatment, an average weight loss of 9.9 kg is obtained.[101]

Patients are able to maintain, on average, about two-thirds of their initial weight loss 9–10 months after behavioural counselling ends.[102] Additionally, interventions that initiate behavioural modification before implementing a weight-loss program result in improved weight maintenance.[103]

Size Acceptance

It is important to help people realize that there is no ideal body size, shape or weight for an individual and that people of all sizes and shapes can reduce their risk of poor health by adopting a healthy lifestyle.[25]

Weight Maintenance and Prevention of Weight Regain

The maintenance of a reduced body weight is difficult. After 6 months, the rate of weight loss usually declines and plateaus.[1] Successful weight maintenance is defined as a weight regain of <3 kg in 2 years and a sustained reduction in waist circumference of at least 4 cm. Patients on a calorie-reduced diet experience a 15–20% drop in metabolic rate.[104] This reduced metabolic rate may also make it easier to regain weight upon returning to a less restrictive diet. To combat this, the American College of Sports Medicine (ACSM) recommends >250 minutes/week of moderate-intensity physical activity to prevent weight regain.[105] Ultimately, dietary therapy, physical activity and behaviour therapy must be continued indefinitely after weight loss; otherwise weight will likely be regained.[1]

Weight Loss Programs

A number of self-help programs such as Weight Watchers, NutriSystem, Overeaters Anonymous and Take Off Pounds Sensibly (TOPS) offer support and motivation (see Resource Tips).

Technology-based weight loss programs offer patients convenient tools (e.g., personal digital assistants (PDAs), mobile phones, tablets or computers) to self-monitor their diet[106] and physical activity[107] and technology engages the younger population, who are comfortable with and often prefer electronic media.[108] Additionally, connective mobile technology allows patients to transmit diet and physical activity information to a healthcare practitioner or coach, who can provide feedback and support. The addition of a PDA and telephone coaching to an intensive group weight loss program demonstrated that the PDA-based group achieved significantly greater weight loss than the standard-care group.[109] Mobile telephone interventions have also been proven to be an effective strategy for promoting weight loss. The interventions studied included contact by text messages (text, pictures or other multimedia) that delivered frequent reminders of nutrition and physical activity goals and recommendations.[110]

Health and fitness apps on smartphones are able to collect data on diet, exercise and sleep habits from user entry and from the phones' built-in tools, such as the Global Positioning System (GPS), accelerometer, microphone, speaker and camera. The apps can analyze the data, develop personalized programs, track effort and results, provide feedback, coaching and motivation, and even share results on social media, which may facilitate behaviour change through social support, camaraderie, competition and accountability.[111] A randomized controlled trial that examined the effect of mobile phone technology on weight loss and diabetes prevention showed that a combined smartphone app and pedometer intervention resulted in significant weight loss vs. control.[112] Another trial examined acceptability and feasibility of a self-monitoring weight management intervention delivered by a smartphone app compared with a website or paper diary and found both adherence and weight loss were greater with the smartphone app.[113] Popular weight management apps include MyFitnessPal, Fitocracy, Fooducate, FitBit, Noom Coach: Weight Loss, Lose It!, MapMyFitness, Nike+ Running, RunKeeper, and Runtastic.[111]

While technology-based weight loss warrants further study to determine effectiveness in changing patients' behaviours and improving their well-being, and to identify which specific aspects (e.g., convenience, personalization, interactivity or cost-effectiveness) make it successful for weight loss, it has potential for a wide range of uses in weight management and health improvement.[111,114]

Surgery

Bariatric or weight-reduction surgery is considered for people with a BMI >40, or BMI 35–40 combined with high-risk comorbid conditions, and whose obesity is refractory to other approaches.[1]

Surgical treatment of obesity is based on 1 of 2 principles:

- A short bowel is created to produce malabsorption of ingested calories (gastric bypass), *or*
- A small stomach is created to prevent large caloric intake at any one time (banded gastroplasty and vertical sleeve gastrectomy).

Bariatric surgery for obesity, such as gastric bypass, gastric banding and sleeve gastrectomy, results in greater improvement in weight loss outcomes and weight-associated comorbidities compared with nonsurgical interventions, regardless of the type of procedures used.[115,116] Bariatric surgery demonstrates more efficient prevention of type 2 diabetes than usual care (lifestyle interventions combined with antiobesity medications), particularly in patients with impaired fasting glucose.[117] It is also associated with a significant reduction of cardiovascular deaths and lower incidence of cardiovascular events in obese adults when compared with usual care.[118]

When comparing different types of bariatric surgeries, long-term outcomes (weight loss, type 2 diabetes control and remission, hypertension and hyperlipidemia) are better with gastric bypass than with gastric band procedures in severely obese adults.[119] Adolescents with severe obesity obtained substantial weight loss and improvement of comorbidities with an acceptable complication rate with all three bariatric procedures[120] and improvements in weight, cardiometabolic health and weight-related quality of life have been maintained for 3 years after gastric bypass or sleeve gastrectomy.[121]

Patients who undergo bariatric surgery are likely to need lifelong medical supervision.[122] Complications of bariatric surgery include wound healing, metabolic disturbances, severe diarrhea, bloating and anorectal pain. Drug-related complications arise postoperatively; the most common are listed below.

Drug-related management after bariatric surgery:[123]

- Potential malabsorption of bisphosphonates, calcium, iron, thiamine, vitamin B_{12} and vitamin D. Other nutrients may be involved, depending on the type of surgery.
- Immediate-release formulations may be more effective than extended-release.
- Monitor for changes in the dose requirements of digoxin, levothyroxine, erythromycin (do not use base formulations), warfarin.
- Hypertension, dyslipidemia and diabetes may improve and require less treatment.
- Diuretics should be discontinued or reduced in dosage for the first 1–2 months postoperatively to avoid dehydration and electrolyte abnormalities.
- Antihyperglycemic therapies should be reduced in dosage postoperatively to avoid hypoglycemia.

Liposuction, a cosmetic surgical procedure, removes fat to reshape the body. It removes some fat cells, but a compensatory hypertrophy of remaining adipose tissue after lipectomy has been demonstrated.[122] There are risks such as blood clots, perforation injuries and skin and nerve damage. Liposuction has no impact on eating habits.

Pharmacologic Therapy

For further discussion of pharmacologic therapy for weight-loss, consult the *Compendium of Therapeutic Choices*: Obesity.

Dietary Products

Meal Replacements

For comparative ingredients of nonprescription products, consult the *Compendium of Products for Minor Ailments*—Nutrition Products: Adult Nutrition Products.

One or 2 meals per day are replaced with a portion-controlled food item such as a shake or bar, e.g., Slim-Fast, Ensure, Boost. As a result, dieters have to make fewer choices. Compared with a conventional reduced-calorie diet, where the weight loss was 3–7% of initial body weight over 3 months to 1 year, patients using meal replacements lost 7–8%.[124]

Fat Substitutes

Fat substitutes are carbohydrate-, protein- or lipid-based. The carbohydrate- and protein-based products provide less than the usual 9 kcal per gram of fat. They allow incorporation of extra water into foods by binding to it, which decreases the calories per serving. They have a moist, thick texture which mimics the richness of fat. Carbohydrate-based fat substitutes include dextrans, maltodextrans, gums, pectin, cellulose and β-glucan. Protein-based products use whey protein combined with egg white (Simpless, available in the United States). The fatty acids in lipid-based fat substitutes are arranged on the glycerol molecule in order to inhibit absorption. Olestra is a lipid-based product available in the United States. Long-term benefits and safety are unknown.

"Low-fat foods" should not be confused with "low-calorie foods"; the calories saved by eating low-fat foods are often negligible, especially if more is eaten in compensation.[25,125] In addition, low-fat foods (dessert/snacks) may be high-calorie due to the addition of extra sugars to compensate for the loss of texture and flavour from fat.

Artificial Sweeteners

Nutritive sweeteners include sorbitol, mannitol and xylitol, which are sugar alcohols. They contain about half the calories of sugar because the body absorbs them more slowly and incompletely. The side effect of this slow absorption is diarrhea. Natural sweeteners are nutritive sweeteners which contain the same number of calories as table sugar. Natural sweeteners include date sugar, grape juice concentrate, honey, maple sugar, maple syrup, molasses and agave nectar. They are promoted as healthier options than processed table sugar or other sugar substitutes, even though many undergo processing and refining. Be aware that honey may contain small amounts of bacterial spores that can produce botulism toxin and should not be given to babies under 1 year old. Choose a natural sweetener based on its taste and uses rather than on its health claims, as glucose and fructose are the end-products of both natural sweeteners and table sugar.

Non-nutritive sweeteners include saccharin, aspartame, acesulfame potassium (acesulfame K), sucralose, cyclamate, neotame and the herb stevia. They are so intensely sweet that tiny amounts can be used, so the calories they provide are undetectable (Table 10). If used as substitutes for higher energy yielding sweeteners, there is a potential to aid in weight management,[128] but if there is no energy restriction (no reduction of calories), the addition of non-nutritive sweeteners to the diet poses no benefit for weight loss or reduced weight gain. Use of non-nutritive sweeteners may also promote a preference for foods and beverages that have a sweeter taste. Some research suggests that artificial sweeteners may actually contribute to weight gain,[129,130] and in the MESA study (Multi-Ethnic Study of Atherosclerosis), daily diet soda consumption was associated with a significantly greater risk of incident metabolic syndrome (high waist circumference and fasting glucose) and type 2 diabetes than nonconsumption.[131] A 2014 study published in Nature showed that artificial sweeteners (saccharin, sucralose, aspartame) induced glucose intolerance by altering the intestinal microbiota. This resulted in a metabolic disorder in both mice and humans.[132] A 2016 systematic review concluded artificial sweeteners do not increase energy intake or body weight.[133] Given the conflicting evidence on their effect on weight management and the lack of evidence on long-term health consequences, more research on artificial sweeteners is required.

Selected Weight-loss Products

For comparative ingredients of nonprescription products, consult the *Compendium of Products for Minor Ailments*—Gastrointestinal Products: Laxatives; Herbal and Natural Health Products: Combinations, Single Entity; Nutrition Products: Weight Control; Vitamin and Mineral Products: Single Entity.

Several weight-loss products have been used to assist patients in achieving weight loss with varying levels of evidence for clinical efficacy (see Table 11).

Table 10: **Artificial Sweeteners**[126,127]

Product	Kilocalories/g	Sweetness Compared with Sugar	Acceptable Daily Intake[a] (mg/kg body weight)	Comments
Acesulfame K	0	200×	15	Caution if sulfa allergy. Contains potassium—caution in potassium-restricted diets.
Aspartame	4 (so sweet that very little is used)	160–220×	40	Contraindicated in patients with phenylketonuria. Allergy possible. No adverse effects normally associated with ingestion of less than 50 mg/kg/day.
Cyclamate	0	30×	11	Acceptable daily intake is up to 4 mg. Large doses cause diarrhea. Photosensitivity has been reported.
Neotame	7	7000–13 000×	18	Chemically related to aspartame. Does not contain phenylalanine; not contraindicated in phenylketonuria.
Saccharin	0	300–500×	5	Schedule III—permitted only as a tabletop sweetener due to risk of carcinogenesis in rats (not shown in humans). Health Canada is reconsidering allowance in foods.
Sucralose	0	600×	15	Used to replace sugar 1:1 in baking. Passes through the body intact. Splenda contains sucralose, dextrose and maltodextrin and may substitute for sugar in baking (1:1). It contains some calories due to the added sugars; may alter drug absorption.
Xylitol, sorbitol, mannitol	Approximately 2 but very little is absorbed, therefore virtually no calories	0.5×	Not available	Not readily absorbed and can cause osmotic diarrhea.
Stevia (*Stevia rebaudiana)*	0	300×	0–4 (as steviol)	In Canada, stevia leaf and its crude extracts are available as food ingredients and NHPs; purified stevia extract is available as a food additive.

[a] Acceptable Daily Intake from the Joint Commission of Experts on Food Additives of the World Health Organization.

Table 11: **Weight-loss Products with Limited Evidence of Efficacy**[25,127]

Class	Product	Mechanism of Action	Dose	Adverse Effects	Comments
Fibre	psyllium *(Plantago psyllium)*	Delayed gastric emptying creates a feeling of fullness and satiety	10 g/day in divided doses po	Cramping, bloating, flatulence, blockage of esophagus, intestine or fecal impaction if not taken with sufficient fluid. Allergy to psyllium.	Clinical trials needed to evaluate efficacy. Similar effect may be obtained by eating high-fibre vegetables and fruits.
	glucomannan *(Amorphophallus konjac)*	Soluble fibre promotes satiety, increases fat metabolism	1.2–3 g/day po	General gastrointestinal discomfort. Esophageal obstruction possible.	Glucomannan use results in weight and fat loss in adults and children in most studies.[134,135] Safety not established.
Natural Health Products	hydroxycitric acid *(Garcinia cambogia)*	Prevents storage of excess calories as fat, may suppress appetite	500 mg TID po	Upper respiratory tract symptoms, nausea, GI discomfort, headache.	Weight loss in trials only slightly higher than placebo or no difference.[136,137] Safety not established.
	green tea	Thermogenic	100–750 mg/day po	Sympathetic stimulation due to caffeine content (see caffeine below). Tannins cause constipation.	Cochrane systematic review showed small, statistically nonsignificant, positive effect on weight loss. More pronounced effect in Japanese population.[138] Catechin content may be more important than caffeine content.
	Hoodia gordonii	Appetite suppressant	400–800 mg/day po	None reported.	Anecdotal evidence.[139]
Stimulants	caffeine	Anorectic, thermogenic, diuretic	200 mg TID po	Sympathetic stimulation, insomnia, nervousness, tachycardia, headache, anxiety, etc.	All studies done in combination with ephedra (banned in Canada).[140,141] Herbal products containing caffeine include tea, guarana and yerba mate.
Minerals	calcium	Unknown mechanism; may increase metabolism of fat or decrease desire to eat	1000–1500 mg/day po	Belching, flatulence. Constipation possible with $CaCO_3$.	Studies have shown: - 1500 mg/day failed to show efficacy in weight loss[142] - 800 mg dairy calcium did not affect energy expenditure or fat burning[143] - weight loss only in people who are calcium deficient[144] - more research needed.
	chromium picolinate	Increases basal metabolic rate (BMR)	100–500 µg BID po	Nausea, vomiting, stomach discomfort.	A Cochrane systematic review found no reliable evidence of the efficacy and safety of chromium

(cont'd)

Table 11: **Weight-loss Products with Limited Evidence of Efficacy[25,127]** *(cont'd)*

Class	Product	Mechanism of Action	Dose	Adverse Effects	Comments
					picolinate in overweight or obese adults.[145]
Topical Anesthetics	benzocaine	Local anesthetic numbs the oral cavity to decrease taste sensation	3–4 mg in gum, lozenge or tablets; chew gum or suck tablets 30 min before meals po	Numbs oral cavity and gastric mucosa. Topical anesthesia may impair swallowing and increase risk of aspiration. Numbness of tongue may increase risk of biting trauma.	Clinical trials needed to assess efficacy.
Various	apple cider vinegar	Unknown	1 oz (30 mL) cider + 1 tsp (5 mL) honey in 1–4 oz (30–120 mL) water before each meal po	Long-term risk of hypokalemia, decreased bone density, may destroy tooth enamel. If undiluted, may harm the esophagus and stomach.	No available studies. Safety not established.
	chitosan	Decreases absorption of fat	1.35 g TID po	Constipation and flatulence. Derived from shellfish (watch allergies).	A Cochrane review concluded minimal effect on body weight.[146]
	conjugated linoleic acid (CLA)	Suggested to reduce body fat	0.7–4.5 g/day po	Diarrhea, nausea and dyspepsia.	Affects body composition rather than body weight.[147] Warrants further research.
	pyruvate	Unknown; purported to increase metabolism and fat utilization	3–5 g/day po	Stomach upset and diarrhea.	Small weight loss of 0.8–1.6 kg compared with placebo.[148] Safety not established.

Orlistat inhibits fat absorption in the intestine by blocking pancreatic lipase. As a result, about 30% of ingested fat is passed in the stool. Side effects include loose and oily stools (especially if a low-fat diet is not consumed), fecal incontinence, abdominal cramping and nausea. Weight loss on average is 2.9% greater than placebo over 6–12 months and continued therapy can maintain the lower weight for up to 2 years. It can reduce the absorption of fat-soluble vitamins (A, D, E and K), and therefore supplementation is recommended.[149]

Liraglutide stimulates insulin secretion, reduces postprandial glucagon levels, slows gastric emptying and reduces appetite. The most common side effects include nausea, vomiting, diarrhea and constipation. In conjunction with diet and lifestyle interventions, patients on liraglutide achieved and maintained an average weight loss of 8 kg through 2 years of therapy. Adjustment of concomitant diabetes medications may be required to prevent potentially severe hypoglycemia.[150,151,152,153]

Inappropriate Medications for Weight Loss

Syrup of ipecac: People with eating disorders sometimes misuse syrup of ipecac to induce vomiting. Repeated use can cause cardiotoxicity and dental erosion due to acidic stomach contents.

Laxatives: Laxatives are used to speed up the passage of food through the GI tract to decrease the absorption of calories. However, they have little or no effect on reducing weight, as the ingested calories have already been absorbed by the time the laxative takes effect. Prolonged use of laxatives causes electrolyte imbalances and suppresses the natural urge to defecate, leading to constipation.

Diuretics: An initial weight loss is due to dehydration but continued use causes electrolyte imbalances.

Ephedra (Ma Huang): The US Food and Drug Administration and Health Canada have issued warnings about the use of ephedra for weight loss, bodybuilding or increasing energy.[154,155] Ephedrine increases the release of norepinephrine, which suppresses appetite, enhances thermogenesis and speeds up metabolism. Side effects include insomnia, nervousness, seizures, stroke, heart attack and even death. Ephedra is authorized by Health Canada for use only as a nasal decongestant in cold products. These products have smaller dosages and are less likely to be abused.[155] Watch for hidden sources of ephedrine in bitter orange (*Citrus aurantium*), country mallow or heartleaf (*Sida cordifolia*).

Thermogenic agents: Thyroid hormone is touted as a treatment for obesity because of its thermogenic properties. However, there are serious and potentially life-threatening consequences of elevating thyroid hormone levels beyond the normal range. Thyroid hormones should be avoided unless there is a confirmed thyroid deficiency.[127]

Monitoring of Therapy

- Evaluate at 6 months to determine success and assess further need for additional weight loss. If necessary, refer to a dietitian, exercise physiologist, psychologist and/or other healthcare practitioner if there is no success in weight reduction.
- Assess whether patient has been able to reach and maintain a healthy weight range (BMI of 18.5–24.9).
- If patient is on medication for obesity, assess medication tolerance and maintenance of improved diet and activity.

Underweight

Underweight is defined as:[4]

- Adults >19 years: BMI <18.5
- Children and adolescents 2–19 years: BMI-for-age <5th percentile
- Children <2 years: weight-for-length <5th percentile

Prevalence

In 2008, the prevalence of underweight in Canada was 2.6% for females and 1.4% for males aged 18 and older.[156] In the United States, the prevalence decreased from an estimated 4% in the early 1960s to approximately 2% in 2003–2006 among all age groups.[157] The WHO focuses on underweight (malnourished) children in underdeveloped countries and states that the prevalence is dropping.[158]

Health Risks

- Malnourishment; in children, slowed growth, delayed development and a high rate of illness can occur
- Osteoporosis
- Infertility, amenorrhea
- Impaired immunocompetence—increased infections

Pathophysiology

The most common reason for being underweight is malnutrition caused by the unavailability of adequate food. The elderly are particularly prone to being malnourished as are infants and adolescents, who are in rapid periods of growth. Those suffering from eating disorders (anorexia nervosa, bulimia nervosa, binge eating—see Eating Disorders), chronic diseases such as HIV/AIDS and those with poor eating habits are likely to be malnourished. Physical, physiological and psychological factors play a role.[159]

Causes of malnutrition include:

- Poverty
- Diseases that reduce appetite, decrease absorption or utilization of nutrients (e.g., cancer) or increase requirements for nutrients
- Drugs that cause nausea and vomiting (see Chapter 36: Nausea and Vomiting) and/or affect absorption, utilization or excretion of nutrients
- Ignorance about good nutrition or food preparation
- Dental problems
- Depression or mental health issues
- Decreased physical ability to buy food or prepare a meal
- Alcoholism
- Eating disorders.

Goals of Therapy

- Achieve and maintain a healthy weight (BMI between 18.5 and 24.9)
- Treat the underlying cause
- Provide adequate nutrient intake
- Prevent complications associated with being underweight

Patient Assessment

- Assess the individual's weight status (BMI) and risk factors above
- Determine any underlying cause
- Assess diet
- Assess physical activity history

Nonpharmacologic Therapy

Patients who are underweight can increase nutrient intake by eating at mealtime, increasing the number and size of servings, increasing nutrient density by adding extra protein, carbohydrate and fat and by eating more frequently. Restricting physical exercise so there is a positive energy balance can be beneficial, as can behaviour modification. It is best to increase body weight gradually (approximately 0.5 kg weekly). Referral to a dietitian for an in-depth diet assessment would be appropriate.

Pharmacologic Therapy

Appetite Stimulants

Oxandrolone, corticosteroids, cyproheptadine, megesterol acetate and dronabinol are appetite stimulants used largely in cancer-associated anorexia (cachexia).

Monitoring of Therapy

- Assess whether patient has been able to reach and maintain a healthy weight (BMI 18.5–24.9)
- If patient is on medication for being underweight, assess tolerance as well as whether patient is sustaining improved diet and activity patterns.

Eating Disorders

Overview

For further discussion of management of eating disorders, consult the *Compendium of Therapeutic Choices*: Eating Disorders.

Anorexia nervosa (see Table 12) is characterized by 3 essential features: persistent restriction of energy intake that leads to significantly low body weight; intense fear of gaining weight or of becoming fat, or persistent behavior that interferes with weight gain despite being at a significantly low weight; and a disturbance in self-perceived weight or shape. Individuals maintain a body weight that is below a minimally normal level for age, sex, development and physical health and do not recognize the seriousness of the low body weight.[160]

Bulimia nervosa (see Table 12) is characterized by recurrent episodes of binge eating, inappropriate compensatory behaviors to prevent weight gain (purging) and self-evaluation that is unduly influenced by body shape and weight. Binge eating involves eating an amount of food within a set time period (e.g., 2 hours) which is larger than what most individuals would eat under similar circumstances and is accompanied by a sense of lack of control over eating. Purging includes self-induced vomiting; misuse of laxatives, diuretics or other medications; fasting; or excessive exercise. A diagnosis of bulimia is made when the binge eating and purging occurs at least once per week for 3 months. Unlike individuals with anorexia, who are excessively thin, individuals with bulimia are typically normal weight or overweight.[160]

Table 12: **Warning Signs of Anorexia and Bulimia Nervosa**[161]

Anorexia	Bulimia
Loss of significant amount of weight	Bingeing, or eating uncontrollably
Continuing to diet (although thin)	Purging by strict dieting, fasting, vigorous exercise, vomiting or abusing laxatives or diuretics in an attempt to lose weight
Feeling fat, even after losing weight	Using the bathroom frequently after meals
Fear of weight gain	Preoccupation with body weight
Cessation of monthly menstrual periods	Depression or mood swings
Preoccupation with food, calories, nutrition and/or cooking	Irregular menstrual periods
Preferring to eat in isolation	Dental problems, swollen cheeks or glands, heartburn or bloating
Exercising compulsively	Bingeing and purging

Binge-eating disorder is also characterized by episodes of binge eating that occur at least once per week for 3 months; however, it is not associated with the use of compensatory behaviors to prevent weight gain. In binge-eating disorder, there is a marked distress regarding the binge eating and the binge eating episodes are associated with eating more rapidly than normal, eating until feeling uncomfortably full, eating large amounts of food when not physically hungry, eating alone due to feeling embarrassed by the amount of food being consumed and feeling disgusted with oneself, depressed or very guilty afterwards.[160]

Health practitioners should lead efforts to prevent eating disorders by learning to promote self-esteem in their patients and teaching patients to focus on health vs. size. Warn patients of the potential dangers of inappropriate methods of weight loss, including medications (see Inappropriate Medications for Weight Loss).

Figure 1: **Algorithm for the Assessment and Stepwise Management of the Overweight or Obese Adult[1]**

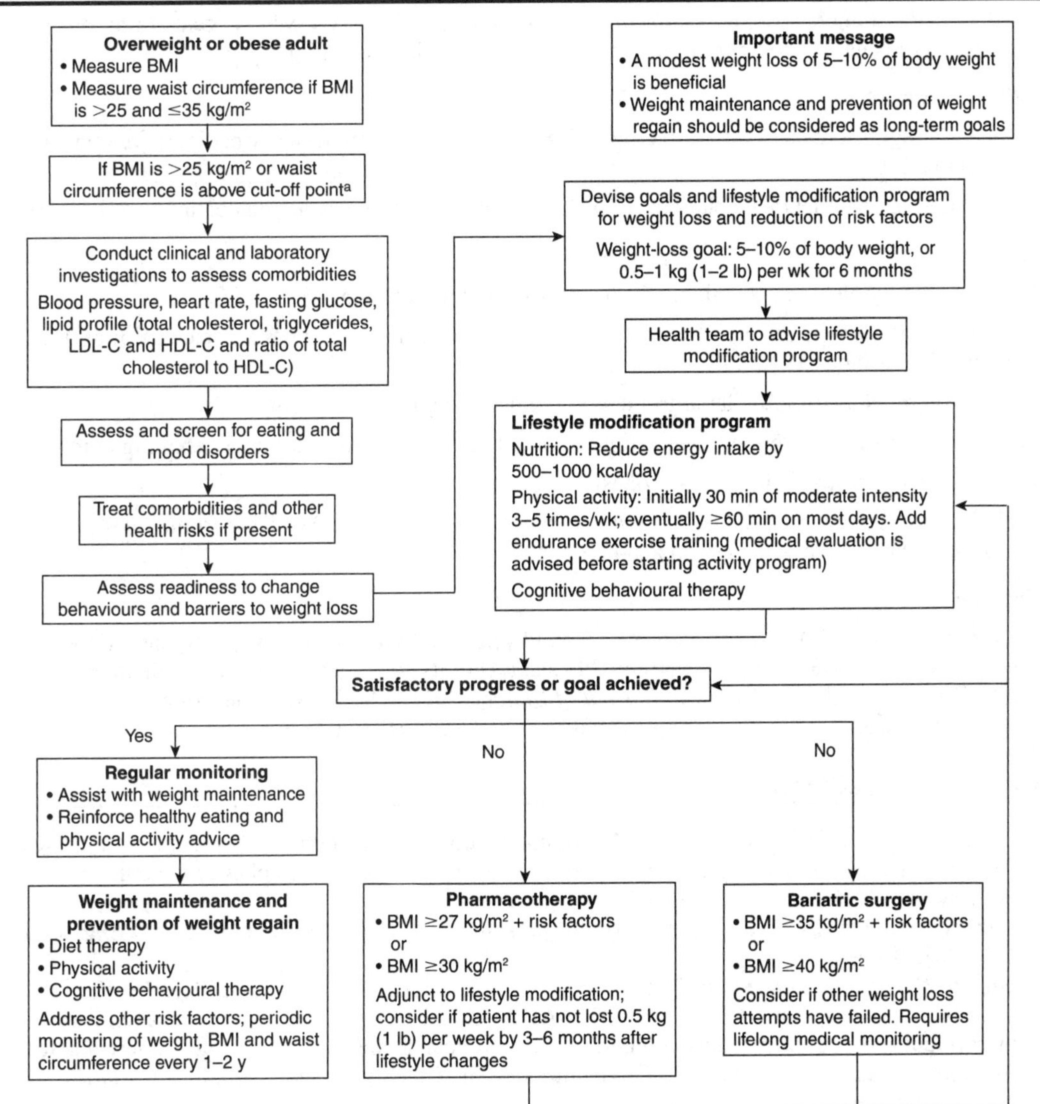

[a] Body mass index (BMI) and waist circumference cut-off points are different for some ethnic groups; see Table 3 for ethnicity-specific waist circumference cut-off points.

Abbreviations: HDL-C = high-density lipoprotein cholesterol; LDL-C = low-density lipoprotein cholesterol

Adapted with permission from Lau DC, Douketis JD, Morrison KM et al. 2006 Canadian clinical practice guidelines on the management and prevention of obesity in adults and children. *CMAJ* 2007;176:SS1-117.

Resource Tips

Calculation of Body Mass Index (BMI)

Canadian Diabetes Association. *Body Mass Index (BMI) calculator*. Available from: www.diabetes.ca/diabetes-and-you/healthy-living-resources/weight-management/body-mass-index-bmi-calculator.

Health Canada. *Body Mass Index (BMI) nomogram*. Available from: www.hc-sc.gc.ca/fn-an/nutrition/weights-poids/guide-ld-adult/bmi_chart_java-graph_imc_java-eng.php.

Eating Disorders

National Eating Disorder Information Centre (NEDIC). Available from: www.nedic.ca. Telephone: 416-340-4156.

National Eating Disorders Association. (NEDA). Available from: www.nationaleatingdisorders.org.

Obesity

Canadian Obesity Network. Available from: www.obesitynetwork.ca.

Health Canada. *Eating well with Canada's food guide*. Available from: www.hc-sc.gc.ca/fn-an/food-guide-aliment/index-eng.php.

Healthy Weight Network. Available from: www.healthyweightnetwork.com.

National Center for Overcoming Overeating. Available from: www.overcomingovereating.com.

Obesity Society. Available from: www.obesity.org.

Public Health Agency of Canada. *Physical activity: Tips to get active*. Available from: www.phac-aspc.gc.ca/hp-ps/hl-mvs/pa-ap/04paap-eng.php.

Physical Activity

Warburton DE, Jamnik VK, Bredin SS et al. The Physical Activity Readiness Questionnaire for everyone (2015 PAR-Q+) and electronic Physical Activity Readiness medical examination (ePARmed-X+). *Health & Fitness Journal of Canada* 2011;4:3-23. Available from: www.eparmedx.com/wp-content/uploads/2013/03/PARQplusJan2015.pdf.

Suggested Readings

Brauer P, Connor Gorber S, Shaw E et al. Recommendations for prevention of weight gain and use of behavioural and pharmacologic interventions to manage overweight and obesity in adults in primary care. *CMAJ* 2015;187:184-95.

Casazza K, Fontaine KR, Astrup A et al. Myths, presumptions, and facts about obesity. *N Engl J Med* 2013;368:446-54.

Freedman HR, King J, Kennedy E. Popular diets: a scientific review. *Obes Res* 2001;9:1S-40S.

Jensen MD, Ryan DH, Apovian CM et al. 2013 AHA/ACC/TOS guideline for the management of overweight and obesity in adults: a report of the American College of Cardiology/American Heart Association Task Force on Practice Guidelines and The Obesity Society. *J Am Coll Cardiol* 2014;63:2985-3023.

Lau DC, Douketis JD, Morrison KM et al. 2006 Canadian clinical practice guidelines on the management and prevention of obesity in adults and children. *CMAJ* 2007;176:S1-117. Available from: www.cmaj.ca/content/suppl/2007/09/04/176.8.S1.DC1/obesity-lau-onlineNEW.pdf.

National Institutes of Health; National Heart, Lung, and Blood Institute; North American Association for the Study of Obesity. *The practical guide: identification, evaluation, and treatment of overweight and obesity in adults*. October 2000. Available from: www.nhlbi.nih.gov/guidelines/obesity/prctgd_c.pdf.

Sharma AM. Obesity. In: Jovaisas B, ed. *Compendium of therapeutic choices: (CTC 7)*. 7th ed. Ottawa: Canadian Pharmacists Association; 2014. p. 398-410.
Strychar I. Diet in the management of weight loss. *CMAJ* 2006;174:56-63.

References

1. Lau DC, Douketis JD, Morrison KM et al. 2006 Canadian clinical practice guidelines on the management and prevention of obesity in adults and children. *CMAJ* 2007;176:SS1-117. Available from: www.cmaj.ca/content/suppl/2007/09/04/176.8.S1.DC1/obesity-lau-onlineNEW.pdf.
2. Brauer P, Connor Gorber S, Shaw E et al. Recommendations for prevention of weight gain and use of behavioural and pharmacologic interventions to manage overweight and obesity in adults in primary care. *CMAJ* 2015;187:184-95.
3. Bales CW, Buhr G. Is obesity bad for older persons? A systematic review of the pros and cons of weight reduction in later life. *J Am Med Dir Assoc* 2008;9:302-12.
4. Centers for Disease Control and Prevention. *CDC growth charts*. Available from: www.cdc.gov/growthcharts. Accessed April 26, 2016.
5. Dietitians of Canada. *WHO growth charts [adapted for Canada]*. Available from: www.dietitians.ca/secondary-pages/public/who-growth-charts.aspx. Accessed April 26, 2016.
6. Janssen I, Mark AE. Elevated body mass index and mortality risk in the elderly. *Obes Rev* 2007;8:41-59.
7. Oreopoulos A, Kalantar-Zadeh K, Sharma AM et al. The obesity paradox in the elderly: potential mechanisms and clinical implications. *Clin Geriatr Med* 2009;25:643-59.
8. Winter JE, MacInnis RJ, Wattanapenpaiboon N et al. BMI and all-cause mortality in older adults: a meta-analysis. *Am J Clin Nutr* 2014;99:875-90.
9. National Institutes of Health; National Institute of Diabetes and Digestive and Kidney Diseases. Weight-control Information Network. *Weight and waist measurement: tools for adults*. Available from: wellness.unl.edu/wellness_documents/weight_and_waist_measurements.pdf. Accessed April 26, 2016.
10. International Diabetes Federation. *The IDF consensus worldwide definition of the metabolic syndrome*. Available from: www.idf.org/webdata/docs/MetS_def_update2006.pdf. Accessed April 26, 2016.
11. Statistics Canada. *Body mass index of children and youth, 2012 to 2013*. Available from: www.statcan.gc.ca/pub/82-625-x/2014001/article/14105-eng.htm. Accessed April 26, 2016.
12. Statistics Canada. *Body composition of adults, 2012 to 2013*. Available from: www.statcan.gc.ca/pub/82-625-x/2014001/article/14104-eng.htm. Accessed April 26, 2016.
13. Twells LK, Gregory DM, Reddigan J et al. Current and predicted prevalence of obesity in Canada: a trend analysis. *CMAJ* 2014;2:E18-26.
14. Williamson DF. Descriptive epidemiology of bodyweight and weight change in U.S. adults. *Ann Intern Med* 1993;119:646-9.
15. Valera B, Sohani Z, Rana A et al. The ethnoepidemiology of obesity. *Can J Cardiol* 2015;31:131-41.
16. Mandl DL, Jason IL. Obesity and eating disorders. In: Herfindal ET, Gourley DR, eds. *Textbook of therapeutics: drug and disease management*. 7th ed. Philadelphia: Lippincott Williams & Wilkins; 2000. p. 1271-88.
17. Anderson TJ, Grégoire J, Hegele RA et al. 2012 update of the Canadian Cardiovascular Society guidelines for the diagnosis and treatment of dyslipidemia for the prevention of cardiovascular disease in the adult. *Can J Cardiol* 2013;29:151-67.
18. Lavie CJ, Milani RV, Ventura HO. Obesity and cardiovascular disease: risk factor, paradox, and impact of weight loss. *J Am Coll Cardiol* 2009;53:1925-32.
19. Suwaidi JA, Wright RS, Grill JP et al. Obesity is associated with premature occurrence of acute myocardial infarction. *Clin Cardiol* 2001;24:542-7.
20. Manson JE, Willet WC, Stampfer MJ et al. Body weight and mortality among women. *N Engl J Med* 1995;333:677-85.
21. Kannel WB, Brand N, Skinner JJ et al. The relation of adiposity to blood pressure and development of hypertension. The Framingham study. *Ann Intern Med* 1967;67:48-59.
22. Pi-Sunyer FX. Medical hazards of obesity. *Ann Intern Med* 1993;119:655-60.
23. Bhaskaran K, Douglas I, Forbes H et al. Body-mass index and risk of 22 specific cancers: a population-based cohort study of 5.24 million UK adults. *Lancet* 2014;384:755-65.
24. Renehan AG, Tyson M, Egger M et al. Body-mass index and incidence of cancer: a systematic review and meta-analysis of prospective observational studies. *Lancet* 2008;371:569-78.
25. American Dietetic Association; South Suburban Dietetic Association (Ill.); Dietitians of Canada. *Manual of clinical dietetics*. 6th ed. Chicago; 2000. p. 365-86.
26. Public Health Agency of Canada. *Diabetes in Canada: facts and figures from a public health perspective*. Available from: www.phac-aspc.gc.ca/cd-mc/publications/diabetes-diabete/facts-figures-faits-chiffres-2011/chap4-eng.php. Accessed April 26, 2016.
27. Singh M, Lee J, Gupta N et al. Weight loss can lead to resolution of gastroesophageal reflux disease symptoms: a prospective intervention trial. *Obesity (Silver Spring)* 2013;21:284-90.
28. Health and Welfare Canada. *Using the food guide*. Ottawa: Health and Welfare Canada; 1992.
29. Juraschek SP, Miller ER, Gelber AC. Body mass index, obesity, and prevalent gout in the United States in 1988-1994 and 2007-2010. *Arthritis Care Res (Hoboken)* 2013;65:127-32.
30. Huttunen R, Karppelin M, Syrjänen J. Obesity and nosocomial infections. *J Hosp Infect* 2013;85:8-16.
31. Huttunen R, Syrjänen J. Obesity and the risk and outcome of infection. *Int J Obes (Lond)* 2013;37:333-40.
32. Boza C, Riquelme A, Ibañez L et al. Predictors of nonalcoholic steatohepatitis (NASH) in obese patients undergoing gastric bypass. *Obes Surg* 2005;15:1148-53.
33. Lee IM, Paffenbarger RS. Change in body weight and longevity. *JAMA* 1992;268:2045-9.
34. Reljman H, Pois HAP, Bergink AP et al. Body mass index associated with onset and progression of osteoarthritis of the knee but hot of the hip: the Rotterdam Study. *Ann Rheum Dis* 2007;66:158-62.
35. Zhou ZY, Liu YK, Chen HL et al. Body mass index and knee osteoarthritis risk: a dose-response meta-analysis. *Obesity (Silver Spring)* 2014;22:2180-5.
36. Waller DK, Shaw GM, Rasmussen SA et al. Prepregnancy obesity as a risk factor for structural birth defects. *Arch Pediatr Adolesc Med* 2007;161:745-50.
37. Stamilio DM, Scifres CM. Extreme obesity and postcesarean maternal complications. *Obstet Gynecol* 2014;124:227-32.

38. Cnattingius S, Villamor E, Johansson S et al. Maternal obesity and risk of preterm delivery. *JAMA* 2013;309:2362-70.
39. Blomberg M. Maternal obesity, mode of delivery, and neonatal outcome. *Obstet Gynecol* 2013;122:50-5.
40. Papachatzi E, Dimitriou G, Dimitropoulos K et al. Pre-pregnancy obesity: maternal, neonatal and childhood outcomes. *J Neonatal Perinatal Med* 2013;6:203-16.
41. Peromaa-Haavisto P, Tuomilehto H, Kössi J et al. Prevalence of obstructive sleep apnoea among patients admitted for bariatric surgery. A prospective multicentre trial. *Obes Surg* 2015 Nov 11. [Epub ahead of print].
42. Krueger H, Turner D, Krueger J et al. The economic benefits of risk factor reduction in Canada: tobacco smoking, excess weight and physical inactivity. *Can J Public Health* 2014;105:e69-78.
43. Apovian CM, Aronne LJ, Bessesen DH et al. Pharmacological management of obesity: an endocrine society clinical practice guideline. *J Clin Endocrinol Metab* 2015;100:342-62.
44. Price RA, Cadoret RJ, Stunkard AJ et al. Genetic contributions to human fatness: an adoption study. *Am J Psychiatry* 1987;144:1003-8.
45. Obesity. A report of the Royal College of Physicians. *J R Coll Physicians Lond* 1983;17:5-65.
46. Dietz WH. Critical periods in childhood for the development of obesity. *Am J Clin Nutr* 1994;59:955-9.
47. Laitinen J, Power C, Jarvelin MR. Family social class, maternal body mass index, childhood body mass index, and age at menarche as predictors of adult obesity. *Am J Clin Nutr* 2001;74:287-94.
48. Patel SR, Hu FB. Short sleep duration and weight gain: a systematic review. *Obesity (Silver Spring)* 2008;16:643-53.
49. Spiegel K, Tasali E, Peney P et al. Brief communication: Sleep curtailment in healthy young men is associated with decreased leptin levels, elevated ghrelin levels, and increased hunger and appetite. *Ann Intern Med* 2004;141:846-50.
50. St-Onge M, McReynolds A, Trivedi ZB et al. Sleep restriction leads to increased activation of brain regions sensitive to food stimuli. *Am J Clin Nutr* 2012;95:818-24.
51. Weinsier RL, Nagy TR, Hunter GR et al. Do adaptive changes in metabolic rate favor weight regain in weight-reduced individuals? An examination of the set-point theory. *Am J Clin Nutr* 2000;72:1088-94.
52. Pijl H, Meinders AE. Bodyweight change as an adverse effect of drug treatment. Mechanisms and management. *Drug Saf* 1996;14:329-42.
53. Domecq JP, Prutsky G, Leppin A et al. Clinical review: drugs commonly associated with weight change: a systematic review and meta-analysis. *J Clin Endocrinol Metab* 2015;100:363-70.
54. Kushner RF, Ryan DH. Assessment and lifestyle management of patients with obesity: clinical recommendations from systematic reviews. *JAMA* 2014;312:943-52.
55. Petry NM, Barry D, Pietrzak RH et al. Overweight and obesity are associated with psychiatric disorders: results from the national epidemiologic survey on alcohol and related conditions. *Psychosom Med* 2008;70:288-97.
56. Markowitz S, Friedman MA, Arent SM. Understanding the relation between obesity and depression: causal mechanisms and implications for treatment. *Clinical Psychology: Science and Practice* 2008;15:1-20.
57. French SA, Story M, Jeffery RW. Environmental influences on eating and physical activity. *Annu Rev Public Health* 2001;22:309-25.
58. Vallis M, Piccinini-Vallis H, Sharma AM et al. Clinical review: modified 5 As: minimal intervention for obesity counseling in primary care. *Can Fam Physician* 2013;59:27-31.
59. Sharma AM, Kushner RF. A proposed clinical staging system for obesity. *Int J Obes (Lond)* 2009;33:289-95.
60. Kuk JL, Ardern CI, Church TS et al. Edmonton Obesity Staging System: association with weight history and mortality risk. *Appl Physiol Nutr Metab* 2011;36:570-6.
61. Doran GT. There's a S.M.A.R.T. way to write management's goals and objectives. *Manage Rev* 1981;70:35-6.
62. Rolls BJ, Bell EA. Dietary approaches to the treatment of obesity. *Med Clin North Am* 2000;84:401-18.
63. Sacks FM, Bray GA, Carey VJ et al. Comparison of weight-loss diets with different compositions of fat, protein, and carbohydrates. *N Engl J Med* 2009;360:859-73.
64. Johnston BC, Kanters S, Bandayrel K et al. Comparison of weight loss among named diet programs in overweight and obese adults: a meta-analysis. *JAMA* 2014;312:923-33.
65. Gow ML, Ho M, Burrows TL et al. Impact of dietary macronutrient distribution on BMI and cardiometabolic outcomes in overweight and obese children and adolescents: a systematic review. *Nutr Rev* 2014;72:453-70.
66. Freedman MR, King J, Kennedy E. Popular diets: a scientific review. *Obes Res* 2001;9:1S-40S.
67. The Atkins diet. *Med Lett Drugs Ther* 2000;42:52.
68. Atkins RC. *Dr. Atkins' new diet revolution*. New York: Avon Books; 1992.
69. Sears B, Lawren B. *Enter the zone: a dietary road map*. New York: Harper Collins; 1995.
70. Steward HL, Morrison CB, Andrews SS et al. *Sugar busters: cut sugar to trim fat*. New York: Ballantine Books; 1998.
71. Ornish D. *Eat more, weigh less*. New York: Harper Paperbooks; 1993.
72. Davis C, Bryan J, Hodgson J et al. Definition of the Mediterranean diet; a literature review. *Nutrients* 2015;7:9139-53.
73. Pi-Sunyer FX. The role of very-low-calorie diets in obesity. *Am J Clin Nutr* 1992;56:240S-3S.
74. Nackers LM, Ross KM, Perri MG. The association between rate of initial weight loss and long-term success in obesity treatment: does slow and steady win the race? *Int J Behav Med* 2010;17:161-7.
75. Astrup A, Rossner S. Lessons from obesity management programmes: greater initial weight loss improves long-term maintenance. *Obes Rev* 2000;1:17-19.
76. Nordmann AJ, Nordmann A, Briel M et al. Effects of low-carbohydrate vs low-fat diets on weight loss and cardiovascular risk factors: a meta-analysis of randomized controlled trials. *Arch Intern Med* 2006;166:285-93.
77. Petersen M, Taylor MA, Saris WH et al. Randomized, multi-center trial of two hypo-energetic diets in obese subjects: high-versus-low-fat content. *Int J Obes (London)* 2006;30:552-60.
78. Hooper L, Abdelhamid A, Moore HJ et al. Effect of reducing total fat intake on body weight: systematic review and meta-analysis of randomised controlled trials and cohort studies. *BMJ* 2012;345:e7666.
79. Ludwig DS, Pereira MA, Kroenke CH et al. Dietary fibre, weight gain, and cardiovascular disease risk factors in young adults. *JAMA* 1999;282:1539-46.
80. Rolls BJ. Carbohydrates, fats and satiety. *Am J Clin Nutr* 1995;61:960S-7S.
81. Burton-Freeman B. Dietary fiber and energy regulation. *J Nutr* 2000;130:272S-5S.
82. Ludwig DS. The glycemic index: physiological mechanisms relating to obesity, diabetes, and cardiovascular disease. *JAMA* 2002;287:2414-23.

83. Foster-Powell K, Holt SH, Brand-Miller JC. International table of glycemic index and glycemic load values: 2002. *Am J Clin Nutr* 2002;76:5-56.
84. Raben A. Should obese patients be counseled to follow a low-glycemic index diet? No. *Obes Rev* 2002;3:245-56.
85. Das SK, Gilhooly CH, Golden JK et al. Long-term effects of 2 energy-restricted diets differing in glycemic load on dietary adherence, body composition, and metabolism in CALERIE: a 1-y randomized controlled trial. *Am J Clin Nutr* 2007;85:1023-30.
86. Sofi F, Cesari F, Abbate R et al. Adherence to Mediterranean diet and health status: meta-analysis. *BMJ* 2008;337:a1344.
87. Shai I, Schwarzfuchs D, Henkin Y et al. Weight loss with a low-carbohydrate, Mediterranean or low-fat diet. *N Engl J Med* 2008;359:229-41.
88. Salas-Salvadó J, Bulló M, Estruch R et al. Prevention of diabetes with Mediterranean diets: a subgroup analysis of a randomized trial. *Ann Intern Med* 2014;160:1-10.
89. Toledo E, Hu FB, Estruch R et al. Effect of the Mediterranean diet on blood pressure in the PREDIMED trial: results from a randomized controlled trial. *BMC Med* 2013;11:207.
90. Babio N, Toledo E, Estruch R et al. Mediterranean diets and metabolic syndrome status in the PREDIMED randomized trial. *CMAJ* 2014;186:E649-57.
91. The Blood Type Diet. Available from: www.dadamo.com. Accessed April 26, 2016.
92. The Dukan Diet. Available from: www.dukandiet.com. Accessed April 26, 2016.
93. The Paleolithic Diet Nutrition Page. Available from: www.paleodiet.com. Accessed April 26, 2016.
94. The Abs Diet. Available from: www.theabsdiet.com. Accessed April 26, 2016.
95. Davis W. *Wheat belly*. Toronto: Harpers Collins; 2012.
96. Ross R, Hudson R, Stotz PJ et al. Effects of exercise amount and intensity on abdominal obesity and glucose tolerance in obese adults: a randomized trial. *Ann Intern Med* 2015;162:325-34.
97. Levy RL, Finch EA, Crowell KD. Behavioral intervention for the treatment of obesity: strategies and effectiveness data. *Am J Gastroenterol* 2007;102:2314-21.
98. Bly T, Hammond M, Thomson R et al. Exploring the use of mindful eating training in the bariatric population. *Bariatric Times* 2007;4:15-7.
99. The Center for Mindful Eating. *Principles of mindful eating*. Available from: thecenterformindfuleating.org/principles. Accessed April 26, 2016.
100. Foreyt JP, Poston WS. The role of the behavioral counselor in obesity treatment. *J Am Diet Assoc* 1998;98:S27-30.
101. Foreyt JP, Goodrick GK. Evidence for success of behavior modification in weight loss and control. *Ann Intern Med* 1993;119:698-701.
102. Wing RR. Behavioral approaches to the treatment of obesity. In: Bray GA, Bouchard C, James WP, eds. *Handbook of obesity*. New York: M. Dekker; 1998. p. 855-73.
103. Kiernan M, Brown SD, Schoffman DE et al. Promoting healthy weight with "stability skills first": a randomized trial. *J Consult Clin Psychol* 2013;81:336-46.
104. Apfelbaum M, Bostsarron J, Lacatis D. Effect of caloric restriction and excessive caloric intake on energy expenditure. *Am J Clin Nutr* 1971;24:1405-9.
105. Donnelly JE, Blair SN, Jakicic JM et al. American College of Sports Medicine Position Stand. Appropriate physical activity intervention strategies for weight loss and prevention of weight regain for adults. *Med Sci Sports Exerc* 2009;41:459-71.
106. Acharya SD, Elci OU, Sereika SM et al. Using a personal digital assistant for self-monitoring influences diet quality in comparison to a standard paper record among overweight/obese adults. *J Am Diet Assoc* 2011;111:583-8.
107. Stephens J, Allen J. Mobile phone interventions to increase physical activity and reduce weight: a systematic review. *J Cardiovasc Nurs* 2013;28:320-9.
108. Baranowski T, Frankel L. Let's get technical! Gaming and technology for weight control and health promotion in children. *Child Obes* 2012;8:34-7.
109. Spring B, Duncan JM, Janke EA et al. Integrating technology into standard weight loss treatment: a randomized controlled trial. *JAMA Intern Med* 2013;173:105-11.
110. Liu F, Kong X, Cao J et al. Mobile phone intervention and weight loss among overweight and obese adults: a meta-analysis of randomized controlled trials. *Am J Epidemiol* 2015;181:337-48.
111. Higgins JP. Smartphone applications for patients' health and fitness. *Am J Med* 2016;129:11-9.
112. Fukuoka Y, Gay CL, Joiner KL et al. A novel diabetes prevention intervention using a mobile app: a randomized controlled trial with overweight adults at risk. *Am J Prev Med* 2015;49:223-37.
113. Carter MC, Burley VJ, Nykjaer C et al. Adherence to a smartphone application for weight loss compared to website and paper diary: pilot randomized controlled trial. *J Med Internet Res* 2013;15:e32.
114. Archer E, Groessi EJ, Sui X et al. An economic analysis of traditional and technology-based approaches to weight loss. *Am J Prev Med* 2012;43:176-82.
115. Colquitt JL, Pickett K, Loveman E et al. Surgery for weight loss in adults. *Cochrane Database Syst Rev* 2014;8:CD003641.
116. Chang SH, Stoll CR, Song J et al. The effectiveness and risks of bariatric surgery: an updated systematic review and meta-analysis, 2003-2012. *JAMA Surg* 2014;149:275-87.
117. Carlsson LM, Peltonen M, Ahlin S et al. Bariatric surgery and prevention of type 2 diabetes in Swedish obese subjects. *N Engl J Med* 2012;367:695-704.
118. Sjostrom L, Peltonen M, Jacobson P et al. Bariatric surgery and long-term cardiovascular events. *JAMA* 2012;307:56-65.
119. Puzziferri N, Roshek TB, Mayo HG et al. Long-term follow-up after bariatric surgery: a systematic review. *JAMA* 2014;312:934-42.
120. Paulus GF, de Vaan LE, Verdam FJ et al. Bariatric surgery in morbidly obese adolescents: a systematic review and meta-analysis. *Obes Surg* 2015;25:860-78.
121. Inge TH, Courcoulas AP, Jenkins TM et al. Weight loss and health status 3 years after bariatric surgery in adolescents. *N Engl J Med* 2016;374:113-23.
122. Greenway FL. Surgery for obesity. *Endocrinol Metab Clin North Am* 1996;25:1005-27.
123. Mechanick JI, Kushner RF, Sugerman HJ et al. American Association of Clinical Endocrinologists, The Obesity Society, and American Society for Metabolic & Bariatric Surgery medical guidelines for clinical practice for the perioperative nutritional, metabolic, and nonsurgical support of the bariatric surgery patient. *Endocr Pract* 2008;14:1-83.
124. Heymsfield SB, van Mierlo CA, van der Knaap HC et al. Weight management using a meal replacement strategy: meta and pooling analysis from six studies. *Int J Obes Relat Metab Disord* 2003;27:537-49.
125. Are reduced fat foods keeping Americans healthier? *Tufts U Health Nutr Lett* 1998;16:4-5.

126. The safety of artificial sweeteners. *Pharmacist's Letter/Prescriber's Letter* 2006;22:220212.
127. Insel PM, Turner RE, Ross D. Energy balance, body composition, and weight management. In: Insel PM, ed. *Nutrition.* 1st ed. Boston: Jones and Bartlett; 2001. p. 283-325.
128. Mattes RD, Popkin BM. Nonnutritive sweetener consumption in humans: effects on appetite and food intake and their putative mechanisms. *Am J Clin Nutr* 2009;89:1-14.
129. Yang Q. Gain weight by "going diet?" Artificial sweeteners and the neurobiology of sugar cravings. *Yale J Biol Med* 2010;83:101-8.
130. Gardner C, Wylie-Rosett J, Gidding SS et al. Nonnutritive sweeteners: current use and health perspectives: a scientific statement from the American Heart Association and the American Diabetes Association. *Circulation* 2012;126:509-19.
131. Nettleton JA, Lutsey PL, Wang Y et al. Diet soda intake and risk of incident metabolic syndrome and type 2 diabetes in the Multi-Ethnic Study of Atherosclerosis (MESA). *Diabetes Care* 2009;32:688-94.
132. Suez J, Korem T, Zeevi D et al. Artificial sweeteners induce glucose intolerance by altering the gut microbiota. *Nature* 2014;514:181-6.
133. Rogers PJ, Hogenkamp PS, de Graaf C et al. Does low-energy sweetener consumption affect energy intake and body weight? A systematic review, including meta-analyses, of the evidence from human and animal studies. *Int J Obes (Lond)* 2016;40:381-94.
134. Birketvedt GS, Shimshi M, Erling T et al. Experiences with three different fiber supplements in weight reduction. *Med Sci Monit* 2005;11:P15-8.
135. Sood N, Baker WL, Coleman CI. Effect of glucomannan on plasma lipid and glucose concentrations, body weight, and blood pressure: systematic review and meta-analysis. *Am J Clin Nutr* 2008;88:1167-75.
136. Mattes RD, Bormann L. Effects of (-)-hydroxycitric acid on appetitive variables. *Physiol Behav* 2000;71:87-94.
137. Heymsfield SB, Allison DB, Vasselli JR et al. Garcinia cambogia (hydroxycitric acid) as a potential antiobesity agent: a randomized controlled trial. *JAMA* 1998;280:1596-600.
138. Jurgens TM, Wehlan AM, Killian L et al. Green tea for weight loss and weight maintenance in overweight or obese adults. *Cochrane Database Syst Rev* 2012:CD008650.
139. Natural Medicines Comprehensive Database. *Hoodia.* Available from: www.naturaldatabase.com. Accessed April 26, 2016. Subscription required.
140. Toubro S, Astrup AV, Breum L et al. Safety and efficacy of long-term treatment with ephedrine, caffeine and an ephedrine/caffeine mixture. *Int J Obes Relat Metab Discord* 1993;17:S69-72.
141. McBride BF, Karapanos AK, Krudysz A et al. Electrocardiographic and hemodynamic effects of multicomponent dietary supplement containing ephedra and caffeine: a randomized controlled trial. *JAMA* 2004;291:216-21.
142. Yanovski JA, Parikh SJ, Yanoff LB et al. Effects of calcium supplementation on body weight and adiposity in overweight and obese adults: a randomized trial. *Ann Intern Med* 2009;150:821-9.
143. Astrup A. The role of calcium in energy balance and obesity: the search for mechanisms. *Am J Clin Nutr* 2008;88:873-4.
144. Major GC, Alarie FP, Dore J et al. Calcium plus vitamin D supplementation and fat mass loss in female very low-calcium consumers: potential link with a calcium-specific appetite control. *Br J Nutr* 2009;101:659-63.
145. Tian H, Guo X, Wang X et al. Chromium picolinate supplementation for overweight or obese adults. *Cochrane Database Syst Rev* 2013;11:CD010063.
146. Jull AB, Ni Mhurchu C, Bennett DA et al. Chitosan for overweight or obesity. *Cochrane Database Syst Rev* 2008;(3):CD003892.
147. Kovacs EM, Mela DJ. Metabolically active functional food ingredients for weight control. *Obes Rev* 2006;7:59-78.
148. Stanko RT, Reynolds HR, Hoyson R et al. Pyruvate supplementation of a low-cholesterol, low-fat diet: effects on plasma lipid concentrations and body composition in hyperlipidemic patients. *Am J Clin Nutr* 1994;59:423-7.
149. Hutton B, Fergusson D. Changes in body weight and serum lipid profile in obese patients treated with orlistat in addition to a hypocaloric diet: a systematic review of randomized clinical trials. *Am J Clin Nutr* 2004;80:1461-8.
150. Astrup A, Rossner S, Van Gaal L et al. Effects of liraglutide in the treatment of obesity: a randomized, double-blind, placebo-controlled study. *Lancet* 2009;374:1606-16.
151. Wadden TA, Hollander P, Klein S et al. Weight maintenance and additional weight loss with liraglutide after low-calorie-diet induced weight loss: the SCALE Maintenance randomized study. *Int J Obes (Lond)* 2013;37:1443-51.
152. Pi-Sunyer X, Astrup A, Fujioka K et al. A randomized, controlled trial of 3.0 mg of liraglutide in weight management. *N Engl J Med* 2015;373:11-22.
153. Astrup A, Carraro R, Finer N et al. Safety, tolerability and sustained weight loss over 2 years with the once-daily human GLP-1 analog, liraglutide. *Int J Obes (Lond)* 2012;36:843-54.
154. Government of Canada. Healthy Canadians. *Health Canada reminds Canadians not to use ephedra/ephedrine products.* Available from: www.healthycanadians.gc.ca/recall-alert-rappel-avis/hc-sc/2008/13279a-eng.php. Accessed April 26, 2016.
155. FDA proposes constraints on ephedrine dietary supplements. *Am J Health Syst Pharm* 1997;54:1578.
156. Statistics Canada. *Percentage distribution by body mass index (BMI) category, by sex, household population aged 18 or older, Canada excluding territories, 2004, 2005 and 2008.* Available from: www.statcan.gc.ca/pub/82-229-x/2009001/status/desc/abm-desc4.1-eng.htm. Accessed April 26, 2016.
157. Centers For Disease Control and Prevention. NCHS Health E-Stats. *Prevalence of underweight among adults: United States, 2003-2006.* Available from: www.cdc.gov/nchs/data/hestat/underweight/underweight_adults.pdf. Accessed April 26, 2016.
158. de Onis M, Frongillo EA, Blössner M. Is malnutrition declining? An analysis of changes in levels of child malnutrition since 1980. *Bull World Health Organ* 2000;78:1222-33.
159. Roland DA. Nutrition in adulthood and the later years. In: Krause MV, Mahan LK, eds. *Food, nutrition and diet therapy: a textbook of nutritional care.* 7th ed. Philadelphia: Saunders; 1984. p. 324.
160. American Psychiatric Association. *Diagnostic and statistical manual of mental disorders: DSM-5.* 5th ed. Washington: American Psychiatric Publishing; 2013.
161. Insel PM, Turner RE, Ross D. Eating disorders. In: Insel PM, ed. *Nutrition.* 1st ed. Boston: Jones and Bartlett; 2001.

Managing Your Weight—What You Need to Know

Hints to help you *lose* weight safely:

- **Set short-term, achievable goals.**
  Don't focus on the 25 kg you want to lose. Start with a smaller goal that is easier to achieve. For example, try to lose 0.5 to 1 kg per week. Over 6 months that will add up to your 25 kg goal (2.2 lb=1 kg).
- **Don't go on a crash diet.**
  Think slow weight loss over a longer period of time. Change your eating habits so that your meals and snacks include a variety of healthy foods. Consult *Eating Well with Canada's Food Guide* (www.hc-sc.gc.ca/fn-an/food-guide-aliment/index-eng.php) to follow a balanced diet.
- **Increase your activity.**
  Pick an exercise routine that suits your lifestyle. Try to do 30 minutes of aerobic exercise (like walking) at least 3 times per week. Look for easy ways to increase your activity (such as using the stairs rather than the elevator; parking further away to increase the walking time to your destination).
- **Don't give up.**
  After you lose a few pounds you may stop losing weight. Your body may be adjusting to the new level of fat and calories. Don't cut back again on the amount you eat.
- **Give yourself a break.**
  If you overeat one day, just get back on the plan the following day.
- **See your healthcare provider if necessary.**
  If you are 30% or more above normal weight for you, your healthcare provider may recommend a medically supervised very-low-calorie diet or drug therapy.
- **Look for social support.**
  Identify a friend or family member who is willing to support you. You can also find support groups in the community or through the Internet.

Hints to help you *gain* weight safely:

- **Set short-term, achievable goals.**
  Increase body weight gradually (0.5 kg per week).
- **Change your eating habits.**
  Increase number and size of servings.
  Increase nutrient density (add extra protein, carbohydrate and fat).
  Eat more frequently.
- **Change your activity level.**
  Think about how you might be able to reduce the calories you need.
- **See your doctor or a dietitian.**

Chapter 44

Drug Use and Abuse in Sports

Lily Lum, BScPharm, CSPI

Olympic athletes of ancient Greece are believed to have used herbs and mushrooms to improve athletic performance.[1,2] Now, in the age of the modern Olympic games, athletes continue to take substances that are not officially permitted (prohibited substances) to boost their performance and give them an advantage to win.[3]

Ergogenic (performance-enhancing) drug use or doping is defined as "the administration of or use by a competing athlete of any substance foreign to the body or of any physiological substance taken in abnormal quantity or taken by an abnormal route of entry into the body with the sole intention of increasing in an artificial manner his/her performance in competition."[1] Sports organizations have developed antidoping policies and drug testing programs in order to protect the health of the athletes and to keep competition fair and drug free.[4] Although drugs carry potential adverse effects, most athletes who use them view the risk-benefit ratio as favourable.[5] Ergogenic aids come from many sources and the list often appears endless as access to such products is easy, especially with use of the Internet. Ergogenic aids may be prescription or nonprescription drugs, recreational drugs such as alcohol and marijuana, nutritional supplements or natural health products.

Nonprescription Drugs

A number of agents found in nonprescription products are used as ergogenic aids (see Table 1).[1,2,4,5,6,7]

Table 1: **Common Ergogenic Aids Found in Nonprescription Products**

Drug/Drug Class	Reason for Use	Adverse Effects	Evidence for Performance Enhancement
Caffeine	Increased alertness; reduced perception of fatigue; increased endurance	Nervousness, insomnia, tremors, diuresis	Inconclusive or conflicting evidence; found in stimulants, combination analgesic products.
Codeine	Treatment of pain allows athlete to participate while injured but has potential to further aggravate injury	Dizziness, lightheadedness, drowsiness, nausea or vomiting, constipation	Inconclusive or conflicting evidence; found in combination analgesic products and cold preparations.
Creatine	Muscle-performance enhancer	Dizziness, diarrhea; liver and renal toxicity at high doses	Evidence to support in power sports but not endurance sports.[8,9,10]
Cyproheptadine	Promotes appetite and weight gain	Drowsiness	No evidence to support; theoretical benefit based on pharmacologic actions.
Sympathomimetics (e.g., phenylephrine, pseudoephedrine)	Increased subjective energy ("energizing" effect), decreased appetite and increased metabolism	Restlessness, nervousness, tachycardia, arrhythmias, hypertension	No evidence to support; theoretical benefit based on pharmacologic actions. Found in many cold preparations.

Prescription Drugs

Many prescription drugs are also used as ergogenic aids (Table 2).[1,2,4,5,6,7] Anabolic steroids are the best known. They are synthetic derivatives of the male sex hormone testosterone.[1] Individuals use anabolic steroids primarily to increase muscle mass and strength. Athletes who take anabolic steroids employ unusual dosing regimens in an attempt to increase the effects of the drugs, prevent detection or decrease the occurrence of drug-related adverse effects. Stacking is a technique where several different anabolic agents (oral and injectable) are used concomitantly in order to produce a synergistic effect. Cycling is a dosing technique with on and off periods of drug use. Pyramiding is another dosing technique where low doses are initiated, increased to a plateau 10–100 times the recommended therapeutic dose and then tapered to the original level.[1,5,11] Much of what is known about the side effects of anabolic steroids involves patients receiving therapeutic doses for treatment of disease. The adverse effects of the high doses used in some doping regimens are not fully understood.

Recreational Drugs

Alcohol and marijuana may be abused by athletes with the misconception that these recreational drugs can reduce anxiety. However, alcohol and marijuana can actually impair athletic performance.[1,4] In sports requiring precision, such as riflery events, alcohol in low doses may reduce essential tremor and is prohibited in competition. In-competition use of Δ9-tetrahydrocannabinol (THC) and all cannabimimetics is prohibited (see Prohibited Substances/Therapeutic Use Exemptions).

Nutritional Supplements and Natural Health Products

There are countless products (e.g., chromium picolinate, creatine) described as nutritional supplements, herbals or natural health products with claims of possessing anabolic properties or other ergogenic effects.[7,18] Because of the known toxicity associated with anabolic steroids, natural health products are perceived as less or not harmful, and they are also more accessible to the public. Natural health products are often promoted in a misleading fashion and usually have no scientific evidence to support their claims of anabolic or performance-enhancing effects.[18] The Canadian Centre for Ethics in Sport (CCES) believes the use of most supplements poses an unacceptable risk for athletes and their athletic careers.[19] Supplements may intentionally contain prohibited substances or may be inadvertently contaminated with prohibited substances.

CCES states that athletes have a personal responsibility to consider all the risks associated with supplements they plan to take.[20] If athletes choose to use supplements, they should take the following precautions to reduce their risk of ingesting a prohibited substance:

- Get a written guarantee through a direct enquiry to the manufacturer that the product is free of any substances on the WADA Prohibited List
- Ask whether the manufacturer is prepared to stand behind its product
- Ask the manufacturer whether any products containing prohibited substances are manufactured at the same plant as the supplement.

The NSF Certified for Sport program (see Resource Tips) can help athletes identify products that have been tested to confirm their content and purity.

Creatine is widely used as an ergogenic aid. It is a naturally occurring compound produced by the liver, kidneys and pancreas from the amino acids glycine, arginine and methionine. Most individuals also consume 1–2 g exogenous creatine daily, primarily from meat and fish.[8]

Creatine is promoted as improving muscle strength and outcomes in short-duration anaerobic events. Studies of its effectiveness are conflicting. It may improve performance in power sports (e.g., weight lifting, sprinting) but has not demonstrated any benefit in endurance sports (e.g., cycling, cross-country running).[8,9]

Table 2: Common Ergogenic Aids Found in Prescription Products

Drug/Drug Class	Reason for Abuse	Adverse Effects	Evidence for Performance Enhancement
Anabolic steroids[11]	Increase muscle mass and strength	Hepatotoxicity; acne; gynecomastia in males; masculinization in females; premature closure of the growth centres of long bones (adolescents); psychiatric effects such as psychosis, aggression, mood disorders[12]	Evidence to support.[9]
$Beta_1$-adrenergic antagonists	Reduce anxiety, hand tremor and heart rate	Dizziness or lightheadedness; unusual tiredness or weakness; sexual dysfunction	No evidence to support; theoretical benefit based on pharmacologic actions.
$Beta_2$-agonists	Anabolic effects	Dizziness, lightheadedness, nervousness, tremor, nausea, increased heart rate	Inconclusive or conflicting evidence (no evidence with inhaled formulations).
Diuretics	Promote excretion of prohibited substances; decrease weight before official weigh-ins in sports with weight classes (e.g., boxing, martial arts)	Dizziness or lightheadedness; photosensitivity (with thiazides)	No evidence to support; theoretical benefit based on pharmacologic actions.
Peptide hormones and analogues: epoetin alfa (erythropoietin), darbepoetin	Increase red blood cell production, increasing aerobic capacity	Chest pain; shortness of breath; increased blood pressure[12]	Conflicting evidence.[7,13,14,15]
Peptide hormones and analogues: human growth hormone	Anabolic effects	If growth hormone is given to children or adults with normal growth who do not need growth hormone, serious unwanted effects may occur including: development of diabetes, abnormal growth of bones and internal organs such as the heart, kidneys and liver, atherosclerosis, and hypertension[12]	Inconclusive or conflicting evidence.
Probenecid	Promote urinary excretion of a prohibited substance	Headache; joint pain, redness, or swelling; loss of appetite; nausea	No evidence to support; theoretical benefit based on pharmacologic actions.
Sildenafil, tadalafil	Increase oxygen supply by causing vasodilation in the lungs	Prolonged erection	Inconclusive or conflicting evidence.[16,17]
Tamoxifen	Reverse gynecomastia caused by steroids	Hot flushes, weight gain in females; sexual dysfunction in males	No evidence to support; theoretical benefit based on pharmacologic actions.

Creatine is taken as a loading dose of 5 g 4 times a day for the first 4–6 days followed by the standard dose of 2 g daily for the next 3 months.[9] Because of the theoretical concerns of dehydration and heat illness during sporting events, it is recommended that athletes taking creatine drink 6–8 glasses of water per day.[9]

Side effects of creatine are usually minimal and include nausea, vomiting, diarrhea, muscle cramps and weight gain (the latter is thought to be due to water retention). The greatest safety concern with long-term use of creatine is its potential effect on renal function.[8,9,21] Several case reports describe compromised renal function with the use of creatine.[9]

Androstenedione is a precursor of testosterone and estrone. There is some evidence that it may elevate testosterone levels and increase strength and muscle mass during resistance training.[8] Information on the side effects of long-term use is not available but these are expected to be similar to those of anabolic steroids.[8] Though it is illegal in Canada, some athletes may obtain supplies from sources in the United States or online.

Prohibited Substances/Therapeutic Use Exemptions

Athletes are not permitted to use prohibited substances because they are believed to enhance performance. If a prohibited substance or method is used by the athlete for a specified, legitimate medical condition, they must apply for a Therapeutic Use Exemption. Some substances are not prohibited but the athlete must submit a Declaration of Use when taking them for medical reasons. Table 3 lists categories of drugs that may be considered prohibited substances in amateur sports.

The list of prohibited substances may vary among different sport organizations and is subject to change. The World Anti-Doping Agency (WADA) annually publishes the WADA Prohibited List which is the international standard that designates what substance and method is prohibited in and out of competition. It also indicates whether a substance is prohibited only in a particular sport. Other substances are included in the WADA Monitoring Program; these are not prohibited but WADA monitors their use to detect potential patterns of misuse by athletes. These lists can be accessed through the CCES website (see Resource Tips).

Table 3: **Substances Prohibited in Amateur Sports**[19]

Prohibited	Examples	Comments
Anabolic androgenic steroids and other anabolic agents	androstenedione dehydroepiandrosterone fluoxymesterone nandrolone stanozolol testosterone	Prohibited at all times Clenbuterol (a $beta_2$-agonist) is included as an anabolic agent.
$Beta_1$-adrenergic antagonists	acebutolol atenolol metoprolol propranolol	Prohibited during competition in certain sports, e.g., billiards, darts, golf. Archery and shooting prohibit beta-blocker use both during and outside competition.
$Beta_2$-agonists	formoterol salbutamol salmeterol terbutaline	When given orally or by injection, $beta_2$-agonists may have anabolic effects. Therapeutic doses of formoterol, salbutamol and salmeterol by inhalation are *not* prohibited.

(cont'd)

Table 3: **Substances Prohibited in Amateur Sports**[19] *(cont'd)*

Prohibited	Examples	Comments
		Terbutaline by inhalation requires a Therapeutic Use Exemption.
Caffeine		Not on the Prohibited List but included in the Monitoring Program since 2004.
Diuretics and masking agents	acetazolamide desmopressin furosemide hydrochlorothiazide probenecid spironolactone triamterene	Prohibited because they are used to promote urinary excretion of a prohibited substance. Exception: pamabrom and topical dorzolamide and brinzolamide.
Glucocorticoids	fluticasone hydrocortisone methylprednisolone prednisone	Prohibited when administered by oral, iv, im or rectal routes. Glucocorticoids administered by iv injection, im injection, oral or rectal routes require a Therapeutic Use Exemption.
Hormone and metabolic modulators	anastrozole clomiphene exemestane fulvestrant insulin letrozole raloxifene tamoxifen	Prohibited at all times. Insulin is permitted only to treat athletes with certified insulin-dependent diabetes. A Therapeutic Use Exemption form must be completed.
Opioids	fentanyl hydromorphone meperidine morphine oxycodone	Some opioids and derivatives such as codeine, dextromethorphan, diphenoxylate and propoxyphene are permitted. Hydrocodone and tramadol are included in the Monitoring Program (2012).
Peptide hormones, growth factors and related substances	chorionic gonadotropin (HCG) luteinizing hormone (LH) in males erythropoietin growth hormone and other growth factors	
Stimulants	ephedrine[a] fenfluramine methylhexaneamine (dimethylamylamine, DMAA) methylphenidate modafinil phentermine pseudoephedrine[a]	Oral decongestants containing phenylephrine are included in the Monitoring Program. Use of decongestant nasal sprays is permitted.

[a] Ephedrine (>10 µg/mL urinary level) and pseudoephedrine (>150 µg/mL urinary level) are prohibited in competition; lesser amounts are permitted but are included in the World Anti-Doping Agency (WADA) 2015 Monitoring Program. Although the urinary threshold should not be attained with therapeutic use of pseudoephedrine, WADA suggests discontinuing the drug 24 hours before competition.[22]

Resource Tips

Canadian Centre for Ethics in Sport (CCES). Available from: www.cces.ca. By phone: 613-521-3340 or 1-800-672-7775. By email: substances@cces.ca.

NSF International Certified for Sport. Available from: www.nsfsport.com.

World Anti-Doping Agency (WADA). Available from: wada-ama.org. By phone: 514-904-9232.

Suggested Readings

Ahrendt DM. Ergogenic aids: counseling the athlete. *Am Fam Physician* 2001;63:913-22.

Calfee R, Fadale P. Popular ergogenic drugs and supplements in young athletes. *Pediatrics* 2006;117:e577-89.

Canadian Centre for Ethics in Sport (CCES). *2015 Substance classification booklet*. Ottawa: CCES; 2015. Available from: www.cces.ca/substance-classification-booklet.

Catlin DH, Murray TH. Performance-enhancing drugs, fair competition, and Olympic sport. *JAMA* 1996;276:231-7.

National Institutes of Health (NIH). National Institute on Drug Abuse (NIDA). *Research Report Series: Anabolic steroid abuse*. August 2006. Available from: www.drugabuse.gov/publications/research-reports/anabolic-steroid-abuse.

References

1. Wagner JC. Enhancement of athletic performance with drugs. An overview. *Sports Med* 1991;12:250-65.
2. Merchant WF. Medications and athletes: increasing your sports medicine knowledge. *Am Drug* 1992;206:6-13.
3. Morente-Sanchez J, Zabala M. Doping in sport: a review of elite athletes' attitudes, beliefs, and knowledge. *Sports Med* 2013;43:395-411.
4. Catlin DH, Murray TH. Performance-enhancing drugs, fair competition, and Olympic sport. *JAMA* 1996;276:231-7.
5. Goldwire MA, Price KO. Sports pharmacy: counseling athletes about banned drugs. *Am Pharmacy* 1995;NS35:24-30.
6. Woolley BH. The latest fads to increase muscle mass and energy. A look at what some athletes are using. *Postgrad Med* 1991;89:195-8, 201-5.
7. Ahrendt DM. Ergogenic aids: counseling the athlete. *Am Fam Physician* 2001;63:913-22.
8. Barnes CL, Kushner JM. Use of creatine and androstenedione to enhance athletic performance. *US Pharm* 2001;26:47-9.
9. Calfee R, Fadale P. Popular ergogenic drugs and supplements in young athletes. *Pediatrics* 2006;117:e577-89.
10. Jenkinson DM, Harbert AJ. Supplements and sports. *Am Fam Physician* 2008;78:1039-46.
11. National Institutes of Health (NIH). National Institute on Drug Abuse (NIDA). *Research Report Series: Anabolic steroid abuse: Why do people abuse anabolic steroids? How are anabolic steroids abused?* August 2006. Available from: www.drugabuse.gov/publications/research-reports/anabolic-steroid-abuse. Accessed May 5, 2015.
12. Pope HG, Wood RI, Rogol A et al. Adverse health consequences of performance-enhancing drugs: an Endocrine Society scientific statement. *Endocr Rev* 2014;35:341-75.
13. Birkeland KI, Stray-Gundersen J, Hemmersbach P et al. Effect of rhEPO administration on serum levels of sTfR and cycling performance. *Med Sci Sports Exerc* 2000;32:1238-43.
14. Pommering TL. Erythropoietin and other blood-boosting methods. *Pediatr Clin North Am* 2007;54:691-9.
15. Heuberger JA, Cohen Tervaert JM, Schepers FM et al. Erythropoietin doping in cycling: lack of evidence for efficacy and a negative risk-benefit. *Br J Clin Pharmacol* 2013;75:1406-21.
16. Hsu AR, Barnholt KE, Grundmann NK et al. Sildenafil improves cardiac output and exercise performance during acute hypoxia, but not normoxia. *J Appl Physiol* 2006;100:2031-40.
17. Guidetti L, Emerenziani GP, Gallotta MC et al. Effect of tadalafil on anaerobic performance indices in healthy athletes. *Br J Sports Med* 2008;42:130-3.
18. Barron RL, Vanscoy GJ. Natural products and the athlete: facts and folklore. *Ann Pharmacother* 1993;27:607-15.
19. Canadian Centre for Ethics in Sport (CCES). *2015 Substance classification booklet*. Ottawa: CCES; 2015. Available from: www.cces.ca/substance-classification-booklet. Accessed September 15, 2015.
20. Canadian Centre for Ethics in Sport (CCES). *Athlete zone: Supplements*. Available from: www.cces.ca/supplements. Accessed September 15, 2015.
21. Lattavo A, Kopperud A, Rogers PD. Creatine and other supplements. *Pediatr Clin North Am* 2007;54:735-60.
22. World Anti-Doping Agency (WADA). *Additional information in regards to the reintroduction of pseudoephedrine to the 2010 Prohibited List*. Available from: www.wada-main-prod.s3.amazonaws.com/resources/files/WADA_Additional_Info_Pseudoephedrine_2010_EN.pdf. Accessed September 15, 2015.

Drugs and Sport—What You Need to Know

Some people think that taking drugs or other substances (such as steroids) will build their muscles, make them look better and improve their sports ability. How many products tell us they can make us faster, slimmer or less tired? Be cautious and avoid such products. They may be harmful.

Which products are safe?

It is now well known that steroids cause serious side effects. Steroids can cause liver problems and mood changes. Men and boys may find that they develop breasts. Women and girls may begin to show male characteristics such as a deeper voice and more body hair.

Ask your healthcare provider for information on the side effects of drugs or other substances. Avoid any product that has not been studied for side effects.

Which products are prohibited in sports?

To find out what substances are prohibited in your sport, check with the World Anti-Doping Agency (WADA) and your national or local organization.

Carefully check the list of ingredients for any medication you are taking. Refer to the annual WADA Prohibited List for information on which substances are prohibited. This list is subject to change each year and is available on the WADA website www.wada-ama.org. If you have any questions about your medications, consult your healthcare provider.

Which drugs are legal?

The majority of drugs require a prescription from your healthcare provider. While it is possible to get some drugs illegally, it is never wise to do that.

What if you have to take drugs for an illness?

Athletes can take some drugs for an illness or medical condition as long as they declare the drug in advance and apply for a Therapeutic Use Exemption. Contact the Canadian Centre for Ethics in Sport (CCES) for more information **before** taking any medications or supplements.

Chapter 45
Low Back Pain

Kelly Grindrod, BSc(Pharm), PharmD, MSc
Jason Kielly, BSc(Pharm), PharmD
Carlo Marra, BSc(Pharm), PharmD, PhD, FCSHP

Pathophysiology

Low back pain is defined as spinal and paraspinal symptoms in the lumbosacral region that can extend to the gluteal muscles, hips and lower extremities.[1,2] With an estimated prevalence of 15–30%, between 50% and 80% of people will experience an episode of low back pain during their lifetime.[3] Globally, low back pain causes more disability than any other disease.[4] This results in significant direct and indirect costs to the healthcare system including direct medical care, disability, decreased productivity while at work and time lost from work.[5]

Despite the high prevalence of disease, the incidence and prognosis of low back pain are difficult to characterize because of the variety of ways low back pain has been defined in studies.[6] Historically, there has been a widely held belief that up to 90% of cases of low back pain will resolve within 2 months. Newer data indicate rapid improvement occurs within 6 weeks of presentation, after which the rate of improvement is slower.[7] Up to 75% of people with low back pain will continue to have some degree of pain after 1 year.[6,7] Most will experience relapses in symptoms, and up to 10% of individuals experience chronic symptoms resulting in significant time away from work.[6,8,9,10]

Factors that increase the risk of low back pain include age (most common between 45 and 64 years), greater height, climbing stairs often and stress.[11] In addition, individuals who develop low back pain have a poorer prognosis if they have a higher level of disability, have sciatica, are older or are in poor general health, have more stress in their lives, have poor relationships with work colleagues or have a heavy physical demand at work.[8,9,10] Other factors that may be associated with low back pain include obesity[12] and smoking.[13] Usual daily activities that include frequent walking, standing, lifting or carrying have been associated with low back pain; however, evidence indicates these activities are not causative on their own.[14,15,16]

Low back pain can be acute (<4 weeks' duration), subacute (4–12 weeks' duration) or chronic (>12 weeks' duration). Low back pain can be categorized as: 1) nonspecific low back pain; 2) low back pain associated with radiculopathy or spinal stenosis; or 3) low back pain associated with other specific spinal causes.[2]

In over 85% of people, the cause of low back pain cannot be reliably identified, though muscular-ligamentous injuries of the low back such as strains and sprains are often suspected.[17] The symptoms, similar to those experienced with other muscle, ligament and tendon disorders, include localized pain of varying severity, spasm, inflammation and immobility.

Radiculopathy results from the dysfunction of the nerve root.[18] Symptoms include pain, sensory impairment, weakness and impaired tendon reflexes. Sciatica, which is the most common type of radiculopathy, is characterized by pain that radiates to the buttocks and down the posterior-lateral aspect of the leg. It may be described as a "shooting pain" originating in the lumbar region (location of the sciatic nerve).

Other specific spinal causes can include cancer, vertebral compression fractures, spinal infections (e.g., herpes zoster), disc herniation, inflammatory arthritis (e.g., ankylosing spondylitis) and referred visceral pain (e.g., prostatitis, endometriosis, abdominal aortic aneurysm).[2]

Goals of Therapy

- Relieve symptoms
- Maintain or improve mobility and quality of life
- Prevent or minimize re-injury

Healthcare practitioners can support the goals of therapy by educating patients and caregivers to help them understand the condition and make informed therapy decisions. Evidence suggests that patient education by primary care providers may reduce the number of primary care visits related to low back pain and provide long-term reassurance for patients with low back pain.[19]

Patient Assessment

An algorithm for assessing patients with low back pain is presented in Figure 1.

The most important aspect of assessing low back pain is ruling out potential serious etiologies that require immediate evaluation by an appropriate healthcare practitioner, including those patients who have experienced a recent trauma, rapid weight loss or fever or those with increasing motor weakness (see Figure 1 for a more complete list). Patients with chronic pain (lasting >12 weeks), sciatic conditions or specific causes for their pain also require further evaluation.

Principles of Therapy

Current pharmacologic therapies for low back pain provide symptomatic relief but are not curative. Therefore, the choice of agent is based on a combination of risk vs. benefit, cost and patient preference. Pharmacologic therapy should always be initiated in combination with nonpharmacologic modalities. If tolerated, pharmacologic therapies should be tried for at least 2–4 weeks to allow the patient to fully assess effectiveness.

Numerous treatment approaches are supported by various levels of evidence of efficacy in the management of low back pain (see Table 1). Much of the available evidence lacks rigor with respect to study methodologies including sample size, randomization, use of placebo, blinding, controlling for confounding variables and population variances (acute, chronic, ±sciatica). Many guidelines are not developed in a systematic, scientifically rigorous manner, do not consider patient preferences, have no established process for updating, and lack overall transparency.[20,21] Nonetheless, systematic reviews, including several by the Cochrane Back Pain group, (see Suggested Readings) and improved evidence-based guidelines are now available to guide the treatment of low back pain.[2,21,22,23,24,25]

Nonpharmacologic Therapy

In nonspecific low back pain, the primary recommendation is to provide patients with information on treatment options and the expected course of disease, and to advise them to maintain usual activity. Advise individuals with low back pain to stay active and only avoid activities that may worsen pain or injury (e.g., heavy lifting, twisting, high impact exercise). Although bed rest was historically recommended, staying active may offer patients better pain relief and function.[26] If possible, patients should be assessed by a physiotherapist to identify appropriate exercise intensity.[27]

Other nonpharmacologic therapies such as back exercises and spinal manipulation have not been shown to improve pain or function in acute nonspecific low back pain but may provide some relief in patients with chronic symptoms.[23,28] Consistent evidence shows that acupuncture and massage are both safe and effective in alleviating some of the symptoms of chronic low back pain.[29] Yoga, pilates and stretching may improve both pain and function in chronic low back pain.[30,31,32,33,34,35] In chronic nonspecific low back pain, exercise programs are at least as effective as other conservative treatments such as the provision of self-care education books, massage, spinal manipulation and back schools (structured programs where individuals are taught how to maximize recovery and minimize recurrences of low back pain).[36,37,38] Certain post-treatment exercise programs may prevent the recurrence of low back pain.[39]

The application of heat may provide short-term relief in acute pain but there is insufficient evidence to recommend the use of cold packs.[40] Other modalities such as therapeutic ultrasound,[41] lumbar supports, corsets, shoe lifts, insoles and orthoses[42] have shown little benefit.

Surgical therapy is considered in individuals with persistent and disabling symptoms from common degenerative spinal changes or spinal stenosis, or in individuals with disabling radiculopathy from a herniated disk.[43]

Behavioural therapy may provide some short-term pain relief in chronic low back pain but does not offer long-term improvements compared with usual care.[44] There is no demonstrated benefit of behavioural therapy when compared to other forms of therapy; however, the combination of behavioural therapy and exercise may decrease disability and pain and improve quality of life compared with exercise alone.[45] A Cochrane systematic review suggests that a multidisciplinary biopsychosocial treatment approach may result in larger improvements in pain and daily function compared with usual care or interventions aimed only at physical factors.[46] Due to the need for stronger evidence, behavioural therapy for chronic low back pain should be incorporated on an individual basis and under the care of a qualified professional.

Table 1: Conservative Treatments for Low Back Pain[a]

Category	Treatment	Acute (<4 wk)	Subacute or Chronic (>4 wk)
Pharmacologic Therapy	Acetaminophen	■	■
	NSAIDs	■	■
	Benzodiazepines, muscle relaxants	■	
	Antidepressants (tricyclic)		■
	Opioids, tramadol	■	■
Nonpharmacologic Therapy	Self-care: Advice to remain active	■	■
	Self-care: Books, handouts	■	■
	Self-care: Application of superficial heat	■	
	Exercise		■
	Massage		■
	Acupuncture		■
	Yoga		■
	Cognitive-behavioural therapy		■
	Progressive relaxation		■
	Intensive interdisciplinary rehabilitation		■

[a] Interventions supported by fair-quality evidence of moderate benefit, or small benefit but no significant harms, costs or burdens.

Adapted with permission from Chou R, Qaseem A, Snow V et al. Diagnosis and treatment of low back pain: a joint clinical practice guideline from the American College of Physicians and the American Pain Society. *Ann Intern Med* 2007;147:478-91. Copyright © 2007 American College of Physicians. All Rights Reserved. Reprinted with the permission of American College of Physicians, Inc.

Encourage patients to remain active; physical therapy exercises and spinal manipulation should be reserved for individuals who fail to improve after an acute episode (>4 weeks).[2]

Pharmacologic Therapy

For further discussion of pharmacologic therapy for low back pain, consult the *Compendium of Therapeutic Choices*: Low Back Pain.

For comparative ingredients of nonprescription products, consult the *Compendium of Products for Minor Ailments*—Analgesic Products: Internal Analgesics and Antipyretics; Herbal and Natural Health Products: Single Entity.

Medication is commonly prescribed for nonspecific low back pain but is primarily intended to relieve pain and discomfort in the short term and to facilitate activity. Long-term therapy may be required in individuals who experience chronic back pain. Common treatments for nonspecific low back pain include acetaminophen, NSAIDs, opioid analgesics, skeletal muscle relaxants and antidepressants. Evidence of efficacy for all agents is generally weak.[24] Table 3 presents selected pharmacologic options for the treatment of low back pain.

Acetaminophen has long been the first-line agent to treat low back pain, but its efficacy is in question.[50,51] Small trials have suggested that acetaminophen does not provide superior pain relief compared with NSAIDs.[52,53] A small randomized controlled trial found that continuous heat wrap therapy may provide better pain relief than regular doses of acetaminophen or ibuprofen.[54] However, acetaminophen has a better safety profile than NSAIDs, so it continues to be recommended as the first-line pharmacologic option for alleviating symptoms associated with back pain.[2]

NSAIDs may provide small improvements in low back pain in patients without sciatica compared with placebo. There is no demonstrated superiority of one NSAID over another.[52]

Combination products containing **acetaminophen**, **caffeine** and **codeine** (8 mg) are options for nonresponsive individuals in the short-term but they have not demonstrated benefit in the management of acute or chronic nonspecific low back pain.

In low back pain, as with other muscular strain disorders, the complexity of spasm physiology makes it difficult to determine the extent to which spasm is contributing to the injury or symptoms. Muscle relaxants such as **methocarbamol** are really sedatives with very little direct muscle-relaxing properties. Despite their popularity, these agents have not been shown to provide relief in low back pain.[55]

Small trials comparing **opioid analgesics** with NSAIDs report conflicting results; opioids may be reserved for individuals who do not respond to acetaminophen or NSAIDs.[24,52] A systematic review suggests there is insufficient evidence to determine the effectiveness of long-term opioid therapy in improving chronic pain and function.[56] There is evidence of short-term efficacy (moderate for pain and small for function) of opioids to treat chronic low back pain compared with placebo. However, the effectiveness and safety of long-term opioid therapy for treatment of chronic low back pain remains unproven.[57] A systematic review of opioids in chronic low back pain showed **tramadol** had a small effect on pain but was also associated with significant side effects such as headache, nausea, somnolence and constipation.[58] Tramadol is not routinely used to treat low back pain as adverse effects limit its use in many patients.

If patients have contraindications to analgesics, have failed all other treatments or have been diagnosed with a spastic component to their disease, direct-acting **muscle relaxants (baclofen, benzodiazepines, cyclobenzaprine** and **tizanidine)** may be used. While these agents are generally not recommended for the management of acute or chronic low back pain, evidence suggests that they are more effective than placebo and may result in additive benefit when used in combination with other agents.[55] However, the side effect profile and potential for long-term abuse render these agents undesirable.

Natural Health Products

There have been numerous claims that agents such as D-phenylalanine, devil's claw, capsicum, ginger, turmeric and white willow bark are effective in managing symptoms of low back pain. A Cochrane review of natural health products for nonspecific low back pain found that low to moderate quality evidence suggests that four herbal medicines (i.e., devil's claw, white willow bark, cayenne and comfrey root extract) may reduce pain in acute and chronic lower back pain.[59] For **devil's claw**, standardized daily doses of 50–100 mg of the active ingredient harpagoside improved pain compared with placebo. **White willow bark**, in standardized daily doses of 120–240 mg of the active ingredient salicin has provided similar benefit. Topically applied **cayenne** and **comfrey** appear to reduce pain more than placebo. These topical agents could be considered as a treatment option for acute (comfrey) and for chronic (cayenne) low back pain. There is no evidence that any of these substances are safe or efficacious for long-term use.[59]

Note that the quantity of active ingredient was standardized for these studies and this cannot be expected with all products currently available in Canada.

Monitoring of Therapy

Table 2 provides a monitoring plan for patients with low back pain.

Advice for the Patient

Advise patients on:

- The importance of using nonpharmacologic measures concurrently with medication
- The importance of maintaining ordinary activities and increasing level of activity based on pain tolerance
- Expected benefits of treatment
- Possible side effects (Table 3) and their management
- When to contact a healthcare practitioner.

Table 2: Monitoring of Therapy for Low Back Pain

Parameter	Degree	Timeframe	Action/Comments
Pain relief	Elimination of pain or progression toward predefined goals as set by patient at the beginning of therapy	Patient or caregiver: Assess daily Healthcare practitioner: Call on day 3, 7, 14 and 28	Patient requires further assessment by appropriate healthcare practitioner if symptoms not relieved after adequate trial of at least 2 analgesics or if new or worsening pain symptoms develop during therapy. ▪ Use visual analog scale or other individual measure (e.g., ability to perform ADLs—walking, gardening) to quantify and characterize pain. ▪ Trial of each analgesic for 2–4 wk at optimal dose to fully assess impact on daily activities/functioning. ▪ Considerations in timing of medications: – Around-the-clock vs. PRN – Take dose of analgesic at least 1 h prior to activities that may exacerbate pain.
Nausea, dyspepsia, abdominal discomfort (NSAIDs)	Minimal or none during therapy	Patient or caregiver: Monitor daily Healthcare practitioner: Call on day 3 and 7	Change therapy if symptoms severe or intolerable. Minimize development by taking medication with food or milk. Consider antacids or H_2RAs to treat dyspepsia.
Hemateme-sis, melena, hematochezia (NSAIDs)	None during therapy	Patient or caregiver: Monitor daily on an ongoing basis Healthcare practitioner: Call on days 3, 7 and 28, then ask when medication is refilled	Assess risk of GI complications (see Chapter 46: Osteoarthritis, Table 3 for risk factors of serious adverse effects with NSAID therapy). If high risk, patient requires further assessment by appropriate healthcare practitioner. Patient should discontinue therapy immediately and seek medical attention if these signs or symptoms develop.
Hypertension (NSAIDs)	Stable during therapy	Healthcare practitioner: Measure BP within 1 wk of starting NSAIDs	Monitor patients with pre-existing hypertension; if BP increases, adjust the dose of the NSAID or that of the antihypertensive.
Renal function and signs of fluid retention (weight gain or edema) in high-risk patients (NSAIDs)	No significant change in renal function	Patient or caregiver: Look for decreased urine production; watch for signs of fluid retention on an ongoing basis, (e.g., edema). Patients with severe heart failure should weigh themselves daily. Healthcare practitioner: In patients >65 y or with other risk factors, consider baseline serum creatinine, repeat at 1 wk and then periodically afterwards.	Assess risk of renal complications (see Chapter 46: Osteoarthritis, Table 3 for risk factors of serious adverse effects with NSAID therapy). Hold NSAID that day if patient cannot eat or drink. Discontinue NSAID if significant changes in serum creatinine, electrolytes or signs of fluid retention occur.
Recurrent low back injury	Avoid or minimize	Patient: Ongoing	Patient to seek medical attention if recurrent episodes occur, to identify and implement potential nonpharmacologic strategies for management and prevention.
Functional ability after acute injury	Avoid immobilization. Patient able to perform ADLs, usual activity to tolerable pain level	Patient: Daily Healthcare practitioner: Call on day 3 and 7	Further assessment by appropriate healthcare practitioner required if unable to perform ADL.

Abbreviations: ADL = activities of daily living; BP = blood pressure; H_2RA = H_2-receptor antagonist

Figure 1: **Assessment of Patients with Low Back Pain**[1,2]

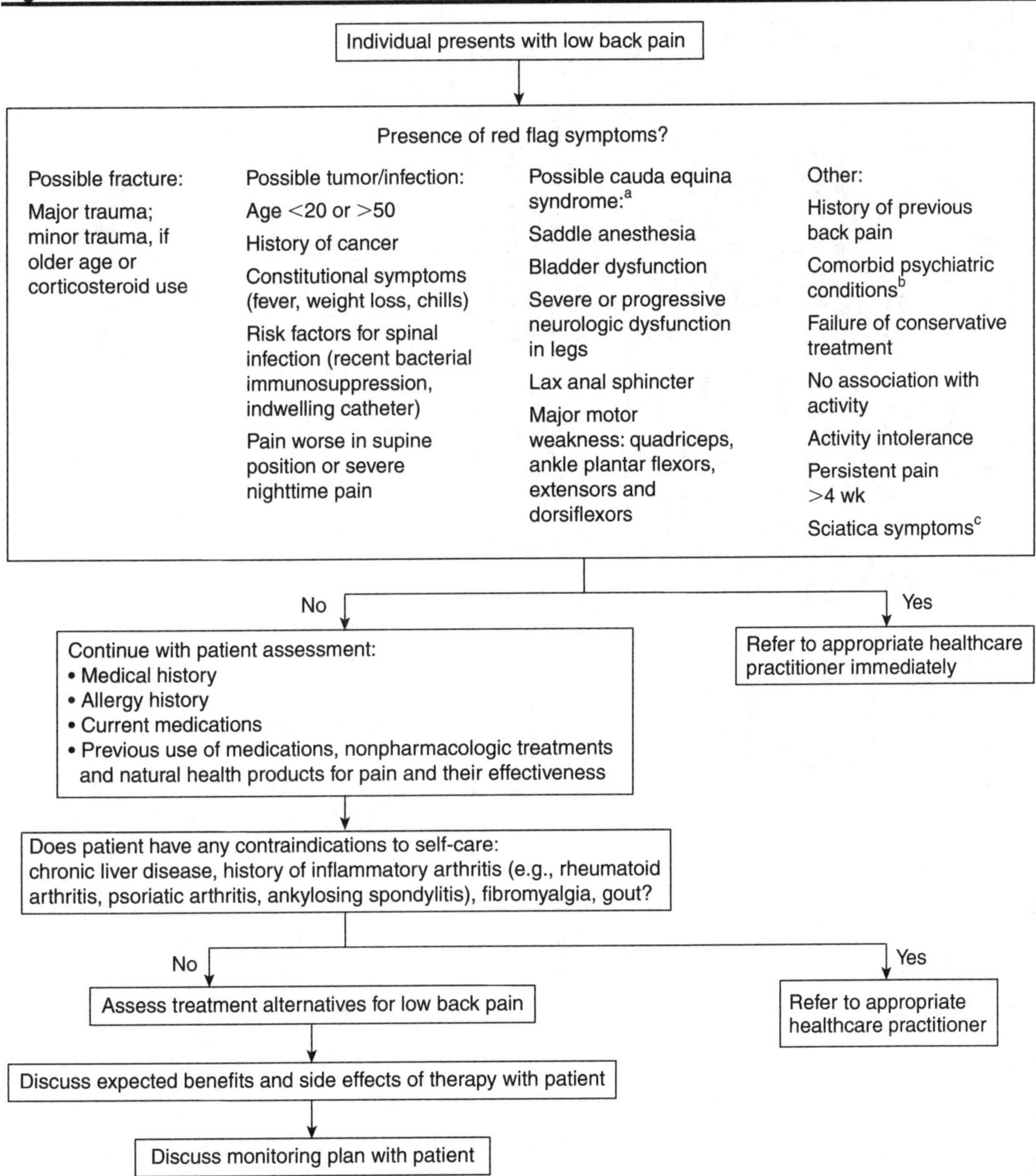
Individual presents with low back pain
Presence of red flag symptoms?
Possible fracture:
Major trauma; minor trauma, if older age or corticosteroid use
Possible tumor/infection:
Age <20 or >50
History of cancer
Constitutional symptoms (fever, weight loss, chills)
Risk factors for spinal infection (recent bacterial immunosuppression, indwelling catheter)
Pain worse in supine position or severe nighttime pain
Possible cauda equina syndrome:[a]
Saddle anesthesia
Bladder dysfunction
Severe or progressive neurologic dysfunction in legs
Lax anal sphincter
Major motor weakness: quadriceps, ankle plantar flexors, extensors and dorsiflexors
Other:
History of previous back pain
Comorbid psychiatric conditions[b]
Failure of conservative treatment
No association with activity
Activity intolerance
Persistent pain >4 wk
Sciatica symptoms[c]
No
Yes
Continue with patient assessment:
• Medical history
• Allergy history
• Current medications
• Previous use of medications, nonpharmacologic treatments and natural health products for pain and their effectiveness
Refer to appropriate healthcare practitioner immediately
Does patient have any contraindications to self-care: chronic liver disease, history of inflammatory arthritis (e.g., rheumatoid arthritis, psoriatic arthritis, ankylosing spondylitis), fibromyalgia, gout?
No
Yes
Assess treatment alternatives for low back pain
Refer to appropriate healthcare practitioner
Discuss expected benefits and side effects of therapy with patient
Discuss monitoring plan with patient

a Cauda equina syndrome: a rare clinical syndrome characterized by dull pain in the lower back and upper buttock region, analgesia in the buttocks, genitalia or thigh, accompanied by a disturbance of bowel and bladder function.
b History of depression, psychological distress or substance abuse can increase likelihood of persistent back pain.
c Sharp/burning pain radiating down posterior-lateral aspect of one or both legs. Symptoms worsen with change of position.

Table 3: **Drug Therapy for Low Back Pain[2,47]**

Class	Drug	Dosage	Adverse Effects	Drug Interactions	Comments	Cost[a]
Analgesics, oral	*acetaminophen* Atasol Preparations, Tylenol, generics	325–1000 mg Q4–6H po SR: 650 mg Q8H po (maximum 4 g/day)	Hepatotoxicity: Increased risk in malnourished patients, those with excessive alcohol intake (e.g., >3 drinks per day) or pre-existing hepatic disease; perform baseline LFTs in high-risk patients.	Acetaminophen has been reported to increase INR in warfarin-treated patients.[48] Check INR if acetaminophen ≥2 g/day is used for ≥3 consecutive days. Adjust warfarin dosage as required. Phenytoin, barbiturates, carbamazepine may increase acetaminophen metabolism and formation of toxic metabolite, thus increased risk of hepatotoxicity; risk may be increased in patients taking high therapeutic doses of acetaminophen and antiepileptic drugs chronically.	Maximal onset of pain relief within 24–48 h. Lower doses may be required in patients with severe hepatic and renal disease. Caution with concurrent use of other products containing acetaminophen (do not exceed 4 g/day). Consider regular schedule in individuals with pain persisting throughout the day. PRN dosing is acceptable for episodic pain of short duration.	$
	acetaminophen/caffeine/ codeine 8 mg ❥ Atasol with Codeine, generics	1–2 tablets Q4–6H po (maximum 4 g/day acetaminophen)	See acetaminophen. Sedation, nausea, vomiting, constipation.	See acetaminophen. Increased adverse effects with concurrent use of other sedating or constipating medications.	See acetaminophen. Recommended for short-term use, e.g., 2–3 days. Elderly are at higher risk for adverse effects.	$

Class	Drug	Dosage	Adverse Effects	Drug Interactions	Comments	Cost[a]
NSAIDs, oral	*ibuprofen* Advil, Advil Liqui-Gels, Motrin, Motrin IB, generics	200–400 mg Q6–8H po; maximum dose for self-care 1200 mg/day	GI: Dyspepsia, epigastric pain, nausea/vomiting, diarrhea, gastric and duodenal ulcers, GI bleeding. Cardiovascular: MI, stroke, heart failure, fluid retention, hypertension. Nephrotoxicity may occur; avoid NSAIDs in patients with severe renal impairment (ClCr <30 mL/min). CNS: Dizziness, drowsiness, headache, tinnitus, confusion (especially in the elderly); CNS effects may be dose related and respond to decreased dosage. Minor or serious skin rashes, pruritus.	Warfarin: Increased bleeding risk via antiplatelet effects and GI complications; monitor INR more frequently during initial period after NSAID started and monitor for signs of bleeding. Increased lithium levels—monitor. NSAIDs inhibit the renal elimination of methotrexate. Avoid NSAIDs in people using high-dose methotrexate (e.g., cancer treatment). For people using intermittent, low-dose methotrexate for arthritis, risk is minimal. Antihypertensives (e.g., beta-blockers, diuretics, ACEIs): May decrease antihypertensive effects; measure baseline BP, remeasure 1–2 wk after starting NSAID and adjust antihypertensive therapy as required. Increased risk of GI bleeding with SSRIs. Increased risk of GI adverse effects with alcohol. Give 30 min after or 8 h before low-dose ASA.	Caution when used in elderly or patients with pre-existing renal disease or comorbid conditions that may affect renal function (e.g., HF, diabetes, hypertension). Advise patients to stop taking NSAID that day if unable to eat or drink. NSAIDs are not a substitute for ASA being taken for MI or stroke prophylaxis. Avoid in patients with ASA or ibuprofen hypersensitivity. Avoid concurrent use of other NSAID-containing products (increased risk of GI-related side effects). PRN dosing is acceptable for episodic pain of short duration; consider regular schedule if pain persists throughout the day. Consider gastroprotection with misoprostol or PPI in high-risk patients. Increased risk of stroke or serious CV events at doses ≥2400 mg/day. Doses ≥2400 mg/day should not be used in patients with a history of CV events or with risk factors for CV disease.[49]	$
	naproxen sodium Aleve, generics	220–440 mg/day po in 1 or 2 divided doses; maximum dose for self-care 440 mg/day	See ibuprofen.	See ibuprofen.	See ibuprofen.	$$

(cont'd)

Table 3: **Drug Therapy for Low Back Pain**[2,47] *(cont'd)*

Class	Drug	Dosage	Adverse Effects	Drug Interactions	Comments	Cost[a]
Skeletal Muscle Relaxants	*chlorzoxazone* Combination products: Acetazone Forte	250–750 mg (chlorzoxazone) TID–QID po Consult and follow directions on combination product labels	Sedation, dizziness, light-headedness, nausea. Hepatotoxicity has been reported.	Increased effects with other CNS sedating medications, anticholinergics.	Onset of action within 12–24 h. No muscle relaxant has demonstrated superior efficacy. Use is generally not recommended due to side effect profile. Should be used only in the short term (2–3 days). Elderly are at increased risk of adverse effects. Available only in combination with acetaminophen (with or without codeine).	$$$
	methocarbamol Robaxin, generics Combination Products: Robax Platinum, Robaxacet, Robaxisal, generics	400–1500 mg (methocarbamol) QID po Consult and follow directions on combination product labels	Sedation, dizziness, light-headedness, nausea.	See chlorzoxazone.	Onset of action within 12–24 h. No muscle relaxant has demonstrated superior efficacy. Use is generally not recommended due to side effect profile. Should be used only in the short term (2–3 days). Elderly are at increased risk of adverse effects. Available as single entity or in combination with ASA or acetaminophen (with or without codeine) or ibuprofen.	$$$
	orphenadrine Orfenace, generics	50–100 mg BID–TID po	Sedation, dizziness, light-headedness, nausea. Anticholinergic effects: Agitation, dry mouth, constipation,	See chlorzoxazone.	Onset of action >24 h. No muscle relaxant has demonstrated superior efficacy. Use is generally not recommended due to side effect profile.	$$$$

Class	Drug	Dosage	Adverse Effects	Drug Interactions	Comments	Cost[a]
			hallucinations, urinary retention, blurred vision. Contraindicated with BPH, angle closure glaucoma, bladder obstruction, stenosing peptic ulcer, myasthenia gravis.		Should be used only in the short term (2–3 days). Elderly are at increased risk of adverse effects.	
Natural Health Products	*devil's claw (harpagophytum procumbens)*	50–100 mg (harpagoside) per day po	Diarrhea, GI upset.	Theoretical interaction with many drugs due to possible inhibition of CYP2C9, 2C19 or 3A4. May enhance anticoagulant effect of warfarin (bruising reported with combination).	Lack of product standardization may result in inter- and intra-product variability.	$$
	white willow bark (salix alba)	120–240 mg (salicin) per day po	Minimal adverse effects reported with oral use. One case of hypersensitivity reported. Theoretical (but unproven) risks associated with tannins include kidney and liver damage, GI intolerance.	Theoretical drug interaction with tannin-containing herbs. Significance of other interactions unknown due to lack of information pertaining to the exact salicylate content.	Onset of action 1–3 wk. Has been studied in chronic low back pain only. Exact mechanism of action unknown, but may possess anti-inflammatory activity. Long-term efficacy and toxicity are unknown. Lack of product standardization may result in inter- and intra-product variability. Constituents include tannins, flavonoids and salicylates (metabolite). Avoid in patients with history of salicylate hypersensitivity.	$$

[a] Cost of 30-day supply, includes drug cost only.

Dosage adjustment may be required in renal impairment.

Abbreviations: ACEI = angiotensin converting enzyme inhibitor; BP = blood pressure; BPH = benign prostatic hyperplasia; CV = cardiovascular; HF = heart failure; INR = international normalized ratio; LFT = liver function tests; PPI = proton pump inhibitor

Legend: $ <$5 $$ $5–10 $$$ $10–20 $$$$ $20–30

Resource Tips

For more information on low back pain, contact: Chronic Pain Association of Canada, P.O. Box 66017 Heritage Postal Station, Edmonton, AB, T6J 6T4. Available from: www.chronicpaincanada.com.

Suggested Readings

Chou R. In the clinic. Low back pain. *Ann Intern Med* 2014;160:ITC6-1.

Chou R, Qaseem A, Snow V et al. Diagnosis and treatment of low back pain: a joint clinical practice guideline from the American College of Physicians and the American Pain Society. *Ann Intern Med* 2007;147:478-91.

Cochrane Library. *Cochrane Back Group*. Available from: onlinelibrary.wiley.com/book/10.1002/14651858/homepage/crg_BACK.html#BACK.

Cohen SP, Argoff CE, Carragee EJ. Management of low back pain. *BMJ* 2008;337:a2718.

References

1. Cohen SP, Argoff CE, Carragee EJ. Management of low back pain. *BMJ* 2008;337:a2718.
2. Chou R, Qaseem A, Snow V et al. Diagnosis and treatment of low back pain: a joint clinical practice guideline from the American College of Physicians and the American Pain Society. *Ann Intern Med* 2007;147:478-91.
3. Andersson GB. Epidemiological features of chronic low-back pain. *Lancet* 1999;354:581-5.
4. Hoy D, March L, Brooks P et al. The global burden of low back pain: estimates from the Global Burden of Disease 2010 study. *Ann Rheum Dis* 2014;73:968-74.
5. Frank JW, Kerr MS, Brooker AS et al. Disability resulting from occupational low back pain. Part 1: What do we know about primary prevention? A review of the scientific evidence on prevention before disability begins. *Spine (Phila Pa 1976)* 1996;21:2908-17.
6. Hestbaek L, Leboeuf-Yde C, Manniche C. Low back pain: what is the long-term course? A review of studies of general patient populations. *Eur Spine J* 2003;12:149-65.
7. da C Menezes Costa L, Maher CG, Hancock MJ et al. The prognosis of acute and persistent low-back pain: a meta-analysis. *CMAJ* 2012;184:E613-24.
8. Cassidy JD, Cote P, Carrol LJ et al. Incidence and course of low back pain episodes in the general population. *Spine (Phila Pa 1976)* 2005;30:2817-23.
9. Hayden JA, Chou R, Hogg-Johnson S et al. Systematic reviews of low back pain prognosis had variable methods and results: guidance for future prognosis reviews. *J Clin Epidemiol* 2009;62:781-96.
10. Pengel LH, Herbert RD, Maher CG et al. Acute low back pain: a systematic review of its prognosis. *BMJ* 2003;327:323.
11. Kopec JA, Sayre EC, Esdaile JM. Predictors of back pain in a general population cohort. *Spine (Phila Pa 1976)* 2004;29:70-7.
12. Shiri R, Karppinen J, Leino-Arjas P et al. The association between obesity and low back pain: a meta-analysis. *Am J Epidemiol* 2010;171:135-54.
13. Shiri R, Karppinen J, Leino-Arjas P et al. The association between smoking and low back pain: a meta-analysis. *Am J Med* 2010;123:87.e7-35.
14. Roffey DM, Wai EK, Bishop P et al. Causal assessment of occupational standing or walking and low back pain: results of a systematic review. *Spine J* 2010;10:262-72.
15. Wai EK, Roffey DM, Bishop P et al. Causal assessment of occupational lifting and low back pain: results of a systematic review. *Spine J* 2010;10:554-66.
16. Wai EK, Roffey DM, Bishop P et al. Causal assessment of occupational carrying and low back pain: results of a systematic review. *Spine J* 2010;10:628-38.
17. Deyo RA, Rainville J, Kent DL. What can the history and physical examination tell us about low back pain? *JAMA* 1992;268:760-5.
18. van der Windt DA, Simons E, Riphagen II et al. Physical examination for lumbar radiculopathy due to disc herniation in patients with low-back pain. *Cochrane Database System Rev* 2010;2:CD007431.
19. Traeger AC, Hübscher M, Henschke N et al. Effect of primary care-based education on reassurance in patients with acute low back pain: systematic review and meta-analysis. *JAMA Intern Med* 2015;175:733-43.
20. van Tulder MW, Tuut M, Pennick V et al. Quality of primary care guidelines for acute low back pain. *Spine (Phila Pa 1976)* 2004;29:E357-62.
21. Arnau JM, Vallano A, Lopez A et al. A critical review of guidelines for low back pain treatment. *Eur Spine J* 2006;15:543-53.
22. Keller A, Hayden J, Bombardier C et al. Effect sizes of non-surgical treatments of non-specific low-back pain. *Eur Spine J* 2007;16:1776-88.
23. Chou R, Huffman LH. Nonpharmacologic therapies for acute and chronic low back pain: a review of the evidence for an American Pain Society/American College of Physicians clinical practice guideline. *Ann Intern Med* 2007;147:492-504.
24. Chou R, Huffman LH. Medications for acute and chronic low back pain: a review of the evidence for an American Pain Society/American College of Physicians clinical practice guideline. *Ann Intern Med* 2007;147:505-14.
25. Machado LA, Kamper SJ, Herbert RD et al. Analgesic effects of treatments for non-specific low back pain: a meta-analysis of placebo-controlled randomized trials. *Rheumatology (Oxford)* 2009;48:520-7.
26. Dahm KT, Brurberg KG, Jamtvedt G et al. Advice to rest in bed versus advice to stay active for acute low-back pain and sciatica. *Cochrane Database Syst Rev* 2010;6:CD007612.
27. Delitto A, George SZ, Van Dillen LR et al. Low back pain. *J Orthop Sports Phys Ther* 2012;42:A1-57.
28. Hayden JA, van Tulder MW, Malmivaara A et al. Exercise therapy for treatment of non-specific low back pain. *Cochrane Database Syst Rev* 2005;3:CD000335.

29. Doherty M, Ernst E, Fisken M et al. Arthritis Research UK. *Practitioner-based complementary and alternative therapies for the treatment of rheumatoid arthritis, osteoarthritis, fibromyalgia and low back pain.* Available from: www.arthritisresearchuk.org/news/press-releases/2013/march/january/new-report-on-complementary-therapies-for-arthritis-reveals-lack-of-scientific-evidence.aspx. Accessed on May 2, 2016.
30. Tilbrook HE, Cox H, Hewitt CE et al. Yoga for chronic low back pain: a randomized trial. *Ann Intern Med* 2011;155:569-78.
31. Bussing A, Ostermann T, Ludtke R et al. Effects of yoga interventions on pain and pain-associated disability: a meta-analysis. *J Pain* 2012;13:1-9.
32. Posadzki P, Ernst E. Yoga for low back pain: a systematic review of randomized clinical trials. *Clin Rheumatol* 2011;30:1257-62.
33. Sherman KJ, Cherkin DC, Wellman RD et al. A randomized trial comparing yoga, stretching and a self-care book for chronic low back pain. *Arch Intern Med* 2011;171:2019-26.
34. Natour J, Cazotti LdeA, Ribeiro LH et al. Pilates improves pain, function and quality of life in patients with chronic low back pain: a randomized controlled trial. *Clin Rehabil* 2015;29:59-68.
35. Cramer H, Lauche R, Haller H et al. A systematic review and meta-analysis of yoga for low back pain. *Clin J Pain* 2013;29:450-60.
36. Furlan AD, Imamura M, Dryden T et al. Massage for low-back pain. *Cochrane Database Syst Rev* 2008;4:CD001929.
37. Rubinstein SM, Terwee CB, Assendelft WJ et al. Spinal manipulative therapy for acute low-back pain. *Cochrane Database Syst Rev* 2012;9:CD008880.
38. Heymans MW, van Tulder MW, Esmail R et al. Back schools for non-specific low-back pain. *Cochrane Database Syst Rev* 2004;4:CD000261.
39. Choi BK, Verbeek JH, Tam WW et al. Exercises for prevention of recurrences of low-back pain. *Cochrane Database Syst Rev* 2010;1:CD006555.
40. French SD, Cameron M, Walker BF et al. Superficial heat or cold for low back pain. *Cochrane Database Syst Rev* 2006;1:CD004750.
41. Ebadi S, Henschke N, Nakhostin Ansari N et al. Therapeutic ultrasound for chronic low-back pain. *Cochrane Database Syst Rev* 2014;3:CD009169.
42. Chuter V, Spink M, Searle A et al. The effectiveness of shoe insoles for the prevention and treatment of low back pain: a systematic review and meta-analysis of randomised controlled trials. *BMC Musculoskelet Disord* 2014;15:140.
43. Chou R, Loeser JD, Owens DK et al. Interventional therapies, surgery and interdisciplinary rehabilitation for low back pain: an evidence-based clinical practice guideline from the American Pain Society. *Spine (Phila Pa 1976)* 2009;34:1066-77.
44. Henschke N, Ostelo RW, van Tulder MW et al. Behavioural treatment for chronic low-back pain. *Cochrane Database Syst Rev* 2010;7:CD002014.
45. Monticone M, Ferrante S, Rocca B et al. Effect of a long-lasting multidisciplinary program on disability and fear-avoidance behaviors in patients with chronic low back pain: results of a randomized controlled trial. *Clin J Pain* 2013;29:929-38.
46. Kamper SJ, Apeldoorn AT, Chiarotto A et al. Multidisciplinary biopsychosocial rehabilitation for chronic low back pain. *Cochrane Database Syst Rev* 2014;9:CD000963.
47. McEvoy GK, Snow EK, Miller J et al., eds. *AHFS drug information*. Bethesda: American Society of Health-System Pharmacists; 2016.
48. Lopes RD, Horowitz JD, Garcia DA et al. Warfarin and acetaminophen interaction: a summary of the evidence and biologic plausibility. *Blood* 2011;118:6269-73.
49. Government of Canada. Healthy Canadians. *New safety information for prescription-strength ibuprofen: Risk of heart attack and stroke at high doses.* Available from: www.healthycanadians.gc.ca/recall-alert-rappel-avis/hc-sc/2015/53055a-eng.php.
50. Machado GC, Maher CG, Ferreira PH et al. Efficacy and safety of paracetamol for spinal pain and osteoarthritis: systematic review and meta-analysis of randomised placebo controlled trials. *BMJ* 2015;350:h1225.
51. Williams CM, Maher CG, Latimer J et al. Efficacy of paracetamol for acute low-back pain: a double-blind, randomised controlled trial. *Lancet* 2014;384:1586-96.
52. Roelofs PD, Deyo RA, Koes BW et al. Non-steroidal anti-inflammatory drugs for low back pain. *Cochrane Database Syst Rev* 2008;1:CD000396.
53. Davies RA, Maher CG, Hancock MJ. A systematic review of paracetamol for non-specific low back pain. *Eur Spine J* 2008;17:1423-30.
54. Nadler SF, Steiner DJ, Erasala GN et al. Continuous low-level heat wrap therapy provides more efficacy than ibuprofen and acetaminophen for acute low back pain. *Spine (Phila Pa 1976)* 2002;27:1012-7.
55. van Tulder MW, Touray T, Furlan AD et al. Muscle relaxants for non-specific low back pain. *Cochrane Database Syst Rev* 2003;4:CD004252.
56. Chou R, Turner JA, Devine EB et al. The effectiveness and risks of long-term opioid therapy for chronic pain: a systematic review for a National Institutes of Health Pathways to Prevention Workshop. *Ann Intern Med* 2015;162:276-86.
57. Chaparro LE, Furlan AD, Deshpande A et al. Opioids compared with placebo or other treatments for chronic low back pain: an update of the Cochrane Review. *Spine (Phila Pa 1976)* 2014;39:556-63.
58. Deshpande A, Furlan A, Mailis-Gagnon A et al. Opioids for chronic low-back pain. *Cochrane Database Syst Rev* 2007;3:CD004959.
59. Oltean H, Robbins C, van Tulder MW et al. Herbal medicine for low-back pain. *Cochrane Database Syst Rev* 2014;12:CD004504.

Low Back Pain—What You Need to Know

Why do so many people have low back pain?

Low back pain is a very common problem because the lower back carries most of your weight. Four out of 5 adults have back pain at some time in their life.

What are the most common causes of low back pain?

The most common causes of low back pain are pulled muscles and spasms, usually as a result of sports or work-related injury. However, lifting too much, lifting in the wrong way or twisting the back can all cause a strain or sprain of the muscles.

Another common cause of low back pain is sciatica. Sciatica is caused by pressure on a nerve within your spinal column. This can happen when a disk slips out of its spot between your backbones. The nerve is squeezed and becomes inflamed. Pain may travel from your back down into your leg.

What usually happens when someone has back pain?

Most people who have back pain find that it gets better gradually over a few weeks. This is similar to what happens when other muscles or ligaments are injured.

If you see a doctor or other health professional when your back is very sore, they will ask you questions to make sure the pain is not caused by something serious. Serious causes are very rare, but it is important to rule them out before deciding on a treatment.

What warning signs should I look for with low back pain?

Contact your doctor if you have back pain plus any of the following conditions:

- Fever
- Past use of steroids, like prednisone
- Unexplained weight loss
- Pain that worsens or does not get better when you stop moving and rest
- Previous history of back injury
- Problems with your bladder or bowel
- Weakness in your legs
- Severe pain restricting complete mobility
- A history of cancer

How is back pain treated?

Most of the time, back pain gets better in 2–4 weeks with very little treatment. Treatment usually consists of:

- Returning to your usual activities as soon as you can
- Reducing the amount of time you rest in bed since it may slow the healing process
- Taking over-the-counter pain medications
- Applying heat

If symptoms don't improve within 3–4 weeks, your doctor may send you to a therapist for special exercises.

How can I prevent back pain?

It is common for back pain to come back. Follow these simple measures to prevent chronic pain:

- If you injured your back at work, talk to your supervisor or an occupational health worker about how to prevent further injuries.
- When lifting an object, always bend your knees, use your leg muscles to lift, tighten your stomach and avoid bending and lifting at the same time.
- Exercise regularly to keep your back muscles strong and flexible.
- Don't slouch; poor posture puts a strain on your lower back.
- Try to keep a positive attitude about your personal and professional life. Studies have shown that people who are unhappy with their professional life are more likely to have low back problems.

Chapter 46
Osteoarthritis

Kelly Grindrod, BSc(Pharm), PharmD, MSc
Jason Kielly, BSc(Pharm), PharmD
Carlo Marra, BSc(Pharm), PharmD, PhD, FCSHP

Pathophysiology

Osteoarthritis (OA) is the most common form of arthritis, affecting an estimated 1 in 10 Canadians.[1] The Global Burden of Disease 2010 study found that knee and hip OA ranked as the eleventh highest contributors to global disability.[2] OA is a progressive disease of the synovial joints. In the past, OA was thought to be due to daily "wear and tear" that resulted from excessive and repetitive force on the cartilage in joints. While this is partially true, OA is now thought to be a systemic disorder due to an imbalance between joint destruction and repair.[3,4,5] This ultimately results in a breakdown of cartilage and bone, leading to symptoms of pain, stiffness and functional disability.[5] OA is more prevalent as we age, affecting nearly half the population over age 70.[6]

Synovial joints are structures in which the opposing bony surfaces are covered with a layer of cartilage. There is also a joint cavity that contains synovial fluid and is lined with synovial membrane.[3] Cartilage acts as a shock absorber and, with synovial fluid, provides a smooth, low-friction surface for movement. Surrounding the joints are the articular capsule, ligaments, muscles and tendons, all of which act to stabilize and protect the joint.

In early disease, the joint maintains function by thickening the cartilage. As the disease progresses, the cartilage softens, becoming pitted and frayed, and pieces may break off into the synovial fluid. This causes further damage and interferes with joint function. The joint may also lose its shape, and the surrounding ligaments, muscles and tendons may start to weaken.

As the cartilage deteriorates, the joint space narrows and the bones start to rub against one another. At this point, the bones may start to remodel, leading to a thickening of the bone ends and the formation of bony outgrowths (osteophytes) and subchondral cysts. These changes may lead to joint deformities. Generally, OA is not associated with inflammation but symptomatic inflammation of the synovial lining and/or joint may occur in severe OA.

The most significant risk factors for OA are advancing age and female gender.[6,7] Other risk factors include obesity,[8] quadriceps muscle weakness,[9] family history,[10,11] joint injury,[12,13,14] and joint overuse or injury associated with certain sports (e.g., soccer)[15] and occupations (e.g., farming).[16]

Goals of Therapy

- Relieve symptoms such as pain and inflammation
- Maintain or improve mobility and quality of life
- Minimize functional disability and improve physical functioning

Healthcare practitioners can educate patients and caregivers to help them understand the condition and make informed decisions about which therapies to choose.

Patient Assessment

Typically, OA occurs in the hands, knees, hips, feet, neck and back (from most to least common).[17] Asymmetrical joint pain is the most common symptom of OA.[18,19] The synovial joints are generally insensitive to pain but can become sensitized in OA as a result of physiologic stress and damage to tissue and nerves. Pain does not arise from the damaged cartilage itself but is caused by the various stresses placed on the muscles, ligaments and tendons in the areas surrounding the cartilage as a result of the damage. The pain is usually felt near the joint during use but it may be referred elsewhere and may be felt at night or during rest with more severe disease.[20,21] Stiffness after inactivity and limited range of motion are other common symptoms. Inflammation may or may not be present. Crepitus may be present with joint movement. Table 1 lists the signs and symptoms of OA.

Table 1: **Clinical Features of Osteoarthritis vs. Rheumatoid Arthritis[19]**

Clinical Parameter	Feature	Osteoarthritis	Rheumatoid Arthritis
Symptoms	Stiffness	Morning or after periods of inactivity; usually lasts <30 min	Significant, prolonged (>60 min) in the morning
	Symptoms localized	Yes—limited to affected joints	No
	Pain	Worsens with activity or after prolonged use (especially with weight-bearing activity)	Worsens after prolonged inactivity; usually improves with activity
Signs	Symmetry	Occasional	Common
	Tenderness	Unusual	Over entire exposed joint spaces
	Inflammation	Unusual	Common
	Instability	Occasional; buckling or joint instability can result in decreased range of movement and falls	Uncommon
	Multisystem disease	No	Often feel systemically unwell (e.g., can have one or more of fatigue, fever, chills, weight loss, hair loss, dry mouth or dry eyes)

Rheumatoid arthritis is a systemic inflammatory disease that often presents with joint pain as one of many symptoms. The scope of this chapter does not include the management of rheumatoid arthritis; however, symptom recognition (Table 1) is important so that patients with suspected rheumatoid arthritis can be appropriately evaluated and treated to control inflammation and delay disease progression.

For more information on the management of rheumatoid arthritis, consult the *Compendium of Therapeutic Choices*: Rheumatoid Arthritis.

Since joint pain can have a number of causes, it is important to rule out more serious conditions requiring medical intervention. In particular, recent history of significant trauma, hot, swollen joints, rapidly worsening pain, joint locking and signs and symptoms of infection should be promptly investigated.[19] Reports of arthralgia have occurred with numerous drugs; however, the numbers are small and often a cause and effect relationship cannot be clearly established.[22]

Figure 1 is an algorithm for assessing patients with joint pain.

Principles of Therapy

Current nonpharmacologic and pharmacologic therapies for OA provide symptomatic relief but are not curative and do not slow disease progression. Several evidence-based guidelines are available for the management of OA.[23,24,25] Choice of treatment is based on a combination of risk vs. benefit assessment, cost and patient preference. Pharmacologic therapy should always be initiated in combination with nonpharmacologic modalities. If tolerated, pharmacologic therapies (except localized therapy) should be tried for at least 1–2 weeks to allow the patient to fully assess their effectiveness. An algorithm for treatment of osteoarthritis can be found in Figure 2.

Nonpharmacologic Therapy

Nonpharmacologic therapy for OA (Table 2) should always be initiated first or started concurrently with drug therapy. The quality of published evidence supporting these modalities is varied.[27] There is reasonably good evidence that self-management education programs can improve mobility and reduce discomfort.[28,29] In addition, evidence suggests that aerobic exercise and strength training,[30,31,32,33,34] weight loss through a combination of diet and exercise,[35] and supports and braces[36,37,38,39,40] may effectively reduce symptoms and improve function. Therapies that actively engage the patient (e.g., aerobic, aquatic and strength exercises) may be more effective than passive therapies (e.g., diathermy, orthotics, magnetic stimulation).[51] Consider referring patients who wish to evaluate these options to a physiotherapist or occupational therapist.[52]

Surgery is usually reserved as a last resort for patients with severe, painful and activity-limiting OA who have tried other pharmacologic and nonpharmacologic modalities.[23,24,25]

Table 2: Nonpharmacologic Therapy for Osteoarthritis[27]

Modalities Supported by Evidence	Purpose/Benefits
Patient education for self-management[28,29]	Educate about treatment options and coping skills Reduce pain and disability
Strength training and aerobic exercise[30,31,32,33,34] (includes land and aquatic exercise)	Reduce pain and disability in knee, hip osteoarthritis (OA) Intensity not important
Weight loss if overweight/obese, through diet and exercise (weight loss of at least 5%)[35]	Decrease load on weight-bearing joints Improve pain and function in knee OA
Joint protection, e.g., splints, taping, braces[36,37,38]	Ensure joint properly positioned during activity and at rest Improve pain and joint function in knee OA
Supportive footwear, e.g., no raised heel; thick, shock-absorbing sole; arch support; adequately sized[36,38,39,40]	Absorbs shock and controls foot pronation Improve pain and physical function
Use of ambulation aids and assistive devices, e.g., canes, walkers[24]	May improve functional status, ambulation Facilitate activities of daily living (ADL)
Social support, e.g., telephone follow up,[28,41,42] education of family members and caregivers[43]	Improve pain and psychological status
Transcutaneous electrical nerve stimulation (TENS)[44]	Improve pain and stiffness in knee OA
Acupuncture[25,45,46]	Improve pain, stiffness, function in knee OA
Heat[47]	Increase blood flow to affected areas

(cont'd)

Table 2: **Nonpharmacologic Therapy for Osteoarthritis**[27] *(cont'd)*

Modalities Supported by Evidence	Purpose/Benefits
	Apply for 10 min prior to strength training exercises for knee OA
Cold[48]	Reduce blood flow to affected area, block nerve impulses to joints, reduce swelling Improve range of motion, function and knee strength Massage ice around affected joint for 20 min, 5 times per wk
Massage[49]	Small trial suggests may improve pain, stiffness and function in knee OA Massage produces counterirritation
Surgery[24,25,50]	Indicated in patients with severe symptomatic OA who have failed nonsurgical strategies and continue to have significant limitations in ADL

Pharmacologic Therapy

Table 5 lists selected oral and topical medications used to treat osteoarthritis.[24,25,50]

For more information on pharmacologic therapy, consult the *Compendium of Therapeutic Choices*: Osteoarthritis.

For comparative ingredients of nonprescription products, consult the *Compendium of Products for Minor Ailments*—Analgesic Products: External Analgesics, Internal Analgesics and Antipyretics.

Acetaminophen

Acetaminophen continues to be the initial drug of choice for symptomatic relief of osteoarthritis.[24,25] The rationale for using acetaminophen has been the fact that it is effective, relatively safe, well tolerated and easily accessible. Most studies of acetaminophen in OA used the maximum daily dose of 1 g QID for a short period (median 6 weeks) and show that it provides moderate pain relief and improvements in function.[55,56] However, 2 meta-analyses showed that acetaminophen likely has a small effect on OA pain and may not be sufficient to treat OA of the knee or hip.[57,58] Maximum therapeutic doses should be tried for an adequate period (1–2 weeks) to assess efficacy. Following this trial, the lowest effective dose should be used.

Acetaminophen overdose is the leading cause of acute liver failure, which led the US Food and Drug Administration to recommend that all products containing acetaminophen be limited to 325 mg of acetaminophen per dosage unit;[59] Health Canada continues to review the data to assess whether similar changes will be made in Canada.[60] Patients taking acetaminophen *must* be counselled to not exceed the recommended daily dose and to be informed of nonprescription and prescription products that contain acetaminophen.[61] Conditions such as chronic alcohol abuse and liver disease preclude the long-term use of maximum therapeutic doses and should be investigated prior to beginning therapy; however, they are not contraindications to acetaminophen therapy.[62,63,64]

Topical Agents

Topical **diclofenac** and topical **capsaicin** are reasonable options for patients with OA of the knee who have suboptimal relief with acetaminophen, or who cannot tolerate or are reluctant to use systemic agents.[24,25] Initial NSAID therapy should be topical rather than oral in persons ≥75 years old.[25] Both agents are effective in those who have OA in only 1 or 2 joints, such as the knee or hand.[65,66,67,68,69] Several systematic reviews have shown that topical NSAIDs are better tolerated than oral NSAIDs and have similar effects on pain and function.[65,66,67] In a Cochrane review, the proportion of patients with osteoarthritis who experienced a 50% reduction in pain over 8–12 weeks compared with placebo was 48% vs. 32% (NNT=6) for topical diclofenac solution and 60% vs. 51% (NNT=11) for topical diclofenac gel.[70] Systematic reviews have also shown topical capsaicin to be efficacious for the treatment of chronic pain. The proportion of patients who experienced a 50% reduction in pain after 4 weeks compared with placebo was 38% vs. 25% (NNT=8) for capsaicin 0.025% and 57% vs. 42% (NNT=6) for capsaicin 0.075%.[68,69]

Zucapsaicin, a synthetic form of capsaicin, is indicated for the management of severe pain from knee osteoarthritis not managed by NSAIDs alone. A 3-month phase III clinical trial showed that in patients with severe pain despite NSAID or COX-2 inhibitor therapy, adding topical zucapsaicin 0.075% cream improved both pain and function compared to zucapsaicin 0.01% (used as the control).[71]

Topical therapies may also be tried as an adjunct to systemic agents where pain relief is not adequate. Both agents should be applied 3–4 times daily. Maximal effect can take up to 2 weeks for topical NSAIDs and 4 weeks for topical capsaicin. Unfortunately, the tingling and burning sensation caused by capsaicin often prevents an adequate trial of this medication.

A systematic review found little evidence to support the use of topical counterirritants such as **salicylates** in chronic musculoskeletal pain.[72] Since they are readily available without a prescription, the potential exists for overuse of these products leading to bleeding from salicylate toxicity or drug interactions with oral anticoagulants.[73]

Early randomized trials of topical herbal preparations suggest that ***Arnica*** or **comfrey** may also provide symptom relief but further research is needed to understand the clinical significance of these findings.[74]

If patients experience pain, swelling or burning from topical analgesics, advise them to stop using the product and seek immediate medical attention.[75]

NSAIDs

Due to their risk of serious adverse effects, nonsteroidal anti-inflammatory drugs (NSAIDs) are considered second-line therapy after failure of acetaminophen in the management of OA pain.[24,25] Although acetaminophen is superior in terms of safety, NSAIDs are often preferred by OA patients due to better pain relief.[76,77] Not surprisingly, patients who discontinue NSAID use due to toxicity are less willing to resume therapy with another NSAID.[76]

Celecoxib is as effective as nonselective NSAIDs for pain control in OA of the hip and knee and is associated with a lower incidence of gastroduodenal ulcers compared with nonselective NSAIDs.[78] Like nonselective NSAIDs, celecoxib can exacerbate pre-existing renal disease. Baseline and periodic monitoring of serum creatinine and electrolytes is recommended for high-risk patients.

Prior to starting long-term NSAID therapy, assess patients for their risk of cardiovascular, GI and renal complications (see Table 3).[78,79,80,81] If a patient has no risk factors, a low-dose of a nonselective NSAID can be started (e.g., ibuprofen 200–400 mg Q8H or naproxen sodium 220 mg Q12H). Over a 1- to 2-week trial, the dose can be titrated until adequate pain relief is achieved or the maximum dose is reached. Avoid long-term therapy if possible, but if continued therapy is needed, use the lowest effective dose. Patients who require chronic NSAID therapy should discuss their use with a healthcare practitioner. Due to the serious adverse effects associated with ASA it is not generally recommended for the self-management of OA.

Avoid most NSAIDs (including COX-2 inhibitors) in patients at increased risk of cardiovascular events. If treatment with an NSAID is essential, patients at high risk of cardiovascular complications should receive naproxen (with low-dose ASA, if indicated). Nonselective NSAIDs may inhibit the antithrombotic effect of ASA by competitively binding to the COX-1 receptor.[82] This theoretical interaction has not been documented with enteric-coated ASA or COX-2 inhibitors. Advise patients to take nonselective NSAIDs at least 30 minutes after or 8 hours before ASA.[83]

There are no definitive data to indicate the superiority or safety of one NSAID over another but both the Canadian Cardiovascular Society[78] and the American Heart Association[79] have released position statements to guide the use of NSAIDs.

Table 3: **Risk Factors for the Development of Serious Adverse Events with NSAID Therapy**

	Cardiovascular Complications	GI Complications	Renal Complications
Age	>65 y	>65 y	>65 y
Medical History	Heart failure CV disease Diabetes Hypertension Myocardial infarction Stroke Rheumatoid arthritis	Alcoholic liver disease *H. pylori* infection Peptic ulcer disease Rheumatoid arthritis Upper GI bleeding	Heart failure Dehydration Hypertension Pre-existing renal disease
Concomitant Medications		Regular use of multiple NSAIDs Antithrombotic, e.g., daily low-dose ASA, warfarin Oral glucocorticoids	ACE inhibitors ARBs Direct renin inhibitors Diuretics

Abbreviations: ARB = angiotensin receptor blocker; CV = cardiovascular

NSAID Risks

While dyspepsia has been reported in up to 60% of patients taking NSAIDs, the actual incidence is likely closer to 5–10%.[84] If dyspepsia occurs for more than 7 days in a month, consider discontinuing NSAID therapy.[85] Minor heartburn can be managed symptomatically with antacids or histamine-2 receptor antagonists (see Chapter 31: Dyspepsia and GERD).

Serious GI complications such as perforated ulcers, hemorrhage and obstruction are estimated to occur at an incidence of less than 1% per year.[86] Prior to starting NSAID therapy, identify patients at risk of serious NSAID-related GI complications and take preventive measures (see Figure 2). **Histamine-2 receptor antagonists** and **antacids** provide relief from dyspeptic symptoms, but not against more serious GI complications. **Misoprostol** and **proton pump inhibitors (PPIs)** such as omeprazole are appropriate options for preventing serious GI complications, though PPIs are much better tolerated.[87,88,89,90,91]

NSAIDs can increase blood pressure in patients with normal or high blood pressure.[92,93] When starting NSAIDs in patients on antihypertensive therapy, measure blood pressure within 1 week of starting treatment to assess whether changes to either NSAID or antihypertensive therapy are warranted. In addition to affecting blood pressure, NSAIDs can cause acute kidney injury, especially when added to antihypertensive therapies like diuretics, ACE inhibitors or angiotensin receptor blockers.[94]

Meta-analyses of both randomized controlled trials and observational studies have shown that NSAIDs increase the risk of thromboembolic cardiovascular events such as MI.[95,96,97] With the exception of naproxen, this risk has been shown with most NSAIDs, including several COX-2 inhibitors and nonselective agents such as ibuprofen and diclofenac. It is still unclear whether the use of low-dose acetylsalicylic acid (ASA) in high-risk patients mitigates this risk.[96,98]

Natural Health Products

For comparative ingredients of nonprescription products, consult the *Compendium of Products for Minor Ailments*—Herbal and Natural Health Products: Combinations, Single Entity.

Endogenous **glucosamine** and **chondroitin** maintain the integrity of cartilage within a joint. Exogenous formulations (glucosamine sulfate, glucosamine hydrochloride, chondroitin sulfate) have been evaluated in the treatment of OA. Their pharmacologic effect is believed to mimic their physiologic effect on cartilage tissue. The proposed mechanisms of action are to stimulate the production of cartilage, prevent cartilage destruction by inhibiting inflammatory mediators and/or enzymes and maintain viscosity of the joint.[99,100]

The majority of available evidence suggests that glucosamine hydrochloride is ineffective for pain reduction in patients with OA. One study of glucosamine hydrochloride plus chondroitin compared with celecoxib in patients with knee OA suggested comparable efficacy in reducing pain scores after 6 months.[101] The study lacked a placebo arm, which is concerning as up to 75% of the effect of analgesics in OA may be due to placebo effect.[102] Glucosamine sulfate may have function-modifying effects in patients with knee OA when administered for more than 6 months, but no pain-reduction benefits were demonstrated after 6 months of therapy.[103] A systematic review evaluating the benefit and harm of chondroitin for OA found that chondroitin, alone or in combination with glucosamine, was better than placebo in improving pain and had lower risk of serious adverse events compared to control.[104] A large-scale randomized controlled trial in knee OA compared the combination of glucosamine HCl (500 mg TID) and chondroitin sulfate (400 mg TID) to either placebo or celecoxib (200 mg daily). Celecoxib was the only intervention that proved efficacious. A small subset of patients with moderate to severe pain experienced some pain relief with the combination of glucosamine and chondroitin.[105] In another randomized controlled trial, glucosamine sulfate (1500 mg once daily) failed to improve pain, function or the number of medications taken in patients with hip OA.[106]

As large-scale randomized controlled trials have not shown glucosamine and chondroitin to have substantial effect, treatment guidelines for OA do not recommend these agents.[25,107,108,109] However, given the great interest that many patients have in "natural" alternatives, it is worthwhile having a discussion with patients about the most recent evidence.

S-adenosyl-L-methionine (SAMe) is a naturally occurring substance that is produced by the body. It may promote the production of cartilage building blocks. A systematic review suggests that SAMe is well tolerated and may improve both pain and function in osteoarthritis.[110] However, a 2009 Cochrane review noted that many of the trials were small, not placebo-controlled and of questionable quality. Reviewers cautioned against using SAMe until adequately sized, randomized, parallel-group trials have been done.[111]

Other complementary and alternative products such as **methylsulphonylmethane** (MSM), **Indian frankincense**, **avocado–soybean unsaponifiables (ASU)** and **rose hip** may also be effective but high quality evidence is lacking.[110,112]

Localized Therapy

The use of **intra-articular corticosteroids** in OA is limited to acute knee pain and patients who have local signs of inflammation and joint effusion. If joints are painful and swollen, aspiration of fluid followed by intra-articular injection of a corticosteroid (e.g., **triamcinolone acetonide** or **methylprednisolone acetate**) is effective in temporarily (4–6 weeks) decreasing pain.[113] It is often used in combination with other therapies, although it can be used as monotherapy. Repeated injections may damage cartilage. The injection should be provided by a qualified healthcare practitioner and the same site should not be injected more than 3–4 times per year.[23]

The efficacy of intra-articular corticosteroids for hand and hip OA has not been studied and use is not routine due to the risk of cartilage damage through repeated injections. Rheumatologists, using radiographic guidance, may provide injections to these joints for certain patients.

Hyaluronan is a linear polysaccharide found in synovial fluid. Meta-analyses investigating the efficacy and safety of hyaluronan injections have found conflicting results.[57,114,115] The effect of repeated courses of hyaluronan injections is unknown. These products are usually reserved for patients who have failed other therapies. Costs are high ($200–400 per treatment course) and they are not routinely covered by insurance plans. The injections can be purchased without a prescription but they must be administered by a qualified healthcare practitioner.

Opioid Analgesics

An opioid analgesic alone or in combination with acetaminophen or NSAIDs may be useful in patients who do not respond to other analgesics, experience acute exacerbations of OA pain, or are not willing or able to receive surgical treatments.[24] Side effects such as sedation, constipation, tolerance and dependence may limit the long-term use of these agents in many patients. However, the high risk of serious adverse effects from NSAIDs in the elderly limits their use in this population and opioids provide an alternative. The American Geriatrics Society recommends a trial of opioids in carefully selected and monitored elderly patients with moderate to severe persistent pain, pain-related functional impairment or diminished quality of life due to pain.[116]

Evidence about the efficacy and safety of opioids in treating osteoarthritis pain has been contradictory. A systematic review of long-term opioid therapy for chronic pain concluded that there is insufficient evidence for improving chronic pain and function, and there is a dose-dependent risk of serious harms including overdose, abuse and fractures.[117] A Cochrane review of the effect of oral or transdermal opioids in knee or hip OA similarly concluded that there is small mean benefit of non-tramadol opioids in OA, but it is associated with a significant risk of adverse events.[118]

Numerous combination analgesic products containing codeine 8 mg are available. The effectiveness of low-dose combination codeine products compared with single ingredient products (e.g., NSAIDs, acetaminophen) for OA has not been adequately studied, but they may be reasonable options for individuals at risk of serious adverse events from NSAIDs.[24,25]

Tramadol is a partial opioid agonist used for acute pain. It may be used as monotherapy or in combination with acetaminophen or NSAIDs for OA of the hip and knee if treatment with these agents has not provided adequate pain relief. Tramadol may have a small effect on pain and function, and the risk of abuse appears to be low.[119]

Antidepressants

Duloxetine is an antidepressant approved for use in osteoarthritis of the knee. A pooled analysis of 2 randomized placebo-controlled trials showed the proportion of patients who experienced ≥ 50% reduction in pain after 13 weeks with duloxetine compared with placebo was 47% vs. 31% (NNT=7). Duloxetine may be used as monotherapy or in combination with acetaminophen or NSAIDs for OA of the hip and knee if treatment with these agents has not provided adequate pain relief. Common side effects include nausea, fatigue and constipation.[120]

Monitoring of Therapy

Table 4 provides a monitoring plan for patients with osteoarthritis.

Table 4: **Monitoring of Therapy for Osteoarthritis**

Parameter	Degree	Timeframe	Action/Comments
Pain relief	Elimination or improvement toward predefined, realistic goals as set by patient	Patient: Assess daily Healthcare practitioner: Call on days 3, 7, 14 and 28	Patient may require further assessment if no symptom relief after adequate trial of at least 2 analgesics or on development of new or worsening pain during therapy. Considerations: ▪ Use visual analog scale or other individual measure to quantify and characterize pain (e.g., ADL—walking, gardening) ▪ Establish acceptable level of pain control and functioning with the patient at the beginning of therapy ▪ Timing of medications: – Around-the-clock vs. PRN – Take analgesic at least 1 h prior to activities that may exacerbate pain.
Nausea, dyspepsia, abdominal discomfort	Minimal or none during therapy	Patient: Monitor daily Healthcare practitioner: Call on days 3 and 7	Change therapy if symptoms severe or intolerable. Minimize development by advising to take with food or milk. Consider antacids or H_2RAs to treat dyspepsia.
Hematemesis, melena, hematochezia	None during therapy	Patient: Monitor daily on an ongoing basis Healthcare practitioner: Call on days 3, 7, 28 then ask when medication is refilled	Assess risk of GI complications (Table 3). If high risk, patient requires further assessment and workup. Patient should discontinue therapy immediately and seek medical attention if these signs or symptoms develop.
Hypertension	Stable during therapy	Healthcare practitioner: Measure BP within 1 wk of starting NSAIDs	Monitor patients with pre-existing hypertension; if BP increases, adjust the dose of the NSAID or antihypertensive.
Renal function and signs of fluid retention (e.g., weight gain or edema) in high-risk patients	No significant change in renal function	Patient: Look for decreased urine production; watch for signs of fluid retention, e.g., edema. Patients with severe heart failure should weigh themselves daily Healthcare practitioner: Call on day 3 to ask about urine production In patients >65 y or with other risk factors, consider taking a baseline serum creatinine, repeat at 1 wk and then periodically	Assess risk of renal complications (Table 3). Hold NSAID that day if patient cannot eat or drink. Discontinue NSAID if significant changes in serum creatinine or electrolytes or if signs of fluid retention occur.

Abbreviations: ADL = activities of daily living; BP = blood pressure; H_2RA = H_2-receptor antagonist

Advice for the Patient

Advise patients on:

- The importance of using nonpharmacologic measures concurrently with medication therapy
- Expected benefits of therapy
- Possible side effects and their management
- When to contact a healthcare practitioner.

Figure 1: **Assessment of Patients with Joint Pain**

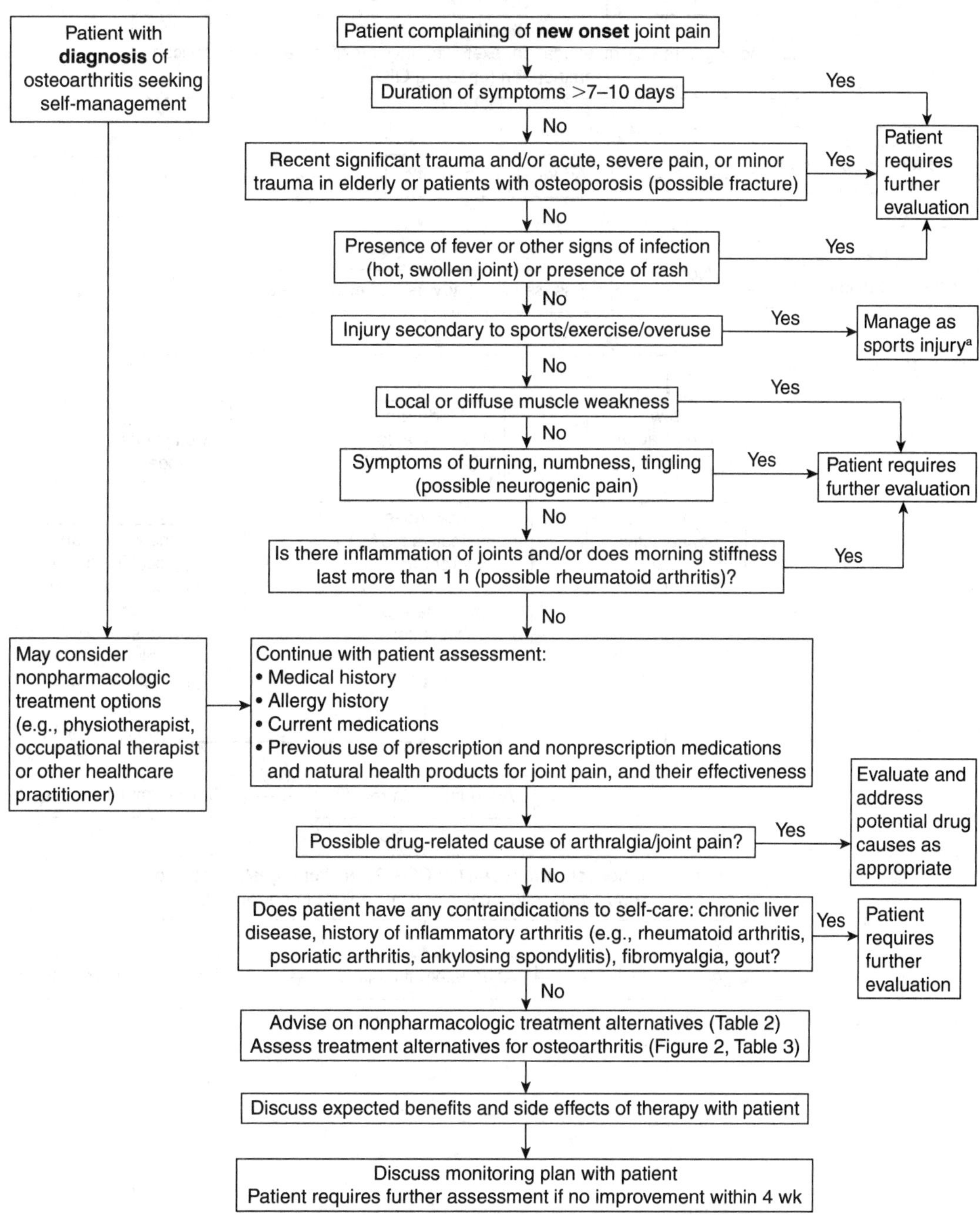

[a] See Chapter 48: Sports Injuries.

Figure 2: **Treatment of Osteoarthritis**

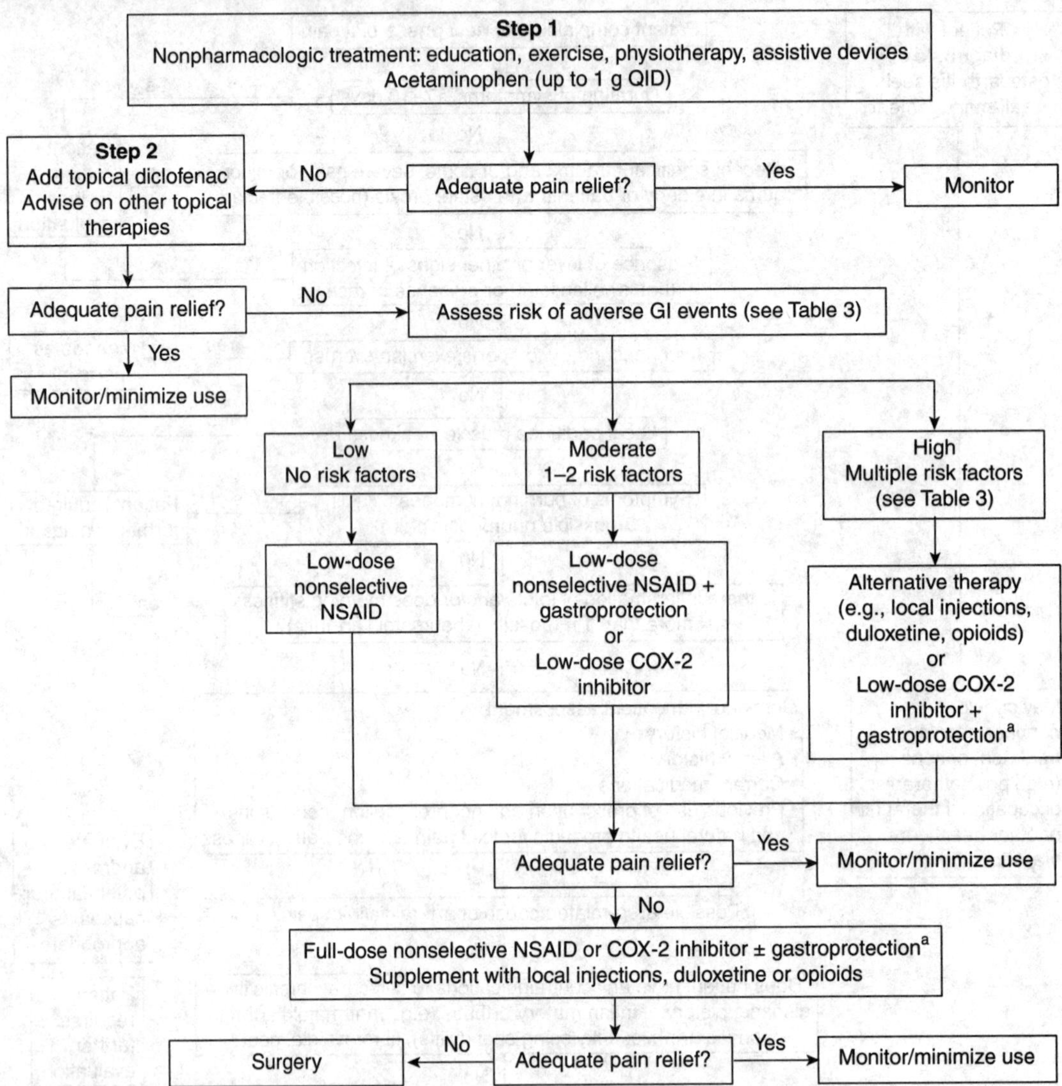

[a] See *Guidelines for prevention of NSAID-related ulcer complications.*[26]

Table 5: Selected Pharmacologic Therapy for Osteoarthritis

Class	Drug	Dosage	Adverse Effects	Drug Interactions	Comments	Cost[a]
Analgesics, oral	*acetaminophen* Atasol Preparations, Tylenol, generics	325–1000 mg Q4–6H po SR: 650 mg Q8H po Maximum: 4 g/day	Hepatotoxicity: increased risk in patients with excessive alcohol intake (>3 drinks/day), malnourishment or pre-existing hepatic disease. Baseline LFTs should be measured in high-risk patients.	Acetaminophen has been reported to increase INR in warfarin-treated patients.[53] Check INR if acetaminophen ≥2 g/day is used for ≥3 consecutive days. Adjust warfarin dosage as required. Phenytoin, barbiturates, carbamazepine may increase acetaminophen metabolism and formation of toxic metabolite (increased risk of hepatotoxicity); risk may be increased in patients taking high therapeutic doses of acetaminophen and antiepileptic drugs chronically.	Maximal onset of pain relief within 24–48 h. Lower doses may be required in patients with severe hepatic and renal disease. Caution with concurrent use of other products containing acetaminophen (do not exceed 4 g/day). Consider continuous therapy in individuals with pain persisting throughout the day. PRN dosing is acceptable for episodic pain of short duration.	$
	acetaminophen/caffeine/ codeine 8 mg generics	1–2 tablets Q4–6H po Maximum: 4 g/day of acetaminophen from all sources	See acetaminophen. Sedation, nausea, vomiting, constipation.	See acetaminophen. Concurrent use of medications that cause CNS depression (e.g., sedatives, tranquilizers, alcohol) or constipation may increase these effects.	Recommended for short-term use only, e.g., 2–3 days. Elderly are at increased risk for adverse effects. Caution with concurrent use of other products containing acetaminophen (do not exceed 4 g/day).	$
Analgesics, topical	*capsaicin* Zostrix, Zostrix HP, generics	Apply sparingly TID–QID for 3–4 wk to achieve maximum therapeutic effect	Tingling, burning or redness (majority of patients).	None known. Concurrent use of other topical medications on areas treated with capsaicin should be avoided.	Pain relief may take up to 2 wk with daily use. Maximum effect can take up to 4 wk. Apply with gloves and wash hands thoroughly after application to avoid irritation of other areas. Tingling/burning usually decreases within 72 h with repeated use; if effect is bothersome, use lower concentration or pretreat with topical lidocaine or EMLA cream.	$$

(cont'd)

Table 5: **Selected Pharmacologic Therapy for Osteoarthritis** *(cont'd)*

Class	Drug	Dosage	Adverse Effects	Drug Interactions	Comments	Cost[a]
					Do not apply near mucous membranes or on broken skin. Do not cover with tight or occlusive dressing. Do not place heating devices (e.g., hot water bottle, heating pad) on skin after applying product.	
	zucapsaicin Zuacta	Apply TID	Transient burning on application.	None known. Concurrent use of other topical medications on areas treated with zucapsaicin should be avoided.	Approved in adults for adjunctive use with oral NSAIDs for severe pain in OA of knee for maximum of 3 months. Avoid contact with eyes or open lesions.	$$$$$
NSAIDs, oral	*ibuprofen* Advil, Advil Liqui-Gels, Motrin, Motrin IB, Motrin Liquid Gels, generics	200–400 mg Q6–8H po Maximum dose for self-care: 1200 mg/day for up to 5 days Usual maximum dose: 2400 mg/day	More common: Dyspepsia, diarrhea. More serious: Ulceration/upper GI bleed, exacerbation of heart failure, MI, stroke, acute renal failure, transient elevated liver enzymes, rare hepatotoxicity.	Warfarin (increased bleeding risk); monitor INR more frequently during initial period after starting drug and watch for signs of bleeding. Increased lithium levels; monitor. Increased methotrexate levels (rare, with high doses MTX); monitor for toxicity. Antihypertensives (e.g., beta-blockers, ACEI, diuretics): may decrease antihypertensive effects. Measure baseline BP, then remeasure in 1–2 wk and adjust antihypertensive therapy as required. Increased risk of GI bleed with SSRIs. Increased risk of GI adverse effects with alcohol.	Renal effects are more likely in the elderly or patients with pre-existing renal disease or comorbid conditions that may affect renal function (e.g., diabetes, heart failure, hypertension). Advise patients to stop taking NSAID if unable to eat or drink that day. Hepatotoxicity is more likely to occur in patients with pre-existing hepatic disease or those with excessive alcohol intake (>3 drinks/day). Consider continuous therapy in individuals with pain persisting throughout the day; PRN dosing is acceptable for episodic pain of short duration. Consider gastroprotection in high-risk patients (see Table 3).	$

Class	Drug	Dosage	Adverse Effects	Drug Interactions	Comments	Cost[a]
				Give 30 min after or 8 h before low-dose ASA.	Avoid in patients with ASA or ibuprofen hypersensitivity. NSAIDs are not a substitute for low-dose ASA therapy for MI or stroke prophylaxis. Avoid concurrent use of more than one NSAID-containing product due to increased risk of GI side effects—the only exception is low-dose ASA for cardiovascular protection. Increased risk of stroke or serious CV events at doses ≥2400 mg/day. Doses ≥2400 mg/day should not be used in patients with a history of CV events or with risk factors for CV disease.[54]	
	naproxen Naprosyn, generics	250–500 mg BID po	See ibuprofen.	See ibuprofen.	Renal effects are more likely in the elderly or patients with pre-existing renal disease or comorbid conditions that may affect renal function (e.g., diabetes, heart failure, hypertension). Advise patients to stop taking NSAID if unable to eat or drink that day. Hepatotoxicity is more likely to occur in patients with pre-existing hepatic disease or those with excessive alcohol intake (>3 drinks/day). Consider continuous therapy in individuals with pain persisting throughout the day; PRN dosing is acceptable for episodic pain of short duration. Consider gastroprotection in high-risk patients (see Table 3). Avoid in patients with ASA or ibuprofen hypersensitivity.	$$

(cont'd)

Table 5: **Selected Pharmacologic Therapy for Osteoarthritis** *(cont'd)*

Class	Drug	Dosage	Adverse Effects	Drug Interactions	Comments	Cost[a]
					NSAIDs are not a substitute for low-dose ASA therapy for MI or stroke prophylaxis. Avoid concurrent use of more than one NSAID-containing product due to increased risk of GI-related side effects—the only exception is low-dose ASA for cardiovascular protection.	
	naproxen sodium Aleve, Anaprox, generics	Immediate-release: 220–550 mg BID po Maximum dose for self-care: 440 mg daily	See ibuprofen.	See ibuprofen.	See naproxen.	$
NSAIDs, topical	*diclofenac diethylamine* Voltaren Emulgel, Voltaren Emulgel Extra Strength	Apply TID–QID Recommended treatment duration of 7 days. If pain does not improve or becomes worse within the recommended duration of use, re-evaluate therapy	Skin dryness or irritation, hypersensitivity. Serious GI toxicity has not been seen to date in clinical trials.	With significantly lower amounts of medication in circulation following topical application (approximately 6% absorbed) vs. oral administration, drug interactions are unlikely with use of topical diclofenac. See ibuprofen for potential interactions.	Available as 1.16% and 2.32% gel. Do not apply near mucous membranes or on broken skin. Do not cover with tight or occlusive dressing. Do not place heating devices (e.g., hot water bottle, heating pad) on skin after applying product.	$

Class	Drug	Dosage	Adverse Effects	Drug Interactions	Comments	Cost[a]
	diclofenac sodium Pennsaid, generics	Apply TID–QID Recommended treatment duration ≤3 months. If pain does not improve or becomes worse within the recommended duration of use, re-evaluate therapy	Skin dryness or irritation, hypersensitivity. Serious GI toxicity has not been seen to date in clinical trials.	With significantly lower amounts of medication in circulation following topical application (approximately 6% absorbed) vs. oral administration, drug interactions are unlikely with use of topical diclofenac. See ibuprofen for potential interactions.	Available as 1.5% lotion. Do not apply near mucous membranes or on broken skin. Do not cover with tight or occlusive dressing. Do not place heating devices (e.g., hot water bottle, heating pad) on skin after applying product.	$$$$
	methyl salicylate Rub A-535, others	Apply TID–QID	Skin irritation.	Warfarin: may increase anticoagulant effect.	Avoid in ASA-allergic patients. Avoid contact with eyes and mucous membranes.	$

[a] Cost of 1 week therapy or smallest available pack size; includes drug cost only.

Dosage adjustment may be required in renal impairment.

Abbreviations: ACEI = angiotensin converting enzyme inhibitor; BP = blood pressure; EMLA = lidocaine–prilocaine topical anesthetic; INR = international normalized ratio; LFT = liver function tests; SR = sustained release

Legend: $ <$10 $$ $10–20 $$$ $20–30 $$$$ $30–40 $$$$$ $40–50

Resource Tips

The Arthritis Society (National Office), 393 University Avenue, Suite 1700, Toronto, Ontario M5G 1E6. Tel.: 416-979-7228. Available from: www.arthritis.ca.

Suggested Readings

British Columbia Ministry of Health Services. GPAC: Guidelines and Protocols Advisory Committee. *Osteoarthritis in peripheral joints: diagnosis and treatment*. Available from: www.bcguidelines.ca/guideline_osteoarthritis.html.

Hochberg MC, Altman RD, April KT et al. American College of Rheumatology 2012 recommendations for the use of nonpharmacologic and pharmacologic therapies in osteoarthritis of the hand, hip and knee. *Arthritis Care Res (Hoboken)* 2012;64:465-74.

References

1. The Arthritis Society. Available from: www.arthritis.ca. Accessed April 21, 2016.
2. Cross M, Smith E, Hoy D et al. The global burden of hip and knee osteoarthritis: estimates from the global burden of disease 2010 study. *Ann Rheum Dis* 2014;73:1323-30.
3. Pritzker KP. Pathology of osteoarthritis. In: Brandt KD, Doherty M, Lohmander LS, eds. *Osteoarthritis*. New York: Oxford University Press; 2000. p. 49-58.
4. Aspden RM. Osteoarthritis: a problem of growth not decay? *Rheumatology (Oxford)* 2008;47:1452-60.
5. Lane NE, Brandt K, Hawker G et al. OARSI-FDA initiative: defining the disease state of osteoarthritis. *Osteoarthritis Cartilage* 2011;19:478-82.
6. Kopec JA, Rahman MM, Berthelot JM et al. Descriptive epidemiology of osteoarthritis in British Columbia, Canada. *J Rheumatol* 2007;34:386-93.
7. Health Canada. *Arthritis in Canada: an ongoing challenge*. Ottawa: Health Canada; 2003. Available from: publications.gc.ca/collections/Collection/H39-4-14-2003E.pdf. Accessed April 21, 2016.
8. Anderson JJ, Felson DT. Factors associated with osteoarthritis of the knee in the first national Health and Nutrition Examination Survey (HANES I). Evidence for an association with overweight, race, and physical demands of work. *Am J Epidemiol* 1988;128:179-89.
9. Slemenda C, Heilman DK, Brandt KD et al. Reduced quadriceps strength relative to body weight: a risk factor for knee osteoarthritis in women? *Arthritis Rheum* 1998;41:1951-9.
10. Spector TD, Cicuttini F, Baker J et al. Genetic influences on osteoarthritis in women: a twin study. *BMJ* 1996;312:940-3.
11. Demissie S, Cupples LA, Myers R et al. Genome scan for quantity of hand osteoarthritis: the Framingham Study. *Arthritis Rheum* 2002;46:946-52.
12. Roos H, Lauren M, Adalberth T et al. Knee osteoarthritis after meniscectomy: prevalence of radiographic changes after twenty-one years, compared with matched controls. *Arthritis Rheum* 1998;41:687-93.
13. Englund M, Lohmander LS. Risk factors for symptomatic knee osteoarthritis fifteen to twenty-two years after meniscectomy. *Arthritis Rheum* 2004;50:2811-9.
14. Ding C, Martel-Pelletier J, Pelletier JP et al. Meniscal tear as an osteoarthritis risk factor in a largely non-osteoarthritic cohort: a cross-sectional study. *J Rheumatol* 2007;34:776-84.
15. Lohmander LS, Ostenberg A, Englund M et al. High prevalence of knee osteoarthritis, pain, and functional limitations in female soccer players twelve years after anterior cruciate ligament injury. *Arthritis Rheum* 2004;50:3145-52.
16. Felson D. Epidemiology of osteoarthritis. In: Brandt KD, Doherty M, Lohmander LS, eds. *Osteoarthritis*. New York: Oxford University Press; 2000.
17. Lawrence RC, Felson DT, Helmick CG et al. Estimates of the prevalence of arthritis and other rheumatic conditions in the United States. Part II. *Arthritis Rheum* 2008;58:26-35.
18. O'Reilly S, Doherty M. Signs, symptoms, and laboratory tests. In: Brandt KD, Doherty M, Lohmander LS, eds. *Osteoarthritis*. New York: Oxford University Press; 2000.
19. Altman R, Asch E, Bloch D et al. Development of criteria for the classification and reporting of osteoarthritis. Classification of osteoarthritis of the knee. Diagnostic and Therapeutic Criteria Committee of the American Rheumatism Association. *Arthritis Rheum* 1986;29:1039-49.
20. Kidd BL. Osteoarthritis and joint pain. *Pain* 2006;123:6-9.
21. Kidd BL. Pathogenesis of joint pain in osteoarthritis. In: Brandt KD, Doherty M, Lohmander LS, eds. *Osteoarthritis*. New York: Oxford University Press; 2000.
22. Bannwarth B. Drug-induced musculoskeletal disorders. *Drug Saf* 2007;30:27-46.
23. McAlindon TE, Bannuru RR, Sullivan MC et al. OARSI guidelines for the non-surgical management of knee osteoarthritis. *Osteoarthritis Cartilage* 2014;22:363-88.
24. Jordan KM, Arden NK, Doherty M et al. EULAR Recommendations 2003: an evidence based approach to the management of knee osteoarthritis: report of a Task Force of the Standing Committee for International Clinical Studies Including Therapeutic Trials (ESCISIT). *Ann Rheum Dis* 2003;62:1145-55.
25. Hochberg MC, Altman RD, April KT et al. American College of Rheumatology 2012 recommendations for the use of nonpharmacologic and pharmacologic therapies in osteoarthritis of the hand, hip and knee. *Arthritis Care Res (Hoboken)* 2012;64:465-74.
26. Lanza FL, Chan FK, Quigley EM et al. Guidelines for prevention of NSAID-related ulcer complications. *Am J Gastroenterol* 2009;104:728-38.
27. Fernandes L, Hagen KB, Bijlsma JW et al. EULAR recommendations for the non-pharmacological core management of hip and knee osteoarthritis. *Ann Rheum Dis* 2013;72:1125-35.

28. Warsi A, LaValley MP, Wang PS et al. Arthritis self-management education programs: a meta-analysis of the effect on pain and disability. *Arthritis Rheum* 2003;48:2207-13.
29. Kroon FP, van der Burg LR, Buchbinder R et al. Self-management education programmes for osteoarthritis. *Cochrane Database Syst Rev* 2014;1:CD008963.
30. Fransen M, McConnell S, Harmer AR et al. Exercise for osteoarthritis of the knee. *Cochrane Database Syst Rev* 2015;1:CD004376.
31. Fransen M, McConnell S, Hernandez-Molina G et al. Exercise for osteoarthritis of the hip. *Cochrane Database Syst Rev* 2014;4:CD007912.
32. Bartels EM, Lund H, Hagen KB et al. Aquatic exercise for the treatment of knee and hip osteoarthritis. *Cochrane Database Syst Rev* 2007;4:CD005523.
33. Juhl C, Christensen R, Roos EM et al. Impact of exercise type and dose on pain and disability in knee osteoarthritis: a systematic review and meta-regression analysis of randomized controlled trials. *Arthritis Rheumatol* 2014;663:622-36.
34. Uthman OA, van der Windt DA, Jordan JL et al. Exercise for lower limb osteoarthritis: systematic review incorporating trial sequential analysis and network meta-analysis. *BMJ* 2013;347:f5555.
35. Messier SP, Loeser RF, Miller GD et al. Exercise and dietary weight loss in overweight and obese older adults with knee osteoarthritis: the Arthritis, Diet, and Activity Promotion Trial. *Arthritis Rheum* 2004;50:1501-10.
36. Duivenvoorden T, Brouwer RW, van Raaij TM et al. Braces and orthoses for treating osteoarthritis of the knee. *Cochrane Database Syst Rev* 2015;3:CD004020.
37. Moyer RF, Birmingham TB, Bryant DM et al. Valgus bracing for knee osteoarthritis: a meta-analysis of randomized trials. *Arthritis Care Res (Hoboken)* 2015;674:493-501.
38. Raja K, Dewan N. Efficacy of knee braces and foot orthoses in conservative management of knee osteoarthritis: a systematic review. *Am J Phys Med Rehabil* 2011;90:247-62.
39. Bennell KL, Bowles KA, Payne C et al. Lateral wedge insoles for medial knee osteoarthritis: 12 month randomised controlled trial. *BMJ* 2011;342:d2912.
40. Parkes MJ, Maricar N, Lunt M et al. Lateral wedge insoles as a conservative treatment for pain in patients with medial knee osteoarthritis: a meta-analysis. *JAMA* 2013;310:722-30.
41. Weinberger M, Tierney WM, Cowper PA et al. Cost-effectiveness of increased telephone contact for patients with osteoarthritis. A randomized, controlled trial. *Arthritis Rheum* 1993;36:243-6.
42. Weinberger M, Tierney WM, Booher P et al. Can the provision of information to patients with osteoarthritis improve functional status? A randomized, controlled trial. *Arthritis Rheum* 1989;32:1577-83.
43. Keefe FJ, Caldwell DS, Baucom D et al. Spouse-assisted coping skills training in the management of knee pain in osteoarthritis: long-term followup results. *Arthritis Care Res* 1999;12:101-11.
44. Rutjes AWS, Nüesch E, Sterchi R et al. Transcutaneous electrostimulation for osteoarthritis of the knee. *Cochrane Database Syst Rev* 2009;4:CD002823.
45. Manheimer E, Linde K, Lao L et al. Meta-analysis: acupuncture for osteoarthritis of the knee. *Ann Intern Med* 2007;146:868-77.
46. Manheimer E, Cheng K, Linde K et al. Acupuncture for peripheral joint osteoarthritis. *Cochrane Database Syst Rev* 2010;1:CD001977.
47. Cetin N, Aytar A, Atalay A et al. Comparing hot pack, short-wave diathermy, ultrasound, and TENS on isokinetic strength, pain, and functional status of women with osteoarthritic knees: a single-blind, randomized, controlled trial. *Am J Phys Med Rehabil* 2008;87:443-51.
48. Brosseau L, Yonge KA, Robinson V et al. Thermotherapy for treatment of osteoarthritis. *Cochrane Database Syst Rev* 2003;4:CD004522.
49. Perlman AI, Sabina A, Williams AL et al. Massage therapy for osteoarthritis of the knee: a randomized controlled trial. *Arch Intern Med* 2006;166:2533-8.
50. Zhang W, Moskowitz RW, Nuki G et al. OARSI recommendations for the management of hip and knee osteoarthritis, Part II: OARSI evidence-based, expert consensus guidelines. *Osteoarthritis Cartilage* 2008;16:137-62.
51. Wang SY, Olson-Kellogg B, Shamliyan TA et al. Physical therapy interventions for knee pain secondary to osteoarthritis: a systematic review. *Ann Intern Med* 2012;157:632-44.
52. Hay EM, Foster NE, Thomas E et al. Effectiveness of community physiotherapy and enhanced pharmacy review for knee pain in people aged over 55 presenting to primary care: pragmatic randomised trial. *BMJ* 2006;333:995.
53. Lopes RD, Horowitz JD, Garcia DA et al. Warfarin and acetaminophen interaction: a summary of the evidence and biologic plausibility. *Blood* 2011;118:6269-73.
54. Government of Canada. Healthy Canadians. *New safety information for prescription-strength ibuprofen: risk of heart attack and stroke at high doses*. Available from: www.healthycanadians.gc.ca/recall-alert-rappel-avis/hc-sc/2015/53055a-eng.php.
55. Towheed TE, Maxwell L, Judd MG et al. Acetaminophen for osteoarthritis. *Cochrane Database Syst Rev* 2006;1:CD004257.
56. Zhang W, Jones A, Doherty M. Does paracetamol (acetaminophen) reduce the pain of osteoarthritis? A meta-analysis of randomised controlled trials. *Ann Rheum Dis* 2004;63:901-7.
57. Bannuru RR, Schmid CH, Kent DM et al. Comparative effectiveness of pharmacologic interventions for knee osteoarthritis: a systematic review and network meta-analysis. *Ann Intern Med* 2015;162:46-54.
58. Machado GC, Maher CG, Ferreira PH et al. Efficacy and safety of paracetamol for spinal pain and osteoarthritis: systematic review and meta-analysis of randomised placebo controlled trials. *BMJ* 2015;350:h1225.
59. U.S. Food and Drug Adminstration. FDA Drug Safety Communication. *Prescription acetaminophen products to be limited to 325 mg per dosage unit; boxed warning will highlight potential for severe liver failure*. Available from: www.fda.gov/Drugs/DrugSafety/ucm239821.htm.
60. Government of Canada. Healthy Canadians. *Reminding Canadians about using acetaminophen safely*. Available from: healthycanadians.gc.ca/recall-alert-rappel-avis/hc-sc/2011/13523a-eng.php.
61. Fosnocht D, Taylor JR, Caravati EM. Emergency department patient knowledge concerning acetaminophen (paracetamol) in over-the-counter and prescription analgesics. *Emerg Med J* 2008;25:213-6.
62. Kuffner EK, Green JL, Bogdan GM et al. The effect of acetaminophen (four grams a day for three consecutive days) on hepatic tests in alcoholic patients–a multicenter randomized study. *BMC Med* 2007;5:13.
63. Heard K, Green JL, Bailey JE et al. A randomized trial to determine the change in alanine aminotransferase during 10 days of paracetamol (acetaminophen) administration in subjects who consume moderate amounts of alcohol. *Aliment Pharmacol Ther* 2007;26:283-90.
64. Dart RC, Kuffner EK, Rumack BH. Treatment of pain or fever with paracetamol (acetaminophen) in the alcoholic patient: a systematic review. *Am J Ther* 2000;7:123-34.
65. Lin J, Zhang W, Jones A et al. Efficacy of topical non-steroidal anti-inflammatory drugs in the treatment of osteoarthritis: meta-analysis of randomised controlled trials. *BMJ* 2004;329:324.

66. Mason L, Moore RA, Edwards JE et al. Topical NSAIDs for chronic musculoskeletal pain: systematic review and meta-analysis. *BMC Musculoskelet Disord* 2004;5:28.
67. Towheed TE. Pennsaid therapy for osteoarthritis of the knee: a systematic review and meta-analysis of randomized controlled trials. *J Rheumatol* 2006;33:567-73.
68. Zhang WY, Li Wan Po A. The effectiveness of topically applied capsaicin. A meta-analysis. *Eur J Clin Pharmacol* 1994;46:517-22.
69. Mason L, Moore RA, Derry S et al. Systematic review of topical capsaicin for the treatment of chronic pain. *BMJ* 2004;328:991.
70. Derry S, Moore RA, Rabbie R. Topical NSAIDs for chronic musculoskeletal pain in adults. *Cochrane Database Syst Rev* 2012;9:CD007400.
71. Schnitzer TJ, Pelletier JP, Haselwood DM et al. Civamide cream 0.075% in patients with osteoarthritis of the knee: a 12-week randomized controlled clinical trial with a longterm extension. *J Rheumatol* 2012;39:610-20.
72. Derry S, Matthews PR, Wiffen PJ et al. Salicylate-containing rubefacients for acute and chronic musculoskeletal pain in adults. *Cochrane Database Syst Rev* 2014;11:CD007403.
73. Joss JD, LeBlond RF. Potentiation of warfarin anticoagulation associated with topical methyl salicylate. *Ann Pharmacother* 2000;34:729-33.
74. Cameron M, Chrubasik S. Topical herbal therapies for treating osteoarthritis. *Cochrane Database Syst Rev* 2013;5:CD010538.
75. U.S. Food and Drug Administration. FDA Drug Safety Communication. *Rare cases of serious burns with the use of over-the-counter topical muscle and joint pain relievers*. Available from: fda.gov/Drugs/DrugSafety/ucm318858.htm. Accessed April 21, 2016.
76. Pincus T, Swearingen C, Cummins P et al. Preference for nonsteroidal antiinflammatory drugs versus acetaminophen and concomitant use of both types of drugs in patients with osteoarthritis. *J Rheumatol* 2000;27:1020-7.
77. Wolfe F, Zhao S, Lane N. Preference for nonsteroidal antiinflammatory drugs over acetaminophen by rheumatic disease patients: a survey of 1,799 patients with osteoarthritis, rheumatoid arthritis, and fibromyalgia. *Arthritis Rheum* 2000;43:378-85.
78. Tannenbaum H, Bombardier C, Davis P et al. An evidence-based approach to prescribing nonsteroidal antiinflammatory drugs. Third Canadian Consensus Conference. *J Rheumatol* 2006;33:140-57.
79. Antman EM, Bennett JS, Daugherty A et al. Use of nonsteroidal anti-inflammatory drugs: an update for clinicians: a scientific statement from the American Heart Association. *Circulation* 2007;115:1634-42.
80. Solomon DH, Karlson EW, Rimm EB et al. Cardiovascular morbidity and mortality in women diagnosed with rheumatoid arthritis. *Circulation* 2003;107:1303-7.
81. Maradit-Kremers H, Crowson CS, Nicola PJ et al. Increased unrecognized coronary heart disease and sudden deaths in rheumatoid arthritis: a population-based cohort study. *Arthritis Rheum* 2005;52:402-11.
82. Meek IL, Vonkeman HE, Kasemier J et al. Interference of NSAIDs with the thrombocyte inhibitor effect of aspirin: a placebo-controlled, ex vivo, serial placebo-controlled serial crossover study. *Eur J Clin Pharmacol* 2013;69:365-71.
83. U.S. Food and Drug Administration. Information for Healthcare Professionals. *Concomitant use of ibuprofen and aspirin*. Available from: www.fda.gov/Drugs/DrugSafety/PostmarketDrugSafetyInformationforPatientsandProviders/ucm125222.htm. Accessed April 21, 2016.
84. Ofman JJ, Maclean CH, Straus WL et al. Meta-analysis of dyspepsia and nonsteroidal antiinflammatory drugs. *Arthritis Rheum* 2003;49:508-18.
85. Institute for Clinical Systems Improvement. *Health care guideline: initial management of dyspepsia and GERD*. 7th ed. Bloomington: ICSI; 2006.
86. Wolfe MM, Lichtenstein DR, Singh G. Gastrointestinal toxicity of nonsteroidal antiinflammatory drugs. *N Engl J Med* 1999;340:1888-99.
87. Saag KG, Olivieri JJ, Patino F et al. Measuring quality in arthritis care: the Arthritis Foundation's quality indicator set for analgesics. *Arthritis Rheum* 2004;51:337-49.
88. Chan FK, Wong VW, Suen BY et al. Combination of a cyclo-oxygenase-2 inhibitor and a proton-pump inhibitor for prevention of recurrent ulcer bleeding in patients at very high risk: a double-blind, randomised trial. *Lancet* 2007;369:1621-6.
89. Rostom A, Dube C, Wells G et al. Prevention of NSAID-induced gastroduodenal ulcers. *Cochrane Database Syst Rev* 2002;4:CD002296.
90. Hooper L, Brown TJ, Elliott R et al. The effectiveness of five strategies for the prevention of gastrointestinal toxicity induced by non-steroidal anti-inflammatory drugs: systematic review. *BMJ* 2004;329:948.
91. Leandro G, Pilotto A, Franceschi M et al. Prevention of acute NSAID-related gastroduodenal damage: a meta-analysis of controlled clinical trials. *Dig Dis Sci* 2001;46:1924-36.
92. Pope JE, Anderson JJ, Felson DT. A meta-analysis of the effects of nonsteroidal anti-inflammatory drugs on blood pressure. *Arch Intern Med* 1993;153:477-84.
93. Johnson AG, Nguyen TV, Day RO. Do nonsteroidal anti-inflammatory drugs affect blood pressure? A meta-analysis. *Ann Intern Med* 1994;121:289-300.
94. Lapi F, Azoulay L, Yin H et al. Concurrent use of diuretics, angiotensin converting enzyme inhibitors, and angiotensin receptor blockers with non-steroidal anti-inflammatory drugs and risk of acute kidney injury: nested case-control study. *BMJ* 2013;346:e8525.
95. Kearney PM, Baigent C, Godwin J et al. Do selective cyclo-oxygenase-2 inhibitors and traditional non-steroidal anti-inflammatory drugs increase the risk of atherothrombosis? Meta-analysis of randomised trials. *BMJ* 2006;332:1302-8.
96. McGettigan P, Henry D. Cardiovascular risk and inhibition of cyclooxygenase: a systematic review of the observational studies of selective and nonselective inhibitors of cyclooxygenase 2. *JAMA* 2006;296:1633-44.
97. Singh G, Wu O, Langhorne P et al. Risk of acute myocardial infarction with nonselective non-steroidal anti-inflammatory drugs: a meta-analysis. *Arthritis Res Ther* 2006;8:R153.
98. White WB, Faich G, Whelton A et al. Comparison of thromboembolic events in patients treated with celecoxib, a cyclooxygenase-2 specific inhibitor, versus ibuprofen or diclofenac. *Am J Cardiol* 2002;89:425-30.
99. Reginster JY, Deroisy R, Rovati LC et al. Long-term effects of glucosamine sulphate on osteoarthritis progression: a randomised placebo-controlled clinical trial. *Lancet* 2001;357:251-6.
100. Lippiello L, Woodward J, Karpman R et al. In vivo chondroprotection and metabolic synergy of glucosamine and chondroitin sulfate. *Clin Orthop Relat Res* 2000;381:229-40.
101. Hochberg MC, Martel-Pelletier J, Monfort J et al. Combined chondroitin sulfate and glucosamine for painful knee osteoarthritis: a multicentre, randomised, double-blind, non-inferiority trial versus celecoxib. *Ann Rheum Dis* 2016;75:37-44.
102. Zou K, Wong J, Abdullah N et al. Examination of overall treatment effect and the proportion attributable to contextual effect in osteoarthritis: meta-analysis of randomised controlled trials. *Ann Rheum Dis* 2016 Feb 16. [Epub ahead of print].
103. Wu D, Huang Y, Gu Y et al. Efficacies of different preparations of glucosamine for the treatment of osteoarthritis: a meta-analysis of randomised, double-blind, placebo-controlled trials. *Int J Clin Pract* 2013;67:585-94.
104. Singh JA, Noorbaloochi S, MacDonald R et al. Chondroitin for osteoarthritis. *Cochrane Database Syst Rev* 2015;1:CD005614.

105. Clegg DO, Reda DJ, Harris CL et al. Glucosamine, chondroitin sulfate, and the two in combination for painful knee osteoarthritis. *N Engl J Med* 2006;354:795-808.

106. Rozendaal RM, Koes BW, van Osch GJ et al. Effect of glucosamine sulfate on hip osteoarthritis: a randomized trial. *Ann Intern Med* 2008;148:268-77.

107. McAlindon TE, LaValley MP, Gulin JP et al. Glucosamine and chondroitin for treatment of osteoarthritis: a systematic quality assessment and meta-analysis. *JAMA* 2000;283:1469-75.

108. Towheed TE, Maxwell L, Anastassiades TP et al. Glucosamine therapy for treating osteoarthritis. *Cochrane Database Syst Rev* 2005;2:CD002946.

109. Richmond J, Hunter D, Irrgang J et al. Treatment of osteoarthritis of the knee (non-arthroplasty). *J Am Acad Orthop Surg* 2009;17:591-600.

110. De Silva V, El-Metwally A, Ernst E et al. Evidence for the efficacy of complementary and alternative medicines in the management of osteoarthritis: a systematic review. *Rheumatology (Oxford)* 2011;50:911-20.

111. Rutjes AW, Nuesch E, Reichenbach S et al. S-Adenosylmethionine for osteoarthritis of the knee or hip. *Cochrane Database Syst Rev* 2009;4:CD007321.

112. Zhang W, Nuki G, Moskowitz RW et al. OARSI recommendations for the management of hip and knee osteoarthritis: part III: changes in evidence following systematic cumulative update of research published through January 2009. *Osteoarthritis Cartilage* 2010;18:476-99.

113. Bellamy N, Campbell J, Robinson V et al. Intraarticular corticosteroid for treatment of osteoarthritis of the knee. *Cochrane Database Syst Rev* 2006;2:CD005328.

114. Bellamy N, Campbell J, Robinson V et al. Viscosupplementation for the treatment of osteoarthritis of the knee. *Cochrane Database Syst Rev* 2006;2:CD005321.

115. Rutjes AW, Juni P, da Costa BR et al. Viscosupplementation for osteoarthritis of the knee: systematic review and meta-analysis. *Ann Intern Med* 2012;157:180-91.

116. American Geriatrics Society Panel on the Pharmacological Management of Persistent Pain in Older Persons. Pharmacological management of persistent pain in older persons. *J Am Geriatr Soc* 2009;57:1331-46.

117. Chou R, Turner JA, Devine EB et al. The effectiveness and risks of long-term opioid therapy for chronic pain: a systematic review for a National Institutes of Health Pathways to Prevention Workshop. *Ann Intern Med* 2015;1624:276-86.

118. da Costa BR, Nüesch E, Kasteler R et al. Oral or transdermal opioids for osteoarthritis of the knee or hip. *Cochrane Database Syst Rev* 2014;9:CD003115.

119. Cepeda MS, Camargo F, Zea C et al. Tramadol for osteoarthritis. *Cochrane Database Syst Rev* 2006;3:CD005522.

120. Hochberg MC, Wohlreich M, Gaynor P et al. Clinically relevant outcomes based on analysis of pooled data from 2 trials of duloxetine in patients with knee osteoarthritis. *J Rheumatol* 2012;39:352-8.

Osteoarthritis—What You Need to Know

What is osteoarthritis?

Osteoarthritis is a disease that results from changes to the joint structure and is the most common kind of arthritis. It usually affects the joints of the fingers and hands, knees, hips, neck and lower back of middle-aged and older people.

What causes osteoarthritis?

Osteoarthritis occurs when the cartilage that normally cushions and protects the joints becomes worn down or works less efficiently. This can happen for many reasons. Osteoarthritis may occur in joints that have been injured in the past or joints that have had heavy use over a long period of time. Some kinds of osteoarthritis are passed from one generation to the next.

What are the signs and symptoms of osteoarthritis?

People with osteoarthritis experience pain, stiffness and poor function in or around the joint. Sometimes a grating sound can be heard when moving the joint.

Osteoarthritis can be diagnosed by your healthcare provider using a combination of x-rays, physical examination and ruling out other types of arthritis.

How is osteoarthritis treated?

Osteoarthritis can be treated with therapy as well as drugs. It is best to try nondrug treatments first. You can combine these treatments with drugs if needed. The goals of treatment are to:

- Decrease pain and discomfort so that you can continue to carry out your usual daily activities
- Protect your joints

Nondrug treatments:

- Consult a physiotherapist and/or occupational therapist for exercises to reduce pain and to strengthen and protect the joints that have osteoarthritis. The therapist may also suggest tools or devices to help you manage everyday tasks.
- If you are overweight, consider losing weight to relieve stress on your joints.
- Learn as much as you can about osteoarthritis. You will find lots of information to help you manage pain and protect your joints.

Self-care measures:

There are several types of medications available for helping with osteoarthritis pain. If you need to use pain medication for more than 7 days in a row, talk to your healthcare provider to see if this is the best treatment for you.

Chapter 47
Osteoporosis

Lalitha Raman-Wilms, PharmD, FCSHP
Anne Marie Whelan, PharmD, FCSHP

Osteoporosis is a common skeletal disorder that results in more than 8.9 million fractures annually worldwide.[1] It is characterized by compromised bone strength, resulting in a fragile skeleton vulnerable to fractures. Bone strength is determined by both bone quantity, measured by bone mineral density (BMD) and quality.[2]

Osteoporosis affects about 1 in 4 women and 1 in 8 men in Canada over 50 years of age.[3] Individuals with osteoporosis can suffer from chronic disabling pain and loss of height from vertebral fractures. In severe cases, kyphosis (curvature of the spine or hunching) can cause shortness of breath and dysphagia. In individuals who have sustained a hip fracture, mortality in the first year has been reported to be as high as 28% in women and 37% in men.[4]

The relationship between fractures and mortality was studied in a subgroup from the Canadian Multicentre Osteoporosis Study. The results demonstrated that men and women ≥50 years with hip or vertebral fractures were more likely to die during the 5 years of follow up, compared with those without these fractures.[5] However, possibly due to better availability of diagnostic and treatment modalities, analysis of Canadian data in those hospitalized for hip fracture between 1985 and 2005 indicate that hip fracture rates show a steady decline, with the greatest decrease seen between 1996 and 2005.[6]

Hip fracture is one of the leading causes of institutionalization in the elderly. A fear of falling and decreased functioning can lead to social isolation, anxiety and depression. Osteoporosis also results in complications such as loss of independence and nursing home admissions, secondary to fractures. The economic implication of hip fractures alone in Canada was an estimated $650 million in 2001, and the annual cost of acute care management associated with osteoporosis is expected to rise to $2.4 billion dollars by 2041.[7]

Pathophysiology

Bone is constantly renewed. The bone-remodelling unit consists of osteoblasts (cells that lay down new bone) and osteoclasts (cells that resorb bone). The coupling of this process ensures that early in life, more bone is laid down as the child grows. Although up to 90% of bone mass is attained in girls at age 18 and in boys at age 20, the coupling process continues and reaches a plateau whereby the amount of bone broken down is balanced by the amount of new bone formed. At this point, usually around the age of 30, individuals attain their peak bone mass or their highest BMD.[8] After the third decade, age-related changes favour resorption, resulting in a gradual loss of 0.3–0.5% of bone mass per year. In women, a decrease in estrogen at menopause leads to accelerated bone loss of 2–3% per year; this loss continues for the first 5–10 years after menopause. Women have a lower peak bone mass compared with men, further increasing their risk of osteoporosis.[8,9]

Most of the body's calcium is stored in bone. Calcium is essential for functions such as muscle contraction and nerve conduction. With insufficient calcium intake, parathyroid hormone (PTH) is released, leading to reduced excretion of calcium from the kidney, increased calcium resorption from bone and vitamin D activation by the kidneys. An increase in vitamin D activation results in increased calcium absorption from the GI tract. This feedback normally helps maintain an adequate serum calcium level. Deficiency in vitamin D can result in secondary hyperparathyroidism and increased calcium resorption from bone.[10]

The World Health Organization has established guidelines for the diagnosis of osteoporosis based on BMD readings at the lumbar spine and femoral neck. Osteoporosis is defined as a BMD of 2.5 standard deviations (SD) or more below the average for young, healthy women (T-score of ≤ -2.5 SD).[1,11] A BMD between −1 and −2.5 signifies osteopenia.[1,11] Diagnosis is usually confirmed by measuring the individual's BMD using dual energy x-ray absorptiometry (DXA), which is considered best practice. In those who have sustained fractures, an x-ray is usually used to confirm the fracture.

Clinically, osteoporosis may present with fractures ± pain associated with fractures. Common sites for fracture include the wrist, spine and hip. Wrist and spinal compression fractures are seen earlier in the disease, while hip fractures usually occur in the seventh or eighth decade of life. Many patients may go undiagnosed, as often the only symptom is nonspecific chronic back pain. The lifetime risk of fracture is about 30–40% for individuals in developed countries.[9]

Goals of Therapy

- Prevent fractures by addressing clinical risk factors that increase fracture risk
- Prevent development or progression of osteoporosis by maximizing and/or maintaining existing BMD
- Minimize the risk of falls

Patient Assessment

Though the main indicator of osteoporosis is low BMD, bone strength is determined by both quantity and quality of bone, and some individuals with normal BMD may sustain osteoporotic fractures. Hence, identification of risk factors for this disease is important in assessing an individual's risk of fracture. In assessing a patient's risk factors for osteoporosis (Figure 1), consider age, family history, medical conditions, diet, smoking, alcohol use and lifestyle. Use Table 1 and Table 2 to identify risk factors for osteoporosis and fractures that would indicate the need to measure BMD.

Some medical conditions and drug therapies are associated with an increased risk of osteoporosis (Table 2). Monitor patients on medications associated with the development of osteoporosis closely. A thorough medication history may identify drugs that increase the risk of osteoporosis in patients with other risk factors (Table 2). Minimization of drug-related risk is a component of the overall management strategy.

A propensity to fall increases the patient's risk of a fracture. Factors that can increase the risk of falls (and fractures) should therefore be assessed. In the elderly, this may include poor eyesight, poor lighting in hallways and loose rugs. Ensuring that nonslip mats are placed in bathtubs and avoiding the use of bath oils in the tub can prevent falls. Drugs such as benzodiazepines, tricyclic antidepressants and antipsychotic agents have been associated with an increased risk of falls.[29,30]

Individuals who have sustained a fracture, have one or more risk factors, or who are at moderate to high risk of fractures based on the 10-year fracture risk assessment (see Assessment of Fracture Risk) require further assessment and consideration of drug therapy.[12]

Table 1: **Osteoporosis Risk Factors: Indications for Bone Mineral Density Measurement**

Older Adults (≥50 y)	Younger Adults (<50 y)
▪ Age ≥65 y (men and women) ▪ Clinical risk factors for fracture (men 50–64 y and menopausal women): – fragility fracture after age 40 – vertebral compression fracture – glucocorticoid use (prednisone-equivalent dose ≥7.5 mg/day for at least 3 months (cumulative) in the previous year) – use of other high-risk medications, e.g., aromatase inhibitors, androgen deprivation therapy – parent with hip fracture – osteopenia identified on x-ray – current smoking – high alcohol intake – low body weight (<60 kg) or major weight loss (>10% of weight at age 25) – rheumatoid arthritis – other disorders strongly associated with osteoporosis (Table 2)	▪ Fragility fracture ▪ Glucocorticoid use (prednisone-equivalent dose ≥7.5 mg/day for at least 3 months in the previous year) ▪ Use of other high-risk medications, e.g., aromatase inhibitors, androgen deprivation therapy ▪ Hypogonadism or premature menopause (<45 y) ▪ Malabsorption syndrome ▪ Primary hyperparathyroidism ▪ Other disorders strongly associated with rapid bone loss or fracture (Table 2)

Adapted with permission from: Papaioannou A, Morin S, Cheung AM et al. 2010 clinical practice guidelines for the diagnosis and management of osteoporosis in Canada: summary. *CMAJ* 2010;182:1864-73.

Table 2: **Medical Conditions and Drugs Commonly Associated with an Increased Risk of Osteoporosis**

Conditions[9,13]	Drugs
Anorexia nervosa	Antiepileptic drugs, e.g., phenytoin[14,15]
Bulimia	Antiretrovirals, e.g., protease inhibitors[16,17,18]
Chronic inflammatory conditions, e.g., inflammatory bowel disease	Chemotherapeutic agents, e.g., aromatase inhibitors, androgen deprivation therapy[12,19,20]
Chronic kidney disease	Corticosteroids, e.g., prednisone[21]
Cushing's syndrome	Cyclosporine[22]
Diabetes, type 1	Heparin (long-term therapy)[23]
Gastrectomy	Levothyroxine (in doses that suppress serum TSH in postmenopausal women)[24]
Hyperparathyroidism, primary	Loop diuretics[22]
Hyperthyroidism (untreated)	Medroxyprogesterone acetate[25]
Hypogonadism (untreated)	Proton pump inhibitors[26,27,28]
Liver disease	SSRIs[22]
Malabsorption syndromes including celiac disease	Thiazolidinediones[22]
Menopause, prior to age 45 (untreated)	Vitamin A[22]
Neoplasia	
Osteogenesis imperfecta in adults	
Thyrotoxicosis	

Assessment of Fracture Risk

Patient assessment for osteoporosis should include the individual's risk factors for osteoporosis, fracture and falls. Two related tools are available for assessing a patient's risk of fractures: the World

Health Organization (WHO) FRAX Risk Assessment Tool[31] and the Canadian Association of Radiologists and Osteoporosis Canada (CAROC) risk assessment tool.[32]

FRAX is an algorithm developed to predict an individual's 10-year fracture risk. It incorporates assessment of clinical risk factors (sex, age, body mass index, prior fracture, parental hip fracture, prolonged glucocorticoid use, rheumatoid arthritis, current smoking, alcohol intake) and (optionally) the femoral neck BMD. This tool is appropriate to use for both men and women and is specific for use in Canadians. It is available from www.shef.ac.uk/FRAX/tool.jsp.[12]

The CAROC guidelines for fracture risk assessment assign an initial risk category based on sex, age and femoral neck BMD. Certain risk factors, i.e., a prior fragility fracture or glucocorticoid use, raise the initial risk category to the next level; having both of these risk factors places the individual in the highest risk category.[12]

The 10-year fracture risk is classified as low (<10%), moderate (10–20%) or high (>20%); this classification can better guide management of osteoporosis. An individual's risk can vary over time, and should be re-evaluated every 5–10 years in those with low risk, and every 1–5 years in those with moderate risk.[12] This tool is available from www.osteoporosis.ca/multimedia/pdf/CAROC.pdf.

Management of Patients Based on Risk-factor Assessment

The 2010 Canadian guidelines recommend:[12]

- All patients at risk of osteoporosis should participate in lifestyle measures such as performing regular weight-bearing exercise, ensuring adequate calcium and Vitamin D intake, initiating fall prevention strategies and stopping smoking
- Patients who are categorized as being at low risk of fracture after their assessment should undertake, as appropriate, the lifestyle measures previously mentioned
- Management strategies for patients at moderate risk should be individualized
- Pharmacologic therapy is recommended for those at high risk of fracture.

Prevention

Strategies for preventing osteoporosis should be considered at a young age. In children, adolescents and young adults, ensuring sufficient exercise and adequate calcium, vitamin D and protein intake will help maximize peak bone mass.[9] In middle-aged and older adults, these same strategies can help maintain bone mass. The diet is the best source of calcium and vitamin D. Calcium and/or vitamin D supplementation is recommended for those whose diet is inadequate to meet daily requirements.

Nonpharmacologic Therapy

For comparative ingredients of nonprescription products, consult the *Compendium of Products for Minor Ailments*—Vitamin and Mineral Products: Single Entity, Solid Combinations.

Adequate dietary calcium, vitamin D and protein intake, in addition to regular exercise and lifestyle changes, such as minimizing caffeine and alcohol intake, are all important in maintaining bone mass.[9] For those with osteoporosis, implement strategies to prevent falls. Referral to an occupational therapist for a home safety assessment may be beneficial in the elderly.

For those in nursing homes, the use of hip protectors and exercise help minimize the risk of fractures.[33] Multiple strategies to prevent falls should be individualized based on the resident's level of risk and lifestyle choices.

Direct exposure of the arms and legs to sunlight (ultraviolet B radiation) for 5–10 minutes allows the skin to synthesize vitamin D; however, the amount is dependent on the time of day (best between

10 a.m. and 3 p.m.), season, latitude (exposure to UVB is greater at latitudes <37°, i.e., closer to the equator), length of exposure and skin sensitivity.[34] The elderly and individuals with increased skin melanin pigmentation require longer periods of sun exposure to make the same amount of vitamin D_3 as a younger individual or one with less skin pigmentation. While it was thought that the application of sunblock decreased the natural production of vitamin D by the skin,[10,34] studies have determined that normal usage of sunscreen does not generally result in vitamin D deficiency but does decrease the incidence of skin cancers.[35] Most Canadians do not get sufficient vitamin D based on sun exposure only and must obtain vitamin D via diet and supplements to prevent deficiency.

Dietary Measures

Adequate intake of calcium and vitamin D are essential, to help increase peak bone mass in the early years and to help maintain bone mass later in life. Daily calcium needs are best met through dietary sources. A baseline **calcium** intake of about 300 mg daily can be assumed, since many foods contain small amounts of calcium.[36] Table 3 lists some calcium-rich foods and their calcium content. Food sources of **vitamin D** include fatty fish (salmon, mackerel), fish liver oils and fortified foods such as milk, bread, breakfast cereals, juices and margarine. Calcium and vitamin D requirements vary by age and gender[37,38] (see Table 6).

Table 3: **Selected Dietary Sources of Calcium**[37]

Food	Portion Size	Calcium[a]
Beans, baked	125 mL	75 mg
Bread, whole wheat	2 slices	40 mg
Broccoli, cooked	185 mL	50 mg
Cheese (cheddar, edam, gouda)	3 cm cube	245 mg
Cheese, mozzarella	3 cm cube	200 mg
Cottage cheese (2%, 1%)	125 mL	75 mg
Figs, dried	10	150 mg
Ice cream	125 mL	80 mg
Milk (2%, 1%, skim, chocolate)	250mL	300 mg
Orange juice, fortified	250 mL	335 mg
Rice or soy beverage, fortified	250 mL	300 mg
Salmon, with bones, canned	105 g	240 mg
Sardines, with bones	55 g	200 mg
Tofu, with calcium sulfate	84 g	130 mg
Yogurt, plain	185 mL	295 mg

[a] Approximate values.

Exercise

Like muscle, bone is living tissue that responds to exercise by becoming stronger. Weight-bearing exercise in the young can help increase peak bone mass; a 2014 meta-analysis found that weight-bearing exercise was most beneficial for improving bone mineral content in prepubertal children.[3,42] In older individuals (including postmenopausal women) regular weight-bearing exercise such as walking or jogging can help maintain bone mass. A Cochrane systematic review demonstrated that weight-bearing and/or non-weight-bearing exercises may prevent bone loss in postmenopausal women.[43] Exercises that strengthen core muscles and improve balance may also be beneficial.[12] Additional benefits of exercising regularly include increased muscle strength and flexibility, which can improve balance and minimize the risk of falls. Exercise, including strength, balance, weight-bearing and agility training, was shown to reduce injurious falls (those requiring medical attention) in a trial of 409 home-dwelling women aged 70–80 years.[44]

Lifestyle Changes

Recommend smoking cessation and minimizing alcohol and caffeine intake when identifying strategies to decrease the risk of osteoporosis.[2] Limiting the amount of caffeine-containing beverages (cola, hot chocolate, coffee, tea) to no more than 3 servings daily can help minimize calcium loss. Excessive alcohol consumption can affect calcium absorption and bone formation, and increase the risk of falls. For general good health, limit alcohol consumption to no more than 2 drinks per day.[45]

Pharmacologic Therapy

For further discussion of pharmacologic therapy for osteoporosis, consult the *Compendium of Therapeutic Choices*: Osteoporosis.

For comparative ingredients of nonprescription products, consult the *Compendium of Products for Minor Ailments*—Vitamin and Mineral Products: Single Entity, Solid Combinations.

Calcium and vitamin D are important considerations in preventing bone loss and are recommended in addition to any antiresorptive or anabolic (or any additional pharmacologic) therapy that may be used (see Table 6).[46]

Calcium Supplements

To determine whether individuals are receiving sufficient calcium from their diet, the following calcium calculator may be helpful: www.osteoporosis.ca/osteoporosis-and-you/nutrition/calculate-my-calcuim. If diet is not sufficient to meet the daily calcium requirements, consider supplementation. Calcium supplements are available in various salt forms (Table 4); the carbonate and citrate salts are commonly used. **Calcium carbonate** is most often recommended as it is inexpensive and is available in many dosage forms. Both natural (e.g., from oyster shells) and synthetically produced sources are equally effective. Individuals who may have decreased acid secretion, such as those on H_2-receptor antagonists (e.g., ranitidine) or proton pump inhibitors (e.g., pantoprazole), should consider supplementation with **calcium citrate**, as its absorption is not affected by these agents. Patients should be aware of the differences in absorption in order to choose the appropriate calcium salt for their needs.

Lead content of natural calcium supplements has been a concern. Although the amount of lead was variable among 17 different calcium carbonate products at doses used in osteoporosis, the lead content did not pose a risk to the patient.[47] In individuals taking calcium at much higher doses (e.g., as a phosphate binder in renal disease), lead content may be a more important concern.[47]

Table 4: **Elemental Calcium Content of Calcium Salts**

Calcium Salt	Elemental Calcium
Calcium carbonate	40%
Calcium citrate	21%
Calcium gluconate	9%
Calcium lactate	13%

Supplemental calcium can significantly slow the rate of bone loss in postmenopausal women.[48,49] Calcium supplementation, without the addition of Vitamin D or antiresorptive agents, has not been shown to decrease fracture risk.[2] In the Women's Health Initiative trial, older postmenopausal women aged 50–79 who were randomized to calcium 1000 mg/day plus vitamin D 400 IU/day showed greater preservation of hip BMD, seen up to 9 years of follow up, and a nonsignificant decrease in hip fractures.[50] Limitations of this study include the age of women (young to sustain hip fractures) and the fact that all women, including those in the control group, had a baseline daily intake of 1200 mg of calcium.

A meta-analysis of randomised controlled trials evaluating the effects of calcium in those >50 years showed small increases in BMD with both dietary and supplemental calcium. The authors concluded that this small increase in BMD may not significantly decrease fracture risk on its own.[51] A systematic review evaluating the effects of calcium in those >50 years showed no association of dietary calcium with risk of fracture and small inconsistent benefits on fracture prevention with calcium supplementation.[52]

Increased cardiovascular events have been reported in patients taking calcium supplements[53,54,55,56] while other studies have indicated no increase.[57,58] The effect of daily calcium supplementation on cardiovascular events is still unclear. Those who have inadequate intake should first consider increasing their dietary calcium, and when appropriate, adding calcium supplements.

In a randomized, double-blind, placebo-controlled study of 3270 elderly institutionalized women, combined use of calcium 1200 mg daily and vitamin D 800 IU daily decreased the risk of nonvertebral fractures.[59] Compared with placebo, supplementation resulted in a relative reduction in incidence of hip fractures after 36 months of 23% (4.19% vs. 5.44%) and of all nonvertebral fractures of 17.2% (7.8% vs. 9.42%).[60] Benefit from supplementation was seen within 12 months of treatment. All women had inadequate calcium intake at baseline (<800 mg/day) and 44% were vitamin D deficient (serum 25-hydroxyvitamin D level of <30 nmol/L). Based on available evidence, Osteoporosis Canada and the Society of Obstetricians and Gynaecologists of Canada (SOGC) recommend optimizing calcium intake in all individuals, for preventing and treating osteoporosis.[12,46]

Vitamin D Analogues

Vitamin D is essential for normal calcium absorption and good bone health. If vitamin D is deficient, less than 10% of calcium is absorbed. As discussed previously (see Nonpharmacologic Therapy), vitamin D is produced in the body usually through exposure to sunlight and is also absorbed from the diet. However, for adults over 50 years of age, and for those who are homebound or institutionalized, a daily vitamin D supplement is recommended.[3]

Vitamin D 800 IU daily, when given with adequate calcium supplementation, has resulted in moderately increased bone mass[61] and decreased fracture risk in elderly men and women.[59] A meta-analysis of randomized, controlled trials in postmenopausal women (mean age 71–85 years) showed that vitamin D 700–800 IU/day was associated with a significant reduction in the risk of hip and nonvertebral fractures.[62] At lower doses of 400 IU/day, a decrease in nonvertebral fracture was observed, but not a decrease in hip fractures. A Cochrane review also suggests that vitamin D alone appears unlikely to prevent fractures; however, vitamin D with calcium may prevent hip fractures in older individuals.[63,64] Vitamin D supplements may increase muscle strength in adults with vitamin D deficiency,[65] and supplements of 800–1000 IU daily reduced the risk of falls in persons >60 years of age.[66]

The Osteoporosis Canada recommendation for those ≥50 years at moderate risk of deficiency is 800–1000 IU of vitamin D daily. Daily supplementation with more than 1000 IU may be required to achieve optimal vitamin D status, and doses up to 2000 IU are considered safe.[12,40] Ensure adequate calcium intake (Table 6) when supplementing with vitamin D.

Measuring serum 25-hydroxyvitamin D is unnecessary in adults at low risk of vitamin D deficiency. Measuring is appropriate prior to initiation of pharmacologic therapy for osteoporosis, in those who have sustained recurrent fractures and in those who continue to lose bone mass with treatment.[12] Levels should be measured after 3–4 months of supplementation and not repeated if serum concentrations >75 nmol/L are achieved.

Vitamin D is available as **cholecalciferol** (vitamin D_3) or **ergocalciferol** (vitamin D_2). **Calcitriol,** an active form of vitamin D, is recommended only in those who may have renal or hepatic impairment and are not able to activate vitamin D.

Bisphosphonates

Antiresorptive or anabolic pharmacologic therapy is recommended if the 10-year absolute fracture risk is greater than 20% (high risk). In those with a moderate risk, management decisions should be individualized.[12,46]

Bisphosphonates increase bone density and decrease fractures and are usually considered first choice. Large RCTs have demonstrated that both **alendronate** and **risedronate** decrease the risk of vertebral and hip fractures.[67] **Etidronate** appears to reduce vertebral fractures; however, clinical trials were not well designed.[68] Injectable **zoledronic acid** also decreases vertebral and hip fractures.[69] Concern raised in one zoledronic acid trial[69] over a possible association with increased risk of atrial fibrillation was not supported by subsequent reviews.[70,71]

Side effects of bisphosphonates may include GI effects such as abdominal pain, dyspepsia and nausea. Rarely, they may cause esophagitis or esophageal ulceration. Osteonecrosis of the jaw (ONJ) has been reported, more commonly in patients with cancer and/or those who have received high doses of iv bisphosphonates; however, case reports and retrospective data have identified ONJ in those taking oral bisphosphonates. The true incidence of bisphosphonate-associated ONJ, particularly in those without cancer or those taking oral bisphosphonates, remains unclear.[72] Atypical fractures of the femur have also been reported, mainly when bisphosphonates were used long term.[73,74,75,76] These adverse effects must be considered when assessing the benefits of treatment for each patient.

Bisphosphonates are an appropriate option for both men and women with osteoporosis.[12,77]

Hormone Therapy

Hormone therapy (HT) reduces fracture risk in postmenopausal women; however, due to potential adverse effects of HT it is usually recommended only for short-term treatment (<5 years) of menopausal symptoms.[46,78] Evidence from RCTs with standard doses of HT (0.625 mg conjugated equine estrogens) supports decreased clinical fractures at all sites in postmenopausal women. The Women's Health Initiative study demonstrated that HT (conjugated equine estrogens with or without a progestogen) decreased clinical fractures at the hip, vertebrae and other sites in postmenopausal women.[46,78]

Other Pharmacologic Choices

Raloxifene decreased vertebral fractures in RCTs.[79,80,81] Reported side effects include leg cramps and vasomotor symptoms. It is also associated with an increase in risk of venous thromboembolism.

Denosumab is a human monoclonal antibody (IgG2) that binds to receptor activator of nuclear factor-kappa B (RANK) ligand and inhibits osteoclast formation, function and survival. It is a first-line option for the treatment of osteoporosis[12] but cost may limit its use to postmenopausal women at high risk of fracture who have failed or are unable to tolerate other therapies.[82,83]

In those with severe osteoporosis or those at high risk of glucocorticoid-induced osteoporosis, **teriparatide** may be considered.[12,46] Teriparatide, a parathyroid hormone (PTH) analogue, is an anabolic agent that causes a steady gain in bone density and reduces the risk of vertebral and nonvertebral (but not hip) fractures.[84] It may also decrease the pain of vertebral fractures.

Calcitonin demonstrated a moderate increase in BMD and decrease in vertebral fractures,[67,85,86] and a nasal formulation was previously available. Since 2013, Health Canada has withdrawn all nasal calcitonin spray following a review of the benefits and safety of this formulation; a small increase in cancer risk has been noted with long-term use.[87]

Sodium fluoride increases bone formation by stimulating osteoblasts. A meta-analysis of 11 RCTs found that fluoride increased spinal BMD, had little effect on hip BMD, and decreased forearm BMD.[88] The relative risk of vertebral fractures was unchanged, but the risk of nonvertebral fractures increased, possibly due to the production of bone of inferior quality. These equivocal results, along with adverse effects such as GI distress and lower extremity pain syndrome, led to the disuse of fluoride as a treatment for osteoporosis.

However, a meta-analysis of 25 studies re-examined the data and found that use of sodium fluoride resulted in increased BMD of the spine and hip, with no reduction in overall fracture risk.[89] In a subgroup analysis, doses of ≤20 mg fluoride equivalents resulted in a statistically significant reduction in vertebral and nonvertebral fractures with a trend toward a greater risk of pain syndrome with the lower dose. Additional controlled trials are needed to clarify efficacy and safety in osteoporosis, especially using lower doses.

Natural Health Products

Many consumers are interested in using alternative therapies, such as natural health products (NHPs), to manage their osteoporosis. A systematic review identified 45 NHPs that claimed to be of benefit for osteoporosis.[90] Calcium and vitamin D are the only NHPs recommended in the 2010 Canadian practice guidelines for the diagnosis and management of osteoporosis.[12]

For the following NHPs, randomized controlled trials (RCTs) investigating bone mineral density and/or fracture rate were identified. Results from these preliminary studies should be confirmed using larger studies conducted over several years, using fracture rates as an outcome and considering such factors as calcium and vitamin D intake.

Dehydroepiandrosterone (DHEA) is a steroid hormone that is produced in the adrenal glands.[91] While not available in Canada, it is widely available on the Internet.

Declining DHEA levels after the mid-twenties have been linked with diseases such as obesity, cardiovascular disease and osteoporosis; therefore, it has been proposed that DHEA may be useful in the management of these diseases.[92] A systematic review identified 2 trials of DHEA conducted in healthy adults over the age of 50,[90] and 2 additional trials were published subsequently.[93,94] Results of the studies were conflicting.[94,95,96] DHEA did increase BMD in the spine in a study of men with osteoporosis.[93] A dose of 50–100 mg/day was used in the studies showing beneficial effect on BMD.

Adverse effects included hair loss, deepening of the voice, insulin resistance, menstrual pattern changes and abdominal pain.[97]

Phytoestrogens, found in sources such as soy and red clover, are nonsteroidal plant compounds that include **isoflavones, lignans** and **coumestans.**[98] Of these, isoflavones are the most commonly used for osteoporosis. Isoflavones such as genistein and daidzein are structurally similar to estrogens and thus can bind to estrogen receptors to produce weak estrogenic activity. A 2006 systematic review concluded that evidence for the use of phytoestrogens in women with osteoporosis was equivocal, with some trials demonstrating a positive effect on BMD and others showing no effect.[90] Other RCTs[99,100,101,102,103,104,105,106] and a 2013 review[107] also produced conflicting results. Interpretation and comparison of these studies is complicated by different phytoestrogen formulations, content and doses used, varying study lengths and concomitant use of calcium and vitamin D.

Studies reporting a positive effect on BMD have used products containing 54–126 mg of isoflavones.[90,99,100,101,104,105] Adverse effects reported included gastrointestinal irritation, constipation, diarrhea, malaise, sleep disturbances, shortness of breath and joint pain.[90]

Ipriflavone is a synthetic isoflavone derivative that may have a similar effect to that of estrogens on bone mineralization, without having direct estrogen-like activity.[108] At least 15 RCTs have examined the use of ipriflavone for the prevention of postmenopausal bone loss. In postmenopausal women with low BMD or osteoporosis, ipriflavone maintained or increased BMD in the distal radius[109,110,111,112,113,114,115] and in the spine.[114,116,117,118,119,120,121,122,123] However, a study of over 450 women reported no significant changes in BMD in the spine, hip or forearm.[124] Limited data are available regarding fracture outcome. One study[115] reported a reduction in vertebral fractures in the ipriflavone group compared with placebo, while another study[124] found that the number of fractures in the treatment and control groups was not different.

Ipriflavone 200 mg TID has been used, with concomitant calcium 500–1000 mg/day. Ipriflavone was generally well tolerated; adverse effects most commonly reported were abdominal pain, nausea, diarrhea and constipation.[113,115]

Vitamin K refers to several fat-soluble vitamins known as quinones. Vitamin K_1 (phytonadione) is found in leafy green vegetables, broccoli and brussels sprouts while Vitamin K_2 (menaquinone) is found in meats and cheeses.[125,126] Vitamin K_2 is also synthesized by bacteria in the gut. Low vitamin K intake and/or serum levels have been associated with lower BMD and fractures in people with osteoporosis.[127] Two systematic reviews reported that phytonadione and menaquinone maintained or improved BMD;[90,128] one of these reviews reported that menaquinone administration reduced vertebral and nonvertebral fracture rates.[128] A 2015 systematic review of menaquinone in postmenopausal women found similar results in that there was an improvement in vertebral BMD and possibly a reduction in fractures.[129] However, there is concern about the quality of the studies in all of these reviews and many were conducted in Asian populations, making it difficult to generalize the results. Three studies report no effect on bone loss rates in postmenopausal women from Europe or Canada with and without low BMD.[130,131,132] One of these trials found that women taking vitamin K_1 had fewer clinical fractures compared with the placebo group.[131]

Vitamin K_2 15 mg TID was most commonly used in the studies. It was well tolerated; GI adverse effects such as nausea and vomiting were reported in some studies.[130,131,133,134]

Black cohosh has been shown to increase levels of markers of bone formation,[135] but a 12-month RCT in menopausal women found no significant effect on BMD compared with placebo.[106]

Monitoring of Therapy

Table 5 lists some measures to reduce modifiable risks and how to monitor their success. In patients at risk of osteoporosis, the expected outcome is to maintain baseline BMD. In those with demonstrated osteoporosis, the goal is to remain free of fractures and prevent further loss of BMD.

Table 5: Monitoring Outcome of Modifiable Risk Reduction Measures

Risk Factor	Recommendation	Considerations
Low calcium intake	Ensure diet is adequate (may refer to dietitian). Add supplements to meet total daily requirements (Table 6).	If supplements recommended, educate patient on proper administration and prevention of constipation and drug interactions. Suggest appropriate dose based on salt form of supplement (Table 4).
Sedentary lifestyle	If osteoporosis is not diagnosed, recommend weight-bearing exercises such as walking. If patient has significant cardiovascular disease or osteoporosis, refer to an appropriate healthcare practitioner.	Exercise should be started gradually and tailored to the individual's health status (e.g., consider conditions such as cardiovascular or respiratory disease).
Inadequate vitamin D intake or >50 years of age	Recommend 800–1000 IU/day of vitamin D. >1000 IU/day may be required to achieve optimal vitamin D status; doses up to 2000 IU/day are safe.[12,40]	If patient is taking a multivitamin, check for amount of vitamin D.

Figure 1: Assessment of Risk for Osteoporosis[12]

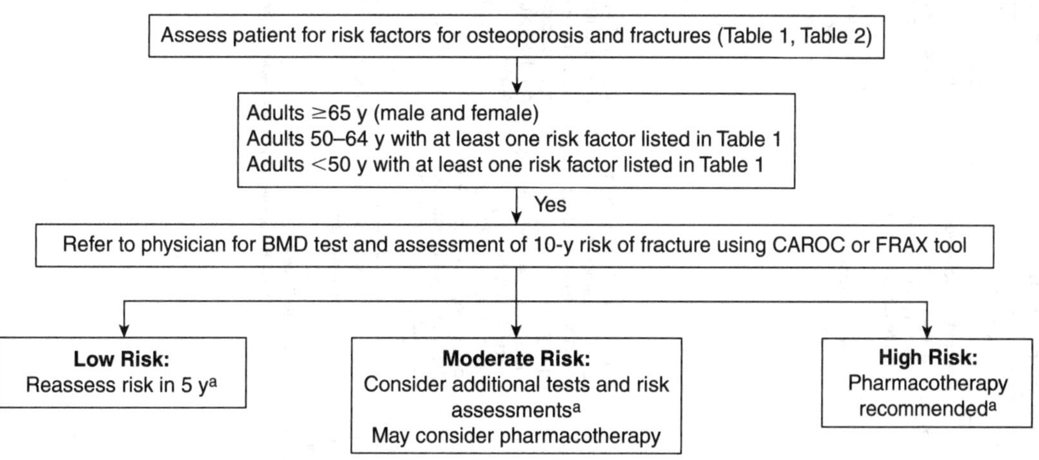

For all levels of risk for osteoporosis, educate patients on:

- Adequate daily intake of calcium and vitamin D through diet (consider referral to a dietician) and supplements
- Physical activity
- Other lifestyle factors (caffeine and alcohol use)
- Fall prevention strategies

[a] For further detail, refer to Papaioannou A, Morin S, Cheung AM et al. 2010 clinical practice guidelines for the diagnosis and management of osteoporosis in Canada: summary.[12]

Abbreviations: BMD = bone mineral density; CAROC = Canadian Association of Radiologists and Osteoporosis Canada

Table 6: **Calcium and Vitamin D Recommendations for Prevention and Treatment of Osteoporosis**[a]

Class	Drug	Dosage[b]	Adverse Effects	Drug Interactions	Comments	Cost[c]
Nutritional Supplements	*calcium* Caltrate, generics	Elemental calcium/day:[d] Men and women 19–50 y (includes pregnant or breastfeeding women): 1000 mg po Men and women >50 y: 1200 mg po	When taken as a supplement: constipation, flatulence, nausea; rarely, hypercalcemia, hypercalciuria, renal calcification, renal stones (at high doses).	Calcium supplements may decrease absorption of bisphosphonates, ciprofloxacin, iron, levothyroxine, tetracycline. Separate administration by 2 h.	Encourage fulfillment of calcium needs through dietary intake first. Select product based on salt type and amount of elemental calcium per tablet. Supplement doses >500 mg/day should be taken in divided doses. Calcium carbonate requires acidic medium for best absorption (take with or after meals); calcium citrate does not.	$
	vitamin D generics	Adults <50 y (healthy, at low risk of deficiency):[e] 400–1000 IU/day (10–25 µg/day) po Adults ≥50 y (at moderate risk of vitamin D deficiency):[e] 800–1000 IU/day (20–25 µg/day) po; doses up to 2000 IU/day (50 µg/day) may be required and are considered safe.[12,40,41]	Vitamin D intoxication (>50 000 IU/day)[10] may result in hypercalcemia, hypercalciuria, renal calcification, renal stones.	Mineral oil can impair absorption of vitamin D. Increases calcium absorption.	Most multivitamins and many calcium supplements contain vitamin D. Also present in fish oils (with vitamin A).	$

[a] For further discussion of pharmacologic therapy for osteoporosis, consult the *Compendium of Therapeutic Choices*: Osteoporosis.
[b] Dosage represents total daily recommended intake, from diet and supplements.
[c] Cost of 30-day supply; includes drug cost only.
[d] For comparison of elemental calcium content of various salts, see Table 4.
[e] Osteoporosis Canada recommendations differ from the Health Canada Recommended Daily Allowances for vitamin D (600 IU/day for ages 1–70 y and 800 IU/day for those >70 y).[39]

Legend: $ <$5

Resource Tips

Osteoporosis Canada. 1200 Eglinton Ave East, Suite 500, Toronto, Ontario M3C 1H9. Telephone: 416-696-2663, Toll-free (in Canada only): 1-800-463-6842 (English) or 1-800-977-1778 (French). Available from: www.osteoporosis.ca.

Suggested Readings

Khan A, Fortier M, Reid R et al. Osteoporosis in menopause. *J Obstet Gynaecol Can* 2014;36:S1-15. Available from: sogc.org/wp-content/uploads/2014/09/JOGC-Sept2014-CPG-312_Eng_Online-Complete.pdf.

Management of osteoporosis in postmenopausal women: 2010 position statement of The North American Menopause Society. *Menopause* 2010;17:25-54.

Papaioannou A, Morin S, Cheung AM et al. 2010 clinical practice guidelines for the diagnosis and management of osteoporosis in Canada: summary. *CMAJ* 2010;182:1864-73.

Whelan AM, Jurgens TM, Bowles SK. Natural health products in the prevention and treatment of osteoporosis: systematic review of randomized controlled trials. *Ann Pharmacother* 2006;40:836-49.

References

1. *WHO Scientific Group on the assessment of osteoporosis at primary health care level: summary meeting report, Brussels, Belgium, 5-7 May 2004*. Available from: www.who.int/chp/topics/Osteoporosis.pdf. Accessed April 26, 2016.
2. Management of osteoporosis in postmenopausal women: 2010 position statement of The North American Menopause Society. *Menopause* 2010;17:25-54.
3. Brown JP, Fortier M, Frame H et al. Canadian Consensus Conference on osteoporosis, 2006 update. *J Obstet Gynaecol Can* 2006;28:S95-112.
4. Jiang HX, Majumdar SR, Dick DA et al. Development and initial validation of a risk score for predicting in-hospital and 1-year mortality in patients with hip fractures. *J Bone Miner Res* 2005;20:494-500.
5. Ioannidis G, Papaioannou A, Hopman WM et al. Relation between fractures and mortality: results from the Canadian Multicentre Osteoporosis Study. *CMAJ* 2009;181:265-71.
6. Leslie WD, O'Donnell S, Jean S et al. Trends in hip fracture rates in Canada. *JAMA* 2009;302:883-9.
7. Wiktorowicz ME, Goeree R, Papaioannou A et al. Economic implications of hip fracture: health service use, institutional care and cost in Canada. *Osteoporos Int* 2001;12:271-8.
8. National Institutes of Health. National Institute of Arthritis and Musculoskeletal and Skin Diseases. *Osteoporosis: Peak bone mass in women*. Reviewed May 2009. Available from: www.niams.nih.gov/Health_Info/Bone/Osteoporosis/bone_mass.asp. Accessed April 26, 2016.
9. World Health Organization. *Prevention and management of osteoporosis: report of a WHO Scientific Group*. Geneva: WHO Technical Report Series 921; 2003. Available from: whqlibdoc.who.int/trs/WHO_TRS_921.pdf. Accessed April 26, 2016.
10. Holick MF. Vitamin D deficiency. *N Engl J Med* 2007;357:266-81.
11. Kanis JA, Melton LJ, Christiansen C et al. The diagnosis of osteoporosis. *J Bone Miner Res* 1994;9:1137-41.
12. Papaioannou A, Morin S, Cheung AM et al. 2010 clinical practice guidelines for the diagnosis and management of osteoporosis in Canada: summary. *CMAJ* 2010;182:1864-73.
13. Papaioannou A, Morin S, Cheung AM et al. *Clinical practice guidelines for the diagnosis and management of osteoporosis in Canada: background and technical report*. Available from: www.osteoporosis.ca/multimedia/pdf/Osteoporosis_Guidelines_2010_Background_And_Technical_Report.pdf. Accessed April 26, 2016.
14. Pack AM, Morrell MJ. Adverse effects of antiepileptic drugs on bone structure: epidemiology, mechanisms and therapeutic implications. *CNS Drugs* 2001;15:633-42.
15. Ray JG, Adachi JR. Anticonvulsants and bone disease: a systematic overview of their association and possible preventive strategies. *Can J Clin Pharmacol* 1998;5:217-23.
16. Brown TT, Qaqish RB. Antiretroviral therapy and the prevalence of osteopenia and osteoporosis: a meta-analytic review. *AIDS* 2006;20:2165-74.
17. Carvalho EH, Gelenske T, Bandeira F et al. Bone mineral density in HIV-infected women taking antiretroviral therapy: a systematic review. *Arq Bras Endocrinol Metab* 2010;54:133-42.
18. Bolland MJ, Wang TKM, Grey A et al. Stable bone density in HAART-treated individuals with HIV: a meta-analysis. *J Clin Endocrinol Metab* 2011;96:2721-31.
19. Michaud LB, Goodin S. Cancer-treatment-induced bone loss, part 1. *Am J Health Syst Pharm* 2006;63:419-30.
20. Michaud LB, Goodin S. Cancer-treatment-induced bone loss, part 2. *Am J Health Syst Pharm* 2006;63:534-46.
21. Kanis JA, Johansson H, Oden A et al. A meta-analysis of prior corticosteroid use and fracture risk. *J Bone Miner Res* 2004;19:893-9.
22. O'Connell MB, Borgelt L, Bowles SK et al. Drug-induced osteoporosis in the older adult. *Aging Health* 2010;6:501-18.
23. Nelson-Piercy C. Heparin-induced osteoporosis. *Scand J Rheumatol Suppl* 1998;107:68-71.
24. Faber J, Galloe AM. Changes in bone mass during prolonged subclinical hyperthyroidism due to L-thyroxine treatment: a meta-analysis. *Eur J Endocrinol* 1994;130:350-6.
25. Guilbert ER, Brown JP, Kaunitz AM et al. The use of depot-medroxyprogesterone acetate in contraception and its potential impact on skeletal health. *Contraception* 2009;79:167-77.
26. Yang YX, Lewis JD, Epstein S et al. Long-term proton pump inhibitor therapy and risk of hip fracture. *JAMA* 2006;296:2947-53.

27. Roux C, Briot K, Gossec L et al. Increase in vertebral fracture risk in postmenopausal women using omeprazole. *Calcif Tissue Int* 2009;84:13-9.
28. Yu EW, Blackwell T, Ensrud KE et al. Acid-suppressive medications and risk of bone loss and fracture in older adults. *Calcif Tissue Int* 2008;83:251-9.
29. Cumming RG, Le Couteur DG. Benzodiazepines and risk of hip fractures in older people: a review of the evidence. *CNS Drugs* 2003;17:825-37.
30. Madhusoodanan S, Bogunovic OJ. Safety of benzodiazepines in the geriatric population. *Expert Opin Drug Saf* 2004;3:485-93.
31. University of Sheffield, UK. World Health Organization Collaborating Centre for Metabolic Bone Diseases. *FRAX: WHO fracture risk assessment tool*. Available from: www.shef.ac.uk/FRAX. Accessed April 26, 2016.
32. Siminoski K, Leslie WD, Frame H et al. Recommendations for bone mineral density reporting in Canada.*Can Assoc Radiol J* 2005;56:178-88.
33. Papaioannou A, Santesso N, Morin SN et al. Recommendations for preventing fractures in long-term care. *CMAJ* 2015;187:1135-44, E450-61.
34. Holick MF. Sunlight and vitamin D for bone health and prevention of autoimmune diseases, cancers, and cardiovascular disease. *Am J Clin Nutr* 2004;80:1678S-88S.
35. Norval M, Wulf HC. Does chronic sunscreen use reduce vitamin D production to insufficient levels? *Br J Dermatol* 2009;161:732-6.
36. Osteoporosis Canada. *Calcium is good—are calcium supplements bad?* Updated May 2012. Available from: www.osteoporosis.ca/index.php/ci_id/9931/la_id/1.htm. Accessed April 26, 2016.
37. Osteoporosis Canada. *Calcium: an important nutrient that builds stronger bones*. Available from: www.osteoporosis.ca/osteoporosis-and-you/nutrition/calcium-requirements. Accessed April 26, 2016.
38. Osteoporosis Canada. *Vitamin D: an important nutrient that protects you against falls and fractures*. Available from: www.osteoporosis.ca/osteoporosis-and-you/nutrition/vitamin-d. Accessed April 26, 2016.
39. Health Canada. *Vitamin D and calcium: updated dietary references intakes*. Available from: www.hc-sc.gc.ca/fn-an/nutrition/vitamin/vita-d-eng.php. Accessed April 26, 2016.
40. Hanley DA, Cranney A, Jones G et al. Vitamin D in adult health and disease: a review and guideline statement from Osteoporosis Canada (summary). *CMAJ* 2010;182:1315-19.
41. Osteoporosis Canada. *Despite recent studies, calcium and vitamin D remain important nutrients for overall bone health*. Available from: www.osteoporosis.ca/despite-recent-studies-calcium-and-vitamin-d-remain-important-nutrients-for-overall-bone-health/. Accessed April 26, 2016.
42. Behringer M, Gruetzner S, McCourt M et al. Effects of weight-bearing activities on bone mineral content and density in children and adolescents: a meta-analysis. *J Bone Miner Res* 2014;29:467-78.
43. Howe TE, Shea B, Dawson et al. Exercise for preventing and treating osteoporosis in postmenopausal women. *Cochrane Database Syst Rev* 2011;7:CD000333.
44. Uusi-Rasi K, Patil R, Karinkanta S et al. Exercise and vitamin D in fall prevention among older women: a randomized clinical trial. *JAMA Intern Med* 2015;175:703-11.
45. Heart and Stroke Foundation. *Excessive alcohol consumption*. Available from: www.heartandstroke.on.ca/site/c.pvI3IeNWJwE/b.3581749/k.9AAF/Heart_Disease_8211_Excessive_alcohol_consumption.htm. Accessed April 26, 2016.
46. Khan A, Fortier M, Reid R et al. Osteoporosis in menopause. *J Obstet Gynaecol Can* 2014;36:S1-15. Available from: sogc.org/wp-content/uploads/2014/09/JOGC-Sept2014-CPG-312_Eng_Online-Complete.pdf.
47. Ross EA, Szabo NJ, Tebbett IR. Lead content of calcium supplements. *JAMA* 2000;284:1425-9.
48. Reid IR, Ames RW, Evans MC et al. Effect of calcium supplementation on bone loss in postmenopausal women. *N Engl J Med* 1993;328:460-4.
49. Aloia JF, Vaswani A, Yeh JK et al. Calcium supplementation with and without hormone replacement therapy to prevent postmenopausal bone loss. *Ann Intern Med* 1994;120:97-103.
50. Jackson RD, LaCroix AZ, Gass M et al. Calcium plus vitamin D supplementation and the risk of fractures. *N Engl J Med* 2006;354:669-83.
51. Tai V, Leung W, Grey A et al. Calcium intake and bone mineral density: systematic review and meta-analysis. *BMJ* 2015;351:h4183.
52. Bolland MJ, Leung W, Tai V et al. Calcium intake and risk of fracture: systematic review. *BMJ* 2015;351:h4580.
53. Bolland MJ, Barber PA, Doughty RN et al. Vascular events in healthy older women receiving calcium supplementation: randomised controlled trial. *BMJ* 2008;336:262-6.
54. Bolland MJ, Avenell A, Baron JA et al. Effect of calcium supplements on risk of myocardial infarction and cardiovascular events: meta-analysis. *BMJ* 2010;341:c3691.
55. Xiao Q, Murphy RA, Houston DK et al. Dietary and supplemental calcium intake and cardiovascular disease mortality: the National Institutes of Health-AARP diet and health study. *JAMA Intern Med* 2013;173:639-46.
56. Michaëlsson K, Melhus H, Warensjö Lemming E et al. Long term calcium intake and rates of all cause and cardiovascular mortality: community based prospective longitudinal cohort study. *BMJ* 2013;346:f228.
57. Lewis JR, Calver J, Zhu K et al. Calcium supplementation and the risks of atherosclerotic vascular disease in older women: results of a 5-year RCT and a 4.5-year follow up. *J Bone Miner Res* 2011;26:35-41.
58. Wang L, Manson JE, Song Y et al. Systematic review: vitamin D and calcium supplementation in prevention of cardiovascular events. *Ann Intern Med* 2010;152:315-23.
59. Chapuy MC, Arlot ME, Duboeuf F et al. Vitamin D3 and calcium to prevent hip fractures in the elderly woman. *N Engl J Med* 1992;327:1637-42.
60. Chapuy MC, Arlot ME, Delmas PD et al. Effect of calcium and cholecalciferol treatment for three years on hip fractures in elderly women. *BMJ* 1994;308:1081-2.
61. Dawson-Hughes B, Harris SS, Krall EA et al. Effect of calcium and vitamin D supplementation on bone density in men and women 65 years of age or older. *N Engl J Med* 1997;337:670-6.
62. Bischoff-Ferrari HA, Willett WC, Wong JB et al. Fracture prevention with vitamin D supplementation: a meta-analysis of randomized controlled trials. *JAMA* 2005;293:2257-64.
63. Avenell A, Gillespie WJ, Gillespie LD et al. Vitamin D and vitamin D analogues for preventing fractures associated with involutional and post-menopausal osteoporosis. *Cochrane Database Syst Rev* 2009;2:CD000227.
64. Avenell A, Mak JC, O'Connell D. Vitamin D and vitamin D analogues for preventing fractures in post-menopausal women and older men. *Cochrane Database Syst Rev* 2014;4:CD000227.

65. Stockton KA, Mengersen K, Paratz JD et al. Effect of vitamin D supplementation on muscle strength: a systematic review and meta-analysis. *Osteoporos Int* 2011;22:859-71.
66. Kalyani RR, Stein B, Valiyil R et al. Vitamin D treatment for the prevention of falls in older adults: systematic review and meta-analysis. *J Am Geriatr Soc* 2010;58:1299-310.
67. Cranney A, Guyatt G, Griffith L et al. Meta-analyses of therapies for postmenopausal osteoporosis. IX: Summary of meta-analyses of therapies for postmenopausal osteoporosis. *Endocr Rev* 2002;23:570-8.
68. Cranney A, Guyatt G, Krolicki N et al. A meta-analysis of etidronate for the treatment of postmenopausal osteoporosis. *Osteoporos Int* 2001;12:140-51.
69. Black DM, Delmas PD, Eastell R et al. Once-yearly zoledronic acid for treatment of postmenopausal osteoporosis. *N Engl J Med* 2007;356:1809-22.
70. Loke YK, Jeevanantham V, Singh S. Bisphosphonates and atrial fibrillation: systematic review and meta-analysis. *Drug Saf* 2009;32:219-28.
71. Sorensen HT, Christensen S, Mehnert F et al. Use of bisphosphonates among women and risk of atrial fibrillation and flutter: population based case-control study. *BMJ* 2008;336:813-6.
72. Crandall CJ, Newberry SJ, Diamant A et al. Comparative effectiveness of pharmacologic treatments to prevent fractures: an updated systematic review. *Ann Intern Med* 2014;161:711-23.
73. Lee S, Yin RV, Hirpara H et al. Increased risk for atypical fractures associated with bisphosphonate use. *Fam Pract* 2015;32:276-81.
74. Dell RM, Adams AL, Greene DF et al. Incidence of atypical nontraumatic diaphyseal fractures of the femur. *J Bone Miner Res* 2012;27:2544-50.
75. Shane E, Burr D, Abrahamsen B et al. Atypical subtrochanteric and diaphyseal femoral fractures: second report of a task force of the American Society for Bone and Mineral Research. *J Bone Miner Res* 2014;29:1-23.
76. Saita Y, Ishijima M, Kaneko K. Atypical femoral fractures and bisphosphonate use: current evidence and clinical implications. *Ther Adv Chronic Dis* 2015;6:185-93.
77. Khan AA, Hodsman AB, Papaioannou A et al. Management of osteoporosis in men: an update and case example. *CMAJ* 2007;176:345-8.
78. Cauley JA, Robbins J, Chen Z et al. Effects of estrogen plus progestin on risk of fracture and bone mineral density: the Women's Health Initiative randomized trial. *JAMA* 2003;290:1729-38.
79. Stone KL, Seeley DG, Lui LY et al. BMD at multiple sites and risk of fracture of multiple types: long-term results from the Study of Osteoporotic Fractures. *J Bone Miner Res* 2003;18:1947-54.
80. Cummings SR, Eckert S, Krueger KA et al. The effect of raloxifene on risk of breast cancer in postmenopausal women: results from the MORE randomized trial. Multiple Outcomes of Raloxifene Evaluation. *JAMA* 1999;281:2189-97.
81. Barrett-Connor E, Mosca L, Collins P et al. Effects of raloxifene on cardiovascular events and breast cancer in postmenopausal women. *N Engl J Med* 2006;355:125-37.
82. Whelan AM, Raman-Wilms, L. Denosumab: a new injectable treatment for postmenopausal osteoporosis. *Pharm J* 2011;144:72-8.
83. CPS online. Ottawa: Canadian Pharmacists Association; 2014. *Prolia* [product monograph]. Available from: e-therapeutics.ca. Subscription required.
84. Cranney A, Papaioannou A, Zytaruk N et al. Parathyroid hormone for the treatment of osteoporosis: a systematic review. *CMAJ* 2006;175:52-9.
85. Overgaard K, Hansen MA, Jensen SB et al. Effect of salcatonin given intranasally on bone mass and fracture rates in established osteoporosis: a dose-response study. *BMJ* 1992;305:556-61.
86. Chesnut CH, Silverman S, Andriano K et al. A randomized trial of nasal spray salmon calcitonin in postmenopausal women with established osteoporosis: the prevent recurrence of osteoporotic fractures study. PROOF Study Group. *Am J Med* 2000;109:267-76.
87. Osteoporosis Canada. *The potential cancer risk with long-term use of calcitonin-containing drugs*. Available from: www.osteoporosis.ca/wp-content/uploads/Potential_Cancer_Risk_with_Long_Term_Use_of_Calcitonin-containing_Drugs_aug_2013.pdf. Accessed April 26, 2016.
88. Haguenauer D, Welch V, Shea B et al. Fluoride for the treatment of postmenopausal osteoporotic fractures: a meta-analysis. *Osteoporos Int* 2000;11:727-38.
89. Vestergaard P, Jorgensen NR, Schwarz P et al. Effects of treatment with fluoride on bone mineral density and fracture risk–a meta-analysis. *Osteoporos Int* 2008;19:257-68.
90. Whelan AM, Jurgens TM, Bowles SK. Natural health products in the prevention and treatment of osteoporosis: systematic review of randomized controlled trials. *Ann Pharmacother* 2006;40:836-49.
91. Pepping J. DHEA: dehydroepiandrosterone. *Am J Health Syst Pharm* 2000;57:2048-50, 2053-4, 2056.
92. Mackowiak E, Tu P. Alternative therapies. DHEA: does it have a role in osteoporosis? Many women seek a natural alternative to HRT. Is DHEA the answer? *US Pharm* 2000;25:62.
93. Sun Y, Mao M, Sun L et al. Treatment of osteoporosis in men using dehydroepiandrosterone sulfate. *Chin Med J (Engl)* 2002;115:402-4.
94. von Muhlen D, Laughlin GA, Kritz-Silverstein D et al. Effect of dehydroepiandrosterone supplementation on bone mineral density, bone markers, and body composition in older adults: the DAWN trial. *Osteoporos Int* 2008;19:699-707.
95. Baulieu EE, Thomas G, Legrain S et al. Dehydroepiandrosterone (DHEA), DHEA sulfate, and aging: contribution of the DHEAge. Study to a sociobiomedical issue. *Proc Natl Acad Sci U S A* 2000;97:4279-84.
96. Morales AJ, Haubrich RH, Hwang JY et al. The effect of six months treatment with a 100 mg daily dose of dehydroepiandrosterone (DHEA) on circulating sex steroids, body composition and muscle strength in age-advanced men and women. *Clin Endocrinol (Oxf)* 1998;49:421-32.
97. Natural Medicines Comprehensive Database. *DHEA*. Available from: www.naturaldatabase.com. Accessed April 26, 2016. Subscription required.
98. Glazier MG, Bowman MA. A review of the evidence for the use of phytoestrogens as a replacement for traditional estrogen replacement therapy. *Arch Intern Med* 2001;161:1161-72.
99. Mori M, Aizawa T, Tokoro M et al. Soy isoflavone tablets reduce osteoporosis risk factors and obesity in middle-aged Japanese women. *Clin Exp Pharmacol Physiol* 2004;3:S39-41.
100. Harkness LS, Fiedler K, Sehgal AR et al. Decreased bone resorption with soy isoflavone supplementation in postmenopausal women. *J Womens Health (Larchmt)* 2004;3:1000-7.
101. Newton KM, LaCroix AZ, Levy L et al. Soy protein and bone mineral density in older men and women: a randomized trial. *Maturitas* 2006;55:270-7.
102. Ye YB, Tang XY, Verbruggen MA et al. Soy isoflavones attenuate bone loss in early postmenopausal Chinese women: a single-blind randomized, placebo-controlled trial. *Eur J Nutr* 2006;45:327-34.

103. Levis S, Strickman-Stein N, Ganjei-Azar P et al. Soy isoflavones in the prevention of menopausal bone loss and menopausal symptoms: a randomized, double-blind trial. *Arch Intern Med* 2001;171:1363-9.
104. Atteritano M, Mazzaferro S, Frisina A et al. Genistein effects on quantitative ultrasound parameters and bone mineral density in osteopenic postmenopausal women. *Osteoporosis Int* 2009;20:1947-54.
105. Marini H, Bitto A, Altavilla D et al. Breast safety and efficacy of genistein aglycone for postmenopausal bone loss: a follow-up study. *J Clin Endocrinol Metab* 2008;93:4787-96.
106. Geller SE, Shulman LP, van Breeman RB et al. Safety and efficacy of black cohosh and red clover for the management of vasomotor symptoms: a randomized controlled trial. *Menopause* 2009;16:1156-66.
107. Nieves JW. Skeletal effects of nutrients and nutraceuticals, beyond calcium and vitamin D. *Osteoporos Int* 2013;24(3):771-86.
108. Melis GB, Paoletti AM, Cagnacci A et al. Lack of any estrogenic effect of ipriflavone in postmenopausal women. *J Endocrinol Invest* 1992;15:755-61.
109. Agnusdei D, Zacchei F, Bigazzi S et al. Metabolic and clinical effects of ipriflavone in established post-menopausal osteoporosis. *Drugs Exp Clin Res* 1989;15:97-104.
110. Agnusdei D, Adami S, Cervetti R et al. Effects of ipriflavone on bone mass and calcium metabolism in postmenopausal osteoporosis. *Bone Miner* 1992;19:S43-8.
111. Passeri M, Biondi M, Costi D et al. Effect of ipriflavone on bone mass in elderly osteoporotic women. *Bone Miner* 1992;19:S57-62.
112. Hanabayashi T, Imai A, Tamaya T. Effects of ipriflavone and estriol on postmenopausal osteoporotic changes. *Int J Gynaecol Obstet* 1995;51:63-4.
113. Adami S, Bufalino L, Cervetti R et al. Ipriflavone prevents radial bone loss in postmenopausal women with low bone mass over 2 years. *Osteoporos Int* 1997;7:119-25.
114. Gennari C, Adami S, Agnusdei D et al. Effect of chronic treatment with ipriflavone in postmenopausal women with low bone mass. *Calcif Tissue Int* 1997;61:S19-22.
115. Agnusdei D, Bufalino L. Efficacy of ipriflavone in established osteoporosis and long-term safety. *Calcif Tissue Int* 1997;61:S23-7.
116. Gambacciani M, Ciaponi M, Cappagli B et al. Effects of combined low dose of the isoflavone derivative ipriflavone and estrogen replacement on bone mineral density and metabolism in postmenopausal women. *Maturitas* 1997;28:75-81.
117. Kovacs AB. Efficacy of ipriflavone in the prevention and treatment of postmenopausal osteoporosis. *Agents Actions* 1994;41:86-7.
118. Valente M, Bufalino L, Castiglione GN et al. Effects of 1-year treatment with ipriflavone on bone in postmenopausal women with low bone mass. *Calcif Tissue Int* 1994;54:377-80.
119. Agnusdei D, Crepaldi G, Isaia G et al. A double blind, placebo-controlled trial of ipriflavone for prevention of postmenopausal spinal bone loss. *Calcif Tissue Int* 1997;61:142-7.
120. Gennari C, Agnusdei D, Crepaldi G et al. Effect of ipriflavone–a synthetic derivative of natural isoflavones–on bone mass loss in the early years after menopause. *Menopause* 1998;5:9-15.
121. Ohta H, Komukai S, Makita K et al. Effects of 1-year ipriflavone treatment on lumbar bone mineral density and bone metabolic markers in postmenopausal women with low bone mass. *Horm Res* 1999;51:178-83.
122. Katase K, Kato T, Hirai Y et al. Effects of ipriflavone on bone loss following a bilateral ovariectomy and menopause: a randomized placebo-controlled study. *Calcif Tissue Int* 2001;69:73-7.
123. Zhang X, Li SW, Wu JF et al. Effects of ipriflavone on postmenopausal syndrome and osteoporosis. *Gynecol Endocrinol* 2010;26:76-80.
124. Alexandersen P, Toussaint A, Christiansen C et al. Ipriflavone in the treatment of postmenopausal osteoporosis: a randomized controlled trial. *JAMA* 2001;285:1482-8.
125. Vermeer C, Schurgers LJ. A comprehensive review of vitamin K and vitamin K antagonists. *Hematol Oncol Clin North Am* 2000;14:339-53.
126. Shearer MJ, Bach A, Kohlmeier M. Chemistry, nutritional sources, tissue distribution and metabolism of vitamin K with special reference to bone health. *J Nutr* 1996;126:1181S-6S.
127. Weber P. Management of osteoporosis: is there a role for vitamin K? *Int J Vitam Nutr Res* 1997;67:350-6.
128. Cockayne S, Adamson J, Lanham-New S et al. Vitamin K and the prevention of fractures: systematic review and meta-analysis of randomized controlled trials. *Arch Intern Med* 2006;166:1256-61.
129. Huang ZB, Wan SL, Lu YJ et al. Does vitamin K2 play a role in the prevention and treatment of osteoporosis for postmenopausal women: a meta-analysis of randomized controlled trials. *Osteoporos Int* 2015;26:1175-86.
130. Knapen MH, Schurgers LJ, Vermeer C. Vitamin K2 supplementation improves hip bone geometry and bone strength indices in postmenopausal women. *Osteoporos Int* 2007;18:963-72.
131. Cheung AM, Tile L, Lee Y et al. Vitamin K supplementation in postmenopausal women with osteopenia (ECKO trial): a randomized controlled trial. *PLoS Med* 2008;5:e196.
132. Emaus N, Gjesdal CG, Almas B et al. Vitamin K2 supplementation does not influence bone loss in early menopausal women: a randomized double-blind placebo-controlled trial. *Osteoporosis Int* 2010;21:1731-40.
133. Ishida Y, Kawai S. Comparative efficacy of hormone replacement therapy, etidronate, calcitonin, alfacalcidol, and vitamin K in postmenopausal women with osteoporosis: the Yamaguchi Osteoporosis Prevention Study. *Am J Med* 2004;117:549-55.
134. Purwosunu Y, Muharram, Rachman IA et al. Vitamin K2 treatment for postmenopausal osteoporosis in Indonesia. *J Obstet Gynaecol Res* 2006;32:230-4.
135. Wuttke W, Gorkow C, Seidlova-Wuttke D. Effects of black cohosh (Cimicifuga racemosa) on bone turnover, vaginal mucosa, and various blood parameters in postmenopausal women: a double-blind, placebo-controlled, and conjugated estrogens-controlled study. *Menopause* 2006;13:185-96.

Osteoporosis—What You Need to Know

Osteoporosis is a condition where a person's bones are thin and can break easily. Both men and women can have osteoporosis but it is more common in women. The risk of getting osteoporosis increases for women after menopause. The risk is also greater for people with a family history of osteoporosis and people who take certain kinds of medicine.

How can you prevent osteoporosis?

Talk to your healthcare provider to find out whether you are at risk for osteoporosis. To prevent osteoporosis, follow these steps:

- Make sure you get enough calcium and vitamin D every day to protect your bones. The best way to get your daily calcium and vitamin D is through your diet. Table 1 shows you how much calcium is recommended. Assume that you are getting about 300 mg a day from any of the foods you eat, since there are small amounts of calcium in many foods. Table 2 lists foods that are a good source of calcium.
- If you don't get enough calcium and vitamin D from food, begin taking a supplement. Your healthcare provider can recommend one that is right for you.
- Strengthening your core muscles will help improve your balance and minimize your risk for falling.
- Get regular exercise, such as moderate to vigorous walking, to help strengthen your bones. Try to exercise at least 3 times a week for 20–30 minutes.
- Limit your alcohol (less than 2 drinks each day) and caffeine intake (3–4 cups of coffee per day). Quitting smoking may also reduce your risk.

Table 1: **How Much Calcium Do You Need?**

Age, years	Recommended intake of elemental calcium (each day)
4–8	1000 mg
9–18	1300 mg
19–50	1000 mg
Pregnant or breastfeeding women	1000 mg
50+	1200 mg

What can you do if you have osteoporosis?

- Make sure you are getting enough calcium and vitamin D every day.
- Before you begin an exercise program, talk to your healthcare provider.
- Talk to your healthcare provider about medicines that can help to make your bones stronger.

Table 2: Selected Foods That Are High in Calcium

Food	Serving Size	Calcium[a]
Beans, baked	one-half cup/125 mL	75 mg
Bread, whole wheat	2 slices	40 mg
Broccoli, cooked	three-quarters cup/185 mL	50 mg
Cheese (cheddar, edam, gouda)	1.25 inches/3 cm cube	245 mg
Cheese, mozzarella	1.25 inches/3 cm cube	200 mg
Cottage cheese (2%, 1%)	one-half cup/125 mL	75 mg
Figs, dried	10	150 mg
Ice cream	one-half cup/125 mL	80 mg
Milk (2%, 1%, skim, chocolate)	1 cup/250mL	300 mg
Orange juice, fortified	1 cup/250 mL	335 mg
Rice or soy beverage, fortified	1 cup/250 mL	300 mg
Salmon, with bones, canned	3.5 ounces/105 g	240 mg
Sardines, with bones	2 ounces/55 g	200 mg
Tofu, with calcium sulfate	3 ounces/84 g	130 mg
Yogurt, plain	three-quarters cup/185 mL	295 mg

[a] Approximate values.

For more information on osteoporosis, contact Osteoporosis Canada at: www.osteoporosis.ca.

Chapter 48

Sports Injuries

Lily Lum, BScPharm, CSPI

Pathophysiology

Participation in sports activities and exercise programs is increasing as people become more health conscious. Although associated with health benefits, sports and exercise can also cause injuries.[1,2]

Individuals in all age groups benefit from regular exercise when it is properly performed. In people over 45 years, the benefits of exercise (e.g., prevention of coronary heart disease and osteoporosis) outweigh the risk of sports-related injuries.

Based on the increasing rate of obesity, Health Canada recommends that children and teenagers participate in at least 60 minutes of moderate- to vigorous-intensity physical activity daily.[3] Participation in sports is also encouraged. However, children and adolescents may be particularly at risk for sports injuries for several reasons. Their bones, muscles, tendons and ligaments are still growing, making them more prone to injury. Young athletes of similar age vary greatly in size and physical maturity; they may try to perform at levels beyond their ability to keep up with peers. Other factors contributing to an increased risk of sports injury include improper technique, poorly fitting protective equipment and training errors.[4,5,6]

Sports-related injuries are varied and can be caused by trauma, overuse of specific parts of the body such as muscles or joints, and environmental factors.[5] Acute injuries such as ligament sprains and muscle strains are usually caused by sudden trauma and are more likely to occur in contact sports. Overuse or chronic injuries are more subtle and are most commonly associated with sports that involve repetitive movements. The 3Fs or "terrible toos" acronym—too fast, too far and too frequent—is often used to describe the cause of overuse injuries.[1] Some of the more common sports-related injuries such as strains and sprains, overuse injuries (e.g., Achilles tendinitis, bursitis, plantar fasciitis, shin splints and tennis elbow) and stress fractures are defined below.

Sports injuries can also be caused by environmental factors; e.g., heat stroke can occur during participation in outdoor sports activities during hot temperatures.[1] For further information, see Chapter 9: Heat-related Disorders.

Common Sports Injuries

Bursitis is the inflammation of a bursa. Bursae are tiny, fluid-containing, sac-like structures that are located wherever there might be friction, such as between bones and the muscles and tendons near joints (Figure 1). When they become inflamed, movement or pressure is painful. Sports-related bursitis occurs most commonly in the elbow, knee and shoulder.

A sprain is an injury to a ligament caused by overstretching or twisting. In the ankle, a common area for sprains, it is mainly the lateral ligaments of the joint that are involved. Symptoms include pain, swelling and tenderness, with subsequent bruising around the injury. Symptomatically, severe sprains may be difficult to differentiate from fractures, and an x-ray may be needed to make a firm diagnosis.[1,5]

Figure 1: **Knee Joint—Sagital Section**

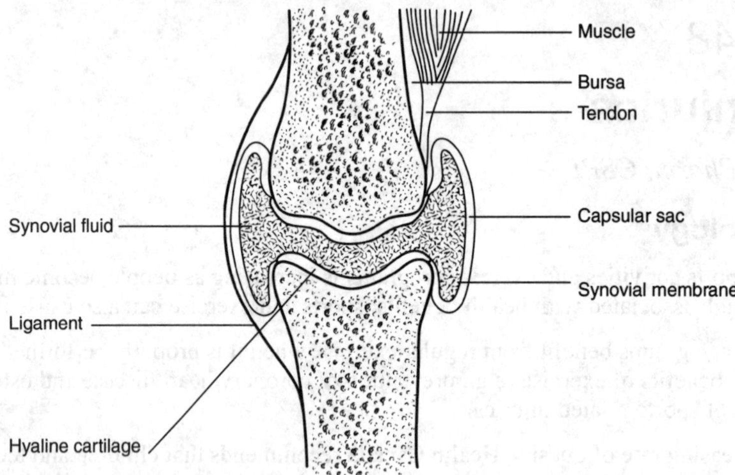

A strain is an injury to a muscle and is also referred to as a torn or pulled muscle. It is usually caused by overstretching and is characterized by pain and swelling. Muscle strains vary in severity, from damage to the fibres with the muscle sheath left intact, to complete rupture of the muscle.[1,7]

Plantar fasciitis is a common condition causing heel pain; it involves inflammation of the plantar fascia, the tough, fibrous band of tissue that runs along the sole of the foot. Inflammation usually occurs following increased or repetitive activity such as jogging.[7,8]

Shin splints, also known as medial tibial stress syndrome, are inflammation of the muscles, tendons and periosteum (bone tissue) around the tibia or shinbone. Pain occurs along the inner edge of the tibia where the muscles attach to the bone. Shin splints are the result of repetitive activity and often occur following sudden changes in frequency, duration or intensity of physical activity. Having flat feet or exercising with inappropriate footwear can contribute to the development of shin splints.[9]

Stress fractures are tiny cracks in bones that often result from repeated, excessive impact. Athletes required to jump repetitively (e.g., gymnasts, basketball players) often get stress fractures.[7,9] They usually occur in the feet, ankles and legs although any bone can suffer a stress fracture. An individual may not even notice when a stress fracture initially occurs. The pain decreases with rest and increases over time, getting worse when pressure is applied during activity. It starts progressively earlier in the workout, becoming so severe that it prohibits exercise and persists even during rest. The area may or may not show signs of tenderness and swelling. Stress fractures can be mistaken for shin splints because both can cause mid-calf discomfort. However, stress fractures are more serious than shin splints, the pain lasts longer and the injury takes longer to heal.

Tendinitis refers to acute inflammation of a tendon, the thick fibrous cord that attaches muscle to bone. Two common examples of tendinitis are Achilles tendinitis and tennis elbow. Achilles tendinitis is inflammation of the Achilles tendon which connects the heel to the calf muscle.[9] A patient with Achilles tendinitis experiences pain and tenderness just above the heel.

Tennis elbow, also known as lateral epicondylitis, is inflammation of the tendons attached to the outside/lateral side of the elbow at the bony prominence of the arm bone.[7] It commonly occurs during racquet sports (such as tennis) and activities that require repetitive, one-sided movements. The patient experiences pain and tenderness outside of the affected area, at and below the elbow joint. With repeated overuse, degenerative micro-tears occur in the tendon, resulting in chronic epicondylosis.

While inflammation may be present with acute tendon injuries such as tendinitis, chronic injuries are more correctly referred to as tendinosis or tendinopathy. The pathology of chronic tendinopathies is related not to inflammation but to degenerative changes occurring in the tendon over time due to microscopic tears that fail to heal properly.

Goals of Therapy

- Provide relief of symptoms
- Promote healing of the injury
- Prevent re-injury or aggravation of the injury

Patient Assessment

An assessment plan for patients suffering from musculoskeletal sports injuries is illustrated in Figure 2. Symptoms of selected non-soft tissue injuries that require immediate medical attention are described in Table 1.

Table 1: Selected Injuries Requiring Immediate Medical Attention[7]

Injury	Symptoms that Warrant Immediate Medical Attention
Eye injury[10]	Blurred vision, loss of vision, moderate to severe eye discomfort or pain
Head injury, e.g., concussion[11]	Confusion, amnesia, headache, loss of consciousness after injury, tinnitus, drowsiness, dizziness, nausea, vomiting, seizures, unusual eye movements or slurred speech
Nosebleed[12]	Bleeding lasting longer than 20 min
Tympanic membrane perforation (ruptured eardrum)[13]	Earache, partial hearing loss, slight bleeding or discharge from ear

Prevention

Proper conditioning and training prevent many sports-related injuries. Muscle pain and stiffness commonly occur 24 hours after unaccustomed intense physical activity.[7] Appropriate warm-up exercises, stretching and cooling down (gradually slowing down before stopping the exercise) should be routinely performed. Warmed-up muscles are more pliable and less likely to tear. Stretching allows the muscles to lengthen so that they can contract and perform more effectively. Cooling down can prevent dizziness and fainting. In a person who exercises vigorously and suddenly stops, blood can pool in the dilated leg veins, causing dizziness and fainting. Cooling down maintains increased circulation and helps clear the build up of lactic acid in the bloodstream.[9] A gradual increase in the intensity and duration of workouts and adequate fluid replacement are also important preventive measures. For more information on hydration in the athlete, see Chapter 42: Sports Nutrition.

Warning signs of impending injury include extreme fatigue, pain and lack of enthusiasm for training.[1] Protective equipment (e.g., helmet, eye protection, mouth guard, knee and wrist pads) and proper footwear are essential for those participating in sports with a high risk of falls (e.g., in-line skating) or those requiring direct contact with playing equipment or other players (e.g., boxing, football).[5,14] Note that eyeglasses or sunglasses do not provide adequate eye protection unless they are specifically designed for use in sporting activities.

Nonpharmacologic Therapy

The 4 essentials of early management of soft-tissue injuries can be remembered using the acronym RICE: **R**est, **I**ce, **C**ompression, **E**levation (Table 2).[1,5,9]

After 48 hours have passed and the initial swelling has subsided, the RICE regimen can be replaced by heat, early mobilization, massage and/or rehabilitation with physical therapy if necessary.[9]

Table 2: **RICE Regimen**

Rest	Immobilization is recommended for at least the first 24 hours to avoid aggravation of the injury. If long-term rest is indicated, the unaffected joint(s) should be exercised to prevent tissue atrophy and loss of coordination. Rest for a prolonged period of time is usually discouraged for muscle injuries.
Ice	The application of cold to an injury reduces local blood flow by constricting blood vessels, limiting the swelling. Apply cold therapy at regular intervals, allowing a few hours between treatments.
Compression	An elasticized bandage applied to an injured area for at least the first 24 hours can reduce swelling, support a weak joint or provide a protective layer for wounds.
Elevation	The injured area should be raised above the level of the heart to help drain fluid and reduce swelling.

Heat vs. Cold Therapy

Should patients apply heat or cold therapy to a sports injury? As a general rule, the application of cold is the preferred immediate treatment (first 24–48 hours) for most acute musculoskeletal injuries.[15] Sources of **cold therapy** include ice bags (putting crushed ice in a thick plastic bag), commercial cold gel packs or bags of frozen peas or corn.[16] Recommendations for duration and frequency of cold therapy application vary considerably.[17] The application time varies depending on the body part and comfort but usually ranges from 10–30 minutes. Apply cold at regular intervals throughout the waking hours of the day, allowing a few hours between treatments. Areas with little body fat (bony areas such as the knee, ankle and elbow) do not tolerate cold as well as fatty areas (such as thighs and buttocks). For bony areas, keep application time to the lower end of the range (10 minutes); double the time when applying to fatty areas. Applying ice directly to the skin or for too long can cause frostbite and tissue damage. A thin towel can be placed between the ice bag and skin to prevent frostbite. Use cold therapy with caution in patients with poor circulation, such as those with diabetes or Raynaud's disease, since these patients already have reduced local blood flow.[16]

Heat therapy (thermotherapy) is recommended after the first 48 hours when the swelling has subsided, and during the chronic rehabilitative phases of the injury.[18] Local heat produces analgesia by affecting free nerve endings, decreases the incidence of painful muscle spasms by relaxing muscles, and reduces joint stiffness by decreasing synovial fluid viscosity. Heat causes vasodilation, producing increased blood flow, which in turn helps provide a greater local supply of nutrients, oxygen, antibodies, leukocytes and enzymes to the injured area. Waste products from the inflammatory process are transported away with the increased blood circulation.[15] Heat may be applied for 20–30 minutes, every 2–4 hours as needed. Contraindications to the use of local heat therapy include patients who are unconscious and those with impaired skin sensitivity, poor circulation or open wounds.[15,18] Sources of local heat therapy include hot water bottles, electric heating pads, commercial heat packs and infrared heat lamps.[15] Patients must take care to avoid burns from the use of heat therapy products. Hot water bottles and heat packs should be wrapped with a towel or cloth for comfort and safety. Heating pads and heat lamps should be kept on low to moderate settings.[18]

Pharmacologic Therapy

Therapies used to treat minor sports injuries are listed in Table 4.

For more information on pharmacologic therapy for sports injuries, consult the *Compendium of Therapeutic Choices*:Sports Injuries.

For comparative ingredients of nonprescription products, consult the *Compendium of Products for Minor Ailments*—Analgesic Products: External Analgesics, Internal Analgesics and Antipyretics.

Oral Analgesics

Oral analgesics such as **acetaminophen** and **NSAIDs** can provide effective relief of musculoskeletal pain.[1,5,9,20] They may be useful for acute as well as chronic injuries. Advise patients to take the lowest effective dose to relieve their pain and inflammation. Acetaminophen or NSAIDs can be given concurrently with opioids for an additive analgesic effect. **Codeine** can be found in combination products for the treatment of moderate or moderately severe pain. When taken alone in usual doses, e.g., 15–30 mg, codeine is no more effective than ASA or acetaminophen.[21] Codeine is regarded as second-line therapy for management of sports injuries. Opioids are often drugs of choice in severe acute pain or cancer pain but have limited use for most sports injuries. For injuries such as bone fractures, which are often extremely painful, short-term use of acetaminophen plus codeine combinations may be warranted.[20] In patients with concussion, avoid opioids so that clouding of the patient's mental status on neurologic exam does not occur.[22]

Muscle Relaxants

Muscle relaxants (e.g., **methocarbamol**, **chlorzoxazone**) are generally intended to provide pain relief when muscle spasm is a component of an acute injury. However, muscle relaxants are not routinely recommended and are not considered first-line therapy in acute musculoskeletal injuries because of their limited effectiveness in providing pain relief.[23] Fatal hepatotoxicity has been reported with chlorzoxazone use.[24]

External Analgesics

External analgesics (e.g., **methyl salicylate**, **menthol**, **camphor**, **capsaicin**) are traditional remedies for the treatment of general aches and pains. Their value is limited but they may be useful during rehabilitation as cooling or heating rubs or as accompaniments to massage therapy.[1,25] Although not often prescribed, patients frequently purchase these products for self-treatment.[20]

Some patients may experience skin reactions such as rash or blisters or rarely, serious burns. External analgesics should not be applied to acute injuries if there is bleeding or if the wounds are open or covered by dressings, since this can further irritate the wound area.[1] They should not be used more than 3 or 4 times a day. External analgesics should not be used concurrently with thermotherapy devices as burns may result.[26] If patients experience pain, swelling or burning from the external analgesic, advise them to stop using the product and seek immediate medical attention.[27]

Topical NSAIDs

Although oral NSAIDs play a well-established role in reducing pain, swelling and inflammation resulting from sports injuries, the use of topical NSAIDs is less well entrenched.[28,29,30] It is theorized that topical application minimizes the risk of side effects associated with systemic therapy (e.g., gastrointestinal toxicity).

A meta-analysis of 86 randomized, placebo-controlled trials of transdermal NSAIDs involving 10 160 patients concluded that topical NSAIDs are effective in relieving pain in acute and chronic conditions.[31] Another meta-analysis of 47 randomised, double-blind, active or placebo-controlled trials involving 3455 patients concluded that topical NSAIDs were effective and safe in treating acute pain in musculoskeletal conditions.[32]

Topical **diclofenac** is available as a 1.5% solution which is indicated for osteoarthritis of the knee, and as a 1.16% or 2.32% gel indicated for the treatment of acute pain caused by injury to joints or muscles.[33] Pharmacists can also extemporaneously compound topical NSAID products. Special commercial bases (e.g., Phlojel, Diffusimax) are available for compounding of topical NSAIDs. NSAIDs commonly incorporated into topical formulations include **diclofenac**, **ibuprofen** and **ketoprofen**.[34,35,36,37,38]

Corticosteroid Injections

Local corticosteroid injection therapy has been used to treat painful conditions involving tendinitis despite limited evidence of effectiveness. The number of local corticosteroid injections is usually limited to 3 per year due to risk of atrophy, tendon rupture and osteoporosis. Corticosteroid injections should be avoided in Achilles tendonitis, where risk of rupture is highest. Other complications of local corticosteroid injections include temporary flare of pain and inflammation, joint infection, nerve damage and loss of skin pigmentation around the injection site.[39,40,41]

Vapocoolants

Some topical anesthetic preparations, known as vapocoolants or refrigerants (e.g., **ethyl chloride**, Spray and Stretch), may be useful when applied topically to control the pain associated with injuries such as sprained ankles and bursitis. Side effects appear to be minimal although cutaneous sensitization may occur. Spray and Stretch (**pentafluoropropane** 95%/**tetrafluoroethane** 5%) is used with the "spray and stretch" technique: the product is sprayed onto the injured area, blocking pain impulses so the muscle can be stretched to its normal length in a pain-free state.[42,43]

Monitoring of Therapy

Table 3 provides a monitoring plan framework for soft tissue sports injuries, which should be individualized.

Table 3: **Monitoring of Therapy for Soft Tissue Sports Injuries**

Symptoms	Monitoring	Endpoint of Therapy	Actions
Pain and swelling from muscle sprain or strain and overuse injuries	Patient: Daily Healthcare practitioner: After 14 days of therapy	Decrease in pain and swelling over a 14-day period. The injured area can gradually be used with minimal discomfort, and daily activities can eventually be performed without pain.	If pain symptoms have not improved after 14 days of self-care, patient requires referral to an appropriate healthcare practitioner for further assessment. If pain is worsening despite drug therapy, patient requires immediate referral to an appropriate healthcare practitioner.

Figure 2: **Assessment of Patients with Musculoskeletal Sports Injurie**

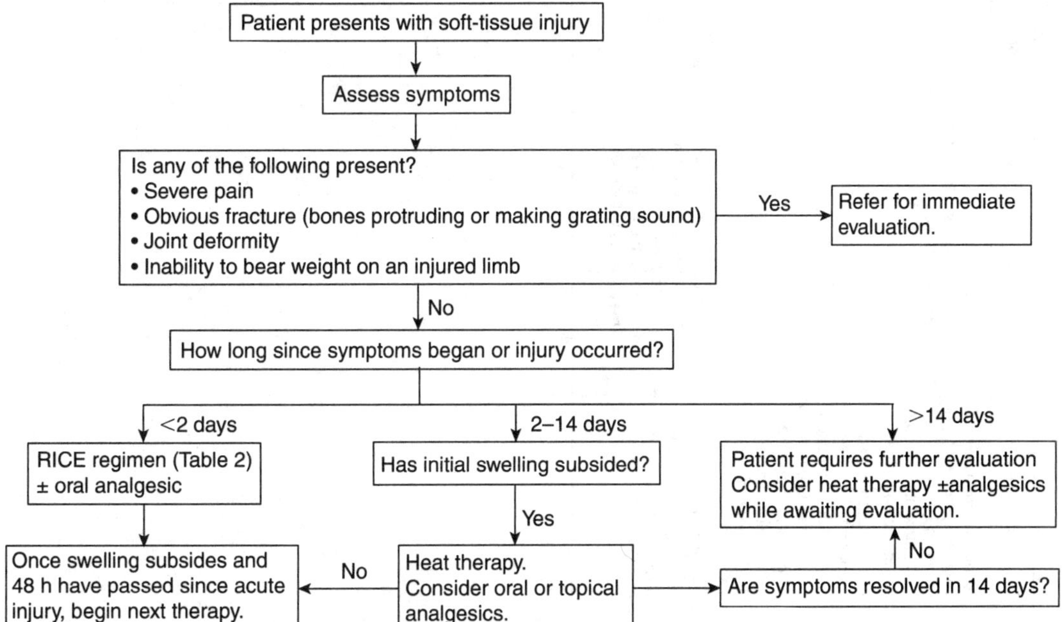

Abbreviations: RICE = **R**est, **I**ce, **C**ompression, **E**levation

Table 4: Selected Drug Therapies for Sports Injuries

Class	Drug	Dosage	Adverse Effects	Drug Interactions	Comments	Cost[a]
Analgesics, oral	*acetaminophen* Atasol Preparations Tylenol generics	325–500 mg Q3H PRN po *or* 325–650 mg Q4H PRN po *or* 650–1000 mg Q6H PRN po Maximum dose: 4 g/day	Hepatotoxicity associated with chronic use, especially at high doses.	Isoniazid, phenytoin may decrease acetaminophen effect and increase hepatotoxicity; decreased effect of zidovudine. Acetaminophen has been reported to increase INR in warfarin-treated patients.[19] Check INR if acetaminophen ≥2 g/day is used for ≥3 consecutive days. Adjust warfarin dosage as required.	Increased risk of hepatotoxicity with chronic alcohol intake.	$
	acetaminophen caffeine codeine 8 mg Atasol with Codeine generics	1–2 tablets Q4H PRN po Maximum: 4 g/day of acetaminophen from all sources	See acetaminophen. Dizziness, drowsiness, nausea, vomiting, constipation.	See acetaminophen Alcohol, CNS depressants (increased CNS effects of codeine).	Use of opioids for a long time or in high doses may cause dependency; stopping the drug abruptly may lead to withdrawal symptoms.	$

Class	Drug	Dosage	Adverse Effects	Drug Interactions	Comments	Cost[a]
NSAIDs, oral	*ASA* Aspirin Coated Aspirin Entrophen generics	325–500 mg Q3H PRN po *or* 325–650 mg Q4H PRN po *or* 650–1000 mg Q6H PRN po	GI: Dyspepsia, epigastric pain, nausea/vomiting, diarrhea, gastric and duodenal ulcers, GI bleeding. Cardiovascular: MI, stroke, heart failure, fluid retention, hypertension. Nephrotoxicity may occur; avoid NSAIDs in patients with severe renal impairment (ClCr <30 mL/min). CNS: Dizziness, drowsiness, headache, tinnitus, confusion (especially in the elderly); CNS effects may be dose related and respond to decreased dosage. Minor or serious skin rashes, pruritus.	Increased risk of bleeding with anticoagulants (e.g., warfarin) or antiplatelet drugs (e.g., clopidogrel); monitor INR more frequently and watch for signs of bleeding; consider alternative therapy. May decrease effect of antihypertensives. May decrease renal clearance of lithium; monitor lithium levels when NSAID added. Increased risk of GI bleeding when used with SSRIs.	Avoid use in third trimester of pregnancy. Avoid in children, particularly those <16 y with chickenpox or flu-like symptoms because of possible association with Reye's syndrome. May require discontinuation prior to surgery to avoid bleeding. Avoid in patients with asthma or at risk of peptic ulcer.	$
	ibuprofen Advil Advil Liqui-Gels Motrin Motrin IB generics	200–400 mg Q4–6H PRN po Maximum dose for self-care: 1200 mg/day Maximum dose: 2400 mg/day	Abdominal discomfort, epigastric pain, nausea, diarrhea, dizziness, drowsiness.	Enhanced effect of anticoagulants; diminished effect of diuretics, antihypertensives; increased serum levels of digoxin, lithium.	Caution in ASA-sensitive patients. Avoid use in third trimester of pregnancy. Avoid in patients with asthma or at risk of peptic ulcer. Increased risk of stroke or serious CV events at doses ≥2400 mg/day. Doses ≥2400 mg/day should not be used in patients with a history of CV events or with risk factors for CV disease.[44]	$

(cont'd)

Table 4: **Selected Drug Therapies for Sports Injuries** *(cont'd)*

Class	Drug	Dosage	Adverse Effects	Drug Interactions	Comments	Cost[a]
	naproxen Naprosyn generics	250–500 mg BID po	See ibuprofen.	See ibuprofen.	See ibuprofen.	$$
	naproxen sodium Aleve generics	220–440 mg Q8–12H PRN po Maximum dose for self-care: 440 mg/day	See ibuprofen.	See ibuprofen.	See ibuprofen.	$
NSAIDs, topical	*diclofenac diethylamine* Voltaren Emulgel Voltaren Emulgel Extra Strength	Apply TID-QID to affected area Patient may require further assessment if no improvement after 7 days	Local irritation, rarely, systemic effects (headache, GI irritation, bronchospasm), hepatotoxicity.	Not recommended in combination with other NSAIDs due to potential of additive side effects. Plasma levels of diclofenac are not significant after topical application resulting in decreased risk of drug interactions; caution with medications that may interact with oral diclofenac.	Available as 1.16% and 2.32% gel. Wash hands after application. Do not apply near mucous membranes or on broken skin. Do not cover with tight or occlusive dressing. Do not place heating devices (e.g., hot water bottle, heating pad) on skin after applying product.	$
	diclofenac sodium Pennsaid generics	Apply TID–QID	Skin dryness or irritation, hypersensitivity. Serious GI toxicity has not been seen to date in clinical trials.	See diclofenac.	Available as 1.5% lotion. Do not apply near mucous membranes or on broken skin. Do not cover with tight or occlusive dressing. Do not place heating devices (e.g., hot water bottle, heating pad) on skin after applying product.	$$$$

[a] Cost of 1 week of therapy or smallest available pack size; includes drug cost only.

Dosage adjustment may be required in renal impairment.

Abbreviations: ASA = acetylsalicylic acid; CNS = central nervous system; GI = gastrointestinal

Legend: $ <$10 $$ $10–20 $$$ $20–30 $$$$ $30–40

Resource Tips

Johns Hopkins Medicine. Health Library. *Overview of sports injuries*. Available from: www.hopkinsmedicine.org/healthlibrary/conditions/adult/mens_health/overview_of_sports_injuries_85,P09509/.

U.S. National Institutes of Health. Department of Health and Human Services. National Institute of Arthritis and Musculoskeletal and Skin Diseases (NIAMS). *Handout on health: Sports injuries*. November 2013. Available from: www.niams.nih.gov/Health_Info/Sports_Injuries/default.asp.

Suggested Readings

Harries M et al., eds. *Oxford textbook of sports medicine*. 2nd ed. Oxford: Oxford University Press; 1998.

Mellion MB, Putukian M, Madden CC, eds. *Sports medicine secrets*. 3rd ed. Philadelphia: Hanley & Belfus; 2003.

Schwellnus M, ed. *The Olympic textbook of medicine in sport*. Chichester, West Sussex: Wiley-Blackwell; 2008.

References

1. Nykamp D. Sports injuries. *US Pharm* 1992;17:34-55.
2. Matheson GO. Balancing sport risk and health benefits. *Phys Sportsmed* 1999;27:3-7.
3. Canadian Society for Exercise Physiology. *Canadian physical activity guidelines*. Available from: www.csep.ca/guidelines. Accessed April 26, 2016.
4. Cassas KJ, Cassettari-Wayhs A. Childhood and adolescent sports-related overuse injuries. *Am Fam Physician* 2006;73:1014-22.
5. Kayne S. Sport and exercise. In: Harman RJ, ed. *Handbook of pharmacy health education*. 2nd ed. London: Pharmaceutical Press; 1998. p. 191-232.
6. U.S. National Institutes of Health. Department of Health and Human Services. National Institute of Arthritis and Musculoskeletal and Skin Diseases (NIAMS). *Handout on health: Sports injuries*. November 2013. Available from: www.niams.nih.gov/Health_Info/Sports_Injuries/default.asp. Accessed April 26, 2016.
7. Johns Hopkins Medicine. Health Library. *Sports injuries: overview of sports injuries*. Available from: www.hopkinsmedicine.org/healthlibrary/conditions/adult/mens_health/sports_injuries_85,P00725/. Accessed April 26, 2016.
8. Edwards C, Stilman P. Musculoskeletal disorders. *Pharm J* 1993;251:733-8.
9. Sports injuries. In: Berkow R, ed. *Merck manual of medical information*. Whitehouse Station: Merck Research Laboratories; 1997. p. 286-302.
10. U.S. National Library of Medicine. National Institutes of Health. MedlinePlus. *Eye emergencies*. Available from: www.nlm.nih.gov/medlineplus/ency/article/000054.htm. Accessed April 26, 2016.
11. Mayo Clinic. *Concussion*. Available from: www.mayoclinic.org/diseases-conditions/concussion/basics/symptoms/con-20019272.
12. U.S. National Library of Medicine. National Institutes of Health. MedlinePlus. *Nosebleed*. Available from: www.nlm.nih.gov/medlineplus/ency/article/003106.htm. Accessed April 26, 2016.
13. Mayo Clinic. *Ruptured eardrum (perforated eardrum)*. Available from: www.mayoclinic.org/diseases-conditions/ruptured-eardrum/multimedia/ruptured-eardrum/img-20007671. Accessed April 26, 2016.
14. Roberts WO. Keeping sports safe: physicians should take the lead. *Phys Sportsmed* 1998;26:25-8.
15. Sherman M. A primer on use of hot or cold therapy. *US Pharm* 1987;12:72-81.
16. Stamford B. Giving injuries the cold treatment. *Phys Sportsmed* 1996;24:99-102.
17. MacAuley D. Do textbooks agree on their advice on ice? *Clin J Sport Med* 2001;11:67-72.
18. Pray WS. Use of local heat for minor injuries. *US Pharm* 1993;18:39-45.
19. Lopes RD, Horowitz JD, Garcia DA et al. Warfarin and acetaminophen interaction: a summary of the evidence and biologic plausibility. *Blood* 2011;118:6269-73.
20. Thornton JS. Pain relief for acute soft-tissue injuries. *Phys Sportsmed* 1997;25:108-14.
21. Drugs for pain. *Med Lett Drugs Ther* 1998;40:79-84.
22. WebMD. Bernhardt DT. *Concussion medication. Overview, treatment, medication*. Available from: emedicine.medscape.com/article/92095-medication. Accessed April 26, 2016.
23. Ontario Musculoskeletal Therapeutics Review Panel. *Ontario treatment guidelines for osteoarthritis, rheumatoid arthritis, and acute musculoskeletal injury*. 1st ed. Toronto: Queen's Printer of Ontario; 2000.
24. Chlorzoxazone hepatotoxicity. *Med Lett Drugs Ther* 1996;38:46.
25. Derry S, Matthews PR, Whiffen PJ et al. Salicylate-containing rubefacients for acute and chronic musculoskeletal pain in adults. *Cochrane Database Syst Rev* 2014;11:CD007403.
26. Injuries to muscles, ligaments and tendons. In: Pray WS. *Nonprescription product therapeutics*. 1st ed. Philadelphia: Lippincott Williams & Wilkins; 1999. p. 295-309.
27. U.S. Food and Drug Administration. *FDA Drug Safety Communication: Rare cases of serious burns with the use of over-the-counter topical muscle and joint pain relievers*. Available from: fda.gov/Drugs/DrugSafety/ucm318858.htm. Accessed April 26, 2016.
28. Heyneman CA. Topical nonsteroidal antiinflammatory drugs for acute soft tissue injuries. *Ann Pharmacother* 1995;29:780-2.
29. More topical NSAIDs: worth the rub? *Drug Ther Bull* 1990;28:27-8.
30. Buchanan NM. Is there a place for topical NSAIDs? *Pharm J* 1997;259:294-5.

31. Moore RA, Tramer MR, Carroll D et al. Quantitative systematic review of topically applied non-steroidal anti-inflammatory drugs. *BMJ* 1998;316:333-8.
32. Massey T, Derry S, Moore RA et al. Topical NSAIDs for acute pain in adults. *Cochrane Database Syst Rev* 2010;(6):CD007402.
33. Cupp, M. New drug: Voltaren emulgel (diclofenac gel). *Pharmacist's Letter/Prescriber's Letter*. Detail-Document #241218. Stockton: Therapeutic Research Center; 2008.
34. Hudson S. Compounding for athletes: successful sports compounds. *Int J Pharm Compound* 1999;3:382-3.
35. What is Diffusimax? Drug Information and Research Centre. *New Drugs/Drug News* 1999;17:3.
36. Allen LV. Ketoprofen gel. *US Pharm* 1993;18:98-100.
37. U.S. Food and Drug Administration. *FDA issues warning letters to marketers of topical ibuprofen drug products*. August 20, 2009. Available from: www.fda.gov/NewsEvents/Newsroom/PressAnnouncements/ucm179689.htm. Accessed April 26, 2016.
38. Patient.co.uk. *Ibuprofen (gel for pain relief (Ibuderm, Ibugel, Ibuleve)*. Available from: patient.info/medicine/ibuprofen-gel-for-pain-relief-ibuderm-ibugel-ibuleve. Accessed April 26, 2016.
39. Pfenninger JL. Injections of joints and soft tissue: part I. General guidelines. *Am Fam Physician* 1991;44:1196-202.
40. Sherman M. Health-care team provides support for tennis elbow. *Can Pharm J* 1982;115:351-3.
41. Mayo Clinic. *Cortisone shots*. Available from: www.mayoclinic.org/tests-procedures/cortisone-shots/basics/risks/prc-20014455. Accessed on April 26, 2016.
42. Drugdex Editorial Staff. Fluorimethane spray availability (drug consult). In: Conner CR, Rumack BH, eds. *Drugdex information system*. Denver: Micromedex [edition expired 2/28/97].
43. Gebauer Company. *Gebauer's Spray and Stretch*. Available from: www.gebauer.com/products/spray-and-stretch/product/. Accessed April 26, 2016.
44. Government of Canada. Healthy Canadians. *New safety information for prescription-strength ibuprofen: risk of heart attack and stroke at high doses*. Available from: www.healthycanadians.gc.ca/recall-alert-rappel-avis/hc-sc/2015/53055a-eng.php.

Sports Injuries—What You Need to Know

Participation in sports and exercise can improve your health but it can also lead to sports injuries.

Some common sports injuries:

- Achilles tendinitis: Painful inflammation of the Achilles tendon (which connects the heel to the calf muscle).
- Muscle strains: Torn or pulled muscles.
- Plantar fasciitis: Heel pain.
- Shin splints: Sore, stiff areas along the shin bones above the ankles.

How to prevent sport injuries:

Keep sports activities and exercise safe. The following tips can help prevent injuries:

- Do warm-up exercises and stretching before you begin any sport or exercise program.
- Slowly increase the intensity and length of your workouts.
- Drink enough fluids.
- Wear appropriate clothing and protective equipment, especially in high-risk sports activities.

What to do if you have a sports injury:

If you get a sports injury, remember **RICE**—Rest, Ice, Compression and Elevation. **RICE** tells you what to do for the first 2 days after an injury or until the swelling goes away.

- **Rest:** Rest the injured area to prevent the injury from getting worse.
- **Ice:** Apply ice every few hours to reduce the swelling. If a bony area such as the knee has been hurt, keep the ice on for only 10 minutes; otherwise keep it on for 20 minutes. Remember to keep a towel between the ice bag and your skin to prevent frostbite.
- **Compression:** Bandage the injury to reduce swelling, support a joint or protect the wound.
- **Elevation:** Raise the injured area (e.g., arm or leg) above the level of the heart to allow the fluid to drain. This will help to reduce swelling.

When to see a healthcare provider:

- If you think you may need medication for pain and swelling, talk to your healthcare provider.
- See your healthcare provider if a sports injury does not get better in 2 weeks or if the pain gets worse even with treatment.

Chapter 49

Assessment of Foot Symptoms

Anne Mallin, RPh, BScPhm, PharmD, CDE

Figure 1: **Assessment of Patients with Foot Symptoms**[1,2,3,4,5,6,7,8,9,10,11,12,13,14,15]

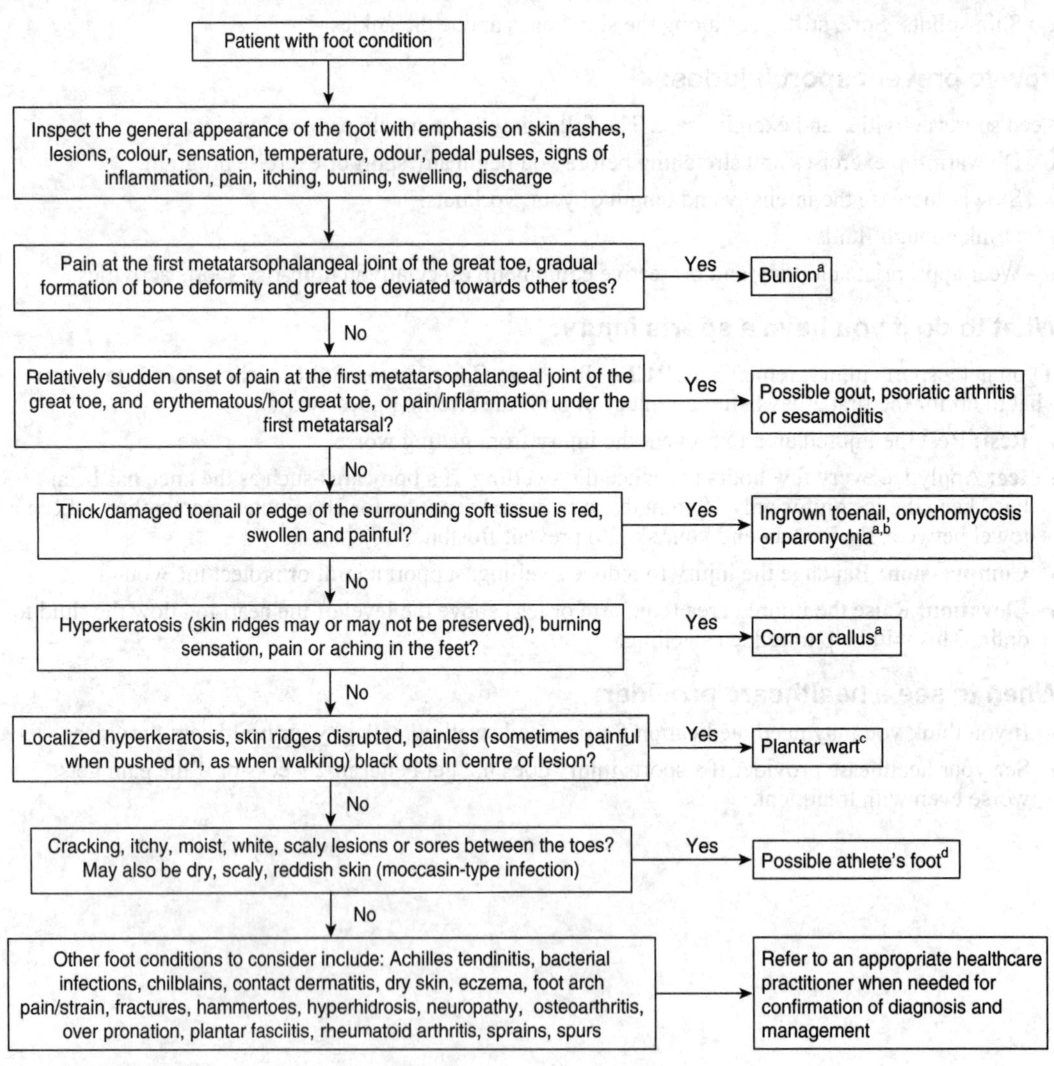
Patient with foot condition
Inspect the general appearance of the foot with emphasis on skin rashes, lesions, colour, sensation, temperature, odour, pedal pulses, signs of inflammation, pain, itching, burning, swelling, discharge
Pain at the first metatarsophalangeal joint of the great toe, gradual formation of bone deformity and great toe deviated towards other toes?
Yes
Bunion[a]
No
Relatively sudden onset of pain at the first metatarsophalangeal joint of the great toe, and erythematous/hot great toe, or pain/inflammation under the first metatarsal?
Yes
Possible gout, psoriatic arthritis or sesamoiditis
No
Thick/damaged toenail or edge of the surrounding soft tissue is red, swollen and painful?
Yes
Ingrown toenail, onychomycosis or paronychia[a,b]
No
Hyperkeratosis (skin ridges may or may not be preserved), burning sensation, pain or aching in the feet?
Yes
Corn or callus[a]
No
Localized hyperkeratosis, skin ridges disrupted, painless (sometimes painful when pushed on, as when walking) black dots in centre of lesion?
Yes
Plantar wart[c]
No
Cracking, itchy, moist, white, scaly lesions or sores between the toes? May also be dry, scaly, reddish skin (moccasin-type infection)
Yes
Possible athlete's foot[d]
No
Other foot conditions to consider include: Achilles tendinitis, bacterial infections, chilblains, contact dermatitis, dry skin, eczema, foot arch pain/strain, fractures, hammertoes, hyperhidrosis, neuropathy, osteoarthritis, over pronation, plantar fasciitis, rheumatoid arthritis, sprains, spurs
Refer to an appropriate healthcare practitioner when needed for confirmation of diagnosis and management

a See Chapter 51: Corns, Calluses, Bunions and Ingrown Toenails.
b See Chapter 64: Fungal Nail Infections (Onychomycosis).
c See Chapter 52: Plantar Warts.
d See Chapter 50: Athlete's Foot.

References

1. Government of Saskatchewan. Ministry of Health. *Learning package. Learning to perform a diabetes foot screen.* Available from: www.health.gov.sk.ca. Accessed July 19, 2012.
2. National Diabetes Education Program. *Feet can last a lifetime: a health care provider's guide to preventing diabetes foot problems.* Available from: www.ndep.nih.gov/media/feet_kit_eng.pdf. Accessed July 19, 2012.
3. Ford-Martin P, Blumer I. *Monofilament test.* Available from: www.netplaces.com/diabetes/the-diabetic-foot/monofilament-test.htm. Accessed July 19, 2012.
4. Diabetes Centre, Royal Prince Alfred Hospital. Diabetic foot disease: an interactive guide. *Foot examination.* Available from: www.sydney.edu.au/medicine/diabetes/foot/Fexam1.html. Accessed July 19, 2012.
5. Edwards C, Stillman P. *Minor illness or major disease?: responding to symptoms in the pharmacy.* 3rd ed. London: Pharmaceutical Press; 2000.
6. American Podiatric Medical Association. *Warts. What are warts?* Available from: www.apma.org/Learn/FootHealth.cfm?ItemNumber=989. Accessed August 30, 2009.
7. Baxter J. Feet not just there to keep your socks on. *New Zealand Pharmacy* 1996 Dec:10-12.
8. Nork SE, Couglin RR. How to examine a foot and what to do with a bunion. *Prim Care* 1996;23:281-97.
9. Singh D, Bentley G, Trevino SG. Callosities, corns, and calluses. *BMJ* 1996;312:1403-6.
10. Ontario Podiatric Medical Association. Naftolin N. *Foot surgery the minimal incision approach.* Available from: www.opma.ca/press/press_details.asp?pID=18. Accessed August 30, 2009.
11. Diabetes Québec. Chapter 23. Foot care and general hygiene. In: Benhamron C, ed. *Understand your diabetes...and live a healthy life.* Montreal: Rogers Media; 2008. p. 205-14.
12. eMedicineHealth. Barton ED, Chatlin BE. *Corns and calluses.* Available from: www.emedicinehealth.com. Accessed September 2, 2009. Registration required.
13. American Podiatric Medical Association. *Nail problems. Barometers of health.* Available from: www.apma.org. Accessed August 30, 2009.
14. American Podiatric Medical Association. *Bunions. What is a bunion?* Available from: www.apma.org/Learn/FootHealth.cfm?ItemNumber=979. Accessed August 30, 2009.
15. Canadian Diabetes Association. *Clinical practice guidelines.* Available from: guidelines.diabetes.ca/. Accessed July 20, 2013.

Chapter 50
Athlete's Foot

Anne Mallin, RPh, BScPhm, PharmD, CDE

Pathophysiology

Athlete's foot (tinea pedis) is a superficial fungal infection of the feet.[1] The fungal species most commonly involved are *Trichophyton rubrum*, *Trichophyton mentagrophytes* and *Epidermophyton floccosum*.[2,3] Up to 70% of the population will acquire this infection at some point in their lives.[4] It occurs most commonly in teenage and adult males and is uncommon in children.[1,3] Not all infected individuals will be aware of or have symptoms of tinea pedis infection.[5]

Tinea pedis is transmitted either directly via contact with an infected person or indirectly through contact with contaminated surfaces (e.g., swimming pool decks, gym change rooms).[5] The infection can be spread to other parts of the body, usually the groin or underarms, by autoinoculation (e.g., touching the infected feet then touching other parts of the body).[6]

Hyperhidrosis may contribute to the presence of athlete's foot. Warm, dark, poorly ventilated, moist environments between the toes promote fungal growth and may contribute to the presence of this condition.[7] Wearing shoes, with or without socks or hosiery, can create such environments. Other risk factors for athlete's foot may include diabetes, immunosuppression, peripheral vascular disease, occluded skin, poor hygiene, obesity and trauma.[8] Susceptibility to the fungus varies among individuals.[5]

Tinea pedis may progress to ulceration if the infection extends into the dermis. Complications may include secondary bacterial infections that may be localized or spreading (e.g., cellulitis, lymphangitis).[8] Patients with diabetes or those who have had saphenous vein grafts for coronary artery bypass are especially prone to secondary bacterial infections.[1]

Goals of Therapy

- Resolve symptoms
- Cure infection
- Prevent recurrence
- Prevent transmission to others

Patient Assessment

Tinea pedis may present in several ways (Table 1). The most common presentation is chronic interdigital infection.[9,10,11,12,13]

Evidence of blisters, pruritic lesions, burning sensations, redness and inflammation in the favoured locations or in a characteristic pattern on the feet may indicate the presence of athlete's foot. The skin may appear macerated and an odour may be present. Severe cases may present with pain, peeling, cracking and/or bleeding.[5] See Athlete's Foot in Photo Section.

Table 1: **Morphologic Variants of Tinea Pedis**

Variant	Lesion Morphology	Typical Location	Special Considerations
Chronic interdigital infection	Fissures, scaling or maceration in the interdigital spaces	Most commonly found on the lateral toe webs, usually between the fourth and fifth or third and fourth toes. From this area, the infection often spreads to the instep or sole of the foot.	Humidity and warmth worsen this condition. Therefore, patients whose feet are prone to excessive sweating should be encouraged to treat their hyperhidrosis along with the fungal infection.
Moccasin-type infection	Chronic, papulosquamous pattern	Generally found on both feet, it is characterized by a mild inflammation and diffuse scaling on the soles of the feet. Often the toenails are affected.	Involvement of the toenails perpetuates the infection such that the toenail infection must be treated by oral antifungal therapy for up to 3–4 months or by surgery.[5]
Vesicular	Small vesicles	Near the instep and on the midanterior plantar surface. Skin scaling is also observed in this area and on the toe webs.	Often caused by *T. mentagrophytes*. More prevalent in the summer.
Acute ulcerative disease	Macerated, denuded, weeping lesions	Sole of the foot.	Hyperkeratosis and a pungent odour are usually present. May be complicated by an overgrowth of opportunistic, gram-negative bacteria such as *Proteus* or *Pseudomonas* and for this reason is often referred to as gram-negative athlete's foot or dermatophytosis complex.

Athlete's foot may be confused with the following conditions: disturbances of the sweat mechanism; contact dermatitis, often due to dyes or adhesives in footwear; eczema; psoriasis or bacterial infections (including erythrasma).[9]

Figure 1 depicts an approach to assessing and managing athlete's foot.

Prevention

Give patients the following instructions:[5,7,9,14,15,16,17]

- Wash feet with soap and water every day
- Dry feet thoroughly, paying special attention to areas between the toes
- Change socks daily (more frequently if feet sweat)
- Wear socks made of natural, absorbent materials or synthetic blends (e.g., acrylic, cotton, polypropylene, wool). Individuals with hyperhidrosis should avoid socks that are made of nylon
- Avoid tight-fitting footwear
- Allow shoes to dry completely before being worn again. This may take 2–3 days and it may be necessary to alternate pairs of shoes on different days
- Do not go barefoot in public places (e.g., swimming pool decks or gym change rooms)—wear foot protection (e.g., sandals, pool shoes)
- Do not share personal items such as towels.

Antiperspirants or absorbent powders (e.g., **talcum** or **aluminum chloride**) can be applied to the feet to decrease sweating.

In addition to the above measures, individuals with a history of athlete's foot may regularly apply a dusting of antifungal powder such as **tolnaftate** once or twice daily on their feet to prevent further recurrences.[18] To prevent coagulation of powder and moisture buildup, antifungal powder should not be placed in shoes.[18,19]

Nonpharmacologic Therapy

Individuals with tinea pedis should follow the guidelines described under Prevention as adjuncts to pharmacologic treatment. Follow these measures to eliminate moisture and reduce recurrence.[14] Absorption of moisture and decreasing moisture buildup can be achieved by separating the toes using cotton balls.

Pharmacologic Therapy

For comparative ingredients of nonprescription products, consult the *Compendium of Products for Minor Ailments*—Foot Care Products: Athlete's Foot.

Treatment of the skin with a topical antifungal agent (e.g., **ciclopirox 1%**, **clotrimazole 1%**, **ketoconazole 2%**, **miconazole 2%**, **terbinafine 1%**) twice daily is the mainstay of therapy (Table 2). Treatment typically continues for up to 4 weeks, including 1–2 weeks after the lesions have disappeared, to prevent recurrences.[20]

Topical terbinafine 1% may have a slightly higher cure rate compared with other topical antifungals.[21] Inflamed infections may benefit from adding a topical anti-inflammatory such as betamethasone or hydrocortisone; some antifungal and topical corticosteroid combinations exist commercially (e.g., **clioquinol 3%/hydrocortisone 1%**, **clioquinol 3%/flumethasone pivalate 0.02%**, **clotrimazole 1%/betamethasone dipropionate 0.05%**). If signs and symptoms persist beyond 6 weeks consider referral to a foot care specialist. The main causes of treatment failure are incorrect diagnosis and inadequate treatment.

Oral **fluconazole**, **itraconazole** or **terbinafine** may be indicated for tinea pedis infections that are resistant to topical treatment.[22] Toenail involvement requires oral treatment.

There is no evidence that **tea tree oil** is effective in the treatment of tinea pedis, and if used it should not be applied to open lesions.[21]

The selection of dosage form is based on individual preference. Generally, ointments remain in contact with the affected area for a longer period of time than creams; however, there is the danger of creating an occlusive barrier, which promotes skin maceration and retards wound healing. Powders may be either nonmedicated or medicated and are also absorbent. Solutions, sprays or foams applied directly to the skin should be allowed to air dry.

Monitoring of Therapy

Rash during therapy may indicate an allergic reaction to the product. The patient should discontinue use of the product and consult with an appropriate healthcare practitioner.

If no improvement is seen within 2 weeks, or if symptoms have not completely disappeared within 6 weeks of treatment, refer the patient to a foot care specialist.

Advice for the Patient

Advise patient to:

- Finish the recommended course of treatment to prevent recurrence, even though symptoms may improve before the treatment course is complete[5]
- Dry the feet last after showering or bathing and use a clean towel every day, to prevent autoinoculation
- Prevent transmission to others by not going barefoot around the home or in public areas until the infection is cured.

Figure 1: **Assessment and Treatment of Patients with Athlete's Foot**

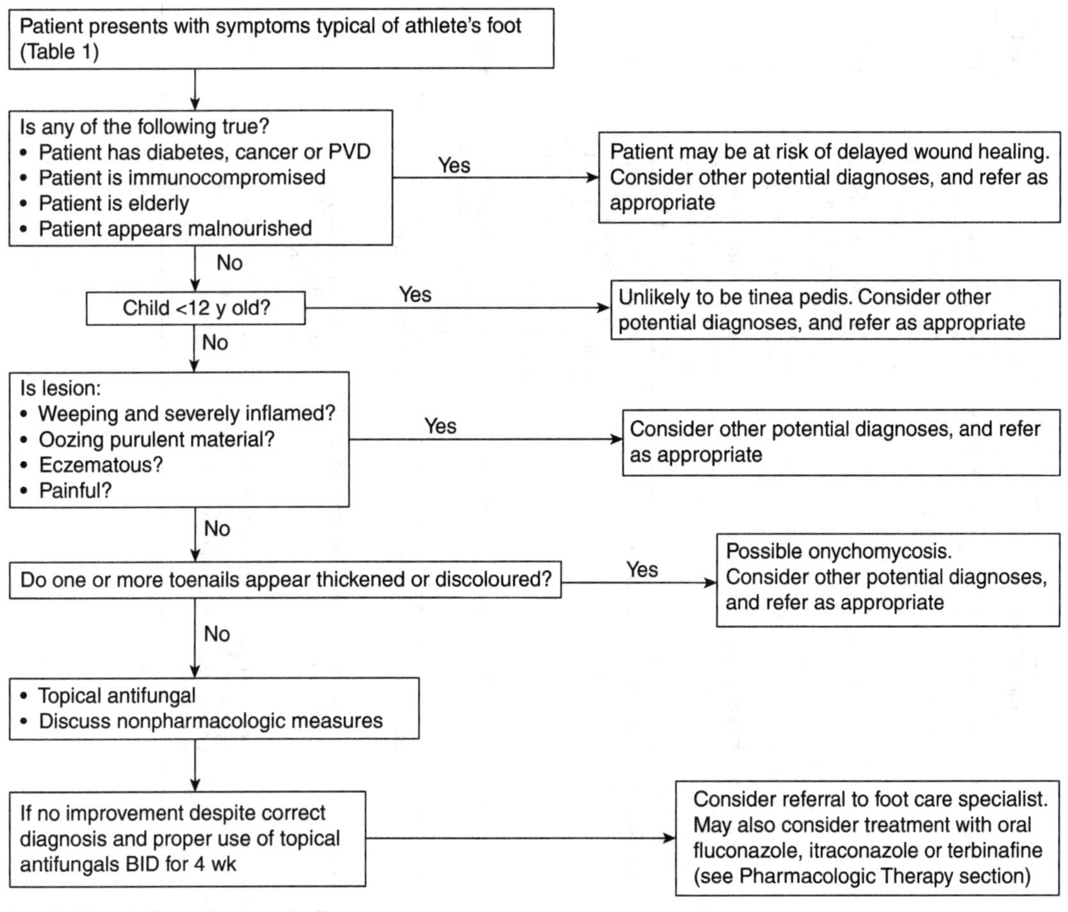

Abbreviations: PVD = peripheral vascular disease.

Table 2: **Pharmacologic Therapy for Athlete's Foot**

Class	Drug	Dosage	Adverse Effects	Comments	Cost[a]
Antifungal/ Corticosteroid Combinations	*clioquinol 3%/flumethasone pivalate 0.02%* Locacorten Vioform	Apply to affected areas BID × 4 wk	Local skin irritation or hypersensitivity (burning, erythema, pruritus, rash, stinging).	Also exhibits antibacterial and anti-inflammatory properties. Particularly useful when inflammation is a prominent feature. Available as cream.	$$$
	clioquinol 3%/ hydrocortisone 1% Vioform HC	Apply to affected areas BID × 4 wk	See clioquinol/flumethasone.	Also exhibits antibacterial and anti-inflammatory properties. Particularly useful when inflammation is a prominent feature. Available as cream.	$$$
	clotrimazole 1%/ betamethasone dipropionate 0.05% Lotriderm	Apply to affected areas BID × 4 wk	See clioquinol/flumethasone.	Particularly useful when inflammation is a prominent feature. Available as cream.	$$
Antifungals, Allylamine	*terbinafine 1%* Lamisil	Apply to affected areas BID × 4 wk	See clioquinol/flumethasone.	Patients treated with shorter durations of therapy (1–2 wk) continue to improve during the 2- to 4-wk period after therapy has been completed. Available as cream and spray.	$$
	terbinafine oral Terbinafine, other generics	250 mg once daily po × 2 wk	GI irritation, headache, skin irritation.	Considered for tinea pedis infections that are resistant to topical treatment.	$$$$
Antifungals, Azole	*clotrimazole 1%* Canesten Topical, generics	Apply to affected areas BID × 4 wk	See clioquinol/flumethasone.	Available as cream.	$
	fluconazole Diflucan One, CanesOral, generics	150 mg once weekly po × 2–6 wk	No clinically meaningful adverse effects at this dosage regimen.	Considered for tinea pedis infections that are resistant to topical treatment.	$/wk
	itraconazole Sporanox Capsules, Sporanox Oral Solution	200 mg BID po × 1 wk	Abdominal pain, constipation, diarrhea, dyspepsia, flatulence, headache, nausea, pruritus, skin rash, worsening heart failure symptoms.	Considered for tinea pedis infections that are resistant to topical treatment.	$70

Class	Drug	Dosage	Adverse Effects	Comments	Cost[a]
	ketoconazole 2% Ketoderm	Apply to affected areas BID × 4 wk	See clioquinol/flumethasone.	Available as cream.	$
	miconazole 2% Micatin, Monistat	Apply to affected areas BID × 4 wk	See clioquinol/flumethasone.	Available as cream, spray powder. Avoid inhaling powder preparations.	$
Antifungals, Hydroxypyridone	*ciclopirox 1%* Loprox	Apply to affected areas BID × 4 wk	See clioquinol/flumethasone.	Available as cream or lotion.	$$
Antifungals, Miscellaneous	*tolnaftate 1%* Tinactin, others	Apply to affected areas BID × 4 wk	See clioquinol/flumethasone.	Available as cream, aerosol, topical powder, spray. Avoid inhaling powder preparations.	$
	undecylenic acid Fungicure, Flexitol Antifungal, others	Apply to affected areas BID × 4 wk	See clioquinol/flumethasone.	Available as cream, liquid, ointment, powder, aerosol spray. Avoid inhaling powder preparations.	$

[a] Cost of specified duration of treatment for oral dose or smallest available pack size unless otherwise specified; includes drug cost only.

Dosage adjustment may be required in renal impairment.

Legend: $ <$10 $$ $10–20 $$$ $20–30 $$$$ $30–40

Resource Tips

Mayo Clinic. Diseases and Conditions. *Athlete's foot*. Available from: www.mayoclinic.com/health/athletes-foot/DS00317.

U.S. National Library of Medicine; National Institutes of Health. MedlinePlus. *Athlete's foot*. Available from: www.nlm.nih.gov/medlineplus/ency/article/000875.htm.

Suggested Readings

Andrews MD, Burns M. Common tinea infections in children. *Am Fam Physician* 2008;77:1415-20.

Gupta AK, Cooper EA. Update in antifungal therapy of dermatophytosis. *Mycopathologia* 2008;166:353-67.

Weinstein A, Berman B. Topical treatment of common superficial tinea infections. *Am Fam Physician* 2002;65:2095-102.

References

1. Fitzpatrick TB, Johnson RA, Wolff K et al. Fungal infections of the skin and hair. In: Fitzpatrick TB et al., eds. *Color atlas and synopsis of clinical dermatology: common and serious diseases*. 4th ed. New York: McGraw-Hill Medical; 2001. p. 684-725.
2. Rinaldi MG. Dermatophytosis: epidemiological and microbiological update. *J Am Acad Dermatol* 2000;43:S120-4.
3. Antifungal agents for common paediatric infections. *Paediatr Child Health* 2000;5:477-91.
4. Zuber TJ, Baddam K. Superficial fungal infection of the skin. Where and how it appears help determine therapy. *Postgrad Med* 2001;109:117-20,123-6, 131-2.
5. MedicineNet. *Athlete's foot*. Available from: www.medicinenet.com. Accessed February 9, 2016. Registration required.
6. American Podiatric Medical Association. *Athlete's foot. What is athlete's foot?* Available from: apma.org/MainMenu/Foot-Health/Brochures/Learn-About-Your-Feet/Athletes-Foot.aspx. Accessed February 9, 2016.
7. Diabetes Québec. Chapter 23. Foot care and general hygiene. In: Benhamron C, ed. *Understand your diabetes...and live a healthy life*. Montreal: Rogers Media; 2008. p. 205-14.
8. Al Hasan M, Fitzgerald SM, Saoudian M et al. Dermatology for the practicing allergist: Tinea pedis and its complications. *Clin Mol Allergy* 2004;2:5.
9. Crawford F, Hart R, Bell-Syer SE et al. Extracts from "Clinical evidence": Athlete's foot and fungally infected toenails. *BMJ* 2001;322:288-9.
10. Beers M, Berkow R, eds. *The Merck manual of diagnosis and therapy*. 17th ed. Whitehouse Station: Merck Research Laboratories; 1999.
11. American Diabetes Association clinical practice recommendations. Foot care in patients with diabetes mellitus. *Diabetes Care* 1997;20:S31.
12. May I see the pharmacist? *Aus Pharm* 1997;16:223.
13. Bedinghaus JM, Niedfeldt MW. Over-the-counter foot remedies. *Am Fam Physician* 2001;64:791-6.
14. Donaldson R. Athlete's foot. *Can Pharm J* 1998 Apr:33.
15. Canadian Podiatric Medical Association. *Common conditions and ailments: athlete's foot*. Available from: www.podiatrycanada.org. Accessed February 9, 2016.
16. eMedicineHealth from WebMD. Cole GW. *Athlete's foot*. Reviewed March 2014, Available from: www.emedicinehealth.com. Accessed February 9, 2016. Registration required.
17. Pickup TL, Adams BB. Prevalence of tinea pedis in professional and college soccer players versus non-athletes. *Clin J Sport Med* 2007;17:52-4.
18. Smith EB, Dickson JE, Knox JM. Tolnaftate powder in prophylaxis of tinea pedis. *South Med J* 1974;67:776-8.
19. Field LA, Adams BB. Tinea pedis in athletes. *Int J Dermatol* 2008;47:485-92.
20. Weinstein A, Berman B. Topical treatment of common superficial tinea infections. *Am Fam Physician* 2002;65:2095-102.
21. Crawford F, Hollis S. Topical treatments for fungal infections of the skin and nails of the foot. *Cochrane Database Syst Rev* 2007;(3):CD001434.
22. Bell-Syer SE, Khan SM, Torgerson DJ. Oral treatments for fungal infections of the skin of the foot. *Cochrane Database Syst Rev* 2012;(10):CD003584.

Athlete's Foot—What You Need to Know

What is athlete's foot?

Athlete's foot is an infection of the skin on the feet. It is caused by a fungus. Anyone can get athlete's foot—not just athletes!

What are the signs of athlete's foot?

If a person has athlete's foot, the soles of the feet may be red and itchy. The skin between the smaller toes may be scaly or peeling. Athlete's foot may be confused with other kinds of skin infections.

How do you treat athlete's foot?

To get rid of athlete's foot, you must kill the fungus that causes it. There are many different products to treat athlete's foot, including creams, ointments, gels, lotions, powders or sprays. Most products are available without a prescription. Your pharmacist can help you choose the product that is best for you.

Usually, the product is applied to the affected areas twice daily for at least 4 weeks. If nonprescription products do not get rid of the athlete's foot, you may benefit from medication that you take by mouth to treat the infection.

See a foot care specialist if:

- You do not see any improvement in your symptoms within 2 weeks;
- Your symptoms are not completely gone within 6 weeks.

Hints to help you get rid of athlete's foot

- Wash your feet daily in lukewarm water with a mild soap that does not contain deodorant.
- Do not soak your feet longer than 10 minutes.
- Rinse your feet well.
- Dry your feet carefully, especially between the toes. Use a soft towel to reduce irritation. If possible, use a clean towel each time you wash your feet.
- Use a nonabsorbent bath mat that can be disinfected.
- Change your shoes and socks daily.
- Wear socks made of natural, absorbent materials or synthetic blends, such as acrylic, cotton, polypropylene or wool.
- Wear shoes that provide good ventilation. Leather or canvas shoes allow moisture (from perspiration) to escape so your feet stay drier.
- Do not go barefoot in places where you could catch athlete's foot or spread it to other people. Wear sandals in pool or shower areas.
- Do not share personal items such as towels.

Chapter 51
Corns, Calluses, Bunions and Ingrown Toenails

Anne Mallin, RPh, BScPhm, PharmD, CDE

Pathophysiology
Corns and Calluses

Corns (clavus, heloma) and calluses (tyloma) occur when keratinization becomes overactive in an attempt to protect the foot from excessive friction or pressure from the skin rubbing against bony areas of the foot.[1,2,3]

Poorly fitting footwear can lead to the presence of corns and calluses by placing pressure on bony areas or causing excess friction. Calluses may also form as a result of weight gain, abnormal gait or foot structure (e.g., bunion, hammertoe). Corns and calluses are not contagious and are observed in most age groups.

Bunions

A bunion (hallux valgus) is a deformed great toe joint (first metatarsophalangeal or MTP joint), where the joint is angled outward with the great toe angled toward the other toes (Figure 1).[3,4] Bursitis with signs and symptoms of pain, swelling and erythema may also be present. Factors causing predisposition include arthritis, which may cause further damage to the joint space, or the foot's bone structure, which may be inherited. When the joint of the little toe is involved it is called a bunionette.

Figure 1: **Bunion**

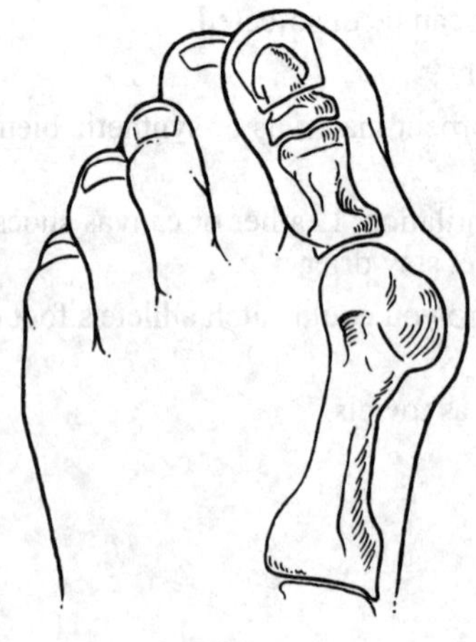

Heredity of foot type, abnormal gait, constant abnormal joint motion and pressure and the wearing of tight-fitting shoes may all contribute to the presence of bunions. They are 10 times more common in women than men, possibly due to the wearing of narrow, pointed-toe shoes.

Ingrown Toenails

It was previously thought that ingrown toenails (onychocryptosis) have nail edges that curve into the soft tissue surrounding the toenails, usually that of the great toes. Another more recent approach suggests that overgrowth of the tissue surrounding the nail bed is responsible for the impact between the nail edge and the tissue.[5,6,7] When the soft tissue and the nail edge impact on each other, the nail edge becomes irritated and often appears red and inflamed. Heredity, improper trimming of toenails, trauma and toe crowding may all contribute to the development of ingrown toenails. The incidence in males is double that of females and is highest between the ages of 10 and 30 years.

Goals of Therapy

- Relieve symptoms
- Remove the cause of the lesion so that it may regress (or not progress in the case of bunions)
- Prevent recurrences

Patient Assessment

When possible, inspect the patient's feet and footwear. Note the presence of lesions, changes in skin colour, sensation, texture or temperature, swelling, pain, rashes, signs of gangrene (dryness, moisture, gas) or obvious abnormalities in foot structure such as bunions or hammertoes.[1,3,8,9,10] Check the fit of the shoe (see Proper Shoe Fit), paying special attention to its length and the width and depth of the toe box.

Corns and Calluses

Corns (helomae) appear as tough layers of compacted, dead skin cells, which may have a central cone (radix) over the bony area or spur. The radix is triangular in shape and points inward. The affected area may also be yellowed.

Hard corns favour the areas over the fifth toe joint and on the soles of the feet, while soft corns are found between the toes, especially between the fourth and fifth. Corns are rarely found under a toenail (see Corns in Photo Section). Hard corns may be confused with plantar warts (verrucae plantaris). However, when the top layer of skin cells is removed, pinpoint bleeding is observed with plantar warts. In addition, skin ridges pass through corns but around plantar warts.

A soft corn is essentially a hard corn that has absorbed moisture from sweat, becoming macerated. Soft corns are often confused with athlete's foot. However, soft corns are often quite painful, whereas athlete's foot tends to be pruritic and usually not painful. Corns may also become inflamed or infected.

Calluses (*tylomae*) have a similar appearance to corns and tend to be well defined. They are of relatively even thickness and do not have a radix. Calluses tend to occur on the soles of the feet, especially on the heel or ball of the foot.

A burning sensation and pain when the affected area is compressed may indicate the presence of a corn or callus.

Bunions

A bunion looks like a bump on the outside edge of the affected foot. Its distinctive appearance along with swelling, pain and redness are characteristic of this foot condition. Individuals with a bunion should receive early treatment to stabilize the joint and reduce arthritic development.

Figure 3 depicts the assessment and management of corns, calluses and bunions.

Ingrown Toenails

Patients usually experience pain generated by the penetration and irritation of the soft tissue surrounding the toenail. Tenderness of the immediate area, erythema and abscess formation may also be present.

Nonpharmacologic Therapy

For comparative features of nonprescription products, consult the *Compendium of Products for Minor Ailments*—Foot Care Products: Insoles, Pads, Moleskins and Toe Protection Products.

Corns, Calluses and Bunions

Identifying and removing the cause of the lesion is the most important step in the treatment of corns, calluses or bunions. In addition to self-examination of the feet, persons with specific medical conditions such as diabetes should be examined by a health practitioner with foot care expertise at each office visit and at least annually. Individuals deemed to be at higher risk should have their feet examined more often.[11] The most common intervention is a change in footwear and this is often the only treatment required (see Proper Shoe Fit).[12,13,14,15] Orthotic devices may be inserted into footwear to provide arch support and to distribute body weight more evenly so that excess pressure is removed from the affected area of the foot.

Devices such as cushions, felt pads and latex foam can be used to protect a corn, callus or bunion.[12] A variety of shapes and sizes are available to accommodate the various lesions. Custom pads can be constructed from moleskin or lambswool. Placing lambswool between the toes affected by a soft corn decreases the pain.

Débridement of a corn or callus using a pumice stone can be performed after soaking the area in warm water for about 10 minutes, with or without sodium bicarbonate (baking soda). Castor, olive, sesame seed or wheat germ oils can be applied to the affected area to soften corns or calluses. The abrasive action of walking on wet sand can assist in the removal of dead skin from the soles of the feet. A foot file (e.g., emery board) can be used on a dry foot. Persons with specific medical conditions such as diabetes should not self-treat for corns or calluses.[11] Excising corns with electrosurgery may result in superior pain relief at 6 months compared with standard sharp débridement with a scalpel or scissors.[16]

When nonsurgical interventions have failed to adequately relieve pain and discomfort, surgery is indicated. The choice of surgical options for bunions is based on a variety of factors.[17]

Ingrown Toenails

Polyurethane foam toecaps are useful as protective devices for ingrown toenails. Determining optimum shoe fit and altering footwear to remove pressure points may prevent recurrences of ingrown toenails (see Proper Shoe Fit below). To prevent toenails from becoming ingrown, trim them straight across and do not round the corners. The corners of nails should project beyond the skin (Figure 2). Instruments such as rounded-end scissors and nail clippers should be handled with care and individuals with impaired vision or poor dexterity should avoid their use altogether to avoid foot injuries. A footcare specialist may excise infected tissue or chemically destroy the nail matrix for effective treatment of ingrown toenails.[18,19]

Figure 2: **Trimming of Ingrown Toenails**

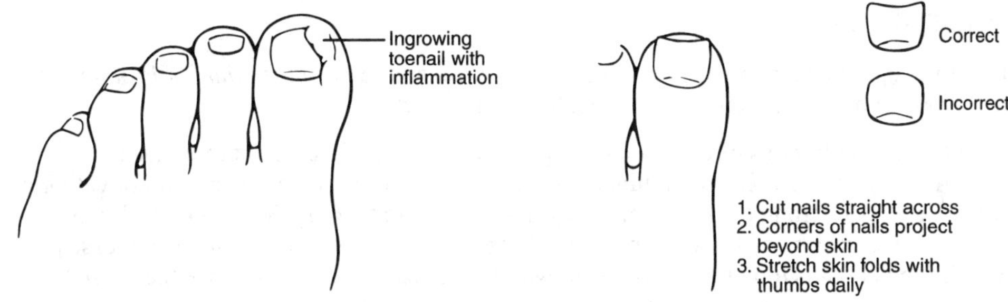
Ingrowing toenail with inflammation
Correct
Incorrect
1. Cut nails straight across
2. Corners of nails project beyond skin
3. Stretch skin folds with thumbs daily

Proper Shoe Fit

Proper shoe fit is especially important in women as they are 4 times more likely than men to develop foot problems.[14,15] Shoe choices should be appropriate for the type of activity (e.g., hiking boots for hikers). If possible, shoes should be purchased at the end of the day when feet are most swollen due to gravity pulling fluid in the body down to the feet.[15] Since one foot is often larger than the other, both shoes should be tried on with stockings. When standing, there should be enough room for the toes to spread in the toe box. The individual should walk around to check for tightness or rubbing within the shoes. If the individual plans to wear orthotics in the shoe, these should be worn during the fitting. Allow one-half inch (1.25 cm) between the end of the shoe and the longest toe so the toes do not bump into the shoe during ambulation. The first MTP joint (located at the base of the great toe) should be in the widest part of the toe box. The heel should fit snugly and the foot should not slip up and down during ambulation. New shoes should be worn approximately one-half hour daily at first to gradually break them in.

The following are desirable characteristics of footwear:

- fastened with buckles, laces or velcro (slip-on shoes should be avoided due to possible slipping of the foot inside the shoe) and made from canvas or leather (to allow for flexibility)
- wide toe box and not pointed to prevent toe crowding
- heels lower than 1.5 inches (3.75 cm) to prevent forward pressure and crowding of the toes
- light weight and flexible under the balls of the feet with good shock-absorbing, cushioned soles (e.g., rubber, crepe).

Pharmacologic Therapy

Prevention

For comparative ingredients of nonprescription products, consult the *Compendium of Products for Minor Ailments*—Skin Care Products: Dermatitis and Dry Skin.

Maintaining moisture balance and removing dead skin cells help prevent formation of corns and calluses.[20] Neutral, unscented, **moisturizing topical products** without acid content may be applied to dry skin on the feet (except between the toes, as it may cause excessive softening) to prevent the formation of corns and calluses or to soften existing lesions. **Hydrating products** with humectants soften the skin (e.g., Nivea, Glaxal Base). **Anti-dehydration products** form a film on the skin to reduce moisture evaporation (e.g., Lubriderm lotion, Cetaphil, Keri lotion, Vaseline Intensive Care lotion, silicone cream). Hydrating products containing keratolytic and exfoliating ingredients should be applied only to the top layer of skin (stratum corneum) and not to broken skin. These products assist with the removal of dead skin cells (e.g., Uremol 10, Dermal Therapy with urea concentrations 10%, 15%, 20% or 25%). **Urea** has the potential to cause burning or tingling sensations when applied to dry or cracked skin.

Corns and Calluses

For comparative ingredients of nonprescription products, consult the *Compendium of Products for Minor Ailments*—Foot Care Products: Corns, Calluses and Warts.

Salicylic acid in concentrations of up to 40% is available for the self-treatment of corns and calluses.[12,20] Although various concentrations of salicylic acid appear to be successful in treating corns and calluses, there is no strong evidence for their effectiveness in treating these foot conditions. Salicylic acid concentrations of 12–40% may be indicated if the cause of the lesion is not easily corrected or if the patient is too uncomfortable to wait for the lesion to regress once the cause has been removed. Some products are described in Table 1.

Plasters and pads tend to adhere to the lesion better than liquid dosage forms. Salicylic acid will damage normal skin, so it is important that it not be applied outside the edge of the corn or callus. When liquid preparations are used, the normal skin surrounding the lesion can be protected with an occlusive application of petrolatum or a mechanical occlusion, such as a bandage with an aperture for application of the product. Liquid collodion vehicles should not be used by the elderly due to risk of poor vision, or by children due to the potential for poisoning by ingestion or inhalation.

Bunions

For comparative ingredients of nonprescription products, consult the *Compendium of Products for Minor Ailments*—Analgesic Products: Internal Analgesics and Antipyretics.

Use of ice packs and **analgesics** such as **acetaminophen** or **nonsteroidal anti-inflammatory drugs** (NSAIDs) may be considered, to reduce pain and swelling of an inflamed bunion.[3,4] If nonpharmacologic approaches or analgesics are inadequate, **intra-articular corticosteroids** may be considered for pain reduction.

Ingrown Toenails

For comparative ingredients of nonprescription products, consult the *Compendium of Products for Minor Ailments*—Analgesic Products: Internal Analgesics and Antipyretics; Skin Care Products: First Aid.

Refer patients with ingrown toenails to a foot care specialist. In the interim, general measures can be employed to control infections or relieve pain and inflammation.[5] Protection from infection can be achieved with the use of **topical antibiotic** creams or ointments. Topical **antiseptics** (e.g., **alcohol** 70% swabs, **povidone-iodine** and **chlorhexidine gluconate** 0.05% dressings) or footbath solutions (e.g., 15 mL of **povidone-iodine** or **chlorhexidine gluconate** 2% or 4% in 1 litre of lukewarm boiled water) can be used to disinfect the skin. **Local anesthetics** (e.g., **benzocaine** 20% solution) or **hypertonic saline** or **magnesium sulfate** (Epsom salts) footbaths 3 or 4 times daily may be useful in reducing pain. Footbaths are typically used for no longer than 10 minutes.

The treatment of choice is partial surgical removal of the nail border with or without destruction of the nail bed matrix.[5] After surgery the area is kept dry overnight with the foot elevated. This is generally followed with daily foot soaks and antibiotic ointment application starting 48 hours after the procedure. Oral **analgesics** (e.g., **acetaminophen** or **NSAIDs**) may be considered, if appropriate. Depending upon the presence and extent of infection, systemic antibiotics may be used; however, the available evidence suggests that oral antibiotics taken before or after surgery do not decrease healing time. Further assessment is required if signs of infection develop or persist (e.g., erythema, swelling, purulent discharge).

Monitoring of Therapy

Corns and Calluses

Clinical improvement should be evident within 10–14 days after initiating treatment with a salicylic acid–containing product. Advise the patient to inspect the affected area at least twice weekly until healing is complete. If no improvement is noted, refer to a foot care specialist. If normal skin surrounding the lesion is damaged by incorrect use of salicylic acid preparations, recommend discontinuation of the product until the normal skin is healed. If the lesion becomes red or inflamed or drains purulent material, refer to a foot care specialist.

Advice for the Patient

Advise the patient regarding:

- foot inspection for lesions
- strategies for preventing future occurrences, including proper fit of footwear
- nonpharmacologic treatment
- proper use of protective devices
- pharmacologic treatment, including proper use of a salicylic acid product, if indicated
- when to seek the attention of a foot care specialist.

Figure 3: **Assessment of Patients with Corns, Calluses and Bunions**

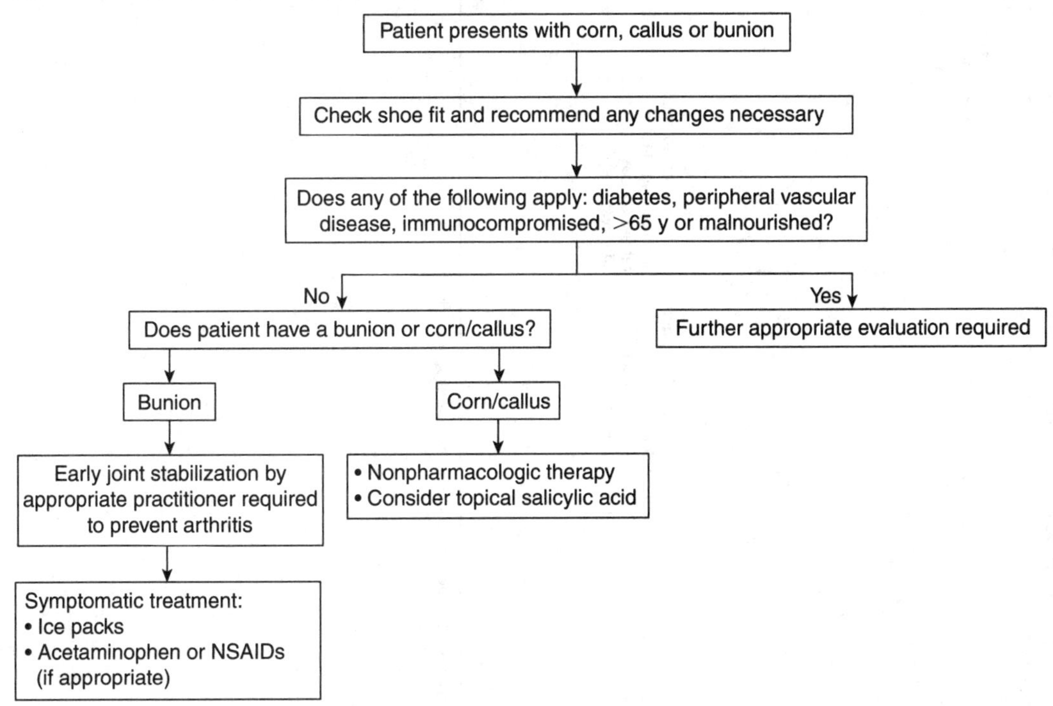

Table 1: **Topical Treatment of Corns and Calluses**

Class	Drug	Dosage	Adverse Effects	Comments	Cost[a]
Keratolytics	*salicylic acid 12–17.6% liquid* Compound W, Soluver, others	Apply daily or BID PRN for up to 14 days	Excessive burning or irritation.	Available as liquid in a collodion-like solution. Apply a small amount to the clean and dry area of the lesion. Not to be used by individuals with diabetes, peripheral vascular disease or impaired circulation. Highly flammable—store at room temperature away from fire or flame. Avoid inhaling fumes or direct eye contact. Do not apply to broken, infected or irritated skin. Wash hands thoroughly after application.	$
	salicylic acid 12–40% pads and plasters Compound W, Soluver Plus, others	Apply medicated plaster and leave in place × 2 days; repeat Q2 days for up to 14 days	Excessive burning or irritation.	Available as pads or plasters for external use. Trim pad or plaster to fit the size and shape of the clean and dry area of the lesion. Not to be used by individuals with diabetes, peripheral vascular disease or impaired circulation. Do not apply to broken, infected or irritated skin. Wash hands thoroughly after application.	$

[a] Cost of smallest available pack size; includes drug cost only.

Legend: $ <$10

Suggested Readings

Bedinghaus JM, Niedfeldt MW. Over-the-counter foot remedies. *Am Fam Physician* 2001;64:791-6.
Heidelbaugh JJ, Lee H. Management of the ingrown toenail. *Am Fam Physician* 2009;79:303-8.

References

1. Singh D, Bentley G, Trevino SG. Callosities, corns, and calluses. *BMJ* 1996;312:1403-6.
2. Knight AL. Selected disorders of the skin. In: Taylor RB, ed. *Family medicine: principles and practice*. 4th ed. New York: Springer-Verlag; 1994. p. 952-3.
3. Silfverskiold JP. Common foot problems. Relieving the pain of bunions, keratoses, corns, and calluses. *Postgrad Med* 1991;89:183-8.
4. American Podiatric Medical Association. *Bunions. What is a bunion?* Available from: www.apma.org/Learn/FootHealth.cfm?ItemNumber=979. Accessed January 28, 2013.
5. Heidelbaugh JJ, Lee H. Management of the ingrown toenail. *Am Fam Physician* 2009;79:303-8.
6. Overgrown toeskin. Available from: www.overgrowntoeskin.ca. Accessed March 25, 2015.
7. Chapeskie H. Ingrown toenail or overgrown toe skin?: Alternative treatment for onychocryptosis. *Can Fam Physician* 2008;54:1561-2.
8. Nork SE, Coughlin RR. How to examine a foot and what to do with a bunion. *Prim Care* 1996;23:281-97.
9. Canadian Podiatric Medical Association. *Foot health*. Available from: www.podiatrycanada.org/foot-health/. Accessed February 2, 2016.
10. Edwards C, Stillman P. *Minor illness or major disease?: the clinical pharmacist in the community*. 3rd ed. London: Pharmaceutical Press; 2000.
11. Canadian Diabetes Association. *Clinical practice guidelines 2013*. Available from: guidelines.diabetes.ca. Accessed March 25, 2015.
12. Bedinghaus JM, Niedfeldt MW. Over-the-counter foot remedies. *Am Fam Physician* 2001;64:791-6.
13. Richards RN. Calluses, corns and shoes. *Semin Dermatol* 1991;10:112-4.
14. Ontario Podiatric Medical Association. Miltchin H. *How to buy the best shoes*. Available from: go.epublish4me.com/ebook/ebook?id=10058746#/14. Accessed February 16, 2016.
15. Ontario Podiatric Medical Association. Koven N, Miltchin H, Wong-Sing J. *Buyers guide to foot wear*. Available from: go.epublish4me.com/ebook/ebook?id=10058746#/14. Accessed February 2, 2016.
16. Bevans JS, Bosson G. A comparison of electrosurgery and sharp debridement in the treatment of chronic neurovascular, neurofibrous and hard corns. A pragmatic randomised controlled trial. *Foot (Edinb)* 2010;20:12-7.
17. Joseph TN, Mroczek KJ. Decision making in the treatment of hallux valgus. *Bull NYU Hosp Jt Dis* 2007;65:19-23.
18. Eekhof JA, Van Wijk B, Knuistingh Neven A et al. Interventions for ingrowing toenails. *Cochrane Database Syst Rev* 2012;4:CD001541.
19. Eekhof JA, Neven AK, Gransjean SP et al. Minor derm ailments: how good is the evidence for common treatments? *J Fam Pract* 2009;58:E2.
20. Barton ED, Chatlin BE. *Corns and calluses*. Available from: www.emedicinehealth.com. Accessed January 28, 2013.

Corns and Calluses—What You Need to Know

What are corns and calluses?

Corns and calluses look like thick, tough layers of skin. Corns are usually found on or between the toes. Calluses, which are found on the soles of the feet, are caused by friction or pressure from the skin rubbing against the bones of the feet. The area may look red or be painful.

How do you treat corns and calluses?

- Make sure your shoes fit properly. They should not crowd your toes nor allow your foot to slip around in the heel. There should be a space of at least one-half inch (1.25 cm) between the tip of your longest toe and the front of the shoe.
- Apply a felt pad with a hole in the centre over a corn to reduce pressure on the area.
- Put a latex foam insole into your shoe or apply moleskin to the affected area to cushion and protect your foot.
- You can use a pumice stone or callus file (e.g., emery board) to remove dry skin build-up. Use the pumice stone on wet skin and the file on dry skin.
- **Never** cut a corn or callus yourself with any instrument.

Nonprescription products are available to help remove the corn or callus. Talk to your pharmacist to see if one is right for you.

Bunions—What You Need to Know

What is a bunion?

A bunion looks like a bump on the outside edge of the foot. It is caused by a deformed great toe joint that causes the great toe to point towards the other toes of the foot.

If you have foot pain, see your healthcare provider.

How do you treat a bunion?

- It is important to relieve pressure on the bunion to reduce pain and to keep it from getting worse.
- Avoid wearing narrow-fitting shoes or shoes with heels over 1.5 inches (3.75 cm) high. You will need a wider shoe to relieve pressure and rubbing.
- Use felt pads (e.g., moleskin) or latex foam to cushion the bunion.
- If the bunion becomes painful or swollen, apply an ice pack for 10 minutes. You can use the ice pack several times during the day.
- Nonprescription pain relievers such as acetaminophen, ibuprofen or naproxen may help with pain and swelling. Talk to your pharmacist for help in choosing a pain reliever.
- If ice packs and pain relievers do not work, a footcare specialist may inject cortisone into the joint.

Some people need a surgical procedure to correct the problem.

Chapter 52
Plantar Warts

Anne Mallin, RPh, BScPhm, PharmD, CDE

Pathophysiology

Warts are benign tumors caused by many human papilloma virus (HPV) types including 1, 2, 4 and 57.[1] Warts found on the soles of the feet are called plantar warts (verrucae plantaris). HPV infects the upper epidermis and causes squamous epithelial cells to proliferate.[2] The infection exists only in humans and is transmitted via contact with another lesion or contaminated surfaces.[3] Infection usually occurs through small cuts or microabrasions.[4] The infection may become clinically evident through the appearance of warts, or it may remain latent or cause subclinical infection where the change in the skin surface is not evident to the naked eye.[1] The incubation period between initial infection and the appearance of warty lesions varies from 1 to 8 months.[5] Up to 30% of warts spontaneously regress within 6 months due to cell-mediated immunity, but those that do not regress in that time period frequently proliferate. Regression within 6 months is more likely in children.

Plantar warts may occur singly or in clusters (mosaic warts). They are uncommon in infancy and are most common in children and young adults. The peak incidence of warts occurs between 12 and 16 years of age.

Risk factors for plantar warts include immunosuppression and exposure to environments where the virus may contaminate surfaces (e.g., swimming pool decks, communal showers).

Goals of Therapy

- Alleviate or prevent pain due to the wart
- Eradicate lesions and prevent their proliferation
- Prevent recurrence
- Prevent transmission to others

Patient Assessment

Most warts are harmless. However, depending upon their size, number and location, they can cause pain and may be a source of embarrassment to the patient.[2,4,6,7]

Plantar warts are often symptomless, producing pain only upon pressure. This pain is usually greater on lateral compression (when the lesion is pinched from the sides) than with direct pressure. They are usually rough, firm hyperkeratoses that, unlike common warts on the hands, grow inwards due to pressure from walking. Warts are usually skin coloured but may often be grey or brown. Thrombosed capillaries may appear as black dots in the centre of the lesion, or these may only be evident as pinpoint bleeding that occurs if the lesion is débrided. Unlike corns, skin striations tend to run around the wart, as opposed to through it. Plantar warts tend to arise on the heel or the ball of the foot where microabrasions are more likely to occur and allow inoculation. See Plantar Warts in Photo Section.

Figure 1 depicts the assessment and treatment of patients with plantar warts.

Prevention

Give patients the following instructions:[4,8,9]

- Avoid walking barefoot in public places and wear foot protection (e.g., sandals, pool shoes) when in areas where transmission may be more common (e.g., swimming pool decks, gym showers, dormitories)
- Change shoes and socks every day
- Keep feet clean and dry
- Avoid touching warts on someone else or on another part of your body
- Do not share socks or footwear
- Use waterproof tape during treatment to prevent transmission of the virus to others.

Nonpharmacologic Therapy

Hyperthermic therapy, immunotherapy, cryosurgery using liquid nitrogen, CO_2 laser, curettage and radiosurgery using electrodes have been used to treat plantar warts with varying success.[9,10] Hyperthermic treatment involves soaking the affected area in hot water for 90 minutes daily for many months.[9] CO_2 laser therapy involves the vapourization of tissue and is thought to be the most effective form of treatment.[11] Clear **duct tape** is not effective.[12] Conflicting data suggest that **cryotherapy** with liquid nitrogen may not be more effective than placebo.[12]

Based on the cryosurgery method using liquid nitrogen, a medical device containing **dimethylether** and **propane** freezes the wart so that it ceases to host the virus and causes a blister to form under it, resulting in the wart falling off approximately 10 days after treatment.[9] Efficacy in inducing cell necrosis may be lower than that achieved with liquid nitrogen as lower cell temperatures are attained with liquid nitrogen (−196°C) than with dimethylether and propane (−57°C).[3] Its role in self-care is yet to be determined.

Pharmacologic Therapy

For comparative ingredients of nonprescription products, consult the *Compendium of Products for Minor Ailments*—Foot Care Products: Corns, Calluses and Warts.

Chemicals applied topically over the long term can trigger an inflammatory response to stimulate the body's immune system to attack the virus. These chemicals may also have the ability to destroy infected tissue. Generally, improvement is evident within 1–2 weeks after the initiation of treatment.[9,10] When home therapy results in increased pain, swelling, bleeding or fever, or improvement is not evident in several weeks, refer the patient to a healthcare practitioner experienced in the treatment of plantar warts for further assessment.[8,9]

Topical application of chemicals such as 2-hydroxybenzoic acid, 2-hydroxypropanoic acid, 5-fluorouracil, cantharidin, dichloroacetic acid, formalin, glutaraldehyde, podophyllin, pyrogallic acid, salicylic acid, trichloroacetic acid and vitamin A, which may be keratolytic, drying or cauterizing, has been used to treat plantar warts.

Table 1 describes some preparations available for self-treatment of plantar warts. The ingredient common to all products is **salicylic acid** in concentrations of 5–40%. The advantages of salicylic acid and other topical chemicals include control over the amount of disability and discomfort and a low risk of scarring. Disadvantages include the length of treatment, which is often several months. Application of liquid preparations that dry on the wart allows for treatment of the affected area only, whereas more solid dosage forms (e.g., pastes, ointments) may spread to normal skin upon weight bearing.[13] Topical salicylic acid is safe and effective for the treatment of warts at all body sites and may be as effective as cryotherapy.[12,14,15]

Vitamin A has been used orally and topically to treat patients with multiple lesions;[9,13] there are no randomized controlled trials to support this approach.

A topical preparation containing **cantharidin** 1%, **podophyllin** 2% or 5% and **salicylic acid** 30% is a vesicant that must be applied by a foot care specialist. After application, the lesion is kept occluded for 3–7 days. During this time a blister forms and the plantar wart becomes necrotic. Treatment with or without curettage may need to be repeated. In some patients, pain may interfere with ambulation. Analgesics (e.g., acetaminophen, ASA, ibuprofen or naproxen sodium) may be considered for pain management.

Cure rates with any method of treatment are 60–70% and up to 60% of plantar warts go into spontaneous remission. Untreated plantar warts can easily spread to other sites.[9,16] Cure rates are higher in children and immunocompetent hosts and when the duration of infection is short. They are lower if the wart has failed to respond to any other type of treatment. Mosaic warts are more resistant to treatment than single lesions.[3,15] Even when treatment appears to have been successful, warts may recur. This may be due to failure to remove tissue in which the virus has caused only latent or subclinical infection.

Monitoring of Therapy

Check with the patient every 4 weeks to see if any improvement has been noted and to encourage adherence. If the lesion persists after 12 weeks of self-treatment, or if skin is damaged and becomes painful or inflamed or drains purulent material, refer the patient to a foot care specialist.

Advice for the Patient

Advise patients regarding:

- covering the wart to prevent transmission to other people
- not removing the plantar wart themselves
- using the chosen preparation properly
- preventing and managing adverse effects of treatment
- when to contact a foot care specialist.

Figure 1: Assessment and Treatment of Plantar Warts

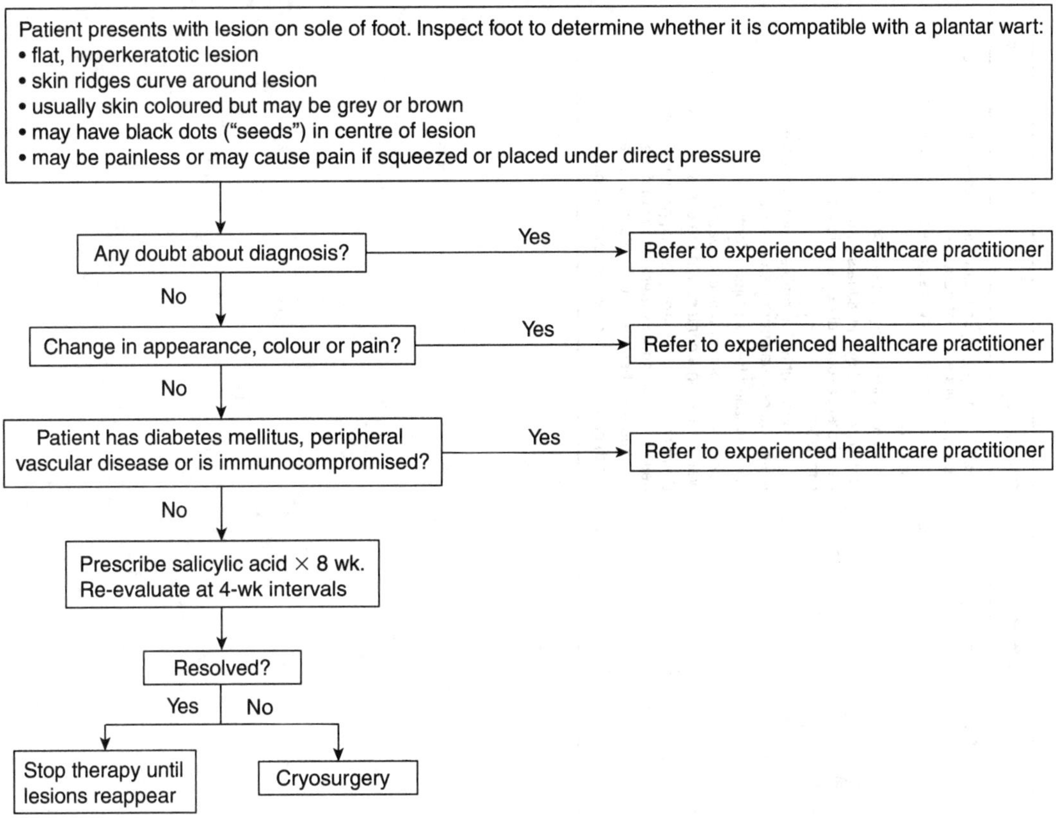

Patient presents with lesion on sole of foot. Inspect foot to determine whether it is compatible with a plantar wart:
- flat, hyperkeratotic lesion
- skin ridges curve around lesion
- usually skin coloured but may be grey or brown
- may have black dots ("seeds") in centre of lesion
- may be painless or may cause pain if squeezed or placed under direct pressure

↓

Any doubt about diagnosis? — Yes → Refer to experienced healthcare practitioner

No ↓

Change in appearance, colour or pain? — Yes → Refer to experienced healthcare practitioner

No ↓

Patient has diabetes mellitus, peripheral vascular disease or is immunocompromised? — Yes → Refer to experienced healthcare practitioner

No ↓

Prescribe salicylic acid × 8 wk.
Re-evaluate at 4-wk intervals

↓

Resolved?

- Yes → Stop therapy until lesions reappear
- No → Cryosurgery

Table 1: Products for Self-treatment of Plantar Warts

Class	Drug	Dosage	Adverse Effects	Comments	Cost[a]
Keratolytic Agents	*salicylic acid 5–17% in collodion-like solution; 15% in a karaya gum, glycol plaster; 12–40% in other plasters* Compound W, Soluver, others	Gel/liquid: Apply 1 drop daily or BID Pads/plasters: Apply once daily Apply salicylic acid products after showering or soaking the affected area at bedtime; repeat daily up to 12 wk	Excessive burning/irritation.	Available as gel, liquid in collodion-like solution, pads, plasters and ointment. Apply to clean and dry area of lesion; for external use only. Trim pads/plasters to fit lesion area. Not to be used by individuals with diabetes, peripheral vascular disease or impaired circulation. Liquid form highly flammable—store at room temperature away from fire or flame. Avoid inhaling fumes of liquid form. Avoid direct contact with the eyes; flush with water × 15 min if contact with the eye(s) occurs. Do not use on birthmarks, moles, genital/facial/hairy warts or mucous membranes or if the affected area becomes red, irritated or inflamed. Wash hands thoroughly after application.	$

[a] Cost of smallest available pack size; includes drug cost only.

Legend: $ <$10

Resource Tips

Mayo Clinic. Diseases and Conditions. *Plantar warts*. Available from: www.mayoclinic.com/health/plantar-warts/ds00509.

U.S. National Library of Medicine; National Institutes of Health. MedlinePlus. *Warts*. Available from: www.nlm.nih.gov/medlineplus/ency/article/000885.htm.

Suggested Readings

Lichon V, Khachemoune A. Plantar warts: a focus on treatment modalities. *Dermatol Nurs* 2007;19:372-5.

References

1. Drake LA, Ceilley RI, Cornelison RL et al. Guidelines of care for warts: human papillomavirus. Committee on Guidelines of Care. *J Am Acad Dermatol* 1995;32:98-103.
2. Verbov J. How to manage warts. *Arch Dis Child* 1999;80:97-9.
3. Sterling JC, Handfield-Jones S, Hudson PM. Guidelines for the management of cutaneous warts. *Br J Dermatol* 2001;144:4-11.
4. Landsman MJ, Mancuso JE, Abramow SP. Diagnosis, pathophysiology, and treatment of plantar verruca. *Clin Podiatr Med Surg* 1996;13:55-71.
5. Bolton RA. Nongenital warts: classification and treatment options. *Am Fam Physician* 1991;43:2049-56.
6. Baxter J. Feet not just there to keep your socks on. *New Zealand Pharmacy* 1996 Dec:10-2.
7. Popovich NG, Newton GD. Minor foot disorders. In: Young LL, Engle JP, Berardi RR et al., eds. *Handbook of nonprescription drugs*. 12th ed. Washington: American Pharmaceutical Association; 2000. p. 781-818.
8. Canadian Podiatric Medical Association. *Common conditions and ailments*. Available from: www.podiatrycanada.org. Accessed February 25, 2016.
9. eMedicineHealth from WebMD. Cole GW. *Plantar warts*. Reviewed July 2015. Available from: www.emedicinehealth.com. Registration required. Accessed February 25, 2016.
10. Ontario Podiatric Medical Association. Goldberg R. *The war on warts*. Available from: go.epublish4me.com/ebook/ebook?id=10058745#/2. Accessed May 3, 2016.
11. Ontario Podiatric Medical Association. Nesbitt L. *Laser foot surgery*. Available from: go.epublish4me.com/ebook/ebook?id=10058746#/2. Accessed May 3, 2016.
12. Kwok CS, Gibbs S, Bennett C et al. Topical treatments for cutaneous warts. *Cochrane Database Syst Rev* 2012;(9):CD001781.
13. Lemont H. Exploring current approaches to plantar warts. *Podiatry Today* 2006;19:68-74. Available from: www.podiatrytoday.com/article/6440. Accessed February 25, 2016.
14. Eekhof JA, Neven AK, Gransjean SP et al. Minor derm ailments: how good is the evidence for common treatments? *J Fam Pract* 2009;58:E2.
15. Gibbs S, Harvey I Local treatments for cutaneous warts. *Cochrane Database Syst Rev* 2006;(3):CD001781.
16. Remedy's Health Communities. Lunsford JM. *Plantar warts*. Modified October 2015. Available from: www.healthcommunities.com/plantar-warts/overview-of-plantar-warts.shtml. Accessed February 25, 2016.

Plantar Warts—What You Need to Know

What is a plantar wart?

A plantar wart is a wart on the bottom of the foot. Plantar warts are caused by a viral infection of the skin. They are usually harmless but can be painful.

Where does the virus come from?

You catch the virus by touching someone else's wart or touching a surface that has the virus on it. The virus is often found on swimming pool decks and in gym showers or dormitories.

What can you do to prevent plantar warts?

- **Do not** go barefoot in public places. Wear sandals or pool shoes when necessary.
- Change your shoes and socks every day.
- Keep your feet clean and dry.
- Avoid touching another person's warts or another part of your body after touching a wart.
- Do not share socks or footwear.
- Use waterproof tape during treatment.

How are plantar warts treated?

A number of wart removal products are available. Most contain a type of acid that, over time, eats away the wart. It can take up to 12 weeks or several months for the wart to go away. People who have diabetes, poor circulation or weak immune systems should **not** use these products without professional advice. Talk to a healthcare provider with footcare experience about the treatment that is best for you.

How to use wart removal products safely:

- Soak the wart in warm water for 5 minutes, then gently rub away loose tissue with a pumice stone, emery board file or rough washcloth.
- Liquid preparations: Protect healthy skin around the wart by applying a thin layer of white petrolatum such as Vaseline. Apply the liquid to the wart 1 drop at a time until the affected area is covered. Let it air dry, then cover with waterproof adhesive tape. If the preparation touches healthy skin, immediately wash it off with soap and water.
- Stick-on plaster: Trim it to the size and shape of the wart before putting it on.
- Disk with a pad: Choose a disk that is the right size, apply it, then cover with the pad supplied.
- **Do not** apply any product to skin that is red, broken or swollen.
- **Do not** use the product more often than recommended in the directions.
- **Do not** use any product for more than 12 weeks.

When should you see your healthcare provider?

See your healthcare provider if the wart is not gone after 12 weeks of treatment or if the healthy skin has been damaged.

Chapter 53

A Summary of Common Skin Conditions

Penny F. Miller, BSc(Pharm), MA

Table 1: Summary of Common Skin Conditions[a,1,2,3,4,5,6]

Body Area	Condition	Signs and Symptoms	Location(s)	Management
Scalp	Tinea capitis See Chapter 65: Fungal Skin Infections	Bald patch(es) with round, scaling lesions; itchy. May be inflamed boggy nodule	Scalp (usually in children)	Patient requires assessment and/or treatment by appropriate healthcare practitioner.
	Head lice See Chapter 69: Parasitic Skin Infections: Lice and Scabies	White spots (nits) clinging to base of hair that are not easily removed; itchy	Scalp, especially sides and posterior aspects (commonly in children)	Recommend self-care.
	Psoriasis See Chapter 71: Psoriasis	Silver scales on an elevated erythematous base (plaques). Pinpoint bleeding spots are evident when scales are scratched off. Symmetric distribution is common	Posterior scalp	Patient requires assessment by appropriate healthcare practitioner for diagnosis; self-care measures may be appropriate depending on severity at diagnosis.
	Dandruff See Chapter 58: Dandruff and Seborrheic Dermatitis	Diffuse, white flakes without redness; mildly itchy	Scalp	Recommend self-care.
	Shingles (Herpes zoster) See Chapter 74: Viral Skin Rashes	Unilateral, painful, grouped blisters with eventual crusts. The lesions are arranged in a linear (dermatomal) pattern along a sensory nerve	Scalp, forehead and face	Patient requires assessment and/or treatment by appropriate healthcare practitioner immediately, due to risk of eye involvement.
	Seborrheic dermatitis See Chapter 58: Dandruff and Seborrheic Dermatitis	Mildly red patches with yellowish, greasy scale. Ill-defined borders	Scalp, eyebrows and nasolabial folds, eyelid margins	Recommend self-care; patient requires assessment and/or treatment by appropriate healthcare practitioner if severe.
Trunk	Shingles (Herpes zoster) See Chapter 74: Viral Skin Rashes	Painful vesicles in a unilateral dermatomal distribution with eventual crusting	Dermatomal distribution, linear from back to chest or abdomen	Patient requires assessment and/or treatment by appropriate healthcare practitioner promptly as treatment should be initiated <72 h from onset of rash.
	Tinea corporis	Round, red, scaly patches with well-defined, raised	Trunk, limbs	Recommend self-care.

(cont'd)

Table 1: **Summary of Common Skin Conditions**[a,1,2,3,4,5,6] *(cont'd)*

Body Area	Condition	Signs and Symptoms	Location(s)	Management
	See Chapter 65: Fungal Skin Infections	edges; central clearing and itchy		
	Phototoxic photosensitivity reaction See Chapter 72: Prevention and Treatment of Sun-induced Skin Damage	Exaggerated sunburn (may be blistered if severe)	Sun-exposed areas	Recommend self-care unless severe; patients then require management by appropriate healthcare practitioner for reassessment of drug therapy if necessary.
	Photoallergic photosensitivity reaction	Red, itchy papules with no sharp borders	Any skin area	Recommend self-care.
	Pityriasis versicolor See Chapter 65: Fungal Skin Infections	Light-coloured patches on tanned skin or darker-coloured patches on untanned skin; fine scale	Chest, back	Recommend self-care.
Face	Acne See Chapter 54: Acne	Comedones, papules, pustules and cysts. Commonly in adolescents	Face	Recommend self-care if mild; patient requires assessment and/or treatment by appropriate healthcare practitioner if moderate-severe.
	Acne rosacea See Chapter 54: Acne	Papules, pustules (no comedones); flushing in blush areas	Face	Patient requires assessment and/or treatment by appropriate healthcare practitioner.
	Perioral dermatitis See Chapter 54: Acne	Discrete, red or flesh-coloured papules and pustules. May be pruritic and burning	Around mouth and nasolabial folds	Patient requires assessment and/or treatment by appropriate healthcare practitioner.
	Folliculitis See Chapter 56: Bacterial Skin Infections: Impetigo, Furuncles and Carbuncles and Chapter 54: Acne	Small red pustules surrounding hair follicles	Bearded (hairy) areas	Recommend self-care.
	Furuncles See Chapter 56: Bacterial Skin Infections: Impetigo, Furuncles and Carbuncles	Painful, red, raised lump (nodules) with pus-filled centre around hair follicle	Bearded (hairy) areas, back of neck	Recommend self-care if only a few, small lesions are present; otherwise patient requires assessment and/or treatment by appropriate healthcare practitioner.
	Carbuncles See Chapter 56: Bacterial Skin	Large, painful, red, raised nodules with pus-filled centre around multiple hair follicles; fever, malaise, adenopathy	Bearded (hairy) areas, back of neck	Patient requires assessment and/or treatment by appropriate healthcare practitioner.

(cont'd)

Table 1: **Summary of Common Skin Conditions**[a,1,2,3,4,5,6] *(cont'd)*

Body Area	Condition	Signs and Symptoms	Location(s)	Management
	Infections: Impetigo, Furuncles and Carbuncles			
	Cold sores (Herpes simplex) See Chapter 90: Cold Sores (Herpes Labialis)	Tingling sensation progressing to tiny, painful, grouped blisters, then crusts	Lips	Recommend self-care; patient requires assessment and/or treatment by appropriate healthcare practitioner if genital involvement or immunocompromised.
	Impetigo See Chapter 56: Bacterial Skin Infections: Impetigo, Furuncles and Carbuncles	Weeping vesicles with honey-coloured crusts. Erythema surrounds lesion. Adenopathy is common	Around nose and mouth (usually)	Recommend self-care if a few small lesions; otherwise, patient requires assessment and/or treatment by appropriate healthcare practitioner.
	Phototoxic photosensitivity reaction See Chapter 72: Prevention and Treatment of Sun-induced Skin Damage	Exaggerated sunburn	Sun-exposed skin areas	Recommend self-care unless severe; patients then require management by appropriate healthcare practitioner for reassessment of drug therapy if necessary.
	Photoallergic photosensitivity reaction	Red, itchy vesicles	Any skin area	Recommend self-care unless severe; patient requires management by appropriate healthcare practitioner for reassessment of drug therapy if necessary.
	Contact dermatitis See Chapter 55: Atopic, Contact, and Stasis Dermatitis	Localized, itchy, red vesicles	Any skin area in contact with allergen	Recommend self-care unless severe.
	Atopic dermatitis See Chapter 55: Atopic, Contact, and Stasis Dermatitis	Red, itchy, weeping vesicles; eventually see chronic changes—lichenified dry skin (thickened, accentuated skin markings)	Infants: face (cheeks) Adolescents and young adults: sides of neck	Patient requires assessment and/or treatment by appropriate healthcare practitioner.
Limbs	Contact dermatitis See Chapter 55: Atopic, Contact, and Stasis Dermatitis	Localized, itchy red vesicles	Hands, wrists or any area exposed to contact allergen	Recommend self-care unless severe.
	Common warts See Chapter 73: Viral Skin Infections:	Skin-coloured, well-defined, small, round, rough-surfaced papules. May see black dots on surface	Hands, fingers, around nails	Recommend self-care.

(cont'd)

Table 1: **Summary of Common Skin Conditions**[a,1,2,3,4,5,6] *(cont'd)*

Body Area	Condition	Signs and Symptoms	Location(s)	Management
	Common and Flat Warts			
	Flat warts See Chapter 73: Viral Skin Infections: Common and Flat Warts	Multiple, smooth, flat or slightly elevated reddish papules	Hands	Patient requires assessment and/or treatment by appropriate healthcare practitioner.
	Psoriasis See Chapter 71: Psoriasis	Red plaques with a silvery scale which reveal bleeding points when removed.	Knees, elbows	Patient requires assessment by appropriate healthcare practitioner for diagnosis; self-care measures may be appropriate depending on severity at diagnosis.
	Scabies See Chapter 69: Parasitic Skin Infections: Lice and Scabies	Red lesions, possibly with thin grey lines; itching that increases at night	Finger webs and wrists; armpits	Patient requires assessment by appropriate healthcare practitioner for diagnosis; recommend self-care for management.
	Atopic dermatitis See Chapter 55: Atopic, Contact, and Stasis Dermatitis	Red, itchy vesicles	Extensor areas in infants; flexural area in adolescents and adults	Patient requires assessment and/or treatment by appropriate healthcare practitioner.
	Cellulitis	Red, hot, hard, painful skin area with systemic symptoms of fever and malaise	Often at site of trauma	Patient requires immediate assessment and/or treatment by appropriate healthcare practitioner.
	Stasis dermatitis See Chapter 55: Atopic, Contact, and Stasis Dermatitis	Red, itchy vesicles, edema followed by brownish, scaly, thickened skin; pain	Lower legs, ankles (in older adults)	Patient requires assessment and/or treatment by appropriate healthcare practitioner.
Nails	Distal and lateral subungual onychomycosis (Tinea unguium) See Chapter 64: Fungal Nail Infections (Onychomycosis)	Thickened; discoloured yellow-brown; debris collection under the nail; separation of nail plate from nail bed	Fungal infection starts in the nail bed just under the tip of the nail (distal end) and spreads proximally towards cuticle	Patient requires assessment and/or treatment by appropriate healthcare practitioner.
	White superficial onychomycosis (Tinea unguium) See Chapter 64: Fungal Nail Infections (Onychomycosis)	Powdery white patches on nail surface. May spread to involve entire nail which becomes roughened and crumbly	Fungal infection starts as patches on top of nail plate	Patient requires assessment and/or treatment by appropriate healthcare practitioner.

(cont'd)

Table 1: **Summary of Common Skin Conditions**[a,1,2,3,4,5,6] *(cont'd)*

Body Area	Condition	Signs and Symptoms	Location(s)	Management
	Paronychia (*Candida* onychomycosis) See Chapter 64: Fungal Nail Infections (Onychomycosis)	Swelling and redness of nail fold. Cuticle may detach from nail plate	Involves nail folds and nails in persons with excessive water exposure	Patient requires assessment by appropriate healthcare practitioner for diagnosis; recommend self-care once diagnosed if mild case.
Genitals	Pubic lice See Chapter 69: Parasitic Skin Infections: Lice and Scabies	Crab lice and eggs detectable; very itchy	Genital area; other hairy areas	Recommend self-care.
	Candidiasis See Chapter 65: Fungal Skin Infections	Red, moist rash with irregular edges and satellite lesions (papules outside the edge of the rash); itchy and sore	Skin folds such as groin (gluteal fold), under breasts, axillae	Recommend self-care.
	Tinea cruris See Chapter 65: Fungal Skin Infections	Red-brown, bilateral, well-demarcated rash; itchy	Inner aspect of thighs and pubic area; scrotum and penis is spared in males. Often associated with tinea pedis	Recommend self-care.
	Psoriasis See Chapter 71: Psoriasis	Bilateral, red, sharply demarcated plaques (scales are absent in intertriginous areas)	Intergluteal folds (groin), axillae	Patient requires assessment by appropriate healthcare practitioner for diagnosis; recommend self-care for management depending on severity at diagnosis.

[a] *Only the most common signs and symptoms, presentations and locations are listed; not inclusive. Systemic symptoms accompanying these rashes or any conditions not responding to self-care management should be referred to an appropriate healthcare practitioner. Viral exanthems and foot conditions not included in this table.*

References

1. Edwards C, Stillman P. *Minor illness or major disease?: responding to symptoms in the pharmacy.* 3rd ed. London: Pharmaceutical Press; 2000.
2. Marks JG, Miller JJ, eds. *Lookingbill and Marks' principles of dermatology.* 5th ed. Philadelphia: Saunders/Elsevier; 2013.
3. Goldsmith LA, Katz SI, Gilchrest BA et al., eds. *Fitzpatrick's dermatology in general medicine.* 8th ed. New York: McGraw-Hill; 2012.
4. Schalock PC, Hsu JT, Arndt, KA, eds. *Lippincott's primary care dermatology.* Philadelphia: Wolters Kluwer/Lippincott Williams & Wilkins; 2011.
5. Habif TP. *Clinical dermatology: a color guide to diagnosis and therapy.* 6th ed. St. Louis: Elsevier; 2016.
6. Habif TP, Campbell JL, Chapman MS et al. *Skin disease: diagnosis and treatment.* 3rd ed. New York: Saunders/Elsevier; 2011.

Chapter 54
Acne

Debra Sibbald, BScPhm, ACPR, MA (Adult Education), PhD (Education)

Pathophysiology

Acne vulgaris, or acne, is a common, multifactorial, androgen-dependent skin disorder, which can vary in presentation and be difficult to treat. Although perceived as benign and self-limiting, acne is associated with important physical and psychological problems. Acne is present in about 80% of people between the ages of 11 and 30. Although primarily a disease of adolescence (prevalence in this age group ranges from 50–95%), it is not limited to teenagers, can begin as early as the neonatal period, and is present in 20–30% of individuals aged 20–40. The intensity and duration vary for each individual, and in most cases acne becomes less active as adolescence ends. It is severe in males in about 15% of cases, which is tenfold greater than females. Acne has an earlier onset and is more persistent in females (12% of women vs. 3% of men in those aged 25–58 years); periodic premenstrual flares may continue until menopause.[1,2] Genetic factors have been recognized: there is a high concordance among identical twins and a tendency towards severe acne in patients with a family history of acne.[3]

Four primary pathogenic factors interact to produce acne lesions:

1. Increased sebum production by the sebaceous gland
2. *Propionibacterium acnes* follicular colonization (and bacterial lipolysis of sebum triglycerides to free fatty acids)
3. Release of inflammatory mediators
4. Alteration in the inflammatory process

Acne usually begins in the prepubertal period when the adrenal glands mature, and progresses as androgen production and sebaceous gland activity increase with gonad development.

There has been an improvement in the understanding of acne development that suggests acne is a disease that involves both innate and adaptive immune systems and inflammatory events.[3] Receptors that regulate sebaceous lipid metabolism work in concert with those regulating epidermal growth and differentiation. Acne is the result of an obstructed sebaceous follicle, called a microcomedone. Patients with seborrhea and acne have a significantly greater number of lobules per sebaceous gland compared with unaffected individuals. Sebaceous glands (Figure 1) increase in size and activity in response to circulating androgens. Sterol regulatory element-binding proteins mediate the increase in sebaceous lipid formation. The composition of sebum is altered, with a reduction in linoleic acid. The pooling of sebum in the follicle provides ideal substrate conditions for proliferation of the anaerobic bacterium *P. acnes*, which produces a lipase that can hydrolyze sebum triglycerides into free fatty acids. This generates a T-cell response, which results in inflammation. Inflammatory responses occur prior to the hyperproliferation of keratinocytes.[4,5]

The development of comedones is independent of the colonization with *P. acnes* and occurs due to the growth change of keratinocytes. The infra-infundibulum increases its keratinization of cells leading to hypercornification and development of the microcomedone, the primary lesion of both noninflammatory and inflammatory acne.[6] Cells aggregate in an expanding mass, which forms a dense keratinous plug. Sebum, produced in increasing amounts by the active gland, becomes trapped behind the keratin plug and solidifies, contributing to open or closed comedone formation. The sebaceous gland also acts as an endocrine organ in response to changes in androgens and other hormones. Oxidized squalene can stimulate the hyperproliferative behaviour of keratinocytes. The closed comedone, or whitehead, is the first clinically visible lesion of acne and takes approximately 5 months to develop. The closed comedone is almost completely obstructed to drainage and has a tendency to rupture.[7,8,9]

As the plug extends to the upper canal and dilates its opening, an open comedone, or blackhead, is formed. Its dark colour is not due to dirt but to either oxidized lipid and melanin or to the impacted mass of horny cells. The cylindrically shaped, open comedone is very stable and may persist for a long time as soluble substances and liquid sebum escape more easily. Acne that is characterized by open and closed comedones is called noninflammatory acne.

Recruitment of polymorphs into the follicle during the inflammatory process, and release of *P. acnes*-generated chemokines, leads to pus formation. The pus eventually bursts on the surface with resolution of the inflammation, or into the dermis. *P. acnes* also produces enzymes which increase the permeability of the follicular wall, causing it to rupture, releasing keratin, hair, lipids and irritating free fatty acids into the dermis. Several different types of inflammatory lesions may form. A superficial aggregation of neutrophils forms a pustule, a raised white lesion filled with pus, usually less than 5 mm in diameter. Superficial pustules usually resolve within a few days without scarring. A deeper, dermal, inflammatory infiltration will produce a nodule, the most severe variant of acne. They are warm, tender, firm lesions, with a diameter of 5 mm or greater. They may be suppurative or hemorrhagic within the dermis, may involve adjacent follicles and sometimes extend down to fat. Nodules and deep lesions may result in scarring. Suppurative nodules can be called cysts because they resemble inflamed epidermal cysts. The cascade of the pathogenesis of acne is shown in Figure 2.

Hyperpigmentation and scarring are 2 sequelae of acne (see Treating Sequelae of Acne). A time delay of up to 3 years between acne onset and adequate treatment correlates to degrees of scarring, and emphasizes the need for earlier therapy.[10,11]

Figure 1: **The Skin**

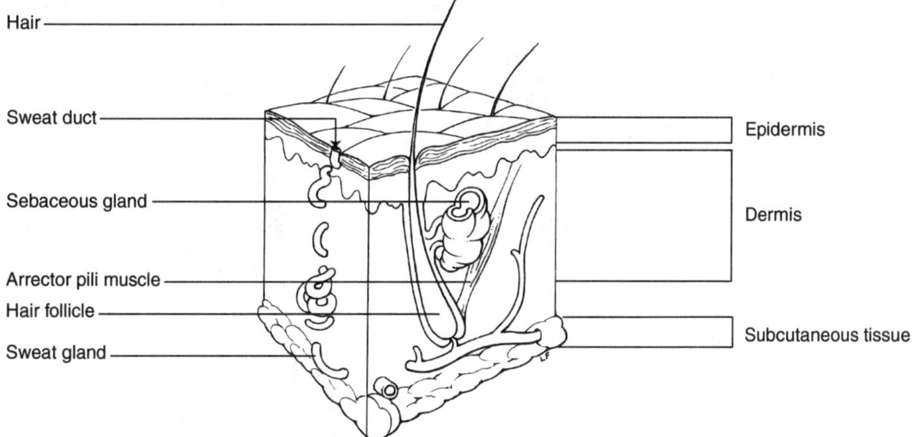

Figure 2: **Pathogenesis of Acne Cascade**

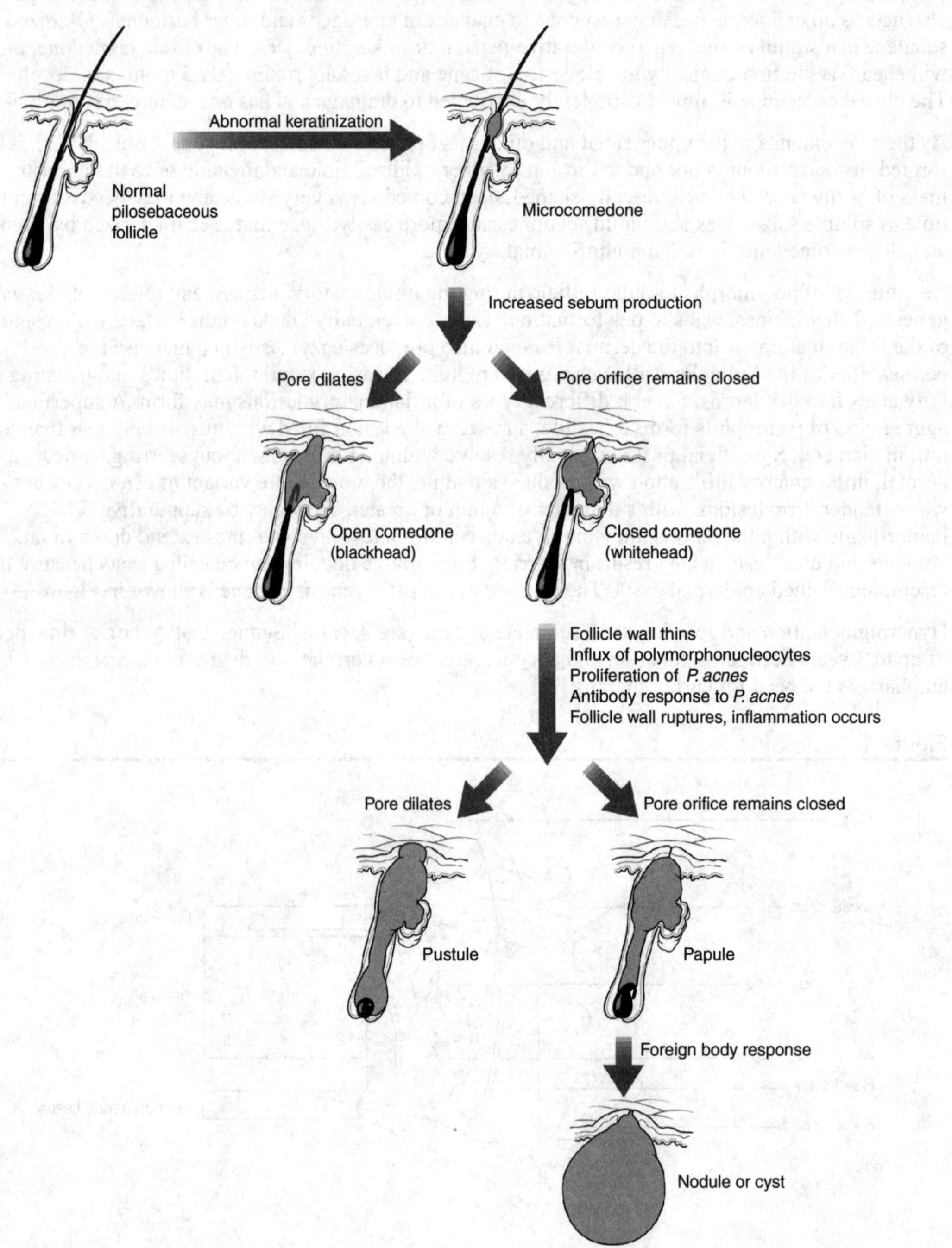

Goals of Therapy

- Alleviate symptoms by reducing the number and severity of lesions
- Slow the progression of signs and symptoms
- Limit disease duration and recurrence
- Prevent long-term disfigurement associated with scarring and hyperpigmentation
- Avoid psychological suffering

Patient Assessment

Information on the assessment of patients with acne can also be found in Figure 3.

Clinical Presentation

Acne can be noninflammatory or inflammatory. Noninflammatory acne is characterized by open and closed comedones. Inflammatory acne is traditionally characterized by papulopustular and/or nodular lesions. Lesions can occur anywhere on the body apart from the palms and soles, and are usually located on the face, back, neck and chest, and may extend to buttocks or extremities. Often resolution of these lesions leaves erythematous or pigmented macules that can persist for months or longer, especially in dark-skinned individuals.

Existing grading systems are very difficult to compare. Two commonly used grading systems are detailed in Table 1.

Table 1: **Severity Grading of Acne Lesions**[3,12]

FDA Investigator Global Assessment (2005)		European Union Guidelines Clinical Classification (2012)
Type 1	Almost clear: Rare noninflammatory lesions (NIL) with no more than 1 papule	Comedonal acne
Type 2	Mild: Some NIL but no more than a few papules or pustules	Mild-moderate papulopustular acne
Type 3	Moderate: Many NIL, some inflammatory lesions (IL), no more than 1 nodule	Severe papulopustular acne, moderate nodular acne
Type 4	Severe: Up to many NIL and IL, but no more than a few nodular lesions	Severe nodular acne, conglobate acne

Risk and Aggravating Factors

Acne can be caused or exacerbated by a variety of factors. One in 5 infants ≤3 months of age may develop papules, pustules and, less commonly, closed or open comedones, primarily on the cheeks, due to placental transfer of maternal androgens (neonatal acne). The acne subsides within a few months with regular maturation. Boys are affected more often than girls because of a transient increase in testosterone secretion during the third and fourth month of intrauterine life. *Malassezia* species (a yeast) may be involved in pathogenesis.[2] Resolution occurs without therapy.[13] Infants with neonatal acne may have more severe teenage acne compared with their peers.[2]

Acneiform eruptions may be provoked by hormonal changes such as androgenic and antiestrogenic progestogens, found in oral contraceptives. Hormonal changes in pregnancy may also change the appearance of acne. Seventy percent of females may complain of premenstrual flares. The pilosebaceous duct opening is significantly smaller between days 15 and 20 of the menstrual cycle, causing duct obstruction which impedes sebum flow and keratin hydration.[14,15] Endocrine-related conditions (e.g., irregular menses, hirsutism, alopecia) may contribute to formation of acne lesions.

The application of some topical agents may promote the formation of acne (contact acne). This can be due to the use of cosmetics or topical medications or to occupational hazards. Comedone formation through mechanically occluded follicles (pomade acne) may occur with the use of oil-based scalp preparations on the forehead and temples, oily lubricants (such as baby oil) in infants and children and the application of topical tar products. Tar folliculitis can be minimized by applying the tar in the direction the hair grows out at the skin surface, leaving the angle beneath the hair free of tar to allow secretion of duct contents. In some postadolescent women, acne can be caused or made worse by the liberal use of oily cosmetics (cosmetic acne). This commonly occurs in a perioral distribution with a clear zone around the lips; acne due to application of hairspray may develop around the hair margins. Closed comedones, papules, pustules and nodules may be induced by contact with occupational materials including acnegenic industrial agents such as coal tar, pitch, mineral oil and petroleum oil (occupational acne). Ingestion, inhalation or transcutaneous penetration of halogenated aromatic hydrocarbons, including the polychlorobiphenyls in paint, varnishes, lacquers, fungicides, insecticides, herbicides, wood preservatives and various oils, produces a distinct form of occupational acne (chloracne). Within a few months of sufficient exposure, open and closed comedones appear on the chest, temples and behind the ears. Inflammatory lesions may follow.[16]

Physical pressure from headbands, violins, chin straps, sports helmets, guitar straps and orthopedic braces has induced localized acne (acne mechanica). Mechanical friction should be eliminated or reduced. Wool or other rough textured fabrics and occlusive clothing may also be irritants.

Acne patients may manipulate their comedones and pustules with finger pressure by picking, excoriating or pinching in an attempt to drain lesions, often subconsciously or during sleep (acne excoriée). Crusting erosions, scarring and hyperpigmentation may result from the ensuing rupture and inflammation.

Diet has been the focus of investigations, with studies indicating a correlation between acne and a Western diet.[3] In the past, it was thought that acne was not influenced by diet, but a balanced diet should be advised for overall health. In studies examining diet and acne, patients could choose to restrict the intake of certain foods they perceived as exacerbating acne (chocolate, cola drinks, milk and milk products).[17,18] Conclusions were based on results of a methodologically flawed study that was conducted over 40 years ago, showing no significant differences in lesion count or sebum characteristics following ingestion of an enriched chocolate bar vs. a control bar without cocoa butter and chocolate liquor.[18] A subsequent small study also showed no differences in count or grade of acne in medical students who were asked to consume the food they thought most likely to worsen acne, for 7 days.[19] The information from these studies was likely over-interpreted to dismiss potential effects of diet on acne.

Beginning in 2005, a series of studies have linked consumption of dairy products with acne, perhaps due to natural hormonal components and/or other bioactive molecules in milk.[20,21,22] The Nurses Health Study, which involved 47 355 women, used retrospective data on diet during high school and found an association between acne and intake of milk.

Insulin-like growth factor (IGF) may play a role in acne.[23,24] IGF is increased by ingestion of high glycemic loads and so could potentially link diet and acne. A Cochrane review concluded there is some low quality evidence from a single trial[25] that a low-glycemic-load diet may reduce total skin lesions in acne.[26] While improvements in acne and insulin sensitivity suggest the role of nutrition-related lifestyle factors in acne pathogenesis, the independent effects of weight loss vs. dietary intervention need to be isolated.[27]

The possible role of dietary factors in acne cannot be dismissed as studies to date have not been sufficiently large or robust. While still controversial, diet may play a role in the development or progression of acne and further studies are ongoing.[26,28,29,30]

Environmental factors including heat and humidity may induce comedones, while pressure, friction and excessive scrubbing or washing can exacerbate existing acne by causing microcomedones to rupture. Hairstyles low on the forehead or neck or occlusive clothing may cause excessive sweating and worsen acne.[31] Sunlight may be palliating. Studies examining the relationship between tobacco smoking and acne show inconsistent results. However, dermatologists have begun to counsel people to quit tobacco smoking as a potential auxiliary treatment for acne.[32]

Emotions such as intense anger and stress can exacerbate acne, causing flares or increasing mechanical manipulation. Two-thirds of affected teenagers wish that they could speak with their healthcare provider about acne, but only one-third actually do.[33]

Differential Diagnosis

Acne is rarely misdiagnosed. The most commonly mistaken conditions include rosacea, perioral dermatitis, gram-negative folliculitis and drug-induced acne.[34]

Acne rosacea, often called adult acne, is a chronic, relapsing condition involving blood vessels, occurring after age 30 in fair-complexioned persons, commonly Celtic. The first sign is easy flushing (redness or erythema), followed by development of inflammatory lesions with edema, papules and pustules appearing on the nose, cheeks, chin and forehead, with telangiectasia (spider veins) appearing as the condition progresses. It may be sensitive to the touch. It differs from acne vulgaris in several ways: onset is not linked to increased androgens or endocrine changes, comedones are not usually present and aggravating factors include alcohol ingestion, spicy foods, smoking, overexposure to sunlight, hot drinks (especially those containing caffeine), temperature extremes, friction, irritating cosmetics and corticosteroid use. It is not curable and progressively worsens, and may ultimately result in rhinophyma (enlarged nose). Treatment with antibiotics, particularly topical metronidazole, may be required.[35]

Perioral dermatitis occurs primarily in young women and adolescents and is characterized by erythema, scaling and papulopustular lesions commonly clustered around the nasolabial folds, mouth and chin. The cause is unknown.[34]

Gram-negative folliculitis (*Proteus, Pseudomonas, Klebsiella*) may complicate acne, presenting as a sudden change to pustules or large inflammatory cysts occurring after long-term treatment of acne with oral antibiotics. Folliculitis may occur due to staphylococci. There is a sudden onset of superficial pustules around the nose, chin and cheeks.[34]

Several conditions include acne as a characteristic component, and understanding the mechanisms involved in these syndromes provides insight into acne pathogenesis. They include polycystic ovary syndrome (elevated androgen levels), PAPA syndrome (pyogenic arthritis, pyoderma gangrenosum, acne—early onset arthritis with increased inflammatory activity) and SAPHO syndrome (synovitis, acne, pustulosis, hyperostosis, osteitis syndrome—sterile inflammatory arthro-osteitis, with *P. acnes* as a possible trigger).[6]

Table 2 summarizes conditions included in the differential diagnosis of acne.

Table 2: **Differential Diagnosis of Acne[a]**

Acne Variant	Comedones: Open	Comedones: Closed	Pustules	Papules	Nodules	Other
Vulgaris	+	+	+	+	+	
Drug-induced		+/–	+	+		
Neonatal		+	+	+/–		
Conglobata			+	++	++	Cysts, abscesses, sinus tracts
Fulminans			+	++	++	Ulcerating cysts
Contact						
pomade		++	+			
cosmetic	+	++	++	+		
occupational (e.g., exposure to oil)		++	+	+		
chloracne	++	++	+	+		
Endocrine			++	+	+	
Excoriated			+	+		Crusts, scars, erosions, hyperpigmentation
Mechanical		++	++	+		
Rosacea			+	+	+/–	Erythema, edema, telangiectasia

[a] Other conditions that present with raised lesions resembling papules or pustules include milia, folliculitis (gram-negative, staphylococcal, *Candida*), impetigo, warts, dental sinuses and epidermoid cysts.

Drug-induced Acne

Certain drugs may cause acneiform eruptions (Table 3). Systemic corticosteroids can cause a pustular inflammatory form of acne, especially on the trunk; onset is abrupt, 2–6 weeks after initiation of therapy. Acne has also been associated with most of the potent topical corticosteroids, but not with hydrocortisone, which lacks the ability to inhibit protein synthesis. Discontinuation of the corticosteroid results in an initial worsening of the appearance due to removal of the anti-inflammatory action of the corticosteroid itself. Caution patients about this reaction, which can be subdued through judicious use of topical hydrocortisone.[38,39,40]

Antiepileptics and tuberculostatics are most commonly implicated in drug-induced acne, followed by lithium. Other metals that can induce acne include cobalt in vitamin B_{12}.[41] Halogens, especially an excess of iodide in seafood, salt and health foods, can worsen acne.

As well, certain minor cosmetic ingredients have been implicated in cosmetic acne, including isopropyl myristate, cocoa butter and fatty acids.[2]

Table 3: **Drug-induced Acne**[36,37]

Drugs that May Produce Acne-like Eruptions (Comedonal and/or Inflammatory)	
Hormones:	**Tuberculostatic Drugs:**
Anabolic steroids	Ethambutol
Androgenic hormones in women	Isoniazid
Corticosteroids	**Miscellaneous:**
Corticotropin (ACTH)	Azathioprine
Oral contraceptives (especially those with high progestin component)	Coal tar
Halogens:	Cyclosporine
Bromides	Dantrolene
Chlorides	Epidermal growth factor receptor (EGFR)
Halothane	Gold salts
Iodides	Lithium salts
Antiepileptic Drugs:	Maprotiline
Phenobarbital	Psoralens
Phenytoin	Quinidine
	Quinine
	Vitamins B_2, B_6 and B_{12}

Drugs that May Produce Inflammatory Papular/Pustular Eruptions or Folliculitis (Occlusion of Hair Follicles)	
Carbamazepine	Isoniazid
Cefazolin	Naproxen
Cephalexin	Norfloxacin
Chloramphenicol	Piperazine
Furosemide	Pyrimethamine
Dactinomycin	Streptomycin
Diltiazem	Sulfamethoxazole/trimethoprim
	Tetracyclines

Quality of Life (QOL) Indicators

QOL indicators represent patients' perceptions of and reactions to their health. This is important in patient assessment as it relates to patients' understanding, expectations, concerns and behaviour regarding acne therapy as a self-care option. Assessing patients' acne-related impairment in QOL may aid in management by evaluating the psychological impact of their acne, which may not correlate with the clinical severity, aid in detection of depression or need for psychological care, and improve therapeutic outcomes. Examples of global scales that have been used to evaluate acne include Skindex[42] and the Dermatology QOL Index;[43] examples of acne-specific scales include the Acne-specific QOL questionnaire[44] and the Acne QOL Scale.[45]

Figure 3 provides an approach to the assessment of patients with acne.

Specialist Consultation for Complicated Acne

Patients may require further investigation, additional therapy or other modalities in the following situations:

- Acne is drug-induced or due to a known endocrinopathy (e.g., polycystic ovarian syndrome as may be suspected with hirsutism, weight gain)
- Acne at a very young age (may need endocrinology consult)
- Moderate to severe acne
- Acne that is nonresponsive to initial therapy
- Presence of scarring, especially if moderate to severe.

Nonpharmacologic Therapy

Figure 4 provides an approach for treating acne with nonprescription medication.

Cleansing: Patients should wash no more than twice daily with a mild soap or soapless cleanser. Patients with acne may wash too frequently, attempting to remove surface oils. There is no evidence this is helpful since surface lipids do not affect acne.[46] Contributory lipids are deep in the follicle and cannot be removed through washing. Antiseptic cleansers, while producing a clean, refreshed feeling, remove only surface dirt, oil and aerobic bacteria. They do not affect *P. acnes*. There is no evidence that one washing regimen is superior to another. Scrubbing should be minimized to prevent follicular rupture. Soaps produce a drying effect on the skin due to detergent action. As medicated cleansers require increased contact time, this drying action is pronounced, especially with peeling agents. Avoid cream-based cleansers.

Shaving: Males should try both electric and safety razors to determine which is more comfortable. When using a safety razor, the beard should be softened with soap and warm water or shaving gel. Shaving should be done as lightly and infrequently as possible, using a sharp blade and avoiding nicking lesions. Strokes should be in the direction of hair growth, shaving each area only once.

Comedone extraction: Comedone extraction by the patient is useful and painless. It results in immediate cosmetic improvement although it has not been widely tested in clinical trials. Pretreatment with a peeler for 4–6 weeks often facilitates the procedure.[40] Following cleansing with hot water, a comedone extractor is placed over the lesion and gentle pressure applied until the contents are expressed. This removes unsightly lesions, preventing progression to inflammation. A correctly sized extractor allows the central keratin plug to extrude through the opening. The small end of a plastic eye dropper, with bulb removed, may also be used. These instruments should be cleaned with alcohol after each use. Some initial reddening may be apparent. If the contents are not expressed with modest pressure, patients should not continue since improper extraction may further irritate the skin. A healthcare practitioner should be consulted if this technique is too difficult for the patient to manage. Since the follicle is difficult to remove completely, comedones may recur between 25–50 days following expression. Fewer than 10% of comedone extractions are a complete success, but the process is useful if done properly.[2]

Ultraviolet light: Although ultraviolet light was recommended in the past for desquamation, it is no longer advised since the carcinogenic and photoaging effects of ultraviolet exposure are well established. Moreover, inflamed skin is more susceptible to the damaging effects of ultraviolet light. Patients using tretinoin may show heightened sensitivity to ultraviolet light.[47] Acne patients should apply sunscreen (SPF ≥15) with an alcohol- or oil-free base and avoid using the acnegenic benzophenones (see Chapter 72: Prevention and Treatment of Sun-induced Skin Damage).

Encourage patients with acne to discontinue or avoid any aggravating factors, to maintain a balanced, low-glycemic-load diet (see Chapter 43: Weight Management) and control stress. Evidence shows that by being empathetic and informative during counselling, the health practitioner may motivate the patient to continue long-term therapy.[31,33,34]

Prevention of Cosmetic Acne

Persistent low-grade acne in women after their mid-twenties is frequently caused by heavy cosmetic use. Adolescent acne in younger women may be exacerbated with makeup overuse. The problem is perpetuated when the resultant blemishes are concealed with more cosmetics.

Advise patients to stop using oil-containing cosmetics and avoid cosmetic programs that advocate applying multiple layers of cream-based cleansers and cover-ups, which are advertised through the media and often available through Internet shopping with promotional bonuses. Three-step basic systems usually combine medicated and nonmedicated ingredients, although it may not be apparent that therapeutic agents are included. They often start with cleansers, in lotions or creams, which may contain a multitude of unnecessary ingredients, including medicated peelers, oils, fragrances and preservatives. Drugs commonly included are subtherapeutic or low doses of salicylic acid, sulfur or benzoyl peroxide. The second step is generally a "toner" or "refresher" that is usually water- or alcohol-based and might contain medicated ingredients such as alpha-hydroxy acids (e.g., glycolic acid, a mild comedolytic) or even glycerin as a humectant. The final product may be called intensive or repairing solution, usually lowest-strength combinations of peelers such as benzoyl peroxide, sulfur or salicylic acid, plus potentially sensitizing fragrances and preservatives, or oil-soluble sunscreens that are not identified on the label. Bases may have significant oil content. There may be additional products to supplement as necessary to the base routine of 3 steps, such as masks or spot treatments. Multiple-step cosmetic programs are often costly, and contain subtherapeutic concentrations of ingredients that are not necessarily first line.[48] They should be avoided in favour of simple cleansers and more effective single-ingredient peelers, at optimal concentrations. Creams and cosmetics used during a beauty salon facial may precipitate acne in susceptible patients.

Patients with acne should wash twice daily with a mild soap or a soapless cleanser, and restrict cosmetics including makeup, moisturizers and sunscreens to oil-free rather than water-based products. Since the spread time of oil-free makeup is lower (i.e., they "sink in" to the skin more quickly), best results are achieved if they are applied to one-quarter of the face at a time. Topical medication should be applied after gentle cleansing.[49]

Cover-up cosmetics for acne are available in several skin tones, in lotion and cream forms. They may be applied as cosmetics 2–3 times daily, over the entire face or to individual lesions. They are usually water-based, nongreasy preparations, often containing peeling agents, antibacterials or hydroquinone. Most contain sulfur. However, nonmedicated, oil-free makeups are preferable to water-based products. Water-based cosmetics may contain significant amounts of oil in the form of undiluted vegetable oils, lanolin, fatty acid esters (butyl stearate, isopropyl myristate), fatty acids (stearic acid), fatty acid alcohols, cocoa butter, coconut oil, red veterinary petrolatum and sunscreens containing benzophenones.[50,51] These are more likely than oil-free products to contribute to pore blockage. The term "noncomedogenic" may refer to either water-based vehicles or products that are free of substances known to induce comedones. They are not necessarily oil-free.

Lipstick, eye shadow, eyeliner, eyebrow pencils and loose face powders are relatively innocuous. Heavier, oil-based preparations, particularly moisturizers and hairsprays, clog pores and accelerate comedone formation.[52]

Since the action of most therapeutic acne agents is to dry the skin, the use of moisturizers should be carefully considered to select the most appropriate product. Active agents such as alpha-hydroxy acids (glycolic, lactic, pyruvic and citric acids) may be present in the cosmetic formulation since they reduce corneocyte adhesion.[2] Patients with acne should use only oil-free products unless absolutely necessary due to treatment with strong drying agents or isotretinoin. Many marketed moisturizers are considered noncomedogenic.

Pharmacologic Therapy

The most critical target for treatment is the microcomedone, because without the follicular occlusion, the whole cascade of acne is arrested. This will involve a combination of preventive measures (to reduce or eliminate risk and aggravating factors) and treatment measures. These should integrate nonpharmacologic and pharmacologic protocols aimed at cleansing as well as targeting all 4 mechanisms involved in acne pathogenesis. Combination therapy to target multiple pathogenic steps is often more effective than monotherapy and may offer secondary advantages of decreasing agent-related side effects and minimizing resistance or tolerance to individual treatments. It takes 8 weeks for a microcomedone to mature, thus any therapy must be continued beyond this duration to assess efficacy.[40] Recommendations should be based on critical evaluation of the literature combined with clinical experience.

Because acne is a chronic disease, lesions typically recur for years. Microcomedones significantly decrease during therapy but rebound almost immediately after therapy is discontinued. Hence, the strategy for treating acne includes an induction phase followed by a maintenance phase, which are further supported by adjunctive treatments and/or cosmetic routines. Maintenance therapy with regular use of appropriate agents reduces the potential for recurrrence of visible lesions. To achieve successful long-term treatment, maintenance therapy must be tolerable, appropriate for the patient's lifestyle and convenient. It will continue for months to years depending on the patient's age. Education about the pathophysiology of acne and the psychosocial benefits of clearer skin may improve patient adherence to consistent therapy which will sustain remission.

Information about treating acne with nonprescription products can also be found in Figure 4 and Table 5. More information about further therapy for acne can be found in *Compendium of Therapeutic Choices*: Acne.

For comparative ingredients of nonprescription products, consult the *Compendium of Products for Minor Ailments*—Skin Care Products: Acne.

Medicated Soaps and Washes

Medicated soaps, washes and foams may contain topical antiseptics or peeling agents such as **salicylic acid**, **sulfur**, **benzoyl peroxide** or **clindamycin**, alone or in combination in low concentrations. Most washes should remain on the skin from 15 seconds to 5 minutes followed by thorough rinsing, limiting the amount of time the active ingredient is in contact with the skin. Other cleansers are applied after washing and left on the skin without rinsing. Quaternary ammonium compounds are cationic detergents that are inactivated quickly in the presence of organic material, such as sebum. The duration of action of these products is short. Evidence of effectiveness of cleansers is limited. One small study found cleansers effective in reducing inflammatory and noninflammatory lesions.[53]

Bacteriostatic soaps such as **hexachlorophene**, **carbanilides** and **salicylanilides (halogenated hydroxyphenols)** have been found to be acnegenic.[46] Few ordinary soaps induce acne. However, patients with acne are particularly susceptible to comedogenic contactants, and if bacteriostatic soaps are applied several times daily for long periods, they may aggravate the skin. Soaps containing **coal tar**, which can induce folliculitis, are not indicated for acne.

Chlorhexidine inhibits in vitro growth of *P. acnes*.[54] A 4% chlorhexidine gluconate preparation in a detergent base has been shown to be as effective as **benzoyl peroxide** washes in patients with mild acne, and both preparations reduced the number of inflammatory and noninflammatory lesions after 8 and 12 weeks, compared with vehicle alone.[55]

Polyester cleansing sponges (e.g., Buf-Puf) are synthetics that abrade the skin surface, removing superficial debris. They are unlikely to unseat comedones, considering the structure of these lesions. The sponges are available in soft or coarse textures, with or without soap. Caution patients against using a circular or rubbing motion that will increase irritation, and instruct them to use single, gentle, continuous strokes on each side of the face, from the midline out towards the ears.

Alcohol-detergent medicated pads, impregnated with **salicylic acid 0.5%**, reduce inflammatory lesions and open comedones in mild to moderate acne. This type of medication is less abrasive, not rinsed off and convenient.[56]

Alcohol-detergent wipes, **swabs** or **"pledgets"** impregnated with antibiotics, such as **clindamycin**, are available. The antibiotic is deposited in low concentrations on the surface of the skin, and may not penetrate to the depths of the pilosebaceous duct. Although patients may like the convenience and perception of using an active agent, these products should not be recommended over simple cleansing.

Cationic (C) bond strips that become activated by water are available. Dirt/oil in the pores is anionic. As the strip dries, the C-bond binds the anionic dirt and removes it when the strip is peeled off.

Abrasives consist of finely divided particles of fused aluminum or plastic together with cleansing and wetting agents. Abrasives peel and remove surface debris and may assist resorption of papules and pustules but despite vigorous rubbing, removal of comedones is not accomplished. Particles such as **sodium tetraborate decahydrate**, dissolve on contact, limiting their usefulness as abrasives.[57] Abrasive cleansers containing polyethylene granules are not more effective than the same cleansing agent without the abrasive granules. These products are not indicated in most cases but may be used in a patient who responds empirically.[58]

Vehicles

The formulation must balance the technical characteristics of maintaining and delivering the drug in an active state together with the need for an elegant product that the patient will enjoy using, so that it is more likely to be applied as required and deliver the full benefit of the active agent. Physically and chemically, the vehicle itself or its contents attempts to do 1 or more of the following: reduce excess oil, control bacteria associated with acne, reduce the effects of hyperkeratinization and unclog pores. Performance, safety and stability should be maximized while addressing technical and commercial factors.

Immiscible liquids might be delivered in oil-in-water or water-in-oil emulsions. In addition to having the undesirable oil content, these vehicles also contain humectants, thickeners, preservatives and fragrance, which may be problematic.

Cleansers often utilize surfactant systems to de-fat the skin surface. Oil is dispersed from the skin into the surfactant system; however, the active ingredient is sometimes trapped and removed on rinsing. As well, the balance between cleanliness and drying or irritation should be taken into account. Most patients prefer products with foaming action, and these must contain additional secondary surfactants to enhance the foam and condition the skin. Soaps are the most widely used cleansing products, but do not lend themselves to efficient delivery of active drug. Two main disadvantages are: as soaps are rinsed off, the deposit of active agent will be small, and the high pH required in soaps may degrade some active ingredients and be less tolerable on sensitive skin. Soapless cleansers are alternatives to soaps.[59]

Solutions are simpler formulations; there is a trend to use them as the soaking liquid for wipe products made with fibrous cloths. Use of these products requires consideration of whether packages are resealable if they contain multiple wipes, and whether the volatility of the solvent will affect storage and availability of the active agent, or cause crystallization. Solutions are used mainly with topical antibiotics, which are often dissolved in alcohol. **Glycolic acid 8%** solution is available for use alone or for incorporation in topical antibiotic preparations. Solutions and washes can be more easily applied to large areas such as the back.[60]

Select nongreasy solutions, gels, lotions and creams as bases for topical acne preparations. Gels are very useful as they are totally oil-free mixtures of water or alcohol, whereas lotions and creams contain some oil phase. Discourage use of moisturizers and oil-based products. Lotions are slightly less drying than gels while creams are more emollient. Many gels contain ethanol or isopropyl alcohol. Isopropyl alcohol is more lipid soluble and may be preferred. Propylene glycol is sometimes present in small amounts to add viscosity and lessen the drying effects of strong peeling agents. Gels are drying but may cause a burning irritation in some patients and may prevent certain kinds of cosmetics from adhering to the skin.[61] Propylene glycol gels are easy to apply and dry without a visible or sticky film.

Nonalcoholic gels may be as effective and less drying than alcoholic solutions. Alcoholic or acetone gels are usually more drying and provide better penetration of the active ingredient.

Consider the patient's skin type and preferences in the choice of vehicle for topical agents: patients with oily skin may prefer vehicles with higher proportions of alcohol (solutions and gels) while those with dry or sensitive skin may prefer nonirritating lotions and creams. Lotions can be used with any skin type and spread well over hair-bearing skin, but will burn or dry if they contain propylene glycol. Also consider the compatibility of vehicles and agents with cosmetics.[62]

Effect of the vehicle alone may be quite substantial in topical therapy. One study estimated vehicle effect to account for an average of 55% (range 35–82%) of reduction in lesion counts for 8 commonly prescribed topical preparations.

How to use topical preparations: To prevent new lesions from developing, topical preparations should not be applied to individual lesions but to the whole area affected by acne, using care around the eyelid, mouth and neck, which chafe easily. Lotions should be applied with a cotton swab once or twice a day after washing or at bedtime if they leave a visible residue. Skincare products may cause dryness and redness, particularly in the early stages of treatment. Should this occur, the product can be applied less frequently, stopped for a while, or switched to different product. Applying a topical vehicle with a high water content a few minutes after applying the medicinal product may reduce irritation. Initial irritation usually subsides as the skin becomes accustomed to the product.

Exfoliants (Peeling Agents)

Exfoliants induce continuous mild drying and peeling by primary irritation, damaging the superficial layers of the skin and inciting inflammation. This stimulates mitosis, thickening the epidermis and increasing horny cells, scaling and erythema. A decrease in sweating results in a dry, less oily surface and may superficially resolve pustular lesions.

Resorcinol, a phenol derivative, has good solubility in both water and alcohol and is heat stable, and is incorporated into a variety of products, including emulsions.[63] Protective packaging is important as resorcinol is reactive to light and oxygen. It is less keratolytic than salicylic acid and may be both bactericidal and fungicidal. It is an irritant and sensitizer and should not be applied to large areas of the skin or on broken skin. It produces a reversible, dark brown scale on some dark-skinned individuals. Products containing resorcinol 1–2% have been used for acne, often in combination with other peeling agents such as sulfur or salicylic acid. The US Food and Drug Administration (FDA) considers resorcinol 2% and resorcinol monoacetate 3%, in combination with sulfur 3–8%, to be safe and effective. These ingredients may enhance the activity of the sulfur.[64]

Salicylic acid is a beta-hydroxy acid that penetrates the pilosebaceous unit (Table 5). It has comedolytic activity, although the concentration in commercial preparations (less than 2–3%) is generally low. While concentrations less than 2% may actually increase keratinization, concentrations between 3 and 6% are keratolytic, softening the horny layer and shedding scales. Salicylic acid's mechanism remains unresolved, attributed to reduced cohesion of corneocytes and shedding of epidermal cells, rather than "lysing" of keratin. It has no effect on mitotic activity of normal epidermis and does not influence disordered cornification.[65] It may also provide mild antibacterial value, as it is active against *P. acnes*. It also offers slight anti-inflammatory activity at concentrations ranging from 0.5–5%. Its efficacy against comedones prevents the development of inflamed lesions; this represents a type of delayed or secondary efficacy.[66]

Salicylic acid products are often used as first-line therapy for mild acne because of their wide availability. They are available in alcohol-detergent–impregnated pads as well as washes, bars and semisolid vehicles. Lower concentrations are sometimes combined with sulfur to produce an additive keratolytic effect. Concentrations of 5–10% can be used for acne, beginning with a low concentration and increasing as tolerance to the irritation develops. It is an effective agent, although as a peeling agent its comparative potency varies according to the model used in measurement. It is slightly less potent than equal-strength benzoyl peroxide when measured with the rabbit ear animal model, and slightly more potent when measured with a biologic microcomedone model.[66] It may have anti-inflammatory properties that help dry inflammatory lesions.[24] Its keratolytic effect may enhance the absorption of other agents. Salicylic acid may cause some degree of local skin peeling and discomfort (burning or reddening) as it is a mild irritant. It is not a sensitizer. Although recognized by the FDA as safe and effective, salicylic acid offers no advantages over other topical agents such as benzoyl peroxide.[64,65,67]

In high concentrations of 20–30% in hydroethanolic vehicles, salicylic acid can be used as a single or multiple peeling agent for comedonal or papular acne and hyperpigmentation. It has been shown to extrude closed and open comedones several days post-peel,[68] and to be effective for inflammatory and noninflammatory acne[69] but must be applied under strict control to offer this adjunctive benefit when treating acne.

Sulfur is used in the precipitated or colloidal form in concentrations of 2–10% since it is practically insoluble in water and must be well dispersed. Stability depends on effective maintenance of the dispersion.[63] Sulfur compounds (e.g., sulfides, thioglycolates, sulfites, thiols, cysteines and thioacetates) are also available and are somewhat weaker. Sulfur-based medications often lessen the severity of acne, presumably because of keratolytic and antibacterial action. Sulfur helps resolve comedones via its exfoliant action. Sulfur's popularity stems from its mild antibacterial action and its ability to quickly resolve pustules and papules, mask and conceal lesions (similar to a thick foundation lotion), and produce irritation leading to skin peeling. Sulfur can cause slight ophthalmic and dermatologic irritation and patients should be cautioned to avoid eye contact. Use should be discontinued if excessive irritation results. Although it is often combined with salicylic acid or resorcinol to increase its effect, use is limited by its offensive odour and the availability of more effective agents.[70] Sulfur meets the criteria of the FDA Advisory Review Panel for nonprescription topical acne products and is considered safe and effective when used alone, but its antibacterial effects are not recognized. Sodium thiosulfate, zinc sulfate and zinc sulfide are not considered safe and effective.

Glycolic acid (an alpha-hydroxy acid) is a humectant that increases water content of the stratum corneum and decreases corneocyte cohesion, and thus may increase desquamation and promote hydration. There is some evidence of efficacy of glycolic acid alone[71] or in combination with other agents[72,73] in the treatment of acne. Glycolic acid is also frequently used in higher strengths (40%) as a chemical peel. Use of a glycolic acid 40% peel at least 5 times (at 2-week intervals), as an adjuvant to the treatment of moderate facial acne, resulted in reduction of noninflammatory lesions in 1 study.[74]

Azelaic acid is another alpha-hydroxy acid effective in the treatment of acne.[3] It has comedolytic and antibacterial effects but does not promote resistant organisms. It is mildly irritating and may cause hypopigmentation. In Canada it is not officially indicated for use in acne.

The **topical retinoids**, which include **tretinoin**, **adapalene**, and **tazarotene**, are the most powerful topical peeling agents. Normal epithelial cell differentiation is a vitamin A–dependent process. Because retinoids reverse the abnormal keratinocyte desquamation found in acne,[47] members of the retinoid family are highly active peelers. They improve acne by inhibiting microcomedone formation, diminishing the number of mature comedones and subsequently of inflammatory lesions, and by normalizing follicular epithelium maturation and desquamation.

Retinoids also have a secondary effect that facilitates acne clearance. By loosening and decreasing corneocytes, they increase skin permeability and facilitate absorption of other agents such as antimicrobials or benzoyl peroxide and penetration of oral antibiotics into the follicular canal. This decreases the overall duration of antibiotic treatment and lessens the possibility of resistance.

Therefore, combination products with oral or topical antimicrobials are useful due to their increased efficacy, faster onset, decreased total antibiotic use (and therefore decreased risk of resistance) and shorter duration of treatment.[47]

Topical retinoids tend to produce remissions that are maintained for extended periods of time, provided the accompanying irritation does not impede patient adherence. Side effects including erythema, xerosis, burning and desquamation are issues for many patients. Application should be at night, 30 minutes after cleansing, starting with every other night for 1–2 weeks to adjust to irritation. During the winter months or for patients with sensitive skin, advise short contact time starting with 2 minutes and adding 30 seconds per dose; discontinue and resume after a 3-day rest if undue irritation results. Doses can be increased after 4–6 weeks use of the lowest concentration and with the least irritating vehicle. Gels and creams are less irritating than solutions. Adapalene and tazarotene are photoirritants not photosensitizers, and sun avoidance and sunscreen use are imperative.[47]

Retinoids may also improve and prevent postinflammatory hyperpigmentation, often seen in darker complexions.

Retinoids are teratogens. Safety of topical retinoids during pregnancy has not been documented and their use remains contraindicated. A meta-analysis showed no increase in major congenital malformations, spontaneous abortions, low birthweight and prematurity in babies exposed to topical retinoids during the first trimester. This information may be useful to reassure women who were inadvertently exposed, but is not adequate to justify use of topical retinoids during pregnancy.[75]

Overall, topical retinoids are the cornerstone of prescription acne treatment and are a safe, effective and economical means of treating all but the most severe cases, and should be the initial first step in moderate acne, alone or in combination with antibiotics and benzoyl peroxide, reverting to retinoids alone for maintenance once adequate results are achieved.

Antibacterials

Choices for antibacterial therapy include benzoyl peroxide, as well as prescription topical and systemic antibiotics and combination products. These drugs kill *P. acnes* and inhibit the production of proinflammatory mediators by organisms that are not killed.[4]

Benzoyl Peroxide

Benzoyl peroxide, a derivative of coal tar, is effective in the treatment of acne.[76] Alone, or in combination, it is part of the standard of care for mild to moderate papular-pustular acne.[77] Benzoyl peroxide is well absorbed through the stratum corneum and concentrates in the pilosebaceous unit. It has 3 principal actions useful in both inflammatory and noninflammatory acne. Firstly, it produces powerful anaerobic antibacterial activity due to slow release of oxygen, expressing bactericidal activity against gram-positive and gram-negative bacteria, yeasts and fungi; this nonspecific antibacterial mechanism does not induce resistance with long-term use.[66] Secondly, it has a rapid (within 2 hours) bactericidal effect that lasts at least 48 hours. As a result, it may decrease the number of inflamed lesions within 5 days. Thirdly, it induces depression of sebum production—this is not a direct effect, nor does it reduce skin surface lipids, but it is effective in reducing free fatty acids, which are comedogenic agents and triggers of inflammation. Topical benzoyl peroxide 5% lowers free fatty acids by 50–60% after daily application for 14 days, and decreases aerobic bacteria by 84% and anaerobic bacteria (primarily *P. acnes*) by 98%.[2] Since its primary effect is antibacterial, it is most effective for predominantly inflammatory acne.

Topical benzoyl peroxide also produces comedolysis. Studies using native microcomedones show an anticomedogenic effect that is slight compared with tretinoin or salicylic acid.[63,78] Many patients with noninflammatory comedonal acne will respond to its peeling action.

Benzoyl peroxide's antiacne effect is augmented by increased blood flow, dermal irritation, local anesthetic properties and promotion of healing.[79,80,81,82]

Cleansers containing benzoyl peroxide are available as liquid washes and solid bars of various strengths. The desquamative and antibacterial effectiveness in a soap or wash is minimized by limited contact time and removal with proper rinsing. Stable lotions are available in concentrations of 2.5, 5 and 10%. Alcohol and acetone gels facilitate bioavailability and may be more effective, while water-based vehicles are less irritating and better tolerated. A benzoyl peroxide 4% hydrophase gel (Solugel) suspends crystals of benzoyl peroxide in a dimethylisosorbide solvent as the water in the base evaporates. The resulting solution is absorbed by the skin, leaving no film. The manufacturer claims the resulting efficacy is equal to benzoyl peroxide 10% with irritation equivalent to that of a 2.5% concentration in aqueous-base gel, and may be an alternative for the patient with easily irritated skin who requires additional potency. This vehicle is easily combined with prepackaged clindamycin or erythromycin powders. Paste vehicles are stiffer and more drying than ointments or creams, facilitating absorption of the active ingredients and allowing them to stay localized.

Benzoyl peroxide 2.5% is equivalent to the 5% and 10% formulations in reducing the number of inflammatory lesions. The lower strength may not be as effective a peeler (which is due to an irritancy reaction) compared with higher strengths. Irritant side effects with the 2.5% gel are less frequent than with the 10% gel but equivalent to the 5% gel. The lowest concentration of benzoyl peroxide should be used for treating patients with easily irritated skin and may lessen irritation when used in combination topical therapy with comedolytic agents.

Benzoyl peroxide is combined with topical antibiotics or retinoids to improve efficacy, allow reduction in dosage of antibiotics or retinoids, decrease irritation, and reduce development of resistance to antibiotics.[83,84,85] Benzoyl peroxide has also been used in combination with other antiacne medications, such as sulfur, chlorhydroxyquinoline or urea, an ingredient used to facilitate drug delivery. No significant improvement has been demonstrated.

Benzoyl peroxide may bleach hair and fabrics such as towels, bedding and clothing. Odour from breakdown of benzoyl peroxide may remain on clothing and bedsheets.

Benzoyl peroxide produces a mild primary irritant dermatitis that settles with continued use, and is more likely to occur in those who have fair complexions or susceptibility to irritation, or who sunburn easily. Irritation is dependent on the concentration and vehicle—higher with alcoholic gels compared with emulsion bases. Contact allergic dermatitis is reported rarely. Cross-reactions with other sensitizers, notably balsam of Peru and cinnamon, are well established. It may cross-sensitize to other benzoic acid derivatives such as topical anesthetics. Concomitant use of an abrasive cleanser may initiate or enhance sensitization.[86]

There is no evidence that the normal use of benzoyl peroxide in the treatment of acne is associated with an increased risk of facial skin cancer in humans, although links have been made in mice experiments. Overall, the cutaneous use of benzoyl peroxide is safe, and is recognized by the FDA as category 3, which means that more information is required to make a final determination of safety and efficacy for nonprescription use.[87,88,89,90]

Preparations of benzoyl peroxide are available in concentrations up to 10%. Recommend the weakest concentration (2.5%) in a water-based formulation or the 4% hydrophase formulation for anyone with a history of skin irritation or who must use combination therapy.[91] There are many suggested routines for initiating therapy. One is to gently cleanse the skin and apply the preparation for 15 minutes the first evening, avoiding the eyes and mucous membranes. A mild stinging and reddening may appear. The time should be doubled each evening until the preparation is left on for 4 hours and subsequently all night. Dryness and peeling will appear after a few days. Once tolerance is achieved, the strength may be increased to 5% or the base changed to acetone or alcohol gels or paste. Alternatively, benzoyl peroxide can be applied for 2 hours for 4 nights, 4 hours for 4 nights, and then left on all night. It is important to wash the product off in the morning. Other drying agents should be discontinued. Patients with very sensitive skin or demonstrated sensitivity to benzoyl peroxide should not use the product, and it should be discontinued if irritation becomes severe upon use. Contact with eyes, lips or mouth should be avoided.

A **sunscreen** (see Chapter 72: Prevention and Treatment of Sun-induced Skin Damage) is recommended if benzoyl peroxide is used. To avoid interactions, apply the sunscreen during the day and the benzoyl peroxide at night.

Comparison of salicylic acid and benzoyl peroxide: While both of these ingredients are used for mild to moderate acne, their mechanisms differ and therefore the type of acne most responsive to each varies. Benzoyl peroxide is a strong antibacterial, while salicylic acid acts primarily through keratolysis. Salicylic acid is equal or slightly superior to benzoyl peroxide in reducing the number of comedones and subsequently the number of inflammatory lesions, since it interferes with an earlier step in pathogenesis—formation of the primary lesion of acne, the microcomedone—and thus could be superior in acting against later steps.[65,67] However, studies did not use identical formulations; the base itself has an effect and influences penetration and duration of action. Salicylic acid is superior to benzoyl peroxide in retarding comedone formation. Benzoyl peroxide, as an antibacterial with some peeling effects, is considered the nonprescription and cosmetic gold standard for milder acne. It is used alone or in combination with other antibacterials or peelers, to increase efficacy and improve tolerability.

Topical and Oral Antibiotics

In addition to reduction of *P. acnes* as the mechanism for efficacy in acne treatment, certain antibiotic drugs are also potent anti-inflammatory agents via other mechanisms. The induction of resistance has made antibiotic therapy problematic in many patients, particularly because therapy is directed at control over a long time period.[92]

Topical and oral **erythromycin** and topical **clindamycin**, well-established acne treatments, have become less effective since the early 1990s due to resistance of *P. acnes*.[92] Addition of **benzoyl peroxide** to the antibiotic regimen is more effective than monotherapy, and mitigates against survival of resistant *P. acnes* populations. Clindamycin is preferred because of its potent action and lack of absorption. It is available as a single-ingredient topical preparation and can also be combined with benzoyl peroxide. Erythromycin is available in combination with tretinoin or benzoyl peroxide. Some topical antibiotic-benzoyl peroxide combinations require refrigeration.

The **tetracycline** antibiotic family has well-understood antibacterial effects and anti-inflammatory effects that target an additional aspect of pathogenesis.[92,93] These agents are used only systemically and include **tetracycline**, **minocycline** and **doxycycline**. Through calcium chelation, they inhibit neutrophil and monocyte chemotaxis; minocycline and doxycycline are 10 times more active than tetracycline. Concentrations below the antibiotic threshold still inhibit inflammation and improve both acne vulgaris and acne rosacea. Resistance is lower with tetracyclines than with erythromycin or clindamycin; cross-resistance occurs between tetracycline and doxycycline but not minocycline.[92] In practice, minocycline appears more effective than doxycycline and is effective in patients who do not respond to doxycycline.[92] This may be due to greater lipophilicity; there is a tenfold greater reduction of *P. acnes* by minocycline compared with doxycycline.[93] However, a Cochrane review showed that although minocycline is an effective treatment for moderate to severe inflammatory acne, there is little evidence to support its superiority to other tetracyclines.[94] There is no conclusive clinical difference although it is more lipophilic, may act more quickly and can be taken once daily. Doxycycline and minocycline differ in side effect profiles. Doxycycline is a photosensitizer, especially at higher doses. Minocycline may cause dose-related dizziness, which resolves with dosage titration. People treated with minocycline are at significantly greater risk of developing an autoimmune syndrome than those receiving tetracycline or no treatment. Hypersensitivity reactions include urticaria, serum sickness–like reactions and generalized drug-induced reactions resembling lupus.[92]

Other antibiotics sometimes useful in acne include **azithromycin**, **ciprofloxacin** and **sulfamethoxazole/trimethoprim**, but these should be reserved for patients who do not respond to conventional treatment.[64,95,96]

Dapsone, a synthetic sulfone, is an anti-inflammatory agent effective for acne when given orally, but not used due to risk of serious systemic side effects. A topical gel formulation of dapsone is now available and currently does not appear to pose the risks associated with systemic dapsone use. Sulfones have both anti-inflammatory and antimicrobial properties that improve both inflammatory and noninflammatory acne, with more prominent effects occurring in inflammatory lesions. Short and long-term safety have been demonstrated.[97,98,99,100] One study showed dapsone gel may be more effective in women than men.[101] It also appears to be safe and effective in combination with adapalene and benzoyl peroxide.[102,103] Topical dapsone is a novel addition to the treatment armamentarium especially for patients exhibiting sensitivities or intolerance to conventional antiacne agents.

Strategies to limit antibiotic resistance are important in acne management. Oral and topical antibiotics should not be used as monotherapy.[77] Concurrent use of oral and topical antibiotics should be avoided, particularly if chemically different, due to increased risk of bacterial resistance. The use of systemic antibiotics should be limited (both indication and duration). Patients with less severe forms of acne should not be treated with oral antibiotics, and where possible such therapy should be limited to the shortest feasible duration. Avoid use of antibiotics for maintenance therapy. Discontinue antibiotics when there is no further improvement or the improvement is only slight. Oral antibiotics should ideally be used for 3 months, but response to antibiotics should be assessed 6–8 weeks into treatment. Nearly 70% of patients with acne require antibiotics for 12 weeks or less if aggressive retinoid therapy is used during that time; therefore, early use of combination therapy with retinoids is encouraged. The complementary modes of action of antimicrobials plus retinoids result in increased speed of response, greater clearing and enhanced efficacy against comedones and inflammatory lesions. If patients relapse, use the original antibiotic for subsequent courses unless there is adequate justification for a change. In addition, isotretinoin use should be initiated earlier in indicated patients, rather than prolonging antibiotic courses.[92] Prolonged oral administration of antibiotics may cause overgrowth of gram-negative organisms, producing a refractory folliculitis and necessitating discontinuation. Adding benzoyl peroxide to oral or topical antibiotic therapy will also reduce development of antibiotic resistance.[77]

Other Systemic Agents

Antisebum agents: No topical agents directly influence the production of sebum. Systemic drugs that influence sebum production include **estrogens**, **antiandrogens (drospirenone, cyproterone acetate)**, **spironolactone** and the retinoid **isotretinoin**.

Oral contraceptives (OCs) are effective for the treatment of acne[104] and several are indicated for this purpose in Canada. OCs with minimal androgenic effects (see Chapter 76: Contraception) and those containing the antiandrogens cyproterone acetate or drospirenone are especially useful in women with other signs of androgen excess. OCs showed equivalent efficacy to oral antibiotics in one meta-analysis.[105] There is a small risk of venous thromboembolic events with the use of any combined OC.[106,107,108] This risk is slightly higher with those that contain cyproterone or drospirenone.[107,108,109] Therefore, consider cyproterone- or drospirenone-containing OCs when other OCs are ineffective or not tolerated. Spironolactone is also used as a form of antiandrogenic hormonal therapy for acne in some patients.

Isotretinoin is the only drug treatment for acne that produces prolonged remission. It is recommended as first-choice therapy for severe papulopustular or moderate nodular acne and for nodular or conglabate acne for many reasons: clinical effectiveness, prevention of scarring and quick improvement of a patient's quality of life, including minimizing depression.[3,77] Although comparative trials are lacking, clinical experience confirms relapse rates after isotretinoin treatment are the lowest among available therapies. Additionally, it is recommended for management of less severe acne that is treatment-resistant (unresponsive to adequate treatment, reasonable courses of antibiotic, or combination peelers and antibiotics administered for 6 weeks to 3 months) or that is producing either physical or psychologic scarring. The risk of potential side effects must be weighed against its ability to prevent lifelong and permanent physical and psychological scarring.

Oral isotretinoin is a natural metabolite of vitamin A. Its mechanism is elusive, as it does not bind to retinoid receptors. It has been shown to reduce sebogenesis and may also inhibit sebaceous gland activity, growth of *P. acnes* and inflammation, and improve follicular epithelial differentiation. Systemic isotretinoin exerts a primary effect on comedogenesis, reducing size and formation of new comedones. Conventional dosing is 0.5–2 mg/kg/day for 12–16 weeks. Initiating with a low dose and titrating will minimize transient exacerbation of acne at the start of therapy. Some patients experience a relapse of acne after the first course of isotretinoin: a second course may be used starting at least 8 weeks after the end of the first course (as acne may continue to improve during this time). Studies have shown that other dosing regimens (low-dose, intermittent) may also be effective.[110,111,112]

Because isotretinoin is a vitamin A derivative, it interacts with many of the biologic systems of the body, and consequently has a significant pattern of adverse effects. The pattern is similar to that seen in hypervitaminosis A. Side effects include those of the mucocutaneous (most common), musculoskeletal and ophthalmic systems, as well as headaches and CNS effects. Most adverse effects, such as cheilitis and dry nose, eyes and mouth, are temporary and resolve after the drug is discontinued. Replace any concurrent topical products that produce a drying effect with moisturizers. Laboratory monitoring during therapy should include triglycerides, cholesterol, transaminases and complete blood counts.

Mood disorders, depression, suicidal ideation and suicides have been reported sporadically in patients taking this drug. Evidence is insufficient to support a causal association. These symptoms are common in patients with acne and in adolescents and young adults, who represent the majority of patients receiving isotretinoin. Prescribers of isotretinoin are advised to note prior psychiatric symptoms, monitor patients at each visit for early recognition and advise patients about a possible risk of depression and suicidal behaviour. This disputed association remains an important area for future research.[113,114]

The teratogenic effects of oral retinoid therapy are well documented. Women must start contraceptive measures 1 month prior to treatment, continue for the duration of treatment and for 1 month after stopping treatment with isotretinoin.

Treating Sequelae of Acne

Pigmentation: Postinflammatory pigmentation is a common consequence of acne that may persist up to 2 years after lesions have resolved. To control this pigmentation, **hydroquinone**, which reversibly damages melanocytes, has been used as a hypopigmenting agent in concentrations of 2–4%, in preparations of clear or tinted gels (which are more drying), and as vanishing or opaque, flesh-tinted creams, with or without alpha-hydroxy acids or sunscreens. Hydroquinone causes fading of epidermal (but not dermal) pigmentation. Onset of response is usually 3–4 weeks, and the depigmentation lasts for 2–6 months. After considering additional data and information on the safety of hydroquinone, the FDA issued a proposed ruling in 2006 stating that nonprescription serums and lotions containing hydroquinone are not generally recognized as safe and effective and are misbranded. The FDA also intends to consider all prescription hydroquinone products to be new drugs requiring an approved new drug application for continued marketing. Hydroquinone has already been banned in Japan, much of the European Union and Africa. While effective in the removal of melanin, hydroquinone may be a carcinogen and causes a blue-black discoloration known as ochronosis.[115]

Scarring: Many patients have acne scarring despite adequate treatments. Atrophic scars can be treated with laser resurfacing. For patients with mild scarring, **alpha-hydroxy acids** may be used, while severe scarring may be corrected with other treatment modalities that require a dermatologist consultation. Dermabrasion, chemical peels (e.g., 70% glycolic acid) and laser therapy have been used. Usually the scar is not completely removed, but a more cosmetically acceptable result is achieved.[25] Keloids and hypertrophic scars can be treated with intralesional triamcinolone, cryotherapy, topical corticosteroids and silicone sheeting.[6] Surgical options for scars include excision, augmentation with collagen or fat, subcision and injection of autologous fibroblasts.[2]

Natural Health Products

A systematic review of complementary and alternative medicines (CAMs) for acne concluded that there is some low-quality evidence from single trials that **tea tree oil** and **bee venom** may reduce total skin lesions in acne. The same review cautioned that there is a lack of evidence to support the use of other CAMs such as aloe vera, copaiba essential oil, dried fruit of *Berberis vulgaris*, seaweed oligosacchrides, acupuncture or wet-cupping in the treatment of acne.[26] Natural health products can cause adverse effects; future studies need to assess safety. Methodological and reporting quality limitations weaken any evidence. The use nonstandardized botanical preparations should be discouraged in favour of traditional quality-controlled preparations that have evidence of efficacy.

Common Drug Therapy Problems with Acne

- Indiscriminate use of topical applications: failure to use systemic treatment when indicated
- Prolonged treatment with antibiotics when unnecessary or ineffective
- Wrong choice of drug
- Failure to use combination therapy
- Improper application of active drug
- Drug side effects

Monitoring of Therapy

Table 4 provides a monitoring framework for patients with acne.

Parameters should be monitored by the patient in a diary. Therapy should be appropriately tapered in response to improvement or resolution. The healthcare practitioner should be responsible for ensuring that the treatment plan remains on schedule and is effective, and that no adverse effects are occurring.

Patient Education

Acne is usually considered self-limiting in that it begins in the teenage years and usually subsides in the mid to late twenties. However, for some it evolves into a chronic condition. Symptoms can be managed with diligent and long-term treatment, focused on control and prevention, if proper education is provided. However, acne is poorly understood by adolescents in terms of many issues: identifying the cause of the disorder and aggravating factors, indications for self-care vs. prescription treatment, concerns regarding safety and duration of treatment and appropriate application of topicals. Review the patient's understanding of each of these important factors in ensuring patient adherence. There is often a need to supplement counselling sessions with written materials that the patient can refer to at home. Both written handouts and audiovisual computerized presentations about acne conferred significant and equivalent benefits in terms of short- and long-term knowledge gains among adolescent patients with acne.[116] Electronic reminders in the form of daily, customized text messages were not associated with significant differences in adherence to topical medications in patients with mild to moderate acne and had no significant effect on therapeutic response.[117]

Table 4: **Monitoring of Therapy for Acne**

Parameter	Timeframe/Degree of Change	Actions[a]
Short-term Effectiveness Endpoints (Acne resolution/control)		
Lesion count	Decrease by 10–25% within 4–8 wk, with control, or more than a 50% decrease within 2–4 months.	If endpoints not achieved, consider further therapy.
Comedones	Resolve by 3–4 months.	
Inflammatory lesions	Resolve within a few wk.	
Anxiety or depression	Achieve control or improvement within 2–4 months.	
Long-term Effectiveness Endpoints		
Progression of severity	No progression of severity.	If endpoints not achieved, consider further therapy.
Recurrent episodes	Lengthening of acne-free periods throughout therapy.	
Scarring or pigmentation	No further scarring or pigmentation throughout therapy.	
Safety Endpoints (treatment side effects)		
For each nondrug or drug measure initiated, list the side effect (safety endpoint) most likely to occur, the degree to which it might be tolerated, if at all, and within what timeframe it might be expected. Indicate how the side effect would impact therapy, i.e., continue and monitor, continue and treat side effect, continue but decrease dose, or discontinue therapy and choose alternative.		

[a] Advise patient to monitor each parameter daily while on drug therapy. Healthcare practitioners should monitor each parameter every 4–8 weeks during therapy (or at next visit).

Figure 3: **Assessment of Patients with Acne**

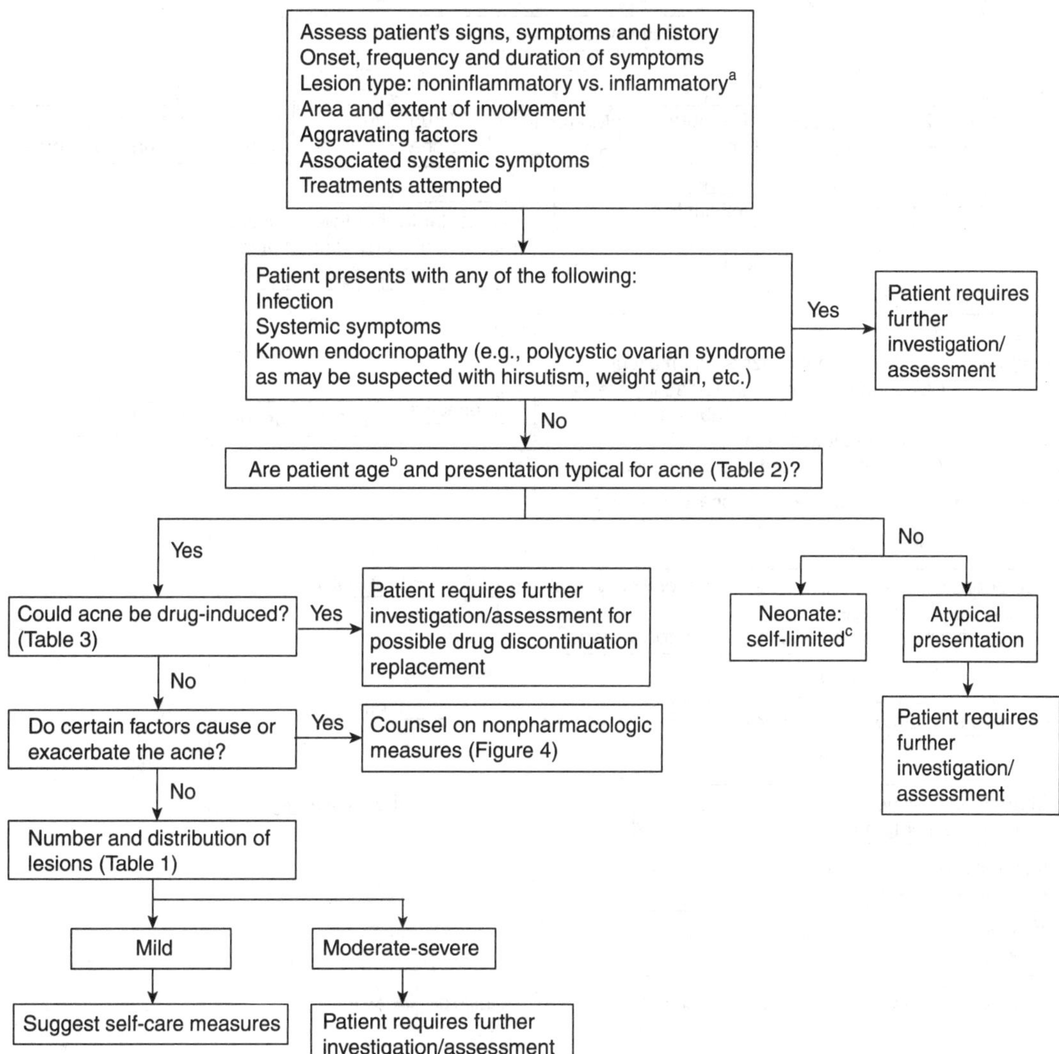

a Noninflammatory (open/closed comedones)/inflammatory (papules, pustules, nodules/cysts).
b Typical ages 12–25 years; onset after puberty may signal acne rosacea.
c Baby oil should be avoided as it may aggravate follicular occlusion.

Figure 4: **Treatment of Acne with Nonprescription Medication**

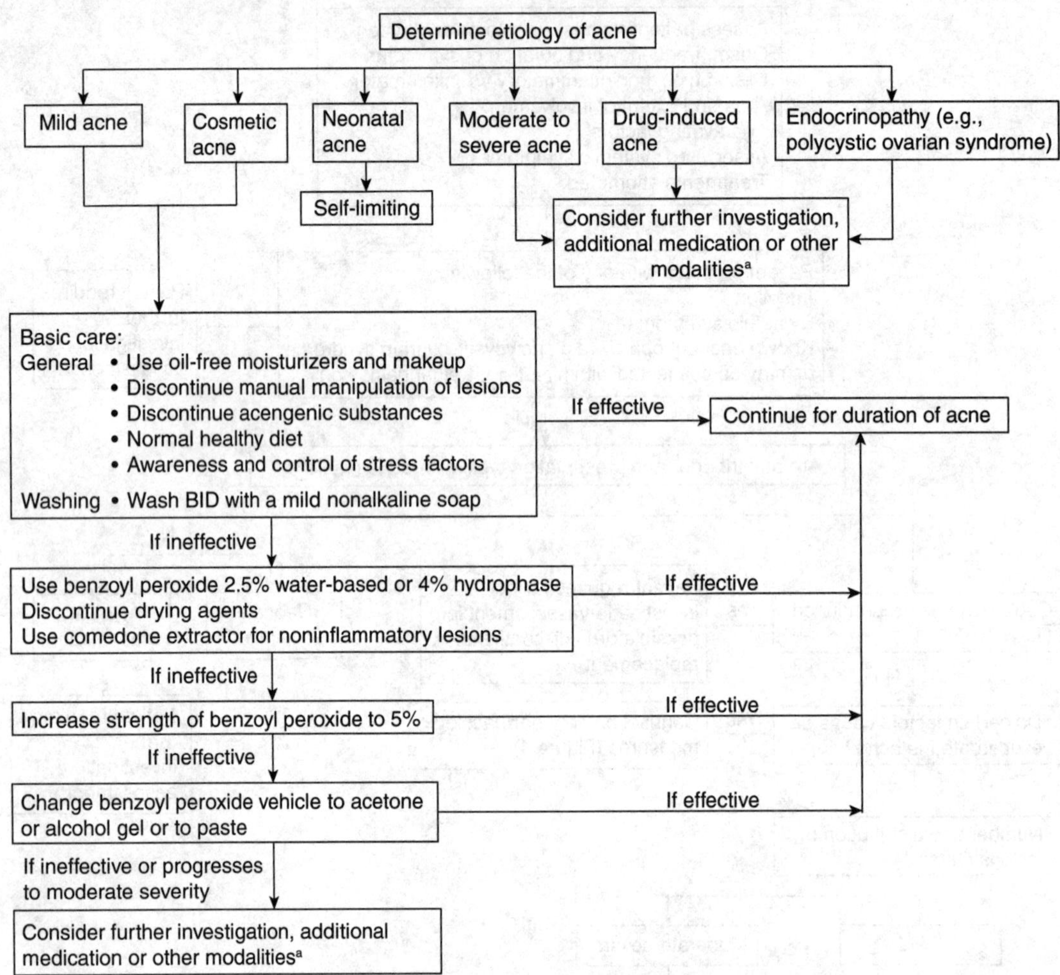

Determine etiology of acne
Mild acne
Cosmetic acne
Neonatal acne
Self-limiting
Moderate to severe acne
Drug-induced acne
Endocrinopathy (e.g., polycystic ovarian syndrome)
Consider further investigation, additional medication or other modalities[a]
Basic care:
General • Use oil-free moisturizers and makeup
• Discontinue manual manipulation of lesions
• Discontinue acengenic substances
• Normal healthy diet
• Awareness and control of stress factors
Washing • Wash BID with a mild nonalkaline soap
If effective
Continue for duration of acne
If ineffective
Use benzoyl peroxide 2.5% water-based or 4% hydrophase
Discontinue drying agents
Use comedone extractor for noninflammatory lesions
If effective
If ineffective
Increase strength of benzoyl peroxide to 5%
If effective
If ineffective
Change benzoyl peroxide vehicle to acetone or alcohol gel or to paste
If effective
If ineffective or progresses to moderate severity
Consider further investigation, additional medication or other modalities[a]

[a] For more information on the management of acne, consult *Compendium of Therapeutic Choices*: Acne.

Table 5: Nonprescription Agents Used to Treat Acne[a]

Class	Drug	Dosage	Onset	Adverse Effects	Comments	Cost[b]
Antibacterial/ exfoliant	*benzoyl peroxide 2.5–10%* Benzagel, Proactive, others	Apply daily or BID	Antibacterial effect: Onset: Rapid; number of inflamed lesions could decrease within 5 days. Duration: Bactericidal effect lasts for at least 48 h. Exfoliant effect: Onset: Must be used for 8–12 wk before improvement noted. Duration of treatment is long term. Dosing schedules adjusted PRN for chronic control. Taper off until natural resolution.	Produces mild irritant dermatitis. Dryness and peeling appear after a few days. Contact allergic dermatitis. May bleach hair or fabric. Odour remains on clothing and bed sheets.	Cross-sensitivity with balsam of Peru, cinnamon and other benzoic acid derivatives (topical anesthetics).	$
Exfoliant	*glycolic acid 2–15%* Neostrata, Reversa, others	Apply BID	Some effect may be seen in 6–7 wk.	Irritating		$$
	salicylic acid 0.5–2% Clean and Clear Moisturizer, Clearasil Wash, others	Apply daily or BID	Must be used for 8–12 wk before improvement noted. Duration of treatment is long term.	Initial irritation. 3–6% is keratolytic, causing softening of horny layer.	Increases penetration of other active ingredients.	$

[a] For more information on drug therapy for acne, consult the *Compendium of Therapeutic Choices*: Acne.

[b] Cost of smallest available pack size; includes drug cost only.

Legend: $ <$10 $$ $10–20

Suggested Readings

Asai Y, Baibergenova A, Dutil M et al. Management of acne: Canadian clinical practice guideline. *CMAJ* 2015. DOI:10.1503 /cmaj.140665

Eichenfield LF, Krakowski AC, Piggott C et al. Evidence-based recommendations for the diagnosis and treatment of pediatric acne. *Pediatrics* 2013;131:S163-86.

Nast A, Dréno B, Bettoli V et al. European evidence-based (S3) guidelines for the treatment of acne. *J Eur Acad Dermatol Venereol* 2012;26:1-29.

Sibbald D. Acne. In: DiPiro JT, ed. *Pharmacotherapy: a pathophysiologic approach*. 9th ed. New York: McGraw-Hill; 2013.

Thiboutot D, Gollnick H, Bettoli V et al. New Insights into the management of acne: an update from the Global Alliance to Improve Outcomes in Acne Group. *J Am Acad Dermatolog* 2009;60:S1-50.

Williams HC, Dellavalle RP, Garner S. Acne vulgaris. *Lancet* 2012;379:361-72.

References

1. Leyden JJ, Shalita AR. Rational therapy for acne vulgaris: an update on topical treatment. *J Am Acad Dermatol* 1986;15:907-15.
2. Batra RS. Acne. In: Arndt KA, Hsu JTS, eds. *Manual of dermatologic therapeutics*. 7th ed. Philadelphia: Wolters Kluwer/Lippincott Williams & Wilkins; 2007. p. 1:3-18.
3. Nast A, Dreno B, Bettoli V et al. European evidence-based (S3) guidelines for the treatment of acne. *J Eur Acad Dermatol Venereol* 2012;26:1-29.
4. Shalita AR. Genesis of free fatty acids. *J Invest Dermatol* 1974;62:332-5.
5. Tucker SB, Rogers RS, Winkelmann RK et al. Inflammation in acne vulgaris: leukocyte attraction and cytotoxicity by comedonal material. *J Invest Dermatol* 1980;74:21-5.
6. Chu A. Acne vulgaris. In: Lebwohl MG, Heyman WR, Berth-Jones J et al., eds. *Treatment of skin disease: comprehensive therapeutic strategies*. 2nd ed. Philadelphia: Mosby Elsevier; 2006. p. 6-12.
7. Winston MH, Shalita AR. Acne vulgaris. Pathogenesis and treatment. *Pediatr Clin North Am* 1991;38:889-903.
8. Plewig G, Kligman AM. The dynamics of primary comedo formation. In: Plewig G, Kligman AM, eds. *Acne: morphogenesis and treatment*. New York: Springer-Verlag; 1975. p. 58-107.
9. Puissegur-Lupo ML. Acne vulgaris. Treatments and their rationale. *Postgrad Med* 1985;78:76-80, 83-4.
10. Layton AM, Henderson CA, Cunliffe WJ. A clinical evaluation of acne scarring and its incidence. *Clin Exp Dermatol* 1994;19:303-8.
11. Thiboutot DM. Acne. An overview of clinical research findings. *Dermatol Clin* 1997;15:97-109.
12. U.S. Department of Health and Human Services, Food and Drug Administration, Center for Drug Evaluation and Research (CDER). *Guidance for industry. Acne vulgaris: developing drugs for treatment*. September 2005. Available from: www.fda.gov/downloads/Drugs/.../Guidances/UCM071292.pdf.
13. Katsambas AD, Katoulis AC, Stavropoulos P. Acne neonatorum: a study of 22 cases. *Int J Dermatol* 1999;38:128-30.
14. Williams M, Cunliffe WJ. Explanation for premenstrual acne. *Lancet* 1973;2:1055-7.
15. Strasburger VC. Acne. What every pediatrician should know about treatment. *Pediatr Clin North Am* 1997;44:1505-23.
16. Taylor JS. Chloracne: a continuing problem. *Cutis* 1974;13:585.
17. Rosenberg EW, Kirk BS. Acne diet reconsidered. *Arch Dermatol* 1981;117:193-5.
18. Fulton JE, Plewig G, Kligman AM. Effect of chocolate on acne vulgaris. *JAMA* 1969;210:2071-4.
19. Anderson PC. Foods as the cause of acne. *Am Fam Physician* 1971;3:102-3.
20. Kim J, Ko Y, Park YK et al. Dietary effect of lactoferrin-enriched fermented milk on skin surface lipid and clinical improvement of acne vulgaris. *Nutrition* 2010;26:902-9.
21. Adebamowo CA, Spiegelman D, Danby FW et al. High school dietary dairy intake and teenage acne. *J Am Acad Dermatol* 2005;52:207-14.
22. Danby FW. Acne and milk, the diet myth, and beyond. *J Am Acad Dermatol* 2005;52:360-2.
23. Thiboutot D. Acne: hormonal concepts and therapy. *Clin Dermatol* 2004;22:419-28.
24. Cappel M, Mauger D, Thiboutot D. Correlation between serum levels of insulin-like growth factor 1, dehydroepiandrosterone sulfate, and dihydritestosterone and acne lesion counts in adult women. *Arch Dermatol* 2005;141:333-8.
25. Smith RN, Mann NJ, Braue A et al The effect of a high-protein, low-glycemic load diet versus a conventional high-glycemic load diet on biochemical parameters associated with acne vulgaris: a randomized, investigator-masked controlled trial. *J Am Acad Dermatol* 2007;57:247-56.
26. Cao H, Yang G, Wang Y et al. Complementary therapies for acne vulgaris. *Cochrane Database Syst Rev* 2015;1:CD009436.
27. Smith RN, Mann NJ, Braue A et al. A low-glycemic-load diet improves symptoms in acne vulgaris patients: a randomized controlled trial. *Am J Clin Nutr* 2007;86:107-15.
28. Burris J, Rietkerk W, Woolf K. Acne: the role of medical nutrition therapy. *J Acad Nutr Diet* 2013;113:416-30.
29. Melnik BC. Diet in acne: further evidence for the role of nutrient signalling in acne pathogenesis. *Acta Derm Venereol* 2012;92:228-31.
30. Bowe WP, Joshi SS, Shalita AR. Diet and acne. *J Am Acad Dermatol* 2010;63:124-41.
31. Shalita AR. Acne vulgaris: pathogenesis and treatment. *Cosmet Toiletries* 1983;98:57-60.
32. Firooz A, Sarhangnejad R, Davoudi SM et al. Acne and smoking: is there a relationship? *BMC Dermatol* 2005;5:2.
33. Malus M, LaChance PA, Lamy L et al. Priorities in adolescent health care: the teenager's viewpoint. *J Fam Pract* 1987;25:159-62.
34. Johnson BA, Nunley JR. Topical therapy for acne vulgaris: How do you choose the best drug for each patient? *Postgrad Med* 2000;107:69-70, 73-6, 79-80.
35. Habif TP. Acne, rosacea, and related disorders. In: Klein EA, Menczer BS, eds. *Clinical dermatology*. Toronto: Mosby; 1990. p. 756.
36. Bruinsma W. *A guide to drug eruptions*. 5th ed. Oosthuizen: European Book Service; 1990. p. 6.

37. UpToDate. Wirth FA. *Approach to acne vulgaris*. Available from: www.uptodate.com. Accessed June 9, 2016. Subscription required.
38. Kelly AP. Acne and related disorders. In: Sams WM, Lynch PJ, eds. *Principles and practice of dermatology*. New York: Churchill Livingstone; 1990. p. 1014.
39. Hull SM, Cunliffe WJ. The use of a corticosteroid cream for immediate reduction in the clinical signs of acne vulgaris. *Acta Derm Venereol* 1989;69:452-3.
40. Brodell RT, O'Brien MJ. Topical corticosteroid-induced acne. Three treatment strategies to break the 'addiction' cycle. *Postgrad Med* 1999;106:225-6, 229.
41. Hitch JM. Acneform eruption induced by drugs and chemicals. *JAMA* 1967;200:879-80.
42. Chren MM, Lasek RJ Quinn LM et al. Skindex, a quality-of-life measure for patients with skin disease: reliability, validity, and responsiveness. *J Invest Dermatol* 1996;107:707-13.
43. Finlay AY, Khan GK. Dermatology Quality of Life Index (DLQI)–a simple practical measure for routine clinical use. *Clin Exp Dermatol* 1994;19:210-6.
44. Girman CJ, Hartmaier S, Thiboutot D et al. Evaluating health-related quality of life in patients with facial acne: development of a self-administered questionnaire for clinical trials. *Qual Lif Res* 1996;5:481-90.
45. Gupta MA, Johnson AM, Gupta AK. The development of an Acne Quality of Life scale: reliability, validity, and relation to subjective acne severity in mild to moderate acne vulgaris. *Acta Derm Venereol* 1998;78:451-6.
46. Plewig G, Kligman AM. Acne detergicans. In: Plewig G, Kligman AM, eds. *Acne: morphogenesis and treatment*. New York: Springer-Verlag; 1975. p. 270-325.
47. Kroshinsky D, Shalita AR. Topical retinoids. In: Webster GF, Rawlings AV, eds. *Acne and its therapy*. New York: Informa Healthcare; 2007. p. 103-12.
48. Green L, Kircik LH, Gwazdauskas J. Randomized, controlled, evaluator-blinded studies conducted to compare the efficacy and tolerability of 3 over-the-counter regimens in subjects with mild or moderate acne. *J Drugs Dermatol* 2013;12:180-5.
49. Epinette WW, Gresit MC, Ozols II. The role of cosmetics in postadolescent acne. *Cutis* 1982;29:500-4, 514.
50. Plewig G, Kligman AM. Acne cosmetica. In: Plewig G, Kligman AM, eds. *Acne: morphogenesis and treatment*. New York: Springer-Verlag; 1975. p. 226-9.
51. Mills OH, Kligman AM. Comedogenicity of sunscreens. Experimental observations in rabbits. *Arch Dermatol* 1982;118:417-9.
52. Walzer RA. Acne: some answers to a complexion problem In: Walzer RA, ed. *Skintelligence: how to be smart about your skin*. New York: ACC; 1981. p. 53-69.
53. Choi YS, Suh HS, Yoon MY et al. A study of the efficacy of cleansers for acne vulgaris. *J Dermatolog Treat* 2010;21:201-5.
54. Stoughton RB. Comparative in vitro bioassay of skin penetration and activity of chlorhexidine preparations and other topical agents against P. acnes: an assessment of their potential use in the treatment of acne vulgaris. ICI: American Inc. *Research Report on File* 1979 Mar;CLR-120.
55. Stoughton RB, Leyden JJ. Efficacy of 4 percent chlorhexidine gluconate skin cleanser in the treatment of acne vulgaris. *Cutis* 1987;39:551-3.
56. Shalita AR. Treatment of mild and moderate acne vulgaris with salicylic acid in an alcohol-detergent vehicle. *Cutis* 1981;28:556-8, 561.
57. Arndt KA. Acne. In: Arndt KA, ed. *Manual of dermatologic therapeutics: with essentials of diagnosis*. 4th ed. Toronto: Little, Brown; 1989. p. 3-13.
58. Fulghum DD, Catalano PM, Childers RC et al. Abrasive cleansing in the management of acne vulgaris. *Arch Dermatol* 1982;118:658-9.
59. Boothroyd S. Topical therapy and formulation principles. In: Webster GF, Rawlings AV, eds. *Acne and its therapy*. New York: Informa Healthcare; 2007. p. 253-74.
60. Thiboutot D. New treatments and therapeutic strategies for acne. *Arch Fam Med* 2000;9:179-87.
61. Russell JJ. Topical therapy for acne. *Am Fam Physician* 2000;61:357-66.
62. Chiou WL. Low intrinsic drug activity and dominant vehicle (placebo) effect in the topical treatment of acne vulgaris. *Int J Clin Pharmacol Ther* 2012:50:434-7.
63. Zouboulis CC. Moderne aknetherapie. *Akt Dermatol* 2003;29:49-57.
64. Sykes NL, Webster GF. Acne. A review of optimum treatment. *Drugs* 1994;48:59-70.
65. Zander E, Weisman S. Treatment of acne vulgaris with salicylic acid pads. *Clin Ther* 1992;14:247-53.
66. Gross G. Benzoyl peroxide and salicylic acid therapy. In: Webster GF, Rawlings AV, eds. *Acne and its therapy*. New York: Informa Healthcare; 2007. p. 117-36.
67. Shalita AR. Comparison of a salicylic acid cleanser and a benzoyl peroxide wash in the treatment of acne vulgaris. *Clin Ther* 1989;11:264-7.
68. Kligman D, Kligman AM. Salicylic acid as a peeling agent for the treatment of acne. *Cosmetic Dermatol* 1997;10:44-7.
69. Bae BG, Park CO, Shin H et al. Salicylic acid peels versus Jessner's solution for acne vulgaris: a comparative study. *Dermatol Surg* 2013;39:248-53.
70. Lin AN, Reimer RJ, Carter DM. Sulfur revisited. *J Am Acad Dermatol* 1988;18:553-8.
71. Abels C, Kaszuba A, Michalak I et al. A 10% glycolic acid containing oil-in-water emulsion improves mild acne: a randomized double-blind placebo-controlled trial. *J Cosmet Dermatol* 2011;10:202-9.
72. Poli F, Ribet V, Lauze C et al. Efficacy and safety of 0.1% retinaldehyde/6% glycolic acid (diacneal) for mild to moderate acne vulgaris. A multicentre, double-blind, randomized, vehicle-controlled trial. *Dermatology* 2005;210:14-21.
73. Baumann LS, Oresajo C, Yatskayer M et al. Comparison of clindamycin 1% and benzoyl peroxide 5% gel to a novel composition containing salicylic acid, capryloyl salicylic acid, HEPES, glycolic acid, citric acid and dioic acid in the treatment of acne vulgaris. *J Drugs Dermatol* 2013;12:266-9.
74. Kaminaka C, Uede M, Matsunaka H et al. Clinical evaluation of glycolic acid chemical peeling in patients with acne vulgaris: a randomized, double-blind, placebo-controlled, split-face comparative study. *Dermatol Surg* 2014;40:314-22.
75. Kaplan YC, Ozsarfati J, Etwel F et al. Pregnancy outcomes following first trimester exposure to topical retinoids: a systematic review and meta-analysis. *Br J Dermatol*. 2015;173(5):1132–41.
76. Mohd Nor NH, Aziz Z. A systematic review of benzoyl peroxide for acne vulgaris. *J Dermatol Treat* 2013;25:377-86.
77. Thiboutot D, Gollnick H, Bettoli V et al. New insights into the management of acne: and update from the Global Alliance to Improve Outcomes in Acne Group. *J Am Acad Dermatol* 2009;60:S1-50.
78. Gollnick H, Schramm M. Topical drug treatment in acne. *Dermatology* 1998;196:119-25.
79. Cotterill JA. Benzoyl peroxide. *Acta Derm Venereol Suppl (Stockh)* 1980;89:57-63.
80. Cunliffe WJ, Holland KT. The effect of benzoyl peroxide on acne. *Acta Derm Venereol* 1981;61:267-9.

81. Lassus A. Local treatment of acne. A clinical study and evaluation of the effect of different concentrations of benzoyl peroxide gel. *Curr Med Res Opin* 1981;7:370-3.
82. Cunliffe WJ, Dodman B, Ead R. Benzoyl peroxide in acne. *Practitioner* 1978;220:479-82.
83. Bowman S, Gold M, Nasir A et al. Comparison of clindamycin/benzoyl peroxide, tretinoin plus clindamycin, and the combination of clindamycin/benzoyl peroxide and tretinoin plus clindamycin in the treatment of acne vulgaris: a randomized, blinded study. *J Drugs Dermatol* 2005;4:611-8.
84. Korkut C, Piskin S. Benzoyl peroxide, adapalene, and their combination in the treatment of acne vulgaris. *J Dermatol* 2005;32:169-73.
85. Bikowski JB. Clinical experience results with clindamycin 1% benzoyl peroxide 5% gel (Duac) as monotherapy and in combination. *J Drugs Dermatol* 2005;4:164-71.
86. Maddin S. Benzoyl peroxide. *Can J Dermatol* 1989;1:92.
87. Report of the Expert Advisory Committee on Dermatology. The carcinogenic activity of benzoyl peroxide. Ottawa: Health Protection Branch. *Information Letter* 1987;711:1-9.
88. Cunliffe WJ, Burke B. Benzoyl peroxide: lack of sensitization. *Acta Derm Venereol* 1982;62:458-9.
89. Tkach JR. Allergic contact urticaria to benzoyl peroxide. *Cutis* 1982;29:187-8.
90. Rietschel RL, Duncan SH. Benzoyl peroxide reactions in an acne study group. *Contact Dermatitis* 1982;8:323-6.
91. Mills OH, Kligman AM, Pochi P et al. Comparing 2.5%, 5%, and 10% benzoyl peroxide on inflammatory acne vulgaris. *Int J Dermatol* 1986;25:664-7.
92. Webster GF. Antimicrobial therapy in acne. In: Webster GF, Rawlings AV, eds. *Acne and its therapy.* New York: Informa Healthcare; 2007. p. 97-102.
93. Leyden JJ. The antimicrobial effects in vivo of minocycline, doxycycline and tetracycline in humans. *J Dermatolog Treat* 1996;7:223-5.
94. Garner SE, Eady EA, Popescu C et al. Minocycline for acne vulgaris: efficacy and safety. *Cochrane Database Syst Rev* 2003;1:CD002086.
95. Bottomley WW, Cunliffe WJ. Oral trimethoprim as a third-line antibiotic in the management of acne vulgaris. *Dermatology* 1993;187:193-6.
96. Ullah G, Noor SM, Bhatti Z et al. Comparison of oral azithromycin with oral doxycycline in the treatment of acne vulgaris. *J Ayub Med Coll Abbottabad* 2014;26:64-7.
97. Draelos ZD, Carter E, Maloney JM et al. Two randomized studies demonstrate the efficacy and safety of dapsone gel, 5% for the treatment of acne vulgaris. *J Am Acad Dermatol* 2007;56:439.e1-10.
98. Lucky AW, Maloney JM, Roberts J et al. Dapsone gel 5% for the treatment of acne vulgaris: safety and efficacy of long-term (1 year) treatment. *J Drugs Dermatol* 2007;6:981-7.
99. Piette WW, Taylor S, Pariser D et al. Hematologic safety of dapsone gel, 5%, for topical treatment of acne vulgaris. *Arch Dermatol* 2008;144:1564-70.
100. Lynde CW, Andriessen A. Cohort study on the treatment with dapsone 5% gel of mild to moderate inflammatory acne of the face in women. *Skinmed* 2014;12:15-21.
101. Tanghetti E, Harper JC, Oefelein MG. The efficacy and tolerability of dapsone 5% gel in female vs male patients with facial acne vulgaris: gender as a clinically relevant outcome variable. *J Drugs Dermatol* 2013;11:1417-21.
102. Fleischer AB, Sahlita A, Eichenfield LF et al. Dapsone gel 5% in combination with adapalene gel 0.1%, benzoyl peroxide gel 4% or moisturizer for the treatment of acne vulgaris: a 12-week, randomized, double-blind study. *J Drugs Dermatol* 2010;9:33-40.
103. Gamble R, Dunn J, Dawson A et al. Topical antimicrobial treatment of acne vulgaris: an evidence-based review. *Am J Clin Dermatol* 2012;13:141-52.
104. Arowojolu AO, Gallo MF, Lopez LM et al. Combined oral contraceptive pills for treatment of acne. *Cochrane Database Syst Rev* 2012;7:CD004425.
105. Koo EB, Petersen TD, Kimball AB. Meta-analysis comparing efficacy of antibiotics versus oral contraceptives in acne vulgaris. *J Am Acad Dermatol* 2014;71:450-9.
106. Reid R; Society of Obstetricians and Gynaecologists of Canada. SOGC clinical practice guideline. No. 252, December 2010. Oral contraceptives and the risk of venous thromboembolism: an update. *J Obstet Gynaecol Can* 2010;32:1192-204.
107. Vinogradova Y, Coupland C, Hippisley-Cox J. Use of combined oral contraceptives and risk of venous thromboembolism: nested case-control studies using the QResearch and CPRD databases. *BMJ* 2015;350:h2135.
108. de Bastos M, Stegeman BH, Rosendaal FR et al. Combined oral contraceptives: venous thrombosis. *Cochrane Database Syst Rev* 2014;3:CD010813.
109. Stegeman BH, de Bastos M, Rosendaal FR et al. Different combined oral contraceptives and the risk of venous thrombosis: systematic review and network meta-analysis. *BMJ* 2013;347:f5298.
110. Agarwal US, Besarwal RK, Bhola K. Oral isotretinoin in different dose regimens for acne vulgaris: a randomized comparative trial. *Indian J Dermatol Venereol Leprol* 2011;77:688-94.
111. Lee JW, Yoo KH;, Park KY et al. Effectiveness of conventional, low-dose and intermittent oral isotretinoin in the treatment of acne: a randomized, controlled comparative study. *Br J Dermatol* 2011;164:1369-75.
112. Berk DR. Effectiveness of conventional, low-dose and intermittent oral isotretinoin in the treatment of acne: a randomized, controlled comparative study: comment. *Br J Dermatol* 2011;165:205.
113. Marqueling AL, Zane LT, Depression and suicidal behavior in acne patients treated with isotretinoin: a systematic review. *Semin Cutan Med Surg* 2005;24:92-102.
114. Sundstrom A, Alfredsson L, Sjolin-Forsberg G et al. Association of suicide attempts with acne and treatment with isotretinoin: retrospective Swedish cohort study. *BMJ* 2010;341:c5812.
115. U.S. Department of Health and Human Services. Food and Drug Administration. *Skin bleaching drug products for over-the-counter human use; proposed rule.* Available from: www.fda.gov/OHRMS/DOCKETS/98fr/78n-0065-npr0003.pdf. Accessed February, 2016.
116. Koch PE, Ryder HF, Dziura J et al. Educating adolescents about acne vulgaris: a comparison of written handouts with audiovisual computerized presentations. *Arch Dermatol* 2008;144:208-14.
117. Boker A, Feetham HJ, Armstrong A et al. Do automated text messages increase adherence to acne therapy? Results of a randomized, controlled trial. *J Am Acad Dermatol* 2012;67:1136-42.

Acne—What You Need to Know

Acne is a common skin disorder that affects most adolescents and some adults. Acne generally appears as pimples or larger pustules on the face, chest, back and upper arms. Severe acne may cause scars. Acne usually goes away by the time a person becomes an adult. However, having acne causes emotional difficulties for many people.

What causes acne?

- Acne is not caused by dirt. Washing your face too often can irritate your skin and may make your acne worse. Wash your skin gently from the jawline to the hairline no more than twice daily with water alone or a mild, nonalkaline soap or soapless cleanser. Do not rub or scrub your skin and avoid rough washcloths.
- Acne is not caused by eating chocolate or greasy foods. However, you should try to eat a healthy, balanced diet, including fruit and vegetables. Cut down on fatty treats for your general health and choose low-glycemic options.
- Stress can make acne worse. Try to reduce stress through exercise or relaxation.
- Some medications and chemicals can cause acne. Talk to your healthcare provider if you have to take medicine daily or if you are exposed to chemicals at work.

How do you treat acne?

- Treat acne as soon as it appears to avoid complications such as scarring. Many different acne medications are available without a prescription.
- Ask a healthcare provider for advice about nonprescription acne medication. Some can irritate your skin or make your acne worse for a short time. Use the medication only once a day until your skin gets used to it.
- Use a nonprescription acne medication for 6–8 weeks. Remember, it may take some time before your skin looks better. Try not to get discouraged!
- Apply acne medication everywhere you have pimples. The medication will work better if you cover all the affected skin, not just the pimples. Use a clean cotton pad for each area that you are going to treat. Throw the pads away after using once.
- See your healthcare provider if
  - you have a lot of acne (pimples or large pustules).
  - you suspect your acne is being caused by a medical condition or by medicine that you have to take.
  - your acne has not improved after using nonprescription medication for 6–8 weeks.
  - you have a sudden change in the appearance or number of acne lesions.

Some Helpful Hints

- Do not use greasy cosmetics, coverstick, moisturizer, hair gel, scalp oil, eye cream or hairspray. All of these products can make your acne last longer—even if you only use them once.
- Do not use makeup regularly. If you must use makeup, choose an oil-free product that has the words "noncomedogenic" or "nonacnegenic" on the label. These words mean that the product will not cause acne. Remove all makeup carefully at bedtime.
- Wash your hair regularly. If you have oily hair, wash it more often. Keep your hair off your face as much as possible. Tie it back while you sleep.

- Do not pick, scratch, pop or squeeze your pimples. Cupping the chin in a hand can cause acne. It is best not to touch your skin at all if you can avoid it. If you have the habit of touching your skin, try to decrease this habit. You may want to keep a daily record of when you touch your skin to help you break this habit.
- Blackheads or whiteheads (comedones) can be removed with a "comedone extractor" (a tool to help press the blackhead out). The small end of a plastic eye dropper, without the bulb part, may also work. After cleaning the area with hot water, the comedone extractor is placed over the blackhead or whitehead and gentle pressure is applied until the contents are pressed out. This removes the blackhead or whitehead and may prevent it from becoming inflamed. If gentle pressure is not enough to remove the comedone, do not continue, as you will irritate the skin. Clean the comedone extractor with alcohol after each use. Blackheads and whiteheads may come back 25–50 days after removal. Treating the area of comedones with a peeling product for 4–6 weeks before using the comedone extractor may give a better result.
- If you shave, try both an electric razor and a safety razor to see which is more comfortable. If you use a safety razor, soften your beard with soap and warm water before you shave. Try to shave less often. Always use a sharp blade and shave lightly. Shave over each area only once in the direction the hair grows.
- A tan can hide acne, but tanning can also damage your skin. To protect your skin, use an oil-free sunscreen with a sun protection factor (SPF) of at least 15. An alcohol lotion or gel sunscreen is the best form for your skin. There are 2 main kinds of sunscreen: chemical and physical. Chemical sunscreens must be absorbed by the skin to be effective, so they should be applied after cleansing but before acne medication. Physical sunscreens (containing zinc or titanium) remain on the surface of the skin to reflect the sun and may stop acne medication from being absorbed (and being effective) if they are applied first, therefore, physical sunscreens should be applied after acne medication. If your acne medication contains benzoyl peroxide, do not use it at the same time as a sunscreen. Apply the sunscreen during the day and the benzoyl peroxide at night.
- Avoid humid environments.
- Wear clothing that allows the skin to breathe.
- Avoid or reduce exposure to environmental factors, such as dirt, dust, petroleum products, cooking oils or chemical irritants.
- If your skin is irritated by a headband, violin, chin strap, guitar strap or orthopedic braces, try cutting a sterile cotton pad to fit underneath.
- Avoid sports equipment such as sports helmets that rub against the skin with friction. If not possible, wear clean absorbent cotton garments or padding underneath equipment or uniforms.
- Follow these suggestions as long as you have acne. Remember to see your healthcare provider if the acne does not improve after 6–8 weeks of treatment.

Chapter 55
Atopic, Contact, and Stasis Dermatitis

Debra Sibbald, BScPhm, ACPR, MA (Adult Education), PhD (Education)

Dermatitis is a nonspecific term describing both acute and chronic skin reactions with corresponding clinical patterns and history. Although the word eczema (boiling over) has been used synonymously with atopic dermatitis, most dermatologists use the term dermatitis to describe an acute, nonspecific skin reaction that exhibits swelling, erythema, scaling, vesicles and crusts. Atopic dermatitis is a chronic inflammatory skin disease caused by mucocutaneous barrier dysfunction. Contact dermatitis is an inflammatory skin reaction caused by exposure to allergens or irritants. Stasis dermatitis is inflammation of the skin of the lower legs caused by chronic venous insufficiency.

Skin changes in dermatitis reflect the pattern of inflammatory response. The appearance is similar in all forms of dermatitis, regardless of cause.

When the reaction is acute, the earliest and mildest changes are erythema (redness) caused by engorgement and dilatation of the small blood vessels and, usually, swelling (edema) resulting from leakage of fluid from blood vessels and accumulation in tissues. If swelling is severe, skin cells form vesicles that fill with edema fluid; this process is called vesiculation or blistering. Breakage of blisters results in oozing or weeping and evaporation of this fluid causes crusting and scaling.

Dermatitis may progress to a chronic stage where the skin becomes dry, fissured and cracked. With prolonged itching and scratching it thickens, and the normal skin markings become more prominent. This process is called lichenification. The skin may show damage from scratching (linear or punctate scarring) and hyperpigmentation or hypopigmentation.[1]

Pathophysiology
Atopic Dermatitis

Atopic dermatitis, allergic rhinitis/conjunctivitis and allergic bronchial asthma belong to the atopic syndrome, or atopic diathesis, which is a mucocutaneous barrier dysfunction.[2] Atopic dermatitis is a chronic inflammatory skin disease associated with cutaneous and mucous membranes hyper-reactivity to environmental triggers that are innocuous to nonatopic individuals.[3] Atopic dermatitis affects 10–20% of the population. The disease is genetically associated, with a risk of 70% if both parents are afflicted, and a higher risk of inheritance from mother than father. While the genetic link may contribute to increased incidence in Asians or black Caribbeans, this is evident only if living in dry, cold climates.[4] It is significantly more common in those of higher socioeconomic status, children from small families and those who live in privately owned properties, possibly reflecting the influence of lifestyle, home furnishing and education.[4]

Eighty to 85% of patients with atopic dermatitis have high levels of total IgE, which correlate with the severity of clinical disease. Children with mild to moderate disease have much lower levels than those with severe disease.[5] The IgE trigger causes an eczema-type reaction rather than a classic urticarial reaction. Eosinophils are involved in producing pro-inflammatory products in the skin and mucous membranes. Twenty percent of patients show normal IgE levels and lack specific sensitization against inhalant and food allergens. Genetic impairment of the epidermal barrier has been proposed as a cause of atopic dermatitis. Evidence supports the classical concept of atopic dermatitis as a continuum that begins with impaired epidermal barrier and penetration of environmental factors causing eczema in about 20% of individuals, primarily female and with normal IgE. Sensitization to allergens and infections progresses to atopic dermatitis, leading to scratching and ensuing tissue damage. This causes sensitization to self-proteins and the "autoallergic" stage of atopic dermatitis which is associated with high levels of IgE and the concomitant risk of development of asthma.[6]

Atopic dermatitis is predominantly a disease of childhood.[4] It begins in infancy but is rarely present at birth, and decreases in intensity with age. In approximately 80% of cases the problem develops during the first year of life, and in up to 90% of cases the onset occurs before 5 years of age.[7] In children younger than 2 years, there may be a stronger male-to-female ratio, but this is reversed after age 2, with a slight female preponderance. Increased disease chronicity in females may be responsible.[4] Incidence of occupational allergic and irritant contact dermatitis is increased in patients with atopic dermatitis. In adults and children, *Staphylococcus aureus* colonization is high, whereas adult skin is more heavily colonized with *Malassezia* yeasts.[8]

Contact Dermatitis

Contact dermatitis is a pattern of inflammatory responses in the skin that occurs through contact with external factors. The clinical picture is a polymorphic pattern of skin inflammation characterized by a wide range of clinical features, including itching, swelling, redness and scaling. Contact dermatitis is a common occupational disease and is also caused by cosmetics, skin care products and other chemicals such as textile dyes in clothing and outdoor plants. Aggravating factors play a large role since the extent and severity varies with: the frequency and duration of exposure; presence of infected, inflamed or burned skin; degree of allergic sensitivity and mechanical factors such as pressure, friction and excessive perspiration, which may intensify the dermatitis.[9] Extremes in temperature, humidity, sweating and occlusion can lower the threshold for irritation.[10] Secondary infection with bacteria or fungi is more likely in dermatitic skin.[10]

Contact dermatitis occurs from infancy onwards and is divided into 2 categories: allergic contact dermatitis (20% of patients) and irritant contact dermatitis (80% of patients). Lower incidence among children is due to limited exposure to allergens.[11]

Allergic contact dermatitis is a delayed or T cell-driven hypersensitivity immune reaction mediated by lymphocytes previously sensitized by exposure to contact allergens, or haptens. Allergenic substances must be processed within the epidermis by the Langerhans cells that migrate to regional lymph nodes. Here, antigen is conjugated with proteins processed by T lymphocytes, which become specifically reactive to the presented antigen, initiating a sequence of cytokine-mediated events and inflammatory response.[12] The reactivity of the skin is a result of balance between T lymphocyte hypersensitivity and suppressor cells which invoke allergen tolerance.[12] Most of these cellular reactions produce sensitization in only a small percentage of those exposed. The incubation period after initial sensitization is 5–21 days and 12–48 hours after subsequent re-exposure, but the reaction may continue to develop for several weeks.[9] Predisposition to develop allergic contact dermatitis is genetic. Allergic contact dermatitis decreases with age since the skin of people over 65 is less reactive to allergens, due to diminished immune function that occurs with age.[11] However, older patients also have impaired epidermal barrier function and slower skin recovery after an insult. In the elderly, eczematous erythroderma (severe widespread redness of the skin) is common.[13] Elderly patients may acquire allergy to topical preparations used to treat stasis or contact dermatitis.[14]

Primary irritant contact dermatitis is a nonallergic reaction resulting from activation of the innate immune system by the direct cytotoxic effect produced by exposure to any substance including chemical, physical or biologic agents, if the concentration and duration of contact are sufficient. Mild irritants such as soaps, detergents and most solvents require repeated or sustained contact to produce inflammation. Strong irritants such as acids and alkalis may injure the skin immediately. Irritant effects may be considerably enhanced by occlusion. The majority of cases are related to occupation, in particular jobs that involve work with water or exposure to irritant substances. Hand dermatitis results from frequent washing of the hands which damages the skin through a combination of mechanisms: increased skin permeability from alkali-induced damage to the keratin, removal of lipids and amino acids from the skin, and alteration of the skin's buffering capacity. Intensification may also be produced by irritants such as waxes, polishes and turpentine and through excoriation or rubbing.[12] Hand dermatitis may affect 1 in 9 adults in any given year, predominating in females with a ratio greater than 5:1.[15] Diaper dermatitis is common and is discussed in Chapter 59: Diaper Dermatitis.

Stasis Dermatitis

Stasis dermatitis results from chronic venous insufficiency and is commonly seen in middle-aged or elderly patients, more frequently in women than in men. Approximately one-third of patients have a previous history of deep vein thrombophlebitis related to trauma, pregnancy, surgery or prolonged illness.[9]

Goals of Therapy

- Eliminate individual trigger factors or contact exposure to irritants and allergens
- Restore barrier function
- Provide symptomatic relief while decreasing skin lesions
- Implement preventive measures focusing on decreasing the number of episodic flares, lengthening symptom-free periods and prevention of excoriations
- Develop coping strategies and expectations for patients/caregivers

Patient Assessment

The pattern of dermatitis and its trigger factors influence the clinical classification and therapy. An approach to assessing patients with dermatitis is shown in Figure 1.

Atopic Dermatitis

Clinical Presentation

Atopic dermatitis presents as an intensely pruritic acute, subacute or chronic eruption seen in characteristic patterns in infants, children and adults. The diagnosis is purely clinical; the symptoms and signs of atopic dermatitis are numerous, but usually nonspecific. Itch is the main symptom. There is no primary skin lesion in atopic dermatitis; the clinical presentation of eczematous skin lesions represents skin changes induced by constant scratching and excoriations.[16] The skin is typically dry and the lesions scaly, though they may be vesicular, weeping or oozing in the acute stage. Clinical presentation supports both debated theories as to the chronology of pruritus and lesions: itch may precede visible skin lesions and/or erythema, and inflammation may evoke pruritus.[17] Various triggers such as stress result in appearance of erythema followed by itch, then vasodilation and inflammation due to scratching. The pruritus may be focal or generalized if skin is dry and may be most intense during the evening and at night. It is usually intermittent and leads to vigorous itch-scratch cycles, commonly with secondary bacterial infection of excoriated lesions.[9]

Although atopic dermatitis can affect any area of the body, it preferentially affects the flexures and the face. Distribution of lesions depends on the age of the patient, with infantile, childhood, adolescent and adult phases. In babies aged less than 6 months, the face and scalp are the sites most commonly affected, and redness and chapping of a baby's cheeks can be the earliest sign.[3] This chapping usually begins at 2–3 months and persists for 2 years. Remission usually occurs between 2 and 4 years of age. Subsequently, a chronically relapsing dermatitis begins, located on the extensor sides of the extremities but also on the flexural areas. The most common sites are the antecubital and popliteal fossae.[3] It can also be located around the mouth, eyelids, neck and hands. The lips can be dry and scaly. Visual signs of chronic atopic dermatitis include less redness, increased dryness and early lichenification (thickened skin, hyperpigmentation and accentuation of skin furrows due to repeated rubbing and scratching). Involvement of the back of the arms and the front of the legs is seen first, and later a transition occurs to the elbows and knee folds. Frictional areas such as wrists and ankles are regular sites, and localization may occur to the toes. Occlusive footwear causing excessive sweating and drying of the feet may exacerbate the condition. Children aged 4–6 years usually develop symmetric eczema on flexural areas, hands, feet, and the back of the thigh. As the child reaches adulthood, recurrent outbreaks diminish or disappear. In adolescents and adults, the involvement may be generalized, but flexural accentuation is the hallmark of clinical disease. Adults typically exhibit lesions on the face, upper body and flexural areas.[18]

In addition to the classical patterns, there are site-specific variants. Eyelid eczema is common in 21% of adolescents and is associated with hay fever and exposure to aeroantigens such as house dust mites. The infra-auricular and retro-auricular sites of the ears are particularly prone to fissuring, as a reaction to minor trauma.[3]

Areas of predisposition may be related to the thickness of the stratum corneum and variations in exposure to irritants and allergens at different body sites: thinnest areas are genitals and eyelids, often subject to rubbing, followed by flexor forearms and posterior auricular.[3] Other parts of the face and flexures have a thin epidermal barrier with decreased barrier function. In the areas most vulnerable to penetration, the disease persists longer.[3]

Other minor features exhibited by atopic patients include recurrent conjunctivitis, cheilitis (chapped lips), infraorbital folds (Dennie-Morgan lines), recurrent infections (especially viral) and impaired cell-mediated immunity.[16] See Atopic Dermatitis in Photo Section.

The diagnosis of atopic dermatitis is based on essential and supporting features. Essential features must be present and include pruritus and dermatitis (typical morphology, age-specific features and chronic or relapsing history). Supporting features are present in most cases and include early onset, family history and high IgE reactivity. Other associated features are too nonspecific to be diagnostic. Conditions which must be included in the differential diagnosis are: scabies, contact dermatitis, ichthyosis, cutaneous T-cell lymphoma, psoriasis, photosensitivity, immune deficiency and erythroderma due to other causes.[19]

Risk and Aggravating Factors

Genetics: Atopic dermatitis patients have an increased personal or family history of atopic syndrome, including type 1 allergies (immediate hypersensitivity), hay fever, asthma and chronic allergic rhinitis/conjunctivitis and are genetically predisposed.[19]

Environmental Allergens: Excessive use of soaps, detergents and shampoos irritate the skin and disturb the skin barrier. Alcohol and astringents in skin care products can be drying and their use should be limited.[20] Central heating, insulation, air conditioning and inadequate ventilation may increase exposure to environmental antigens such as house dust mites, molds, pollens and furry pets. Global warming and increased use of fertilizer may enhance density and allergenic potency of pollen from trees and grains.[2] The influence of these environmental and lifestyle factors may account for increased incidence in individuals of higher socioeconomic status.[4]

Climate: The influence of climate is shown in Asians with atopic syndrome who live in humid tropical climates and do not manifest cutaneous symptoms until they move to colder, drier countries.[2] A seasonal variation is due to several contributing factors: environmental allergens cause relapses in summer, while climatic influences may cause clearing in summer sun and worsening in the dry, cold air of winter. Dryness of the skin (xerosis) with water content below 10% is crucial for induction of itch and scratching.[17] Heat worsens the skin condition.

Sweating: Any stimulus to sweating (thermal, emotional) is a typical hallmark and the most common trigger of itch. Acetylcholine may be involved and there may be a decreased threshold for sweat stimulation.[17]

Physiologic Stress: Stress associated with demanding modern lifestyles appears to enhance skin irritability and contributes to the itch-scratch cycle and sleep disturbances.[7,2] The alteration in skin appearance due to scratching escalates the emotional reaction to coping with the disease.[21]

Dietary Influences: There are convincing data that food hypersensitivity plays a significant role in the symptomatology of atopic dermatitis.[22] More than 50 food allergens have been characterized. In general, high-protein foods are considered more allergenic; water-soluble glycoproteins are particularly resistant to food processing, cooking and digestion.[23] Foods triggering the majority of food-allergic reactions have been ranked differently depending upon the population and country studied.[24] While ranking is continually debated, for infants and children a currently accepted list of food allergens includes milk, egg, wheat, soy, peanut, tree nuts, fish and shellfish.[25] For adolescents and adults, food allergens include peanut, tree nut, fish and shellfish.[26] The persistence of food allergy is variable and depends on the specific food allergen. Outgrowing milk allergy may be more prolonged than reported previously (79% by age 16), and it also may take longer for children to outgrow egg allergy (68% by age 16). In contrast, only 20% of children with peanut allergy and 9% with tree nut allergy eventually develop tolerance.[23]

Irritants: Disinfectants, solvents and allergens in skin care products play an important role. Issues of irritation extend to clothing fabrics and products. Intolerance to wool is a hallmark of atopy. Coarse-textured fabrics, liquid or sheet fabric softeners (which cause fibres to plump up and stay erect) and bleach should be avoided.

Infections: Atopic patients have an increased propensity for cutaneous viral infections including herpes simplex, molluscum contagiosum and warts, fungal infections such as dermatophytosis, pityriasis (tinea) versicolor and candidiasis, and bacterial infections such as *S. aureus*.[24]

Itch-scratch cycle: Severe pruritus elicits reflexive scratching, resulting in a vicious cycle of itch and scratch.

Contact Dermatitis

Clinical Presentation

Cutaneous responses are dependent on the particular chemical, the duration and nature of the contact, and individual host susceptibility. Despite different pathogeneses, the allergic and irritant forms have similar clinical appearances, especially in the chronic forms. The clinical presentation of contact dermatitis is determined by the severity and acuteness of the inflammation. The area involved usually reflects the pattern of the contacting substance and may have sharp, well-demarcated linear margins or unusual geographic shapes. It may spread to distant sites through lymphocytes. Contact substances may be transferred from the primary site by touch to distant areas, especially the eyelids and neck, which are very reactive sites. The face may display a reaction to substances applied to the scalp. Allergic contact dermatitis and irritant contact dermatitis are predominant causes of periorbital dermatitis.[27] Scalp, palms and sole areas are more resistant. The distribution of the lesions may provide clues to the irritant or allergen trigger.

Acute reactions are often red, edematous papules in the early phase, which become vesicles and bullae that ooze if the reaction is severe enough. Chronic reactions produce an entirely different clinical picture in which primary lesions are minimal, and secondary changes such as dryness, lichenification, pigment changes, hyperkeratosis or thickening, excoriation and fissuring predominate. As with other forms of acute and chronic dermatitis, itching is the primary symptom.[28]

Irritant Contact Dermatitis: Acute irritant contact dermatitis reactions usually reach their peak within minutes to hours after exposure and then start to heal. Symptoms of an acute reaction to mild irritants include burning, stinging and soreness at the site and physical signs of the reaction include erythema, vesiculation and oozing. Strong irritants produce blistering, erosions and ulcers. Acute reactions will have sharply demarcated borders and will generally be asymmetrical. Cumulative irritant contact dermatitis is a consequence of multiple subthreshold skin insults without sufficient time in between for complete restoration of skin barrier function. It may be due to a variety of stimuli or frequent repetition of one factor, especially if occupational. Clinical symptoms will develop only after cumulative damage exceeds the threshold, and the lesions may be less well demarcated. Hand dermatitis occurs principally on the fingers, web spaces and dorsa of the hand. Palms are spared and dryness, erythema and scaling are early features. It often begins on the fourth finger, beneath a ring.[9] Long-term glove occlusion and the accumulation of barrier damage from hand washing, even when mild hand cleansers are employed, may lead to cumulative skin irritation.[29]

Allergic Contact Dermatitis: This is a pruritic eczematous reaction which in its mild form is similar to exposure to an irritant. A typical allergic reaction consists of grouped or linear tense vesicles and blisters, and in severe involvement, marked edema, particularly on the face and in periorbital and genital areas. The acute form can also have a diffuse patchy distribution depending on the allergen (for example, body washes and shampoos that get rinsed over the body) and/or the development of disseminated auto-sensitization (acute, generalized dermatitis arising in response to a prior localized inflammatory reaction). The suspected diagnosis is based on clinical symptoms, a plausible contact to allergens and a suitable history of dermatitis. Differential diagnoses should be considered only after careful exclusion of any causal contact sensitization. Careful diagnosis by patch testing is of great importance. Modifications of the standardized test procedure are the strip patch test and the repeated open application test.[30]

Common Contact Allergens

A list of contact allergens is presented in Table 1. The most common contact allergens include plants of the *Rhus* genus, nickel, rubber, ethylenediamine (a stabilizer in many topical preparations) and paraphenylenediamine (an ingredient in black hair dye and industrial chemicals).[31] Nearly any chemical can produce contact dermatitis. Small molecules are most likely to be sensitizers since they penetrate the epidermis more readily. The possibility of cross-sensitization with other chemicals is an important consideration. The most notable are listed in Table 2. Cross-sensitization may prohibit use of critically important systemically administered drugs.[9]

Allergens of Note

Plants

Toxicodendron plants, also known as *Rhus* and poison ivy account for the largest number of cases of allergic contact dermatitis. The typical warning to avoid contact is "Leaflets three, let it be." The leaves, stems, seeds, flowers, berries and roots of plants contain milky sap that turns into a black varnish-like substance on exposure to air. Once the solvent evaporates, the allergen (urushiol) remains and is antigenic indefinitely, even if the plant has died.[32] Sensitization is immediate with the formation of a complex protein in the skin that is not removed through washing. Sensitization and dermatitis occur after 7–10 days, and re-exposure produces a reaction within 8 hours to 2 days. Streaks of erythema or papules, vesicles and bullae in linear arrangement are a characteristic clinical presentation and accompany itching and edema as key features.[12] Urushiol is nonvolatile. Smoke may carry the poison in dispersed form.[32] See Table 1 and Table 2.

Table 1: **Common Causes of Contact Dermatitis**

Type of Dermatitis	Substance	Source
Allergic contact dermatitis	Aloe vera	Topical medications and cosmetics
	Bacitracin	Topical antibiotic creams, eye and ear preparations
	Balsam of Peru	Cough syrups, flavourings
	Benzocaine	Topical antibiotic creams, eye and ear preparations
	Cetylstearyl alcohols	Topical medications, cosmetics, paste bandages
	Chromium salts	Potassium dichromate electroplating, cement, leather tanning agents, detergents, dyes
	Cobalt chloride	Cements, metal plating, pigments in paints
	Ethylenediamine	Dyes, fungicides, medications
	Formaldehyde	Germicides, plastics, clothing, glue, adhesives
	Fragrances	Topical medications, baby products, cosmetics, household products
	Lanolin	Topical medications, bath oils and cosmetics
	Latex	Rubber products, e.g., gloves, catheters, balloons, plants, medical devices, tires, conveyor belts
	Methylisothiazolinone	Baby wipes
	Neomycin	Topical antibiotic creams, eye and ear preparations
	Nickel	Metal alloys, hairpins, jewelry, zippers, hair dyes
	Paraphenylenediamine	Hair and clothing dyes, chemical photographic use
	Potassium dichromate	Cement, leather, household cleansers, bleaches
	Quaternium 15	Preservative in topical medications and cosmetics
	Rhus genus	Poison ivy, poison oak, mangos
	Rosins (gum and wood)	Topical medications
	Rubber accelerators (mercaptos/ carbamates/thiurams)	Rubber products (ostomy products, bandages, latex products, toys, condoms, diaphragms, goggles, pacifiers)
	Topical antihistamines	Topical medications
Irritant contact dermatitis	Acids	Solvents
	Alkalis	Surfactants
	Enzymes	Wet cement
	Oxidants	Hydrogen peroxide, household bleach

Table 2: **Cross-sensitizers with Common Contact Allergens[32,33]**

Sensitizers	Cross-sensitizers
Ethylenediamine	Aminophylline, ethylenediamine antihistamines
Latex	Bananas, kiwi, pineapple, chestnuts, avocados, apricots, cherries, grapes, passion fruit, potatoes, peaches, tomatoes (occasionally other fruits and nuts). Alert healthcare practitioners prior to procedures.
Local anesthetics (ester type, e.g., benzocaine)	Para-amino-containing compounds (widely used in topicals): parabens, some oral hypoglycemics, sulfonamides, thiazide diuretics
Neomycin	Aminoglycosides (gentamicin, tobramcyin), framycetin
Rhus	Lacquers from China and Japan, mangos, cashews and ginkgo

Latex

Natural rubber latex, sourced in southeast Asia, is a leading cause of immunologic contact urticaria, and can cause IgE-mediated skin-related findings as well as acute respiratory symptoms and even anaphylaxis. Delayed contact allergy may exist more commonly than previously noted, particularly in atopic individuals. Immediate latex allergy (irritant contact dermatitis) is not the same as the more common, less severe T cell-mediated delayed hypersensitivity reaction seen clinically as allergic contact dermatitis.[33]

Added ingredients to rubber products may cause allergic contact dermatitis: accelerators in the rubber product make it more functional, antioxidants and antiozonants (parapheylenediamine) delay degradation, and other chemicals increase softness and pliability. Allergic contact dermatitis is due to carbamates and thiurams in rubber gloves, mercaptos and parapheylenediamine in shoes, industrial materials and tires, and thioureas in neoprene (used in medical and sporting goods).[33] See Table 1 and Table 2.

Metals

Metals are the most common contact allergens; nickel is the most common cause of metal allergy and in most series ranks as the most commonly positive of all screening allergens.[34] Nickel allergy can result in both cutaneous and systemic manifestations.[35] Reactions to gold, chrome and cobalt are also frequently seen. Cross-sensitization to other metals can occur, e.g., nickel and palladium. Cobalt, nickel and chromium may induce co-reactions and other substances may contain them (cobalt in cement). Usually, the metals must be in solution for allergic contact, but can be liberated by sweat. Nickel, palladium and titanium are the most common metal allergens in contact dermatitis due to eyeglass frames.[36] Metals can also be ingested (dietary nickel) or due to sources such as orthopedic implants.[34] Irritant contact dermatitis to metals is common in workers exposed to metal salts, dust or fumes.[34]

Antibiotics

Topical antibiotics used long-term on skin with impaired protective barrier leads to increased risk of hypersensitivity. Groups at a high risk of contact sensitivity include: patients with chronic venous insufficiency, chronic ulcers or chronic otitis externa, or individuals with occupational exposure to antibiotics (e.g., human medicine and veterinary medicine practitioners, pharmaceutical industry workers, cattle breeders). When long-term therapy with topical antibiotics in these patients fails to result in improvement, allergic reactions to topical antibiotics should be considered. Cross-sensitivity, which is frequently associated with topical aminoglycoside antibiotics, poses a significant problem.[37]

Bacitracin is an antibiotic used in several types of consumer products, including cosmetics and ophthalmic and skin ointments. Bacitracin was the ninth most common contact allergen detected in 2003, causing more than 9% of positive reactions among 5812 patients with suspected contact dermatitis.[38] Because bacitracin is used on wounds and is often inappropriately applied to fungal infections, the diagnosis of contact dermatitis can often be elusive. Reactions may be attributed to a slow-healing wound or worsening infection that is treated, ironically, with more topical antibiotic agents. Due to the significant prevalence of bacitracin allergy, the American Contact Dermatitis Society warns it should not be used routinely.[38] Clinical affect, scientific evidence, and need for medical cost containment all advocate the discontinuation of routine usage of bacitracin in clean wounds. Table 3 reports changes in common allergic responses, which reflects routine usage.

Antihistamines

Topical antihistamines have been reported to cause contact dermatitis. Doxepin cream was the most commonly implicated topical preparation. A causal relationship is often difficult to recognize because the reaction may be similar to the disease being treated with the antihistamine preparation. Cross-reactivity within the same class of medication is likely but not certain.[39]

Preservatives

Many preservatives can cause allergic contact dermatitis (e.g., parabens, formaldehyde). Methylisothiazolinone is a preservative commonly found in baby wipes. Incidence of allergy to this chemical is rising with increasing use and some jurisdictions are calling for a ban on its use. It has been suggested that it is common enough to be included in the standardized series of allergens used in patch testing.[40] In Canada, concentration of methylisothiazolinone used alone is limited to 100 ppm, however this is 25 times the limit allowed when it is used in combination with methylchloro-isothiazolinone (see Chapter 59: Diaper Dermatitis for more information).[41]

Emulsifiers

Sorbitan sesquioleate and/or sorbitan monooleate are emulsifiers in many topical corticosteroid products. One study and its follow up found incidence rates for allergic contact dermatitis due to these chemicals of 8.9% and 4.1% respectively. The authors suggest that given the presence of sorbitans in many topical corticosteroid formulations, allergy to these chemicals should be considered when patients do not improve as expected with topical corticosteroid therapy.[42]

Table 3: **Most Common Patch-test Responses in Patients with Suspected Contact Dermatitis[38]**

Substance	Percentage of Patients Exhibiting Reaction
Nickel sulfate	16.2%
Balsam of Peru	12.3%
Neomycin	11.5%
Fragrance mix	10.9%
Thimerosal	10.8%
Sodium gold thiosulfate	10.5%
Formaldehyde	9.2%
Quaternium 15	9.2%
Bacitracin	9.2%
Cobalt chloride	7.6%

Risk and Aggravating Factors

Consort Contact Dermatitis: Skin-to-skin contact can result in transfer of potential contact allergens from one sex partner to the other and may result from lubricants, hygiene products, seminal fluids, and rubber in diaphragms and condoms.[14]

Impaired Cell-mediated Immunity: Risk is reduced with impairment of cell-mediated immunity, such as AIDS, lymphomas or atopic dermatitis. Atopic patients are more likely to develop pustular reactions when exposed to nickel.[14]

Diet: It has been suggested that diet may play a role in allergic contact dermatitis. Approximately 30–50% of patients with latex allergy have hypersensitivity to certain fruits. Presence in food of nickel (e.g., from water, cooking utensils) or balsam of Peru (e.g., wine, candy chocolate, curry) can aggravate allergic contact dermatitis; eliminating these items from the diet may alleviate symptoms.[43]

Ethnicity: The incidence of contact dermatitis in Caucasians is greater than blacks due to their greater skin reactivity; however, blacks experience a higher incidence of paraphenylenediamine allergy. Caucasians have a looser packing of skin layers and fewer intercellular lipids, making their skin more permeable to irritants and allergens.[44]

Gender: Although women develop contact dermatitis more often than men, it is primarily because women are more frequently exposed to irritants, allergens and wet work, and not because of differences in skin reactivity.[44]

Body Site: Eyelid contact dermatitis may be due to mascara, cosmetic preservatives, nail polish, hair cosmetics, eyeliner, ophthalmic medications, adhesives in false eyelashes, eyelash curlers, paper products, plants, airborne materials and dyes. The chest and abdomen are sites for allergy to metals and elastic objects, and genital areas are susceptible to dermatitis from hygiene products, contraceptives, condoms and seminal fluid. Nails exhibit contact dermatitis from acrylate applications, hardeners, enamels, hydroquinone in bleaching creams, weed killers, insecticides and physical trauma.[45]

Climate: Seasonal variation occurs with increased prevalence during winter months and exposure to cold, dry air.[31]

Occupation: Individuals at risk of contact dermatitis are often those who are exposed to these substances occupationally or as part of their daily routine. Exposure to organic solvents together with detergents may increase the risk of acquiring occupational contact dermatitis.[46] *Rhus* dermatitis is seen less often in dark-skinned individuals, more commonly in younger persons, and is a hazard for outdoor workers and enthusiasts.

Latex allergy (from rubber gloves and other sources) is common in healthcare practitioners. The medical community is also at risk of contact dermatitis due to occupational substances, including mucolytics, dressings, adhesive removers, gowns, scrub solutions, formaldehyde and glutaraldehyde, mercury (dentists) as well as active drugs such as anesthetics, essential oils, antibiotics and inactive ingredients including aluminum, petrolatum, oils (olive, castor and sesame) and lanolin.[47]

Other occupations that can increase the risk of contact dermatitis include photography, textile work, printing industry, agricultural work, office work (carbon sources), bakery work and hairdressing.[48] Hand dermatitis as a subtype of contact dermatitis is often seen in healthcare practitioners, hairdressers and dishwashers, especially in those who have atopic dermatitis. Susceptibility is greater among younger people. Bakers and chefs may experience food contact dermatitis due to sorbic acid preservatives, antioxidants, flavour ingredients (peppermint, cinnamon, anise, coriander, garlic, sesame, cashew) and food additives, such as dyes, and benzoyl peroxide.[49] Plant allergy may include extracts used in medications such as balsam of Peru, rosin and benzoin.[50]

Ultraviolet Light: Photocontact dermatitis requires exposure to UV light and may occur due to irritant or allergic causes. Irritant reactions (phototoxic) can occur in anyone due to substances like psoralens, whereas photoallergic contact dermatitis occurs only after an individual with sensitivities is exposed to an allergen. Fragrances and sunscreen chemicals are causes of photocontact dermatitis.[51]

Stasis Dermatitis

Clinical Presentation

Stasis dermatitis, which occurs due to venous insufficiency, is seen on the lower leg. Acute changes consist of inflammation, edema, pigmentation and ulceration. The eruption may be erythematous and oozing, with marked inflammation. Chronic stasis results in scaling, discoloration and lichenification and is accompanied by edema due to venous disease. This may result in fibrosis, producing hardening and induration of soft tissue. Pigmentation is invariably present in the early stages due to dermal extravasation of red blood cells following small venule rupture. Superficial ulceration may result from acute inflammation and may heal or progress to deeper ulcers. Superficial venous varicosities may also be present.[9]

Differential Diagnosis of Dermatitis

Table 4 outlines other conditions that should be considered in the differential diagnosis of eczematous dermatitis.

Table 4: **Differential Diagnosis of Eczematous Dermatitis**

Infections and infestations		Papulosquamous conditions	
	Scabies (see Chapter 69: Parasitic Skin Infections: Lice and Scabies)		Psoriasis (see Chapter 71: Psoriasis)
	Candidiasis (see Chapter 65: Fungal Skin Infections)		Seborrheic dermatitis (see Chapter 58: Dandruff and Seborrheic Dermatitis)
	Herpes (see Chapter 74: Viral Skin Rashes)		Neoplasms
	Tinea (see Chapter 65: Fungal Skin Infections)		Cutaneous T cell lymphoma
	Staphylococcus aureus infections (impetigo) (see Chapter 56: Bacterial Skin Infections: Impetigo, Furuncles and Carbuncles)		Photosensitivity (see Chapter 72: Prevention and Treatment of Sun-induced Skin Damage)
Metabolic diseases		Immunodeficiencies	
Fatty acid deficiencies			

Differentiating Features of Atopic, Contact and Stasis Dermatitis

Table 5 outlines the differentiating features of common dermatitis subtypes.

Drug-induced Dermatitis

Eczematous eruptions can also occur with many drugs given either topically or systemically. Cross-sensitivity may occur with structurally related drugs administered by either route. Common sensitizers include antibiotics, phenothiazines and the ester group of anesthetics. As a rule, the eruption starts shortly after administration of the drug, if previous sensitization has occurred. Patch testing with the responsible drug will give positive results. Table 6 lists drugs that commonly evoke eczematous reactions.[52]

Table 5: **Differentiating Features of Subtypes of Dermatitis**

Condition	Duration/Location	Description	Trigger Factors	Goals of Therapy
Atopic dermatitis	2 months; chest, face, neck, diaper area	Cycles of itching and scratching. Red, raised blisters with oozing, dry skin	Extreme heat or cold, rapid temperature changes, sweating, irritant or occlusive clothing (wool or nylon), soaps and detergents, greases, environmental allergens, anxiety, infections	Decrease trigger factors and pruritus Suppress inflammation Lubricate skin Alleviate anxiety
	2 y; scalp, neck, extremities			
	4–10 y; scattered—neck, wrist, elbow, knee	Less acute and oozing; dry papules, thickening, periorbital edema and erythema		
	12–20 y; flexor areas, hands	Dry, thickened, hyperpigmented plaques		
Contact dermatitis (irritant and allergic)	Irritant/allergic: In contact area Allergic: May generalize	Unusual patterns resembling contacting substance Acute: Red, blisters, oozing, may erode Chronic: Dry, thick, fissured	Irritant: Time and concentration of irritant Allergic: Sensitization to allergen	Decrease contact exposure to irritants and allergens If dry, wet it If wet, dry it
Dry skin	Lower legs (shins), dorsa of hands, forearms	Mild to moderate: Dry skin with fine scale; diffuse or round patches Severe: Cracks and fissures in diamond pattern with redness	Increasing age, decreased humidity, increased indoor heat, cold, dry, winter air, contact with soaps and irritants, hypothyroidism	Replace water in the skin and the environment
Hand dermatitis	Irritant: Sides of the fingers, less often throughout palms Allergic: Back of the hands	Redness, dryness, chapping; small vesicles; excess sweating	Repeated contact with primary irritants, soap and water, solvents and detergents Family history of atopic dermatitis or psoriasis	Decrease contact exposure
Stasis dermatitis	Lower leg, proximal to medial Malleolus	Acute: Inflammation, edema, pigmentation and ulceration Chronic: Scaling, discoloration, lichenification	Venous insufficiency, and edema, upright posture, hot, humid environment, sensitizers	Decrease triggers, bed rest and elevation, compression of leg

Severe or Complicated Dermatitis

Atopic dermatitis that is acute and vesicular, or if moderate to severe (defined as: generalized to more than 30% of the body surface area (BSA), continues to involve larger body areas, remains unresponsive, becomes secondarily infected or interferes with activities of daily life or sleep patterns) requires further assessment and treatment by an appropriate healthcare practitioner. Parameters for assessing severity of atopic dermatitis include: Eczema Area Severity Index (EASI)[55] score (a tool used to measure the severity and extent of atopic dermatitis in order to assess clinical response to treatment), quality of life measurement tools (e.g., Dermatology Life Quality Index),[55] sleep disturbances, itch (diary), redness, scale, dryness and amount of emollient used. If there is uncertainty about the diagnosis, of if there is suspicion of wide spread herpes simplex, an appropriate healthcare practitioner should be consulted.[56]

Contact or stasis dermatitis that spreads to distant sites or becomes generalized to more than 30% of BSA, is acute and nonresponsive within a few days, includes edema that persists or increases within a few days, is chronic and nonresponsive within 7–10 days or interferes with quality of life is considered severe or complicated and requires further assessment and treatment by an appropriate healthcare practitioner. To identify the cause of allergic contact dermatitis, practitioners generally use the patch test during which standard concentrations of known substances are applied to the skin and the reactions monitored. Provocative and open use tests may be used after patch testing to distinguish an allergic from an irritant response. Other tests include prick tests and intradermal tests.[57]

Table 6: **Drugs that Commonly Cause Eczematous Eruptions[52]**

Antibiotics	chloramphenicol clioquinol gentamicin neomycin penicillin streptomycin sulfonamides
Antihistamines	promethazine
Antipsychotics	phenothiazines, e.g., chlorpromazine, fluphenazine, perphenazine, prochlorperazine, trifluoperazine
Beta-blockers	metoprolol propranolol timolol
Calcium channel blockers[53,54]	amlodipine diltiazem felodipine nifedipine verapamil
Diuretics	thiazide diuretics
Sulfonylureas	chlorpropamide tolbutamide
Miscellaneous	aminophylline carbamazepine chloral hydrate cyanocobalamin fluorouracil idoxuridine minoxidil nitroglycerin nystatin procainamide quinine quinidine

Nonpharmacologic Therapy

Atopic and Contact Dermatitis

Avoidance of irritants and aggravating factors is key. A thorough history is essential to identify the cause, especially any previous treatments that may have exacerbated symptoms or cross-reacted with the irritant or allergen.

Environmental factors that can modulate the effect of irritants include temperature, humidity and texture of fabrics. Intense sun exposure should be avoided. Temperature in home and work environments should be temperate with moderate humidity to minimize sweating and reduce problems related to heat and perspiration. Air conditioning in the summer and a cool air humidifier in the winter may be helpful. If a humidifier is not available, a bowl of water in the room will enhance ambient humidity.

New **clothing** should be laundered prior to wearing to remove formaldehyde and other chemicals.[20] Occlusive clothing should be avoided and loose-fitting cotton or cotton blend garments substituted for nylon, and corduroy for wool. Many blended fabrics are well tolerated. Texture or roughness, rather than fabric type (natural vs. synthetic) determine tolerability and skin irritancy.[20,58,59] Liquid fabric softeners or dryer sheets should be avoided because plumping up fibres and making them erect increases irritancy. Bleach in the rinse also irritates and should be avoided. A dilute vinegar rinse can be substituted. Use of liquid rather than powder detergent can result in more complete rinsing; adding a second rinse cycle may facilitate removal of residual powder detergent.

Swimming may be a better tolerated sport than those involving intense perspiration or physical contact and may improve dermatitis. Bathing may also remove allergens from the skin surface and reduce colonization by *S. aureus*. Despite a drying or irritating effect, swimming in chlorinated pools results in clinical improvement in some atopic patients. Rather than simply rinsing off after swimming, gentle cleansers should be used to effectively remove the chlorine or bromine, and then moisturizer should be applied.[20]

Wearing **cotton gloves** or **mittens** prevents scratching and secondary infections and allows healing of affected hands. They can be used as a barrier against irritants such as newsprint when reading the paper, and can also allow children to play or perform normal activities, with good acceptance. Keeping fingernails clean and short is essential.

A **diet** that excludes specific foods is not recommended for patients with atopic dermatitis without confirmed food allergy.[56] Intervention is indicated in only about 10–15% of atopic children, when the disease is of sufficient severity and there is a strong suspicion that certain food(s) aggravate the condition. Restrictions in diet should not have a greater effect on quality of life than the disease. Risks of dietary restriction must be kept in mind: such diets may lead to malnutrition and deficiencies, carry the risk of anaphylactic reactions upon rechallenge to a restricted food, and challenge the psychological and social well-being of the child.[7] If foods aggravate atopic dermatitis, they represent only a fraction of the expression of the disease. Exclusion of foods in pregnancy or breastfeeding to prevent development of atopic dermatitis is not recommended.[56] The benefit of breastfeeding is recognized; patients should be advised that exclusive breastfeeding for the first 3 months or more may help prevent the development of atopic dermatitis where there is a family history of atopy.[20] Hydrolyzed formulas should not be offered to infants in preference to breast milk for prevention of atopic dermatitis. The introduction of any specific solid food (soft, mashed consistency to prevent choking) should not be delayed beyond 6 months of age. Later introduction of peanut, fish or egg does not prevent, and may even increase, the risk of developing food allergy. Skin or specific IgE blood testing before a first ingestion is discouraged due to the high false-positive rate. Regular ingestion (several times weekly) of newly introduced foods is important to maintain tolerance.[60] Maternal use of **probiotics** during pregnancy and maternal and/or infant use during breastfeeding may be helpful in reducing the development of atopic dermatitis in the child.[61,62,63,64] Strain and dose of probiotic is not consistent across studies. There is insufficient evidence to recommend the use of probiotics for treatment of established eczema.[65,66]

Wet dressing solutions used in atopic and contact dermatitis may include ordinary tap water or saline, in addition to pharmacologic solutions containing astringent and/or antiseptic compounds. The action of a wet dressing is primarily physical, and thus water or physiologic saline are the solutions of choice as they are convenient, inexpensive and pose no problems of sensitivity or damage to healing wounds. Note that the technique used in applying wet dressings determines the effect on the skin: used as compresses, they are drying, whereas used as soaks, they are hydrating. The rule of thumb for application of wet dressings is "If it is wet, dry it (compress); if it is dry, wet it (soak)."

Wet dressings as compresses cool and dry the skin through evaporation. They reduce inflammatory blood flow, cleanse the skin of exudates, crusts and debris and help maintain drainage of infected areas through vasoconstriction. They are indicated in acute eczematous conditions with oozing and crusting, which can be seen in atopic, contact or stasis dermatitis. The solution should be tepid or room temperature, although cold solution is effective in relieving itch in skin that is otherwise not symptomatic. A nonirritating gauze or thin cloth is soaked with solution, then wrung gently so it remains wet but not dripping. The compress is applied to the skin, removed, remoistened and reapplied every few minutes for 20–30 minute periods, 4–6 times daily ("a minute on, a minute off"). After removal, a lotion may be applied to the skin, but avoid occlusion with an ointment. Powders are not applied to any exudative lesion as they crust, causing bleeding on removal and increased risk of infection.

Wet dressings as soaks soften hardened crusts in scaling conditions usually apparent in chronic atopic, contact or stasis dermatitis, and can hydrate the skin. To apply a soak, saturate the cloth and apply to the area for 15–20 minutes without removal. This procedure occludes and breaks down underlying tissue. Soaks are never used for acute, exudating dermatitis as they may macerate the skin, further damaging barrier function. Chronic contact dermatitis that is dry or fissured should be soaked for 5 minutes rather than compressed before application of an occlusive emollient.

Wet-wrap therapy with or without a topical corticosteroid can be recommended for patients with moderate to severe atopic dermatitis and/or recalcitrant disease to decrease disease severity and water loss during flares. It may be performed on an ambulatory or inpatient basis. Most use a technique of a topical agent covered by a wetted first layer of tubular bandages, gauze, or a cotton suit, followed by a dry second/outside layer. For more generalized disease, 2 layers of nonirritating clothing can be similarly prepared. Rationale includes occluding the topical agent for increased penetration, decreasing water loss, and providing a physical barrier against scratching. The wrap can be worn for several hours up to 24 hours at a time, depending on patient tolerance. Most suggest several days of use, although a few studies continued for up to 2 weeks. Use of topical corticosteroids under the wet wraps seems to be more efficacious than using only moisturizers with the wraps. Care should be taken if mid- to higher-potency corticosteroids are applied under the wraps, as absorption is increased and may cause hypothalamic-pituitary-adrenal axis suppression, especially if used widely on the skin. Temporary decreases in early morning serum cortisol levels have been reported, although short courses of use have not been associated with prolonged adrenal suppression. The potential for increased risk of infection has been raised with the use of mid- to higher-potency topical corticosteroids in wet-wrap therapy, although the data are sparse and conflicting regarding its actual occurrence.[67]

In the case of atopic dermatitis, control of trigger factors and anxiety is a major strategy. Control of exposure to environmental inhaled allergens is important. Direct contact with allergens and irritants should be reduced. Limit soap cleansing to axillae and groin, using mild soaps, creams or soapless cleansers (Table 8). Restrict showers to once weekly, if possible. Use bathing to rehydrate the skin and follow with liberal use of emollients to prevent evaporation. Water temperature should be warm, not hot.

If contact dermatitis is acute, some principles should be kept in mind. The affected area should be washed immediately and thoroughly. If wet or oozing, compresses with saline or tap water can be applied (1 minute on, 1 minute off for 20–30 minutes) 4–6 times daily. Protect the damaged skin against secondary infection until the acute stage subsides. Do not allow debris due to oozing, scaling and crusting to accumulate (see Nonpharmacologic Therapy, Wet Dressings).

Patients with contact dermatitis should avoid touching the following with bare hands: fruit juices, raw meat, fish and vegetables, especially raw onions and garlic; detergents, turpentine and kerosenes; hair tonics and shampoos. Remove rings when washing hands, as trapped soap may produce flares. Use an unscented soap or hand cleanser free of colour, antiseptics, deodorants, vitamins and tar. Wash hands with lukewarm water and use soap sparingly. Rinse hands thoroughly and dry with clean towel, especially between fingers. Wash as infrequently as possible, no more than 2–3 times daily. Hands can be protected with plastic or vinyl gloves worn with cotton liners, but rubber gloves should be avoided. In hand dermatitis, avoid activity that involves friction, pressure, squeezing or twisting. A low nickel diet for vesicular hand dermatitis can be helpful in select nickel-sensitive cases.[68] Avoid adhesive bandages. Chronic hand dermatitis often becomes secondarily infected, especially if fissured, and should be managed appropriately. Despite lack of evidence, small, noninfected fissures can be closed with **cyanoacrylate glue** (e.g., Superglue). Occlusive dressings such as kitchen plastic wrap (overnight) may expedite healing.

Stasis Dermatitis

Local treatment of stasis dermatitis varies with the state of inflammation. Apply only those topical medications considered essential as patients with stasis dermatitis are readily sensitized; 80% of patients with chronic stasis dermatitis are at risk of contact dermatitis. Ointment bases are the most common inciting agents.[69]

The reduction of edema is important and achieved through bed rest and elevation of the extremity. After edema subsides, compressive support in the form of an elastic bandage should be applied. After the dermatitis is healed, advise the life-long use of elastic compression stockings.[9]

Pharmacologic Therapy

For comparative ingredients of nonprescription products, consult the *Compendium of Products for Minor Ailments*—Cough, Cold and Allergy Products; Skin Care Products: Dermatitis and Dry Skin, First Aid.

For further information on the pharmacologic treatment of atopic dermatitis, consult *Compendium of Therapeutic Choices*: Atopic Dermatitis.

Bath Products

In most dermatitis conditions, dryness at some stage initiates or exacerbates the symptoms. The primary means of correcting dryness is to add water to the skin and then to apply a hydrophobic substance to keep it there. The benefits of hydration and moisturizers to help restore and maintain normal barrier function cannot be overemphasized. Since wet skin is more permeable to water, it is essential that the skin be covered within the first few minutes to prevent evaporation. Appropriate use of hydration together with occlusive bases or moisturizers will help re-establish and maintain the skin's barrier function. Bathing can have differing effects on the skin depending on the manner in which it is carried out. Bathing with water can hydrate the skin and remove scale, crust, irritants, and allergens, which can be helpful for patients with atopic dermatitis. However, if the water is left to evaporate from the skin, greater transepidermal water loss occurs.[70] Bathing is suggested for patients with atopic dermatitis as part of treatment and maintenance; however, there is no standard for the frequency or duration of bathing appropriate for atopic dermatitis. However, it is generally recommended that up to once-daily bathing be performed to remove serous crust; the duration should be limited to short periods of time (e.g., 5–10 minutes) with use of warm water. Moisturizers should be applied soon after bathing to improve skin hydration. Hydration of the face or neck can be achieved by applying a wet washcloth or towel to the involved area. Isolated areas such as hands and feet can be treated with soaks in basins. For the treatment of patients with atopic dermatitis, there is insufficient evidence for clear recommendations on the addition of oils, emollients and most other additives to bath water, or the use of acidic spring water.[71]

Despite lack of evidence it is generally thought that **bath oils** applied during or after bathing may help to reduce the rate of water loss through the epidermis; however, they are less effective than lotions and creams applied directly to wet skin since they are diluted with water and are in contact with the skin for a short time period, and most of the deposited oil is wiped off when towel drying. If added at the beginning of the bath, they may prevent rather than enhance hydration and thus should be added near the end of the bath to trap water in the skin. Bath oils give a false sense of lubrication and can make the bathtub slippery. Most bath oils combine mineral or vegetable oils with surfactants that disperse oil through the bath. Concentrations of surfactants (e.g., sodium lauryl sulfate) above 4% reduce the affinity of oil for the skin. Avoid products with fragrance and lanolin. Oil used as a single ingredient will float on top of the water. Bath oil capsules enclose small amounts of oil in soft, flexible gelatin capsules that dissolve in hot water but may necessitate a higher water temperature than desirable and often contain a higher percentage of fragrance. **Olive oil** is an inexpensive natural product that may be applied directly to rehydrated skin after bathing.

Avoid **bath salts**. They are highly fragranced and soften water by raising the alkalinity. This may cause itching or redness on sensitive skin. Avoid detergent bubble baths if skin is dry or itchy.

Colloidal oatmeal preparations contain starch and protein and are effective antipruritics. Addition of oatmeal products may be soothing but does not promote increased water absorption. For dry skin, they are not as effective as oils in trapping water to maintain hydration unless the oilated versions are used. Bathing in colloidal oatmeal baths is useful when large body areas are involved.[68]

Soaps are made from animal or vegetable fat and alkali and consist of surfactants that interact with stratum corneum proteins and lipids in a manner that causes damage, dry skin, and irritation. Most soaps are alkaline in pH, whereas the skin's normal pH is 4–5.5. Fatty acid plus sodium or potassium hydroxide produce a water-soluble soap. Toilet soaps are usually made from palmitic, stearic or oleic acids. Hard sodium soaps are suitable for bars, flakes and powders while more soluble potassium soaps are used for liquid preparations. Softer and more water-soluble, **transparent soaps** (or glycerin soaps) do not last long or lather well. They claim to be less drying or irritating than alkaline **opaque** soaps. However, objective clinical evaluations are lacking.

Soapless cleansers are surfactants and synthetic detergents often recommended for better tolerance, although this is based on only a few clinical studies. They lack lipid and are available in lotion and gel forms. Soapless lotions can be applied liberally and have a foaming action. Removed gently, they leave a thin film on the skin to aid in water retention. No good evidence demonstrates that addition of neutral fats or cold cream to the soapless cleanser counteracts the drying effect. It is improbable that a simple cleansing agent can achieve the 2 opposing tasks (cleansing of the skin and deposition of fat on the skin), especially since the soap is rinsed off. Limited use of soapless cleansers (that are neutral to low pH, hypoallergenic and fragrance free) is recommended.

Excessive washing may remove lipids and water that normally keep the stratum corneum soft and pliable. Choice of soap depends on the type of dermatitis. Avoid soap in acute atopic or contact dermatitis. For chronic dermatitis and for dry skin, a mild, nonalkaline soap, an aqueous cream or a soap-free cleanser can be used alternately (Table 8). Soap is applied only to intact skin, without rubbing or massaging. Sufficient water should be used to rinse away all traces of soap.

Moisturizers

Breakdown of the skin barrier, the first event in the development of atopic dermatitis, results in xerosis (dry skin), one of the cardinal clinical features. This provides a rationale for the use of a complete moisturizing therapy regimen to combat xerosis and transepidermal water loss (TEWL) in atopic dermatitis and related skin barrier breakdown conditions such as irritant contact dermatitis.[72] The main purpose of moisturizer therapy is to restore the epidermal barrier, which is composed of corneocytes, extracellular proteins, and a lipid-rich matrix (ceramides, fatty acids, and cholesterol). Barrier damage is directly correlated to the severity of dermatitis. Use of moisturizers leads to the integrity of the epidermal barrier and a consequent reduction of both TEWL and penetration of irritant substances.

Patients with atopic dermatitis require ongoing moisturizer therapy. Clinical trials have shown that they lessen symptoms and signs of atopic dermatitis, including pruritus, erythema, fissuring, and lichenification.[71] Moisturizers can themselves result in some reduction in inflammation and atopic dermatitis severity. There is strong evidence that their use can also reduce the need for pharmacologic intervention. Moisturizers are first-line therapy for mild disease and an important part of the treatment regimen for moderate and severe disease. They also play a key role in maintenance treatment and prevention of flares.[71]

Skin protection creams or "barrier" creams (usually silicone-based) may be used in the occupational setting to help prevent irritant contact dermatitis. The protective efficacy depends on the amount of product applied per unit skin surface area. The actual amounts applied and the resulting dose per unit area have been reported to be lower than recommended. Some products may show no protective efficacy when used at doses close to those practically applied at workplaces.[73] In 1 study, 2 of 6 protective creams failed to prevent solvent-induced cumulative skin irritation, which emphasizes the lack of comparative efficacy among barrier creams.[74] Antioxidant creams have been shown to effectively protect the skin from chemical-induced irritation.[75] Unfortunately low adherence to skin protective measures that combine creams and other approaches has been reported after 1 year.[76]

Moisturizers are generally classified by their mechanism of action as emollients, occlusives, or humectants. Newer agents containing ceramides may be classed as barrier repair agents.

Emollients

Emollients are semisolid bases designed to control dryness by slowing evaporation and lubricating the stratum corneum. They may contain glycol, glyceryl stearate, and soy sterols which lubricate and soften the skin. These products cannot keep skin soft and flexible without the required concentration of water in the skin and function only to trap existing moisture. Very little water from emollients is absorbed by the skin; most water in the emollients evaporates when the product is applied and therefore they should be applied while the skin is still damp from bathing. Emollients include lotions, creams and ointments. Most are oil-in-water or water-in-oil emulsions. The higher the oil content, the greater the occlusion and the less drying through evaporation. Ointments are therefore the most occlusive and have the fewest additives, though in a hot, humid environment their use may lead to trapping of sweat with subsequent irritation of the skin. Users may not tolerate oil or water-in-oil products because the greasy texture increases discomfort. Greasy applications are unsuitable for acute oozing dermatitis. In contrast, evaporating water from oil-in-water creams or more liquid oil-in-water lotions produces a cooling effect which alleviates pruritus. A smaller amount of oil content is left as a residual film to protect hydration. Lotions contain more water than creams and may be drying due to the effects of evaporation. Obtain products in the largest size available because they usually need to be applied several times a day on a long-term basis.

Scrutinize the emollient product for other ingredients, as some preservatives, stabilizers, emulsifiers and fragrances may aggravate atopic, allergic or stasis dermatitis (e.g., lanolin, parabens, cresols, sodium lauryl sulfate, cetylstearyl alcohols and fragrance). Choose an emollient for its drying or lubricating properties as suitable for the stage of dermatitis. For an acute, wet dermatitis that has been compressed, apply a lotion after oozing stops, to facilitate dryness. In less acute, drier dermatitis, an oil-in-water emulsion base is appropriate. In chronic, very dry or scaly dermatitis, a water-in-oil emulsion gives maximum lubrication. Hairy areas may require gels or lotions.

Occlusives

Occlusive agents (petrolatum, dimethicone, mineral oil) form a layer on the skin that retards evaporation of water. **Petrolatum** provides an occlusive effect but is cosmetically unacceptable as it feels greasy and does not wash off easily. It is sometimes used as a sealer after hydrating the skin; however, it is effective only when used in conjunction with hydration. Due to its highly occlusive properties, it can cause maceration and overgrowth of bacteria or yeast if used on acutely inflamed and oozing lesions. Petrolatum is discussed further as an alternative for diaper dermatitis (see Chapter 59: Diaper Dermatitis).

Humectants/Hydrating Agents

Humectants are ingredients with hygroscopic properties to attract and hold water in the skin. Emollients to which humectants have been added may be called **hydrating agents**. Examples include alpha-hydroxy acids, glycerin, phospholipids, propylene glycol and urea. Some ingredients such as urea also soften keratin. Because they draw water and hydrate the skin, they are more efficacious for dry skin than emollients, which merely trap water present on the skin. Regular use of hydrating agents decreases the need for topical corticosteroids.[77,78]

Alpha-hydroxy acids (e.g., lactic, citric, glycolic, malic, pyruvic and glucuronic acids) may increase biosynthesis of mucopolysaccharides, contributing to the natural control of keratinization. Concentrations of 2–5% applied twice daily are best for use on larger areas or on the whole body as these compounds may produce irritation at concentrations of 10% or higher.[79] Alpha-hydroxy acids affect keratinization at the lowest levels of the stratum corneum, where they affect corneocyte cohesion and new stratum corneum formation. In addition, they increase dermal mucopolysaccharides and collagen formation. Products such as lactic acid have been shown to increase skin surface lipids, extensibility and firmness of the skin, improving skin barrier function.[20]

Glycerin is a humectant that helps keep the product moist and facilitates spreading. In optimal concentrations of 50% or less, glycerin helps retard water evaporation, keeping it in close contact with the skin. There is no evidence that glycerin is absorbed through the skin.

Phospholipid products contain **lecithin**, which hydrolyzes to yield oleic, palmitic and stearic fatty acids. Lecithin is a water-binding agent that occurs naturally in the skin. Each phospholipid molecule forms a complex with 15 molecules of water. Water is drawn to and kept in the skin for hydration, keeping it soft and resilient. These preparations may also contain mineral oil, glycerin and lanolin.

Propylene glycol is a viscous, colourless, odourless, hygroscopic liquid used as a solvent and vehicle for water-insoluble or unstable compounds. The pH may vary from 4–8 with these products and an acid pH may result in an irritant reaction. A small percentage of patients may be hypersensitive to propylene glycol.

Urea works mainly by drawing water into the stratum corneum, though there are claims of keratolytic, antifungal, antipruritic, anesthetic and anti-infective properties. It is used mainly in atopic dermatitis for xerosis, as application on open, excoriated areas results in burning and discomfort. It can improve skin barrier function and reduce skin susceptibility to irritants. The concentration of urea determines its effect. Concentrations of 10% hydrate dry skin and 15% accelerate fibrin digestion. Concentrations of 20–30% are antipruritic, break down keratin, decrease the thickness of the stratum corneum and are used in scaling conditions such as ichthyosis. Concentrations of 40% are proteolytic and may be used to dissolve and peel dystrophic nails. Urea is sometimes combined with other active ingredients, such as corticosteroids, anthralin and benzoyl peroxide, to accelerate skin penetration. Combinations with hydrocortisone are useful for the dry itching skin of atopic dermatitis.[80]

Barrier Repair Products

Recognition of the role of disrupted ceramide content in barrier dysfunction led to the development of barrier repair therapies that aim to restore appropriate ceramide balance. In one study, a ceramide-dominant product was as effective as a mid-potency topical corticosteroid after 28 days.[81] The use of barrier repair products containing key stratum corneum lipids, including ceramides may make it possible to reduce the use of topical corticosteroids and immunosuppressive agents such as tacrolimus and pimecrolimus.

Tar Preparations

Topical **coal tar** derivatives have been used for many years in the treatment of inflammatory skin diseases. Coal tar activates the aryl hydrocarbon receptor signaling pathway, resulting in enhanced epidermal differentiation, increased levels of filaggrin, and inhibition of a major atopic dermatitis cytokine pathway.[82] Prior to the widespread use of corticosteroids, crude coal tar extracts were used to reduce inflammation in atopic dermatitis. Despite limited evidence of efficacy, tar preparations[71] may be used to reduce the need for corticosteroids in chronic maintenance therapy of atopic dermatitis. Their effect is not felt to be as potent as corticosteroids but they are long lasting with few side effects. Coal tar is primarily used in scalp preparations, compounded in cream bases that are generally used at night to increase adherence. Patients should cover the head with a shower cap to limit staining, and rinse out in the morning. Coal tar products should not be used on inflamed skin due to irritating effects. Cosmetically, they are less acceptable due to staining and unpleasant smell.[20]

Topical Corticosteroids

Topical corticosteroids are the mainstay of treatment for atopic dermatitis and first-line treatment for patients with allergic contact dermatitis. They reduce inflammation and pruritus and are useful for both the acute and chronic phases of atopic and contact dermatitis. Their mechanism is complex, affecting multiple resident and infiltrating cells primarily by suppressing inflammatory genes.

A large number of topical corticosteroids are available, ranging in potency from low to extremely high. A variety of factors should be considered when choosing a particular topical corticosteroid, including patient age, areas of the body to which the medication will be applied, and other patient factors such as degree of xerosis, patient preference, and cost of medication. Low-potency choices are recommended for areas of thinner skin (particularly the face and eyelids) and high-potency products are indicated for thickened and lichenified lesions in other locations. Choice of **vehicle** for the corticosteroid is also important. Vehicles include lotions, solutions, gels, sprays, foams, and oils. In general, ointments are considered more potent and more occlusive and contain less preservatives than creams and lotions. Creams are better tolerated in excessive heat or humidity; lotions are less effective and contribute to xerosis. Solutions are used on the scalp or hairy areas, but the alcohol content may irritate inflamed or excoriated lesions.

As a general rule, the lowest potency corticosteroid that is effective should be used. Therapy should not exceed a 2-week course. Lack of response to low-potency agents such as **hydrocortisone** may indicate the need for stronger corticosteroids except on the face and in skin folds, where low-potency agents like hydrocortisone remain the drugs of choice.[83,84] Using a topical corticosteroid too low in potency may sometimes result in persistence or worsening of atopic dermatitis. In such cases, after a 2-week trial, institute a stepped-care approach, beginning with a mid-to-high potency corticosteroid until control is achieved, and then reducing to a lower-potency agent. Discontinuing a mid- to high-potency corticosteroid without tapering to a lower-potency corticosteroid may result in rebound flaring of atopic dermatitis. Some patients may not respond to corticosteroid therapy due to superinfection.[20] When topical corticosteroids are used, any coexisting infection should be treated promptly.

If there are areas of significantly inflamed skin, soaking the affected area in plain water for 20 minutes followed by the immediate application of topical corticosteroids, without toweling dry, is a helpful treatment measure. This "soak and smear" technique can improve response in cases where the topical corticosteroid alone is inadequate.[71,85] Severe or complicated dermatitis may require treatment with stronger corticosteroids. Resistant cases may sometimes respond to the addition of occlusion to the application of the corticosteroid, but this approach should be used with caution and is generally reserved for dermatitis of the hands or feet.

Patients with atopic dermatitis should be advised to continue with moisturizer therapy during treatment with topical corticosteroids. Topical corticosteroids should be used once daily although if insufficient for control, twice daily can be used. Twice weekly maintenance therapy is recommended in patients with moderate to severe atopic dermatitis experiencing frequent relapses and is more effective than use of moisturizers alone for prevention of flares.[71] There is insufficient evidence to know whether it is more beneficial to apply moisturizers before or after topical corticosteroids. A small, randomized study showed no difference over 2 weeks between patients who applied moisturizer before topical corticosteroids and those who did the reverse.[86] Many sources suggest moisturizer be applied 30 minutes before topical corticosteroid but this is based on low-level evidence or consensus recommendations and is not universally accepted. Practicality and patient adherence are key factors to consider when deciding on order of application.[87]

Physical examination for cutaneous side effects is recommended during long-term, potent corticosteroid therapy. Consider the potential for both topical and systemic side effects, including possible hypothalamic-pituitary-adrenal axis suppression, particularly in children. Patient fears of side effects associated with the use of topical corticosteroids for atopic dermatitis should be recognized and addressed to improve adherence and avoid undertreatment. Despite widespread use, with correct education, adverse effects are infrequent with appropriately used mid- to high-potency corticosteroids. Over time, antiproliferative effects (e.g., skin thinning), poor wound healing, hypopigmentation, secondary infections and acne may occur, particularly on the face and in the intertriginous areas. Perioral dermatitis may occur on the face, characterized by erythema, scaling and follicular papules and pustules around the mouth or eye creases. Discontinue the corticosteroid if this occurs, and taper using hydrocortisone. **Hydrocortisone** is always the drug of choice in these sites. Use of "steroid sparers" such as emollients, occlusives and hydrators help to reduce total corticosteroid exposure, thereby reducing the risk of adverse effects.

It is possible to develop an allergic sensitivity to corticosteroid preparations themselves which appears paradoxical due to the anti-inflammatory effects of the corticosteroids. However, delayed-type reaction to corticosteroids do occur.[88] Reported incidence rates in positive patch test results ranged from 0.5%–3% for various topical corticosteroids in one study.[89] Nonresponding eczema, development of subacute contact dermatitis, systemically reactivated allergic contact dermatitis or maculopapular exanthems can be a clinical symptom of a delayed-type hypersensitivity reaction to corticosteroids. The anti-inflammatory nature of corticosteroids makes the diagnosis of allergy more difficult, but it should be considered in patients suffering from intractable dermatitis. Immediate-type hypersensitivity reactions to corticosteroids remain uncommon.

Systemic Corticosteroids

Systemic agents are reserved for severe, acute cases, such as extensive poison ivy/oak; when treating poison ivy/oak, a prolonged course of oral therapy with a slow taper is often required. In general, prolonged use of oral agents for other causes is to be avoided due to adverse effects including diabetes, hypertension, growth retardation, lymphopenia, bone loss, glaucoma/cataracts, and development of Cushing syndrome.[90]

Topical Calcineurin Inhibitors

Topical calcineurin inhibitors (TCIs) such as **tacrolimus** and **pimecrolimus** are analogues of cyclosporine and have anti-inflammatory effects. They are highly effective in improving dermatitis and pruritus. Tacrolimus was effective in the treatment of corticosteroid-resistant allergic contact dermatitis in one study[91] and as effective as a moderate-potency corticosteroid in another.[92] Tacrolimus and pimecrolimus have both been shown to be effective for treatment of atopic dermatitis in children and adults.[71,93] There is some evidence that tacrolimus may have a greater effect than pimecrolimus over time.[93,94,95,96] Topical calcineurin inhibitors may not be as effective as moderate- to high-potency topical corticosteroids in the treatment of atopic dermatitis.[93] Use of TCI therapy 2–3 times weekly between atopic dermatitis flares is recommended on flare-prone areas to help prevent relapses and decrease the amount of topical corticosteroid needed.[71]

The most common adverse effect reported for TCIs is burning and stinging at the application site, particularly if the skin is acutely inflamed. Treatment with topical corticosteroids to reduce inflammation prior to instituting TCI therapy may help minimize these reactions.[71] Concerns about increased risk of infections due to immunosuppression may warrant avoiding use on actively infected skin. There is insufficient evidence to support concerns about any link between use of TCIs and risk of malignancy. Routine bloodwork is not recommended.[56,71]

TCIs are usually considered second-line therapy when topical corticosteroid therapy is ineffective or not tolerated. The major advantage of TCIs is their safety profile and tolerability. They are recommended as steroid-sparing options for long-term topical treatment. They may be safely used in sensitive or thin-skinned areas such as the face, anogenital region and skin folds. [71]

Topical Anti-Infectives

Atopic individuals are predisposed to skin infections because of a compromised physical barrier. *S. aureus* is found in more than 90% of atopic dermatitis. A systematic review examined 26 randomized controlled trials that used a variety of antistaphylococcal treatments in the management of atopic dermatitis, including oral antibiotics, antibacterial soaps, topical antibiotics or antiseptics, special textiles and combinations of topical corticosteroids with antibacterials. While reduction of *S. aureus* counts on the skin was reported with some interventions, no trials showed improvement in eczema control. The poor quality of many of the studies and low patient numbers make this evidence difficult to interpret.[97] Topical antimicrobial preparations are not generally recommended in the treatment of atopic dermatitis. They can be associated with contact dermatitis, and there is concern that their use could promote wider antimicrobial drug resistance. Oral antibiotics are not indicated for routine treatment in noninfected atopic dermatitis.[71]

Bleach baths may be helpful in cases of moderate to severe disease with frequent bacterial infections, particularly for maintenance because the majority of patients do not show clearance of the bacteria. Development of bacterial resistance is less of a concern with use of dilute bleach compared with the use of topical and systemic antibiotics. Topical hypochlorite products are also available but are more expensive and have not been studied specifically.[71]

Treatment with antifungal agents is sometimes used to address dermatophyte pathogens such as *Malassezia* in atopic dermatitis, but the response to these is less effective than treatment with topical corticosteroids.[20]

Antihistamines

Pruritus is the hallmark of atopic dermatitis and a frequent symptom of contact dermatitis. The itch-scratch cycle complicates atopic dermatitis and should be aborted. Oral antihistamines act by blocking H_1-receptors, thereby reducing pruritus caused by histamine. However, pruritus associated with atopic dermatitis is thought to be caused by mediators other than histamine, which is not the key factor.[98]

Certain subgroups of patients may benefit from antihistamines for other reasons. The first subgroup are those with sleep disturbances. The benefit of antihistamines comes from their side effects. **First-generation antihistamines** cause drowsiness which may help patients with atopic or contact dermatitis (adults and children) by promoting sleep or affecting sleep disturbances in the presence of pruritus. In these situations, first-generation antihistamines should be used before going to sleep.[98] For a second subgroup with comorbid conditions of the atopic diathesis, including allergic rhinitis, chronic urticaria, dermographism or allergen-induced asthma, **second-generation antihistamines** such as **loratadine** and **desloratadine** can be tried. **Fexofenadine** has demonstrated a small but significant reduction in pruritus in atopic dermatitis, and may be the first option for patients who do not fall into the previous 2 subgroups.[99] See Chapter 22: Allergic Rhinitis for more information regarding oral antihistamines.

Topical antihistamines are strong contact sensitizers. In addition, due to the ionization that occurs topically, they are not efficacious when applied to normal skin unless to mucous membranes. They have demonstrated little utility and for these reasons, and due to the increased efficacy of other agents, they should be avoided.

An approach to the treatment of atopic dermatitis is shown in Figure 2. An approach to the treatment of contact dermatitis is shown in Figure 3.

Natural Health Products

Natural remedies may not be harmless and should not be recommended over traditional, standardized and proven therapies. At this time, there are little data to support the majority of complementary therapies tried for atopic dermatitis management. Chinese herbal therapy (or traditional Chinese medicine) has been the most extensively studied. Anti-eczematous efficacy of traditional Chinese herbal medicines was found in one study.[100] While it may have some benefit for lesions, the results from randomized controlled trials of oral therapy are conflicting, and reports of serious hepatotoxicity raise potential safety concerns. Some preparations have been reported to cause fatal toxic reactions, and adulteration with other substances such as corticosteroids has also been reported.[101,102] The individualized and dynamic nature of this intervention (a different herb is added or subtracted depending on the patient) also poses challenges to performing controlled studies. Acupuncture alone or in conjunction with traditional Chinese medicine decreases signs and symptoms of atopic dermatitis, but the evidence is confined to small studies of limited quality.[103,104]

The disturbed epidermal barrier function of atopic dermatitis has been linked to altered metabolism of unsaturated fatty acids. This is the theoretical rationale for treatment with **essential fatty acids** such as **gamma-linolenic acid** (evening primrose oil). Use is characterized by a low incidence of side effects but also low efficacy in adults, with results in children no better than placebo. Two potential problems associated with use of evening primrose oil are its high cost and the lack of product standardization; adulterated brands may simply contain corn oil. Its use is clinically unsubstantiated and should not be recommended.[7] A Cochrane review found no improvement in symptoms of atopic eczema or quality of life with use of **borage oil** or **evening primrose oil** compared with placebo.[105]

Massage therapy may improve symptoms of atopic dermatitis and associated patient and parental anxiety levels. While it is a safe intervention, studies to date are small and of limited quality, precluding recommendation at this time.[106,107] Other complementary therapies lacking sufficient evidence include: aromatherapy, homeopathy, naturopathy,[108] acupressure[109] and autologous blood injections.[110]

In the case of allergic contact dermatitis due to nickel sensitivity, some effects of nickel may be eliminated or reduced by supplementing with divalent essential metals as there is some evidence that nickel dermatitis improved following oral administration of zinc sulfate.[111,112]

Monitoring of Therapy

Table 7 provides a monitoring framework for patients with dermatitis, which should be individualized. Parameters should be monitored by the patient or the caregiver, and a diary can be used. Therapy should be appropriately tapered in response to improvement or resolution. The healthcare practitioner should be responsible for ensuring that the treatment plan remains on schedule and is effective, and no adverse effects are occurring. Changes in symptoms due to treatment can be correlated with alterations in trigger factors such as irritants and foods. Stress, anxiety or depression levels should be tracked if they are suspected aggravating factors, and may lessen as skin symptoms improve.

Table 7: Monitoring of Therapy for Atopic, Contact or Stasis Dermatitis

Type of Dermatitis	Parameter	Timeframe/Degree of Change	Actions[a]
Acute	Inflammation (redness, swelling, pain, warmth)	Decrease by 50% within 7–10 days	Taper therapy in response to resolution: if endpoints not achieved, consider additional or different therapy.
	Surface area involved	No progression	
	Extension to other sites or generalization	None	
	Blister formation	No new blisters after 1–2 days	
	Itch/scratching	Control to tolerable level within 7–10 days	
	Disruption of sleep or daily activities	Restoration of normal patterns within 2–3 wk	
	Stress, anxiety, depression	Re-establish normal pattern within 2–3 wk	
Chronic	Changes in inflammation, scaling, dryness, itch, scratching	Control by 4–8 wk	If endpoints not achieved, consider additional or different therapy.
	Progression of severity	No progression of severity	
	Recurrent episodes	Lengthening of symptom-free periods throughout therapy	
	Lichenification	No further lichenification throughout therapy	
Acute and chronic	Allergic reactions	None	If allergic reaction occurs, discontinue therapy.
	Severe dryness, irritation (e.g., redness, inflammation, stinging)	Minimal Should disappear, diminish or be controlled with continued use	If severe, decrease dose, concentration or frequency of use. If still no improvement, consider different therapy.

[a] Patients should monitor all parameters daily while on drug therapy. Healthcare practitioners should monitor all parameters after 7–10 days for acute dermatitis and after 2–3 weeks for chronic dermatitis.

Figure 1: **Assessment of Patients with Dermatitis**

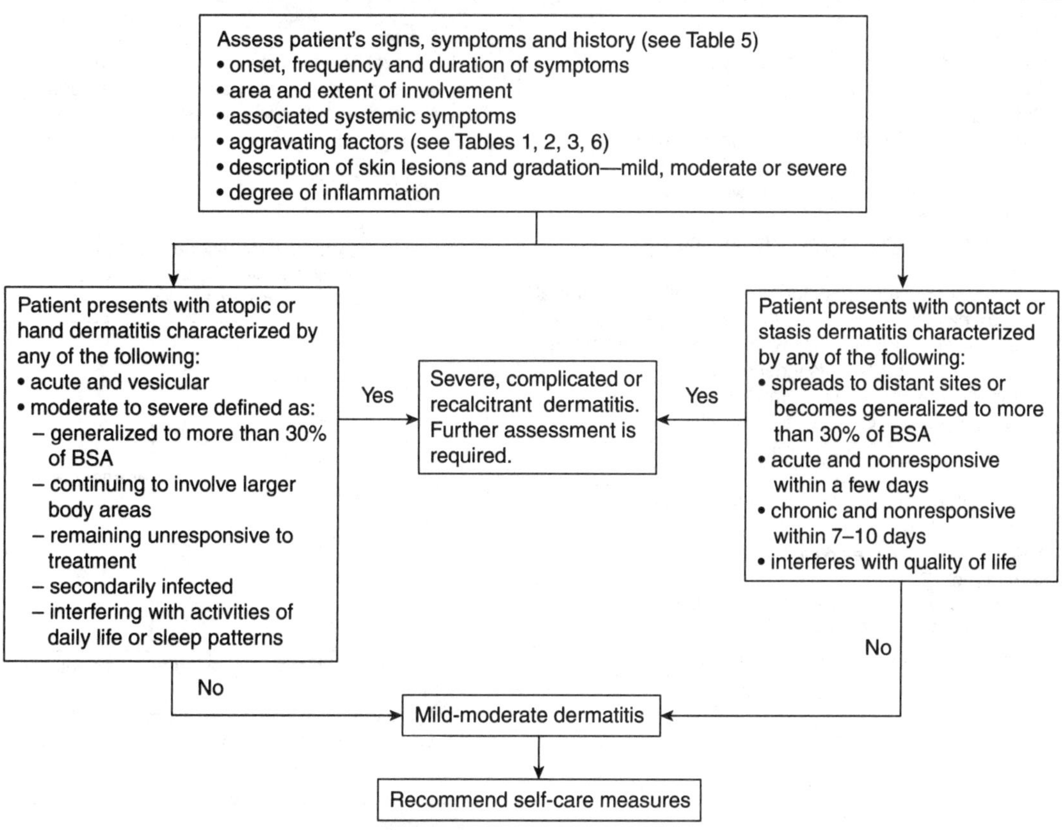
Assess patient's signs, symptoms and history (see Table 5)
• onset, frequency and duration of symptoms
• area and extent of involvement
• associated systemic symptoms
• aggravating factors (see Tables 1, 2, 3, 6)
• description of skin lesions and gradation—mild, moderate or severe
• degree of inflammation
Patient presents with atopic or hand dermatitis characterized by any of the following:
• acute and vesicular
• moderate to severe defined as:
– generalized to more than 30% of BSA
– continuing to involve larger body areas
– remaining unresponsive to treatment
– secondarily infected
– interfering with activities of daily life or sleep patterns
Yes
Severe, complicated or recalcitrant dermatitis. Further assessment is required.
Yes
Patient presents with contact or stasis dermatitis characterized by any of the following:
• spreads to distant sites or becomes generalized to more than 30% of BSA
• acute and nonresponsive within a few days
• chronic and nonresponsive within 7–10 days
• interferes with quality of life
No
No
Mild-moderate dermatitis
Recommend self-care measures

Abbreviations: BSA = body surface area

Figure 2: **Treatment of Atopic Dermatitis**

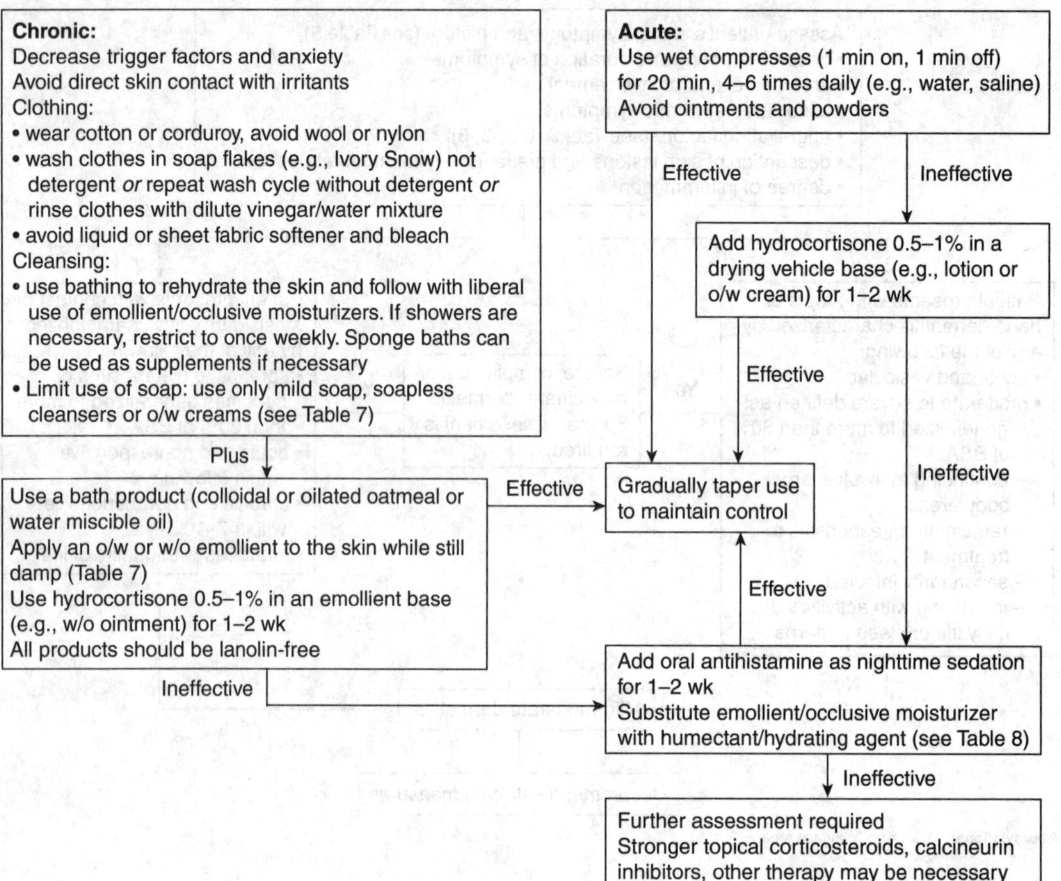
Chronic:
Decrease trigger factors and anxiety
Avoid direct skin contact with irritants
Clothing:
• wear cotton or corduroy, avoid wool or nylon
• wash clothes in soap flakes (e.g., Ivory Snow) not detergent or repeat wash cycle without detergent or rinse clothes with dilute vinegar/water mixture
• avoid liquid or sheet fabric softener and bleach
Cleansing:
• use bathing to rehydrate the skin and follow with liberal use of emollient/occlusive moisturizers. If showers are necessary, restrict to once weekly. Sponge baths can be used as supplements if necessary
• Limit use of soap: use only mild soap, soapless cleansers or o/w creams (see Table 7)
Plus
Use a bath product (colloidal or oilated oatmeal or water miscible oil)
Apply an o/w or w/o emollient to the skin while still damp (Table 7)
Use hydrocortisone 0.5–1% in an emollient base (e.g., w/o ointment) for 1–2 wk
All products should be lanolin-free
Effective
Ineffective
Acute:
Use wet compresses (1 min on, 1 min off) for 20 min, 4–6 times daily (e.g., water, saline)
Avoid ointments and powders
Effective
Ineffective
Add hydrocortisone 0.5–1% in a drying vehicle base (e.g., lotion or o/w cream) for 1–2 wk
Effective
Ineffective
Gradually taper use to maintain control
Effective
Add oral antihistamine as nighttime sedation for 1–2 wk
Substitute emollient/occlusive moisturizer with humectant/hydrating agent (see Table 8)
Ineffective
Further assessment required
Stronger topical corticosteroids, calcineurin inhibitors, other therapy may be necessary

Figure 3: **Treatment of Contact Dermatitis**

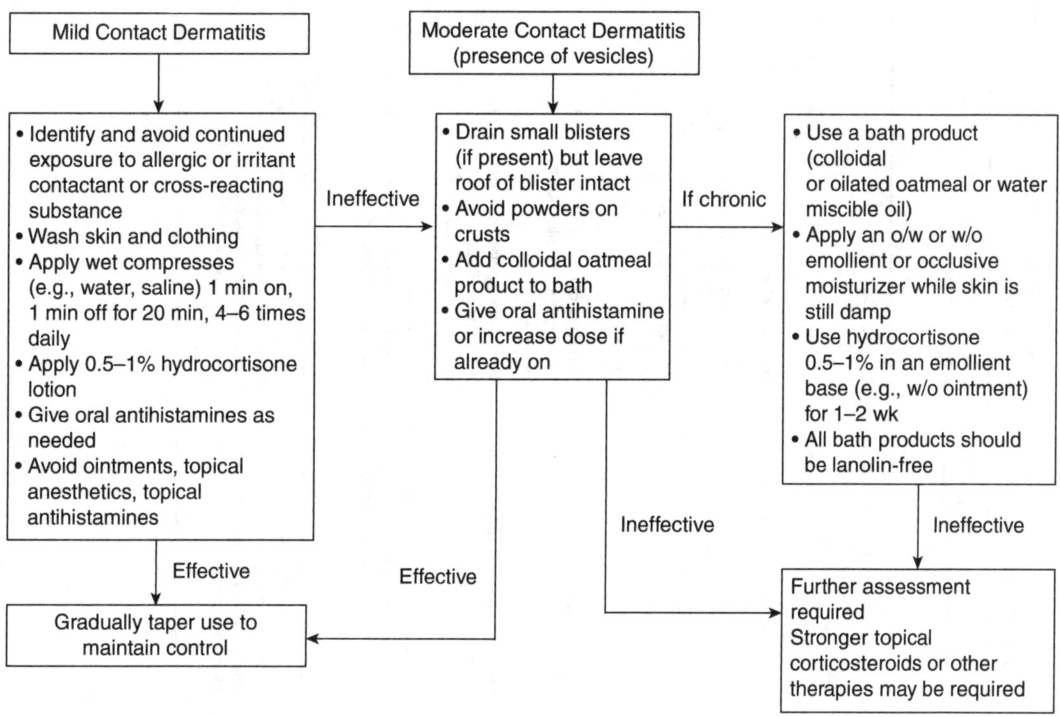

Table 8: Selected Self-care Topical Products for Dermatitis[a]

Class	Drug	Dosage	Adverse Effects	Comments	Cost[b]
Barrier repair products	*ceramides/cholesterol/free fatty acids* EpiCeram Skin Barrier Emulsion, others	Apply thin layer to affected area BID or prn	After application, a temporary tingling sensation may occur (lasting 10–15 min).	Do not apply within 4 h prior to radiation therapy.	$$
Bath Products	*bath oils* Keri Oil, others	After bath apply 5 mL of oil in 50 mL water with a cotton swab while the skin is still damp	Allergic sensitization may occur due to lanolin, fragrance and other contact sensitizers. May make the bathtub slippery.	Acts as a barrier to reduce water loss.	$
	colloidal oatmeal Aveeno Bath Preparations, generics	As per product instructions; must be properly dispersed in water to be effective	Can clump and clog drain.	Provides relief for itching skin. May contain oils and can act as an emollient.	$
Cleansers	*opaque soaps* Lowila, others	Rinse well after washing In atopic patients, restrict to axillae and groin	Drying.	May contain moisturizers. Use fragrance-free soap if possible.	$
	soapless cleansers Spectro Jel, others	Apply and rinse	Minor irritation seen rarely.	Thin layer of product is left on skin allowing for retention of water.	$
	transparent soaps Pears, Neutrogena, others	Rinse well after washing In atopic patients, restrict to axillae and groin	May be less drying than opaque soaps.	More water soluble but not as effective as other cleansers. Use fragrance-free soap if possible.	$
Corticosteroids, topical	*hydrocortisone 0.5%, 1% cream, lotion, ointment* Cortate, Emo-Cort, Prevex HC, generics	Apply thin layer sparingly BID–TID PRN Reassess after 2 wk	Mild to severe skin irritation. Rarely, hypersensitivity reactions.	Temporary relief of redness, pain, swelling and itch.	$
Emollients[c]	*emollients Examples: glycol, glyceryl stearate, soy sterols* Glaxal Base, Keri Lotion, Lubriderm, Neutrogena Cream	Apply PRN several times daily, preferably while skin is damp	Allergic sensitization may occur if contains lanolin, selected preservatives, fragrance and other contact sensitizers.	Retards evaporation of water. As oil content increases becomes more occlusive. Use fragrance-free products if possible.	$

Class	Drug	Dosage	Adverse Effects	Comments	Cost[b]
Humectants/ Hydrating agents[c]	*humectants Examples: alpha-hydroxy acids (glycolic acid, lactic acid), glycerin, phospholipids (lecithin), propylene glycol, urea* Dermal Therapy, Lac-Hydrin, Neostrata, Uremol	Apply PRN several times daily, preferably while skin is damp	See emollients.	Humectants are usually incorporated into an emollient base to form hydrating agents. The emollient base prevents water evaporation and the humectants attract water into skin.	$
Occlusives[c]	*occlusives Examples: petrolatum, dimethicone, mineral oil* Barriere, Complex 15, Moisturel, Prevex, Vaseline	Apply PRN several times daily	Well tolerated, usually less stinging than with emollient creams or lotions or humectant-containing hydrating agents	Used to protect against irritants such as chemicals, detergents, polishes and water. Also useful for prevention and treatment of occupational hand eczema.	$

[a] For more information on the use of topical corticosteroids consult the *Compendium of Therapeutic Choices*: Atopic Dermatitis.

[b] Cost of smallest available pack size; includes drug cost only.

[c] Most moisturizers contain combinations of emollients, humectants and occlusives.

Legend: $ <$10 $$ $10–20

Suggested Readings

Cury Martins J, Martins C, Aoki V et al. Topical tacrolimus for atopic dermatitis. *Cochrane Database Syst Rev* 2015;7:CD009864.

Eichenfield LF, Tom WL, Chamlin SL et al. Guidelines of care for the management of atopic dermatitis: section 1. Diagnosis and assessment of atopic dermatitis. *J Am Acad Dermatol* 2014;70:338-51.

Eichenfield LF, Tom WL, Berger TG et al. Guidelines of care for the management of atopic dermatitis: section 2. Management and treatment of atopic dermatitis with topical therapies. *J Am Acad Dermatol* 2014;71:116-32.

Lynde C, Guenther L, Diepgen TL et al. Canadian hand dermatitis management guidelines. *J Cutan Med Surg* 2010;14:267-84.

Saji D, Asiniwasis R, Skotnicki-Grant S. A look at epidermal barrier function in atopic dermatitis: physiologic lipid replacement and the role of ceramides. *Skin Therapy Lett* 2012;17:6-9.

Scottish Intercollegiate Guidelines Network. *Management of atopic eczema in primary care: a national clinical guideline*. Edinburgh: SIGN; 2011. Available from: www.sign.ac.uk/pdf/sign125.pdf.

Sidbury R, Davis DM, Cohen DE et al. Guidelines of care for the management of atopic dermatitis: section 3. Management and treatment with phototherapy and systemic agents. *J Am Acad Dermatol* 2014;71:327-49.

Sidbury R, Tom WL, Bergman JN et al. Guidelines of care for the management of atopic dermatitis: section 4. Prevention of disease flares and use of adjunctive therapies and approaches. *J Am Acad Dermatol* 2014;71:1218-33.

References

1. Sams WM, Lynch PJ, eds. *Principles and practice of dermatology.* 2nd ed. New York: Churchill Livingstone; 1996. p. 419-26.
2. Proksch E, Folster-Holsts R, Jensen JM. Epidermal barrier in atopic dermatitis. In: Bieber T, Leung DY, eds. *Atopic dermatitis*. 2nd ed. New York: Informa Healthcare; 2009. p. 69-86.
3. Cork MJ, Danby S, Vasilopoulos Y et al. Epidermal barrier dysfunction in atopic dermatitis. In: Reitamo S, Luger TA, Steinhoff M, eds. *Textbook of atopic dermatitis*. London: Informa Healthcare; 2008. p. 35-57.
4. Flohr C, Williams HC. Epidermiology. In: Bieber T, Leung DY, eds. *Atopic dermatitis*. 2nd ed. New York: Informa Healthcare; 2009. p. 11-35.
5. Flohr C, Johansson SG, Wahlgren CF et al. How atopic is atopic dermatitis? *J Allergy Clin Immunol* 2004;114:150-8.
6. Bieber T. Atopic dermatitis: one or several diseases? In: Bieber T, Leung DY, eds. *Atopic dermatitis*. 2nd ed. New York: Informa Healthcare; 2009. p. 1-9.
7. Ruzicka T. Atopic eczema between rationality and irrationality. *Arch Dermatol* 1998;134:1462-9.
8. Katsarou, A, Armenaka, M. Atopic dermatitis in older patients: particular points. *J Eur Acad Dermatol Venereol* 2011;25:12-8.
9. Sternbach G, Callen JP. Dermatitis. *Emerg Med Clin North Am* 1985;3:677-92.
10. Zug KA, McKay M. Eczematous dermatitis: a practical review. *Am Fam Physician* 1996;54:1243-50, 1253-4.
11. Belsito DV. The diagnostic evaluation, treatment, and prevention of allergic contact dermatitis in the new millennium. *J Allergy Clin Immunol* 2000;105:409-20.
12. Rietschel RL, Fowler JF. *Fisher's contact dermatitis*. 6th ed. Hamilton: BC Decker; 2008. p. 1:1-10.
13. Prakash AV, Davis MD. Contact dermatitis in older adults: a review of the literature. *Am J Clin Dermatol* 2010;11:373-81.
14. Rietschel RL, Fowler JF. *Fisher's contact dermatitis*. 6th ed. Hamilton: BC Decker; 2008. p. 4:38-65.
15. Landow K. Hand dermatitis. The perennial scourge. *Postgrad Med* 1998;103:141-2, 145-8, 151-2.
16. Charlesworth EN. Allergic skin disease: atopic dermatitis as a prototype. *Prim Care* 1998;25:775-90.
17. Stander S, Luger TA. Pathophysiology of pruritus. In: Bieber T, Leung DY, eds. *Atopic dermatitis*. 2nd ed. New York: Informa Healthcare; 2009. p. 229-57.
18. Remitz A, Reitamo S. The clinical manifestations of atopic dermatitis. In: Reitamo S, Luger TA, Steinhoff M, eds. *Textbook of atopic dermatitis*. London: Informa Healthcare; 2008. p. 1-12.
19. Eichenfield LF, Tom WL, Chamlin SL et al. Guidelines of care for the management of atopic dermatitis: section 1. Diagnosis and assessment of atopic dermatitis. *J Am Acad Dermatol* 2014;70:338-51.
20. Boguniewicz M, Nicol N. General management of patients with atopic dermatitis. In: Reitamo S, Luger TA, Steinhoff M, eds. *Textbook of atopic dermatitis*. London: Informa Healthcare; 2008. p. 147-64.
21. Heuth G, Schneider G. Psychosomatic aspects of atopic dermatitis. In: Reitamo S, Luger TA, Steinhoff M, eds. *Textbook of atopic dermatitis*. London: Informa Healthcare; 2008. p. 131-7.
22. Wang J, Sampson HA. Food allergens and atopic dermatitis. In: Bieber T, Leung DY, eds. *Atopic dermatitis*. 2nd ed. New York: Informa Healthcare; 2009. p. 271-85.
23. Heine RG, Hill DJ, Hosking CS. Role of food allergens in atopic dermatitis. In: Reitamo S, Luger TA, Steinhoff M, eds. *Textbook of atopic dermatitis*. London: Informa Healthcare; 2008. p. 85-100.
24. Sampson HA, Scanlon SM. Natural history of food hypersensitivity in children with atopic dermatitis. *J Pediatr* 1989;115:23-7.

25. Ellman LK, Chatchatee P, Sicherer SH et al. Food hypersensitivity in two groups of children and young adults with atopic dermatitis evaluated a decade apart. *Pediatr Allergy Immunol* 2002;13:295-8.
26. Bock SA, Atkins FM. The natural history of peanut allergy. *J Allergy Clin Immunol* 1989;83:900-4.
27. Feser A, Mahler V. Periorbital dermatitis: causes, differential diagnoses and therapy. *J Dtsch Dermatol Ges* 2010;8:159-66.
28. Pariser RJ. Allergic and reactive dermatoses. How to identify and treat them. *Postgrad Med* 1991;89:75-80, 85.
29. Antonov D, Kleesz P, Elsner P et al. Impact of glove occlusion on cumulative skin irritation with or without hand cleanser-comparison in an experimental repeated irritation model. *Contact Dermatitis* 2013;68:293-9.
30. Becker D. Allergic contact dermatitis. *J Dtsch Dermatol Ges* 2013;11:607-19
31. Klaus MV, Wieselthier JS. Contact dermatitis. *Am Fam Physician* 1993;48:629-32.
32. Rietschel RL, Fowler JF. *Fisher's contact dermatitis*. 6th ed. Hamilton: BC Decker; 2008. p. 21:405-53.
33. Rietschel RL, Fowler JF. *Fisher's contact dermatitis*. 6th ed. Hamilton: BC Decker; 2008. p. 29:581-603.
34. Rietschel RL, Fowler JF. *Fisher's contact dermatitis*. 6th ed. Hamilton: BC Decker; 2008. p. 32:641-99.
35. Tammaro A, Narcisi A, Persechino S et al. Topical and systemic therapies for nickel allergy. *Dermatitis* 2011;22:251-5.
36. Situm M, Lugovic-Mihic L, Bulat V et al. Dermatological aspects of contact dermatitis from eyeglass frames and optical materials. *Coll Antropol* 2013;37:19-24.
37. Gorgievska Sukarovska B, Turcic P, Marasovic D et al. Allergic contact dermatitis to antibacterial agents. *Acta Dermatovenerol Croat* 2009;17:70-6.
38. Bates B. Contact dermatitis treatment may reveal bacitracin sensitivity: contact allergen of the year. *Skin Allergy News* 2004 Feb.
39. Shakouri AA, Bahna SL. Hypersensitivity to antihistamines. *Allergy Asthma Proc* 2013;34:488-96.
40. Yu SH, Sood A, Taylor JS. Patch testing for methylisothiazolinone and methylchlorothiazolinine-methylsiothiazolinone contact allergy. *JAMA Dermatol* 2016;152:67-72.
41. Cross C. Ubiquitous preservative blamed for rash of skin allergies. *CMAJ* 2013;185:E712.
42. Cressey BD, Kumar N, Scheinman PL. Contact allergy to sorbitans: a follow-up study. *Dermatitis* 2012;23:158-61.
43. Kaimal S, Thappa DM. Diet in dermatology: revisited. *Indian J Dermatol Venereol Leprol* 2010;76:103-15.
44. Robinson MK. Population differences in skin structure and physiology and the susceptibility to irritant and allergic contact dermatitis: implications for skin safety testing and risk assessment. *Contact Dermatitis* 1999;41:65-79.
45. Rietschel RL, Fowler JF. *Fisher's contact dermatitis*. 6th ed. Hamilton: BC Decker; 2008. p. 5:66-87.
46. Schliemann S, Schmidt C, Elsner P. Tandem repeated application of organic solvents and sodium lauryl sulphate enhances cumulative skin irritation. *Skin Pharmacol Physiol* 2014;27:158-63.
47. Rietschel RL, Fowler JF. *Fisher's contact dermatitis*. 6th ed. Hamilton: BC Decker; 2008. p. 9:125-74.
48. Rietschel RL, Fowler JF. *Fisher's contact dermatitis*. 6th ed. Hamilton: BC Decker; 2008. p. 24:484-519.
49. Rietschel RL, Fowler JF. *Fisher's contact dermatitis*. 6th ed. Hamilton: BC Decker; 2008. p. 22:454-83.
50. Rietschel RL, Fowler JF. *Fisher's contact dermatitis*. 6th ed. Hamilton: BC Decker; 2008. p. 10:175-89.
51. Rietschel RL, Fowler JF. *Fisher's contact dermatitis*. 6th ed. Hamilton: BC Decker; 2008. p. 28:566-80.
52. Bruinsma W. *A guide to drug eruptions*. 5th ed. Oosthuizen: File of Medicines; 1990. p. 6,30-1.
53. Joly P, Benoit-Corven C, Baricault S et al. Chronic eczematous eruptions of the elderly are associated with chronic exposure to calcium channel blockers: results from a case-control study. *J Invest Dermatol* 2007;127:2766-71.
54. Summers EM, Bingham CS, Dahle KW et al. Chronic eczematous eruptions in the aging: further support for an association with exposure to calcium channel blockers. *JAMA Dermatol* 2013;149:814-8.
55. Augustin M, Radtke MA. Quality of life in atopic dermatitis patients. In: Reitamo S, Luger TA, Steinhoff M, eds. *Textbook of atopic dermatitis*. London: Informa Healthcare; 2008.
56. Scottish Intercollegiate Guidelines Network. *Management of atopic eczema in primary care: a national clinical guideline*. Edinburgh: SIGN; 2011. Available from: www.sign.ac.uk/pdf/sign125.pdf.
57. Rietschel RL, Fowler JF. *Fisher's contact dermatitis*. 6th ed. Hamilton: BC Decker; 2008. p. 2:11-29.
58. Diepgen TL, Saltzer B, Tepe A et al. A study of skin irritations caused by textiles under standardised sweating conditions in patients with atopic eczema. *Melliand Deutisch/English* 1995;17:21-2.
59. Bendsoe N, Bjornberg A, Asnes H. Itching from wool fibres in atopic dermatitis. *Contact Dermatitis* 1987;17:21-2.
60. Chan ES, Cummings C; Canadian Paediatric Society, Community Paediatrics Committee and Allergy Section. Dietary exposures and allergy prevention in high-risk infants: a joint statement with the Canadian Society of Allergy and Immunology. *Paediatr Child Health* 2013;18:545-54.
61. Rautava S, Kainonen E, Salminen S et al. Maternal probiotic supplementation during pregnancy and breast-feeding reduces the risk of eczema in the infant. *J Allergy Clin Immunol* 2012;130:1355-60.
62. Foolad N, Brezinski EA, Chase EP et al. Effect of nutrient supplementation on atopic dermatitis in children: a systematic review of probiotics, prebiotics, formula, and fatty acids. *JAMA Dermatol* 2013;149:350-5.
63. Cuello-Garcia CA, Brozek JL, Fiocchi A et al. Probiotics for the prevention of allergy: a systematic review and meta-analysis of randomized controlled trials. *J Allergy Clin Immunol* 2015;136:952-61.
64. Panduru M, Panduru NM, Salavastru CM et al. Probiotics and primary prevention of atopic dermatitis: a meta-analysis of randomized controlled studies. *J Eur Acad Dermatol Venerol* 2015;29:232-42.
65. Bath-Hextall FJ, Jenkinson C, Humphreys R et al. Dietary supplements for established atopic eczema. *Cochrane Database Syst Rev* 2012;2:CD005205.
66. Boyle RJ, Bath-Hextall FJ, Leonardi-Bee J et al. Probiotics for treating eczema. *Cochrane Database Syst Rev* 2008;4:CD006135.
67. Andersen RM, Thyssen JP, Maibach HI. The role of wet wrap therapy in skin disorders—a literature review. *Acta Derm Venereol* 2015;95:933-9.
68. Rietschel RL, Fowler JF. *Fisher's contact dermatitis*. 6th ed. Hamilton: BC Decker; 2008. p. 34:722-30.
69. Ryan TJ. The management of the consequences of chronic venous stasis. *Clin Exp Dermatol* 1982;7:423-8.
70. Chiang C, Eichenfield LF. Quantitative assessment of combination bathing and moisturizing regimens on skin hydration in atopic dermatitis. *Pediatr Dermatol* 2009;26:273-8.
71. Eichenfield LF, Tom WL, Berger TG et al. Guidelines of care for the management of atopic dermatitis: section 2. Management and treatment of atopic dermatitis with topical therapies. *J Am Acad Dermatol* 2014;71:116-32.
72. Cork MJ, Danby S. Skin barrier breakdown: a renaissance in emollient therapy. *Br J Nur* 2009;18:872, 874, 876-7.

73. Schliemann S, Petri M, Elsner P. Preventing irritant contact dermatitis with protective creams: influence of the application dose. *Contact Dermatitis* 2014;70:19-26.
74. Schliemann S, Kleesz P, Elsner P. Protective creams fail to prevent solvent-induced cumulative skin irritation—results of a randomized double-blind study. *Contact Dermatitis* 2013;69:363-71.
75. Schempp CM, Meinke MC, Lademann J et al. Topical antioxidants protect the skin from chemical-induced irritation in the repetitive washing test: a placebo-controlled, double-blind study. *Contact Dermatitis* 2012;67:234-7.
76. Kutting B, Baumeister T, Weistenhofer W et al. Effectiveness of skin protection measures in prevention of occupational hand eczema: results of a prospective randomized controlled trial over a follow-up period of 1 year. *Br J Dermatol* 2010;162:362-70.
77. Lucky AW, Leach AD, Laskarzewski P et al. Use of an emollient as a steroid-sparing agent in the treatment of mild to moderate atopic dermatitis in children. *Pediatr Dermatol* 1997;14:321-4.
78. Grimalt R, Mengeaud V, Cambazard F et al. The steroid-sparing effect of an emollient therapy in infants with atopic dermatitis: a randomized controlled study. *Dermatology* 2007;214:61-7.
79. Van Scott EJ, Yu RJ. Control of keratinization with alpha-hydroxy acids and related compounds. I. Topical treatment of ichthyotic disorders. *Arch Dermatol* 1974;110:586-90.
80. Farber EM, South DA. Urea ointment in the nonsurgical avulsion of nail dystrophies. *Cutis* 1978;22:689-92.
81. Sugarman JL, Parish LC. Efficacy of lipid-based barrier repair formulation in moderate-to-severe pediatric atopic dermatitis. *J Drugs Dermatol* 2009;8:1106-11.
82. van den Bogaard EH, Bergboer JG, Vonk-Bergers M et al. Coal tar induces AHR-dependent skin barrier repair in atopic dermatitis. *J Clin Invest* 2013;123:917-27.
83. Snell ES. The pharmacological properties of corticosteroids in relation to clinical efficacy. *Br J Dermatol* 1976;94:15-23.
84. Sneddon IB. Clinical use of topical corticosteroids. *Drugs* 1976;11:193-9.
85. Gutman AB, Kligman AM, Sciacca J et al. Soak and smear: a standard technique revisited. *Arch Dermatol* 2005;141:1556-9.
86. Ng SY, Begum S, Chong SY. Does order of application of emollient and topical corticosteroids make a difference in the severity of atopic eczema in children? *Pediatr Dermatol* 2016;33:160–4
87. Smoker A, Voegeli D. Topical steroid or emollient—which to apply first? A critical review of the science and debate. *Dermatol Nurs* 2014;13:15-26.
88. Basedow S, Eigelshoven S, Homey B. Immediate and delayed hypersensitivity to corticosteroids. *J Dtsch Dermatol Ges* 2011;9:885-8.
89. Pratt MD, Belsito DV, DeLeo VAet al. North American Contact Dermatitis Group patch-test results, 2001-2002 study period. *Dermatitis* 2004;15:176-83.
90. Fonacier LS, Aquino MR, Mucci T. Current strategies in treating severe contact dermatitis in pediatric patients. *Curr Allergy Asthma Rep* 2012;12:599-606.
91. Pacor ML, Di Lorenzo G, Martinelli N et al. Tacrolimus ointment in nickel sulphate-induced steroid-resistant allergic contact dermatitis. *Allergy Asthma Proc* 2006;27:527–31.
92. Katsarou A, Makris M, Papagiannaki K et al. Tacrolimus 0.1 % vs mometasone furoate topical treatment in allergic contact hand eczema: a prospective randomized clinical study. *Eur J Dermatol* 2012;22:192-6.
93. Cury Martins J, Martins C, Aoki V et al. Topical tacrolimus for atopic dermatitis. *Cochrane Database Syst Rev* 2015;7:CD009864.
94. Abramovits W, Fleischer AB, Jaracz E et al. Adult patients with moderate atopic dermatitis: tacrolimus ointment versus pimecrolimus cream. *J Drugs Dermatol* 2008;71153-8.
95. Fleischer AB, Abramovits W, Breneman D et al. Tacrolimus ointment is more effective than pimecrolimus cream in adult patients with moderate to very severe atopic dermatitis. *J Dermatolog Treat* 2007;18:151-7.
96. Kempers S, Boguniewicz M, Carter E et al.. A randomized investigator-blinded study comparing pimecrolimus cream 1% with tacrolimus ointment 0.03% in the treatment of pediatric patients with moderate atopic dermatitis. *J Am Acad Dermatol* 2004;51:515-25.
97. Bath-Hextall FJ, Birnie AJ, Ravenscroft JC et al. Interventions to reduce Staphylococcus aureus in the management of atopic eczema: an updated Cochrane review. *Br J Dermatol* 2010;163:12-26.
98. Maurer M, Worm M, Zuberbier T. Antihistamines in atopic dermatitis. In: Reitamo S, Luger TA, Steinhoff M, eds. *Textbook of atopic dermatitis*. London: Informa Healthcare; 2008. p. 198-206.
99. Kawashima M, Tango T, Noguchi T et al. Addition of fexofenadine to a topical corticosteroid reduces the pruritus associated with atopic dermatitis in a 1-week randomized, multicentre, double-blind, placebo-controlled, parallel-group study. *Br J Dermatol* 2003;148:1212-21.
100. Sheehan MP, Atherton DJ. A controlled trial of traditional Chinese medicinal plants in widespread non-exudative atopic eczema. *Br J Dermatol* 1992;126:179-84.
101. Ferguson JE, Chalmers RJ, Rowlands DJ. Reversible dilated cardiomyopathy following treatment of atopic eczema with Chinese herbal medicine. *Br J Dermatol* 1997;136:592-3.
102. Chan TY, Chan JC, Tomlinson B et al. Chinese herbal medicines revisited: a Hong Kong perspective. *Lancet* 1993;32:1532-4.
103. Pfab F, Huss-Marp J, Gatti A et al. Influence of acupuncture on type I hypersensitivity itch and the wheal and flare response in adults with atopic eczema—a blinded, randomized, placebo-controlled, crossover trial. *Allergy* 2010;65:903-10.
104. Salameh F, Perla D, Solomon M et al. The effectiveness of combined Chinese herbal medicine and acupuncture in the treatment of atopic dermatitis. *J Altern Complement Med* 2008;14:1043-8.
105. Bamford JT, Ray S, Musekiwa A et al. Oral evening primrose oil and borage oil for eczema. *Cochrane Database Syst Rev* 2013;4:CD004416.
106. Schachner L, Field T, Hernandez-Reif M et al. Atopic dermatitis symptoms decreased in children following massage therapy. *Pediatr Dermatol* 1998;15:390-5.
107. Anderson C, Lis-Balchin M, Kirk-Smith M. Evaluation of massage with essential oils on childhood atopic eczema. *Phytother Res* 2000;14:452-6.
108. Itamura R. Effect of homeopathic treatment of 60 Japanese patients with chronic skin disease. *Complement Ther Med* 2007;15:115-20.
109. Lee KC, Keyes A, Hensley JR et al. Effectiveness of acupressure on pruritus and lichenification associated with atopic dermatitis: a pilot trial. *Acupunct Med* 2012;30:8-11.
110. Pittler MH, Armstrong NC, Cox A et al. Randomized, double-blind, placebo-controlled trial of autologous blood therapy for atopic dermatitis. *Br J Dermatol* 2003;148:307-13.
111. Santucci B, Cristaudo A, Mehraban M, et al. ZnSO4 treatment of NiSO4-positive patients. *Contact Dermatitis* 1999;40:281–2.
112. Weissmann K, Menné T. Nickel allergy and drug interaction. In: Maibach HI, Menné T, editors. Nickel and the skin: immunology and toxicology. Boca Raton: CRC Press Inc; 1989. p. 179–86.

Atopic and Contact Dermatitis—What You Need to Know

What is dermatitis?

Dermatitis is the name used for a number of similar skin conditions. Atopic dermatitis refers to dry, itchy and sensitive skin. The irritation may go away for a while then come back. Contact dermatitis refers to an itchy rash caused by an allergic reaction or something that irritates the skin.

How do you treat dermatitis?

It is important to treat the rash or irritation as soon as possible so that it does not spread or become infected from scratching. There are many products that can help relieve itching, dryness and irritation. Your healthcare provider can help you select the best product for you.

See your healthcare provider if:

- the rash does not improve after a week of recommended treatment
- pain, redness (inflammation) or itching has increased
- you have oozing blisters, fever or diarrhea
- the rash comes back frequently.

Tips for Treating Dermatitis:

- Eat a healthy, balanced diet. Avoid foods that you know cause problems for you.
- Try to avoid things that irritate your skin or make you itchy.
- Be aware that stress may make your symptoms worse. Try to reduce stress through exercise or relaxation.
- Use a cool air humidifier so the air in your house is less dry.

Clothing:

- Wear cotton or corduroy clothes. Avoid wool or nylon clothing.
- Use plastic or vinyl gloves with cotton liners for any wet work. Avoid latex products.

Laundry:

- Wash clothes in soap flakes (e.g., Ivory Snow), not detergent. If you have to use detergent, wash clothes a second time in clear water (no detergent).
- Do not use bleach in your laundry.
- Do not use liquid or sheet fabric softener.

Cleansing:

- Cleanse your skin every day to control symptoms. Follow the suggestions below.
- Use daily baths to rehydrate the skin followed by moisturizers to avoid evaporation and drying. Do not take more than one shower each week. Have a sponge bath or quick shower on other days.
- Use warm water, not hot.
- Use only a small amount of mild soap or a soapless cleanser.
- Try using a bath product such as colloidal or oilated oatmeal (e.g., Aveeno) or bath oil designed to mix with water.
- Apply a lubricating lotion (moisturizer) to your skin while it is still damp.
- Do not use products that contain lanolin. Check the label to be sure.

- If you have dry skin, you can use an moisturizer that contains any of the following ingredients: urea, lactic acid, alpha-hydroxy acid or phospholipids. These ingredients help to relieve dry skin. Check the product label.

To relieve itching:

- Use hydrocortisone 0.5 or 1% in an emollient base. Ask the pharmacist for advice about this kind of product.
- Keep nails short.
- Try not to scratch or rub your skin. Use worry beads or a small beanbag to keep your hands busy.
- To keep small children from scratching at night, put socks or mittens on their hands.

If itching keeps you awake, try taking an oral antihistamine at night for one week.

Chapter 56

Bacterial Skin Infections: Impetigo, Furuncles and Carbuncles

Penny F. Miller, BSc(Pharm), MA

The skin has a remarkable ability to protect against the external environment. A number of protective mechanisms are involved. The uppermost layer of the epidermis, the stratum corneum, provides a physical barrier to invading organisms, and its constant shedding also protects against entrenchment of microorganisms. Sebaceous glands secrete oily sebum providing an acidic pH of 5.5 that is unfavourable for microbial growth. The normal flora of the skin competes with potential pathogenic organisms. An effective immune system includes Langerhans' cells in the epidermis and mast cells and macrophages in the dermis. Still, infections do occur, usually as a result of a break in the integrity of the skin. Other predisposing conditions for microbial invasion include excessive exposure to water through sweating, bathing, occlusion, increased skin temperature or scrubbing the skin. Common bacterial skin infections include impetigo, furuncles and carbuncles.

Impetigo

Pathophysiology

Impetigo is a very common and highly contagious skin infection involving the uppermost portion of the epidermis. Most cases occur in preschool-aged children but it can affect any age group. The infection is usually spread through direct contact with the lesions or infected exudates and develops quickly at sites of minor trauma; however, it can also develop on normal skin with no apparent contactant. Predisposing factors for impetigo include varicella, insect bites, burns, scabies, atopic dermatitis, diabetes, hypogammaglobulinemia and HIV infection.[1] The spread of impetigo is promoted by factors such as crowding, poor personal hygiene and warm, humid conditions. Impetigo is most often caused by *Staphylococcus aureus*. Nonbullous impetigo can also be caused by *Streptococcus pyogenes* (also known as group A beta-hemolytic *Streptococcus*). In a minority of cases, other strains such as group C and group G streptococci may be involved.[2,3,4] About 30% of the population is colonized with *S. aureus* in the anterior nares and 10% in the perineum, which serve as a reservoir for infection. Patients who are colonized with *S. aureus* on their skin may be at risk of recurrent infection.

There are 2 distinct clinical presentations of impetigo. Nonbullous impetigo presents as papules that progress to small vesicles (blisters) surrounded by erythema (a reddened area). Over a few days, these lesions become pustules that exude and eventually dry to leave a honey-coloured, adherent crust. Lesions are often multiple, involve the central face or extremities, and may be associated with local adenopathy. The lesions may be tender and slightly itchy. The less common form, bullous impetigo, is almost exclusively caused by an exfoliating toxin-producing *S. aureus* phage group II.[5] These toxins cause loss of cell adhesion in the superficial epidermis, causing blisters.[6] The lesions begin as a superficial vesicle then become very large, flaccid, transparent blisters (bullae) filled with a clear yellow fluid that rupture after 3–5 days and leave a thin varnish-like crust.[5] There is no surrounding erythema. These lesions are typically found on the trunk, extremities, axilla and intertriginous (skin-fold and diaper) areas most commonly affecting neonates and young infants.[1] Rarely (up to 5% of cases), streptococcal impetigo leads to acute glomerulonephritis as an immunologic response to the presence of a nephritogenic strain of *S. pyogenes*. Topical and/or oral antibiotic treatment of impetigo due to group A streptococcus does not prevent poststreptococcal glomerulonephritis. Other infrequent complications of impetigo include cellulitis, lymphangitis, guttate psoriasis, osteomyelitis, septic arthritis, pneumonia, septicemia and staphylococcal scalded skin syndrome.[7] Rheumatic fever is not a risk following streptococcal impetigo.[8] See photo section, Impetigo.

Goals of Therapy

- Treat causative organisms
- Relieve symptoms and resolve lesions
- Prevent the spread of infection

Patient Assessment

Table 1 provides a description and differential diagnosis of impetigo and furuncles and carbuncles.

Table 1: **Characteristics and Differential Diagnosis of Selected Bacterial Skin Infections[9,10,11]**

Condition	Distribution	Lesion	Differential Diagnosis
Nonbullous impetigo	Face, arms or legs	Primary lesions are vesicles and pustules. Secondary lesions occurring later are yellow or honey-coloured crusts, with erosions and erythema surrounding the lesion.	Ecthyma: A crust but unlike impetigo, it is a deeper infection through the dermis causing ulcers and is usually found on the lower extremities. Tinea corporis: Inflammatory pustules but unlike impetigo, has a central clearing and develops more slowly. See Chapter 65: Fungal Skin Infections. Herpes simplex, herpes zoster, varicella and other blistering disorders such as contact dermatitis may be misdiagnosed as impetigo. However, unlike impetigo, these conditions have vesicles that are initially clear rather than honey-coloured. Herpes usually recurs in the same location on the skin. See Chapter 74: Viral Skin Rashes. Contact or atopic dermatitis typically produce marked pruritus. See Chapter 55: Atopic, Contact, and Stasis Dermatitis.
Bullous impetigo	Moist, intertriginous areas (axillae, neck folds, diaper area) Occasionally, trunk and extremeties	Superficial vesicles rapidly progress to large, flaccid bullae with no surrounding erythema. Upon rupture of bullae, oozing clear yellow fluid dries to leave a varnish-like crust.	Bullous pemphigoid: Vesicles and bullae rapidly appear on itchy urticarial plaques. Stevens-Johnson syndrome is a vesiculobullous disease affecting skin, mouth, eyes and genitalia. Thermal burns are localized. See Chapter 57: Burns. Insect bites are itchy and grouped. See Chapter 67: Insect Bites and Stings.
Furuncles and carbuncles	Hairy areas: Face, back of neck, buttocks and axillae	Primary lesions are inflammatory nodules around hair follicles. Secondary lesions are pustular with drainage.	Acne vulgaris: Pus-filled nodules and cysts on the face and upper trunk, but other acne lesions such as comedones, papules and pustules are present. See Chapter 54: Acne. Hidradenitis suppurativa: Recurrent pustules and exudative sinus tracts in the areas of apocrine glands, namely, the axillae and groin of young women after puberty.

Impetigo is considered a self-limiting infection that typically heals without scarring over a 2- to 3-week time frame. Antibiotic therapy provides a quicker resolution and prevents the spread of this contagious infection.[12,13]

The toxin produced by the strain of *S. aureus* that causes bullous impetigo may spread through the blood to cause a serious disorder called generalized staphylococcal scalded skin syndrome. This is more likely to occur in young children, people with renal impairment or in those who are immunocompromised.[5] Patients with bullous impetigo, recurrent bouts of impetigo, or an infection of unknown etiology, require assessment and treatment by an appropriate healthcare provider.

Nonpharmacologic Therapy

Prior to application of a topical antibacterial, impetigo crusts should be removed with warm water or saline compresses or soap-and-water washes. Compresses applied for 10–15 minutes and repeated 3–4 times daily, using a clean compress for each application, may hasten the healing process.[9,10,11] Patients should not manipulate the lesions as the infection could spread.

Pharmacologic Therapy

For comparative ingredients of nonprescription products, consult the *Compendium of Products for Minor Ailments*—Skin Care Products: First Aid.

Topical antibiotic therapy is considered the treatment of choice for patients with uncomplicated impetigo localized to 2 or 3 small areas. Topical therapy eradicates isolated disease and limits transmission. Compared with oral therapy, topical antibiotics have fewer side effects and a lower risk of bacterial resistance.[13] A variety of topical antibiotics are available but only **mupirocin** and **fusidic acid** have been shown to be as effective as oral antibiotics in localized infections and they are considered first-line options.[13,14,15]

Mupirocin acts by reversible inhibition of bacterial isoleucyl-transfer RNA synthetase.[9] It is effective against gram-positive organisms only. Mupirocin does not exhibit cross-resistance with other antibiotics. There are documented cases of mupirocin-resistant streptococci[15] and staphylococci[16] and therefore widespread use for minor infections is discouraged.

Fusidic acid is a protein synthesis inhibitor effective against gram-positive organisms only. Resistance is also reported with this agent.[12,13,15,17]

Topical antibiotics containing various combinations of **polymyxin B**, **bacitracin**, **gramicidin** and **neosporin** have been shown to be inferior to mupirocin and fusidic acid (see Table 4).[13,14,18,19,20]

Systemic antibiotic therapy should be considered if the condition is widespread, the patient is immunocompromised or has valvular heart disease, there are signs of fever or bacteremia or there is a lack of improvement after 24–48 hours of topical therapy.[21] Oral therapy is also recommended as a means of decreasing transmission in outbreaks. Empiric therapy should involve a 7-day regimen with coverage for both streptococci and beta-lactamase–producing *S. aureus*. If cultures reveal streptococci as the sole pathogens, penicillin should be used. Because most *S. aureus* strains are MSSA (methicillin-susceptible *S. aureus*), **amoxicillin/clavulanate**, **cefadroxil**, **cephalexin** and **cloxacillin** are recommended options. If infection with MRSA (methicillin-resistant *S. aureus*) is confirmed or suspected, **doxycycline**, **clindamycin** or **sulfamethoxazole/trimethoprim** (SMX/TMP) is recommended; however, culture and antibiotic susceptibility testing may be warranted to identify resistant strains of MRSA. Although there are few reports of clinical failure, empiric use of SMX/TMP is limited by inadequate coverage of streptococci.[3] **Erythromycin** and other macrolides are not recommended as resistance rates are rising and GI adverse effects are frequent.[3,13,14]

Recurrent impetigo may occur when there is *S. aureus* carriage in the anterior nares or perineum. Recurrent cases require culture and, if positive, treatment with a 5-day eradication regimen consisting of topical mupirocin applied to the nares 2–3 times daily and daily washing with topical chlorhexidine or hexachlorophene (particularly the perineum and axilla).[3,21]

Topical solutions including saline, **hexachlorophene**, **povidone-iodine** and **chlorhexidine** are inferior to topical antibiotic therapy and are not recommended as sole therapy for impetigo.[13,22]

Monitoring of Therapy

Table 2 presents a monitoring framework for patients with impetigo. Lesions should begin to heal within 2–3 days of starting therapy, and the patient is no longer infectious about 48 hours after the initiation of treatment. Lesions usually heal without scarring. Further assessment and/or treatment is advised if lesions spread, or if fever or other systemic symptoms arise. Given the increasing rate of community-acquired MRSA, in nonresponsive cases a swab of the lesion or wound for culture and sensitivity is recommended.

Table 2: **Monitoring of Therapy for Impetigo**

Symptoms	Monitoring	Endpoint of Therapy	Actions
Vesicles and crusts	Patient: Daily while on therapy	Clearing of all lesions by 7–10 days. Return of normal skin appearance within 2–3 wk.	If worsening or no improvement by day 3, consider further assessment and/or treatment.
Bullous lesions	Patient: Daily while on therapy Healthcare practitioner: After 3 days if no improvement with therapy	Clearing of all lesions. Return of normal skin appearance within 2–3 wk.	If worsening or no improvement by day 3, consider further assessment and/or treatment.
Reddish-brown or "cola" coloured urine (possible indicator of post-streptococcal glomerulonephritis)	Patient: Daily while on therapy and for weeks following	No renal problems.	Patient requires immediate assessment for renal evaluation.
Postinflammatory pigmentary skin change	Patient: Weekly after therapy is completed	Resolution several months after clearing of initial infection.	Patient requires further evaluation and/or treatment if persisting.
Allergy to topical agents	Patient: Daily while on therapy Healthcare practitioner: After 1 wk or next pharmacy visit	No allergy.	Stop therapy. Patient requires further assessment and/or treatment.
Irritation caused by topical agents	Patient: Daily while on therapy Healthcare practitioner: After 1 wk or next pharmacy visit	Little to no irritation that subsides with continued use.	Stop therapy if no improvement in irritation after several doses.

Furuncles and Carbuncles

Pathophysiology

Furuncles (boils) and carbuncles usually begin near hair follicles as a superficial folliculitis which consists of yellowish pustules, then spreads to deeper layers of skin. Furuncles are most common in adolescence and early adulthood; carbuncles occur more often in older males.[11,23]

Furuncles spread into the dermis to produce a painful and erythematous swelling with a central pustule. Pus often drains spontaneously. Carbuncles penetrate deeper over a larger area than furuncles with involvement of numerous adjacent follicles and extension into the subcutaneous fat. Hairy areas subjected to irritation from perspiration or friction, such as the bearded area of the face, back of neck, buttocks and axillae, are common sites of infection (see Figure 1).[11,23]

Figure 1: **Folliculitis, Furuncle and Carbuncle**

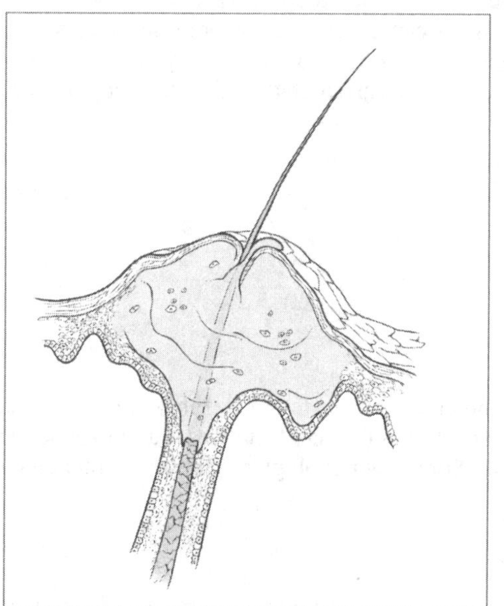

Folliculitis

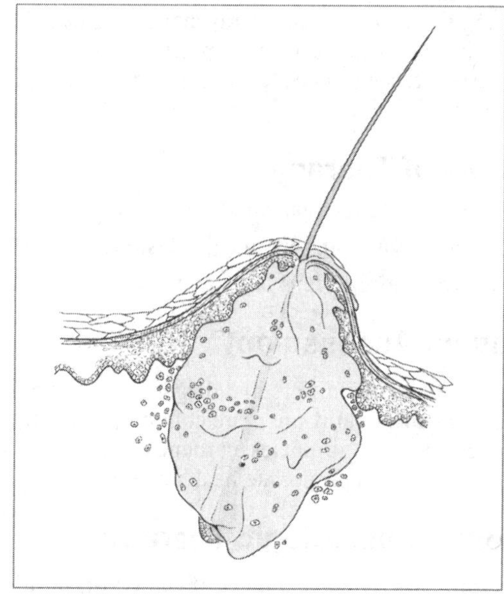

Furuncle

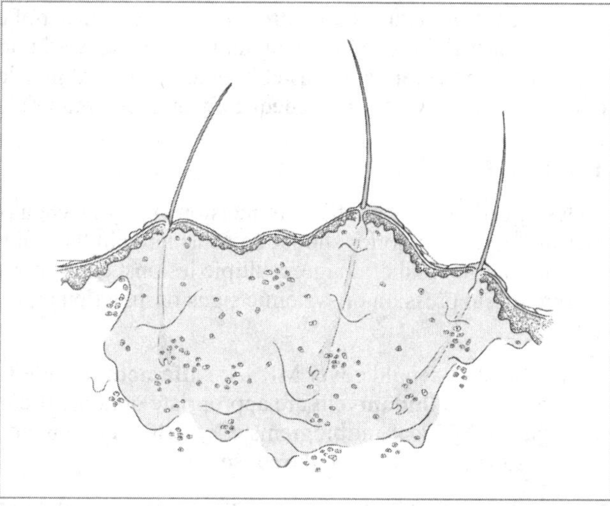

Carbuncle

Furuncles and carbuncles are usually attributable to methicillin-susceptible *or* methicillin-resistant *S. aureus*. Additional pathogens implicated in hair follicle infections include *Pseudomonas*, as in the usually benign "hot-tub folliculitis", oral anaerobes as seen among intravenous drug users, and *Mycobacterium* associated with whirlpool footbaths at nail salons.[24,25]

Predisposing factors for these infections include obesity, suppressed immune states, heat, friction, occlusion and excessive sweating. Close contact with individuals with furunculosis appears to be a risk factor for transmission.[26] Risk factors for MRSA infection include sharing sports equipment, recent hospitalization, residing in a long-term care facility, recent antibiotic therapy, HIV infection, men having sex with men and intravenous drug use.[23] Furuncles can progress to become carbuncles or cellulitis. Carbuncles have the potential to cause bacteremia with resultant morbidity or mortality.[7] Recurrent cases can occur especially if *S. aureus* is present in a carrier state in the anterior nares or perineum.[7,23]

Goals of Therapy

- Treat causative organisms
- Relieve symptoms and resolve lesions
- Prevent more serious infections

Patient Assessment

A description and differential diagnosis of furuncles and carbuncles is found in Table 1. Fever, malaise and local adenopathy are more common in patients with carbuncles than furuncles. Patients who have a fever, recurrent furuncles, carbuncles or an infection of unknown etiology require assessment and/or treatment by an appropriate healthcare provider.

Nonpharmacologic Therapy

A furuncle is a fluctuant mass of walled-off purulent material that normally ruptures and drains pus spontaneously. Warm water or saline compresses applied for 20–30 minutes 3 or 4 times daily may promote spontaneous drainage and help relieve discomfort.[10,11] Washing the area with soap and water or chlorhexidine 4% four times daily to reduce the *S. aureus* colony counts is advised.[27,28] To prevent transmission, lesions should be covered with a sterile dressing and not touched. Personal items contacting the lesion should be washed daily in hot water and not shared. Carbuncles, and furuncles that are large or unresponsive to warm compresses, usually require surgical incision and drainage.[11] Some spontaneously draining lesions may not drain adequately and may require incision and drainage.

Pharmacologic Therapy

Many patients with furuncles or carbuncles benefit from incision and drainage alone;[3] the role of ancillary antibiotics is unclear.[29] Oral antibiotics should be considered in the following situations: inadequate clinical response to incision and drainage, multiple lesions, extensive surrounding cellulitis, associated comorbidities, immunosuppression or systemic signs of infection (fever, tachypnea, tachycardia, leukocytosis).[3]

Empiric treatment with oral antibiotics should cover MRSA; **sulfamethoxazole/trimethoprim** (SMX/TMP), **doxycycline**, **minocycline** and **clindamycin** are appropriate options. If culture results are available, therapy should be guided by local antibiograms. **Cephalexin** or **cloxacillin** is appropriate for infections where cultures have shown MSSA to be the cause.[3,30]

Parenteral antibiotic therapy is indicated in immunocompromised patients and in patients who fail initial antibiotic therapy combined with incision and drainage and exhibit signs of severe systemic infection such as temperature >38°C, tachycardia >90 beats per minute, tachypnea >24 breaths per minute, white blood cell count >12 000 or <400 cells/µL, or hypotension.[3] For more information on the treatment of bacterial skin infections with oral or parenteral antibiotics, consult the *Compendium of Therapeutic Choices*: Bacterial Skin Infections.

Some patients have recurrent furuncles or carbuncles. It is unknown whether the risk of recurrent infection is decreased or whether the prevalence of resistance is increased with use of antibiotics in addition to incision and drainage.[23,31,32] Recurrent furuncles or carbuncles should be treated for 5–10 days with antibiotics active against the identified pathogen. In addition, local causes of recurrent infection such as foreign material, pilonidal cyst or hidradenitis suppurativa should be ruled out. Adult patients with recurrent abscesses since childhood should be evaluated for neutrophil disorders. Encourage meticulous personal and environmental hygiene measures. Recommend MRSA decolonization when there are multiple documented recurrences of MRSA infection or if ongoing transmission is occurring among household members or other close contacts despite optimal hygiene. Intranasal application of **mupirocin** ointment twice daily for 5 days each month for 3 months combined with **chlorhexidine** antiseptic washes daily for 5–14 days is recommended in spite of weak supportive evidence.[3,30] Dilute bleach baths may be considered as a means of reducing *S. aureus* infections,[3,30] although limited evidence has not demonstrated significant clinical benefit in atopic dermatitis patients[33] or children with recurrent skin and soft tissue infections.[34]

Monitoring of Therapy

After spontaneous or surgical drainage, healing usually occurs within a week. Large lesions may heal with a scar. Patients with recurrent infections may have underlying systemic illnesses that require investigation and management. A monitoring framework for patients with furuncles or carbuncles can be found in Table 3.

Table 3: **Monitoring of Therapy of Furuncles/Carbuncles**

Symptoms	Monitoring	Endpoint of Therapy	Actions
Boils and pus	Patient: Daily while on therapy	No more drainage of pus, and lesions heal over several weeks.	If no improvement or worsening by day 3, patient requires further assessment and/or treatment.
Fever	Patient: Daily while on therapy Healthcare practitioner: After 48 h	Return to normal body temperature.	If no improvement by day 2, patient requires further assessment and/or treatment.
Pain on palpation	Patient: Daily while on therapy	Relief of pain as the lesion heals.	If no improvement or worsening by day 3, patient requires further assessment and/or treatment.
Recurrent lesions	Patient: Watch for any new lesions for weeks and months following the initial lesions	No recurrent infections.	Patient requires culture of anterior nares and perineum. Patient may require assessment and/or treatment for underlying causes of recurrence.
Allergy to topical agents	Patient: Daily while on therapy Healthcare practitioner: After 1 wk or next visit	No allergy.	Stop therapy. Patient requires further assessment and/or treatment.
Irritation caused by topical agents	Patient: Daily while on therapy Healthcare practitioner: After 1 wk or next visit	Little to no irritation that subsides with continued use.	Stop therapy if no improvement in irritation after several doses.

Table 4: Topical Antibacterial Agents for the Treatment of Impetigo

Class	Drug	Dosage[a]	Adverse Effects	Comments	Cost[b]
Antibiotics, topical	*bacitracin* Bacitracin USP, generics	Apply 1–3 times daily for up to 7 days or until all lesions are healed	Common cause of allergic contact dermatitis	Less effective than fusidic acid or mupirocin. Spectrum: Gram-positive only. Stable only in petrolatum (ointment).	$
	fusidic acid Fucidin	Apply BID–TID × 5 days or until all lesions are healed	Rare: Mild irritation, allergic contact dermatitis	First-line treatment option. Spectrum: Gram-positive only.	$$$
	mupirocin Bactroban, generics	Apply BID–TID × 5 days or until all lesions are healed	Infrequent: burning, stinging Rare: Allergic contact dermatitis	First-line treatment option. Spectrum: Gram-positive only.	$$
	bacitracin/neomycin/polymyxin B Neosporin Ointment, generics	Apply TID × up to 7 days or until all lesions are healed	Neomycin and bacitracin components are common causes of allergic contact dermatitis	Less effective than fusidic acid or mupirocin. Spectrum: Gram-positive and gram-negative. Rarely nephrotoxic when applied to large denuded areas.	$
	bacitracin/gramicidin/polymyxin B Polysporin Products, generics	Apply TID × up to 7 days or until all lesions are healed	Bacitracin component is a common cause of allergic contact dermatitis	Less effective than fusidic acid or mupirocin. Spectrum: Gram-positive and gram-negative. Rarely nephrotoxic when applied to large denuded areas.	$

[a] Reassess if there is a lack of improvement after 48 hours of topical therapy.

[b] Cost of 15 g; includes drug cost only.

Legend: $ <$5 $$ $5–10 $$$ $10–15

Suggested Readings

Hartman-Adams H, Banvard C, Juckett G. Impetigo: diagnosis and treatment. *Am Fam Physician* 2014;90:229-35.

Liu C, Bayer A, Cosgrove SE et al. Clinical practice guidelines by the Infectious Diseases Society of America for the treatment of methicillin-resistant Staphylococcus aureus infections in adults and children. *Clin Infect Dis* 2011;52:e18-55.

Stevens DL, Bisno AL, Chambers HF et al. Practice guidelines for the diagnosis and management of skin and soft tissue infections: 2014 update by the Infectious Diseases Society of America. *Clin Infect Dis* 2014;59:e10-52.

References

1. Hartman-Adams H, Banvard C, Juckett G. Impetigo: diagnosis and treatment. *Am Fam Physician* 2014;90:229-35.
2. DermNet NZ. *Impetigo*. Available from: www.dermnetnz.org/bacterial/impetigo.html. Accessed April 20, 2016.
3. Stevens DL, Bisno AL, Chambers HF et al. Practice guidelines for the diagnosis and management of skin and soft tissue infections: 2014 update by the Infectious Diseases Society of America. *Clin Infect Dis* 2014;59:e10-52.
4. Baddour LM. *Impetigo*. Available from: www.uptodate.com. Accessed July 2015. Subscription required.
5. Amagai M, Matsuyoshi N, Wang ZH et al. Toxin in bullous impetigo and staphylococcal scalded skin syndrome targets desmoglein 1. *Nat Med* 2000;6:1275-7.
6. Amagai M, Yamaguchi T, Hanakawa Y et al. Staphylococcal exfoliative toxin B specifically cleaves desmoglein 1. *J Invest Dermatol* 2002;118:845-50.
7. Morelli JG. Cutaneous bacterial infections. In: Kliegman R, ed. *Nelson textbook of pediatrics*. 18th ed. Philadelphia: Saunders; 2007.
8. Bisno AL, Stevens DL. Streptococcal infections of skin and soft tissues. *N Engl J Med* 1996;334:240-5.
9. Burd RM, Sladden M. Impetigo. In: Lebwohl MG, Heymann WR, Berth-Jones J et al., eds. *Treatment of skin disease: comprehensive therapeutic strategies*. 4th ed. Edinburgh: Elsevier/Saunders; 2014.
10. Marks JG, Miller JJ. *Lookingbill and Marks' principles of dermatology*. 5th ed. London: Saunders/Elsevier; 2013.
11. Craft N. Superficial cutaneous infections and pyodermas. In: Goldsmith LA, Katz SI, Gilchrest BA et al., eds. *Fitzpatrick's dermatology in general medicine*. 8th ed. New York: McGraw-Hill; 2012.
12. Feaster T, Singer JI. Topical therapies for impetigo. *Pediatr Emerg Care* 2010;26:222-7.
13. Koning S, van der Sande R, Verhagen AP et al. Interventions for impetigo. *Cochrane Database Syst Rev* 2012;1:CD003261.
14. George A, Rubin G. A systematic review and meta-analysis of treatments for impetigo. *Br J Gen Pract* 2003;53:480-7.
15. Bangert S, Levy M, Hebert AA. Bacterial resistance and impetigo treatment trends: a review. *Pediatr Dermatol* 2012;29:243-8.
16. Hetem DJ, Bonten MJ. Clinical relevance of mupirocin resistance in Staphylococcus aureus. *J Hosp Infect* 2013;85:249-56.
17. Sutton JB. Efficacy and acceptability of fusidic acid cream and mupirocin ointment in facial impetigo. *Curr Ther Res* 1992;51:673-8.
18. Noah S. A primer in topical antibiotics for the skin and eyes. *J Drugs Dermatol* 2008;7:409-15.
19. Wilkinson RD, Carey WD. Topical mupirocin versus topical neosporin in the treatment of cutaneous infections. *Int J Dermatol* 1988;27:514-5.
20. Bass JW, Chan DS, Creamer KM et al. Comparison of oral cephalexin, topical mupirocin and topical bacitracin for treatment of impetigo. *Pediatr Infect Dis J* 1997;16:708-10.
21. Anti-infective Review Panel. *Anti-infective guidelines for community-acquired infections*. Toronto: MUMS Guideline Clearinghouse; 2013.
22. Ruby RJ, Nelson JD. The influence of hexachlorophene scrubs on the response to placebo or penicillin therapy in impetigo. *Pediatrics* 1973;52:854-9.
23. Baddour LM. *Skin abscesses, furuncules and carbuncles*. Available from: www.uptodate.com. Accessed July 2015. Subscription required.
24. Gira AK, Reisenauer AH, Hammock L et al. Furunculosis due to Mycobacterium mageritense associated with footbaths at a nail salon. *J Clin Microbiol* 2004;42:1813-7.
25. Summanen PH, Talan DA, Strong C et al. Bacteriology of skin and soft-tissue infections: comparison of infections in intravenous drug users and individuals with no history of intravenous drug use. *Clin Infect Dis* 1995;20:S279-82.
26. Lopez FA, Lartchenko S. Skin and soft tissue infections. *Infect Dis Clin North Am* 2006;20:759-72.
27. Zimakoff J, Rosdahl VT, Petersen W et al. Recurrent staphylococcal furunculosis in families. *Scand J Infect Dis* 1988;20:403-5.
28. Raz R, Miron D, Colodner R et al. A 1-year trial of nasal mupirocin in the prevention of recurrent staphylococcal nasal colonization and skin infection. *Arch Intern Med* 1996;156:1109-12.
29. Gorwitz RJ. The role of ancillary antimicrobial therapy for treatment of uncomplicated skin infections in the era of community-associated methicillin-resistant Staphylococcus aureus. *Clin Infect Dis* 2007;44:785-7.
30. Liu C, Bayer A, Cosgrove SE et al. Clinical practice guidelines by the Infectious Diseases Society of America for the treatment of methicillin-resistant Staphylococcus aureus infections in adults and children. *Clin Infect Dis* 2011;52:e18-55.
31. Schmitz GR, Bruner D, Pitotti R et al. Randomized controlled trial of trimethoprim-sulfamethoxazole for uncomplicated skin abscesses in patients at risk for community-associated methicillin-resistant Staphylococcus aureus infection. *Ann Emerg Med* 2010;56:283-7.
32. Duong M, Markwell S, Peter J et al. Randomized, controlled trial of antibiotics in the management of community-acquired skin abscesses in the pediatric patient. *Ann Emerg Med* 2010;55:401-7.
33. Huang JT, Abrams M, Tlougan B et al. Treatment of Staphylococcus aureus colonization in atopic dermatitis decreases disease severity. *Pediatrics* 2009;123:3808-14.
34. Kaplan SL, Forbes A, Hammerman WA et al. Randomized trial of "bleach baths" plus routine hygienic measures vs routine hygienic measures alone for prevention of recurrent infections. *Clin Infec Dis* 2014;58:679-82.

Impetigo—What You Need to Know

What is impetigo?

Impetigo is a contagious skin infection caused by bacteria. Children get impetigo more often than adults, but adults can get it too.

Impetigo usually appears around the nose and mouth. It can also show up on other parts of the body where the skin has been broken, such as cuts, scrapes or insect bites.

What causes impetigo?

We all have bacteria living on our skin and in our nose. Most of the time they don't cause any trouble. However, if bacteria get into a cut, an infection can result. Two types of bacteria can cause impetigo: Group A streptococcus (called "strep") and *Staphylococcus aureus* (called "staph"). The medicine chosen to treat the infection depends on the type of bacteria that are causing the problem.

What are the signs of impetigo?

- Impetigo starts as small blisters that grow larger every day. They ooze fluid that dries up to form a crust. The crust is yellow-brown, or honey-coloured.
- Impetigo may also appear as a very large blister but this is less common.
- Impetigo may be itchy but it is generally not painful.

How does impetigo spread?

A person can get impetigo by touching the infected area or by using the same towel, cup or glass as an infected person.

What is the treatment for impetigo?

- Antibiotic ointments that contain polymyxin B and bacitracin or gramicidin can be bought from the pharmacist. Use if there are only 1 or 2 recent, small spots. If the spots spread, see your healthcare provider; you may need a different antibiotic.
- How to use antibiotic ointment:
  - Remove any crusts from the skin before applying the antibiotic ointment. Use a clean cloth soaked in warm soapy water or saline (salt) solution. Apply the warm cloth to the area for 10–15 minutes then gently scrub off the crusts.
  - Apply the ointment directly to the infected area 3 times a day until the spots are healed. This may take 5–7 days.
  - Cover the draining sores lightly with gauze and tape to avoid spreading the infection.

When should you see your healthcare provider?

- If the impetigo is more than just a few small spots. You may need a different antibiotic.
- If the skin does not begin to heal after 3 days of treatment.
- If the infected person develops a fever.
- If the infected area gets worse—becomes red, warm or painful.

How can you prevent impetigo from spreading?

- Avoid close contact with people who have impetigo.
- Keep any scratches or cuts very clean and covered with bandages.

- Tell children not to touch or pick the sores. Touching the sores can spread the infection.
- Be sure to wash hands well with alcohol-based cleansers or soap and warm water after treating the impetigo.
- Wash and change the infected person's clothes, towels and bedding daily for the first 2 days of antibiotic treatment.
- After 2 days of antibiotic treatment, the impetigo will no longer be contagious.

Boils and Carbuncles—What You Need to Know

What are boils?

Boils are skin infections that causes painful, red, pus-filled swellings around the base of hair strands. Boils are also called furuncles. If the infection spreads, you may get very large boils or groups of boils, called carbuncles.

How do you get boils?

- Boils are caused by bacteria called *Staphylococcus aureus* ("staph"). The bacteria live on the skin in the rectum, genitals and lining of the nose. Most of the time, these bacteria do not cause any problems. However, if your skin is broken or scraped, the bacteria can get under the skin and cause an infection. The infection usually grows in the hair follicle (the skin pocket where a hair strand grows).
- People with diseases such as diabetes, kidney or liver disease are more likely to get boils because their resistance to disease is low.

What are the symptoms?

- The first sign of infection is a tiny white- or yellow-headed pimple at the base of a hair strand. This condition is called folliculitis. The infection can spread wider and deeper into the skin to cause a painful, red swelling (lump) that is about 1 or 2 cm wide. This is a boil or furuncle.
- After several days, the centre of the boil becomes soft and filled with pus. Eventually, this pus will drain and relieve the pain.
- Carbuncles cause similar symptoms but they are more severe.
- Boils most commonly occur in hairy, moist areas of the body such as the back of the neck, face, armpits and buttocks.

How do you treat boils?

- A single boil can usually be treated at home. See a healthcare provider if you develop carbuncles.
- Apply a warm compress (a clean washcloth soaked in warm water) to the boil for 20–30 minutes. Do it 3 times a day. It will help the boil to come to a "head."
- Clean the boil with antiseptic soap and cover it with a loose gauze dressing.
- The boil will usually burst and drain on its own. It may take several days for it to drain completely. Be sure to keep it covered to prevent the infection from spreading.
- The boil will be very painful until it drains. **Do not** squeeze the boil—the bacteria may spread into your blood and cause a more serious infection.

When should you see your healthcare provider?

- If the boil has come to a head and needs to be opened for it to drain. **Do not** do this yourself.
- If carbuncles form you may need a prescription for antibiotics.
- If you feel sick and you have a fever.
- If your boils come back or other family members also develop boils.

How can you prevent the spread of boils?

- The pus is contagious. It can spread the infection to other parts of the skin or to other people.
- Wash your hands with alcohol-based hand cleansers or antibacterial soap after touching the boils.

- Shower and wash your hair every day with antibacterial soap. This will help to decrease bacteria on the skin and reduce the chance of boils spreading.
- Wash washcloths, towels or clothes that touched the boils in hot soapy water. Dry them in the hot cycle of the dryer.
- Do not share facecloths and towels.
- Antibiotic ointments or creams will not heal boils but they may help prevent the boils from spreading.

Chapter 57
Burns

Nancy Kleiman, BSP, MBA

Pathophysiology

Burns encompass a spectrum of tissue injury (see Table 1) with cell death and protein denaturation caused by:[1,2]

- heat (thermal burns), e.g., flame, scalding liquids, hot objects, gases
- radiation, e.g., sun, ultraviolet (UV) lamps, lasers
- electricity, e.g., lightning, home appliances
- chemical exposures, e.g., caustic cleaners, solvents, laboratory reagents.

The potential seriousness of the burn is related to:[1,2]

- body location and skin thickness
- temperature of the causative agent
- type of causative agent
- duration of exposure to causative agent
- extent of the burn
- depth of the burn (particularly affects healing time and potential sequelae of scarring and contractures).

Table 1: Characteristics of Burn Wounds[1,2,3]

Old Nomenclature	Class	Examples	Appearance	Healing
First-degree	Superficial (epidermis only)	Sunburn; very brief thermal contact; low-intensity heat	Dry; pink; blanches with pressure; painful; some edema; no blisters; skin remains intact so infection is not a concern	3–5 days; no scarring
Second-degree	Superficial partial thickness (epidermis, upper dermis)	Scald (spill, splash); brief flame; thermal contact or exposure to dilute chemicals	Moist; weeping; red; small blisters; blanches with pressure; extreme pain	7–21 days; scarring unusual; potential pigment changes
	Deep partial thickness (epidermis, deep dermis with some hair follicle, sweat gland damage)	Scald; oil or grease; flame; prolonged exposure to dilute chemicals	Wet or waxy; dry; colour variable (red, patchy white); blisters may be present; no blanching with pressure; pain only with pressure	>21 days; risk of scarring and contracture
Third-degree	Full thickness (epidermis, dermis to subcutaneous layer)	Scald (immersion); steam; flame; concentrated chemicals; high-voltage electrical	Dry; waxy white to leathery gray to charred and black; no blanching with pressure; painless (due to destruction of nerves)	Never heals spontaneously; requires surgery/grafts; high risk of scarring; contractures; systemic and skin infection; fluid loss

Patient factors that increase the risk of burn wound infections or delayed burn healing include:[1,2]

- age (very young or elderly)
- underlying medical conditions such as diabetes or vascular disease
- malnutrition
- smoking
- drug therapy that suppresses the immune system.

See Superficial, Deep Partial Thickness, and Full Thickness Burns in Photo Section.

The extent and seriousness of partial-thickness to full-thickness burns, and thus their appropriate treatment, is determined in part by estimating the total body surface area (TBSA) affected by the burn. One way of measuring the extent of the burn is referred to as the "rule of nines"[3] (see Table 2). This estimation is best done by an experienced burn specialist in a hospital setting. Superficial burns are *not* included in TBSA calculations of burn wounds and are generally self-treatable. Partial- and full-thickness burns in adults that are >10% TBSA, or in children that are >5% TBSA, should be assessed in a hospital setting.[4]

Table 2: **Assessing Extent of a Burn—Rule of Nines[3,5]**

Body Part	% of Body Surface Area (Adult)	% of Body Surface Area (Infant/small child)
Head	9	18
Both arms	18	18
Anterior trunk	18	18
Posterior trunk	18	18
Both legs	36	28
Palm of hands	1	1

Goals of Therapy

- Minimize further damage from the suspected causative agent
- Promote healing and restoration of damaged tissue
- Prevent infection/complications
- Control pain

Patient Assessment

Self-management is appropriate for most superficial burns or superficial partial-thickness burns (a few small blisters with limited distribution on the body). Patients with burns of any size that are more serious than the mildest partial-thickness burn (minimal blistering) should be seen in an emergency care setting. Appropriate referral minimizes the risk of infection, fluid and electrolyte loss and scarring.

Assess patients to determine whether there is concomitant trauma (e.g., electrical injury causing cardiac dysrhythmias).

Patients who have burns with minimal blistering should be seen in an emergency care setting if they involve thin skin areas (e.g., face, ears, eyelids, inner surface of arm, perineum) or occur in individuals presumed to have thin skin (e.g., children less than 2 years or adults older than 55 years).[1,2]

Electrical burns and chemical burns involving concentrated acid and alkali products should also be assessed and treated in an emergency care setting even if they appear to be minor, since the injury may be deeper than the initial appearance of the burn suggests and can progress to deep tissue necrosis within 24 hours.[2]

Patients with underlying conditions that put them at risk of infection or delayed healing, such as diabetes, chronic alcohol abuse, immunocompromised states (including drug-induced immunosuppression), require close monitoring and follow up.[1,2]

Assessment of burn patients is summarized in Figure 1.

Nonpharmacologic Therapy

Thermal burns are treated by removal of the causative agent to minimize further tissue damage. Cooling can limit the extent of injury and provide some pain relief, and should be started as soon as possible.[2] Thermal burns can be cooled for up to 30 minutes with tepid (cool to touch) tap water irrigations, immersion in tepid water, or application of cool tap water compresses for up to 20 minutes (12°C).[3,5] If the burn is serious enough to require medical attention, continue with cool compresses during transport. Plastic cling wrap can be used over the burn during transport to protect the area against fluid and heat loss and from infection.[4] Ice application is not recommended because it can cause vasoconstriction that may worsen the injury and lead to frostbite.[4,5]

Chemical burns are treated by removing the causative agent and clothing that has become saturated with the chemical. Irrigate the burn area with copious amounts of lukewarm or cool water and transport the patient to the emergency room for further treatment.[5]

Electrical burns are treated by first removing the source of electricity if safely possible, and then immediately transporting the person to the emergency room for further treatment as these burns are often more serious than they appear.[5]

Radiation burns are commonly caused by sun exposure and are treated in a similar manner to a thermal burn.

First Aid for Burns

First-aid treatment of burns is dependent on the type of burn and the causative agent. Superficial or superficial partial-thickness burns caused by thermal agents or the sun are generally self-treatable, while deep partial-thickness or full-thickness burns, or those with chemical or electrical causes, require immediate medical attention.

To apply first aid for superficial burns:

- Stop the process or cause of the burn by either removing the causative agent or removing the patient from the source of the burn
- Cool the burn area by running cool tap water (8–25°C) over the area for 20 minutes.[4] Cooling the burn helps to reduce pain and inflammation[6] and may reduce the severity of tissue damage[7]
- Remove jewelry or anything restrictive from the burned area quickly in case the area swells
- Leave small blisters intact. If blisters break, gently clean the area with mild soap and water and cover with nonadherent gauze dressing
- The use of **disinfectants** to clean burn wounds is not recommended because they may impair wound healing[2]

- Tap water and mild soap can be used to gently clean secretions and remove wound debris with each dressing change
- Seek medical attention if the burn is >10% TBSA for adults or >5% TBSA for children, in those <2 or >55 years old or if there is involvement of face, ear, eyelid, palms, feet, inner surface of arms or perineum.

Pharmacologic Therapy

For more information on therapy for burns, consult the *Compendium of Therapeutic Choices*: Burns.

For comparative ingredients of nonprescription products, consult the *Compendium of Products for Minor Ailments*—Analgesic Products: Internal Analgesics and Antipyretics; Skin Care Products: Anesthetics, Dermatitis and Dry Skin, First Aid.

Antibacterial Agents

Topical antibiotics are not recommended for routine use on minor burns unless infection is present.[4] It is important to monitor the patient for signs of infection and to treat if needed.[6] **Silver sulfadiazine** (SSD), a broad spectrum topical antibiotic, has historically been used to prevent burn wound infections. However, limited poor quality evidence suggests that the use of SSD on superficial or partial thickness burns may lead to poorer healing outcomes than other topical treatments.[8,9]

Oral antibiotics are not effective in preventing burn wound infections and should be used only when there is a known active infection.[10]

Pain and Itch Control

Usual doses of nonprescription **analgesics** (e.g., **acetaminophen**, **ibuprofen**) are often sufficient to control pain in minor burns. **ASA** should be avoided in superficial partial-thickness or deep partial-thickness burns because platelet inhibition poses a risk of bleeding in the presence of open wounds.[2] Deeper burns with open areas often require opioids for adequate pain management.[2]

Local anesthetics are a common ingredient in topical products marketed for the relief of minor pain and itching associated with superficial burns. There is no evidence to substantiate their effectiveness. **Lidocaine** and **benzocaine** commonly cause contact dermatitis, while **pramoxine** has low sensitizing potential. There is a risk of systemic absorption if local anesthetics are applied to blistered or large areas of skin. **Camphor**, **menthol** and **phenol** are counterirritants thought to have a cooling effect on the burned area and to provide some relief from itching. However, there is no evidence available for the use of counterirritants in the treatment of minor burns.

Deep partial-thickness and full-thickness burn wounds can take 6 months to 2 years to heal completely. Itching is common during the healing phase, particularly in partial thickness burns. **Moisturizing lotions** and **colloidal oatmeal baths** may provide symptomatic relief of itch in less severe burns. Systemic antihistamines such as **diphenhydramine**, **cetirizine** and **hydroxyzine** may be helpful in some patients whose itching is more bothersome.[2] Some evidence indicates that **gabapentin** may be an option for patients with itch that has not responded to moisturizers and antihistamines.[11] Avoid the use of topical antihistamines in this situation since the risk of sensitization and allergic contact dermatitis increases with prolonged use. The area will also be more sensitive to sun and extremes of heat and cold. High SPF (30 or greater) **sunscreens** should be used until the wound has healed completely, to prevent permanent hyperpigmentation from repeated injury due to sun radiation.[1,2] See Chapter 72: Prevention and Treatment of Sun-induced Skin Damage.

Other Agents

Topical **honey** appears to result in healing of partial thickness burns 4–5 days more quickly than some conventional treatments, though differences in rates of adverse events or infection are unclear. There is also uncertainty about the replicability and applicability of this evidence.[12]

A systematic review determined that evidence is inconclusive regarding whether **aloe vera** gel or dressings improve outcomes for acute wounds including burns.[13] Some patients experience mild side effects of burning sensation, contact dermatitis or mild itching with topical application.[14]

Tetanus prophylaxis is recommended for deep partial-thickness and full-thickness burns if it has been more than 10 years since the last booster. The Public Health Agency of Canada recommends that tetanus prophylaxis also be implemented if it is uncertain when the patient's last booster was given, or if the patient has not received the full 3 doses of the primary immunization series.[15]

Monitoring of Therapy

Table 3 provides a monitoring plan for burn therapy.

Table 3: **Monitoring of Therapy for Burns**

Symptom	Monitoring	Endpoint	Actions
Pain	Monitor pain level every 4–6 h for the first few days and then daily. Monitor the level of pain based on a scale of 0–10 where 0 is no pain and 10 is the worst possible pain. Assess whether pain interferes with sleep or usual activities.	The patient's worst pain score should be less than 5. Higher pain scores interfere with sleep, daily activities and mood.	Patients whose pain is not responding adequately to regular (Q4–6H) doses of nonprescription analgesics may require further assessment and/or treatment. Opioid analgesics will be required if burn is more severe.
Burn healing	Monitor daily for 2–3 days, then weekly until healing is complete (usually 2 wk). Monitor every 4–6 wk to assess scar formation.	Sunburn erythema should be markedly reduced by 48 h. Peeling is normal. In partial-thickness burns, when healing is complete, the wound appears pink or red with tiny opalescent islands of epithelium throughout and no secretions.	Patients require further assessment and/or treatment if healing is not complete within 7 days or if there is a significant risk or sign of scarring.
Itching	Monitor every 4–6 h for itching on a daily basis for 5–7 days. Consider oral antihistamines for itching not responding to supportive measures such as moisturizing lotions, cool compresses or bathing.	Itching does not interfere with sleep or normal activities.	If itching does not respond to oral diphenhydramine or appears to worsen despite treatment, patient requires further assessment and/or treatment.
Infection (swelling; surrounding redness that is tender to touch; red streaks from the wound; pus; fever; swollen or tender lumps in the groin or armpit)	Monitor daily at each dressing change for signs of infection.	No signs or symptoms of infection noted before healing is complete. Risk is low after this point.	If signs and symptoms of infection are observed at the burn site, patient requires further assessment and/or treatment.

Figure 1: **Assessment of Patients with Burns**

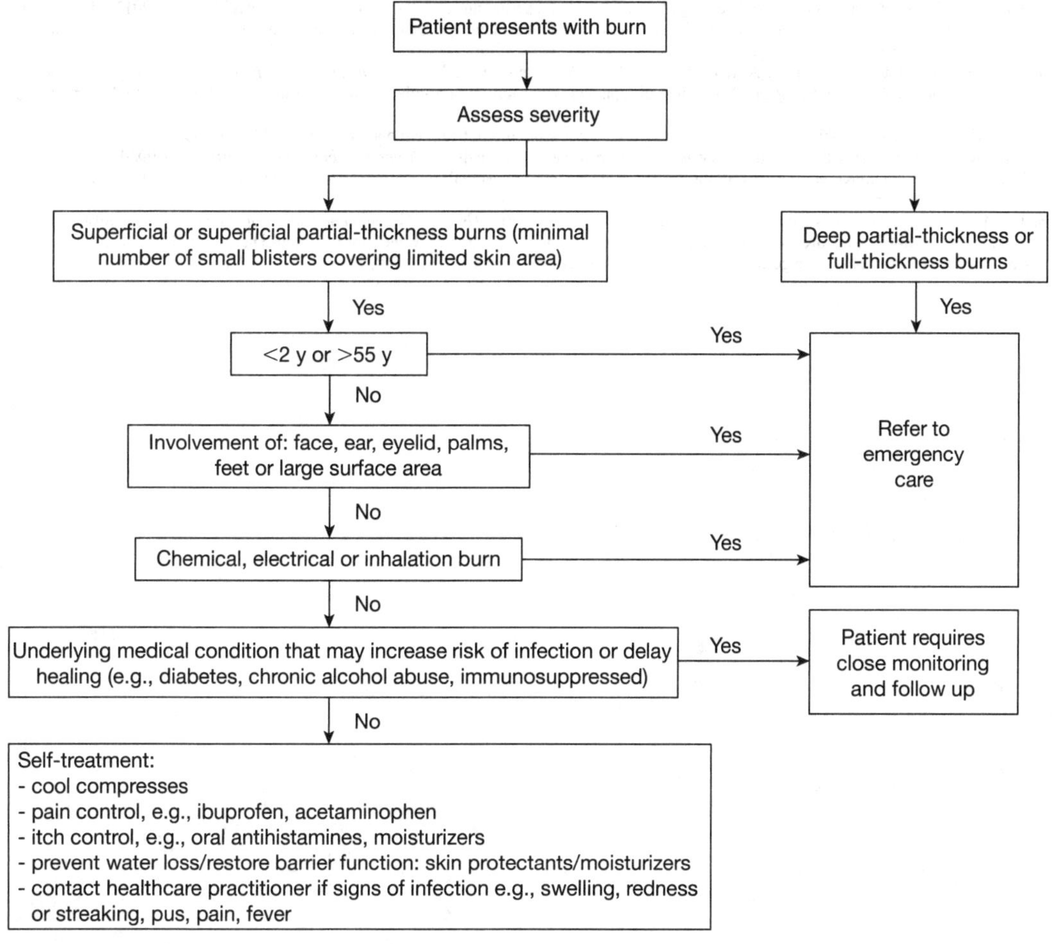

Suggested Readings

Health Canada. Clinical Practice Guidelines for Nurses in Primary Care. Adult care—Chapter 9—Skin. *Dermatological emergencies. Skin wounds*. Available from: www.hc-sc.gc.ca/fniah-spnia/services/nurs-infirm/clini/adult/skin-peau-eng.php.

References

1. Clayton MC, Solem LD. No ice, no butter. Advice on management of burns for primary care physicians. *Postgrad Med* 1995;97:151-5,159-60,165.
2. Morgan ED, Bledsoe SC, Barker J. Ambulatory management of burns. *Am Fam Physician* 2000;62:2015-26, 2029-30, 2032.
3. Enoch S, Roshan A, Shah M. Emergency and early management of burns and scalds. *BMJ* 2009;338:b1037.
4. NSW Ministry of Health; Agency for Clinical Innovation. Connolly S. *Clinical practice guidelines: burn patient management*. Chatswood: ACI; 2011. Available from: www.aci.health.nsw.gov.au/__data/assets/pdf_file/0019/162631/Clinical_Practice_Guidelines_2012.pdf. Accessed March 8, 2016.
5. Health Canada. Clinical Practice Guidelines for Nurses in Primary Care. Adult care—Chapter 9—Skin. *Dermatological emergencies. Skin wounds*. Available from: www.hc-sc.gc.ca/fniah-spnia/services/nurs-infirm/clini/adult/skin-peau-eng.php. Accessed March 8, 2016.
6. Baker M. Burns: classification and community management. *InnovAiT* 2012;5:520-6. Available from: ino.sagepub.com/content/5/9/520.full.pdf+html. Accessed March 8, 2016.

7. The Global Evidence Mapping Initiative. Early cooling of burns: evidence summary. Australasian Cochrane Centre. Available at: http://www.alfred.org.au/Assets/Files/Burns%20Cooling%20Summary.pdf. Accessed April 29, 2016.
8. Wasiak J, Cleland H, Campbell F et al. Dressings for superficial and partial thickness burns. *Cochrane Database Syst Rev* 2013;3:CD002106.
9. Rosanova M, Stamboulian D, Lede R. Systematic review: which topical agent is more efficacious in the prevention of infections in burn patients? *Arch Argent Pediatr* 2012;110:298-303.
10. Victorian Adult Burns Service at the Alfred (Australia). Burns Management Guidelines. *Management of a patient with a minor burn injury.* Available from: www.vicburns.org.au/management-of-a-patient-with-a-minor-burn-injury/minimising-infection.html. Accessed March 8, 2016.
11. Zachariah JR, Rao AL, Prabha R et al. Post burn pruritus: a review of current treatment options. *Burns* 2014;38:621-9.
12. Jull AB, Cullum N, Dumville JC et al. Honey as a topical treatment for wounds. *Cochrane Database Syst Rev* 2015;3:CD005083.
13. Dat AD, Poon F, Pham KB et al. Aloe vera for treating acute and chronic wounds. *Cochrane Database Syst Rev* 2012;2:CD008762.
14. Combest WL. Aloe vera. *US Pharm* 2000;25:64-74.
15. Part 4. Active vaccines. In: National Advisory Committee on Immunization (NACI). *Canadian immunization guide*. 7th ed. Ottawa: Public Health Agency of Canada, Infectious Disease and Emergency Preparedness Branch, Centre for Infectious Disease and Control; 2006. Available from: www.phac-aspc.gc.ca/publicat/cig-gci/p04-tet-eng.php. Accessed March 8, 2016.

Burns—What You Need to Know

When should you see a healthcare provider?

See a healthcare provider for **all** of the following kinds of burns:

- Burns in thin skin areas (e.g., inner surface of arm, groin area, face), particularly if there are blisters.
- Burns to children less than 2 years or adults older than 55 years. The skin tends to be thinner in both these groups and a burn may be more serious than it originally appears.
- Burns to people who have conditions that increase the chance of infection or slow healing times (e.g., diabetes, chronic alcohol abuse, those on chemotherapy agents, HIV treatment).
- Electrical burns, inhalation and chemical burns as the burn may be more severe than appears on the surface.
- Burns where the pain is not controlled with cooling or appropriate doses of nonprescription pain relievers.

The only types of burns that are self-treatable are sunburns and minor burns that look like sunburns (red, painful, no blisters or small blisters in only a few areas).

First Aid for Burns

- Carefully remove clothing that is burnt, hot or contaminated by chemicals. Remove jewelry from the affected area.
- **Cool the burn**—this is the most important first aid measure.
  - Use water that is cool to your skin but not cold. **Do not use ice (risk of frostbite).**
  - Hold the burned area under cool running tap water (medium force) or in a clean container filled with cool tap water for at least 20 minutes.
  - If it is not possible to place the burned area under cool running water, apply a cloth or sterile gauze pad soaked in cool tap water for 15–30 minutes at a time.
  - If it is deemed necessary to seek medical attention, a clean piece of plastic cling wrap can be applied to the area until arrival. This will keep the area clean and does not stick to the wound.
- **Do not** use butter, grease, powder or other home remedies on a burn. These products could make it worse and increase the risk of infection.
- **Do not** try to neutralize chemical burns by putting a different kind of chemical on the burn. This could make it worse by causing further damage to the tissue.

Follow-up Treatment

- Minor burns are often painful. Cooling with tap water helps relieve the pain for short periods of time. Pain relievers such as acetaminophen or ibuprofen can help to relieve the pain for longer periods of time. **Do not** use ASA (also known as Aspirin) for burns as these products may delay healing.
- Minor burns are sometimes itchy. Avoid scratching as this can lead to open areas and increase the risk of infection. Apply moisturizing creams often to keep the area moist and relieve some of the dryness that may lead to itching. If a moisturizing cream is not relieving the itching, products containing pramoxine with some menthol or camphor for cooling may be helpful. An oral antihistamine (e.g., diphenhydramine, cetirizine) can be used for more severe itching that is affecting sleep patterns.

- For minor burns where the skin is not broken:
  - It is not necessary to apply a gauze bandage or antibiotic cream to minor burns.
  - Minor burns will usually heal in 3–6 days. Peeling is normal.
- Burned areas will be more sensitive to sunlight for up to 1 year, so it is important to wear a sunscreen with an SPF of at least 30.
- For burns where the skin is broken:
  - The risk of infection increases if the skin is broken (examples—deeper burns, blisters that break, scratching itchy burns)
  - The area should immediately be cleaned gently with tap water and mild soap. Cover the burn loosely with a sterile bandage or sterile gauze dressing
  - The bandage or dressing should be changed every day until the area is dry. Clean the area gently with tap water and mild soap each time the dressing is changed
  - Seek medical attention if any signs of infection are observed.
    Watch for:
    - an increase in redness, swelling and tenderness at the site
    - yellowish discharge (pus)
    - fever and tender lumps in the armpit or groin.

Chapter 58
Dandruff and Seborrheic Dermatitis

Debra Sibbald, BScPhm, ACPR, MA (Adult Education), PhD (Education)

Pathophysiology

Dandruff and seborrheic dermatitis are papulosquamous cutaneous disorders, which are the most commonly encountered group of skin problems. They are characterized by palpable, usually erythematous, eruptions that typically all have a variable degree of scaling.[1] They may be difficult to distinguish from one another.

Seborrheic dermatitis and dandruff (pityriasis simplex capitis) are manifestations of different severities of a similar origin. Both cause scaling on the scalp often associated with itching. Dandruff is a noninflammatory form with increased desquamation. Seborrheic dermatitis is an inflammatory erythematous and scaling eruption primarily in "seborrheic areas", those with high numbers of sebaceous glands—scalp, face and upper trunk.

Uncommon in childhood, dandruff usually begins between ages 10 and 20 years, and affects up to 40% of men and women over age 30.[2] It is primarily a cosmetic problem. Turnover rate of skin cells may be twice the normal rate. It is associated with a dry environment but *Malassezia* yeast may be present in some cases and play an inflammatory role. Although a relatively stable condition, it may be exacerbated by poor hygiene or a dry winter environment.

Seborrheic dermatitis is found in about 3% of the population, affecting persons of all ages.[2] Both infantile and adult forms exist. Flares occur when sebaceous glands are most active (first 3 months of life and after puberty). The adult form, which is chronic, usually occurs between 30 and 50 years of age. A male predominance is seen at all ages, regardless of race, probably because androgens control sebaceous gland activity. In adolescents and adults, it is commonly manifested as "dandruff" or as an erythema of the nasolabial folds, ranging in intensity from barely perceptible to marked, waxing and waning from the teens throughout adulthood.[3] It may be a cutaneous marker of HIV and AIDS, especially when severe, atypical or therapy-resistant. The incidence in patients with HIV may be as high as 85%.[4]

Despite its frequency, considerable controversy exists regarding the pathogenesis of seborrheic dermatitis. Some postulate that it is a fungal disease caused by the lipophilic *Malassezia* yeasts, based on the observation of their presence in affected skin and the therapeutic response to antifungal agents. Others propose that *Malassezia* infection is secondary to a primary inflammatory dermatosis that results in increased cell turnover, scaling and inflammation in the epidermis (similar to psoriasis). It also has been traditionally considered to be a form of dermatitis because *Malassezia* is present in healthy skin, the pathogenic mycelial form of *Malassezia* yeasts is absent, and it has a chronic course. In addition, the lipase activity of *Malassezia* produces free fatty acids and reactive oxygen radicals which have antibacterial activity that alters the normal skin flora, contributing to dermatitis. As a result of these theories, proposed treatments vary, ranging from topical antifungals and antimicrobial peptides to topical corticosteroids and calcineurin inhibitors.[5]

Other factors contribute to the uncertainty around the etiology of seborrheic dermatitis. Though sebaceous glands are more active at the times of life that seborrheic dermatitis presents (neonatal and postpubertal periods), there is no direct relationship between the amount or composition of sebum and the condition.[6] Hormonal factors have also been implicated. The occurrence of seborrheic dermatitis in the neonatal period and remission by 6–12 months suggests a response to maternal androgen stimulation; recurrence postpuberty is further evidence of a response to androgen stimulation.[4] Atmospheric humidity and stress play a role as triggers.

Goals of Therapy

Dandruff:

- Reduce or eliminate scales (dry flakes of skin) and flaking
- Prevent recurrence by improving scalp hygiene
- Eliminate or reduce environmental triggers

Seborrheic dermatitis:

- Control not cure
- Reduce fungus and the resulting scaling and inflammation
- Relieve symptoms such as pruritus
- Educate on the importance of control through good hygiene
- Eliminate or reduce environmental triggers

Patient Assessment

A systematic approach to the assessment of dandruff and seborrheic dermatitis consists of assessing a patient's signs, symptoms and history for the following:

- Onset, frequency and duration of symptoms
- Area and extent of involvement
- Associated systemic symptoms
- Aggravating factors
- Description of skin lesions
- Attempted treatments

Ensure further assessment if the diagnosis is in doubt, if there is sudden onset in a young patient in which HIV is suspected or if the patient is not responding to treatment. Patients should also be appropriately assessed if the condition is widespread or generalized.[4]

Symptoms of Dandruff and Seborrheic Dermatitis

Lesions of seborrheic dermatitis and dandruff are often asymptomatic with a mild clinical course. Variations in the intensity of episodes are common and may be precipitated by tiredness, stress or cold weather. In seborrheic dermatitis, pruritus varies, being common in scalp and ear canal involvement, and may be intense. Dandruff is usually asymptomatic, although itching may develop.

Signs of Dandruff

Dandruff results in increased shedding of small flakes of scale from an otherwise normal scalp showing minimal erythema with no or limited inflammation. The scales are silver-grey, in patches or diffuse, and may separate fully or become detached only after combing. It is usually symmetrical, and absent in the bald area of male pattern baldness. There is no evidence of other skin disease on the scalp or elsewhere.[2,7,8] Dandruff does not present with scalp erythema. The characteristic scales are easy to diagnose yet often confused with other scaling conditions of the scalp such as seborrheic dermatitis, tinea capitis and psoriasis.[2]

Signs of Seborrheic Dermatitis

Seborrheic dermatitis is an inflammatory, erythematous, greasy, scaling eruption often confused with dandruff (see Seborrheic Dermatitis in Photo Section). It is characterized by sharply demarcated yellow to brown, greasy or bran-like scaling patches and plaques. In adolescents and adults, seborrheic dermatitis typically affects symmetric areas of the skin rich in sebaceous glands, including hairy areas of the head, such as scalp, scalp margin, eyebrows, eyelashes, mustache and beard. Other common sites are the forehead, nasolabial folds, external ear canals and postauricular creases. Seborrheic dermatitis of the trunk may appear in the presternal area and in infants, in body folds, including the axillae, navel, groin, inframammary and anogenital areas.[4]

Seborrheic dermatitis typically presents as mild, greasy scales on the scalp that may be thick and may accumulate, with erythematous plaques and scaling of the nasolabial folds, behind the ears and elsewhere. The borders of erythema and scaling may be seen at or beyond the frontal hairline. It begins in small patches, rapidly spreading, with diffuse fine scales that can be white, off-white or yellow, with no signs of acute dermatitis, such as oozing or weeping.[9] Exudation may be seen in facial seborrheic dermatitis from time to time. It typically flares and resolves in a cyclic or seasonal fashion, often in response to stress.[1]

Profuse powdery scales of the eyebrows may compromise wearing of contact lenses. The eyelids alone may be affected, developing honey-coloured crusting called marginal blepharitis. There is erythema and scaling of eyelid margins and cilia, often associated with mild granular conjunctivitis or ocular irritation. Involvement in other sites may not be present. Marginal blepharitis may also be associated with ocular rosacea.

Paranasal involvement is typically seen in young women, who may not have dandruff. The most common type of facial seborrheic dermatitis in males is a follicular erythematous form involving the upper lip, beard, scalp, back, flanks and abdomen. Plaques may present with thick, adherent silvery scales (as seen with psoriasis) which usually spare the face, called sebopsoriasis.[1] Ear involvement may complicate otitis externa. On the trunk, 2 forms may appear—follicular (more common) or macular (rare).

In infants, the entire scalp may be covered with thick, dry, adherent, yellowish-brown scales overlying erythema, often called "cradle cap". It may also involve the central face, forehead and ears. A widespread erythema with cheesy exudate sometimes presents in the flexural folds, manifesting as diaper dermatitis in infants or an intertriginous genital eruption in adults. These may generalize.[9] Cradle cap is self-limiting, appears in the first to fourth week and usually disappears after the first 3 months of life.

In both children and adults, persistent generalized seborrheic dermatitis may be associated with HIV infection. There is a predominance of inflammatory and hyperkeratotic lesions, with involvement of trunk, groin and extremities, and occasionally erythroderma, alopecia and hyper- or hypopigmentation.[9]

In chronic cases, nonscarring alopecia may occur secondary to inflammation and scratching. This alopecia should be reversible with treatment.[6]

Failure to respond to therapy may indicate coexisting diseases such as fungal infections, psoriasis or HIV infection.

Scalp seborrheic dermatitis must be distinguished from atopic dermatitis, tinea capitis and psoriasis. Atopic dermatitis in adults tends to affect the antecubital (inner elbow) and popliteal (behind the knee) fossae. In infants, atopic dermatitis has the same sites of predilection as seborrheic dermatitis: face, diaper areas and extensor limbs. Seborrheic dermatitis may present with axillary involvement, lack of scratching and absence of oozing and weeping. The distinction between seborrheic dermatitis and psoriasis may be clarified by psoriasiform lesions elsewhere on the body or pitting of the nails. Facial seborrheic dermatitis can be confused with rosacea, which displays central facial erythema, or forehead only, or with systemic lupus erythematosus which exhibits a butterfly-like rash. Seborrheic dermatitis of the groin may resemble dermatophytosis, psoriasis and candidiasis, but tends to be bilaterally symmetric, with reddish-brown patches that respond quickly to therapy. A very rare condition confused with seborrheic dermatitis in infants is histiocytosis X, associated with systemic signs such as fever.[9]

Seborrheic Dermatitis: Risk and Aggravating Factors

Incidence of extensive and severe seborrheic dermatitis is significantly increased (30–83%) in HIV-positive patients and patients with AIDS. They are more prone to an atypical explosive onset of seborrheic dermatitis, with more severe and generalized involvement.

Patients with CNS disorders (e.g., Parkinson's disease, cranial nerve palsies, major truncal paralyses) also appear to be prone to the development of seborrheic dermatitis, tend to develop more extensive disease and are frequently refractory to treatment. Sebum excretion may be increased secondary to either overactivity of the parasympathetic nervous system or action of androgens or melanocyte-stimulating hormone.[6]

Other diseases associated with seborrheic dermatitis include depression, mood disorders and pityriasis versicolor.[6]

Areas of increased skin temperature on facial skin are sites predisposed to seborrheic dermatitis.[6]

Genetics, as well as other comorbid diseases, may predispose specific populations to seborrheic dermatitis, and an increased incidence of allergy within the family is usually present.[6]

Environmental factors such as low humidity and temperature, as well as stress, may provoke flares of seborrheic dermatitis.[1] Bright light suppresses melatonin while UVA and UVB light inhibit the growth of *Malassezia restricta*; many patients report improvement in seborrheic dermatitis during the summer.[10]

Drug-induced Seborrheic Dermatitis

A number of drugs have been implicated in causing or aggravating seborrheic dermatitis (see Table 1). When deciding whether to discontinue the offending agent, consider individual circumstances such as the severity of the seborrheic dermatitis, the need for the drug, and the availability of alternative medications.

Table 1: **Drugs Known to Trigger Seborrheic Dermatitis**[11,12,13,14]

Arsenic	Danazol	Lithium	Stanozolol[a]
Auranofin	Ethionamide	Methyldopa	Thiothixene
Aurothioglucose	Gold	Methoxsalen[a]	Trioxsalen[a]
Buspirone	Griseofulvin[a]	Penicillamine	
Chlorpromazine	Haloperidol	Phenothiazines	
Cimetidine	Interferon, alfa	Psoralens	

[a] This medication is not currently marketed in Canada.

Differential Diagnosis

A summary of differential diagnosis and management of dandruff and seborrheic dermatitis is provided in Table 2.

Table 2: Characteristics, Differential Diagnosis and Management of Dandruff and Seborrheic Dermatitis

Condition	Form	Characteristics	Differential Diagnosis	Action
Dandruff	Scalp	Dry, white scales scattered diffusely over scalp	Seborrheic dermatitis Psoriasis; see Chapter 71: Psoriasis Atopic dermatitis; see Chapter 55: Atopic, Contact, and Stasis Dermatitis Tinea capitis; see Chapter 65: Fungal Skin Infections	Self-care management.
Seborrheic Dermatitis	Scalp	Greasy, yellowish scales over erythematous patches	Dandruff Psoriasis; see Chapter 71: Psoriasis Atopic dermatitis; see Chapter 55: Atopic, Contact, and Stasis Dermatitis Tinea capitis; see Chapter 65: Fungal Skin Infections	Self-care management. Requires further assessement by appropriate healthcare practitioner if moderate to severe.
	Facial	Greasy, yellowish scales over erythematous patches, involvement of nasolabial folds, eyebrows, eyelashes, lips, retroauricular areas	Atopic dermatitis (infants); see Chapter 55: Atopic, Contact, and Stasis Dermatitis Rosacea; see Chapter 54: Acne Systemic lupus erythematosus Contact dermatitis; see Chapter 55: Atopic, Contact, and Stasis Dermatitis	Requires further assessement by appropriate healthcare practitioner.
	Groin	Bilaterally symmetric, with reddish-brown fine scaling patches	Atopic dermatitis (infants); see Chapter 55: Atopic, Contact, and Stasis Dermatitis Dermatophytosis; see Chapter 65: Fungal Skin Infections Psoriasis; see Chapter 71: Psoriasis Candidiasis; see Chapter 65: Fungal Skin Infections	Requires further assessement by appropriate healthcare practitioner.

Dandruff and seborrheic dermatitis are often confused with psoriasis, especially when present on the scalp. Table 3 clarifies the differences among the 3 conditions.

Nonpharmacologic Therapy

Infantile seborrheic dermatitis (cradle cap) is self-limiting and a conservative approach should be taken. A mild, nonmedicated shampoo should be used initially for frequent washing. Scales may be softened with a surfactant-containing bath oil, gently brushed free with a baby brush and washed clear. In scale removal, it is important to avoid irritation with strong shampoos or mechanical measures. Cradle cap responds well to the use of emollients and moisturizers. One study showed that a nonmedicated topical cream or placebo cream applied twice daily for up to 14 days were equally effective in reducing erythema crusting, scaling and oiliness.[15] Infants do not respond to dietary avoidance or vitamin supplementation.

Table 3: **Comparative Features of Dandruff, Seborrheic Dermatitis and Psoriasis**

Feature	Dandruff	Seborrheic Dermatitis	Psoriasis
Lesions	On nonerythematous base with fine, diffuse scales	Erythema with mild greasy yellow scales, plaques with indistinct margins	Annular well-demarcated silvery, scaly plaques, with erythematous base; bleed easily
Common sites	Scalp	Central face, scalp, mid-chest	Scalp, elbows, knees, sacrum
Palms and soles	No	No	Common
Nails	No	No	Pitting, thickening, dystrophy
Hair and scalp	Yes	Yes; hair may thin	Thick scales common
Intertrigo (skin fold involvement)	No	Inverse type, glans penis, mostly infants	Common
Pruritus	Due to dryness	Varies; more common with involvement of scalp or ear canal	Sometimes
Associated systemic symptoms	None	May generalize in infants; worse in patients with HIV infection	May generalize; psoriatic arthritis

Eyelids affected with seborrheic blepharitis can be treated with warm to hot compresses and washing with baby shampoo, followed by gentle cotton tip debridement of thick scales.

Patients may also cut their hair shorter or trim their beards to decrease symptoms.[16]

Dandruff may improve in a moist environment. Stop use of hair sprays and pomades. Encourage use of a cool air humidifier.

For adult seborrheic dermatitis, the first steps are to discontinue aggravating factors and control stress. Seborrheic dermatitis often improves in the summer months and in sunlight.[16] Irritating soaps, heavy gels, hairsprays and greasy creams should be avoided. Excessive hot water may dry out the skin. Dry air can provoke symptoms; placing a cool air humidifier or dish of water in the room adds moisture to the environment.[17]

Nonmedicated shampoos: The main measure to remove scales and ease itching in dandruff or seborrheic dermatitis is frequent cleansing with a nonmedicated, nonresidue shampoo (preferably one indicated for dry hair) and rinsing thoroughly to remove dirt, oil and scales. Frequent shampooing is key to controlling symptoms while contributing to the cosmetic appearance of hair. Patients should use a nonmedicated shampoo at least 3 times weekly. Even more frequent shampooing or a longer period of lathering may also be helpful in the case of dandruff. Shampoos with surfactants (e.g., sodium lauryl sulfate) and detergents are better able to remove unsightly scales and will lead to clinical improvement and decreased scaling.[18] Frequency of shampooing can be decreased or increased according to response. Once-weekly shampooing may be more reasonable for institutionalized patients.[4] Patients who develop itching may decrease shampooing due to the drying effects. Decreased frequency of shampooing can lead to further scale accumulation. The shampoo vehicle is important for both nonmedicated cleansing products and medicated shampoos. The effect of the vehicle on appearance of the hair affects adherence in the treatment of dandruff or seborrheic dermatitis.[19]

Pharmacologic Therapy

For comparative ingredients of nonprescription products, consult the *Compendium of Products for Minor Ailments*—Skin Care Products: Acne, Dandruff and Seborrheic Dermatitis, and Dermatitis and Dry Skin.

General Use of Medicated Shampoos

To ensure adherence, the shampoo has to be both highly effective and cosmetically appealing. Effective therapies are based on antifungal action, with associated anti-inflammatory and keratolytic action. Antiseptic activity is less important.[7] Various regimens are recommended (see Table 5).

Shampoos may be used on the scalp, beard and chest but may flare the disease if used on the face or other intertrigious areas if left on for extended periods. To be effective, the shampoo must be massaged into the scalp for 4–5 minutes, rinsed thoroughly and repeated. Instruct patients to part their hair in small sections, and apply and massage the medicated shampoo or scalp treatment into the scalp at the hair roots. This should be repeated until the entire scalp has been treated. Medicated therapies should be left in contact with the scalp or beard for 2–20 minutes depending on the product. For more severe cases, therapies can be left on overnight under a shower cap, to allow the treatment to interact with the skin of the scalp. Moisturizing, nonmedicated shampoos or conditioners can be used afterward to prevent desiccation of the hair.[4]

If the scalp is covered with diffuse, dense scales, the scales may be removed prior to using a medicated shampoo by applying warm oil (**mineral** or **olive**), or a more easily rinsed surfactant-containing bath oil, to the scalp for several hours or overnight and then rinsing.[4]

Antifungals

Antifungal agents that decrease colonization by lipophilic yeasts (*Malassezia* species) are effective in the treatment of dandruff and seborrheic dermatitis and are generally considered first-line therapy in both conditions. Seborrheic dermatitis in adults tends to be chronic and recurrent. Treatment is directed toward control rather than cure. Seborrheic dermatitis tends to relapse after 2–3 weeks if treatments are not carried out repetitively. This reflects the slow proliferation rate of *Malassezia*. Shampoos are used if scalp is affected and creams or lotions for face, ears and trunk. Treatment effect of antifungals on overall quality of life remains unknown. Better study design, outcome measures, and reporting are needed to improve the evidence base for antifungal treatment of seborrheic dermatitis.[20]

Topical **ketoconazole** is the most widely studied azole against *Malassezia*; however, other azoles have been used with success.[21] Very few studies of antifungals have assessed symptom clearance for longer than 4 weeks. At therapeutic concentrations, ketoconazole is fungistatic.[22] As a cytostatic, it also slows cell turnover.[16] Approximately 80% of patients show good response within 4 weeks. Topical ketoconazole causes fewer side effects than topical corticosteroid treatment.[20] Long-term safety is favourable with chronic use and efficacy is maintained.

Ciclopirox olamine has demonstrated similar efficacy to ketoconazole and can be used as an alternative treatment.[20,23] Various concentrations of **ciclopirox olamine** shampoo or gel are effective (1% is optimal) and safe in the treatment of seborrheic dermatitis of the scalp, alone or in combination with **zinc pyrithione**.[24,25,26,27]

Selenium sulfide is fungicidal against numerous strains of *Malassezia*[28] and may have fungistatic action on the scalp.[3] It is classified as a keratolytic by the FDA and slows scale production and epidermal proliferation. Although the use of selenium sulfide 2.5% suspension in seborrheic dermatitis of the scalp has improved dandruff, folliculitis, pain and dryness, symptoms recur in more than 50% of patients after stopping treatment.[29] It should be used no more than twice weekly, as excessive use could cause oily hair and hair loss.[3] It is more effective with longer contact time. Mild cases of scalp seborrheic dermatitis may be controlled with selenium sulfide alone. It is also used in combination with other topical therapy.

Zinc pyrithione has a somewhat similar mechanism of action to selenium sulfide. It has cytostatic properties and is classified as keratolytic, but it also affects membrane transport, macromolecular synthesis, cell structure and function.[30] It reduces counts of *Malassezia*.[3,7] Weekly shampooing with zinc pyrithione 1% significantly reduced dandruff in one study, but resolution of symptoms was not complete after 9 treatments.[7] Response rates may decrease over time, but this is due to nonadherence rather than tachyphylaxis.[31] Zinc pyrithione shampoo significantly returned stratum corneum ultrastructure to normal, suggesting it can control dandruff.[32] Like selenium sulfide, it is more effective with longer contact time and may be effective alone for mild cases of scalp seborrheic dermatitis, but is also used in combination with other topical therapy.

Propylene glycol 15% solution applied to the scalp reduces the numbers of yeast and, as a result of its hygroscopic effects, improves seborrheic dermatitis in 90% of treated patients. It is commercially available or can be compounded.[33]

Many other topical antifungals have been used with varying success. These include clotrimazole, fluconazole, miconazole and itraconazole.[20]

Oral antifungals are reserved for severe or refractory cases due to increased risk of side effects and drug interactions. Various medications have been studied including fluconazole, itraconazole, ketoconazole and terbinafine. Ketoconazole therapy was associated with more relapses compared with other treatments in one systematic review.[34] Pulsed dosing of itraconazole (200 mg/day for 2 consecutive days/month) showed significantly higher efficacy and lower recurrence rates over 4 months compared with placebo in patients with moderate to severe seborrheic dermatitis.[35] Other evidence is generally of low quality and reported clinical efficacy varies considerably among studies.

Anti-inflammatory Agents

Topical corticosteroids area also effective for decreasing the symptoms of seborrheic dermatitis[36] and dandruff as they reduce pruritus and inflammation. They may be added to antifungal treatment if the response is not adequate or the lesions are extensive or severe. Topical corticosteroids are intended for temporary use. They should be discontinued when itching and erythema resolve, and maintenance therapy with antifungals should then be adequate.[4] Low-potency corticosteroids such as **hydrocortisone** 1% should be used on the face or folds. Stronger topical corticosteroids may be used on other body areas if the response to hydrocortisone is insufficient. Severe and thick scales on the scalp can respond to overnight application of topical corticosteroids followed by shower cap occlusion. Long-term use of potent agents is discouraged for controlling seborrheic dermatitis as relapse rates are often high[37] and their use may lead to undesirable side effects such as atrophy, telangiectasia, poor wound healing, perioral dermatitis and pustular acne. The form of topical corticosteroid selected is determined by the patient and the treatment site. Ointments, due to their occlusive nature, are preferred for use on areas that are resistant to absorption or are dry or scaly. Avoid ointments if acne is present. Creams are used in moist areas due to their drying effect, while lotions and solutions are best for the scalp and hairy areas or for large areas that require a minimal application. The potency of the same corticosteroid is affected by the vehicle: ointment>cream>lotion.[4] For more information on the effect of vehicles, see Chapter 55: Atopic, Contact, and Stasis Dermatitis and Chapter 71: Psoriasis. In severe cases, keratolytics such as salicylic acid or coal tar preparations may be used to remove dense scales, before applying topical corticosteroids.

Ocular corticosteroids should be avoided in seborrheic blepharitis.

Topical calcineurin inhibitors are immunomodulators used in the treatment of seborrheic dermatitis as second-line agents. **Tacrolimus** and **pimecrolimus** have anti-inflammatory activity and tacrolimus has also demonstrated antifungal properties. These agents have efficacy comparable to standard antifungal and topical corticosteroid treatments in decreasing severity of erythema, scaling and pruritus.[38] Tacrolimus ointment and pimecrolimus cream lack the side effects associated with corticosteroid use and require significantly fewer applications to achieve comparable clinical response in adults with facial seborrheic dermatitis.[39] They have also been used in combination with topical corticosteroids.[40,41,42,43] There is some evidence that intermittent (e.g., twice-weekly) use may maintain remission in facial seborrheic dermatitis.[44] Topical tacrolimus used together with zinc pyrithione may be an alternative to topical corticosteroids in treating scalp seborrheic dermatitis.[45] Concerns of a link between use of topical calcineurin inhibitors and malignancy have not been substantiated by available evidence.[35]

Topical tacrolimus ointment and pimecrolimus cream are alternatives to topical corticosteroids in the treatment of seborrheic blepharitis. Use of topical calcineurin inhibitors on the eyelids has an established long-term safety profile. Tacrolimus ointment is reportedly more effective and better tolerated than pimecrolimus cream. Additional studies are needed to address the efficacy of calcineurin inhibitors compared with topical corticosteroids.[46]

Keratolytic Agents

Traditionally, keratolytics have been used for dandruff and seborrheic dermatitis. Current mainstays of therapy are antifungals for dandruff and antifungals plus anti-inflammatories for seborrheic dermatitis; however, keratolytics may be added on to other topical therapy if the response has been inadequate. Their keratolytic effect may also increase penetration of other topical medications and lead to increased effectiveness.

Salicylic acid and **sulfur** have minimal proven antifungal activity but are mildly effective because of their keratolytic and antiseptic activities. They are used alone or combined with other active ingredients. **Salicylic acid** provides a keratolytic effect by loosening the bonds between keratinocytes in the skin, which helps detach flakes and increases the penetration of other drugs.[1,7] **Sulfur** exhibits antifungal, antibacterial and keratolytic activity.[32] Products containing salicylic acid *and* sulfur are more potent, but are proportionally more irritating and therefore proper use is important.[3] Bar, cleansing lotion and shampoo forms include salicylic acid 2–3% and sulfur 3–5%. All products should be lathered into the scalp with continued rubbing for at least 5 minutes, and then rinsed thoroughly. Young children may be at more risk of unwanted side effects because of increased absorption of salicylic acid through the skin. Salicylic acid should not be applied to large areas of the body or used for long periods of time in this population.[18] Discontinue other drying preparations such as cosmetics, soaps or alcohol-containing products. Generally, products containing salicylic acid and sulfur should be used no more than twice a week.

Coal tar is mildly effective for seborrheic dermatitis because it reduces local swelling and inflammation, relieves itching and is keratolytic and antiseptic. However, it has minimal antifungal activity, making it a poor alternative to anti-*Malassezia* agents.[7] Coal tar reduces cell proliferation and requires time to lengthen cell differentiation and normalize epidermal differentiation, resulting in a slow decline in visible scales. It is available in shampoo, ointment, lotion, gel and bath forms that are used once daily to once weekly on the beard, face, body or scalp. Avoid the eye area to prevent irritation and apply a sunblock when outdoors. Irritation generally subsides following discontinuation or when the frequency of use is reduced. Coal tar preparations may also contain alcohol that will cause burning and irritation of acutely inflamed skin. Coal tar products are messy, can stain blond or grey hair and clothing, have an unpleasant odour and can possibly cause tar acne, contact dermatitis[18] and photosensitivity.[17]

Other Treatments

Many other alternative treatments have been used for severe or refractory cases or as novel approaches. Some of these are noted below.

Topical **metronidazole** has been studied vs. placebo or antifungals with mixed results.[47,48,49,50]

Sodium sulfacetamide 10% lotion alone or in combination with a topical corticosteroid has been used in the treatment of seborrheic dermatitis, including seborrheic blepharitis. There are no comparative trials for the use of this agent.[8]

Limited low-quality evidence has shown **lithium gluconate** 8% ointment to be more effective than ketoconazole 2% emulsion for inducing complete remission in seborrheic dermatitis, with comparable safety. Lithium also showed better results on symptoms of burning and dryness. Systemic absorption of topical lithium is low.[36,51,52] This product is not commercially available in Canada but can be compounded. It should be considered a last resort for recalcitrant cases.

Ultraviolet light inhibits *Malassezia* yeasts. Many patients note improvement during the summer months. UVB phototherapy has been shown to be effective in severe seborrheic dermatitis.[53,54] However, some patients have developed seborrheic dermatitis subsequent to psoralens UVA (PUVA) therapy.[6,55] Phototherapy may be ineffective if patients have thick hair.

Other therapies such as nicotinamide 4% cream,[56] a shampoo containing lipohydroxy acid and salicylic acid[57] and a solution containing urea, lactic acid and propylene glycol[58] have shown some efficacy in small preliminary studies.

Comparative Efficacy

Most studies are small and short (4 weeks or less), not appropriately blinded and do not compare more than 1 or 2 ingredients or use controls. They also may restrict area of application to face and scalp or body alone. Outcomes are not similar and do not examine *Malassezia* action as well as short- and long-term clearance. Lack of strong evidence affects recommendations for comparative efficacy. Adequate trials should be more than 200–300 participants; follow-up time should be at least 1 year, and outcomes should be well validated in terms of areas of application.[20,36] Overall, antifungals (particularly ketoconazole and ciclopirox olamine) produce better or equal clinical responses in the treatment of seborrheic dermatitis in the short term compared with other agents and have a specific action against *Malassezia*. From highest to lowest, efficacy of these compounds can be ranked as: 1) antifungals or moderate-potency corticosteroids; 2) hydrocortisone or calcineurin inhibitors; 3) selenium sulfide; 4) zinc pyrithione; 5) keratolytics; and 6) coal tar.[7] Antifungals can be used long term without decreased response whereas topical corticosteroids must be used intermittently in combination with other agents. Calcineurin inhibitors, as second-line agents, can also be used intermittently in combination with other agents for maintenance.

Figure 1 provides a suggested approach for the treatment of dandruff and seborrheic dermatitis of the scalp. Figure 2 provides a suggested approach for the treatment of nonscalp seborrheic dermatitis. See Table 5 for information on therapies for dandruff and seborrheic dermatitis.

Natural Health Products

Evidence showing that natural health products and homeopathic products are efficacious is limited. Further, the use of herbal preparations that are nonstandardized should be discouraged in favour of traditional quality-controlled preparations.[59]

Quassia amara gel 4% has been compared with topical ketoconazole 2% and topical ciclopirox oalamine 1% for facial seborrheic dermatitis with significant advantage in efficacy after 4 weeks.[60]

Heartsease (*Viola tricolor*) and oat straw (*Avenae stramentum*) are herbal formulations that are purported to be effective for mild cases of seborrheic dermatitis. *Viola tricolor* is applied externally as a poultice or in an infusion to the area at a dose of 15 mL TID. *Avenae stramentum* is administered in a bath soak (100 g).

Tea tree oil (*Melaleuca alternifolia*) leaves contain terpinen-4-ol, which has some in vitro activity against *M. furfur*. Solutions of 5–10% are used as external antifungals.[61] Tea tree oil 5% was effective and well tolerated in the treatment of dandruff compared with placebo.[62]

Leaf extract of the plant *Solanum chrysotrichum* possesses biologic activity against dermatophytes and yeast. Various steroidal saponins with antimycotic activity have been isolated from the active extract. Therapeutic effectiveness and tolerability of the standardized extract from *S. chrysotrichum* for local treatment of pityriasis capitis associated with the yeast *Malassezia* showed no significant difference compared with ketoconazole 2%.[63]

Monitoring of Therapy

Table 4 presents a monitoring framework for patients with dandruff and seborrheic dermatitis. The parameters should be monitored by the patient in a diary. Scales will improve quite quickly with cosmetic treatment and hygiene control; thickness of scales will improve more slowly and erythema will take longest to respond.

The side effects of drug therapy should also be monitored. Discontinue therapy if allergic reactions occur. If the condition worsens due to irritation, alter therapy. Failure to meet the end points should result in alteration of dosage or drug therapy. Therapy should be appropriately tapered in response to improvement or resolution.

Table 4: **Monitoring of Therapy for Dandruff and Seborrheic Dermatitis**

Parameter	Timeframe/Degree of Change	Actions[a]
Effectiveness endpoints (resolution/control; relief of symptoms)		
Scales	Decrease by 50% within 7–10 days	Taper therapy in response to resolution: if end points not achieved, consider additional or different therapy.
Thickness of plaque	Decrease by 50% within 6–8 wk and by 75% within 8–12 wk	
Redness	Decrease by 50% within 8–12 wk and by 75% within 12–16 wk	
Surface area involved	Decrease by 50% within 6–8 wk and by 75% within 8–12 wk	
Extension to other sites or generalization	None	
Itch/scratching	Decrease to tolerable level within 1–2 wk	
Disruption of sleep or daily activities	Restoration of normal patterns within 2–3 wk	
Stress, anxiety, depression	Restoration of normal patterns within 2–3 wk	
Progression of severity	No progression of severity	
Recurrent episodes	Lengthening of symptom-free periods throughout therapy	
Safety endpoints (treatment side effects)		
Allergic reactions	None	If they occur, discontinue therapy. If severe, decrease dose, concentration or frequency of use. If still no improvement, consider different therapy.
Severe dryness, irritation (redness, inflammation, stinging)	Minimal Should disappear, diminish or be controlled with continued use	

[a] Advise patients to monitor each parameter daily while on drug therapy. Healthcare practitioners should monitor each parameter after 2–3 wk or at the next visit.

Figure 1: Treatment of Dandruff and Seborrheic Dermatitis of the Scalp

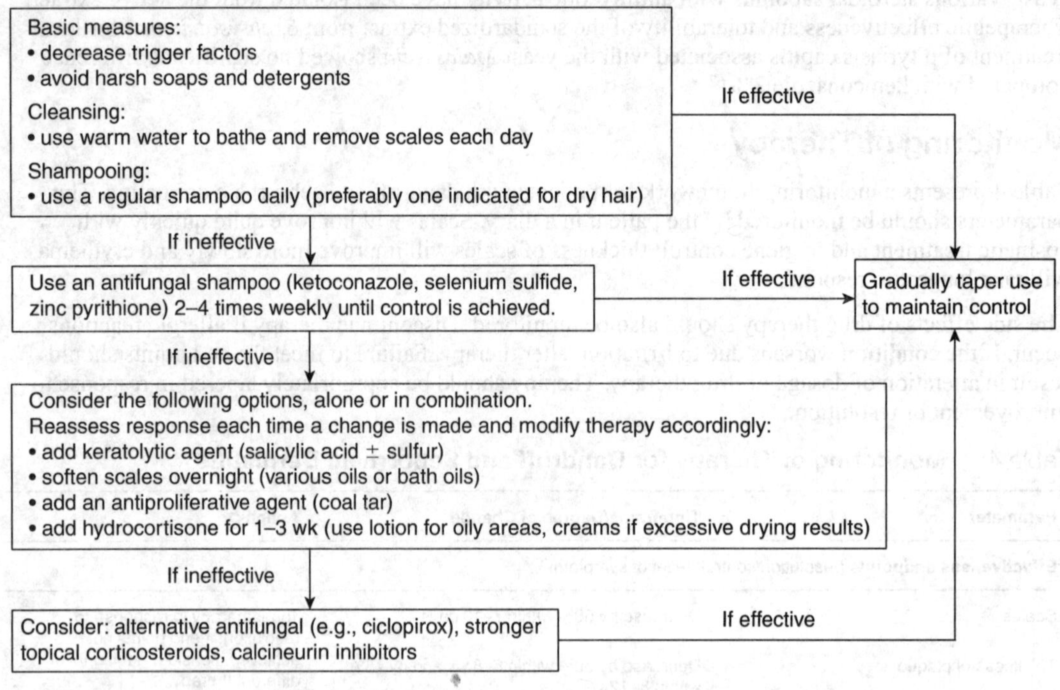

Basic measures:
• decrease trigger factors
• avoid harsh soaps and detergents
Cleansing:
• use warm water to bathe and remove scales each day
Shampooing:
• use a regular shampoo daily (preferably one indicated for dry hair)
If effective
If ineffective
Use an antifungal shampoo (ketoconazole, selenium sulfide, zinc pyrithione) 2–4 times weekly until control is achieved.
If effective
Gradually taper use to maintain control
If ineffective
Consider the following options, alone or in combination.
Reassess response each time a change is made and modify therapy accordingly:
• add keratolytic agent (salicylic acid ± sulfur)
• soften scales overnight (various oils or bath oils)
• add an antiproliferative agent (coal tar)
• add hydrocortisone for 1–3 wk (use lotion for oily areas, creams if excessive drying results)
If ineffective
Consider: alternative antifungal (e.g., ciclopirox), stronger topical corticosteroids, calcineurin inhibitors
If effective

Figure 2: Treatment of Nonscalp Seborrheic Dermatitis

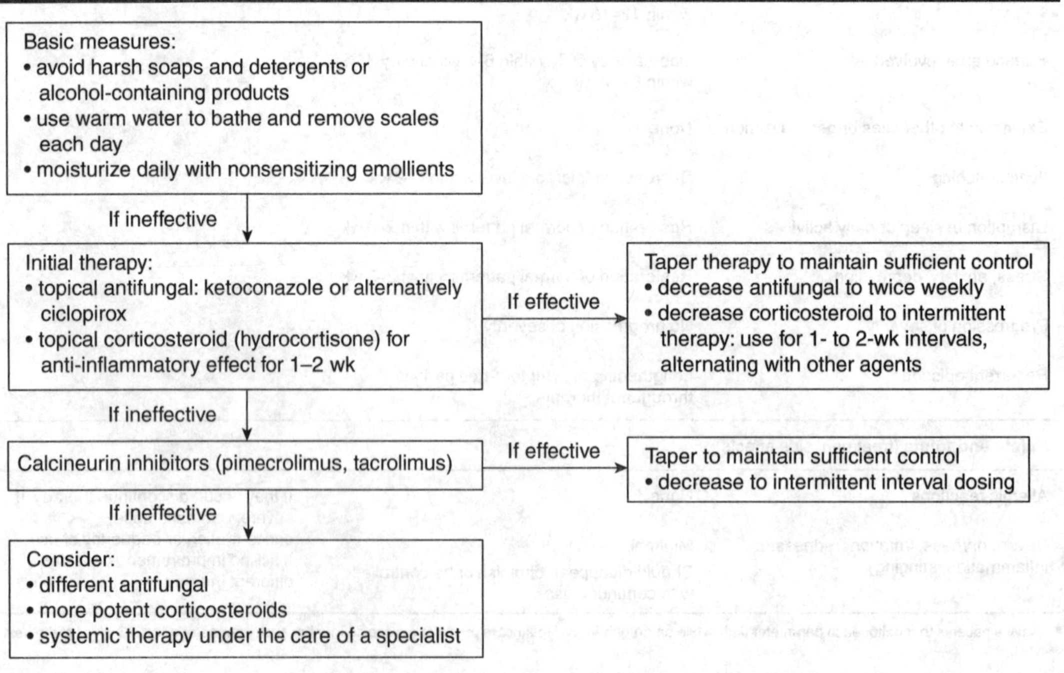

Basic measures:
• avoid harsh soaps and detergents or alcohol-containing products
• use warm water to bathe and remove scales each day
• moisturize daily with nonsensitizing emollients
If ineffective
Initial therapy:
• topical antifungal: ketoconazole or alternatively ciclopirox
• topical corticosteroid (hydrocortisone) for anti-inflammatory effect for 1–2 wk
If effective
Taper therapy to maintain sufficient control
• decrease antifungal to twice weekly
• decrease corticosteroid to intermittent therapy: use for 1- to 2-wk intervals, alternating with other agents
If ineffective
Calcineurin inhibitors (pimecrolimus, tacrolimus)
If effective
Taper to maintain sufficient control
• decrease to intermittent interval dosing
If ineffective
Consider:
• different antifungal
• more potent corticosteroids
• systemic therapy under the care of a specialist

Table 5: Therapy for Dandruff and Seborrheic Dermatitis

Class	Drug	Dosage	Onset	Adverse Effects	Comments	Cost[a]
Antifungals, topical	*ciclopirox olamine* Loprox (cream, lotion), Stieprox (shampoo)	Scalp: Shampoo: Use 2–3 times weekly or as often as necessary Application Instructions: Wet hair and part a small section. Rub into scalp at the roots. Repeat until entire head has been treated. Leave on for at least 5 min then rinse Body: Cream, lotion: Rub gently into affected area BID. Can be applied to beard, face and body Prophylaxis/maintenance: Treat once every 1–2 wk	Requires 2–3 wk to see onset of effect and 4 wk to see full effect. Maintain use at the interval necessary to keep the condition under control.	Uncommonly: Pruritus, burning sensation.	Alternative to ketoconazole. If using antifungal in a patient already on corticosteroid treatment, maintain corticosteroid for 2–3 wk to allow time for onset of effect of antifungal, then withdraw the corticosteroid (to prevent rebound flare of symptoms).	Cream/ Lotion:$ Sham-poo:$$
	ketoconazole Ketoderm (cream), Nizoral (shampoo)	Scalp: Shampoo: Use 2–4 times weekly Application Instructions: Wet hair and part a small section. Rub into scalp at the roots. Repeat until entire head has been treated. Leave on for at least 5 min then rinse Body: Cream: Rub gently into afffected area once daily. Can be applied to beard, face and body Prophylaxis/maintenance: Treat once every 1–2 wk	See ciclopirox.	<1% systemic absorption. Minimal scalp and skin irritation, itching, stinging. May cause greasy or dry hair or scalp. Less irritating than selenium sulfide.	First-line treatment. Avoid eye area. If using antifungal in a patient already on corticosteroid treatment, maintain corticosteroid for 2–3 wk to allow time for onset of effect of antifungal, then withdraw the corticosteroid (to prevent rebound flare of symptoms).	$

(cont'd)

Table 5: Therapy for Dandruff and Seborrheic Dermatitis *(cont'd)*

Class	Drug	Dosage	Onset	Adverse Effects	Comments	Cost[a]
	selenium sulfide Selsun, Selsun Blue, others	Scalp: Shampoo 1%, Lotion 2.5%: 2 applications per wk for 2 wk and afterwards use at less frequent intervals; do not use more than 3 times per wk Application Instructions: Wet hair and part a small section. Rub into scalp at the roots. Repeat until entire head has been treated. Leave on for at least 5 min then rinse	Requires 2–4 wk to see effect. Maintain use at the interval necessary to keep the condition under control.	Excessive use may cause oily hair and hair loss. Will sting if applied to broken skin. May discolour bleached, tinted or permanent-waved hair. Avoid use of these hair products within 2 days of treatment with selenium sulfide. Avoid contact with any jewelry as it may be damaged.	Second-line therapy. Cannot be used on damaged or inflamed skin. Avoid eye area.	$
	zinc pyrithione Head and Shoulders Shampoo, Z-Plus Shampoo, others	Scalp: Shampoo: Use 2–3 times weekly or as often as necessary Application Instructions: Wet hair and part a small section. Rub into scalp at the roots. Repeat until entire head has been treated. Leave on for at least 5 min then rinse	See selenium sulfide.	May discolour hair if metal-based tints are used. Safe to use after perm solutions.	Second-line therapy.	$
Calcineurin inhibitors	*pimecrolimus* Elidel	Body: Rub a thin layer into affected area BID Maintenance dose: Once daily, 2 days per week	See selenium sulfide.	Mild and transient skin burning at onset of therapy. Lacks the long-term side effects of topical corticosteroids.	Second-line therapy.	$70
	tacrolimus Protopic	Body: Rub a thin layer into affected area BID Maintenance dose: Once daily, 2 days per wk	See selenium sulfide.	See pimecrolimus.	Second-line therapy.	$70

Class	Drug	Dosage	Onset	Adverse Effects	Comments	Cost[a]
Corticosteroids, topical[b]	*hydrocortisone* Cortate, Emo-Cort, Prevex HC , generics	Scalp or Body: Rub gently into affected area BID–TID	Treat for 1–2 wk to see effect. Reassess use after 2 wk and continue intermittently if needed. Alternate with emollients or other agents for maintenance if necessary.	Well tolerated.	Useful for suppressing initial inflammation. Stronger topical corticosteroids may be used on body areas other than face and folds if the response to hydrocortisone is insufficient.	$
Corticosteroids, topical (formulated for scalp)[b]	*betamethasone valerate lotion* Valisone Scalp Lotion, generics	Scalp: Apply a thin film BID–TID to completely cover affected area	See hydrocortisone.	Burning/irritation at application site, pruritus, dryness, atrophy.	Moderate-potency topical corticosteroid. Severe and thick scales on the scalp can respond to overnight application of topical corticosteroids.	$
	betamethasone valerate foam Luxiq	Scalp: Apply a thin film BID to completely cover affected area	See hydrocortisone.	Burning/irritation at application site, pruritus, dryness, atrophy.	See betamethasone.	$80
Corticosteroid, topical/keratolytic combination (formulated for scalp)	*betamethasone valerate/salicylic acid* Diprosalic, generics	Scalp: Apply a thin film once daily–BID	See hydrocortisone.	Corticosteroid: burning, itching, irritation, acneiform eruptions, skin atrophy, striae. Keratolytic: erythema, scaling, local irritation.	See betamethasone.	$$

(cont'd)

Table 5: **Therapy for Dandruff and Seborrheic Dermatitis** *(cont'd)*

Class	Drug	Dosage	Onset	Adverse Effects	Comments	Cost[a]
Keratolytic agents	*coal tar* Denorex, Liquor Carbonis Detergens, Targel, others	Scalp: Once daily to once weekly as needed More effective with prolonged contact time	Requires 2–4 wk to see effect. Follow by interval necessary to keep the condition under control.	Folliculitis (especially of hairy regions), acne, contact dermatitis, photosensitivity, unappealing odour, stains skin and hair.	Second-line treatment. Additive antimitotic activity with UVA and UVB. Products may contain crude coal tar or tar distillates (which are 10–20% as potent as crude coal tar). Also available in commercial products combined with salicylic acid and/or sulfur.	$
	salicylic acid Dermarest, Sebcur, others	Scalp: At least twice weekly, massaging thoroughly into affected area	See coal tar.	Irritation, redness or peeling. Irritating to mucous membranes and eyes.	Salicylic acid enhances penetration of topical agents through stratum corneum. Also available in commercial products combined with coal tar and/or sulfur.	$
	sulfur Sulfur8, others	Scalp: At least twice weekly, massaging thoroughly into affected area	See coal tar.	See salicylic acid.	Many commercial products contain various combinations of coal tar, salicylic acid, sulfur.	$$

[a] Cost of 30 g for cream or smallest available pack size unless otherwise specified; includes drug cost only.

[b] For a comprehensive list of topical corticosteroids, see Corticosteroids: Topical (CPhA Monograph).

Legend: $ <$10 $$ $10–20

Suggested Readings

Johnson BA, Nunley JR. Treatment of seborrheic dermatitis. *Am Fam Physician* 2000;61:2703-10, 2713-4.

Kastarinen H, Oksanen T, Okokon EO et al. Topical anti-inflammatory agents for seborrhoeic dermatitis of the face or scalp. *Cochrane Database Syst Rev* 2014;5:CD009446.

Naldi L, Rebora A. Clinical practice. Seborrheic dermatitis. *N Engl J Med* 2009;360:387-96.

Okokon EO1, Verbeek JH, Ruotsalainen JH et al. Topical antifungals for seborrhoeic dermatitis *Cochrane Database Syst Rev* 2015;5:CD008138.

References

1. Gardner SS, McKay M. Seborrhea, psoriasis and the papulosquamous dermatosis. *Prim Care* 1989;16:739-63.
2. Shuster S. The aetiology of dandruff and the mode of action of therapeutic agents. *Br J Dermatol* 1984;111:235-42.
3. Tooley P. Dandruff: an irritating problem. *Practitioner* 1990;234:593-6.
4. Johnson BA, Nunley JR. Treatment of seborrheic dermatitis. *Am Fam Physician* 2000;61:2703-10, 2713-4.
5. Dessinioti C, Katsambas A. Seborrheic dermatitis: etiology, risk factors, and treatments: facts and controversies. *Clin Dermatol* 2013;31:343-51.
6. Wattanakrai P. Seborrheic dermatitis and dandruff. In: Arndt KA, Tsu JT. *Manual of dermatologic therapeutics*. 7th ed. Philadelphia: Wolters Kluwer/Lippincott Williams & Wilkins; 2007. p. 29:180-4.
7. McGrath J, Murphy GM. The control of seborrhoeic dermatitis and dandruff by antipityrosporal drugs. *Drugs* 1991;41:178-84.
8. Sobell JM, Geist DE. Psoriasis. In: Arndt KA, Tsu JT. *Manual of dermatologic therapeutics*. 7th ed. Philadelphia: Wolters Kluwer/Lippincott Williams & Wilkins; 2007. p. 27:164-73.
9. Janniger CK, Schwartz RA. Seborrheic dermatitis. *Am Fam Physician* 1995;52:149-55, 159-60.
10. Maietta G, Rongioletti R, Rebora A. Seborrheic dermatitis and daylight. *Acta Derm Venereol* 1991;71:538-9.
11. Zone J, Ward J, Boyce E et al. Penicillamine-induced pemphigus. *JAMA* 1982;247:2705-7.
12. Greenberg RD. Acne vulgaris associated with antigonadotropic (Danazol) therapy. *Cutis* 1979;24:431-3.
13. Litt JZ, Pawlak WA. *Drug eruption reference manual*. 4th ed. Cleveland: Wal-Zac Enterprises; 1995. p. 1-13.
14. Collins CD, Hivnor C. Seborrheic dermatitis. In: Goldsmith LA, Katz SI, Gilchrest BA et al. *Fitzpatick's dermatology in general medicine*. 8th ed. New York: McGraw-Hill; 2012. p. 259-66.
15. David E, Tanuos H, Sullivan T et al. A double-blind, placebo-controlled pilot study to estimate the efficacy and tolerability of a nonsteroidal cream for the treatment of cradle cap (seborrheic dermatitis). *J Drugs Dermatolog* 2013;12:448-52.
16. Pandya AG. Seborrheic dermatitis or tinea capitis: don't be fooled. *Int J Dermatol* 1998;37:827-8.
17. Arndt KA et al., eds. *Primary care dermatology*. Boston: Saunders; 1997.
18. Arndt KA. *Manual of dermatologic therapeutics: with essentials of diagnosis*. 5th ed. Boston: Little, Brown; 1995.
19. Draelos ZD, Kenneally DC, Hodges LT et al. A comparison of hair quality and cosmetic acceptance following the use of two anti-dandruff shampoos. *J Investig Dermatol Symp Proc* 2005;10:201-4.
20. Okokon EO1, Verbeek JH, Ruotsalainen JH et al. Topical antifungals for seborrhoeic dermatitis. *Cochrane Database Syst Rev* 2015;5:CD008138.
21. Cauwenbergh G. International experience with ketoconazole shampoo in the treatment of seborrhoeic dermatitis and dandruff. In: Shuster S, Blatchford N, eds. *Seborrhoeic dermatitis and dandruff: a fungal disease*. London: Royal Society of Medicine Services; 1988. p. 35-42.
22. Borgers M. Ultrastructural correlates of antimycotic treatment. *Curr Top Med Mycol* 1988;2:1-39.
23. Ratnavel RC, Squire RA, Boorman GC. Clinical efficacies of shampoos containing ciclopirox olamine (1.5%) and ketoconazole (2.0%) in the treatment of seborrhoeic dermatitis. *J Dermatolog Treat* 2007;18:88-96.
24. Altmeyer P, Hoffmann K. Efficacy of different concentrations of ciclopirox shampoo for the treatment of seborrheic dermatitis of the scalp: results of a randomized, double-blind, vehicle-controlled trial. *Int J Dermatol* 2004:43:9-12.
25. Gupta AK, Nicol KA. Ciclopirox 1% shampoo for the treatment of seborrheic dermatitis. *Int J Dermatol* 2006;45:66-9.
26. Lorette G, Ermosilla V. Clinical efficacy of a new ciclopiroxolamine/zinc pyrithione shampoo in scalp seborrheic dermatitis treatment. *Eur J Dermatol* 2006;16:558-64.
27. Abeck D; Loprox Shampoo Dosing Study Group. Rationale of frequency of use of ciclopirox 1% shampoo in the treatment of seborrheic dermatitis: results of a double-blind, placebo-controlled study comparing the efficacy of once, twice, and three times weekly usage. *Int J Dermatol* 2004;43:13-6.
28. Butterfield W, Roberts MM, Dave VK. Sensitivities of Pityrosporum sp. to selected commercial shampoos. *Br J Dermatol* 1987;116:233-5.
29. Fredriksson T. Controlled comparison of Clinitar shampoo and Selsun shampoo in the treatment of seborrhoeic dermatitis of the scalp. *Br J Clin Pract* 1985;29:25-8.
30. Chandler CJ, Segel IH. Mechanism of the antimicrobial action of pyrithione: effects on membrane transport, ATP levels, and protein synthesis. *Antimicrob Agents Chemother* 1978;14:60-8.
31. Schwartz JR, Rocchetta H, Asawanonda P et al. Does tachyphylaxis occur in long-term management of scalp seborrheic dermatitis with pyrithione zinc-based treatments? *Int J Dermatol* 2009;48:79-85.
32. Warner RR, Schwartz JR, Boissy Y et al. Dandruff has an altered stratum corneum ultrastructure that is improved with zinc pyrithione shampoo. *J Am Acad Dermatol* 2001;45:897-903.
33. Faergemann J. Propylene glycol in the treatment of seborrheic dermatitis of the scalp: a double-blind study. *Cutis* 1988;42:69-71.
34. Gupta AK, Richardson M, Paquet M. Systematic review of oral treatments for seborrheic dermatitis. *J Eur Acad Dermatol Venereol* 2014;28:16-26.
35. Ghodsi SZ, Abbas Z, Abedeni R. Efficacy of oral itraconazole in the treatment and relapse prevention of moderate to severe seborrheic dermatitis: a randomized, placebo-controlled trial. *Am J Clin Dermatol* 2015;16:431-7.

36. Kastarinen H, Oksanen T, Okokon EO et al. Topical anti-inflammatory agents for seborrhoeic dermatitis of the face or scalp. *Cochrane Database Syst Rev* 2014;5:CD009446.
37. Faergemann J. Seborrhoeic dermatitis and Pityrosporum orbiculare: treatment of seborrhoeic dermatitis of the scalp with miconazole-hydrocortione (Daktacort), miconazole and hydrocortisone. *Br J Dermatol* 1986;114:695-700.
38. Ang-Tiu CU, Meghrajani CF, Maano CC. Pimecrolimus 1% cream for the treatment of seborrheic dermatitis: a systematic review of randomized controlled trials. *Expert Rev Clin Pharmacol* 2012;5:91-7.
39. Papp KA, Papp A, Dahmer B et al. Single-blind, randomized controlled trial evaluating the treatment of facial seborrheic dermatitis with hydrocortisone 1% ointment compared with tacrolimus 0.1% ointment in adults. *J Am Acad Dermatol* 2012;67:e11-5.
40. Warshaw EM, Wohlhuter RJ, Liu A et al. Results of a randomized, double-blind, vehicle-controlled efficacy trial of pimecrolimus cream 1% for the treatment of moderate to severe facial seborrheic dermatitis. *J Am Acad Dermatol* 2007;57:257-64.
41. Firooz A, Solhpour A, Gorouhi F et al. Pimecrolimus cream, 1%, vs hydrocortisone acetate cream, 1%, in the treatment of facial seborrheic dermatitis: a randomized, investigator-blind, clinical trial. *Arch Dermatol* 2006;142:1066-7.
42. Rigopoulos D, Ioannides D, Kalogeromitros D et al. Pimecrolimus cream 1% vs. betamethasone 17-valerate 0.1% cream in the treatment of seborrhoeic dermatitis. A randomized open-label clinical trial. *Br J Dermatol* 2004;151:1071-5.
43. Cicek D, Kandi B, Bakar S et al. Pimecrolimus 1% cream, methylprednisolone aceponate 0.1% cream and metronidazole 0.75% gel in the treatment of seborrhoeic dermatitis: a randomized clinical study. *J Dermatol Treat* 2009;20:344-9.
44. Kim TW, Mun JH, Jwa SW et al. Proactive treatment of adult facial seborrhoeic dermatitis with 0.1% tacrolimus ointment: randomized, double-blind, vehicle-controlled, multi-centre trial. *Acta Derm Venereol* 2013;93:557-61.
45. Shin H, Kwon OS, Won CH et al. Clinical efficacies of topical agents for the treatment of seborrheic dermatitis of the scalp: a comparative study. *J Dermatol* 2009;36:131-7.
46. Kiiski V, Remitz A, Reitano S et al. Long-term safety of topical pimecrolimus and topical tacrolimus in atopic blepharoconjunctivitis. *JAMA Dermatol* 2014;150:571-3.
47. Ozcan H, Seyhan M, Yologlu S. Is metronidazole 0.75% gel effective in the treatment of seborrhoeic dermatitis? A double-blind, placebo controlled study. *Eur J Dermatol* 2007;17:313-6.
48. Koca R, Altinyazar HC, Esturk E. Is topical metronidazole effective in seborrheic dermatitis? A double-blind study. *Int J Dermatol* 2003;42:632-5.
49. Siadat AH, Iraji F, Shahmoradi Z et al. The efficacy of 1% metronidazole gel in facial seborrheic dermatitis: a double blind study. *Indian J Dermatol Venereol Leprol* 2006;72:266-9.
50. Seckin D, Gurbuz O, Akin O. Metronidazole 0.75% gel vs. ketoconazole 2% cream in the treatment of facial seborrheic dermatitis: a randomized, double-blind study. *J Eur Acad Dermatol Venereol* 2007;21:345-50.
51. Dreno B, Chosidow O, Revuz J et al. Lithium gluconate 8% vs ketoconazole 2% in the treatment of seborrhoeic dermatitis: a multicentre, randomized study. *Br J Dermatol* 2003;148:1230-6.
52. Dreno B, Moyse D. Lithium gluconate in the treatment of seborrhoeic dermatitis: a multicenter, randomised, double-blind study versus placebo. *Eur J Dermatol* 2002;12:549-52.
53. Pirkhammer D, Seeber A, Hönigsmann H et al. Narrow-band ultraviolet B (ATL-01) phototherapy is an effective and safe treatment option for patients with severe seborrhoeic dermatitis. *Br J Dermatol* 2000;143:964-8.
54. Ranki A, Puska P, Mattinen S et al. Effect of PUVA on immunologic and virologic findings in HIV-infected patients. *J Am Acad Dermatol* 1991;24:404-10.
55. Tegner E. Seborrhoeic dermatitis of the face induced by PUVA treatment. *Acta Derm Venereol* 1983;63:335-9.
56. Fabbrocini G, Cantelli M, Monfrecola G. Topical nicotinamide for seborrheic dermatitis: an open randomized study. *J Dermatolog Treat* 2014;25:241-5.
57. Seite S, Rougier A, Talarico S. Randomized study comparing the efficacy and tolerance of a lipohydroxy acid shampoo to a ciclopiroxolamine shampoo in the treatment of scalp seborrheic dermatitis. *J Cosmet Dermatol* 2009;8:249-53.
58. Emtestam L, Svensson A, Rensfeldt K. Treatment of seborrhoeic dermatitis of the scalp with a topical solution of urea, lactic acid, and propylene glycol (K301): results of two double-blind, randomised, placebo-controlled studies. *Mycoses* 2012;55:393-403.
59. Gruenwald J, Brendler T, Jaenicke C et al., eds. *PDR for herbal medicines*. 1st ed. Montvale: Medical Economics; 1998.
60. Diehl C, Ferrari A. Efficacy of topical 4% Quassia amara gel in facial seborrheic dermatitis:a randomized, double-blind, comparative study. *J Drugs Dermatol* 2013;12:312-5.
61. Nenoff P, Haustein UF, Brandt W. Antifungal activity of the essential oil of Melaleuca alternifolia (tea tree oil) against pathogenic fungi in vitro. *Skin Pharmacol* 1996;9:388-94.
62. Satchell AC, Saurajen A, Bell C et al. Treatment of dandruff with 5% tea tree oil shampoo. *J Am Acad Dermatol* 2002;47:852-5.
63. Herrera-Arellano A, Jimenez-Ferrer E, Vega-Pimentel AM et al. Clinical and mycological evaluation of therapeutic effectiveness of Solanum chrysotrichum standardized extract on patients with Pityriasis capitis (dandruff). A double blind and randomized clinical trial controlled with ketoconazole. *Planta Med* 2004;70:483-8.

Seborrheic Dermatitis—What You Need to Know

What is seborrheic dermatitis?

Seborrheic dermatitis is a common skin problem, which appears as a red rash and greasy scales on the scalp, face, eyebrows, eyelids, and mid-chest. Infants may have seborrheic dermatitis on the scalp ("cradle cap"), in body folds or in the diaper area. Seborrheic dermatitis in infants usually goes away after about 6 months.

Seborrheic dermatitis is common in men, the elderly and persons who have oily skin, Parkinson's disease or HIV infection. A number of factors cause seborrheic dermatitis, including yeast, hormones and stress.

Cleansing the skin:

- It's important to keep your body clean.
- Use warm water (not hot or cold) to bathe or shower each day to help remove scales.
- Avoid using harsh soap on your skin or strong detergents on your clothes.

Shampooing:

- You may use a regular shampoo daily to remove scales. Having scales does not mean that your hair is too dry. Use a medicated shampoo 2–3 times weekly, or as directed, to keep seborrheic dermatitis under control.
- **How to use a medicated shampoo:**
  - Wet your hair. Work on small sections at a time.
  - Rub some medicated shampoo into your scalp at the roots. Repeat until the entire head has been treated.
  - Leave the shampoo on for at least 5 minutes. Rinse it out.
  - Repeat if necessary.
- **How to manage infant's cradle cap:**
  - First try a mild, nonmedicated baby shampoo.
  - If scales are thick, soften them before shampooing by rubbing on warm oil or bath oil. Gently brush with a baby hairbrush. Then use shampoo, and rinse well.

Moisturizing:

- Keep your skin well lubricated at all times to reduce dryness and scratching.
- You can use an emollient cream as a cleanser and a moisturizer.
- Apply creams smoothly in the direction that hairs lie flat.
- Use a sunscreen to protect your skin from sun damage and keep it moist.

Triggers:

- Reduce or control factors that may aggravate seborrheic dermatitis, such as sweating, high temperatures and depression.
- Use a cool air humidifier.
- Maintain a healthy diet.
- Exercise moderately and get enough rest.
- Reduce stress by pursuing hobbies and increasing leisure or vacation time.

Medications:

- Ask your healthcare provider about medications that can make seborrheic dermatitis worse.
- Ask your healthcare provider about cosmetics, natural health products or nonprescription products before trying them.

Do not stop taking your prescribed medications without checking with your healthcare provider.

Chapter 59
Diaper Dermatitis

Debra Sibbald, BScPhm, ACPR, MA (Adult Education), PhD (Education)

Pathophysiology

Diaper dermatitis ("diaper rash") is a highly prevalent condition causing discomfort to patients, affecting caregivers and frustrating healthcare practitioners.[1] It is a form of area-specific contact dermatitis and can be irritant or allergic.

Irritant diaper dermatitis is the result of progressive barrier compromise, and in mild forms is characterized by dryness, scaling, abnormal desquamation and erythema. In severe cases there are eruptions, papules, vesicles, intense erythema and ulcerations. Reported frequencies vary depending on methodologies, but most are of an irritant etiology. Prevalence in infants ranges from 25–53% varying with population, and up to 75% in diaper-wearing incontinent elderly nursing home patients.[1] Seborrheic dermatitis is a predisposing factor for infants.[2]

Diaper dermatitis is the cumulative result of several features of the diaper environment which predispose the skin to damage, especially overhydration and contact with skin irritants (including urine, feces, associated enzymes and bile salts). Other factors play a role, including: mechanical friction (skin-to-diaper and skin-to-skin), increased skin pH (contributing to decreased barrier function and increased reactivity to irritants), diet (fecal composition), age (urinary frequency), gestational age (inherent barrier maturation), antibiotic therapy, diarrhea and underlying medical conditions. Risk is higher in infants who are diapered with cotton diapers plus plastic covers, fed cow's milk (vs. breast milk), or malnourished.[1]

Diapers

Diapered-skin pH is higher due to effects of occlusion and increased skin permeability, leading to increased skin hydration and risk of diaper rash.[3] Controversy persists about whether cloth or disposable diapers better minimize diaper dermatitis, because variables such as duration of wetness and frequency of diaper changes are not controlled in many studies. Reusable cloth diapers may contribute to dermatitis if not adequately washed and rinsed of harsh cleansing chemicals. Airtight plastic occlusion to prevent leakage of urine and stool increases the risk of excessive hydration and maceration of skin; modern disposable diapers minimize this by wicking urine and water away from the skin surface to outer diaper layers. Prolonged wearing of any diaper promotes damage to the skin.[4]

Friction and Contact Irritation

A primary causative factor is repeated friction as the infant or immobilized patient shifts in the bed or chair. Body folds increase areas of skin-to-skin contact. More frictional injury occurs if the skin is wet, producing chafing and shiny erythema and allowing other irritants to harm the skin.[4]

Urine and Ammonia

The level of ammonia in infant urine is not sufficient to cause or initiate diaper dermatitis but may aggravate an existing inflammatory process.[1] Damaged skin is more susceptible to irritating effects of ammonia, which is liberated by urease enzymes from cutaneous or colonic bacteria.[5] Urine hydrates the skin and makes it more vulnerable to frictional injury.[4]

Feces and Alkaline pH

The most important factors in the pathogenesis of diaper dermatitis are now considered to be the alkaline pH of the urine and the role of fecal bacteria. Perineal skin breakdown can occur in infants and older patients when pancreatic enzymes and bile salts cannot be adequately deactivated in the colon. The resultant lipases, proteolytic enzymes and ureases present in the feces may induce contact irritant dermatitis by attacking the epidermis and raising the surface pH to alkaline range. Fecal protease activity is pH dependent and increases to a maximum at pH 7.[1] Ammonia also raises the pH of the skin, making it more susceptible to damage or infection. An alkaline pH also facilitates the development of *Candida albicans*. Loose and watery stools, common in infants, contribute to excessive hydration and frictional forces.[4] Cow's milk–fed infants are more likely to develop diaper dermatitis because these formulas are colonized by a greater number of urease-producing bacteria.[2] Breastfed infants, whose feces are less copious, less alkaline and less caustic, may have less diaper rash. Foods ingested by either infants or breastfeeding mothers that increase the urinary and fecal pH (e.g., high-protein diets) may contribute to diaper rash.

Microorganisms

Candida infection is associated with diaper wearing. This is partly due to the fact that moist environments support microbial growth.[1] More importantly, the GI tract is an important reservoir for *C. albicans*, a secondary invader of dermatitic skin. Feces containing *C. albicans* are held against the skin, providing a mechanism for infection. *C. albicans* is present in 70–80% of patients with diaper dermatitis, compared with 10–12.5% in those without diaper dermatitis.[4,6,7] *Candida* is most frequently found in the periphery of intense diaper dermatitis, particularly in pustules.

Colonization of dermatitic skin by *Staphylococcus aureus* can occur frequently, and can be suspected in a severely inflamed dermatitis with follicular pustules.

Goals of Therapy

- Avoidance of causative factors
- Relief of symptoms
- Resolution of dermatitis
- Prevention of complications and recurrences

Patient Assessment

Clinical Presentation

Diaper dermatitis is a "geographic" diagnosis (strictly confined to the diaper area), occurring in patients of any age who wear diapers. Onset of diaper dermatitis is gradual but may not be clinically apparent until an abrupt appearance of observable skin changes in the few hours between diaper changes. The location of diaper rash is the area covered by the specific boundaries of the diaper: around the lower abdomen and the lumbar back at about the level of the umbilicus and below, around the upper thighs, encompassing the genitalia, perineum and buttocks.[1] It may be more extensive on the front or back if the diaper wearer lies primarily in one position.

Irritant Diaper Dermatitis

Irritant contact dermatitis or chafing rash is the most common type of primary diaper dermatitis. Clinically, diaper dermatitis appears as moist, sometimes scaly and erythematous, often shiny patches over the convex surfaces of the diaper area, including the buttocks, genitalia, lower abdomen and upper thighs. Irritant diaper dermatitis usually spares the inguinal skin folds (creases). It may appear dusky purple on darker skin. The spectrum of severity ranges from mild, with erythema, to severe, with a shiny, deep erythema, followed by the development of erythematous papules, vesicles and oozing and widespread shallow erosions and ulcers.[8] It can be asymptomatic or tender. It may resolve spontaneously or wax and wane, but is treated regardless.

Candida Diaper Dermatitis

Candida diaper dermatitis is the second most common diaper dermatitis after irritant diaper dermatitis. *Candida* from intestinal flora contaminates any type of diaper dermatitis present for greater than 3 days and the levels increase with clinical severity of the dermatitis. The most common presentation is an initial diffuse erythematous patch progressing over days to confluent tomato-red plaques, papules, pustules, peripheral scale and small erythematous satellite papules, which are most likely to be culture-positive for *Candida.* It is classically described as a beefy red rash with satellite pustules, with early maceration of the anal mucosa and perianal skin. It almost always involves the inguinal creases. Pustules may not be seen due to maceration under the diaper.[8,9] Oral thrush may also be present.

Allergic Diaper Dermatitis

An allergic reaction may resemble the irritant presentation but typically consists of grouped or linear tense vesicles and blisters and, in severe involvement, marked edema, particularly in genital areas.

Risk and Aggravating Factors

Irritants and friction: Chemical and mechanical irritants from urine, feces, cleansing products and cleansing methods contribute to and aggravate diaper dermatitis. Excessive rubbing and over-cleaning can cause mechanical stripping and barrier damage. Frequent vigorous cleansing with detergents or soaps can actually induce contact dermatitis and can easily aggravate already inflamed, damaged skin.

Chemicals: Various ingredients in skin care products may aggravate or cause diaper dermatitis. See Chemical/Drug-induced Diaper Dermatitis.

Comorbid Conditions: Infants with atopic or seborrheic dermatitis or psoriasis, the incontinent immobilized patient, and the incontinent elderly are at greater risk of diaper dermatitis.[10] Diaper dermatitis can also be a manifestation of other diseases such as Kawasaki's syndrome, granuloma gluteale infantum and cytomegalovirus. Unusual manifestations of diaper dermatitis may occur in infants born to immunocompromised mothers. Untreated or infected diaper dermatitis can progress to skin ulceration, infection of the penis or vulva, and urinary tract infections.

Differential Diagnosis

A summary of the possible differential diagnoses related to diaper dermatitis is provided in Table 1.

Chemical/Drug-induced Diaper Dermatitis

The risk of chemical or drug-induced diaper dermatitis, which may be allergic or irritant contact dermatitis, is greater in infants than in other patients due to the thin epidermis, high surface-to-volume ratio and differences in systemic metabolism and detoxification in very young children, particularly those with inflamed skin. Elderly diapered patients with atrophic skin are similarly more susceptible to injury from topical agents.[5]

Table 1: **Differential Diagnosis of Diaper Dermatitis**

Diagnosis	Symptoms
Primary irritant diaper dermatitis	Erythematous, often shiny, patches over the convex surfaces of the diaper area, usually sparing the inguinal skin folds.
Candida diaper dermatitis	Early maceration of the anal mucosa and perianal skin, progressing over days to confluent tomato-red plaques, papules, pustules, peripheral scale and satellite papules, almost always involving the inguinal creases. Lack of sebum by age 4 months or oral antibiotic therapy for otitis media may be factors. May have thrush in oral cavity.
Miliaria rubra (prickly heat, heat rash)	Clear superficial vesicles without inflammation in newborns, or in older infants, tiny red papules and papulovesicles, sometimes pruritic due to eccrine sweat duct occlusion. Also found in overlapping skin folds in infants, especially neck and axillary folds. May be caused by occlusion from plastic outer coverings of diapers.
Allergic contact dermatitis (see Chapter 55: Atopic, Contact, and Stasis Dermatitis)	More common in infants over 12 months. Failure to respond to treatment for irritant dermatitis. Allergy to component of topical preparation. More severe in flexural areas since topical agent may concentrate in folds.
Seborrheic dermatitis (see Chapter 58: Dandruff and Seborrheic Dermatitis)	Well-circumscribed, erythematous, greasy scaly plaques with flexural accentuation, typically asymptomatic. May involve scalp, neck, face, axillae and retroauricular areas as well. Occurs in the first 6 months of life and extremely common in the aged.
Atopic dermatitis (see Chapter 55: Atopic, Contact, and Stasis Dermatitis)	Usually not in the groin, but atopic individuals are more susceptible to irritant dermatitis, which may present as acute dermatitis or chronic lichenification. History of pruritus, eczema, especially in flexural areas, asthma or allergic rhinitis. Later onset (after 2 months) and family history of atopy.
Psoriasis (see Chapter 71: Psoriasis)	Less common. Brilliant erythematous plaques in the diaper area, lack of silvery scale due to hydrating effect of diapers. Family history of psoriasis and typical lesions elsewhere on the body. Lack of response to topical steroids and antiyeast medications.
Scabies (see Chapter 69: Parasitic Skin Infections: Lice and Scabies)	Excoriations and ill-defined papular eruptions in the diaper area. Burrows on palms, soles, axillary and genital areas, nipples, umbilicus and finger webs. Itching persists 3–4 wk after treatment.
Bullous impetigo (see Chapter 56: Bacterial Skin Infections: Impetigo, Furuncles and Carbuncles)	Large flaccid bullae filled with straw-coloured liquid in the first few weeks of life. Ruptured bullae leave red, denuded areas and honey-coloured crusts.
Histiocytosis	Rare. Recalcitrant diaper dermatitis with erythematous papules surmounted by scale; may be hemorrhagic. Involvement of scalp and retroauricular areas. Systemic symptoms of hepatosplenomegaly, anemia and lymphadenopathy.
Acrodermatitis enteropathica	Disorder of zinc metabolism leading to perioral, perineal and sacral skin erosions and erythematous, well-demarcated scaly plaques. Infants may also have alopecia, growth failure, diarrhea and irritability.
Congenital syphilis	Copper-coloured erythematous macules and papules and moist erosions in the diaper region, denuded sacral areas. May have anemia, hepatosplenomegaly, jaundice, bone involvement.

Products containing boric acid are not recommended due to toxicity.[11,12] Benzalkonium chloride is used in skin products as a disinfectant or preservative and has been implicated in allergic dermatitis in infants; its use should be avoided.[13] Volatile alcohol (ethyl and isopropyl), fragrance and cleansing products containing surface active agents (surfactants) may aggravate dermatitis. Surfactants vary in inherent irritancy as reported in Table 2. Residual surfactant can remain on the skin when copious rinsing is not practical. There is a rising incidence of allergy, currently reported as 1.5–6%, to a common preservative in baby wipes called methylisothiazolinone, due to increased use. Some associations have called for a ban on its use.[14]

In addition to the topical medications listed in Table 3 which directly cause contact dermatitis, medications can contribute to diaper dermatitis through secondary effects. Oral medications can affect the motility and flora of the GI tract (e.g., antibiotics) or the autonomic control of urination and defecation, especially if given frequently. Some foods, such as caffeine and citrus juices, are irritating when eliminated from the body. One study reported a higher incidence of diaper rash in infants given antibiotics or oral glucose 50% solution.[15]

Table 2: Relative Irritancy of Surfactants Found in Skin Care Products[1]

Relative Irritancy	Surfactants
High	Sodium lauryl sulfate Sodium dodecyl sulfate Sodium alkyl sulfate Sodium or potassium cocoate Sodium or potassium tallowate Sodium palmitate Sodium or potassium stearate Linear alkyl benzene sulfate Triethanolamine laurate Sodium olefin sulfonate Benzalkonium chloride Dodecyl trimethyl ammonium bromide
Moderate	Sodium ethoxylates Sodium laureth sulfate Ammonium laureth sulfate
Low	Sodium cocoyl isethionate Sodium alkyl glycerol ether sulfonate Sodium cocoyl sulfosuccinate Disodium stearyl sulfosuccinate

Table 3: Chemical/Drug-induced Diaper Dermatitis

Substances that may Cause Contact Dermatitis in the Diaper Area[5]	
Antihistamines, topical	Methylisothiazolinone
Bacitracin	PABA derivatives, e.g., benzocaine
Balsam of Peru	Parabens
Ethylenediamine	Penicillins
Lanolin	Sulfonamides
Neomycin	Thimerosal
Substances to Avoid in the Diaper Area due to Toxicity[5]	
Sensitizer or Toxin	**Effect**
Alcohol	Dehydration
Benzocaine and resorcinol	Contact sensitivity, methemoglobinemia
Camphor	Seizures
Potent topical corticosteroids	Cushing's syndrome, atrophic changes, acne, superinfections
Topical salicylates (methyl salicylate)	Salicylate intoxication, metabolic acidosis

An approach to assessment of the patient with diaper dermatitis can be found in Figure 1.

Severe or Complicated Diaper Dermatitis

Assess patients further for other possibilities including contact sensitivity, infection or alternative diagnosis when:

- a correctly identified rash fails to improve after a week of recommended treatment
- pain, itching or inflammation has increased
- oozing blisters or pus are present
- the dermatitis has not healed in 7–10 days
- the dermatitis has an acute onset
- the dermatitis is chronic or recurs frequently
- there is a complicated secondary infection, urinary tract infection or infection of the penis or vulva
- there are systemic symptoms, e.g., fever, diarrhea, nausea, vomiting, rash or skin lesions elsewhere on the body
- there are signs of immunodeficiency, deep ulceration, or abuse or neglect
- the dermatitis is associated with another disease state
- the patient shows behavioural changes.

A diaper rash grading scale with associated description to quantify severity has been proposed. It uses ratings of very slight, slight, moderate, moderate to severe and severe, to assess skin integrity (ulceration and scaling), erythema (macules and continuous), rash (papules and edema) and the percentage of the area affected.[16]

Prevention

Prevention (and treatment) of diaper dermatitis is important for the duration of time the patient wears diapers. Appropriate skin care practices support skin barrier function and protect the buttocks skin from feces and urine. There is no evidence that any single method is effective alone.[17]

Combination methods should address all causative factors, combining nonpharmacologic and pharmacologic measures according to the following acronym:

A. air, absorptives, antifungals, anti-inflammatories
B. barriers
C. cleansing, compressing
D. diaper
E. education

The first step is to discontinue aggravating factors (see Risk and Aggravating Factors).

Air: It is important to allow "air" drying to diminish the damaging effects of occlusion and maceration, by removing the diaper for as long as possible during cleansing, treatment and changes. Avoid practices that may cause chapping and burns, such as drying the buttocks area with a hair dryer, even on the lowest setting, or exposure to infrared lamps. Adult incontinence products with absorbent cores and breathable outer covers marketed for adults increase aeration. Breathable covers also create conditions unfavourable to *C. albicans* survival.[1] Absorptives, antifungals and anti-inflammatories are discussed in Pharmacologic Therapy.

Barriers: **Powders** are potentially dangerous due to risk of inadvertent inhalation and are best avoided. **Cornstarch** reduces friction. It may absorb some moisture, although inefficiently compared with pastes, and it does not wick moisture away from the skin surface. It may serve as a culture medium for *C. albicans*, promoting or aggravating diaper dermatitis.[18] **Talc** is a finely milled form of hydrous magnesium silicate which is more a lubricant than an absorbent. It reduces friction, and adheres well to the skin. However, respiratory problems may develop from aspiration of cornstarch or talc unless it is applied to a cotton puff or to the hands and dabbed on.[19] Metabolic alkalosis has been reported in an infant whose diaper rash was treated with baking soda.[20] When powders are applied to broken or oozing skin, a crust may form leading to infection.

Cleansing should be gentle, and the frequency of washing should be decreased. A soft cloth should be used. The area should be well rinsed if possible. Cleansing should occur after urination or defecation. Rinsing with water and wiping with cotton wool balls is sufficient to remove urine.[21] Mild soaps should be used for feces removal. After cleansing, the area should be blotted dry. An alternative to soap is a soapless cleanser or an oil-in-water lotion. This is especially important for the atopic child whose skin is further irritated by frequent washing with soap and water. Irritant surfactants should be avoided.

Diaper wipes are composed of a substrate with cleansing agents and/or emollients. In studies among healthy infants, cleansing with a diaper wipe resulted in significantly lower erythema and surface roughness compared with water used with a cotton washcloth or cotton wool balls.[22,23] Avoid commercial diaper wipes if they contain chemicals such as alcohol, fragrance, lanolin, methylisothiazolinone or soap, especially if they add to skin irritation. Wipes without sensitizers were as well tolerated as water in daily cleansing in infants with atopic dermatitis.[22] Most wipes should be discontinued if the skin is broken.

Combination products for managing adult incontinence offer another approach for improving diaper skin conditions through cleansing. Use of a system including an adult brief (diaper) and 2 wipes for cleansing/protection in a waterproof pouch resulted in a greater frequency of using wipes for cleansing and decreased the time for care.[24]

Compressing: If there is oozing and crusting with acute inflammation, compressing with wet dressings (tap water, normal saline, astringents) or oatmeal baths has been recommended. However, no studies compare astringents to plain tap water or normal saline, which have less risk of further damage to the skin.

Compresses cool and dry the skin through evaporation. They reduce inflammatory blood flow, cleanse the skin of exudates, crusts and debris, and help maintain drainage of infected areas through vasoconstriction. They are indicated in acute eczematous conditions with oozing and crusting, which can be seen in acute diaper dermatitis. The solution should be tepid or room temperature, although cold solution is effective to relieve itch in skin that is otherwise not symptomatic. A nonirritating gauze or thin cloth is soaked with solution, then wrung gently so it remains wet but not dripping. The compress is applied to the skin, removed, remoistened and reapplied every few minutes ("a minute on, a minute off") for 20- to 30-minute periods, 4–6 times daily. After using a compress, a lotion may be applied to the skin; however, avoid occlusion with an ointment. Instructions for compressing are different from instructions for soaking. Although the same solutions are used, opposite effects are produced: soaks are used for chronic dry dermatitis and will rehydrate the skin. If used in weeping conditions, they will macerate and cause harm (see Chapter 55: Atopic, Contact, and Stasis Dermatitis, Wet Dressings). Powders are not applied to any exudative lesion because they crust, causing bleeding on removal and increased risk of infection. Oilated or nonoilated oatmeal baths may soothe diaper dermatitis. Irritant contact dermatitis has been reported from overuse of acid pH cleansers.[25]

Diapers: As a barrier and an absorptive device, an appropriately chosen diaper can prevent and ameliorate diaper dermatitis. Inappropriately chosen diapers may exacerbate this condition. Diapers should be changed as frequently as possible to reduce occlusion, decrease contact time of urine and feces with skin, reduce mechanical irritation and trauma and discourage onset of secondary infection.

The practice of double-diapering to reduce the frequency of diaper changes is not recommended. The apparently unsoiled part of the diaper should never be used to wipe or clean the diaper area. Plastic pants should be avoided with cloth diapers.

Infant diapers have evolved from the use of cloth (covered with plastic, impermeable overpants), to disposable diapers with a cellulose core and a plastic outer cover, to disposable diapers with highly absorbent polymers (known as absorbent gelling material and referred to as AGM diapers) and to AGM diapers with a permeable or "breathable" outer cover.[1] A comparison of the technologies showed that reusable cloth diapers absorb urine but do not reduce humidity or remove skin surface moisture, especially when used with plastic pants. Disposable diapers with AGM absorb urine/moisture and wick it vertically away from the skin, reducing maceration and mixing of urine with feces and prevent rewetting over time. The net effect is decreased humidity compared with cloth. Infants wearing breathable disposable diapers experienced significantly less diaper dermatitis including confirmed infection with *Candida* compared with standard, nonbreathable disposable diapers in a series of double-blind clinical trials. Severe dermatitis was reduced by 38–50%.[26] However, a systematic review found that there was insufficient good-quality evidence to draw any conclusions about use of disposable diapers and prevention of diaper dermatitis.[27]

Choice of diaper is highly personal and steeped in controversy. Some consider cloth more economical, comfortable and environmentally friendly. Others prefer the convenience of disposable diapers. Diapers may also be therapeutic for atopic children, as the "tropical" environment may effectively rehydrate dry, atopic skin.[28]

Care of cloth diapers: Cloth diapers should be washed with mild detergent, avoiding water softeners or harsh soaps, and may be rinsed of bleach (if it has been used in the wash) by running through an additional rinse cycle. A cup of vinegar in the final rinse water lowers the pH of the diapers. Commercial diaper services rinse diapers of harsh chemicals, sterilize them and iron them to kill bacteria, fungi and yeasts.

Education: Patients and caregivers must understand both prevention and treatment of diaper dermatitis (see Diaper Rash—What You Need to Know).

Nonpharmacologic Therapy

Diaper dermatitis represents a persistent challenge to the epidermal barrier. Although episodes of dermatitis may resolve, barrier function usually remains compromised and further minor skin damage increases the risk of injury and future episodes. Skin condition should be examined at every diaper change or incontinence episode, and patients should be assessed for risk factors and contributing issues.

Hydration should be minimized through the use of diaper products that wick moisture away from the skin surface, minimizing contact with wetness, frequent diaper changes, selection of properly sized diapers and ensuring the skin surface is dried after cleansing.

Cleansing should be gentle, using soft cloths with minimal rubbing and avoiding products with known irritants, fragrance or alcohol.

Pharmacologic Therapy

For comparative ingredients of nonprescription products, consult the *Compendium of Products for Minor Ailments*—Baby Care Products: Diaper Rash.

Topical treatments should be used as preventive and active therapy. Treatment should begin at the first appearance of signs and symptoms such as slight erythema, dryness, dermatitis or abnormal skin anywhere in the diaper area. Re-evaluate and modify plan if condition worsens or does not show improvement.

An approach to prevention and treatment of diaper dermatitis is presented in Figure 2.

Barrier Products

Vehicles as Delivery Systems: The type of vehicle and manner of use in the clinical setting are important considerations. Ideally, topical treatments for diaper dermatitis should provide a semipermeable film or layer over the damaged skin to facilitate barrier repair, provide a physical shield between the skin and the irritants, remain in place on the skin (not removed by feces), maintain the acid mantle (acidic pH) and allow for ease of cleansing the skin (minimize stripping).[1] The success of therapy for diaper dermatitis depends as much on the choice of vehicle as on the choice of active ingredients.

Thicker products (pastes, creams and ointments) are usually water-in-oil emulsions that have low water content or are anhydrous. Lotions and emulsion creams cool and protect mechanically. Ointments protect, soften and lubricate. Powders, either loose or incorporated into pastes, protect the skin mechanically, absorb fluid and decrease friction. However, if the powder is within a hydrophobic material or lipid (e.g., zinc oxide powder in petrolatum), external water cannot be absorbed.[29] Pastes combine the actions of both powders (absorb, protect, decrease friction) and the ointment bases (soften, lubricate) into which they are incorporated. Pastes and petrolatum-based barriers can be occlusive.

Barrier bases are the mainstay of topical diaper dermatitis therapy and can be of 2 types: those that provide a water-impermeable barrier only, and those that provide a barrier and are also water-absorptive. Since the 2 essential contributions to the development of the dermatitis are loss of barrier function and overhydration, barrier-absorptive bases are preferred as they both lessen the overhydration and create a barrier. Both types of products provide a physical barrier to shield the skin from outside irritants, protect surfaces that are healing, and lubricate against maceration and friction. Barrier base products usually contain a mixture of ingredients including zinc oxide, petrolatum, mineral oil, eucerin, lanolin, or a silicone base in the vehicle, with or without absorptive ingredients such as talc, cornstarch or kaolin. Some may also contain astringents such as hamamelis (witch hazel), which may be a sensitizer, or vitamins such as A, or A and D in the form of cod liver oil. Preservative and fragrance may be present. Some of these added constituents are of dubious value, or may be contact sensitizers. Avoid first aid products not approved for diaper dermatitis as they may contain other harmful ingredients such as an unnecessary antibiotic or a sensitizing anesthetic.

The use of barriers is recommended as both prevention and treatment of diaper dermatitis. Use will help prevent dermatitis in all diaper wearers with risk factors present, and especially in newborns with frequent urination and defecation, those with sensitive skin or patients with coexisting conditions. Thicker, absorptive barriers are suggested for treatment of an existing dermatitis.

Barrier-only products that are suitable for use in diaper dermatitis are either oleaginous hydrocarbon bases (petrolatum), absorption bases (anhydrous lanolin, anhydrous Eucerin) or silicone bases. **Petrolatum** (yellow or decolourized white) is a translucent, oil-phase greasy preparation with no capacity to absorb moisture. It traps moisture present on the skin surface and may lead to maceration if applied to overhydrated skin. As a mineral-derived product, it may be irritating to inflamed skin. Though widely recommended and anecdotally effective for prevention of diaper dermatitis, evidence is lacking. One study showed no significant difference in preventing diaper rash when petrolatum jelly was compared with controls.[15] **Anhydrous lanolin**, a sheep wool–fat product, and **anhydrous Eucerin**, a wool fat alcohol extraction that is less sticky and has less odour, are 2 translucent, oil-phase "absorption" bases (so called due to their ability to absorb water if needed in compounding). However, these wool-derived substances are strong contact allergens and should be avoided in patients who have allergic contact dermatitis, open or inflamed skin or atopic dermatitis. Lanolin-like products may be components of commercial combination bases, wipes or oils for diaper dermatitis; labels should be scrutinized carefully when selecting products for patients who could be sensitized. Wool fat absorption bases are therefore less widely suitable than oleaginous bases for diaper dermatitis. Silicone-based products containing **dimethicone** or **dimethylpolysiloxane** are synthetic bases that are water-repellent only, and soothe by protecting against irritants. **Ceramide** products used as protectants have not been compared with other barriers. In principle, they assist in maintaining normal barrier function and reduce transepidermal water loss by increasing the ceramide/cholesterol ratio, which is reduced in irritated skin. They do not absorb excess moisture.

Bases that are both barrier and absorptive are usually creams or pastes with various percentages of **zinc oxide**. Zinc oxide, a mild antiseptic, is astringent and also functions as an absorptive powder as concentrations increase. Moderate concentrations of zinc oxide (e.g., 15%) are usually creams that are easy to spread and good for daily maintenance to prevent diaper dermatitis. Higher concentrations, (up to 40%), are stiff, have enhanced absorptive and astringent properties, and are suitable for treatment of diaper dermatitis. Pastes are especially useful for diaper dermatitis associated with diarrhea or increased stool output.[30] They may need to be spread gently with a tongue depressor or spatula, and removed with mineral oil. Although zinc absorption through the skin has been reported in a child with acrodermatitis enteropathica, zinc is a naturally occurring essential mineral and part of daily dietary requirements.[31] A plain zinc oxide barrier is preferable to those that may sensitize due to the presence of other constituents, such as aloe vera. Vitamin A and a vitamin B_5 derivative (dexpanthenol) are popular additives to diaper rash barrier products, but no benefit has been demonstrated compared with zinc oxide, lanolin and petrolatum alone.[32]

Glycerin is an active humectant at concentrations of 20–45%. Frequently, lower concentrations of glycerin are present to ensure shelf-life of a product only and are inactive as humectants.

A Cochrane review examined the evidence on **vitamin A**, a component of the skin protectant cod liver oil, for treatment and/or prevention of diaper dermatitis. One study investigating 114 newborns reported no differences in diaper dermatitis for an ointment with vitamin A compared with the vehicle;[33] it should not be recommended.

Topical films: Solutions and sprays that dry to form a semipermeable barrier film on the skin are alternatives. They are intended to remain in place to protect the skin from direct contact with irritants and to facilitate skin barrier repair. They can be useful alternatives to topical creams whose effectiveness can be limited by poor persistence of effect and removal with diaper changes. The films can minimize skin stripping from cleansing procedures. One example is Cavilon No-Sting Barrier Film, delivered from a volatile silicone solvent to form a semipermeable film, which is flammable. It can be used on infants older than 1 month (not for use on preterm infants). Another film is Sureprep No-Sting Protective Barrier Wipe, delivered to the skin from a nonflammable water-based solution. Trials of these products lacked sufficient numbers of subjects to conclusively determine the effectiveness and the time course of improvement relative to conventional barrier creams.[34,35]

Topical Antifungals

Topical antifungal preparations with antiyeast activity are usually necessary in diaper dermatitis showing signs of barrier compromise such as inflammation; it is likely critically colonized with *Candida* due to transfer from the bowel via feces. This may occur before classic signs of a *Candida* infection (diaper dermatitis which is beefy red with a lacy, scaly border and satellite pustules, involving the creases) appear. Topical imidazoles are the treatment of choice. Topical **miconazole** or **clotrimazole** are generally 70–90% effective against *Candida* within 1 week of treatment. The polyene antifungal **nystatin** is another antiyeast preparation with slightly less efficacy than the imidazoles (approximately 70% effectiveness). Nystatin typically requires longer treatment (about 2 weeks) for symptoms to resolve. Nystatin is known to cause staining of fabric. Topical miconazole was reported to be well tolerated and significantly more effective than zinc oxide/petrolatum for treatment of diaper dermatitis complicated by candidiasis.[36,37] A randomized, controlled study found clinical response to clotrimazole superior to nystatin in infants with diaper dermatitis.[38]

Topical **ciclopirox** provided a significant reduction in severity and an increase in cure rate among infants with diaper dermatitis in 1 study.[39] It is often recommended because of additional broad-spectrum antibacterial and anti-inflammatory effects. It is considered superior to nystatin and inferior to imidazoles in terms of clinical efficacy.

One small study found that topical application of a liquid menthol product prior to topical clotrimazole therapy significantly improved erythema and pustules and time to complete healing, compared with clotrimazole alone.[40]

Antifungal preparations function to keep the antifungal at the skin surface, where it can release the medication to attack the yeast in the stratum corneum. They should be applied first, followed by the barrier cream. Once the inflammation has subsided, discontinue the antiyeast preparation and continue treatment with the barrier cream.

Topical Corticosteroids

Corticosteroids: Topical **hydrocortisone** 0.5–1 % can be applied to the occluded area under the diaper. Use caution in children under 2 years of age. Hydrocortisone can be added to the regimen for short periods of 1–2 weeks only, if severe inflammation exists. It can be used with a barrier cream if the diaper dermatitis is an irritant dermatitis, or with an antiyeast preparation for prevention or treatment of *Candida*. If used as a cream or ointment with an antiyeast cream in a polyethylene glycol base, apply the corticosteroid first.

More potent corticosteroids are not recommended as absorption due to heat and moisture can cause serious side effects. Hydrocortisone 1% is sometimes added extemporaneously as a powder to commercial antifungal preparations to facilitate adherence. Equal parts of hydrocortisone and antifungal creams should *not* be mixed as the resultant product contains half the required concentration of each active agent, and half the required concentration of preservative. This may lead to a lack of therapeutic response and the possibility of resistance arising with continued use. Once inflammation subsides, the corticosteroid should be discontinued.

Combinations of antifungals and mid- to high-potency corticosteroids (e.g., nystatin and triamcinolone, clotrimazole and betamethasone dipropionate) are not recommended because of the risk of corticosteroid-induced skin atrophy and the ability of the occlusive environment to enhance penetration.[41]

Pharmacologic options for the prevention and treatment of diaper dermatitis are summarized in Table 5.

Natural Health Products

Natural health products for diaper dermatitis may include mixtures of oils of sandalwood, peppermint and lavender, calendula cream, chickweed root, powdered comfrey root, goldenseal root powder, sweet almond oil, and beeswax heated in a cast-iron pan and strained through cheesecloth before applying to the diaper rash.[9] Evidence is sparse. One study found olive or sunflower oil had a negative effect on the lipid structure of the skin barrier in neonates, though the clinical importance of this finding is unknown.[42] Another study showed both topical *Calendula officinalis* ointment and topical aloe vera cream improved severity of diaper dermatitis in infants; however, calendula was significantly more effective. No adverse effects were reported.[43] Significant improvement over 5 days was found in a preliminary trial in infants with moderate erythema with or without maceration who were treated with **honey, olive oil** and **beeswax**, and the number of candidiasis cases decreased.[44] A derivative of guaiac and chamomile oil, guaiazulene, had beneficial effects compared with placebo when applied to high-risk neonates with diaper dermatitis recalcitrant to extended antifungal therapy.[45] Topical human breast milk has been compared with zinc oxide barrier cream (40%) with no significant difference except that zinc oxide showed a better decrease in lesion score.[46] In another study topical human breast milk was as effective as hydrocortisone 1% ointment after one week in treatment of infants with diaper dermatitis.[47] Natural health products are sold with few instructions, may not be regulated as to purity or potential toxicity and should not be recommended.[48]

Monitoring of Therapy

Table 4 provides a monitoring framework for patients with diaper dermatitis. Parameters should be monitored by the patient or the caregiver. Taper therapy appropriately in response to improvement or resolution. The healthcare practitioner should be responsible for ensuring that the treatment plan remains on schedule, is effective, and that no adverse effects are occurring. The patient or caregiver should be contacted within 2–3 weeks to determine progress. If allergic reactions occur, discontinue therapy. If the condition worsens due to irritation, alter therapy. Severe inflammation should be minimal and should disappear after continued use.

Table 4: **Monitoring of Therapy for Diaper Dermatitis**

Parameter	Expected Change/Timeframe	Actions[a]
Effectiveness endpoints (dermatitis resolution/control; relief of symptoms): short-term		
Inflammation (redness, swelling, pain, warmth)	Decrease by 80% within 1–2 wk	Taper therapy in response to resolution; if end points not achieved, consider further therapy.
Surface area involved	No progression	
Extension to body folds, other local sites or generalization to whole body area	None	
Blister formation and oozing	No new blisters, cessation of oozing after 1–2 days	
Appearance of border scale or satellite pustules	None	
Disruption of sleep behaviour	Restoration of normal pattern within 2–3 wk	
Effectiveness endpoints (dermatitis resolution/control; relief of symptoms): long-term		
Progression of severity	No progression of severity	If end points not achieved, consider further therapy.
Recurrent episodes	Lengthening of symptom-free periods throughout therapy	
Safety endpoints (treatment side effects)		
Allergic reactions	None	If allergic reaction occurs, discontinue therapy.
Severe dryness, irritation (e.g., redness, inflammation, stinging)	Minimal Should disappear, diminish or be controlled with continued use	If severe, decrease dose, concentration or frequency of use. If still no improvement, consider alternative treatment.

[a] Patient or caregiver should monitor all parameters daily while on drug therapy. Healthcare practitioners should monitor all parameters after 1–2 weeks of therapy or at next visit.

Figure 1: Assessment of Diaper Dermatitis

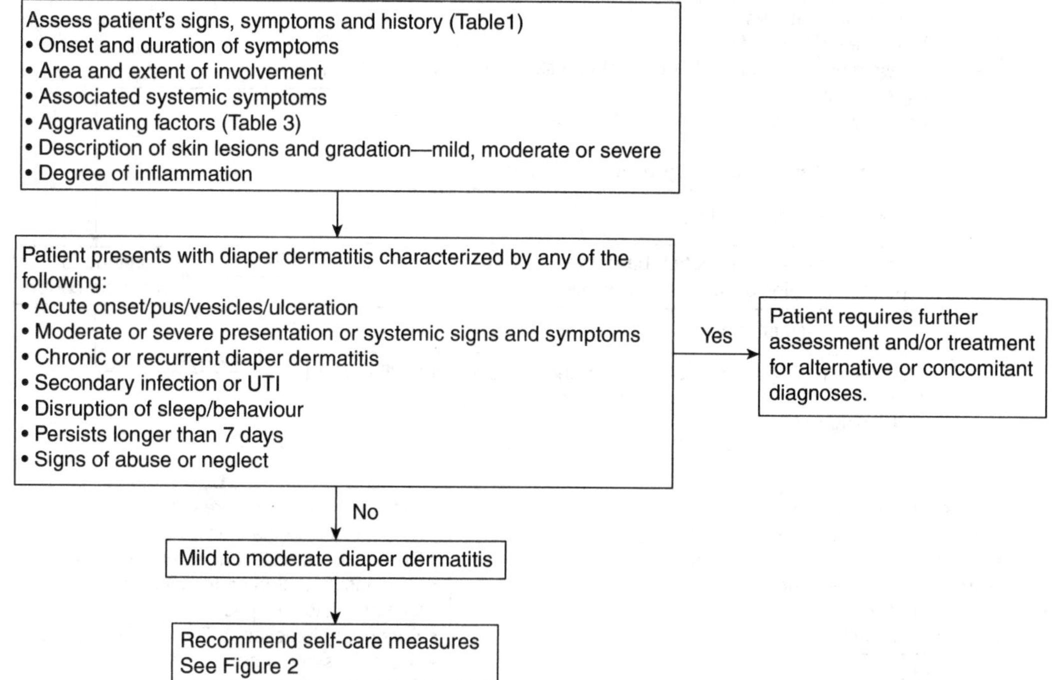

Assess patient's signs, symptoms and history (Table1)
• Onset and duration of symptoms
• Area and extent of involvement
• Associated systemic symptoms
• Aggravating factors (Table 3)
• Description of skin lesions and gradation—mild, moderate or severe
• Degree of inflammation
Patient presents with diaper dermatitis characterized by any of the following:
• Acute onset/pus/vesicles/ulceration
• Moderate or severe presentation or systemic signs and symptoms
• Chronic or recurrent diaper dermatitis
• Secondary infection or UTI
• Disruption of sleep/behaviour
• Persists longer than 7 days
• Signs of abuse or neglect
Yes
Patient requires further assessment and/or treatment for alternative or concomitant diagnoses.
No
Mild to moderate diaper dermatitis
Recommend self-care measures
See Figure 2

Figure 2: **Treatment of Diaper Dermatitis**

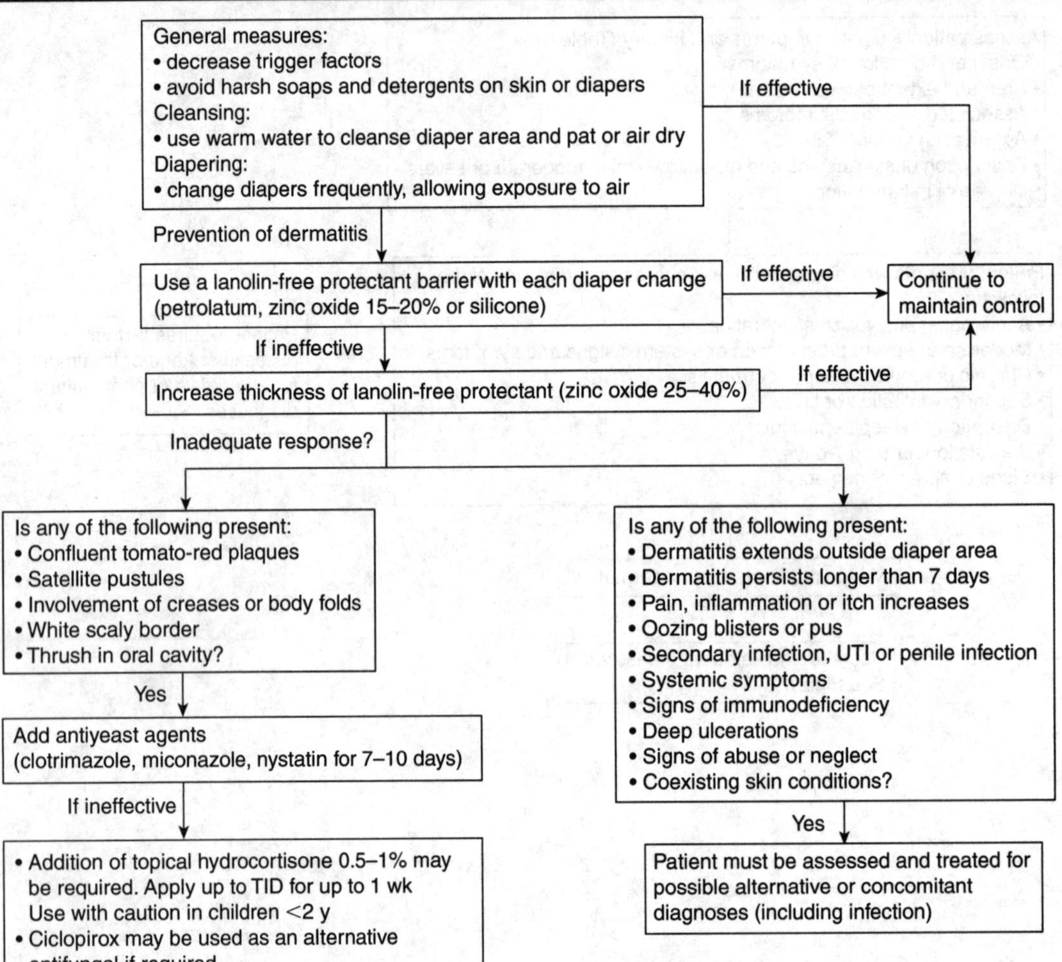

General measures:
• decrease trigger factors
• avoid harsh soaps and detergents on skin or diapers
Cleansing:
• use warm water to cleanse diaper area and pat or air dry
Diapering:
• change diapers frequently, allowing exposure to air
If effective
Prevention of dermatitis
Use a lanolin-free protectant barrier with each diaper change (petrolatum, zinc oxide 15–20% or silicone)
If effective
Continue to maintain control
If ineffective
Increase thickness of lanolin-free protectant (zinc oxide 25–40%)
If effective
Inadequate response?
Is any of the following present:
• Confluent tomato-red plaques
• Satellite pustules
• Involvement of creases or body folds
• White scaly border
• Thrush in oral cavity?
Yes
Add antiyeast agents (clotrimazole, miconazole, nystatin for 7–10 days)
If ineffective
• Addition of topical hydrocortisone 0.5–1% may be required. Apply up to TID for up to 1 wk Use with caution in children <2 y
• Ciclopirox may be used as an alternative antifungal if required
Is any of the following present:
• Dermatitis extends outside diaper area
• Dermatitis persists longer than 7 days
• Pain, inflammation or itch increases
• Oozing blisters or pus
• Secondary infection, UTI or penile infection
• Systemic symptoms
• Signs of immunodeficiency
• Deep ulcerations
• Signs of abuse or neglect
• Coexisting skin conditions?
Yes
Patient must be assessed and treated for possible alternative or concomitant diagnoses (including infection)

Table 5: **Pharmacologic Therapy for Prevention and Treatment of Diaper Dermatitis**

Class	Drug	Dosage	Onset/Duration	Adverse Effects	Comments	Cost[a]
Antifungal	*ciclopirox olamine*[b] *1%* Loprox	Massage into affected area and surrounding skin BID	Onset: Clinical improvement and relief of pruritus within 1 wk Duration: Continue for minimum of 4 wk	Transient pruritus, mild burning at application site	Broad-spectrum antifungal. If using in combination with barrier product, apply antifungal first. Manufacturer states that safety and efficacy have not been established in children <10 y; however, ciclopirox has been studied in this age group and is used in practice.	$$
	clotrimazole 1% Canesten, generics	Massage into affected area and surrounding skin BID	Onset: Clinical improvement and relief of pruritus within 1 wk Duration: Continue for minimum of 1–2 wk	Blistering, irritation, burning, pruritus, stinging.	Some anti-inflammatory and gram-positive antibacterial action. Cross-sensitivity with other azole derivatives. If using in combination with barrier product, apply antifungal first.	$$
	miconazole nitrate[c] *2%* Micatin, Monistat Derm, generics	Massage into affected area and surrounding skin BID	See clotrimazole.	See clotrimazole.	See clotrimazole.	$$
	nystatin generics	Massage into affected area and surrounding skin BID–TID	Onset: Within 24–72 h after initiation of therapy. Duration: Continue for minimum of 2 wk	Irritation (rash, urticaria) primarily due to preservatives (parabens) in some formulations. May stain clothing.	Effective only against *Candida*. If using in combination with barrier product, apply antifungal first.	$
Barrier Products	*silicone-based products (dimethicone or dimethylpolysiloxane)* Barriere Cream, Moisturel Cream	Apply PRN in a thick layer	Onset: Skin protection is immediate Duration: Skin protection lasts about 3 hours.	Not irritating. Formulations that contain additives such as lanolin, preservatives or fragrance may be sensitizing.	Water-repellent only. Soothe by protecting against irritants.	$

(cont'd)

Table 5: **Pharmacologic Therapy for Prevention and Treatment of Diaper Dermatitis** *(cont'd)*

Class	Drug	Dosage	Onset/Duration	Adverse Effects	Comments	Cost[a]
	zinc oxide 15%, 40% Zincofax, generics	Apply PRN in a thick layer	See silicone-based products.	See silicone-based products.	Astringent and antiseptic actions as well as absorbent and protectant properties. Effective preventive measure at lower concentrations (15%). Highly effective treatment at concentrations >25%. Mineral oil may be used to remove the product if necessary. If using in combination with antifungal product, apply antifungal first.	$
Corticosteroids, topical	*hydrocortisone 0.5%, 1%* Cortate, Emo-Cort, Prevex HC, generics	Massage a thin layer into the affected area up to TID PRN Should not be used for more than 1 wk	Onset for pruritus relief is immediate; inflammation relief takes about 2 days.	Mild to severe skin irritation. Rarely, hypersensitivity reactions.	Effective anti-inflammatory agent. Use caution in treatment of children <2 y due to increased risk of absorption. Apply before polyethylene glycol–based antifungal products if being used in combination.	$

[a] Cost of 15 g; includes drug cost only.

[b] Manufacturer states that safety and effectiveness have not been established in children <12 y; however, ciclopirox has been studied in children and is used in this population in clinical practice.

[c] Manufacturer states that this product is not to be used in children <2 y; however, it is widely used in clinical practice.

Legend: $ <$3 $$ $3–6

Suggested Readings

Coughlin CC, Eichenfield LF, Frieden IJ. Diaper dermatitis: clinical characteristics and differential diagnosis. *Pediatr Dermatol* 2014;31:19-24.

Coughlin CC, Frieden IJ, Eichenfield LF. Clinical approaches to skin cleansing of the diaper area: practice and challenges. *Pediatr Dermatol* 2014;3:1-4.

Klunk C, Domingues E, Wiss K. An update on diaper dermatitis. *Clin Dermatol* 2014;32:477-87.

Lavender T, Furber C, Campbell M et al. Effect on skin hydration of using baby wipes to clean the napkin area of newborn babies: assessor-blinded randomised controlled equivalence trial. *BMC Pediatr* 2012;12:59.

Shin HT. Diagnosis and management of diaper dermatitis. *Pediatr Clin North Am* 2014;61:367-82.

References

1. Visscher MO. Recent advances in diaper dermatitis: etiology and treatment. *Ped Health* 2009;3:81-98.
2. Reider N, Fritsch PO. Other eczematous eruptions. In: Bolognia JL Jorizzo JL Schaffer JV, eds. *Dermatology.* 3rd ed. Philadelphia: Elsevier Saunders; 2012. p. 219-31.
3. Visscher MO, Hoath SB. Diaper dermatitis. In: Chew A, Maibach HI, eds. *Irritant dermatitis*. New York: Springer; 2006. p. 37-51.
4. Leyden JJ. Diaper dermatitis. *Dermatol Clin* 1986;4:23-8.
5. Schanzer MC, Wilkin JK. Diaper dermatitis. *Am Fam Physician* 1982;25:127-32.
6. de Wet PM, Rode H, van Dyk A et al. Perianal candidosis–a comparative study with mupirocin and nystatin. *Int J Dermatol* 1999;38:618-22.
7. Montes LF, Pittillo RF, Hunt D et al. Microbial flora of infant's skin. Comparison of types of microorganisms between normal skin and diaper dermatitis. *Arch Dermatol* 1971;103:400-6.
8. Sires UI, Mallory SB. Diaper dermatitis. How to treat and prevent. *Postgrad Med* 1995;98:79-84, 86.
9. Boiko S. Treatment of diaper dermatitis. *Dermatol Clin* 1999;17:235-40.
10. Makrides HC, MacFarlane TW. An investigation of the factors involved in increased adherence of C. albicans to epithelial cells mediated by E. coli. *Microbios* 1983;38:177-85.
11. Weston WL, Lane AT, Weston JA. Diaper dermatitis: current concepts. *Pediatrics* 1980;66:532-6.
12. Siegel E, Wason S. Borix acid toxicity. *Pediatr Clin North Am* 1986;33:363-7.
13. Scheinfeld N. Diaper dermatitis: a review and brief survey of eruptions of the diaper area. *Am J Clin Dermatol* 2005;6:273-81.
14. Dross C. Ubiquitous preservative blamed for rash of skin allergies *CMAJ* 2013;185:E712.
15. Alonso C, Larburu I, Bon E et al. Efficacy of petrolatum jelly for the prevention of diaper rash: a randomized clinical trial. *J Spec Pediatr Nurs* 2013;18:123-32.
16. Jordan WE, Lawson KD, Berg RW et al. Diaper dermatitis: frequency and severity among a general infant population. *Pediatr Dermatol* 1986;3:198-207.
17. Blume-Peytavi U, Hauser M, Lunnemann L et al. Prevention of diaper dermatitis in infants—a literature review. *Pediatr Dermatol* 2014;31:413-29.
18. Belsito DV. The diagnostic evaluation, treatment, and prevention of allergic contact dermatitis in the new millennium. *J Allergy Clin Immunol* 2000;105:409-20.
19. Mofenson HC, Greensher J, DiTomasso A et al. Baby powder–a hazard! *Pediatrics* 1981;68:265-6.
20. Gonzalez J, Hogg RJ. Metabolic alkalosis secondary to baking soda treatment of a diaper rash. *Pediatrics* 1981;67:820-2.
21. Furber C, Bedwell C, Campbell M et al. The challenges and realties of diaper area cleansing for parents. *J Obstet Gynecol Neonatal Nursi* 2012;41:E13-25.
22. Ehretsmann C, Schaefer P, Adam R. Cutaneous tolerance of baby wipes by infants with atopic dermatitis, and comparison of the mildness of baby wipe and water in infant skin. *J Eur Acad Dermatol Venereol* 2001;15:16-21.
23. Odio M, Streicher-Scott J, Hansen RC. Disposable baby wipes: efficacy and skin mildness. *Dermatol Nurs* 2001;13:107-12, 117-8, 121.
24. Al-Samarrai NR, Uman GC, Al-Samarrai T et al. Introducing a new incontinence management system for nursing home residents. *J Am Med Dir Assoc* 2007;8:253-61.
25. Patrizi A, Neri I, Marzaduri S et al. Pigmented and hyperkeratotic napkin dermatitis: a liquid detergent irritant dermatitis. *Dermatology* 1996;193:36-40.
26. Akin F, Spraker M, Aly R et al. Effects of breathable disposable diapers: reduced prevalence of Candida and common diaper dermatitis. *Pediatr Dermatol* 2001;18:282-90.
27. Baer EL, Davies MW, Easterbrook KJ. Disposable nappies for preventing napkin dermatitis in infants. *Cochrane Database Syst Rev* 2006;(3):CD004262.
28. Wong DL, Brantly D, Clutter LB et al. Diapering choices: a critical review of the issues. *Pediatr Nurs* 1992;18:41-54.
29. Juch RD, Rufli T, Surber C. Pastes: what do they contain? How do they work? *Dermatology* 1994;189:373-7.
30. Kramer D, Honig PJ. Diaper dermatitis in the hospitalized child. *J Enterostomal Ther* 1988;15:167-70.
31. Parra CA, Smalik AV. Percutaneous absorption of zinc in acrodermatitis enteropathica. *Dermatologica* 1981;163:413-6.
32. Bosch-Banyeras JM, Catala M, Mas P et al. Diaper dermatitis. Value of vitamin A topically applied. *Clin Pediatr (Phila)* 1988;27:448-50.
33. Davies MW, Dore AJ, Perissinotto KL. Topical vitamin A, or its derivatives, for treating and preventing napkin dermatitis in infants. *Cochrane Database Syst Rev* 2005;(4):CD004300.
34. Baatenburg de Jong H, Admiraal H. Comparing cost per use of 3M Cavilon No Sting Barrier Film with zinc oxide oil in incontinent patients. *J Wound Care* 2004;13:398-400.
35. Visscher M. *Use of a water-based skin barrier film to treat skin breakdown*. Presented at the National Association of Neonatal Nurses Annual Educational Conference. Fort Lauderdale: NANN; 2008 Sep 24-27.

36. Spraker MK, Gisoldi EM, Siegfried EC et al. Topical miconazole nitrate ointment in the treatment of diaper dermatitis complicated by candidiasis. *Cutis* 2006;77:113-20.
37. Concannon P, Gisoldi E, Phillips S et al. Diaper dermatitis: a therapeutic dilemma. Results of a double-blind placebo controlled trial of miconazole nitrate 0.25%. *Pediatr Dermatol* 2001;18:149-55.
38. Hoeger PH, Stark S, Jost G. Efficacy and safety of two different antifungal pastes in infants with diaper dermatitis: a randomized, controlled study. *J Eur Acad Dermatol Venereol* 2010;24:1094-8.
39. Gallup E, Plott T. A multicenter, open-label study to assess the safety and efficacy of ciclopirox topical suspension 0.77% in the treatment of diaper dermatitis due to Candida albicans. *J Drugs Dermatol* 2005;4:29-34.
40. Sabzghabaee AM, Nili F, Ghannadi A et al. Role of menthol in treatment of candidal napkin dermatitis. *World J Pediatr* 2011;7:167-70.
41. Ward DB, Fleischer AB, Feldman SR et al. Characterization of diaper dermatitis in the United States. *Arch Pediatr Adolesc Med* 2000;154:943-6.
42. Cooke A, Cork MJ, Victor S et al. Olive oil, sunflower oil or no oil for baby dry skin or massage: a pilot, assessor-blinded, randomized controlled trial (the oil in baby SkincaRE [OBSeRvE] Study). *Acta Derm Venereol* 2016;96:323-30.
43. Panahi Y, Sharif MR, Sharif A ET AL. A randomized comparative trial on the therapeutic efficacy of topical aloe vera and Calendula officinalis on diaper dermatitis in children. *ScientificWorldJournal* 2012;2012:810234.
44. Al-Waili NS. Clinical and mycological benefits of topical application of honey, olive oil and beeswax in diaper dermatitis. *Clin Microbiol Infect* 2005;11:160-3.
45. Gunes T, Akin MA, Sarici D et al. Guaiazulene: a new treatment option for recalcitrant diaper dermatitis in NICU patients. *J Matern Fetal Neonatal Med* 2013;26:197-200.
46. Gozen D, Caglar S, Bayraktar S et al. Diaper dermatitis care of newborns human breast milk or barrier cream. *J Clin Nurs* 2014;23:515-23.
47. Farahani LA, Ghobadzadeh M, Yousefi P. Comparison of the effect of human milk and topical hydrocortisone 1% on diaper dermatitis. *Pediatr Dermatol* 2013;30:725-9.
48. Vann A. The herbal medicine boom: understanding what patients are taking. *Cleve Clin J Med* 1998;65:129-34.

Diaper Rash—What You Need to Know

What is diaper rash?

Diaper rash is a skin irritation that can be caused by different things, such as friction or too much moisture on the skin. You should treat it immediately to prevent it from spreading or becoming infected.

What can you do to prevent diaper rash?

- For breastfed infants—mothers should eat a healthy, balanced diet. Try to avoid food that may irritate the baby's digestive system and cause diarrhea (examples—caffeine, citrus fruit, spicy foods).
- **Do not** use harsh soap, detergent or perfumed products on baby's skin.
- Wash diapers in hot water and soap flakes (example—Ivory Snow), not detergent. If you have to use detergent, wash diapers a second time in clear water (no detergent).
- **Do not** use bleach or fabric softener (liquid or sheets).
- **Do not** use lotion or other products that contain lanolin.

How to care for diaper rash:

- Never double-diaper or use plastic pants.
- Avoid wiping the diaper area with any part of a soiled diaper.
- Change diapers often.
- Use warm water to cleanse the diaper area and pat or air dry.
- Use only a small amount of mild soap or a soapless cleanser.
- Avoid using diaper wipes or other products that contain perfume or lanolin.
- Ask your healthcare provider for advice about creams to protect the skin.
- Use a lanolin-free barrier cream every time you change the diaper (examples—petrolatum, zinc oxide 15–20% or silicone). If these products don't work, you can use a thicker lanolin-free barrier paste, such as zinc oxide 25–40%.
- **Do not** use powder. Any powder, including talc, baby powder or cornstarch can cause serious breathing problems if the baby inhales the particles.
- Clean the skin properly every day to control symptoms.

Consult a healthcare provider if the rash:

- continues for longer than 1 week
- becomes more painful, inflamed or itchy
- spreads to other areas
- develops blisters, pus-filled spots, open sores, a scaly border or extends into the body folds.

Chapter 60
Dressings

Marie Berry, BScPharm, BA, LLB

Dressings are intended to protect a wound from damage and contamination, and in some cases promote healing. The simplest dressing is gauze covering a wound, held in place by adhesive tape. Minor cuts and scrapes are often covered by self-adhesive strips that combine both gauze and adhesive tape in a prepackaged format.

Wounds may be chronic (e.g., ulcerations secondary to conditions such as diabetes, peripheral vascular ulcers and pressure ulcers or "bed sores"). Wounds may be extensive, such as a deep wound or one that has had tissue torn from it. All wounds, including minor or postsurgical wounds, require dressings that are specific for the type of wound.

First and foremost, dressings help to stop bleeding and protect the wound from debris, microorganisms and further damage.[1] However, dressings may serve other purposes. An ideal dressing maintains a moist environment while removing excess exudate to prevent maceration. Wounds that are painful benefit from dressings that "soothe" nerve endings, e.g., hydrogels, hydrocolloids, sheet gels. Table 1 lists some of the common characteristics of dressings.

Table 1: **Characteristics of an Ideal Dressing**

Provides a moist environment—a moist environment will accelerate epidermal migration and dermal repair.
Provides thermal insulation—a drop in temperature below 37°C delays mitotic activity for up to 4 h.
Is highly absorptive—excess exudate can macerate healthy tissue.
Is impermeable to bacteria—bacteria and other microorganisms can colonize a wound.
Is free of contaminants—sterile technique is paramount in the application of sterile dressings.
Is nonadherent—dressings that adhere to wounds can cause further tissue damage.
Is nontoxic—some antiseptics and hypochlorites are toxic to tissue.

Dressing Types

Gauze

Gauze acts as an absorbent and protectant. It is made by weaving bleached cotton into an open-mesh cloth. Natural waxes and impurities are removed from the cotton to increase its absorbing capacity. Gauze is classified either according to its mesh or to the number of threads per inch. Self-adherent gauze clings to itself; available as pads or rolls, it can be used to wrap a wound without adhesive tape, e.g., head wound. Viscous rayon and regenerated cellulose are also used in bandages, sometimes in conjunction with gauze.

Nonadherent gauze is easily removable, yet still protective. It is preferred as the primary dressing, next to the wound, because of increased comfort. When removed, nonadherent gauze does not leave gauze threads on the wound surface, nor does it disturb the wound surface by "pulling" or removing any of the surface. It is prepared by impregnating viscous rayon with an oil-in-water emulsion or by covering the gauze with a perforated plastic film.

Adhesive Tape

Adhesive tape is used to secure a gauze dressing to a wound. Several kinds are available, including waterproof, cloth, clear and paper, in a variety of widths. The choice of tape depends upon the size and type of wound, potential skin sensitivities and personal preference. In general, hypoallergenic and easy-to-remove adhesive tapes are preferred. For maximal adhesion, apply tape to dry skin. For wounds that require protection from water or even dirt, a waterproof tape is preferred. Paper or cloth tape reduces the risk of skin damage for wounds that require frequent dressing changes.

Adhesive tape is a fabric or film evenly coated with a pressure-sensitive adhesive mixture. Today, most adhesives are acrylate-based; historically, they were rubber-based. Acrylate-based adhesives tend to produce fewer allergic reactions, and thus are generally termed hypoallergenic. While some reports estimate adhesive tape allergies occur in 0.3% of patients, true allergic reactions represent a small fraction of reactions to adhesive tape.[2] Rather, the irritation may be considered a non-allergic tape reaction caused by factors such as the mechanics of tape removal (repeated removal or skin stripping, removal from a hair-covered area of skin). Combined with an existing dermatitis or a fragile skin surface, adhesive tape reactions may be severe.

Bandages

Bandages are most commonly a combination of gauze and adhesive tape. They may be self-adhesive or require further adhesive material.[3] Self-adhesive bandages are convenient alternatives to gauze and tape and include those with adhesive borders on all sides; however, the correct size needs to be chosen for the wound. The bandage should be large enough to cover the wound completely, yet not too large. If the bandage is too small, the adhesive may adhere to the wound, making removal difficult, or alternatively, a portion of the wound will be exposed. If the bandage is too large, the wound will not be covered securely, impairing healing, and the bandage itself may "bunch" and come loose from the wound. For wounds on body areas that are difficult to bandage, such as fingertips and knuckles, specially shaped bandages are available. Butterfly closures are self-adhesive bandages that pull and hold the edges of small wounds together to encourage healing. Butterfly closures are not a substitute for stitches in larger wounds.

Medicated Dressings

Gauze bandages may be impregnated with therapeutic agents. Medicated gauze allows easy removal and provides a delivery system for antibiotics and antiseptics. Petrolatum gauze is easily removed and acts as a protectant for the underlying skin.

Antiseptic-impregnated gauze contains **chlorhexidine** or **povidone-iodine** and is used to treat and prevent infection and ease removal of the dressing. Gauze impregnated with zinc compounds acts as a protectant and assists in preventing infection. However, there is some controversy regarding the use of antiseptics on wounds.[4] Antiseptic use is not a substitute for appropriate and effective wound cleansing and debridement. Systemic absorption may complicate the use of antiseptics on wounds covering large areas (e.g., burns). Dressings containing water or saline aid in débridement (the removal of foreign material as well as dead tissue) and prevent dehydration. Antibiotics, such as **framycetin** sulfate, may be added to gauze to prevent and treat infections.[5]

Protective Dressings

Protective dressings are either mechanical or physical or a combination of both. Compared with physical dressings which simply provide a physical barrier, mechanical dressings perform other functions. Some act as tissue adhesives, absorbents for exudate and wound débridement agents. Most require a secondary dressing of gauze and adhesive tape to secure them. Table 2 lists suitable dressings based on the wound to be treated.

- **Antimicrobials** are used for draining, exuding and non-healing wounds where reduction and prevention of infection is desired. Often these dressings are an integral part of other types of dressings. Staining of the wound and surrounding skin along with stinging and sensitization can occur; however, development of resistant organisms has not yet been reported.
- **Alginates** are made from seaweed and create a moist environment while absorbing exudate and blood. They also have hemostatic properties in that they are able to stop bleeding. Some are higher in galuronic acid, which means they retain their shape and can be lifted off the wound in one piece. Others are higher in mannuronic acid and less likely to retain their shape. They are easily washed out of the wound with sterile saline. An alginate can absorb up to 20 times its weight; however, they can dehydrate the wound bed and a secondary dressing is often needed to keep an alginate in place.
- **Collagen** dressings are made from collagen, which is found in skin, bones, ligaments and cartilage. During wound healing, collagen promotes the deposition and organization of new tissue in the wound bed. Available as sheets, pads, particles, solutions and gels, these dressings are used in partial thickness burns, donor sites and ulcers (including pressure ulcers).
- **Composites** combine 2 or more physically distinct products or types in a single dressing to serve multiple functions. These are becoming more commonly used because of their practicality.
- **Cyanoacrylate** compounds are tissue adhesives used to close small wounds. Collodion is a viscous solution of pyroxolin in ether and alcohol. Flexible collodion contains camphor and castor oil. Traditionally, both have also been used to seal small wounds.[6]
- **Films** are semipermeable, polyurethane membrane dressings that vary in thickness and size. They can be used alone or in conjunction with other dressings. They can prevent bacterial contamination but do not absorb exudate so should not be used in wounds with moderate to large amounts of drainage. However, they do allow fluid to evaporate while keeping the wound moist. They should not be used alone with infected wounds. Films dressings are comfortable and resistant to shearing.
- **Foam** dressings are the product of advanced polymer technology. They do not adhere to the wound, yet absorb exudate. Hydrophilic polyurethane dressings can absorb several times their weight in exudate. Some have an adhesive border and some have a film coating to provide an additional bacterial barrier. They can be used as either a primary or secondary dressing on a wide variety of wounds, ranging from partial to full thickness wounds with minimal, moderate or heavy draining.
- **Hydrocolloids** consist of a mixture of pectins, gelatins and sodium carboxymethylcellulose. Ideal for sloughing or necrotic wounds, they provide an occlusive environment and remove exudate by mixing with it. These dressings are impermeable to bacteria and other contaminates while minimizing skin trauma and moulding well to the wound.
- **Hydrogels** are matrices containing a high percentage of water and are available as both sheets and gels. The sheets are polysaccharides cross-linked with polyacrylamide and are ideal for shallow wounds like burns. Gels are more suitable for deeper wounds. Because of their high water content, they do not absorb exudate, but they do help maintain a moist healing environment. If they are self-adhesive, they may be used as a primary dressing; however, a secondary dressing is sometimes needed to keep the hydrogel dressing in place.

Choice of Dressing

The choice of dressing depends upon the characteristics of the wound, patient characteristics and cost. Primary factors are wound etiology, classification, size and shape, and the amount and type of healing that has occurred. The appearance of the wound edges and surrounding skin influence the dressing size and adhesive choice. The presence of an exudate or infection must also be considered.

The presence of exudate is a barrier to healing because it inhibits cell growth, contributes to bacterial imbalance, increases necrotic tissue development and reduces the migration of key cells needed for healing (e.g., keratinocytes, fibroblasts, endothelial cells). Compression therapy, mechanical devices such as some débridement materials and absorptive dressings are used to reduce exudate.

The potential need for débridement can affect the choice of dressing. An occlusive dressing maintains a moist environment which results in autolytic or self-débridement. Wet-to-dry dressings and irrigation will mechanically débride a wound, but may remove healthy as well as dead tissue. Due to risk of skin sensitivity and the availability of more effective methods, chemical or enzyme débridement is now reserved for specific, problematic wounds. Physical débridement (using tweezers to remove debris) is an important step in preparing a wound for dressing application.

Patient comfort and preference as well as the anatomical location of the wound will affect the choice of dressing. Factors such as the patient's circulation, nutritional and medical status are considerations, as are the availability and durability of the dressing itself.

For comparative features of nonprescription products, consult the *Compendium of Products for Minor Ailments*—Skin Care Products: Dressings.

Table 2: **Wound Dressings**

Wound Description/ Symptom	Types of Suitable Dressings	Examples of Products[a]
Black surface, hard eschar requiring rehydration and/ or débridement	Hydrogel	Duoderm Hydrogel
	Hydrocolloid	Duoderm CGF, Comfeel Plus
Soft black surface requiring removal	Cadexomer iodine dressings	Iodosorb
Green surface which may be malodorous, requiring infection control	Film dressings	Opsite
	Antiseptic-impregnated gauze (e.g., povidone-iodine)	Betadine
	Anti-infective–impregnated dressings (e.g., framycetin sulfate)	SofraTulle
Yellow surface	Hydrogel	Duoderm Hydrogel
	Hydrocolloid	Duoderm CGF, Comfeel Plus
Clinical infection requiring treatment of infection and control of exudate and odour	Film dressings	Opsite
	Antiseptic-impregnated gauze (e.g., povidone-iodine)	Betadine
	Anti-infective–impregnated dressings (e.g., framycetin sulfate)	SofraTulle
Granulating surface requiring creation of moist environment and management of exudate	Alginates	Aquacel, Algisite, Kaltostat
	Foam dressings	Allevyn
	Film dressings	Opsite

(cont'd)

Table 2: **Wound Dressings** *(cont'd)*

Wound Description/ Symptom	Types of Suitable Dressings	Examples of Products[a]
	Hydrocolloid	Duoderm CGF, Comfeel Plus
Epithelializing surface requiring creation of moist environment	Film dressings	Opsite
	Foam dressings	Allevyn
	Thin hydrocolloid	DuoDerm Extra Thin, Comfeel Plus Transparent
Pain requiring dressings that protect nerve endings	Hydrogels, hydrocolloids and sheet gels are good choices	Duoderm CGF, Comfeel Plus
	Hydrophilic dressings such as sugar paste or cadexomer iodine exert an osmotic pull and may increase the pain	
Odour, most often caused by gram-negative bacteria such as *Pseudomonas*	Silver sulfadiazine and framycetin reduce colonization. Povidone-iodine has antiseptic activity, but is quickly deactivated in the presence of pus; therefore, an iodine cadexomer dressing may be preferred since it allows for a slower release of antiseptic, extending the antiseptic activity	Flamazine, SofraTulle, Iodosorb
Excessive exudate requiring a balance between the need for a moist environment and prevention of maceration	Foam and hydrocolloid dressings are good choices to absorb exudate. Some types of wounds (e.g., venous ulcers) and wounds in some types of medical conditions (e.g., hypertension coupled with venous disease) produce more exudate. In these situations, compression bandages may also be useful to help reduce exudate by decreasing venous pressure and controlling edema	Allevyn, Duoderm CGF, Comfeel Plus
Bleeding needs to be controlled	Alginates have hemostatic properties	Aquacel, Algisite, Kaltostat
Infection may need to be controlled by systemic antibiotic treatment	Antiseptic- or antibiotic-impregnated gauze may be useful	Bactigras, SofraTulle

[a] These products are listed as examples only and do not imply recommendation of one brand over another.

Potential Problems when Applying a Dressing

The most commonly used dressings are self-adhesive bandages. Their application is straightforward; however, care must be taken to ensure the gauze pad is not contaminated through handling. Proper use and application of any dressing are essential for maximum effectiveness.

Principles of optimal use of dressings include:

- Use the correct size. A dressing should be large enough to cover the wound, yet not so large that it bunches. If 2 or more dressings are needed to cover the wound, the edges should be overlapped to ensure complete wound coverage
- Use sterile technique to apply the dressing with clean hands or gloves. The dressing surface and wound itself should not be touched. Table 3 describes the steps in applying a dressing
- Whatever is applied to the wound will eventually have to be removed. Greasy substances are best avoided as they may be difficult to remove, causing more damage to the wound. Lint from loosely woven gauze can also be problematic

- The wound must be cleaned prior to applying any dressing. Applying a dressing to a contaminated wound increases the risk of infection. Flushing the wound with water or sterile saline may be sufficient
- If a wound requires débridement or control of bleeding, it should be performed before a dressing is applied, unless the dressing is specifically designed for débridement or control of bleeding
- Sutures may be needed; dressings, even butterfly closures, do not replace necessary sutures
- Always consider potential complications such as excessive bleeding and infection. SHARP is an acronym for signs of infection—swelling, heat, ache, redness, pus. A malodorous wound is usually infected
- Remember that some patients have a higher risk of complications. Individuals with diabetes have impaired peripheral circulation and wound-healing ability. Nutritional deficiencies may delay healing, and the use of some medications (e.g., anticoagulants, NSAIDs) may increase the risk of bleeding
- Dressings require changing at different intervals. It is a misconception that once a dressing is applied, there is no need to change it. Manufacturer instructions and wound care protocols need to be consulted regarding whether a dressing requires changing and the interval recommended.

Table 3: **Application of a Dressing**

Wash hands and work in a clean area—wearing gloves is an option; the table or countertop may need to be cleaned with a disinfectant.
Assess wound—if wound is deep or bleeding excessively, seek medical attention.
Control bleeding—allow the wound to bleed slightly, then apply gentle pressure to stop bleeding; a puncture wound should not be squeezed because the puncturing object may be pushed further into the wound.
Clean wound—remove large foreign particles, débride if necessary by flushing with water, and wash with soap and water.
Check for symptoms of infection—swelling, heat, ache, redness or pus (SHARP), and if present, seek medical attention.
Apply dressing—cover the wound with a dry, sterile gauze dressing using commercially available materials whenever possible; ensure the dressing extends beyond the edges of the wound, use adhesive tape to secure the dressing and do not impede circulation by bandaging the wound too tightly.

Suggested Readings

Advances in Skin and Wound Care. Available from: journals.lww.com/aswcjournal/pages/default.aspx.
Kirsner RS. Wound healing. In: Bolognia JL et al., eds. *Dermatology*. New York: Mosby; 2003.
Ovington LG, Eastman SR. Moist wound healing. *US Pharm* 2001:99-108.

References

1. Jeter KF, Tintle TE. Wound dressings of the nineties: indications and contraindications. *Clin Podiatr Med Surg* 1991;8:799-816.
2. Smith SM, Zirwas MJ. Nonallergic reactions to medical tapes. *Dermatitis* 2015;26:38-43.
3. Bolton L, van Rijswijk L. Wound dressings: meeting clinical and biological needs. *Dermatol Nurs* 1991;3:146-61.
4. Drosou A, Falabella A, Kirsner RS. Antiseptics on wounds: an area of controversy. *Wounds* 2003;15:1-7.
5. Brown CD, Zitelli JA. A review of topical agents for wounds and methods of wounding. Guidelines for wound management. *J Dermatol Surg Oncol* 1993;19:732-7.
6. Edlich RF, Reddy VR. 5th Annual David R. Boyd, MD Lecture: Revolutionary advances in wound repair in emergency medicine during the last three decades. A view toward the new millennium. *J Emerg Med* 2001;20:167-93.

Chapter 61

Drug-induced Skin Reactions

Sandra Knowles, BScPhm

Pathophysiology

Approximately 6% of all hospital admissions are the result of adverse drug reactions (ADRs).[1] Drug-induced skin eruptions are the most frequently observed adverse reactions to medications. In the Boston Collaborative Drug Surveillance Program, the prevalence of cutaneous ADRs in hospitalized patients was 2.2%.[2] Maculopapular eruptions and urticaria/angioedema are the most frequently reported drug rashes.[3]

The morphology of cutaneous eruptions (Table 1 and Table 3) may be broadly classified as exanthematous, urticarial, blistering or pustular. Within each of these categories, the presence of a fever or other accompanying symptoms other than itch signals a more serious reaction, which requires immediate referral to an appropriate healthcare practitioner (Table 2).[17]

Table 1: Dermatologic Terminology[4]

Ballet	A vesicle greater than 0.5 cm in diameter
Desquamation	Peeling of the skin
Erythema	Abnormal redness of the skin
Exanthem	An eruptive disease
Macule	A circumscribed, flat lesion less than 0.5 cm in diameter that differs from surrounding skin because of its colour
Morbilliform	Measles-like eruption
Papule	A solid, circumscribed, elevated lesion less than 0.5 cm in diameter
Plaque	An elevated, flat lesion greater than 0.5 cm in diameter
Purpura	Impalpable (macular) unblanchable purple spots
Pustule	A vesicle or bulla (usually less than 1 cm in diameter) filled with purulent exudate
Urticaria	Hives or an eruption of itching wheals
Vesicle	Blister; small, circumscribed, elevation of the skin filled with clear fluid less than 0.5 cm in diameter
Wheal	A transitory, elevated papule or plaque caused by edema of the skin

Exanthematous Eruptions

Simple Eruptions

Exanthematous eruptions, also known as morbilliform or maculopapular eruptions, are the most common cutaneous ADRs. These eruptions have been reported to account for approximately 95% of all drug-induced cutaneous eruptions.[18] They usually start as erythematous macules and papules on the trunk, become confluent and later spread symmetrically to the face and limbs; there is no evidence of blistering or pustulation. Resolution occurs with a change in colour from bright red to a brownish red. This colour change may be followed by scaling or desquamation. Pruritus is a frequent clinical symptom but is not necessarily present. Simple eruptions usually begin within 7–10 days of starting therapy and resolve within 7–14 days after discontinuation of the drug.[19]

Complex Exanthems

Drug rash eosinophilia and systemic symptoms (DRESS), also known as the drug hypersensitivity syndrome reaction, is a complex drug reaction that includes fever, skin eruption (usually exanthematous), eosinophilia and internal organ involvement such as hepatitis, nephritis or agranulocytosis, although the internal organ involvement may be asymptomatic.[20] The syndrome usually begins with fever 2–3 weeks after initial drug exposure, and patients often initially complain of malaise.[17] In patients with a history of DRESS, re-exposure to the offending agent may lead to symptoms within 1 day. DRESS is not related to dose or serum concentration of the drug. Although symptoms resolve in most patients after discontinuation of the drug, in rare instances some patients develop autoimmune disease and/or production of autoantibodies after resolution of DRESS.[21,22] This can include development of type 1 diabetes, autoimmune thyroid disease or lupus erythematosus (see Hypersensitivity Syndrome Reaction in Photo Section).

Urticarial Eruptions

Simple Eruptions

Urticaria, characterized by extremely pruritic, red, raised wheals of varying sizes and shapes, and angioedema (affecting deep dermal and subcutaneous tissues) are reversible types of edema affecting the skin. In general, individual lesions of urticaria last for less than 24 hours, although new lesions continually develop. Many medications can cause urticaria, angioedema or both; other causal agents are food, physical factors (e.g., cold, pressure), infections and idiopathic factors.[23] Medications account for only 5–10% of urticaria cases. Adverse reactions to ACE inhibitors, manifesting as angioedema, may occur within hours of starting the drug but can occur as late as 1 week to several months into therapy.[24]

Complex Eruptions

Serum sickness–like reactions are defined by fever, rash (usually urticarial) and arthralgias occurring 1–3 weeks after drug initiation. In contrast to true serum sickness, serum sickness–like reactions are not associated with immune complex formation, vasculitis or renal lesions. See Serum Sickness–like Reaction in Photo Section.

Table 2: **Clinical Features of Severe Cutaneous Drug Reactions**[16]

Fever	Palpable purpura
Enlarged lymph nodes	Skin tenderness
Arthralgias or arthritis	Blisters or epidermal detachment
Shortness of breath, wheezing, hypotension	Mucous membrane erosions
Confluent and diffuse erythema	Angioedema or swelling of tongue
Facial edema or involvement of central part of face	

Table 3: Characteristics of Drug Eruptions

Type of Eruption	Description	Onset after Initial Exposure	Clinical Features	Common Drug Causes	Treatment	Testing
Exanthematous	Without fever: Simple	7–10 days	Rash only	Antiepileptic drugs, beta-lactam antibiotics, sulfonamide antibiotics[2]	Symptomatic therapy (e.g., antihistamines, soothing baths, topical corticosteroids)	Mononucleosis
	With fever: Drug rash with eosinophilia and systemic symptoms (DRESS) also known as drug hypersensitivity syndrome reaction	14–21 days (up to 3 months)	Fever, rash, eosinophilia, internal organ involvement (may be asymptomatic)	Allopurinol,[5] antiepileptic drugs (carbamazepine, lamotrigine, phenobarbital, phenytoin),[6] dapsone, nevirapine, sulfonamide antibiotics	Systemic cortico-steroids, symptomatic therapy	CBC, liver enzymes, urinalysis, thyroid function tests
Urticarial	Without fever: Urticaria and/or angioedema	Minutes to hours	Urticaria ± angio-edema	ASA,[7] ACE inhibitors,[8] penicillins, NSAIDs,[7] opioids, radiocontrast media, sulfonamide antibiotics	Symptomatic relief (e.g., antihistamines, topical corticosteroids); angioedema requires immediate therapy with epinephrine	Skin test for penicillin, if suspected as causal agent
	With fever: Serum sickness–like reaction	7–21 days	Fever, rash, arthralgias ± lymph-adenopathy	Bupropion,[9] cefaclor,[10] minocycline,[11] penicillins, rituximab,[12] sulfonamide antibiotics	Symptomatic treatment (including antipyretic, antihistamine); short course of oral corticosteroids in patients with severe symptoms	
Blistering	Without fever: Bullous fixed drug eruption	Hours to days	Solitary erythematous macules that may blister and that recur in the same skin area after readministration of drug	Acetaminophen, barbiturates, NSAIDs, sulfonamide antibiotics, tetracycline	Symptomatic therapy (e.g., moisturizer, topical corticosteroid)	

(cont'd)

Table 3: **Characteristics of Drug Eruptions** *(cont'd)*

Type of Eruption	Description	Onset after Initial Exposure	Clinical Features	Common Drug Causes	Treatment	Testing
	With fever: SJS, TEN	7–14 days	Targets ± epidermal detachment, mucous membrane involvement	Allopurinol,[13] antiepileptic drugs (barbiturates, carbamazepine, lamotrigine, phenytoin), NSAIDs (especially piroxicam),[14] sulfonamide antibiotics	Supportive measures, intravenous immune globulin (IVIG), cyclosporine	CBC, liver enzymes, urinalysis, skin biopsy
Pustular	Without fever: Acneiform	7–21 days	Atypical areas: arms, legs. No comedones	Androgens, antiepileptic drugs, corticosteroids (systemic), epidermal growth factor receptor inhibitors (e.g., cetuximab, erlotinib, gefitinib), isoniazid, lithium	Topical tretinoin (if drug cannot be discontinued)	
	With fever: AGEP	≤10 days	Many pustules on diffuse erythematous base. Fever. 50% have other cutaneous lesions. 25% have mucosal erosions	Beta-lactam antibiotics, calcium channel blockers, quinolones,[15] macrolide antibiotics	Symptomatic therapy, corticosteroids if severe	CBC, skin biopsy

Abbreviations: AGEP = acute generalized exanthematous pustulosis; CBC = complete blood count; SJS = Stevens-Johnson syndrome; TEN = toxic epidermal necrolysis

Blistering Eruptions

Simple Eruptions

Fixed drug eruptions usually appear as pruritic, erythematous, bright red or dusky red macules that may evolve into an edematous plaque. In some patients multiple lesions may be present. Blistering and erosion may occur on mucosal surfaces, especially the genitalia and lips, and some patients may complain of burning or stinging on the affected skin sites. Fixed drug eruptions recur in the same skin area after readministration of the causative medication.[25]

Complex Eruptions

Serious dermatologic eruptions include Stevens-Johnson syndrome (SJS) and toxic epidermal necrolysis (TEN). The typical course of SJS or TEN consists of extreme illness, including fever and malaise, with generalized tender or painful erythema of the skin followed by extensive epidermal necrosis and sloughing of skin or mucous membrane leading to marked loss of fluids and electrolytes[17]. Diagnosis of SJS versus TEN is based on the extent of epidermal detachment: for SJS <10% of body surface area, SJS/TEN overlap 10–30% and TEN >30%. These conditions predispose the patient to pneumonia and septicemia; mortality as high as 30% has been reported when these complications occur (see Toxic Epidermal Necrolysis in Photo Section).

Pustular Eruptions

Simple Eruptions

Drug-induced acne may appear in atypical areas, such as arms and legs, and comedones are usually absent (see Acneiform Eruption in Photo Section). An acneiform eruption often occurs following treatment with epidermal growth factor receptor inhibitors (e.g., gefitinib, erlotinib, cetuximab). The acneiform rash is often accompanied by paronychia, dry skin and skin fissures. The eruption is dose dependent, with respect to both incidence and severity.[26]

Complex Eruptions

Acute generalized exanthematous pustulosis (AGEP) is characterized by acute onset, fever, and a cutaneous eruption with nonfollicular pustules. Generalized desquamation occurs 2 weeks after the initial reaction (see Acute Generalized Exanthematous Pustulosis in Photo Section).

Other Skin Eruptions

Photosensitivity[27]

Photosensitivity is an adverse cutaneous response to normally harmless doses of ultraviolet radiation. Ultraviolet A (UVA) rays are responsible for the majority of photosensitivity reactions. There are 2 types of photosensitivity reactions: phototoxicity and photoallergy.

Phototoxicity, the more common type, refers to an increased reactivity of the skin to ultraviolet (UV) radiation. This can occur on the first exposure to a drug, is dose related and is confined to exposed areas of the skin (e.g., face, neckline, back of the hands, arms, forearms and tops of feet). It generally resembles an exaggerated sunburn. These reactions do not contraindicate continued treatment with the drug, or its reintroduction, as long as effective protection against sunlight is ensured. Drugs associated with phototoxicity include amiodarone, fluoroquinolones, methotrexate, phenothiazines and tetracyclines. See Chapter 72: Prevention and Treatment of Sun-induced Skin Damage, Table 1: Medications That May Cause Phototoxic Reactions.

Photoallergic reactions involve the immune system and therefore require prior sensitization to the drug. Photoallergy is delayed, usually occurring within 24–48 hours of exposure. Pruritus may occur prior to the onset of the cutaneous eruption. The lesions are often eczematous (e.g., with erythema, vesicles and scaling) and may spread beyond exposed areas. Carbamazepine, chloroquine, NSAIDs, and sulfonamides have been reported to cause photoallergic reactions.

Contact Dermatitis

Contact dermatitis is an inflammatory reaction of the skin that results from direct contact with a causative agent.[28] Most cases are either allergic contact dermatitis (e.g., poison ivy, nickel) or irritant contact dermatitis (e.g., chemicals, hot peppers). See Chapter 55: Atopic, Contact, and Stasis Dermatitis.

Goals of Therapy

- Attempt to determine causality of the drug eruption
- Control symptoms associated with the drug eruption (e.g., pruritus)
- Provide patient education about drugs to avoid and those which can be used in the future
- For patients with photosensitivity reactions, provide information regarding preventive measures (e.g., avoiding UV radiation, wearing broad-spectrum sunscreen)
- Report all unexpected or serious ADRs or reactions to recently marketed drugs to Health Canada, through the Canada Vigilance Program or through one of the Canada Vigilance Regional Offices

Patient Assessment

Stepwise assessment of patients with possible drug-induced skin reactions is described in Figure 1.

Patients with a drug eruption require referral to an appropriate healthcare practitioner. Although the rash may be self-limiting and require only self-care measures, patients may require alternative therapy (e.g., a patient develops a nonspecific maculopapular rash 7 days after starting lamotrigine for a seizure disorder, the lamotrigine is discontinued, and now an alternative drug is needed for the seizure disorder). Many drug eruptions are more complex in that they are also associated with systemic signs. A patient who develops any systemic symptom such as malaise, fever or shortness of breath requires immediate medical care since this may signal a more serious reaction.[29]

Since many skin diseases mimic drug reactions, it is important to carefully evaluate other causes of the cutaneous eruption. For example, guttate psoriasis may develop in a person being treated with penicillin for streptococcal infection, but the skin lesions are those of psoriasis and not a drug reaction. Differential diagnoses often include viral exanthems (e.g., infectious mononucleosis, rubella or roseola, see Chapter 74: Viral Skin Rashes), bacterial infections (see Chapter 56: Bacterial Skin Infections: Impetigo, Furuncles and Carbuncles), Kawasaki disease, collagen vascular disease and neoplasia. Disease states can also act as cofactors in the development of a cutaneous eruption. For example, the presence of infectious mononucleosis raises the risk of ampicillin- or amoxicillin-induced exanthematous eruptions from 3–7% to 60–100%. As well, between 44% and 83% of HIV-infected individuals experience a dermatologic adverse reaction with sulfamethoxazole/trimethoprim, whereas these events occur in less than 10% of the general population.[30]

Cutaneous reactions to drugs frequently occur in complicated clinical scenarios that may include exposure to multiple agents, in which case a timeline should be developed. It is important that a detailed history be obtained for evaluation of an adverse drug reaction. This includes dosage, rechallenge and dechallenge, and onset of reaction. A history of prior exposure to the drug and related compounds is also important. If a patient has become sensitized to a drug they have received previously, on re-exposure to that drug the rash may appear sooner. New drugs initiated within the preceding 3 months are more likely causative agents, as are drugs that have been used intermittently, including nonprescription medications and natural health products.[31] Although excipients do not cause ADRs in most individuals, there are isolated case reports of excipients causing skin reactions.[32]

The final step in the assessment of a patient with a cutaneous eruption is to determine the probability of each potential drug cause. A cutaneous eruption is commonly mislabelled as a drug reaction. This misdiagnosis may unnecessarily limit the future use of a particular medication or any related compound. It is important to document the possible drug reaction in the patient's medical and pharmacy records to ensure that future therapies are not pharmacologically and/or chemically related to the suspect drug.

Nonpharmacologic Therapy

Many drug-induced skin eruptions, such as urticaria, are often pruritic. Dry skin and overheating can exacerbate pruritus. Overbathing, hot water, harsh soaps and bubble bath preparations dry and irritate the skin and should be avoided.[33] A simple physical measure is cooling the skin by tepid showering. Four tablespoons of baking soda in the bath may also help to relieve pruritus associated with urticaria. Tap water compresses can be used on blistering lesions; moisten gauze or other thin cloth in warm tap water and apply for 20 minutes 4–6 times daily. Alternatively, compresses can be applied intermittently, 1 minute on 1 minute off, for 20 minutes. Oral lesions can be treated with warm water or saline rinses. Advise patients to avoid factors that may enhance pruritus, such as wearing of tight elasticized apparel or coarse woolen fabrics.

Pharmacologic Therapy

Discontinuation of the offending drug is considered paramount in the management of patients with cutaneous eruptions. However, in some cases the drug may be continued and the reaction "treated through".[34] This decision is influenced by the severity and probable course of the reaction, disease for which the drug was prescribed, ease or difficulty with which the reaction can be managed and the availability of chemically unrelated drugs with similar pharmacologic properties.[35]

Table 4 addresses pharmacologic management of drug-induced skin reactions.

For comparative ingredients of nonprescription products, consult the *Compendium of Products for Minor Ailments*—Analgesic Products: External Analgesics; Cough, Cold and Allergy Products; Skin Care Products: Dermatitis and Dry Skin.

Both traditional **H_1-antagonist antihistamines** and **nonsedating antihistamines** are effective in the treatment of pruritus associated with urticaria.[36] See Chapter 22: Allergic Rhinitis for adult and pediatric doses of oral antihistamines. The addition of **H_2-antagonist antihistamines** (e.g., **ranitidine**, **famotidine**) has been used in some patients with chronic urticaria with some initial benefit;[36] however, patients with acute drug-induced urticaria do not generally require additional therapy with H_2-antagonist antihistamines. Patients whose symptoms do not improve within 5–7 days require further assessment and/or treatment. The use of **topical antihistamines**, such as those containing **diphenhydramine**, is not recommended due to risk of allergic contact dermatitis as well as increased systemic absorption when applied to open lesions. Patients with urticarial lesions should avoid NSAIDs or ASA since these agents may exacerbate urticaria; they are common causes of drug-induced urticaria.

Bathing with **colloidal oatmeal** bath preparations is helpful for pruritus. Unscented **moisture cream** or white **petrolatum** should be applied to the skin while it is slightly damp to retard water evaporation. Topical agents may be kept in a refrigerator because the physical cooling enhances their antipruritic effect.

Topical cream or lotion **astringents**, such as plain **calamine lotion** or **zinc oxide** cream, can also be used. The use of **cooling salves** such as **menthol** 0.25–0.5% or **camphor** 0.25–0.5% cream may be helpful although they may occasionally be irritating. Another local treatment is half-strength **hydrogen peroxide** rinses for oral lesions.

Counsel patients with photosensitivity reactions to stay out of the sun until the reaction resolves, or to wear sunscreen and protective clothing. Exposed areas should be covered with a sunscreen that protects in the UVA range with a minimum SPF of 15–30. See Chapter 72: Prevention and Treatment of Sun-induced Skin Damage for a further discussion of sunscreens. Mild to moderate phototoxic reactions can be managed as ordinary sunburn (e.g., oral analgesics, cooling compresses or baths, emollient lotions).[27]

Topical corticosteroids are often used in the management of patients with drug-induced skin eruptions. Choice of potency and vehicle will depend on the body area affected and the extent and severity of the reaction. Only **hydrocortisone** 0.5–1% should be used on the face and intertriginous folds. Ointments are more occlusive and are preferred for dry or scaly lesions, whereas creams are used in moist areas since they are more drying. Lotions are useful for the scalp and other hairy areas or for application to large body areas. The topical corticosteroid should be applied sparingly, with gentle massage, onto the affected area 2–4 times a day. If the skin lesions persist or worsen after 5–7 days of topical corticosteroid therapy, the patient should seek further assessment and/or treatment. For more detailed information on the use of topical corticosteroids, see Chapter 55: Atopic, Contact, and Stasis Dermatitis.

Systemic corticosteroids are often used at a dose of 1–2 mg/kg/day of prednisone (or equivalent), in patients with severe systemic symptoms (e.g., life-threatening internal organ involvement) in conjunction with their cutaneous eruption; a slow taper is necessary, often requiring weeks to months.[37] For patients with SJS/TEN, intravenous immunoglobulin or cyclosporine has been used.[38]

Monitoring of Therapy

Provide symptomatic therapy for patients with drug-induced skin lesions. After discontinuation of the offending medication, most drug-induced cutaneous eruptions will resolve in 5–7 days. In patients with serious drug-induced reactions, symptoms generally begin to abate within days, but this may vary from weeks to months. Many patients require further assessment; some patients may require a change in therapy, drug testing or follow up (e.g., liver function tests). Any patient who has a fever or other accompanying symptoms such as malaise should be assessed by an appropriate healthcare practitioner.

Advice for the Patient

Provide the patient with information regarding the adverse drug reaction. This includes the drug involved in the reaction (if known), the patient's predisposition to possible recurrence on exposure to the drug, potential cross-reaction to other drugs (e.g., ASA and NSAIDs) and genetic predisposition of family members, if applicable. No genetic basis has been found for most adverse drug reactions, including penicillin-allergic reactions. However, for serious reactions such as DRESS, serum sickness-like reactions to cefaclor and serious dermatologic reactions (e.g., SJS and TEN), the risk in first-degree relatives of patients who have had reactions is substantially higher, and counselling family members is a crucial part of the management process. Studies have shown that genetic susceptibility may also increase the risk of developing SJS/TEN. In a Han Chinese population, HLA-B*1502 and HLA-A*3101 were strongly associated with carbamazepine-induced Stevens-Johnson syndrome.[39] In response to these studies, the US Food and Drug Administration (FDA) and Health Canada recommend genetic screening for patients of Asian ancestry before initiation of carbamazepine therapy, and avoidance of carbamazepine in patients who test positive.[40] In addition, advise the patient to enroll in the Medic Alert program.

Figure 1: Assessment of Patients with Possible Drug-induced Skin Reactions

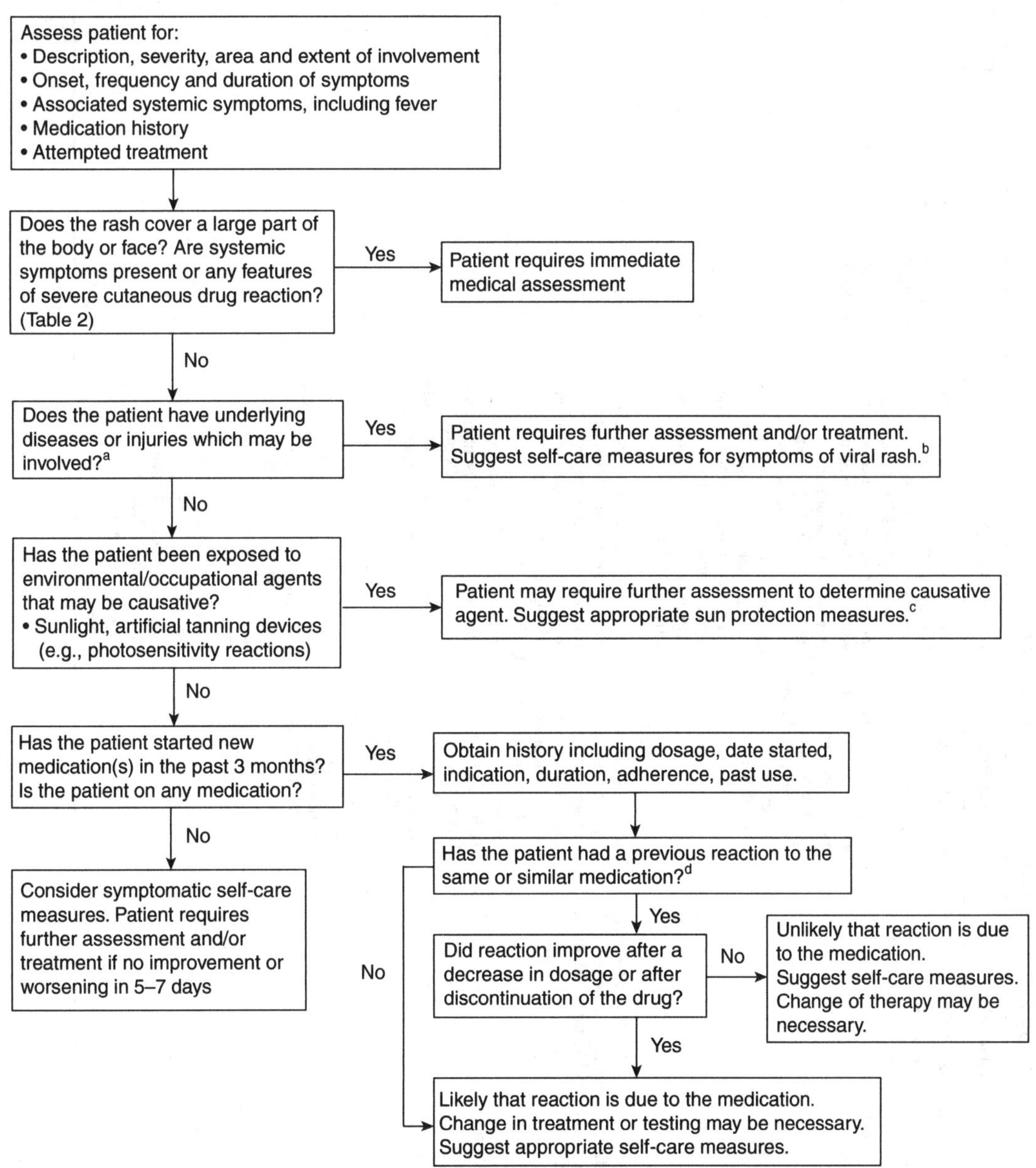

a Examples of underlying diseases include infectious mononucleosis (ampicillin-related reactions), HIV (sulfamethoxazole/trimethoprim), and infectious etiologies, e.g., viral skin rash, bacterial infections.
b See Chapter 74: Viral Skin Rashes.
c See Chapter 72: Prevention and Treatment of Sun-induced Skin Damage.
d At this point perform a literature search to determine whether this reaction has been reported in association with this drug.

Table 4: Pharmacologic Therapy for Drug-induced Skin Reactions

Class	Drug	Dosage	Adverse Effects	Drug Interactions	Comments	Cost[a]
Analgesics	*acetaminophen* Atasol Preparations, Tempra, Tylenol, Tylenol Children's, generics	325–1000 mg Q4–6H po SR: 650 mg Q8H po (maximum 4 g/day)	Hepatotoxicity: Increased risk in malnourished patients, those with excessive alcohol intake (>3 drinks per day) or pre-existing hepatic disease. Baseline LFTs should be measured in high-risk patients.	Acetaminophen has been reported to increase INR in warfarin-treated patients. Check INR if acetaminophen ≥2 g/day is used for ≥3 consecutive days. Adjust warfarin dosage as required. Phenytoin, barbiturates, carbamazepine may increase acetaminophen metabolism and formation of toxic metabolite, thus increase risk of hepatotoxicity; risk may be increased in patients taking high therapeutic doses of acetaminophen and antiepileptic drugs chronically.	Useful for treatment of mild to moderate phototoxic reactions that can be managed as for ordinary sunburn. Avoid ASA and NSAIDs in urticarial lesions.	$
	ibuprofen Advil, Advil Children/ Pediatric, Advil Junior Strength, Advil Liquid Gels, Motrin, Motrin (Children's), Motrin IB, Motrin Liquid Gels, generics	200–400 mg Q6–8H po; maximum dose for self-care: 1200 mg/day	Local GI effects (dyspepsia, diarrhea), GI complications (ulceration/upper GI bleed); exacerbation of HF, acute renal failure. Increased LFTs: Transient; hepatotoxicity is rare; more likely to occur in patients with pre-existing hepatic disease or in patients with excessive alcohol intake (>3 drinks per day).	Warfarin (increased bleeding risk via antiplatelet effects and GI complications); monitor INR more frequently during initial period after NSAID started and watch for signs of bleeding. Increased lithium levels—monitor. Methotrexate—NSAIDs inhibit the renal elimination of MTX. Avoid NSAIDs in people using high dose MTX (e.g., cancer). For people using intermittent low-dose MTX for arthritis, risk is minimal. Antihypertensives (e.g., beta-blockers, diuretics, ACEI): may decrease antihypertensive effects; measure baseline BP, remeasure 1–2 wk after starting NSAID and adjust antihypertensive therapy as required. Increased risk of GI bleed with SSRIs. Increased risk of GI adverse effects with alcohol. Give 30 min after or 8 h before low-dose ASA.	See acetaminophen.	$

Class	Drug	Dosage	Adverse Effects	Drug Interactions	Comments	Cost[a]
	naproxen sodium Aleve, Maxidol, generics	220–440 mg/day po in 1 or 2 divided doses; maximum dose for self-care: 440 mg/day	See ibuprofen.	See ibuprofen.	See acetaminophen.	$
Antihistamines, H_1 antagonists[b]	*cetirizine* Reactine, generics	Adults and children >12 y: 5–10 mg/day; maximum 20 mg/day Children: 6–12 y: 5–10 mg/day 2–5 y: 2.5–5 mg/day 12–23 months: 2.5 mg once daily; maximum 2.5 mg BID 6–11 months: 0.25 mg/kg Q12H	Minimal to no anticholinergic or CNS effects; however, may cause drowsiness in some individuals especially at higher doses. Headache.	Increased CNS depression: alcohol, sedatives, tranquilizers, barbiturates. Increased anticholinergic side effects: TCAs, scopolamine.	Patients whose symptoms do not improve within 5–7 days require further assessment and/or treatment.	$
	diphenhydramine Benadryl Preparations, generics	Adults and children ≥12 y: 25–50 mg Q4–6H po; maximum 300 mg/day Children: 6–11 y: 12.5–25 mg Q4–6H; maximum 150 mg/day 2–5 y: 6.25 mg Q4–6H maximum 37.5 mg/day	CNS: Sedation, fatigue, dizziness, impairment of cognition and performance (the patient may be unaware of impairment). Anticholinergic: Dryness of the mouth and eyes, constipation, inhibition of micturition, potential precipitation of angle-closure glaucoma, thickening of bronchial secretions.	Increased CNS depression: alcohol, sedatives, tranquilizers, barbiturates. Increased anticholinergic side effects: TCAs, scopolamine. May increase levels of CYP2D6 substrates, e.g., metoprolol, venlafaxine.	Use with caution in the elderly as they may be more susceptible to side effects such as sedation and syncope. Avoid in patients with angle-closure glaucoma (increased IOP), urinary obstruction (prostatic hypertrophy), bladder neck obstruction (can cause urinary retention), GI obstruction. Observe infants and young children for paradoxical excitation. Patients whose symptoms do not improve within 5–7 days require further assessment and/or treatment.	$

Table 4: **Pharmacologic Therapy for Drug-induced Skin Reactions** *(cont'd)*

Class	Drug	Dosage	Adverse Effects	Drug Interactions	Comments	Cost[a]
	loratadine Claritin, Claritin Liquid Capsules, generics	Adults and children ≥10 y (>30 kg): 10 mg once daily Children 2–9 y (≤30 kg): 5 mg once daily	Minimal to no anticholinergic or CNS effects. Headache.	QT_c prolongation reported with concomitant use of loratadine and amiodarone. Caution is advised. P-gp inhibitors (e.g., erythromycin, ketoconazole) may increase loratadine levels while P-gp inducers (e.g., carbamazepine, dexamethasone) may decrease loratadine levels; clinical effect probably minimal.	See cetirizine.	$
Antiseptic	*hydrogen peroxide*	Mix half-and-half with water and gargle then spit, as required	Well tolerated.	No clinically significant drug interactions.	Useful for oral lesions.	$
Astringents	*calamine lotion* generics	Apply generously PRN	Well tolerated.	No clinically significant drug interactions.	Store in refrigerator as physical cooling enhances antipruritic effect.	$
	zinc oxide cream/paste Zincofax, generics	Apply generously PRN	See calamine.	No clinically significant drug interactions.	See calamine.	$
Bath emollients	*colloidal oatmeal* Aveeno Oatmeal Bath	Add to bath water PRN	Well tolerated.	No clinically significant drug interactions.	Apply unscented moisture cream or white petrolatum to the skin while it is still slightly damp to avoid water evaporation.	$
Counterirritants	*menthol and/or camphor-containing salves* Rub A-535, others	0.25–5% in various bases: apply PRN	May occasionally be irritating.	No clinically significant drug interactions.	Provide a cooling sensation on the skin. Store in refrigerator as physical cooling enhances their effect.	$

Class	Drug	Dosage	Adverse Effects	Drug Interactions	Comments	Cost[a]
Corticosteroids, systemic	*prednisone* generics	1–2 mg/kg/day po × 7–10 days May need to continue for longer time periods if symptoms reoccur	Acne, glucose intolerance, weight gain, mood swings and agitation, cataracts, myopathy, hypertension, osteoporosis, aseptic necrosis of large joints, adrenal suppression, increased susceptibility to infection	Clearance may decrease with estrogens; may increase digitalis toxicity secondary to hypokalemia. Phenobarbital, phenytoin, and rifampin may increase metabolism which may necessitate increased maintenance dose. Increased risk of hypokalemia with coadministration of diuretics.	Only used for select patients with systemic symptoms in association with a cutaneous eruption (e.g., DRESS).	$
Corticosteroids, topical[c]	*hydrocortisone 0.5%, 1%* Cortate, Emo-Cort, Prevex HC, generics	Apply sparingly with gentle massage BID–QID PRN More potent products may be used in areas other than face or folds if required	Striae, telangiectasia, atrophy, purpura.	No clinically significant drug interactions.	Cream: useful in moist areas (due to possible drying effect). Ointment: preferred for dry or scaly lesions. Lotion: useful for scalp and other hairy areas or for application to large body areas. Patients whose symptoms do not improve within 5–7 days require further assessment and/or treatment.	$
Emollients[d]	*emollients (e.g., unscented moisture creams or white petrolatum)*	Apply generously PRN	Possible temporary stinging on application.	No clinically significant drug interactions.	After bathing, apply unscented moisture cream or white petrolatum to the skin while it is still slightly damp to avoid water evaporation. Useful for treatment of mild to moderate phototoxic reactions that can be managed as for ordinary sunburn.	$

[a] Cost of 1 dose or 30 g of cream unless otherwise specified; includes drug cost only.
[b] For information on other antihistamines, see Chapter 22: Allergic Rhinitis.
[c] For information on other topical corticosteroids, consult the *Compendium of Therapeutic Choices*: Atopic Dermatitis
[d] For more information on emollients, see Chapter 62: Dry Skin.
Dosage adjustment may be required in renal impairment.
Abbreviations: ACEI = angiotension converting enzyme inhibitors; CNS = central nervous system; CYP = cytochrome P450; GI = gastrointestinal; IOP = intraocular pressure; MTX = methotrexate
Legend: $ <$3

Suggested Readings

Cotliar J. Approach to the patient with a suspected drug eruption. *Semin Cutan Med Surg* 2007;26:147-54.

Mockenhaupt M. Severe drug-induced skin reactions: clinical pattern, diagnostics and therapy. *J Dtsch Dermatol Ges* 2009;7:142-60.

References

1. Pirmohamed M, James S, Meakin S et al. Adverse drug reactions as cause of admission to hospital: prospective analysis of 18,820 patients. *BMJ* 2004;329:15-9.
2. Bigby M, Jick S, Jick H et al. Drug-induced cutaneous reactions. A report from the Boston Collaborative Drug Surveillance Program on 15,438 consecutive inpatients, 1975 to 1982. *JAMA* 1986;256:3358-63.
3. Heinzerling LM, Tomsitz D, Anliker MD. Is drug allergy less prevalent than previously assumed? A 5-year analysis. *Br J Dermatol* 2012;166:107-14.
4. Segal AR, Doherty KM, Leggott J et al. Cutaneous reactions to drugs in children. *Pediatrics* 2007;120:e1082-96.
5. Lee HY, Ariyasinghe JT, Thirumoorthy T. Allopurinol hypersensitivity syndrome: a preventable severe cutaneous adverse reaction? *Singapore Med J* 2008;49:384-7.
6. Knowles SR, Dewhurst N, Shear NH. Anticonvulsant hypersensitivity syndrome: an update. *Expert Opin Drug Saf* 2012;11:767-78.
7. Knowles SR, Drucker AM, Weber EA et al. Management options for patients with aspirin and nonsteroidal antiinflammatory drug sensitivity. *Ann Pharmacother* 2007;41:1191-200.
8. Dykewicz MS. Cough and angioedema from angiotenin-converting enzyme inhibitors: new insights into mechanisms and management. *Curr Opin Allergy Clin Immunol* 2004;4:267-70.
9. McCollom RA, Elbe DH, Ritchie AH. Bupropion-induced serum sickness-like reaction. *Ann Pharmacother* 2000;34:471-3.
10. Kearns GL, Wheeler JG, Childress SH et al. Serum sickness-like reactions to cefaclor: role of hepatic metabolism and individual susceptibility. *J Pediatr* 1994;125:805-11.
11. Knowles SR, Shapiro L, Shear NH. Serious adverse reactions induced by minocycline. Report of 13 patients and review of the literature. *Arch Dermatol* 1996;132:934-9.
12. Todd DJ, Helfgott SM. Serum sickness following treatment with rituximab. *J Rheumatol* 2007;34:430-3.
13. Halevy S, Ghislain PD, Mockenhaupt M et al. Allopurinol is the most common cause of Stevens-Johnson syndrome and toxic epidermal necrolysis in Europe and Israel. *J Am Acad Dermatol* 2007;58:25-32.
14. Mockenhaupt M, Viboud C, Dunant A et al. Stevens-Johnson syndrome and toxic epidermal necrolysis: assessment of medication risks with emphasis on recently marketed drugs. The EuroSCAR-study. *J Invest Dermatol* 2008;128:35-44.
15. Sidoroff A, Dunant A, Viboud C et al. Risk factors for acute generalized exanthematous pustulosis (AGEP)-results of a multinational case control study (EuroSCAR). *Br J Dermatol* 2007;157:989-96.
16. Roujeau JC, Stern RS. Severe adverse cutaneous reactions to drugs. *N Engl J Med* 1994;331:1272-85.
17. Mockenhaupt M. Severe drug-induced skin reactions: clinical pattern, diagnostics and therapy. *J Dtsch Dermatol Ges* 2009;7:142-60.
18. Gerson D, Sriganeshan V, Alexis JB. Cutaneous drug eruptions: a 5-year experience. *J Am Acad Dermatol* 2008;59:995-9.
19. Stern RS. Clinical practice. Exanthematous drug eruptions. *N Engl J Med* 2012;366:2492-501.
20. Cacoub P, Musette P, Descamps V et al. The DRESS syndrome: a literature review. *Am J Med* 2011;124:588-97.
21. Kano Y, Ishida T, Hirahara K et al. Visceral involvements and long-term sequelae in drug-induced hypersensitivity syndrome. *Med Clin North Am* 2010;94:743-59.
22. Brown RJ, Rother KI, Artman H et al. Minocycline-induced drug hypersensitivity syndrome followed by multiple autoimmune sequelae. *Arch Dermatol* 2009;145:63-6.
23. Lipozencic J, Wolf R. Life-threatening severe allergic reactions: urticaria, angioedema, and anaphylaxis. *Clin Dermatol* 2005;23:193-205.
24. Pavletic AJ. Late angio-edema in patients taking angiotensin-converting-enzyme inhibitors. *Lancet* 2002;360:493-4.
25. Lee AY. Fixed drug eruptions. Incidence, recognition, and avoidance. *Am J Clin Dermatol* 2000;1:277-85.
26. Wu PA, Balagula Y, Lacouture, ME et al. Prophylaxis and treatment of dermatologic adverse events from epidermal growth factor receptor inhibitors. *Curr Opin Oncol* 2011;23:343-51.
27. Moore DE. Drug-induced cutaneous photosensitivity: incidence, mechanism, prevention and management. *Drug Saf* 2002;25:345-72.
28. Wolff K, Johnson R, Suurmond D. Contact dermatitis. In: Wolff K, Johnson RA, eds. *Fitzpatrick's color atlas and synopsis of clinical dermatology*. 5th ed. New York: McGraw-Hill; 2005.
29. Cotliar J. Approach to the patient with a suspected drug eruption. *Semin Cutan Med Surg* 2007;26:147-54.
30. Davis CM, Shearer WT. Diagnosis and management of HIV drug hypersensitivity. *J Allergy Clin Immunol* 2008;121:826-32.
31. Lim YL, Thirumoorthy T. Serious cutaneous adverse reactions to traditional Chinese medicines. *Singapore Med J* 2005;46:714-7.
32. Caliskaner Z, Ozturk S, Karaayvaz M. Not all adverse drug reactions originate from active component: coloring agent-induced skin eruption in a patient treated with rifampicin. *Allergy* 2003;58:1077-9.
33. Tan JK. Pruritus. In: Jovaisas B, ed. *Compendium of therapeutic choices: CTC7*. 7th ed. Ottawa: Canadian Pharmacists Association; 2014. p. 1151-62.
34. Valeyrie-Allanore L, Sassolas B, Roujeau JC. Drug-induced skin, nail and hair disorders. *Drug Saf* 2007;30:1011-30.
35. Drake LA, Dinehart SM, Farmer ER et al. Guidelines of care for cutaneous adverse drug reactions. American Academy of Dermatology. *J Am Acad Dermatol* 1996;35:458-61.
36. Deacock SJ. An approach to the patient with urticaria. *Clin Exp Immunol* 2008;153:151-61.
37. Funck-Brentano E, Duong TA, Bouvresse S et al. Therapeutic management of DRESS: a retrospective study of 38 cases. *J Am Acad Dermatol* 2015;72:246-52.
38. Kirchhof MG, Miliszewski MA, Sikora S et al. Retrospective review of Stevens-Johnson syndrome/toxic epidermal necrolysis treatment comparing intravenous immunoglobulin with cyclosporine. *J Am Acad Dermatol* 2014;71:941-7.

39. Pavlos R, Mallal S, Ostrov D et al. Fever, rash and systemic symptoms: understanding the role of HLA in severe cutaneous drug allergy. *J Allergy Clin Immunol Pract* 2014;2:21-33.

40. Government of Canada. Healthy Canadians. *Patients of Asian ancestry using epilepsy drug carbamazepine may be at increased risk of serious skin reactions*. Ottawa: Health Canada; 2008. Available from: http://healthycanadians.gc.ca/recall-alert-rappel-avis/hc-sc/2008/13283a-eng.php Accessed April 14, 2016.

Skin Reactions to Medications—What You Need to Know

Skin rashes may be caused by infections or other diseases. However, some rashes can be caused by an allergic reaction to a prescribed medicine.

You should stop taking the suspected medicine right away. The rash may continue to get worse for one to two days. It should begin to get better after five to seven days. See your healthcare provider if:

- the rash does not improve or gets worse
- you have a fever or feel like you have the flu (loss of appetite, nausea).

What should you do if you have a bad reaction to a medicine?

Contact your healthcare provider to inform them about your rash. Find out about other medicines that may cause a similar reaction. If you see a new healthcare provider, be sure to tell them about your reaction. Consider registering in the Medic Alert program.

How can you treat the rash?

For rashes that are itchy:

- Cool the skin with a lukewarm shower several times a day. You can also try a bath, adding an oatmeal bath preparation or four tablespoons of baking soda to the water.
- Ask your healthcare provider for advice about creams or lotions to relieve the itch. Ointments can be used for dry areas and creams are recommended for moist areas. Lotions are useful for the scalp and other hairy areas. Examples of nonprescription products are:
  - plain calamine lotion or zinc oxide cream
  - hydrocortisone 0.5 or 1% cream, ointment or lotion. Follow the directions on the package or ask the pharmacist for advice on how to use these products
  - moisturizing cream (use an unscented form).
- Keep creams and ointments in the refrigerator. The coolness will help control the itch.
- Avoid tight clothing or rough fabrics.
- Avoid getting your body overheated. Dress lightly.
- Check with your healthcare provider to see whether you can take an antihistamine to relieve the itching. Some antihistamines may interfere with other medicines or medical conditions.
- Use of antihistamines in creams is not recommended.

Chapter 62
Dry Skin

Nancy Kleiman, BSP, MBA

Pathophysiology

The skin and its appendages (e.g., sweat glands, sebaceous glands, hair follicles) serve several important functions. They protect against minor injury, help control body temperature and water loss, prevent invasion by microorganisms and prevent radiation damage from sun exposure. The skin is composed of 3 main layers: epidermis (which includes the stratum corneum), dermis and subcutaneous[1] (Figure 1). The stratum corneum is the upper layer of the skin and acts as the main barrier to water loss and protects from foreign material. The stratum corneum is composed of dead cells, corneocytes and intercellular lipids. The lipid component consists of ceramides, cholesterol and free fatty acids. Ceramides are found in high concentrations in healthy skin and act as a barrier to protect the skin and to maintain hydration.[2]

If the skin barrier is compromised there is an increase in transepidermal water loss (TEWL) and a decrease in ceramides and other lipids in the skin. Research in the treatment of dry skin conditions focusses on the effects of TEWL and decreased ceramide content.[3]

The term "dry skin" (also known as xeroderma or xerosis) is commonly used to describe skin that may be rough to the touch and have mild scaling, flaking or peeling of the upper layers, and is often very itchy, with possible cracking if severe enough.[4] Dry skin most often affects the skin of the thighs, lower legs, sides of the abdomen and the arms. The incidence of dry skin increases with age but can occur at any age depending on skin type, environmental factors, medical conditions and chronic skin conditions.[4] Dry skin is not related to lack of oils in the skin but rather to water loss from the skin's surface. Dry skin has many potential causes, some of which are listed in Table 1.

Figure 1: **The Skin**

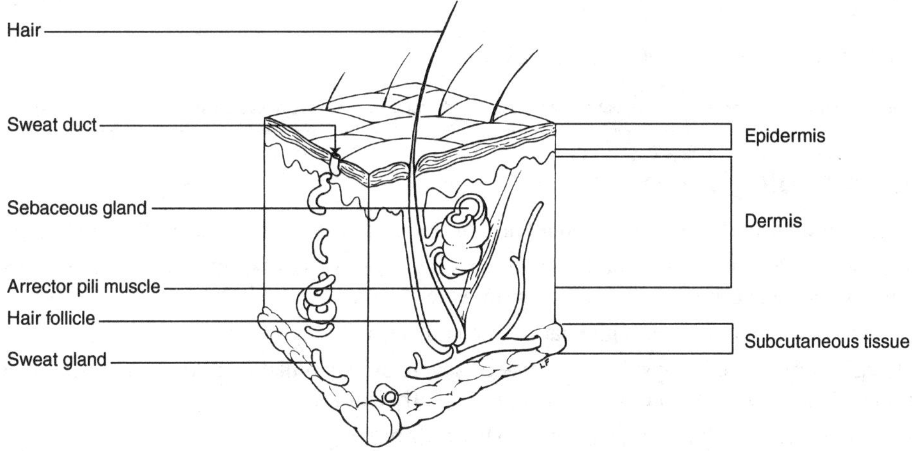

Goals of Therapy

- Alleviate the unpleasant feel of rough, scaly skin
- Restore skin hydration and reduce transepidermal water loss
- Facilitate repair of the barrier function and maintain the integrity of the stratum corneum
- Relieve itching associated with dry skin
- Educate the patient on self-treatment to prevent further damage

Patient Assessment

Dry skin is generally managed with nonprescription therapy by improving skin hydration and addressing any contributing factors if possible (see Table 1).

Assessment should differentiate between dry skin and other skin conditions (e.g., atopic dermatitis, psoriasis, fungal infections). Patients require further assessment and/or treatment if the condition does not respond to initial treatment for dry skin. Treatment failure may indicate an underlying medical disease or condition. An approach to the patient with concerns about dry skin is presented in Figure 2.

Table 1: **Factors Contributing to Dry Skin**[5,6,7,8,9,10,11]

Genetic abnormalities in keratocyte composition or function (e.g., ichthyosis)
Bathing or showering in hot water too frequently or for long periods of time.
Swimming in chlorinated pools
Use of harsh (alkaline pH), perfumed, deodorant or antibacterial soaps
Over-exposure to sun (e.g., photoaging)
Normal skin aging (decreased activity in the sebaceous and sweat glands)
Low humidity (e.g., cold/windy or very hot climates, electric heat, fireplaces, air conditioning, recycled air in airplanes)
Medical conditions (e.g., hypothyroidism, chronic renal failure, diabetes, liver disease)
Exposure to UV radiation (e.g., sun) or chemicals
Abrasion
Certain skin conditions (e.g., atopic dermatitis, acne, psoriasis)
Medications known to cause dry skin (e.g., anticholinergics, chemotherapy agents, niacin, systemic retinoids, vitamin A)

Nonpharmacologic Therapy

Several self-care measures will reduce the feeling of dry, rough skin.[4,5,11,12] Offer the following advice:

- Avoid excessive bathing or long baths or showers; have brief 3- to 5-minute baths or showers 2–3 times per week; take sponge baths using warm water to maintain hydration
- Use tepid rather than hot water while bathing or showering
- Avoid harsh or perfumed soaps; limit the use of soaps; use soap that is mild and nonperfumed or use a mild cleanser with a pH close to skin pH (slightly acidic)
- Pat the skin dry (rather than rubbing vigorously) after bathing

- Add bath products at the end of a bath or after a bath. Skin hydration is increased if bath products are added after a bath or applied directly to damp skin and gently patted dry. Bath oils can be added to the bath, but there is increased risk of slipping, particularly in older persons
- Apply a moisturizer after bathing (see Table 2); apply while the skin is still damp (within 3 minutes after bathing); apply several times a day (3–4 times daily)
- Avoid licking dry lips as this can further irritate the lips or worsen the condition. Apply a lip balm frequently for dry, chapped lips
- Increase humidity indoors. Cool mist humidifiers increase the humidity indoors and will minimize water evaporation from the skin. Humidity should be between 40% and 50% in winter (30% in summer)
- Wear gloves, face masks and scarves when outdoors in cold or windy weather to protect the skin from the drying effects of cold and wind
- Avoid wool clothing that may be irritating to the skin. Cotton clothing next to the skin is less irritating
- Avoid caffeine, spices and alcohol, which may contribute to dehydration if ingested in large quantities or used on a regular basis
- Avoid swimming in chlorinated pools
- Avoid products that contain ingredients that may sensitize the skin (e.g., lanolin, propylene glycol, fragrances, vitamin E, aloe vera), particuarly in those with with very sensitive skin or in the elderly
- Maintain adequate fluid intake from food and water.[13]

Pharmacologic Therapy

For comparative ingredients of nonprescription products, consult the *Compendium of Products for Minor Ailments*—Skin Care Products: Dermatitis and Dry Skin, First Aid.

Therapeutic moisturizers should be noncomedogenic, nonirritant and hypoallergenic. Moisturizing agents include occlusives, humectants, emollients, bath products and barrier repair agents. The value of herbal products (e.g., **aloe vera**) as moisturizers is unclear and they may cause skin sensitization. Emollient ointments act as a barrier and minimize water loss.[5,6] They have longer lasting effects than creams or lotions, but are greasy and not ideal for use on the face. Creams and lotions are more cosmetically appealing and easier to spread, but their duration of effect is shorter than ointments.[4,12] Lotions are generally oil-in-water emulsions and easier to spread than creams. To enhance adherence, consider patient preference when selecting a product. Sunscreens are now added to many moisturizing agents to prevent sun-induced skin damage. Information on moisturizer ingredients can also be found in Table 2.

Short-term use of low-potency **topical corticosteroids** in addition to emollients, is recommended by some experts for dry skin that is extremely red, inflamed and swollen. This is used as a temporary measure only. Once the inflammation improves, the topical corticosteroids are stopped and the emollients continued.[8]

Table 2: **Moisturizer Ingredients for Dry Skin**[5,6,14]

Type	Action	Examples	Comments
Occlusives	Physically block surface of stratum corneum to prevent further water loss, which promotes barrier repair. Minimizes water loss to the external environment.	Beeswax, dimethicone, lanolin, mineral oil, paraffin, petrolatum, soybean oil, zinc oxide	Petrolatum is not cosmetically appealing (greasy, difficult to spread and remove). Lanolin may cause contact dermatitis: avoid in patients with sensitive skin. Occlusives are generally not well tolerated on facial skin or in hot, humid climates due to their greasy nature. Silicones often found in "oil-free" products. To avoid the greasy feel of silicone products, warm the product in the hand, use a thin layer and rub in gently but well. Apply TID–QID or more often if required.
Humectants	Draw water from the dermis to the epidermis and from the environment (providing humidity is 70–80%) into the stratum corneum. Retain water already present.	Alpha-hydroxy acid (AHA), glycerin, glycolic acid, lactic acid, propylene glycol, sodium hyaluronate, sorbitol, urea	Used in combination with occlusives they will enhance water holding ability of the skin. Glycerin in high concentrations may increase water loss by drawing water away from the skin and may be irritating. Should not be used alone, or in those with sensitive skin. Lactic acid (>12%) and urea (>10%) are keratolytic and used for treatment of more severe skin conditions. Lower concentrations are recommended as moisturizing agents (lactic acid ≤12% and urea ≤10%). Urea may cause stinging and burning on open skin in any concentration. Apply BID–TID PRN.
Emollients	Fill the spaces between cells in the stratum corneum, sealing moisture into the skin which makes it feel smoother and softer.	Castor oil, cocoa butter, ceramides, coconut oil, fatty acids, lanolin, lipids, mineral oil, palm oil, vitamins A and E, wool fat	Combining with emulsifiers (stearic acid, stearyl alcohol, cetyl alcohol) may improve the oil/water balance of the product. May be combined with occlusives to decrease water loss. Apply TID–QID PRN.
Bath oils	Provide a layer of oil on the skin that prevents moisture evaporation.	Coal tar, colloidal oatmeal, liquid paraffin	Best applied at the end of the bath or shower or immediately after using a wet compress. Safety hazard if added to bath water (increased chance of slipping). Colloidal oatmeal relieves itching and enhances the barrier function of the skin.
Barrier repair agents	Normalize skin barrier by replacing ceramides; decreasing transepidermal water loss (TEWL); decreasing triggers for inflammation.	Ceramides/cholesterol/free fatty acids combinations	Nonsteroidal barrier repair cream. Used to treat dry skin and associated pruritus in atopic, irritant and radiation dermatitis.

Monitoring of Therapy

Mild to moderate dry skin can be self-managed by patients educated on nonpharmacologic methods of treatment and prevention. The patient should monitor the skin daily for 7–10 days after starting treatment for improvement in symptoms, and seek medical attention if the condition worsens or shows no improvement.

Table 3 provides a plan for monitoring therapy for dry skin.

Table 3: Monitoring of Therapy for Dry Skin

Symptom	Monitoring	Endpoint	Actions
Rough, scaly skin	Monitor daily for 7–10 days for signs of improvement with treatment (moisturizers or nonpharmacologic methods).	Skin feels smoother, no longer red, rough or irritated.	If irritation worsens, consider allergy to moisturizer ingredient and discontinue.
Itching	Monitor daily for 7–10 days for decrease in symptoms with treatment (moisturizers or nonpharmacologic methods). Monitor for signs of infection if scratching has caused open areas.	Itching has decreased or is controlled (no scratching, redness or signs of infection).	If itching increases or does not decrease in severity, consider the addition of a second moisturizer from a different group. Signs of infection (pus, pain, redness) require further assessment and/or treatment.
Dry, flaky skin	Monitor daily while using moisturizing products. Monitor for signs of improvement.	Dry, flaky skin has decreased or skin is soft and hydrated.	If skin continues to be dry and flaky, consider alternative treatment.

Figure 2: Assessment of Patients with Dry Skin

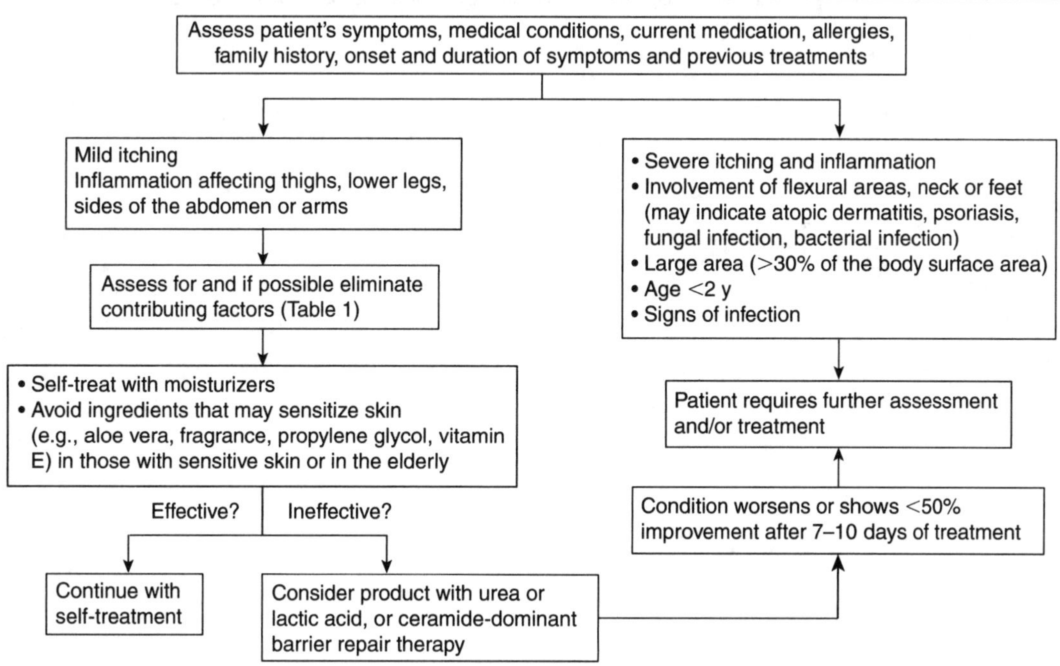

Suggested Readings

Green L. Emollient therapy for dry and inflammatory skin conditions. *Nurs Stand* 2011;26:39-46.

Guenther L, Lynde CW, Andriessen A et al. Pathway to dry skin prevention and treatment. *J Cutan Med Surg* 2012;16:23-31.

Reddy M. Skin and wound care: important considerations in the older adult. *Adv Skin Wound Care* 2008;21:424-36.

References

1. Bond CA. Skin disorders. In: Koda-Kimble MA, Young LY, eds. *Applied therapeutics: the clinical use of drugs*. 5th ed. Vancouver: Applied Therapeutics; 1992. p. 64-1-6.
2. Novotny J, Hrabalek, A, Vavrova K. Synthesis and structure-activity relationships of skin ceramides. *Curr Med Chem* 2010;17:2301-24.
3. Bikowski J. Case studies assessing a new skin barrier repair cream for the treatment of atopic dermatitis. *J Drugs Dermatol* 2009;8:1037-41.
4. Reddy M. Skin and wound care: important considerations in the older adult. *Adv Skin Wound Care* 2008;21:424-36.
5. Proksch E. The role of emollients in the management of diseases with chronic dry skin. *Skin Pharmacol Physiol* 2008;21:75-80.
6. Fitzpatrick TB, Bernhard JD, Cropley TG. The structure of skin lesions and fundamentals of diagnosis. In: Freedberg IM, Fitzpatrick TB et al., eds. *Fitzpatrick's dermatology in general medicine*. 5th ed. New York: McGraw-Hill; 1999. p. 155-64.
7. Lynde CB, Kraft JN, Lynde CW. Skin care as an adjunct treatment for skin disease. *Skin Therapy Lett* 2007;2:1-8. Available from: www.skinpharmacies.ca/2_1_en.pdf. Accessed April 13, 2016.
8. Guenther L, Lynde CW, Andriessen A et al. Pathway to dry skin prevention and treatment. *J Cutan Med Surg* 2012;16:23-31.
9. Hurlow H, Bliss DZ. Dry skin in older adults. *Geriatr Nurs* 2011;32:257-62.
10. Andriessen A. Prevention, recognition and treatment of dry skin conditions. *Br J Nurs* 2013;22:26-30.
11. White-Chu EF, Reddy M. Dry skin in the elderly: complexities of a common problem. *Clin Dermatol* 2011;29:37-42.
12. Butler N. National guidelines at a glance: atopic eczema. *SA Pharmaceutical Journal* June 2009:32-7.
13. Popkin BM, D'Anci KE, Rosenberg IH. Water, hydration, and health. *Nutr Rev* 2010;68:439-58.
14. Wan DC, Wong VW, Longaker MT et al. Moisturizing different racial skin types. *J Clin Aesthet Dermatol* 2014;7:25-32.

Dry Skin—What You Need to Know

Normal skin may become dry as a result of aging, certain medical conditions, medications, a dry climate, wind and cold. The skin becomes dry because of a decrease in moisture on the skin's surface.

What can be done to prevent dry skin?

- Use a humidifier to moisturize the air in dry climates (especially important during the winter).
- Keep the room temperature at the lowest comfortable level in the winter and avoid electric heat when possible.
- Baths and showers can dry out the skin. Bathe or shower every 2–3 days using warm, not hot, water. Sponge baths with warm water (not hot) in between showers will help to keep the moisture in the skin.
- Soap makes dry skin worse, so use a mild soap, without perfumes, or a mild cleanser. Avoid using soap on dry skin areas unless you need to remove visible dirt or oil.

What can be done to treat dry skin?

- Applying a moisturizing cream or lotion to the body within the first 3 minutes after a bath or shower will improve skin moisture.
- Gently pat skin dry with a soft towel (do not rub as this will further irritate the skin).
- Add bath oils during the last few minutes of a bath, or apply to the skin while it is still wet and then pat dry. Bath oils can be a hazard as the tub will be slippery and there is a risk of falling if added directly into the tub.
- Apply a moisturizing lotion or cream to the skin at least twice a day (morning and night) or more often if the skin feels very rough and dry. If regular use of moisturizers has not relieved the dry skin, a product containing urea or lactic acid can be used. Note: Urea or lactic acid can irritate cuts or scrapes on the skin.
- Apply a lip balm frequently for dry, chapped lips. Licking the lips can further irritate the lips or worsen the condition.

Chapter 63
Frostbite

Nancy Kleiman, BSP, MBA

Pathophysiology

Frostbite refers to acute freezing of the tissue caused by temperatures below the freezing point of intact skin. Frostbite is caused by formation of ice crystals in the tissue, leading to tissue damage.[1,2] Formation of extracellular, and later intracellular, ice crystals results in cellular dehydration and physical damage to cell membranes and vascular structures. This leads to progressive microvascular collapse and initiates a series of events that in serious frostbite leads to progressive ischemia, thrombosis and tissue necrosis.[3,4] The severity of injury and degree of irreversible damage is related to the duration of exposure and length of time the tissue remains frozen, rather than solely to air temperature.

Factors that increase the risk of frostbite include:[1,3,5]

- Wind, high humidity and temperatures below –3°C
- Drug use: Alcohol and sedatives dull mental awareness of cold and impair judgment that would prevent exposure to cold. Alcohol also inhibits shivering and causes vasodilation. Medications with sedative or muscle relaxing effects may inhibit shivering and increase the risk of frostbite
- General: Psychiatric illness, vagrancy, inadequate or constrictive clothing, previous history of cold injury, and immobilization may increase the risk of frostbite. Infants have a higher ratio of body surface area to mass and the elderly have a decreased capacity for metabolic heat production and vasoconstriction; therefore, they are at higher risk of developing frostbite
- Neurologic conditions: Peripheral neuropathy, hypothalamic disease and spinal cord damage may lead to impairment of cutaneous vasoconstriction
- Cardiovascular conditions: Peripheral vascular disease, vascular disease and nicotine use are predisposing factors for frostbite
- Endocrine conditions: Hypothyroidism, hypoglycemia and adrenal insufficiency can increase the risk of frostbite by decreasing metabolic heat production. Diabetic neuropathy may impair cold awareness.

Frostbite most often affects the hands, fingers, feet, toes, nose, cheeks and ears.[3,4] It is difficult to assess the severity of frostbite while the skin is still frozen as all frozen tissue is hard, pale and numb. Classification of frostbite is based on rewarmed/thawed tissue. Different degrees of frostbite can occur within different parts of the same extremity.[6,7] The full extent of injury may not be apparent for days after the freezing episode. Close observation during this time is warranted.[8]

Frostnip is a superficial nonfreezing injury in which cooling of tissues to less than 10°C results in a blue-white discoloration of skin, loss of sensation and transient numbness and tingling. Ice crystals (appearing as frost) form on the surface of the cheeks, ears or nose. Symptoms resolve quickly with rewarming (covering with clothing, breathing on the affected area and moving to a warmer location). There may be erythema and mild edema, but there is no tissue damage.[2,4,9,10]

First-degree frostbite involves partial-thickness skin freezing and presents with a numb central white plaque with peripheral erythema. There may be mild edema, but no blistering. Second-degree frostbite involves full thickness skin freezing and presents with significant edema with erythema and large blisters filled with a clear or milky fluid appearing within 24–48 hours. The skin under the blisters remains soft and perfused. The affected area generally remains sensitive to heat and cold.[2,6,9,11,12]

In third-degree frostbite there is skin and subcutaneous tissue freezing with tissue necrosis. The affected area may appear deep purple or red with dark, hemorrhagic blisters that turn into a hard black eschar (scab) over 2 weeks. Fourth-degree frostbite involves deep tissue necrosis extending to the level of muscle and bone. It presents with the affected area being cold and waxy, firm and numb (even after rewarming) with deep red, mottled skin which eventually becomes gangrenous.[6,9,11,12] The most serious injuries result in mummification and autoamputation at 22–45 days.[3,4]

First- and second-degree frostbite are generally considered superficial frostbite in that minimal or no tissue damage is anticipated. Third- and fourth-degree frostbite are considered deep frostbite and tissue loss is anticipated.[9,12]

Long-term sequelae of frostbite can include tingling and burning sensations from ischemic neuritis lasting for weeks. Cold sensitivity, loss of sensation, pigmentation changes, nail deformities or hyperhidrosis may persist for years.[3,10]

Two other cold-related injuries that do not involve freezing are chilblains (also known as pernio or perniosis) from repetitive exposure to mild, dry cold, and trench foot from prolonged exposure to wet cold.[10] In chilblains, persistent vasospasm and vasculitis results in pruritus, redness and mild edema of the face, hands, feet and shins, which can progress to the development of plaques, bluish nodules and ulceration. In trench foot, neurovascular damage occurs in the absence of ice crystal formation. Feet initially appear pale and cyanotic, and feel cold, numb and tingly. After rewarming, the skin remains very painful to touch, and blisters are common and may ulcerate. Pain, cold sensitivity and hyperhidrosis may last for years.[10]

Goals of Therapy

- Identify associated hypothermia and prevent further heat loss
- Minimize tissue damage during rewarming
- Control pain
- Prevent infection in damaged tissues

Patient Assessment

All patients with suspected frostbite should also be assessed for symptoms of hypothermia such as shivering (although this decreases as hypothermia worsens), dizziness, hunger, nausea, slurred speech or mumbling, confusion, irrational behaviour and drowsiness. If hypothermia is suspected, urgent medical care is required. For further discussion of hypothermia, consult the *Compendium of Therapeutic Choices*: Thermoregulatory Disorders in Adults.

Except in the case of mild (first-degree) frostbite (affected area is pink, warm, has no blisters after thawing and pain is controlled with nonprescription analgesics), emergency hospital care for all patients is preferred for the following reasons:[6,7,12]

- severity of the injury is difficult to assess while tissue is still frozen; proper rewarming and post-warming assessment is required
- full extent of the injury may not become apparent for several days and may be more severe than the original appearance suggested; close observation is recommended during this time

- some treatment options for severe frostbite (e.g., thrombolytics, vasodilators) should be instituted within 24 hours of injury.

If immediate referral is not possible, provide instructions for rewarming if appropriate, and observation (see Nonpharmacologic Therapy). Assessment of patients with frostbite is presented in Figure 1.

Prevention

Frostbite and related cold injuries can generally be prevented with planning prior to exposure to the cold. Ensuring adequate tissue perfusion and minimizing heat loss are the main components of frostbite prevention.

Measures to reduce the risk of frostbite include:[9,13]

- maintaining adequate hydration and nutrition
- minimizing restriction in blood flow by avoiding immobility or constrictive clothing or footwear
- avoiding environmental conditions below −15°C, even with low wind speeds
- dressing appropriately; wear a warm hat and heavy warm mittens (preferred over gloves), increase insulation by layering clothes appropriately, choose synthetic fabrics, fleece, silk or wool blends, and avoid cotton as it retains moisture
- avoiding perspiration or wet extremities (keep hands and feet dry)
- avoiding drugs or alcohol as they may impair awareness of changing physical and environmental conditions
- using chemical hand and foot warmers (these must not be placed directly against the skin or constrict blood flow in any way)
- recognizing frostnip or superficial frostbite before it progresses: an extremity at risk of frostbite (e.g., numb, poor dexterity, pale colour) should be warmed in the axilla or on the abdomen
- minimizing duration of exposure to cold
- using caution while exercising; it can increase core and peripheral temperatures and perfusion, but can also lead to exhaustion and collapse
- applying emollients on the skin is *not* preventive and may even increase risk of frostbite.

Nonpharmacologic Therapy

Until emergency medical care is available, the following first aid measures can be undertaken:[2,3,9,10]

- move the patient to a warm location as soon as possible. Unless absolutely necessary, the person should not walk on frostbitten toes or feet
- do not thaw the area if there is any risk of refreezing, which can worsen tissue damage
- remove jewelry or constrictive clothing from the affected area
- do not rub the area (even to dry it) as friction can increase tissue damage
- remove wet clothing once the patient is in a warm environment
- institute passive rewarming (warm environment, blankets, tucking affected area into armpit, groin or against abdomen) until active rewarming can be started. If active rewarming cannot be undertaken, allow passive thawing to occur
- institute rapid active rewarming as soon as possible by immersing in warm water (40–42°C; comfortably warm bath) for 15–30 minutes until the skin feels soft and pliable and appears red
- after rewarming, elevate the affected area to minimize edema
- fingers and toes may be separated by dry sterile dressings/gauze

- ensure the patient is adequately hydrated
- if blisters develop, leave them intact to decrease risk of infection, unless they are restricting range of motion
- if blisters rupture, cover with clean dry gauze until emergency medical care is available
- patients should not smoke as nicotine may cause vasoconstriction and reduce blood flow.

Frostnip responds quickly to rewarming with no sequelae.[4,10] Chilblains are treated conservatively with warmth, elevation of the area and application of soothing moisturizers.[4] Trench foot is treated by rewarming the skin, elevating the area and wrapping the patient in loose, soft material to maintain constant warmth.

Pharmacologic Therapy

For comparative ingredients of nonprescription products, consult the *Compendium of Products for Minor Ailments*—Analgesic Products: Internal Analgesics and Antipyretics; Skin Products: First Aid.

Frostbitten areas may become very painful during the rewarming process. Adequate pain relief should be provided. **NSAIDs** (e.g., ibuprofen, naproxen sodium) are recommended as their mechanism of action (decreasing production of prostaglandins and thromboxanes which lead to vasoconstriction and can worsen dermal ischemia) may prevent further tissue damage as well as relieve pain.[1,3,9] Some guidelines recommend the routine use of ibuprofen at a dose of 12 mg/kg/day divided BID for its prostaglandin inhibitory effects (even in the absence of pain).[9] **Acetaminophen** can be used to relieve pain for patients unable to take NSAIDs.[2] In serious frostbite, **opioid analgesics** may be required for pain not responding adequately to nonprescription analgesics.

Limited observational evidence shows **aloe vera** may improve frostbite outcomes by reducing prostaglandin and thromboxane formation in more serious frostbite where blisters have formed.[14] Although it does not penetrate far into tissue and may be beneficial only for superficial areas, some guidelines recommend aloe vera gel be applied to thawed tissue at each dressing change or Q6H despite the limited evidence, as the risks associated with its use are low.[9] A systematic review showed there is inconclusive evidence regarding whether **aloe vera** gel or dressings improve healing in acute or chronic wounds.[15]

Frostbite injuries are not particularly prone to infection and use of **systemic antibiotics** for infection prophylaxis is controversial; however, they are sometimes used in cases of significant tissue loss.[1,3] Although evidence is not available regarding effectiveness, some sources recommend **topical antibiotics** be applied in cases where blisters have been debrided or have ruptured, as the area may be at a higher risk of infection.[5]

Frostbite injuries that include blisters are prone to tetanus and therefore **tetanus prophylaxis** is indicated.[2]

Other therapies aimed at increasing tissue perfusion (with varying amounts of evidence to support their use) may be considered in some patients admitted to hospital. These may include **low-molecular-weight dextran**, **thrombolytics**, **vasodilators** and **pentoxifylline**. Other measures that may improve healing include hydrotherapy and hyperbaric oxygen.[7,9,12]

Monitoring of Therapy

Table 1 provides information on monitoring of therapy for frostbite.

Table 1: Monitoring of Therapy for Frostbite

Symptom	Monitoring	Endpoint	Actions
Tissue appearance (Hard, whitish, frozen-looking tissue)	Monitor continuously until area has rewarmed (15–30 min in warm water). Monitor over the next 24–48 h for blistering or signs of infection. Monitor for 4–7 days for wound healing and signs of infection.	Rewarmed tissue will be warm, red and pliable. It may be swollen. Areas of superficial frostbite will develop normal colour and warmth with no blisters within 24 h.	Patients require further assessment and treatment if there are signs of infection (pus, increased redness, fever, increased pain). If blisters rupture, cover with nonadherent gauze and consider need for topical antibiotics.[a]
Numbness and tingling	Monitor for symptoms of numbness and tingling during rewarming. Monitor for 24–48 h for increase in numbness or tingling with superficial frostbite. Monitor for 2–4 weeks for signs of improvement or worsening of numbness or tingling to the area frozen.	Symptoms of tingling and pain are tolerable by patient during rewarming. In superficial frostbite, tingling and numbness subside without treatment within 24–48 h. In deep tissue frostbite, tingling and numbness may persist for weeks after freezing.	Patients with superficial frostbite with continued numbness and tingling for 24–48 h need further assessment and/or treatment as the frostbite may be worse than initially thought. Patients with tingling and numbness longer than 2 wk should have already been assessed as the frostbite is likely deep tissue frostbite.
Pain	Monitor pain every 4–6 h for 24 h. If pain increases or is not resolved with nonprescription treatment within 24 h treatment with opioid analgesics is required.	Pain relief for patient during and after the rewarming process. Pain relief within 24 h for superficial frostbite.	Treat with pain relievers according to type of frostbite: NSAIDs or acetaminophen for superficial frostbite. If pain relief has not improved with nonprescription pain relievers (as in deep tissue frostbite) further assessment for possible treatment with opioids is necessary.

[a] Evidence to support use of topical antibiotics in this scenario is lacking; however, they are often used in practice.

Figure 1: **Assessment of Patients with Frostbite**

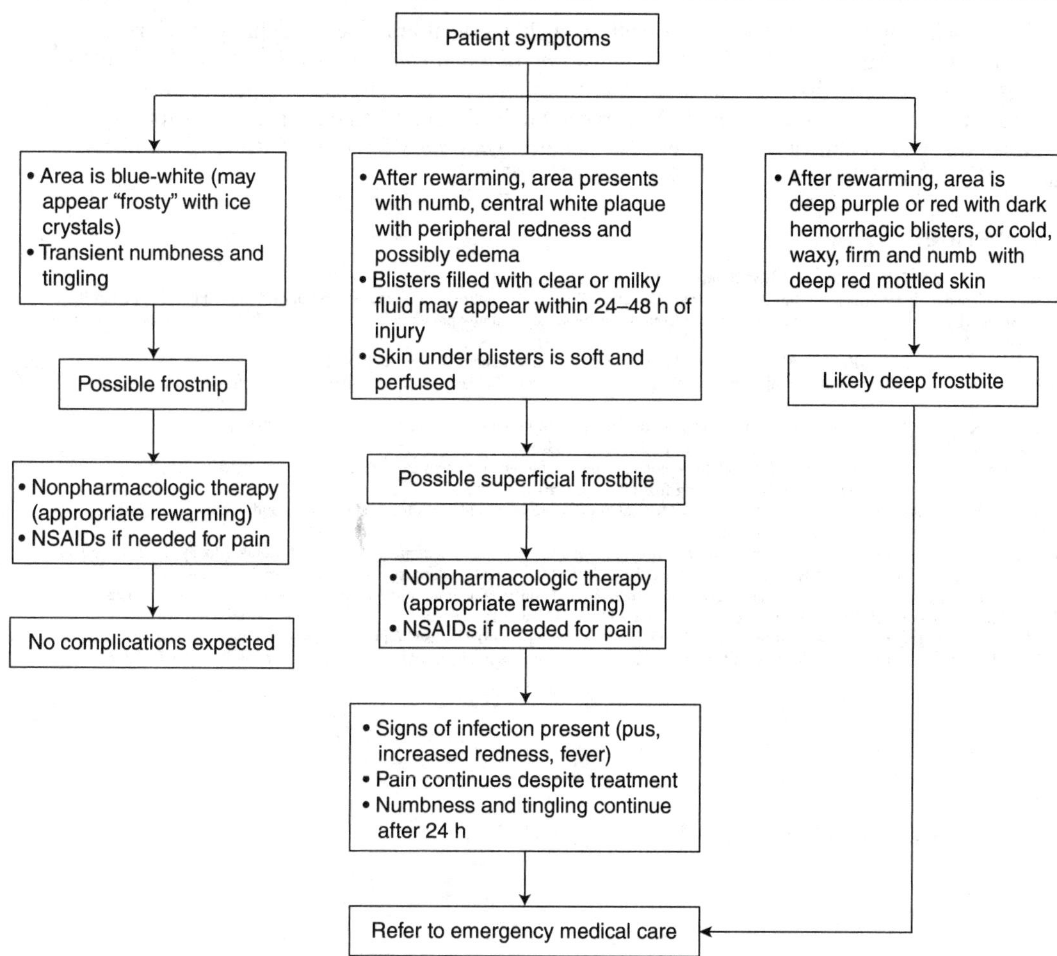

Suggested Readings

Health Canada. First Nations and Inuit Health Branch. Clinical Practice Guidelines for Nurses in Primary Care. Adult care. Chapter 9. Skin. *Dermatological emergencies. Frostbite*. Available from: www.hc-sc.gc.ca/fniah-spnia/services/nurs-infirm/clini/adult/skin-peau-eng.php#tc20.

McIntosh SE, Opacic M, Freer L et al. Wilderness Medical Society practice guidelines for the prevention and treatment of frostbite: 2014 update. *Wilderness Environ Med* 2014;25:S43-54.

Patel NN, Patel DN. Frostbite. *Am J Med* 2008;121:765-6.

References

1. Patel NN, Patel DN. Frostbite. *Am J Med* 2008;121:765-6.
2. Health Canada. First Nations and Inuit Health Branch. Clinical Practice Guidelines for Nurses in Primary Care. Adult care. Chapter 9. Skin. *Dermatological emergencies. Frostbite*. Available from: www.hc-sc.gc.ca/fniah-spnia/services/nurs-infirm/clini/adult/skin-peau-eng.php#tc20. Accessed March 8, 2016.
3. Murphy JV, Banwell PE, Roberts AH et al. Frostbite: pathogenesis and treatment. *J Trauma* 2000;48:171-8.
4. Kanzenbach TL, Dexter WW. Cold injuries. Protecting your patients from the dangers of hypothermia and frostbite. *Postgrad Med* 1999;105:72-8.
5. Biem J, Koehncke N, Classen D et al. Out of the cold: management of hypothermia and frostbite. *CMAJ* 2003;168:305-11.
6. Hutchsion RL. Frostbite of the Hand. *J Hand Surg Am* 2014;39:1863-8.
7. Handford C, Buxton P, Russell K et al. Frostbite: a practical approach to hospital management. *Extrem Physiol Med* 2014;3:7.
8. Hallam MJ, Cubison T, Dheansa B et al. Managing frostbite. *BMJ* 2010;341:c5864.
9. McIntosh SE, Opacic M, Freer L et al. Wilderness Medical Society practice guidelines for the prevention and treatment of frostbite: 2014 update. *Wilderness Environ Med* 2014;25:S43-54.
10. Danzl DF. Frostbite. In: Rosen P, Barkin R, eds. *Emergency medicine: concepts and clinical practice*. St. Louis: Mosby; 1998. p. 953-62.
11. Petrone P, Asensio JA, Marini CP. Management of accidental hypothermia and cold injury. *Curr Probl Surg* 2014;51:417-31.
12. Ingram BJ, Raymond TJ. Recognition and treatment of freezing and nonfreezing cold injuries. *Curr Sports Med Rep* 2013;12:125-30.
13. Varnado M. Frostbite. *J Wound Ostomy Continence Nurs* 2008;35:341-6.
14. McCauley RL, Hing DN, Robson MC et al. Frostbite injuries: a rational approach based on the pathophysiology. *J Trauma* 1983;23:143-7.
15. Dat AD, Poon F, Pham KB et al. Aloe vera for treating acute and chronic wounds. *Cochrane Database Syst Rev* 2012;2:CD008762.

Frostbite—What You Need to Know

What is frostbite?

Frostbite is the term used for frozen tissues caused by crystallization of water in the tissues. Tissues that are affected by frostbite must be handled carefully to prevent permanent damage to the tissue. Serious frostbite requires medical attention.

Adults can more easily develop frostbite if they drink excessive amounts of alcohol, dress inappropriately for the cold or have medical conditions that affect blood flow to their skin (such as diabetes).

Watch carefully for signs of frostbite on body parts that are commonly exposed to cold—cheeks, nose, ears, hands, fingers, feet and toes.

What can you do to prevent frostbite?

- Prevent frostbite by wearing layers of warm clothing, a hat, scarf and gloves when you are outside in very cold weather. Wind and high humidity increase the risk of frostbite; always consider wind chill when going out into the cold for longer periods of time.
- Watch carefully for signs of frostbite:
  - numbness and tingling in any body part
  - skin that looks pale.
- If signs of frostbite are noticed, go indoors immediately to warm up and remove wet clothing and socks.
- If unable to find shelter immediately, cover the area and warm it by holding your hand over it. Do not rub the area.

What are the signs of serious frostbite?

- Skin that is frozen feels hard, wooden and numb. The colour is waxy white, yellow or blue-white depending on the severity of the frostbite.
- Frostbite in the hands or feet may lead to clumsiness or difficulty gripping objects. Deep tissue frostbite may lead to an inability to move parts of the body that have been affected.

What is the treatment for superficial or mild frostbite?

- Remove any wet or tight clothing from the area. Cover the area with dry clothing and get indoors as soon as possible.
- **Do not** rub or massage frostbitten skin or put snow on it.
- **Do not** hold near direct heat such as a fire or heating pad.
- Warm the area by placing the frozen areas in warm water (not hot) or applying warm compresses for 15–30 minutes if appropriate. **Do not** rub the area while it is under water. If warm water is not available, wrap the frozen area gently in warm blankets. Continue rewarming the skin until it is pink and feels warm and soft.
- Prevent refreezing and **do not** rewarm if there is a risk of refreezing the area.
- Once the area is thawed, keep it elevated and open to the air if possible. Do not cover the area or apply topical products to the area, unless blisters break.
- Do not break blisters. If a blister breaks, cover with a nonstick gauze and look for signs of infection (pus, increased redness, increased pain). If signs of infection occur, see your healthcare provider.

- Separate toes and fingers if affected and wrap the person in a soft, loosely fitting blanket during transport.
- It is normal to feel pain and tingling when the frozen area is thawed. Nonprescription pain relievers such as ibuprofen and naproxen sodium are good choices. Acetaminophen can be used if the person cannot take these drugs.

Chapter 64
Fungal Nail Infections (Onychomycosis)

Penny F. Miller, BSc(Pharm), MA

Onychomycosis is a fungal infection of the nails. It can cause discomfort, pain and disfigurement, resulting in functional and occupational limitations that can significantly impact quality of life.[1] Treatment is prolonged and reinfection is common.

Pathophysiology

The nail is a specialized outgrowth of skin. The visible hard nail (nail plate) grows from a small area located in the half-moon white region (nail matrix) near the cuticle (Figure 1). The nail plate grows toward the tip of the toe or finger and is attached longitudinally to the nail bed. Fungal invasion of the nail matrix can drastically change the appearance of the nail.

Figure 1: Anatomy of the Toenail Showing Right Large Toe

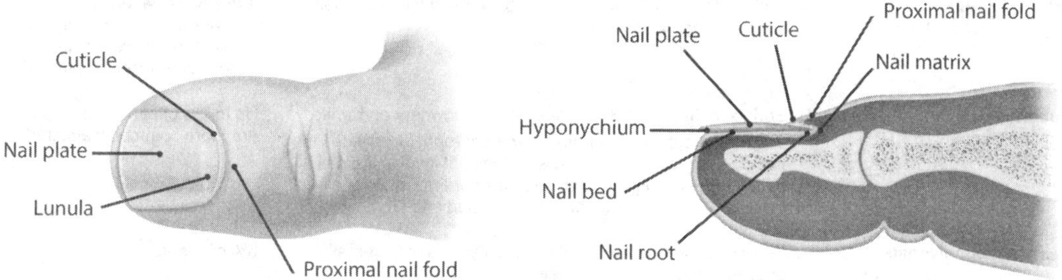

Reproduced with permission from Renee L. Cannon, 2001

Onychomycosis is estimated to affect 6.5% of the Canadian population, with increasing prevalence in older individuals.[2] It is more common in persons with other nail problems (e.g., psoriasis or trauma), occupations requiring occlusive footwear, peripheral vascular insufficiency or immunosuppressed states (e.g., diabetes, HIV infection or immunosuppressive therapy).[3,4] In one-third of cases, there is an association with the presence of tinea pedis (athlete's foot).[5,6]

Onychomycosis is caused primarily by dermatophytes, occasionally by yeasts (mainly *Candida*) and rarely by nondermatophyte moulds. When dermatophytes are the specific cause of the nail infection, this is called tinea unguium.[7] The usual causative dermatophyte is *Trichophyton rubrum*. Occasionally, other dermatophytes such as *Trichophyton mentagrophytes* var interdigitale and *Epidermophyton floccosum* are involved.[8,9]

Onychomycosis is a chronic infectious condition that rarely remits spontaneously and usually progresses to affect other nails or skin areas. In patients with diabetes or immunosuppression, these infected areas can serve as a reservoir of fungi that may cause reinfection or serve as a portal of entry for bacteria, leading to secondary bacterial infections such as cellulitis.[10]

Onychomycosis is classified into 5 subtypes, which are described in Table 1.

Table 1: **Characteristics of Onychomycosis Subtypes**

Type of Onychomycosis	Characteristics	Comments
Distal and lateral subungual onychomycosis (DLSO)	Thickening and white-to-brown discoloration of the distal and/ or lateral edge of the nail, with modest or no change to the nail's shape. The dermatophyte *Trichophyton rubrum* invades the nail bed and the underside of the nail plate beginning at the hyponychium, then migrates to the cuticle/nail matrix. Crumbling yellow debris (subungual hyperkeratosis) is usually evident under the nail edge. Progressive invasion of the nail plate causes a worsening dystrophic nail and onycholysis (nail plate separates from the nail bed).	Most common: 90% of cases. Intercurrent tinea pedis is frequent. Infected toenails more common than fingernails.
Endonyx subungual onychomycosis	Infection with *Trichophyton soudanense* and *Trichophyton violaceum* starts from the pulp as in DLSO, but penetrates the distal nail plate to form milky white patches and indentations. There is no involvement of the nail bed so there is no subungual hyperkeratosis or onycholysis.	Rare and often considered a subtype of DLSO.
Proximal subungual onychomycosis (PSO)	Whitening and crumbling begins at the proximal area beneath the nail bed (at the cuticle). The infecting dermatophyte *Trichophyton rubrum* enters through the proximal nail fold and penetrates the newly formed nail plate, then migrates distally.	Up to 6% of cases. Most common in immunosuppressed patients; often a marker for AIDS.
Total dystrophic onychomycosis (TDO)	Nail is thickened, opaque, yellow-brown and the entire nail plate and matrix are infected.	Any severe variety of onychomycosis can progress to the state where the nail plate is completely destroyed.
Superficial white onychomycosis (SWO)	Surface of the nail has patches that are powdery and white. The dermatophyte *Trichophyton mentagrophytes* invades the nail plate directly from above and does not involve the nail bed. As the disease progresses, the entire nail plate can be involved and the nail becomes roughened and crumbly.	Up to 7% of cases. Children are more commonly affected.
Yeast onychomycosis	Yeast is a common cause of onychomycosis of fingernails and, less frequently, of toenails. *C. albicans* is involved in 70% of cases. Can manifest in several forms.	5% of cases.
Chronic paronychia	Erythematous swelling of the nail fold with secondary onycholysis. Nail plates become discoloured (brown or bluish-black). In severe cases, the digits can appear to have a bulbous or drumstick appearance and the entire thickness of the nail may be involved. Pressure on and movement of the nail is painful.	Affects persons who have occupations requiring frequent immersion of hands in water.
Distal nail candidal infection	Initial subungual hyperkeratosis with a yellowish grey mass that lifts off the nail plate. This leads to onycholysis.	Associated with some forms of peripheral vascular disease.
Chronic mucocutaneous candidiasis	Can lead to gross thickening of the nails (amounting to a candida granuloma) and additional involvement of mucous membranes. Candida invades the entire thickness of the nail into the nail plate to cause brittle nails.	Associated with immunosuppressed states.
Secondary candidal onychomycosis	Severe pre-existing dystrophic changes to the nail are worsened when candida invades the nail plate and nail bed. Clinical signs vary.	Occurs in nails damaged from trauma or diseases such as psoriasis.

Goals of Therapy

- Eradicate or reduce fungal infection
- Improve appearance of nail
- Prevent spread of fungal infection
- Prevent recurrences of fungal infection
- Prevent secondary bacterial infections

Patient Assessment

Characteristics and differential diagnosis of onychomycosis can be found in Table 1 and Table 2. Nail dystrophy has many causes, making diagnosis based on clinical appearance difficult; fungi are responsible 50% of the time. In addition, since treatment of onychomycosis is long term and an extended time period is needed for the nail to grow out, an accurate diagnosis is necessary. Fingernails take about 6 months to grow out while toenails take about 12 months. It is necessary to submit a collection of specimens (e.g., subungual debris and nail clippings) to a laboratory for culture and microscopy to confirm the diagnosis and identify the causative fungus.[11]

Table 2: **Differential Diagnosis of Fungal Nail Infections**

Differential Diagnosis to Consider	Clinical Features
Bacterial paronychia	Painful red swollen area of the nail fold or cuticle which occurs suddenly in contrast to the slow onset seen with candidal paronychia. Bacterial paronychia is often also associated with pus-filled vesicles.
Drugs, e.g., cancer chemotherapy, fluoroquinolones, naproxen, oral contraceptives, tetracyclines	Onycholysis.
Eczema	Transverse ridges. Nail folds affected. History of eczema.
Lichen planus	Nails have prominent longitudinal ridges. Nail atrophy. Oral ulcers, itchy papules on wrists, shins and torso.
Malignant melanoma	Vertical pigmented bands form in the nail bed.
Onychogryphosis (senile)	Thickened, curved nail (claw-like), often seen in elderly persons with vascular insufficiency.
Psoriasis	Symmetrical nail involvement. Nail pitting and “oil staining”. Yellow-gray or silvery white nails. Thick, silvery scales on skin of elbows and knees. Terminal interphalangeal joint arthritis.
Squamous cell carcinoma	Papilloma or warty involvement of paronychia, erosions and scaling.
Trauma	Single nail affected, nail colour change is homogeneous, nail shape is altered.
Yellow-nail syndrome	Nails grow slowly, are yellow-green, thick and curved. Associated with a defective lymphatic drainage in lungs causing pulmonary infections.

Nonpharmacologic Therapy

Persons with onychomycosis should be treated for any associated tinea pedis. Nonpharmacologic treatments include wearing footwear and cotton socks that minimize humidity, drying feet and interdigital spaces thoroughly after washing, and avoiding fungal transmission from shared public spaces such as swimming pools. Nails should be kept clean and cut short. Infected persons should not share nail clippers or footwear.[12] Preventing further trauma to toenails by wearing nonrestrictive footwear or orthotics (which require fitting) may be helpful. People who have their hands immersed in water for long periods of time can wear rubber gloves to protect their fingernails. Applying emollients to cracked skin may reduce further entry points for fungus. Chronic health conditions such as diabetes or peripheral vascular disease that predispose persons to nail infections should be well controlled.[5,13,14] Although nail débridement is sometimes tried, evidence of its efficacy is lacking.[5,15]

Pharmacologic Therapy

For further discussion of pharmacologic therapy for fungal nail infections, consult the *Compendium of Therapeutic Choices*: Fungal Nail Infections.

For comparative ingredients of nonprescription products, consult the *Compendium of Products for Minor Ailments*—Skin Care Products: Antifungals.

In 90% of onychomycosis cases, the infecting dermatophyte is *T. rubrum* and in 80% of cases, toenails are affected. Most patients have the distal and lateral subungual subtype in which the fungus hides under the nail plate; therefore, response to topical therapies is not expected unless the formulation allows for penetration through the nail plate.[11,16] Although the evidence is inconsistent, topical therapies may be useful adjuncts in combination with oral therapy or as prophylaxis to prevent recurrence.

Topical Therapy

Topical agents (e.g., **ciclopirox 8%, efinaconazole 10%, propylene glycol 66.4%/urea 20%/lactic acid 10%**) are recommended for very early, mild cases of DLSO with only distal involvement, SWO or when there are contraindications to systemic therapy.[11] Cases with involvement of the lunula (crescent-shaped area at the base of the nail) or onycholysis should not be treated topically. Limited evidence suggests that topical agents have equally poor cure rates.[15,17] Ciclopirox 8% lacquer is applied to the affected nails once daily for 21 weeks (fingernails) or 48 weeks (toenails). The complete cure rate is 7% with a relapse rate of 40% three months after finishing treatment.[18] Efinaconazole 10% solution is applied as 2 drops (great toenail) or 1 drop (other toenails) once daily for 48 weeks. The complete cure rate is 15%.[19] The combination product of propylene glycol 66.4%/urea 20%/lactic acid 10% is applied once daily to the nail and under the tip of the nail for 6 months.[20] Although evidence is lacking, filing the upper surface of the thickened nail (vigorous débridement) may increase the extent of penetration for a topical preparation and may increase the likelihood for successful topical therapy.[13,21]

Systemic Therapy

Oral agents for onychomycosis treatment include the allylamine **terbinafine** and the azole antifungals **fluconazole, itraconazole, ketoconazole** and **voriconazole**. Terbinafine is considered the drug of choice for dermatophyte onychomycosis based on its higher efficacy, tolerability and lower risk of drug interactions.[11] For candidal onychomycosis, itraconazole is considered first-line treatment based on its high activity against *Candida* and shorter treatment course compared with terbinafine.[11] Fluconazole has relatively reduced efficacy and is considered an alternative if there is intolerance to the other agents.[22] Voriconazole is an option only for recalcitrant nail infections as clinical trial data are limited. There is insufficient evidence to support the use of oral ketoconazole.

Doses and regimens of oral agents shown to be effective for onychomycosis include **terbinafine** 250 mg daily and **itraconazole** 200 mg daily for 12 weeks for toenails and 6 weeks for fingernails. Other regimens include "pulse dosing" of itraconazole 200 mg twice daily for 1 week per month, or terbinafine 500 mg once daily for 1 week per month, with 2 cycles for fingernails and 3 for toenails.[11,23,24,25] These antifungals are incorporated into the nail plate via the nail matrix and by diffusion from the nail bed. Their antifungal activity is retained in the nail bed for months after cessation of therapy.[26] Four months of continuous therapy with terbinafine or itraconazole typically results in a 55% or 26% complete cure rate, respectively.[27,28] The relapse rate with either agent is approximately 30%.[29] **Fluconazole** 150–300 mg once weekly may be effective if used for a duration of 12–16 weeks for fingernail onychomycosis or 18–26 weeks for toenail onychomycosis.[30,31] There is no evidence that continuous or intermittent regimens produce significantly different cure rates or adverse events.

Chemical or Surgical Avulsion

In unresponsive cases, chemical or surgical avulsion combined with topical **ketoconazole 2%** cream or **ciclopirox 8%** lacquer applied under occlusion with polyethylene wrap may be performed by a podiatrist or dermatologist.[32] Risks associated with nail avulsion include pain, possible wound infection and scarring.

Laser and Light Therapy

Device-based therapy involving lasers, photodynamic therapy, iontophoresis and ultrasound are promising alternatives for patients unable or unwilling to use conventional pharmacologic options. Evidence regarding the efficacy and safety of these techniques is accumulating.[33,34]

Monitoring of Therapy

A monitoring plan for patients with onychomycosis is provided in Table 3. Resolution of the fungal infection takes months, while it can take up to 18 months for the appearance of the nail to return to normal, particularly in persons with poor circulation. The nail may never appear normal in some cases. Continued monitoring for recurrence of a nail infection or a concurrent skin infection is important. While the patient is taking continuous daily doses of itraconazole, liver function tests should be performed at baseline then monthly.[35] Hepatic enzyme elevations double the upper level of normal occur in 4% of patients, at which time the drug should be discontinued. Monitoring liver function in healthy patients is usually unnecessary when using terbinafine or pulsed itraconazole regimens for the treatment of onychomycosis. However, baseline liver function tests and complete blood count are advised in patients with heavy alcohol consumption, hepatitis or hematological abnormalities.[36] If the patient has active or chronic liver disease, oral antifungals should be avoided.[37,38]

Table 3: **Monitoring of Therapy for Onychomycosis**

Symptoms	Monitoring	Endpoint of Treatment	Actions
Measure distance of outgrowth of disease-free nail (normal growth rate is 1.5–2 mm/month)	Patient: Monthly Healthcare practitioner: Every 1–2 months	Cessation of growth of diseased nail (6 wk for fingernails, 12 wk for toenails). Normal appearance of nail (at 12 months)	Further assessment is required if no improvement in nail appearance at expected endpoint.
Fatigue, jaundice, anorexia, nausea, vomiting, dark urine or pale stools due to oral antifungals	Patient: Daily Healthcare practitioner: Monthly	Absence of symptoms	Discontinue oral antifungal and perform liver function tests.
Paronychia (*Candida albicans*)	Patient: Weekly	No new lesions	Treat with topical nonprescription anti-yeast

(cont'd)

Table 3: **Monitoring of Therapy for Onychomycosis** *(cont'd)*

Symptoms	Monitoring	Endpoint of Treatment	Actions
	Healthcare practitioner: Monthly		agents (clotrimazole, miconazole, nystatin).
Irritation caused by topical agents	Patient: Daily while on therapy Healthcare practitioner: Monthly	Little or no irritation that subsides with continued use	Stop therapy if no improvement after several doses or if severe.
Secondary bacterial infections: cellulitis	Patient: Daily Healthcare practitioner: Monthly	No new lesions	Further assessment required if signs of pain, swelling, redness or drainage around nails.

Suggested Readings

de Berker D. Clinical practice. Fungal nail disease. *N Engl J Med* 2009;360:2108-16.

Gupta AK, Uro M, Cooper EA. Onychomycosis therapy: past, present, future. *J Drugs Dermatol* 2010;9:1109-13.

References

1. Roseeuw D. Achilles foot screening project: preliminary results of patients screened by dermatologists. *J Eur Acad Dermatol Venereol* 1999;12:S6-9.
2. Gupta AK, Jain HC, Lynde CW et al. Prevalence and epidemiology of onychomycosis in patients visiting physicians' offices: a multicenter canadian survey of 15,000 patients. *J Am Acad Dermatol* 2000;43:244-8.
3. Gupta AK, Konnikov N, MacDonald P et al. Prevalence and epidemiology of toenail onychomycosis in diabetic subjects: a multicentre survey. *Br J Dermatol* 1998;139:665-71.
4. Burzykowski T, Molenberghs G, Abeck D et al. High prevalence of foot diseases in Europe: results of the Achilles Project. *Mycoses* 2003;46:496-505.
5. Szepietowski JC, Reich A, Garlowska E et al. Factors influencing coexistence of toenail onychomycosis with tinea pedis and other dermatomycoses: a survey of 2761 patients. *Arch Dermatol* 2006;142:1279-84.
6. de Berker D. Clinical practice. Fungal nail disease. *N Engl J Med* 2009;360:2108-16.
7. Verma S, Heffernan P. Superficial fungal infections. In: Fitzpatrick TB, Wolff K et al., eds. *Fitzpatrick's dermatology in general medicine*. 7th ed. New York: McGraw-Hill; 2008.
8. Sigurgeirsson B, Baran R. The prevalence of onychomycosis in the global population: a literature study. *J Eur Acad Dermatol Venereol* 2014;28:1480-91.
9. Coleman NW, Fleckman P, Huang JI. Fungal nail infections. *J Hand Surg Am* 2014;39:985-8.
10. Elewski BE. Onychomycosis. Treatment, quality of life, and economic issues. *Am J Clin Dermatol* 2000;1:19-26.
11. Ameen M, Lear JT, Madan V et al. British Association of Dermatologists' guidelines for the management of onychomycosis 2014. *Br J Dermatol* 2014;171:937-58.
12. Gupta AK, Daniel CR. Onychomycosis: strategies to reduce failure and recurrence. *Cutis* 1998;62:189-91.
13. Scher RK, Baran R. Onychomycosis in clinical practice: factors contributing to recurrence. *Br J Dermatol* 2003;149:5-9.
14. Gupta AK, Tu LQ. Onychomycosis therapies: strategies to improve efficacy. *Dermatol Clin* 2006;24:381-6.
15. Ferrari J. Fungal toenail infections. *Clin Evid (Online)* 2008;pii:1715.
16. Kyle AA, Dahl MV. Topical therapy for fungal infections. *Am J Clin Dermatol* 2004:5:443-51.
17. Crawford F, Hollis S. Topical treatments for fungal infections of the skin and nails of the foot. *Cochrane Database Syst Rev* 2007;3:CD001434.
18. Gupta AK, Fleckman P, Baran R. Ciclopirox nail lacquer topical solution 8% in the treatment of toenail onychomycosis. *J Am Acad Dermatol* 2000;43:S70-80.
19. Elewski BE, Rich P, Pollak R et al. Efinaconazole 10% solution in the treatment of toenail onychomycosis: two phase III multicenter, randomized, double-blind studies. *J Am Acad Dermatol* 2013;68:600-8.
20. Emtestam L, Kaaman T, Rensfeldt K. Treatment of distal subungual onychomycosis with a topical preparation of urea, propylene glycol and lactic acid: results of a 24-week, double-blind, placebo-controlled study. *Mycoses* 2012;55:532-40.
21. Roberts DT, Evans EG. Subungual dermatophytoma complicating dermatophyte onychomycosis. *Br J Dermatol* 1998;138:189-90.
22. Havu V, Heikkilä H, Kuokkanen K et al. A double-blind, randomized study to compare the efficacy and safety of terbinafine (Lamisil) with fluconazole (Diflucan) in the treatment of onychomycosis. *Br J Dermatol* 2000;142:97-102.
23. Gupta AK, Ryder JE, Johnson AM. Cumulative meta-analysis of systemic antifungal agents for the treatment of onychomycosis. *Br J Dermatol* 2004;150:537-44.
24. Warshaw EM, Fett DD, Bloomfield HE et al. Pulse versus continuous terbinafine for onychomycosis: a randomized, double-blind, controlled trial. *J Am Acad Dermatol* 2005;53:578-84.

25. Gupta AK, Paquet M, Simpson F et al. Terbinafine in the treatment of dermatophyte toenail onychomycosis: a meta-analysis of efficacy for continuous and intermittent regimens. *J Eur Acad Dermatol Venereol* 2013;27:267-72.

26. Meinhof W. Kinetics and spectrum of activity of oral antifungals: the therapeutic implications. *J Am Acad Dermatol* 1993;29:S37-41.

27. Evans EG, Sigurgeirsson B. Double blind, randomised study of continuous terbinafine compared with intermittent itraconazole in treatment of toenail onychomycosis. The LION Study Group. *BMJ* 1999;318:1031-5.

28. Crawford F, Young P, Godfrey C et al. Oral treatments for toenail onychomycosis: a systematic review. *Arch Dermatol* 2002;138:811-6.

29. Sigurgeirsson B, Olafsson JH, Steinsson JB et al. Long-term effectiveness of treatment with terbinafine vs itraconazole in onychomycosis: a 5-year blinded prospective follow-up study. *Arch Dermatol* 2002;138:353-7.

30. Gupta AK, Drummond-Main C, Paquet M. Evidence-based optimal fluconazole dosing regimen for onychomycosis treatment. *J Dermatolog Treat* 2013;24:75-80.

31. de Sá DC, Lamas AP, Tosti A. Oral therapy for onychomycosis: an evidence-based review. *Am J Clin Dermatol* 2014;15:17-36.

32. Baden HP. Treatment of distal onychomycosis with avulsion and topical antifungal agents under occlusion. *Arch Dermatol* 1994;130:558-9.

33. Bristow IR. The effectiveness of lasers in the treatment of onychomycosis: a systematic review. *J Foot Ankle Res* 2014;7:34.

34. Ortiz AE, Avram MM, Wanner MA. A review of lasers and light for the treatment of onychomycosis. *Lasers Surg Med* 2014;46:117-24.

35. Chang CH, Young-Xu Y, Kurth T et al. The safety of oral antifungal treatments for superficial dermatophytosis and onychomycosis: a meta-analysis. *Am J Med* 2007;120:791-8.

36. Gupta AK, Ryder JE, Lynch LE et al. The use of terbinafine in the treatment of onychomycosis in adults and special populations: a review of the evidence. *J Drugs Dermatol* 2005;4:302-8.

37. Gupta AK, Chwetzoff E, Del Rosso J et al. Hepatic safety of itraconazole. *J Cutan Med Surg* 2002;6:210-3.

38. Elewski B, Tavakkol A. Safety and tolerability of oral antifungal agents in the treatment of fungal nail disease: a proven reality. *Ther Clin Risk Manag* 2005;1:299-306.

Fungal Infections of the Nail—What You Need to Know

What are fungal nail infections?

- This is an infection of the nails commonly caused by the same fungus that causes athlete's foot. The toenails of adults are infected most often. Fingernails are less often infected.
- Fungal nail infections can also be caused by a different yeast-like fungus called *Candida*. This yeast can also cause diaper rash or mouth thrush.

How do you get a fungal nail infection?

- Fungi grow well in warm, damp areas. Public swimming pools or gym showers are places where you may get these fungi. Skin and nails that are damp from swimming or from wearing closed-in shoes make you more likely to get a fungal toenail infection.
- People who have their hands are in water for long periods of time as part of their jobs are more likely to get a (yeast) fingernail infection.
- Diabetics and adults over age 60 are more likely to get these infections.

What are the signs of a fungal nail infection?

- Fungi live under the nail. The first sign of an infection is a white section under the tip of the nail that slowly spreads. Soon the nail becomes loosened from the nail bed. As the infection spreads, there may be a collection of material under the nail. The nail becomes yellow-brown, thickened and brittle, and crumbles. If the infection is not treated, the entire nail may fall off.
- Footwear may cause pain in the toenail and the nail looks unhealthy.
- Yeast nail infections may cause swelling and redness of the skin around the nail. The nail appears white and lifts up from the nail bed.

What is the treatment for a fungal nail infection?

- If you think you have a fungal nail infection, it is important to see a healthcare provider to make sure. There are many medicines to treat fungal nail infections.
- A medicine in tablet form may need to be taken for 6 weeks or for several months in order to work.
- It will take about 1 year for the nail to grow out and look normal.
- About 1 in 3 persons with nail infections will not be cured with the first treatment and will require more treatment.
- Medicine that you put on the nail (as a nail lacquer) may be used if the fungal infection is mild or is a yeast infection.
- Sometimes, medication that you put on the nail is used at the same time as medicine that you take by mouth. Medicines that you take by mouth have caused liver damage in some people so blood tests will be needed.

How can you stop fungal nail infections from coming back?

- Keep nails trimmed short. Do not use the same file or trimmer on healthy nails.
- Dry feet well after swimming or using public showers. Wear shower shoes in public areas. Foot powders may help absorb wetness.
- Wear shoes that are not tight and allow the feet to breathe.
- Wear 100% cotton socks and change them every day and whenever they are damp.
- Wear waterproof gloves for wet work (such as washing dishes).

When should you see a healthcare provider?

- If your toes or fingers become swollen, red, painful or drain pus. This may be a bacterial infection that will need antibiotics.
- If you have fungal infections that are not clearing up or you are getting other infections on your skin.
- To make sure the medicine you take by mouth is working and not causing any harm.
- If you develop any side effects from your medications such as rash, nausea, vomiting, fatigue, abdominal pain or dark-coloured urine.

Chapter 65

Fungal Skin Infections

Penny F. Miller, BSc(Pharm), MA(Ed)

Superficial fungal infections are very common skin diseases affecting the majority of people at some point in their lifetime. Numerous fungi are capable of invading the epidermis, hair, nails and mucosa. Three genera of dermatophytes (*Trichophyton*, *Epidermophyton* and *Microsporum*) and yeastlike fungi, *Candida* or *Malassezia furfur*, are responsible for most infections.[1,2] This chapter is divided into 3 sections: Dermatophyte Infections, Yeast Infections: Pityriasis Versicolor (Tinea Versicolor), and Yeast Infections: Cutaneous Candidiasis. Table 1 provides information on the characteristics and differential diagnosis of fungal skin infections.

Table 1: **Characteristics and Differential Diagnosis of Fungal Skin Infections**[1,3,4,5]

Condition	Distribution	Lesions	Differential Diagnosis
Infections caused by dermatophytes (see Dermatophyte Infections)[a]			
Tinea Barbae	Beard	Reddened areas with perifollicular papules and pustules or swollen, inflamed mass with pus and hair loss.	Folliculitis (bacterial or candidal): small pustules around hair follicles. Perioral dermatitis: papules and pustules surrounding the mouth and chin. Often includes a history of topical steroid use. See Chapter 54: Acne. Acne vulgaris: pustules and blackheads affecting other areas of the face as well. See Chapter 54: Acne. Acne rosacea: pustules and dilated or broken blood vessels with facial flushing involving cheeks. See Chapter 54: Acne. Contact dermatitis: itchy vesicles and papules that become scaly, thickened and itchy when chronic. See Chapter 55: Atopic, Contact, and Stasis Dermatitis.
Tinea Capitis	Scalp	May be quite varied from an irregular-shaped scaly patch with broken hairs or a very inflamed soft, swollen mass called a kerion with hair loss.	Seborrheic dermatitis: yellow, greasy scales; often involves the hairline and face. See Chapter 58: Dandruff and Seborrheic Dermatitis. Impetigo: honey-coloured crusts. See Chapter 56: Bacterial Skin Infections: Impetigo, Furuncles and Carbuncles. Psoriasis: symmetric distribution of silvery scales on reddened base. See Chapter 71: Psoriasis. Alopecia areata: small nonscaly patches of sudden hair loss. See Chapter 66: Hair Care and Hair Growth.
Tinea Corporis	Exposed areas, namely, trunk, limbs and face	Typically annular (round), erythematous patch; scaly with a vesicular border and central clearing.	Psoriasis: thick and silvery scales often in a symmetrical arrangement. See Chapter 71: Psoriasis. Seborrheic dermatitis: yellow, greasy scales affecting face, scalp and central chest. See Chapter 58: Dandruff and Seborrheic Dermatitis. Nummular eczema: smaller lesions usually affecting arms, legs and neck. Contact dermatitis: acute onset of itchy vesicles. SeeChapter 55: Atopic, Contact, and Stasis Dermatitis.

(cont'd)

Table 1: **Characteristics and Differential Diagnosis of Fungal Skin Infections**[1,3,4,5] *(cont'd)*

Condition	Distribution	Lesions	Differential Diagnosis
			Lyme disease: an initial erythematous circular lesion (erythema migrans) with a central clearing at the site of the tick bite. It lacks scales. See Chapter 67: Insect Bites and Stings. Pityriasis rosea: acute onset of small scaled lesions in a Christmas tree distribution on the trunk. A single salmon-coloured patch that can be mistaken for tinea corporis appears on the trunk 2 weeks preceding this rash.
Tinea Cruris	Symmetrical, involving the upper inner thigh and groin The penis and scrotum are usually spared	Annular, erythematous patch, with scales and central clearing. The borders are well defined.	Yeast Infections: Cutaneous Candidiasis: Very red with poorly defined borders and has satellite lesions (vesicles, papules) outside the borders of the rash. The scrotum or penis may be involved. Erythrasma: Overgrowth of normal skin bacterium, *Corynebacterium minutissimum*; presents as bilateral, irregular-shaped, brown plaques with scales found in intertriginous (skin fold) areas. Psoriasis: Symmetrical erythematous patches. See Chapter 71: Psoriasis. Seborrheic dermatitis: Usually also involves the scalp, face and central chest. See Chapter 58: Dandruff and Seborrheic Dermatitis.
Tinea Manuum	Palmar surface of the hand more often than the back of the hand Only one hand may be involved if it occurs in conjunction with tinea pedis	Usually dry, mild diffuse scales on an erythematous base.	Allergic or contact dermatitis: Acute onset and very pruritic. See Chapter 55: Atopic, Contact, and Stasis Dermatitis. Atopic dermatitis usually involves other skin areas. See Chapter 55: Atopic, Contact, and Stasis Dermatitis. Psoriasis: Silvery scale. Involved nails are pitted. See Chapter 71: Psoriasis.
Infections caused by yeast (see Yeast Infections: Pityriasis Versicolor (Tinea Versicolor) and Yeast Infections: Cutaneous Candidiasis)			
Yeast Infections: Pityriasis Versicolor (Tinea Versicolor)	Back, chest, upper arms	Multiple white-pink to brown macules with an overlying fine scale.	Vitiligo: Nonscaly, chalk-white lesions. Seborrheic dermatitis: Yellow, greasy scales involving the chest as well as the scalp. See Chapter 58: Dandruff and Seborrheic Dermatitis. Tinea Corporis: Well-defined borders.
Yeast Infections: Cutaneous Candidia-sis	Moist areas, skin folds, particularly the groin	A "beefy red" edematous area with irregular edges and many small papules (satellite lesions) outside of the borders.	Tinea Corporis or Tinea Cruris: Well-defined borders, no satellite lesions and the scrotum is not involved. Contact dermatitis: Will not have satellite lesions. See Chapter 55: Atopic, Contact, and Stasis Dermatitis. Psoriasis: Symmetrical with well-defined borders and no satellite lesions. See Chapter 71: Psoriasis.

[a] Tinea pedis is discussed in Chapter 50: Athlete's Foot.

Dermatophyte Infections

Pathophysiology

The dermatophytes (an umbrella term that includes the genera *Microsporum*, *Trichophyton* and *Epidermophyton*) survive on dead keratin and do not invade living tissue. They affect the top layer of the epidermis, hair, nails and skin. Mucosal tissues are spared as they lack a keratin layer. Infections are transmitted through direct contact with infected persons or fomites, or occasionally infected soil or animals. Many predisposing factors can contribute to dermatophyte infections including conditions that increase moisture such as occlusive clothing or shoes and warm humid climates. Impaired immunity states (e.g., diabetes, HIV infection, chemotherapy) or genetic predisposition can also increase susceptibility to dermatophyte infection. Dermatophyte infections are commonly called ringworm or tinea which means fungus. Classification of tinea infections is based on their anatomic location rather than the fungal species.[1,2] See Chapter 50: Athlete's Foot for an in-depth discussion of tinea pedis.

Tinea Corporis

The classic presentation affects the smooth and bare (glabrous) areas of the trunk or limbs (excluding the face, hands, feet and groin) and begins as a flat, circular, scaly spot with a clearing central portion and a raised vesicular red border that advances circumferentially outward.[1,2] See Tinea Corporis in Photo Section. Outbreaks of tinea corporis can occur in athletes who have skin-to-skin contact, such as wrestlers, where it is called tinea corporis gladiatorum.[6,7]

Tinea Cruris

Tinea cruris or "jock itch" involves the groin area (medial and upper parts of the thigh and the pubic area). Occasionally the anal cleft is affected. Unlike yeast infections, the scrotum and penis are spared. The infection occurs most often in men during the summer months. Often a reservoir for the infection is found on the feet.[6] The lesions are usually bilateral, scaly with red-brown centres and a clearly defined, raised border. Pruritus is common.[1,2,6]

Tinea Manuum

An infrequent infection, tinea manuum may present as the classic pattern of limited erythema and scaling of the dorsal surface of the hands. Another form affecting the palmar hand surfaces produces diffuse dryness and hyperkeratosis of only one palm and is associated with tinea pedis, referred to as "two feet–one hand syndrome".[1,2]

Tinea Capitis

Tinea capitis is a dermatophyte infection involving the scalp hair follicles and adjacent skin. Children are primarily affected. The most common form, "black dot tinea capitis", often appears as an annular patch of itchy, scaling skin and hair loss. Hairs may eventually break off flush with the scalp surface, and debris in the follicle formerly occupied by hair appears as black dots.[6]

A less common type of tinea capitis contracted from cats and dogs, called "gray patch tinea capitis", causes hairs in the affected area to turn gray as a result of loss of the hair sheath. The hairs break 1 or 2 millimetres above the scalp and the remaining hair stubs have a frosted appearance. The initial erythematous, scaling patch eventually subsides.

Tinea scalp infections may result in a hypersensitivity response where some patients develop a boggy inflammatory mass called a kerion that can result in scarring and permanent hair loss.

Tinea of the scalp is common in low socioeconomic and crowded environments, and the causative dermatophyte species vary among different countries. It is contagious via direct contact with infected persons, animals or contaminated clothing (e.g., hats, combs). Affected shedded hairs can harbour viable organisms for more than 1 year.[1,2]

Tinea Barbae

Coarse hair of the beard area and occasionally the mustache area in adult men may become infected with tinea. Typically this is a disease spread by animals to farm workers. The lesions are usually unilateral and may appear as typical scaly patches, follicular pustules or erythematous kerions.[1,8]

Tinea pedis/athlete's foot is discussed in Chapter 50: Athlete's Foot.

Goals of Therapy

- Eradicate causative organism
- Resolve the lesion and symptoms
- Prevent spread of the infection
- Prevent secondary complications

Patient Assessment

Assess patient's signs, symptoms and history including:

- location and distribution of lesions
- aggravating factors, affect on activities and quality of life
- treatments attempted.

Characteristics and differential diagnosis of fungal skin infections can be found in Table 1. Topical antifungal treatment is effective for tinea corporis, tinea cruris and tinea pedis.[4]

Further assessment and/or treatment is required in those patients who are:[5]

- experiencing an infection with unclear etiology
- immunocompromised (e.g., high dose or prolonged immunosuppressant drug therapy, advanced or uncontrolled diabetes, acquired immunodeficiency syndrome)
- experiencing tinea capitis, tinea barbae or tinea unguium (tinea of the nails) for systemic therapy since topical agents do not penetrate the hair follicles or nails well
- responding poorly or are intolerant to topical therapy
- experiencing an extensive, disabling, multifocal or inflammatory disease.

Topical therapy can be attempted for tinea manuum but because of the thickness of palmar skin and frequent association with infected fingernails, systemic therapy is often necessary.

Nonpharmacologic Therapy

Skin should be kept clean and dry to discourage fungal proliferation. Using an electric hairdryer on the cool setting will aid in drying the skin; avoid excessive rubbing with towels. Loose-fitting cotton clothing that allows adequate ventilation is encouraged. Nonmedicated powders can be used to absorb excess perspiration but cornstarch should be avoided since it may provide nourishment for fungi, thereby delaying resolution. Clothing and linens of the infected person should be laundered separately from those of other family members.[3,4]

Pharmacologic Therapy

Topical pharmacologic options available for the treatment of dermatophyte skin infections include: **clotrimazole**, **ketoconazole**, **miconazole**, **terbinafine**, **tolnaftate** and **undecylenic acid**.[9] Topical antifungal treatment is effective for tinea corporis, tinea cruris and tinea pedis.[10,11] The azoles (clotrimazole, ketoconazole, miconazole) are generally more effective than tolnaftate.[12,13] A systematic review provided low-quality evidence that the topical azoles, terbinafine and ciclopirox achieve comparable clinical and mycological cure rates (all have an NNT of 2), but treatment duration is shorter with terbinafine.[14] Terbinafine treatment for 1 week has produced similar cure rates to those reported for azole treatment for 4 weeks.[15,16]

Nystatin is ineffective in the treatment of dermatophytosis.[9] Undecylenic acid is effective but there are insufficient data to compare its efficacy with that of other topical antifungals.[13,17]

Because they are rubbed into the skin, creams and lotions are considered to be more effective than sprays or powders, which are often used adjunctively. Lotions and powders are preferred in intertriginous areas where creams may be more occlusive and could lead to maceration. Liberal use of antifungal powder (e.g., tolnaftate) may help to absorb skin perspiration and prevent rubbing.

Optimal dosage regimens and durations of treatment for various fungal infections have not been determined due to lack of quality evidence, except in the case of terbinafine treatment of tinea corporis and tinea cruris which is recommended to be applied once daily for 1 week.[14] Treatment with other antifungals is usually for a minimum of 2 weeks or until 1 week after the skin clears. Tinea cruris may respond in 2 weeks while tinea corporis typically requires 4 weeks of treatment.

Patients with widespread disease or persistent recurrence or who are immunocompromised may require treatment with systemic antifungals (e.g., oral terbinafine, itraconazole, fluconazole).

Before the advent of effective antifungal agents, keratolytics such as **Whitfield's ointment** (**salicylic acid** 3% and **benzoic acid** 6%) were used to produce desquamation of the fungus-containing epidermis. There is insufficient evidence to determine whether Whitfield's ointment is effective.[14] The preparation can be irritating and if used over a large surface area, can lead to salicylate toxicity.[18] Safer and more effective antifungal agents are preferred.

Topical corticosteroids may suppress the signs of the fungal infection by altering the appearance of the lesions, which are then called “tinea incognito”. Corticosteroids may also decrease the local immunologic reaction in persistent or recurrent infections or accelerate fungal growth resulting in the invasion of deeper tissues.[19] However, in severe inflammatory cases, a low-potency topical corticosteroid may be used in combination with the topical antifungal for a short period until itch and irritation are relieved, after which the antifungal is continued alone for the remainder of the treatment period.[14] The combination of corticosteroid and antifungal agent should be avoided in occluded areas and on the face.[20]

More information regarding topical therapy for fungal skin infections can be found in Table 3.

Monitoring of Therapy

Table 2 provides a monitoring plan for patients with fungal skin infections.

Yeast Infections: Pityriasis Versicolor (Tinea Versicolor)

Pathophysiology

Pityriasis versicolor is an infection of the stratum corneum of the skin where sebaceous glands are present, especially the upper trunk. Since the term tinea refers to diseases caused by dermatophytes, the preferred term for this infection which is caused by yeast (and not dermatophytes) is is pityriasis (meaning scaling). *Malassezia* species (formerly called *Pityrosporum orbiculare* or *Pityrosporum ovale*) normally colonize the skin but cause an opportunistic infection in association with hereditary factors, immunodeficiency, malnutrition, oily skin, hyperhidrosis or use of corticosteroids or oral contraceptives.[24] It affects about 3% of the general population and occurs most commonly in postpubertal adults and in warm, humid climates.[25,26] The term versicolor denotes a variety of colours or changing colours.

The most common presentation is multiple white to reddish-brown macules that may coalesce to form large patches of various colours ranging from white to tan. A fine scale is apparent when scratched. The lesions tend to be darker than the surrounding skin in fair-skinned patients and lighter in dark-skinned patients. This is primarily a cosmetic problem where the lesions do not tan along with the surrounding normal skin. Recurrence rates are as high as 60–80%.[27] See Pityriasis Versicolor in Photo Section. It is not considered contagious and is not due to poor hygiene.[25]

Goals of Therapy

- Reduce or eliminate yeast elements
- Reduce or eliminate skin lesions and symptoms
- Prevent recurrences of infection

Patient Assessment

Characteristics and differential diagnosis of pityriasis versicolor can be found in Table 1. Patients with pityriasis versicolor usually have only cosmetic manifestations; pruritus is unusual. Self-care measures are appropriate for those with pityriasis versicolor. If the etiology of the infection is unclear, patients require further assessment to confirm diagnosis.[26,28]

Nonpharmacologic Therapy

Because yeasts thrive in moist environments, controlling excess heat and humidity may be helpful. Avoid application of oil to the skin, as *Malassezia* species can overgrow in such an environment.

Pharmacologic Therapy

More information regarding topical therapy for fungal skin infections can be found in Table 3.

Pityriasis versicolor can be successfully treated with a number of topical antifungal agents. Those used most commonly include: topical azoles (**clotrimazole**, **ketoconazole**, **miconazole**) and **selenium sulfide** 2.5% suspension.

Ketoconazole is the most extensively studied treatment approach. In one meta-analysis, topical ketoconazole was associated with a mycological eradication rate of 65% compared with 45% for terbinafine.[29] Another study found ketoconazole 2% shampoo produced clinical cure rates of about 70%.[30] Other azoles such as clotrimazole and miconazole, as well as the hydroxypyridone **ciclopirox olamine**, appear to have equivalent efficacy.[29,31,32,33]

Selenium sulfide suspension has traditionally been used and remains effective.[34,35] It appears to be as efficacious as topical azoles and is more cost effective when the condition is widespread.[25]

Topical **terbinafine** has been used but has inferior evidence of efficacy.[31,32,33]

Other topical agents such as **sulfur** 2%, **salicylic acid**, **zinc pyrithione** 1% or 2% shampoo, **benzoyl peroxide** or extemporaneously compounded **propylene glycol** 50% have demonstrated limited efficacy in older trials.[18,25,36,37,38]

Oral therapy for patients with extensive infection or those who are intolerant of or unable to use topical therapy includes **fluconazole** (400 mg single dose or 300 mg weekly for 2 weeks) or **itraconazole** (200 mg daily for 5–7 days).[25,26,32,39] Oral terbinafine is ineffective.[31] Oral ketoconazole is not recommended due to the risk of hepatotoxicity.[40]

Preventive Therapy

Pityriasis versicolor has a high rate of recurrence; prophylactic treatment with topical or oral therapy on an intermittent basis is often necessary. Preventive treatment with once- to twice-monthly applications of **selenium sulfide** suspension can reduce the recurrence rate to less than 15%. Soaps or shampoos containing **zinc pyrithione**, **salicylic acid** or **sulfur** can also be used.[9] **Itraconazole** 200 mg taken once monthly has also been used successfully.[41]

Monitoring of Therapy

A monitoring plan for patients with fungal skin infections is provided in Table 2. Resolution of scaling with pityriasis versicolor occurs promptly but the pigmentary changes may take weeks to months to resolve.

Yeast Infections: Cutaneous Candidiasis

Pathophysiology

Candida yeasts are part of the normal flora of the oropharynx, intestinal tract and vagina. Infections arise when skin pH is increased, competing bacteria are removed by antibiotic treatments, glucose content in sweat increases (as in diabetes) and/or the surrounding environment is warm and moist.[42,49] With impaired host defenses, infections may not only affect skin, nails or mucous membranes but may also rarely lead to systemic infections. Risk factors for cutaneous candidiasis include diabetes mellitus, malignancy, obesity, tropical environment, neutropenia, HIV infection, psoriasis, contact dermatitis and use of corticosteroids, antibiotics, cytotoxic or immunosuppressant agents.[26,42,43] See Candidiasis Intertrigo in Photo Section.

The most common form of *Candida albicans* infection is intertrigo. Any skin fold area such as the gluteal fold, axillae (armpits), interdigital spaces, area under breasts or abdominal folds can be affected. These occluded areas create moist, warm environments ideal for *C. albicans* to flourish.[26] Intertrigo is often colonized with bacteria which can lead to a secondary bacterial infection. This may result in cellulitis, especially in patients with diabetes. In addition, the macerated skin can break down to cause fissures and ulcers, particularly in the deep folds of obese persons, leading to pain and disability.[44,45]

Candidal paronychia occurs in individuals who have their hands in water excessively. This condition consists of painful, reddened and swollen nail folds. Chronic infection can lead to transverse depressions of the nail plate and brownish discoloration and eventual separation of the nail plate from the nail bed (onycholysis).[31,46] See Chapter 64: Fungal Nail Infections (Onychomycosis).

Goals of Therapy

- Eradicate or reduce the yeast elements
- Eliminate or reduce lesions and symptoms
- Prevent spread of infection
- Prevent recurrences

Patient Assessment

A description and differential diagnosis of cutaneous candidiasis is provided in Table 1. The lesions are red, macerated patches with irregular scalloped borders. Papules and pustules called satellite lesions form outside of the borders. Symptoms of pruritus and soreness are common.[9]

Patients with widespread, systemic or persistent, recurrent infection or those who are immunocompromised require further assessment and/or treatment by an appropriate healthcare practitioner.

Nonpharmacologic Therapy

Hygiene measures such as daily bathing and avoidance of tight-fitting clothing aid in skin dryness, making a less desirable environment for yeasts. Useful measures for keeping the area dry include using cool water compresses (1 minute on, 1 minute off) for 15–20 minutes 3 times daily. The affected area should be air dried afterwards. Applying nonmedicated powders several times daily helps to reduce the moisture in skin folds and may help prevent the infection.[47] Although 1 study did not find enhanced yeast growth,[48] it is recommended that the use of cornstarch be avoided as this may promote the growth of *Candida*.[6]

Pharmacologic Therapy

Many topical antifungal agents are effective for the treatment of cutaneous candidiasis including: **azole antifungals** (e.g., **clotrimazole**, **ketoconazole**, **miconazole**) **nystatin**, **ciclopirox olamine** and **terbinafine** (see Table 3). **Tolnaftate** and **undecylenic acid** are ineffective.

If there is pronounced inflammation, low- to mid-potency **topical corticosteroids** may be used sparingly once or twice daily for short periods (1–2 weeks) in conjunction with an antifungal.[42,49] Stronger topical corticosteroids should be avoided as the occlusive effect of skin folds can increase absorption of the corticosteroid and accelerate skin atrophy and striae.[46]

Monotherapy with drying antifungal powders (e.g., **miconazole spray**) is less effective than monotherapy with antifungal creams or ointments due to comparatively decreased skin penetration.[49]

In widespread cutaneous disease and immunocompromised patients, **oral** azole antifungals (e.g., **fluconazole**, **itraconazole**) may be indicated. **Oral terbinafine** may not be as effective as oral azole antifungals.[50]

More information regarding topical therapy for fungal skin infections can be found in Table 3.

Monitoring of Therapy

Substantial improvement should be evident within 1 week of topical treatment. If topical corticosteroids are used (with antifungals) to control an inflammatory intertrigo, patients should be monitored closely for the development of a hidden bacterial infection or striae.[45]

Persistent candidal infection may be a sign of immunosuppression and these patients should undergo further investigation. Table 2 suggests a monitoring plan for patients with fungal infections.

Natural Health Products

A number of herbal therapies have been used for a variety of fungal skin infections, including: goldenseal, purple coneflower (*Echinacea*), slippery elm bark. St. John's wort and tea tree oil (*Melaluca*). There is insufficient evidence to recommend the use of any of these herbs.[51,52] One study of tea tree oil in tinea pedis showed some benefit.[53]

Table 2: **Monitoring of Therapy for Fungal Skin Infections**

Symptoms	Monitoring	Desired Outcome	Actions
Lesions specific for each fungal infection	Patient: Daily for lesions decreasing in size and no more new lesions developing Healthcare Practitioner: Next visit	Clearing of all lesions within 4 wk	If no improvement or spreading of lesions by 1 wk, patient requries further assessment and/or treatment.
Pain, swelling, redness or drainage	Patient: Daily for any evidence of new onset of these symptoms Healthcare Practitioner: Next visit	No development of these symptoms	Patient requires further assessment and/or treatment if these symptoms develop, as they may indicate a bacterial superinfection.
Recurrent lesions	Patient: Watch for recurrence of any new lesions for weeks or months following initial infection	No new lesions	Patient requires further assessment to rule out any underlying predisposing conditions. Emphasize preventive measures.
Inflammation being treated with corticosteroids	Patient: Daily	Resolution of inflamed areas	If no improvement or lesion is worsening by 1 wk, patient requires further assessment and/or treatment. Emphasize correct use of cool compresses.
Allergy	Patient: Daily while on therapy	No allergy	Stop therapy. Patient requires further assessment and/or treatment.
Irritation caused by topical agents	Patient: Daily while on therapy Healthcare Practitioner: After 1 wk or next pharmacy visit	Little to no irritation that subsides with continued use	Stop therapy if no improvement in irritation secondary to the topical agent after several doses.

Table 3: Topical Antifungal Agents[21,22]

Class	Drug	Dosage	Adverse Effects	Comments	Cost[a]
Allylyamines	*terbinafine 1% cream, spray* Lamisil	Tinea corporis/cruris: Once daily × 1 wk Pityriasis versicolor: Once daily–BID × 1–2 wk Cutaneous candidiasis: Once daily–BID × 2 wk	Irritation, burning, erythema, contact dermatitis	Effective for treatment of infections caused by dermatophytes or yeasts. In dermatophyte infections: less frequent application and shorter duration of treatment than other topical antifungals.	$$
Azoles	*clotrimazole 1% cream* Canesten Topical, generics	Tinea corporis: BID × 4 wk Tinea cruris: BID × 2–4 wk Pityriasis versicolor: BID × 2 wk Cutaneous candidiasis: BID × 2–3 wk	Irritation, erythema, itching, stinging. Rare: hypersensitivity reactions.	Effective in treatment of infections caused by dermatophytes or yeasts.	$
	ketoconazole 2% cream, shampoo Ketoderm, Nizoral	Tinea corporis: Once daily × 3–4 wk Tinea cruris: Once daily × 2–4 wk Pityriasis versicolor: Shampoo (used as a lotion): Scrub into affected area then rinse off after 5 min Single dose or once daily × 3 days Cream: Once daily × 2–3 wk Cutaneous candidiasis: Once daily × 2–3 wk	Itching, burning, stinging, skin sensitivity, itching, contact dermatitis.	Effective for treatment of infections caused by dermatophytes or yeasts. Various regimens have been studied and found to be effective. Regimens with longer durations of treatment may lead to longer time before recurrence.[23]	$
	miconazole 2% cream Micatin Derm, Monistat Derm, generics	Tinea corporis: BID × 4 wk Tinea cruris: BID × 2–4 wk Pityriasis versicolor: BID × 2 wk Cutaneous candidiasis: BID × 2–3 wk	Irritation, erythema, itching, stinging. Rare: hypersensitivity reactions.	Effective for treatment of infections caused by dermatophytes or yeasts.	$
Hydroxypyridone	*ciclopirox olamine 1% cream, lotion, shampoo* Loprox, Stieprox	Tinea corporis/cruris: Cream or lotion: BID × 4 wk Pityriasis versicolor: Cream or lotion: BID × 2 wk Shampoo: Twice weekly × 2 wk	Itching, burning, stinging, skin sensitivity, contact dermatitis.	Effective for treatment of infections caused by dermatophytes or yeasts.	$$
Polyenes	*nystatin 100 000 units/g cream, ointment* generics	Cutaneous candidiasis: BID–TID × 2–3 wk	Rarely irritation.	Ineffective in treatment of dermatophytoses.	$

(cont'd)

Table 3: **Topical Antifungal Agents[21,22]** *(cont'd)*

Class	Drug	Dosage	Adverse Effects	Comments	Cost[a]
Thiocarbamates	*tolnaftate 1% cream, spray* Tinactin	Tinea corporis or cruris: BID × 2–4 wk	Local skin irritation.	Ineffective in treatment of cutaneous candidiasis.	$
Other antifungal agents	*selenium sulfide 2.5% suspension* Selsun	Pityriasis versicolor: Apply to affected areas and lather with a small amount of water. Allow product to remain on skin for 10 min, then rinse the body thoroughly. Use once daily × 1–2 wk Prevention: Once to twice monthly	Skin irritation.		$
	undecylenic acid 1% gel, liquid Fungicure	Tinea corporis: BID × 4 wk Tinea cruris: BID × 2 wk	Itching, burning, stinging.	Ineffective in treatment of cutaneous candidiasis.	$

[a] Cost of smallest available pack size; includes drug cost only.

[b] Application instructions (unless otherwise stated): skin should be clean and dry. Apply in a thin layer to the affected area and 2–3 cm beyond its border, and rub in lightly.

Legend: $ <$10 $$ $10–20

Suggested Readings

Gupta AK, Einarson TR, Summerbell RC et al. An overview of topical antifungal therapy in dermatomycoses. A North American perspective. *Drugs* 1998;55:645-74.

Hainer BL. Dermatophyte infections. *Am Fam Physician* 2003;67:101-8.

Janniger CK, Schwartz RA, Szepietowski JC et al. Intertrigo and common secondary skin infections. *Am Fam Physician* 2005;72:833-8.

UpToDate. Goldstein AO, Goldstein BG. *Dermatophyte (tinea) infections*. Available from: www.uptodate.com. Subscription required.

References

1. Verma S, Heffernan MP. Superficial fungal infection: dermatophytosis, onychomycosis, tinea nigra, piedra. In: Fitzpatrick TB, Wolff K et al., eds. *Fitzpatrick's dermatology in general medicine*. 7th ed. New York: McGraw-Hill; 2008.
2. Habif TP. Superficial fungal infections. In: Habif TP. *Clinical dermatology: a color guide to diagnosis and therapy*. 4th ed. New York: Mosby; 2004.
3. Hooper BJ, Goldman MP. *Primary dermatologic care*. St. Louis: Mosby; 1999.
4. Goldstein BG, Goldstein AO. *Practical dermatology*. 2nd ed. St. Louis: Mosby; 1997. p. 71-7.
5. Lookingbill DP, Marks JG. *Principles of dermatology*. 3rd ed. Philadelphia: Saunders; 2000.
6. UpToDate. Goldstein AO, Goldstein BG. *Dermatophyte (tinea) infections*. Available from: www.uptodate.com. Accessed July 2015. Subscription required.
7. Pleacher MD, Dexter WW. Cutaneous fungal and viral infections in athletes. *Clin Sports Med* 2007;26:397-411.
8. Hainer BL. Dermatophyte infections. *Am Fam Physician* 2003;67:101-8.
9. Kyle AA, Dahl MV. Topical therapy for fungal infections. *Am J Clin Dermatol* 2004:5:443-51.
10. Drake LA, Dinehart SM, Farmer ER et al. Guidelines of care for superficial mycotic infections of the skin: tinea corporis, tinea cruris, tinea faciei, tinea manuum, and tinea pedis. Guidelines/Outcomes Committee. American Academy of Dermatology. *J Am Acad Dermatol* 1996;34:282-6.
11. Gilbert DN, Chambers HF, Eliopoulos GM et al. *Sanford guide to antimicrobial therapy*. 45th ed. Hyde Park: Antimicrobial Therapy; 2015.
12. Crawford F, Hollis S. Topical treatments for fungal infections of the skin and nails of the foot. *Cochrane Database Syst Rev* 2007;(3):CD001434.
13. Hart R, Bell-Syer SE, Crawford F et al. Systematic review of topical treatments for fungal infections of the skin and nails of the feet. *BMJ* 1999;319:79-82.
14. El-Gohary M, van Zuuren EJ, Fedorowicz Z et al. Topical antifungal treatments for tinea cruris and tinea corporis. *Cochrane Database Syst Rev* 2014;8:CD009992.
15. Budimulja U, Bramono K, Urip KS et al. Once daily treatment with terbinafine 1% cream (Lamisil) for one week is effective in the treatment of tinea corporis and cruris. A placebo-controlled study. *Mycoses* 2001;44:300-6.
16. Schopf R, Hettler O, Brautigam M et al. Efficacy and tolerability of terbinafine 1% topical solution used for 1 week compared with 4 weeks clotrimazole 1% topical solution in the treatment of interdigital tinea pedis: a randomized, double-blind, multi-centre, 8-week clinical trial. *Mycoses* 1999;42:415-20.
17. Crawford F, Hart R, Bell-Syer S et al. Topical treatments for fungal infections of the skin and nails of the foot. *Cochrane Database Syst Rev* 2000;(2):CD001434.
18. Gupta AK, Einarson TR, Summerbell RC et al. An overview of topical antifungal therapy in dermatomycoses. A North American perspective. *Drugs* 1998;55:645-74.
19. Alston SJ, Cohen BA, Braun M. Persistent and recurrent tinea corporis in children treated with combination antifungal/corticosteroid agents. *Pediatrics* 2003;111:201-3.
20. Erbagci Z. Topical therapy for dermatophytoses: should corticosteroids be included? *Am J Clin Dermatol* 2004;5:375-84.
21. Gupta AK, Sauder DN, Shear NH. Antifungal agents: an overview. Part I. *J Am Acad Dermatol* 1994;30:677-98.
22. Gupta AK, Sauder DN, Shear NH. Antifungal agents: an overview. Part II. *J Am Acad Dermatol* 1994;30:911-33.
23. Gupta AK, Foley KA. Antifungal treatment for pityriasis versicolor. *J Fungi* 2015;1:13-29.
24. Gupta AK, Cooper EA, Ryder JE et al. Optimal management of fungal infections of the skin, hair, and nails. *Am J Clin Dermatol* 2004;5:225-37.
25. Schwartz RA. Superficial fungal infections. *Lancet* 2004;364:1173-82.
26. Janik MP, Heffernan MP. Yeast infections: candidiasis and tinea (pityriasis) versicolor. In: Fitzpatrick TB, Wolff K et al., eds. *Fitzpatrick's dermatology in general medicine*. 7th ed. New York: McGraw-Hill; 2008.
27. Faergemann J. The role of Malassezia yeasts in skin disease. *Mikol Lek* 2004;11:129-33.
28. eMedicine from WebMD. Burkhart CG, Gottwald L. *Tinea versicolor*. Available from: emedicine.medscape.com. Updated July 21, 2014. Accessed July 2015. Registration required.
29. Hu SW, Bigby M. Pityriasis versicolor: a systematic review of interventions. *Arch Dermatol* 2010;146 1132-40.
30. Lange DS, Richards HM, Guarnieri J et al. Ketoconazole 2% shampoo in the treatment of tinea versicolor: a multicenter, randomized, double-blind, placebo-controlled trial. *J Am Acad Dermatol* 1998;39:944-50.
31. Savin R. Diagnosis and treatment of tinea versicolor. *J Fam Pract* 1996;43:127-32.
32. Hald, M, Arendrup MC, Svejgaard EL et al. Evidence-based Danish guidelines for the treatment of Malassezia related skin diseases. *Acta Derm Venereol* 2015;95:12-9.
33. Drake LA, Dinehart SM, Farmer ER et al. Guidelines of care for superficial mycotic infections of the skin: Pityriasis (tinea) versicolor. Guidelines/Outcomes Committee. American Academy of Dermatology. *J Am Acad Dermatol* 1996;34:287-9.
34. Hull CA, Johnson SM. A double-blind comparative study of sodium sulfacetamide lotion 10% versus selenium sulfide lotion 2.5% in the treatment of pityriasis (tinea) versicolor. *Cutis* 2004;73:425-9.

35. Hersle K. Selenium sulphide treatment of tinea versicolor. *Acta Derm Venereol* 1971;51:476-8.
36. Gupta AK, Batra R, Bluhm R et al.. Pityriasis versicolor. *Dermatol Clin* 2003;21:413-29.
37. Fredriksson T, Faergemann J. Double-blind comparison of a zinc pyrithione shampoo and its shampoo base in the treatment of tinea versicolor. *Cutis* 1983;31:436-7.
38. Gupta A, Bluhm R, Summerbell R. Pityriasis versicolor. *J Eur Acad Dermatol Venereol* 2002;16:19-33.
39. Gupta AK, Lane D, Paquet M. Systematic review of systemic treatments for tinea versicolor and evidence-based dosing regimen recommendations. *J Cutan Med Surg* 2014;18:79-90.
40. U.S. Food and Drug Administration. FDA Drug Safety Communication. *FDA limits usage of Nizoral (ketoconazole) oral tablets due to potentially fatal liver injury and risk of drug interactions and adrenal gland problems*. Available from: www.fda.gov/Drugs/DrugSafety/ucm362415.htm. Accessed: February 8, 2016.
41. Faergemann J, Gupta AK, Al Mofadi A et al. Efficacy of itraconazole in the prophylactic treatment of pityriasis (tinea) versicolor. *Arch Dermatol* 2002;138:69-73.
42. Guidelines of care for superficial mycotic infections of the skin: mucocutaneous candidiasis. Guidelines/Outcomes Committee. American Academy of Dermatology. *J Am Acad Dermatol* 1996;34:110-5.
43. Ramos-E-Silva M, Lima CM, Schechtman RC et al. Superficial mycoses in immunodepressed patients (AIDS). *Clin Dermatol* 2010;28:217-25.
44. Vanhooteghem O, Szepetiuk G, Paurobally D et al. Chronic interdigital dermatophytic infection: a common lesion associated with potentially severe consequences. *Diabetes Res Clin Pract* 2011;91:23-5.
45. eMedicine from Web MD. Selden ST. *Intertrigo*. Updated September 3, 2014. Available from : emedicine.medscape.com. Accessed July 2015. Registration required.
46. eMedicine from Web MD. Scheinfeld NS. *Cutaneous candidiasis*. Updated January 12, 2015. Available from : emedicine.medscape.com. Accessed July 2015. Registration required.
47. Hay RJ. The management of superficial candidiasis. *J Am Acad Dermatol* 1999;40:S35-42.
48. Leyden JJ. Corn starch, Candida albicans, and diaper rash. *Pediatr Dermatol* 1984;1:322-5.
49. UpToDate. Parker ER. *Candidal intertrigo*. Available from: www.uptodate.com. Accessed July 2015. Subscription required.
50. McClellan KJ, Wiseman LR, Markham A. Terbinafine. An update of its use in superficial mycoses. *Drugs* 1999;58:179-202.
51. Gardiner R, Kemper KJ. Herbs in pediatric and adolescent medicine. *Pediatr Rev* 2000;21:44-57.
52. Natural Medicines Comprehensive Database. Available from: www.naturaldatabase.com. Accessed July 2015. Subscription required.
53. Satchell AC, Saurajen A, Bell C et al. Treatment of interdigital tinea pedis with 25% and 50% tea tree oil solution: a randomized, placebo-controlled, blinded study. *Australas J Dermatol* 2002;43:175-8.

Fungal (Tinea) Infections—What You Need to Know

What is tinea?

Tinea is a kind of fungus that can grow on your skin, hair or nails. Tinea lives in soil, on animals and on people. It grows quickly in damp areas. As long as the fungus stays on the surface of the skin it will not cause any problems. However, if it gets into a cut or scrape on the skin, it can cause a fungal infection.

As the fungus grows it spreads out in a circle leaving normal-looking skin in the middle. At the outside of these ring-shaped spots, there is a raised red border that looks a bit like a worm under the skin. Because of the way it looks, a tinea (fungal) infection is often called "ringworm". However, there really isn't a worm under the skin.

You can get a fungal infection anywhere on your body or on your scalp. If you get a fungal infection in the groin area, it is called jock itch. Jock itch is more common for men because they often wear athletic equipment. If you get a fungal infection on your feet (usually between the toes) it is called athlete's foot.

How do you get a fungal infection?

You may be exposed to tinea in a number of ways:

- by touching a person who has a fungal infection
- by walking barefoot in a damp area like a public shower or locker room
- by touching an animal that has a fungal infection.

What are the signs of a fungal infection?

- Skin that is itchy, light red or scaly.
- Small ring-shaped spots on the body that grow larger as the infection spreads. The skin at the outside of the ring is red and scaly. Inside the ring the skin looks normal.
- If the infection is on the head, it may look like dandruff with patchy, scaly spots and stubby hair.
- If the infection is in the groin area, the skin may be moist and itchy. It may also feel hot.

What is the treatment for tinea (fungal) infections?

- Tinea can be treated with antifungal creams, lotions or shampoos. Ask your healthcare provider for advice about these products.
- Wash and dry the affected area well. Apply an antifungal product to the rash twice a day. Spread it on the rash and about 2–3 cm outside its borders.
- Treat jock itch for 2 weeks and ringworm of the body for 4 weeks.

How can you prevent the spread of tinea?

- Keep the skin clean, cool and dry. This will discourage growth of the fungus.
- Change your socks and underwear every day, especially in warm weather.
- Wear clean cotton clothing that allows fresh air to circulate.
- Apply powder to absorb sweat and prevent rubbing.

When should you see your doctor?

- If the ringworm continues to spread after 1 week of treatment with an antifungal product.
- If the rash has not gone away after 2 weeks of treatment for jock itch, or 4 weeks for ringworm of the body.
- If the rash comes back after treatment.
- If you have an infection on your scalp or nails. You will need a prescription medication to get rid of the infection.

Chapter 66
Hair Care and Hair Growth

Nancy Kleiman, BSP, MBA

Pathophysiology

Humans are born with a fixed number of hair follicles. Approximately 100 000 hair follicles are on the scalp alone. Two types of hair are found on a human body: vellous and terminal. Vellous hair is fine, soft hair that is nonpigmented and covers the body. Terminal hair is generally long, course hair that is pigmented and covers the scalp, face, axillae and pubic area. Terminal hair grows on the face, chest, legs and arms in response to androgens at puberty. Decreased estrogen levels can also allow androgens to stimulate terminal hair growth in menopausal women.[1]

Hair growth occurs in 4 stages on the scalp:

1. The active growing phase or anagen stage lasts 2–6 years and determines hair length. Normally about 80–90% of follicles are in this stage at any one time on a human scalp
2. The transitional phase or catagen stage can last 2–3 weeks after which the follicle degenerates and growth stops. On a normal scalp approximately 1–3% of the follicles are in this stage
3. The third stage is the resting phase or telogen stage which lasts 3–4 months. Approximately 5–10% of follicles are in this stage on a normal scalp
4. The last stage of hair growth is the shedding phase or exogen phase where the hair is shed and the cycle of growth begins again. Normally about 75–100 scalp hairs are shed each day or about 0.1% of scalp hair.

Repeated chemical treatments, poor grooming habits and exposure to the environment can cause hair texture to change and result in hair breakage. This progressive degeneration of the hair shaft is called "weathering" and contributes to structural weakening of the hair, making it tangle easier and appear rough.[2]

Hair Loss (Alopecia)

Androgenic alopecia sometimes referred to as androgenetic alopecia is the most common type of hair loss. It is commonly referred to as male-pattern baldness or female-pattern baldness.

Characteristics of androgenic alopecia include:

- A hereditary form of androgen-induced diffuse hair loss that presents as a reduction in hair thickness as well as hair loss
- The exact influence of genetics on androgenetic alopecia is unknown. The androgen receptor gene is located on the x chromosome and passed from mother to son; however, family studies have also shown marked resemblance of hair loss between fathers and sons[3]
- The actual number of hair follicles remains the same and the growth cycle is constant but the anagen or growth stage is somewhat shorter producing a shorter, thinner hair shaft. This thinner hair shaft covers less scalp, the area becomes progressively becomes larger, and balding appears, particularly in men
- In men, hair thinning starts in the crown area, gradually progressing to the mid-scalp area

- Female-pattern baldness is also referred to as androgenetic alopecia but it appears that androgens player a smaller role than in male-pattern baldness
- Hair loss in women is milder than in men and presents as central thinning or "widening of the part line".

Telogen effluvium is an abnormal number of hair follicles prematurely entering the telogen or resting phase. Characteristics of telogen effluvium include:

- Excessive hair shedding and thinning occurs in the scalp, possibly followed about 3–4 months later by hair loss in pubic and underarm areas. More than 300 hairs are lost per day (normal is 75–100 per day)
- Causes can include hormonal changes during pregnancy, severe psychological stress, injury or stress from infections, serious illness or major surgery, endocrine disorders, iron deficiency and crash diets
- In about one-third of the cases no cause can be definitely determined
- Hair loss generally begins 1–3 months after the causative event
- Hair loss can last up to 6 months after correcting the causative factor.

Anagen effluvium is the loss of hair over the entire scalp. Characteristics of anagen effluvium include:

- Can be caused by chemotherapy, radiation to the head, certain medications (see Table 1) and heavy metal toxicity
- Hair loss is usually sudden and severe, affecting most of the anagen scalp hairs simultaneously
- Normal hair growth is generally rapidly restored once the underlying cause is removed.

Alopecia areata is an autoimmune inflammatory disorder that affects the hair follicles and nail matrix. Characteristics of alopecia areata include:

- Occurs at any age but commonly affects children and younger adults
- Can be associated with pre-existing autoimmune disorders such as thyroid conditions, systemic lupus erythematosus and vitiligo
- There is also a family history connection as those with early onset often have a close family member with the condition
- Physical stress, emotional stress and some types of infections can also cause this condition
- Typically presents as smooth round or oval patches on the scalp but also can appear on any other hairy areas of the body
- There is no clinical evidence of inflammation or scarring in the affected area
- Nail pitting or ridging can also occur and may be a function of the disease itself
- Generally self-limiting and hair can spontaneously regrow. Chronic, extensive forms are often associated with a family history of hair loss that may not regrow. This chronic hair loss can occur in children with an onset prior to 5 years of age.

Inflammatory scalp conditions caused by bacterial infections, parasitic infections and dermatitis can cause hair loss. Compulsive self-inflicted hair loss (trichotillomania) can also cause patchy hair loss. These conditions usually present with erythema, scale, itch or irritation.

Table 1: **Drugs Associated with Hair Loss[a,1]**

ACE inhibitors (captopril, enalapril)	Antiparkinson agents (levodopa)
Androgens (systemic and oral testosterone)	Beta-blockers (metoprolol, propranolol)
Anticoagulants (warfarin)	Cholesterol-lowering agents (clofibrate)
Antiepileptic drugs (valproic acid)	H_2-antagonists (cimetidine)
Antimanic agents (lithium)	Heavy metals (mercury, lead)
Antimitotic agents (colchicine)	Oral contraceptives
Antineoplastics	Oral retinoids (isotretinoin)

[a] Specific drugs listed are given as examples only; other medications in the same class may have similar effects.

Excessive Hair Growth

Hirsutism is the production of excessive terminal hair in a male-pattern distribution in women. It is usually a consequence of increased androgen activity in women caused by an underlying medical problem such as polycystic ovary syndrome, androgen-secreting tumors, Cushing syndrome, acromegaly or thyroid dysfunction. Androgenic medications (danazol, testosterone) may also be a cause of hirsutism and must be considered when diagnosing this condition.[4] Many peri- and postmenopausal women experience increased facial hair growth due to hormone fluctuations.[5]

Hypertrichosis is excessive hair growth that is either hereditary or caused by medications such as glucocorticoids, phenytoin, minoxidil or cyclosporine. Hypertrichosis is not caused by increased androgen activity but can be aggravated by it.[4]

Goals of Therapy

Goals of therapy for hair loss:

- Correct or treat underlying conditions that may be causing hair loss
- Maintain healthy-appearing hair by decreasing the rate of thinning and increasing coverage in areas of loss
- Consider changing medications if causative factor
- Manage psychological factors such as self-esteem and mood changes

Goals of therapy for excessive hair growth:

- Correct or treat underlying conditions that may be causing excessive hair growth
- Remove or control growth of, excess body hair
- Consider changing medications if causative factor
- Manage psychological factors such as self-esteem and mood changes

Patient Assessment

The assessment process is an opportunity to educate patients about the various factors that contribute to hair growth changes and effective treatment methods to either reverse or cosmetically cover the condition. Patients require further investigation when they present with unusual changes in hair growth and/or significant concerns about their hair changes. An approach to the patient with hair-related concerns is presented in Figure 1 and Figure 2.

Nonpharmacologic Therapy

Hair Care

Hair colour, texture, body and curliness is genetically determined. Shiny hair that has a smooth texture and clean cut ends and has not been damaged by chemical treatments is considered "healthy hair".[6] When the cuticle is damaged, hair can appear dull, feel rough and brittle and have split ends.

To maintain healthy hair and minimize damage:

- Have hair cut by a professional to remove ends that are damaged
- Use appropriate shampoos designed for the type of hair (dry, damaged or chemically treated hair) and condition hair regularly (according to the recommended frequency for the specific product)
- Minimize exposure to harsh chemical treatments such as permanents, dyes, bleaches and straighteners[6]
- Avoid excessive brushing. Use a brush with natural, round-ended bristles, and brush gently. Use a wide-toothed comb to detangle or comb wet hair
- Minimize use of blow dryers, curling and straightening irons.[6] Use a lower setting on a blow dryer, and use a diffuser to blow dry chemically treated hair.

The frequency of hair washing may be influenced by length of hair, culture, sex, social pressures, economics and individual preference; daily washing is not harmful. Various hair care products can be used to cosmetically enhance the hair's appearance (See Table 2).

Hair Loss

Nonpharmacologic options for patients with hair loss include cosmetic hair products such as sprays, foams and lotions that make the hair look thicker.[10] Hair extensions, wigs and hair pieces are also becoming more acceptable and improving in quality, providing a minimally invasive method to cover hair loss areas.

Follicle transplants can be considered when there has been limited success with medical treatments. The procedure is done on an outpatient basis under local anesthesia. The transplanted hair will grow over 3- to 6-month period postprocedure.

A number of devices for home use that administer low-level laser therapy (supposedly to stimulate metabolic processes needed for hair growth) are being investigated and aggressively marketed. Industry sponsored studies appear promising, but there is no independent evidence of effectiveness and anecdotal reports so far are disappointing.[11,12]

Excessive Hair Growth

Weight loss may lead to decreased androgen levels and subsequent improvement in excessive hair growth in obese women, particularly in those women with polycystic ovary syndrome.[13]

Excess hair can be routinely controlled with physical removal by shaving, waxing, plucking or the application of depilatory creams, or camouflaged by bleaching. These forms of physical removal are all associated with the regrowth of the hair and will often be used in combination with more permanent hair removal methods. Hair does not grow back any faster, thicker or denser than normal.[14]

Table 2: **Hair Care Products**[2,6,7,8,9]

Product	Action	Uses	Comments
Shampoo	Detergent component helps remove oil, dirt, sweat, fungal elements and hair care products (styling gels, hair spray). Primarily cleans the scalp but also prevents hair shaft damage. Baby shampoos contain amphoteric detergents that are less irritating to eyes.	Routine use as part of a personal hygiene regimen to maintain healthy hair.	Shampoos are formulated for hair that is considered to be normal, greasy, dry or chemically treated. Daily use is not harmful provided the product is well formulated.
Conditioner	Contains cationic polymers (balance the negativity of damaged hair), film formers (fill hair shaft defects) or proteins (thought to restore protein to damaged hair). Lubricates and moisturizes hair leaving it soft, smooth and hydrated, which decreases static. Reduces static electricity and restores manageability by reducing friction on the hair shaft.	Restores appearance, softness and manageability of hair. Decreases friction, frizz and tangles. Reconditions hair after chemical treatments and physical trauma such as blow drying and brushing.	Instant conditioners are applied immediately after shampooing and left on for a short period of time. Deep conditioners, used for very dry hair are creams that are left on for 20–30 min and may or may not require heat to increase penetration.
Styling gels, sprays, mousses, sculpting gels and waxes	Contain large-molecular-weight polymers, proteins, and/or resins to hold hair in place or coat hair, adding thickness and texture. Silicone-containing products provide sheen, lubricate and increase resistance to humidity, making hair more manageable.	Creates changes in hair volume or style. May be useful for those with thinning hair, low hair density or if increased volume is desired.	Can be used to improve appearance of hair loss (add volume, make hair look fuller, keep hair in place to cover thin areas). Mousses aid in styling, are soft to touch and can be easily removed. Styling lotions are applied to wet hair and hold style when blow drying.
Hair colouring agents	Dyes that cause a gradual hair colouring use metallic dyes that cause a chemical reaction on the hair shaft. Temporary colours are water-soluble dyes consisting of large molecules that are deposited on the hair shaft. Semipermanent dyes are mainly synthetic. They consist mainly of low-molecular-weight coal tar dyes that penetrate the hair shaft easily. Permanent colour results from an oxidation process within the hair shaft and is irreversible.	Alter the colour of hair through various methods. Gradual dyes change grey hair incrementally over a few weeks to brown or black. Temporary dyes are used to cover small amounts of grey, brighten natural or coloured hair or remove yellow tones from grey hair. Semipermanent dyes are used to cover grey, produce highlights or to change hair tones. Permanent dyes are used to cover grey or change hair colour.	Gradual dyes must be used continuously for colour change to remain, and are inexpensive. Hair can become stiff, dull and brittle and colour quality is often poor. Temporary dyes are safe and gentle. They are available as rinses, gels, mousses or sprays that are easily washed out. Semipermanent dyes can cause contact dermatitis. These dyes last 4–6 wk depending on the condition of the hair. Natural vegetable dyes such as henna have largely been replaced by synthetic formulations for use as semipermanent dyes. Permanent dyes are re-applied every 4–6 wk depending on rate of hair growth. These dyes contain ammonia and/or peroxide and can damage hair.
Permanents, straighteners/ relaxers	Changes the chemical structure of hair shaft by altering disulfide bonds. Chemical hair straightening also involves mechanically straightening the hair once it has been treated.	Used to either curl or add wave to hair or to straighten hair that is naturally curly.	Process must be repeated every 6–12 wk based on individual's hair. May damage hair if too strong, left on too long, used too frequently. Often irritates the scalp.

Shaving removes hair at the skin level and is suitable for most areas, but the hair grows back quickly. This method does not affect the rate of hair growth and is a safe and inexpensive way to control regular hair growth.[15]

Cold waxing involves application of wax-impregnated strips that are pressed on the skin then pulled off in the direction opposite to hair growth. Warm waxing involves wax that is heated to 37°C and then spread over the area in the direction of hair growth. The waxed area is covered with strips and allowed to cool. The strips are then pulled off against the direction of hair growth. Hot waxing consists of melted wax spread over the desired area against the direction of hair growth and allowed to cool. It is then quickly pulled off.[16] Waxing allows the area to be free of hair for several days but is painful when performed by someone not trained in the field.

Plucking can be effective for small areas (eyebrows, upper lip and chin), but is time consuming, painful and temporary.[16,17]

Threading is a process by which twisted cotton thread is used to pull the hair from the follicle. It is used to temporarily remove hair from small areas. Training and experience are necessary to obtain a good result.

Bleaching lightens hair so that it is not as noticeable. Several products are available; all contain hydrogen peroxide and many contain ammonia (accelerates the bleaching action). Bleaching is fast, generally painless and reserved for small areas. Results can last up to 4 weeks. Side effects include skin irritation and hair discoloration.[17]

Depilatory creams act by separating the hair from the follicles. Hair regrowth can begin within a few days of treatment. These methods are best used for weekly hair removal or in combination with laser treatment. Contact dermatitis (allergic and irritant) can occur with the use of these products because of the alkaline nature as well as the added fragrances. Some find the products messy and the odour offensive which limits their use.[17]

Laser systems and intense pulsed light sources (IPL) both work on the same principle, selectively targeting specific areas without affecting the surrounding tissue. Melanin pigment in the hair follicles absorbs the wavelength selected, effectively destroying the hair follicle via thermal damage and impairing future hair growth.[17] A Cochrane review that examined studies of laser and IPL procedures concluded that permanent hair removal is not a realistic expectation.[18] More realistically, long-term stable reduction in hair regrowth lasting 4–12 months can be accomplished with these procedures.[17,18] Side effects can include mild to moderate pain, skin redness, pigment changes and burned hairs. These side effects are dependent on the type of laser used for treatment.[17] **Topical anesthetics** containing **lidocaine** and **prilocaine** are commonly used prior to laser treatment to decrease pain from the procedure. Consumers may apply these products in larger amounts and to a larger area than is recommended, increasing the risk of serious side effects,[19] such as CNS toxicity, methemoglobinemia and cardiovascular collapse. Systemic effects may manifest as headache, drowsiness, respiratory depression, confusion, convulsions, hypotension and cardiac arrhythmias.[19] Laser and IPL treatments are expensive and must be administered by a trained professional on a regular basis to maintain hair removal.[4] A number of hand-held, home-use laser and light devices can be purchased for personal use. Non-industry–sponsored evidence of safety and effectiveness is not available.[12]

Electrolysis is an option for the removal of unwanted hair. A small needle or metal probe is inserted into the hair follicle and low-level electrical current is used to destroy the follicle. It is important that the procedure be performed by a trained and certified professional. The designations C.P.E. (Certified Professional Electrologist) and C.C.E. (Certified Canadian Electrologist) indicate the electrologist has satisfied a board of examiners and is a member in good standing.

Pharmacologic Therapy

Hair Loss

Information about the management of hair loss can also be found in Table 4.

Topical Therapy for Hair Loss

For comparative ingredients of nonprescription products, consult the *Compendium of Products for Minor Ailments*—Skin Care Products: Hair Growth.

Minoxidil has been shown to be effective for the treatment of male-pattern[26] and female-pattern hair loss.[27] The mechanism of action of minoxidil is unclear but it is thought to stimulate the conversion of small hair follicles to larger follicles. Minoxidil prolongs the duration of the anagen phase and increases hair count and weight.[28,29] Minoxidil 2% solution is approved for male-pattern hair loss only and minoxidil 5% foam is approved for both male- and female-pattern hair loss. Minoxidil is most effective when started early, prior to the area becoming completely bald. Hair growth is visible within 2 months or more with a maximum effect within a year.[28,30] Daily application is required indefinitely to maintain hair growth.[1] Transitory increased hair shedding may occur during the first 1–2 months of treatment due to telogen (resting phase) follicles being stimulated to re-enter anagen (growing phase). Patients should be advised that this may occur and that it will normalize within a few weeks to months.[26] The most common side effect is contact dermatitis at the application site, which is possibly caused by propylene glycol.[31] Compounding minoxidil using butylene glycol instead of propylene glycol may decrease this side effect.[31] Minoxidil 5% foam formulation is propylene glycol–free, causes less scalp irritation and improves adherence.[32] This formulation is more cosmetically pleasing as it is less greasy, and it is easier to apply to the scalp only and avoid the hair. Systemic absorption of minoxidil is minimal but tachycardia and decreased blood pressure have been reported. Use caution when recommending this treatment for patients with cardiovascular disease or low blood pressure.[28] Although systemic absorption of topical minoxidil is minimal, safety in pregnancy has not been established and it is not recommended.[33] Transfer of topically applied minoxidil into breast milk is expected to be minimal and pose low risk to the nursing infant.[34]

Systemic Therapy for Hair Loss

Finasteride halts or reverses the progression of mild to moderate hair loss in men by inhibiting 5-alpha reductase–mediated conversion of testosterone to dihydrotestosterone.[26] Effectiveness rates for slowing progression of male androgenetic alopecia or producing partial regrowth of hair range from 60–90% of patients. Regular daily use for 3–6 months may be required to see reduced hair loss and up to 12 months to see noticeable regrowth. Hair loss resumes when therapy is stopped. The most common side effects experienced by men using finasteride are decreased libido, decreased semen volume and erectile dysfunction. These side effects may decrease with continued treatment and may or may not be reversible when treatment is discontinued. Finasteride may reduce prostate specific antigen (PSA) levels by up to 50% depending on the dose and age of the patient. This should be considered when interpreting PSA levels in patients taking finasteride.[3,26,35] Evidence for use of finasteride in females is limited and conflicting.[27] Finasteride should never be used or handled by women who are pregnant or may become pregnant as it may cause feminization of the male fetus.[10] Since finasteride concentration in semen is very low, there is no risk to a fetus via intercourse.[26]

Another 5-alpha reductase inhibitor, **dutasteride**, has also been shown to be effective in male androgenetic alopecia[3] but is not officially indicated for this condition. Side effects and precautions are similar to those for finasteride.

Hormone therapy with **combined oral contraceptives**, **cyproterone**, **drospirenone**, **flutamide** and **spironolactone** has been studied for female-pattern hair loss. Evidence is sparse and of limited quality and therefore no recommendations can be made.[26,27] Other therapies being investigated include **onabotulinumtoxinA** and prostaglandin analogues such as **latanoprost** and **bimatoprost**.[20,21]

Combining therapies may help increase efficacy. Combinations that have been studied include finasteride plus minoxidil,[26,36] finasteride plus ketoconazole shampoo (may help reduce androgenetic alopecia–associated follicular inflammation and is also an anti-androgen),[37] and topical or systemic therapy in combination with transplant procedures.

In the specific case of alopecia areata, many treatments have been tried with varying success. These include topical minoxidil, topical, oral and locally injected corticosteroids, anthralin, azelaic acid and topical sensitizers such as dinitrochlorobenzene or diphenylcyclopropenone (to stimulate an immune response).[38,39]

Excessive Hair Growth in Women

Information about assessment and management of excessive hair growth can also be found in Table 5.

Hormonal treatments for hirsutism either suppress androgen levels or block the effects of androgens on hair follicles. First-line therapy for hirsutism unless contraindicated is **combination oral contraceptives** (COCs). Those containing **ethinyl estradiol** and a minimally androgenic progestogen (e.g., **desogestrel, norgestimate**) can slow progression but not reverse excess hair growth and generally require 9–12 months for maximal effect.[4,13,14] COCs containing the antiandrogens **cyproterone acetate** or **drospirenone** are also effective and may be preferred.[4,13,14,22] The antiandrogens **spironolactone**, **flutamide** and **cyproterone acetate** are also effective. These agents have been used as monotherapy but are generally recommended in addition to COCs for moderate to severe hirsutism that has not responded to COCs alone.[13,22] **Finasteride** has shown inconsistent results in studies[22] but is considered a second-line antiandrogen by some experts.[13,23] There is evidence that **eflornithine** cream reduces the rate of hair growth in women by suppressing the mitotic activity in the follicle.[22,40,41] While it may be tried alone for mild cases,[13] it is generally recommended as adjunctive therapy with hair removal techniques such as laser therapy. Improvement is expected after 4–8 weeks of treatment but may take up to 24 weeks in some patients. Discontinuing use of the product results in hair regrowth within 8 weeks of stopping treatment.[14]

Monitoring of Therapy

Monitoring plans for patients should be individualized; hair loss and its psychological effects are different for each person. The degree of hair loss (mild to moderate or severe) should also be considered when determining initial treatment and monitoring outcomes. Table 3 provides a monitoring plan framework for both hair loss and excessive growth.

Table 3: **Monitoring of Therapy for Hair Conditions**

Symptom	Monitoring	Desired Outcome	Actions
Hair thinning	Monitor for improvement for a minimum of 6–12 months after treatment started.	Reduced thinning, progression slowed and improved scalp coverage.	Continue therapy indefinitely if patient satisfied with results. Patient must weigh benefits vs. cost of long-term treatment.
Excess hair shedding	Monitor for increased shedding for 2–8 wk after treatment started. Monitor for excess hair shedding (>300/day) for 1–3 months (possible	Normal rate of hair loss (75–100 hairs per day) within 4–6 months after treatment started.	If shedding does not resolve in 4–6 months after removal of trigger or beginning of therapy, patient requires further assessment and/or treatment.

(cont'd)

Table 3: **Monitoring of Therapy for Hair Conditions** *(cont'd)*

Symptom	Monitoring	Desired Outcome	Actions
	diagnosis of telogen effluvium. See Pathophysiology).		
Excess hair growth	Monitor hair regrowth after removal. Shaving, waxing, plucking, bleaching, depilatories: Monitor daily. Laser therapy and electrolysis procedures should be monitored for 4–12 months.	Cosmetically acceptable appearance.	Cosmetic management of excess hair is usually required. Topical anesthetics should be used with caution prior to laser treatment. Serious reactions should be assessed and/or treated appropriately.
Skin irritation from topical agents	Monitor daily for skin reactions to cosmetic treatment as well as topical treatment.	Minimal to no skin irritation.	Stop using product. Treat symptomatically with low-potency topical corticosteroids.

Figure 1: **Assessment and Management of Hair Loss**

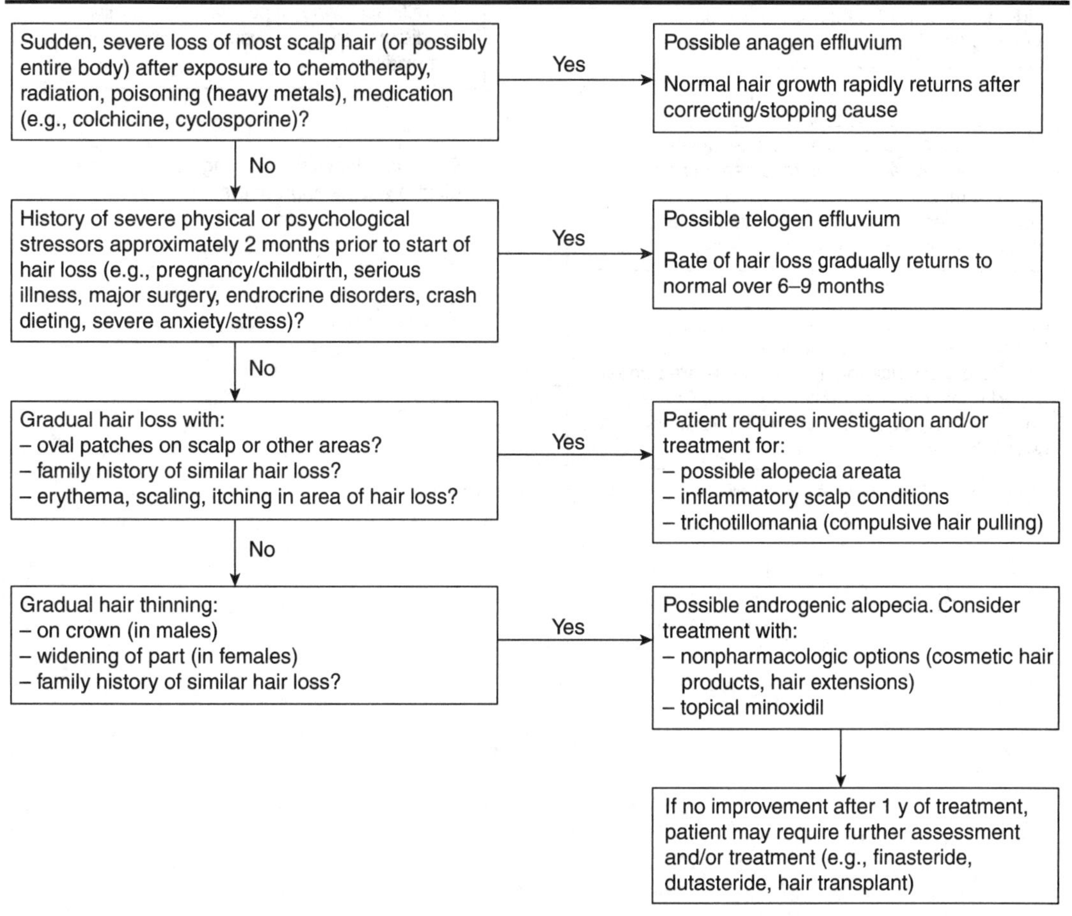

Figure 2: **Assessment and Management of Excessive Hair Growth**

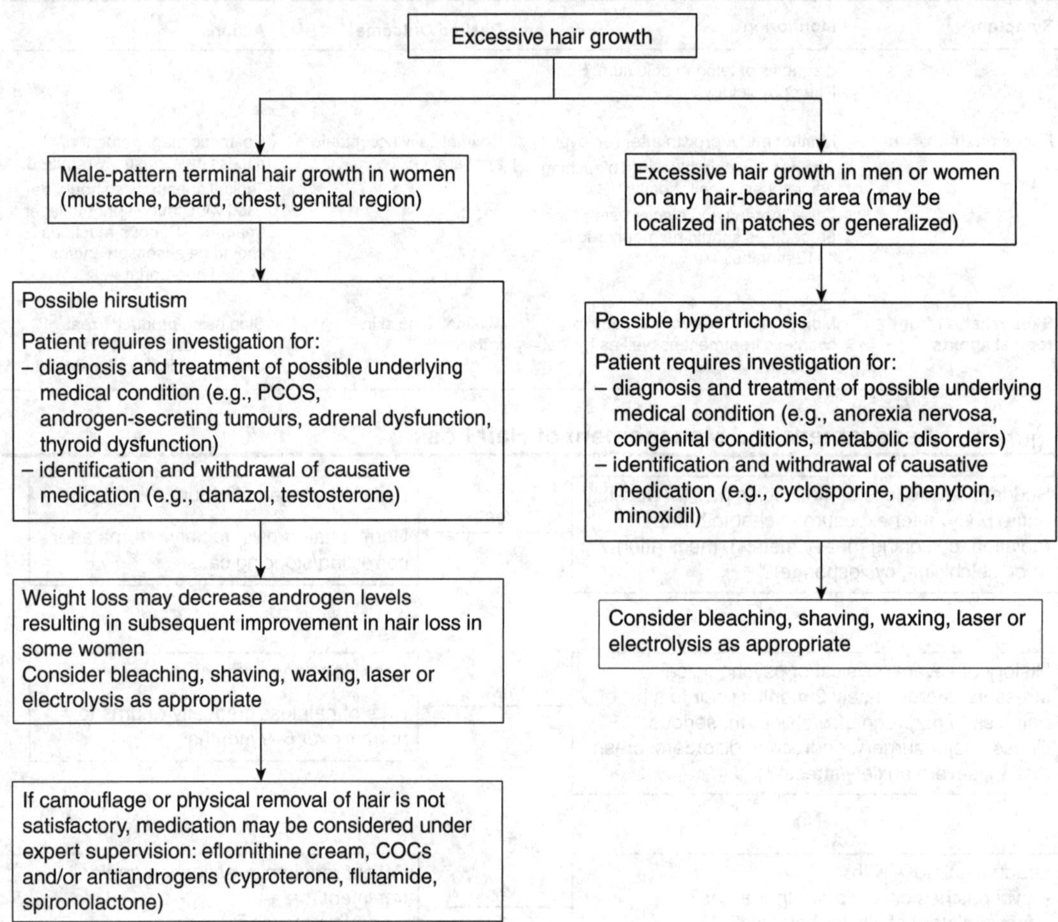

Excessive hair growth
Male-pattern terminal hair growth in women (mustache, beard, chest, genital region)
Excessive hair growth in men or women on any hair-bearing area (may be localized in patches or generalized)
Possible hirsutism
Patient requires investigation for:
– diagnosis and treatment of possible underlying medical condition (e.g., PCOS, androgen-secreting tumours, adrenal dysfunction, thyroid dysfunction)
– identification and withdrawal of causative medication (e.g., danazol, testosterone)
Possible hypertrichosis
Patient requires investigation for:
– diagnosis and treatment of possible underlying medical condition (e.g., anorexia nervosa, congenital conditions, metabolic disorders)
– identification and withdrawal of causative medication (e.g., cyclosporine, phenytoin, minoxidil)
Weight loss may decrease androgen levels resulting in subsequent improvement in hair loss in some women
Consider bleaching, shaving, waxing, laser or electrolysis as appropriate
Consider bleaching, shaving, waxing, laser or electrolysis as appropriate
If camouflage or physical removal of hair is not satisfactory, medication may be considered under expert supervision: eflornithine cream, COCs and/or antiandrogens (cyproterone, flutamide, spironolactone)

Abbreviations: COCs = combined oral contraceptives; PCOS = polycystic ovary syndrome.

Table 4: Therapy for Male- and Female-pattern Hair Loss (Androgenic Alopecia)[a,1,20,21,31]

Class	Drug	Dosage	Adverse Effects	Drug Interactions	Comments	Cost
5-Alpha-reductase Inhibitors	*dutasteride* Avodart, Dutasteride, other generics	0.5 mg daily (some studies have used up to 2.5 mg daily)	Men: Decreased libido and semen volume, erectile dysfunction, headaches, dry skin. There is some concern that due to dutasteride's increased half-life compared with finasteride, side effects may potentially be more severe or long-lasting.	Combination with strong CYP3A4 inhibitors (e.g., ketoconazole, ritonavir) may increase serum concentration of dutasteride. Monitor for increased adverse reactions, e.g., erectile dysfunction, decreased libido.	Not a Health Canada–approved indication. No evidence for use in women (a few case reports only).	$
	finasteride Propecia, generics	1 mg daily po	Men: Decreased libido and semen volume, erectile dysfunction, headaches, dry skin.	No known clinically significant drug interactions.	Limited evidence for use in women. Can cause feminization of a developing fetus; contraindicated in pregnancy. Concentration in semen is very low: no risk to fetus via sexual contact of mother with a male taking finasteride.	$$
Antifungals, azole	*ketoconazole shampoo* Nizoral	2% shampoo: Lather in and leave on for 3–5 min before rinsing, twice weekly to once every 2 wk depending on response	Uncommonly: Application site irritation.	No known clinically significant drug interactions with topical use of ketoconazole.	Not a Health Canada–approved indication. Very limited evidence of efficacy (in combination with finasteride) but little risk of harm.	$
Piperidinopyrimidines, topical	*minoxidil 2% solution* Rogaine Topical Solution	Apply 1 mL (20 mg) BID Total daily dose not to exceed 2 mL (40 mg) Leave on scalp for at least 4 h to maximize absorption	Scalp irritation, itching, dryness, change in hair colour. Temporary hair loss may occur within the first 2–6 wk of use. Discontinue if lasts >2 wk. Systemic absorption is minimal with correct application and usual doses.	Not expected since systemic absorption is minimal.	Apply to dry scalp starting at the centre of the affected area. Avoid applying directly to the hair as a greasy, flaky appearance can result.	$$

(cont'd)

Table 4: **Therapy for Male- and Female-pattern Hair Loss (Androgenic Alopecia)**[a,1,20,21,31] *(cont'd)*

Class	Drug	Dosage	Adverse Effects	Drug Interactions	Comments	Cost
	minoxidil 5% foam for men Rogaine Foam	Apply one-half capful (1g foam/50 mg minoxidil) BID Total daily dose not to exceed 2 g foam (100 mg minoxidil) Leave on scalp for at least 4 h to maximize absorption	See minoxidil.	See minoxidil.	Massage lightly into the affected areas of the scalp, avoiding direct application to the hair.	$$$
	minoxidil 5% foam for women Rogaine Women's Foam	Apply one-half capful (1 g foam/50 mg minoxidil) once daily Total daily dose not to exceed 1 g foam (50 mg minoxidil) Leave on scalp for at least 4 h to maximize absorption	See minoxidil.	See minoxidil.	See minoxidil.	$$$

[a] Cost of 30-day supply or smallest available pack size; includes drug cost only.

Legend: $ <$15 $$ $15–30 $$$ $30–45

Table 5: Therapy for Excessive Hair Growth in Women[13,20,21,22,23,24]

Class	Drug	Dosage	Adverse Effects	Drug Interactions	Comments	Cost[a]
Antiandrogens	*cyproterone acetate* Androcur, generics	25–100 mg daily po × 10 days (either days 1–10 or 5–15 of menstrual cycle)	Menstrual irregularities, decreased libido, nausea, depression, fatigue, weight gain.	Metabolized by CYP3A4, strong inhibitors or inducers of this enzyme may alter levels and/or effect of cyproterone.	Not a Health Canada–approved use. May be used to treat moderate to severe hirsutism, including in combination with COCs.	$
	flutamide generics	250 mg BID po (study doses have ranged from 62.5–750 mg per day)	Breast tenderness, menstrual irregularities. Risk of hepatotoxicity: Monitor liver function	May increase anticoagulant effect of warfarin.	Not a Health Canada–approved use. May be used to treat moderate to severe hirsutism, including in combination with COCs.	$$$$
	spironolactone Aldactone, generics	50–200 mg once daily po	Mild diuretic, lethargy, hyperkalemia, hypotension, breast tenderness, menstrual irregularities.	Increases serum K+ when combined with ACE inhibitors, angiotensin receptor blockers, K+ supplements, cyclosporine, tacrolimus, other potassium-sparing diuretics.	Not a Health Canada–approved use. Commonly used to treat moderate to severe hirsutism associated with PCOS. Sometimes combined with COCs for increased efficacy.	$

(cont'd)

Table 5: **Therapy for Excessive Hair Growth in Women**[13,20,21,22,23,24] *(cont'd)*

Class	Drug	Dosage	Adverse Effects	Drug Interactions	Comments	Cost[a]
Contraceptives, oral—combined ethinyl estradiol and antiandrogen	*ethinyl estradiol 35 µg/ cyproterone 2 mg* Diane-35, generics	1 tablet daily po × 21 days, off 7 days and repeat cycle	Major: Thromboembolism (rare), stroke, retinal artery thrombosis, MI, benign liver tumour, cholelithiasis, hypertension. Watch for danger signals: ACHES—**a**bdominal pain, **c**hest pain, **h**eadaches, **e**ye problems, **s**evere leg pain. Advise patient to consult physician. Common: Breakthrough bleeding/spotting, amenorrhea, nausea/ vomiting, bloating, chloasma, breast tenderness, mood changes such as depression, headaches. May increase risk of VTE compared with levonorgestreol-containing COCs.	May increase cyclosporine levels or hepatotoxicity; may decrease lamotrigine levels. Significant pharmacokinetic interaction with rifampin, griseofulvin (advise backup barrier method during therapy). Monitor INR with concurrent oral anticoagulant use. Carbamazepine, modafinil, phenytoin, protease inhibitors, phenobarbital, St. John's wort, topiramate may decrease ethinyl estradiol/progestin serum concentrations. Reports of COC failure with concomitant ampicillin, amoxicillin, tetracycline, erythromycin, sulfamethoxazole/ trimethoprim or nitrofurantoin.	Considered first-line treatment for general hirsutism. Not a Health Canada–approved use. Health Canada has prepared a Suggested prescriber/counselling checklist for Diane-35 and its generics[25] to facilitate documentation of discussion of risks.	$
	ethinyl estradiol 30 µg/ drospirenone 3 mg Yasmin, Zamine, Zarah	1 tablet daily po × 21 days, off 7 days and repeat cycle	See ethinyl estradiol/ cyproterone.	See ethinyl estradiol/ cyproterone.	Considered first-line treatment for general hirsutism. Not a Health Canada–approved use.	$
	ethinyl estradiol 20 µg/ drospirenone 3 mg Yaz, MYA	1 tablet daily po × 21 days, off 7 days and repeat cycle	See ethinyl estradiol/ cyproterone.	See ethinyl estradiol/ cyproterone.	See ethinyl estradiol/ drospirenone.	$
	ethinyl estradiol 20 µg/ drospirenone 3 mg/ levomefolate calcium 0.451 mg Yaz Plus	1 tablet daily po × 21 days, off 7 days and repeat cycle	See ethinyl estradiol/ cyproterone.	See ethinyl estradiol/ cyproterone.	See ethinyl estradiol/ drospirenone.	$

Class	Drug	Dosage	Adverse Effects	Drug Interactions	Comments	Cost[a]
Contraceptives, oral—combined ethinyl estradiol and minimally androgenic progestin	*ethinyl estradiol 30 µg/ desogestrel 0.15 mg* Marvelon, Apri, Freya, Mirvala, Reclipsen	1 tablet daily po × 21 days, off 7 days and repeat cycle	Major: Thromboembolism (rare), stroke, retinal artery thrombosis, MI, benign liver tumour, cholelithiasis, hypertension. Watch for danger signals: ACHES—**a**bdominal pain, **c**hest pain, **h**eadaches, **e**ye problems, **s**evere leg pain. Advise patient to consult physician. Common: Breakthrough bleeding/spotting, amenorrhea, nausea/ vomiting, bloating, chloasma, breast tenderness, mood changes such as depression, headaches.	See ethinyl estradiol/ cyproterone.	See ethinyl estradiol/ drospirenone.	$
	ethinyl estradiol 25 µg/ desogestrel 0.1 mg/ 0.125 mg/0.15 mg Linessa	1 tablet daily po × 21 days, off 7 days and repeat cycle	See ethinyl estradiol/ desogestrel.	See ethinyl estradiol/ cyproterone.	See ethinyl estradiol/ drospirenone.	$
	ethinyl estradiol 35 µg/ norgestimate 0.25 mg Cyclen	1 tablet daily po × 21 days, off 7 days and repeat cycle	See ethinyl estradiol/ desogestrel.	See ethinyl estradiol/ cyproterone.	See ethinyl estradiol/ drospirenone.	$
	ethinyl estradiol 35 µg/ norgestimate 0.18 mg/ 0.215 mg/0.25 mg Tri-Cyclen	1 tablet daily po × 21 days, off 7 days and repeat cycle	See ethinyl estradiol/ desogestrel.	See ethinyl estradiol/ cyproterone.	See ethinyl estradiol/ drospirenone.	$
	ethinyl estradiol 25 µg/ norgestimate 0.18 mg/ 0.215 mg/0.25 mg Tri-Cyclen Lo, Tricira Lo	1 tablet daily po × 21 days, off 7 days and repeat cycle	See ethinyl estradiol/ desogestrel.	See ethinyl estradiol/ cyproterone.	See ethinyl estradiol/ drospirenone.	$

(cont'd)

Table 5: **Therapy for Excessive Hair Growth in Women**[13,20,21,22,23,24] *(cont'd)*

Class	Drug	Dosage	Adverse Effects	Drug Interactions	Comments	Cost[a]
Ornithine decarboxylase inhibitors	*eflornithine 13.9% cream* Vaniqa	Apply thinly to affected areas of face and neck BID	Burning, stinging, tingling, redness at application site.	No clinically significant drug interactions.	Wait 5 min after other hair removal techniques before applying. Allow to dry before applying cosmetics or sunscreen. Often used in conjunction with laser therapy.	$$$

[a] Cost of 30-day supply or smallest available pack size; includes drug cost only.

Dosage adjustment may be required in renal impairment.

Abbreviations: COCs = combined oral contraceptives

Legend: $ <$25 $$ $25–50 $$$ $50–75 $$$$ $75–100

Suggested Readings

Blumeyer A, Tosti A, Messenger A et al. Evidence-based (S3) guideline for the treatment of androgenetic alopecia in women and in men. *J Dtsch Dermatol Ges* 2011;9:S1-57.

Gray J. Hair care and hair care products. *Clin Dermatol* 2001;19:227-36.

Hohl A, Ronsoni MF, de Oliveira M. Hirsutism: diagnosis and management. *Arq Bras Endocrinol Metab* 2014;58:97-107.

Koulouri O, Conway GS. Management of hirsutism. *BMJ* 2009;338:b847.

References

1. Disorders of hair follicles and related disorders. In: Wolff K, Johnson RA, eds. *Fitzpatrick's color atlas and synopsis of clinical dermatology*. 6th ed. New York: McGraw-Hill Medical; 2009.
2. Sinclair RD. Healthy hair: what is it? *J Investig Dermatol Symp Proc* 2007;12:2-5.
3. Cranwell W, Sinclair R. Male androgenetic alopecia. In: De Groot LJ, Beck-Peccoz P, Chrousos G et al., eds. *Endotext* [Internet]. South Dartmouth: MDText.com; 2000. Available from: www.ncbi.nlm.nih.gov/books/NBK278957/.
4. Rosenfield RL. Clinical practice. Hirsutism. *N Engl J Med* 2005;353:2578-88.
5. Blume-Peytavi U, Atkin S, Gieler U et al. Skin academy: hair, skin, hormones and menopause—current status/knowledge on the management of hair disorders in menopausal women. *Eur J Dermatol* 2012;22:310-8.
6. Gray J. Hair care and hair care products. *Clin Dermatol* 2001;19:227-36.
7. Bolduc C, Shapiro J. Hair care products: waving, straightening, conditioning, and coloring. *Clin Dermatol* 2001;19:431-6.
8. Gavazzoni Dias MF. Hair cosmetics: an overview. *Int J Trichology* 2015;7:2-15.
9. Draelos ZD. Shampoos, conditioners, and camouflage techniques. *Dermatol Clin* 2013;31:173-8.
10. University of Texas at Austin, School of Nursing, Family Nurse Practitioner Program. *Treatment of female pattern hair loss in primary care*. May 2011. Available from: www.guideline.gov/content.aspx?id=34048.
11. DermNet NZ. Ranaweera A. *Low dose laser therapy for hair loss*. Available from: www.dermnetnz.org/procedures/laser-for-hair-loss.html. Accessed September 3, 2015.
12. Hession MT, Markova A, Graber EM. A review of hand-held, home-use cosmetic laser and light devices. *Dermatol Surg* 2015;41:307-20.
13. Somani N, Turvy D. Hirsutism: an evidence-based treatment update. *Am J Clin Dermatol* 2014;15:247-66.
14. Smith D, Tan C. Hirsutism: investigation and management. *Endocrinologist* 2007;17:335-40.
15. Koulouri O, Conway GS. Management of hirsutism. *BMJ* 2009;338:b847.
16. Kunte C, Wolff H, Gottschaller C et al. Therapy of hypertrichosis. *J Dtsch Dermatol Ges* 2007;5:807-10.
17. Wanitphakdeedecha R, Alster TS. Physical means of treating unwanted hair. *Dermatol Ther* 2008;21:392-401.
18. Haedersdal M, Gotzsche PC. Laser and photoepilation for unwanted hair growth. *Cochrane Database Syst Rev* 2006;4:CD004684.
19. Government of Canada. Healthy Canadians. *Safety information regarding topical anesthetics with serious adverse events—for health professionals*. Available from: www.healthycanadians.gc.ca/recall-alert-rappel-avis/hc-sc/2009/14544a-eng.php. Accessed April 27, 2016.
20. Atanaskova Mesinkovska N, Bergfeld WF. Hair: what is new in diagnosis and management? Female pattern hair loss update: diagnosis and treatment. *Dermatol Clin* 2013;31:119-27.
21. Rogers NE, Avram MR. Medical treatments for male and female pattern hair loss. *J Am Acad Dermatol* 2008;59:547-66.
22. van Zuuren EJ, Fedorowicz Z, Carter B et al. Interventions for hirsutism (excluding laser and photoepilation therapy alone). *Cochrane Database Syst Rev* 2015;4:CD010334.
23. Hohl A, Ronsoni MF, de Oliveira M. Hirsutism: diagnosis and management. *Arq Bras Endocrinol Metab* 2014;58:97-107.
24. Blume-Peytavi U. How to diagnose and treat medically women with excessive hair. *Dermatol Clin* 2013;31:57-65.
25. Health Canada. *Suggested prescriber/counselling checklist for Diane-35 (cyproterone acetate/ethinyl estradiol) and its generics*. Available from: www.hc-sc.gc.ca/dhp-mps/alt_formats/pdf/medeff/advisories-avis/review-examen/checklist-verification-diane-35-eng.pdf. Accessed April 29, 2014.
26. Blumeyer A, Tosti A, Messenger A et al. Evidence-based (S3) guideline for the treatment of androgenetic alopecia in women and in men. *J Dtsch Dermatol Ges* 2011;9:S1-57.
27. van Zuuren E, Fedorowicz Z, Carter B et al. Interventions for female pattern hair loss. *Cochrane Database Syst Rev* 2012;5:CD007628.
28. Messenger AG, Rundegren J. Minoxidil: mechanisms of action on hair growth. *Br J Dermatol* 2004;150:186-94.
29. Herskovitz I, Tosti A. Female pattern hair loss. *Int J Endocrinol Metab* 2013;11:e9860.
30. Johnson & Johnson Inc. *Rogaine topical 2% solution, Rogaine foam 5%, Women's Rogaine foam 5%* [product monograph]. Available from: www.rogaine.ca. Accessed May 7, 2014.
31. Ross EK, Shapiro J. Management of hair loss. *Dermatol Clin* 2005;23:227-43.
32. Olsen EA, Whiting D, Bergfeld W et al. A multicenter, randomized, placebo-controlled, double-blind clinical trial of a novel formulation of 5% minoxidil topical foam versus placebo in the treatment of androgenetic alopecia in men. *J Am Acad Dermatol* 2007;57:767-74.
33. Briggs GG, Freeman RK, Yaffe SJ. *Drugs in pregnancy and lactation: a reference guide to fetal and neonatal risk*. 10th ed. Philadelphia: Lippincott Williams & Wilkins; 2014.
34. Drugs and Lactation Database (LactMed). *Minoxidil*. Bethesda: National Library of Medicine. Available from: toxnet.nlm.nih.gov/cgi-bin/sis/htmlgen?LACT. Accessed April 27, 2016.
35. DermNet NZ. Birchall NM. *Finasteride*. Available from: www.dermnetnz.org/treatments/finasteride.html.
36. Hu R, Xu F, Sheng Y et al. Combined treatment with oral finasteride and topical minoxidil in male androgenetic alopecia: a randomized comparative study in Chinese patients. *Dermatol Ther* 2015;28:303-8.
37. Khanpur S, Suman M, Reddy BS. Comparative efficacy of various treatment regimens for androgenetic alopecia in men. *J Dermatol* 2002;29:489-98.
38. Hordinsky M, Donati A. Alopecia areata: an evidence-based treatment update. *Am J Clin Dermatol* 2014;15:231-46.
39. Spano F, Donovan JC. Alopecia areata: Part 2: treatment. *Can Fam Physician* 2015;61:757-61.

40. Jackson J, Caro JJ, Caro G et al. The effect of eflornithine 13.9% cream on the bother and discomfort due to hirsutism. *Int J Dermatol* 2007;46:976-81.
41. Wolf JE, Shander D, Huber F et al. Randomized, double-blind clinical evaluation of the efficacy and safety of topical eflornithine HCl 13.9% cream in the treatment of women with facial hair. *Int J Dermatol* 2007;46:94-8.

Hair Concerns—What You Need to Know

Tips to keep your hair looking healthy:

- Wash hair regularly to remove dirt, oil, sweat and hair care products. People with oily hair may need to shampoo daily. People who have dry hair should shampoo less often to allow the natural scalp oils to condition the hair.
- Have your hair cut by a professional to remove ends that are damaged.
- Use shampoos designed for your type of hair (dry, damaged or chemically treated hair) and condition hair regularly according to the product's instructions.
- Minimize use of harsh chemical treatments such as perms, dyes, bleaches and straighteners.
- Avoid excessive brushing. Use a brush with natural, round-ended bristles, and brush gently. Use only a wide-toothed comb on wet hair.
- Minimize use of blow dryers, curling and straightening irons. Use a lower setting on a blow dryer, and use a diffuser to blow dry chemical-treated hair.

Tips to treat thinning hair:

- The most common cause of hair thinning is male-pattern/female-pattern baldness. This type of hair loss is genetic—it runs in families. It can start any time from the teens to middle age. For women, it is more common after menopause.
- Nonprescription products containing minoxidil can be used to treat thinning hair. Follow the instructions carefully to get the best results.
- Apply minoxidil directly to the area on the scalp that is affected. Hands should be washed immediately after applying the product. The scalp should remain dry for 4 hours after applying minoxidil to ensure maximum absorption.
- It will take at least 2 months before any results will be seen. Full results may not be seen for a year.
- An increase in the amount of hair that falls out may start within 2–6 weeks of beginning to use minoxidil. This is normal and will decrease with continued use. If it continues longer than 2 weeks, stop using the product. Minoxidil must be used continuously to maintain hair growth.

Chapter 67
Insect Bites and Stings

Nancy Kleiman, BSP, MBA

Pathophysiology

Arthropods have exoskeletons, multisegmented bodies and paired, jointed appendages. Arthropods include spiders, scorpions, ticks, fleas, lice, caterpillars, centipedes, ants, bees, wasps, mosquitoes and flies. Arthropods may bite (e.g., spiders, ticks, centipedes, mosquitoes, ants, black flies, horse flies) or sting (e.g., bees, wasps, fire ants, scorpions), emit a toxic secretion (e.g., caterpillars) or have irritant hairs (e.g., some caterpillars or spiders).[1] The most common injury when coming into contact with arthropods is a localized, self-limiting skin reaction. Occasionally, serious sequelae can result from systemic effects of envenomation or from significant allergic reactions. Deaths from arthropod exposures are rare in North America and usually result from anaphylaxis.[1]

Spiders

Most spiders are venomous but few deliver sufficient venom in a human bite to cause systemic symptoms. Most spider bites cause an initial stinging sensation followed by localized swelling, itching and inflammation.[2] Spiders in the black widow family (*Lactrodectus* species) can be found throughout the United States and in the western and southeastern parts of Canada close to the US border.[2] The bite of the black widow can lead to pain within 30–60 minutes followed by sweating, nausea, blurred vision, muscle cramps, and swelling and redness at the site. Treatment is symptomatic. Hospitalization may be necessary if more severe symptoms (tachycardia, chest pain, respiratory depression, infection at the site) occur.[2] The brown recluse spider is found in the Southeastern United States. Its bite can cause redness, itching and pain within 6 hours. The venom contains enzymes that can cause tissue destruction; untreated bites can lead to tissue necrosis.[2]

Ticks

Ticks attach to their victims with specialized mouth parts and feed until they are engorged with blood. The most common reaction to tick bites is a red papule at the bite site, but swelling, blistering, bruising, itching or secondary skin infection may develop.[3]

A number of different ticks can be carried by pets.[3] Remove ticks from pets before they enter the yard or home. Removal of ticks from pets is important to humans as ticks can carry diseases such as Lyme disease and Rocky Mountain spotted fever.[3,4] The risk to animals is minimal in most cases, but infection can occur if mouth parts remain in the skin of the animal.

In Canada, the black-legged tick (deer tick) and the Western black-legged tick are the species known to carry the spirochete *Borrelia burgdorferi*, which causes Lyme disease. Not all black-legged ticks carry Lyme disease but the number is increasing. The black-legged tick is endemic in southeastern and southcentral Manitoba, parts of eastern, southern and northwestern Ontario, southern New Brunswick, Grand Manan Island and a number of areas on the east coast of Nova Scotia. The Western black-legged tick is endemic in the southern mainland of British Columbia and southern tip of Vancouver Island. Health Canada maintains a map of current and predicted areas of concern (www.phac-aspc.gc.ca/id-mi/tickinfo-eng.php).[4,5] The tick must be attached to the skin for at least 36 hours to transmit the bacterium that causes Lyme disease.[4,6]

Lyme disease typically presents with a rash called erythema migrans that expands outward from the bite site in a ring pattern or bull's eye[6] (see Lyme Disease Lesion in Photo Section). The rash can appear from 3–30 days after exposure. It begins at the site of the bite and gradually becomes larger over several days. Flu-like symptoms such as fever, chills, lethargy, fatigue and headache can occur.[6] If left untreated, the infection can spread over several weeks and lead to more severe symptoms such as Bell's palsy, severe headaches, neck stiffness and joint pain.[6] If left untreated for several months, more severe complications can occur; arthritis is the most common and neurologic complications (pain, numbness, tingling and memory loss) are less common.[4,6] Treatment with antibiotics can cure Lyme disease in most cases. Antibiotics used for treatment are **doxycycline**, **amoxicillin** and **cefuroxime axetil**, and therapy continues for several weeks.[6]

A number of tick species (species depends on geographical area) carry the *Rickettsia* bacterium, which can lead to Rocky Mountain spotted fever. In Canada, the Rocky Mountain wood tick is the major carrier of this disease and is found in Western Canada. This disease is relatively rare but has been reported throughout the Americas including the United States, Mexico, Panama, Costa Rica, Argentina, Brazil, Columbia and Bolivia. Prevalence in Canada is much less than that of Lyme disease. The tick requires an attachment period between 4 and 6 hours to transmit the bacterium.[7] Rocky Mountain spotted fever is characterized by a sudden onset of fever, nausea, vomiting, headache and myalgias within 3 days.[7,8] Two to five days after onset of fever, a maculopapular rash appears on the wrists and ankles, expanding over the next 7 days along the extremities.[7] Without treatment, patients may become severely ill and require hospitalization. **Doxycycline** is the usual drug of choice for treatment, with **tetracycline** and **chloramphenicol** being alternatives.[7]

Prompt removal of ticks minimizes systemic reactions and risk of tick-borne diseases. See Nonpharmacologic Therapy for information on how to remove a tick.

Mosquitoes

Biting insects such as mosquitoes deposit salivary secretions into the skin that commonly cause local histamine reactions with redness, swelling and intense itchiness. Reddened, itchy papules develop within hours then subside slowly over a few days. Some people may develop antibodies that contribute to formation of large welts that last several days. Anaphylaxis is rare.[9]

A number of viral and parasitic diseases can be carried by infected mosquitoes, the most relevant in Canada being West Nile virus. The Public Health Agency of Canada closely monitors and reports on West Nile virus, particularly in peak times from May to October. West Nile virus infection has been reported in British Columbia, Alberta, Saskatchewan, Manitoba, Ontario and Quebec. Reports outside these provinces are thought to be related to travel. West Nile virus can be transmitted to humans via the bite of a mosquito that has previously fed on an infected bird. The virus can also be transmitted through blood transfusions or organ/tissue transplants. There is evidence that pregnant women can pass the virus to their unborn child. Transmission may also be through breast milk, though level of risk is unknown. The virus is not known to be transmitted by touching or kissing between people or between animals and people.[9]

Many people infected with West Nile virus do not become sick. Symptoms usually appear within 2–15 days of being infected. Mild cases present with flu-like symptoms (fever, body aches, headache) and possibly rash or swollen lymph glands. Symptoms of more severe illness can include the sudden onset of headache, high fever, stiff neck, vomiting, confusion and muscle weakness. Movement disorders, parkinsonism, polio-like syndrome and muscle degeneration can also occur. Elderly, immunocompromised or chronically ill persons are more likely to become severely ill after being infected; meningitis, encephalitis or acute flaccid paralysis can be fatal. There is no specific treatment for West Nile virus. Patients with severe symptoms are managed with supportive therapy.[9]

Preventive measures (see Prevention) are especially important in areas of high risk and for those at risk of developing severe illness.

Bed Bugs

Bed bugs feed on blood by piercing the skin, which can cause red itchy lesions at the location of the bite. Bites are typically in clusters of 3–5 and may appear in a zigzag pattern. There may be tiny specks of blood on bedding or pyjamas. Allergic reactions (redness, swelling, hives) can occur in some patients. Bed bugs are attracted to humans by warmth and carbon dioxide. They generally feed just before dawn and hide during the daylight hours in seams of mattresses, crevices in box springs or walls, or behind headboards. Adult bed bugs have an average life span of 6–12 months but are able to survive up to a year without feeding.[10,11] Infestations of bed bugs are increasing, as is the interest in whether bed bugs can transmit infections from one person to another. Although bed bugs are known to be carriers of over 40 microorganisms and potentially plausible mechanisms for transmission have been identified, studies in HIV, hepatitis B and methicillin-resistant *Staphylococcus aureus* have been unable to definitively state that bed bugs can act as vectors of disease.[12,13,14] One study suggested that severe infestations of bed bugs may lead to blood loss and subsequent iron-deficiency anemia, particularly in high-risk populations (alcohol abuse, poor diet, cognitive impairment, mental illness or poverty).[15]

Adult bed bugs are light yellow to reddish brown, oval shaped and approximately 5 mm in length. They are easily visible. Using a magnifying glass to thoroughly check headboards, mattresses, box springs, baseboards, furniture and curtains may be helpful to identify an infestation. Live bedbugs can sometimes be seen by using a flashlight just before dawn when they are most active, but also larger and slow-moving due to feeding.[11] See Bed Bug and Bed Bug Infestation in Photo Section. Chemical repellents have not been proven to be effective for prevention of bed bug infestation or bites. It is prudent to carefully check hotel rooms or new environments (seams of mattresses, crevices in box springs, behind headboards, under baseboards and behind hanging pictures) or any garage sale or second-hand items brought into the home. A combination of chemical pesticides (professionally applied) and nonchemical methods (vacuuming, application of heat or steam for at least 2 hours, exposure to temperatures <–5ºC for at least 5 days, mattress encasements, discarding of furniture) offers the best chance of eradication and must include follow-up confirmation.[10,11]

Stinging Insects

Stinging insects of the order *Hymenoptera*, are known to cause the majority of severe insect-related reactions. There are 3 families of insects known to cause a reaction: bees (bumblebees, honeybees), vespids (yellow jackets, wasps and hornets) and stinging ants (fire ants). The venom of bees and vespids contain multiple protein allergens which lead to a severe reaction in those who are susceptible.[16] The most common reaction to a sting from a hymenoptera insect is a local reaction with an onset of 4–48 hours (pain, redness and swelling at site). Occasionally there may be an extensive local reaction with swelling over a large area (e.g., the whole limb) peaking at 48 hours and subsiding over the next 3–10 days.[16] Systemic reactions (headache, fever, nausea and vomiting within 12–24 hours) are more likely with multiple stings from the same insect as well as repeated stings within a few months (same summer).[16,17]

The most serious reaction to insect stings is anaphylaxis, which can occur within minutes or up to 72 hours after the initial sting.[17] Systemic reactions can involve cutaneous, vascular and/or respiratory systems. The patient may initially experience generalized warmth, flushing and itchiness. This can progress to hives, airway edema with throat tightness and difficulty breathing, bronchospasm and, in severe cases, shock with hypotension.[16] **Venom immunotherapy (VIT)** greatly reduces the risk of developing severe systemic reactions in affected individuals[18] (see Emergency Treatment).

Goals of Therapy

- Prevent bites and stings
- Prevent diseases or reactions caused by bites or stings
- Ensure patient receives appropriate care when warranted in the case of more serious reactions
- Provide symptomatic relief for localized reactions

Patient Assessment

Self-management is appropriate for most arthropod bites or stings in Canada because localized skin reactions (itching, redness and swelling of bite area) are the most common consequence. Mild allergic reactions (hives, rash and mild swelling at the bite site) can also be self-treated.[1] Patients require further medical treatment if they experience extensive local reactions (swelling beyond the bite site), multiple stings or an anaphylactic reaction (difficulty breathing, swelling of throat, large areas of swelling, or fainting). Suspected anaphylaxis is a medical emergency and requires immediate treatment and follow-up medical care. An assessment plan for patients with arthropod bites and stings is presented in Figure 1.

Prevention

Prevention of stings from stinging insects is accomplished by avoiding situations where the insect may feel threatened (e.g., near nesting areas, approaching hives, removal of nests) as stinging insects sting in self-defence.[19] Preventive measures include avoiding the use of scented cosmetics, perfumes and hairsprays that can attract insects, avoiding or using caution when eating outdoors and ensuring that drinks are covered to avoid swallowing wasps or bees. Limiting the time spent outdoors at dawn and dusk will also decrease the chances of a sting. Clothing that covers as much skin as possible and tucking in pant legs when near nesting areas will also decrease the risk of being stung.[20]

Prevention of bites from biting insects can be accomplished by avoiding infested areas such as tall grasses, marshes, swamps or bushy areas and avoiding being outdoors at dawn and dusk as mosquitoes are most active during these times. Eliminating sources of standing water, such as rain barrels, clogged gutters and bird baths is the most effective way to reduce the local mosquito population.[20]

To protect against ticks, pants and shirts should be tight at the ankles and wrists, or tucked into socks and gloves. Light-coloured clothing makes ticks more visible for quick removal which will help to prevent attachment to the skin. This in turn helps to prevent the transmission of disease and lessen local reactions. It is important when going indoors after possible exposure to ticks to inspect clothing and tick-prone areas of skin such as the ankle, wrist and neck areas and quickly remove if present.[20]

Use of mosquito netting and clothing that covers exposed areas of the body are recommended for infants less than 6 months of age and travellers to areas where mosquito-borne illness is endemic.[9]

Insect Repellents

Insect repellents can deter biting insects such as mosquitoes, black flies and ticks, but not stinging insects.[20] Insect repellents should be applied lightly directly to clothing and exposed skin, preferably outdoors or in a well-ventilated area. The repellent should not be applied directly to the face (apply to the hands and then use hands to apply to face) nor sprayed into or near the eyes or mouth. Avoid application to the hands of children who may then inadvertently transfer it to their eyes or mouth. Repellent activity and duration of effect are highly variable, depending on the chemical and its concentration, the individual's activity level, the environment and the insect.[20] See Table 1 for more information on insect repellents.

The insecticide **permethrin** can be used for protection against tick bites. Permethrin has insect repellent activity and immobilizes ticks after ≤15 minutes of contact. It is sprayed directly onto clothing, tents or sleeping bags and the effect can last for up to 20 washes. Permethrin spray is not available in Canada but permethrin-impregnated clothing can be obtained from online retailers and is effective and long-lasting (no loss in effectiveness after 100 washes in one study).[21]

Nonpharmacologic Therapy

First, remove the insect or stinger to decrease the local reaction. Stingers from the honeybee are barbed and remain embedded in the skin. The stinger should be removed as soon as possible to stop the injection of venom into the wound.[19] The stinger can be removed by gently scraping side to side with a fingernail, tweezers or credit card.[17,19] The bite or sting site should then be cleansed with warm water and soap to help prevent secondary infection. Ice or cool compresses applied to the site provide symptomatic relief and reduce swelling.[17] Home remedies such as baking soda poultices or toothpaste, vinegar and salt applied to the site may relieve symptoms, but have not been well studied.[17]

Ticks are best removed by using tweezers[25] that are able to grasp the tick close to where the head contacts the skin. It is important to avoid twisting or pulling the tick out too quickly as this could cause the head to break off and remain in the skin. Clean the area with soap and water once the tick has been completely removed as this will decrease some of the irritation at the site.[4]

Pharmacologic Therapy

For comparative ingredients of nonprescription products, consult the *Compendium of Products for Minor Ailments*—Analgesic Products: Internal Analgesics and Antipyretics; Cough, Cold and Allergy Products; Insect Repellents; Skin Care Products: First Aid.

A variety of treatments can be used to relieve symptoms from local reactions to bites and stings. For pain, consider usual doses of **oral analgesics** such as **acetaminophen**, **ASA** or **ibuprofen**. **Oral antihistamines** are more effective than topical products in relieving pain, itching and inflammation caused by insect stings.[19] **First-generation antihistamines** (e.g., **diphenhydramine**, **chlorpheniramine**) and **second-generation antihistamines** (e.g., **loratadine, cetirizine**) are equally effective in relieving the itching and inflammation from insect bites and stings. First-generation antihistamines tend to cause more sedation and have a shorter duration of action than second-generation agents which must be considered when recommending therapy.[19] See Chapter 22: Allergic Rhinitis for further information on antihistamines and doses to be used in treatment.

Topical products marketed for symptomatic relief of bites and stings may contain **local anesthetics** (e.g., **benzocaine, lidocaine, pramoxine**), **astringents** (e.g., **calamine, zinc oxide**), counterirritants (e.g., **camphor**, **menthol**) or **ammonia/baking soda** combination (e.g., Afterbite). **Topical anesthetics** reduce the conduction of sensory nerve impulses in the skin, resulting in reversible loss of sensation. They have a short duration of action and give only minor relief immediately after the sting or bite occurs.[19] These products may provide temporary relief but evidence of effectiveness or comparative efficacy among topical products is lacking. Apply as recommended (Table 3) for 2 or 3 days until the symptoms subside.[26]

Topical **diphenhydramine** is not recommended for the relief of itching as it can cause allergic contact dermatitis and sensitization.[19]

Studies on the efficacy of topical **corticosteroids** for the treatment of insect bites and stings are limited but they may be recommended to relieve the associated itchiness, swelling and redness.[19,27,28] Table 3 provides more information on topical antipruritics.

Table 1: **Insect Repellents**[20,22,23,24]

Ingredient	Action	Dosage	Adverse Effects	Comments
DEET (N,N-diethyl-m-toluamide)	Vapour thought to have offensive smell or taste to insects and repels mosquitoes. Effective against mosquitoes, black flies, ticks, chiggers and fleas. Duration of effect depends on concentration: 30% DEET = 5–8 h 20% DEET = 4–6.5 h 15% DEET = 3.5–5.5 h 10% DEET = 2.5–4.5 h 5% DEET = 1.5–2.5 h	Concentration: 5–30% Apply sparingly to clothing or exposed skin according to Health Canada guidelines: <6 months: Not recommended 6 months–1 y: ≤10%; maximum once daily 2–11 y: 10%; maximum TID ≥12 y: 5–30%; maximum TID Available as lotion, pump and aerosol sprays, towelette	Irritating to mucous membranes and open wounds. Contact dermatitis (rash, redness, itching) has been reported. Absorbed through intact skin, and systemic effects are related to the amount absorbed. If ingested may lead to seizures, hypotension, angioedema or death.	Second choice in children 6 months–12 y (icaridin 20% first choice). If travelling to area with high risk of arthropod-associated disease, up to 10% may be applied to children <6 months. DEET ≤10% should not be used for exposures longer than 1–2 h as it may not be effective in preventing tick bites. Sunscreen should be applied first and allowed to penetrate before DEET application. No evidence that the use of DEET by pregnant or breastfeeding women poses a health hazard to unborn babies or breastfed infants/children. Avoid excessive or prolonged use.
icaridin (also known as picaridin)	Believed to affect the insect's ability to detect the host by concealing attractants emitted by hosts or by changing the insect's ability to smell them. Effective against mosquitoes, ticks and black flies. Duration of effect: 10% = 5 h for mosquitoes and 7 h for ticks. 20% = 7 h for mosquitoes and 8 h for ticks and blackflies.	Concentration: 10–20% Apply directly to skin—avoid eye contact <6 months: Not recommended ≥6 months: Up to 20% Reapply 10% after 5 h, up to QID Reapply 20% after 7 h, up to BID Available as spray, aerosol or towelette	Low toxicity. Nonirritating to the skin, but should be kept out of eyes and mouth. No allergic reactions reported.	Icaridin (20%) recommended as first choice in children 6 months–12 y. If travelling to area with high risk of arthropod-associated disease, up to 10% may be applied to children <6 months. No human data re. safety in pregnancy and breastfeeding (no toxicity seen in animal studies).
p-menthane 3,8-diol (PMD; oil of lemon eucalyptus)	Effective against mosquitoes, biting flies and gnats (not effective against ticks). Duration of effect is about 2 h.	Concentration: 10% <3 y: Not recommended ≥3 y: Maximum BID Available as lotion	None known.	Considered a second choice (first-choice: DEET or icaridin) for ≥3 y.

(cont'd)

Table 1: **Insect Repellents**[20,22,23,24] *(cont'd)*

Ingredient	Action	Dosage	Adverse Effects	Comments
oil of citronella	Thought to have an offensive smell or taste to insects. Tested against mosquitoes only. Duration of effect is 20 min to 2 h.	Concentration: 5–15% Apply to exposed skin as needed <2 y: Not recommended Available as lotion, spray or towelette	Low toxicity. Skin irritation (redness, rash, itchiness) may occur. Hypersensitivity reactions possible.	Frequent reapplication needed. Lack of safety data but no health risks associated with use.
soybean oil	Thought to mask attractants emitted by host and/or by cooling skin surface temperature. Duration of effect is 1–4 h against mosquitoes and up to 8 h against black flies. Effectiveness against ticks approximately equal to DEET 10%.	Concentration: 2% Apply to exposed skin as needed Available as mist/spray formulation	Very low toxicity. Skin irritation reported rarely. Low potential for hypersensitivity reactions. No systemic absorption through skin.	No age restriction on use.

Emergency Treatment

For comparative ingredients of nonprescription products, consult the *Compendium of Products for Minor Ailments*—Skin Care Products: First Aid.

Anaphylaxis is a severe allergic reaction that occurs in those previously exposed to the allergen. It can be life-threatening and requires immediate emergency attention. Symptoms can occur within minutes or up to several hours after exposure. Respiratory reactions may appear as throat or chest tightness, cough or swelling of the tongue. Cutaneous reactions may appear as hives or welts and severe itching, as well as flushing or redness of the skin. Gastrointestinal reactions may manifest as difficult or painful swallowing, nausea, vomiting or abdominal cramping. Other reactions may include lightheadedness, sweating or arrhythmias.[29] Give **epinephrine** as soon as possible. Epinephrine alleviates symptoms by reducing vasodilation and vascular permeability, decreasing bronchospasm, and enhancing coronary blood flow and blood pressure. Transport the patient to hospital immediately. A second dose of epinephrine may be administered within 5–20 minutes if the patient has not responded adequately to the first dose. Up to 20% of insect bite anaphylactic reactions are biphasic. The second reaction is most likely to occur within 4–6 hours of the initial reaction but the range is 1–30 hours.[30] **Oral antihistamines** should not be used as first-line therapy in an emergency situation. They should be considered secondary medication, to help with hives and itching.[31] Epinephrine for self-injection is commercially available in various formats. Information and complete instructions for use are found in the specific product monographs.

All patients who have reactions to venom should undergo allergy testing no sooner than 4–6 weeks after a sting; testing earlier may cause a false-negative result.[32] Immunotherapy with escalating doses of venom is effective in reducing subsequent reactions.[33]

Monitoring of Therapy

Table 2 provides a monitoring framework for management of arthropod stings and bites.

Table 2: **Monitoring of Therapy for Insect Bites and Stings**[16,19,27,29]

Symptom	Monitoring	Endpoint	Actions
Pain/fever	Monitor for increased pain or fever daily for 7 days after bite or sting (monitor for signs of infection). Monitor the degree and duration of pain and fever relief for effectiveness with each analgesic dose. Pain should subside within 24 h.	Pain reduced to a tolerable level for the patient. No fever present.	Treatment with acetaminophen or ibuprofen (according to recommended dosing). Patients with significant symptoms past 24–48 h (intolerable pain and high fever) or fever or pain that persists for >7 days require further treatment.
Itching	Monitor daily for degree and duration of relief with each application. Relief should occur within minutes of treatment with topical agents and within 1 h for oral agents.	Itching reduced to a tolerable level for the patient (does not affect daily activities or sleep patterns).	Treatment with topical corticosteroids (according to recommended dosing), topical anesthetics up to QID or oral diphenhydramine (according to recommended dosing). Patients with itching that persists for >7 days despite appropriate treatment, require further assessment and/or treatment.
Swelling, redness	Monitor daily for signs of increased swelling or redness at site (signs of infection). Swelling and redness should subside within 24–48 h of bite or sting.	Minimal swelling or redness at site.	Treatment with topical corticosteroids (according to recommended dosing), or oral diphenhydramine (according to recommended dosing). Patients with extensive swelling occurs (e.g., if whole limb is involved) require further assessment and/or treatment.
Local infection (unusual swelling, redness or tenderness at bite site, pus or fever)	Monitor daily for up to 7 days for signs of infection.	No signs or symptoms of infection.	Topical antibiotics can be used to treat minor infection. Patients with signs and symptoms of local infection that do not respond to topical antibiotics within 48 h require further assessment and/or treatment.
Suspected anaphylaxis[a]	Monitor for signs and symptoms of anaphylaxis within 30 min or less of exposure.	Symptoms subside and do not recur or worsen during 6 h of observation.	Treat with epinephrine. All cases of suspected anaphylaxis require emergency medical attention.

[a] Mild: Generalized itching, flushing, hives, angioedema; Moderate: Dizziness, nausea, vomiting, abdominal cramps, chest or throat tightness, hoarseness; Severe: Hypotension, breathing difficulties, hypoxia, confusion, incontinence

Figure 1: **Assessment of Patients with Insect Bites and Stings**

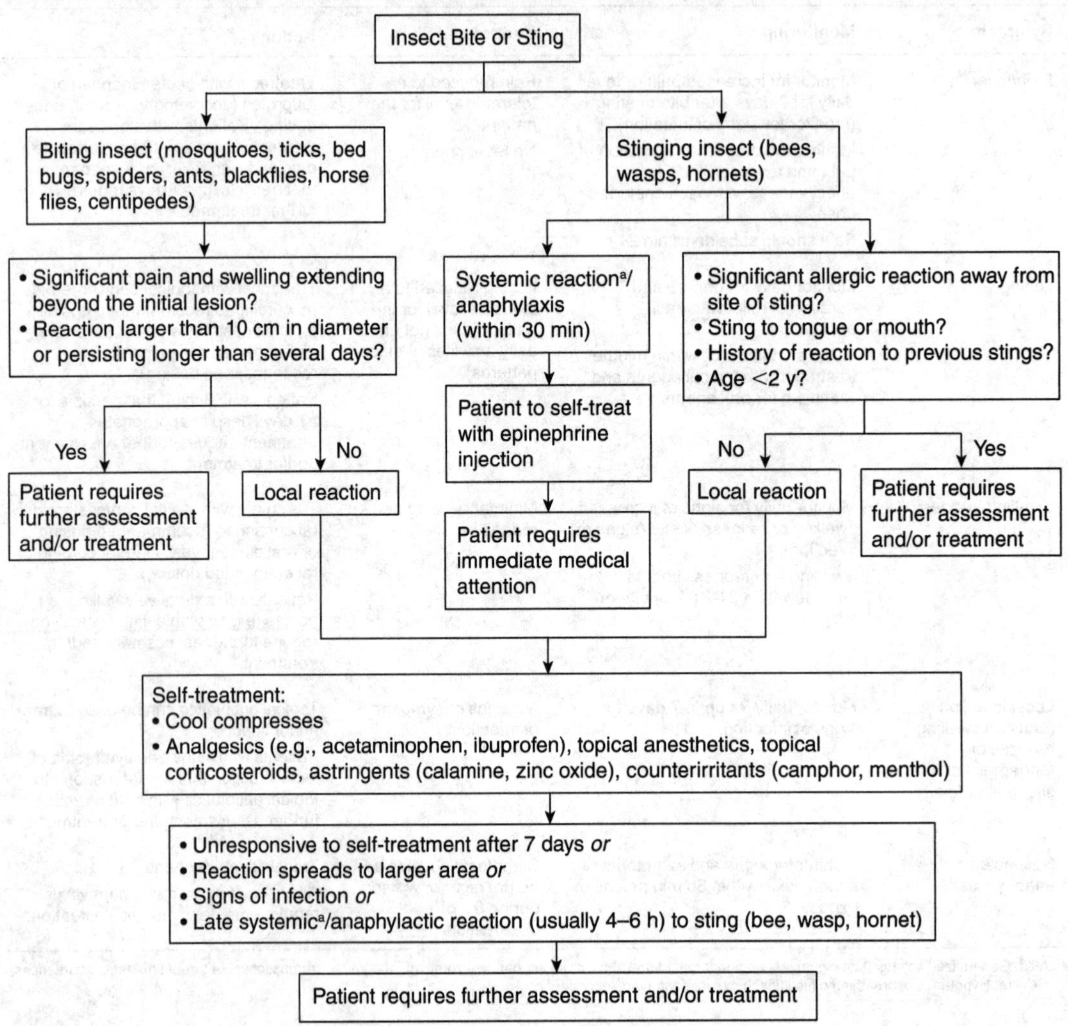

[a] Systemic symptoms: Generalized itching, flushing, sneezing, watery eyes, hives, nausea, vomiting, muscle cramps, dizziness, fainting, hoarseness, lump in throat, difficulty breathing, changes in heart rate (faster or slower).

Table 3: Topical Therapy for Insect Bites and Stings[19,26,28]

Class	Drug	Dosage	Mechanism of Action	Adverse Effects	Comments	Cost[a]
Anesthetics, topical (amides)	*lidocaine* Maxilene, Solarcaine, Xylocaine Jelly, Xylocaine Ointment, Xylocaine Viscous, generics	0.5–9.6%: Apply as needed up to 5 times daily; use sprays no more than twice per hour	Reduce the conduction of sensory nerve impulses in the skin, resulting in reversible loss of sensation.	Skin irritation and sensitization possible but uncommon when applied correctly. Poor absorption through intact skin. Systemic effects possible if absorption through open skin.	Lower concentrations preferred for self-care. Avoid frequent application or application to large open wounds or large areas of broken skin. Keep out of reach of small children since methemoglobinemia can occur with accidental ingestion.	$
Anesthetics, topical (esters)	*benzocaine*[b] Anbesol, Lanacane Medicated Cream, Orajel	7.5–20%: Apply TID–QID PRN for itching; maximum 7 days	See lidocaine.	See lidocaine.	Contraindicated in those with known hypersensitivity. Keep out of reach of small children since methemoglobinemia can occur with accidental ingestion.	$
Anesthetics, topical (others)	*pramoxine*[c] Aveeno Anti-Itch, Gold Bond Medicated Cream, Pramox HC Cream, Lotion, generics	1%: Apply QID PRN	See lidocaine.	Local irritation with burning, stinging possible, especially of mucous membranes.	Avoid application near eyes or nose. Preferred choice of topical anesthetic because of low potential for sensitization and low toxicity. No cross-allergenicity with esters or amides.	$
Corticosteroids, topical	*hydrocortisone* Cortate, Emo-Cort, Prevex HC, generics	0.5%, 1%: Apply TID–QID PRN; maximum 7 days	Antipruritic and anti-inflammatory.	Prolonged use can cause acneiform eruptions, irritation and cracking of the skin.	Do not use if signs of infection are present. Caution with use near eyes or on any areas of broken skin (including those caused by scratching).	$
Counterirritants	*camphor or menthol-containing salves*[d,e]	0.13–10.5% (most are <1%): Apply sparingly PRN	Cooling sensation from rubefacient effect. Mild local analgesia and anti-itch effects from local irritant effect. Irritants stimulate local sensory nerves reducing transmission of pain signals.	Skin irritation (burning, redness) at higher concentrations. Readily absorbed through intact and broken skin. Systemic toxicity includes nausea, vomiting, headache, dizziness, tremors.	Lower concentration products preferred. Do not apply to large areas of skin or open wounds. Keep out of reach of small children (especially high-concentration products).	$

(cont'd)

Table 3: Topical Therapy for Insect Bites and Stings[19,26,28] *(cont'd)*

Class	Drug	Dosage	Mechanism of Action	Adverse Effects	Comments	Cost[a]
Protectants	*calamine lotion* generics	1–16%: Apply liberally PRN	Skin protectants and mild astringents (reduce edema, inflammation). Soothing effect on irritated skin.	Well tolerated, no hypersensitivity reactions, no systemic absorption.		$
Others	*ammonia/baking soda* Afterbite	3.5% ammonia: Apply sparingly PRN	Localized cooling effect and relief of itching.	Some skin irritation with burning. Inhalation may cause sneezing and coughing.	Avoid exposure to eyes, mouth and mucous membranes. Not recommended for children <2 y.	$

[a] Cost of smallest available pack size; includes drug cost only.
[b] Single-entity products are marketed for teething pain only, but could be used. Benzocaine is a component of some first aid products.
[c] No single-entity products available. Pramoxine is a component of some first aid products.
[d] Extemporaneously compounded preparations can be used.
[e] Camphor and/or menthol are components of many first aid products.

Legend: $ <$5

Suggested Readings

Government of Canada. *For health professionals: Lyme disease*. Available from: healthycanadians.gc.ca/diseases-conditions-maladies-affections/disease-maladie/lyme/professionals-professionnels/index-eng.php.

Government of Canada. *For health professionals treating West Nile virus*. Available from: http://healthycanadians.gc.ca/diseases-conditions-maladies-affections/disease-maladie/west-nile-nil-occidental/professionals-professionnels-eng.php

Government of Canada. *Insect repellents*. Available from: healthycanadians.gc.ca/product-safety-securite-produits/pest-control-products-produits-antiparasitaires/pesticides/about-au-sujet/insect_repellents-insectifuges-eng.php?_ga=1.136545712.1489682248.1448374858.

Management of insect bites. *Pharmacist's Letter/Prescriber's Letter* 2008;24:240815.

References

1. Russell FE. Venomous arthropods. *Vet Hum Toxicol* 1991;33:505-8.
2. Quan D. North American poisonous bites and stings. *Crit Care Clin* 2012;28:633-59.
3. University of Guelph. Pest Diagnostic Clinic. *Ticks of Eastern Canada*. Available from: www.guelphlabservices.com/files/PDC/003Ticks.pdf. Accessed August 7, 2014.
4. Government of Canada. *For health professionals: Lyme disease*. Available from: healthycanadians.gc.ca/diseases-conditions-maladies-affections/disease-maladie/lyme/professionals-professionnels/index-eng.php. Accessed August 7, 2014.
5. Public Health Agency of Canada. *Public health reminder: Lyme disease*. Available from: www.phac-aspc.gc.ca/phn-asp/2015/lyme-eng.php. Accessed October 19, 2015.
6. Centers for Disease Control and Prevention. *Lyme disease*. Available from: www.cdc.gov/lyme/. Accessed August 7, 2014.
7. Dantas-Torres F. Rocky Mountain spotted fever. *Lancet Infect Dis* 2007;7:724-32.
8. Public Health Agency of Canada. Infectious Diseases. *Rickettsia Rickettsii* Available at: http://www.phac-aspc.gc.ca/lab-bio/res/psds-ftss/rickettsia-rickettsii-eng.php. Accessed April 20, 2016.
9. Government of Canada. *West Nile virus*. Available from: healthycanadians.gc.ca/health-sante/disease-maladie/wnv-vno-eng.php. Accessed October 10, 2015.
10. Goddard J, deShazo R. Bed bugs (Cimex lectularius) and clinical consequences of their bites. *JAMA* 2009;301:1358-66.
11. Studdiford JS, Conniff KM, Trayes KP et al. Bedbug infestation. *Am Fam Physician* 2012;86:653-8.
12. Delaunay P, Blanc V, Del Giudice P et al. Bedbugs and infectious diseases. *Clin Infect Dis* 2011;52:200-10.
13. Lowe CF, Romney MG. Bedbugs as vectors for drug-resistant bacteria. *Emerg Infect Dis* 2011;17:1132-4.
14. Brouqui P. Arthropod-bourne diseases associate with political and social disorder. *Annu Rev Entomol* 2011;56:357-74.
15. Pritchard MJ, Hwang SW. Cases: Severe anemia from bedbugs. *CMAJ* 2009;181:287-8.
16. Golden DB. Insect sting anaphylaxis. *Immunol Allergy Clin North Am* 2007;27:261-72.
17. Diaz JH. Hymenopterid bites, stings, allergic reactions, and the impact of hurricanes on hymenopterid-inflicted injuries. *J La State Med Soc* 2007;159:149-57.
18. Golden DB, Moffitt J, Nicklas RA et al. Stinging insect hypersensitivity: a practice parameter update 2011. *J Allergy Clin Immunol* 2011;125:852-4.
19. Nathan A. Advising on insect bites and stings. *Pharm J* 2007;278:577-60.
20. Government of Canada. *Insect repellents*. Available from: http://healthycanadians.gc.ca/product-safety-securite-produits/pest-control-products-produits-antiparasitaires/pesticides/about-au-sujet/insect_repellents-insectifuges-eng.php Accessed August 7, 2014.
21. Due C, Fox W, Medlock JM et al. Tick bite prevention and tick removal. *BMJ* 2013;347:f7123.
22. Committee to Advise on Tropical Medicine and Travel (CATMAT). An Advisory Committee Statement (ACS). Statement on personal protective measures to prevent arthropod bites. *Can Commun Dis Rep* 2012;38:1-18. Available from: www.phac-aspc.gc.ca/publicat/ccdr-rmtc/12vol38/acs-dcc-3/index-eng.php.
23. Health Canada. *Registration Decision RD2012-05, Icaridin (Archived)* Available at: http://www.hc-sc.gc.ca/cps-spc/pest/part/consultations/_prd2011-10/prd2011-10-eng.php. Accessed April 20, 2016.
24. Onyett H; Canadian Paediatric Society, Infectious Diseases and Immunization Committee. Preventing mosquito and tick bites: a Canadian update. *Paediatr Child Health* 2014;19:326-32.
25. AkIn Belli A, Dervis E, Kar S et al. Revisiting tick detachment techniques in human-biting ticks. *J Am Acad Dermatol* 2016 Mar 2. [Epub ahead of print.]
26. Management of insect bites. *Pharmacist's Letter/Prescriber's Letter* 2008;24:240815.
27. Bonifazi F, Jutel M, Bilo BM et al. Prevention and treatment of hymenoptera venom allergy: guidelines for clinical practice. *Allergy* 2005;60:1459-70.
28. Management of simple insect bites: where's the evidence? *Drug Ther Bull* 2012;50:45-8.
29. Brown A. Current management of anaphylaxis. *Emergendas* 2009;21:213-23.
30. Tole JW, Lieberman P. Biphasic anaphylaxis: review of incidence, clinical predictors, and observation recommendations. *Immunol Allergy Clin North Am* 2007;27:309-26.
31. Waserman S, Chad Z, Francoeur MJ et al. Management of anaphylaxis in primary care: Canadian expert consensus recommendations. *Allergy* 2010;65:1082-92.
32. Golden DB, Kagey-Sobotka A, Norman PS et al. Insect sting allergy with negative venom skin test responses. *J Allergy Clin Immunol* 2001;107:897-901.
33. Boyle RJ, Elremeli M, Hockenhull J et al. Venom immunotherapy for preventing allergic reactions to insect stings. *Cochrane Database Syst Rev* 2012;10:CD008838.

Insect Bites and Stings—What You Need to Know

Use an insect repellent to prevent bites from mosquitoes, black flies and ticks. Insect repellents do not work against stinging insects such as bees and wasps.

How to protect children from insect bites and stings

- The best way to protect infants and small children is by using netting over beds and strollers and dressing them in long-sleeved, tightly woven clothing.
- DEET is the most effective insect repellent but it should not be used on children under 6 months. A repellent that has less than 10% DEET can be used once a day on children older than 6 months and up to 2 years. Older children can use a repellent containing less than 10% DEET up to 3 times in 1 day.
- Icaridin effectively protects against mosquitoes, ticks and black flies for up to 8 hours depending on the strength of the product used. It is safe to use in children over 6 months of age.
- **Do not** use repellents containing citronella or lavender oil on children less than 2 years of age. There is not enough information to know whether they can harm small children. Duration of action is 30 minutes to 2 hours.
- To use insect repellent safely on children:
  - Apply the product lightly and only to exposed skin. **Do not** apply to open wounds or irritated skin. **Do not** apply to a child's hands or face.
  - Wash insect repellent off when protection is no longer needed.

How to protect adults from insect bites and stings

- DEET and icaridin are effective insect repellents with minimal toxic effects.
- Women who are pregnant or breastfeeding should try to avoid using insect repellents. Choose nonchemical methods instead, such as wearing pants and long sleeves. If an insect repellent is needed, use one that has less than 10% DEET and apply it sparingly. Pregnant and breastfeeding women can use products that contain soybean oil. Studies have shown these products are very safe. These products do not protect against ticks.
- To use insect repellent safely:
  - Choose an insect repellent that contains no more than 30% DEET or 20% icaridin. Follow the instructions on the product bottle.
  - Do not use products that contain permethrin on skin. These products should only be used on clothing, tents or equipment.
  - Apply repellent lightly and only to exposed skin. Do not apply to open wounds or irritated skin. Be careful when applying to the face.
  - Apply sunscreen first, allow to penetrate for 20 minutes and then apply the insect repellent.
  - Wash hands after applying repellent. Wash insect repellent off when protection is no longer needed.

Use aerosol products (sprays, mists) in a well-ventilated area. If you accidentally get the product in your eyes or mouth, rinse them well with plenty of warm water.

How to protect yourself when travelling

- In areas where mosquito-borne illness (such as malaria or West Nile virus) is common:
  - Wear light-coloured, tightly woven clothing that covers arms and legs.

  - Apply an insect repellent that contains 30% DEET or 20% icaridin to all exposed skin, including neck, wrists and ankles.
  - At night, burn a mosquito coil around your sleeping area, and protect yourself with a mosquito net.
  - Spray clothing, tents and netting with an insecticide such as permethrin to help keep mosquitoes away.
- In areas where ticks are common:
  - Wear light-coloured clothing that is tight at the wrists and ankles. You can also tuck clothing into gloves and socks.
  - Apply an insect repellent that contains 30% DEET or 20% icaridin to all exposed skin.
  - Spray clothing and boots with an insecticide such as permethrin to help keep ticks away.
  - Inspect your skin for ticks immediately before going indoors after exposure to tick areas and every day after. Remove ticks immediately. Use tweezers to grab the tick and pull gently until the tick detaches. This may take up to a minute of steady pulling. **Do not** apply heat, poison or other substances to the tick. These methods do not work and may be harmful.

How to treat insect bites or stings

- When you get a bite or sting, wash the spot with warm water and soap.
- Apply ice or a cool compress (such as a wet cloth) to relieve the irritation. To prevent frostbite, **do not** apply ice for longer than 10 minutes at a time.
- For pain, use a pain reliever such as acetaminophen, ASA or ibuprofen.
- For itching, use anti-itch lotions, creams or sprays. You can also use a nonprescription corticosteroid cream, e.g., hydrocortisone 0.5% or 1%. Oral antihistamines can be used to relieve itching, particularly if there is swelling. Topical antihistamines are not recommended.
- Avoid scratching the bite area. You may damage your skin and cause an infection.
- If the symptoms do not improve over 24–48 hours **or** if the symptoms are worse, see a health professional.
- It is not common to have a serious reaction to an insect bite or sting unless you have an allergy. Seek medical attention **immediately** if you develop any of the following symptoms within a few minutes to 30 minutes after being bitten:
  - a red flush or itching all over your body
  - chest or throat tightness (difficulty breathing)
  - hives
  - nausea, vomiting
  - abdominal cramps
  - dizziness, fainting
  - hoarse voice or swelling in the throat
  - changes in heart rate (fast or slow)

Contact a doctor if:

- a rash develops around the bite
- the bite reaction spreads to a large area (whole arm or leg)
- an unusual reaction around a bite develops (such as a purplish colour or blisters).

Those with a past history of severe allergic reactions may want to take the following precautions:

- Wear a MedicAlert bracelet or bracelet identifying the reaction
- Carry epinephrine injection (Allerject, EpiPen) for emergency use
- Carry oral antihistamine (diphenhydramine tablet)

Chapter 68
Minor Cuts and Wounds

Nancy Kleiman, BSP, MBA

Pathophysiology

A wound is a disruption in the normal skin structure and functioning due to mechanical trauma and injury. Partial-thickness wounds affect the epidermis and outer dermal layers, while deeper, full-thickness wounds penetrate through the subcutaneous tissues (fat layer) exposing structures such as muscle or bone.[1] Blunt trauma can produce a superficial bruise or deeper hematoma as a result of leakage of blood from small venules and arterioles.[2]

Wounds are classified as acute or chronic:

- Acute wounds can occur from burns, bites, abrasions, scrapes, minor lacerations and punctures, and acute wounds tend to heal quickly with minor treatment
- Chronic wounds occur when healing has been delayed or impaired due to various conditions (e.g., immunocompromised states, diabetes) or have not proceeded through the healing process correctly.[1] This chapter does not discuss management of chronic wounds. See Chapter 55: Atopic, Contact, and Stasis Dermatitis and consult the *Compendium of Therapeutic Choices*: Pressure Ulcers and Diabetic Foot Infections.

Wound healing begins at the time of injury and generally proceeds through 3 phases:

- The first phase is the inflammatory phase which begins at the time of injury and lasts up to 6 days. This phase is characterized by the release of inflammatory mediators resulting in vasoconstriction, redness, pain, platelet aggregation and clot formation, and manifests as redness, edema and a higher level of drainage from the wound[1]
- The second phase is the proliferative phase which lasts from 4–24 days depending on the type of wound, cause and depth. This phase is characterized by the formation of new tissue, wound contraction and the formation of new epithelium; the wound remains red and raised
- The third and final phase is the maturation phase. Within 4–5 days of injury, collagen forms early scar tissue that holds the wound edges together and strengthens it.[2,3] Collagen continues to strengthen the wound for up to 2 years depending on the type of wound.[1] Minor wounds usually heal without scarring. Large or deep wounds may leave a visible ridge or puckering of excess collagen at the healed wound site.

Wound Complications

The most common complications of wounds are infection and scarring.

Infection

All wounds are contaminated with bacteria to some extent, and infection is possible if the wound is not dealt with appropriately and promptly. Gram-negative and gram-positive bacteria (including tetanus) and fungi may be involved in wound infections. Infection with *Clostridium tetani* (found in soil) via a contaminated wound can be fatal. Patients with wounds that are unclean should be given a **tetanus vaccination** to prevent infection with this bacterium if their vaccination status is not adequate (see Pharmacologic Therapy).[1]

Minor infection presents with redness, inflammation, tenderness to touch and warmth in the immediate area of the wound. Other symptoms of wound infection may appear as discharge, delayed healing, abnormal odour, wound breakdown and increased pain.[1] These symptoms may indicate a more serious infection.

Wound factors that may increase the risk of infection include:[1,2]

- Presence and type of foreign matter in the wound (débridement removes dead or contaminated material that can harbor bacteria)
- Location of the wound (near a site of potential contamination such as the anal area); one study also found wounds on the lower extremities to be at higher risk of infection[4]
- Injury to underlying structures such as bone or muscle (deep wound that is difficult and slow to heal and at higher risk of bacterial invasion and infection)
- Presence of devitalized tissue (increases the risk of harbouring bacteria in the wound)
- Although historically it was believed that wounds that were closed (sutured) >12 hours after time of injury were more likely to become infected, there is some evidence that time lapse before wound closure is not as important as previously thought.[4]

Patient factors related to infection risk include:[1,2]

- Age (epidermis and subcutaneous layer become thinner with increased age)
- Underlying medical conditions (e.g., diabetes can affect wound healing if there is poor glycemic control and presence of peripheral vascular disease)
- Malnutrition (deficiencies of protein, zinc and vitamins A and C may slow or impair the healing process)
- Smoking
- Drug therapy (e.g., long-term corticosteroid use inhibits cell growth, chemotherapy medications may affect the immune system and delay healing, anticoagulants slow the clotting rate and increase the healing time of wounds).

Scarring

Scarring occurs when there is a large deposit of collagen and glycoprotein at the wound site and is a natural part of the healing process. Moist healing environments have been shown to decrease the extent of scarring and improve the healing of wounds by accelerating inflammatory and proliferative phases of repair.[5] Discoloration can occur if the area is exposed to the sun, but can be decreased with the use of sunblock for up to 6 months after the injury heals.[1] **Silicone gels** and **sheets** applied topically hydrate the scar and are used for 3–6 months.[6]

Goals of Therapy

- Provide an environment that optimizes wound healing and prevents cosmetic deformity
- Prevent infection
- Minimize further trauma to the area
- Minimize patient discomfort

Patient Assessment

Superficial wounds that are small and accompanied by limited bleeding are suitable for self-management. Patients require further assessment and/or treatment in the following situations: wounds that continue to bleed, deep puncture wounds, gaping wounds, wounds that expose fat, muscle or bone, animal bites, wounds with visible foreign material or dirt, wounds causing severe pain, wounds in patients with underlying medical conditions or drug therapy that puts them at risk of infection or delayed healing (see Wound Complications), and those with large, complicated or chronic wounds.[2] See Figure 1.

Nonpharmacologic Therapy

Self-treatment of minor wounds includes the following steps:

1. **Cleanse the wound:** Remove dirt and debris from the wound as soon as possible to prevent infection and promote healing.[1] Once debris has been removed, carefully wash the wound with water. Drinkable tap water is as effective for wound cleaning as saline or purified water, with no increased risk of infection or decrease in wound healing[7]
2. **Stop the bleeding:** Apply a clean dressing or gauze to the wound area for 10 minutes. If the bleeding does not stop within 10 minutes (or 15 minutes if anticoagulated) the patient should seek emergency medical attention. Monitor those on anticoagulants for up to 15 minutes, as the clotting time will be longer, and refer if the bleeding does not stop within that time period. Visible pieces of dirt or other foreign material that remain after irrigation can be gently picked out of the wound with tweezers that have been cleaned with rubbing alcohol, or by brushing gently with clean gauze. These steps protect the wound from infection and tissue destruction and help the wound to heal faster[1]
3. **Apply a dressing:** Choose a dressing that maintains a moist wound bed (see Chapter 60: Dressings) to protect the wound from possible infection and improve the healing process. Minor cuts, paper cuts or skin cracks can be closed using tissue adhesives or liquid bandage. Larger cuts, where the edges won't stay together, the edges are jagged or the wound is deep, may need stitches.

Débridement: The removal of foreign material such as dead or contaminated tissue from the wound should be performed only by an appropriately trained healthcare practitioner and under sterile conditions.[1]

Pharmacologic Therapy

Cleansing and Antiseptic Agents

Use of antiseptics is appropriate only when the risk of infection is high (see Wound Complications). They should be applied only around the wound area, not directly onto the wound (see Table 1).

For comparative ingredients of nonprescription products, consult the *Compendium of Products for Minor Ailments*—Skin Care Products: First Aid.

Topical Antibacterials

Prophylaxis: **Topical antibiotics** are recommended for prevention of complications in wounds that are at higher risk of becoming infected (see Wound Complications), improperly cleansed wounds or chronic wounds.[12] Evidence shows that use of topical **bacitracin**[13] and **bacitracin/neomycin/ polymyxin B** combination[13,14] result in significantly lower infection rates than plain petrolatum or placebo ointment for minor wounds. **Antibacterial bandages** have not been proven to be more effective for wound care than regular bandages and are more expensive.[12] **Silver sulfadiazine** was previously believed to play a role in reducing microbes in wounds. However, despite limitations in available evidence, there appears to be a risk of delayed wound healing associated with silver sulfadiazine, and alternative wound regimens should be considered when feasible.[15]

Treatment: Superficial, mildly infected wounds may be treated with topical antibiotics such as **fusidic acid**, **mupirocin** or various combinations of **bacitracin/gramicidin/polymyxin B/neomycin** (see Wound Complications).[16,17] There is insufficient evidence to recommend one topical antibiotic over another except in the case of methicillin-resistant *Staphylococcus aureus* (MRSA) infection where mupirocin is recommended.[18] Consider topical antibiotics only when medically necessary and use responsibly to prevent resistant strains from developing.[19] If used, discontinue as soon as signs and symptoms of infection are no longer present. Consider further assessment and/or treatment if clinical improvement is not evident within 3–5 days of topical antibiotic therapy or if signs and symptoms of infection worsen at any time.

Table 1: **Cleansing and Antiseptic Agents**[1,8,9,10,11]

Treatment	Uses	Advantages	Disadvantages
Saline solution	Cleansing agent for the initial removal of dirt and debris from a wound.	Not harmful to tissue.	Not always available; drinkable tap water is just as effective for cleansing wounds.[7]
Hydrogen peroxide 3%	An oxidizing agent that has antiseptic, disinfectant and deodorant properties used to clean wounds.	Effervescent action cleanses wounds. Has some mild antibacterial activity.	May cause tissue toxicity and impair wound healing through irritation of the tissue and destruction of regenerating epithelium. Has limited bactericidal effect. Little benefit over soapy water.
Isopropyl alcohol 70%	Bactericidal in concentrations of 70–90% and used as a disinfectant for wounds and prior to injections.	Can decrease bacteria counts for 20–40 min after contact. Some fungicidal activity.	Not to be used on open wounds. High potential for drying the skin. Irritating to tissue.
Iodine	Used as a disinfectant and antiseptic for contaminated wounds, wound bed management and prevention of infection.	Aqueous solution is preferable as it is less irritating and drying than alcohol base.	Stains skin and clothing. May irritate tissue and impair wound healing. May cause allergic sensitization.
Povidone-iodine	Used as a disinfectant and antiseptic for contaminated wounds and pre-operative preparation of the skin.	Nonirritating to skin. Rapid bactericidal activity. Broad-spectrum.	Contraindicated in patients with iodine or shellfish allergy. May be absorbed systemically: can be harmful if used on large areas or for prolonged periods of time. Use with caution in patients with thyroid disorder. Infection and tissue damage increased if used in combination with surfactants. May impair wound healing.

More information on topical antibacterials can be found in Table 3.

Other Therapy

Systematic reviews have determined that evidence is inconclusive regarding whether **aloe vera** gel[20] or topical **honey**[21] improve outcomes for acute wounds. Some patients experience mild side effects of burning sensation, contact dermatitis or mild itching with topical application of aloe vera.[22] Prevention of wound infection with **oral antibiotics** is generally recommended only in cases of animal or human bites, deep puncture wounds and wounds involving the palms and fingers.[17] Treatment of wound infections with oral antibiotics is recommended for infections involving deeper tissues (including puncture and bite wounds)[17] and may also be considered if an infection persists for more than 2 weeks with topical antibiotic use and correct wound management.[1] For further information on use of oral antibiotics in the treatment of bacterial skin infections, consult the *Compendium of Therapeutic Choices*: Bacterial Skin Infections.

Tetanus is a potential complication of any wound in those whose tetanus immunization is incomplete or has lapsed.[12,17] Even patients with apparently minor, clean wounds should receive a **tetanus booster** if: their immunization is incomplete (less than 3 doses), they are uncertain when they received their last tetanus shot or their last tetanus shot was more than 10 years ago. Patients with dirty or complicated wounds require tetanus prophylaxis if more than 5 years have elapsed since their last tetanus booster.[12] Consider **rabies vaccination** in cases of bites from unprovoked animal attacks, especially where wild animals such as raccoons, skunks, foxes or bats are involved.[3]

Monitoring of Therapy

A monitoring plan for patients with minor cuts and wounds is provided in Table 2.

Table 2: **Monitoring of Therapy for Minor Cuts and Wounds**

Sign/Symptom	Monitoring	Endpoint	Actions
Bleeding	Monitor bleeding: Should stop within 10 min (15 min if on anticoagulants).	Bleeding significantly slows or stops within 10–15 min of direct pressure.	Patient requires emergency medical treatment if blood is spurting or significant bleeding persists after 10 min of direct pressure (15 min if anticoagulated).
Infection, e.g., swelling, surrounding redness that is tender to touch, red streaks from the wound, pus or fever	Monitor daily at dressing change for at least 48 h.	No signs or symptoms of infection present at 48 h.	Assess for further treatment if signs and symptoms of infection are present at or before 48 h.
Wound healing	Monitor daily at dressing change for 4–14 days (depending on wound type, depth and location).	Normally, healing wounds appear pink or red with tiny opalescent islands of epithelium throughout and no drainage.	If wound continues to weep, remains raw and red or does not appear to be closing within 2–4 wk, further assessment is required.

Figure 1: **Assessment of Patients with Minor Acute Wounds**

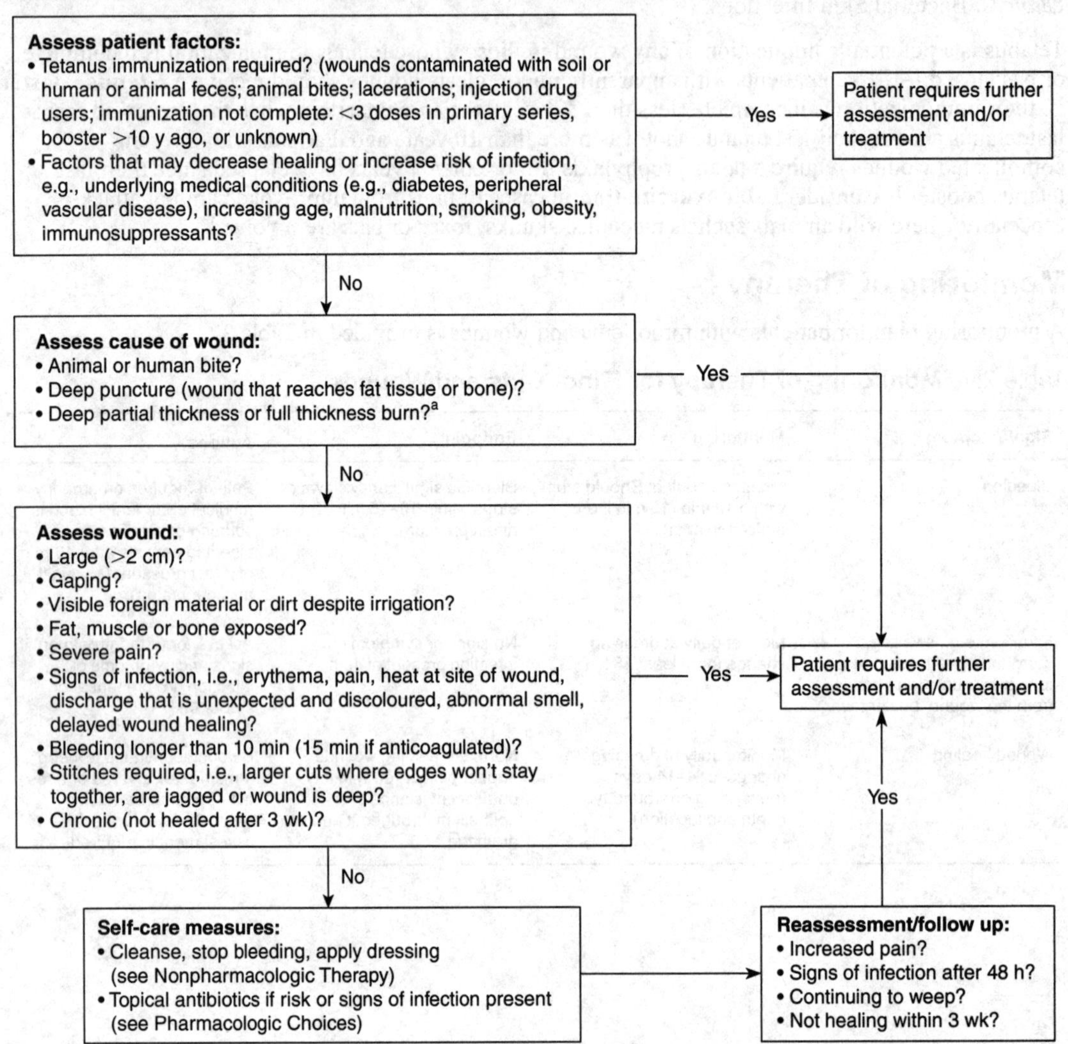
Assess patient factors:
• Tetanus immunization required? (wounds contaminated with soil or human or animal feces; animal bites; lacerations; injection drug users; immunization not complete: <3 doses in primary series, booster >10 y ago, or unknown)
• Factors that may decrease healing or increase risk of infection, e.g., underlying medical conditions (e.g., diabetes, peripheral vascular disease), increasing age, malnutrition, smoking, obesity, immunosuppressants?
Yes
Patient requires further assessment and/or treatment
No
Assess cause of wound:
• Animal or human bite?
• Deep puncture (wound that reaches fat tissue or bone)?
• Deep partial thickness or full thickness burn?[a]
Yes
No
Assess wound:
• Large (>2 cm)?
• Gaping?
• Visible foreign material or dirt despite irrigation?
• Fat, muscle or bone exposed?
• Severe pain?
• Signs of infection, i.e., erythema, pain, heat at site of wound, discharge that is unexpected and discoloured, abnormal smell, delayed wound healing?
• Bleeding longer than 10 min (15 min if anticoagulated)?
• Stitches required, i.e., larger cuts where edges won't stay together, are jagged or wound is deep?
• Chronic (not healed after 3 wk)?
Yes
Patient requires further assessment and/or treatment
Yes
No
Self-care measures:
• Cleanse, stop bleeding, apply dressing (see Nonpharmacologic Therapy)
• Topical antibiotics if risk or signs of infection present (see Pharmacologic Choices)
Reassessment/follow up:
• Increased pain?
• Signs of infection after 48 h?
• Continuing to weep?
• Not healing within 3 wk?

[a] See Chapter 57: Burns.

Table 3: Topical Antibacterials for Minor Cuts and Wounds

Class	Drug	Dosage	Adverse Effects	Comments	Cost[a]
Antibacterials, miscellaneous	*bacitracin* Bacitracin USP, generics	Apply daily–TID	Common: Localized itching and burning. Relatively common sensitizer.	Spectrum: Mostly gram-positive, minimal gram-negative. Common co-reactions with neomycin (not a true cross-reaction). Possible cross-reaction with polymyxin B. Resistance uncommon but can develop with prolonged use.	$
	fusidic acid Fucidin	Apply BID–TID	Dryness, itching, burning, local irritation.	Spectrum: Gram-positives.	$$$
	mupirocin Bactroban, generics	Apply BID–TID	Dryness, itching, burning, local irritation.	Spectrum: Gram-positives including some strains of MRSA (resistance is developing).	$$
Antibacterial combinations	*bacitracin/gramicidin/polymyxin B* Polysporin Products, generics	Apply daily–TID	Common: Localized itching and burning. Bacitracin component is a relatively common sensitizer.	Spectrum: Gramicidin: Gram-positives. Polymyxin B: Gram-negatives. Ingredients are combined to provide broad antibacterial coverage. Resistance uncommon but can develop with prolonged use.	$
	bacitracin/neomycin/polymyxin B Neosporin Ointment, generics	Apply daily–TID	See bacitracin/gramicidin/polymyxin B.	Spectrum: Neomycin: Gram-positives and gram-negatives. Ingredients are combined to provide broad antibacterial coverage. Resistance uncommon but can develop with prolonged use.	$

[a] Cost of 15 g; includes drug cost only.

Legend: $ <$5 $$ $5–10 $$$ $10–15

Suggested Readings

Canadian Association of Wound Care. Available from: www.cawc.net.

Dufour A. Wound care. CE lesson. *Pharmacy Practice* 2007;CE1-8.

Health Canada. First Nations and Inuit Health Branch (FNIHB) Clinical Practice Guidelines for Nurses in Primary Care. Adult care. Chapter 9. Skin. *Dermatological emergencies. Skin wounds of traumatic origin*. Available from: www.hc-sc.gc.ca/fniah-spnia/services/nurs-infirm/clini/adult/skin-peau-eng.php#sw1.

Singer AJ, Dagum AB. Current management of acute cutaneous wounds. *N Engl J Med* 2008;359:1037-46.

References

1. Dufour A. Wound care. CE lesson. *Pharmacy Practice* 2007;CE1-8.
2. Lammers RL. Principles of wound management. In: Roberts JR, Hedges JR, eds. *Clinical procedures in emergency medicine*. 3rd ed. Philadelphia: Saunders; 1998. p. 533-9.
3. Eastman SR. Basics of wound care. *US Pharm* 1996;21:91-8.
4. Quinn JV, Polevoi SK, Kohn MA. Traumatic lacerations: what are the risks for infection and has the "golden period" of laceration care disappeared? *Emerg Med J* 2014;31:96-100.
5. Korting HC, Schollmann C, White RJ. Management of minor acute cutaneous wounds: importance of wound healing in a moist environment. *J Eur Acad Dermatol Venereol* 2011;25:130-8.
6. Shields K. Scar reduction products. *Pharmacist's Letter* 2004;20(200704).
7. Fernandez R, Griffiths R. Water for wound cleansing. *Cochrane Database Syst Rev* 2012;2:CD003861.
8. Pray S. Caring for minor wounds. *US Pharm* 2006;31:16-23.
9. Sweetman SC, ed. *Martindale: the complete drug reference*. 35th ed. London: Pharmaceutical Press; 2007.
10. World Wide Wounds. Collier M. *Recognition and management of wound infections*. Available from: www.worldwidewounds.com/2004/january/Collier/Management-of-Wound-infections.html. Accessed August 7, 2014.
11. Sibbald RG, Orsted HL, Coutts PM et al. Best practice recommendations for preparing the wound bed: update 2006. *Wound Care Canada* 2006;41:15-29. Available from: cawc.net/images/uploads/wcc/4-1-vol4no1-BP-WBP.pdf.
12. Health Canada. First Nations and Inuit Health Branch (FNIHB) Clinical Practice Guidelines for Nurses in Primary Care. Adult care. Chapter 9. Skin. *Dermatological emergencies. Skin wounds of traumatic origin*. Available from: www.hc-sc.gc.ca/fniah-spnia/services/nurs-infirm/clini/adult/skin-peau-eng.php#sw1. Accessed April 14, 2016.
13. Dire DJ, Coppola DO, Dwyer DA et al. Prospective evaluation of topical antibiotics for preventing infections in uncomplicated soft-tissue wounds repaired in the ED. *Acad Emerg Med* 1995;2:4-10.
14. Maddox JS, Ware JC, Dillon HC. The natural history of streptococcal skin infection: prevention with topical antibiotics. *J Am Acad Derm* 1985;13:207-12.
15. Wasiak J, Cleland H, Campbell F et al. Dressings for superficial and partial thickness burns. *Cochrane Database Syst Rev* 2013;3:CD002106.
16. Lipsky BA, Berendt AR, Deery HG et al. Diagnosis and treatment of diabetic foot infections. *Clin Infect Dis* 2004;39:885-910.
17. Worster B, Zawora MQ, Hsieh C. Common questions about wound care. *Am Fam Physician* 2015;91:86-92.
18. Liu C, Bayer A, Cosgrove SE et al. Clinical practice guidelines by the infectious diseases society of America for the treatment of methicillin-resistant Staphylococcus Aureus infections in adults and children. *Clin Infect Dis* 2011;52:1-38.
19. Elston DM. Topical antibiotics in dermatology: emerging patterns of resistance. *Dermatol Clin* 2009;27:25-31.
20. Dat AD, Poon F, Pham KB et al. Aloe vera for treating acute and chronic wounds. *Cochrane Database Syst Rev* 2012;2:CD008762.
21. Jull AB, Cullum N, Dumville JC et al. Honey as a topical treatment for wounds. *Cochrane Database Syst Rev* 2015;3:CD005083.
22. Combest WL. Aloe vera. *US Pharm* 2000;25:64-74.

Minor Cuts and Wounds—What You Need to Know

Tips to treat minor cuts and wounds:

- Clean the wound with soap and drinkable tap water to remove dirt and debris from the wound area. Do not use hydrogen peroxide or rubbing alcohol directly on the wound as they can be irritating and interfere with healing.
- If possible, use running water or water under gentle pressure to clean the wound. A squirt bottle containing water or a large syringe with no needle can be used.
- Stop the bleeding by applying gentle pressure to the wound using a sterile gauze or clean dressing. Apply pressure for 10 minutes (15 minutes if the person is taking blood thinners) and if the bleeding does not stop refer the patient for further medical treatment.
- Remove any pieces of dirt or other material (such as glass, metal or gravel) from the wound. Use a pair of tweezers soaked in rubbing alcohol or rub gently with a clean gauze pad.
- The dressing should be changed daily or more often if it appears dirty or damp. Some dressings can be left on longer and are designed to be able to monitor the wound without disturbing it.
- When changing the dressing, monitor for signs of infection such as:
  - red, puffy areas around the wound that are tender to touch
  - red streaks coming from the wound
  - throbbing pain in the wound area
  - pus (creamy yellowish-grey fluid) in the wound

  Other signs of infection include fever, chills or tender lumps or swelling in your armpit, groin or neck.

The dressing can be removed after 48 hours if the wound is healing well.

Chapter 69
Parasitic Skin Infections: Lice and Scabies

Penny F. Miller, BSc(Pharm), MA

Lice (Pediculosis)
Pathophysiology

Lice are tiny, blood-sucking insects that are specific parasites of humans. Outbreaks in institutions such as schools and long-term care facilities are common with an estimated prevalence of 1–3% in elementary school-aged children.[1] Three species of lice exist: head lice (*Pediculus humanus capitis*), body lice (*Pediculus humanus corporis*) and pubic lice (*Phthirus pubis* or "crabs").

Lice are 1–4 mm long with 3 pairs of legs that end with claws. Head and pubic lice live on the skin, whereas body lice live in the seams of clothing. The adult female life cycle is up to 30 days and she lays 7–10 eggs daily. The body louse lays her eggs in clothing, while head and pubic lice lay their eggs at the base of hair shafts, cemented to the hair in egg casings called nits. Eggs hatch 8–10 days later and undergo 3 nymph stages to eventually mature into adult forms within 8–15 days (head and body) or 14–22 days (pubic). Lice are obligate human parasites and survival time off the human host varies: 4 days for head lice, 3 days for body lice, and 3 days for pubic lice. Female lice can mate and begin to lay viable eggs approximately 1.5 days after becoming adults. Nits can survive away from the human host for up to 10 days. In contrast to head and pubic lice, the body louse is a vector of human diseases such as typhus, relapsing fever, trench fever and endocarditis.

Transmission of head lice is by hair-to-hair contact and by fomites such as clothing or hair accessories. Pubic lice are transmitted via sexual or close body contact and fomites such as bed linens and towels. Body lice move from host to host only through shared clothing and linens. Poor hygiene has a major role only in the epidemiology of body lice.[2,3,4,5,6]

Head Lice

Pruritus, particularly around the back and sides of the scalp, is the main symptom of lice infestation. Physical examination of the scalp should detect nits (eggs) attached to the base of hair shafts in the warmer parts of the scalp (back and sides). The height of the nits above the scalp indicates how long the infestation has been present on the growing hair. Itchy papules can develop as a hypersensitivity reaction to the louse saliva or fecal material. Secondary bacterial infection may occur as a result of scratching.[2,3,4,5,7]

Body Lice

The body louse lives and lays eggs in the seams of clothing and usually emerges at night to take a blood meal from the host. Consequently, nocturnal pruritus is a common symptom. Erythematous papules with a central puncture point (bite sites) are evident often around the waist and axillae where seams of clothing contact the skin. Occasionally, bite sites reveal sky-blue or slate-coloured macules known as maculae ceruleae, the result of injected louse anticoagulant saliva during feeding. Hypersensitivity reactions to the bites can develop and the resultant pruritus is accompanied by excoriations that may become secondarily infected. Lice and eggs are found in clothing seams.[2,3,4,5]

Pubic Lice

Nits attached at the base of pubic hair follicles are more difficult to find than those of head lice. The lice may appear as small, yellow-brown to grey dots. Small brown specks on undergarments result from lice excreta. With heavy infestations, bite sites may reveal a blue-gray skin discoloration (maculae ceruleae). Pruritus in the genital area is the main symptom; hypersensitivity reactions and secondary infections are also possible.

Eyelashes, eyebrows, beards and other hairy areas can also be infested with pubic lice. Itching, burning and eye irritation can occur when the eyelashes are involved.[2,3,4,5,8]

Goals of Therapy

- Exterminate head, body or pubic lice
- Relieve pruritus
- Prevent secondary bacterial infections
- Prevent spread of the infestation

Patient Assessment

Patients with recurrent or unresponsive head lice or pubic lice require further assessment and/or treatment by an appropriate healthcare practitioner. Characteristics of the 3 types of lice are compared in Table 1.

Table 1: **Assessment of Lice**[4,9]

Characteristic	Head Lice	Body Lice	Pubic Lice
Type of primary lesions	Papules	Papules	Papules
Type of secondary lesions	Excoriations, crusts; pustules with secondary infections Enlarged cervical and nuchal lymph nodes	Linear excoriations, crusts; pustules with secondary infections	Excoriations, crusts; blue-grey pigmentation; pustules with secondary infections
Distribution of lesions and pruritus	Scalp	Waist and axillae (trunk)	Pubic area (uncommonly, eyelashes, eyebrows, beard or axillae)
Presence of lice or nits	Scalp hair	Seams of clothing	Pubic hair (also eyelashes, eyebrows, beard or axillae)
Transmission	Head-to-head contact; sharing hats or combs	Clothing or bedding; conditions of poor hygiene	Sexual exposure to an infected person
Differential diagnosis	Dandruff Seborrheic dermatitis Accumulation of hair cosmetics	Seborrheic dermatitis Flea bites or other insect bites Eczema Impetigo Folliculitis	Seborrheic dermatitis Folliculitis Dermatophytosis
Host	Children	Persons with poor hygiene	Sexually active adults

The diagnosis of head lice is established by identifying live lice, which can be difficult since lice crawl quickly and avoid light. The most reliable method of detecting head lice is called "wet combing with conditioner".[10,11]

This method requires that white coloured hair conditioner is maximally applied to all of the hair, first combing from the base of the hair to the end with a regular comb, then with a nit comb. The remaining material in the comb should be checked for live lice which should be discarded in tissue; the combing procedure should be repeated 5 times for each area of hair.[12]

Nonpharmacologic Therapy

Contact with infected persons promotes the spread of the infestation. Avoid sharing personal items such as clothing, combs, hats and bedding of an infected person.

Clothes, linens, scarves and hats should be dry cleaned, washed in hot water and dried in the hot cycle for 15 minutes, or stored in plastic bags for 2 weeks. Furniture should be vacuumed. Combs and brushes should be soaked in hot water for 5–10 minutes or washed with a pediculicide shampoo.[4,7,11,13]

A combing method known as "bug busting" requires combing of wet hair for 30 minutes every third or fourth day using a fine-toothed comb, for 2 weeks. This method is considered unfeasible on a widespread basis but may be an option for motivated caregivers of children with short, straight or wavy hair. Trials comparing wet combing with placebo, permethrin or malathion as a primary treatment for head lice have yielded conflicting results, possibly because of varying insecticide resistance.[9,14,15,16]

It is well known that body lice die via desiccation when exposed to hot air (51°C) for 5 minutes. In an attempt to use this method for the treatment of head lice, the LouseBuster was developed. It is a high-volume, hot-air blower with a hand piece supporting a coarse-tooth comb device. One trial investigated 6 methods of delivery of hot air treatments and found the LouseBuster to be the most effective.[17] One 30-minute application of hot air resulted in nearly 100% mortality of eggs and 80% mortality of hatched lice. However, since only 11 children treated with this method had follow up and subjects with a high probability of reinfestation were excluded, valid conclusions on clinical effectiveness cannot be made. The machine is expensive and requires special training to use.[18] A regular blow dryer should be avoided as it can cause live lice to be airborne and spread to others nearby.[19]

Pharmacologic Therapy

The best choice of a pediculicide depends on local resistance patterns, safety considerations and ease of administration. See Table 5 for more information.

For comparative ingredients of nonprescription products, consult the *Compendium of Products for Minor Ailments*—Skin Care Products: Pediculicides.

Head Lice

The insecticides **permethrin** and **pyrethrins with piperonyl butoxide** and the physically acting agents **isopropyl myristate/cyclomethicone** and **dimeticones (dimethicones)** have demonstrated efficacy and lack of toxicity in the treatment of head lice.[14,16] Table 5 provides information on the mechanism of action, precautions, directions for use, efficacy, safety and adverse effects of these 4 treatments for head lice. **Lindane** is also an effective pediculicide; however, there are concerns about possible neurotoxicity, bone marrow suppression and carcinogenicity following percutaneous absorption.[4,32,33] Lindane is no longer available in Canada.

Family members and close contacts should be examined and treated if infested. Bed mates should be treated prophylactically.[7,11,34]

After treatment, nits will remain attached to the hair. The female louse secretes a cement-like fixative to hold her eggs in place on the hair strand. This fixative material works as a simple holdfast and not a chemical adhesive. To loosen louse nits, lubricants such as hair conditioners can assist in sliding the eggshells along the hair shaft. Commercial nit removal products have no proven efficacy.[35,36] Several other methods of removing nits have been suggested. The glue by which nits are attached can be loosened by soaking the hair with **white vinegar** (3–5% **acetic acid**), wrapping the hair in a towel (soaked in the vinegar) for 30–60 minutes and rinsing with water afterwards. Although the clinical benefit has not been documented,[31] the nits may then be more easily removed with a fine-toothed metal nit comb.[5]

The "no-nit" policy requiring children be free of nits before returning to school has not been effective in mitigating outbreaks. Consequently, it is recommended that parents of an affected child be notified, and that the child not be sent home early but receive treatment with an effective pediculicide that evening, and return to school the next morning.[7,11,20,34]

Head Lice Treatment Failures

Treatment failure can occur due to misdiagnosis, improper use of pediculicide (e.g., hair not saturated from scalp to ends or product not left on hair long enough), not repeating the treatment after 7–10 days, reapplication too soon after initial application, inadequate manual removal of nits, repeated exposure to lice (reinfestation) or resistance to a pediculicide.

Some pediculicides rely on neurotoxic effects to kill lice. Resistance to pyrethrins and permethrin has developed in countries with heavy pediculicide usage such as France, Czech Republic, Ireland, the United Kingdom and the United States.[37] Formal collection of resistance patterns has not been done in Canada so the prevalence of resistance is unknown. In countries with documented resistance, the appropriate choice has been dependent on local resistance patterns, which continue to change.[38,39,40]

When a properly applied treatment fails, try switching to a product of a different pharmacologic class.[3] A number of alternative therapies have been investigated for difficult cases unresponsive to the usual agents. **Permethrin** 5% cream (officially indicated only for scabies treatment) left on the hair overnight covered with a plastic shower cap[41] or oral **ivermectin** 200 µg/kg repeated in 7–10 days[42] (available through the Special Access Programme in Canada) or the combination of oral **sulfamethoxazole/trimethoprim** (10 mg/kg per day of trimethoprim usually twice daily for 10 days) plus **permethrin** 1% applied for 10 minutes on day 1 and day 7 may be effective for cases resistant to all topical pediculicides.[43] Ivermectin is not recommended in children weighing <15 kg.[6] Itching does not necessarily mean that a reinfestation has occurred. Itching can be caused by an inflammatory response to the pediculicide and may persist for several days after treatment. An **oral antihistamine** or low-potency **topical corticosteroid** may be required for relief.[4]

Suffocation-based treatments with occlusive agents may only partially impede lice ventilation. Examples of occlusive agents are petroleum jelly (Vaseline), Cetaphil cleanser, and mayonnaise. Instead of lungs, lice have air channels throughout their body such as in the prothorax and abdomen areas, allowing the diffusion of oxygen. These air channels can be closed by structures called spiracles and any occlusive agent would need to block 100% of the spiracles for asphyxiation to occur. The musculature of these spiracles responds much like a human cough to clear the airways and therefore smothering lice is difficult.[44,45]

Pubic Lice

The pediculicides used to treat head lice are effective for pubic lice (see Table 5). The recommended regimens are **permethrin** 1% cream rinse or **pyrethrins with piperonyl butoxide** applied to affected areas then washed off after 10 minutes, with retreatment in 7–9 days.[8]

If eyelashes are infested, nits and lice can be removed with tweezers, followed by an application of **white petrolatum** twice daily for 10 days to asphyxiate the remaining lice. More data are needed to determine the efficacy of occlusive agents such as petroleum jelly, olive oil or mayonnaise.[46]

Sexual contacts within the previous month should be treated if infested. Again, itching caused by the pediculicide can be treated with an **oral antihistamine** or **topical corticosteroid**.[4]

Body Lice

Pediculicides are unnecessary. Simple hygienic measures, including bathing and laundering of infested clothing and linens in hot water, are effective management. Alternative strategies for items that cannot be washed include dry cleaning or storing the items in a sealed plastic bag for 2 weeks.[5]

If lice are adherent to body hairs, pediculicides may be helpful.[4,5]

Natural Health Products

Several natural health products are used as alternative pediculicides (e.g., anacyclus pyrethrum, anamirta, chrysanthemum flowers, delphinium, field scabious, henna, tea tree oil, black pepper, ranunculus). There is insufficient clinical evidence of efficacy for any of these herbs.[14,47]

Lavender oil and **tea tree oil** are often used in toiletries and in products to treat head lice. They have been associated with cases of prepubertal gynecomastia in boys with normal endogenous steroid levels.[48]

Monitoring of Therapy

After treatment of head and pubic lice, the dead nits will still be attached to the hair. They can be removed with fingertips, tweezers or a fine-toothed (nit) comb. Observe for any recurrence of lice and nits. Further assessment and/or treatment is required for patients with recurrent or unresponsive head lice or pubic lice following 2 treatments with recommended therapy.

For body lice infestations, inspect clothing and other personal items for the presence of lice.

A secondary bacterial skin infection with redness and pus may develop and may require topical antibacterial treatment. A monitoring plan for patients with pediculosis can be found in Table 2.

Table 2: **Monitoring of Therapy for Lice**[4,9]

Symptoms	Monitoring	Endpoint of Treatment	Actions
Detection of live lice	Patient: Daily for 2 wk	Absence of live lice 24 h after applying pediculicide	Treat again with pediculicide 7–10 days after initial application to eradicate any recently hatched immature nymphs. Presence of adult lice may indicate resistance and need for change of therapy.
Presence of nits	Patient: Daily for 2 wk	Absence of nits	Vinegar, nit comb to physically remove dead nits.
Pruritus	Patient: Daily for 2 wk	Relief of pruritus	Oral antihistamines, topical corticosteroids.
Inflammatory pustules	Patient: Daily for 2 wk	Clearing of any lesions and return to normal appearance of the skin within 1 wk of treatment	If mild, topical antibiotics (e.g., bacitracin/polymyxin B). If unresponsive or extensive, systemic antibiotics may be necessary.

Scabies

Pathophysiology

Scabies is a highly contagious infestation of the skin with the human mite, *Sarcoptes scabiei* var *hominis*. It can occur across all socioeconomic levels, but women and children have a higher number of infestations than men. Cycles of epidemics every 7–15 years occur in crowded living conditions and in institutions.[49,50]

Scabies infestations are most commonly transmitted through close personal contact, particularly sexual contact. Spread by fomites such as furniture and towels is rare unless they were in contact with patients who had a very high parasite load.[51] The impregnated female mite, which has a rounded body and 4 pairs of legs, burrows (creates a tunnel) into the uppermost layer (stratum corneum) of the epidermis, depositing feces along its path, and lays 2 or 3 eggs daily. She remains in the burrow and continues to lay eggs for her lifespan of 4–6 weeks.[52] Three or 4 days later, the eggs hatch into larvae with 6 legs that travel from the burrow to the skin surface where they mature into adult mites within 14–17 days. On warm skin, mites are capable of crawling 2.5 cm per minute. The smaller male mite lives predominantly on the skin surface and dies shortly after mating with the female mite. Patients typically harbour an average of 10–12 mites.[4,5,53]

Scabies can survive off the human host for an average of 2–36 hours at room temperature (21°C and relative humidity of 40–80%). In a cool, humid environment, survival is increased to about 19 days.[54]

With a first infection, intense pruritus that is worse at night occurs after 3–4 weeks as a result of sensitization to the mites, eggs or feces. After a reinfestation, pruritus may occur within 24–48 hours. Burrows (white or grey wavy lines) may be apparent, and an immune response to the scabies mite results in erythematous papules or vesicles. The face and scalp are spared in adults but not in infants and young children. Scratching leads to excoriations that may become secondarily infected with *Staphylococcus aureus* or *Streptococci pyogenes* leading to pustules, furunculosis and impetigo. In areas of high prevalence, scabies is a risk factor for developing acute poststreptococcal glomerulonephritis.[50,51,52] See Scabies in Photo Section.

Immunocompromised hosts such as patients with HIV infection or lymphoma or institutionalized elderly persons may develop an atypical, hyperkeratotic and more contagious form of scabies called crusted scabies (also referred to as Norwegian scabies). Patients present with pronounced thickened skin patches especially affecting the scalp, hands and feet but may be generalized. The lesions may be malodorous, and pruritus is minimal. Infested persons have huge numbers of mites (e.g., hundreds of thousands) and this infection carries a high mortality rate due to secondary infection and sepsis.[50,52]

Goals of Therapy

- Exterminate the scabies mite
- Relieve the pruritus
- Prevent secondary bacterial infections
- Prevent the spread of the infestation

Patient Assessment

Intense pruritus that worsens at night is the most common presenting symptom. Affected patients exhibit silvery lines known as burrows on the hands (especially the web spaces), flexor surfaces of the wrists and genitalia, but occasionally other sites such as the axillae, buttocks and nipples may be involved. Papules may be present on the trunk. Children may have atypical lesions but they are often concentrated on hands, feet, scalp and body folds.[7] Table 3 provides characteristics and differential diagnosis of scabies.

Suspect scabies in all patients with a pruritic rash, especially if it worsens at night. Papules appearing on the genitalia and breasts when other household members have similar signs and symptoms strengthen the diagnosis. However, a definitive diagnosis should be made by an appropriate healthcare practitioner prior to treatment.[52]

Definitive diagnosis is made by mounting scrapings from nonexcoriated burrows, papules or vesicles in potassium hydroxide onto a slide and examining under direct microscopy. Any sign of a mite, eggs or fecal material is a positive test.[57,58]

Table 3: **Characteristics and Differential Diagnosis of Scabies[55,56]**

Condition	Lesions	Distribution	Differential Diagnosis
Scabies	Primary lesions are linear or wavy burrows (2–5 mm long) with papules and vesicles near burrows. Secondary lesions as a result of excessive scratching are excoriations or eczema. Secondary infections with impetigo or pustules are possible.	Fingerwebs, wrists, sides of hands and feet, axillae, groin, breasts, belt line.	Flea or insect bites: Lesions are usually single or multiple papules. Atopic dermatitis: Distribution is behind knees or in fold of elbows. Seborrheic dermatitis: Scales in a distribution involving the scalp and face. Impetigo: Exhibits honey-coloured exudates and crusting; this may appear as a secondary infection.

Nonpharmacologic Therapy

Clothes and linens should be washed in soap and hot water (60°C) and machine dried using the hot cycle, dry cleaned, or stored in plastic bags for 5–7 days. All surfaces, rugs, furniture and unwashable items should be vacuumed. Avoid body contact with others until completion of treatment and follow up. Children may return to school the day after treatment is completed.[59] Fingernails should be closely trimmed to prevent skin injury resulting from excessive scratching.[60]

Pharmacologic Therapy

There is insufficient evidence to determine the effectiveness of the traditional recommendation to treat close contacts of patients with scabies prophylactically.[61] However, the Public Health Agency of Canada recommends preventive treatment of sexual partners within the last month[62] and the Canadian Pediatric Society recommends treatment of all household contacts whether symptomatic or not.[63] The US Centers for Disease Control recommends that close contacts within the month preceding the infestation should be examined and treated if infested.[60]

For comparative ingredients of nonprescription products, consult the *Compendium of Products for Minor Ailments*—Skin Care Products: Scabicides.

Topical Therapy

Permethrin 5% is an insecticide that appears to be more effective than all other scabicides,[64,65,66] and it is the preferred treatment for adults and children >2 months of age.[60,62] Comparative trials of other scabicides including **crotamiton** and **sulfur** have produced equivocal results suggesting there is no most effective second-line agent.[64,67] Topical permethrin may be more effective at reducing persistent itch than **crotamiton**.[65] There are limited human studies of permethrin in pregnancy;[68] however, less than 2% of the topical dose of permethrin is absorbed and it is considered the drug of choice for treating scabies in pregnant and breastfeeding women.[62,69]

Topical **sulfur** has many mechanisms of action including keratolytic, fungicidal, parasiticidal and antibacterial activity. Its germicidal activity may be the result of conversion to pentathionic acid by epidermal cells or by certain microorganisms. In organisms without lungs, such as insects or plants, sulfur prevents respiration. There is limited evidence of efficacy[64,70] but it is often recommended in a petrolatum base as the preferred therapy in infants <2 months of age due to low risk of toxicity.[62,63] Odour and mess associated with application reduce adherence and limit use. Sulfur is considered a second-line agent.

Crotamiton 10% cream is an antiparasitic agent with an unknown mechanism of action. It reduces itch via a counterirritant effect (creates a cooling sensation as it evaporates from the skin). Crotamiton is less effective than permethrin[71] and resistance has been reported.[65,72] It is considered a second-line agent.

Lindane is an effective scabicide; however, there are concerns about possible neurotoxicity, bone marrow suppression and carcinogenicity following percutaneous absorption.[4,32,33] Lindane is no longer available in Canada.

Information on topical therapies for the treatment of scabies can be found in Table 6.

Systemic Therapy

Severe or resistant forms of scabies such as crusted (Norwegian) forms, infections in persons with HIV or outbreaks in institutions are more difficult to treat and the failure rate is significant with the usual treatments. Oral **ivermectin** is often recommended in these situations. Ivermectin is a broad-spectrum antiparasitic agent commonly used worldwide for various parasitic infections. No serious drug-related adverse events have been reported. Adverse effects include fever, headache, chills, arthralgia, rash, eosinophilia and anorexia. Many of these symptoms are thought to result from the death of parasites rather than adverse effects from the drug. Low levels of ivermectin are detected in the CNS as it concentrates in the liver and fat tissue. No significant drug interactions have been reported. It is not recommended for children <15 kg or in pregnancy and breastfeeding since safety is unknown.[76] Oral ivermectin is available in Canada only through Health Canada's Special Access Programme.

Resistant or severe scabies can be treated with oral ivermectin 200 µg/kg orally, repeated in 2 weeks.[60] In the treatment of crusted (Norweigan) scabies, oral ivermectin 200 µg/kg as a single dose has limited evidence of efficacy but is considered likely to be beneficial.[65] To prevent resistance and improve efficacy, a combination of ivermectin 200 µg/kg on days 1, 2, 8, 9 and 15 (and days 22 and 29 in severe, unresponsive cases) along with topical permethrin 5% cream daily for 7 days then twice weekly until cure is achieved, is often recommended.[60] A concern about increased deaths in elderly people receiving this combination[77] has not been confirmed with further study.

Institutional epidemics of scabies occur frequently in hospitals, nursing homes, residential facilities, and other isolated communities. Control of an epidemic can best be achieved by treating the entire population at risk. Ivermectin 200 ug/kg (repeated in 7–14 days) can be considered in these settings, especially if treatment with topical scabicides fails or is too difficult to coordinate. Epidemics should be managed in consultation with a specialist.[60,78,79,80]

Monitoring of Therapy

The appearance of new burrows at any stage after treatment is an indication for further treatment. Itch resulting from an immune allergic response to the mite can persist for up to 4 weeks and may be relieved with topical corticosteroids and/or oral antihistamines or crotamiton.[81,82] Mites separated from the host die in 72 hours. Table 4 presents a monitoring plan for patients with scabies.

Table 4: **Monitoring of Therapy for Scabies**[83,84]

Symptoms	Monitoring	Endpoint of Treatment	Actions
Burrows	Patient: Daily for the following 2 wk Healthcare practitioner: Next visit	Clearing of burrows over the following 2 wk and return to normal skin appearance.	If new burrows are detected, then retreatment with a scabicide is necessary. Ensure nonpharmacologic measures are utilized.
Papules	Patient: Daily for the following 2 wk Healthcare practitioner: Next visit	Clearing of papules and return to normal skin appearance.	If new papules are detected, then retreatment with a scabicide is necessary after 7–10 days. Ensure nonpharmacologic measures are utilized.
Pruritus	Patient: Daily for several wk Healthcare practitioner: Next visit	Itching should resolve within several (up to 4) wk. Itching beyond 4 wk requires reinvestigation of the cause.[82]	If itching persists for several weeks, then antihistamines, topical corticosteroids or crotamiton may be tried as antipruritic agents.[72,85]
Pustules, impetigo	Patient: Daily for several wk Healthcare practitioner: Next visit	This secondary infection should improve with 3 days of topical antibacterial (bacitracin/polymyxin B) treatment.	If no improvement or worsening within 3 days of treatment, patient requires further assessment and/or treatment.

Table 5: **Topical Therapy for the Treatment of Head Lice[11,20,21,22,23,24,25,26,27,28]**

Class	Drug	Mechanism of Action	Administration Instructions	Adverse Effects	Comments	Cost[a]
Pediculicides	*dimeticone 50%* NYDA	Noninsecticidal, physically acting agent; penetrates spiracles causing suffocation or inhibition of water excretion resulting in gut rupture from osmotic stress. Cure rate: 97% Ovicidal activity: 100% but second application still recommended due to imperfect application.[6]	Spray carefully all over dry hair. Massage in until hair is completely wetted with solution. Avoid contact with eyes. Leave solution on hair. After 30 min, comb the hair with a lice comb. Allow the solution to dry on the hair for at least 8 h and then wash. Repeat after 8–10 days.	Mild itching, ocular irritation	Not recommended for infants or children younger than 2 y. Resistance to product is unlikely due to physical mode of action. No data on safety during pregnancy and breastfeeding. Mixture is volatile; keep away from open flame, sources of ignition, lit cigarettes.	$$$
	isopropyl myristate/ cyclomethicone Resultz	Noninsecticidal, physically acting agent; dissolves the louse exoskeleton, leading to death from dehydration. Cure rate: 57–93%[29,30]	Apply to dry hair and scalp (30–60 mL for short hair, 60–90 mL for shoulder-length hair, 90–120 mL for long hair). Allow product to remain on hair and scalp for 10 min. Rinse off with warm water. Repeat in 7 days.	Local irritation with mild erythema and scalp pruritus If contact with eyes, immediately flush well with water.	Not recommended for infants or children younger than 2 y. Resistance to product is unlikely due to physical mode of action. No data on safety during pregnancy and breastfeeding.	$$
	permethrin 1% Kwellada-P Creme Rinse, Nix Creme Rinse	Synthetic pyrethroid; disrupts sodium channels, to delay repolarization causing respiratory paralysis of louse. Cure rate: 96–100% Ovicidal activity: 70–80%	Wash hair with conditioner-free shampoo, rinse with water and towel dry. Apply permethrin to saturate the hair and scalp (one-half to 1 bottle for adults and children with long hair); leave on for 10 min then rinse. May repeat after 7 days if live lice are observed.	Mild, transient itching, redness and swelling. Uncommon adverse effects include burning, stinging, rash, tingling and numbness.	Drug of choice for most patients. Contraindicated in patients with chrysanthemum allergy. Permethrin resistance may result in treatment failure. Compatible with pregnancy and breastfeeding.	$

(cont'd)

Table 5: Topical Therapy for the Treatment of Head Lice[11,20,21,22,23,24,25,26,27,28] *(cont'd)*

Class	Drug	Mechanism of Action	Administration Instructions	Adverse Effects	Comments	Cost[a]
	pyrethrins/piperonyl butoxide R&C Shampoo	Naturally occurring pyrethroid: disrupts sodium channels, to delay repolarization causing respiratory paralysis of louse. Piperonyl butoxide is added to inhibit pyrethrin breakdown. Cure rate: 45% after 1 application; 94% after 2 applications.	Apply to thoroughly saturate dry hair and massage scalp/skin; leave on for 10 min. Add a little water; work the shampoo into the hair and skin to form a lather. Rinse thoroughly. Repeat treatment in 7 days.	Contact dermatitis due to the petroleum distillates used for solvent purposes in the formulation.	Contraindicated in patients allergic to ragweed, chrysanthemums or other pyrethrin products. Compatible with pregnancy and breastfeeding.	$

[a] Cost of smallest available pack size; includes drug cost only.

Legend: $ <$10 $$ $10–20 $$$ $20–30

Table 6: Topical Therapy for the Treatment of Scabies

Class	Drug	Administration Instructions	Adverse Effects	Comments	Cost[a]
Scabicides	*crotamiton 10%* Eurax cream	Massage into all skin areas, from the neck down to the soles of the feet; every bit of skin must be treated, including the fingernails, waist and genitalia. In infants and young children, the entire head and neck should also be treated; repeat in 24 h. Do not wash off until 48 h after last application.	Local irritation.	Less effective than permethrin.[71] Considered second-line treatment. Resistance has been reported.[65,72] Multiple applications recommended.[73] Not recommended for patients with exudative or vesicular dermatitis. Low toxicity and beneficial antipruritic effect. Possible second-line treatment during pregnancy and breastfeeding.[69]	$$
	permethrin 5%[b] Kwellada-P Lotion, Nix Dermal Cream	Massage into all skin areas, from the neck down to the soles of the feet; every bit of skin must be treated, including the fingernails, waist and genitalia. In infants and young children, the entire head and neck should also be treated. Leave on for 8–14 h without interruption, then wash off (shower may be the best way).	Pruritus, edema and erythema.	Drug of choice for scabies in adults and children >2 months.[57,64,66,65] Resistance of scabies to permethrin is rare.[73,74] Contraindicated in patients allergic to chrysanthemums. Second administration 1 wk after first often recommended.[3] Recommended during pregnancy and breastfeeding.[60,68,75]	Cream: $$ Lotion: $$$
	sulfur 5–10%[c]	Apply to all skin areas[d] QHS for 5–7 days. Infants <2 months: 8–10% in petrolatum. Apply to all skin areas[d] QHS for 3 days.[63]	Local irritation or dermatitis with repeated applications.	Limited study data to support use.[64,70] Considered a second-line treatment. Not popular because it is malodorous, requires multiple applications and stains clothing. Extemporaneously compounded. Possible second-line treatment during pregnancy and breastfeeding.[69]	$

[a] Cost of smallest available pack size; includes drug cost only.

[b] Lower strengths are not effective as scabicides.

[c] Extermoraneously compounded preparations can be used.

[d] As for permethrin.

Legend: $ <$10 $$ $10–20 $$$ $20–30

Suggested Readings

Chosidow O. Clinical practices. Scabies. *N Engl J Med* 2006;354:1718-27.

Gunning K, Pipitt K, Kiraly B et al. Pediculosis and scabies: treatment update. *Am Fam Physician* 2012;86:535-41.

Head lice infestations: a clinical update. *Paediatr Child Health* 2008;13:692-6. [Reaffirmed February 1, 2014].

Ko CJ, Elston DM. Pediculosis. *J Am Acad Dermatol* 2004;50:1-12.

References

1. Harris J, Crawshaw JG, Millership S. Incidence and prevalence of head lice in a district health authority area. *Commun Dis Public Health* 2003;6:246-9.
2. Burkhart CN, Burkhart CG. Scabies, other mites, and pediculosis. In: Goldsmith LA, Katz SI, Gilchrest BA et al. *Fitzpatrick's dermatology in general medicine*. 8th ed. New York: McGraw-Hill; 2012.
3. Chosidow O. Scabies and pediculosis. *Lancet* 2000;355:819-27.
4. Goldstein BG, Goldstein AO. *Pediculosis*. Available from: www.uptodate.com/login. Subscription required.
5. Ko CJ, Elston DM. Pediculosis. *J Am Acad Dermatol* 2004;50:1-12.
6. Feldmeier H. Treatment of pediculosis capitis: a critical appraisal of the current literature. *Am J Clin Dermatol* 2014;15:401-12.
7. Head lice infestations: a clinical update. *Paediatr Child Health* 2008;13:692-704.
8. Leone PA. Scabies and pediculosis pubis: an update of treatment regimens and general review. *Clin Infect Dis* 2007;44:S153-9.
9. Infestations and bites. In: Habif TP. *Clinical dermatology: a color guide to diagnosis and therapy.* 6th ed. St. Louis: Elsevier; 2015.
10. Jahnke C, Bauer E, Hengge UR et al. Accuracy of diagnosis of pediculosis capitis: visual inspection vs wet combing. *Arch Dermatol* 2009;145:309-13.
11. Devore CD, Schutze GE; Council on School Health and Committee on Infectious Diseases. Head lice. *Pediatrics* 2015;135:e1355-65.
12. Nova Scotia. Health Promotion and Protection. *Guidelines for treatment of pediculosis capitis (head lice)*. August 2008. Available from: novascotia.ca/dhw/publications/Public-Health-Education/Head_Lice_Guidelines_for_Treatment.pdf. Accessed August 23, 2015.
13. Izri A, Chosidow O. Efficacy of machine laundering to eradicate head lice: recommendations to decontaminate washable clothes, linens, and fomites. *Clin Infect Dis* 2006;42:e9-10.
14. Burgess I, Silverston P. Head lice. *BMJ Clin Evid* 2015 Jan 14;2015. pii: 1703.
15. Mumcuoglu KY, Barker SC, Burgess IF et al. International guidelines for effective control of head louse infestations. *J Drugs Dermatol* 2007;6:409-14.
16. Burgess IF. Head lice. *BMJ Clin Evid* 2011 May 16;2011. pii: 1703.
17. Goates BM, Atkin JS, Wilding KG et al. An effective non-chemical treatment for head lice: a lot of hot air. *Pediatrics* 2006;118:1962-70.
18. Tebruegge M, Pantazidou A, Curtis N. What's bugging you? An update on the treatment of head lice infestation. *Arch Dis Child Educ Pract Ed* 2011;96:2-8.
19. Frankowski BL, Bocchini JA; Council on School Health and Committee on Infectious Diseases. Head lice. *Pediatrics* 2010;126:392-403.
20. Head lice infestations: a clinical update. *Paediatr Child Health* 2008;13:692-6. [Reaffirmed February 1, 2014].
21. American Society of Health-System Pharmacists. *AHFS drug information*. Bethesda: American Society of Health-System Pharmacists; 2015.
22. Lebwohl M, Clark L, Levitt J. Therapy for head lice based on life cycle, resistance, and safety considerations. *Pediatrics* 2007;119:965-74.
23. Burgess IF, Brown CM, Lee PN. Treatment of head louse infestation with 4% dimeticone lotion: randomised controlled equivalence trial. *BMJ* 2005;330:1423.
24. Burgess IF, Lee PN, Matlock G. Randomised, controlled, assessor blind trial comparing 4% dimeticone lotion with 0.5% malathion liquid for head louse infestation. *PLoS One* 2007;2:e1127.
25. Kurt O, Balcioglu IC, Burgess IF et al. Treatment of head lice with dimeticone 4% lotion: comparison of two formulations in a randomised controlled trial in rural Turkey. *BMC Public Health* 2009;9:441.
26. Burgess IF. The mode of action of dimeticone 4% lotion against head lice, Pediculus capitis. *BMC Pharmacol* 2009;9:3.
27. Richling I, Bockeler W. Lethal effects of treatment with a special dimeticone formula on head lice and house crickets (Orthoptera, Ensifera: Acheta domestica and Anoplura, phthiraptera: Pediculus humanus). Insights into physical mechanisms. *Arzneimittelforschung* 2008;58:248-54.
28. Heukelbach J, Pilger D, Oliveira FA et al. A highly efficacious pediculicide based on dimeticone: randomized observer blinded comparative trial. *BMC Infect Dis* 2008;8:115.
29. Burgess IF, Lee PN, Brown CM. Randomized, controlled, parallel group of clinical trials to evaluate the efficacy of isopropyl myristate/cyclomethicone solution against head lice. *Pharm J* 2008;280:371-5.
30. Kaul N, Palma KG, Silagy SS et al. North American efficacy and safety of a novel pediculicide rinse, isopropyl myristate 50% (Resultz). *J Cutan Med Surg* 2007;11:161-7.
31. Burkhart CN, Burkhart CG, Pchalek I et al. The adherent cylindrical nit structure and its chemical denaturation in vitro: an assessment with therapeutic implications for head lice. *Arch Pediatr Adolesc Med* 1998;152:711-2.
32. Nolan K, Kamrath J, Levitt J. Lindane toxicity: a comprehensive review of the medical literature. *Pediatr Dermatol* 2012;29:141-6.
33. Loomis D, Guyton K, Grosse Y et al. Carcinogenicity of lindane, DDT, and 2,4-dichlorophenoxyacetic acid. *Lancet Oncol* 2015;16:891-2.
34. Frankowski BL, Weiner LB; Committee on School Health the Committee on Infectious Diseases. Head lice. *Pediatrics* 2002;110:638-43.
35. Burgess IF. Do nit removal formulations and other treatments loosen head louse eggs and nits from hair? *Med Vet Entomol* 2010;24:55-61.
36. Lapeere H, Brochez L, Verhaeghe E et al. Efficacy of products to remove eggs of Pediculosis humanus capitis (Phthiraptera: Pediculidae) from the human hair. *J Med Entomol* 2014;51:400-7.
37. Downs AM, Stafford KA, Harvey I et al. Evidence of double resistance to permethrin and malathion in head lice. *Br J Dermatol* 1999;141:508-11.

38. Meinking TL, Serrano L, Hard B et al. Comparative in vitro pediculicidal efficacy of treatments in a resistant head lice population in the United States. *Arch Dermatol* 2002;138:220-4.
39. Meinking TL, Entzel P, Villar ME et al. Comparative efficacy of treatments for pediculosis capitis infestations. *Arch Dermatol* 2001;137:287-92.
40. Durand R, Bouvresse S, Berdjane Z et al. Insecticide resistance in head lice: clinical, parasitological and genetic aspects. *Clin Microbiol Infect* 2012;18:338-44.
41. Schachner LA. Treatment resistant head lice: alternative therapeutic approaches. *Pediatr Dermatol* 1997;14:409-10.
42. Burkhart CN, Burkhart CG. Another look at ivermectin in the treatment of scabies and head lice. *Int J Dermatol* 1999;38:235.
43. Hipolito RB, Mallorca FG, Zuniga-Macaraig ZO et al. Head lice infestation: single drug versus combination therapy with one percent permethrin and trimethoprim/sulfamethoxazole. *Pediatrics* 2001;107:E30.
44. Burkhart CG, Burkhart CN. Asphyxiation of lice with topical agents, not a reality…yet. *J Am Acad Dermatol* 2006;54:721-2.
45. Perlman D. Cetaphil cleanser (Nuvo lotion) cures head lice. *Pediatrics* 2005;116:1612.
46. Takano-Lee M, Edman JD, Mullens BA et al. Home remedies to control head lice: assessment of home remedies to control the human head louse, Pediculus humanus capitis (Anoplura: Pediculidae). *J Pediatr Nurs* 2004;19:393-8.
47. Burgess I. Head lice. What are the effects of treatment for head lice? Herbal treatments and aromatherapy. *Clin Evid* 2001 Jan;(6).
48. Burgess IF. Current treatments for pediculosis capitis. *Curr Opin Infect Dis* 2009;22:131-6.
49. Chosidow O. Clinical practices. Scabies. *N Engl J Med* 2006;354:1718-27.
50. Goldstein BG, Goldstein AO. *Scabies*. Available from: www.uptodate.com/login. Subscription required.
51. Heukelbach J, Feldmeier H. Scabies. *Lancet* 2006;367:1767-74.
52. McCarthy JS, Kemp DJ, Walton SF et al. Scabies: more than just an irritation. *Postgrad Med J* 2004;80:382-7.
53. Golant AK, Levitt JO. Scabies: a review of diagnosis and management on mite biology. *Pediatr Rev* 2012;33:e1-e12.
54. Arlian LG, Runyan RA, Achar S et al. Survival and infectivity of Sarcoptes scabiei var. canis and var. hominis. *J Am Acad Dermatol* 1984;11:210-5.
55. Hooper BJ, Goldman MP. *Primary dermatologic care*. St. Louis: Mosby; 1999.
56. Goldstein BG, Goldstein AO. *Practical dermatology*. 2nd ed. St. Louis: Mosby; 1997. p. 71-7.
57. Davis JS, McGloughlin S, Tong SY et a. A novel clinical grading scale to guide the management of crusted scabies. *PLoS Negl Trop Dis* 2013;7:e2387.
58. Shimose L, Munoz-Price LS. Diagnosis, prevention, and treatment of scabies. *Curr Infect Dis Rep* 2013;15:426-31.
59. Scabies management. *Paediatr Child Health* 2001;6:775-86.
60. Workowski KA, Bolan GA; Centers for Disease Control and Prevention. Sexually transmitted diseases treatment guidelines, 2015. *MMWR Recomm Rep* 2015;64:1-137.
61. FitzGerald D, Grainger RJ, Reid A. Interventions for preventing the spread of infestation in close contacts of people with scabies. *Cochrane Database Syst Rev* 2014;2:CD009943.
62. Section 5–Management and treatment of specific infections. Ectoparasitic infestations (pubic lice, scabies). In: Public Health Agency of Canada. *Canadian guidelines on sexually transmitted infections*. Available from: www.phac-aspc.gc.ca/std-mts/sti-its/cgsti-ldcits/section-5-3-eng.php. Accessed February 2, 2016.
63. Banerji A; Canadian Paediatric Society. Position Statement. Scabies. *Paediatr Child Health* 2015;20:395-8. Available from: www.cps.ca/documents/position/scabies. Accessed February 2, 2016.
64. Strong M, Johnstone P. Interventions for treating scabies. *Cochrane Database Syst Rev* 2007;3:CD000320.
65. Johnstone P, Strong M. Scabies. *BMJ Clin Evid* 2014 Dec 22;2014. pii:1707.
66. Goldust M, Babae Nejad S, Rezaee E et al. Comparative trial of permethrin 5% versus lindane 1 % for the treatment of scabies. *J Dermatolog Treat* 2013 Jan 20. [Epub ahead of print].
67. Clinical Effectiveness Group, British Association for Sexual Health and HIV (BASHH). *United Kingdom national guideline on the management of scabies infestation*. London: BASHH; 2008 Feb 15. 6 p.
68. Mytton OT, McGready R, Lee SJ et al. Safety of benzyl benzoate lotion and permethrin in pregnancy: a retrospective matched cohort study. *BJOG* 2007;114:582-7.
69. Ferreira E, Martin B, Morin C. *Grossesse et allaitement: guide thérapeutique*. 2nd ed. Montréal: CHU Sainte-Justine; 2013.
70. Sharquie KE, Al-Rawi JR, Noaimi AA et al. Treatment of scabies using 8% and 10% topical sulfur ointment in different regimens of application. *J Drugs Dermatol* 2012;11:357-64.
71. Pourhasan A, Goldust M, Rezaee E. Treatment of scabies, permethrin 5% cream vs. crotamiton 10% cream. *Ann Parasitol* 2013;59:143-7.
72. Roos TC, Alam M, Roos S et al. Pharmacotherapy of ectoparasitic infections. *Drugs* 2001;61:1067-88.
73. Mounsey KE, McCarthy JS. Treatment and control of scabies. *Curr Opin Infect Dis* 2013;26:133-9.
74. Meinking TL, Taplin D. Safety of permethrin vs lindane for the treatment of scabies. *Arch Dermatol* 1996;132:959-62.
75. Kennedy D, Hurst V, Konradsdottir E et al. Pregnancy outcome following exposure to permethrin and use of teratogen information. *Am J Perinatol* 2005;22:87-90.
76. Panahi Y, Poursaleh Z, Goldust M. The efficacy of topical and oral ivermectin in the treatment of human scabies. *Ann Parasitol* 2015;61:11-6.
77. Barkwell R, Shields S. Deaths associated with ivermectin treatment in scabies. *Lancet* 1997;349:1144-5.
78. DermNet NZ. *Institutional scabies*. Available from: www.dermnetnz.org/arthropods/institutional-scabies.html. Accessed February 4, 2016.
79. Ortega-Loayza AG, McCall CO, Nunley JR. Crusted scabies and multiple dosages of ivermectin. *J Drugs Dermatol* 2013;12:584-5.
80. Bouvresse S, Chosidow O. Scabies in healthcare settings. *Curr Opin Infect Dis* 2010;23:111-8.
81. Mumcuoglu KY, Gilead L. Treatment of scabies infestations. *Parasite* 2008;15:248-51.
82. Hengge UR, Currie BJ, Jager G et al. Scabies: a ubiquitous neglected skin disease. *Lancet Infect Dis* 2006;6:769-79.
83. Lin AN, Reamer RJ, Carter DM. Sulfur revisited. *J Am Acad Dermatol* 1988;18:553-8.
84. Karthikeyan K. Treatment of scabies: newer perspectives. *Postgrad Med J* 2005;81:7-11.
85. Johnston G, Sladden M. Scabies: diagnosis and treatment. *BMJ* 2005;331:619-22.

Lice—What You Need to Know

What are lice?

- Lice are tiny, wingless insects that live mainly on hairy parts of the human body. Lice feed on human blood.
- There are 3 kinds of lice: **head lice**, **body lice** and **pubic lice**. The female louse lays eggs (called nits) that attach to the base of hairs in the scalp and eyelashes (**head lice**) or pubic area (**pubic lice**). **Body lice** live in the seams of clothing and lay their eggs there. Eggs hatch in 8–10 days. Each louse lives for about a month and produces more eggs. Lice can survive away from humans for several days.
- It is very common for children to get **head lice** and it is not related to poor hygiene. However, **body lice** affect people who do not keep themselves and their clothes clean (poor hygiene). **Pubic lice** are spread by contact with an infected sexual partner.

How do lice spread?

- Lice are spread by close contact with someone who has lice or by sharing personal items such as combs, brushes, hats, towels and bedding with an infected person.

What are the signs of lice?

- The most common sign is itching in the areas where the louse bites. Frequent scratching may cause redness and infection with pus.
- You may see nits, which are tiny white dots attached to the hair. Nits cannot be brushed off easily.
- Pubic lice may cause the affected skin area to turn bluish grey.
- Body lice can spread serious diseases such as typhus, trench fever and relapsing fever.

What is the treatment for head lice and pubic lice?

- If one person in the family has lice, there is a good chance that others will have them too. Treat all affected family members and close contacts at the same time to prevent re-infection.
- Use the same treatment for head lice and pubic lice. Talk to a healthcare provider about the best treatment.
- Follow the directions on the product carefully. Avoid getting the product in your eyes. If you do get the product in your eyes, rinse them immediately with plenty of warm water.
- You should use a second treatment after 7–10 days to make sure the lice and any hatched eggs are gone.
- After the treatment, the dead nits will still be attached to your hair. To make it easier to remove them you can wet the hair with vinegar and water or apply a product that contains formic acid (8%). Ask your pharmacist about this product.
- You can remove nits in 3 ways:
  - Use your fingers to gently pull out any hairs that have nits;
  - Use tweezers to pull nits off the hair;
  - Use a fine-toothed (nit) comb. Start at the scalp and comb to the end of the hair. Clean the comb with soap and hot water when you are finished.
- Wash clothes, bedding, blankets, towels, hats and scarves in hot water—use the hot cycle for the clothes dryer. Soak combs and brushes in hot water and soap for at least 15 minutes.

- Dry clean items that cannot be washed *or* seal them up in a plastic bag for at least 2 weeks. Vacuum all rugs and furniture.

What is the treatment for body lice?

- Body lice live in clothing or bedding that is in contact with the skin. Lice are only found on the skin when they are feeding. It is not usually necessary to use any medication to kill them.
- Wash clothes in hot water—use the hot cycle for the dryer. Dry clean items that cannot be washed *or* seal them up in a plastic bag for at least 10 days.
- Bathe or shower every day.

When should you see your healthcare provider?

- If 2 treatments do not get rid of the lice, see your healthcare provider. You may need a different medication.
- It is normal to be itchy for several weeks after treatment. See your healthcare provider if you continue to have a lot of itching.
  If you develop a skin infection with redness and pus, see your healthcare provider.

Scabies—What You Need to Know

What is scabies?

Scabies is a skin infection caused by a small mite called *Sarcoptes scabiei*. Scabies mites live on the skin of an infected person. They can also live for 2 or 3 days in clothing, bedding or dust.

What causes scabies?

Female mites burrow into the top surface of a person's skin to live. They lay eggs that hatch after 3 to 4 days. The mites mature in about 14 days and repeat the cycle.

Scabies is spread by coming in close contact with someone who has scabies mites—for example, by sharing the same bed or clothing, or from sexual partners.

What are the signs of scabies?

- **Short, wavy, threadlike lines on the skin** in the following areas:
  - webs of the fingers
  - inner side of the wrists or elbows
  - underarms and breasts
  - genitals (private parts) and buttocks
  - infants may have these lines on the face and head
- **Itchiness** at night or when the body is warm. The itching is caused by your body reacting to the presence of scabies mites and eggs under your skin.
  - You may be infected for several weeks before you begin to get itchy.
  - You may continue to feel itchy for several weeks after you have been treated.
  - Try not to scratch the affected areas. Scratching may cause infection. Watch for redness, swelling and pus.

How is scabies treated?

- Scabies is treated with a pesticide or scabicide lotion or cream. Ask your pharmacist for information about these products.
- Read the directions that come with the product completely before you use it. Follow the directions exactly.
- The usual treatment is to apply the cream or lotion to the entire skin surface from the neck down, including under the nails. For children under 2 years, you must apply the scabicide to the head as well. Leave the product on for the time shown in the directions. Wash it off in the shower.
- One treatment is usually all you need. Repeating the treatment may irritate the skin further.

How can you prevent the spread of scabies?

- Treat all family members and close contacts at the same time even if they have no symptoms of scabies. Make sure you have the right product to treat infants or pregnant or breastfeeding women.
- Remember that scabies mites can live in clothing and bedding for 2 or 3 days.
- Wash all clothing, bedding and towels that have been in contact with the infected person during the past week. Do not shake these items. Fold them up and wash them right away in hot water.
- Wash the infected person's underwear and sleepwear every day in **hot** water.

- Items that cannot be washed should be dry cleaned, *or* dried in a hot dryer cycle *or* stored in plastic bags for 14 days.
- Vacuum rugs and furniture.

When should you see your healthcare provider?

See your healthcare provider if any of the following things happen:

- **The condition gets worse after treatment.** You may need a second treatment or you may be re-infected.
- **The itching continues for more than a few weeks.** Itching is not relieved by hydrocortisone cream or oral antihistamines. Remember that the itch normally lasts for several weeks after treatment.
- **If you develop a skin infection** with redness and pus. You may need antibiotic treatment.

Chapter 70

Perspiration and Body Odour

Nancy Kleiman, BSP, MBA

Pathophysiology

Sweating is essential for regulating body temperature. Sweat production increases in response to an increase in body temperature and produces a cooling of the body.[1] Normal body temperature is regulated through receptors in the hypothalamus that monitor the core temperature, and skin receptors that monitor the external temperature. Sweat glands consist of a secretory coil in the dermis and a duct that transports sweat to the skin surface (Figure 1). Failure of this regulating system to reduce body heat can lead to heat exhaustion, heat stroke, hyperthermia and in extreme cases death.[2] Excessive local or systemic sweating is called hyperhidrosis and can be socially and psychologically disabling.[3]

There are 3 main types of sweat glands: eccrine, apocrine and apoeccrine.[2]

- Eccrine sweat glands are primarily responsible for body cooling. They cover the skin surface, with the greatest numbers on the palms, soles, face, head and trunk. Eccrine sweat is primarily hypotonic (sodium, chloride and bicarbonate are reabsorbed through the eccrine duct) which conserves electrolytes during excessive sweating.[2]
- Apocrine glands are larger than eccrine glands, open into hair follicles and are primarily found in the underarm, nipple and genital areas.[2] Apocrine glands become functional at the time of puberty. Apocrine sweat is a milky, viscid, odourless secretion containing fatty substances, but develops an odour once it reaches the skin's surface.
- Apoeccrine glands have structural features of both eccrine and apocrine glands. Like the eccrine gland, they have a long duct and open directly onto the skin's surface. They are found only in the underarm area of adults and also develop at puberty. Apoeccrine glands secrete nearly 10 times as much sweat as eccrine glands.[2]

Physiologic sweating is a natural reaction to thermal and emotional stimuli. Hot environments, over-clothing and exercise all trigger the hypothalamic sweat centre to increase heat loss through cutaneous vasodilation and generalized sweat production, especially on the face and trunk. Sweating around the lips and forehead is a physiologic response to eating hot or spicy foods. Emotional stimuli such as anxiety, embarrassment, fear, anger, excitement or mental stress can cause sweating from the palms, soles, underarms and forehead.[4] Hyperhidrosis is classified as primary or secondary as described below.[3]

- Primary hyperhidrosis is excessive sweating beyond that required for body cooling and is believed to be due to a dysfunction in the autonomic nervous system. It is estimated to affect about 1–3% of the general population and can occur at any age. The axillae are the most commonly affected area (73%) followed by the hands (46%), feet (41%), scalp (23%) and groin (9%).[5] Children generally present with palmoplantar hyperhidrosis whereas axillary hyperhidrosis is more common after onset of puberty. Hyperhidrosis is uncommon in the elderly.[6,7,8] Primary hyperhidrosis is not usually associated with odour but sweating can be excessive to the point of affecting a person's quality of life (e.g., cold sweat is dripping off the hands or face and damaging papers or books; clothing can become wet leading to an increased risk of infection due to the constant dampness in a concentrated area of the skin).[3]

- Secondary hyperhidrosis is more generalized and occurs over the entire body. It is typically associated with menopausal changes and diseases such as diabetes, hyperthyroidism and obesity but can also occur in respiratory failure, chronic infectious diseases, some psychiatric disorders, malignancy, fever, and alcohol or drug withdrawal.[1,3,9] Hyperhidrosis may also be secondary to the use of medications such as ASA, insulin, morphine, fluoxetine and acetaminophen.[3,7,9]

Figure 1: **The Skin**

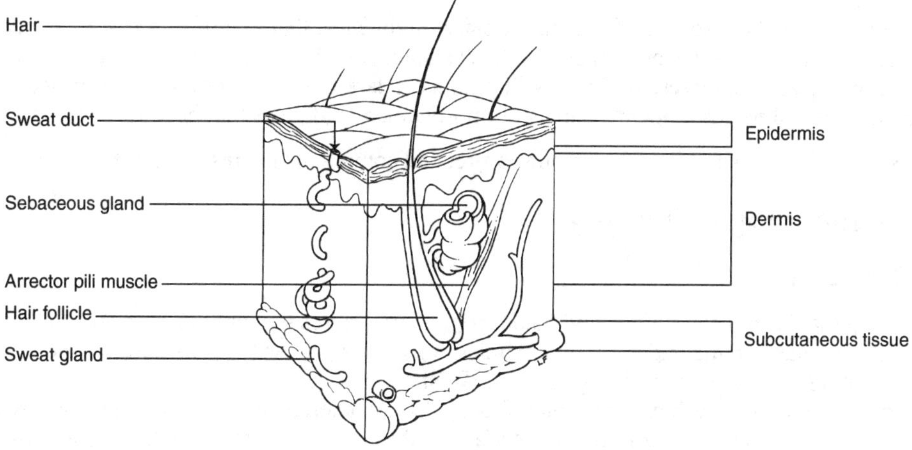

Bromhidrosis is a chronic condition involving sweat that has an offensive odour. Sweat from the eccrine glands is usually odourless, although occasionally excretion in sweat of odour-causing chemicals like garlic, onions and fish can produce an odour. Body odour is generally produced by the action of bacterial decomposition of fatty substances in apocrine sweat. The odour produced from feet is often associated with footwear that does not allow air to circulate, causing excessive sweating and growth of bacteria.[3] Predisposing factors for bromhidrosis include hyperhidrosis, obesity and poor body hygiene.[1]

Goals of Therapy

- Control socially undesirable body odour
- Control underarm wetness resulting from normal, physiologic sweating
- Reduce the quantity of sweat excretion in hyperhidrosis to a tolerable level that permits participation in work and social situations
- Prevent complications of hyperhidrosis involving the feet—odour, blisters and skin infection

Patient Assessment

Concerns about body odour and underarm wetness resulting from normal, physiologic sweating can often be managed with self-treatment. Patients with excessive sweating that has not been controlled with regular use of antiperspirants or deodorants, increased sweating of recent onset in adults, or sweating that occurs in an unusual pattern with no explanation should be assessed in order to eliminate neurologic (spinal injuries, Parkinson's), cardiovascular (heart failure), endocrine or metabolic disorders (hyperthyroidism, diabetes, menopause) and to identify potential drug causes[3] (see Pathophysiology).

Criteria for diagnosing primary hyperhidrosis can include:[7,10]

- Onset of symptoms <25 years of age increases suspicion but it can occur at any age
- At least 6 months' duration
- Sweating occurs in the absence of normal thermal or emotional stimuli and more than once per week
- Occurs in one or more sites (axillary, palmoplantar, scalp, groin) and affects daily life
- Positive family history (genetic connection)

Sweat production can be assessed with a simple starch-iodine test that identifies areas of concern. An iodine solution is applied to the area of skin to be evaluated, and left to dry. A starch (potato or corn) is sprinkled over the area being tested. Sweat will produce a dark blue discoloration. This process can be repeated after several weeks to identify areas of improvement and areas that need further treatment.[11]

An assessment plan for patients with perspiration-related complaints is presented in Figure 2.

Nonpharmacologic Therapy

General Measures

Wear clothing that is cool and porous and made from natural fibres that are more breathable than synthetics, particularly in the underarm area. Underarm shields primarily act as barriers and absorb sweat, preventing wetness from staining clothing. Wash clothing in hot water to remove body odour before wearing again. If possible, avoid spicy foods, alcohol, exercising in hot weather and stressful situations that can trigger strong emotions.[3,4,6] Water and electrolytes lost through excessive sweating should be replaced regularly.

Personal Hygiene

To manage body odour, a regular bath or shower using soap and water will help to prevent buildup of bacteria, sweat and dead skin cells that interact to produce body odour. A daily bath or shower may be necessary for some people. When a full bath or shower is not possible, sponging in the underarm and genital areas can help control the major source of body odour. Shaving the armpits can reduce the propagation of body odour by reducing the surface area for bacterial action.[3] If underarm skin is irritated, avoid soap products that cause further irritation and use unscented cleansers instead.

Foot Care

Foot care is important for patients with excessive foot sweating (plantar hyperhidrosis) and/or odour. Feet should be washed regularly using a skin cleanser and dried thoroughly. Daily washing may be needed for odour control followed by application of an absorbent foot powder twice a day. Non-occlusive footwear made of natural materials, such as leather shoes or sandals, should be worn with cotton or wool socks. Alternating with different pairs of shoes each day will allow them to dry thoroughly. Socks should be changed twice daily to ensure the feet remain dry and are not at risk of fungal infections (athlete's foot).[3] See Chapter 50: Athlete's Foot.

Iontophoresis

Iontophoresis uses a water bath apparatus to introduce a mild electrical current of soluble ions into the skin: it is thought to work by blocking the sweat ducts at the skin surface or by inducing an electrical change in the sweat glands and disrupting secretion.[3] Iontophoresis is often used for hyperhidrosis of the hands and feet not responding to conservative therapy.[3,7] Evidence to confirm efficacy is limited[12,13,14] but it is widely recommended. Commercially available devices can be used at home. The process is time consuming and not practical for some, depending on the area being treated.[1] Up to 4 treatments per week may be needed initially, each lasting 30 minutes.[7] Side effects are minor and consist of dry or cracked skin, tingling or burning and rarely redness and small blisters. If any of these side effects occur, the voltage can be decreased. An emollient can be applied for dry skin or a low-potency topical corticosteroid can be used to treat inflammation/redness.[3] Iontophoresis in contraindicated in anyone who is pregnant, has an orthopedic prosthesis or has a pacemaker.[11]

Surgery

Surgery is considered only when all other options for treatment have failed (see Pharmacologic Therapy) and permanent elimination of sweating is desired. There are 2 types of surgical options. One approach involves removal of the axillary sweat glands by excision, liposuction, curretage or laser. Removal of axillary glands is generally performed in a dermatologist's office under local anesthesia[15] and is considered an emerging therapy as the evidence base is limited.[6] A second method, endoscopic thoracic sympathectomy (ETS), is a major surgical procedure involving cutting nerves that signal sweat glands. It is mainly used to treat palmoplantar hyperhidrosis. In addition to the risk of surgical complications with ETS, a major disadvantage is that compensatory hyperhidrosis may be induced in other areas of the body (usually back, abdomen, thighs, chest) which can be worse than the original condition.[3,6,11,16]

Other Nonpharmacologic Options

Microwave energy is readily absorbed by tissues with a high water content and is used in a new treatment being used for primary hyperhidrosis. The miraDry device is used in some clinics in Canada but requires further studies to confirm efficacy and long-term safety. The procedure takes about 1 hour to complete and must be repeated after 3 months.[15]

Treatment with various laser techniques may be beneficial for some patients with axillary hyperhidrosis. Evidence is limited to small studies.[17]

Pharmacologic Therapy

Topical Therapy

For comparative ingredients of nonprescription products, consult the *Compendium of Products for Minor Ailments*—Antiperspirant and Deodorant Products.

First-line treatments used to manage perspiration and body odour problems in most cases are antiperspirants and deodorants as described in Table 2. The mainstay of treatment is daily use of antiperspirants as part of a personal hygiene regimen.

Antiperspirants reduce sweating by either mechanically obstructing the eccrine gland pores, causing the sweat to thicken and clump, or by causing atrophy of the secretory cells. Once plugged, the sweat glands receive a signal to reduce or stop perspiration, and this effect can last for 24 hours or longer.[1,3] Antiperspirants can be applied to any problematic body area (hands, feet, face, back, chest groin), though irritation may be more common in more sensitive areas. The most commonly used antiperspirants contain various types of **aluminum salts**. Skin irritation is the most common side effect and may be caused by the active ingredient, or by perfumes or preservatives used as additives.[3] **Aluminum chloride** is used in the treatment of hyperhidrosis when standard aluminum products do not control symptoms effectively. Initially the product is applied every 24–48 hours until the condition is controlled, at which time application every 1–3 weeks can be considered.[3] All antiperspirants are more effective if applied at bedtime when sweat glands are less active. More active ingredient can enter the sweat duct and create better plugs. Irritation can be minimized or avoided by making sure the skin is completely dry (using a cool blow dryer if need be) before application. Never occlude skin (e.g., with plastic wrap) while using antiperspirants as it does not increase efficacy but may increase irritation.[18]

There is no evidence of any connection between use of aluminum-containing antiperspirants and Alzheimer's disease (or any other dementias) or breast cancer.[18,19,20]

Deodorants do not prevent sweating but mask body odour with fragrance or by reducing the bacterial population in the area. **Aluminum**- or **zinc**-containing deodorants have antibacterial action. **Alum** has been used traditionally as a water purifier; "natural" or "crystal" deodorants usually contain **potassium alum** or **ammonium alum** crystals. Other products that have been used as deodorants are vinegar, sodium bicarbonate and isopropyl alcohol.[3]

Products used to control foot odour contain combinations of **zinc oxide**, **sodium bicarbonate**, **corn starch**, **aluminum** and **alcohol**.

Astringents like **formaldehyde**, **glutaraldehyde**, **methenamine** and **tannic acid** were once used to treat hyperhidrosis by plugging the pores. These chemicals are no longer used because of contact sensitivity or skin discoloration.[3]

Other Therapy

OnabotulinumtoxinA injection blocks the release of acetylcholine from cholinergic fibres and is beneficial in the treatment of hyperhidrosis. It is approved for treatment of primary hyperhidrosis of the axillae where it reduces sweat production by 75–100%.[6] Although not approved for use on other sites it has been also used clinically for hands, feet, face and groin.[21,22] It is used as first-line treatment for moderate to severe primary hyperhidrosis of the axillae or for milder cases when topical treatment has failed after 1 month of continuous treatment.[23] Sweat reduction should be noticed after 2–4 days and should be significant after 2 weeks.[23] The procedure consists of a number of injections (average of 10–15 per axilla) and the effects last from 4–12 months, after which treatment is repeated. It is painful (topical anesthetics are therefore used) and expensive. Research into administration via microneedles, resulting in less pain, is ongoing.[3,7] Use of onabotulinumtoxinA is not recommended during pregnancy and breastfeeding and in patients with neuromuscular disorders.

Anticholinergics may be helpful in certain cases. **Glycopyrrolate** is safe and effective when used topically, particularly for craniofacial hyperhidrosis for which there is the most evidence.[24,25,26] It has also been used orally.[27] Hyperhidrosis is not a Health Canada–approved indication.

Oxybutynin has been used orally in patients with multifocal primary hyperhidrosis, compensatory hyperhidrosis (e.g., following ETS surgery), or in those for whom topical treatments, iontophoresis and onabotulinumtoxinA (or combinations of these) have not been satisfactory.[3,23,27,28] Use for hyperhidrosis is not a Health Canada–approved indication. Oral anticholinergics are not recommended in patients with glaucoma, impaired gastric emptying or urinary retention and may interfere with thermoregulation in situations where patients are at risk of becoming overheated as it may limit their ability to sweat for cooling purposes.

Monitoring of Therapy

Table 1 provides a monitoring plan framework which should be individualized.

Table 1: **Monitoring of Therapy for Perspiration and Body Odour**

Symptom	Monitoring	Endpoint	Actions
Underarm wetness	Monitor daily for 2–3 wk while using antiperspirants (try standard followed by aluminum chloride if needed) as well as a daily personal hygiene routine.	Dry axillae in resting, non-stressed state at comfortable room temperature after 2–3 wk of intervention.	If aluminum chloride effective, reduce frequency to level required to maintain effect. If patient cannot tolerate aluminum chloride products (mild or stronger strengths) or is not responding after a 2- to 3-wk treatment trial, other treatment options should be considered.
Hand sweating	Monitor daily while using antiperspirants (try standard followed by aluminum chloride if needed) applied to the palms of the hands for 1–3 wk.	Hand sweating reduced to a tolerable level after 4 wk of intervention.	If hand sweating interferes with social or occupational activities, refer to a physician. If patient cannot tolerate aluminum chloride or is not responding after a 3-wk trial, other treatment options should be considered.
Foot sweating	Monitor daily while using a regular foot care routine including nonpharmacologic therapy as indicated previously. Monitor daily for 1–3 wk while using antiperspirants and/or absorbent foot powders.	Foot sweating reduced to a tolerable level after 3 wk of treatment.	If patient cannot tolerate products containing aluminum chloride or is not responding to treatment after a 3-wk trial, other treatment options should be considered.
Body odour	Monitor daily while using a personal hygiene routine that includes washing with soap and water, changing clothing as required and regular use of antiperspirants.	Offensive body odour eliminated after 1–2 wk of intervention.	If personal hygiene measures and antiperspirants are ineffective after 1–2 wk, other treatment options should be considered.
Skin irritation from antiperspirants	Ensure correct use (to completely dry skin) and if irritation continues, use a different brand or a lower concentration aluminum product or a deodorant that is aluminum-free. Treat symptomatically with low-potency topical corticosteroid cream twice daily for no more than 14 days if irritation severe.	Antiperspirant tolerated with minimal or no irritation.	If irritation continues, stop antiperspirant and consider other treatment options. Further therapy may be necessary for severely irritated skin.
Side effects of anticholinergic drugs	Monitor daily for dry mouth, urinary hesitancy, mydriasis, photophobia).	Side effects tolerable.	Discontinue use in consultation with healthcare practitioner if side effects affect quality of life.

Figure 2: **Assessment of Patients with Perspiration and/or Body Odour Complaints**

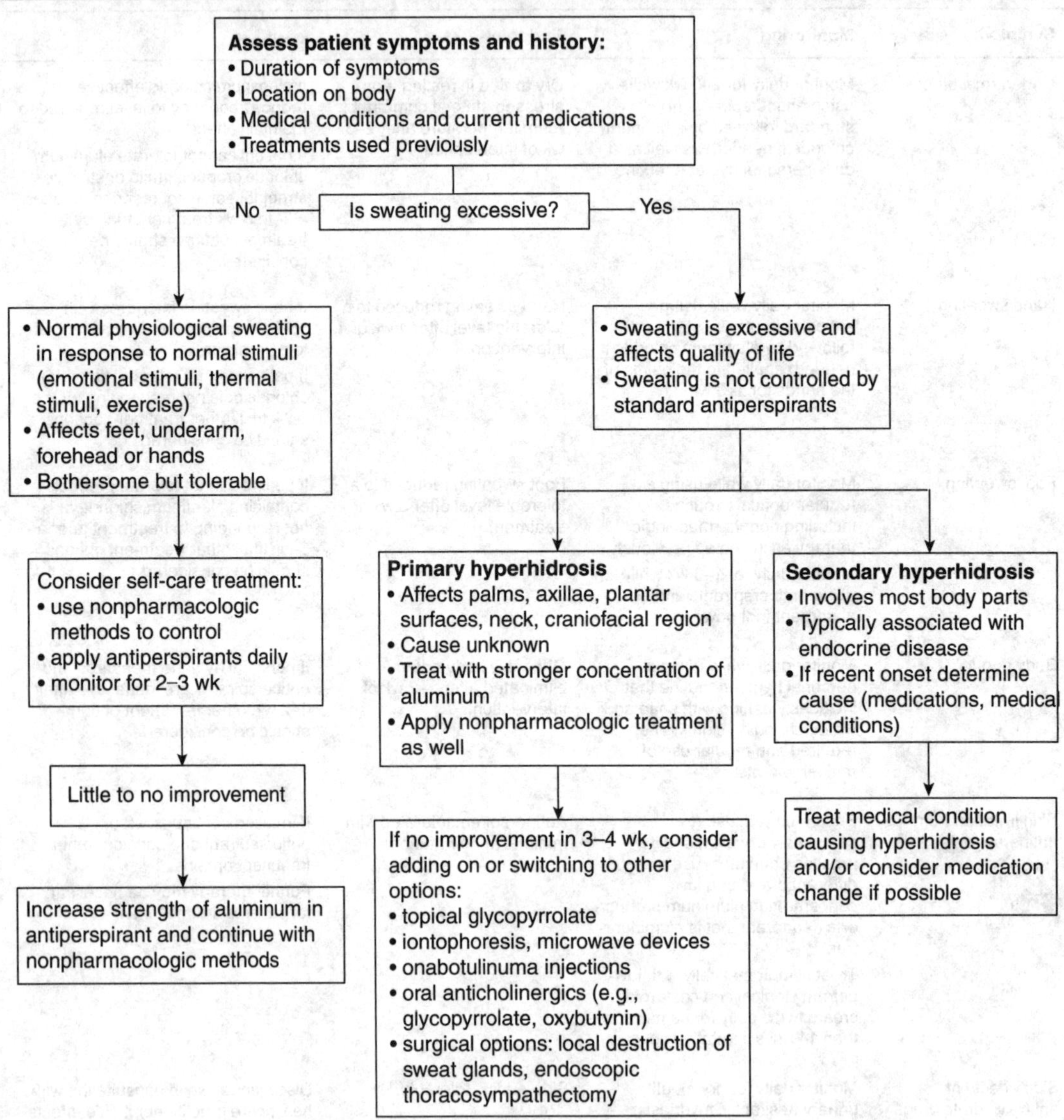

Table 2: **Therapy for the Management of Perspiration and Body Odour**[6,10,27,29,30,31]

Class	Drug	Dosage	Adverse Effects	Drug Interactions	Comments	Cost[a]
Anticholinergics	*glycopyrrolate*[b] Avert Capsules, Secure Pads	Capsules: 1–8 mg daily in 1–3 divided doses po Pads: 0.5–4% impregnated pads wiped onto cleaned, affected area once daily, or on a PRN basis before excessive sweating triggers only	Oral: Mydriasis, dry mouth, dizziness, constipation, urinary retention. Topical: Mild headache	Oral: Caution with concommitant use of other anticholinergics (increased risk of adverse effects); may decrease serum levels of haloperidol, levodopa; may increase bioavailability of atenolol, metformin; effect of glycopyrrolate may be decreased by acetylcholinesterase inhibitors. Topical: No information available.	Often used for craniofacial hyperhidrosis. Topical pads: Avoid contact with eyes, nose and mouth. Not a Health Canada–approved indication.	$
	oxybutynin generics	2.5–20 mg daily in 1–3 divided doses po	Dry mouth (most common), mydriasis, constipation, nausea, dizziness, urinary retention	Caution with concommitant use of other anticholinergics (increased risk of adverse effects); oxybutynin effects increased by strong CYP3A4 inhibitors.	Generally reserved for use in recalcitrant cases or in multifocal hyperhidrosis or compensatory hyperhidrosis. Not a Health Canada–approved indication.	$
Antiperspirants	*aluminum salts, various (e.g., aluminum zirconium tetrachlorohydrex glycine, aluminum chlorohydrate) in solid, spray formats* Arrid, Speed Stick, others	Apply to completely dry skin on affected area daily to BID (if once daily, HS preferred)	Local irritation.	Not applicable.	Avoid application on freshly shaved or abraded skin to reduce irritation.	$$
	aluminum chloride Certain Dri, Drysol, others	6.25%–20%: Apply to completely dry skin on affected area at HS × 3 days or until desired effect reached and then taper to 2–3 times weekly to maintain effect. Choose weaker strengths for sensitive areas such as forehead, and stronger strengths for palms and soles	Local irriation. Correct application and starting with weaker strengths can minimize irritation.	Not applicable.	A cool blow dryer may be used to completely dry the skin prior to application. No evidence that occlusion of the area with plastic wrap improves efficacy, but may increase irritation.	$$$

(cont'd)

Table 2: **Therapy for the Management of Perspiration and Body Odour**[6,10,27,29,30,31] *(cont'd)*

Class	Drug	Dosage	Adverse Effects	Drug Interactions	Comments	Cost[a]
Botulinum Toxins	*onabotulinumtoxinA* Botox	50 U injected intradermally at evenly distributed sites approximately 1–2 cm apart in the affected part of the axilla (average 10–15 injections per axilla); repeated when effect wears off (usually 4–6 months)	Localized pain, inflammation, swelling, bleeding, bruising, muscle weakness. Headache, hot flush, abnormal skin odour, subcutaneous nodules.	Theoretically, drugs interfering with neuromuscular transmission may potentiate the effect of onabotulinumtoxinA. Caution with aminoglycoside antibiotics (amikacin, gentamicin, neomycin, streptomycin, tobramycin) and neuromuscular blocking agents (anticholinesterases, lincosamides, magnesium, polymyxins, quinidine, succinylcholine, tubocurarine).	Pre-procedure local anesthesia generally needed to reduce pain during administration.	$375/100 unit vial
Deodorants	*potassium alum/ ammonium alum* Crystal Body Deodorant, others	Crystal format: Moisten crystal then apply to affected area	Possible local irritation.	Not applicable.	Mask/neutralize body odour only.	$$
	zinc salts (water soluble: zinc chloride, zinc gluconate, zinc lactate), zinc oxide, corn starch Dr. Scholl's Powder, Odor Eaters, others	Apply to affected area daily	Possible local irritation.	Not applicable.	Tend to be contained in foot powders and sprays.	$$

[a] Cost of 1-day supply or smallest available pack size unless otherwise specified; includes drug cost only.

[b] Limited availability: does not require a prescription and can be ordered at www.pharmacy.ca.

Legend: $ <$3 $$ $3–6 $$$ $6–9

Suggested Readings

Nyamekye I. Current therapeutic options for treating primary hyperhidrosis. *Eur J Vasc Endovasc Surg* 2004;27:571-6.

Pariser DM, Ballard A. Topical therapies in hyperhidrosis care. *Dermatol Clin* 2014;32:485-90.

Perera E, Sinclair R. Hyperhydrosis and bromhidrosis. *Aust Fam Physician* 2013;42:266-9.

Schlereth T, Dieterich M, Birklein F. Hyperhidrosis–causes and treatment of enhanced sweating. *Dtsch Arztebl Int* 2009;106:32-7.

References

1. Nyamekye I. Current therapeutic options for treating primary hyperhidrosis. *Eur J Vasc Endovasc Surg* 2004;27:571-6.
2. Mauro T, Goldsmith L. Biology of eccrine, apocrine and apoeccrine sweat glands. In: McGraw-Hill AccessMedicine. *Dermatology.* Subscription required. Accessed June 18, 2009.
3. Clark C. Sweating and hyperhidrosis. *Pharmaceutical J* 2006;276:757-60.
4. Leung AK, Chan PY, Choi MC. Hyperhidrosis. *Int J Dermatol* 1999;38:561-7.
5. Lear W, Kessler E, Solish N et al. An epidemiological study of hyperhidrosis. *Dermatol Surg* 2007;33:S69-75.
6. Benson RA, Palin R, Holt PJ et al. Diagnosis and management of hyperhidrosis. *BMJ* 2013;347:f6800.
7. Singh S, Davis H, Wilson P. Axillary hyperhidrosis: a review of the extent of the problem and treatment modalities. *Surgeon* 2015;13:279-85.
8. Hornberger J, Grimes K, Naumann M et al. Recognition, diagnosis, and treatment of primary focal hyperhidrosis. *J Am Acad Dermatol* 2004;51:274-86.
9. Paisley AN, Buckler HM et al. Investigating secondary hyperhidrosis. *BMJ* 2010;341:c4475.
10. Pariser DM, Ballard A. Topical therapies in hyperhidrosis care. *Dermatol Clin* 2014;32:485-90.
11. Wang R, Solish N, Murray CA. Primary focal hyperhidrosis: diagnosis and management. *Dermatol Nurs* 2008;20:467-70.
12. Dahl JC, Glent-Madsen L. Treatment of hyperhidrosis manuum by tap water iontophoresis. *Acta Derm Venereol* 1989;69:346-8.
13. Reinauer S, Neusser A, Schauf G et al. Iontophoresis with alternating current and direct current offset (AC/DC iontophoresis): a new approach for the treatment of hyperhidrosis. *Br J Dermatol* 1993;129:166-9.
14. Stolman LP. Treatment of excess sweating of the palms by iontophoresis. *Arch Dermatol* 1987;123:893-6.
15. Glaser DA, Galperin TA. Local procedural approaches for axillary hyperhidrosis. *Dermatol Clin* 2014;32:533-40.
16. American Academy of Dermatology. *Hyperhidrosis: overview and treatment.* Available from: www.aad.org/dermatology-a-to-z/diseases-and-treatments/e—h/hyperhidrosis/hyperhidrosis-diagnosis-and-treatment.
17. Canadian Agency for Drugs and Technology in Health. *Laser therapy for hyperhidrosis: a review of the clinical effectiveness and guidelines.* April 29, 2015. Available from: www.cadth.ca/laser-therapy-hyperhidrosis-review-clinical-effectiveness-and-guidelines. Accessed April 7, 2016.
18. International Hyperhidrosis Society. *Antiperspirants: tips for best results-OTC.* Available from: www.sweathelp.org.
19. Exley C. Does antiperspirant use increase the risk of aluminum-related disease, including Alzheimer's disease? *Mol Med Today* 1998;4:107-9.
20. Darbre PD. Aluminum, antiperspirants and breast cancer. *J Inorg Biochem* 2005;99:1912-9.
21. Weinberg T, Solish N, Murray C. Botulinum neurotoxin treatment of palmar and plantar hyperhidrosis. *Dermatol Clin* 2014;32:505-15.
22. Glaser DA, Galperin TA. Botulinum toxin for hyperhidrosis of areas other than the axillae and palms/soles. *Dermatol Clin* 2014:32:517-25.
23. Gee S, Yamauchi PS. Non-surgical management of hyperhydrosis. *Thorac Surg Clin* 2008;18:141-55.
24. Hyun MY, Son IP, Lee Y et al. Efficacy and safety of topical glycopyrrolate in patients with facial hyperhidrosis: a randomized, multicentre, double-blinded, placebo-controlled, split-face study. *J Eur Acad Dermatol Venereol* 2015;29:278-82.
25. Kim WO, Kil HK, Yoon DM et al. Treatment of compensatory gustatory hyperhidrosis with topical glycopyrrolate. *Yonsei Med J* 2003;44:579-82.
26. Kim WO, Kil HK, Yoon KB et al. Topical glycopyrrolate for patients with facial hyperhidrosis. *Br J Dermatol* 2008;158:1094-7.
27. del Boz J. Systemic treatment of hyperhidrosis. *Actas Dermosifiliogr* 2015;106:271-7.
28. Schollhammer M, Brenaut E, Menard-Andivot N et al. Oxybutinin as a treatment for generalized hyperhidrosis: a randomized, placebo-controlled trial. *Br J Dermatol* 2015;173:1163-8.
29. Kanlayavattanakul M, Lourith N. Body malodours and their topical treatment agents. *Int J Cosmet Sci* 2011;33:298-311.
30. Walling HW, Swick BL. Treatment options for hyperhidrosis. *Am J Clin Dermatol* 2011;12:285-95.
31. Wolosker N, Teivelis MP, Krutman M et al. Long-term efficacy of oxybutynin for palmar and plantar hyperhidrosis in children younger than 14 years. *Pediatr Dermatol* 2015;32:663-7.

Perspiration or Body Odour—What You Need to Know

Good personal hygiene is important to prevent body odour:

- Bathe or shower using soap or antibacterial skin cleanser daily if possible to prevent buildup of bacteria, sweat and dead skin cells. If daily cleansing is not possible, sponge baths daily will help to control odour.
- Wear clean clothes that are made from natural fabrics and are breathable to reduce odour.
- Apply an antiperspirant to the underarm area each day, even on days you don't have a bath or shower.

To treat feet that are sweaty and/or have an odour:

- Wash feet regularly and dry thoroughly to prevent odour and fungal infections. Feet may need to be washed each day to control foot odour.
- Use an absorbent foot powder once or twice daily to help control moisture and odour.
- Wear footwear that lets the feet breathe, such as leather shoes or sandals along with cotton or wool socks.
- Alternate shoes daily to allow a thorough drying in between wearings.
- Apply an antiperspirant to the bottoms of the feet if sweating is not controlled with the above measures.

If you have extremely sweaty hands, feet or underarms:

- Talk to a pharmacist or doctor about trying a stronger antiperspirant that contains a higher concentration of aluminum chloride than regular antiperspirants.
- To reduce irritation from antiperspirants that contain aluminum chloride:
  - thoroughly dry the area before application of the antiperspirant using a towel or blow dryer on low heat.
  - apply stronger antiperspirants at night and wash off first thing in the morning.
  - once sweating is controlled, reduce the use of the stronger concentration of aluminum chloride to once or twice a week. Use a regular antiperspirant to control odour during the day.
- If the product irritates the skin, talk to a pharmacist or doctor for other options.

Chapter 71
Psoriasis

Debra Sibbald, BScPhm, ACPR, MA (Adult Education), PhD (Education)

Pathophysiology

Psoriasis is a chronic inflammatory, skin disorder characterized by palpable, erythematous plaques and papules, often with a silver scale. It belongs to the group of papulosquamous cutaneous disorders, which are the most commonly encountered skin problems.[1] They may be difficult to distinguish from one another.

Psoriasis is a common medical condition in which psychosocial issues create a significant burden. In Canada it is estimated that 1–3 % of the population has psoriasis. Although the onset is seen at any age from infancy to old age, incidence peaks at 2 ages: 16–22 years for the more severe, type I psoriasis, and 57–60 years for the less severe, type II psoriasis. Approximately 25% of affected patients have severe conditions. Men and women are affected equally. The disorder occurs in all ethnic groups. Increased frequency in certain ethnic groups and geographical areas is likely related to both genetic and environmental factors. It is more common in colder northern climates than tropical regions, and Caucasians are more affected than other groups.[2] Exogenous and endogenous factors such as upper respiratory infection, psychological stress, humidity and cold weather are known to influence the clinical course of psoriasis regionally. Diets high in protein, unsaturated fat, and essential fatty acids and low in carbohydrate, ascorbic acid and tocopherols may account for reduced prevalence of psoriasis in groups such as Inuit. This has led to the suggestion that fish oil may be appropriate supplementary therapy.[3]

Psoriasis is probably inherited via a multifactorial rather than a simple gene pattern. Genetic and environmental factors determine the clinical manifestations. About 30% of patients with psoriasis have a positive family history. If both parents are psoriasis sufferers, there is a 70% chance of contracting the disorder. Although family history is more closely associated with earlier onset psoriasis, it will not predict the age of onset, severity of disease, or coexistence of psoriatic arthritis.

Up to one-third of psoriasis patients may have coexisting psoriatic arthritis. Although the erythrocyte sedimentation rate (ESR) is often elevated, the generalized subtype may be distinguishable from rheumatoid arthritis by the absence of rheumatoid factors or other autoantibodies.

Psoriasis is a T-lymphocyte–mediated systemic inflammatory disease involving both acquired and innate immunity from a complex interplay between multiple genetic factors and environmental influences. Epidermal hyperplasia, vascular changes and the clinical signs of psoriasis all result from chronic T-cell-mediated inflammation within the psoriatic plaque.[4] An antigenic stimulus activates dermal dendritic cells, which secrete pro-inflammatory cytokines including interferon alpha and interleukins (IL-23 and IL-12). This leads to activation of CD4 and helper T cells (TH-1, TH-17), and formation of additional cytokines and growth factors. Lymphoid structures form in the dermis. Positive therapeutic interventions can reverse the psoriatic phenotype without residual damage; however, in psoriatic arthritis, the damage is significant and irreversible.

As a result of pathogenic T-cell production, psoriatic epidermal cells proliferate sevenfold faster than normal epidermal cells. The dividing epidermal cell cycle is shortened from 163 hours to 37 hours, a higher proportion of basal layer keratinocytes enter the active cell cycle, and psoriatic keratinocytes travel from the basal cell layer to the surface in 3–4 days, much more rapidly than the normal 26–28 days. Decreased keratinocyte transit time does not allow for normal maturation and keratinization. This is reflected clinically by characteristic silvery scaling, a thickened epidermis with increased mitotic activity and by the presence of immature nucleated keratin cells in the stratum corneum.[4] Lesion-free skin is actually considered to be affected, because epidermal proliferation is elevated in this apparently normal skin of patients with psoriasis. Leukocyte chemotaxis may lead to local pustule formation and a generalized inflammatory response results in erythroderma.[5,6]

Lifestyle factors associated with development of psoriasis include smoking and alcohol consumption.[7] A high rate of alcoholism is seen some studies of patients with psoriasis; alcohol and smoking contribute to worsening.[8] Obesity and other features of the metabolic syndrome (e.g., dyslipidemia, hypertension, glucose intolerance) are more prevalent in patients with psoriasis.[7] Stress and anxiety frequently precede flares. Psychosocial problems plague patients with psoriasis, who have visible signs and symptoms that can have a profound effect on quality of life. Patients are self-conscious in public places, refusing to participate in health clubs or sporting activities. Clothes have to be chosen carefully so they will not allow shedding scale to be detected. Psoriasis may also inhibit intimate relationships and sexual activity.

Psoriasis and psoriatic arthritis have been associated with human immunodeficiency virus (HIV) infection. Exacerbation of psoriasis or difficult-to-control psoriasis in an at-risk individual warrants HIV status investigation.[4]

The course of psoriasis is prolonged and unpredictable. In most patients, the disease remains as discrete localized plaques. However, extensive or even generalized involvement may develop, compromising quality of life. Spontaneous clearing is rare. Unexplained exacerbation or improvement is common. Psoriasis resolves without scarring, but may leave temporary hypopigmentation.[9,10] It is a disease of control rather than cure, with relapses occurring unpredictably after weeks or months of remission.

Goals of Therapy

- Eliminate or reduce trigger factors
- Reduce or eliminate signs of psoriasis such as scale and plaques
- Relieve associated symptoms; alleviate pruritus and minimize excoriations
- Reduce the frequency of flares or extend symptom-free intervals
- Treat comorbid conditions (psoriatic arthritis, hypertension, dyslipidemia, diabetes, depression)
- Minimize treatment-associated adverse effects
- Maintain or improve quality of life

Patient Assessment

Clinical Presentation

Psoriasis can present with wide-ranging severity affecting vastly different parts of the body. Limited areas may be involved or diffuse generalized disease can be present. Most lesions are asymptomatic. Pruritus may occur in 20–25% of patients. Patients with generalized psoriasis may have facial, trunk or flexural involvement, which may be scattered, discrete, guttate or large plaques. Those with generalized disease may demonstrate all signs and symptoms of exfoliative dermatitis, including loss of thermoregulation, warm skin, a feeling of chilliness, shivering, increased protein catabolism and cardiovascular stress.[4] Ten percent of patients with psoriasis may have either migratory stomatitis or glossitis.

Diagnosis is usually based on the typical appearance and history of the lesions. A positive family history, detection of lesions in characteristic sites undetected by the patient, or presence of nail changes and psoriatic arthritis may also assist diagnostically.

Nails are affected in 50% of patients and careful total skin examination may reveal nail punctate pits or distal destruction of a nail with loss of color and thickening, and subungual collections of keratotic material, showing psoriatic involvement of the nail matrix or nail bed, respectively. A yellow-brown discolouration of the nail is characteristic. Patients with distal interphalangeal joint involvement or arthritis mutilans usually have adjacent nail involvement.[5]

Psoriatic arthritis occurs in up to one-third of patients. Patients commonly present with asymmetric oligoarthritis (1–4 joints affected) but can also present with symmetric polyarthritis. Oligoarticular or polyarticular pain, tenderness, and morning stiffness, especially in the small joints of the hands and feet, are early manifestations. Intense pain may be present in large joints and in the cervical or lumbosacral spine.[4]

Comorbidities in the form of cardiovascular disease, metabolic syndrome and other inflammatory disorders are common in psoriasis.

Types of Psoriasis

Psoriasis presents in various clinical forms based on morphology: plaque psoriasis is most common (90%). Other forms of psoriasis include inverse, guttate, pustular and erythrodermic psoriasis, which are less common. Plaque and inverse psoriasis are chronic conditions whereas guttate, pustular and erythrodermic psoriasis are acute or subacute variants.

Chronic plaque psoriasis presents with the classic lesion: a well-demarcated, thickened, red plaque with a loosely adherent immature silvery-white scale, which tends to become confluent. It occurs either as single lesions or as generalized disease over a wider area. The character of the lesion may vary from minimal redness to thick, scaly red plaques. Scaling can be made noticeable by scratching the surface of a lesion. If the covering scale is removed, a salmon-pink to erythematous lesion is exposed, sometimes with punctate bleeding from prominent dermal capillaries (Auspitz sign). Appearance of lesions varies with the location affected. In the classic form, plaques are thick with silvery scale and acute lesions tend to be small and drop-shaped. They occur typically on the extensor surface of the arms and legs, elbows, knees, sacrum, buttocks and scalp, but the ears, extremities, palms and soles are also common sites. Scalp involvement may vary from diffuse scaling on an erythematous scalp to thickened plaques with exudation, microabscesses and fissures. Lesions often extend onto the face, particularly along the hairline. Hair loss over time is the most frequent manifestation of psoriasis and an important psychological handicap. It may resemble seborrhea, and an inspection of the entire skin is important in a differential diagnosis.[11]

Inverse psoriasis represents 2–6% of psoriasis. The lesions occur in flexural areas (such as skin folds in the groin or axillae). Moisture and friction in these areas contribute to thinner, shiny or glossy well-demarcated red plaques with less scale and possible breakdown or cracking of the skin. Initial presentation may be localized to a single site. Lesions may be moist and often fissured.[12] The degree of impact on the patient does not correlate to total body surface area involved. Differential diagnosis is important to rule out erythrasma or seborrhea.

Guttate psoriasis, named for its drop-like appearance, presents as a sudden eruption of pinpoint, dark red and subsequently scaling lesions on the trunk and limbs, often preceded by a viral or streptococcal infection in children or young adults. It may be induced by superantigen stimulation of T cells and occurs characteristically as an initial presentation of psoriasis in genetically susceptible patients. Diagnosis may be confirmed by a throat swab and an antistreptolysin O titer (ASOT) even in unrecognized or asymptomatic cases. Despite treatment of the initial symptomatic streptococcal infection, guttate psoriasis may take many months to resolve, and recurrent upper respiratory infections may induce flares.[13,14]

Pustular psoriasis may be generalized (acute) or localized (subacute). In the generalized form, patients with or without a previous history develop systemic symptoms including fever, leukocytosis and general malaise. Average age of onset is 50 years. Pregnancy, infection or recent use of systemic corticosteroids may be triggers. The sterile pustules often start in localized plaques and may generalize quickly without systemic treatment. Individual lesions are often painful erythematous plaques with rows or clusters of tender, bright yellow, nonfollicular pustules. This is an acute emergency requiring systemic therapy and may be resistant to treatment.[13] The localized pustular form of psoriasis is often seen on the trunk and proximal extremities. It may respond to topical treatment but systemic agents are often necessary. Chronic pustular psoriasis limited to the palms and soles is more common in women who smoke. Deep painful pustules, clustered in erythematous plaques, extend from the palms and soles around the sides of the hands and feet to the dorsal surface.[5,15]

Erythrodermic psoriasis presents as a nonspecific, fiery erythema over 75% of the body with desquamation and edema. This unstable acute form may develop from chronic forms of psoriasis and may be associated with serious systemic illness. Provoking factors include sudden withdrawal of potent therapies (especially systemic corticosteroids), drug reactions, trauma or illness.

Risk and Aggravating Factors

A wide variety of environmental triggers may precipitate the first psoriatic skin lesions in a genetically susceptible individual, or induce flares in patients in remission. These include excessive alcohol ingestion, smoking, obesity, stress and pregnancy.

Infections are a common precipitating factor in about 25% of patients and more than 50% have exacerbations within 3 weeks after an upper respiratory infection (bacterial, viral, HIV). The guttate variant is often associated with infections of group A beta-hemolytic *Streptococcus*.

Trauma may precipitate psoriasis. The Koebner phenomenon is the appearance of psoriatic lesions at the site of injury within a day to several weeks (average 10–14 days) after localized trauma. This response may be induced by various types of trauma including rubbing, venipuncture, acupuncture, bites, surgery and mechanical pressure.

Climate can influence psoriasis. While most patients with psoriasis (80%) improve with warm seasons and ultraviolet light, a small percentage (approximately 10%) worsen in the summer, and relapses may be triggered paradoxically by ultraviolet light exposure. Ninety percent of patients report worsening in cold weather.

A summary of differential diagnosis and management of psoriasis is provided in Table 1.

Differential Diagnosis

Psoriasis is often confused with dandruff and seborrhea, especially when present on the scalp. See Chapter 58: Dandruff and Seborrheic Dermatitis, Table 3: Comparisons among Dandruff, Seborrhea and Psoriasis, for a comparison of the differences between the 3 conditions with respect to other determinants.

Table 1: **Psoriasis: Differential Diagnosis**

Form	Characteristics	Differential Diagnosis	Action
Chronic Forms of Psoriasis			
Plaque	Classic form: Sharply defined erythematous papules which coalesce; covered with distinctive silver scale when untreated Auspitz sign—punctate bleeding points when scale removed Localized: Extensors (arms and legs), scalp, ears, palms, soles Generalized: (face, trunk, flexures) or one site with/without nails, nail pits—loss of colour, thickening, distal destruction	Nummular eczema Atopic dermatitis Drug reactions T-cell lymphoma	Diagnosis should be confirmed by qualified practitioner Self-care management if mild
Inverse (flexural)	In body folds and flexures No scale Demarcated erythema	Intertrigo areas (skin folds) Tinea in males (active border) Candida in females (satellite pustules) Contact dermatitis—allergic or irritant (location of contact)	Diagnosis should be confirmed by qualified practitioner
Scalp	Silvery scale, discrete margins, extends beyond the scalp margins; may accompany any form or may be the only visible sign	Seborrhea	Diagnosis should be confirmed by qualified practitioner Self-care management if mild
Acute and Subacute Forms of Psoriasis			
Guttate	Small, discrete, erythematous papular lesions; appears suddenly after upper respiratory tract infection (streptococcal) in children or young adults; may be the initial presentation; takes months to resolve	Pityriasis rosea Secondary syphilis Pityriasis lichenoides	Diagnosis should be confirmed by qualified practitioner
Pustular	Local (palms and soles): Chronic in women who smoke; stable but troublesome Systemic: Uncommon but serious, starts with systemic signs and symptoms such as fever, leukocytosis, general malaise, followed by pustules (2–3 mm) on erythematous skin; may generalize and require hospitalization; corticosteroids are contraindicated	Chronic dyshidrotic eczema—itch is predominant vs pain in psoriasis	Diagnosis should be confirmed by qualified practitioner
Erythrodermic	Generalized erythema without any characteristic lesions	Atopic dermatitis Drug reactions can present as severe skin disorders	Diagnosis should be confirmed by qualified practitioner

Drug-induced Psoriasis

Drugs aggravating psoriasis include alcohol, antimalarials, beta-blockers, lithium, NSAIDs and oral corticosteroids; beta-blockers have been implicated in stimulating an initial episode (Table 2).[6,9,10]

Table 2: **Drugs Known to Trigger Psoriasis**

ACE inhibitors	Chloroquine	Glyburide	Penicillamine
Acebutolol	Chlorthalidone	Gold	Phenylbutazone
Amiodarone	Cimetidine	Hydroxychloroquine	Pindolol
Amoxicillin	Clomipramine	Ibuprofen	Propranolol
Ampicillin	Clonidine	Indomethacin	Pyrazolones
Arsenic	Cyclosporine	Interferon-alfa	Sotalol
ASA	Diclofenac	Ketoprofen	Sulfamethoxazole-trimethoprim
Atenolol	Digoxin	Labetalol	Sulfonamides
Auranofin	Dipyridamole	Levamisole	Tacrine
Aurothioglucose	Enalapril	Lithium	Terbinafine
Beta-blockers	Fluoxetine	Metoprolol	Tetracycline
Bisoprolol	Gemfibrozil	Nadolol	Timolol
Captopril	Glipizide	NSAIDs	Trazodone
Chlorambucil		Omeprazole	

Assessing Severity of Psoriasis

Only mild, chronic forms of plaque and scalp psoriasis can be managed with self-care after an appropriate diagnosis. All other types of psoriasis require investigation, diagnosis and treatment under the care of an appropriate healthcare practitioner (Table 1).

Parameters for assessment of the severity of psoriasis include:

- Body surface area (BSA): The total BSA involved is an important factor in determining severity of psoriasis. The area covering the patient's palm and thumb from wrist to fingertips is estimated to be 1% of total BSA. The National Psoriasis Foundation considers up to 3% BSA as mild psoriasis, 3–10% as moderate and >10% as severe
- Location of lesions: Location of lesions can determine the social or economic impact of the disease. Hands, forearms and particularly face involvement may be disabling. Caution with selection of topical agents is warranted when treating lesions in areas in which there may be greater absorption of medication (e.g., face, eyelids, self-occluded areas) or in locations where thickness of the skin diminishes penetration of medication (e.g., palmoplantar areas)
- Types of lesions: Scale, erythema, thickness of plaques (see Table 1).

Various tools are used by healthcare practitioners to determine severity of disease, impact on quality of life and response to treatment. The 2 most established tools for assessing severity are the Psoriasis Area and Severity Index (PASI) and the Dermatology Life Quality Index (DLQI). These tools and others are summarized as follows:

- Psoriasis Area and Severity Index (PASI): Quantitative tool to measure body surface area involvement, scaling, erythema and thickness of plaques in order to assess clinical changes in response to treatment[16]
- Dermatology Life Quality Index (DLQI): A global scale used to measure the health-related quality of life of adult patients suffering from a skin disease.[17] Quality of life indicators represent patients' perceptions and reactions to their health. Assessing patients' impairment in everyday living is an essential outcome measure in evaluating the impact of psoriasis on quality of life. Another quality of life instrument called Skindex-29 may have greater sensitivity to clinical severity, particularly in mild psoriasis[18,19]
- Physician's Global Assessment (PGA): A key three-item (erythema, induration, and scaling) measure frequently used to classify severity as clear, nearly clear, mild, moderate, severe or very severe. Validity has been substantiated with correlations to the Psoriasis Area and Severity Index (PASI)[20]

- Simplified Psoriasis Index (SPI): Used in specialist settings, this appears to be a valid and reliable psoriasis assessment tool[18]
- Visual analogue scale: Reported to be a useful method for patients to assess psoriasis severity[21]
- Nail Assessment in Psoriasis and Psoriatic Arthritis (NAPPA) and Nail Psoriasis Severity Index (NAPSI): Both of these tools appear to be valid, reliable and practical options for assessing patient-relevant nail psoriasis outcomes.[22]

Nonpharmacologic Therapy

An integral component of psoriasis prevention and control is to address environmental and lifestyle risk factors, to limit progression and reduce frequency and severity of relapses. Patients must be aware of triggers such as streptococcal infections, drugs, trauma or injury, low humidity and emotional stress.[23]

Smoking cessation, minimizing alcohol intake and maintaining a healthy diet are advised, to counteract metabolic syndrome and cardiovascular risk factors.

A restricted diet, with or without the addition of physical exercise, can reduce psoriasis severity and improve health-related quality of life in overweight or obese patients with psoriasis.[18,24]

Activities that promote relaxation and mindfulness have been shown to reduce flares.[25] Computerized or online cognitive behavioural therapy (CCBT) for people with psoriasis appears to reduce anxiety and increase quality of life.[18,26]

Advise patients to avoid skin irritants such as soap. Bathing and use of a cool air humidifier can be beneficial. Aqueous creams can serve as cleansers and emollients as skin should stay moist. Caution patients about removing scale, which could trigger a flare. Nonmedicated products such as emollients help retain moisture in the skin by forming a film over the surface and can be used liberally without concern of side effects. A study evaluating the effect of an emollient on patients with mild plaque psoriasis during and after standard local corticosteroid therapy reported that use of an emollient can limit relapses after the end of 1 month of corticosteroid therapy, and maintain the improvement in skin symptoms.[27]

Pharmacologic Therapy

For further information regarding the treatment of psoriasis, consult the *Compendium of Therapeutic Choices*: Psoriasis.

For comparative ingredients of nonprescription products, consult the *Compendium of Products for Minor Ailments*—Skin Care Products: Dermatitis and Dry Skin, Psoriasis.

Pharmacologic treatments that address management of pathophysiological factors such as modulation of immune abnormalities and cell turnover are combined with nonpharmacologic measures (see Nonpharmacologic Therapy).

Topical treatment is first-line therapy for patients with mild, localized plaque psoriasis when total body surface affected is <5%.[28] Topical therapy is primarily directed toward altering the immune mechanism of the disease, with secondary attention to reduction and removal of scale, inflammation and dryness.

Systemic agents, alone or in combination with topical treatment, are reserved for more moderate to severe, widespread symptoms.

Patients with more resistant psoriasis may benefit from combination, rotational or sequential therapy. Combination therapy is used to maximize clinical results from agents acting by different mechanisms and to minimize side effects. Rotational therapy decreases cumulative toxicity by switching between medications with differing toxicity but is more commonly used with systemic therapies. Sequential therapy is instituted when medications are used in a set sequence to maximize the initial speed of improvement while minimizing long-term toxicity.

Due to the chronicity of the disease, once control is achieved it is important to reduce treatment to the least potent and least toxic regimens that maintain control.

Endorsed treatment guidelines that outline current standards of care are published by American,[28,29,30,31] British,[32] Canadian[33] and European[34] consensus groups.

Adherence: Approximately 40% of patients with psoriasis report nonadherence to treatment, and 50% of psoriasis prescriptions are reported to be unfilled. Reasons include frustration with efficacy, inconvenience, fear of side effects, cost, cosmetic distaste, and unclear or complicated instructions. Approaches to enhancing adherence include involving the patient in decision making, choosing acceptable vehicles, use of fast-acting agents early in the course of therapy and transitioning to longer-acting, safer options for long-term management, intermittent use of corticosteroids with corticosteroid sparers, and use of clear, written instructions. Keeping in contact with the patient to address concerns is important and should be initially done early, especially if treatment is time consuming and difficult, such as with scalp psoriasis.[35] A psoriasis symptom diary demonstrated favorable psychometric properties and is a brief, useful tool for measuring symptoms and the impact of chronic plaque psoriasis.[36] Text message interventions are a promising tool, leading to an increase in adherence to therapy, positive changes in self-care behaviours and better patient-physician relationships fostering improved clinical outcomes and better control of the disease.[37]

Application of appropriate amounts of topical agents can be aided by the use of tools that help to estimate quantities for each application depending on age and body parts affected. To determine the quantity of topical agents required for treatment, the fingertip unit is a practical approach. One fingertip unit is approximately 0.5 g (estimated to be the amount squeezed from a tube with a standard 5 mm nozzle from the fingertip to the first crease of an adult finger). This amount is sufficient to cover one hand (front and back) or about 2% of BSA. The trunk (front and back) is about 30% BSA; to cover the entire trunk once, about 15 fingertip units, or 7.5 g, would be required.[38] A tool that can be used for estimating the amount of cream required to treat specific body areas is based on the Rule of Nines (see Figure 1).

Type of Vehicle

The vehicles in which active topical ingredients are applied may have considerable influence on therapy. Topical therapies are available as creams, foams, gels, liquid solutions, lotions, ointments and drug-impregnated tapes. The appropriate vehicle depends on the location of the lesions, the patient's symptoms and the patient's preference.

Ointment vehicles are occlusive which makes them generally more effective at maintaining hydration of the skin and facilitating drug absorption. They may be preferred in the evening when patients have more time to apply medication and are less worried about staining. Fissured lesions on the palms and soles may improve with the use of ointment vehicles. Creams spread more easily and quickly, are more quickly absorbed and do not produce a greasy effect on clothes. Patients may prefer these for work or school, reserving ointments for use at night. Lotions and foams are easier to apply and remove from the skin and more soothing for itching skin, but are more drying. Gels provide drying and cooling effects, are cosmetically acceptable, and diffuse throughout and remove easily from the scalp while concentrating drug delivery by evaporation. Patients with fissures or cracked lesions will complain of stinging pain if alcohol-based solutions or foams are used.

Figure 1: **Amount of Cream Required for TID Application × 10 Days**[a]

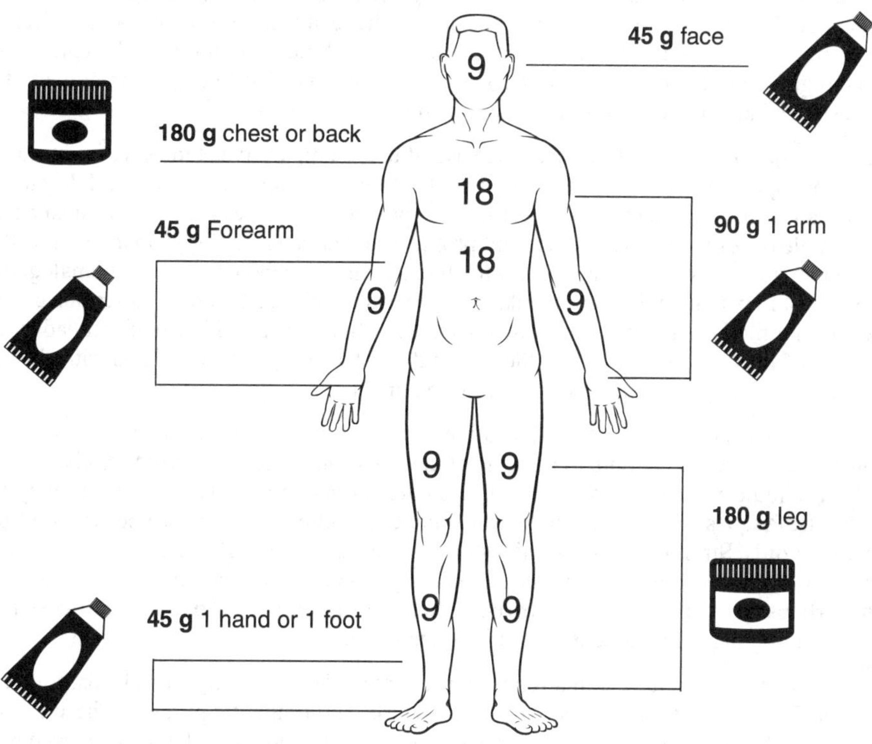

[a] Rule of Nines: 9 g of cream covers 9% of skin area daily (based on TID application).

The location of the psoriasis may assist in selection of vehicle. For the scalp, gels, foams, solutions and lotions are typically better, except in some black patients with curly hair who may respond best to gels and liquids specifically. In intertriginous areas such as axillae, groin and inframammary folds, lotions or creams are more comfortable than ointments. Climate also influences choice: lotions and creams are better tolerated than ointments in warm moist environments, while ointments are preferred in dry or cold climates.

Enhancement of penetration of active drug can be accomplished in various ways. An **occlusive base** may enhance penetration of active drug and inhibit cell division. Medicated creams, lotions and gels can be occluded to enhance drug penetration and potency if required. This is accomplished by covering the medicated area with plastic wrap, plastic baggies, thin plastic gloves, or with fabric such as a sock or cotton gloves. This technique is often used with corticosteroids for psoriasis involving soles, hands and extremities. **Keratolytics** such as salicylic acid or sulfur may remove scale that is limiting penetration. Specific agents such as **urea** or **propylene glycol** may promote penetration by enhancing permeability of the stratum corneum.[39]

Chronic Plaque Psoriasis of Trunk and Extremities

See also Table 4 and Figure 2 for management of chronic plaque psoriasis.

Topical Therapy

Topical corticosteroids are an integral component of psoriasis treatment because they are effective and well tolerated despite adverse effects. Corticosteroids have anti-inflammatory, antiproliferative, immunosuppressive and vasoconstrictive effects, as a result of binding to intracellular corticosteroid receptors and regulation of gene transcription. They are considered first line in the treatment of mild plaque psoriasis, and an adjunct to systemic therapy in more severe forms.[28,40]

Advantages of corticosteroids are fast onset and ease of use. Comparative studies have not shown superiority with respect to potency, frequency of application or formulation. In general, higher potency corticosteroids are considered more effective than low-potency agents, especially for thicker plaques. Occlusion with gloves or plastic wrap overnight provides added benefit. A systematic review that examined randomized trials comparing topical treatments with placebo or vitamin D_3 analogues (alone or in combination) in patients with chronic plaque psoriasis concluded that corticosteroids perform at least as well as vitamin D_3 analogues, and are associated with a lower incidence of local adverse events. There is little evidence concerning the risk of dermal atrophy for individuals with chronic plaque psoriasis receiving long-term corticosteroid treatment.[41]

Choice of potency depends on severity and location of the disease. Pediatric and elderly patients have thinner skin and are more susceptible to atrophic effects of stronger corticosteroids. Only **hydrocortisone** should be used on the face or in the intertriginous folds to avoid skin atrophy and other side effects. Plaques of psoriasis on the trunk and extremities are often treated with mid-potency topical corticosteroids. Stronger topical corticosteroids such as those 9–12 times more potent than hydrocortisone may be necessary for shorter periods (e.g., 2-week intervals) on the palms and soles. Ultrapotent corticosteroids may increase the risk of adrenal suppression. Apply the corticosteroid in a thin layer, since only that which touches the skin is absorbed.

Cutaneous adverse effects include skin atrophy, acne, contact dermatitis, hypertrichosis, folliculitis, hypopigmentation, perioral dermatitis, striae, telangiectases and traumatic purpura. These are unlikely while corticosteroids are being applied to active lesions. Systemic adverse effects have been reported not only with ultrapotent corticosteroids but also with extended or widespread use of mid-potency agents. Systemic adverse effects include hypothalamic-pituitary-adrenal (HPA) axis suppression. Less commonly, Cushing's syndrome, osteonecrosis of the femoral head, cataracts and glaucoma may occur.[28,33] Potential benefits may warrant use of topical corticosteroids in pregnant women despite potential risks.[33]

Topical corticosteroids seldom produce long remissions, and psoriasis tends to rebound promptly when they are withdrawn with a mean remission time of 2 months. Once clinical response is achieved, options for tapering to maintain control include less frequent use of the corticosteroid, switching to a less potent agent, intermittent therapy (e.g., 2–3 times weekly) or pulse dosing (e.g., 3 consecutive doses at 12-hour intervals, once weekly). Topical corticosteroids should be supplemented or substituted with corticosteroid-sparing agents such as plain petrolatum, salicylic acid, tar, anthralin, calcipotriol or tazarotene to decrease the frequency of corticosteroid application.

Corticosteroid-sparing agents are products used in combination with corticosteroids, intermittently and alternately, to reduce risk of side effects from corticosteroids. Corticosteroids are relatively fast in onset; corticosteroid-sparers may take longer to work but enhance long-term maintenance and therefore should be initiated at the same time as the corticosteroid.

One of the simplest corticosteroid-sparing agents is **petrolatum**. It can be used to replace 1 out of every 4 applications of corticosteroid initially. As psoriasis improves after 2–6 weeks, gradually increase the number of applications until it almost completely replaces topical corticosteroids. Petrolatum has an antiproliferative effect on epidermal cells and will help diminish surrounding skin irritation from other corticosteroid-sparing agents if applied in a ring around psoriatic plaques.

Salicylic acid is a keratolytic agent useful in the treatment of mild to moderate psoriasis. It is a good adjunct to other topical medications, but not used as monotherapy because it only removes scale. It is available in concentrations of 2–10% in various vehicles including gels, creams and shampoos. Since salicylic acid breaks down keratin topically, it increases percutaneous absorption of topical corticosteroids. This may be a safe and effective alternative when other treatment modalities are too toxic or not an option. Salicylic acid will increase the penetration of hydrocortisone approximately threefold, and desoximetasone, triamcinolone-acetate and fluocinonide twofold or more.[42] Efficacy is increased with other such combinations; e.g., combination with mometasone furoate showed more significant response after 21 days than with the corticosteroid alone.[43] It has been suggested that salicylic acid–topical corticosteroid combinations be used as first-line therapy on psoriasis plaques that are thick, scaly or recalcitrant to topical corticosteroids alone. A caveat is that salicylic acid should be used with caution in patients with greater than 20% BSA involvement.[44] It may cause salicylate toxicity in these cases; signs of toxicity include tinnitus, fatigue and GI symptoms, reversible when salicylic acid is discontinued. Hypoglycemia in patients with diabetes is a risk with application of salicylic acid to large body surface areas; alternative keratolytic acids such as lactic acid or urea should be considered.[42] Salicylic acid can be added to most topical corticosteroids in concentrations of 3–5%; apply a 1-month expiry date to cream formulations. Salicylic acid is also used in combination (urea 10%/salicylic acid 5% ointment) as a corticosteroid-sparing alternative. Salicylic acid has been used successfully in combination with anthralin. It should not be used with calcipotriol, since it will inactivate calcipotriol upon contact. It also blocks UVB and should not be applied prior to ultraviolet therapy.[42] Salicylic acid use should be avoided in children; however, it may be used for limited and localized plaque psoriasis in pregnancy.[28]

Lactic acid is another less common topical keratolytic agent used in the treatment of psoriasis. It is an alpha-hydroxyacid reserved as a second-line agent in patients with diabetes when salicylic acid treatment is a concern. Lactic acid is effective, proven to enhance desquamation of normal skin, and can be used on a larger surface area.[42]

Crude coal tar is the liquid byproduct of the distillation of bituminous coal and contains more than 10 000 ingredients whose exact mechanism of action is yet unknown. It is a useful agent in mild psoriasis as it decreases epidermal hyperproliferation, is anti-inflammatory and antipruritic, and may be antimicrobial. It is a frequently used, inexpensive, safe and effective topical preparation, producing clearing with long remissions. Concentrations of 0.5–10% are used in ointments, creams, lotions, shampoos, gels, solutions and soaps. Modified tar extracts incorporated into solutions and gels are less effective, although cosmetically superior and ideal for scalp psoriasis. Crude coal tar 4% is equivalent to the tar distillate, liquor carbonis detergens (LCD) 10–20%. Shampoo products often contain both coal tar and salicylic acid to maximize efficacy. Coal tar 5–10% can be added to corticosteroid ointments and creams if a 1-month expiry date is affixed. Most applications are designed for once-daily use at night, but may be used more often if the patient is willing. The photosensitizing action of tar enhances its efficacy in psoriasis: pretreatment for 2 hours is followed by ultraviolet B light treatments in ambulatory clinics (Goeckerman routine).[45,46] A systematic review found one study showing that daily coal tar shampoo was no more effective than placebo; however, most patients had moderate to severe psoriasis[41] and therefore the results may not be generalizable to patients with mild disease for which topical therapy is the mainstay of treatment. Another study found coal tar to be significantly less effective than betamethasone valerate in patients with stable mild to moderate psoriasis.[47] Coal tar appears to have comparable clinical efficacy to calcipotriol, but calcipotriol has a faster onset of action and is better tolerated.[33]

Coal tar may be a reasonable option for long-term maintenance and treatment of mild to moderate psoriasis. It is safe to use and is inexpensive and widely available in shampoos and solutions ideally suited for use on the scalp; however, it also has obvious disadvantages and side effects. These include staining of clothes and furniture, messy application, unpleasant odour, contact sensitivity, burning sensations, photosensitivity and tar folliculitis. Application in circular motions may cause folliculitis or acne; this can be diminished by applying the tar in downward linear strokes in the direction hairs sit flat against the skin which minimizes inflammation and irritation in the hair follicles. The higher the tar concentration, the greater the irritancy. Though tar is effective, patients may find it difficult to adhere to treatment due to its side effects and prolonged treatment durations of 2–4 weeks. There are no reported systemic side effects despite decades of use. The FDA has concluded that coal tar in concentrations and formulations used in nonprescription products (0.5–5%) does not pose a risk of carcinogenicity.[42] Due to lack of evidence of safety and concerns of potential mutagenic effects, some sources recommend avoiding coal tar during pregnancy,[48] while others feel it is likely safe during the second and third trimesters.[33,49] Coal tar should be avoided during breastfeeding due to risk of absorption by the infant via skin-skin or skin-mouth contact.[50]

Anthralin is a less commonly used topical treatment for psoriasis; however, it is appropriate and effective in specific situations. The mechanisms of action of **anthralin** (dithranol) are multiple. It is antiproliferative as it normalizes keratinocyte differentiation by promoting keratinocyte apoptosis, decreasing cell respiration and inhibiting inflammation. It may have a direct effect on mitochondria, reduce mitotic acitivity and prevent T-lymphocyte activation.[51] Anthralin is most useful for thinning plaques and is associated with a remission time of 3.9 months.[52] It was superior to calcipotriol in a study of 106 patients.[53] Conventionally, anthralin is applied once daily to skin or scalp, allowed to remain overnight, and followed by bathing or shampooing the next morning. Short-contact therapy (15–30 minutes followed by washing) is also effective and may be less irritating than once-daily use.[53] Effects may be increased in ambulatory patients through the addition of ultraviolet light (Ingram routine).[42] In this method, anthralin is applied, covered with talcum powder then gauze, wiped off after an interval of time, followed by a tar bath and then ultraviolet light. This is effective but time-consuming and therefore usually reserved for unresponsive psoriasis. Problems with anthralin include burning, stinging, dryness and most importantly, staining of skin, clothes and furniture and discolouration of blond hair. Careful application to affected areas only is important, as surrounding skin is easily irritated through contact. Lesions can be ringed with zinc oxide paste or petrolatum to protect surrounding skin. If compounding with dry anthralin powder, avoid skin contact by wearing gloves. Alternating combinations of tar then anthralin are less irritating, and addition of corticosteroid to uninvolved surrounding skin also reduces irritation. Triethanolamine, a neutralizing agent, placed on unaffected skin 1–2 minutes before anthralin is removed, and again after towel drying, also reduces staining and inflammation. Other adverse effects include folliculitis and allergic contact dermatitis, but these are uncommon. There are no systemic or long-term side effects and anthralin has been used safely for many years; staining is the major limitation. Anthralin is contraindicated on the face, in flexures or on the genitals, where irritation is excessive. It may be alternated with topical corticosteroids. Safety of anthralin in pregnancy has not been confirmed.

Calcitriol and **calcipotriol** are vitamin D_3 analogues, which enhance keratinocyte differentiation and inhibit proliferation and cytokines. Response is slow; a period of 2 months is usually required to see best effects. These agents maintain effectiveness without tachyphylaxis.[16] A systematic review found efficacy of vitamin D_3 analogues similar to corticosteroids when used on the body. Combination treatment with both vitamin D_3 analogues and corticosteroids was more effective than either treatment alone. Corticosteroids also seemed to be better tolerated than vitamin D_3 analogues.[54]

Tazarotene, a receptor-selective topical retinoid, is a corticosteroid-sparing agent that appears to inhibit keratinocyte proliferation, regulate differentiation and modify inflammatory infiltration in the plaque. It is effective in clearing psoriatic plaque lesions and achieving remission.[28] Retinoids are less effective than corticosteroids as topical treatments.[41]

Topical calcineurin inhibitors are a treatment option for patients with limited psoriatic manifestations. **Tacrolimus** ointment and **pimecrolimus** cream are derivatives of cyclosporin that inhibit calcineurin, thereby blocking the synthesis of inflammatory cytokines and further activation of T cells that contribute to psoriasis. They are not approved for the treatment of psoriasis, but are considered useful for treating thin skin or fold areas, despite minimal published data on use or effectiveness. They are reserved as an option for recalcitrant plaques of the face, genitals and intertriginous areas, where use of potent topical corticosteroids or irritating agents are of concern.[33,55]

Systemic Therapy

If psoriatic symptoms are more severe and/or too extensive for topical therapy, systemic therapy is preferred, with topical therapies remaining as useful adjuncts. Methotrexate, cyclosporine and acitretin are the oral agents traditionally used. Biologic response modifiers are effective and have relatively good tolerability but their high cost means other systemic therapy is generally tried first.[33]

Ultraviolet radiation, which inhibits epidermal mitosis, can be very useful in more severe, extensive or resistant cases of psoriasis, in addition to topical therapy, such as tar or anthralin. Phototherapy uses either UVA or UVB light. UVA is given with a photosensitizer, such as oral or topical **psoralens**, to enhance efficacy. This is called PUVA (psoralen + UVA). UVB is used alone as either broadband (BB-UVB) or narrowband (NB-UVB); the latter is preferred. BB-UVB is also given as photochemotherapy with topical agents such as crude coal tar or anthralin for enhanced efficacy. NB-UVB is commonly used with adjunctive topical treatments such as emollients, calcipotriene, corticosteroids, retinoids and tar.[56] Although NB-UVB is slightly less effective than PUVA (which benefits the majority of patients and has the potential to induce long remissions), NB-UVB is generally preferred due to less toxicity, no need for photosensitizer medication and ease of administration. Adverse effects of phototherapy include erythema pruritus, xerosis, hyperpigmentation and blistering, especially with higher dosages. Oral psoralens can cause nausea and vomiting. Long-term PUVA use can induce photoaging and a potential for increased cataract formation (psoralens bind to lens proteins). The concern of carcinogenesis linked to long-term light therapy (dose-related), especially PUVA, has led to recommended limits on total cumulative dose.[28,31,33]

Methotrexate, a folic acid antagonist, is an immunosuppressant effective in treating both psoriasis and psoriatic arthritis; it is given once weekly. There is significant associated liver and bone marrow toxicity.[57] Methotrexate's efficacy is greater than acitretin and equal or slightly inferior to cyclosporine. With appropriate monitoring for adverse effects, methotrexate can be used for years with sustained efficacy.[33]

Cyclosporine is a systemic calcineurin inhibitor, efficacious for both inducing remission and as maintenance therapy for patients with moderate to severe plaque psoriasis. It is also effective in treating pustular, erythrodermic and nail psoriasis. It is associated with significant side effects, particularly renal toxicity and hypertriglyceridemia, and therefore should be reserved for intermittent use only (up to 12 weeks at a time) to decrease risk of toxicity.[33]

Acitretin is an oral retinoid (vitamin A acid derivative) used in pustular or erythrodermic psoriasis. It has no immunosuppressive effects and its efficacy in psoriasis is probably due to modulation of cellular differentiation in the epidermis leading to re-establishment of a more normal pattern of cell growth. It is generally reserved for patients with moderate to severe disease who have not responded to other therapy and is commonly combined with topical vitamin D_3 analogues or phototherapy. Adverse effects include severe mucocutaneous drying, hypertriglyceridemia, and risk of teratogenicity that can remain a concern for up to 3 years after stopping acitretin.

Biologic response modifiers are the most effective agents for treatment of psoriasis but they are much more expensive than traditional systemic agents. Those approved in Canada for treatment of psoriasis include **adalimumab**, **etanercept**, **infliximab**, **secukinumab** and **ustekinumab**. Coverage by drug plans is often reserved for patients who have failed 2 traditional systemic agents (including phototherapy). Biologics may be used in combination with another systemic agent, especially methotrexate, if the response to monotherapy is inadequate. Biologic response modifiers provide a selective, immunologically directed intervention with fewer major organ toxicities. Adverse effects include increased risk of infections and development or worsening of autoimmune diseases or malignancies.[57,58]

Apremilast is an oral phosphodiesterase 4 inhhibitor that has immunosuppressant effects resulting in decreased inflammatory cytokines. It appears to be less effective than cyclosporine and biologic response modifiers and is expensive. It is relatively well tolerated and does not require routine bloodwork.[59,60]

Flexures and Face

Absorption of topical corticosteroid through the skin is greatly increased in flexure areas and the face; only **hydrocortisone** should be used in these areas. Psoriasis in the flexures (inverse psoriasis) poses unique therapeutic challenges since the impact does not relate to total body surface area. Topical hydrocortisone is the mainstay of therapy. If psoriatic lesions in the flexures become infected with tinea or *Candida*, hydrocortisone powder can be added to **topical imidazole** (e.g., **clotrimazole**, **miconazole**) creams, or the 2 creams (hydrocortisone and the imidazole) can be used in succession. Imidazoles have anti-inflammatory, antifungal and some gram-positive antibacterial effects. Stronger agents are sometimes used for recalcitrant cases.[12] The topical calcineurin inhibitors **pimecrolimus** and **tacrolimus** are effective and well tolerated in psoriasis of the face and flexures, though they are not approved for this indication.[33]

Scalp

Scalp treatments should involve 4 stages: descaling, active clearing, stabilization and long-term maintenance. They include the use of shampoos as vehicles for active agents and to remove scale, tar preparations with or without salicylic acid, anthralin, topical corticosteroids, vitamin D_3 analogues or tazarotene gel. A systematic review found that topical corticosteroids alone or combined with vitamin D_3 analogues were both more effective than vitamin D_3 analogues alone. Since safety profiles were similar and combination products provided only a slim benefit over corticosteroids alone, monotherapy with topical corticosteroids is a reasonable, less expensive approach.[61]

Scalp treatments can be applied on a damp scalp after towel drying, or on a dry scalp; the agent must reach the scalp lesions, not just the hair. Water-washable vehicles are preferred. Bath oil with surfactant can be used to assist in scale removal and as a vehicle for coal tar or other active agents, usually overnight. Active medications are often applied at night and shampooed out in the morning. Therapeutic agents must be left on the scalp after the shampoo and not used before. The topical product should be rubbed in to leave a thin film, not leaving a thick or visible coating.

Keratolytics, which decrease scale, should be left on for a minimum of 5–10 minutes, or overnight, and covered with a shower cap. After rinsing, corticosteroid lotions or gels can be applied, reserving higher potencies for pulse therapies of 2 weeks in resistant cases. Cytostatic antifungal preparations such as ketoconazole, selenium sulfide and zinc pyrithione are generally not suitable for treatment of psoriatic scalps. Use of imidazole antifungals remains controversial, since *Malassezia* fungus may be present in persistent nonresponsive psoriasis; use should be determined by positive culture.[11]

Palmoplantar

Palmoplantar psoriasis can be limited in extent (generally 4% of total body area) but have devastating impact due to pain, debilitation and social stigmatization, interfering with dexterity and mobility. Therapy must address alteration in quality of life. Protective measures such as shielding lesions from physical triggers are essential. Altered barrier function enables the Koebner phenomenon (see Risk and Aggravating Factors), adding to aggravation of lesions. Avoid harsh cleansers and contact with chemicals, solvents, fruit and vegetable juices. Protective cotton gloves should be worn. Emollients, especially in oil or ointment bases, help maintain barrier function, but suboptimal, less-greasy vehicles may be used to improve patient acceptance, provided they lack irritants (e.g., lanolin, fragrance, preservatives, see Chapter 55: Atopic, Contact, and Stasis Dermatitis). Topical corticosteroids are the mainstay of treatment, used with nighttime occlusion or keratolytic agents. Topical calcipotriol or tazarotene may be used; phototherapy may be used if topical agents are ineffective (PUVA more effective than UVB).[62]

For more information on the treatment of psoriasis, consult the *Compendium of Therapeutic Choices*: Psoriasis.

Psoriasis and Vaccinations

With the exception of acitretin, vaccine administration may be problematic with the use of systemic agents for psoriasis because of their immunosuppressive effects. An inadequate immune response may decrease effectiveness of an inactivated vaccine or lead to infection with live attenuated vaccines. Vaccination should take place before starting immunosuppressants if possible; wait 14 days after vaccination with an inactivated vaccine to ensure immunogenicity and 4 weeks after a live vaccine to reduce the risk of infection caused by the vaccine strain. If a patient already taking immunosuppressants (except high-dose systemic corticosteroids) requires an inactivated or live vaccine, the immunosuppressant should be stopped for 3 months prior to vaccination. High-dose systemic corticosteroids should be stopped for 4 weeks prior to vaccination.[63] Immunosuppressants should be held during serious or febrile illnesses including pneumonia, wound infections and cellulitis, but can be continued through uncomplicated upper respiratory tract infections or cystitis.[40]

Complementary and Alternative Therapies

The use of complementary and alternative medicine (CAM) among patients with psoriasis is common, with a prevalence of 43–69% in various studies. Most of these patients use natural health products, special diets or dietary supplements in conjunction with their usual antipsoriatic medications and not as replacements.[64] Natural health products such as aloe vera, beta-carotene, zinc, selenium, vitamin B complex, flax seed oil, yellow dock, horsetail, lavender and ginger (in the bath), as well as acupuncture, ayurveda and magnets (see Appendix I: Complementary and Alternative Therapies), have been promoted in the media or on Internet sites. Since these treatments lack controlled studies of their efficacy, side effects or interactions with recommended treatments, they should not be recommended. Psoriasis sufferers, due to distress over their condition, may turn in desperation to the Internet and other nonregulated sources of information. "Miracle cures" touted on the Internet may in fact worsen a patient's condition. A systematic review found the quality of most CAM studies was low.

Agents or interventions with documented clinical efficacy included:[64]

- *Mahonia aquifolium* (Oregon grape) contains berberine as the primary active constituent in the rhizome and root. This alkaloid inhibits keratinocyte growth and proliferation, and has antibacterial and antifungal activities. In 2 clinical trials *Mahonia aquifolium* was efficacious in reducing disease severity compared with placebo
- Fish oils have demonstrated efficacy in comparative trials. Long-chain polyunsaturated fatty acids, eicosapentaenoic acid (EPA) and docosahexaenoic acid (DHA), compete with arachidonic acid for cyclooxygenase and lipoxygenase, reducing proinflammatory molecules in psoriatic plaques. One study comparing EPA plus etretinate with etretinate monotherapy found significantly greater efficacy with the combination of EPA plus etretinate[65]
- Climatotherapy refers to the practice of traveling to sunbathe and/or bathe in the Dead Sea. Two studies using high- or low-concentration saline spa baths plus UVB showed response was significantly better with the saline spa bath plus UVB combination. Bathing in geothermal seawater combined with narrow band UVB therapy in psoriasis induced faster clinical and histological

improvement, produced longer remission time and permited lower UVB doses than UVB therapy alone[64,66]

- Stress-reduction techniques show inconsistent benefit. One randomized study demonstrated that both meditation or meditation plus imagery were efficacious as adjunctive treatments for patients with scalp psoriasis. A second showed the addition of a mindfulness-based stress-reduction audiotape played during light treatments reduced response times for patients receiving UVB but not PUVA therapy.[64]

Monitoring of Therapy

Table 3 presents a monitoring framework for patients. Parameters should be monitored by the patient in a diary. Scale will improve quite quickly with cosmetic treatment and hygiene control; thickness of scale will improve more slowly and erythema will take longest to respond.

Table 3: **Monitoring of Therapy for Psoriasis**

Parameter	Monitoring frequency	Time Frame/Degree of Change (resolution/control; relief of symptoms)	Actions
Scale	Patient: Daily while on drug therapy Healthcare practitioner: After 2–3 wk or next visit	Decrease by 50% within 7–10 days	Taper therapy in response to resolution; if end points not achieved, consider further therapy.
Thickness of plaque	Patient: Daily while on drug therapy Healthcare practitioner: After 2–3 wk or next visit	Decrease by 50% within 6–8 wk and by 75% within 8–12 wk	
Redness	Patient: Daily while on drug therapy Healthcare practitioner: After 2–3 wk or next visit	Decrease by 50% within 8–12 wk and by 75% within 12–16 wk	
Surface area involved	Patient: Daily while on drug therapy Healthcare practitioner: After 2–3 wk or next visit	Decrease by 50% within 6–8 wk and by 75% within 8–12 wk	
Extension to other sites or generalization	Patient: Daily while on drug therapy Healthcare practitioner: After 2–3 wk or next visit		
Itch/scratching	Patient: Daily while on drug therapy Healthcare practitioner: After 2–3 wk or next visit	Decrease to tolerable level within 1–2 wk	
Disruption of sleep or daily activities	Patient: Daily while on drug therapy Healthcare practitioner: After 2–3 wk or next visit	Restoration of normal patterns within 2–3 wk	
Stress, anxiety, depression	Patient: Daily while on drug therapy Healthcare practitioner: After 2–3 wk or next visit	Restoration of normal patterns within 2–3 wk	
Progression of severity	Patient: Daily while on drug therapy Healthcare practitioner: After 2–3 wk or next visit	No progression of severity	
Recurrent episodes	Patient: Daily while on drug therapy Healthcare practitioner: After 2–3 wk or next visit	Lengthening of symptom-free periods throughout therapy	
Allergic reactions	Patient: Daily while on drug therapy Healthcare practitioner: After 2–3 wk or next visit		If they occur, discontinue therapy.
Severe dryness, irritation (e.g., redness, inflammation, stinging)	Patient: Daily while on drug therapy Healthcare practitioner: After 2–3 wk or next visit	Minimal Should disappear, diminish or be controlled with continued use	If severe, decrease dose, concentration or frequency of use. If still no improvement, consider alternative treatment.

Monitor the side effects of drug therapy. If allergic reactions occur, discontinue therapy. If the condition worsens due to irritation, therapy should be altered. Failure to meet the listed end points should result in alteration of dosage or drug therapy. Therapy should be appropriately tapered in response to improvement or resolution.

Figure 2: **Suggested Approach for the Treatment of Psoriasis**

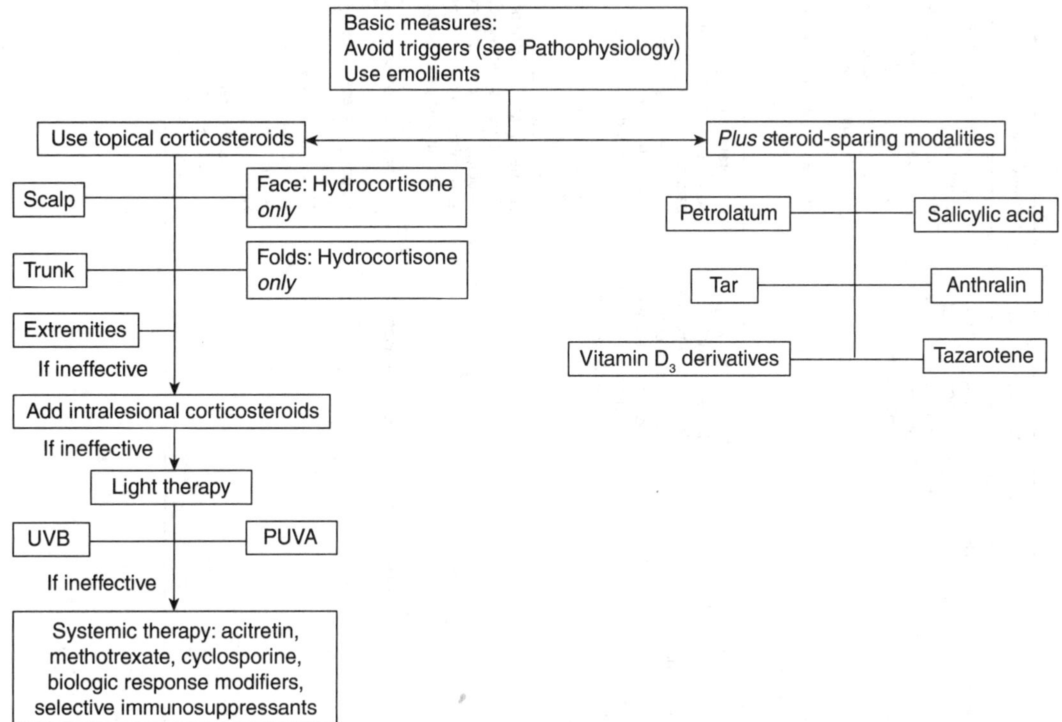

Table 4: Topical Psoriasis Therapies

Class	Drug	Dosage	Onset	Adverse Effects	Comments	Cost[a]
Anthracene derivatives	*anthralin*[b] *cream, ointment*	Short-contact anthralin therapy (SCAT): 0.1–2% formulations are applied to affected area for 15–30 min then washed off Traditional dosage: 0.05–3%. Apply HS and wash off in the morning. Start with lowest strength and increase gradually if tolerated	Onset: Requires 4 wk to see effect Remission: Long	Burning, stinging, irritation. Staining of skin, clothes, furniture. Discolouration of blonde hair.	Ingram routine = anthralin plus UVB. Protect skin around affected area with petrolatum or zinc oxide to minimize irritation. Avoid use on face, flexures or genitals due to irritation. If compounding with dry anthralin powder, gloves should be worn.	$$$
Corticosteroids, topical	*clobetasone 17–butyrate 0.05% cream* Spectro EczemaCare Medicated Cream	Apply BID–TID Limit use to 2–3 wk of therapy on an intermittent basis Once control achieved, maintenance dosing of once daily, 2–3 times per week may be sufficient	Onset: Quick Remission: Short	Burning, stinging, dryness, pruritus. Striae, telangiectasia, atrophy and purpura can occur but are unlikely when being applied to active lesions.	Moderate-potency corticosteroid for use in mild psoriasis on body areas *other than* face, folds and genitals (low-potency products recommended for these areas). To minimize risk of adverse effects intermittent use is recommended, often in an alternating fashion with non-steroidal topical therapies. Stronger corticosteroids may be required on thick-skinned areas such as palms or soles.	$$
	hydrocortisone 0.5%, 1% cream, lotion, ointment Cortate, Emo-Cort, Prevex HC, generics	See clobetasone.	See clobetasone.	See clobetasone.	Low-potency corticosteroid for use in mild psoriasis including on face, folds, genitals. Ointments are less cosmetically acceptable but generally more potent. Absorption greatest for creases and genitals, least from palms and soles. Use occlusion with caution.	$

Class	Drug	Dosage	Onset	Adverse Effects	Comments	Cost[a]
Keratolytic Agents	*coal tar cream, emulsion, gel, liquid, ointment, shampoo* Denorex, Liquor Carbonis Detergens, Targel, others	Use daily Soaks for scale removal: Start with 5% and increase as tolerated—soak 5–10 min Overnight to soften scale: Apply prior to corticosteroids Tar is more effective with prolonged contact time	Onset: 4 wk for full effect Sustained results with continued application	Acne, contact dermatitis, photosensitivity, unappealing odour. Stains skin and hair: cover with cotton/gloves. Apply in linear direction of hair growth to avoid folliculitis—do not rub in circular motion.	The tar distillate, liquor carbonis detergens (LCD), is 20% crude coal tar. Additive antimitotic activity with UVA and UVB. Coal tar plus UVB = Goeckerman routine. Contraindicated for diffuse, acutely inflamed or open wounds. When added to corticosteroid creams: 1-month expiry date.	$
	salicylic acid[b] *3–10% cream, gel, lotion, shampoo*	Lotion, cream, gel: Daily–BID Shampoo: Use on scalp at least twice weekly massaging thoroughly Use at the interval necessary to maintain control of condition	Onset: Requires 2–4 wk to see effect	Irritation, redness or peeling. Irritating to mucous membranes and eyes.	Although approved for single use, most products contain salicylic acid in combination with sulfur, and/or coal tar. Salicylic acid enhances penetration of topical agents through stratum corneum.	$$$

[a] Cost of 50 g or 50 mL; includes drug cost only.
[b] Extemporaneously compounded preparations can be used.
Abbreviations: UVA = ultraviolet A ; UVB = ultraviolet B
Legend: $ <$10 $$ <$10–20 $$$ $20–30

Resource Tips

A number of self-help support groups exist that can be accessed through the Internet.

National Institute of Arthritis and Musculoskeletal and Skin Diseases. *Psoriasis. Questions and answers about psoriasis*. Available from: www.niams.nih.gov/Health_Info/Psoriasis/default.asp.

National Psoriasis Foundation. getinfo@psoriasis.org. 1-800-723-9166. Available from: www.psoriasis.org.

The Psoriasis Association, which is a self-help organization founded in 1968, provides support and information on all aspects of the condition. Available from: www.psoriasis-association.org.uk.

Suggested Readings

Canadian Dermatology Association. Canadian Psoriasis Guidelines Committee. *Canadian guidelines for the management of plaque psoriasis*. June 2009. Available from: http://www.dermatology.ca/wp-content/uploads/2012/01/cdnpsoriasisguidelines.pdf

Menter A, Korman NJ, Elmets CA et al. Guidelines of care for the management of psoriasis and psoriatic arthritis. Section 3. Guidelines of care for the management and treatment of psoriasis with topical therapies. *J Am Acad Dermatol* 2009;60:643-59.

National Institute for Health and Care Excellence (NICE). *Psoriasis: assessment and management*. NICE guidelines (CG153). Manchester: NICE; 2012. Available from: www.nice.org.uk/guidance/cg153.

Samarasekera EJ, Sawyer L, Wonderling D et al. Topical therapies for the treatment of plaque psoriasis: systematic review and meta-analyses. *Br J Dermatol* 2013;168:954-67.

References

1. Gardner SS, McKay M. Seborrhea, psoriasis and the papulosquamous dermatoses. *Prim Care* 1989;16:739-63.
2. Parisi R, Symmons DP, Griffiths CE et al. Global epidemiology of psoriasis: a systematic review of incidence and prevalence. *J Invest Dermatol* 2013;133:377-85.
3. Raychaudhuri SP, Farber EM. The prevalence of psoriasis in the world. *J Eur Acad Dermatol Venereol* 2001;15:16-7.
4. Sobell JM, Geist DE. Psoriasis. In: Arndt KA, Hsu JT, eds. *Manual of dermatologic therapeutics*. 7th ed. Philadelphia: Wolters Kluwer/Lippincott Williams & Wilkins; 2007. p. 164-73.
5. Weller PA. Psoriasis. *Med J Aust* 1996;165:216-21.
6. Kadunce DP, Krueger GG. Pathogenesis of psoriasis. *Dermatol Clin* 1995;13:723-37.
7. Patel RV, Shelling ML, Prodanovich S et al. Psoriasis and vascular disease—risk factors and outcomes: a systematic review of the literature. *J Gen Intern Med* 2011;26:1036-49.
8. Kirby B, Richards HL, Mason DL et al. Alcohol consumption and psychological distress in patients with psoriasis. *Br J Dermatol* 2008;158:138-40.
9. Young DW, Downey DJ. Psoriasis: therapeutic aspects. *N Z Med J* 1993;106:63-4.
10. Guidelines for management of patients with psoriasis. Workshop of the Research Unit of the Royal College of Physicians of London; Department of Dermatology, University of Glasgow; British Association of Dermatologists. *BMJ* 1991;303:829-35.
11. Van de Kerkhof PC, Kleinpenning MM, Gerritsen RM. Scalp psoriasis. In: Koo JY, Lee CS, Lebwohl M, eds. *Mild-to-moderate psoriasis*. 2nd ed. New York: Informa Healthcare; 2009. p. 197-207.
12. Lee RA, Van Voorhees AS. Inverse psoriasis. In: Koo JY, Lee CS, Lebwohl M, eds. *Mild-to-moderate psoriasis*. 2nd ed. New York: Informa Healthcare; 2009. p. 209-23.
13. Lauritz B. The management of psoriasis. *Aust Fam Physician* 1982;11:704-8, 711.
14. Christophers E, Kiene P. Guttate and plaque psoriasis. *Dermatol Clin* 1995;13:751-6.
15. Prytowsky JH, Cohen PR. Pustular and erythrodermic psoriasis. *Dermatol Clin* 1995;13:757-70.
16. Wu JJ, Weinstein GD. General guidelines for administration of topical agents in the treatment of mild-to-moderate psoriasis. In: Koo JY, Lee CS, Lebwohl M, eds. *Mild-to-moderate psoriasis*. 2nd ed. New York: Informa Healthcare; 2009. p. 11-21.
17. Katugampola RP, Lewis VJ, Finlay AY. The Dermatology Life Quality Index: assessing the efficacy of biological therapies for psoriasis. *Br J Dermatol* 2007;156:945-50.
18. National Institute for Health and Care Excellence (NICE). *Psoriasis: Evidence update November 2014*. Manchester: NICE; 2014. Available from: www.nice.org.uk/guidance/cg153/evidence/evidence-update-188313949.
19. Chren MM, Lasek RJ Quinn LM et al. Skindex, a quality-of-life measure for patients with skin disease: reliability, validity, and responsiveness. *J Invest Dermatol* 1996;107:707-13.
20. Cappelleri JC, Bushmakin AG, Harness J et al. Psychometric validation of the physician global assessment scale for assessing severity of psoriasis disease activity. *Qual Life Res* 2013;22:2489-99.
21. Flytstrom I, Stenberg B, Svensson A et al. Patients' visual analogue scale: a useful method for assessing psoriasis severity. *Acta Derm Venereol* 2012;92:347-8.

22. Augustin M, Blome C, Costanzo A et al. Nail assessment in psoriasis and psoriatic arthritis (NAPPA): development and validation of a tool for assessment of nail psoriasis outcomes. *Br J Dermatol* 2014;170:591-8.
23. Farber EM, Nall L. An appraisal of measures to prevent and control psoriasis. *J Am Acad Dermatol* 1984;10:511-7.
24. Naldi L, Conti A, Cazzaniga S et al. Diet and physical exercise in psoriasis: a randomized controlled trial. *Br J Dermatol* 2014;170:634-42.
25. Kabat-Zinn J, Wheeler E, Light T et al. Influence of a mindfulness mediations-based stress reduction intervention on rates of skin clearing in patients with moderate to severe psoriasis undergoing phototherapy (UVB) and photochemotherapy (PUVA). *Psychosom Med* 1998;60:625-32.
26. Bundy C, Pinder B, Bucci S et al. A novel, web-based, psychological intervention for people with psoriasis: the electronic Targeted Intervention for Psoriasis (eTIPs) study. *Br J Dermatol* 2013;169:329-36.
27. Seite S, Khemis A, Rougier A et al. Emollient for maintenance therapy after topical corticotherapy in mild psoriasis. *Exp Dermatol* 2009;18:1076-8.
28. Menter A, Korman NJ, Elmets CA et al., Guidelines of care for the management of psoriasis and psoriatic arthritis. Section 3. Guidelines of care for the management and treatment of psoriasis with topical therapies. *J Am Acad Dermatol* 2009;60:643-59.
29. Gottlieb A, Korman NJ, Gordon KB et al. Guidelines of care for the management of psoriasis and psoriatic arthritis: Section 2. Psoriatic arthritis: overview and guidelines of care for treatment with an emphasis on the biologics. *J Am Acad Dermatol* 2008;58:851-64.
30. Menter A, Korman NJ, Elmets CA et al. Guidelines of care for the management of psoriasis and psoriatic arthritis: Section 4. Guidelines of care for the management and treatment of psoriasis with traditional systemic agents. *J am Acad Dermatol* 2009;61:451-85.
31. Menter A, Korman NJ, Elmets CA et al. Guidelines of care for the management of psoriasis and psoriatic arthritis: Section 5. Guidelines of care for the treatment of psoriasis with phototherapy and photochemotherapy. *J Am Acad Dermatol* 2010;62:114-35.
32. National Clinical Guideline Centre (UK). *Psoriasis: assessment and management of psoriasis*. London: Royal College of Physicians; 2012.
33. Canadian Dermatology Association. Canadian Psoriasis Guidelines Committee. *Canadian guidelines for the management of plaque psoriasis*. June 2009. Available from: www.dermatology.ca/psoriasisguidelines.
34. Pathirana D, Ormerod AD, Saiag P et al. European S3-guidelines on the systemic treatment of psoriasis vulgaris. *J Eur Acad Dermatol Venereol* 2009;23:1-70.
35. Feldman SR. General approach to psoriasis treatment. In: Koo JY, Lee CS, Lebwohl M, eds. *Mild-to-moderate psoriasis*. 2nd ed. New York: Informa Healthcare; 2009. p. 5-9.
36. Strober BE, Nyirady J, Mallya UG et al. Item-level psychometric properties for a new patient-reported psoriasis symptom diary. *Value Health* 2013;16:1014-22.
37. Balato N, Megna M, Di Costanzo L et al. Educational and motivational support service: a pilot study for mobile-phone-based interventions in patients with psoriasis. *Br J Dermatol* 2013;168:201-5.
38. Long CC, Finlay AY. The finger-tip unit–a new practical measure. *Clin Exp Dermatol* 1991;16:444-7.
39. Hodge L, Comaish JS. Psoriasis: current concepts in management. *Drugs* 1977;13:288-96.
40. Hsu S, Papp KA, Lebwhol MG et al. Consensus guidelines for the management of plaque psoriasis. *Arch Dermatol* 2012;148:95-102.
41. Samarasekera EJ, Sawyer L, Wonderling D et al. Topical therapies for the treatment of plaque psoriasis: systematic review and meta-analyses. *Br J Dermatol* 2013;168:954-67.
42. Fitzmaurice S, Becker E, Koo JY et al. Treatment of mild-to-moderate psoriasis with coal tar, anthralin, salicylic acid and lactic acid. In: Koo JY, Lee CS, Lebwohl M, eds. *Mild-to-moderate psoriasis*. 2nd ed. New York: Informa Healthcare; 2009. p. 91-102.
43. Koo J, Cuffie CA, Tanner DJ et al. Mometasone furoate 0.1%-salicylic acid 5% ointment versus mometasone furoate 0.1% ointment in the treatment of moderate-to-severe psoriasis: a multicenter study. *Clin Ther* 1998;20:283-91.
44. Lebwohl M. The role of salicylic acid in the treatment of psoriasis. *Int J Dermatol* 1999;38:16-24.
45. Silverman A, Menter A, Hairston JL. Tars and anthralins. *Dermatol Clin* 1995;13:817-33.
46. Muller SA, Perry HO. The Goeckerman treatment in psoriasis: six decades of experience at the Mayo Clinic. *Cutis* 1984;34:265-8, 270.
47. Thawornchaisit P, Harnchareon K. A comparative study of tar and betamethasone valerate in chronic plaque psoriasis: a study in Thailand. *J Med Assoc Thai* 2007;90:1997-2002.
48. Schaefer C, Peters P, Miller RK, eds. *Drugs during pregnancy and lactation: treatment options and risk assessment*. 3rd ed. Waltham: Academic Press; 2015.
49. Weatherhead S, Robson SC, Reynolds NJ. Management of psoriasis in pregnancy. *BMJ* 2007;334:1218-20.
50. Drugs and Lactation Database (LactMed). Bethesda: U.S. National Library of Medicine. Available from: toxnet.nlm.nih.gov/cgi-bin/sis/htmlgen?LACT. Accessed April 16, 2015.
51. Kraft S, Maibach HI, Shroot B. Dithranol. In: Roenigk HH, Maibach HI, eds. *Psoriasis*. 3rd ed. New York: M. Dekker; 1998. p. 435-52.
52. Koo J, Lebwohl M. Duration of remission of psoriasis therapies. *J Am Acad Dermatol* 1999;41:51–9.
53. van de Kerkhof PC, van der Valk PG, Swinkels OQ et al. A comparison of twice-daily calcipotriol ointment with once-daily short-contact dithranol cream therapy: a randomized controlled trail of supervised treatment of psoriasis vulgaris in a day-care setting. *Br J Dermatol* 2006;155:800-7.
54. Mason AR, Mason J, Cork M et al. Topical treatments for chronic plaque psoriasis. *Cochrane Database Syst Rev* 2013;3:CD005028.
55. Lebwohl MG, Landry CA Topical calcineurin inhibitors. In: Koo JY, Lee CS, Lebwohl M, eds. *Mild-to-moderate psoriasis*. 2nd ed. New York: Informa Healthcare; 2009. p. 83-90.
56. Mehta D, Lim HW. Ultraviolet B phototherapy for psoriasis: review of practical guidelines. *Am J Clin Dermatol* 2016;17:125-33.
57. Nguyen TU, Gottlieb A. Combination therapy. In: Koo JY, Lee CS, Lebwohl M, eds. *Mild-to-moderate psoriasis*. 2nd ed. New York: Informa Healthcare; 2009. p. 139-64.
58. Menter A, Gottlieb A, Feldman SR et al. Guidelines of care for the management of psoriasis and psoriatic arthritis: Section 1. Overview of psoriasis and guidelines of care for the treatment of psoriasis with biologics. *J Am Acad Dermatol* 2008;58:826-50.
59. Poole RM, Ballantyne AD. Apremilast: first global approval. *Drugs* 2014;74:825-37.
60. Papp K, Reich K, Leonardi CL et al. Apremilast, an oral phosphodiesterase 4 (PDE4) inhibitor, in patients with moderate to severe plaque psoriasis: results of a phase III, randomized, controlled trial (Efficacy and Safety Trial Evaluating the Effects of Apremilast in Psoriasis [ESTEEM] 1). *J Am Acad Dermatol*2015;73:37-49.
61. Schlager JG, Rosumeck S , Werner RN et al. Topical treatments for scalp psoriasis. *Cochrane Database Syst Rev* 2016;2:CD009687.
62. Krulig E, Gordon KN. Palmarplantar psoriasis. In: Koo JY, Lee CS, Lebwohl M, eds. *Mild-to-moderate psoriasis*. 2nd ed. New York: Informa Healthcare; 2009. p. 183-95.
63. Public Health Agency of Canada. *Canadian Immunization Guide*. Available at: http://www.phac-aspc.gc.ca/publicat/cig-gci/p03-07-eng.php

64. Smith N, Weymann A, Tausk FA et al. Complementary and alternative medicine for psoriasis: a qualitative review of the clinical trial literature. *J Am Acad Dermatol* 2009;61:841-56.
65. Danno K, Sugie N. Combination therapy with low-dose etretinate and eicosapentaenoic acid for psoriasis vulgaris. *J Dermatol* 1998;25:703-5.
66. Eysteinsdottir JH, Olafsson JH, Agnarsson BA et al. Psoriasis treatment: faster and long-standing results after bathing in geothermal seawater. A randomized trial of three UVB phototherapy regimens. *Photodermatol Photoimmunol Photomed* 2014;30:25-34.

Psoriasis—What You Need to Know

What is psoriasis?

Psoriasis is a common skin condition that comes and goes but never goes away completely (chronic condition). It appears in various forms. The most common form of psoriasis is scaly red patches on the scalp, arms, legs and trunk. The nails may also be affected.

What causes psoriasis?

A number of things can trigger psoriasis:

- Heredity—you are more likely to have psoriasis if a parent or close relative has it
- High level of stress in your life
- Drinking too much alcohol over a long period of time
- Being overweight
- Smoking
- Environmental factors like low humidity (dryness)
- Injury to the skin.

Some medications can make psoriasis worse:

- Ask your healthcare provider about medications that may make psoriasis worse:
  - beta-blockers
  - lithium
  - antimalarial drugs
  - oral corticosteroids (taken by mouth)
  - nonsteroidal anti-inflammatory drugs such as ASA
- Do not stop taking your prescribed medications without checking with your healthcare provider.
- Ask your healthcare provider about cosmetics, herbal remedies, nonprescription products or alternative therapies before you try them.

How should you care for your skin?

Cleanse:

- Bathe or shower every day.
- Use warm water, not hot.
- Do not use harsh soaps on your skin.

Moisturize:

- Keep your skin well lubricated at all times to reduce dryness and scratching.
- Apply a lubricating cream (emollient) to your skin while it is still damp. You may also use this cream as a cleanser.
- Apply creams smoothly in the direction hair grows (hair will lie flat).
- Use a sunscreen to protect your skin from sun damage and keep it moist.

Laundry:

- Wash clothes in soap flakes (e.g., Ivory Snow), not detergent. If you have to use detergent, wash clothes a second time in clear water (no detergent).
- Do not use bleach in your laundry.
- Do not use liquid or sheet fabric softener.

Prevent itching and scratching:

- Keep nails short—try not to scratch the affected skin.
- Avoid tight clothing that rubs your skin. Loose-fitting clothes will reduce rubbing.
- Avoid rough synthetics, nylon or wool fabrics. Look for cotton or corduroy clothing.
- Use a cool air humidifier in your home.

What can you do to control psoriasis?

- Avoid or reduce things that can trigger a flare or make it worse:
  - alcohol
  - smoking
  - increased weight
  - physical injury
  - sunburn
- Eat a healthy diet every day with lots of fruit, vegetables and fibre.
- Take part in moderate exercise on a regular basis.
- Reduce stress in your life. Take up a hobby; try to increase the amount of time you have for relaxation or vacation.
- See your healthcare provider if you have pain in your joints or if your nails are affected.

Chapter 72

Prevention and Treatment of Sun-induced Skin Damage

Nancy Kleiman, BSP, MBA

Pathophysiology

The skin and its appendages (e.g., sweat glands, sebaceous glands and hair follicles) serve several important functions. They protect against minor injury, help control body temperature and water loss, prevent invasion by microorganisms, and prevent radiation damage from sun exposure. The skin is composed of 3 main layers: epidermis (which includes the stratum corneum), dermis and subcutaneous layer (Figure 1).[1]

Figure 1: **The Skin**

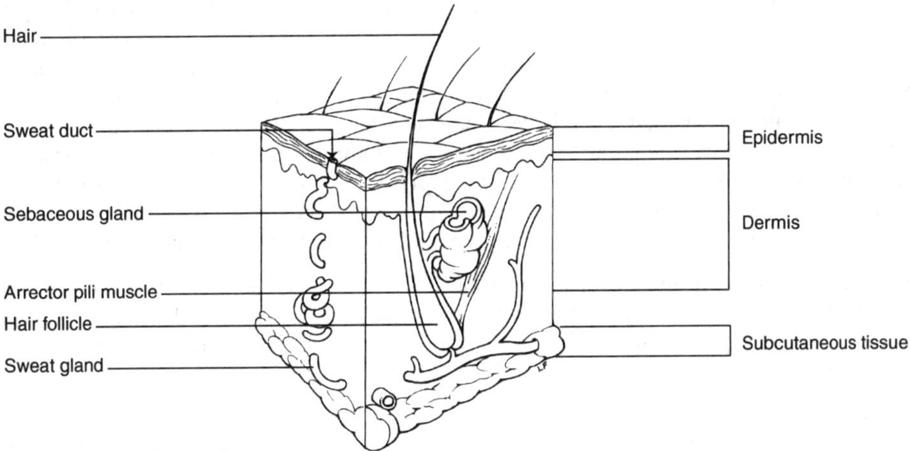

Ultraviolet Radiation

Ultraviolet light is divided into 3 categories: ultraviolet-A (UVA; 320–400 nm), ultraviolet-B (UVB; 290–320 nm) and ultraviolet-C (UVC; 270–290 nm).[2]

- Longwave **UVA** radiation penetrates the dermis and subcutaneous fat. UVA is a less potent carcinogen than UVB or UVC, but is a significant contributor to skin cancer risk because more reaches the Earth than other types of ultraviolet (UV) radiation. UVA is present all day and can penetrate through clouds, windows and clothing. UVA radiation penetrates deep into the skin. There is a strong indication that UVA is responsible for phototoxicity, photoaging, immunosuppression, epidermal thickening, reduced skin barrier function and skin cancers.[3] UVA is also responsible for reactions from **photosensitizing drugs** such as amiodarone, doxycycline, hydrochlorothiazide, naproxen and voriconazole.[4]

- **UVB** damages the stratum corneum and epidermal layers. It is the main cause of sunburn and plays a role in both skin cancer and photoaging.[3] Acute exposure increases blood flow to the skin and activates inflammatory pathways, resulting in reddened skin and sunburn. However, even at doses too low to cause skin reddening, UVB can cause local and systemic immunosuppression, direct damage to DNA and other skin cell abnormalities that increase the risk of skin cancer.[2] UVB is strongest between 10 a.m. and 4 p.m. and at high altitudes, and is intensified by wind, humidity, high temperatures and reflective surfaces (e.g., water, sand, snow, concrete).[2]
- **UVC** does not reach the surface of the Earth as it is filtered by the surrounding ozone layer.

The UV index is provided by Environment Canada and predicts the strength of the sun's UV rays. Higher UV readings indicate a higher risk of sunburn as the rays are stronger. UV indexes of 3 or more are reported daily.

Sun-induced Skin Damage

Sun-induced skin damage includes sunburn, photoaging, pigmentary changes, actinic keratosis and skin cancer.

Sunburn is an inflammatory response of the skin to UV radiation. Sunburn is preventable and generally self-treatable. Refer to Chapter 57: Burns, for assessment and treatment of burns.

Photoaging refers to the effects of long-term exposure to the sun and is commonly referred to as "premature skin aging".[5] The effects can be seen many years before normal age-related changes are noted in non-sun-exposed areas. The difference between the signs of normal aging and photoaging can readily be seen by comparing non-sun-exposed areas of the body with skin on the face, arms and hands. Skin changes in photoaging differ from those in normal skin aging. In photoaged skin, changes in the stratum corneum and epidermal cells result in rough, coarse, dull-appearing skin with fine and deep wrinkles. In more advanced photoaging, deposition of abnormal elastic fibres, decreased collagen and pigment changes in the upper dermis result in deeply wrinkled, yellowish skin. Vascular changes in the dermis can cause telangiectasias and easy bruising. A change in the properties of water-retentive glycosaminoglycan contributes to the dry, rough, leathery appearance of photoaged skin.[6]

Pigmentary changes result from chronic exposure to UV radiation. Hypermelanosis is characterized by an increase in pigmentation, slowly progressing to irregular areas on the skin that range in colour from light to dark brown. It appears primarily on sun-exposed areas, particularly the face, and is commonly referred to as "age spots".[7]

Actinic keratosis is a common sun-induced lesion caused by chronic exposure to sun and is more prevalent in males and in light-skinned individuals. Onset is typically after the age of 50. It generally appears on the face, back of the hands, forearms and legs as a firm, scaling lesion with slight erythema. If left untreated, actinic keratosis can progress to squamous cell carcinoma.[8] See Actinic Keratosis in Photo Section.

Nonmelanoma Skin Cancer: Squamous cell carcinoma risk is related to chronic, cumulative lifetime sun exposure; therefore, people with visibly photoaged skin are at greater risk. Commonly found on the face, ears, neck, forearms, back of the hands and legs, it initially appears as an abnormal scaling or crusty lesion that may be raised and wart-like. The lesions may bleed or erode over time, leading to firm tumors.[5] Basal cell carcinoma is related to sun exposure during childhood and adolescence and is commonly found on the face. It appears as small, dome-shaped lesions that may have a shiny surface (much like a pimple that does not heal) that slowly expand over time and develop central ulceration.[8]

Melanoma Skin Cancer: Malignant melanoma appears to be related to intense and intermittent sun exposure in childhood and adolescence. It is the rarest type of cancer, but is responsible for the majority of skin cancer deaths. Risk is increased in blond or red-headed individuals who have skin that tans poorly and burns easily, in those with a large number of moles, with chronic exposure to the sun or in those with a history of sunburns as a child. It appears as a flat brown or black spot (commonly in a mole or other dark spot) with irregular edges, that can grow larger if left untreated.[8]

Goals of Therapy

- Prevent acute sun-induced skin damage (sunburn)
- Prevent phototoxic reactions from medications
- Provide relief of pain resulting from sunburn
- Minimize the risk of infection in severe sunburns
- Prevent long-term sun-induced skin damage (including photoaging and some types of skin cancer)
- Reduce the visible effects of photoaging on the skin

Patient Assessment

If the concern is sun-induced skin damage, determine whether the goal is prevention (selection and use of sunscreens) or treatment. Figure 2 presents an assessment of patients requesting sun protection.

Prevention of Sun-induced Skin Damage

Nonpharmacologic Therapy

There are many ways to prevent the acute and chronic effects of sun exposure. Avoiding direct sun exposure from 10 a.m. to 4 p.m. when UVB rays are strongest as well as when the UV Index is high decreases the risk of sunburn.[2] A person should seek shade as much as possible while outside. Wearing protective clothing such as long-sleeved shirts, pants and gloves decreases exposure. Cotton or linen clothing that is tightly woven, loose fitting and lightweight provides some protection. Clothing that is wet, white or loosely woven provides very little protection (darker colours give better protection).[2] Wide-brimmed hats of tightly woven fabric will protect the face, ears and parts of the neck from sun exposure, and long-term use will reduce the risk of skin cancers by 40%.[2] Sunglasses should be worn to protect the eyes from sun damage. Children under the age of 6 months should be protected from the sun at all times by keeping them shaded and completely covered.

Tanning salons should be avoided; the protection provided against environmental UV exposure (such as sunburn on tropical holidays) is minimal. Tanning bed use increases the risk of basal and squamous cell carcinoma[11] as well as melanoma.[12] The World Health Organization (WHO) recommends that no one under the age of 18 use tanning facilities. If used, time limits should be observed and protective eyewear should be worn at all times during the session.

Phototoxic reactions are dose-related sunburn-like reactions that occur in all people with sufficient light and drug exposure. Those taking medications that may cause phototoxic reactions should use extra precautions to prevent acute and chronic sun damage (see Table 1). Radiation in the UVA range causes most drug-related phototoxic reactions. In contrast, photoallergic reactions are delayed hypersensitivity reactions after light exposure, and occur only in a small percentage of individuals. Unlike phototoxic reactions, photoallergic reactions may extend beyond the area exposed to light.

Pharmacologic Therapy

For comparative ingredients of nonprescription products, consult the *Compendium of Products for Minor Ailments*—Skin Care Products: Sunscreens.

Sunscreens effectively reduce skin tanning and sunburn. Sunscreen use can also reduce photoaging and development of actinic keratosis, and promote regression of existing actinic keratosis.[2] It is estimated that regular sunscreen use for the first 20 years could decrease the lifetime risk of skin cancer by about 85%.[14] Daily sunscreen use for 4.5 years decreased the incidence of squamous cell cancer[15] and reduced new primary melanomas by 50% and invasive melanomas by 73%.[16] Sunscreens are an adjunct only, and should be used to protect the skin rather than prolong the time that can be spent in the direct sun. Sunscreens should always be used in conjunction with protective clothing in order to fully protect exposed skin.[17]

The Canadian Dermatology Association recommends that sunscreens should:[18]

- have an SPF of at least 30
- be nonirritating, noncomedogenic and hypoallergenic
- be minimally or nonperfumed
- offer broad-spectrum UVA protection.

Sunless tanning products contain **chemical tanning agents** such as **dihydroxyacetone** (DHA), a dye that colours the skin when applied topically to produce an artificial tan. The colour change is temporary, lasting several days, and must be reapplied every few days to maintain an even colour. Tanning agents have a very low sun protection factor (SPF) value of 3–4 unless marketed in combination with sunscreen products. Dihydroxyacetone is considered nontoxic and is regulated as a cosmetic rather than as a drug.[19]

Table 1: **Medications that May Cause Phototoxic Reactions[a,13]**

Antimicrobials	Azole antifungals (itraconazole, voriconazole), ceftazidime, quinolones (ciprofloxacin, norfloxacin, ofloxacin), sulfonamides, tetracyclines (doxycycline, tetracycline), trimethoprim
Antineoplastics	Dacarbazine, EGF inhibitors (cetuximab, erlotinib, gefitinib, lapatinib, panitumumab), 5-fluorouracil, paclitaxel, vinblastine
Diuretics	Furosemide, hydrochlorothiazide
NSAIDs	Diclofenac, ibuprofen, indomethacin, ketoprofen, naproxen, piroxicam, sulindac, tiaprofenic acid
Psychiatric medications	Alprazolam, chlordiazepoxide, chlorpromazine, desipramine, fluphenazine, imipramine, perphenazine, prochlorperazine, trifluoperazine
Retinoids, systemic	Acitretin, alitretinoin, isotretinoin
Retinoids, topical[b]	Adapalene, tazarotene, tretinoin
Statins	
Others	Amiodarone, coal tar derivatives (topical), diltiazem, methoxsalen, quinidine, quinine, sulfites, tolbutamide, verteporfin

[a] Radiation in the UVA range causes most drug-related phototoxic reactions.
[b] After continued use due to thinning of the stratum corneum.

Abbreviations: EGF = epidermal growth factor; NSAID = nonsteroidal anti-inflammatory drug

Sunscreen Labelling

Sunscreens should be used to protect the skin and not to prolong sun exposure. They should be broad spectrum meaning contain recognized ingredients that protect against both UVA and UVB (see Table 2). Sunscreens should have an SPF of at least 15 and preferably 30. SPF is defined as the least amount of energy needed to produce erythema (primarily UVB) with sunscreen, divided by the least amount of energy needed to produce erythema without sunscreen. Sunscreens with the "broad spectrum" designation and SPF ≥15 may use the following statement: "If used as directed with other sun protection measures, decreases the risk of skin cancer and early skin aging caused by the sun".

Sunscreens with an SPF <15 or not designated as "broad spectrum" must use the following statement: "This product has been shown only to help prevent sunburn, not skin cancer or early skin aging".[20,21]

Water-resistant products may be labelled only as "Water/Sweat Resistant (40 minutes)" or "Water/Sweat Resistant (80 minutes)".[20,21]

Sunscreen Application

Sunscreens are combinations of several different active ingredients and may contain physical blockers as well as chemical sunscreens (see Table 2). Physical barriers such as **titanium dioxide** and **zinc oxide** reflect and scatter UV radiation while chemical agents absorb UV light. Physical barrier products currently available have been micronized to be more cosmetically appealing than older products.[5]

Table 2: **Sunscreen Ingredients**[13,22,23]

Class/ *Chemical Name (synonyms)*	Wavelength	Benefits	Comments
Anthranilates *meradimate (menthyl anthranilate, menthyl-2-aminobenzoate)*	UVB (weak) UVA (incomplete protection, 300–340 nm)		Allergic reactions are rare.
Benzimidazoles *ensulizole (2-phnylbenzimidazole-5-sulfonic acid, PBSA, Eusolex 232, Parsol HS)*	UVB (minimal UVA) 290–320 nm	Well tolerated Photostable	Water soluble Allergic reactions are rare.
Benzophenones *dioxybenzone (benzophenone-8)* *oxybenzone (benzophenone-3, Escalol 567, Eusolex 4360)* *sulisobenzone (benzophenone-4, 2-hydroxy-4-methoxybenzone-5-sulfonic acid)*	UVB Lower UVA 260–380 nm depending on chemical	May advertise as broad-spectrum UVB/UVA protection; cover most of UVB plus lower-mid UVA range.	Some skin sensitization, allergic reactions. Must be combined with titanium dioxide and/or zinc oxide for stability.
Benzotriazoles *bisoctrizole (methylene bis-benzotriazolyl-tetramethylbutylphenol, Tinosorb M)*	UVB UVA (broad spectrum, maximum absorption 360 nm)	Characteristics of organic and inorganic filters.	Allergic reactions are rare.
Benzylidene camphor derivatives *enzacamene (4-methylbenzylidene camphor, MBC, Eusolex 6300, Parsol 5000)*	UVB Maximum absorption at 300 nm	Photostable	Water soluble
terephthalylidene dicamphor sulfonic acid (ecamsule, Mexoryl SX)	UVB UVA (broad spectrum, maximum absorption 345 nm)	Good photostability	Easily removed through perspiration or swimming (need to be combined with products that do not wash off). Allergic reactions are rare.
Cinnamates *cinoxate (2-ethoxyethyl p-methoxycinnamate)* *octinoxate (octyl methoxycinnamate, 2-ethylhexylmethoxycinnamate, EMC, OMC, Escalol 557, Parsol MCX)* *octocrylene (2-ethylhexyl-2-cyano-3,3-diphenylacrylate, OCR, Eusolex)*	UVB May have some UVA 280–320 nm	Photostabilize dibenzoylmethanes (avobenzone). Octocrylene: Some coverage in low UVA range which allows products to claim UVB/UVA protection.	Easily removed by abrasion, perspiration or swimming (need to be combined with products that do not wash off). Require frequent application. Allergic reactions are rare.

(cont'd)

Table 2: **Sunscreen Ingredients**[13,22,23] *(cont'd)*

Class/ ***Chemical Name (synonyms)***	**Wavelength**	**Benefits**	**Comments**
Dibenzoylmethanes *avobenzone (t-butylmethoxy-dibenzoylmethane, Eusolex 9020, Parsol 1789)*	UVA (broad spectrum, 320–400 nm)	Better UVA protection than benzophenones and Mexoryl SX.	60% decrease in efficacy after 1 h of exposure to the sun (combined with Mexoryl to enhance photostability). May cause allergic reactions/contact dermatitis. Photo unstable.
Hydroxybenzotriazoles *drometriazole trisiloxane (silatriazole, Mexoryl XL)*	UVB UVA (broad spectrum, 320–360 nm)	Photostable	Allergic reactions are rare.
Hydroxyphenyltriazines *bemotrizinol (anizotriazine, bis-ethylhexyloxyphenolmethoxyphenyl triazine. Tinosorb S)*	UVB UVA (broad spectrum, maximum absorption 343 nm)	Included in products to improve the photostability of sunscreens containing avobenzone.	
Para-aminobenzoic Acid (PABA) esters *padimate O (octyl dimethyl PABA)*	UVB 260–320 nm	Resistant to water and sweating and adhere well to skin even after swimming.	Can cause skin irritation and photosensitivity reactions. Rarely included in products due to frequency of sensitivity issues (contact dermatitis). Can stain clothing. Avoid in those sensitive to sulfonamides, thiazides and sulfonylureas.
Physical blocks (inorganic agents) *titanium dioxide* *zinc oxide*	UVB, UVA (full spectrum) zinc oxide: 290–400 nm titanium dioxide: 290–340 nm	Can be used by all ages (infants >6 months). Less risk of sensitization than chemical sunscreens. Photostable. Reflect and scatter UV and visible light. Clear formulations of micronized particles are cosmetically more appealing.	Titanium should not be used on children under 6 months or applied to open wounds. May cause or worsen acne by clogging skin pores.
Salicylates *homosalate (homomenthyl salicylate, HMS)* *octisalate (octyl salicylate, 2-ethylhexyl salicylate, Escalol 587)* *triethanolamine salicylate (trolamine salicylate)*	UVB only (weak) 260–320 nm	Skin irritation is rare. Very stable; included in other products to improve stability and augment UVB protection.	Easily removed by abrasion, perspiration or swimming.

To ensure full effectiveness, sunscreens should be applied uniformly and liberally over the entire area of sun exposure, including lips, ears and tops of the feet. Sunscreen should be applied 15–30 minutes prior to exposure with reapplication 15–30 minutes later to maximize protection.[2] Sunscreens should also be reapplied after swimming, sweating or towelling off. It is recommended that 2 mg of sunscreen per cm^2 of skin be applied to the body to ensure that the SPF protection claimed by the manufacturer is reached.[8,24,25] An easier way to measure the appropriate amount of sunscreen is referred to as the "teaspoon rule." It is recommended that a person apply 0.5–1 teaspoonful on the face and neck; 1–1.5 teaspoonfuls to arms, shoulders and torso and 2–2.5 teaspoonfuls to the legs and the tops of the feet.[24]

Many individuals do not apply enough sunscreen to attain the stated SPF of the product. Ensure that patients are aware of the proper application methods and that sunscreen should be reapplied after sweating or being in water. Lip balms should also be used on a regular basis to protect lips from the sun. Sunscreen vehicles also affect the application of the product. Lotions and creams are the most common vehicles used and are formulated as oil-in-water or water-in-oil emulsions; inadequate application may occur because the products may be greasy and less desirable than other formulations. Gels are preferred by patients with oily skin but are easily removed when swimming or sweating. Products that are in a spray formulation are convenient and easy to apply. The disadvantage is that sprays are often applied with a thin layer of coverage, areas are missed completely or the spray is not rubbed in sufficiently for full effectiveness.[26]

Sunscreen and Vitamin D

Vitamin D synthesis requires UVB exposure. In theory, 90% of the required vitamin D can be produced this way. In practice, the production of vitamin D is highly variable depending upon which area of skin is exposed to the sun and for how long, latitude, skin pigmentation, age, and season.[27] There has been some concern that the increased use of sunscreens decreases the synthesis of Vitamin D. The debate continues as to the impact of the use of sunscreens on the production of vitamin D and the American Academy of Dermatology suggests supplementation.[26]

Sunscreen Safety

Limited animal and laboratory studies about the safety of some sunscreen ingredients or additives have attracted media attention. These have included carcinogenicity of retinyl palmitate, hormone disruption by oxybenzone and absorption of nanoparticles of zinc and titanium. However, many national dermatology associations have responded to these concerns with statements reassuring consumers that evidence from use in humans shows that approved sunscreen ingredients are safe to use and protect against skin cancer.[28,29,30]

Treatment of Sun-induced Skin Damage

Nonpharmacologic Therapy

Treatment of sunburns, both minor and severe, includes relieving the discomfort caused by the burn. Application of cool tap water compresses will relieve some pain associated with minor sunburn. Patients should avoid further exposure to the sun to prevent further burning, which could lead to an increase in the severity of the sunburn. If further exposure to the sun cannot be avoided, the individual should wear protective clothing, apply a sunscreen and limit the amount of time in the sun during peak times (10 a.m. to 4 p.m.).

Pharmacologic Therapy

For comparative ingredients of nonprescription products, consult the *Compendium of Products for Minor Ailments*—Analgesic Products: Internal Analgesics and Antipyretics; Skin Care Products: First Aid.

Therapy for Sunburn

Skin protectants such as **petrolatum** and hydrophilic ointments provide symptomatic relief of minor sunburns and redness. These products protect the area from irritation caused by friction from clothing and moisturize and rehydrate the skin. Bath and baby oils have minimal effect and peanut and corn oil are ineffective.[31]

Analgesics are used short term to relieve the pain and mild inflammation caused by sunburn. They should be taken either just before or immediately after exposure as inflammation generally occurs within the first 24 hours. Anti-inflammatory agents such as **ibuprofen**, **naproxen sodium** or **acetylsalicylic acid** (ASA) are recommended. **Acetaminophen** can also be used for pain relief if anti-inflammatories cannot be used.[31]

Topical aloe vera has traditionally been promoted for its wound-healing ability. A systematic review found that there is inconclusive evidence to determine whether aloe vera gel or dressings improve outcomes in acute wounds including burns.[32] The amount of active ingredient in aloe vera products varies according to growing conditions, age of the plant, harvesting and extraction methods used.[33] Some patients may experience burning sensation, contact dermatitis or mild itching with topical use.

Therapy for Photoaging

Topical retinoids can improve the appearance of sun-damaged skin. Mechanisms involved are thought to include: increased synthesis and inhibited degradation of collagen leading to less pronounced wrinkles, initiation of epidermal proliferation causing increased smoothness of the skin and decreased melanin content, and enhanced keratinocyte shedding leading to improvement in skin discolouration. They have also been shown to block skin degradation following sun exposure. Improvement is typically seen after several weeks of treatment. Continued treatment over 6–12 months results in skin that is smoother and less sallow, has reduced fine and coarse wrinkles, and is less mottled.[34,35,36] Currently in Canada, only tazarotene cream is approved for this indication; however, in practice other available topical retinoids (tretinoin, adapalene) are also used. Adverse effects include burning, irritation, redness and dryness which usually subside over time. A titrated approach to treatment can minimize these reactions.

Commercial skin care products containing **retinol** have limited efficacy because the skin is able to convert only small amounts of retinol to retinoic acid. Products containing **vitamin A** do not contain sufficient concentrations of retinoids to effectively treat photoaging and are likely added for their moisturizing properties.[37]

Alpha-hydroxy acids (**glycolic acid** and **lactic acid**) are widely available in low concentrations (usually 5–12 %) in many commercial products marketed for photoaged skin. Although scientific evidence of clinical effectiveness is limited,[38,39] anecdotal evidence is widely accepted. These products may help reduce the appearance of minor photodamage by reducing fine lines, and improve skin firmness and tone by removing dead cells from the surface of the skin. Higher concentrations are required for deeper effects and must be administered under supervision of a dermatologist (see Chemical Peels).

Antioxidants including **vitamin C** and **coenzyme Q10 derivatives** are included in many products purported to improve the signs of photoaging. Other compounds being investigated for their ability to reverse the signs of photoaging include soy isoflavones, green tea polyphenols, lutein, carotenoids, ginseng and peptides. In some cases there are (mostly) commercial in vitro studies showing promising results, but uncertainty around their clinical effectiveness remains because of the lack of independent, published in vivo evidence and questions about their effectiveness/stability in combination with other compounds and in the low concentrations that are available without a prescription.[40]

Chemical peels contain **alpha-hydroxy acids**, **salicylic acid**, **trichloroacetic acid** or **phenol**. Chemical peels induce controlled damage to the skin at various skin depths. Regeneration and re-epithelialization of the epidermis and dermis results in firmer skin with a more even skin tone. Chemical peels can be superficial, medium or deep depending on the extent of the photodamage. **Glycolic acid** chemical peels involve concentrations ranging from 20–70% which are administered in a step-wise fashion over several weeks or months. Chemical peels improve skin texture, reduce wrinkles and decrease the number of actinic keratoses.[5,41]

Mottled Hyperpigmentation: Various treatments are used to lighten darkened skin areas that appear with photoaging, leading to an more even skin tone. Topical treatment with **hydroquinone** may help to reduce visibility and degree of mottled pigmentation. Hydroquinone does not affect the upper layer of the skin but interacts with melanin production in the lower layers of the epidermis. Skin improves over 3 weeks to 3 months. Recurrence is prevented by limiting sun exposure and using a sunscreen, particularly on areas that have been treated.[34] Skin irritation, redness and allergic or contact dermatitis have been reported. Hydroquinone can occasionally cause reversible discoloration of the fingernails and has been rarely associated with exogenous ochronosis (persistent blue-black pigmentation of the skin) particulary in dark-skinned individuals.[42] Some countries have banned hydroquinone due to concerns about carcinogenicity and renal toxicity after oral administration in mice and rats,[43,44] but the relevance to topical use in humans is uncertain as the product has been used seemingly safely for decades. Other compounds used for skin lightening include **topical retinoids** (reduce epidermal pigmentation by an unclear mechanism) and **topical corticosteroids** (reduce production of melanin). Various combinations of these ingredients have been used with success when monotherapy has been unsuccessful.

OnabotulinumtoxinA does not reverse photodamage but appears to rejuvenate the skin by relaxing the underlying musculature. The effects of treatment typically last 3 months.[5] **Hyaluronic acid** is a soft tissue filler injected into wrinkles to improve the appearance of the skin. Results usually last 6–9 months in areas with more movement and up to 1 year in areas of limited mobility. **Photodynamic therapy** (exposure to UV light after use of a photosensitizer) and **laser therapy** are also used for the treatment of photoaging.

Figure 3 presents an assessment of patients requesting treatment for nonacute sun-induced skin damage (also see Table 4).

Monitoring of Therapy

Table 3 provides a plan for the monitoring of therapy for sun-induced skin damage.

Table 3: **Monitoring of Therapy for Sun-induced Skin Damage**

Symptom	Monitoring	Endpoint	Actions
Early photodamage (fine wrinkles, dry skin)	Monitor for changes in skin appearance (rough, dry skin with surface or deep wrinkles). Monitor regularly for signs of mottling or pigment changes ("liver" spots or "age" spots).	Skin feels softer, smoother, fine wrinkles less apparent. Skin does not show signs of pigment change.	Prevention is the most effective treatment (continual use of sunscreens with SPF 30 or more). Tretinoins, chemical peels and antioxidants may reverse or improve signs.
Sunburn	Monitor for 24–48 h after unprotected sun exposure for worsening or improvement of burn. Monitor pain 24–48 h. Monitor for 7 days for signs of infection (particularly if blistered).	Sunburn lessens or disappears after 48 h. Pain relief is adequate. No signs of infection after 48 h.	Cool compresses to relieve pain. Analgesics for pain relief (acetaminophen, ibuprofen). Skin protectants such as petrolatum to protect and moisturize. Avoid further exposure. Signs of infection require assessment and treatment if appropriate.
Actinic keratosis	Monitor regularly for dry, scaly lesions on chronically sun-exposed areas (particularly age ≥50 y). Monitor closely for signs of change (size, shape or colour).	No signs of actinic keratosis, e.g., firm scaling lesion with slight erythema.	Avoid chronic exposure to sun. Further investigation required if changes in the area (rule out squamous cell carcinoma, basal cell carcinoma or melanomas). Wear sunscreens regularly and cover area to protect from further sun exposure.

Figure 2: Assessment of Patients Requesting Protection from Sun-induced Skin Damage

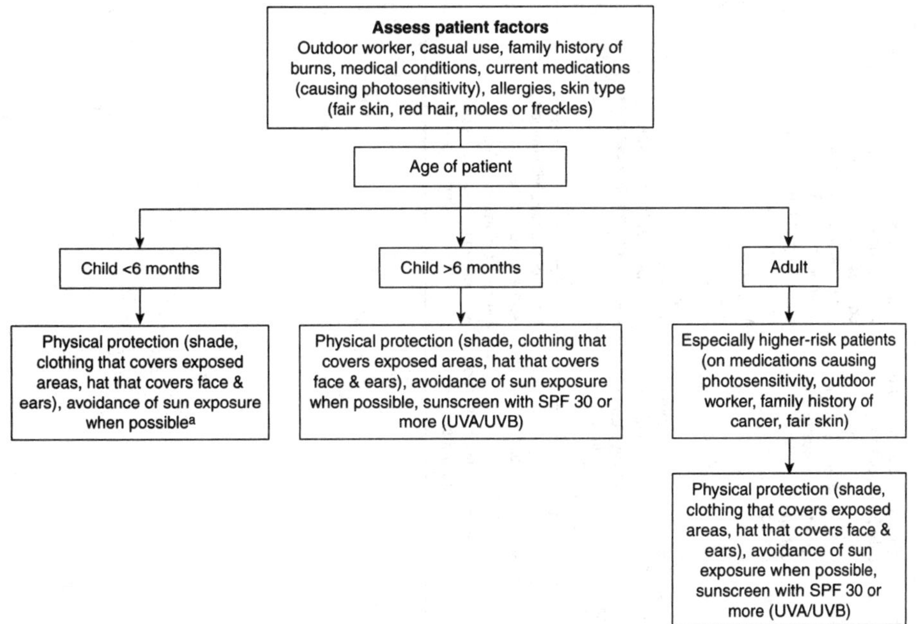

[a] If sun exposure is unavoidable notwithstanding these measures, a broad-spectrum SPF 30 sunscreen for babies can be applied to the small exposed areas (e.g., face, back of hands).[9] Inorganic (physical) sunscreens containing zinc oxide and/or titanium dioxide are minimally absorbed and less likely to cause sensitization.[10]

Abbreviations: SPF = sun protection factor; UVA = ultraviolet-A; UVB = ultraviolet-B

Figure 3: Assessment of Patients Requesting Treatment for Nonacute Sun-induced Skin Damage

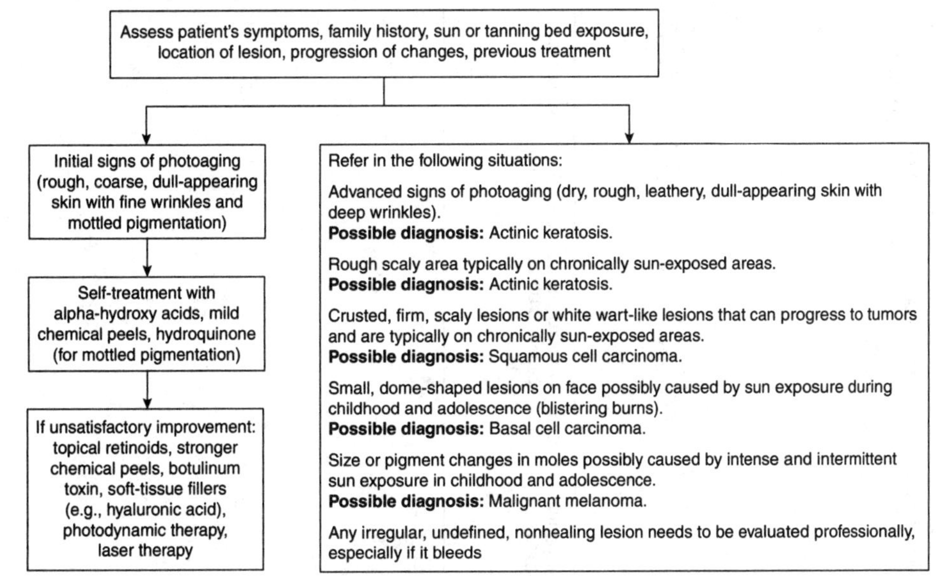

Table 4: Topical Therapy for Photoaged Skin

Class	Drug	Dosage	Mechanism of Action	Adverse Effects	Comments	Cost[a]
Alpha-hydroxy acids	*glycolic acid* Biobase-G, Neostrata HQ Gel, others	5–10% cream/lotion: Apply daily to BID	Removes dead cells from surface of skin, leading to less visible lines and wrinkles and a smoother appearance.	Initially (but decreasing with time): burning, stinging, redness. Increases sensitivity to UV light: always use in conjunction with sunscreen.	Higher concentrations (20–70%) used in superficial chemical peels under expert supervision may provide deeper effects, including thickening of the epidermis and depigmentation. May cause hyperpigmentation: avoid use in dark-skinned patients.	$
	lactic acid Dermalac, others	5–12% cream/lotion: Apply daily to BID	Removes dead cells from surface of skin, leading to less visible lines and wrinkles and a smoother appearance.	Mild redness, dryness. Increases sensitivity to UV light: always use in conjunction with sunscreen.	May cause hyperpigmentation: avoid use in dark-skinned patients.	$
Depigmenting agents	*hydroquinone* Esoterica, Ultraquin, others	2–4%: Apply thinly BID	Decreases melanin production, leading to lighter skin tone over 3 wk to 3 months.	Skin irritation, redness and risk of contact dermatitis. Reversible discolouration of the fingernails.	Often combined with glycolic acid and sunscreen. Use in conjunction with sunscreen decreases risk or recurrence of dark pigment.	$

Class	Drug	Dosage	Mechanism of Action	Adverse Effects	Comments	Cost[a]
Retinoids	*adapalene* Differin, Differin XP	0.1% cream, 0.3% gel: Apply QHS	Decreases fine lines, improves skin texture, tone, elasticity, mottled pigmentation. Slows progression of photoaging.	Scaling, redness, burning and dermatitis, which often subsides with continued use. May cause increased sensitivity to the sun: apply at bedtime and use broad-spectrum sunscreen (SPF ≥15) during the day.	A minimum of 4 months of treatment is required to see any positive results. Not a Health Canada–approved indication.	$$$
	tazarotene Tazorac Cream	0.1% cream: Apply QHS	Decreases fine lines, improves skin texture, tone, elasticity, mottled pigmentation. Slows progression of photoaging.	Scaling, redness, burning and dermatitis, which often subsides with continued use. May cause increased sensitivity to the sun: apply at bedtime and use broad-spectrum sunscreen (SPF ≥15) during the day.	A minimum of 4 months of treatment is required to see any positive results.	$$
	tretinoin Retin-A, Retin-A Micro, Stieva-A	0.01%, 0.02%, 0.05%, 0.1% cream: Apply QHS	Decreases fine lines, improves skin texture, tone, elasticity, mottled pigmentation. Slows progression of photoaging.	Scaling, redness, burning and dermatitis, which often subsides with continued use. May cause increased sensitivity to the sun: apply at bedtime and use broad-spectrum sunscreen (SPF ≥15) during the day.	See adapalene.	$

[a] Cost of 25 g or 25 mL; includes drug cost only.

Legend: $ <$20 $$ $20–40 $$$ $40–60

Suggested Readings

Antoniou C, Kosmadaki M, Stratigos AJ et al. Sunscreens–what's important to know. *J Eur Acad Dermatol Venereol* 2008;22:1110-8.

Government of Canada. *Sunscreens*. Available from: healthycanadians.gc.ca/health-sante/environment-environnement/sun-soleil/screen-ecrans-eng.php.

Lautenschlager S, Wulf HC, Pittelkow MR. Photoprotection. *Lancet* 2007;370:528-37.

Poon F, Kang S, Chien AL. Mechanisms and treatments of photoaging. *Photodermatol Photoimmunol Photomed* 2015;31:65-74.

Ramirez R, Schneider J. Practical guide to sun protection. *Surg Clin North Am* 2003;83:97-107.

References

1. Bond CA. Skin disorders. In: Koda-Kimble MA, Young LY, eds. *Applied therapeutics: the clinical use of drugs*. Vancouver: Applied Therapeutics; 1992. p. 64-1-6.
2. Kullavanijaya P, Lim HW. Photoprotection. *J Am Acad Dermatol* 2005;52:937-58.
3. Wondrak GT, Jacobson MK, Jacobson EL. Endogenous UVA-photosensitizers: mediators of skin photodamage and novel targets for skin photoprotection. *Photochem Photobiol Sci* 2006;5:215-37.
4. Drucker AM, Rosen CF. Drug-induced photosensitivity: culprit drugs, management and prevention. *Drug Saf* 2011;34:821-37.
5. Rabe JH, Mamelak AJ, McElgunn PJ et al. Photoaging: mechanisms and repair. *J Am Acad Dermatol* 2006;55:1-19.
6. Lawrence N. New and emerging treatments for photoaging. *Dermatol Clin* 2000;18:99-112.
7. Cayce KA, McMichael AJ, Feldman SR. Hyperpigmentation: an overview of the common afflictions. *Dermatol Nurs* 2004;16:401-6, 413-6.
8. MacKie RM. Long-term health risk to the skin of ultraviolet radiation. *Prog Biophys Mol Biol* 2006;92:92-6.
9. Environment and Climate Change Canada. *Sun protection for babies*. Available from: www.ec.gc.ca/uv/default.asp?lang=En&n=2B3B8766-1. Accessed April 2016.
10. Paller AS, Hawk JL, Honig P et al. New insights about infant and toddler skin: implications for sun protection. *Pediatrics* 2011;128:92-102.
11. Wehner MR, Shive ML, Chren MM et al. Indoor tanning and non-melanoma skin cancer: systematic review and meta-analysis. *BMJ* 2012;345:e5909.
12. Boniol M, Autier P, Boyle P et al. Cutaneous melanoma attributable to sunbed use: systematic review and meta-analysis. *BMJ* 2012;345:e4757.
13. Guenther L. Sunburn. In: *Compendium of therapeutic choices: CTC 7*. 7th ed. Ottawa: Canadian Pharmacists Association; 2014.
14. Iannacone MR, Hughes MC, Green AC. Effects of sunscreen on skin cancer and photoaging. *Photodermatol Photoimmunol Photomed* 2014;30:55-61.
15. Green A, Williams G, Neale R et al. Daily sunscreen application and betacarotene supplementation in prevention of basal-cell and squamous-cell carcinomas of the skin: a randomised controlled trial. *Lancet* 1999;354:723-9.
16. Green AC, Williams GM, Logan V et al. Reduced melanoma after regular sunscreen use: randomized trial follow-up. *J Clin Oncol* 2011;29:257-63.
17. Pour NS, Saeedi M, Semnani KM et al. Sun protection for children: a review. *J Pediatr Rev* 2015;3:e155. Available from: jpediatricreview.com/en/articles/155.html.
18. Canadian Dermatology Association. Available from: www.dermatology.ca. Accessed March 8, 2016.
19. Fu JM, Dusza SW, Halpern AC. Sunless tanning. *J Am Acad Dermatol* 2004;50:706-13.
20. Hexsel CL, Bangert SD, Hebert AA et al. Current sunscreen issues: 2007 Food and Drug Administration sunscreen labelling recommendations and combination sunscreen/insect repellent products. *J Am Acad Dermatol* 2008;59:316-23.
21. Health Canada. Health Products and Food Branch. *Sunscreen monograph*. July 2013. Available from: webprod.hc-sc.gc.ca/nhpid-bdipsn/atReq.do?atid=sunscreen-ecransolaire⟨=eng. Accessed February 11, 2014.
22. Antoniou C, Kosmadaki M, Stratigos AJ et al. Sunscreens–what's important to know. *J Eur Acad Dermatol Venereol* 2008;22:1110-8.
23. Lautenschlager S, Wulf HC, Pittelkow MR. Photoprotection. *Lancet* 2007;370:528-37.
24. Ramirez R, Schneider J. Practical guide to sun protection. *Surg Clin North Am* 2003;83:97-107.
25. Petersen NB. Wulf C. Application of sunscreens theory and reality. *Photodermatol Photoimmunol Photomed* 2014;30:96-101.
26. Sambandan DR, Ratner D. Sunscreens: an overview and update. *J Am Acad Dermatol* 2011;64:748-58.
27. Norval M, Wulf HC. Does chronic sunscreen use reduce vitamin D production to insufficient levels? *Br J Dermatol* 2009;161:732-6.
28. Canadian Dermatology Association. *Dermatologists reassure Canadians: Sunscreens are safe and effective*. June 2011. Available from: www.dermatology.ca/wp-content/uploads/2012/01/Sunscreen-June2011EN.pdf. Accessed August 24, 2015.
29. American Academy of Dermatology. *Is sunscreen safe?* Available from: www.aad.org/spot-skin-cancer/learn-about-skin-cancer/prevent-skin-cancer/is-sunscreen-safe. Accessed August 24, 2015.
30. Australasian College of Dermatologists. *Sun protection & sunscreens*. Available from: www.dermcoll.edu.au/atoz/sun-protection-sunscreens/. Accessed August 24, 2015.
31. Han A, Maibach HI. Management of acute sunburn. *Am J Clin Dermatol* 2004;5:39-47.
32. Dat AD, Poon F, Pham KB et al. Aloe vera for treating acute and chronic wounds. *Cochrane Database Syst Rev* 2012;2:CD008762.
33. Maenthaisong R, Chaiyakunapruk N, Niruntraporn S et al. The efficacy of aloe vera used for burn wound healing: a systematic review. *Burns* 2007;33:713-8.
34. Osterwalder U, Herzog B. Sun protection factors: worldwide confusion. *Br J Dermatol* 2009;161:13-24.
35. Poon F, Kang S, Chien AL. Mechanisms and treatments of photoaging. *Photodermatol Photoimmunol Photomed* 2015:31;65-74.
36. Han A, Chien AL, Kang S. Photoaging. *Dermatol Clin* 2014;32:291-9.
37. Draelos ZD. Therapeutic moisturizers. *Dermatol Clin* 2000;18:597-607.
38. Smith WP. Epidermal and dermal effects of topical lactic acid. *J Am Acad Dermatol* 1996;35:388-91.

39. Stiller MJ, Bartolone J, Stern R et al. Topical 8% glycolic acid and 8% L-lactic acid creams for the treatment of photodamaged skin. A double-blind vehicle-controlled clinical trial. *Arch Dermatol* 1996;132:631-6.
40. Bradley EJ, Griffiths CE, Sherratt MJ et al. Over-the-counter anti-ageing topical agents and their ability to protect and repair photoaged skin. *Maturitas* 2015;80:265-72.
41. Chemical peels In: Wolverton SE, ed. *Comprehensive dermatologic drug therapy.* 3rd ed. Edinburgh: Saunders Elsevier; 2013.
42. Nagler A, Hale CS, Meehan SA et al. Exogenous ochronosis. *Dermatol Online J* 2014;20.
43. Shibata MA, Hirose M, Tanaka H et al. Induction of renal cell tumors in rats and mice, and enhancement of hepatocellular tumor development in mice after long-term hydroquinone treatment. *Jpn J Cancer Res* 1991;82:1211-9.
44. Hard GC, Whysner J, English JC et al. Relationship of hydroquinone-associated rat renal tumors with spontaneous chronic progressive nephropathy. *Toxicol Pathol* 1997;25:132-43.

Skin Damage from the Sun—What You Need to Know

Sunlight causes damage to the skin that can be seen right away, such as redness or sunburn. It also causes damage that can't be seen right away, even when the skin does not change colour. This damage can show up many years later as skin cancer, or as signs of aging, especially on the face (such as wrinkles, dryness, dullness, yellowing or an uneven skin color).

What can you do to prevent skin damage from the sun?

Here are some suggestions to help prevent immediate skin damage (such as sunburn) and delayed effects of sun exposure (such as wrinkles and skin cancer):

- Avoid direct exposure to the sun from 10 a.m. to 4 p.m. when the sun's rays are the strongest. Staying in the shade offers some protection but caution should still be exercised as sunlight also goes through leafy trees and umbrellas and is reflected from surfaces outside the shaded area.
- Protect the skin from sun damage or burning by wearing clothing that covers areas exposed to the sun (broad-brimmed hat, sunglasses, long-sleeved shirt and long pants). Cotton or linen clothing that is tightly woven, loose fitting and lightweight will provide some protection. Clothing that is wet, white or loosely woven provide very little protection. Avoid tanning lamps and sun lamps as they use UVA radiation and are not considered safe to use on a regular basis (exceptions are for medical use such as patients with psoriasis). There is an increased risk of getting wrinkles and/or skin cancer with the use of tanning lamps or sun lamps.
- **Do not** stay in the sun for long periods of time to get a tan. Tanning increases the risk of skin damage, including wrinkles. A tan does not offer protection from further sun damage.
- Avoid sun exposure in infants less than 6 months of age as they are very vulnerable to sunburn. Infants should be kept in a well shaded area and covered with clothing that will offer complete protection from the sun. Sunscreens have not been proven safe in infants less than 6 months of age.
- Use a sunscreen with an SPF of 30 or more to protect the skin from the sun and from the possibility of permanent skin damage or skin cancer later in life.
- Use sunscreen even during cloudy weather as sun is still able to get through clouds. Sunscreens should be worn while boating, as the sun reflects off the water, increasing sun exposure.

Correct application of sunscreens

Sunscreens can help protect skin but do not completely prevent skin damage from sunlight. These tips will help to get the most benefit from sunscreen:

- Apply a sufficient thickness to offer protection. Thin application will not offer the SPF value indicated on the product. Sunscreens should be applied 30 minutes before exposure and reapplied 15–30 minutes later to maximize protection and ensure enough has been applied to the body.
- Sunscreens should be applied to all exposed areas, ensuring that the ears, nose, lips, back of the neck and hairline are covered as well.
- Sunscreens should be applied to the skin 15–30 minutes before going into the water to allow it time to be absorbed. Sunscreens should be reapplied after swimming, towelling off or sweating, to prevent burning. Sunscreens should be reapplied every 2 hours to ensure that the skin is constantly protected.
- To get the full effect of the labelled sun protection factor (SPF) it must be applied correctly and in the correct quantity (approximately 30 mL to cover the entire body). An average-size adult should use at least the following amounts:
  - one-half to 1 teaspoonful (2.5–5 mL) on the face and neck

- 1–1.5 teaspoonfuls (5–7.5 mL) to arms, shoulders and torso
- 2–2.5 teaspoonfuls (10–12.5 mL) to the legs and the tops of the feet.

Chapter 73
Viral Skin Infections: Common and Flat Warts

Penny F. Miller, BSc(Pharm), MA

Pathophysiology

Warts are common viral infections of the skin and mucus membranes caused by any of 150 or more distinct deoxyribonucleic acid (DNA) viruses in the human papillomavirus (HPV) family. Since warts resemble small hills on the skin, they are named "verruca" which means "a steep place". Children and young adults are most commonly affected. Handlers of meat, poultry and fish have a high incidence of warts. An estimated 12% of the population is affected at any given time, with the highest prevalence (up to 20%) in school-aged children.[1] Warts are usually spread through broken skin by direct skin-to-skin inoculation of the virus from an infected person. The degree of exposure to HPV at home and in school contributes to wart development in elementary school children.[2] Time between inoculation and the appearance of a lesion is variable, ranging from 2–9 months for common warts. Cell-mediated immune responses to the virus are important in host resistance.[3] Immunosuppressed states and organ transplants are predisposing factors for more extensive or recalcitrant warts.[4] Several forms of warts are self-treatable: common warts (hands), flat warts (face) and plantar warts (foot).[3] See Chapter 52: Plantar Warts.

Common Warts

Common warts are caused by HPV types 2, 4, 27 and 29. They appear as single or grouped hyperkeratotic papulonodules most often seen on the knees, fingers, hands and around the nails. They can occur anywhere on the skin. The lesions typically are small, hard, raised growths with a rough surface that looks like cauliflower. Spontaneous remission occurs in about two-thirds of affected patients within 2 years. Recurrence is common.[5] See Common Warts in Photo section.

Flat Warts

Flat warts (also called plane warts) are caused by HPV types 3, 10, 28 and 29 and frequently present as several flesh-coloured, small papules with a smooth surface, affecting the face or neck. The skin and dorsa of hands may also be involved. They may arise after scratching or trauma and appear in a linear arrangement.[3]

Goals of Therapy

- Remove the virus-containing wart with minimal destruction of normal tissue
- Prevent spread of the wart

Patient Assessment

A description and differential diagnosis of warts can be found in Table 1. Nongenital warts may cause pain and may bleed if irritated; otherwise they produce no symptoms and are harmless.

Table 1: **Characteristics and Differential Diagnosis of Common and Flat Warts**[3,6,7,8]

Condi-tion	Distribution	Lesion	Differential Diagnosis
Common warts	Hands, surrounding or beneath the nails, or sites of trauma	Flesh-toned or grey-brown dome-shaped papule, studded with black dots occurring singly or in groups	Callus: Has skin lines. Seborrheic keratosis: Greasy, pigmented (dirty yellow to black colour) appearance, affects middle-aged and elderly persons. Molluscum contagiosum: Small, flesh-coloured, firm, domed papule with a central pore indentation. A cheesy white material can be expressed. It affects primarily children and sexually active young adults. Comedone (whitehead): Contents can be expressed. Occurs in the presence of other acne lesions, e.g., pustules (pimples). Skin tags: Flesh-coloured papules that lack the roughness of warts. Squamous cell carcinoma: Asymptomatic skin-coloured to reddish-brown firm tumor on damaged skin. Usually there is a central ulceration. It occurs in sun-exposed areas and appears later in life.
Flat warts (plane warts)	Face, backs of hands, shins	Skin-coloured or light brown, smooth, flat or slightly elevated papules occurring in multiples	Epidermal nevi (linear birth marks present since birth). Lichen planus: Lesions resemble flat warts but may be symmetrical and accompanied by lacy oral lesions.

Patients presenting with warts on the face or genitals and those with recalcitrant or widespread lesions require assessment by an appropriate healthcare practitioner. Patients with conditions associated with neuropathies, such as diabetes or circulatory disorders, should not self-medicate with caustic substances because they are unable to judge the effects of the therapy and are more likely to have poor healing.[5,6]

Nonpharmacologic Therapy

Based on the natural course of warts, one-half of primary school children with warts will have resolution 1 year later. Resolution rates are higher in young children and those with non-Caucasian skin types, independent of the number and/or size of warts. Consider discussing a **wait-and-see approach** with the patient and/or family.[9] Warts clear more slowly in adults, often persisting for 5–10 years.[4]

Patients should avoid scratching or biting the wart. This will prevent the development of pain or bleeding and will reduce the spread of the virus. Patients should not share personal items such as towels that have been in contact with the wart. Watchful waiting in children is appropriate since two-thirds of untreated warts will disappear within 2 years.[5] However, warts can enlarge and multiply if untreated.[6]

A small number of trials have examined the use of duct tape to impede viral survival by creating an occlusive environment. In one study using silver-coloured duct tape applied in cycles of 6 days on, 1 night off, with soaking and debriding of the wart, an 85% resolution rate was reported.[10] Other more rigorous trials using clear duct tape with acrylic-based adhesive rather than rubber-based adhesive found no benefit.[11,12] It is not clear what role, if any, colour or adhesive type plays in the effectiveness of duct tape. Since there is no clear evidence of effectiveness and adverse effects such as redness, itching, eczema and bleeding have been reported, the use of duct tape remains controversial.[4,11,13]

Curretage and dessication (surgical removal) may be useful for isolated lesions. Local application of anesthetic by injection or topically is required to ease the pain of the procedure. Atrophic or hypertrophic scarring may result and recurrence rates can be as high as 30%.[14,15,16]

Pharmacologic Therapy

For comparative ingredients of nonprescription products, consult the *Compendium of Products for Minor Ailments*—Foot Care Products: Corns, Calluses and Warts.

Topical therapy is used to remove the virus-containing wart with minimal destruction of normal tissue. The type of therapy depends on the location, degree of symptoms and the patient's immune status and level of cooperation. Scarring can occur with more destructive therapies. Therapy may take several weeks or months.

Evidence supports the use of salicylic acid or cryotherapy for the local treatment of common and flat warts.[17,18,19] Recalcitrant warts (those not responding to 3 months of therapy with salicylic acid or cryotherapy) often require cryotherapy every 10–14 days combined with salicylic acid or curettage and electrodessication.[4] Up to one-third of nongenital warts become recalcitrant.[20]

Salicylic Acid

Common and flat warts can be self-treated topically with **salicylic acid**, which has produced a cure rate of 52% vs. 23% with placebo.[19] Salicylic acid is an effective keratolytic that causes a slow destruction of the virus-infected epidermis. In addition, an immune response is stimulated by the resulting mild irritation of the epidermis.[4] Salicylic acid is commercially available in a variety of strengths and dosage forms that may be combined with **lactic acid**. Strengths of about 17% in liquid (collodion) form are useful for common warts and multiple warts, whereas strengths of 20–40% as plasters are preferred for thicker skin areas such as the plantar surface (Table 4).[1] Salicylic acid is suitable for use on any cutaneous site except the face. Instructions for use can be found in Warts—What You Need to Know.

Cryotherapy

A **dimethyl-ether/propane** mixture is available for home cryotherapy but does not appear to be effective in achieving the low temperatures necessary for cellular necrosis.[4,22] Physician-administered cryotherapy with **liquid nitrogen** every 2 weeks can produce a cure rate of 49% after 13 weeks.[23] Melamine foam sponge applicators rather than cotton swab applicators may be the optimal method of application of liquid nitrogen in this setting.[24] Freezing temperatures to −196°C cause cell necrosis and may induce local inflammation where an effective cell-mediated response clears the virus. Cryotherapy has comparable efficacy to topical salicylic acid but causes more adverse effects including pain, blistering, scarring, skin irritation, changes in skin pigmentation and crusting.[13,17] Caution is necessary when cryotherapy is applied near cutaneous nerves, tendons and nail apparatus or in patients with impaired circulation.[4]

Other Treatments

Because recommended wart management (salicylic acid, cryotherapy) is not consistently effective and is dependent on patient adherence over long treatment courses, many other treatment options have been attempted. Evidence of benefit and safety of these approaches is less rigorous than for salicylic acid and cryotherapy, and they are considered second- or third-line options. The British Association of Dermatologists guidelines for the management of cutaneous warts has divided these approaches into 4 categories based on their mechanism of action: destructive (salicylic acid and cryotherapy fall into this category), virucidal, antimitotic and immunologic. These guidelines also provide information on the quality of available evidence and strength of recommendation.[4] Selected therapies from each category are discussed briefly below.

Destructive Therapy

Lasers produce a controlled thermal destruction of the warts. Unlike CO_2 lasers which cause generalized tissue destruction, pulsed dye lasers and KTP (potassium titanyl phosphate) lasers are selectively absorbed by hemoglobin in the dermal blood vessels and destroy only the wart vessel vasculature with additional thermal injury to the HPV virus. Treatment is painless (no local anesthesia required) and no burning tissue smell is produced. Cure rates up to 89% have been reported.[25,26]

Photodynamic therapy involves applying a photosensitizer, 5-aminolevulinic acid (ALA) 20%, to the wart and leaving it on for 3–8 hours followed by exposing the lesion to visible-light irradiation. This induces photooxidation in abnormal cells. Keratolytics and paring before phototherapy are recommended. Burning, itching and occasionally severe pain may occur. Cure rates of 56–75% have been reported.[27]

Cantharidin (0.7%) is a blistering agent produced by beetles that is used in recalcitrant cases with multiple lesions or in young children. Application in the office is painless but pain and blisters occur up to 48 hours after application. Repeated applications at intervals of 1–3 weeks are occasionally needed. Healing without scars occurs in 5–10 days. Reported cure rates are as high as 80% in common, plantar and periungal warts. Cantharidin is highly toxic if ingested.[28,29]

Virucidal Therapy

Glutaraldehyde 10% paint applied daily after paring for 3 months produced cure rates of 80% for periungual and 60% for palmar warts in a small study of young children.[30] Deep necrosis can occur upon repeated application or with higher concentrations.[31]

Formaldehyde 3–4% solution as a 15- to 20-minute soak daily for 8 weeks (along with paring) produced a cure rate of 80% for plantar warts in children in one study. Allergic reactions may occur.[32]

Antimitotic/Antiproliferative Therapy

Bleomycin sulphate (0.1–1 U/mL) intralesional injection is a chemotherapeutic agent that inhibits DNA synthesis in cells and viruses. It may be used for recalcitrant warts by injecting directly into the wart over 1–3 treatments. Local anaesthesia is necessary since this is painful during and up to 2 days after treatment. Bleomycin treatment can result in significant systemic drug exposure and should not be used in children, pregnant women, immunosuppressed patients or those with vascular disease. Cure rates range from 65–85%.[33,34]

Podophyllotoxin 0.5% solution is the active ingredient of podophyllin, an antimitotic agent. This solution can be applied at home once or twice daily 3–4 days per week for up to 4–6 weeks. Pain, burning, erosions, pruritis and bleeding may occur. If applied to large areas (>10 cm^2) or in high concentrations, systemic absorption may result in neurotoxic effects, limiting use. It has been a standard treatment for anogential warts, with limited trial data in cutaneous warts. Cure rates using 25% podophyllin in paraffin for plantar warts were 67%. It is contraindicated in pregnancy.[35,36]

The topical retinoid **tretinoin** (0.025–0.1% cream) disrupts epidermal proliferation and differentiation to reduce wart volume. Applied once or twice daily for 6–12 weeks, it causes skin irritation and dryness that may contribute to an inflammatory reaction to produce an immunomodulatory effect on the virus. Studies suggest a cure rate of 85% in children with flat warts[37] and 29% in organ transplant recipients.[38] There is some evidence of efficacy for **oral retinoids**. Studies have reported cure rates of 100%[39] and 73%[40] for treatment of recalcitrant facial warts with **isotretinoin**. **Etretinate** produced clearance of 80% of all warts in a study in children[41] and **acitretin** reduced the bulk of lesions but had a high recurrence rate in another study.[42]

5-Fluorouracil 5% cream blocks RNA and DNA synthesis and damages dividing basal layer cells. It can be applied under occlusion to common warts and flat warts affecting the hands and feet, once daily for 4–12 weeks. Inflammation with occasional erosions and hyper- or hypopigmentation can occur. Local sun protection is required to prevent an exaggerated response. Cure rates of 60% have been reported.[4,43,44,45,46]

Immunotherapy

Contact immunotherapy involving topical application of contact allergens including squaric acid dibutylester (SABDE), dinitrochlorobenzene (DNCB), or diphenylcyclopropenone (DPCP) has shown efficacy in recalcitrant cases. DNCB has mutagenic potential and therefore is rarely used.[29] Contact immunotherapy begins with high concentrations applied to a small area of the skin to induce sensitization. This local, delayed (type IV) hypersensitivity reaction triggers the local immune response to the virus. Two weeks later, lower concentrations that are titrated are applied twice weekly for 10 weeks. Erythema, edema, pruritis, burning, pigment changes and desquamation may occur. Treatment should be stopped if diffuse eczema or urticaria develop. Cure rates of up to 86% have been reported. Proper storage is important; DPCP should not be exposed to light and SABDE must be refrigerated.[47,48,49]

Intralesional immunotherapy uses antigens such as *Candida*, mumps, *Trichophyton* or tuberculin to stimulate host cell-mediated immunity. This may be used as a nonscarring method in patients with multiple recalcitrant lesions or facial lesions. Resolution of multiple warts may be achieved by injecting only 1 wart, due to the general immune-stimulating effect.[4,50] Reported cure rates range from 47–87%.[50,51] Due to limited evidence of safety and efficacy, this therapy is currently only recommended to be undertaken by experienced dermatologists.[4]

Imiquimod 5% cream is a topical immunomodulator that enhances cell-mediated immunity. It is a painless, nonscarring option for treatment of recalcitrant or facial lesions. The cream can be applied overnight 3 times weekly or up to twice daily, with improvement noted within weeks to months. Duration of treatment can be as long as 16 weeks. Local pain, pruritus and irritation are usually mild. Imiquimod is used in the treatment of genital warts, but efficacy in the treatment of cutaneous warts has not been established. Some small open-label studies have suggested it may be effective (estimated average cure rate of 44%). Dosing, frequency of application and how to optimally combine imiquimod with other modalities are all unanswered questions.[20,52,53,54]

Cimetidine, an oral H_2 receptor antagonist, has been used in the treatment of warts. The proposed mechanism of action is increasing cell-mediated immunity by blocking T-suppressor cells on H_2 receptors. A dose of 30–50 mg/kg/day in 4 divided doses for up to 3 months was effective in open label studies,[55,56,57] but ineffective in small randomized controlled trials.[58,59,60]

A dermatologist referral is necessary if there are symptomatic, recalcitrant warts, multiple warts in immunocompromised patients, facial lesions unresponsive to topical therapy, or in cases where the diagnosis is uncertain.[61]

A summary of treatment recommendations for common and flat warts can be found in Table 2.

Table 2: **Treatment Recommendations for Common and Flat Warts**[4,21,62,63]

Clinical Situation	First-line Therapy	Second-line Therapy	Third-line Therapy	Comments
Common warts, adults	Salicylic acid 17–40% with occlusion following paring until cleared (up to 3–4 months)	Cryotherapy Q2–3 wk until cleared (maximum of 6 treatments)	Bleomycin, contact immunotherapy, 5-FU, pulsed dye laser	Other treatments with low-level evidence: cantharidin, imiquimod, podophyllin, glutaraldehyde, formaldehyde, photodynamic therapy.
Common warts, children	Salicylic acid 17–40% with occlusion until cleared (up to 3–4 months)	Gentle cryotherapy (milder freeze) Q2–3 wk until cleared (maximum of 6 treatments)	Formaldehyde solution, glutaraldehyde, pulsed dye laser, systemic retinoids, topical immunotherapy	Warts are short-lived with clearing in 1–2 y. Painful treatments are not well tolerated.
Flat/plane warts	Salicylic acid 2–10% without occlusion. Cautious use of 12–17% paints. Treat until cleared (up to 3–4 months)	Gentle cryotherapy (milder freeze) Q2–3 wk until cleared (maximum of 6 treatments)	Topical retinoids, cantharidin, 5-FU, formaldehyde, glutaraldehyde, imiquimod, photodynamic therapy, topical immunotherapy	Caution with destructive/caustic agents as they may cause scarring at sites involving hands and face.
Common or flat warts, immunosuppressed patients	Salicylic acid 2–10% without occlusion. Treat until satisfactory improvement (up to 3–4 months). See Comments	Cautious use of destructive methods to avoid damage to surrounding skin	Imiquimod, contact immunotherapy, pulsed dye laser, intralesional bleomycin, surgery, topical retinoid, systemic retinoid	Treatment helps to reduce the size of warts and any associated functional or cosmetic problems. Clinical cure is difficult to attain.

Monitoring of Therapy

Table 3 presents a monitoring framework for patients with warts.

Table 3: **Monitoring of Therapy for Warts**

Symptoms	Monitoring	Desired Outcome	Actions
Wart size (treatment with salicylic acid)	Patient: Daily, watching for dead skin and reduction in the size of the wart Healthcare practitioner: Review response in 2–3 wk	Reduction in the size of wart within 2–3 wk. Disappearance of wart within 4 or more wk. Return of normal healthy skin	Review application technique and evaluate dosage form if no improvement in 2–3 wk. Patient requires further assessment and/or treatment if there is no improvement in the wart after 12 wk of treatment.
Wart colour or shape suggesting it may not be a wart	Patient: Daily, watching for any unexpected dramatic change in colour or shape Healthcare practitioner: Next visit	Disappearance of wart/lesion	Patient requires further assessment and/or treatment if there is any unusual change in colour or shape of the lesion. Need to rule out cancers.
Bleeding after minimal trauma	Patient: Daily Healthcare practitioner: Next visit	Absence of bleeding	Patient requires further assessment and/or treatment if there is any unexplained bleeding. Need to rule out cancers.
Signs of infection such as redness, pain and pus	Patient: Daily Healthcare practitioner: Next visit	Absence of infection	Patient requires further assessment and/or treatment if signs are suggestive of a secondarily infected lesion.

(cont'd)

Table 3: **Monitoring of Therapy for Warts** *(cont'd)*

Symptoms	Monitoring	Desired Outcome	Actions
Warts that are growing quickly	Patient: Daily	Absence of enlarging or new warts	Patient requires further assessment.
Allergy	Patient: Daily while on therapy Healthcare practitioner: Next visit	No allergy	Stop therapy. Patient requires further assessment and/or treament.
Irritation caused by topical agents	Patient: Daily while on therapy Healthcare practitioner: Next visit	Minimal irritation that subsides with continued use	Stop therapy if no improvement after reinforcing method of application. Patient requires further assessment and/or treament.

Table 4: Salicylic Acid Treatment for Common and Flat Warts[a]

Class	Drug	Dosage	Adverse Effects	Comments	Cost
Keratolytic	*salicylic acid* Compound W, Soluver, others	Use 40% for thick-skinned areas and 17% for thin warts or thin-skinned areas Assess response after 2–3 wk Apply for up to several months. Continue treatment for 1–2 wk after clinical removal of wart to ensure complete elimination of virus	Painless application. Stop treatment for a few days if treated area becomes painful and excessively irritated.	Useful for common and flat warts in adults and children. Cure rate 52%.[17] Best supportive evidence of efficacy.[17,21] Lactic acid 17% combination is effective.[5]	$8

[a] Cost of smallest available pack size; includes drug cost only.

Suggested Readings

Lynch MD, Cliffe J, Morris-Jones R. Management of cutaneous viral warts. *BMJ* 2014;348:g3339.
Mulhem E, Pinelis S. Treatment of nongenital cutaneous warts. *Am Fam Physician* 2011;84:288-93.

References

1. Kyriakis K, Pagana G, Michailides C et al. Lifetime prevalence fluctuations of common and plane viral warts. *J Eur Acad Dermatol Venereol* 2007;21:260-2.
2. Bruggink SC, Eekhof JA, Egberts PF et al. Warts transmitted in families and schools: a prospective cohort. *Pediatrics* 2013;131:928-34.
3. Androphy EJ, Lowy DR. Warts. In: Goldsmith LA et al. *Fitzpatrick's dermatology in general medicine*. 8th ed. New York: McGraw-Hill Professional; 2012.
4. Sterling JC, Gibbs S, Haque Hussain SS et al. British Association of Dermatologists' guidelines for the management of cutaneous warts 2014. *Br J Dermatol* 2014;171:696-712.
5. Goldstein BG, Goldstein AO. *Cutaneous warts*. Available from: www.uptodate.com. Subscription required.
6. Goldstein BG, Goldstein AO. *Practical dermatology.* 2nd ed. St. Louis: Mosby; 1997. p. 71-7.
7. Hooper BJ, Goldman MP. *Primary dermatologic care*. St. Louis: Mosby; 1999.
8. Lookingbill DP, Marks JG. *Principles of dermatology.* 3rd ed. Philadelphia: W.B. Saunders; 2000.
9. Bruggink SC, Eekhof JA, Egberts PF et al. Natural course of cutaneous warts among primary school children: a prospective cohort study. *Ann Fam Med* 2013;11:437-41.
10. Focht DR, Spicer C, Fairchok MP. The efficacy of duct tape vs cryotherapy in the treatment of verruca vulgaris (the common wart). *Arch Pediatr Adolesc Med* 2002;156:971-4.
11. de Haen M, Spigt MG, van Uden CJ et al. Efficacy of duct tape vs placebo in the treatment of verruca vulgaris (warts) in primary school children. *Arch Pediatr Adolesc Med* 2006;160:1121-5.
12. Wenner R, Askari SK, Cham PM et al. Duct tape for the treatment of common warts in adults: a double-blind randomized controlled trial. *Arch Dermatol* 2007;143:309-13.
13. Craw L, Wingert A, Lara-Corrales I. Are salicylic acid formulations, liquid nitrogen or duct tape more effective than placebo for the treatment of warts in paediatric patients who present to ambulatory care clinics? *Paediatr Child Health* 2014;19:126-7.
14. Baruch K. Blunt dissection for the treatment of plantar verrucae. *Cutis* 1990;46:145-7, 151-2.
15. Pringle WM, Helms DC. Treatment of plantar warts by blunt dissection. *Arch Dermatol* 1973;108:79-82.
16. Leung L. Treating common warts—options and evidence. *Aust Fam Physician* 2010;39:933-7.
17. Kwok CS, Gibbs S, Bennett C et al. Topical treatments for cutaneous warts. *Cochrane Database Syst Rev* 2012;9:CD001781.
18. Dall'oglio F, D'Amico V, Nasca MR et al. Treatment of cutaneous warts: an evidence-based review. *Am J Clin Dermatol* 2012;13:73-96.
19. Kwok CS, Holland R, Gibbs S. Efficacy of topical treatments for cutaneous warts: a meta-analysis and pooled analysis of randomized controlled trials. *Br J Dermatol* 2011;165:233-46.
20. Leung L. Recalcitrant nongenital warts. *Aust Fam Physician* 2011;40:40-2.
21. Bacelieri R, Johnson SM. Cutaneous warts: an evidence-based approach to therapy. *Am Fam Physician* 2005;72:647-52.
22. Gaspar ZS, Dawber RP. An organic refrigerant for cryosurgery: fact or fiction? *Australas J Dermatol* 1997;38:71-2.
23. Bruggink SC, Gussekloo J, Berger MY et al. Cryotherapy with liquid nitrogen versus topical salicylic acid application for cutaneous warts in primary care: randomized controlled trial. *CMAJ* 2010;182:1624-30.
24. Canadian Agency for Drugs and Technologies in Health. *Cryotherapy systems for wart removal: a review of the clinical effectiveness, cost-effectiveness, and guidelines*. Available from: https://www.cadth.ca/cryotherapy-systems-wart-removal-review-clinical-effectiveness-cost-effectiveness-and-guidelines Accessed March 9, 2016.
25. Gooptu C, James MP. Recalcitrant viral warts: results of treatment with the KTP laser. *Clin Exp Dermatol* 1999;24:60-3.
26. Ross BS, Levine VJ, Nehal K et al. Pulsed dye laser treatment of warts: an update. *Dermatol Surg* 1999;25:377-80.
27. Stender IM, Na R, Fogh H et al. Photodynamic therapy with 5-aminolaevulinic acid or placebo for recalcitrant foot and hand warts: randomised double-blind trial. *Lancet* 2000;355:963-6.
28. Kartal Durmazlar SP, Atacan D, Eskioglu F. Cantharidin treatment for recalcitrant facial flat warts: a preliminary study. *J Dermatolog Treat* 2009;20:114-9.
29. Wolverton SE, ed. *Comprehensive dermatologic drug therapy.* 3rd ed. Edinburgh: Saunders Elsevier; 2013.
30. Hirose R, Hori M, Shukuwa T et al. Topical treatment of resistant warts with glutaraldehyde. *J Dermatol* 1994;21:248-53.
31. Fujisawa Y, Furuta J, Kawachi Y et al. Deep plantaris ulceration secondary to the topical treatment of wart with glutaraldehyde. *J Dermatol* 2009;36:618-9.
32. Vickers CF. Treatment of plantar warts in children. *Br Med J* 1961;2:743-5.
33. Lewis TG, Nydorf ED. Intralesional bleomycin for warts: a review. *J Drugs Dermatol* 2006;5:499-504.
34. Munn SE, Higgins E, Marshall M et al. A new method of intralesional bleomycin therapy in the treatment of recalcitrant warts. *Br J Dermatol* 1996;135:969-71.
35. Duthie DA, McCallum DI. Treatment of plantar warts with elastoplast and podophyllin. *Br Med J* 1951;2:216-8.
36. Filley CM, Graff-Richard NR, Lacy JR et al. Neurologic manifestations of podophyllin toxicity. *Neurology* 1982;32:308-11.
37. Kubeyinje EP. Evaluation of the efficacy and safety of 0.05% tretinoin cream in the treatment of plane warts in Arab children. *J Dermatolog Treat* 1996;7:21-2.
38. Euvrard S, Verschoore M, Touraine JL et al. Topical retinoids for warts and keratoses in transplant recipients. *Lancet* 1992;340:48-9.
39. Olguin-Garcia MG, Jurado-Santa Cruz F, Peralta-Pedrero ML et al. A double-blind, randomized, placebo-controlled trial of oral isotretinoin in the treatment of recalcitrant facial flat warts. *J Dermatolog Treat* 2015;26:78-82.
40. Al-Hamamy HR, Salman HA, Abdulsattar NA. Treatment of plane warts with a low-dose oral isotretinoin. *ISRN Dermatol* 2012:163929.
41. Gelmetti C, Cerri D, Schiuma AA et al. Treatment of extensive warts with etretinate: a clinical trial in 20 children. *Pediatric Dermatol* 1987;4:254-8.
42. Choi YL, Lee KJ, Kim WS et al. Treatment of extensive and recalcitrant viral warts with acitretin. *Int J Dermatol* 2006;45:480-2.
43. Hursthouse MW. A controlled trial on the use of topical 5-fluorouracil on viral warts. *Br J Dermatol* 1975;92:93-6.

44. Iscimen A, Aydemir EH, Goksugur N et al. Intralesional 5-fluorouracil, lidocaine and epinephrine mixture for the treatment of verrucae: a prospective placebo-controlled,single-blind randomized study. *J Eur Acad Dermatol Venereol* 2004;18:455-8.
45. Gibbs S, Harvey I, Sterling J et al. Local treatments for cutaneous warts: systematic review. *BMJ* 2002;325:461.
46. Gibbs S, Harvey I, Sterling JC et al. Local treatments for cutaneous warts. *Cochrane Database Syst Rev* 2003;3:CD001781.
47. Micali G, Nasca MR, Tedeschi A et al. Use of squaric acid dibutylester (SADBE) for cutaneous warts in children. *Pediatr Dermatol* 2000;17:315-8.
48. Buckley DA, Keane FM, Munn SE et al. Recalcitrant viral warts treated by diphencyprone immunotherapy. *Br J Dermatol* 1999;141:292-6.
49. Higgins E, du Vivier A. Topical immunotherapy: unapproved uses, dosages, or indications. *Clin Dermatol* 2002;20:515-21.
50. Horn TD, Johnson SM, Helm RM et al. Intralesional immunotherapy of warts with mumps, Candida, and Trichophyton skin test antigens: a single-blinded, randomized and controlled trial. *Arch Dermatol* 2005;141:589-94.
51. Amirnia M, Khodaeiani E, Masoudnia S et al. Intralesional immunotherapy with tuberculin purified protein derivative (PPD) in recalcitrant wart: a randomized, placebo-controlled, double-blind clinical trial including an extra group of candidates for cryotherapy. *J Dermatol Treat* 2016;27:173-8.
52. Grussendorf-Conen EI, Jacobs S, Rubben A et al. Topical 5% imiquimod long-term treatment of cutaneous warts resistant to standard therapy modalities. *Dermatology* 2002;205:139-45.
53. Hengge UR, Esser S, Schultewolter T et al. Self-administered topical 5% imiquimod for the treatment of common warts and molluscum contagiosum. *Br J Dermatol* 2000;143:1026-31.
54. Ahn CS, Huang WW. Imiquimod in the treatment of cutaneous warts: an evidence-based review. *Am J Clin Dermatol* 2014;15:387-99.
55. Mitsuishi T, Iida K, Kawana S. Cimetidine treatment for viral warts enhances IL-2 and IFN-gamma expression but not IL-18 expression in lesional skin. *Eur J Dermatol* 2003;13:445-8.
56. Glass AT, Solomon BA. Cimetidine therapy for recalcitrant warts in adults. *Arch Dermatol* 1996;132:680-2.
57. Orlow SJ, Paller A. Cimetidine therapy for multiple viral warts in children. *J Am Acad Dermatol* 1993;28:794-6.
58. Rogers CJ, Gibney MD, Siegfried EC et al. Cimetidine therapy for recalcitrant warts in adults: is it any better than placebo? *J Am Acad Dermatol* 1999;41:123-7.
59. Yilmaz E, Alpsoy E, Basaran E. Cimetidine therapy for warts: a placebo-controlled, double-blind study. *J Am Acad Dermatol* 1996;34:1005-7.
60. Karabulut AA, Sahin S, Eksioglu M. Is cimetidine effective for nongenital warts: a double-blind, placebo-controlled study. *Arch Dermatol* 1997;133:533-4.
61. Lynch MD, Cliffe J, Morris-Jones R. Management of cutaneous viral warts. *BMJ* 2014;348:g3339.
62. Boull C, Groth D. Update: treatment of cutaneous viral warts in children. *Pediatr Dermatol* 2011;28:217-29.
63. Lipke MM. An armamentarium of wart treatments. *Clin Med Res* 2006;4:273-93.

Warts—What You Need to Know

What are warts?

- Warts are small, round, hard bumps on the skin that have a rough surface (like a cauliflower). They may be white, pink or brown and they may have little black dots inside.
- Warts are most often found on fingers, hands and the bottom of the feet. They can grow on any part of the body.
- Warts usually do not cause pain except when they are on the bottom of the feet.

What causes warts?

- Warts are caused by a virus called the human papilloma virus (HPV). This virus can be spread from person to person by touching the wart. Some people get warts easily while others never do. It is not known why this happens.

How are warts treated?

- Most warts go away without any treatment but it can take a long time for a wart to disappear.
- Using a wart treatment is a good idea if:
  - the wart is painful
  - it bleeds if it is bumped or rubbed by clothing
  - it makes you feel embarrassed
  - you want to prevent warts from spreading to other areas of the body or to other people
- Wart treatments kill the skin that contains the virus. Ask your healthcare provider for advice about the best wart treatment for you.

Tips for Using a Wart Treatment

Follow these steps for treating warts:

- Soak the wart in warm water for about 10 minutes. Then dry the skin lightly.
- Apply petroleum jelly (Vaseline) to protect the normal skin around the wart.
- Carefully apply a wart treatment solution (salicylic acid) directly to the wart. You may need to use a toothpick to apply some solutions. Let the liquid dry for 5 minutes.
- Cover the wart with thick, adhesive, medical tape. This keeps the skin moist so the medicine can get into the wart and work better.
- After 24 hours, remove the tape. The top of the wart should have turned gray, which means the treatment solution has started to destroy the wart. Remove the gray, dead skin by filing it away with an emery board or pumice. You can get these at any grocery store or drugstore.
- Always wash your hands after touching the wart.
- Repeat the treatment steps once a day until the wart is gone. It may take several weeks or even months.
- If the wart becomes sore, stop the treatment for a few days.

When should you visit your healthcare provider?

- See your healthcare provider if you have warts on your face, genitals (private parts) or around your fingernails. Don't use wart treatments in these areas.
- See your healthcare provider if you still have warts after 8 weeks of home treatment.

What treatments will your healthcare provider suggest?

- Your healthcare provider may suggest any of the following treatments:
  - a chemical solution that is stronger than home treatments
  - liquid nitrogen to freeze the wart
  - burning the wart off with electricity
  - cutting the wart out or removing it with a laser
- The wart may fall off within a few days. You may need more than one treatment.
- Some of these treatments may be painful or leave a scar.

Will the warts come back?

- Treatment does not work every time. The virus may still be in your skin even if it looks like the wart is gone.
- If you get more warts, treat them in the same way as before. Be very careful to follow the directions exactly.

How can you prevent the spread of the virus that causes warts?

- Do not scratch, bite or chew the warts.
- Avoid sharing towels.
- Do not share nail files or pumice stones used to pare down the wart.
- Cover warts with waterproof plastic tape when using public swimming pools or public showers.
- Avoid shaving areas where warts are present.

Chapter 74
Viral Skin Rashes

Sandra Knowles, BScPhm

Viral infections are frequently associated with the development of exanthems, especially in the pediatric population. These exanthems are generally nonspecific and often lack characteristic features. Many of the viral exanthems are associated with low-grade fever, myalgias, headache, rhinorrhea, or gastrointestinal symptoms. This chapter addresses the following topics: rubeola, rubella, erythema infectiosum (parovirus infection/fifth disease), roseola infantum (sixth disease), Gianotti-Crosti syndrome, hand, foot and mouth disease, varicella (chickenpox) and herpes zoster (shingles). It should be noted that many other viral eruptions (e.g., herpes simplex, eruption associated with respiratory and enteric viruses) are not discussed.

Pathophysiology

Characteristics of selected viral skin rashes can be found in Table 1.

Rubeola (Measles)

Measles vaccination resulted in a 74% drop in measles-associated deaths between 2000 and 2012 worldwide. However, there were still 139 300 fatalities in 2010, mostly in low-income countries.[1] Measles virus (paramyxovirus) is spread primarily via respiratory droplets. Koplik spots, which are small gray-blue specks on an erythematous base, appear in the prodromal period. These are found on the buccal mucosa during the prodrome but disappear within 48 hours after the onset of rash. They are generally diagnostic for measles although they may be associated with the human parvovirus B19 (erythema infectiosum). Two to 3 days after Koplik spots appear, a purplish red, maculopapular eruption appears on the scalp, face and neck that spreads downwards. Complications of measles most often include otitis media and rarely bronchopneumonia, encephalitis, myocarditis and pericarditis.[2]

Rubella (German Measles)

Although the prodrome and skin eruption are milder than in typical measles, rubella has devastating effects on the developing fetus if contracted during the first trimester of pregnancy. The most common features of congenital rubella syndrome are sensorineural deafness, cataracts, congenital heart disease and CNS abnormalities.[3] The rubella virus (RNA togavirus) is spread by respiratory droplets. Although in March 2005 the Center for Disease Control in the United States announced the elimination of endemic rubella and congenital rubella syndrome in the United States,[4] more than 450 000 people contract rubella each year, most of them children in third world countries.[5]

Erythema Infectiosum (Parovirus Infection/Fifth Disease)

Erythema infectiosum is a childhood exanthem caused by human parvovirus B19 and thought to be spread by respiratory droplet secretions. It is most common between 4 and 10 years of age. Over 50% of infections are asymptomatic. The eruption occurs in 3 stages: sudden onset of macular erythema on the face giving a "slapped cheek" appearance; after 1 day, erythematous macular eruption that can last up to 7 days occurs on the extensor extremities; a reticulated or lacy erythema appears on the extensor extremities that can last up to 3 weeks. The third stage can recur secondary to friction and sun exposure.[5] See Erythema Infectiosum (Parovirus/Fifth Disease) in Photo Section. Associated findings include arthralgia or arthritis in up to 10% of patients, typically involving the small joints of the hands, wrists, knees or ankles and is generally self-limiting. It is more common in adults, especially women. Fetal infection with parvovirus B19 can lead to anemia with subsequent fetal hydrops, spontaneous miscarriage and stillbirth. The second trimester, especially between 20 and 28 weeks, is the period of highest risk.[3]

Roseola Infantum (Sixth Disease)

Roseola infantum is a skin rash caused by human herpesvirus 6 (HHV-6) or 7 (HHV-7). The mode of transmission of roseola is unknown. After an incubation period of 5–15 days, children present with a high fever without an associated illness that lasts approximately 3–5 days. Febrile convulsions occur in approximately 10% of patients. Rapid defervescence is followed by the onset of a rash which begins on the chest and generalizes into a pink, maculopapular eruption that lasts 24–48 hours. Most infections occur between 6 months and 3 years of age, with a peak at 6–7 months.[5,6]

Gianotti-Crosti Syndrome (Papular Acrodermatitis of Childhood)

The skin eruption of Gianotti-Crosti syndrome is characterized by erythematous, flat-topped papules symmetrically distributed on the face, buttocks and extremities of children. The trunk is usually spared and the lesions are most commonly nonpruritic. The eruption is self-limiting, with spontaneous resolution in 3 weeks. Associated features may include lymphadenopathy, hepatomegaly and occasionally splenomegaly. The eruption is associated with a variety of infectious agents including Epstein-Barr virus, cytomegalovirus and hepatitis B. As well, various immunizations such as influenza, diphtheria and measles have been associated with Gianotti-Crosti syndrome.[7] See Gianotti-Crosti Syndrome in Photo Section.

Hand, Foot and Mouth Disease

The incubation period of hand, foot and mouth disease is 4–6 days with a high rate of contagion. Following an absent or mild prodrome, lesions appear in the oral mucosa and affect the palms and soles. Characteristic grey-white vesiculopustules are often asymptomatic, although oral lesions may be painful. Hand, foot and mouth disease is caused by enteroviruses, mostly coxsackie A16. The virus is spread by direct contact with nose and throat discharges and feces of infected people.[8,9] See Hand, Foot and Mouth Disease in Photo Section.

Varicella (Chickenpox)

Chickenpox is a highly infectious disease caused by the varicella zoster virus (VZV); over 90% of unvaccinated people become infected if exposed.[10] It is transmitted via inhalation of respiratory secretions or contact with skin lesions. Varicella lesions are intensely pruritic and appear as scattered eruptions which vesiculate, rupture and then crust. The vesicles are often described as looking like "drops of water".[8] Secondary bacterial infection of the lesions and otitis media are the most common complications of varicella, occurring in 5–10% of children. Healthy children rarely develop serious complications such as pneumonitis, encephalitis, cerebellar ataxis and Reye's syndrome. Complications are more common and severe in adults or immunocompromised individuals (adults or children). Maternal varicella infection in pregnancy can lead to complications ranging from asymptomatic latency to severe congenital defects.[11] The incidence of embryopathy and fetopathy after maternal varicella infection in the first 20 weeks of pregnancy is estimated to be 2%.[12] In addition, perinatal mortality is high: nearly 30% of infants with clinical lesions die during the first month of life.[13] See Chickenpox (Varicella) in Photo Section.

Herpes Zoster (Shingles)

Herpes zoster is caused by reactivation of the varicella zoster virus that has remained latent in the sensory ganglia after a previous primary infection with chickenpox. Herpes zoster is primarily a disease of elderly people but it can occur across all age groups, especially in immunocompromised individuals. The cause of reactivation is unknown, although physical trauma, ultraviolet light or stress at a time when the host's immune system is suppressed may play a role.[14] Approximately 15% of those who have had the primary varicella infection develop herpes zoster. The dermatomal distribution of herpes zoster can vary although the thoracic area is involved in more than half of cases. Only 1–8% of patients develop recurrences. Although patients with herpes zoster (shingles) are less contagious than those with varicella (chickenpox), susceptible household contacts can develop varicella after exposure to herpes zoster, usually by means of direct contact with the lesions.[15] The most common complication of herpes zoster is postherpetic neuralgia; the pain is described as continuous aching, itching or burning.[11] See Herpes Zoster in Photo Section.

Goals of Therapy

- Minimize patient discomfort
- Shorten duration of symptoms when possible
- Prevent complications

Patient Assessment

An assessment for pediatric patients with a skin eruption is found in Figure 1. Prior to recommending a product for symptomatic relief, evaluate the severity of the patient's condition.

Patients require further assessment by an appropriate healthcare practitioner when:

- The causative factor/organism is uncertain
- Fever and/or malaise is associated with the skin eruption
- The patient has an underlying condition, such as diabetes, cancer or HIV infection, or the patient is on chronic corticosteroid therapy or other immunosuppressive therapy.

Note that many other eruptions induced by viral infections (e.g., herpes simplex, eruptions associated with respiratory and enteric viruses) are not included in Figure 1.

Prevention

Hand hygiene is one of the most effective methods of preventing transmission of pathogens. As many viral skin rashes are spread via respiratory droplets, respiratory hygiene (cough etiquette) should also be used to help prevent transmission.[16]

Vaccines have been developed for the prevention of herpes zoster, measles, rubella and varicella. For current recommendations on immunization schedules for infants and children for the **measles, mumps** and **rubella** vaccine, see the Canadian Immunization Guide.[17] The **varicella virus vaccine** is recommended for primary vaccination of healthy persons 12 months of age or older who are susceptible to the disease.[17] Although **herpes zoster vaccine** is safe and immunogenic in patients 50 years of age and older, the greatest benefit is observed in those 60 years and older. It is recommended for prevention of herpes zoster and its complications, in persons 60 years and older without contraindications.[18,19] High-risk patients, such as those with cancer or HIV infection, should avoid exposure to patients with viral skin eruptions. All women of child-bearing age should be tested for rubella antibodies and vaccinated if necessary, prior to pregnancy. The varicella virus vaccine is contraindicated during pregnancy; pregnant women not previously infected with chickenpox should avoid contact with infected individuals.[17]

Table 1: **Characteristics of Selected Viral Skin Rashes**

Disease	Prodromal Features	Skin Eruption[a]	Incubation Period	Infectious Period	Differential Diagnosis	Prevention	Treatment	Most Common Season of Occurrence
Rubeola (Measles)	3–4 days of fever, cough, coryza, photophobia, conjunctivitis, Koplik spots	Erythematous macules and papules appear initially behind ears and along hairline and spread downward. Fade by day 5 of eruption	8–12 days	1–2 days before prodrome until 4 days after skin eruption	Morbilliform rash: Similar to drug eruptions and viral exanthems; Koplik spots generally diagnostic	Measles vaccine	Supportive care (e.g., antipyretics)	Winter/ spring
Rubella (German Measles)	Children: Usually none or mild fever and lymphadenop- athy Adolescents/ adults: Fever, malaise, sore throat, nausea, painful occipital lymphadenop- athy	Starts on face and neck as mild pink erythematous macules and papules, and generalizes over 1–2 days. Lesions fade within 2–3 days	14–21 days	5–7 days prior to eruption until 3–5 days after	Nonspecific viral exanthems, drug eruptions	Rubella vaccine	Supportive care (e.g., antipyretics)	Spring
Erythema Infectiosum (Parovirus Infection/Fifth Disease)	Children: Mild fever, sore throat and malaise Adults: Flu-like symptoms, arthralgias and arthritis	Red erythematous macules on cheeks with "slapped cheek" appearance followed by maculopapular eruption on proximal extremities, which fades from centre out producing reticulated "lacy" pattern. Resolves in 1 wk	4–14 days	Prior to onset of eruption (only considered mildly contagious)	Systemic lupus erythematosus (butterfly pattern over the bridge of the nose)	None	Supportive care	Winter/ spring

(cont'd)

Table 1: **Characteristics of Selected Viral Skin Rashes** *(cont'd)*

Disease	Prodromal Features	Skin Eruption[a]	Incubation Period	Infectious Period	Differential Diagnosis	Prevention	Treatment	Most Common Season of Occurrence
Roseola Infantum (Sixth Disease); (Human herpes virus 6 or 7 infection)	High fever for 3–4 days	Lesions start on chest and rapidly generalize into a pink maculopapular eruption. Fade within 24–48 h	7–15 days	During illness	Measles, scarlet fever, rubella	None	Supportive care	Spring/fall
Gianotti-Crosti Syndrome (Papular Acrodermatitis of Childhood)	Upper respiratory infection in one-third of patients	Sudden eruption of flat-topped, nonpruritic erythematous papules that are symmetrically distributed over face, buttocks and extremities. Resolves in 2–8 wk	Unknown	Unknown	Lichen planus, drug eruption, pityriasis rosea	None	Usually none required	Spring/early summer
Hand, Foot and Mouth Disease	Absent or mild and occur 1–2 days before lesions. Low-grade fever, anorexia, malaise, sore mouth	Blisters or ulcers surrounded by red halos form in the back of mouth and on tongue, palms, soles, and buttocks	4–6 days	From first appearance until blister-like lesions disappear	Unique disease based on incubation period and distribution of lesions	None	Good oral hydration	Summer/fall
Varicella (Chickenpox)	None to fever, malaise, cough, sore throat	Erythematous macules which develop central vesicles and 2 days later pustules and crusts. Total healing 16 days	10–21 days	Two days prior to eruption until 5 days after	Insect bites during early stages. Kaposi's varicelliform eruption (eczema herpeticum)	Varicella vaccine	Children: Supportive care Adults: Antivirals (e.g., acyclovir, famciclovir)	Sporadic

Disease	Prodromal Features	Skin Eruption[a]	Incubation Period	Infectious Period	Differential Diagnosis	Prevention	Treatment	Most Common Season of Occurrence
Herpes Zoster (Shingles)	Children: None Adults: Dull ache up to 1 wk prior to eruption	Occur in a dermatomal distribution and consist of grouped vesicles and bullae on an erythematous base. Persist for 10–14 days	Not applicable	Until primary crusts have healed	Insect bites, herpes simplex virus	Zoster vaccine, live attenuated	Children: None Adults: Antivirals within 48–72 h of initial appearance of lesions	Sporadic

[a] See Chapter 61: Drug-induced Skin Reactions, Table 1: Dermatologic Terminology.

Nonpharmacologic Therapy

Minimizing patient discomfort is key, and often the only treatment that can be offered to patients with a viral skin eruption.

Many viral skin eruptions are associated with intense pruritus. Since it is exacerbated by dry skin, using a simple emollient is often helpful. A humidifier can also be used, although in some patients high humidity may also cause pruritus secondary to sweat retention. Recommend good hygiene practices including gentle cleansing and drying of lesions as well as trimming of fingernails, to prevent bacterial infection that may develop from scratching the pruritic lesions. The sensation of itching is generally increased if the skin is warm. Therefore, cooling the skin by tepid showering or bathing can often bring relief. As well, rubbing an ice cube over the rash or covering the rash with a clean cloth soaked in cold water will provide temporary relief.

Avoiding factors that may enhance pruritus, such as wearing of tight elasticized apparel or coarse woolen fabrics, is also important. **Cornstarch** or **sodium bicarbonate** baths have been used to relieve itching in patients with chickenpox. Add 2 cups of cornstarch mixed with 4 cups of water to a bathtub full of water. Bathing is recommended once or twice daily for approximately 15–20 minutes. The skin should be gently patted, not rubbed, when drying.

Remind patients to stay well hydrated by drinking plenty of fluids, which can include popsicles and gelatin.

Pharmacologic Therapy

For comparative ingredients of nonprescription products, consult the *Compendium of Products for Minor Ailments*—Analgesic Products: External Analgesics; Skin Care Products: Dermatitis and Dry Skin, First Aid.

Colloidal oatmeal bath preparations may help to relieve pruritus. To be effective the product should be well dispersed in the bathtub water. For dispersion, the patient should fill a strainer with oatmeal bath preparation and hold under the faucet as water fills the tub. Unscented moisture cream or white petrolatum should be applied to the skin while it is slightly damp to retard water evaporation.

Local agents are useful for relieving pruritus and for reducing bacterial colonization of damaged skin. Cool compresses (e.g., gauze or other thin cloth moistened with water) applied for 20 minutes 4–6 times daily can be used, especially for weeping, oozing lesions. **Calamine lotion** can be applied after removal of the wet compresses. Other traditional topical agents including **menthol**, **camphor** and **phenol** are no longer recommended. Concern has been raised over possible phenol toxicity, which has been described in patients with extensive bullous poison ivy who developed renal toxicity.[20] The American Academy of Pediatrics recommends that camphor not be used in children due to adverse effects associated with even minor systemic absorption.[21]

Local anesthetics block conduction along axonal membranes, thereby relieving itching as well as pain. However, topical local anesthetics (e.g., benzocaine) are not recommended due to risk of sensitization, especially if applied to broken or fissured skin.[22] **Pramoxine** has less risk of sensitization than other local anesthetics, and may be used topically as an antipruritic. Topical **lidocaine** has demonstrated efficacy for relief of neuropathic pain (including postherpetic neuralgia), in several low-quality studies.[23] However, the typical large size of the area to be treated and the need for occlusion limit the routine use of local anesthetics in this situation.

Topical corticosteroids may relieve the itching associated with the skin lesions but are not frequently used as most viral-induced skin eruptions are self-limiting and topical corticosteroids do not improve the natural history of the disease. Mild topical corticosteroids such as 0.5 or 1% **hydrocortisone**, can be used on the face and intertriginous folds. Ointments are more occlusive and are preferred for dry or scaly lesions, whereas creams are used in moist areas since they are more drying. Lotions are useful for the scalp and other hairy areas or for application to large body areas. Topical corticosteroids should not be used on bacterial- or fungal-infected skin since the corticosteroid may mask the symptoms of the dermatologic infection and allow the infection to progress. If the skin lesions persist or worsen after 5–7 days of topical corticosteroid therapy, the patient should seek further assessment and/or treatment. There is some evidence that medium-potency **topical corticosteroids** may decrease the duration of lesions of Gianotti-Crosti syndrome when applied once daily for 1–2 weeks. However, patients should be monitored closely, as there have been reports of worsening symptoms with the use of topical corticosteroids.[24] For further discussion on the use of topical corticosteroids, consult the *Compendium of Therapeutic Choices*: Atopic Dermatitis.

Capsaicin 0.025% cream is a topical preparation made from the naturally occurring substance found in hot chili peppers. Applied to the affected area at least 3–4 times daily, it is effective in the treatment of postherpetic neuralgia.[25] Local burning, stinging and irritation are common although they usually disappear with repeated application.

Although H_1-blocking **antihistamines** have been used for the treatment of pruritus especially associated with urticaria, they are often not effective for viral-induced skin lesions. However, sedating or first-generation antihistamines are often used at bedtime to improve sleep.[26] See Chapter 22: Allergic Rhinitis for adult and pediatric doses of oral antihistamines. Topical diphenhydramine is usually not recommended because of the risk of sensitization resulting in contact dermatitis.[26]

Many viral diseases are associated with a fever, especially in the prodromal stages. **Antipyretics** can be recommended to provide symptomatic relief; however, they do not reduce risk of recurrent febrile seizures.[27]

Acetaminophen is recommended as the first-line antipyretic agent in children with chickenpox (see Chapter 7: Fever for adult and pediatric doses of antipyretics). Although acetaminophen was found to delay the clearance of the varicella zoster virus, as shown by delayed scabbing of the lesions,[28] the clinical significance of this is not known. The use of NSAIDs in children with chickenpox may increase the risk of necrotizing soft tissue infections and secondary infections caused by invasive streptococci.[29,30,31]

Avoid **ASA** because of the possible association of Reye's syndrome with salicylate administration[32] especially in children and teenagers with viral infections.[33] Reye's syndrome is an acute, noninflammatory enecephalopathy and hepatotoxicity that follows an acute viral illness.[34] In some countries ASA use is still recommended in children. Parents who travel abroad should be warned regarding this potential risk.[35] There are no case reports of Reye's syndrome in patients with herpes zoster receiving ASA for cardiovascular prophylaxis; many clinicians elect to continue ASA during the acute illness. If analgesics are required in these patients, recommend acetaminophen or ibuprofen as there is no association between these agents and the development of Reye's syndrome.

Mild analgesics (e.g., NSAIDs other than ASA, acetaminophen) are sometimes recommended for the treatment of acute pain associated with herpes zoster, but are often not effective. The pain in acute herpes zoster is frequently moderate to severe and warrants the use of opioid analgesics.[36]

For patients with mouth lesions, recommend warm water rinses or saline rinses (5–15 mL of table salt in 125–250 mL of warm tap water.) Hydrogen peroxide (half-strength) has also been used as a mouth rinse. Frequent oral hygiene with a soft-bristled toothbrush is recommended. Patients should avoid alcohol- and glycerin-based mouthwashes; petrolatum jelly can be applied to lips as needed.

Antiviral therapy may be used in select patients:

- Chickenpox: If initiated within 24 hours of rash onset, **acyclovir** may decrease the total number of new lesions formed and lower the need for antipruritic and analgesic treatment. In immunocompetent children, acyclovir is not generally recommended. However for immunocompetent adults and all immunocompromised hosts, treatment with acyclovir is suggested.[37] Although no randomized control trial evidence is available and it is not an approved indication, **valacyclovir** and **famciclovir** have been used for the treatment of chickenpox in healthy adults.[10]

- Acute herpes zoster: Antiviral therapy with **acyclovir, valacyclovir** or **famciclovir** speeds resolution of the acute lesional events and perhaps reduces the risk of prolonged pain. In patients 50 years of age and over or any patient with moderate to severe acute pain, antiviral therapy should be initiated if the duration of the rash is less than 72 hours. However, antiviral treatment should be considered even in patients who present more than 72 hours after rash onset, particularly in the presence of new vesicle formation or complications.[14]

For further discussion of pharmacologic therapy for chickenpox and acute herpes zoster, consult the *Compendium of Therapeutic Choices*: Herpesvirus Infections.

For further information on topical therapy for viral skin rashes, see Table 3.

Natural Health Products

Although **witch hazel** (hamamelis water) has traditionally been used for skin irritations, bruises and hemorrhoids, clinical data to support its efficacy in these conditions are limited.[38]

Monitoring of Therapy

A monitoring plan for patients with viral rashes is outlined in Table 2. Additional advice should be provided regarding:

- Time frame during which patients are considered infectious
- Assessment by appropriate healthcare practitioner for possible use of antivirals in patients with herpes zoster and varicella (especially adults and those who are immunocompromised).

Table 2: **Monitoring of Therapy for Viral Skin Rashes**

Symptoms	Monitoring	Endpoint of Therapy	Actions
Pruritus associated with skin eruption	Patient: Daily while on therapy Healthcare practitioner: After 2 days of therapy or next pharmacy visit	To decrease itching within 24–48 h	If therapy ineffective after 24–48 h and treatment still required, patient requires further assessment.
Fever	Patient: BID while on therapy Healthcare practitioner: After 2 days or next visit	To decrease fever within 4–6 h of therapy	If fever persists for more than 48 h, patient requires further assessment and/or treatment.
Pain, especially with herpes zoster	Patient: Daily Healthcare practitioner: Within 24 h of initiating therapy	To decrease pain to acceptable levels for the patient within 24 h	If pain persists despite appropriate analgesic medication, patient requires further assessment and/or treatment.
Sedation (due to antihistamine therapy: this may be a desired effect of therapy)	Patient: Daily Healthcare practitioner: After 3 days or next visit	No sedation, especially if patient driving or using heavy machinery	

Figure 1: **Assessment of Pediatric Patient with Skin Eruption[a]**

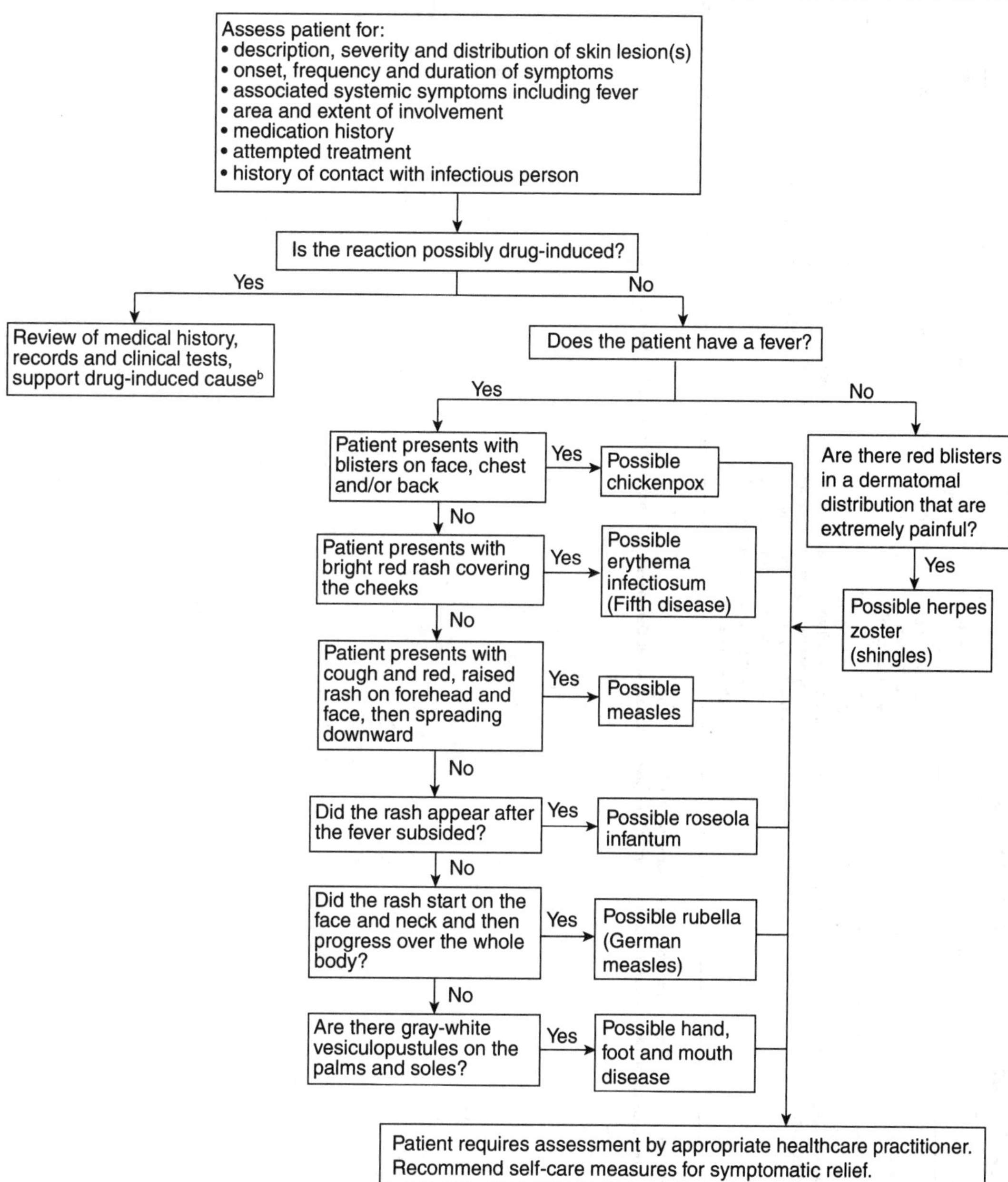

Assess patient for:
• description, severity and distribution of skin lesion(s)
• onset, frequency and duration of symptoms
• associated systemic symptoms including fever
• area and extent of involvement
• medication history
• attempted treatment
• history of contact with infectious person
Is the reaction possibly drug-induced?
Yes
No
Review of medical history, records and clinical tests, support drug-induced cause[b]
Does the patient have a fever?
Yes
No
Patient presents with blisters on face, chest and/or back
Yes
Possible chickenpox
No
Patient presents with bright red rash covering the cheeks
Yes
Possible erythema infectiosum (Fifth disease)
No
Patient presents with cough and red, raised rash on forehead and face, then spreading downward
Yes
Possible measles
No
Did the rash appear after the fever subsided?
Yes
Possible roseola infantum
No
Did the rash start on the face and neck and then progress over the whole body?
Yes
Possible rubella (German measles)
No
Are there gray-white vesiculopustules on the palms and soles?
Yes
Possible hand, foot and mouth disease
Are there red blisters in a dermatomal distribution that are extremely painful?
Yes
Possible herpes zoster (shingles)
Patient requires assessment by appropriate healthcare practitioner. Recommend self-care measures for symptomatic relief.

[a] Many viral-induced eruptions (e.g., herpes simplex, eruption associated with respiratory and enteric viruses) are not included in this assessment.
[b] See Chapter 61: Drug-induced Skin Reactions.

Table 3: Topical Treatments for Viral Skin Rashes

Class	Drug	Dosage	Adverse Effects	Comments	Cost[a]
Analgesics, topical	*capsaicin* Zostrix, generics	Apply to affected area at least TID–QID	Local burning, stinging and irritation are common but disappear with repeated application.	Used for treatment of postherpetic neuralgia.	$$
Corticosteroids, topical[b,c]	*hydrocortisone 0.5%, 1% cream, lotion, ointment* Cortate, generics	Apply to affected area TID–QID for up to 7 days	Striae, telangiectasia, atrophy, purpura. When used around the eye for longer periods of time, ocular side effects may rarely occur. Systemic effects include suppression of HPA axis although clinically relevant features are very rare.	Useful for noninfected, non-weeping lesions. Cream: Moist areas. Ointment: Dry or scaly lesions.	$

[a] Cost of 30 g; includes drug cost only.

[b] Since viral exanthems are self-limiting, topical corticosteroids are generally not recommended.

[c] For further information on other topical corticosteroids, consult the *Compendium of Therapeutic Choices*: Atopic Dermatitis and Corticosteroids: Topical (CPhA Monograph).

Legend: $ <$5 $$ $5–10

Suggested Readings

Folster-Holst R, Kreth H. Viral exanthems in childhood-infectious (direct) exanthems. Part 1: Classic exanthems. *J Dtsch Dermatol Ges* 2009;7:309-16.

Folster-Holst R, Kreth H. Viral exanthems in childhood-infectious (direct) exanthems. Part 2: Other viral exanthems. *J Dtsch Dermatol Ges* 2009;7:414-9.

References

1. World Health Organization. *Measles*. Fact sheet no 286. Reviewed March 2016. Available from: www.who.int/mediacentre/factsheets/fs286/en/index.html.
2. Moss WJ, Griffin DE. Measles. *Lancet* 2012;379:153-64.
3. Dyer JA. Childhood viral exanthems. *Pediatr Ann* 2007;36:21-9.
4. Centers for Disease Control and Prevention (CDC). Elimination of rubella and congenital rubella syndrome-United States, 1969-2004. *MMWR Morb Mortal Wkly Rep* 2005;54:279-82.
5. Folster-Holst R, Kreth H. Viral exanthems in childhood-infectious (direct) exanthems. Part 1: Classic exanthems. *J Dtsch Dermatol Ges* 2009;7:309-16.
6. Scott LA, Stone MS. Viral exanthems. *Dermatol Online J* 2003;9:4.
7. Nelson JS, Stone MS. Update on selected viral exanthems. *Curr Opin Pediatr* 2000;12:359-64.
8. Folster-Holst R, Kreth H. Viral exanthems in childhood-infectious (direct) exanthems. Part 2: Other viral exanthems. *J Dtsch Dermatol Ges* 2009;7:414-9.
9. Wong SS, Yip CC, Lau SK et al. Human enterovirus 71 and hand, foot and mouth disease. *Epidemiol Infect* 2010;138:1071-89.
10. Breuer J, Fifer H. Chickenpox. *Clin Evid (Online)* 2011;pii:0912.
11. McCrary ML, Severson J, Tyring SK. Varicella zoster virus. *J Am Acad Dermatol* 1999;41:1-14.
12. Sauerbrei A, Wutzler P. The congenital varicella syndrome. *J Perinatol* 2000;20:548–54.
13. Mandelbrot L. Fetal varicella—diagnosis, management and outcome. *Prenat Diagn* 2013;32:511–8.
14. Sampathkumar P, Drage LA, Martin DP. Herpes zoster (shingles) and postherpetic neuralgia. *Mayo Clin Proc* 2009;84:274-80.
15. Schmader KE, Oxman MN. Varicella and herpes zoster. In: Goldsmith LA et al., eds. *Fitzpatrick's dermatology in general medicine*. 8th ed. New York: McGraw Hill Medical; 2012.
16. World Health Organization. *Infection control standard precautions in health care*. 2006. Available from: www.who.int/csr/resources/publications/4EPR_AM2.pdf.
17. Public Health Agency of Canada. National Advisory Committee on Immunization (NACI). *Canadian immunization guide*. Evergreen ed. Available from: www.phac-aspc.gc.ca/publicat/cig-gci/index-eng.php. Accessed april 12, 2016.
18. Gagliardi AM, Gomes Silva BN, Torloni MR et al. Vaccines for preventing herpes zoster in older adults. *Cochrane Database Syst Rev* 2012;10:CD008858.
19. Public Health Agency of Canada. An Advisory Committee Statement (ACS). National Advisory Committee on Immunization: (NACI). *Update on the use of herpes zoster vaccine*. January 2014. Available from: publications.gc.ca/collections/collection_2014/aspc-phac/HP40-92-2014-eng.pdf. Accessed June 6, 2015.
20. Millikan LE. Pruritus: unapproved treatments or indications. *Clin Dermatol* 2000;18:149-52.
21. Camphor revisited: focus on toxicity. Committee on Drugs. American Academy of Pediatrics. *Pediatrics* 1994;94:127-8.
22. Warshaw EM, Schram SE, Belsito DV et al. Patch-test reactions to topical anesthetics: retrospective analysis of cross-sectional data, 2001 to 2004. *Dermatitis* 2008;19:81-5.
23. Derry S, Wiffen PJ, Moore RA et al. Topical lidocaine for neuropathic pain in adults. *Cochrane Database Syst Rev* 2014;7:CD010958
24. Belazarian LT, Lorenzo ME, Pearson AL et al. Exanthematous viral diseases. In: Goldsmith LA et al., eds. *Fitzpatrick's dermatology in general medicine*. 8th ed. New York: McGraw Hill Medical; 2012.
25. Bernestine JE, Korman NJ, Bickers DR et al. Topical capsaicin treatment of chronic postherpetic neuralgia. *J Am Acad Dermatol* 1989;21:265-70.
26. Tan JK. Pruritus. In: Jovaisas B, ed. *Compendium of therapeutic choices: CTC7*. 7th ed. Ottawa: Canadian Pharmacists Association; 2014.
27. Lux AL. Antipyretic drugs do not reduce recurrences of febrile seizures in children with previous febrile seizure. *Evid Based Med* 2010;15:15-6.
28. Doran TF, De Angelis C, Baumgardner RA et al. Acetaminophen: more harm than good for chickenpox? *J Pediatr* 1989;114:1045-8.
29. National Pharmacy Association. Use of NSAIDs in children with chickenpox. https://www.npa.co.uk/news-and-events/news-item/use-nsaids-children-chickenpox/ April 14, 2016.
30. Mikaeloff Y, Kezouh A, Suissa A. Nonsteroidal anti-inflammatory drug use and the risk of severe skin and soft tissue complications in patients with varicella or zoster disease. *Br J Clin Pharmacol* 2007;65:203-9.
31. Souyri C, Olivier P, Grolleau S et al. Severe necrotizing soft-tissue infections and nonsteroidal anti-inflammatory drugs. *Clin Exp Dermatol* 2008;33:249-55.
32. Starko KM, Ray CG, Dominguez LB et al. Reye's syndrome and salicylate use. *Pediatrics* 1980;66:859-64.
33. Waldman RJ, Hall WN, McGee H et al. Aspirin as a risk factor in Reye's syndrome. *JAMA* 1982;247:3089-94.
34. Beutler AI, Chesnut GT, Mattingly JC et al. FPIN's Clinical Inquiries. Aspirin use in children for fever or viral syndromes. *Am Fam Physician* 2009;80:1472.
35. Donaldson M, Fleming P. Reye's syndrome in children travelling abroad. *Lancet* 1988;2:1073.
36. Schmader KE, Dworkin RH. Natural history and treatment of herpes zoster. *J Pain* 2008;9:S3-9.
37. Tunbridge AJ, Breuer J, Jeffery KJ. Chickenpox in adults–clinical management. *J Infect* 2008;57:95-102.
38. Natural Medicines. *Witch hazel*. Available from: naturalmedicines.therapeuticresearch.com. Subscription required.

Shingles—What You Need to Know

What is shingles?

Shingles is a viral disease (called herpes zoster) that is caused by the same virus as chickenpox. Shingles is most common in people over the age of 50 or people who have a weak immune system.

What causes shingles?

You can only get shingles if you had chickenpox in the past. At the time you had chickenpox, the virus was stored in nerve cells in your spinal cord. The virus remains in a resting phase in these nerve cells for years. Stress or illness can cause it to become active again. The virus travels down the nerves to the skin to produce shingles.

What are the signs of shingles?

Patients usually complain of pain first. Then they get an itchy red rash with small, fluid-filled blisters. In some patients, the pain continues long after the rash has gone away.

How is shingles treated?

See your healthcare provider to discuss treatment of shingles. You will probably need a prescription. The medicine works best if you start it in the first 3 days after you get the rash.

Hints to be more comfortable:

- Use calamine lotion to stop the itching. A shower or a cool bath (with or without oatmeal) may also help.
- If your itching bothers you a lot, you can take an antihistamine. Ask your healthcare provider which one is best for you.
- Keep the rash clean and dry. Trim fingernails to prevent scratching. Scratching can cause skin infections.
- Wear loose cotton clothing if possible. Avoid wool clothing.
- You can take acetaminophen or ibuprofen to treat pain and fever. Do not take acetylsalicylic acid (Aspirin, ASA); it may cause a serious condition called Reye's syndrome.
- If you develop eye problems, call your healthcare provider immediately.

Hand, Foot and Mouth Disease—What You Need to Know

What is Hand, Foot and Mouth Disease?

Hand, foot and mouth disease (also known as HFMD) is a contagious infection caused by different viruses that occurs most commonly in the summer and fall. Infants and young children under 5 are most likely to get this disease but older children and adults can also get it. A person who has HFMD usually recovers in 7–10 days with no problems.

What are the signs and symptoms of hand, foot and mouth disease?

The signs that a person may have HFMD include:

- Fever, less hungry than usual, sore throat, feeling tired
- Painful sores may develop in the mouth 1–2 days after the fever starts
- A skin rash that is not itchy, with flat red spots can develop on the palms of the hands and soles of the feet; some people may also have a rash on the knees, elbows and buttocks.

How is hand, foot and mouth disease spread?

A person with HFMD is most likely to spread the disease to someone else during the first week of their illness, but they may still be able to give it to another person weeks after they are feeling better. HFMD can be spread by close contact (e.g., kissing, sharing cups, spoons), coughing and sneezing, contact with blister fluid, contact with feces (e.g., changing a diaper) and by touching objects or surfaces that have the virus on them. In some cases, people with HFMD do not have any symptoms themselves yet they are still able to spread the disease.

What is the treatment for hand, foot and mouth disease?

No treatment is needed. However, if the child is feeling uncomfortable:

- You can give children acetaminophen or ibuprofen for fever and pain. Do not give children acetylsalicylic acid (Aspirin, ASA) because of the risk of developing Reye's syndrome, a serious condition.
- Offer the child plenty of food and liquids. If there are sores in the mouth, cold, bland liquids such as milk and water, or cold foods such as flavoured ice pops and ice cream, may help. Do not give fruit juice or spicy foods as they may sting.

Parovirus Infection (Fifth Disease)—What You Need to Know

What is parovirus infection (fifth disease)?

Parovirus Infection (also known as Fifth disease) is a common childhood infection caused by a virus. Young children are most likely to get this virus but older children and adults can also get it. A person who has parovirus infection/fifth disease usually recovers with no complications.

What are the signs of parovirus infection (fifth disease)?

- Mild fever, headache, sore throat and achiness
- Bright red rash that appears first on the cheeks—it often looks like the child has been slapped
- Cheeks feel firm and burning hot
- A rash comes out on other parts of the body after 1–4 days—the rash can last up to 6 weeks
- Older children and adults may have swollen or painful joints

How is parovirus infection (fifth disease) spread?

The virus spreads easily and is most contagious at the beginning. The person seems to have a cold and can spread the virus by coughing and sneezing. Once the rash appears, there is no danger of spreading the virus. Children may go back to school if they feel well enough.

If you are pregnant, there is a very small chance that being around children who have parovirus infection (fifth disease) may affect your unborn child. To reduce this chance, wash your hands often. Do not share food or drinks.

What is the treatment for parovirus infection (fifth disease)?

No specific treatment is needed. However, if the child is feeling uncomfortable then:

- Apply cold compresses to burning hot cheeks.
- Rub an ice cube over the rash for no more than 1 minute at a time or cover the rash with a clean cloth soaked in cold water. This will help for a short time.
- You can give children acetaminophen or ibuprofen for fever. Do not give children acetylsalicylic acid (Aspirin, ASA) because of the risk of developing Reye's syndrome, a serious condition.

Chickenpox—What You Need To Know

What is chickenpox?

Chickenpox is a common and highly contagious infection caused by a virus (varicella zoster). It usually affects children. People usually get chickenpox only once.

Chickenpox can be extremely serious for some people. For example:

- pregnant women who have not had chickenpox before (and their unborn babies)
- people with low resistance to disease (for example – people who have leukemia or diseases of the immune system, including HIV).

There is a chickenpox vaccine. It can be used to protect children and adults who have not had chickenpox before.

What are the signs of chickenpox?

- A slightly raised temperature, cough and tiredness for a few days.
- An itchy rash with small blisters that dry up and form scabs in 2–4 days.
- The spots usually appear over a period of 3–5 days.

How does chickenpox spread?

- Chickenpox is spread by direct contact with the blisters (touching them) or from an infected person's cough or sneeze.
- People with chickenpox are infectious from 2 days before the rash appears until all the blisters have dried up (about 5–10 days later).
- It takes 2–3 weeks after a person is exposed to chickenpox for the spots to appear.

What is the treatment for chickenpox?

- You can prevent chickenpox for most children and adults by getting the chickenpox vaccine. Ask your healthcare provider for more information.
- For most healthy children, no specific treatment is needed. Follow the hints below to help relieve the itching and keep the child comfortable.
- Patients with low resistance to disease should begin antiviral drugs (such as acyclovir) right away. This treatment may also be used for adults (in whom chickenpox may be more serious and last longer) and in some healthy children. Ask your healthcare provider for more information.

Hints to keep comfortable:

- To stop the itching, apply calamine lotion to the blisters. A cool shower or bath can also help. Try adding an oatmeal bath product or half a cup of baking soda to the bath water.
- If the itching is very bad, you can use an antihistamine. Ask your healthcare provider for information about which products are safe for the infected person.
- Keep the rash clean and dry.
- Trim fingernails to prevent scratching, which can cause skin infection.
- Wear loose clothing (cotton is good—avoid wool).

- Acetaminophen can be used to treat fever. Ibuprofen and naproxen are not recommended because of the risk of developing serious skin infections in children with chickenpox. Acetylsalicylic acid (Aspirin, ASA) is not recommended because of the risk of developing Reye's syndrome, a serious condition.
- For mouth sores, rinse with warm water.

When should you see a healthcare provider?

See your healthcare provider if:

- you are pregnant
- you see signs of a skin infection (redness, swelling, a feeling of heat in a specific area);
- the person develops a severe cold or cough. Some people, especially adults, may get pneumonia.

Photo Section Highlights

1. Healthy Stoma (Chapter 37: Ostomy Care)
2. Peristomal Skin Excoriation (Chapter 37: Ostomy Care)
3. Athlete's Foot (Chapter 50: Athlete's Foot)
4. Corns (Chapter 51: Corns, Calluses, Bunions and Ingrown Toenails)
5. Plantar Warts (Chapter 52: Plantar Warts)
6. Atopic Dermatitis (Chapter 55: Atopic, Contact and Stasis Dermatitis)
7. Actinic Keratosis (Chapter 72: Prevention and Treatment of Sun-induced Skin Damage)
8. Erythema Infectiosum (Parovirus/Fifth Disease) (Chapter 74: Viral Skin Rashes)
9. Gianotti-Crosti Syndrome (face) (Chapter 74: Viral Skin Rashes)
10. Gianotti-Crosti Syndrome (body) (Chapter 74: Viral Skin Rashes)
11. Chickenpox (Varicella) (Chapter 74: Viral Skin Rashes)
12. Hand, Foot and Mouth Disease (Chapter 74: Viral Skin Rashes)
13. Herpes Zoster (Chapter 74: Viral Skin Rashes)
14. Acute Generalized Exanthematous Pustulosis (Chapter 61: Drug-induced Skin Reactions)
15. Hypersensitivity Syndrome Reaction (Chapter 61: Drug-induced Skin Reactions)
16. Serum Sickness–like Reaction (Chapter 61: Drug-induced Skin Reactions)
17. Folliculitis (Chapter 56: Bacterial Skin Infections: Impetigo, Furuncles and Carbuncles)
18. Candidiasis (Intertrigo) (Chapter 65: Fungal Skin Infections)
19. Scabies (Chapter 69: Parasitic Skin Infections: Lice and Scabies)
20. Tinea Corporis (Chapter 65: Fungal Skin Infections)
21. Common Warts (Chapter 73: Viral Skin Infections: Common and Flat Warts)
22. Lyme Disease Lesion (Chapter 67: Insect Bites and Stings)
23. Leukoplakia (Chapter 89: Aphthous Ulcers (Canker Sores))
24. Aphthous Ulcer (Chapter 89: Aphthous Ulcers (Canker Sores))
25. Establishing Successful Latch (Chapter 40: Infant Nutrition)
26. Seborrheic Dermatitis (Chapter 58: Dandruff and Seborrheic Dermatitis)
27. Acneiform Eruption (Chapter 61: Drug-induced Skin Reactions)
28. Toxic Epidermal Necrolysis (Chapter 61: Drug-induced Skin Reactions)
29. Impetigo (Chapter 56: Bacterial Skin Infections: Impetigo, Furuncles and Carbuncles)
30. Pityriasis Versicolor (Chapter 65: Fungal Skin Infections)
31. Bed Bug (Chapter 67: Insect Bites and Stings)
32. Bed Bug Infestation (Chapter 67: Insect Bites and Stings)
33. Superficial Burn (scalded thigh) (Chapter 57: Burns)
34. Deep Partial Thickness Burn (4 year old child's hand) (Chapter 57: Burns)
35. Full Thickness Burn (woman's finger) (Chapter 57: Burns)
36. Cold Sore (Chapter 90: Cold Sores (Herpes Labialis))

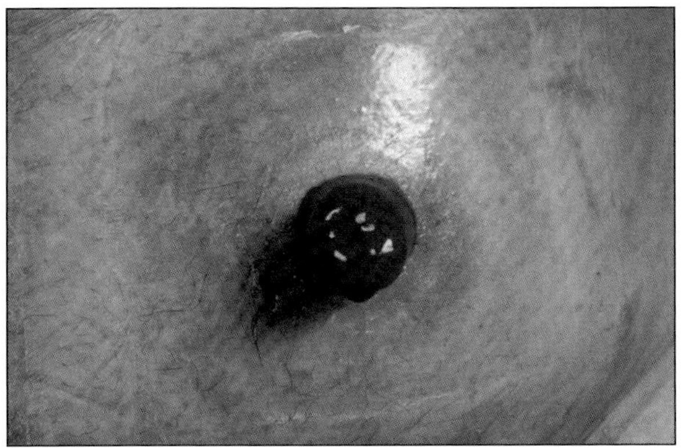

1. **Healthy Stoma**
(Chapter 37: Ostomy Care)
Courtesy of Convatec

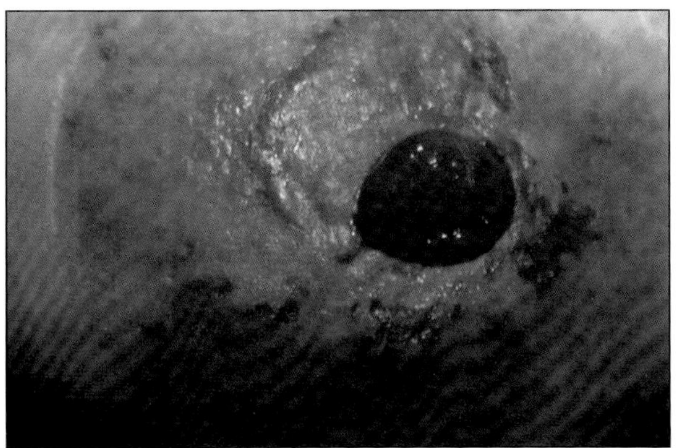

2. **Peristomal Skin Excoriation**
(Chapter 37: Ostomy Care)
Courtesy of Convatec

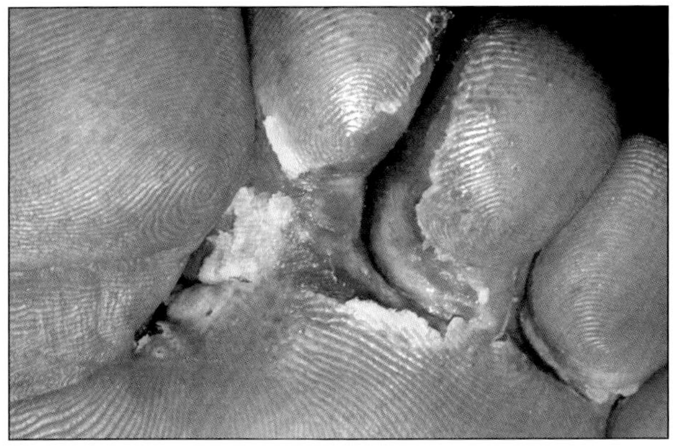

3. **Athlete's Foot**
(Chapter 50: Athlete's Foot)
Science Photo Library

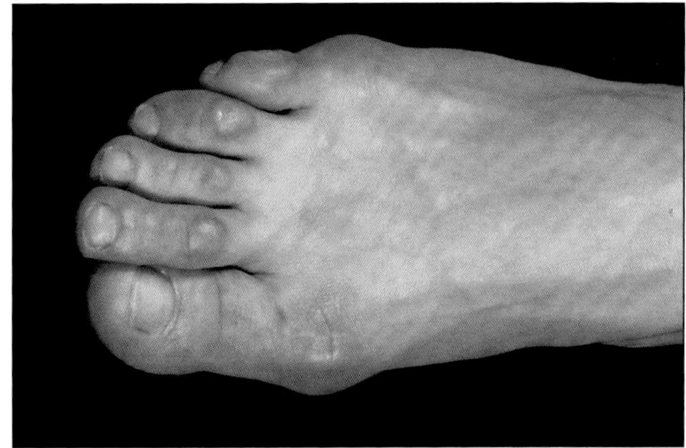

4. **Corns** (Chapter 51:
Corns, Calluses, Bunions and Ingrown Toenails)
Jolyot/Science Photo Library

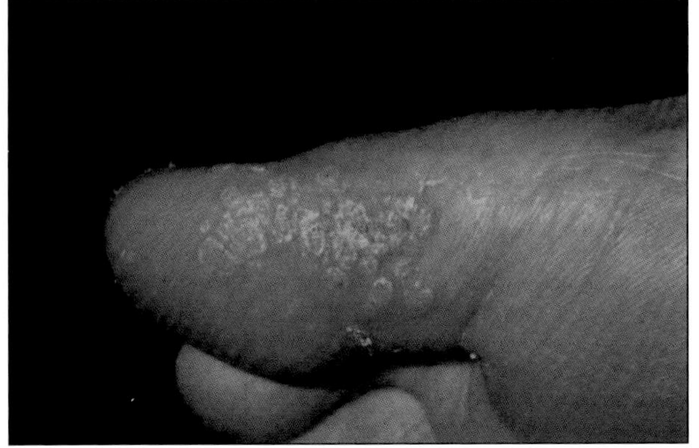

5. **Plantar Warts**
(Chapter 52: Plantar Warts)
Dr. P. Marazzi/Science Photo Library

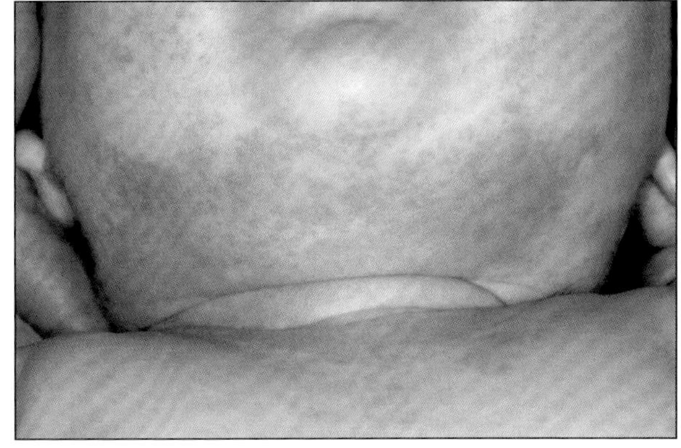

6. **Atopic Dermatitis**
(Chapter 55: Atopic, Contact and Stasis Dermatitis)
Dr. P. Marazzi/Science Photo Library

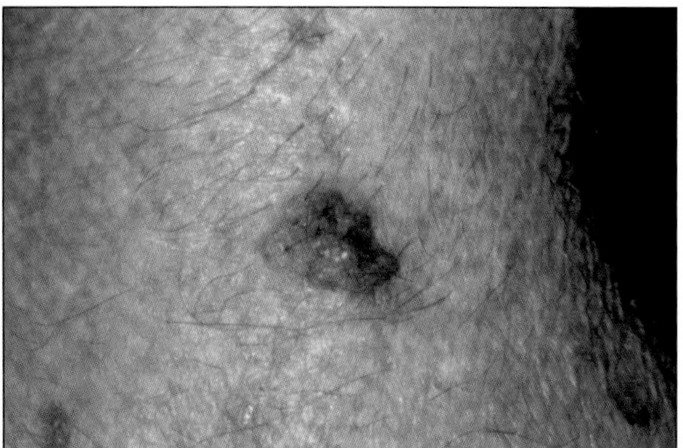

7. **Actinic Keratosis** (Chapter 72: Prevention and Treatment of Sun-induced Skin Damage)
Dr. P. Marazzi/Science Photo Library

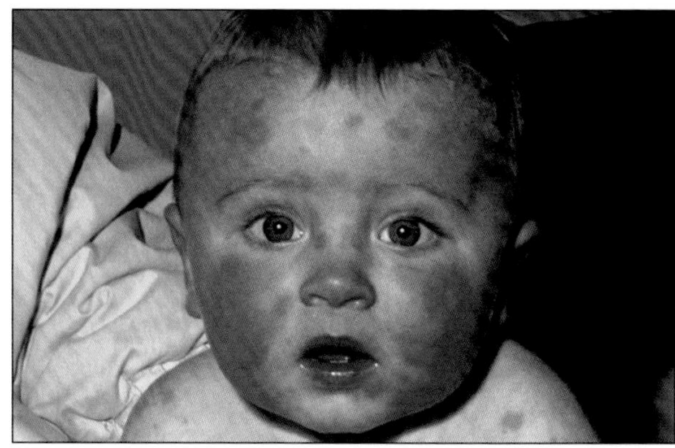

8. **Erythema Infectiosum (Parovirus/Fifth Disease)** (Chapter 74: Viral Skin Rashes)
Dr H.C.Robinson/Science Photo Library

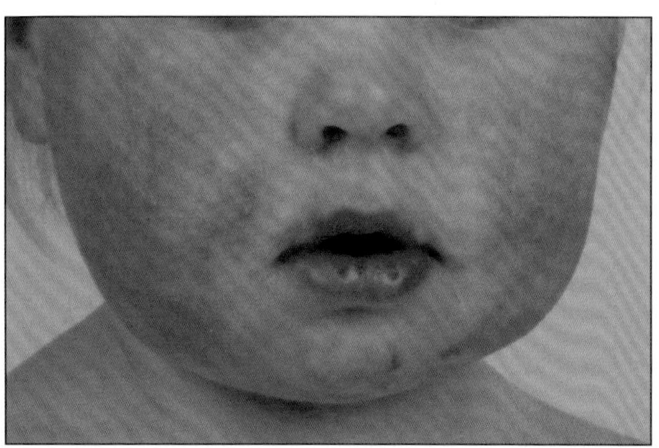

9. **Gianotti-Crosti Syndrome (face)** (Chapter 74: Viral Skin Rashes)
DermNet New Zealand

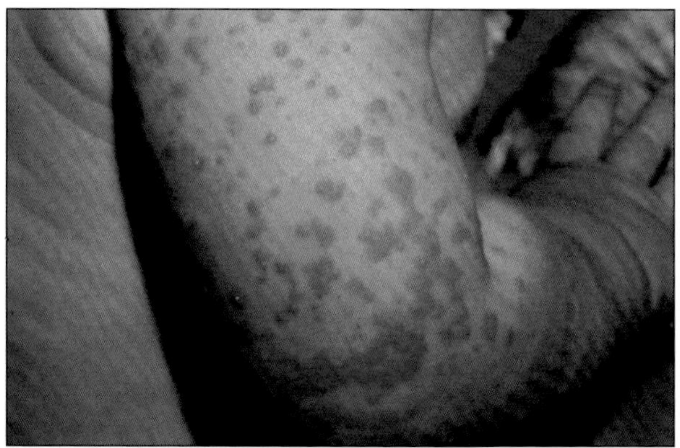

10. **Gianotti-Crosti Syndrome (body)** (Chapter 74: Viral Skin Rashes)
DermNet New Zealand

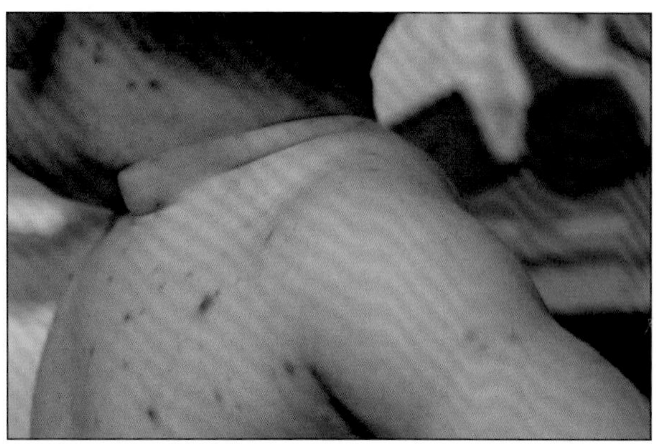

11. **Chickenpox (Varicella)** (Chapter 74: Viral Skin Rashes)
iStockphoto

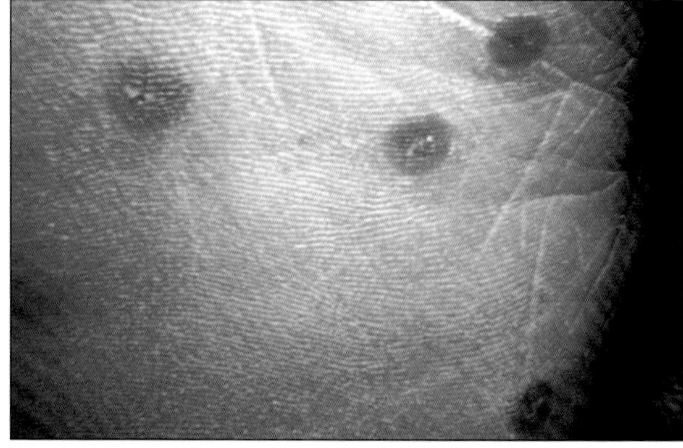

12. **Hand, Foot and Mouth Disease** (Chapter 74: Viral Skin Rashes)
Centers for Disease Control and Prevention

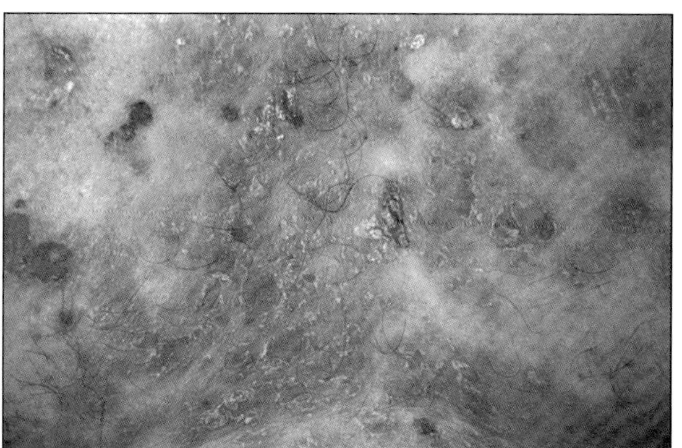

13. **Herpes Zoster**
(Chapter 74: Viral Skin Rashes)
Centers for Disease Control and Prevention

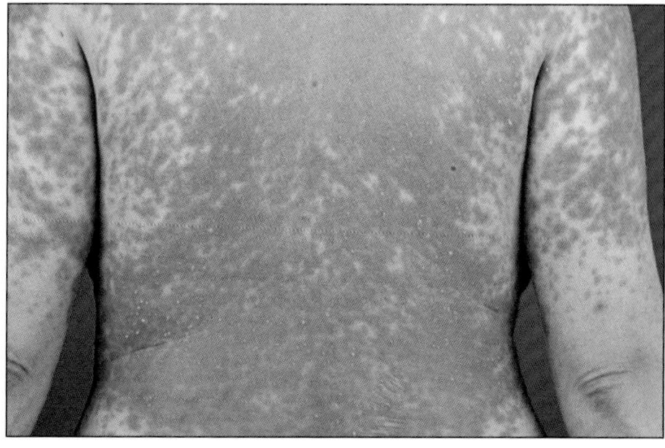

14. **Acute Generalized Exanthematous Pustulosis**
(Chapter 61: Drug-induced Skin Reactions)
DermNet New Zealand

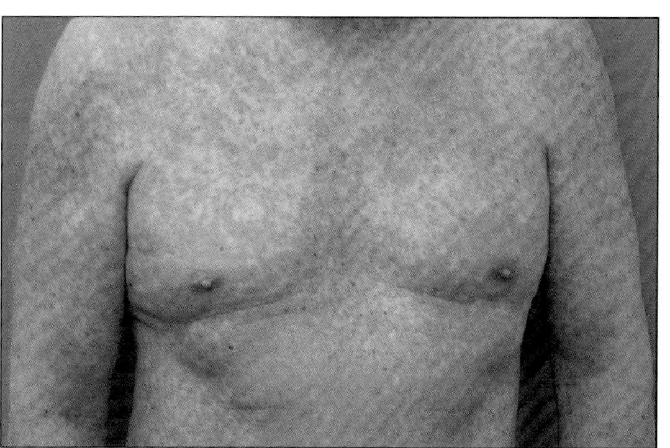

15. **Hypersensitivity Syndrome Reactions**
(Chapter 61: Drug-induced Skin Reactions)
DermNet New Zealand

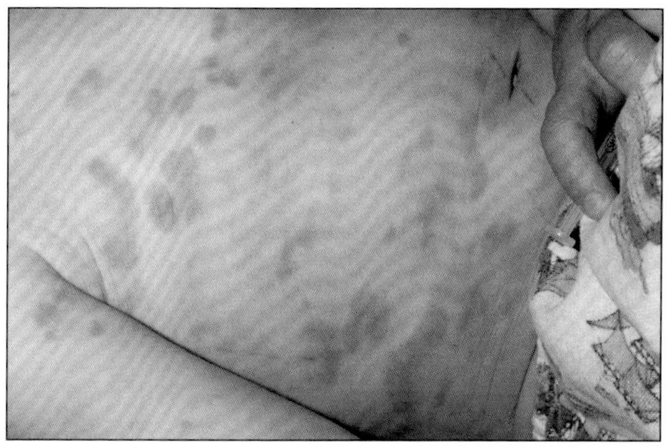

16. **Serum Sickness–like Reaction**
(Chapter 61: Drug-induced Skin Reactions)
DermNet New Zealand

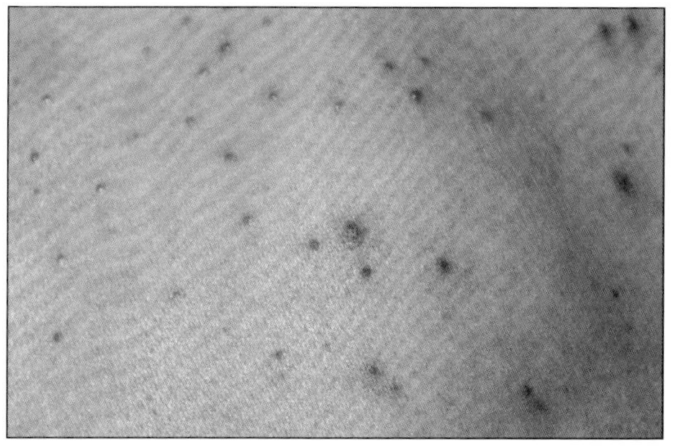

17. **Folliculitis** (Chapter 56: Bacterial Skin Infections: Impetigo, Furuncles and Carbuncles)
iStockphoto

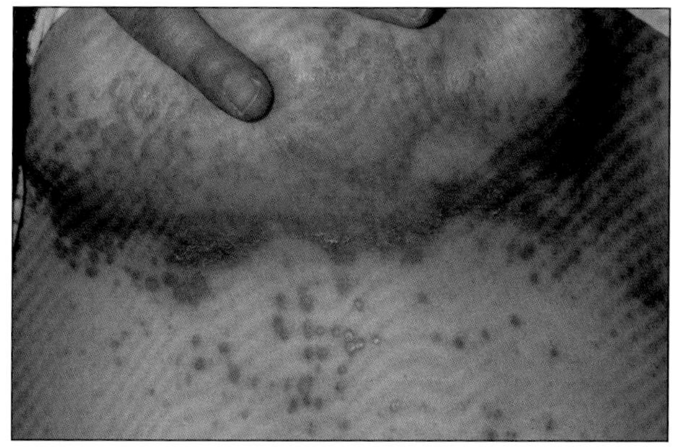

18. **Candidiasis (Intertrigo)**
(Chapter 65: Fungal Skin Infections)
Custom Medical Stock Photo/Science Photo Library

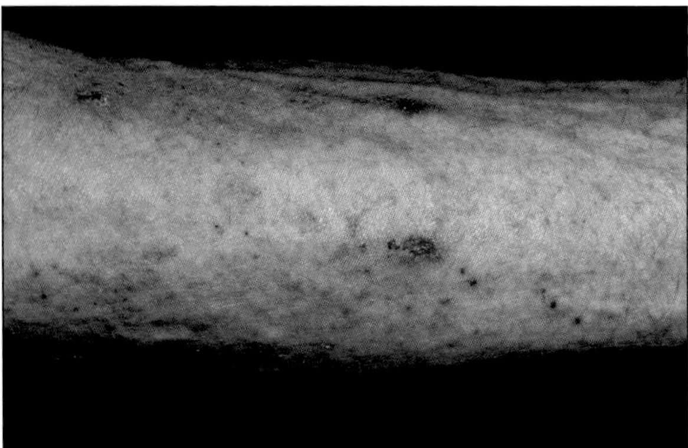

19. **Scabies** (Chapter 69: Parasitic Skin Infections: Lice and Scabies)
Dr P. Marazzi/Science Photo Library

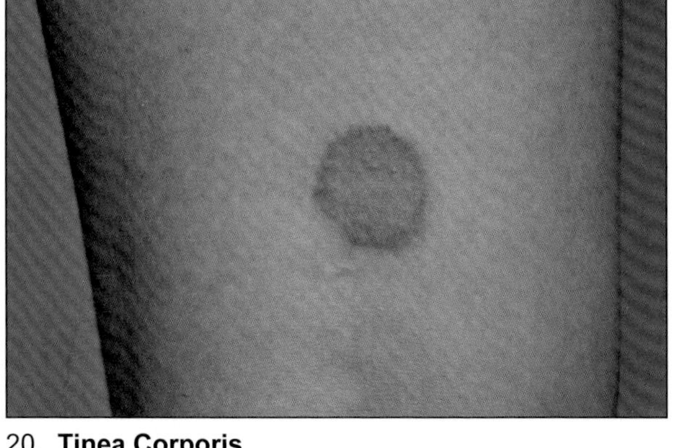

20. **Tinea Corporis** (Chapter 65: Fungal Skin Infections)
iStockphoto

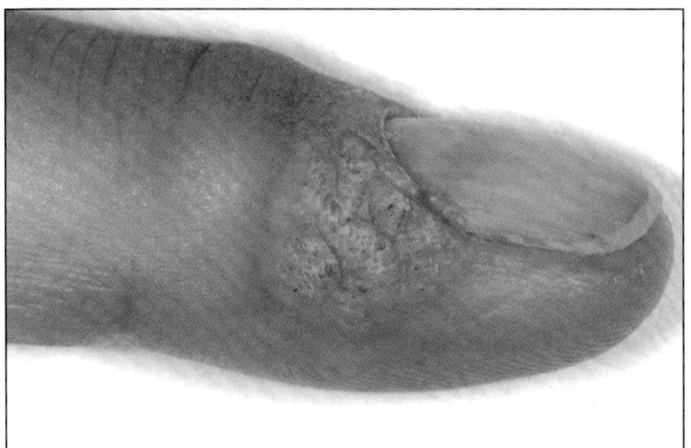

21. **Common Warts** (Chapter 73: Viral Skin Infections: Common and Flat Warts)
Dr P. Marazzi/Science Photo Library

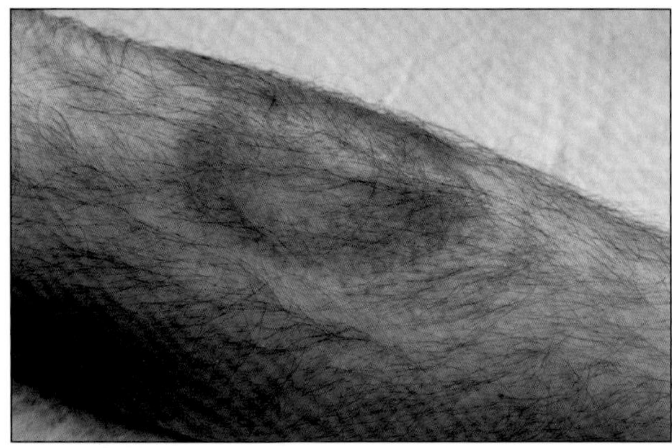

22. **Lyme Disease Lesion** (Chapter 67: Insect Bites and Stings)
iStockphoto

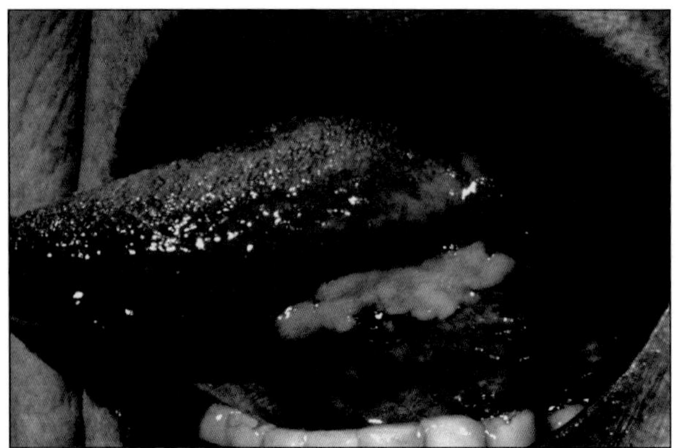

23. **Leukoplakia** (Chapter 89: Aphthous Ulcers (Canker Sores))
Custom Medical Stock Photo/Science Photo Library

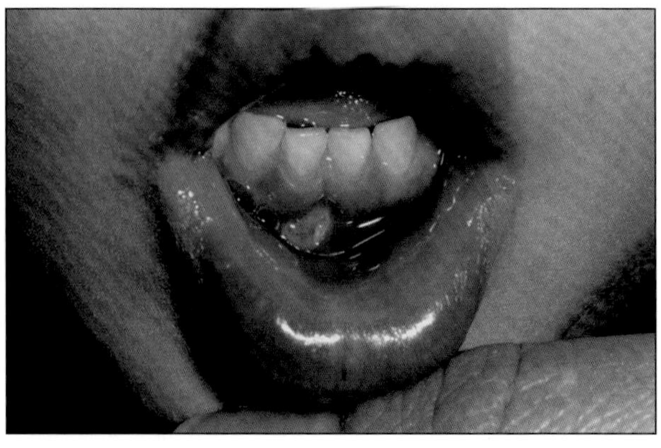

24. **Aphthous Ulcer** (Chapter 89: Aphthous Ulcers (Canker Sores))
Dr P. Marazzi/Science Photo Library

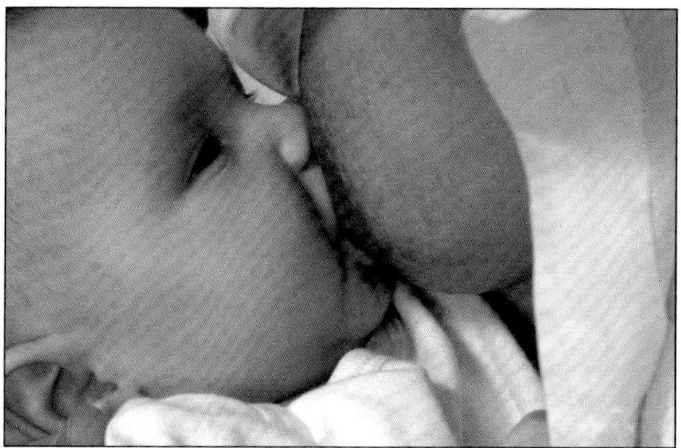

25. **Establishing Successful Latch** (Chapter 40: Infant Nutrition)
iStockphoto

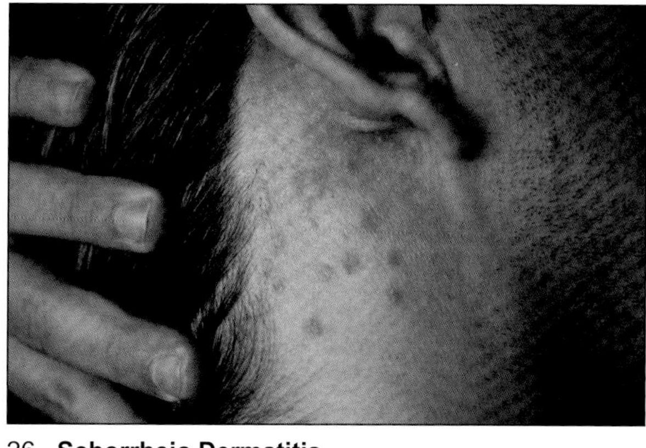

26. **Seborrheic Dermatitis** (Chapter 58: Dandruff and Seborrheic Dermatitis)
iStockphoto

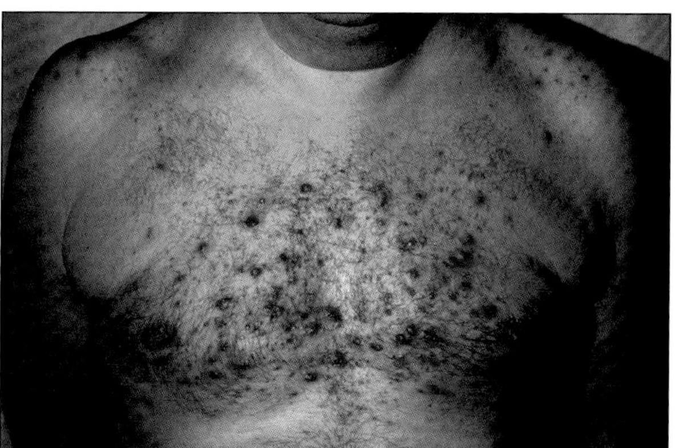

27. **Acneiform Eruption** (Chapter 61: Drug-induced Skin Reactions)
DermNet New Zealand

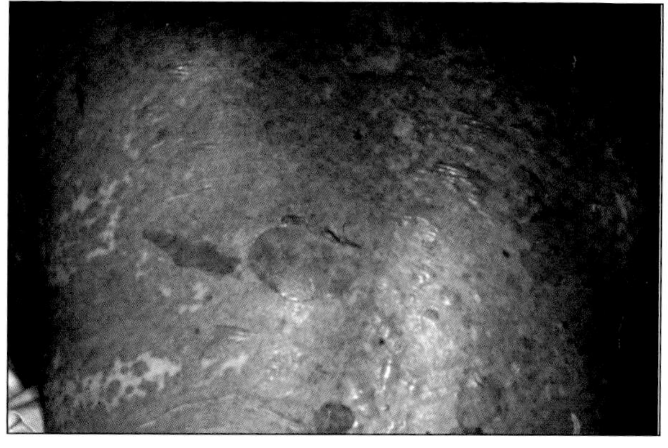

28. **Toxic Epidermal Necrolysis** (Chapter 61: Drug-induced Skin Reactions)
DermNet New Zealand

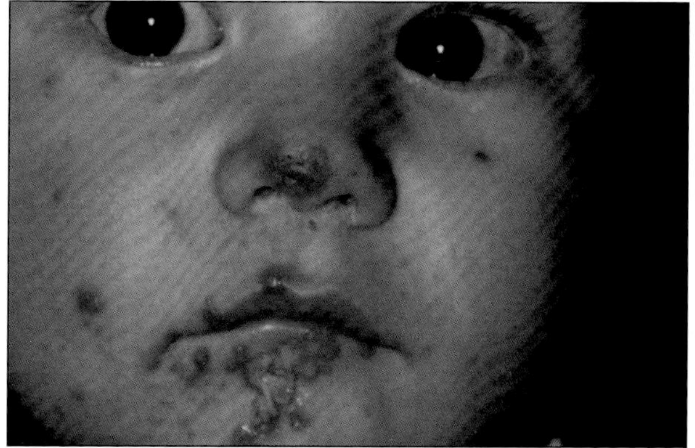

29. **Impetigo** (Chapter 56: Bacterial Skin Infections: Impetigo, Furuncles and Carbuncles)
Dr P. Marazzi/Science Photo Library

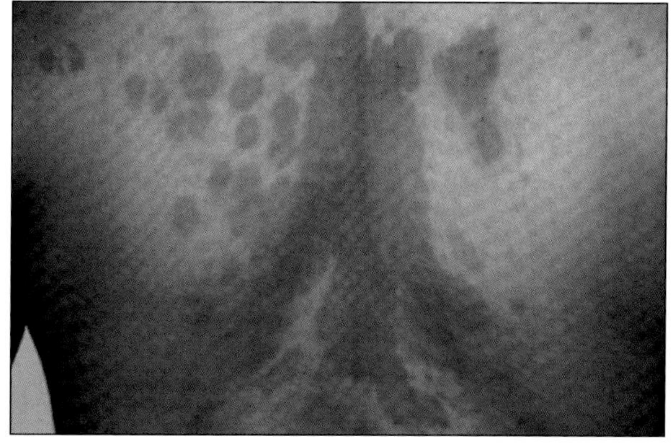

30. **Pityriasis Versicolor** (Chapter 65: Fungal Skin Infections)
Science Photo Library

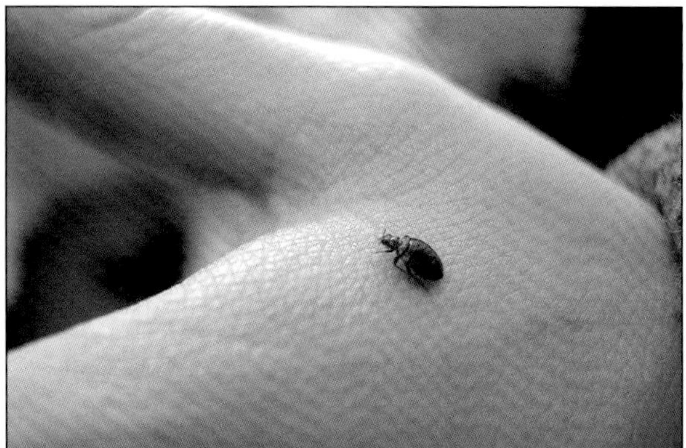

31. **Bed Bug**
(Chapter 67: Insect Bites and Stings)
Centers for Disease Control and Prevention

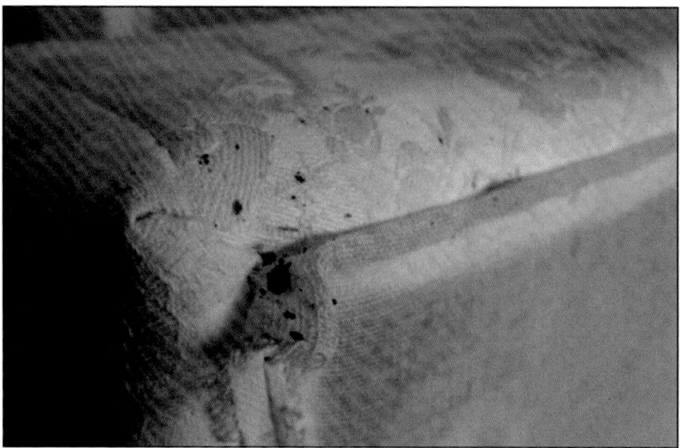

32. **Bed Bug Infestation**
(Chapter 67: Insect Bites and Stings)
Centers for Disease Control and Prevention

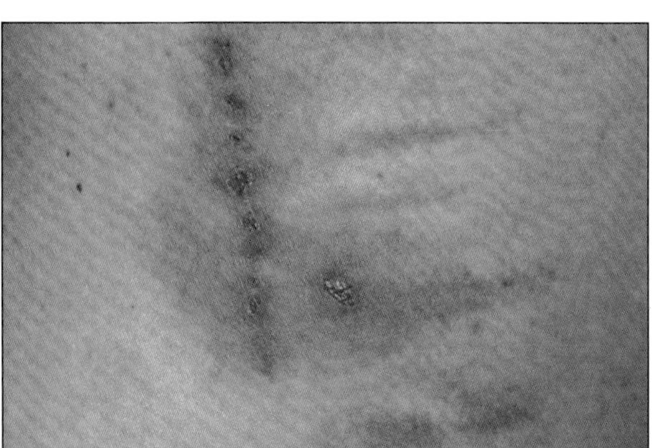

33. **Superficial Burn (scalded thigh)**
(Chapter 57: Burns)
Dr P. Marazzi/Science Photo Library

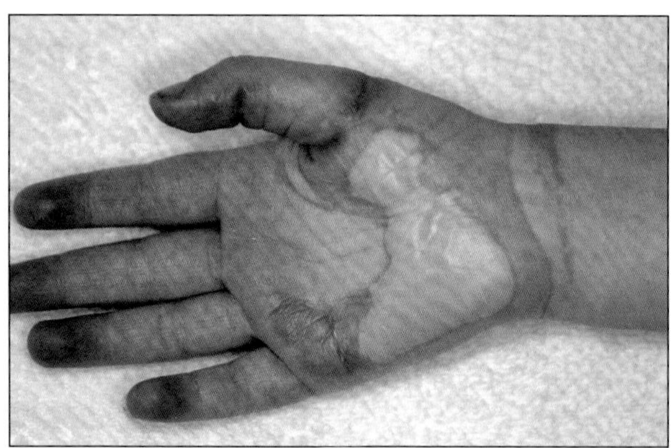

34. **Deep Partial Thickness Burn (4 yr old child's hand)** (Chapter 57: Burns)
Science Photo Library

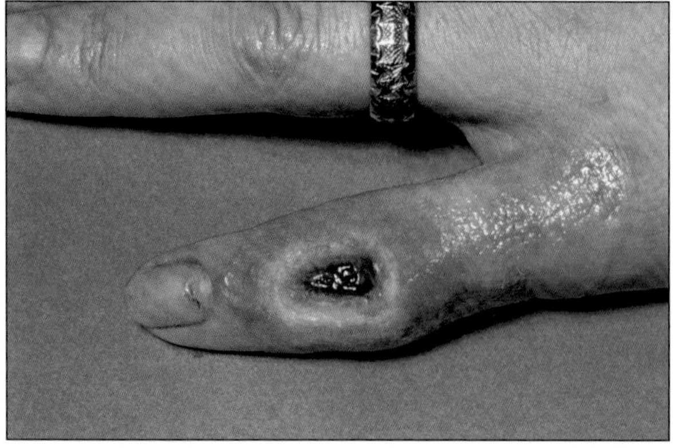

35. **Full Thickness Burn (woman's finger)**
(Chapter 57: Burns)
St Stephen's Hospital/Science Photo Library

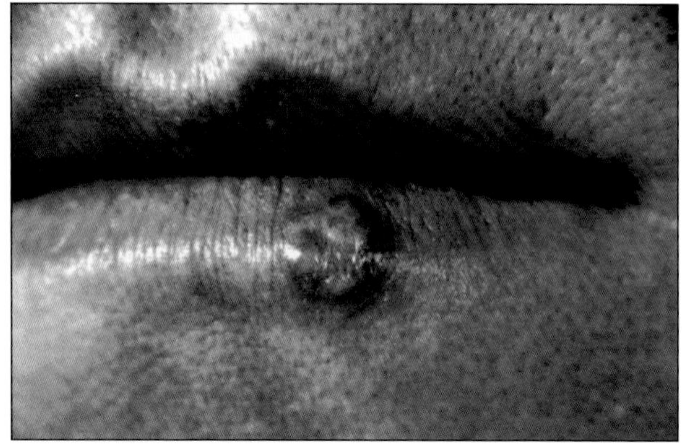

36. **Cold Sore**
(Chapter 90: Cold Sores (Herpes Labialis))
Centers for Disease Control and Prevention

Chapter 75

Benign Prostatic Hyperplasia and Associated Lower Urinary Tract Symptoms

Cheryl A. Sadowski, BSc(Pharm), PharmD

Lower urinary tract symptoms (LUTS) has become an umbrella term encompassing a broad range of urinary symptoms experienced by men and women.[1] This global term includes all urinary symptoms associated with storage, voiding and/or postmicturition.[1] This chapter focuses on those symptoms associated with benign prostatic hyperplasia (BPH). Chapter 83: Urinary Incontinence covers common types of urinary incontinence in women and men, not in association with BPH.

Pathophysiology

BPH is used to describe the histologic changes associated with prostatic enlargement which may or may not be associated with urethral obstruction.[2] It is the most common benign neoplasm in the aging human male.

The prostate is a walnut-sized gland at the base of the bladder that completely surrounds the male urethra (Figure 1). Its functions include contributing fluid to the ejaculate and constriction of the prostatic urethra during ejaculation (to prevent retrograde ejaculation). The prostate normally goes through 2 main periods of growth. The first is during puberty, when the prostate doubles in size. The second begins around age 25 years and may be the cause of BPH much later in life.[3] Symptoms of BPH rarely become apparent before age 40 years. The prevalence of BPH, measured histologically, is 8% for men in their thirties, 20% for men in their forties and up to 90% in men in their seventies.[4,5]

Figure 1: Male Reproductive Anatomy

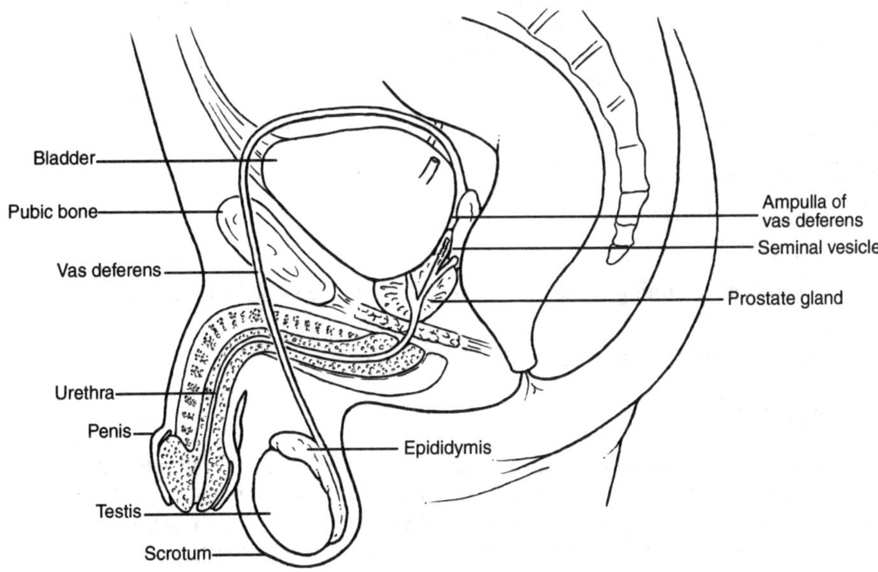

No single pathological mechanism occurs in BPH, but rather a synergy of events.[6] The pathophysiology of BPH is incompletely understood but appears to be related to androgens, aging, prostatic inflammation and genetics.[7,8,9,10] Increases in circulating androgens are considered partly responsible for an alteration in basal cell hyperplasia and increases in stromal and epithelial mass.[11,12] However, testosterone is only partly to blame, as some men do not respond to antiandrogen treatments.[12] Dihydrotestosterone (DHT), a potent metabolite of testosterone, is believed to be the main androgen responsible for both normal and hyperplastic prostate growth.[13,14,15] Testosterone is metabolized to DHT by the enzyme 5-alpha-reductase. Early in the process, BPH manifests as microscopic nodules in the periurethral area, followed by progressive nodular proliferation that may lead to bladder outlet obstruction and subsequent symptoms of BPH.[14,15]

Due to an age-related decline in detrusor muscle strength and prostatic enlargement, the urinary flow rate declines from >15 mL/sec (normal) to <10 mL/sec.[16] A normal prostate is approximately 20–30 mL in volume. Smooth-muscle fibres may compose up to 40% of the volume of a prostate affected by BPH. The bladder neck, stroma and capsule are richly innervated with alpha-1A adrenergic receptors that control smooth muscle contraction.[15,17]

LUTS associated with BPH can be divided into 3 categories: storage (irritative), voiding (obstructive), and postmicturition symptoms (Table 1). For most men, the symptoms appear gradually, over many years. In others, symptoms appear acutely. If left untreated, BPH may contribute to impaired bladder emptying and lead to hydronephrosis, bladder stones and recurrent urinary tract infections.[18,19] Other complications include impaired sleep, decreased quality of life and a higher risk of erectile dysfunction.[20,21] These complications may or may not be prevented with treatment. In many men, particularly those with mild symptoms, watchful waiting is an appropriate approach to treatment.[21,22] Usually an International Prostate Symptom Score (IPSS) ≤7 dictates watchful waiting, but some men with scores up to 19 (moderate symptoms) may choose watchful waiting if they are not particularly bothered by the symptoms (Table 2).[16,23] Progression rates may be variable and are difficult to predict.

Table 1: **Urinary Symptoms of BPH**[18,24]

Voiding (Obstructive symptoms)	Storage (Irritative symptoms)	Postmicturition
Weak urinary stream Hesitancy (difficulty initiating stream) Intermittency Straining Terminal dribbling Urinary retention	Urinary frequency Nocturia Pain during micturition Urinary urgency	Sensation of incomplete bladder emptying Postvoid dribbling

Goals of Therapy

- Alleviate symptoms of BPH
- Improve quality of life
- Prevent complications, including acute urinary retention, acute renal failure and urinary tract infections
- Minimize adverse effects of treatment

Patient Assessment

Patients with suspected BPH should undergo a focused evaluation. Not all patients with BPH are symptomatic, and many may not receive a diagnosis for many years.[25,26] Due to the high rates of BPH with aging and other comorbidities, such as diabetes and erectile dysfunction, ask men over 50 and those with these conditions about their medical history and symptoms of BPH.[26,27,28,29,30,31,32]

Table 2: International Prostate Symptom Score for BPH Assessment[26,33]

Questions to be answered	Not at all	Less than 1 time in 5	Less than half the time	About half the time	More than half the time	Almost always
Circle 1 number on each line						
1. Incomplete emptying: Over the past month, how often have you had a sensation of not emptying your bladder completely after you finished urinating?	0	1	2	3	4	5
2. Frequency: Over the past month, how often have you had to urinate again less than 2 h after you finished urinating?	0	1	2	3	4	5
3. Intermittency: Over the past month, how often have you found you stopped and started again several times when you urinated?	0	1	2	3	4	5
4. Urgency: Over the past month, how often have you found it difficult to postpone urination?	0	1	2	3	4	5
5. Weak stream: Over the past month, how often have you had a weak urinary stream?	0	1	2	3	4	5
6. Straining: Over the past month, how often have you had to push or strain to begin urination?	0	1	2	3	4	5
7. Nocturia: Over the past month, how many times, most typically, did you get up to urinate from the time you went to bed at night until the time you got up in the morning?	0	1	2	3	4	5
Sum of 7 circled numbers:[a]						

Quality of life due to urinary symptoms							
If you were to spend the rest of your life with your urinary condition just the way it is now, how would you feel about that?	**Delighted**	**Pleased**	**Mostly satisfied**	**Mixed**	**Mostly dissatisfied**	**Unhappy**	**Terrible**

[a] Symptoms are classified as: Mild = Score 0–7; Moderate = Score 8–19; Severe = Score 20–35

Reproduced with permission from Lippincott Williams & Wilkins. Barry MJ, Fowler FJ, O'Leary MP et al. The American Urological Association symptom index for benign prostatic hyperplasia. *J Urol* 1992;148:1549-57.

Men assessed for BPH will undergo many of the tests as for other types of LUTS (see Chapter 83: Urinary Incontinence). However, details about BPH symptoms can be gleaned from using the International Prostate Symptom Scale (IPSS) questionnaire specific to BPH (Table 2). This is a simple scale that can be completed by the patient or his healthcare practitioner for quantifying the severity of BPH symptoms. This index should be performed at the onset of therapy and periodically thereafter to monitor the success of treatment. It is not validated as a tool to diagnose BPH.

Physical examination should include the abdomen, external genitalia and prostate (e.g., digital rectal exam). Blood work that could identify underlying comorbidities (e.g., diabetes) and a urinalysis are also important.[18,26,31,32,33] The measurement of prostate specific antigen (PSA) should be considered, especially in men with a positive family history of prostate cancer and those of African descent, but it is controversial because elevated PSA is not specific to the diagnosis of prostate cancer.[19,34] The AUA Guidelines no longer recommend measuring a serum creatinine to evaluate renal function in men with BPH.[35] Additional testing (e.g., urodynamics, bladder scanning) may be done to assess changes in lower urinary tract function.[19] The purpose of these additional tests is to monitor the progression of BPH and to help rule out cancer, bladder stones, urinary tract infections and other comorbidities that could mimic urinary retention in men.[19,33,34,36]

Several medications may exacerbate symptoms of BPH (Table 3). These drugs primarily act through anticholinergic properties and inhibit bladder contraction; others possess stimulant sympathomimetic properties and increase urethral resistance.[37]

Treatment

Treatment is recommended only when BPH becomes bothersome, poses a health risk or is associated with complications (e.g., recurrent urinary infections, renal insufficiency).[32,35,38] Mild BPH does not require treatment and in approximately 15% of cases, symptoms will stabilize or resolve without treatment.[38,39,40] Treatment of BPH can include lifestyle changes, drug therapy or surgery.

Nonpharmacologic Therapy

Lifestyle Changes

The following may be helpful in reducing BPH symptoms:[21,25,32,41]

- Medical
  - blood pressure control
  - body weight reduction
  - management of constipation
- Behavioural
  - smoking cessation
  - increased exercise
  - caffeine and alcohol reduction
  - regular or timed urination
  - redistribution of liquid consumption to earlier in the day
  - double-voiding or penile milking techniques
- Medication
  - adjustment of medication dosage or timing (e.g., diuretics)
- Psychosocial
  - self-help groups[42,43]

Watchful Waiting

Offer watchful waiting (also termed "informed surveillance") to patients with mild symptoms (IPSS score ≤7) which are not particularly bothersome.[16,32,33,35] Reassess these patients at yearly intervals or earlier if there is a change in the symptom complex.[23] These patients should still be counselled to make lifestyle changes, such as limiting late day fluid consumption, taking diuretics earlier in the day, and avoiding stimulants (e.g., caffeine).[17,21]

Surgical Procedures

Transurethral resection of the prostate (TURP) remains the gold standard, with almost 90% of men reporting reduced symptom scores. However, due to risks associated with this procedure, less invasive therapies continue to be developed but none has replaced it to any great extent. Minimally invasive procedures do not remove tissue but cause necrosis by heat. Most procedures require spinal or general anesthesia and all (Table 4) have a risk of erectile dysfunction, retrograde ejaculation and incontinence.

Pharmacologic Therapy

For comparative ingredients of nonprescription products, consult the *Compendium of Products for Minor Ailments*—Herbal and Natural Health Products: Combinations, Single Entity.

For further discussion of pharmacologic therapy for BPH and related symptoms, consult the *Compendium of Therapeutic Choices*: Lower Urinary Tract Symptoms and Benign Prostatic Hyperplasia.

The main pharmacologic options used for treating BPH include the 5-alpha-reductase inhibitors (**dutasteride**, **finasteride**) and alpha-adrenergic receptor antagonists (**alfuzosin**, **doxazosin**, **silodosin**, **tamsulosin** and **terazosin**).[25] Due to their distinct pharmacologic actions, these medication classes may be used together, with the alpha-antagonists working within 1–2 weeks and the 5-alpha-reductase inhibitors working within 3–6 months.[47,48,49] Combination treatment seems to be most effective for patients with prostate volumes >30–40 mL, with greater reduction in IPSS scores and higher urinary flow rates compared with monotherapy. In addition to higher costs, adverse events are approximately 50% greater in dual vs. monotherapy, which leads to higher rates of treatment discontinuation.[50] Consider combination therapy only when monotherapy is not meeting the treatment goals. Medications are effective in approximately 60% of men.[25,51] The phosphodiesterase-5 inhibitor **tadalafil** has been increasingly used for the treatment of LUTS due to BPH and has shown improvement in symptoms and quality of life in men with or without concomitant ED.[32,52]

5-Alpha-reductase Inhibitors

Dutasteride and **finasteride** reduce intraprostatic DHT concentrations by inhibiting 5-alpha-reductase (type 2). This shrinks the prostate by 25%, reduces serum PSA by 50%, prevents further prostatic growth and acute urinary retention, lowers the risk of required prostate surgery and reduces the IPSS by 4–5 points (up to 7 points when combined with an alpha-blocker).[7,16,50,53] This class of medications appears to work best when the prostate volume is ≥40 mL.[54] Long-term usage is required because progressive clinical benefits are not manifest until 3–6 months after initiation of therapy.[55]

Up to 5% of patients taking these medications experience adverse effects such as decreased libido, erectile dysfunction, breast tenderness and gynecomastia.[7,36,53,56]

Table 3: Examples of Drugs that May Exacerbate Symptoms of BPH

Androgens
testosterone
Anticholinergics
benztropine
flavoxate
glycopyrrolate
hyoscine
oxybutynin
scopolamine
tiotropium (inhaled)
tolterodine
Antidepressants
amitriptyline
doxepin
nortriptyline

Antihistamines
brompheniramine
chlorpheniramine
cyproheptadine
dimenhydrinate
diphenhydramine
hydroxyzine
Antipsychotics
fluphenazine
loxapine
olanzapine
Muscle relaxants
baclofen
cyclobenzaprine

Sympathomimetics
phenylephrine
pseudoephedrine
terbutaline
Miscellaneous
caffeine
ipratropium
NSAIDs
pizotifen
procyclidine
selegiline

Table 4: Surgical Procedures for Managing BPH

Procedure	Indication	Comments
Transurethral resection of the prostate (TURP)[44]	For moderately enlarged prostates	The gold standard. A diathermy loop removes the inner (periurethral) zones of the prostate. Advantages: Fewer work days lost and fewer days in hospital than with open surgery. Highest degree of symptom improvement (80–90%) of all procedures. Symptom improvement is long lasting. Disadvantages: Requires spinal or general anesthetic. Requires catheterization for 1–3 days post-operatively. Complications: Up to 20% of patients have morbidity related to TURP. Failure to void, bleeding (5%), clot retention, retrograde ejaculation.
Transurethral electrovaporization of the prostate (TUVP)	For moderately enlarged prostates	Less bleeding than with TURP, but higher rates of irritative symptoms and re-catheterization. Can be done as day surgery. Requires spinal or general anesthesia.
Transurethral incision of the prostate (TUIP)	For smaller prostates (<30 mL)	Lower incidence of complications including retrograde ejaculation and fewer days in hospital than with open surgery or TURP. Symptomatic improvement is similar to TURP. Takes only minutes to perform procedure. Requires spinal or general anesthesia.
Open prostatectomy	For large prostates (>80 mL) or patients with specific concomitant conditions (e.g., bladder diverticula or stones)	Most thorough excision of adenoma of all the procedures. Higher rates of urinary incontinence and bladder neck stenosis. Requires spinal or general anesthesia.
Urethral stent	Patients unfit for surgery or high-risk patients with chronic urinary retention. Temporary stenting for patients who have undergone minimally invasive procedures and require short-term relief	Can be done as outpatient procedure. Usually done under regional or topical anaesthesia. Complications: Failure 20–30%, urinary tract infections, pain.

(cont'd)

Table 4: **Surgical Procedures for Managing BPH** *(cont'd)*

Procedure	Indication	Comments
Minimally Invasive Procedures[45,46]		
Transurethral microwave thermotherapy (TUMT) Transurethral needle ablation (TUNA)	Ideally used in men with smaller prostate volumes (30–100 mL), no history of retention, no previous prostate surgery	Can be done as an outpatient procedure using analgesia and/or sedation. Require catheterization following the procedure. Repeat or more invasive treatment is usually required in approximately 30% of men. Risk of retrograde ejaculation lower than for invasive procedures. Usually lower response in symptoms and quality of life versus TURP, with higher retreatment rates.
Ablative Procedures		
Holmium laser enucleation of the prostate (HoLEP) Holmium laser resection of the prostate (HoLRP) Holmium laser ablation of the prostate (HoLAP) Photoselective vaporization of the prostate (PVP)	Any prostate size Men on anticoagulants, or those with cardiac or renal disease	Can be done as outpatient procedure, less blood loss than with most other procedures. Earlier discharge from hospital versus other procedures. Risk of retrograde ejaculation similar to invasive procedures. Requires spinal or general anesthesia.

Alpha-adrenergic Antagonists

Stromal and fibromuscular tissues are under alpha-adrenergic control. Alpha-blockers antagonize the binding of norepinephrine to the alpha receptors in the prostate gland and bladder neck. This results in smooth muscle relaxation and improved urine flow through the bladder outlet but does not reduce the size of the prostate gland.[16,57,58,59] Benefit is seen within the first 2 weeks, with the full effect realized after titration to full therapeutic dose.[60,61] There is no evidence of tachyphylaxis. All alpha-adrenergic antagonists used for BPH symptoms have been found to be equally effective when dosed therapeutically.[62,63,64] This class of medications reduces the IPSS by 6 points and improves symptoms associated with voiding in approximately 60–80% of patients, although men with larger prostates may have less response.[7,25,32,58]

Adverse effects associated with alpha-adrenergic antagonists (dizziness, headache and peripheral edema) are attributed to the effect on alpha receptors in vascular and central nervous tissue, and occur in up to 15% of patients.[30,35,65] Less common side effects include rhinitis and ejaculatory dysfunction (e.g., retrograde ejaculation).[66] There is also a risk of ophthalmic complications after cataract surgery, as alpha receptors are also found on the iris.[67] To minimize adverse effects such as dizziness or postural hypotension, the second-generation agents (**doxazosin**, **terazosin**) are taken at bedtime, started at low doses and titrated upward over several weeks. **Alfuzosin**, **silodosin** and **tamsulosin** are more specific for the alpha-$_{1A}$ receptors found in the prostate gland and as such are usually not associated with significant hypotensive episodes and do not require dose titration.

Phosphodiesterase-5 Inhibitors

Low-dose daily **tadalafil** is currently the only phosphodiesterase-5 inhibitor (PDE5-I) indicated for use in BPH with or without erectile dysfunction. PDE-5 enzyme exists in prostatic tissue, bladder detrusor and vascular smooth-muscle cells of the urinary tract.[68] Tadalafil causes smooth muscle relaxation and may provide some antiproliferative effects in the prostate. Improvement in symptoms may occur as early as 1–4 weeks.[32] PDE5-Is have been shown to reduce IPSS scores by 4–6 points after 12 weeks of treatment.[69,70,71] Expected side effects include headache, dyspepsia and dizziness.

Antimuscarinics

These medications (e.g., **darifenacin, fesoterodine, oxybutynin, solifenacin, tolterodine**)[72] are used to treat the storage-related symptoms of BPH by decreasing the overactive bladder component. The AUA Guidelines recommend using these drugs with caution if the postvoid residual is >250 mL.[35] They are beneficial when used with an alpha-blocker, improving the IPSS by as much as 4 points, reducing postvoid residual volume and reducing voiding frequency.[7,73,74] Adverse effects (e.g., urinary retention, dry mouth, constipation) can be minimized by using these medications intermittently or in low doses.[75]

Natural Health Products

Natural health products that have been widely promoted for BPH treatment include **saw palmetto, African plum tree** (*Pygeum africanum*), **stinging nettle** and **pumpkin seeds** (Table 5). The evidence for their effectiveness is variable and their role in treating BPH remains unclear.[76,77,78] The AUA, the European Association of Urology, and the International Consultation for Urological Diseases guidelines do not recommend the use of any phytotherapies.[35,36,79] However, many men self-medicate with these products and some respond well subjectively.

Monitoring of Therapy

To ensure effectiveness and tolerability of medications, patients should be evaluated within a few months of starting treatment and monitored regularly thereafter. Improvements in the IPSS may be especially helpful in confirming clinical benefit.

Patients taking an alpha-adrenergic antagonist with or without a 5-alpha-reductase inhibitor should be questioned about the success and potential side effects of their therapy at every visit. Advise patients about how to slowly titrate their alpha-adrenergic antagonist dosing regimen to avoid adverse effects (e.g., dizziness, postural hypotension) and to monitor for symptom change weekly.

Table 5: Natural Health Products Used in Benign Prostatic Hyperplasia[a,b]

Class	Drug	Dosage	Mechanism of Action	Adverse Effects	Cost[c]
Natural Health Products	*cernilton*	500 mg TID po	Inhibition of 5-alpha-reductase, alpha-receptor antagonist, smooth muscle relaxation, inhibition of growth through interference with androgen metabolism	Mild nausea	$
	pumpkin seed	10 g of seeds per day or equivalent	Inhibition of 5-alpha-reductase	None known	$
	pygeum africanum	50 mg BID po, 100 mg daily po, or 100 mg BID po (extract)	Inhibition of 5-alpha-reductase, antiandrogenic effects, inhibits growth factors, reduces inflammatory mediators[80]	GI upset ranging from nausea to severe pain	$
	saw palmetto	160 mg (lipophilic extract) BID po or 1–2 g (berries) once daily po	Inhibition of 5-alpha-reductase, antiandrogenic effects, anti-inflammatory, triggers prostatic cell apoptosis, smooth muscle relaxation[80,81]	Headache, GI upset, hypertension, impotence, decreased libido	$
	soy isoflavones	25–50 g/day po	Inhibition of 5-alpha-reductase, androgenic blocking	Nausea	$
	stinging nettle	150–300 mg (root extract) once daily po	Inhibits the binding of sex hormone-binding globulin to its receptors, binds epidermal growth factor	GI upset	$

[a] Effectiveness and role in treating BPH is unclear. Use only if mild symptoms and if patient has chosen the watchful waiting approach.

[b] For more information on pharmacologic therapy for BPH, consult the *Compendium of Therapeutic Choices*: Lower Urinary Tract Symptoms and Benign Prostatic Hyperplasia.

[c] Cost of 30-day supply; includes drug cost only.

Legend: $ <$15

Resource Tips

National Institute of Diabetes and Digestive and Kidney Diseases (NIDDK). *Prostate enlargement: benign prostatic hyperplasia.* Available from: www.niddk.nih.gov/health-information/health-topics/urologic-disease/benign-prostatic-hyperplasia-bph/Pages/facts.aspx.

The Prostate Centre at the Princess Margaret Hospital. Available from: /www.prostatecentre.ca.

Urological Sciences Research Foundation. *International Prostate Symptom Score (IPSS)*. Available from: www.usrf.org/questionnaires/AUA_SymptomScore.html.

Urology Care Foundation. The Official Foundation of the American Urological Association. *Urologic conditions*. Available from: www.urologyhealth.org.

Suggested Readings

D'Silva KA, Dahm P, Wong CL. Does this man with lower urinary tract symptoms have bladder outlet obstruction?: The Rational Clinical Examination: a systematic review. *JAMA* 2014;312:535-42.

Hollingsworth JM, Wilt TJ. Lower urinary tract symptoms in men. *BMJ* 2014;349:g4474.

McVary KT, Roehrborn CG, Avins AL et al. Update on AUA guideline on the management of benign prostatic hyperplasia. *J Urol* 2011;185:1793-803.

Pagano E, Laudato M, Griffo M et al. Phytotherapy of benign prostatic hyperplasia. A minireview. *Phytother Res* 2014;28:949-55.

Sarma A V, Wei JT. Clinical practice. Benign prostatic hyperplasia and lower urinary tract symptoms. *N Engl J Med* 2012;367:248-57.

References

1. Chapple CR, Wein AJ, Abrams P et al. Lower urinary tract symptoms revisited: a broader clinical perspective. *Eur Urol* 2008;54:563-9.
2. Abrams P. New words for old: lower urinary tract symptoms for "prostatism". *BMJ* 1994;308:929-30.
3. Cunha GR. Role of mesenchymal-epithelial interactions in normal and abnormal development of the mammary gland and prostate. *Cancer* 1994;74:1030-44.
4. Arrighi HM, Metter EJ, Guess HA et al. Natural history of benign prostatic hyperplasia and risk of prostatectomy. The Baltimore Longitudinal Study of Aging. *Urology* 1991;38:4-8.
5. Berry SJ, Coffey DS, Walsh PC et al. The development of human benign prostatic hyperplasia with age. *J Urol* 1984;132:474-9.
6. Gur S, Kadowitz PJ, Hellstrom WJ. Guide to drug therapy for lower urinary tract symptoms in patients with benign prostatic obstruction: implications for sexual dysfunction. *Drugs* 2008;68:209-29.
7. Sarma AV, Wei JT. Clinical practice. Benign prostatic hyperplasia and lower urinary tract symptoms. *N Engl J Med* 2012;367:248-57.
8. Bostanci Y, Kazzazi A, Momtahen S et al. Correlation between benign prostatic hyperplasia and inflammation. *Curr Opin Urol* 2013;23:5-10.
9. Fullhase C, Hakenberg O. New concepts for the treatment of male lower urinary tract symptoms. *Curr Opin Urol* 2015;25:19-26.
10. Izumi K, Mizokami A, Lin WJ et al. Androgen receptor roles in the development of benign prostate hyperplasia. *Am J Pathol* 2013;182:1942-9.
11. Bostwick DG. Prostatic intraepithelial neoplasia (PIN): current concepts. *J Cell Biochem Suppl* 1992;16H:10-9.
12. Nicholson TM, Ricke WA. Androgens and estrogens in benign prostatic hyperplasia: past, present and future. *Differentiation* 2011;82:184-99.
13. Scofield S, Kaplan SA. Voiding dysfunction in men: pathophysiology and risk factors. *Int J Impot Res* 2008;20:S2-10.
14. McConnell JD. Prostatic growth: new insights into hormonal regulation. *Br J Urol* 1995;76:5-10.
15. Timms BG, Hofkamp LE. Prostate development and growth in benign prostatic hyperplasia. *Differentiation* 2011;82:173-83.
16. Roehrborn CG. Male lower urinary tract symptoms (LUTS) and benign prostatic hyperplasia (BPH). *Med Clin North Am* 2011;95:87-100.
17. Patterson RF, Goldenberg SL. Benign prostatic hyperplasia (BPH). In: Teichman JMH. *20 common problems in urology.* New York: McGraw-Hill; 2001. p. 185-98.
18. Nickel JC, Herschorn S, Corcos J et al. Canadian guidelines for the management of benign prostatic hyperplasia. *Can J Urol* 2005;12:2677-83.
19. D'Silva KA, Dahm P, Wong CL. Does this man with lower urinary tract symptoms have bladder outlet obstruction?: The Rational Clinical Examination: a systematic review. *JAMA* 2014;312:535-42.
20. Bruskewitz RC. Quality of life and sexual function in patients with benign prostatic hyperplasia. *Rev Urol* 2003;5:72-80.
21. Hollingsworth JM, Wilt TJ. Lower urinary tract symptoms in men. *BMJ* 2014;349:g4474.
22. Wiygul J, Babayan RK. Watchful waiting in benign prostatic hyperplasia. *Curr Opin Urol* 2009;19:3-6.
23. McVary KT, Roehrborn CG, Avins AL et al. Update on AUA guideline on the management of benign prostatic hyperplasia. *J Urol* 2011;185:1793-803.
24. Abrams P, Cardozo L, Fall M et al. The standardisation of terminology of lower urinary tract function: report from the Standardisation Sub-committee of the International Continence Society. *Am J Obstet Gynecol* 2002;187:116-26.
25. Wilt TJ, N'Dow J. Benign prostatic hyperplasia. Part 2–management. *BMJ* 2008;336:206-10.
26. Wilt TJ, N'Dow J. Benign prostatic hyperplasia. Part 1–diagnosis. *BMJ* 2008;336:146-9.
27. Barry MJ, Fowler FJ, O'Leary MP et al. The American Urological Association symptom index for benign prostatic hyperplasia. The Measurement Committee of the American Urological Association. *J Urol* 1992;148:1549-57.

28. Rosen RC, Giuliano F, Carson CC. Sexual dysfunction and lower urinary tract symptoms (LUTS) associated with benign prostatic hyperplasia (BPH). *Eur Urol* 2005;47:824-37.
29. Gacci M, Corona G, Vignozzi L et al. Metabolic syndrome and benign prostatic enlargement: a systematic review and meta-analysis. *BJU Int* 2015;115:24-31.
30. Davidson JH, Chutka DS. Benign prostatic hyperplasia: treat or wait? *J Fam Pract* 2008;57:454-63.
31. Burden H, Warren K, Abrams P. Diagnosis of male incontinence. *Curr Opin Urol* 2013;23:509-14.
32. Rosenberg MT, Staskin D, Riley J et al. The evaluation and treatment of prostate-related LUTS in the primary care setting: the next STEP. *Curr Urol Rep* 2013;14:595-605.
33. AUA Practice Guidelines Committee. AUA guidelines on management of benign prostatic hyperplasia (2003). Chapter 1: Diagnosis and treatment recommendations. *J Urol* 2003;170:530-47.
34. Juliao AA, Plata M, Kazzazi A et al. American Urological Association and European Association of Urology guidelines in the management of benign prostatic hypertrophy: revisited. *Curr Opin Urol* 2012;22:34-9.
35. McVary KT, Roehrborn CG, Avins AL et al. Update on AUA guideline on the management of benign prostatic hyperplasia. *J Urol* 2011;185:1793-803.
36. Madersbacher S, Alivizatos G, Nordling J et al. EAU 2004 guidelines on assessment, therapy and follow-up of men with lower urinary tract symptoms suggestive of benign prostatic obstruction (BPH guidelines). *Eur Urol* 2004;46:547-54.
37. American Geriatrics Society 2015 Beers Criteria Update Expert Panel. American Geriatrics Society 2015 Updated Beers Criteria for potentially inappropriate medication use in older adults. *J Am Geriatr Soc* 2015;63:2227-46.
38. Moyad MA, Lowe FC. Educating patients about lifestyle modifications for prostate health. *Am J Med* 2008;121:S34-42.
39. McConnell JD; Benign Prostatic Hyperplasia Guideline Panel. *Benign prostatic hyperplasia: diagnosis and treatment*. Rockville: U.S. Dept. of Health and Human Services, Public Health Service, Agency for Health Care Policy and Research; 1994.
40. Djavan B, Fong YK, Harik M et al. Longitudinal study of men with mild symptoms of bladder outlet obstruction treated with watchful waiting for four years. *Urology* 2004;64:1144-8.
41. Brown CT, Yap T, Cromwell DA et al. Self management for men with lower urinary tract symptoms: randomised controlled trial. *BMJ* 2007;334:25.
42. Speakman MJ, Kirby RS, Joyce A et al. Guideline for the primary care management of male lower urinary tract symptoms. *BJU Int* 2004;93:985-90.
43. Logan YT, Belgeri MT. Monotherapy versus combination drug therapy for the treatment of benign prostatic hyperplasia. *Am J Geriatr Pharmacother* 2005;3:103-14.
44. Armstrong N, Vale L, Deverill M et al. Surgical treatments for men with benign prostatic enlargement: cost effectiveness study. *BMJ* 2009;338:b1288.
45. Lourenco T, Pickard R, Vale L et al. Minimally invasive treatments for benign prostatic enlargement: systematic review of randomised controlled trials. *BMJ* 2008;337:a1662.
46. d'Ancona FC. Nonablative minimally invasive thermal therapies in the treatment of symptomatic benign prostatic hyperplasia. *Curr Opin Urol* 2008;18:21-7.
47. Roehrborn CG. Clinical management of lower urinary tract symptoms with combined medical therapy. *BJU Int* 2008;102:13-7.
48. Greco KA, McVary KT. The role of combination medical therapy in benign prostatic hyperplasia. *Int J Impot Res* 2008;20:S33-43.
49. Barry MJ, Williford WO, Chang Y et al. Benign prostatic hyperplasia specific health status measures in clinical research: how much change in the American Urological Association symptom index and the benign prostatic hyperplasia impact index is perceptible to patients? *J Urol* 1995;154:1770-4.
50. Fullhase C, Chapple C, Cornu JN et al. Systematic review of combination drug therapy for non-neurogenic male lower urinary tract symptoms. *Eur Urol* 2013;64:228-43.
51. McNaughton-Collins M, Barry MJ. Managing patients with lower urinary tract symptoms suggestive of benign prostatic hyperplasia. *Am J Med* 2005;118:1331-9.
52. Radomski SB. Update on medical therapy for male LUTS. *Can Urol Assoc J* 2014;8:S148-50.
53. Azzouni F, Mohler J. Role of 5α-reductase inhibitors in benign prostatic diseases. *Prostate Cancer Prostatic Dis* 2012;15:222-30.
54. Clifford GM, Farmer RD. Medical therapy for benign prostatic hyperplasia: a review of the literature. *Eur Urol* 2000;38:2-19.
55. Andriole G, Bruchovsky N, Chung LW et al. Dihydrotestosterone and the prostate: the scientific rationale for 5 alpha-reductase inhibitors in the treatment of benign prostatic hyperplasia. *J Urol* 2004;172:1399-403.
56. Strittmatter F, Gratzke C, Stief CG et al. Current pharmacological treatment options for male lower urinary tract symptoms. *Expert Opin Pharmacother* 2013;14:1043-54.
57. Andersson KE. Alpha-adrenoceptors and benign prostatic hyperplasia: basic principles for treatment with alpha-adrenoceptor antagonists. *World J Urol* 2002;19:390-6.
58. Kaplan SA. Current role of alpha-blockers in the treatment of benign prostatic hyperplasia. *BJU Int* 2008;102:3-7.
59. Abraham N, Goldman HB. An update on the pharmacotherapy for lower urinary tract dysfunction. *Expert Opin Pharmacother* 2015;16:79-93.
60. Reich O, Gratzke C, Stief CG. Techniques and long-term results of surgical procedures for BPH. *Eur Urol* 2006;49:970-8.
61. Milani S, Djavan B. Lower urinary tract symptoms suggestive of benign prostatic hyperplasia: latest update on alpha-adrenoceptor antagonists. *BJU Int* 2005;95:29-36.
62. Lepor H, Kazzazi A, Djavan B. α-Blockers for benign prostatic hyperplasia: the new era. *Curr Opin Urol* 2012;22:7-15.
63. Beduschi MC, Beduschi R, Oesterling JE. Alpha-blockade therapy for benign prostatic hyperplasia: from a nonselective to a more selective alpha 1A-adrenergic antagonist. *Urology* 1998;51:861-72.
64. Yuan J, Liu Y, Yang Z et al. The efficacy and safety of alpha-1 blockers for benign prostatic hyperplasia: an overview of 15 systematic reviews. *Curr Med Res Opin* 2013;29:279-87.
65. Schwinn DA, Roehrborn CG. Alpha1-adrenoceptor subtypes and lower urinary tract symptoms. *Int J Urol* 2008;15:193-9.
66. Welliver C, Butcher M, Potini Y et al. Impact of alpha blockers, 5-alpha reductase inhibitors and combination therapy on sexual function. *Curr Urol Rep* 2014;15:441.
67. Bell CM, Hatch WV, Fischer HD et al. Association between tamsulosin and serious ophthalmic adverse events in older men following cataract surgery. *JAMA* 2009;301:1991-6.
68. Andersson KE, de Groat WC, McVary KT et al. Tadalafil for the treatment of lower urinary tract symptoms secondary to benign prostatic hyperplasia: pathophysiology and mechanism(s) of action. *Neurourol Urodyn* 2011;30:292-301.

69. McVary KT, Roehrborn CG, Kaminetsky JC et al. Tadalafil relieves lower urinary tract symptoms secondary to benign prostatic hyperplasia. *J Urol* 2007;177:1401-7.
70. Roehrborn CG, McVary KT, Elion-Mboussa A et al. Tadalafil administered once daily for lower urinary tract symptoms secondary to benign prostatic hyperplasia: a dose finding study. *J Urol* 2008;180:1228-34.
71. Gacci M, Corona G, Salvi M et al. A systematic review and meta-analysis on the use of phosphodiesterase 5 inhibitors alone or in combination with α-blockers for lower urinary tract symptoms due to benign prostatic hyperplasia. *Eur Urol* 2012;61:994-1003.
72. Kaplan SA, Roehrborn CG, Abrams P et al. Antimuscarinics for treatment of storage lower urinary tract symptoms in men: a systematic review. *Int J Clin Pract* 2011;65:487-507.
73. Filson CP, Hollingsworth JM, Clemens JQ et al. The efficacy and safety of combined therapy with alpha-blockers and anticholinergics for men with benign prostatic hyperplasia: a meta-analysis. *J Urol* 2013;190:2153-60.
74. Hao N, Tian Y, Liu W et al. Antimuscarinics and alpha-blockers or alpha-blockers monotherapy on lower urinary tract symptoms–a meta-analysis. *Urology* 2014;83:556-62.
75. Xin Z, Huang Y, Lu J et al. Addition of antimuscarinics to alpha-blockers for treatment of lower urinary tract symptoms in men: a meta-analysis. *Urology* 2013;82:270-7.
76. MacDonald R, Tacklind JW, Rutks I et al. Serenoa repens monotherapy for benign prostatic hyperplasia (BPH): an updated Cochrane systematic review. *BJU Int* 2012;109:1756-61.
77. Barry MJ, Meleth S, Lee JY et al. Effect of increasing doses of saw palmetto extract on lower urinary tract symptoms: a randomized trial. *JAMA* 2011;306:1344-51.
78. Ma CH, Lin WL, Lui SL et al. Efficacy and safety of Chinese herbal medicine for benign prostatic hyperplasia: systematic review of randomized controlled trials. *Asian J Androl* 2013;15:471-82.
79. Abrams P, Chapple C, Khoury S et al. Evaluation and treatment of lower urinary tract symptoms in older men. *J Urol* 2013;189:S93-S101.
80. Pagano E, Laudato M, Griffo M et al. Phytotherapy of benign prostatic hyperplasia. A minireview. *Phytother Res* 2014;28:949-55.
81. Tacklind J, MacDonald R, Rutks I et al. Serenoa repens for benign prostatic hyperplasia. *Cochrane Database Syst Rev* 2012;12:CD001423.

Enlarged Prostate—What You Need to Know

What is the prostate?

The prostate is a walnut-sized gland that is part of the male reproductive system. It makes the fluid that you see in semen when you ejaculate. The prostate surrounds the urethra, the tube through which urine passes out of the body.

What is the most common prostate problem?

Many older men experience a condition called benign prostatic hyperplasia (BPH). Benign means that the condition is not caused by infection or cancer. Hyperplasia means enlargement. BPH is not usually a serious condition but it can be a bother. It may also cause some discomfort. Symptoms of BPH are most common for men in their 60s and older. It is very rare before age 40.

What are the symptoms of BPH?

Common signs of BPH include:

- a weak urine stream that stops and starts
- leaking or dribbling of urine between trips to the bathroom
- feeling the need to urinate more often (especially at night)
- feeling like the bladder never completely empties, even after urination

BPH occurs when the enlarged prostate starts to push against the urethra, restricting the flow of urine. The bladder wall then begins to thicken and become irritable. The bladder starts to contract even when it contains only small amounts of urine. Over time, the bladder weakens and loses its ability to empty itself completely, leaving urine behind.

The signs of BPH usually come on slowly. But it can appear quickly as a result of certain medications (for example, decongestants), cold temperatures, alcohol and being immobile for a long time.

If you have symptoms of BPH, see your healthcare provider.

Is BPH the same as prostate cancer?

BPH is not the same as prostate cancer. It does not increase the chance of getting prostate cancer. However, some of the symptoms are the same.

What is the treatment for BPH?

Your may receive a rectal exam or ultrasound. Men with possible BPH are often referred to a specialist (called a urologist) for diagnosis and treatment.

No treatment is necessary for mild BPH and symptoms can be managed without medications or disappear without treatment. Herbal products containing saw palmetto, stinging nettle, pygeum (African plum tree) or pumpkin seeds may help a mild case of BPH. Treatment is necessary only when BPH puts your health at risk or when it becomes very bothersome. Treatment of BPH can include surgery or prescribed medications.

What can you do if you have BPH?

- Talk to your pharmacist before trying any over-the-counter medication. Some ingredients such as pseudoephedrine (a decongestant in Sudafed) and dimenhydrinate (an antihistamine in Gravol) can make BPH worse. These ingredients can cause urinary retention and are not recommended for anyone with BPH.
- Try to take your time when emptying your bladder.
- Try to limit fluid intake in the evening. Stay away from fluids that tend to dehydrate you, such as alcohol and caffeine.

Chapter 76
Contraception

Anne Marie Whelan, PharmD, FCSHP

A woman can become pregnant from puberty until menopause, so contraception is an important health issue for many women during these reproductive years. There were a total of 386,044 births in Canada in 2013–14[1] and 82,869 induced abortions,[2] suggesting that many pregnancies in Canada may be unplanned. Unplanned pregnancies have been associated with negative health and social outcomes for both mothers and children.[3,4,5]

Healthy sexual practices, including the use of contraception, are important for countering these unplanned pregnancies. Unsafe sexual behaviours may lead not only to unplanned pregnancy but also to infertility and human immunodeficiency virus (HIV) or other sexually transmitted infections (STIs). However, the Canadian Contraception Study (CCS), conducted in 2002, reported that among Canadians aged 15–44, 9% were not using any method of contraception.[6] The study also found that many women are not familiar with some of the contraceptive methods available to them. Less than 50% of respondents were familiar with spermicides, cervical caps, the rhythm method or the female condom.[6]

Many options are available for effective contraception, some of which, such as condoms, have the added advantage of providing protection against HIV and other STI transmission. However, the 2002 CCS found that among Canadians aged 15–18 who were coitally experienced, 17% had "sometimes" used a condom in the past 6 months and 17% reported not using a condom ever in the past 6 months.[7] These data highlight the need for contraceptive counselling and enhanced public education starting at a young age.[8] Healthcare practitioners are in an excellent position to help women and men with their contraceptive choices by taking into consideration desired outcomes as well as advantages and disadvantages of various methods. This chapter focuses on nonhormonal contraceptive methods but also includes a discussion of hormonal contraceptive methods and emergency contraception.

Pathophysiology

The female reproductive cycle comprises 2 main phases, the follicular or preovulatory phase and the luteal or postovulatory phase. The first day of menses marks the beginning of the follicular phase, during which follicle-stimulating hormone promotes the maturation of several ovarian follicles. After about 7 days, one follicle dominates and development of the other follicles stops. As the dominant follicle continues to grow, estrogen levels increase and the follicle develops luteinizing hormone (LH) receptors. The estrogen causes proliferation of the endometrial lining, and at midcycle stimulates the pituitary gland to release a surge of LH. This LH surge causes final maturation of the follicle and the release of the ovum into the Fallopian tube.

Release of the ovum from the follicle marks the beginning of the luteal phase. Once the follicle ruptures and releases the ovum, the remaining cells of the follicle become the corpus luteum, which secretes large amounts of estrogen and progesterone. Progesterone causes secretory changes to the endometrium which are necessary for implantation. If conception occurs, the corpus luteum continues to maintain the hormone production necessary for the early stages of pregnancy. If the ovum is not fertilized, the corpus luteum degenerates and levels of estrogen and progesterone drop quickly. This fall in hormones causes menses and the cycle starts over again.[9]

The luteal phase lasts 14 ± 2 days and is the more consistent of the 2 phases. The follicular phase can vary by several days, making it difficult to predict when ovulation will occur. The usual menstrual cycle lasts 28 days; however, it can vary from 25–35 days.[9]

Once the ovum is released from the dominant follicle, it is viable (can be fertilized) for up to 24 hours. Upon ejaculation sperm can be viable for up to 5 days, resulting in approximately 6 days when a woman is at her most fertile.[10] If pregnancy is not desired, it is important that she use an effective method of birth control, especially during the days of her cycle she is most likely to be fertile.

Nonhormonal Contraceptive Methods

See Table 1 for a summary of the failure rates, advantages and disadvantages of each nonhormonal method of contraception.

Natural Methods

Coitus Interruptus (Withdrawal)

Coitus interruptus is a method of contraception whereby the penis is withdrawn from the vagina before ejaculation occurs.[11] This method is an option for couples who do not want to or cannot use other contraceptive methods. It also allows the male to participate actively in the control of conception.[32]

Fertility Awareness-based Methods

Fertility awareness-based methods (FABMs) of contraception are methods that rely on the physical signs and symptoms that vary throughout a woman's menstrual cycle in response to hormonal changes.[10] Women can monitor these signs and symptoms and predict when they are most likely to be fertile. Pregnancy is prevented by abstaining from intercourse or by using another method of contraception during the time they are most likely fertile. Natural family planning refers to the use of the FABMs as the only method of contraception. Abstinence is practised during times of predicted fertility to prevent pregnancy.[10] Examples of some of the different types of FABMs are discussed below.

Calendar Methods

These methods require tracking days in the calendar to determine the woman's most likely fertile days. There are 2 different ways to do this.

Calendar Rhythm Method: The woman must record the length of her cycle for 6–12 months and then identify the length of her shortest and longest cycle. She then subtracts 18 from the length of her shortest cycle: this number will be the earliest day that she is most likely to be fertile in her next cycle. She then subtracts 11 from the length of her longest cycle: this number will be the latest day that she is most likely to be fertile in her next cycle. To prevent pregnancy she must abstain from intercourse or use another contraceptive method during her predicted fertile days. For example, if the shortest cycle in the previous 6 months was 28 days and the longest cycle was 30 days, she would subtract 18 from 28 (=10) and 11 from 30 (=19) indicating that she is most likely to be fertile from days 10–19 of her next cycle.

Standard Days Method: The woman begins counting on the first day of her cycle (day 1 of menses). She is most likely to be fertile from days 8–19 and should abstain from intercourse or use another contraceptive method during these days. The Standard Days Method should be used only by women who have regular cycles of 26–32 days in duration. Colour-coded strands of beads, called Cycle Beads, or smart-phone/online applications may be used to help the woman keep track of the days of her menstrual cycle.[14,33]

Basal Body Temperature Method

This method is based on changes to the basal body temperature (temperature of the body at rest) that occur during the menstrual cycle. During the follicular phase the basal temperature is stable. There is a slight drop in basal temperature about 12–24 hours before ovulation, followed by a sharp rise in temperature due to the progesterone secreted by the corpus luteum after ovulation. Three days of sustained elevated temperature suggests that ovulation has likely occurred and the post-ovulation infertile time period has started. As it is difficult to predict the start of the fertile period, some experts suggest that women should abstain from intercourse or use another method of contraception from day 1 of menses until the 3 days of elevated temperature have occurred.[34] The basal temperature remains elevated until menses. Basal thermometers (similar to regular thermometers but with a wider calibration set) are required to easily distinguish the slight variations in temperature. The temperature is taken orally, rectally or vaginally before the woman rises for the day. It should be taken at the same time and by the same route each day. The woman should avoid speaking, eating, drinking or smoking before taking a reading. Factors that can affect basal temperature include fever or infection, travel, emotional changes and certain medications, e.g., hormones, corticosteroids. Digital basal thermometers are preferred over mercury thermometers as they are easier to use and read, and the readings are stored in memory until needed.[35,36,37]

Some digital basal thermometers combine data about menstrual cycle history with the measured temperatures to provide information about the timing of fertility and can be used with smartphone or online apps.

Cervical Mucus Methods

Cervical mucus can be used as an indicator of fertility as it changes over the course of the menstrual cycle. Cervical mucus is almost nonexistent after menses. During the follicular phase it is opaque, white or yellowish in colour, viscous and sticky. The mucus increases in volume and takes on the appearance of uncooked egg whites (clear, thin and stretchable) as ovulation approaches. After ovulation the mucus becomes opaque and viscous until menses. Changes in cervical mucus are the result of an increase in estrogen. Around the time of ovulation, the character of the mucus provides a favourable environment for sperm.[14]

There are 2 different methods of evaluating mucus. With the TwoDay Method, women look for the presence or absence of any mucus every day and ask: 1) Did I have cervical mucus today? and 2) Did I have cervical mucus yesterday? Answering "yes" to one or both questions (e.g., presence of mucus the day before and/or that day) indicates fertility that day, thus the woman should abstain from intercourse or use another method of contraception that day. With the Billings Ovulation Method, the woman checks her cervical mucus every day after menses finishes. She should consider herself fertile as soon as she notices any secretions. The end of the fertile period is the fourth day after the last appearance of abundant, clear and stretchy secretions.[14]

Symptothermal Method

The symptothermal method of contraception uses both the changes in cervical mucus and changes in basal temperature to determine the fertile period.[35,36,37]

Lactational Amenorrhea Method

Maximal suckling at the breast in women who almost exclusively breastfeed their babies provides a natural contraceptive effect. This greatly reduces the risk of pregnancy for the first 6 months postpartum if the baby is breastfed on demand, supplemental bottle feeding is avoided and only minimal supplements are provided by cup or spoon. However, if menstruation has resumed, breastfeeding is reduced, bottle feeding or food supplements are introduced, or the baby has reached 6 months of age, another method of contraception is required.[15]

Fertility Monitors/Ovulation Prediction Tests

For comparative features of nonprescription products, consult the *Compendium of Products for Minor Ailments*—Home Testing Products: Fertility Test Kits.

Fertility monitors or ovulation prediction tests (see Chapter 80: Pregnancy and Fertility Testing) are used by women to help determine their fertile and infertile periods by examining urine and saliva for changes that occur naturally throughout the menstrual cycle. Although primarily marketed for patients with infertility, these monitors can be used by all women to obtain a better understanding of their menstrual cycles and to help identify periods of fertility and infertility for the purpose of contraception. Devices can be purchased from some pharmacies and various websites.

Urinary LH tests test urine for **LH**, alone or in combination with **estrone-3–glucuonide (E3G)** as the presence of LH and E3G in the urine is indicative of a fertile period in a woman's cycle.[38]

Saliva microscopy consists of examining saliva for the presence of sodium chloride, which increases in response to increasing estrogen levels, indicating a fertile period. If sodium chloride is present in dried saliva, it will crystallize and appear as a "fern". A sample of saliva is placed on a glass microscope slide, dried, and inspected. Small dots indicate low fertility while small ferns and large ferns indicate intermediate and high fertility, respectively.[38]

Barrier Methods

For comparative features of nonprescription products, consult the *Compendium of Products for Minor Ailments*—Contraceptive Products: Male Condoms, Vaginal Barrier Devices.

Diaphragm

A diaphragm is a small, reusable, soft silicone dome with a covered flexible spring at the outer edge that is inserted into the vagina (see Figure 1). Proper use of the diaphragm creates a barrier at the cervix and prevents the sperm from entering the uterus, reducing the chance of pregnancy. Traditionally, it was used in conjunction with a spermicidal gel containing **Nonoxynol-9 (N-9)**.[17] However, there is currently no spermicidal gel available in Canada that contains N-9. Acid-buffering gels are now available for use with the diaphragm. These gels form a physical barrier and lower the pH, thus reducing sperm mobility (for further information see Spermicides).[39]

Figure 1: **Diaphragm**

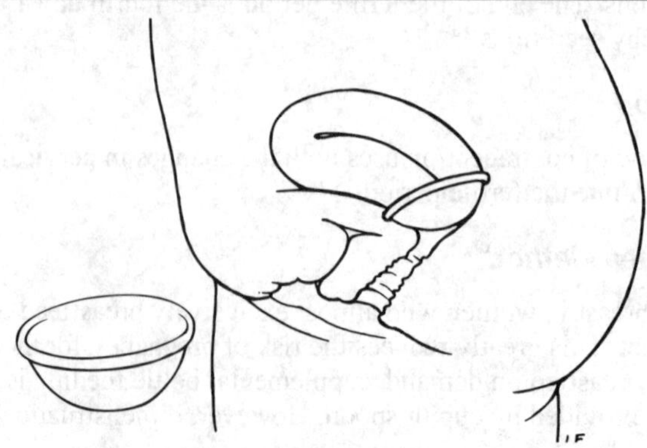

There are currently three types of diaphragms available in Canada. The Milex Wide-Seal Arcing Style and the Milex Wide-Seal Omniflex Style come in a variety of sizes and must be fitted for the individual woman by a trained healthcare practitioner. Annual replacement is recommended.[39,40] The Caya SILCS is available in one size only that is designed to fit most women. It can last up to 2 years.[39,41,42]

The diaphragm must be inserted prior to intercourse and should stay in place for at least 6 hours after intercourse, but it must be removed within 24 hours to reduce the risk of toxic shock syndrome. To apply the gel, the diaphragm is held dome-side down (like a cup) and approximately one teaspoonful of gel squeezed into the dome. A little of the gel is applied to the rim of the diaphragm with a finger. To insert the diaphragm, it must first be folded and then inserted into the vaginal canal. The diaphragm is pushed along the back of the vagina as far as it will go. The front rim is tucked up along the roof of the vagina behind the pubic bone and the back rim of the diaphragm is below and behind the cervix. This is usually done with the woman standing with one foot propped up, squatting or lying on her back. When the diaphragm is properly in place (see Figure 1) the woman should not feel it, nor should the male partner be aware of its presence. The tension between the diaphragm and vaginal wall holds the diaphragm in place. The Arcing[43] and Omniflex[44] diaphragms also create suction with the vaginal mucosa which provides additional action to keep them in place. If intercourse has not occurred within 2 hours of insertion of the diaphragm, more gel should be added.[39,42] An additional application of gel is required with each repeated act of intercourse but must be applied using an applicator, without removing the diaphragm.[21,39]

The diaphragm can be removed by hooking the index finger behind the front rim and pulling down and out. Alternatively, the woman can assume a squatting position and push downward with her abdominal muscles (bearing down as one would for a bowel movement). Once removed, it should be washed with mild soap and water, rinsed, dried with a towel and stored in its container.[21]

Cervical Cap

The cervical cap is a reusable, dome-shaped device that is inserted into the vagina to fit snugly over the cervix (see Figure 2).[17] Like the diaphragm, the cervical cap is a barrier that blocks the passage of sperm from the vagina through the cervix and was traditionally used in conjunction with a spermicidal gel. A groove on the inside of the cap creates a seal that helps to keep the cap in place with support of the vaginal wall.

Figure 2: Cervical Cap

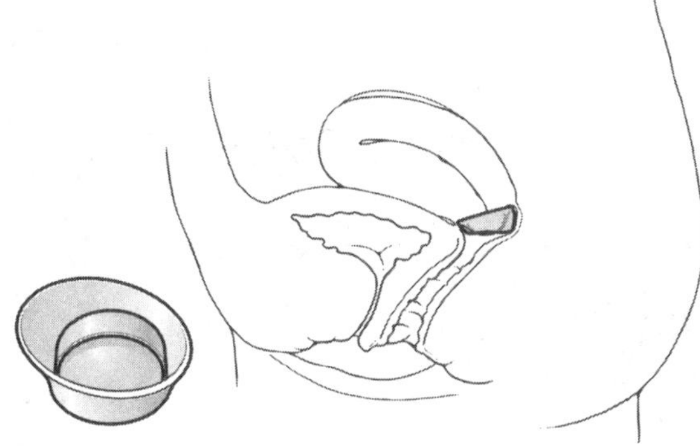

The silicone FemCap is currently the only cervical cap available in Canada although other types have been available in the past and may still be in use.[45] The FemCap is available in 3 sizes; the correct size is ordered not by fit but based on whether the user has ever been pregnant and/or had a vaginal delivery. The smallest size is for women who have never been pregnant. Women who have been pregnant but not delivered vaginally (e.g., have miscarried, terminated a pregnancy or delivered by Caesarian section) use the medium size, while the largest one is used by those who have had vaginal delivery of a full-term baby. The FemCap can be purchased online and should be replaced yearly.[39,45]

When using a cervical cap, it should be filled about one-third full with acid-buffering gel. The rim of a cervical cap should *not* be covered with gel. The rim should be squeezed between the thumb and forefinger and the cap inserted into the vagina. The cap is pushed as deep into the vagina as possible. Suction is produced by pressing on the dome and twisting the cap like the lid on a jar. Proper fitting is verified by running a finger along the rim and firmly tugging down on the dome. The cap should remain in place and there should be a sensation of the cervix being pulled. While not a concern with the FemCap as it is made of silicone, oil-based products (e.g., Vaseline) are not recommended if a vaginal lubricant is required when using a latex cervical cap as they can decrease the integrity of the latex. Additional gel may be inserted if repeat intercourse occurs; however, this should be done without removing the cap.

To remove it, the cap is tilted to one side and a finger is hooked under the rim to pull it out. The cap should be left in place for at least 8 hours after intercourse; it should be worn for no longer than 48 hours at a time. Once removed, the cap is washed with mild soap and warm water.[21]

Contraceptive Sponge

Contraceptive single-use sponges, pieces of soft foam filled with spermicide, have been available in Canada on and off for a number of years (see Figure 3). Sponges are inserted into the vagina so that they cover the cervix. They function by 2 mechanisms: as a physical barrier by blocking the entrance to the uterus and by spermicidal activity.

Perhaps the most well known is the Today Sponge (containing **nonoxynol-9**), discontinued in the early 1990s but reintroduced in Canada in 2011 and available in some pharmacies.

Figure 3: **Contraceptive Sponge**

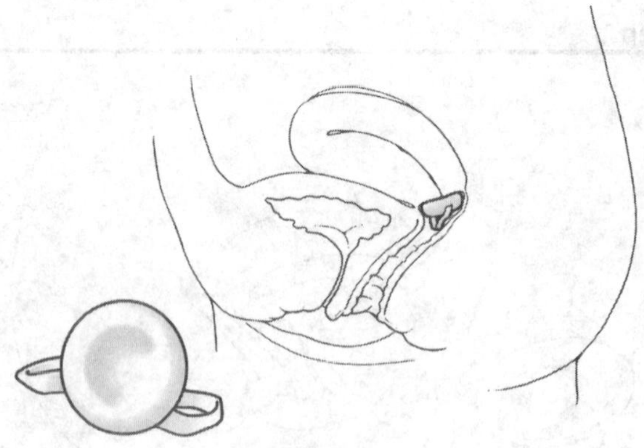

The Today Sponge is available in 1 size only. It can be inserted at any time before sexual intercourse and must be kept in place for at least 6 hours after the last act of intercourse. It provides contraceptive protection for 24 hours no matter how many times intercourse occurs. If intercourse occurs when the sponge has been in place for 24 hours, the sponge should not be removed for 6 hours. Thus, the maximum length of insertion for the sponge is 30 hours. Leaving the sponge in longer than 30 hours increases the risk of vaginal irritation and infections. The Today Sponge has a woven polyester loop on one side that aids in removal. Once removed, the sponge should be discarded.[46]

Female Condom

The female condom (branded as FC2) is a single-use barrier contraceptive that protects against pregnancy as well as against HIV and other STI transmission (see Figure 4). FC2 replaces the first-generation polyurethane female condom sold under the brand name Reality. The second-generation female condom is made from nitrile (a synthetic rubber). The new condom performs as effectively as the original polyurethane condom.[23,47] The female condom is a pouch coated with a silicone-based nonspermicidal lubricant with rings at each end to help keep the condom in place within the vagina. The closed end is inserted into the vagina and covers the cervix. The ring on this end helps anchor it in place like a diaphragm. The open end hangs out of the vagina. The ring on the open end is placed against the body and helps prevent the condom from entering the vagina. Inserting the condom a few minutes before intercourse and/or adding extra lubricant may reduce the noise, but it can be inserted up to 8 hours prior to intercourse.[23,39] After intercourse the condom should be twisted to seal in the semen and then gently removed and discarded. A new condom must be used for repeated intercourse.[17]

Figure 4: **Female Condom**

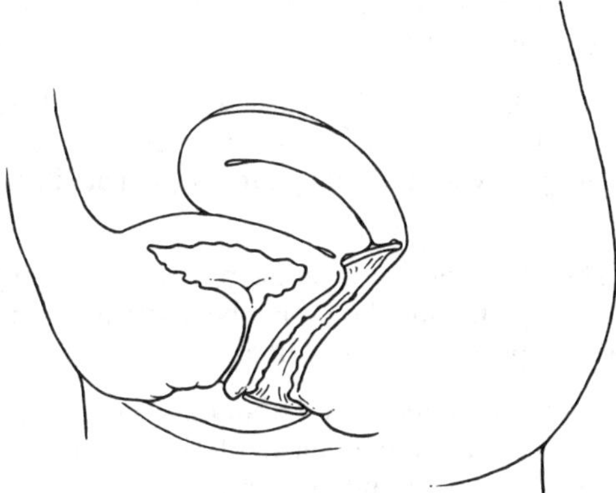

Male Condom

The history of condoms goes back to medieval times when sheaths of linen or animal intestine were used as contraceptives. Today the single-use condom is a sheath of processed lamb cecum ("lambskin"), latex, polyisoprene or polyurethane that fits over an erect penis (see Figure 5). It provides a receptacle that prevents semen from reaching the vagina and cervix. The use of latex condoms as a component of "safer sex" is widely publicized and encouraged as a means of reducing the risk of transmission of STIs, including HIV.[26]

Theoretically, condoms should be completely effective in preventing pregnancy, but in reality they are not. Condom failure may be attributed to either breakage or slippage. The incidence of breakage has been reported to be between 0.5% and 2.5%, and that of slippage between 0.6% and 2%.[48,49,50,51]

Figure 5: **Male Condom**

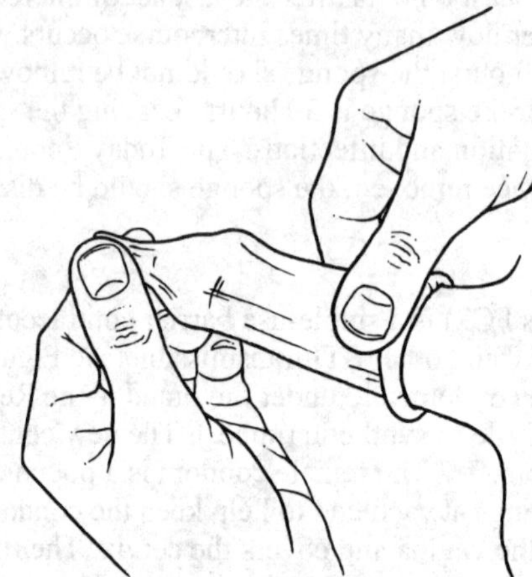

Risk factors associated with breakage and/or slippage include opening the package with sharp objects, unrolling condoms before putting them on, lack of sex education or experience in using condoms and lengthy or intense intercourse.[48,49,50,51,52] The use of lubricants has been associated with increased slippage in vaginal intercourse and reduced slippage in anal intercourse.[48] Alcohol and drugs are also associated with an increased incidence of condom failure (both breakage and slippage).[48,49,50,51,52] Some of these risks may be attenuated by providing appropriate counselling.

Other risk factors for breakage and/or slippage include low income and low education of the user as well as a larger penile circumference.[48,49,50,51,52]

The other leading cause of condom failure relates to user attitudes that lead to inconsistent use, e.g., reduction in physical sensations, uncomfortable feeling, interruption in sexual activity, perception that sexual activity must be less vigorous, fear of sending a message that either the user or partner is unclean.

Condoms should not be used after the expiry date on the product packaging. They should be kept in a cool, dry place, out of the sunlight. Condoms should not be disposed of in the toilet after use; they should be wrapped in tissue and disposed of in the garbage.[26]

Latex condoms are made from natural rubber latex. Laboratory studies reveal that they are an effective physical barrier to microorganisms such as those causing HIV and other STIs. Latex condoms are available with a variety of features: reservoir end, lubricated (wet or dry), lubricated with spermicide (nonoxynol-9), thin latex, extra strength, tapered, contoured, ribbed, studded, textured internal surface, coloured and flavoured. Most are produced in a standard size although smaller and larger sizes are also available.[26]

A 2008 review concluded that latex condoms provide considerable protection against the transmission of STIs that spread primarily through infected secretions (HIV, gonorrhea, chlamydia and trichomoniasis).[53] Only partial protection is afforded by condoms against infections transmitted through skin or mucous membrane (herpes simplex, human papillomavirus).[53] A 2009 meta-analysis produced a similar conclusion, reporting that using a condom provided only moderate protection against transmission of herpes simplex virus 2 (HSV-2).[54]

Oil-based lubricants (e.g., massage oil, Vaseline) should never be used with latex condoms as they cause the latex to deteriorate. Water-based lubricants (e.g., Astroglide, K-Y Jelly) will not cause latex condoms to break down and therefore are safe to use. Latex condoms are more elastic than lambskin and as a result are more likely to remain in place on the penis during intercourse and on withdrawal.

An estimated 1–6% of the American population is allergic to latex. Repeated exposure to certain proteins in the latex is thought to be the cause of allergies. The most common symptom for both men and women is genital inflammation with redness, itching and burning. In more severe cases, intraepidermal edema leads to the formation of vesicles. Once the vesicles rupture, the skin weeps, oozes and crusts. An old recommendation to manage latex allergy advised couples to use a lambskin condom in conjunction with a latex condom for contraception and STI protection. If the woman was allergic, a lambskin condom was worn over a latex condom; if the man was allergic, a lambskin condom was worn under the latex condom.[55] The current recommendation is to use polyurethane or polyisoprene male condoms, or nitrile female condoms, in place of latex condoms.[26,39,56]

Lambskin condoms are made from the intestinal cecum of lambs and may be referred to as "natural skin," "natural membrane" or "lambskin" condoms. Elasticity is poor and they may slip off the penis during intercourse or on withdrawal. Oil- or water-based lubricants or vaginal medications can be used with these condoms. It is claimed that they provide better transmission of body heat and therefore greater sensitivity than latex condoms. Lambskin condoms do not provide the same level of protection against HIV or other STI transmission as latex condoms because they have small pores that allow passage of the microorganisms. Lambskin condoms should be avoided by those who have allergies to lanolin or wool.[26]

Polyurethane condoms are latex-free and are stronger than latex so the condoms are thinner, allowing for greater sensation. Unlike latex condoms, either oil- or water-based lubricants or vaginal medications can be used with polyurethane condoms. However, they are not as stretchy as latex, so breakage and slippage rates are higher.[57] Polyurethane condoms have similar efficacy to latex condoms with regard to preventing pregnancy. Effectiveness for STI prevention has not been well studied; however, they are believed to offer the same level of protection against HIV and other STI transmission as latex condoms.[26]

Polyisoprene condoms are made from a synthetic rubber that is chemically the same as latex, except that the proteins causing latex allergy have been removed. Only water-based lubricants or vaginal medications should be used with these condoms, as oil-based products may reduce the integrity of the condoms. Polyisoprene condoms effectively prevent both pregnancy and HIV or other STI transmission.[57] They are considered to be as strong and safe as latex condoms. Compared with polyurethane, polyisoprene is softer, more form-fitting, thicker, more resistant to breakage and allows more stretch.[57,58]

Spermicides

For comparative ingredients of nonprescription products, consult the *Compendium of Products for Minor Ailments*—Contraceptive Products: Spermicidal Products and Devices.

Spermicides are products that are inserted vaginally and contain chemicals that kill or immobilize sperm. Traditionally, commercially available products have contained the surfactant **nonoxynol-9** (N-9); however, only a few products containing N-9 remain on the market in Canada. N-9 makes sperm unviable by making the sperm cell membranes permeable to moisture, resulting in swelling and destruction of the membranes.[27,59] Spermicides containing N-9 were available in various dosage forms and could be used alone or in combination with condoms, cervical caps, diaphragms or intrauterine devices. Sponges and films containing spermicide also act as physical barriers in preventing conception.

Spermicidal agents containing N-9 were once believed to reduce the transmission of HIV and other STIs;[60] however, this is now refuted. Frequent use of N-9 can cause irritation and lesions to genital mucosa, which is thought to increase the risk of transmission of infections.[59,61] The World Health Organization (WHO) and the Contraceptive Research and Development (CONRAD) Program in the United States reviewed the evidence in 2001 and concluded that N-9 does not protect against the transmission of HIV, gonorrhea, trichomonas, chlamydia, bacterial vaginosis or candidiasis.[62]

Current recommendations include:

- N-9 should not be used for the prevention of HIV or other STIs
- women who have multiple acts of intercourse daily should not use N-9 products
- spermicide-coated condoms should not be recommended; however, condoms lubricated with N-9 can be used if the alternative is no condom at all
- the benefits and risks of use of N-9 should be evaluated before using it for contraception.[63,64]

Due to concerns regarding N-9 there is now more interest in other spermicidal agents. In some countries other surfactants such as octoxynol, menfegol and benzalkonium chloride are used in spermicidal products.[21] **Contragel green** is a jelly produced in Germany by Kessel-Marketing GmbH and distributed in Canada as an acid-buffering barrier gel. It contains a combination of ingredients including lactic acid, sodium lactate, methylcellulose and sorbic acid. **Caya Diaphragm Gel**, similar to Contragel, is also approved for sale in Canada as an acid-buffering barrier gel. The methylcellulose forms a physical barrier while some evidence suggests that lactic acid reduces the pH of the vagina, limiting sperm motility.[65,66] These gels are not intended to be used alone but rather in combination with barrier methods such as diaphragms and cervical caps.[67]

Spermicidal foam and film containing N-9 are currently available in Canadian pharmacies. Advise women using contraceptive foam to mix the product well by shaking the container about 20 times before use and to follow the directions on the package insert regarding the amount required. While the woman is lying down, the applicator is inserted into the vagina as deeply as possible, then the plunger is pushed to release the dose. Intercourse should take place within the prescribed time for the particular product being used (usually 30–60 minutes after insertion). More foam should be inserted if more than the prescribed time has passed since the first dose was inserted, and for every time the couple engages in intercourse.[21] After intercourse any residual spermicide should not be removed (e.g., by douching) for at least 6 hours.[17] Contraceptive foams may be used alone or in combination with a barrier method.[21]

VCF, a **vaginal contraceptive film**, is manufactured by Apothecus Pharmaceutical Corp. and contains N-9 in a film base.[68,69] VCF dissolves completely and quickly into a gel after insertion high into the vagina against the cervix. It can be inserted from 15 minutes to 3 hours before intercourse. If more than 3 hours have elapsed without intercourse, or intercourse is repeated, another film should be inserted.[70] The gel acts as a barrier to block sperm from entering the cervix and the N-9 is spermicidal. To insert the film, the VCF is removed from the packaging, folded in half, placed on the tip of the second or third finger and then inserted into the vagina and applied against the cervix. Women do not need to douche after intercourse as the gel will disappear on its own. However, if douching is desired, the woman should wait at least 6 hours after intercourse to avoid washing away spermicide too early.[17] Contraceptive films may be used alone or in combination with a barrier method.[21]

Copper Intrauterine Device

The copper intrauterine device (IUD) is a small T-shaped device that is inserted into the uterus to prevent pregnancy (see Figure 6).[71,72] Though the precise mechanism of action of the IUD is unknown, it is generally accepted that copper IUDs impede the ascent of sperm to the Fallopian tubes or reduce the ability of sperm to fertilize an ovum. A foreign body reaction to the IUD in the uterus causes both cellular and biochemical changes that may be toxic to sperm. Sperm function is impaired by the increase in copper ions, enzymes, prostaglandins and white blood cells in the fluid in the uterus and

Fallopian tubes.[73] Copper IUDs must be inserted by a trained healthcare practitioner and should be replaced as per the manufacturer's recommendation (e.g., 30 months to 10 years).[31,74,75] Long-acting reversible contraception such as a copper IUD is preferred in young women at high risk of contraceptive failure due to incorrect or inconsistent use.[76,77,78]

Figure 6: **Intrauterine Device**

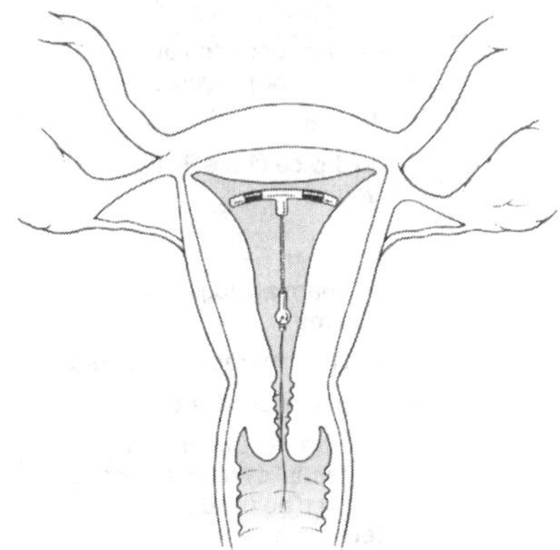

Table 1: **Nonhormonal Contraception Failure Rates, Advantages and Disadvantages**

Method	Failure with Correct and Consistent Use	Failure with Typical Use	Advantages	Disadvantages
Withdrawal[11]	4%	22%	▪ No cost ▪ No device or medication required ▪ No HCP interaction required ▪ No potential adverse effects ▪ Always available	▪ Correct and consistent use may be challenging and ejaculate could be deposited in the vagina if penis is not withdrawn in time ▪ No protection from HIV or other STI transmission
Fertility awareness–based methods (FABMs)[a, 10,11,13,14,15]			▪ No pharmacologic agent required ▪ No HCP interaction required ▪ No potential adverse effects ▪ Women's knowledge of menstrual cycle is increased and can be used to determine fertile period to aid conception if desired ▪ May be supported by religious organizations	▪ Continuous charting and monitoring required ▪ Several months may be required to gain understanding of fertility signs and symptoms ▪ Abstinence or another method of contraception must be used consistently during fertile period ▪ Ovulation may occur outside the calculated fertile times ▪ No protection from HIV or other STI transmission
Rhythm	0.1–9%	25%	▪ No pharmacologic agent required ▪ No HCP interaction required ▪ No potential adverse effects ▪ Women's knowledge of menstrual cycle is increased	▪ Continuous charting and monitoring required ▪ Several months may be required to gain understanding of fertility signs and symptoms

(cont'd)

Table 1: **Nonhormonal Contraception Failure Rates, Advantages and Disadvantages** *(cont'd)*

Method	Failure with Correct and Consistent Use	Failure with Typical Use	Advantages	Disadvantages
			and can be used to determine fertile period to aid conception if desired ▪ May be supported by religious organizations ▪ No cost ▪ No device or medication required	▪ Abstinence or another method of contraception must be used consistently during fertile period ▪ Ovulation may occur outside the calculated fertile times ▪ No protection from HIV or other STI transmission ▪ Difficult to predict fertile days if cycles are irregular
Standard days	4.8–5%	8–25%	▪ No pharmacologic agent required ▪ No HCP interaction required ▪ No potential adverse effects ▪ Women's knowledge of menstrual cycle is increased and can be used to determine fertile period to aid conception if desired ▪ May be supported by religious organizations ▪ Aids such as cycle beads only possible device required	▪ Continuous charting and monitoring required ▪ Several months may be required to gain understanding of fertility signs and symptoms ▪ Abstinence or another method of contraception must be used consistently during fertile period ▪ Ovulation may occur outside the calculated fertile times ▪ No protection from HIV or other STI transmission ▪ Difficult to predict fertile days if cycles are irregular
Basal body temperature	1%	No data for typical use	▪ No pharmacologic agent required ▪ No HCP interaction required ▪ No potential adverse effects ▪ Women's knowledge of menstrual cycle is increased and can be used to determine fertile period to aid conception if desired ▪ May be supported by religious organizations ▪ Thermometer only device required	▪ Continuous charting and monitoring required ▪ Several months may be required to gain understanding of fertility signs and symptoms ▪ Abstinence or another method of contraception must be used consistently during fertile period ▪ Ovulation may occur outside the calculated fertile times ▪ No protection from HIV or other STI transmission ▪ Temperature may be affected by illness, infection or jet lag
TwoDay	4%	14%	▪ No pharmacologic agent required ▪ No HCP interaction required ▪ No potential adverse effects ▪ Women's knowledge of menstrual cycle is increased and can be used to determine fertile period to aid conception if desired ▪ May be supported by religious organizations ▪ No cost	▪ Continuous charting and monitoring required ▪ Several months may be required to gain understanding of fertility signs and symptoms ▪ Abstinence or another method of contraception must be used consistently during fertile period ▪ Ovulation may occur outside the calculated fertile times ▪ No protection from HIV or other STI transmission

(cont'd)

Table 1: **Nonhormonal Contraception Failure Rates, Advantages and Disadvantages** *(cont'd)*

Method	Failure with Correct and Consistent Use	Failure with Typical Use	Advantages	Disadvantages
			▪ No device or medication required	▪ Secretions may be altered by douching, semen, lubricants or vaginal infections
Billings ovulation	0.5–3%	3–22.3%	▪ No pharmacologic agent required ▪ No HCP interaction required ▪ No potential adverse effects ▪ Women's knowledge of menstrual cycle is increased and can be used to determine fertile period to aid conception if desired ▪ May be supported by religious organizations ▪ No cost ▪ No device or medication required	▪ Continuous charting and monitoring required ▪ Several months may be required to gain understanding of fertility signs and symptoms ▪ Abstinence or another method of contraception must be used consistently during fertile period ▪ Ovulation may occur outside the calculated fertile times ▪ No protection from HIV or other STI transmission ▪ Secretions may be altered by douching, semen, lubricants or vaginal infections
Symptothermal	0.3%	0.2–20%	▪ No pharmacologic agent required ▪ No HCP interaction required ▪ No potential adverse effects ▪ Women's knowledge of menstrual cycle is increased and can be used to determine fertile period to aid conception if desired ▪ May be supported by religious organizations ▪ Thermometer only device required	▪ Continuous charting and monitoring required ▪ Several months may be required to gain understanding of fertility signs and symptoms ▪ Abstinence or another method of contraception must be used consistently during fertile period ▪ Ovulation may occur outside the calculated fertile times ▪ No protection from HIV or other STI transmission ▪ Temperature may be affected by illness, infection or jet lag ▪ Secretions may be altered by douching, semen, lubricants or vaginal infections
Lactational amenorrhea	0–8%	No data for typical use	▪ No pharmacologic agent required ▪ No HCP interaction required ▪ No potential adverse effects ▪ May be supported by religious organizations ▪ No cost ▪ No device or medication required	▪ No protection from HIV or other STI transmission ▪ Must breastfeed baby on demand, avoid any bottle feeds and provide only minimal supplemental food
Fertility monitors/ ovulation prediction tests[14,16]	5.3–8.3%	No data for typical use	▪ No pharmacologic agent required ▪ No HCP interaction required ▪ No potential adverse effects	▪ Continuous charting and monitoring required ▪ Several months may be required to gain understanding of fertility signs and symptoms

(cont'd)

Table 1: **Nonhormonal Contraception Failure Rates, Advantages and Disadvantages** *(cont'd)*

Method	Failure with Correct and Consistent Use	Failure with Typical Use	Advantages	Disadvantages
			▪ Women's knowledge of menstrual cycle is increased and can be used to determine fertile period to aid conception if desired	▪ Abstinence or another method of contraception must be used consistently during fertile period ▪ Ovulation may occur outside the calculated fertile times ▪ No protection from HIV or other STI transmission ▪ Cost
Diaphragm[17,18]	6%	16%	▪ Provides immediate protection ▪ Ability to insert in advance to avoid interfering with sexual encounter ▪ Ability to leave in place up to 24 h	▪ May be difficult to insert and/or remove ▪ May be dislodged during intercourse ▪ Not proven to protect against HIV or other STI transmission ▪ May increase the risk of TSS ▪ Fitted diaphragms require refitting after childbirth or weight change (5-10 kg) ▪ Use of N-9 spermicides with a diaphragm may increase risk of UTI
Cervical cap[17,19]	9% in women who have not given birth 26% in women who have given birth	20% in women who have not given birth 40% in women who have given birth[b]	▪ Provides immediate protection ▪ Ability to insert in advance to avoid interfering with sexual encounter ▪ Ability to leave in place up to 48 h, allowing spontaneous intercourse ▪ Requires less acid-buffering gel than a diaphragm	▪ May be difficult to insert and/or remove[c] ▪ May be dislodged during intercourse ▪ No protection from HIV or other STI transmission ▪ May increase the risk of TSS ▪ Not as effective in women who have had a vaginal birth ▪ Not suitable for every woman as size, shape and position of cervix determine proper fit ▪ Unpleasant odour may occur if used for longer than 48 h
Contraceptive sponge[17,21,22]	9% in women who have not given birth 20% in women who have given birth	20% in women who have not given birth 40% in women who have given birth	▪ Provides immediate protection ▪ Ability to insert in advance to avoid interfering with sexual encounter ▪ Offers protection for 24 h even with repeated intercourse ▪ Small, comfortable, easy to carry ▪ No HCP interaction required	▪ May be difficult to insert and/or remove ▪ No protection from HIV or other STI transmission ▪ May increase the risk of TSS; should not be used in women with history TSS ▪ May produce a vaginal discharge, itching or odor ▪ Should not be used during menses ▪ N-9 in the sponge may increase risk of UTI
Female con-dom[17,23,24,25]	5%	21%	▪ Provides immediate protection ▪ Ability to insert up to 8 h in advance to avoid interfering with sexual encounter	▪ May be difficult to learn to use correctly ▪ Part of the condom hangs outside the vagina

(cont'd)

Table 1: **Nonhormonal Contraception Failure Rates, Advantages and Disadvantages** *(cont'd)*

Method	Failure with Correct and Consistent Use	Failure with Typical Use	Advantages	Disadvantages
			▪ Offers protection against HIV and other STI transmission ▪ May be used with oil- or water-based lubricants as not latex based ▪ May be used during menses ▪ May be used in women with history TSS or UTI ▪ May be used in latex-allergic individuals ▪ No HCP interaction required	▪ The condom makes noise during intercourse ▪ Should not be used concurrently with male condoms as they may stick together and result in slippage or breakage
Male condom[26]	2%	18%	▪ Inexpensive ▪ Convenient to obtain ▪ Easy to use and carry ▪ Provides immediate protection ▪ Offers protection against HIV and other STI transmission (latex, polyisoprene and polyurethane varieties only) ▪ No HCP interaction required	▪ May be difficult to put on correctly and may not stay in place ▪ May break or slip and decrease effectiveness ▪ May negatively affect sexual encounters through embarrassment, interruption to put on, inability to maintain an erection, reduced sensation, and need for prompt withdrawal after intercourse
N-9 spermicides (alone)[17,27,28]	18%	29%	▪ Easy to use and carry ▪ Provides immediate protection ▪ No HCP interaction required ▪ Do not cause systemic effects	▪ May negatively affect sexual encounters as repeated application is required before each act of intercourse ▪ Messy, may have unpleasant odour and/or taste ▪ May irritate vagina and/or penis ▪ No protection from HIV or other STI transmission. May increase the risk of HIV transmission. ▪ Use with a diaphragm may increase risk of UTI
Copper IUD[29,30,31]	0.6%	0.8%	▪ Provides protection from 30 months up to 10 y (depending on device) ▪ No interference with sexual encounters	▪ No protection from HIV or other STI transmission ▪ Trained HCP required to insert and remove the IUD ▪ Initial cost may be high, although may be cost-effective over time ▪ May cause periods to become heavier or menstrual cramps to increase ▪ Complications are rare but may include irregular bleeding or spotting, infection, perforation of the uterus or expulsion

[a] Determining failure rates with FABMs has proven to be difficult as the published studies have serious methodological limitations (such as high discontinuation rates and excluding data during the learning phase which results in favoring the method being studied).[10,12] Despite these limitations, reviews[10,13] report the percentages of unintended pregnancy as presented here.

[b] A Cochrane review concluded that the FemCap was not as effective as a diaphragm in preventing pregnancy.[20]

[c] Cervical caps may be more difficult to insert than a diaphragm.

Abbreviations: HCP = healthcare practitioner; IUD = intrauterine device; N-9 = nonoxynol-9; STI = sexually transmitted infection; TSS = toxic shock syndrome; UTI = urinary tract infection

Hormonal Contraceptive Methods

For more information on hormonal contraceptive therapy, consult the *Compendium of Therapeutic Choices:* Contraception.

Estrogen and Progestogen Combinations

Products containing combinations of estrogen and progestogen work primarily by inhibiting ovulation.[79,80] Other mechanisms that may contribute to the action of combined products include thickening of the cervical mucus which impedes sperm from entering the cervix, interference with fertilization by altering tubal motility of the ovum, and inflammation and atrophy of the endometrial lining.[79]

Combination oral contraceptive pills (COCs) contain varying amounts of ethinyl estradiol and different amounts and types of progestogens. Many brand-name and generic options are available. The pills are usually taken in a cyclical manner: active pills are taken for 21 days followed by a 7-day hormone-free interval. The hormone-free interval consists of placebo pills, or no pills at all. COCs that have a shortened pill-free interval (4 days) and extended cycles (pill-free intervals every 84 days) are also available. Failure rates range from 0.3% when used correctly and consistently, to 9% with typical use.[81] COCs may also be given continuously (no pill-free days).[82]

The **transdermal contraceptive patch** (Evra) contains ethinyl estradiol and the progestogen norelgestromin. It is applied in a cyclical manner: one patch is applied once weekly for 3 weeks followed by a 1-week hormone-free interval. Failure rates range from 0.3% when used correctly and consistently, to 9% with typical use.[81] Patches may also be administered continuously (no hormone-free days).[82]

The **vaginal contraceptive ring** (NuvaRing) contains ethinyl estradiol and the progestogen etonorgestrel. It is also used in a cyclical manner: one ring inserted into the vagina and left in place for 3 weeks, followed by a 1-week hormone-free interval. Failure rates range from 0.3% when used correctly and consistently, to 9% with typical use.[81] Vaginal rings may also be administered continuously (no hormone-free days).[82]

Progestogen-only Contraceptives

The **progestogen-only pill** or mini-pill (Micronor) contains **norethindrone**; it works primarily by causing changes to the cervical mucus making it less hospitable to sperm.[80] The progestogen-only pill is taken daily with no hormone-free interval. As the mechanism of action is time-dependent, it is important that the progestogen-only pill be taken at the same time each day; a delay greater than 3 hours is considered a missed pill. Failure rates range from 0.3% when used correctly and consistently, to 9% with typical use.[81]

Depot **medroxyprogesterone acetate** (DMPA) injection (Depo-Provera) contains medroxyprogesterone acetate which is absorbed slowly from the injection site. The primary mechanism of action of DMPA is to suppress ovulation.[80] It is injected intramuscularly every 12–13 weeks. Failure rates range from 0.2% when used correctly and consistently, to 6% with typical use.[81]

The **levonorgestrel intrauterine system** (LNG-IUS) contains levonorgestrel on a vertical stem. Like the copper IUD it offers the same "foreign body" mechanism of action plus the levonorgestrel causes thickening of the cervical mucus, an antiproliferative effect on the endometrium and possible suppression of ovulation in some women. There are 2 products available in Canada. The Mirena IUS releases LNG 20 µg/day and should be replaced every 5 years.[83] The Jaydess IUS releases LNG 6 µg/day and should be replaced every 3 years.[84] Failure rates ranged from 0–1.2% for Mirena[83] and 0.4–0.9% for Jaydess.[84] Jaydess has a smaller and narrower insertion tube than Mirena and therefore it may be an option for women with small and/or narrow uterine cavities. Long-acting reversible contraception such as a levonorgestrel IUS is preferred in young women at high risk of contraceptive failure due to incorrect or inconsistent use.[76,77,78]

Emergency Contraception

For more information on emergency contraception, consult the *Compendium of Therapeutic Choices:* Contraception.

Table 4 lists selected products for emergency contraception.

For comparative ingredients of nonprescription products, consult the *Compendium of Products for Minor Ailments*—Contraceptive Products: Emergency Contraceptives.

Emergency contraception (EC) is a means of avoiding unplanned pregnancies. EC must be used after having unprotected sex but before implantation occurs. It offers no protection against HIV or other STI transmission. EC is meant to be used after an isolated act of intercourse and should not be relied upon as a routine method of contraception because it is not as effective as contraceptives used on a regular basis. Examples of situations that warrant EC include unprotected intercourse, a broken condom, displacement of a diaphragm or cervical cap during intercourse, sexual assault, missed doses of regular birth control or other errors in the use of a regular contraceptive method.[90]

Methods of EC include the use of hormones or IUDs. Hormonal methods are the most commonly used. **Levonorgestrel** is the progestogen-only method. **Estrogen/progestogen** combinations are also known as the Yuzpe method. **Ulipristal** is an anti-progestogen used for EC.[91,92]

Hormonal EC is normally used within 72 hours of unprotected intercourse and is more effective the earlier it is used. There is some evidence that hormonal EC may be somewhat effective beyond the 72-hour period, up to 5 days after intercourse. Insertion of an IUD can be used as a method of EC up to 7 days after unprotected intercourse.[87,91]

A Cochrane review concluded that ulipristal was marginally more effective than levonorgestrel, and levonorgestrel was more effective than the Yuzpe method. The copper IUD was noted as being the most effective EC method, offering the added benefit of providing ongoing contraception.[93]

Copper Intrauterine Device (IUD)

The postcoital insertion of a copper IUD is a highly effective means of EC.[94] To avoid the risk of use after implantation, insertion within 5 days of unprotected intercourse was typically recommended.[95] However, evidence suggests that the copper IUD is effective if inserted within 2–10 days of unprotected intercourse.[87,91,95] The 2015 Canadian Contraception Consensus by the Society of Obstetricians and Gynaecologists of Canada (SOGC) recommends copper IUDs be used for EC up to 7 days after unprotected intercourse, provided pregnancy has been ruled out and there are no other contraindications to use.[39]

Another benefit of the use of a copper IUD for EC is that it can be left in place and used as an effective contraceptive method for the life of the device. Obtaining an IUD for this indication is not as easy as the Yuzpe or levonorgestrel options. Insertion of an IUD requires a trained professional and a pelvic examination.

Mechanism of Action

The popularity of the copper IUD as a choice for EC may have been negatively affected due to the belief that IUDs function as an abortifacient.[96] This is based on one of the proposed mechanisms of action: that IUDs function by preventing implantation of a fertilized ovum. A scientific statement from the WHO argued that it was unlikely that the efficacy of IUDs was based mainly or exclusively on their ability to interfere with implantation.[97] They added that IUDs most likely interfere with steps in the reproductive process that occur before fertilization of the ovum, e.g., direct toxic effect on the sperm. After reviewing the available evidence, the American College of Obstetricians and Gynecologists also concluded that IUDs do not function as an abortifacient.[98]

Efficacy

The copper IUD is a highly effective means of EC, reducing the risk of pregnancy by 99%.[87]

Adverse Effects

IUDs can cause vaginal bleeding and uterine cramping. Insertion of the IUD can be painful.[87]

Progestogen-only (Levonorgestrel)

Mechanism of Action

The precise mechanism of action of LNG in EC has not been clearly elucidated but is believed to be multifactorial. If LNG is given in the first half of the menstrual cycle it will prevent or postpone ovulation.[90] The progestogen also causes thickening of the cervical mucus, which will alter sperm mobility and migration. LNG may interfere with implantation by altering the endometrium but data are conflicting. It has also been suggested that LNG alters Fallopian tube motility but currently no data support this suggestion. The mechanism of action is likely a combination of the above, and may depend somewhat on when LNG is given in relation to the time of unprotected intercourse and the phase of the menstrual cycle. LNG has no effect on an existing pregnancy.[90]

Efficacy

Several studies have evaluated the efficacy of LNG as a method of emergency contraception. Eight studies including over 9500 women reported a reduction in rate of pregnancies ranging from 59–94%.[87] In one of the largest multicentre comparative clinical trials (including almost 2000 women), the LNG method produced a slightly better response than the Yuzpe method.[85] Pregnancy rates were 3.2% and 1.1% with the Yuzpe and LNG methods, respectively. Efficacy was highly dependent on the timing of the first dose relative to the time of unprotected intercourse. If the first dose was given within 24 hours, pregnancy rates were 2% and 0.4% for Yuzpe and LNG, respectively. At 25–48 hours post-intercourse, pregnancy rates rose to 4.1% and 1.2%, and at 49–72 hours to 4.7% and 2.2% respectively.

The efficacy of levonorgestrel may be reduced with increased body weight or BMI.[99] In March 2014, Health Canada issued an advisory to inform women and healthcare practitioners that levonorgestrel emergency contraceptives are less effective in women weighing 75–80 kg and ineffective in women weighing more than 80 kg.[88] In May 2014, SOGC responded to Health Canada's advisory and concluded that, until further evidence is available, women who do not have access to or do not wish to use alternative emergency contraceptive methods (such as copper IUDs) should not be discouraged from using levonorgestrel-only emergency contraception as it may still provide some benefit.[89] The European Medicines Agency completed an extensive review and recommends that emergency contraceptives containing levonorgestrel continue to be used irrespective of body weight as the benefits outweigh the risks.[100,101]

Adverse Effects

There is a lower incidence of adverse effects reported with the levonorgestrel regimen compared with the Yuzpe method. In a comparative trial, adverse effects of the levonorgestrel and Yuzpe groups were nausea (23.1% vs. 50.5%), vomiting (5.6% vs. 18.8%), dizziness (11.2% vs. 16.7%), fatigue (16.9%

vs. 28.5%), headache (16.8% vs. 20.2%), breast tenderness (10.8% vs. 12.1%) and lower abdominal pain (17.6% vs. 20.9%).[85] If vomiting occurs within 2 hours of administration, some practitioners recommend the dose be repeated.[92]

Irregular spotting and breakthrough bleeding have been reported in studies as ranging in incidence from 3–37%.[86] Menses should occur within 1 week of the normally expected time after administration of LNG. If menses does not occur, the woman should be assessed for possible pregnancy.[90]

Despite levonorgestrel not being recognized as a major teratogen, pregnancy is still considered a contraindication to its use for EC. Levonorgestrel has no known adverse effects on clotting factors, so its use in women with a history of thromboembolism and migraine with aura is safer than the Yuzpe method.[102]

Administration and Instructions for Use

LNG is packaged both as a single 1.5 mg tablet and as two 0.75 mg tablets, to be taken together to make a 1.5 mg dose. The tablets (1 or 2 depending on the product) should be taken as soon as possible (within 72 hours) after unprotected intercourse.[103] As noted previously, LNG may be taken up to 120 hours after unprotected intercourse although the efficacy will be lower than when it is taken earlier.[87] Women should be advised of the common adverse effects. If menses does not occur within 3 weeks of the dose, assess for possible pregnancy. Administration of LNG will not protect against future acts of unprotected intercourse. Therefore, her customary method of contraception should be resumed (see Table 2). Alternatively, she may abstain from sex or use backup contraception until menses occurs, then restart contraception after the next menstrual period starts as per usual "start" instructions; she should continue to abstain from sex or use backup contraception until the method is effective. Women may be referred as needed to an appropriate healthcare practitioner for additional counseling regarding ongoing contraceptive methods and/or STI services.

Estrogen-progestogen Combinations

The use of an estrogen/progestogen combination for emergency contraception was first described by Yuzpe et al. in 1974.[105] Various brands of oral contraceptives can be used to obtain the correct dose of hormones (see Table 3). As this method is less effective and has more side effects than levonorgestrel or ulipristal, SOGC recommends that it be used only when other methods are not available.[106]

Table 2: **Resumption of Contraception After Emergency Contraception (EC)**[87,104]

Contraceptive Method	When to Resume
Barrier methods	With next sexual intercourse.
Combination hormonal methods (oral, patch, ring)	Initiate new pack/product 1 day after EC. Abstain from sex or use backup contraception for 7 days until the method is effective.
Medroxyprogesterone acetate injection (DMPA)	Perform a pregnancy test the day after EC to rule out a pre-existing pregnancy. If negative, inject DMPA and abstain from sex or use backup contraception for 7 days. Repeat pregnancy test 2–3 wk after injection.
Progestin-only pill	Continue the day after EC. Abstain from sex or use backup contraception for 48 h.
Copper intrauterine device	Insert after start of next menses. Abstain from sex or use backup contraception before IUD is inserted and, once inserted, until it is effective as per manufacturer's recommendation.
Levonorgestrel intrauterine system	Insert the day after EC. Abstain from sex or use backup contraception for 7 days until the method is effective.

Table 3: **Examples of Estrogen/Progestogen Combinations for Emergency Contraception**

Brand Name	Estrogen	Progestin	1st Dose	2nd Dose
Alesse	ethinyl estradiol 20 µg	levonorgestrel 100 µg	5 tablets po	5 tablets po
MinOvral	ethinyl estradiol 30 µg	levonorgestrel 150 µg	4 tablets po	4 tablets po
Triquilar	ethinyl estradiol 30 µg	levonorgestrel 125 µg	4 yellow tablets po	4 yellow tablets po

Mechanism of Action

Several possible mechanisms of action have been proposed for the Yuzpe method. These mechanisms depend on the point in the menstrual cycle at which the hormones are administered. EC will either delay ovulation, or result in anovulation if taken before ovulation occurs.[91] The progestogen component will also cause thickening of the cervical mucus.[90]

Efficacy

Failure rates reported in trials using the Yuzpe method have ranged from 0.2–7.4%.[107] A meta-analysis of 8 studies estimated that the Yuzpe method probably prevented 74% of pregnancies.[108] The efficacy of the Yuzpe method is higher when taken closer to the time of unprotected intercourse and decreases over time. A WHO Task Force study showed that delaying the first dose of the Yuzpe method from 12–24 hours after intercourse increased the risk of pregnancy by up to 50%.[107]

Adverse Effects

Nausea (50%) and vomiting (20%) are the most commonly reported adverse effects of the Yuzpe method.[87] For this reason, the use of an antinauseant (e.g., dimenhydrinate) 1 hour before the hormone doses is recommended. If vomiting occurs up to 2 hours after administration of the hormone dose, some practitioners recommend that the dose be repeated.[87]

Other possible side effects include headache, dizziness, fatigue, mood changes, menstrual irregularities, vaginal bleeding and abdominal pain.[94]

Regular menses should occur on the expected day, but the Yuzpe method can delay menses by a few days. Approximately 11.5% of women experience a delay of greater than 3 days beyond expected menses.[109]

Pregnancy is the only contraindication to the Yuzpe method; past history of thromboembolism and migraine with aura are relative contraindications.[108,110] Pregnancy itself probably poses a far greater risk of thromboembolism to women with a previous history of embolic events than the Yuzpe method.[94] The risk of thromboembolism due to pregnancy in this population has been estimated to be 60 per 100 000 women.[94] The risk of thromboembolism due to the Yuzpe method is unknown, but 3 cases of venous thromboembolism have been reported in the United Kingdom after approximately 4 million uses.[110]

Administration and Instructions for Use

The first dose of the Yuzpe method (4–5 tablets, depending on the oral contraceptive product being used—see Table 3) should be taken as soon as possible (within 72 hours) after unprotected intercourse. As noted previously, this method may be used up to 120 hours after unprotected intercourse although the efficacy will be lower. The second dose of the Yuzpe method should be given 12 hours after the first dose.[87] If menses does not occur within 3 weeks of the dose, assess for possible pregnancy.

Administration of the EC will not protect against future acts of unprotected intercourse. Therefore, a woman should abstain from intercourse or use a method of contraception until her next menses occurs. Her customary method of contraception may be resumed as per the suggestions in Table 2. Women may be referred as needed to an appropriate healthcare practitioner for additional counselling regarding ongoing contraceptive methods and/or STI services.

Ulipristal

In 2015, ulipristal acetate 30 mg was approved in Canada for prevention of pregnancy when taken within 120 hours (5 days) of unprotected intercourse or known or suspected contraceptive failure.[111]

Mechanism of Action

Ulipristal is a selective progesterone receptor modulator that prevents progesterone from occupying its receptor by competitive inhibition. The primary mechanism of action for emergency contraception is believed to be inhibition or delay of ovulation.

Efficacy

Two multicenter clinical trials found ulipristal significantly reduced the risk of pregnancy after unprotected intercourse from an estimated expected rate of 5.5% to observed rates of 2.1% and 1.78%. Pregnancy rates did not rise significantly when ulipristal was taken later (up to 120 hours after unprotected intercourse) compared with immediately after.[112]

As with levonorgestrel, the efficacy of ulipristal may be reduced with increased body weight or BMI. A subgroup analysis of pooled data from the two phase III clinical trials shows no significant reduction in observed pregnancy rate compared with the expected pregnancy rate for women with a BMI >30 kg/m^2 and an extensive review by the European Medicines Agency (EMA) determined there are limited and inconclusive data on the effect of high body weight/high BMI on the contraceptive efficacy of ulipristal.[112] The EMA recommends that emergency contraceptives containing ulipristal continue to be used irrespective of weight as the benefits outweigh the risks.[100,101]

Adverse Effects

The most common adverse reactions reported in the trials were headache, nausea, abdominal pain, dysmenorrhea, fatigue and dizziness. While limited human data do not suggest a safety concern with ulipristal exposure during pregnancy, it is contraindicated in women with known or suspected pregnancy. Due to its high-affinity binding to the progesterone receptor, use of ulipristal may reduce the contraceptive action of progestogen-containing hormonal contraceptive methods. After use of ulipristal, a reliable barrier method of contraception should be used with subsequent acts of intercourse that occur in that same menstrual cycle.[112]

Administration and Instructions for Use

Ulipristal is available as a single 30 mg tablet. The tablet should be taken as soon as possible (within 120 hours) after unprotected intercourse or known or suspected contraceptive failure. Women should be advised of potential adverse effects. If menses does not occur within 3 weeks of the dose, assess for possible pregnancy. Administration of ulipristal will not protect against future acts of unprotected intercourse. Women should abstain from intercourse or use a barrier method of contraception until the next menses occurs. If a woman wishes to start or continue hormonal contraception after taking ulipristal, it is recommended that she wait 5 days as ulipristal may reduce the efficacy of the hormonal contraceptive. Abstinence or backup contraception is advised for those 5 days and the first 14 days after the hormonal contraceptive is initiated. Women may be referred as needed to an appropriate healthcare practitioner for additional counselling regarding ongoing contraceptive methods and/or STI services.[106,112]

Surgical Methods of Contraception

Procedures

Surgical methods of contraception (sterilization) are one of the most effective methods of contraception. In women, this is most commonly achieved by cutting or occluding the Fallopian tubes, thus blocking fertilization.[113] Failure rates are 0.5% when used correctly (adherence to postprocedural instructions) and are the same with typical use.[81] In men, the vas deferens is blocked or occluded (vasectomy) so that sperm can no longer pass into the ejaculate and out of the body.[113] Failure rates range from 0.1% when used correctly (adherence to postprocedural instructions) to 0.15% with typical use.[81]

Table 4: Selected Products for Emergency Contraception

Class	Drug	Dosage	Adverse Effects	Drug Interactions	Comments	Cost[a]
Contraceptives, emergency postcoital: intrauterine device (IUD)	*copper IUD* Flexi-T, Nova-T	Use within 7 days of unprotected intercourse as an emergency contraceptive	Major: Salpingitis, uterine perforation, cervical perforation, endometrial embedding, menorrhagia, pain, infection, ectopic pregnancy.	None	Interferes with implantation after fertilization. Can be used as ongoing method of contraception.	$70–180
Contraceptives, emergency postcoital: oral progestin	*levonorgestrel* Contingency One, Next Choice, NorLevo, Option 2, Plan B	1.5 mg po (1 x 1.5 mg tablet or 2 × 0.75 mg tablets taken together) as soon as possible after unprotected intercourse (most effective if taken within 72 h)	Nausea, abdominal pain, fatigue, headache, dizziness, breast tenderness (incidence is generally lower than with Yuzpe method);[85] spotting, breakthrough bleeding.[86]	Carbamazepine, griseofulvin, modafinil, phenobarbital, phenytoin, protease inhibitors, St. John's wort, topiramate may decrease levonorgestrel serum concentrations.	May be taken up to 120 h after unprotected intercourse but efficacy will be lower.[87] Heath Canada advisory regarding reduced effectiveness in women weighing 75–80 kg and lack of effectiveness in women weighing ≥80 kg.[88] SOGC recommends women who do not have access to or do not wish to use alternative emergency contraceptive methods should not be discouraged from using levonorgestrel-only emergency contraception as it may still provide some benefit.[89]	$16

(cont'd)

Table 4: **Selected Products for Emergency Contraception** *(cont'd)*

Class	Drug	Dosage	Adverse Effects	Drug Interactions	Comments	Cost[a]
Contraceptives, emergency postcoital: oral selective progesterone receptor modulator	*ulipristal* Ella	30 mg po within 120 h of unprotected intercourse or known or suspected contraceptive failure	Nausea (9%), headache (9%), dysmenorrhea (5%), abdominal pain (5%), fatigue (3.5%), dizziness (3.3%).	CYP3A4 inducers (e.g. rifampicin, phenytoin, phenobarbital, carbamazepine, St. John's wort, barbiturates, carbamazepine, topiramate) may decrease serum concentrations and result in decreased efficacy. CYP3A4 inhibitors increase serum concentrations. Ulipristal binds to the progesterone receptor with high affinity and may interfere with the action of progestogen-containing medicinal products. Contraceptive action of combined hormonal contraceptives and progestogen-only contraception may be reduced. Concomitant use of ulipristal and emergency contraception containing levonorgestrel is not recommended.	Not intended for use as a routine contraceptive. Efficacy not evaluated in women with a BMI ≥35 kg/m^2.	$26

[a] Cost of 1 dose; includes drug cost only.

Resource Tips

Action Canada for Sexual Health & Rights. Available from: www.sexualhealthandrights.ca.

Society of Obstetricians and Gynaecologists of Canada. SexualityandU.ca. Available from: www.sexualityandu.ca.

Suggested Readings

Black A, Guilbert E et al. SOGC Clinical Practice Guideline. Canadian Contraception Consensus (Part 1 of 4). *J Obstet Gynaecol Can* 2015;37:S1-28. Available from: sogc.org/wp-content/uploads/2015/11/gui329Pt1CPG1510E.pdf.

Black A, Guilbert E et al. SOGC Clinical Practice Guideline. Canadian Contraception Consensus (Part 2 of 4). *J Obstet Gynaecol Can* 2015;37:S1-39. Available from: sogc.org/wp-content/uploads/2015/11/gui329Pt2CPG1511E.pdf.

Black A, Guilbert E et al. SOGC Clinical Practice Guideline. Canadian Contraception Consensus (Part 3 of 4): Chapter 7–intrauterine contraception. *J Obstet Gynaecol Can* 2016;38:182-222. Available from: www.jogc.com/article/S1701-2163%2815%2900024-9/pdf.

Pallone SR, Bergus GR. Fertility awareness-based methods: another option for family planning. *J Am Board Fam Med* 2009;22:147-57.

References

1. Statistics Canada. *Births, estimates, by province and territory.* Available from: www.statcan.gc.ca/tables-tableaux/sum-som/l01/cst01/demo04a-eng.htm. Accessed April 21, 2016.
2. Canadian Institute for Health Information. *Induced abortions reported in Canada in 2013*. Available from: www.cihi.ca/en/quick-stats. Accessed April 21, 2016.
3. Altfeld S, Handler A, Burton D et al. Wantedness of pregnancy and prenatal health behaviors. *Women Health* 1997;26:29-43.
4. Wellings K, Wadsworth J, Johnson A et al. Teenage fertility and life chances. *Rev Reprod* 1999;4:184-90.
5. Botting B, Rosato M, Wood R. Teenage mothers and the health of their children. *Popul Trends* 1998;(93):19-28.
6. Fisher W, Boroditsky R, Morris B. The 2002 Canadian Contraception Study: part 1. *J Obstet Gynaecol Can* 2004;26:580-90.
7. Fisher W, Boroditsky R, Morris B. The 2002 Canadian Contraception Study: part 2. *J Obstet Gynaecol Can* 2004;26:646-56.
8. Committee on Adolescence. Contraception for adolescents. *Pediatrics* 2014;134:e1244-56.
9. Hall JE. The female reproductive system: infertility and contraception. In: Fauci AS et al., eds. *Harrison's principles of internal medicine*. 17th ed. New York: McGraw-Hill; 2008.
10. Pallone SR, Bergus GR. Fertility awareness-based methods: another option for family planning. *J Am Board Fam Med* 2009;22:147-57.
11. Kowal D. Coitus interruptus (withdrawal). In: Hatcher RA, Trussell J, Nelson AL et al., eds. *Contraceptive technology.* 20th rev. ed. New York: Ardent Media; 2011. p. 409-15.
12. Grimes DA, Gallo MF, Halpem V et al. Fertility awareness-based methods for contraception. *Cochrane Database Syst Rev* 2004;(4):CD004860.
13. Smoley BA, Robinson CM. Natural family planning. *Am Fam Physician* 2012;86:924-8.
14. Jennings VH, Burke AF. Fertility awareness-based methods. In: Hatcher RA, Trussell J, Nelson AL et al., eds. *Contraceptive technology.* 20th rev. ed. New York: Ardent Media; 2011. p. 417-34.
15. Kennedy KI, Trussell J. Postpartum contraception and lactation. In: Hatcher RA, Trussell J, Nelson AL et al., eds. *Contraceptive technology.* 20th rev. ed. New York: Ardent Media; 2011. p. 483-511.
16. Freundl G, Frank-Herrmann P, Godehardt E et al. Retrospective clinical trial of contraceptive effectiveness of the electronic fertility indicator Ladycomp/Babycomp. *Adv Contracept* 1998;14:97-108.
17. Cates W, Harwood B. Vaginal barriers and spermicides. In: Hatcher RA, Trussell J, Nelson AL et al., eds. *Contraceptive technology.* 20th ed. New York: Ardent Media; 2011. p. 391-408.
18. Society of Obstetricians and Gynaecologists of Canada. SexualityandU.ca. *Contraceptive methods: Barrier methods*. Available from: www.sexualityandu.ca/health-care-professionals/barrier-methods. Accessed April 21, 2016.
19. Society of Obstetricians and Gynaecologists of Canada. SexualityandU.ca. *Non-hormonal methods: Cervical cap*. Available from: www.sexualityandu.ca/birth-control/non-hormonal-methods. Accessed April 21, 2016.
20. Gallo MF, Grimes DA, Schulz KF. Cervical cap versus diaphragm for contraception. *Cochrane Database Syst Rev* 2002;(4):CD003551.
21. Cates W, Raymond EG. Vaginal spermicides. In: Hatcher RA, Trussell J, Nelson AL et al., eds. *Contraceptive technology.* 18th rev. ed. New York: Ardent Media; 2004. p. 355-60.
22. Society of Obstetricians and Gynaecologists of Canada. SexualityandU.ca. *Contraceptive methods: Sponge*. Available from: www.sexualityandu.ca/health-care-professionals/contraceptive-methods/sponge. Accessed April 21, 2016.
23. *FC2 Condom Research*. Available from: www.fc2femalecondom.com/condom-research/ Accessed April 21, 2016.
24. *FC2 FAQS*. Available from: www.fc2femalecondom.com/faqs/. Accessed April 21, 2016.
25. Centers for Disease Control and Prevention (CDC). U.S. Medical Eligibility Criteria for Contraceptive Use, 2010. *MMWR Recomm Rep* 2010;59(RR-4):1-86.
26. Warner L, Steiner MJ. Male condoms. In: Hatcher RA, Trussell J, Nelson AL et al., eds. *Contraceptive technology.* 20th ed. New York: Ardent Media; 2011. p. 371-89.

27. Society of Obstetricians and Gynaecologists of Canada. SexualityandU.ca. *Birth control FAQs: Sponges & spermicides*. Available from: www.sexualityandu.ca/faqs/birth-control#sponges-spermicides. Accessed April 21, 2016.
28. Hooton TM, Scholes D, Hughes JP et al. A prospective study of risk factors for symptomatic urinary tract infection in young women. *N Engl J Med* 1996;335:468-74.
29. Society of Obstetricians and Gynaecologists of Canada. SexualityandU.ca. *Birth control—non-hormonal methods: intrauterine contraceptive device (the copper IUD)*. Available from: www.sexualityandu.ca/birth-control/birth_control_methods_contraception/non-hormonal-methods. Accessed April 21, 2016.
30. University of Michigan Health System. *Advantages and disadvantages of intrauterine devices (IUDs)*. Available from: www.uofmhealth.org/health-library/tw9523. Accessed April 21, 2016.
31. Medisafe Distribution Inc. *Liberté IUDs*. Available from: medisafecanada.com/products/liberte-iuds/. Accessed April 21, 2016.
32. Dude A, Neustadt A, Martins S et al. Use of withdrawal and unintended pregnancy among females 15-24 years of age. *Obstet Gynecol* 2013;122:595-600.
33. Cycle Technologies. *CycleBeads*. Available from: www.cyclebeads.com/. Accessed April 21, 2016.
34. Grimes DA, Gallo MF, Grigorieva V et al. Fertility awareness-based methods for contraception: systematic review of randomized controlled trials. *Contraception* 2005;72:85-90.
35. Parenteau-Carreau S. The sympto-thermal methods. *Int J Fertil* 1981;26:170-81.
36. Rice FJ, Lanctot CA, Garcia-Devesa C. Effectiveness of the sympto-thermal method of natural family planning: an international study. *Int J Fertil* 1981;26:222-30.
37. de Leizaola MA. [Prospective study of the efficacity of a recent symptomatic-thermal method of natural family planning]. *J Gynecol Obstet Biol Reprod (Paris)* 1998;27:174-80. [French].
38. Scolaro KL, Lloyd KB, Helms KL. Devices for home evaluation of women's health concerns. *Am J Health Syst Pharm* 2008;65:299-314.
39. Black A, Guilbert E et al. SOGC Clinical Practice Guideline. Canadian Contraception Consensus (Part 2 of 4). *J Obstet Gynaecol Can* 2015;37:S1-39. Available from: sogc.org/wp-content/uploads/2015/11/gui329Pt2CPG1511E.pdf.
40. CooperSurgical. *Wide-seal silicone diaphragm kits*. Available from: www.coopersurgical.com/ourproducts/familyplanning/diaphragms/Pages/csland.aspx?LC=Diaphragms. Accessed April 21, 2016.
41. Trimedic Supply Network Ltd. *Caya contoured diaphragm*. Available from: trimedic-inc.com/caya_products.html. Accessed April 21, 2016.
42. MEDintim Personal Healthcare. *Caya contoured diaphragm: instruction manual*. Available from: www.medintim.de/assets/Caya/rzmanualcayadeenaufritnl151026NDWEB.pdf. Accessed April 21, 2016.
43. Cooper Surgical. *Milex arcing style diaphragm*. Available from: www.coopersurgical.com/Products/Detail/Milex-Arcing-Style-Diaphragm. Accessed April 21, 2016.
44. Cooper Surgical. *Milex omniflex style diaphragm*. Available from: www.coopersurgical.com/Products/Detail/Milex-Omniflex-Style-Diaphragm. Accessed April 21, 2016.
45. FemCap Canada. *What is the FemCap?* Available from: www.femcapcanada.ca/femcap-details/. Accessed April 21, 2016.
46. Mayer Laboratories, Inc. *Today Sponge: consumer information leaflet*. Available from: www.todaysponge.com/pdf/todaysponge-pi2.pdf. Accessed April 21, 2016.
47. Beksinska M, Smit J, Mabude Z et al. Performance of the Reality polyurethane female condom and a synthetic latex prototype: a randomized crossover trial among South African women. *Contraception* 2006;73:386-93.
48. Smith AM, Jolley D, Hocking J et al. Does additional lubrication affect condom slippage and breakage? *Int J STD AIDS* 1998;9:330-5.
49. Spruyt A, Steiner MJ, Joanis C et al. Identifying condom users at risk for breakage and slippage: findings from three international sites. *Am J Public Health* 1998;88:239-44.
50. Rosenberg MJ, Waugh MS. Latex condom breakage and slippage in a controlled clinical trial. *Contraception* 1997;56:17-21.
51. Lindberg LD, Sonenstein FL, Ku L et al. Young men's experience with condom breakage. *Fam Plann Perspect* 1997;29:128-31, 140.
52. Smith AM, Jolley D, Hocking J et al. Does penis size influence condom slippage and breakage? *Int J STD AIDS* 1998;9:444-7.
53. Mindel A, Sawleshwarkar S. Condoms for sexually transmissible infection prevention: politics versus science. *Sex Health* 2008;5:1-8.
54. Martin ET, Krantz E, Gottlieb SL et al. A pooled analysis of the effect of condoms in preventing HSV-2 acquisition. *Arch Intern Med* 2009;169:1233-40.
55. Region of Peel. Peel Public Health. Healthy sexuality. *Birth control methods: condoms*. Available from: www.peelregion.ca/health/sexuality/birth-control/methods-condom.htm. Accessed April 21, 2016.
56. Levy DA, Moudiki P, Leynadier F. Deproteinised latex condoms are well tolerated by latex allergic patients. *Sex Transm Infect* 2001;77:202-3.
57. Silverberg C. *Latex versus non-latex condoms*. Available from: sexuality.about.com/od/contraception/a/latexfreecondom.htm. Accessed April 21, 2016.
58. Stacey D. *SKYN—Non latex condoms*. Available from: contraception.about.com/od/malecondom/g/SKYN.htm?p=1. Accessed April 21, 2016.
59. Iyer V, Poddar SS. Update on nonoxynol-9 as vaginal spermicide. *Eur J Contracept Reprod Health Care* 2008;13:339-50.
60. Malow RM, Ziskind D, Jones DL. Use of female controlled microbicidal products for HIV risk reduction. *AIDS Care* 2000;12:581-8.
61. Roddy RE, Cordero M, Cordero C et al. A dosing study of nonoxynol-9 and genital irritation. *Int J STD AIDS* 1993;4:165-70.
62. World Health Organization. WHO/CONRAD technical consultation on nonoxynol-9, World Health Organization, Geneva, 9-10 October 2001: summary report. *Reprod Health Matters* 2002;10:175-81.
63. Public Health Agency of Canada. Nonoxynol-9 and the risk of HIV transmission. *HIV/AIDS Epi Update*; May 2004.
64. Francoeur D, Hanvey L, Miller R et al. Barriers methods. In: Black A, Francoeur D, Rowe T et al., eds. *Canadian contraceptive consensus: part 3 of 3*. Ottawa: SOGC; 2004. p. 362.
65. Shedlovsky L, Belcher D, Levenstein I. Titrations of human seminal fluid with acids and alkalis and their effects on the survival of sperm motility. *Am J Physiol* 1942;136:535.
66. Baker JR. The spermicidal powers of chemical contraceptives: II. Pure substances. *J Hyg (Lond)* 1931;31:189-214.
67. RDO Medical UK Ltd. *Effectiveness: How effective is ContraGel?* Available from: contragel.co.uk/contragel-contraceptive-effectiveness.html. Accessed April 21, 2016.
68. Mauck CK, Baker JM, Barr SP et al. A phase I comparative study of three contraceptive vaginal films containing nonoxynol-9. Postcoital testing and colposcopy. *Contraception* 1997;56:97-102.
69. Mauck CK, Allen S, Baker JM et al. An evaluation of the amount of nonoxynol-9 remaining in the vagina up to 4 h after insertion of a vaginal contraceptive film (VCF) containing 70 mg nonoxynol-9. *Contraception* 1997;56:103-10.
70. *VCF vaginal contraceptive film* [product monograph]. Oyster Bay: Apothecus Pharmaceutical Corp.; 2009.

71. Rivera R, Yacobson I, Grimes D. The mechanism of action of hormonal contraceptives and intrauterine contraceptive devices. *Am J Obstet Gynecol* 1999;181:1263-9.
72. Andersson K, Odlind V, Rybo G. Levonorgestrel-releasing and copper-releasing (Nova T) IUDs during five years of use: a randomized comparative trial. *Contraception* 1994;49:56-72.
73. Dean G, Schwarz EB. Intrauterine contraceptives (IUCs). In: Hatcher RA, Trussell J, Nelson AL et al., eds. *Contraceptive technology.* 20th ed. New York: Ardent Media; 2011. p.147-91.
74. Bayer Inc. *Intrauterine device Nova-T.* Available from: omr.bayer.ca/omr/online/nova-t-pi-en.pdf. Accessed April 21, 2016.
75. Trimedic Supply Network Ltd. *Flexi-T IUD advantage.* Available from: www.trimedic-inc.com/flexi-t_iud_advantage.html. Accessed April 21, 2016.
76. Winner B, Peipert JF, Zhao Q et al. Effectiveness of long-acting reversible contraception. *N Engl J Med* 2012;366:1998-2007.
77. Committee on Adolescent Health Care Long-Acting Reversible Contraception Working Group, The American College of Obstetricians and Gynecologists. Committee opinion no. 539: adolescents and long-acting reversible contraception: implants and intrauterine devices. *Obstet Gynecol* 2012;120:983-8.
78. Tang JH, Lopez LM, Mody S et al. Hormonal and intrauterine methods for contraception for women aged 25 years and younger. *Cochrane Database Syst Rev* 2012;11:CD009805.
79. Nelson AL, Cwiak C. Combined oral contraceptives (COCs). In: Hatcher RA, Trussell J, Nelson AL et al., eds. *Contraceptive technology.* 20th rev. ed. New York: Ardent Media; 2011. p. 249-341.
80. Fisher WA, Black A. Contraception in Canada: a review of method choices, characteristics, adherence and approaches to counselling. *CMAJ* 2007;176:953-61.
81. Trussell J, Guthrie KA. Choosing a contraceptive: efficacy, safety and personal considerations. In: Hatcher RA, Trussell J, Nelson AL et al., eds. *Contraceptive technology.* 20th rev. ed. New York: Ardent Media; 2011. p. 45-74.
82. Edelman A, Micks E, Gallo MF et al. Continuous or extended cycle vs. cyclic use of combined hormonal contraceptives for contraception. *Cochrane Database Syst Rev* 2014;(7):CD004695.
83. CPS online. Ottawa: Canadian Pharmacists Association; 2014. *Mirena* [product monograph]. Available from: www.e-therapeutics.ca. Accessed April 21, 2016. Subscription required.
84. CPS online. Ottawa: Canadian Pharmacists Association; 2014. *Jaydess* [product monograph]. Available from: www.e-therapeutics.ca. Accessed April 21, 2016. Subscription required.
85. Task Force on Postovulatory Methods of Fertility Regulation. Randomised controlled trial of levonorgestrel versus the Yuzpe regimen of combined oral contraceptives for emergency contraception. *Lancet* 1998;352:428-33.
86. Raymond EG, Goldberg A, Trussell J et al. Bleeding patterns after use of levonorgestrel emergency contraceptive pills. *Contraception* 2006;73:376-81.
87. Trussell J, Schwarz EB. Emergency contraceptives. In: Hatcher RA, Trussell J, Nelson AL et al., eds. *Contraceptive technology.* 20th rev. ed. New York: Ardent Media; 2011. p. 113-45.
88. Government of Canada. Healthy Canadians. *Emergency contraceptive pills to carry warnings for reduced effectiveness in women over a certain body weight.* March 2014. Available from: healthycanadians.gc.ca/recall-alert-rappel-avis/hc-sc/2014/38701a-eng.php.
89. Society of Obstetricians and Gynaecologists of Canada. Position statement [in response to Health Canada's Emergency contraceptive pills to carry warnings for reduced effectiveness in women over a certain body weight]. May 2014. Available from: sogc.org/wp-content/uploads/2014/05/medStatementEC_BMI_1400502E.pdf.
90. Allen RH, Goldberg AB. Emergency contraception: a clinical review. *Clin Obstet Gynecol* 2007;50:927-36.
91. Bastianelli C, Farris M, Benagiano G. Emergency contraception: a review. *Eur J Contracept Reprod Health Care* 2008;13:9-16.
92. Dunn S, Guilbert E. Emergency contraception. *J Obstet Gynaecol Can* 2012;34:870-8.
93. Cheng L, Che Y, Gulmezoglu AM. Interventions for emergency contraception. *Cochrane Database Syst Rev* 2012;8:CD001324.
94. LaValleur J. Emergency contraception. *Obstet Gynecol Clin North Am* 2000;27:817-39.
95. Cleland K, Zhu H, Goldstuck N et al. The efficacy of intrauterine devices for emergency contraception: a systematic review of 35 years of experience. *Hum Reprod* 2012;27:1994-2000.
96. Sivin I. IUDs are contraceptives, not abortifacients: a comment on research and belief. *Stud Fam Plann* 1989;20:355-9.
97. Mechanism of action, safety and efficacy of intrauterine devices. Report of a WHO Scientific Group. *World Health Organ Tech Rep Ser* 1987;753:1-91.
98. American College of Obstetricians and Gynecologists. *The intrauterine device.* ACOG Technical Bulletin 104. Washington: ACOG; 1987.
99. Glasier A, Cameron ST, Blithe D et al. Can we identify women at risk of pregnancy despite using emergency contraception? Data from randomized trials of ulipristal acetate and levonorgestrel. *Contraception* 2011;84:363-7.
100. European Medicines Agency. *Assessment report. For emergency contraceptive medicinal products containing levonorgestrel or ulipristal.* 2014; EMA/464144/2014. Available from: www.ema.europa.eu/docs/en_GB/document_library/EPAR_-_Assessment_Report_-_Variation/human/001027/WC500176357.pdf.
101. European Medicines Agency. *Levonorgestrel and ulipristal remain suitable emergency contraceptives for all women, regardless of bodyweight.* 2014; EMA/440549/2014. Available from: www.ema.europa.eu/docs/en_GB/document_library/Press_release/2014/07/WC500170056.pdf.
102. Glasier A. Safety of emergency contraception. *J Am Med Womens Assoc* 1998;53:219-21.
103. CPS online. Ottawa: Canadian Pharmacists Association; 2015. *Plan B* [information for the patient]. Available from: www.e-therapeutics.ca.
104. International Consortium for Emergency Contraception. *Emergency contraceptive pills: medical and service delivery guidelines.* 3rd ed. 2012. Available from: www.cecinfo.org/custom-content/uploads/2014/01/ICEC_Medical-and-Service-Delivery-Guildelines-English_June-2013.pdf.
105. Yuzpe AA, Thurlow HJ, Ramzy I et al. Post coital contraception–A pilot study. *J Reprod Med* 1974;13:53-8.
106. Black A, Guilbert E et al. SOGC Clinical Practice Guideline. Canadian Contraception Consensus (Part 1 of 4). *J Obstet Gynaecol Can* 2015;37:S1-28. Available from: sogc.org/wp-content/uploads/2015/11/gui329Pt1CPG1510E.pdf.
107. Ho PC. Emergency contraception: methods and efficacy. *Curr Opin Obstet Gynecol* 2000;12:175-9.
108. Trussell J, Rodriguez G, Ellertson C. Updated estimates of the effectiveness of the Yuzpe regimen of emergency contraception. *Contraception* 1999;59:147-51.
109. Ho PC, Kwan MS. A prospective randomized comparison of levonorgestrel with the Yuzpe regimen in post-coital contraception. *Hum Reprod* 1993;8:389-92.

110. Trussell J, Rodriguez G, Ellertson C. New estimates of the effectiveness of the Yuzpe regimen of emergency contraception. *Contraception* 1998;57:363-9.
111. CPS online. Ottawa: Canadian Pharmacists Association; 2015. *Fibristal* [product monograph]. Available from: www.e-therapeutics.ca. Accessed April 21, 2016. Subscription required.
112. HRA Pharma. *ellaOne* [product monograph]. Available from: www.hra-pharma.com/index.php/en/our_products/womens_health/emergency_contraception/ellaone.
113. Roncari d, Hou MY. Female and male sterilization. In: Hatcher RA, Trussell J, Nelson AL et al., eds. *Contraceptive technology.* 20th rev. ed. New York: Ardent Media; 2011. p. 435-82.

Nonhormonal Birth Control—What You Need to Know

What is nonhormonal birth control?

Nonhormonal birth control methods are diaphragms, cervical caps, contraceptive sponges, male and female condoms, spermicides and copper intrauterine devices (IUDs).

Talk to your healthcare provider about different birth control methods. They can help you decide which is best for you. They can also give you information about:

- how to use each kind of birth control properly
- how to protect yourself from pregnancy and sexually transmitted infections (STIs)

Tips on using nonhormonal birth control:

Male Condoms

- When latex, polyisoprene or polyurethane condoms are used correctly, they protect against pregnancy and STIs.
- If you are allergic to latex, talk to your pharmacist about other choices such as polyurethane or polyisoprene condoms.
- Always check the expiry date before using a condom. Don't use a condom if the expiry date has passed. It may not be effective.
- Store condoms in a cool dry place. **Do not** store them in a wallet or a car for a long time.
- Be careful when using condoms. Fingernails and jewelry can tear them.
- For lubrication, use only water-based products such as K-Y jelly. Oil-based products can weaken latex and polyisoprene condoms and make them less effective.
- If the condom doesn't come with a reservoir at the end, make sure to leave some room between the tip of the penis and the tip of the condom to collect sperm when you ejaculate.
- After having sex, withdraw the penis right away. Hold the rim of the condom so that it doesn't slip off when you withdraw.
- If a condom breaks, the female partner should insert some spermicide into the vagina. She might want to talk to her healthcare provider about emergency contraception as well.
- Wrap used condoms in tissue and throw them in the garbage, not the toilet.

Female Condoms

- Female condoms are safe for people who are allergic to latex.
- Female condoms protect against pregnancy and STIs.
- The closed end of the condom goes inside the vagina, up near the cervix. The open end fits around the outside of the vagina.
- Do not use male condoms and female condoms at the same time.

Diaphragm

- A diaphragm is a dome that fits over the cervix to stop sperm from reaching the uterus.
- A diaphragm protects against pregnancy, but not STIs. For protection against STIs, use a condom along with the diaphragm.
- You have to be fitted for some diaphragms by a trained health professional; one diaphragm is available in a single size designed to fit most women.

- Before inserting a diaphragm, put about a teaspoon of acid-buffering gel inside the dome and a bit on the rim.
- You can insert a diaphragm up to 6 hours before having sex. Leave it in place for at least 6 hours after having sex.
- If you have sex more than once while wearing your diaphragm, insert acid-buffering gel into the vagina before each time (without removing the diaphragm).
- **Do not** leave a diaphragm in place for more than 24 hours. You could get toxic shock syndrome.
- **Do not** use a diaphragm during your period or for 6 weeks after having a baby. There is a risk of getting toxic shock syndrome.
- You may need a different size diaphragm after having a baby. Go for refitting about 6–8 weeks after the baby is born.

Cervical Cap

- A cervical cap looks like a diaphragm but is smaller.
- A cervical cap protects against pregnancy, but not STIs. For protection against STIs, use a condom along with the cervical cap.
- The cervical cap fits snugly over the cervix and has to be in the right position to work best. Talk to your doctor or pharmacist about how to get it in the right position.
- Before inserting a cervical cap, fill the inside of the cap to about one-third full with acid-buffering gel, but do not put any on the rim.
- You must leave the cervical cap in place for 6–8 hours after having sex. You can leave it in place for up to 48 hours. You do not have to insert more acid-buffering gel if you have sex more than once during that time.
- **Do not** use a cervical cap during your period or for 6 weeks after having a baby. There is a risk of getting toxic shock syndrome.

Contraceptive Sponge

- A contraceptive sponge protects against pregnancy, but not STIs. For protection against STIs, use a condom along with the contraceptive sponge.
- Look at the package to find out how long before intercourse the sponge can be inserted and how long it can be left in place.
- It must be kept in place for at least 6 hours after intercourse.
- You can have sex more than once while the sponge is in place. Be sure to leave it in place for 6 hours after the last time.

Contraceptive Film

- Contraceptive film protects against pregnancy, but not STIs. For protection against STIs, use a condom along with contraceptive film.
- Contraceptive film contains spermicide. It dissolves into a gel once inside the vagina.
- Insert the film into the vagina 15 minutes to 3 hours (for VCF contraceptive film) before you have sex. Insert a new film every time you have sex.
- The gel disappears on its own after sex. Douching is not necessary and not recommended.

Emergency Contraception (Birth Control)—What You Need to Know

What is emergency contraception?

Emergency contraception (EC) means using a birth control method after you have had unprotected sex, or when another method of birth control fails. There are two main types of emergency contraception—the "morning after pill" (levonorgestrel only, combination oral contraceptive pills, or ulipristal) and insertion of an intrauterine device (IUD). EC prevents pregnancy but it does not *end* a pregnancy that has already occurred (that is, it will *not* work if a woman is already pregnant).

Regularly using emergency contraception as the only method of preventing pregnancy is not advisable. Routine use of other contraceptive methods is more effective. Talk to your healthcare provider about a regular method of birth control. They can tell you about different methods—how effective they are, what the risks are, and how to prevent sexually transmitted diseases.

Information about emergency contraceptive pills (ECP)

- Some ECPs contain a combination of estrogen and progestogen, others contain progestogen only and a third contains ulipristal, which acts on the progesterone receptors.
- ECPs are called the "morning after pill" but they can be used for up to 72–120 hours after unprotected sex.
- Taking ECPs can greatly decrease your chances of getting pregnant after unprotected sex. The sooner they are taken, the better they work, so take them as soon as possible after unprotected sex and follow the directions exactly.
- The **progestogen-only** pills are available in a pharmacy without a prescription. Take the correct number of tablets (1 or 2 depending on the product) at once, with or without food. If you vomit within 2 hours of taking the pill(s), contact your healthcare provider as a repeat dose may be required. Progestogen-only pills may be less effective if your weight is higher than 75 kg (165 lbs). Talk to your healthcare provider; they may suggest alternative emergency contraceptive methods.
- The **ulipristal** pills require a prescription and can be obtained by seeing a healthcare provider. Take 1 tablet, with or without food. If you vomit within 3 hours of taking the ulipristal pill, contact your healthcare provider as a repeat dose is required. Ulipristal may be less effective if your weight is higher than 75 kg (165 lbs). Talk to your healthcare provider; they may suggest alternative emergency contraceptive methods.
- The **combination estrogen/progestogen** pills require a prescription and can be obtained by seeing a healthcare provider. Take these pills in 2 doses, 12 hours apart (for example–10:00 in the morning and 10:00 at night). The timing of the second dose is very important and you should set an alarm or other reminder to remember. As the combination pills can make you sick to your stomach, you should take a medication to prevent nausea (e.g., dimenhydrinate or Gravol) 30–60 minutes before each dose. This method is less effective and has more side effects than the progestogen-only or ulipristal pills and is recommended only when those are not available.
- After taking ECPs, your period should arrive on time (when you would normally expect it), or it might be a few days early or late. If it is more than a week late, or if it arrives more than 3 weeks after you take the pills, you need to have a pregnancy test. Perform a home test or see your healthcare provider.
- Remember—ECPs do not protect you from sexually transmitted infections.
- Talk to your healthcare provider about when to restart your usual method of birth control or when to start a new method.

Chapter 77
Dysmenorrhea

Thomas E.R. Brown, BScPhm, PharmD

CPhA acknowledges the contribution of Katrina Mulherin as a previous author of this chapter.

Reproductive Physiology

Female reproductive physiology revolves around the menstrual cycle. The average length of a menstrual cycle is 28 days, but it can range from 23–35 days. On average, a woman will menstruate 400 times from menarche to menopause.

Female reproduction is regulated by the hypothalamic-pituitary-ovarian (HPO) axis. A normal menstrual cycle begins with the pulsatile release of gonadotropin-releasing hormone (GnRH) from the hypothalamus. The release of GnRH stimulates the pituitary to release follicle-stimulating hormone (FSH) and luteinizing hormone (LH). The rate and amplitude of GnRH pulses from the hypothalamus determine which hormone (FSH or LH) is released by the pituitary. The first day of the menstrual cycle is identified as the first day of menstruation, when recruitment of follicles in the ovary begins. At the start of each new menstrual cycle, FSH stimulates a group of follicles in the ovary. These follicles produce and secrete estradiol. This is known as the follicular phase of the menstrual cycle. By around the seventh day, one follicle becomes dominant, continues to grow and secretes estradiol. Estradiol causes the hypothalamus to decrease GnRH release and therefore FSH declines. This decline causes nondominant follicles to undergo atresia, i.e., they cease to grow and eventually die. Estradiol concentrations rise throughout the follicular phase and peak just prior to ovulation.

The follicular phase of the menstrual cycle in the ovary corresponds to the proliferative phase in the endometrium. Estradiol released through stimulation of the follicles in the ovaries causes the endometrial lining to proliferate.

Ovulation occurs around day 14 of the menstrual cycle. At this time the pituitary increases the secretion of LH. A surge in LH signals the dominant follicle to rupture and release the egg into the Fallopian tube (ovulation). The ruptured follicle undergoes luteinization and becomes the corpus luteum. Progesterone and estradiol are produced and secreted by the corpus luteum.[1] This second half of the menstrual cycle is referred to as the luteal phase. Progesterone and estradiol concentrations rise during the luteal phase. The corpus luteum has a 14-day lifespan; therefore, if fertilization does not occur, the corpus luteum undergoes atresia and progesterone and estradiol concentrations fall.

The luteal phase of the menstrual cycle corresponds to the secretory phase in the endometrium. Progesterone stimulates glandular cells in the endometrium to produce glycogen, mucus and prostaglandins. These changes in the endometrial tissue are known as secretory changes.

If fertilization and implantation do not occur by around day 23 of the menstrual cycle, the corpus luteum regresses, progesterone and estradiol concentrations decline, the endometrium undergoes involution and menstruation begins.

Pathophysiology

Dysmenorrhea is defined as painful menstruation, and can be primary or secondary. Primary dysmenorrhea is attributed to uterine contractions with no underlying pathology whereas secondary dysmenorrhea is due to pelvic disease such as endometriosis, inflammatory disease or uterine polyps.[2] The main focus of this chapter is primary dysmenorrhea.

Prevalence

The reported prevalence of dysmenorrhea ranges from 6–80%, with the most common being 50%. The peak incidence is in women between 20 and 24 years of age, and it decreases with age. Dysmenorrhea is the most common cause of missed school or workdays in young women. Approximately 10% of women will suffer from severe symptoms.[2]

Etiology

Dysmenorrhea occurs as prostaglandins are released from lysing endometrial cells in the luteal phase of an ovulatory cycle. During anovulatory cycles, the endometrial tissue contains smaller amounts of prostaglandins; therefore, these cycles are usually painless.[2] Prostaglandins have a direct effect on the endometrium and surrounding tissues, resulting in the signs and symptoms of dysmenorrhea.[2]

The role of prostaglandins in the pathogenesis of dysmenorrhea is well established. Women with dysmenorrhea have higher concentrations of PGF_2-alpha and PGE_2 in their menstrual fluid than women who do not complain of pain on menstruation.[2] Moreover, administering these prostaglandins by infusion induces the same discomfort and symptoms experienced by women with dysmenorrhea.

Women with dysmenorrhea have increased uterine activity, resulting in increased resting tone, increased strength and frequency of contractions and/or dysrhythmic contractions.[2]

Dysmenorrhea usually begins 6–12 months after menarche and occurs only with ovulatory cycles. It tends to decrease with age and after childbirth.[3,4]

Risk Factors

Onset of dysmenorrhea has been linked with age <30 years, BMI <20, early menarche (<12 years of age), longer cycles and duration of bleeding, heavy or irregular menstrual flow, premenstrual syndrome (PMS), pelvic inflammatory disease, sterilization, sexual assault[4] and smoking.[5] Protective factors may include use of oral contraceptives, exercise, higher parity and fish intake.

Clinical Presentation

The diagnosis of dysmenorrhea is based on the presence of symptoms, a normal pelvic exam and the patient's response to therapy.[3] Individuals who do not respond to a proven therapy should be investigated for causes of secondary dysmenorrhea.[2] Menstrual pain occurs a few hours before or just after menstruation begins and usually lasts for 48–72 hours. The pain is described as cramping and is most intense over the lower abdomen, but it may radiate to the back and inner thighs.[5] Associated symptoms include nausea and vomiting, fatigue, diarrhea and headache.[2]

Goals of Therapy

- Relieve symptoms
- Minimize time lost from work, school and other activities
- Identify patients who may have secondary dysmenorrhea and require further medical assessment

Patient Assessment

Assess patients with dysmenorrhea to confirm that their complaints are consistent with the etiology, signs and symptoms of primary dysmenorrhea (Figure 1). Cues that additional patient evaluation is required include onset of pain more than 2 years postmenarche, symptoms that occur outside the first

3 days of menses, changes in the severity or pattern of the pain or in the characteristics of the menstrual fluid (e.g., degree of flow, odour, colour, flow pattern). Response to a proven therapy for primary dysmenorrhea is usually a confirmation of the diagnosis; therefore, if a trial fails the patient requires further assessment.

Nonpharmacologic Therapy

There is some evidence that exercise may reduce symptoms of dysmenorrhea;[6,7] however, large, well-designed trials are lacking. Regular aerobic exercise can also decrease stress, which may be a contributing factor.[3] A small (n=92) randomized trial suggests particular yoga poses may be beneficial in relieving dysmenorrhea.[8] The high degree of safety of these poses makes this an attractive nonpharmacologic treatment. It is unclear whether diet is associated with dysmenorrhea; however, decreasing fat intake may be of some benefit.[9]

Warm baths or applying a heating pad, heat patch or hot water bottle to the abdomen may reduce discomfort. In a randomized controlled study, heating pads provided pain relief equivalent to the use of ibuprofen. When both heating pads and ibuprofen were used together there was no more pain relief than with either agent used alone; however, pain relief occurred faster when both therapies were combined.[10,11]

A single trial examining the use of a sericite belt (source of infrared rays) with a heat pack found a statistically significant decrease in visual analog scale pain score for patients using the belt. The clinical significance of this finding is doubtful and the trial design may have led to heat packs rather than the belt causing the beneficial effect.[12]

Behavioral interventions such as massage with aromatic oils (lavender, clary sage, marjoram oils 2:1:1 and rose aboolue, rose otto, clary sage, rose geranium and ginger 0.5:0.1:1:1:1),[13,14] relaxation therapy, biofeedback, pain management sessions and coping skills have been studied; however, good quality trials are lacking.[15] Surgical ablation of the pelvic nerve pathways requires further study and is not recommended.[16] Spinal manipulation has not been shown to provide benefit in dysmenorrhea.[17]

High-frequency transcutaneous electric nerve stimulation (TENS) may have some utility in the treatment of dysmenorrhea.[18,19] A Cochrane systematic review (10 trials in 944 subjects) examining the effectiveness of acupressure and acupuncture found some evidence for benefit; however, due to the small number of subjects and studies, further investigation is needed.[20]

For most women, drug therapy is required and nonpharmacologic measures are used adjunctively.[3]

Pharmacologic Therapy

For more information on pharmacologic management of dysmenorrhea, consult the *Compendium of Therapeutic Choices*: Dysmenorrhea.

Pharmacologic agents that decrease the amount of prostaglandins in endometrial tissue or inhibit prostaglandin synthesis are considered first-line therapies for the treatment of dysmenorrhea.

Nonsteroidal Anti-inflammatory Drugs (NSAIDs)

For comparative ingredients of nonprescription products, consult the *Compendium of Products for Minor Ailments*—Analgesic Products: Internal Analgesics and Antipyretics.

NSAIDs reduce the pain of dysmenorrhea by decreasing prostaglandin concentrations in endometrial and menstrual fluid. NSAIDs commonly used in dysmenorrhea are included in Table 1.

Moderate or excellent pain relief is achieved more often with NSAIDs vs. placebo.[21] Many NSAIDs have been used in the management of dysmenorrhea. Some NSAIDs have theoretical advantages in terms of site of action such as acetic acids (e.g., indomethacin), propionic acids (e.g., ibuprofen, naproxen) and fenamates (e.g., mefenamic acid) which reduce prostaglandin concentrations in endometrial and menstrual fluid.[3] Mefenamic acid not only inhibits the formation of prostaglandins but also blocks prostaglandins at the receptor site. The clinical significance of these pharmacologic differences is questionable and head-to-head comparisons of NSAIDs lend little support for recommending one agent over another in terms of efficacy.[21]

The NSAID should be administered with food at the onset of pain or menses and continued for 72 hours, as the peak concentration of prostaglandins occurs in the first 48 hours.[22] An initial loading dose may help obtain faster relief of symptoms. Women who do not obtain adequate relief of symptoms may try starting NSAIDs 1 or 2 days prior to expected menses. NSAIDs should be used for 3 cycles before being declared a treatment failure.[23] If symptoms are not relieved or if pain becomes worse, refer the patient to an appropriate healthcare professional for further assessment.

In terms of safety, NSAIDs have higher overall rates of adverse events (combined GI disturbance, CNS effects and hypersensitivity reactions) compared with placebo. When these events are analyzed separately only CNS adverse effects have been shown to be statistically significant. This finding is based predominantly on 2 trials using indomethacin and naproxen.[21] Safety comparisons among NSAIDs do not indicate the superiority of any agent in this patient population.[21]

NSAIDs have well-documented drug interactions and contraindications which may not be relevant with occasional, short-term use of these agents. In dysmenorrhea, use is generally limited to 3 days; however, the risks may outweigh the benefits and professional judgment must be used.

In several studies, neither acetaminophen nor ASA was better in providing pain relief than placebo.[24,25] Two trials have shown ASA to be inferior to indomethacin and fenoprofen in terms of pain relief.[21] Caution is advised regarding the use of ASA in adolescents or young adults because of the possible association with Reye's syndrome when ASA is used for conditions such as influenza or varicella. Three trials comparing acetaminophen with NSAIDs indicate that NSAIDs provide superior pain relief in dysmenorrhea.[21] Acetaminophen may have value as additive therapy to NSAIDs and in women with intolerance or contraindications to NSAIDs.[26]

Hormonal Contraceptives

If NSAIDs are contraindicated, if they fail or if birth control is also required, a **combined oral contraceptive** (COC) is often used to treat dysmenorrhea. COCs relieve dysmenorrhea symptoms by reducing the amount of prostaglandins in menstrual fluid (because they reduce the actual amount of fluid), and by inhibiting ovulation (dysmenorrhea occurs only in ovulatory cycles).[3] COCs are up to 90% effective in relieving dysmenorrhea symptoms.[27] This evidence is garnered from older formulations of medium- to high-dose estrogens (50–150 µg ethinyl estradiol) plus first- and second-generation progestogens (norgestrel, levonorgestrel or norethindrone). There are insufficient data on low-dose estrogens (≤35 µg ethinyl estradiol) plus first-, second- or third-generation agents (desogestrel, gestodene) or newer progestogens (drospirenone) to suggest they are as effective as the older formulations.[28] However, due to safety concerns, low-dose estrogen preparations (≤35 µg ethinyl estradiol) are currently used. Formulations containing ≥50 µg ethinyl estradiol are no longer available in Canada. Safety data for use of COCs in this specific population (women with dysmenorrhea) are lacking.[27]

According to one randomized, double-blind, controlled trial, continuous COC regimens (3 months) do not appear to offer any benefit beyond cyclic 28-day regimens.[29] While a difference in efficacy between continuous and cyclic regimens may exist, the evidence is weak.[30]

Comparative efficacy of NSAIDs vs. COCs for treating dysmenorrhea is unknown.[27]

The combination of a COC and an NSAID may also be beneficial. About 10% of women do not respond to treatment with NSAIDs, COCs or both.[31]

Levonorgestrel-containing intrauterine systems (IUS) and oral and parenteral **progestogens** may have some benefit in dysmenorrhea.[32] However, larger-scale confirmatory trials are required before use can be recommended.

For further discussion of hormonal contraceptives, consult the *Compendium of Therapeutic Choices*: Contraception.

Other

Pamabrom is a mild diuretic that is marketed in combination with acetaminophen for relief of dysmenorrhea. There are no trials to support the use of this agent in women with dysmenorrhea.

Beta 2-adrenoceptor agonists have been used to treat dysmenorrhea in the past. A 2012 Cochrane systematic review examining these medications (isoxsuprine, terbutaline oral spray, ritodrine or orciprenalin) in dysmenorrhea found little evidence to support their use. Given the lack of data to support efficacy and the known side effect profile of beta 2-adrenoceptor agonists, they are not recommended for use in dysmenorrhea.[33]

Natural Health Products

For comparative ingredients of nonprescription products, consult the *Compendium of Products for Minor Ailments*—Herbal and Natural Products: Single Entity; Vitamin and Mineral Products: Single Entity, Solid Combinations.

Cholecalciferol (vitamin D_3) supplementation may alleviate dysmenorrhea in women with low vitamin D levels. In a small randomized placebo-controlled trial of menstruating women with low vitamin D levels, a single oral dose of 1 mL cholecalciferol (300 000 IU/mL) 5 days before the anticipated commencement of the next menstrual cycle decreased pain intensity and the requirement for NSAID use. Further corroboration of this small trial is required.[34]

Alternative approaches for managing dysmenorrhea include **magnesium** supplements,[24] **omega-3 fatty acids**,[35] transdermal **nitroglycerin**, **vitamin B_1**,[36,37] **vitamin B_6**, **vitamin E**,[37,38,39] shirazi thymus vulgaris[40] and valerian root.[23,37,41,42] These therapies require further study to determine their role in treating dysmenorrhea.

Chinese herbal medicine (individually-designed formulae or standard) has shown positive effects on pain and overall symptoms, and has reduced requirement for further medication.[43] However, the nature of these individualized treatments and variations among the agents used in trials poses difficulty in evaluating Chinese herbal medicines. While the quality of current studies precludes recommendation of these therapies, further investigation seems warranted.

Women who do not respond to standard therapy should discuss these options with their healthcare practitioner.

Monitoring of Therapy

Efficacy: If a patient fails to respond to a 3-cycle trial of an NSAID and/or a combined oral contraceptive in conjunction with nonpharmacologic measures, further assessment is required.

Safety: Inform patients taking medication for dysmenorrhea about common adverse effects and the timeframe associated with them. Instruct patients to report any signs of serious adverse effects to their healthcare practitioner.

Figure 1: **Treatment of Dysmenorrhea**

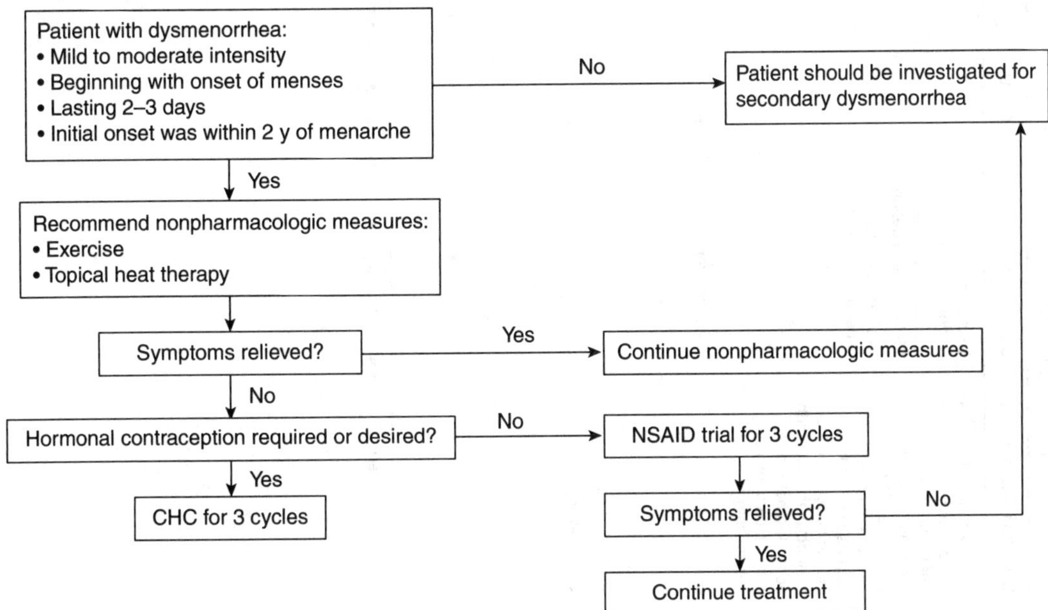

Abbreviations: NSAID = nonsteroidal anti-inflammatory drug; CHC = combined hormonal contraceptive

Table 1: NSAIDs commonly used for Dysmenorrhea

Class	Drug	Dosage	Adverse Effects	Drug Interactions[a]	Comments	Cost[b]
NSAIDs	*ibuprofen* Advil, Advil Liqui-Gels, Motrin, Motrin IB, Motrin Liquid Gels, generics	200–400 mg Q6–8H po; start with onset of pain or menses and continue for 2–3 days Maximum dose for self-care: 1200 mg/day po Usual maximum dose: 2400 mg/day po	Very common (>10%): dyspepsia, nausea/vomiting. Common (5–10%): nonspecific rash, pruritus, dizziness, headache. NSAIDs may be nephrotoxic and should not be used in severe renal impairment.	Anticoagulants (increase risk of bleeding); SSRIs (may increase risk of GI bleeding); decrease effect of antihypertensives, diuretics; may increase lithium levels; may increase levels of methotrexate (with high doses methotrexate); may inhibit phenytoin metabolism.	Take with food to minimize GI upset. Caution in asthmatic or ASA-sensitive patients. Avoid in patients at risk of peptic ulcer and in renal impairment.	$
	naproxen Naprosyn, generics	Loading dose 500 mg po; then 250 mg Q6–8H po or 500 mg BID po Maximum daily dose: 1250 mg/day po	See ibuprofen.	See ibuprofen.	See ibuprofen.	$$
	naproxen sodium Aleve, generics	220–440 mg Q8–12H po; start with onset of pain or menses and continue for 2–3 days Maximum dose for self-care: 440 mg/day po Usual maximum dose: 1375 mg/day po	See ibuprofen.	See ibuprofen.	See ibuprofen.	$

[a] NSAIDs have well-documented drug interactions and contraindications that may not be relevant with occasional, short-term use of these agents. In dysmenorrhea, use is generally limited to 3 days; however, the risks may sometimes outweigh the benefits and professional judgment must be used.

[b] Cost per day; includes drug cost only.

Legend: $ <$1 $$ $1–2

Resource Tips

American College of Obstetricians and Gynecologists. Patient Education Pamphlet. *FAQ: Frequently asked questions. Gynecologic problems. Dysmenorrhea.* Available from: www.acog.org/~/media/For%20Patients/faq046.pdf.

Lefebvre G, Pinsonneault O, Antao V et al. Primary dysmenorrhea consensus guideline. *J Obstet Gynaecol Can* 2005;27:1117-46.

Suggested Readings

Dawood MY. Primary dysmenorrhea: advances in pathogenesis and management. *Obstet Gynecol* 2006;108:428-41.

Borgelt LM, Gunning KM. Disorders related to the menstrual cycle. In: Koda-Kimble MA, Alldredge BK, Corelli RL et al., eds. *Koda-Kimble and Young's applied therapeutics: the clinical use of drugs*. 10th ed. Philadelphia: Wolters Kluwer; Lippincott Williams & Wilkins; 2013. p. 1149-74.

Khan KS, Champaneria R, Latthe PM. How effective are non-drug, non-surgical treatments for primary dysmenorrhea? *BMJ* 2012;344:e3011.

Laufer LR, Gambone JC. Menstrual cycle-influenced disorders. In: Hacker NF, Moore JG, eds. *Essentials of obstetrics and gynecology*. 5th ed. Philadelphia: WB Saunders; 2010. p. 386-9.

Lefebvre G, Pinsonneault O, Antao V et al. Primary dysmenorrhea consensus guideline. *J Obstet Gynaecol Can* 2005;27:1117-46.

Osayande AS, Mehulic S. Diagnosis and initial management of dysmenorrhea. *Am Fam Physician* 2014;89:341-6.

References

1. Gambone JC. Female reproductive physiology. In: Hacker NF, Moore JG, eds. *Essentials of obstetrics and gynecology*. 5th ed. Philadelphia: WB Saunders; 2010. p. 34-45.
2. Laufer LR, Gambone JC. Menstrual cycle-influenced disorders. In: Hacker NF, Moore JG, eds. *Essentials of obstetrics and gynecology*. 5th ed. Philadelphia: WB Saunders; 2010. p. 386-9.
3. Hansen LB, Gunning K. Disorders related to the menstrual cycle. In: Koda-Kimble MA, Young LY et al., eds. *Applied therapeutics: the clinical use of drugs*. 9th ed. Philadelphia: Wolters Kluwer;Lippincott Williams & Wilkins; 2009. p. 47-20-47-24.
4. Latthe P, Mignini L, Gray R et al. Factors predisposing women to chronic pelvic pain: systematic review. *BMJ* 2006;332:749-55.
5. Dawood MY. Primary dysmenorrhea: advances in pathogenesis and management. *Obstet Gynecol* 2006;108:428-41.
6. Daley AJ. Exercise and primary dysmenorrhoea: a comprehensive and critical review of the literature. *Sports Med* 2008;38:659-70.
7. Brown J, Brown S. Exercise for dysmenorrhoea. *Cochrane Database Syst Rev* 2010;2:CD004142.
8. Rakhshaee Z. Effect of three yoga poses (cobra, cat and fish poses) in women with primary dysmenorrhea: a randomized clinical trial. *J Pediatr Adolesc Gynecol* 2011;24:192-6.
9. Barnard ND, Scialli AR, Hurlock D et al. Diet and sex-hormone binding globulin, dysmenorrhea, and premenstrual symptoms. *Obstet Gynecol* 2000;95:245-50.
10. Akin MD, Weingand KW, Hengehold DA et al. Continuous low-level topical heat in the treatment of dysmenorrhea. *Obstet Gynecol* 2001;97:343-9.
11. Potur DC and Komurcu N. The effects of local low-dose heat application on dysmenorrhea. *J Pediatr Adolesc Gynecol* 2014;27:216-21.
12. Lee CH, Roh JW, Lim CY et al. A multicenter, randomized, double-blind, placebo-controlled trial evaluating the efficacy and safety of a far infrared-emitting sericite belt in patients with primary dysmenorrhea. *Complement Ther Med* 2011;19:187-93.
13. Ou MC, Hsu TF, Lai AC et al. Pain relief assessment by aromatic essential oil massage on outpatients with primary dysmenorrhea: a randomized, double-blind clinical trial. *J Obstet Gynaecol Res* 2012;38:817-22.
14. Kim Y, Myenong S, Yang Y et al. Self-aromatherapy massage of the abdomen for the reduction of menstrual pain and anxiety during menstruation in nurses: a placebo-controlled clinical trial. *Eur J Integr Med* 2011;3:e165.
15. Proctor ML, Murphy PA, Pattison HM et al. Behavioural interventions for primary and secondary dysmenorrhoea. *Cochrane Database Syst Rev* 2007;3:CD002248.
16. Proctor ML, Latthe PM, Farquhar CM et al. Surgical interruption of pelvic nerve pathways for primary and secondary dysmenorrhoea. *Cochrane Database Syst Rev* 2005;4:CD001896.
17. Proctor ML, Hing W, Johnson TC et al. Spinal manipulation for primary and secondary dysmenorrhoea. *Cochrane Database Syst Rev* 2006;3:CD002119.
18. Proctor M, Farquhar C, Stones W et al. Transcutaneous electrical nerve stimulation for primary dysmenorrhoea. *Cochrane Database Syst Rev* 2002;1:CD002123.
19. Wu LL, Su CH, Liu CF. Effects of noninvasive electroacupuncture at Hegu (L14) and Sanyinjiao (SP6) acupoints on dysmenorrhea randomized controlled trial. *J Alt Comp Med* 2012;18:137-42.
20. Smith CA, Zhu X, He L et al. Acupuncture for dysmenorrhoea. *Cochrane Database Syst Rev* 2011;1:CD007854.

21. Marjoribanks J, Proctor M, Farquhar C et al. Nonsteroidal anti-inflammatory drugs for dysmenorrhoea. *Cochrane Database Syst Rev* 2010;1:CD001751.
22. Chan WY, Dawood MY, Fuchs F. Prostaglandins in primary dysmenorrhea. Comparison of prophylactic and nonprophylactic treatment with ibuprofen and use of oral contraceptives. *Am J Med* 1981;70:535-41.
23. Lefebvre G, Pinsonneault O, Antao V et al. Primary dysmenorrhea consensus guideline. *J Obstet Gynaecol Can* 2005;27:1117-46.
24. Janbu T, Lokken P, Nesheim BI. Effect of acetylsalicylic acid, paracetamol and placebo on pain and blood loss in dysmenorrheic women. *Acta Obstet Gynecol Scand Suppl* 1979;87:81-5.
25. Zhang WY, Li Wan Po A. Efficacy of minor analgesics in dysmenorrhoea: a systematic review. *Br J Obstet Gynaecol* 1998;105;780-9.
26. Clarity Informatics Ltd (UK). Prodigy Clinical Topics. *Dysmenorrhoea—management.*
27. Wong CL, Farquhar C, Roberts H et al. Oral contraceptive pill as treatment for primary dysmenorrhoea. *Cochrane Database Syst Rev* 2009;2:CD002120.
28. Harada T, Momoeda M, Terakawa N et al. Evaluation of a low-dose oral contraceptive pill for primary dysmenorrhea: a placebo-controlled, double-blind, randomized trial. *Fertil Steril* 2011;95:1928-31.
29. Dmitrovic R, Kunselman AR, Legro RS. Continuous compared with cyclic oral contraceptives for the treatment of primary dysmenorrhea: a randomized controlled trial. *Obstet Gynecol* 2012;119:1143-50.
30. Edelman A, Micks E, Gallo MF et al. Continuous or extended cycle vs. cyclic use of combined hormonal contraceptives for contraception. *Cochrane Database Syst Rev* 2014;7:CD004695.
31. Coco AS. Primary dysmenorrhea. *Am Fam Physician* 1999;60:489-96.
32. Wildemeersch D, Schacht E, Wildemeersch P. Treatment of primary and secondary dysmenorrhea with a novel frameless intrauterine levonorgestrel-releasing drug delivery system: a pilot study. *Eur J Contracept Reprod Health Care* 2001;6:192-8.
33. Fedorowicz Z, Nasser M, Jagannath VA et al. Beta2-adrenoceptor agonists for dysmenorrhoea. *Cochrane Database Syst Rev* 2012;5:CD008585.
34. Lasco A, Catalano A, Benvenga S. Improvement of primary dysmenorrhea caused by a singe oral dose of vitamin D: results of a randomized, double-blind, placebo-controlled study. *Arch Int Med* 2012;172:366-7.
35. Rahbar N, Asgharzadeh N, Ghorbani R. Effect of omega-3 fatty acids on intensity of primary dysmenorrhea. *Int J Gynaecol Obstet* 2011;117:45-7.
36. Aghakhani N, Merhzad M, Rahbar N et al. Effects of fish oil capsules and vitamin B1 Tablets on duration and pain severity of dysmenorrhea. *Pain Practice*. 6th World Congress of the World Institute of Pain; 2012 Feb 4-6; Miami Beach, Florida.
37. Pattanittum P, Kunyanone N, Brown J et al. Dietary supplements for dysmenorrhoea. *Cochrane Database Syst Rev* 2016;3:CD002124.
38. Ziaei S, Faghihzadeh S, Sohrabvand F et al. A randomised placebo-controlled trial to determine the effect of vitamin E in treatment of primary dysmenorrhoea. *BJOG* 2001;108:1181-3.
39. Kashanian M, Lakeh MM, Ghasemi A et al. Evaluation of the effect of vitamin E on pelvic pain reduction in women suffering from primary dysmenorrhea. *J Reprod Med* 2013;58:34-8.
40. Direkvand-Moghadam A, Khosravi A. The impact of a novel herbal Shirazi Thymus Vulgaris on primary dysmenorrhea in comparison to the classical chemical ibuprofen. *J Res Med Sci* 2012;17:668-70.
41. Miabi P, Dolatia M, Mojab F et al. Effects of valerian on the severity and systemic manifestations of dysmenorrhea. *Int J Gynaecol Obstet* 2011;115:285-8.
42. Proctor ML, Murphy PA. Herbal and dietary therapies for primary and secondary dysmenorrhoea. *Cochrane Database Syst Rev* 2001;3:CD002124.
43. Zhu X, Proctor M, Bensoussan A et al. Chinese herbal medicine for primary dysmenorrhoea. *Cochrane Database Syst Rev* 2007;4:CD005288.

Painful Menstrual Periods—What You Need to Know

Why do some women have painful menstrual periods?

Most women have some pain with their periods. The pain can start a few hours before or right at the beginning of your period. It can last 2–3 days. It is common to have abdominal cramps or pain in the back and legs. You may also have a headache or feel very tired. Some women have nausea, vomiting or diarrhea. These problems can keep you from doing your normal activities.

Painful periods (called **dysmenorrhea**) are usually not serious. However, painful periods can sometimes be caused by an infection or ovarian cysts (fluid-filled sacs in the ovary). Pain can also be caused by endometriosis (a problem with the lining of the uterus).

How can you manage painful menstrual periods?

Here are some things you can do to feel better:

- Try using a heating pad, heat patch or hot water bottle on your belly. You can also take a warm bath.
- Some women find that taking ibuprofen or naproxen during their period helps to make their periods less painful. A reasonable trial of these medications is to use them during 3 menstrual cycles. However, some people should not take these medications. Ask your healthcare provider for advice.
- Regular aerobic exercise may help prevent symptoms. Some yoga poses may also help alleviate symptoms.

When should you see your healthcare provider?

- If over-the-counter pain relievers don't work or they make you feel worse.
- If the amount of pain you have with your menstrual period has increased.
- If you have the same kind of pain when you are not having your period.
- If you have a discharge or change in the amount or type of bleeding from your vagina.

You may be examined for ovarian cysts or endometriosis. You can also ask your healthcare provider about using birth control pills to make your periods less painful.

Chapter 78
Male Sexual Dysfunction

Tom Smiley, BScPhm, PharmD

Sexual dysfunction refers to difficulties engaging in sexual intercourse which may be due to physical or psychologic factors or both. This chapter focuses on erectile dysfunction and premature ejaculation.

Erectile Dysfunction

The Canadian Urology Association defines erectile dysfunction (ED) as the preferred clinical term to describe persistent or recurrent inability to achieve and maintain a penile erection of sufficient rigidity to permit satisfactory sexual activity for at least 3 months.[1]

It is estimated that approximately 50% of Canadian men between the ages of 40 and 88 have some degree of ED.[2] The prevalence of ED increases with age, tripling between the ages of 40 and 70 years.[3] About two-thirds of men over the age of 70 years experience ED according to the large landmark cross-sectional Massachusetts Male Aging Study (MMAS).[4]

Pathophysiology

The male erection is a vascular event that is initiated by neuronal action and maintained by a complex interplay between vascular and neurologic events.[5] Parasympathetic input causes relaxation of trabecular smooth muscle and dilation of the helicine arteries of the penis. This leads to expansion of the lacunar spaces and entrapment of blood in the cavernous spaces. Increasing pressure within these spaces causes the penis to become erect, resulting in compression of the venules against the tunica albuginea. The tunica albuginea must have sufficient stiffness to compress the venules penetrating it, blocking venous outflow and maintaining tumescence and rigidity.[5] Erectile dysfunction secondary to smooth muscle pathophysiology may be a consequence of insufficient nitric oxide for smooth muscle relaxation (e.g., associated with endothelial disease), an inadequate number of smooth muscle cells (e.g., cell apoptosis from diabetes or neuropathy) and/or tunical degeneration (caused by Peyronie's disease).[6]

Factors that play a role in promoting ED are usually categorized as being organic, psychogenic or drug-related.[7]

ED is most often associated with organic causes. Within this etiologic classification, atherosclerosis is most prominent.[8] Psychogenic causes of ED may include anxiety, depression or psychosis with a potential loss of self-confidence. Many interrelationships between depression and ED may be possible. The occurrence of either condition may cause, result from, or exacerbate the other.[9] In the MMAS, men who scored highest on depression scales had an almost 90% probability of moderate or complete ED compared with 25% for the least depressed.[4] Depression and ED also share a number of risk factors, including smoking, obesity, dyslipidemia and sedentary lifestyle.[9]

Risk factors and potential mechanisms of ED are presented in Table 1 and drug causes of ED are presented in Table 2.

Goals of Therapy

- Restore erectile capacity

Table 1: **Risk Factors and Mechanisms of Erectile Dysfunction**

Risk Factor	Mechanism or Cause
Metabolic syndrome	Endothelial dysfunction and down-regulation of nitric oxide synthase
Lower urinary tract symptoms of benign prostatic hyperplasia (BPH)	Possible decrease in nitric oxide in the penis, bladder and prostate
Cardiovascular disease	Possible endothelial dysfunction in penile vasculature
Tobacco smoking	Possible endothelial dysfunction, associated atherosclerosis and sympathetic overactivity
Central neurologic conditions, e.g., Parkinson's disease, hemorrhagic or ischemic stroke, tumors, Alzheimer's disease	Disruption of neural control or proerectile processes
Spinal cord injury	Dependent on the extent and location of the spinal lesion; nonsustained reflex erections commonly maintained
Endocrinologic conditions such as hypogonadism, hypothyroidism, hyperthyroidism, hyperprolactinemia	Disruption of testosterone-mediated up-regulation of nitric oxide synthase; low testosterone levels from hyperprolactinemia-influenced changes in the hypothalamic-pituitary axis
Diabetes mellitus	Vasculopathy from endothelial dysfunction and autonomic neuropathy

Adapted with permission from McVary KT. Erectile dysfunction. *N Engl J Med* 2007;357:2472-81.

Patient Assessment

Refer patients with ED to an appropriate healthcare provider to evaluate the psychological and organic factors causing ED. A thorough history including assessment of modifiable causes of ED such as blood pressure, blood glucose, smoking, alcohol and drug use is imperative for a proper diagnosis. Men with psychogenic erectile dysfunction (except when caused by severe depression) usually have normal nocturnal and early morning erections. If the patient indicates the presence of rigid erections (often when awakening), the efferent neurologic and circulatory systems that mediate erections are intact, and the dysfunction is probably psychogenic in nature.[10]

An estimated 25% of ED cases may be attributable to medications prescribed for other conditions.[11] It is important to perform a detailed medication history, identify potential causative agents and recommend alternative medications that have little or no risk of inducing erectile dysfunction (see Table 2). In some instances, either waiting to see if tolerance to the sexual side effect develops or reducing the dose of the offending agent is attempted before switching to another medication. If a decision is made to remove an offending agent, advise the patient of any potential risks associated with an abrupt discontinuation, and recommend an appropriate withdrawal schedule.

Management of erectile dysfunction consists of psychotherapy/behavioural therapy, medical treatment or (most commonly) a combination of the two (see Figure 1).

Nonpharmacologic Therapy

Psychotherapy/Behavioural Therapy

Careful attention to psychological factors and attempts to alleviate sexual anxieties should be a part of the therapeutic intervention in all patients with erectile dysfunction. Psychotherapy/behavioural therapy alone may be beneficial for patients in whom no organic causes are detected, or in cases where patients refuse medical/surgical interventions. Focus should be on treating coexistent problems such as issues related to the loss of a partner, dysfunctional relationships, psychotic disorders or substance abuse.[3,12,13] This approach has been reported to relieve depression and anxiety and improve sexual function; however, outcome data have not been quantified and success of specific techniques is poorly documented.

Vacuum Constriction Devices

For comparative features of nonprescription products, consult the *Compendium of Products for Minor Ailments*—Male Sexual Health Products: Vacuum Constrictive Devices for Erectile Dysfunction.

Vacuum constriction devices are effective in all cases of erectile dysfunction, irrespective of the pathogenesis of ED.[14] However, vacuum therapy may not be tolerated by most patients and is not usually considered a first-line option.

Erection is induced by creating a vacuum around the penis, and it is maintained by using a constriction band. The devices are difficult for some patients to use and may impair ejaculation, which can cause some discomfort. Some men may experience petechiae (reddish pinpoint-sized dots) and ecchymosis (bruising).[15,16] Petechiae are caused by placing the penis under negative pressure too rapidly, and ecchymosis is due to the penis being held under vacuum pressure too long. The major drawback of these devices is the necessity for precoital application, making acceptance by the sexual partner of major importance. Refer patients to their urologist for proper selection of a vacuum constriction device.

Table 2: **Drugs Commonly Associated with Erectile Dysfunction**

Drug Class	Examples[a]	Possible Alternative Treatment or Course of Action
5-alpha reductase inhibitors	Dutasteride, finasteride	Consult urologist
Antiandrogens	Bicalutamide, flutamide, nilutamide	Consult oncologist
Antiepileptic drugs	Carbamazepine, phenytoin	Consult neurologist
Antidepressants	Lithium, MAO inhibitors, tricyclic antidepressants, SSRIs	Bupropion, mirtazapine
Antihypertensive drugs	Beta-blockers, calcium channel blockers, clonidine, hydralazine, methyldopa	ACE inhibitors, angiotensin receptor blockers
Antipsychotic agents	Butyrophenones, phenothiazines, risperidone	Consult psychiatrist
Cytotoxic agents	Methotrexate	Treatment varies according to condition
Diuretics	Spironolactone, thiazides	Furosemide
H_2-receptor antagonists	Cimetidine, ranitidine	Proton pump inhibitors
Opioids	Hydromorphone, morphine, oxycodone	Acetaminophen, NSAIDs
Antiparkinsonian agents	Levodopa	Consult neurologist
Other	Alcohol, cocaine, corticosteroids, cyclophosphamide, digoxin, luteinizing hormone-releasing hormone agonists	Consult appropriate specialist

[a] Not a comprehensive list.

Figure 1: **Management of Erectile Dysfunction**

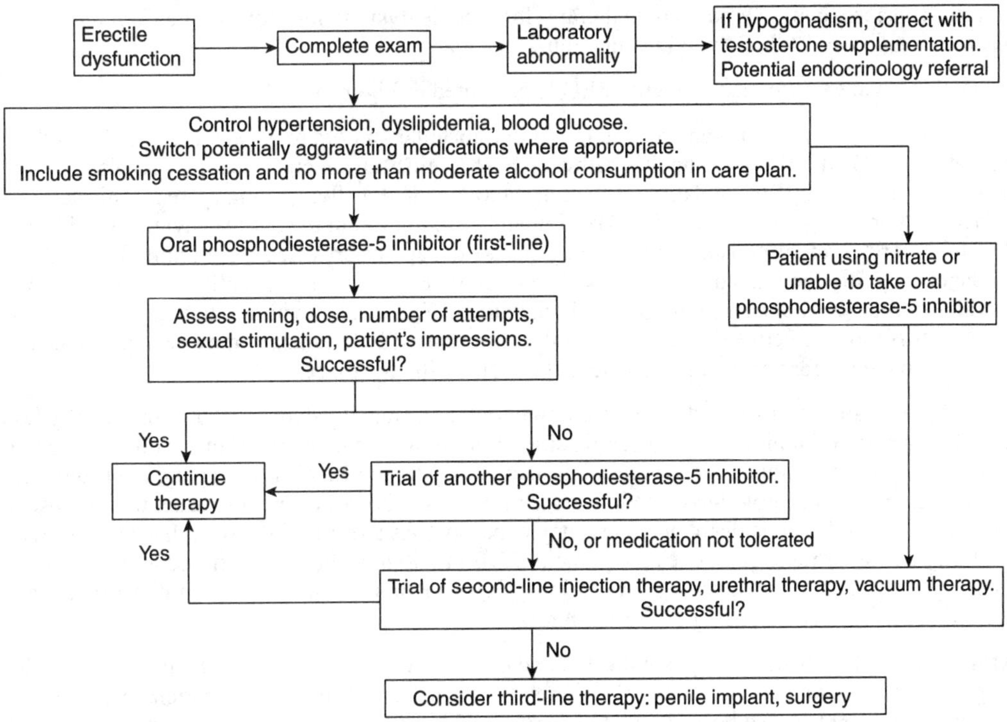

Erectile dysfunction → Complete exam → Laboratory abnormality → If hypogonadism, correct with testosterone supplementation. Potential endocrinology referral

Complete exam → Control hypertension, dyslipidemia, blood glucose. Switch potentially aggravating medications where appropriate. Include smoking cessation and no more than moderate alcohol consumption in care plan.

→ Oral phosphodiesterase-5 inhibitor (first-line)

→ Assess timing, dose, number of attempts, sexual stimulation, patient's impressions. Successful?

- Yes → Continue therapy
- No → Trial of another phosphodiesterase-5 inhibitor. Successful?
  - Yes → Continue therapy
  - No, or medication not tolerated → Trial of second-line injection therapy, urethral therapy, vacuum therapy. Successful?

→ (from Control hypertension box) Patient using nitrate or unable to take oral phosphodiesterase-5 inhibitor → Trial of second-line injection therapy, urethral therapy, vacuum therapy. Successful?

Trial of second-line injection therapy, urethral therapy, vacuum therapy. Successful?
- Yes → Continue therapy
- No → Consider third-line therapy: penile implant, surgery

Vascular Surgery

Surgery of the penile venous system, generally involving venous ligation, has been effective in patients with demonstrated venous leakage.[3] However, evidence from longer-term follow-up studies shows decreased effectiveness of this procedure. Arterial revascularization procedures have a limited role and should be restricted to the clinical investigation setting in medical centres with experienced personnel.[1,3] Surgery is performed in isolated cases and usually for the correction of congenital or trauma-induced vascular abnormalities.[12]

Penile Prostheses

Penile prosthesis placement is indicated for a motivated patient with ED who desires reconstitution of penile function adequate for intercourse and in whom first- and second-line treatments have failed.[17] The most basic prosthesis is the semi-rigid rod prosthesis which consists of 2 rod-like cylinders that are implanted in the corpora cavernosa. A prosthesis may have a mechanically jointed backbone or have a malleable one that allows the phallus to be dressed upward or downward. The surgery permanently alters the corpora, ending most hope of return to natural erections. There is also a risk of repeat surgery with all of the devices.[3]

Most patients using penile prostheses have found them to be satisfactory. Those with penile fibrosis find the device to be especially helpful.[14] In a study of more than 200 men, over 88% said they would recommend the device to a relative or a friend.[18]

The high initial cost of the device is a consideration.[14] Perineal pain may be experienced upon insertion, and it may last for 1–2 months.[14] Sepsis may occur in 2–16% of cases. However, according to a 2-year study the removal rate was only 4.4%.[14]

Pharmacologic Therapy

For further discussion of pharmacologic therapy for erectile dysfunction, consult the *Compendium of Therapeutic Choices*: Male Sexual Dysfunction.

A general overview of the management of ED is presented in Figure 1.

Phosphodiesterase-5 (PDE5) is an enzyme found in trabecular smooth muscle, which catalyzes the degradation of cGMP.[8] By blocking this pathway, **PDE5 inhibitors** increase cellular levels of cGMP and promote erection by up-regulation of the nitric oxide-cGMP cell-signaling system. This action enhances and prolongs smooth muscle relaxation and vasodilation in the corpus cavernosum.[19] Oral PDE5 inhibitor therapy is considered first-line because the agents are effective, minimally invasive and associated with minimal adverse effects. The three PDE5 inhibitors currently available on the Canadian market are **sildenafil**, **tadalafil** and **vardenafil**. There is no evidence to suggest that one of these agents is more effective than another for the treatment of ED. Tadalafil may be dosed once daily, eliminating the need for predicting when sexual activity will take place.

PDE5 inhibitors are well tolerated, with discontinuation rates due to adverse events consistently less than 5%.[8] Each PDE5 inhibitor has a specific side-effect profile that differs from the others, and that could vary among individuals. Headaches and flushing appear to be a class effect and are usually mild and transient. Priapism (prolonged erections over more than 4 hours) occurs infrequently with use of PDE5 inhibitors and is considered an emergency condition. As a result of the overall effectiveness and tolerability of these drugs, guidelines recommend PDE5 inhibitors should be offered to most patients presenting with ED and without contraindications, e.g., concomitant nitrate use.[20] Table 3 presents counselling tips for patients using PDE5 inhibitors.

Testosterone replacement therapy is indicated and effective only for ED caused by diagnosed male hypogonadism (approximately 6% of ED sufferers).[21] In men suffering from hypogonadism, testosterone therapy has also been shown to improve libido and may positively influence bone mass.[22] In a meta-analysis of 16 studies, testosterone treatment was associated with improvement in ED in men with hypogonadism 57% of the time versus 16.7% of the time in men using placebo.[23] The highest response rate was achieved with transdermal testosterone therapy, with 80.9% of participants responding, compared with a 51.3% response rate with intramuscular therapy and 53.2% with oral therapy.

Testosterone replacement therapy is available in oral capsule form as testosterone undecanoate, topically as a transdermal patch or a gel, or as an injection in the form of testosterone cypionate or testosterone enanthate. It should be discontinued in patients who do not respond to treatment within 3 months.[6]

Intracavernous injection is a second-line therapy to be used if PDE5 inhibitor therapy is contraindicated or not tolerated. These injections contain **alprostadil** (synthetic prostaglandin E_1), either alone, or in combination with **papaverine** and **phentolamine** ("triple P" therapy). They are effective in treating erectile dysfunction of vascular, neurogenic or psychogenic causes. Good results are attained in 70–80% of patients.[24,25,26,27] The drugs are self-injected into the corpus cavernosum through the lateral aspect of the shaft of the penis, after cleansing the area with alcohol. Complications from intracavernosal injection may include penile pain, priapism or fibrotic changes at the injection site.

Transurethral therapy, sometimes referred to as MUSE (medicated urethral system for erections), consists of alprostadil pellets inserted into the urethra with a special device. This therapy is effective in approximately 43% of patients. The most common adverse effects include penile pain (32%) and urethral pain or burning (12%).[28,29,30]

Table 3: **Counselling Tips for Patients Using Phosphodiesterase-5 Inhibitors**

Sexual stimulation is necessary for the drug to work. The drug is not an aphrodisiac.
Onset to effect is 30–60 min for sildenafil, vardenafil and tadalafil (if not using once-daily dosing) for most men. It is advisable to take the medication at least 1 h before planned sexual activity to increase potential for success.
High-fat meals may delay the time to onset of action with sildenafil and vardenafil.
Success increases with each use of the drug, even up to 6–8 attempts. Do not assume the drug is not going to work if complete success is not experienced.
If the first dose of the drug is ineffective, a higher dose may be necessary.
Side effects are usually mild and temporary and may include headache, flushing or stomach upset.
Prolonged erection (lasting more than 4 h) is a medical emergency.
Scheduled patient follow up is important (see Monitoring of Therapy). Remind patients to contact their healthcare provider should the medication lose its effectiveness or if cardiovascular status changes. Advise patients that options exist if complete success is not achieved upon first use of the medication.

Monitoring of Therapy

- Routinely ask patients using any type of therapy for ED about tolerability and effectiveness.
- For PDE5 inhibitors, follow up with the patient 1 or 2 weeks after initial drug trial to discuss effectiveness and any side effects. Consider timing of medication administration in evaluating whether the medication is working. If the medication is well-tolerated but not effective, and timing is not an issue, consider recommending an increased dose to the prescriber (if not at maximum recommended dose). Further monitoring at the time of medication refills should assess continued effectiveness and tolerability of the drug as well as the patient's cardiovascular status.
- Monitor patients taking testosterone replacement therapy 1–3 months after initiating therapy and then at least annually for testosterone levels, clinical response and adverse effects.[16]

Premature Ejaculation

Pathophysiology

The International Society for Sexual Medicine defines premature ejaculation (PE) as a male sexual dysfunction characterized by ejaculation which always or nearly always occurs prior to or within about 1 minute of vaginal penetration, or a clinically significant reduction in latency time, often to about 3 minutes or less (acquired premature ejaculation), and the inability to delay ejaculation on all or nearly all vaginal penetrations, with negative personal consequences, such as distress, bother, frustration and/or the avoidance of sexual intimacy.[31] There is insufficient evidence to extend this definition to situations other than intravaginal sexual activity (e.g., men having sex with men).[31]

PE may be the most common male sexual dysfunction reported by patients with a prevalence of approximately 30%.[31,32] The causes of PE are largely unknown and no biological factor has been shown to be definitively causative in the majority of men with PE.[31]

Organic factors are implicated in a relatively small proportion of cases of PE. These include trauma to the sympathetic nervous system, prostatic hypertrophy, prostatitis, urethritis, alcoholism, diabetes, arteriosclerosis, cardiovascular disease, venous leakage and polyneuritis. Premature ejaculation has been described following withdrawal from antipsychotics and opiates.[33,34,35] It is associated with the use of desipramine and sympathomimetics (e.g., pseudoephedrine), and with alcohol-related peripheral neuropathy.[36]

Goals of Therapy

- Improve sexual functioning of the patient
- Improve quality of relationship between patient and sexual partner

Patient Assessment

The assessment of PE should be multidimensional to reach a sound treatment decision. This includes self-reporting as well as behavioural, physiological and medical evaluations. Refer patients to an appropriate healthcare provider for the proper diagnosis of PE. Medical evaluation of PE should include inquiry into genitourinary symptoms, symptoms of generalized or localized neurological disease, previous abdominal or pelvic trauma and use of medications.

Nonpharmacologic Therapy

Various nonpharmacologic treatments exist for men suffering from PE. Frequently, men will have to use a combination of 4–5 techniques to obtain the desired results. These techniques can be taught to the individual or to the couple.

Examples of individual procedures include:[37]

- physiologic relaxation training (e.g., focusing on breathing, body awareness and muscle relaxation exercises)
- sensual awareness training (e.g., teaching the man to become aroused by his own sensations instead of partner interaction)
- pubococcygeal muscle control training
- pelvic floor rehabilitation training
- pacing techniques (e.g., stop-start technique, pause-squeeze technique)
- testicular restraint technique.

Examples of techniques taught to couples include:[37]

- sensate focus pleasuring exercises
- partner genital exploration/relaxation exercises
- pacing techniques
- intercourse acclimatization.

The "pause-squeeze" technique by Masters and Johnson[38] is considered by some specialists to offer the best results. In this technique the partner puts one thumb on the frenulum of the penis, with the first and second fingers of the same hand just above and before the coronal ridge. A firm grasping pressure is applied for four seconds and then released. The pressure is applied front-to-back with the specific pressure proportional to the degree of erection present: a firm squeeze with an erect penis; a moderate squeeze when the penis is more flaccid. The squeeze may lead to a temporary, 10–25% decrease in the erection. This technique is less effective when it is self-applied.[38] The pause-squeeze technique is part of an elaborate treatment regimen that the couple must follow. Initially this technique is used during mutual masturbation. After several days of practice the couple is instructed to transfer this process to coitus. Later, a basilar squeeze technique may be taught, where the partner applies the squeeze technique to the base of the penis, to minimize interruptions to lovemaking.

The testicular restraint technique is a physiological aid to help delay orgasm by preventing the testicles from ascending into the perineum. Some men can benefit from cuffing the testicles and gently pulling down. Alternatively, Velcro-type devices and leather straps can be used to achieve the same effects. These items are available at most stores that sell sexual aids.[37]

If the health professional is not comfortable discussing behavioural therapy for PE with the patient, referral to a sex therapist, psychologist or psychiatrist is recommended.

Pharmacologic Therapy

For further discussion of pharmacologic therapy for premature ejaculation, consult the *Compendium of Therapeutic Choices*: Male Sexual Dysfunction.

For comparative ingredients of nonprescription products, consult the *Compendium of Products for Minor Ailments*—Male Sexual Health Products: Premature Ejaculation.

Topical **lidocaine/prilocaine** cream may be used to delay ejaculation.[39,40,41] The mixture available in Canada contains 2.5% of each ingredient. If topical anesthetics are used, advise the patient to apply the cream to the penis 20 minutes before intercourse[40] and encourage application of a condom to reduce transfer of the anesthetic to the vagina during intercourse.[41]

The International Society for Sexual Medicine recommends daily dosing of **citalopram** (20–40 mg), **clomipramine** (12.5–50 mg), **fluoxetine** (20–40 mg), **paroxetine** (10–40 mg) or **sertraline** (50–200 mg) for the management of PE.[31] Alternatively, on-demand dosing of **clomipramine**, **fluoxetine**, **paroxetine** or **sertraline** 3–6 hours before intercourse is also effective, albeit to a lesser extent.[31] Response to treatment usually starts within 5–10 days of regular daily dosing with antidepressants and full therapeutic benefit may require 2–3 weeks of continuous treatment.

The International Society of Sexual Medicine guidelines do not recommend on-demand or daily dosing of PDE5 inhibitors in the treatment of lifelong PE in men with normal erectile function, as there is conflicting evidence regarding the safety and efficacy of this practice and more high-quality evidence is required.[31]

Weak evidence suggests that **tramadol** may be an effective option for the treatment of PE when other therapies have failed.[42] Caution must be observed due to the risk of addiction and side effects. It should not be combined with an SSRI due to risk of serotonin syndrome. Further research is needed to assess the efficacy and safety of tramadol in the treatment of PE.[31]

Monitoring of Therapy

Inquire during regular visits about the success or failures associated with the therapy. The International Society of Sexual Medicine guidelines recommend the question associated with the Clinical Global Impression of Change: "Compared to before starting treatment, would you describe your premature ejaculation problem as: much worse, worse, slightly worse, no change, slightly better, better, or much better?"[31]

Resource Tips

International Society of Men's Health (ISMH). Available from: www.ismh.org.

Remedy's Health Communities. Available from: www.healthcommunities.com/health-topics/sexual-health.shtml.

The Sex Information and Education Council of Canada (SIECCAN). 235 Danforth Avenue, Toronto, Ontario, M4K 1N2. (Tel.) 416-466-5304; (Fax) 416-778-0785. Available from: www.sieccan.org.

Suggested Readings

Althof SE, McMahon CG, Waldinger MD et al. An update of the International Society of Sexual Medicine's guidelines for the diagnosis and treatment of premature ejaculation (PE). *Sex Med* 2014;2:60-90.

Bella AJ, Lee JC, Carrier S et al. 2015 CUA Practice guidelines for erectile dysfunction. *Can Urol Assoc J* 2015;9:23-9.

References

1. Bella AJ, Lee JC, Carrier S et al. 2015 CUA Practice guidelines for erectile dysfunction. *Can Urol Assoc J* 2015;9:23-9.
2. Grover SA, Lowensteyn I, Kaouache M et al. The prevalence of erectile dysfunction in the primary care setting: importance of risk factors for diabetes and vascular disease. *Arch Intern Med* 2006;166:213-9.
3. NIH Consensus Conference. Impotence. NIH Consensus Development Panel on Impotence. *JAMA* 1993;270:83-90.
4. Feldman HA, Goldstein I, Hatzichristou DG et al. Impotence and its medical and psychosocial correlates: results of the Massachusetts Male Aging Study. *J Urol* 1994;151:54-61.
5. Lue TF. Erectile dysfunction. *N Eng J Med* 2000;342:1802-13.
6. McVary KT. Clinical practice. Erectile dysfunction. *N Engl J Med* 2007;357:2472-81.
7. Steggall MJ. Erectile dysfunction: physiology, causes and patient management. *Nurs Stand* 2007;21:49-56.
8. Fazio L, Brock G. Erectile dysfunction: management update. *CMAJ* 2004;170:1429-37.
9. Nurnberg HG, Seidman SN, Gelenberg AJ et al. Depression, antidepressant therapies, and erectile dysfunction: clinical trials of sildenafil citrate (Viagra) in treated and untreated patients with depression. *Urology* 2002;60:58-66.
10. Finger WW, Lund M, Slagle MA. Medications that contribute to sexual disorders. A guide to assessment and treatment in family practice. *J Fam Pract* 1997;44:33-43.
11. Miller TA. Diagnostic evaluation of erectile dysfunction. *Am Fam Physician* 2000;61:95-104, 109-10.
12. Wilson JD, McConnell JD. Alterations in reproductive and sexual function. In: Isselbacher KJ, Harrison TR, eds. *Harrison's principles of internal medicine*. 13th ed. New York: McGraw-Hill; 1994. p. 262-5.
13. Montague DK, Barada JH, Belker AM et al. Clinical guidelines panel on erectile dysfunction: summary report on the treatment of organic erectile dysfunction. The American Urological Association. *J Urol* 1996;156:2007-11.
14. Ralph D, McNicholas T. UK management guidelines for erectile dysfunction. *BMJ* 2000;321:499-503.
15. Obson JB. *A patient's guide for the treatment of impotence*. Augusta: Obson Medical System, Charter Publishing Company; 1992.
16. Salvatore FT, Sharman GM, Hellstrom WJ. Vacuum constriction devices and the clinical urologist: an informed selection. *Urology* 1991;38:323-7.
17. Santucci RA. *Penile prosthesis implantation*. Available from: www.medscape.com. Registration required.
18. Carson CC, Mulcahy JJ, Govier FE. Efficacy, safety and patient satisfaction outcomes of the AMS 700CX inflatable penile prosthesis: results of a long-term multicenter study. AMS 700CX Study Group. *J Urol* 2000;164:376-80.
19. Rosen RC, Kostis JB. Overview of phosphodiesterase 5 inhibition in erectile dysfunction. *Am J Cardiol* 2003;92:9M-18M.
20. Montague DK, Jarow JP, Broderick GA et al. Chapter 1: The management of erectile dysfunction: an AUA update. *J Urol* 2005;174:230-9.
21. Salonia A, Briganti A, Deho F et al. Pathophysiology of erectile dysfunction. *Int J Androl* 2003;26:129-36.
22. Levine LA. Diagnosis and treatment of erectile dysfunction. *Am J Med* 2000;109:3S-12S.
23. Jain P, Rademaker AW, McVary KT. Testosterone supplementation for erectile dysfunction: results of a meta-analysis. *J Urol* 2000;164:371-5.
24. Schramek R, Plas EG, Hubner WA et al. Intracavernous injection of prostaglandin E1 plus procaine in the treatment of erectile dysfunction. *J Urol* 1994;152:1108-10.
25. Virag R, Shoukry K, Floresco J et al. Intracavernous self-injection of vasoactive drugs in the treatment of impotence: 8-year experience with 615 cases. *J Urol* 1991;145:287-91.
26. Edwards S, ed. Intracavernous injections for impotence. *New Drugs/Drug News* 1995;13:3-4.
27. Govier FE, McClure RD, Weissman RM et al. Experience with triple-drug therapy in a pharmacological erection program. *J Urol* 1993;150:1822-4.
28. Padma-Nathan H, Keller T, Proppiti R et al. Hemodynamic effects of intraurethral alprostadil: the medicated urethral system for erection (MUSE). *Int J Impot Res* 1994;6:A42.
29. Porst H. Transurethral alprostadil with MUSE (medicated urethral system for erection) vs intracavernous alprostadil–a comparative study in 103 patients with erectile dysfunction. *Int J Impot Res* 1997;9:187-92.
30. Williams G, Abbou CC, Amar ET et al. Efficacy and safety of alprostadil therapy in men with erectile dysfunction. MUSE Study Group. *Br J Urol* 1998;81:889-94.
31. Althof SE, McMahon CG, Waldinger MD et al. An update of the International Society of Sexual Medicine's guidelines for the diagnosis and treatment of premature ejaculation (PE). *Sex Med* 2014;2:60-90.
32. Carson C, Gunn K. Premature ejaculation: definition and prevalence. *Int J Impot Res* 2006;18:S5-13.
33. Keitner GI, Selub S. Spontaneous ejaculation and neuroleptics. *J Clin Psychopharmacol* 1983;3:34-6.
34. Blachly PH. Management of the opiate abstinence syndrome. *Am J Psychiatry* 1966;122:742-4.
35. Buffum J. Pharmacosexology: the effects of drugs on sexual function: a review. *J Psychoactive Drugs* 1982;14:5-44.
36. Williams W. Secondary premature ejaculation. *Aust N Z J Psychiatry* 1984;18:333-40.
37. Metz ME, Pryor JL. Premature ejaculation: a psychophysiological approach for assessment and management. *J Sex Marital Ther* 2000;26:293-320.
38. Masters WH, Johnson VE. *Human sexual inadequacy*. London: Churchill; 1970.
39. Atan A, Basar MM, Tuncel A et al. Comparison of efficacy of sildenafil-only, sildenafil plus topical EMLA cream, and topical EMLA-cream-only in treatment of premature ejaculation. *Urology* 2006;67:388-91.

40. Atikeler MK, Gecit I, Senol FA. Optimum usage of prilocaine-lidocaine cream in premature ejaculation. *Andrologia* 2002;34:356-9.
41. Sahin H, Bircan MK. Re: efficacy of prilocaine-lidocaine cream in the treatment of premature ejaculation. *J Urol* 1996;156:1783-4.
42. Martyn-St James M, Cooper K, Kaltenthaler E et al. Tramadol for premature ejaculation: a systematic review and meta-analysis. *BMC Urol* 2015;15:6.

Erectile Dysfunction—What You Need to Know

What is erectile dysfunction?

Erectile dysfunction (ED) is the inability to get or maintain an erection sufficient for intercourse that is sexually satisfying for both partners. About two to three million men in Canada have ED. Unfortunately, very few of these men seek medical attention. Up to two-thirds don't talk to their healthcare provider or partner about it. It is more common as men get older. About 1 in 20 men at the age of 40 and about 1 in 5 at the age of 65 experience ED. However, it should not be viewed as a normal part of aging.

What causes erectile dysfunction?

ED may be caused by physical or psychological problems, or a combination of the two.

The majority of cases are due to *physical* causes such as:

- Disease such as diabetes, atherosclerosis (hardening of the arteries caused by high blood pressure and high cholesterol), kidney disease, chronic alcoholism, multiple sclerosis and blood vessel diseases
- Problems with nerve impulses in the brain, spinal cord or area of the penis
- Fibrous tissue in the penis
- Damage to the veins or arteries of the penis
- Medication
- Smoking
- Hormone imbalance

Psychological causes are identified in about 20% of cases (1 in 5). These causes include:

- Stress
- Anxiety
- Feelings of guilt
- Low self-esteem
- Fear of sexual failure (performance anxiety)

How is erectile dysfunction treated?

Treatment for ED depends on the cause. Your healthcare provider may suggest any of the following treatments:

- Adjustment of any medications which may be causing your ED
- Therapy to help you deal with psychological causes
- If another disease is causing your ED, the healthcare provider may make changes to your treatment for that condition
- Mechanical devices that help cause erections
- Pumps that are surgically implanted in the penis
- Drugs that are taken orally (swallowed)
- Drugs that are placed inside the penis

When should you see your healthcare provider?

Beyond the sexual relation consequences of ED, it may be a symptom of other conditions such as heart disease or diabetes. If you have ED, talk to your healthcare provider and partner right away. You will need a complete medical examination to find out what is causing the problem and how to treat it. There are now many treatment options.

Premature Ejaculation—What You Need to Know

What is premature ejaculation?

Premature ejaculation means that a man ejaculates before he wants this to happen. It may happen with very little sexual stimulation before, upon or shortly after penetration. Premature ejaculation is the most common male sexual problem. It affects about 29% of all men. It causes stress for the man and can affect his relationships.

What causes premature ejaculation?

There are many possible causes, both physical and psychological. See your healthcare provider to discuss this problem.

- Physical causes include:
  - medical conditions such as prostate disease and spinal cord injury
  - certain medications
- Psychological causes include:
  - early sexual experiences such as masturbating quickly to avoid being caught by parents
  - performance anxiety
  - depression or other psychiatric conditions

How is premature ejaculation treated?

Your healthcare provider:

- will examine you and ask you questions in order to make a proper diagnosis.
- may refer you to a specialist such as a neurologist, urologist or psychiatrist.
- may suggest that you work with a specially trained sex therapist to learn how to control ejaculation.
- may recommend a local anesthetic ointment to reduce sensation in the penis to help delay ejaculation.
- may recommend other drugs, such as antidepressants, that have been found effective for delaying ejaculation.

New research is helping diagnose premature ejaculation and find effective treatments. Ask your healthcare provider which treatment is best for you.

Chapter 79
Menopause and Perimenopause

Thomas E.R. Brown, BScPhm, PharmD

Pathophysiology

Definition

Menopause is the cessation of menses for at least 12 consecutive months.[1] This may be a naturally occurring event or it can be related to the removal or destruction of the ovaries. On average, natural menopause occurs at 51 years of age.[1] A menopause that occurs before the age of 40 is defined as a premature menopause, and menopause occurring after 55 years of age is considered a late menopause.[1] Perimenopause refers to the time leading up to menopause, typically characterized by missed menstrual periods with or without symptoms of hypoestrogenism.[1] Perimenopause has an average duration of 4 years with a range of 2–8 years. The climacteric is an older term that encompasses the perimenopause, menopause and postmenopause.

Physiology

At the time of menopause, the ovary has no follicles left that respond to the stimulation of follicle-stimulating hormone (FSH).[2] The lack of follicular stimulation and development signals the end of the regular menstrual cycle and the monthly fluctuations of both estradiol and progesterone concentrations.[2] Without follicular development and the designation of a graafian (dominant) follicle, estradiol concentrations remain low and ovulation does not occur; therefore, progesterone concentrations remain low as well.[2] As a result, endometrial proliferation occurs rarely and there are no secretory changes. The pituitary gland increases the production and release of both FSH and luteinizing hormone (LH) in an attempt to entice the ovary to initiate follicular development.[2] The ovary cannot respond; therefore, FSH and LH concentrations remain elevated while estradiol and progesterone concentrations remain low.[2]

The postmenopausal female continues to produce estrogen in the adipose tissue as a result of the conversion of androstenedione (from the adrenal gland) to estrone.[2] The amount of estrone produced depends on the amount of adipose tissue present. Estrone has a weaker effect on the endometrium than estradiol; therefore, proliferation of endometrial tissue is rare, except in women who are obese.

During perimenopause, cessation of menses, along with the increase in FSH and LH and decrease in estradiol and progesterone, occurs gradually over several months to years.[2] The ovary becomes slow to respond to FSH and LH. Therefore, it can take longer for follicular development and endometrial proliferation to occur; however, unlike in menopause, the follicles in the ovary are still able to respond and ovulation does still occur.[2]

Perimenopausal women may suffer from vasomotor symptoms as well as vaginal dryness. The approach to therapy in these individuals is similar to menopausal women. However, it is important to note that many of the therapies have been studied only in postmenopausal women. Perimenopausal women can also suffer from premenstrual symptoms (see Chapter 81: Premenstrual Syndrome) and must still consider the possibility of becoming pregnant.

Clinical Presentation

For the most part, menopause can be diagnosed based on the absence of menses for 12 consecutive months and the symptoms an individual is experiencing. Blood tests are seldom of value in diagnosing menopause.

There are several different signs and symptoms of hypoestrogenism and their onset can vary widely among women. They can start in the perimenopausal period or present several years after menopause.[1] Initially, a woman may experience changes in menstrual function such as irregular and/or heavy periods,[3] and she may also experience vasomotor symptoms. Vasomotor symptoms are often referred to as either hot flashes or hot flushes. If they occur during sleep they are referred to as night sweats. Approximately 85% of women experience some form of vasomotor symptom and in 25% the symptoms can be severe. Night sweats can lead to insomnia, fatigue and irritability. Changes in menstrual function and vasomotor symptoms may begin in the perimenopause. The menstrual irregularities end at the time of menopause; however, the peak incidence of hot flashes occurs at the time of menopause with maximum symptoms occurring within the first 2 years after the last period. Although most postmenopausal women (60%) experience vasomotor symptoms for less than 7 years, symptoms may persist for 15 years or more in up to 15% of women.[1]

Urogenital aging occurs after menopause and consists of vaginal dryness, pain with intercourse and urinary incontinence.[1] Other symptoms of menopause can include changes in the skin (e.g., increased wrinkling), decreased libido, loss of memory and sleep disturbances (difficulty sleeping, fragmented sleep). It is uncertain whether these symptoms are a result of decreased hormone concentrations or secondary to vasomotor and urogenital symptoms. Mood disturbances (depression, anxiety) may also accompany menopause but most appear to resolve by the age of 60.

Long-term Implications

The 3 main causes of illness and disability in developed countries for postmenopausal women are cardiovascular disease, cancer, and osteoporosis associated fractures.[1] With respect to osteoporosis, the most rapid bone loss occurs in the first 15 years following menopause, after which bone loss continues at a much slower rate. For more information on age-related bone health, see Chapter 47: Osteoporosis.

Premature menopause (before the age of 40) may result from premature ovarian failure or damage to ovarian function and is associated with osteoporosis, sexual dysfunction and premature cardiovascular disease.[1] Compared with natural menopause, induced menopause (from surgery, radiation or chemotherapy) may also have different physiologic effects on the rate of loss of bone mass, atherosclerosis, vulvovaginal atrophy and libido as the ovarian sources of both androgen and estrogen are reduced prematurely and simultaneously.[1]

Goals of Therapy

- Relieve undesirable vasomotor or urogenital symptoms of perimenopause and menopause
- Prevent or minimize menopause-related bone loss
- Help the woman maintain the highest possible quality of life

The healthcare practitioner can support the goals of therapy by educating women on all aspects of menopause, including long-term health implications and options for their treatment or prevention.

Patient Assessment

It is important to determine what symptoms a woman is experiencing and the degree to which these symptoms are bothersome (Figure 1). Women with mild symptoms may try nonpharmacologic approaches and women experiencing only mild vaginal symptoms may try vaginal lubricants or moisturizers. Women with more debilitating symptoms should be informed regarding the risk and benefits of hormone therapy (HT) and nonhormonal therapies.

Nonpharmacologic Therapy

Exercise

A small study on the effects of exercise and vasomotor symptoms concluded that exercise decreases hot flashes; however, HT was significantly more effective[4] and a Cochrane review including this trial concluded that the evidence is insufficient to demonstrate the benefit of exercise on vasomotor symptoms.[5] However, the benefits of regular exercise extend beyond menopausal symptom management to positive impact on both physical and mental health, including improvements in serum lipid levels, weight and stress levels and protection from coronary vascular disease, osteoporosis, diabetes and breast cancer. For these reasons, women aged 18–64 are advised to accumulate at least 150 minutes of moderate to vigorous aerobic physical activity per week in bouts of 10 minutes or more and to perform muscle- and bone-strengthening activities using major muscle groups at least 2 days per week.[1]

Sexual Activity

Increasing blood flow to the pelvic region may relieve vaginal dryness and pain on intercourse. This is usually done through sexual stimulation. Therefore, in women who are experiencing vaginal dryness, increasing sexual activity, rather than avoiding it due to discomfort, may be beneficial.[6] To increase lubrication, sexual intercourse itself is not necessary if it is uncomfortable; any form of sexual activity will help restore vaginal moisture.

Pelvic Floor Exercises

Kegel exercises may be of value in women who are experiencing incontinence.[7] Kegel exercises involve alternating contraction and relaxation of the pelvic muscles. The contraction is similar to trying to stop urinating and should be held for 4–8 seconds. When done correctly, the abdominal and leg muscles are not recruited. Kegel exercises can be done several times a day.

Lifestyle and Dietary Measures

Smoking cessation may reduce the occurrence of vasomotor symptoms. Dietary measures such as decreasing fat intake and increasing fruit, vegetables and whole grains, along with weight loss where appropriate, may reduce vasomotor symptoms.[8] Ingestion of spicy foods, alcohol or caffeine can exacerbate vasomotor symptoms. Therefore, the simplest strategy to reduce the number of hot flashes and night sweats is to avoid spicy foods and to limit alcohol and caffeine intake.

There has been considerable discussion about the potential benefit of ingesting **phytoestrogens** to relieve menopausal symptoms. These are plant-based substances that may have weak estrogenic and/or antiestrogenic activity. There are 2 main types of phytoestrogens: lignans and isoflavones. They are found in a variety of food substances; the richest dietary source of lignans is flax seed and the richest source of isoflavones is soy products, e.g., tofu and tempeh.[9] Observational studies comparing Western and Asian women have shown that Asian women have less vasomotor menopausal symptoms.[10] This may be attributed to differences in the amounts of dietary phytoestrogens ingested by these 2 populations.[11] However, it is difficult to confirm this through prospective studies. The results of studies looking at increasing the amount of phytoestrogens through diet have been variable and the amount of phytoestrogens that need to be consumed remains unknown.[12,13] A meta-analysis of oral phytoestrogen intervention for postmenopausal symptoms concluded the phytoestrogens reduced the frequency of hot flashes without serious adverse effects.[14]

Temperature Control

Vasomotor symptoms can be exacerbated by a warm environment. To minimize this possibility, the indoor temperature should be kept comfortably cool, and it is recommended that a woman dress in layers so that clothes may be removed as needed to maintain comfort.

Psychoeducational Interventions

A 2008 systematic review of 14 studies (of fair to poor quality) involving 475 women investigated psychoeducational interventions to alleviate hot flashes.[15] Five of the studies evaluated the following strategies: education, counselling, cognitive-behavioural strategies and mindfulness-based stress reduction and all showed improvements in vasomotor symptoms. Nine of the trials evaluated relaxation techniques and 5 of these studies showed improvement in hot flashes, but the evidence was considered insufficient as the results were inconsistent and the trial quality was poor. A 2014 Cochrane review further determined the available evidence on relaxation techniques as treatment for vasomotor symptoms in postmenopausal women was of low quality and insufficient to show effectiveness.[16]

Two studies examining cognitive behavioural therapy (CBT) as treatment for vasomotor symptoms in breast cancer survivors[17] and menopausal women[18] showed both group and self-guided CBT were superior to usual-care (usual-care patients received information about VMS, advice on treatment options and symptom management, and instructions for paced breathing and relaxation). Citing this evidence, the North American Menopause Society recommended CBT as an effective nonhormonal management option for menopause-associated vasomotor symptoms in their 2015 position statement.[19] The manuals for both group[20] and self-guided[21] CBT are available to patients and healthcare practitioners.

Acupuncture

Uncontrolled trials evaluating acupuncture have shown improvement in vasomotor symptoms; however, the results have been inconsistent. Controlled trials have shown no effect of acupuncture on reducing hot flashes.[22,23] A Cochrane review found insufficient evidence to determine whether acupuncture is effective for controlling menopausal vasomotor symptoms but cautioned that the available evidence was of low or very low quality.[24]

Pharmacologic Therapy

For further discussion of pharmacologic therapy for menopause and perimenopause, consult the *Compendium of Therapeutic Choices*: Menopause.

Therapy for Urogenital Symptoms

For more information on the management of urinary incontinence, see Chapter 83: Urinary Incontinence.

For comparative ingredients of nonprescription products, consult the *Compendium of Products for Minor Ailments*—Feminine Care Products: Vaginal Lubricants and Moisturizers.

There are nonhormonal treatment options to alleviate the dryness and discomfort of vaginal atrophy. **Vaginal lubricants** (e.g., K-Y Jelly) are used prior to intercourse to provide lubrication. Bioadhesive **vaginal moisturizers**, including polycarbophil gels (e.g., Replens) and hyaluronic acid gels (e.g., Gynatrof), are used continuously to increase vaginal moisture. A randomized, controlled trial comparing Replens to conjugated equine estrogen vaginal cream showed that both products increased vaginal moisture and helped restore the vaginal epithelium.[25] A systematic review that compared vaginal estrogen with nonhormonal moisturizers found patients with 2 or more symptoms of vulvovaginal atrophy were substantially more improved using vaginal estrogens, but those with just one symptom or only minor complaints had similar symptom resolution with either estrogen or nonhormonal moisturizer.[26]

Information on nonhormonal therapy for vaginal dryness can also be found in Table 1.

Therapy for Vasomotor Symptoms

Natural Health Products

For comparative ingredients of nonprescription products, consult the *Compendium of Products for Minor Ailments*—Herbal and Natural Health Products: Combinations, Single Entity.

Many of the studies evaluating the efficacy of natural health products for the treatment of menopausal symptoms have limitations such as small size, lack of control group or other poor design factors. Additionally, lack of standardization of natural health product composition (roots, extracts, herb mixtures) and variability in doses used make comparisons between trials difficult.

Black cohosh is the most commonly used natural health product for the treatment of vasomotor symptoms in Germany. One large study using black cohosh demonstrated improvements in menopausal symptoms; however, 3 small trials failed to show any improvement in vasomotor symptoms.[27,28] The Herbal Alternatives for Menopause Trial, a 1-year randomized, double-blind, placebo-controlled trial, showed no benefit of black cohosh compared with placebo in diminishing hot flashes and night sweats.[29] A Cochrane review of trials of black cohosh concluded that there is insufficient evidence to support its use for menopausal symptoms.[30] Side effects reported with black cohosh include GI upset and decreased blood pressure. Several cases of hepatotoxicity have been reported but their association with black cohosh is uncertain.[31] The safety of black cohosh use in women with breast cancer is not known.

Studies evaluating **phytoestrogen supplements** have shown variable results. A systematic review examined a total of 14 trials of **soy**- or **red clover**–based isoflavones for vasomotor symptoms.[27] The results for soy were mixed and the composition and dose of soy supplements varied across the studies, making any recommendations regarding soy use difficult. No benefit was shown with the use of red clover.[27,28] A meta-analysis of oral phytoestrogen intervention for postmenopausal symptoms concluded the phytoestrogens reduced the frequency of hot flashes without serious adverse effects,[14] while a Cochrane review of trials of phytoestrogen supplements found no evidence of serious adverse effects but no conclusive evidence of efficacy in alleviating hot flashes or night sweats.[13] A strong placebo effect was noted in most trials.

Studies have failed to show a beneficial effect of **oil of evening primrose**, **dong quai**, **ginseng** or other natural health products for reducing hot flashes.[19,27,28,32]

Hormone Therapy

The gold standard for treating symptoms of menopause is **estrogen**. Estrogen may be administered by oral, transdermal or vaginal routes. There are several differences between oral and transdermal estrogens. Oral estrogens cause an increase in HDL-cholesterol, a decrease in LDL-cholesterol and an increase in triglycerides. Transdermal estrogens primarily lower LDL-cholesterol with little change in HDL-cholesterol and no effect on triglycerides. Transdermal estrogen also has less impact on the coagulation cascade and gallbladder compared to oral estrogen. Therefore, transdermal therapy should be preferentially offered to women at high risk of venous thromboembolism, women with malabsorption, women with spontaneous or estrogen-induced hypertriglyceridemia, and obese women with metabolic syndrome.[1] Smoking induces liver enzyme activity; therefore, smokers may achieve higher concentrations of estrogens from a transdermal system compared with oral therapy.

Progestogens are combined with estrogen to reduce the risk of endometrial cancer. Therefore, in a woman who has had a hysterectomy, estrogens are often used alone. Progestogens can be administered either cyclically (12–14 days each month) or continuously, whereas estrogen is usually given continuously. Estrogens with cyclic progestogens will often produce a menstrual bleed, whereas estrogen with continuous progestogen should induce amenorrhea after 6–8 months of therapy.

Different types of progestogens are available.[33] Oral **micronized progesterone** (Prometrium) does not blunt the positive effects of estrogen on HDL-cholesterol, whereas both **medroxyprogesterone** and **norethindrone** can blunt estrogen's positive effect. Oral micronized progesterone may also cause sedation; therefore, it should be taken at bedtime.

Vaginal therapy (vaginal cream, vaginal tablets or vaginal ring) provides estrogen directly to vaginal tissues and alleviates symptoms of atrophy; it may be used for the treatment of urogenital aging. Vaginal estrogen is preferred when urogenital symptoms are the only concern and may be required if symptoms persist while the woman is taking systemic estrogen. Specifically in the case of urinary incontinence, there is modest evidence that vaginal estrogen lessened incontinence while systemic estrogen worsened it.[1,34]

While vaginal therapy results in less systemic absorption than oral therapy, studies reported increased serum estradiol levels with vaginal application of estrogen (especially conjugated equine estrogen cream, compared with the tablet or ring formulations), indicating that some systemic estrogen absorption occurs.[35] However, many studies of vaginal estrogen have shown no evidence of endometrial proliferation after 6–24 months of use; therefore, concomitant progestogen therapy or endometrial surveillance is not generally recommended for endometrial protection in asymptomatic (nonbleeding) women receiving an appropriate dose of vaginal estrogen therapy.[1] Patients using vaginal estrogens should be advised to adhere to the dosage and administration guidelines and to report any bleeding or spotting to their healthcare practitioner for further evaluation.

Combined hormonal contraceptives provide effective menstrual cycle control as well as relief of vasomotor symptoms and are an option for perimenopausal women who require supplemental estrogen.

Alternatives to estrogen for the treatment of vasomotor symptoms include progestogen therapy alone, **clonidine**, SSRIs (e.g., **paroxetine**, **fluoxetine**, **sertraline**, **citalopram** or **escitalopram**), SNRIs (e.g., **venlafaxine** or **desvenlafaxine**) and **gabapentin**. Evidence supporting efficacy of these agents varies from well-controlled trials to case reports and adverse effects may be significant.[1,36,37]

Prevention of Osteoporosis

For comparative ingredients of nonprescription products, consult the *Compendium of Products for Minor Ailments*—Vitamin and Mineral Products: Single Entity, Solid Combinations.

To prevent bone loss, intake of **calcium** 1200 mg daily (ideally from dietary sources) and supplementation of **vitamin D** 800–2000 IU daily is recommended for women >50 years of age (see Table 2).[38,39] For more information on prevention of osteoporosis, consult Chapter 47: Osteoporosis.

Monitoring of Therapy

Both nonpharmacologic and pharmacologic therapies may require several weeks to months of use before efficacy can be established. The length of therapy is variable. Vasomotor symptoms resolve within 5 years of menopause for the majority of women; it is therefore reasonable to continue therapy for up to 5 years. Urogenital atrophy may continue to be problematic indefinitely.

Every woman must make a subjective decision about the intrusiveness or tolerability of a given symptom and participate fully in the decision-making process regarding therapy. Armed with accurate, current information, she can make both short- and long-term decisions about symptom control and prevention of heart disease, osteoporosis and other menopause or age-related health issues. Monitoring can include asking the patient at each visit about the efficacy and side effects of her therapy, checking for interactions if she begins (or has already started) a new therapy and answering any questions she may have.

Figure 1: **Assessment of Patients with Menopausal Symptoms**

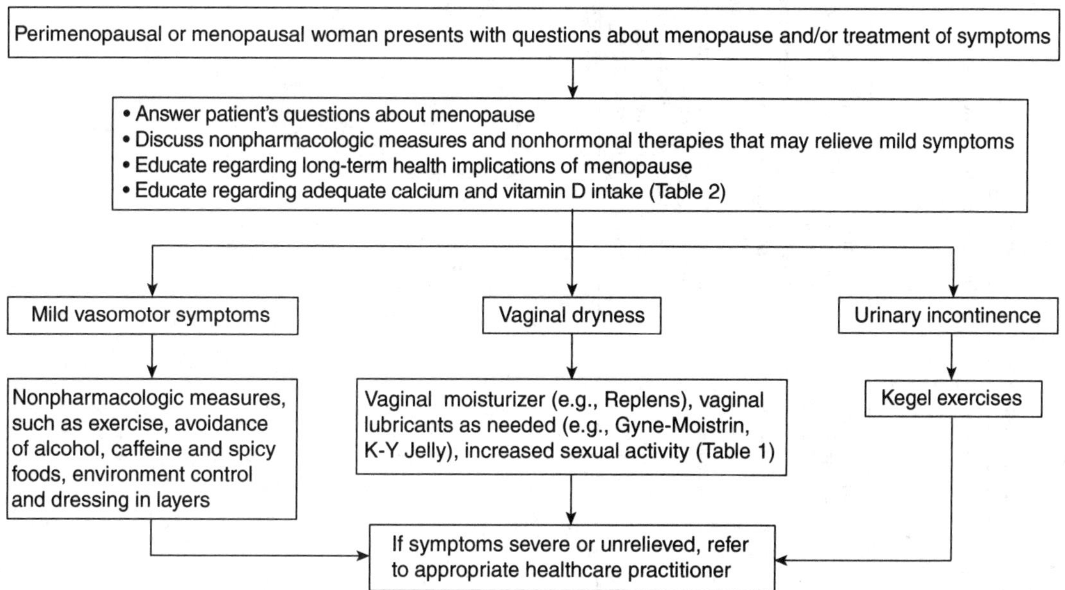

Table 1: Nonhormonal Topical Therapies for Vaginal Dryness

Class	Drug	Dosage	Adverse Effects	Drug Interactions	Comments	Cost[a]
Lubricants, vaginal	*vaginal gels or jelly* Astroglide, Gyne-Moistrin, K-Y Jelly, others	Apply as needed vaginally	Specialty lubricants (e.g., flavoured, scented) may contain ingredients that cause local irritation.	None known	Use prior to intercourse to provide lubrication.	$
Moisturizers, vaginal	*hyaluronic acid* Gynatrof, Zestica, others	Use vaginally QHS for at least 2–3 wk. May be used for longer periods	None known	May alter the absorption of vaginally administered hormones, including contraceptive vaginal rings.	The duration of use depends on evolution of symptoms. May be used every other day. Safe for use with latex, polyurethane and polyisoprene condoms.	$$
	polycarbophil gel Replens	Apply vaginally every 3 days on a continuous basis	None known	None known	Use to increase vaginal moisture and restore epithelium. Not to be used as occasional lubricant. Not to be used as a substitute for a vaginal lubricant prior to intercourse.	$

[a] Cost of smallest available pack size; includes drug cost only.

Legend: $ <$10 $$ $10–20

Table 2: **Nutritional Requirements to Prevent Bone Loss**

Class	Drug	Dosage	Adverse Effects	Drug Interactions	Comments	Cost[a]
Nutritional Supplements	*calcium* Caltrate, generics	1200 mg/day po from all sources (dietary and supplements)	When taken as a supplement: constipation, flatulence, nausea; rarely, hypercalcemia, hypercalciuria, renal calcification, renal stones (at high doses).	May decrease absorption of bisphosphonates, iron, levothyroxine, quinolones, tetracycline. Separate administration by 2 h.	Doses >500 mg/day should be divided. Select product based on salt type and amount of elemental calcium per tablet. Calcium carbonate requires acidic medium for best absorption (take with or after meals). Supplements are available as tablets, chewable forms, effervescent and liquid formulations.	$
	vitamin D generics	800–2000 IU/day po from all sources (dietary and supplements). Up to 2000 IU/ day po does not require monitoring by a healthcare practitioner[38]	Vitamin D intoxication (>50 000 IU/day)[40] may result in hypercalcemia, hypercalciuria, renal calcification, renal stones.	Increases calcium absorption.	Most multivitamins and many calcium supplements contain vitamin D. Also present in fish oils. Cholecalciferol (D_3) or ergocalciferol (D_2) may be used.	$

[a] Cost of 30-day supply; includes drug cost only.

Legend: $ <$5

Resource Tips

North American Menopause Society. Available from: www.menopause.org.

Society of Obstetricians and Gynaecologists of Canada. menopauseandu.ca. Available from: www.menopauseandu.ca in English or www.mamenopause.ca in French.

Suggested Readings

North American Menopause Society. The 2012 hormone therapy position statement of: The North American Menopause Society. *Menopause* 2012;19:257-71.

Position statement: non-hormonal management of menopause-associated vasomotor symptoms: 2015 position statement of the North American Menopause Society. *Menopause* 2015;22:1155-72.

Reid R, Abramson BL, Blake J et al. Managing menopause. *J Obstet Gynaecol Can* 2014;36:S1-80. Available from: sogc.org/wp-content/uploads/2014/09/gui311CPG1505Erev.pdf.

Shifren JL, Grass ML; NAMS Recommendations for Clinical Care of Midlife Women Working Group. The North American Menopause Society recommendations for clinical care of midlife women. *Menopause* 2014;21:1038-62.

Stuenkel CA, Davis SR, Gompel A et al. Treatment of symptoms of the menopause: an Endocrine Society clinical practice guideline. *J Clin Endocrinol Metab* 2015;100:3975-4011.

References

1. Reid R, Abramson BL, Blake J et al. Managing menopause. *J Obstet Gynaecol Can* 2014;36:S1-80. Available from: sogc.org/wp-content/uploads/2014/09/gui311CPG1505Erev.pdf.
2. Wren B. Menopause. In: Hacker NF, Moore JG, eds. *Essentials of obstetrics and gynecology.* 3rd ed. Philadelphia: WB Saunders; 1998. p. 602-9.
3. Paramsothy P, Harlow SD, Greendale GA et al. Bleeding patterns during the menopausal transition in the multi-ethnic Study of Women's Health Across the Nation (SWAN): a prospective cohort study. *BJOG* 2014;121:1564-73.
4. Lindh-Astrand L, Nedstrand E, Wyon Y et al. Vasomotor symptoms and quality of life in previously sedentary postmenopausal women randomised to activity or estrogen therapy. *Maturitas* 2004;48:97-105.
5. Daley A, Stokes-Lampard, H, Thomas A. Exercise for vasomotor menopausal symptoms. *Cochrane Database Syst Rev* 2014;11:CD006108.
6. Leiblum S, Bachmann G, Kemmann E et al. Vaginal atrophy in the postmenopausal woman. The importance of sexual activity and hormones. *JAMA* 1983;249:2195-8.
7. Bo K, Hagen RH, Kvarstein B et al. Pelvic floor muscle exercise for the treatment of female stress incontinence: III. Effects of two different degrees of pelvic floor muscle exercises. *Neurol Urodyn* 1990:489-502.
8. Kroenke CH, Caan BJ, Stefanick ML et al. Effects of dietary intervention and weight change on vasomotor symptoms in the Women's Health Initiative. *Menopause* 2012;19:980-8.
9. Murkies AL, Wilcox G, Davis SR. Clinical review 92: Phytoestrogens. *J Clin Endocrinol Metab* 1998;83:297-303.
10. Tham DM, Gardner CD, Haskell WL. Clinical review 97: Potential health benefits of dietary phytoestrogens: a review of the clinical epidemiological and mechanistic evidence. *J Clin Endocrinol Metab* 1998;83:2223-35.
11. Lock M. Ambiguities of aging: Japanese experience and perceptions of menopause. *Cult Med Psychiatry* 1986;10:23-46.
12. Davis SR. Phytoestrogen therapy for menopausal symptoms? *BMJ* 2001;323:354-5.
13. Lethaby A, Marjoribanks J, Kronenberg F et al. Phytoestrogens for menopausal vasomotor symptoms. *Cochrane Database Syst Rev* 2013;12:CD001395.
14. Chen MN, Lin CC, Liu CF. Efficacy of phytoestrogens for menopausal symptoms: a meta-analysis and systematic review. *Climacteric* 2015;18:260-9.
15. Tremblay A, Sheeran L, Aranda SK. Psychoeducational interventions to alleviate hot flashes: a systematic review. *Menopause* 2008;15:193-202.
16. Saensak S, Vutyavanich T, Somboonporn W et al. Relaxation for perimenopausal and postmenopausal symptoms. *Cochrane Database Syst Rev* 2014;7:CD008582.
17. Mann E, Smith MJ, Hellier J et al. Cognitive behavioural treatment for women who have menopausal symptoms after breast cancer treatment (MENOS 1): a randomised controlled trial. *Lancet Oncol* 2012;133:309-18.
18. Ayers B, Smith M, Hellier J et al. Effectiveness of group and self-help cognitive behavior therapy in reducing problematic menopausal hot flushes and night sweats (MENOS 2): a randomized controlled trial. *Menopause* 2012;19:749-59.
19. Position statement: non-hormonal management of menopause-associated vasomotor symptoms: 2015 position statement of the North American Menopause Society. *Menopause* 2015;22:1155-72.
20. Hunter M, Smith M. *Managing hot flushes and night sweats with group cognitive behaviour therapy: an evidence-based treatment manual for health professionals*. New York: Routledge; 2015.
21. Hunter M, Smith M. *Managing hot flushes and night sweats: a cognitive behavioural self-help guide to the menopause*. New York: Routledge; 2014.
22. Lee MS, Shin BC, Ernst E. Acupuncture for treating menopausal hot flushes: a systematic review. *Climacteric* 2009;12:16-25.
23. Carpenter JS, Neal JG. Other complementary and alternative medicine modalities: acupuncture, magnets, reflexology, and homeopathy. *Am J Med* 2005;118:109-17.

24. Dodin S, Blanchet C, Marc I et al. Acupuncture for menopausal hot flushes. *Cochrane Database Syst Rev* 2013;7:CD007410.
25. Nachtigall LE. Comparative study: Replens versus local estrogen therapy in menopausal women. *Fertil Steril* 1994;61:178-80.
26. Rahn DD, Carberry C, Sanses TV et al. Vaginal estrogen for genitourinary syndrome of menopause: a systematic review. *Obstet Gynecol* 2014;124:1147-56.
27. Nedrow A, Miller J, Walker M et al. Complementary and alternative therapies for the management of menopause-related symptoms: a systematic evidence review. *Arch Intern Med* 2006;166:1453-65.
28. Low Dog T. Menopause: a review of botanical dietary supplements. *Am J Med* 2005;118:98-108.
29. Newton KM, Reed SD, LaCroix AZ et al. Treatment of vasomotor symptoms of menopause with black cohosh, multibotanicals, soy, hormone therapy, or placebo: a randomized trial. *Ann Intern Med* 2006;145:869-79.
30. Leach MJ, Moore V. Black cohosh (Cimicifuga spp.) for menopausal symptoms. *Cochrane Database Syst Rev* 2012;9:CD007244.
31. Painter D, Perwaiz S, Murty M. Black cohosh products and liver toxicity: update. *Canadian Adverse Reaction Newsletter* 2010;20:1-2. Available from: www.hc-sc.gc.ca/dhp-mps/medeff/bulletin/carn-bcei_v20n1-eng.php#_Black_cohosh_products.
32. Herbal medicines for menopausal symptoms. *Drug Ther Bull* 2009;47:2-6.
33. The Writing Group for the PEPI Trial. Effects of estrogen or estrogen/progestin regimens on heart disease risk factors in postmenopausal women. The Postmenopausal Estrogen/Progestin Interventions (PEPI) trial. *JAMA* 1995;273:199-208.
34. Cody JD, Jacobs ML, Richardson K et al. Oestrogen therapy for urinary incontinence in post-menopausal women. *Cochrane Database Syst Rev* 2012;10:CD001405.
35. Suckling J, Lethaby A, Kennedy R. Local oestrogen for vaginal atrophy in postmenopausal women. *Cochrane Database Syst Rev* 2006;4:CD001500.
36. Nelson HD, Vesco KK, Haney E et al. Nonhormonal therapies for menopausal hot flashes: systematic review and meta-analysis. *JAMA* 2006;295:2057-71.
37. Shams T, Firwana B, Habib F et al. SSRIs for hot flashes: a systematic review and meta-analysis of randomized trials. *J Gen Intern Med* 2014;29:204-13.
38. Papaioannou A, Morin S, Cheung AM et al. 2010 clinical practice guidelines for the diagnosis and management of osteoporosis in Canada: summary. *CMAJ* 2010;182:1864-73.
39. Khan A, Fortier M, Reid R et al. Osteoporosis in menopause. *J Obstet Gynaecol Can* 2014;36:S1-15. Available from: sogc.org/wp-content/uploads/2014/09/JOGC-Sept2014-CPG-312_Eng_Online-Complete.pdf.
40. Holick MF. Vitamin D deficiency. *N Engl J Med* 2007;357:266-81.

Menopause and Perimenopause—What You Need to Know

What is menopause?

Menopause is the time in a woman's life when her menstrual periods stop, indicating the end of her childbearing years. It is a normal part of life for every woman. The average age for a woman to have her last period is 51.

The arrival of menopause is a gradual process that can take a number of years. The period of time before menstruation stops is called "perimenopause." It may begin 2–8 years before your final period.

You will see changes in your body during perimenopause and menopause, but menopause does not mean the end of your sex life. There are a lot of things you can do to stay healthy and to have an active sex life.

What are the common symptoms of menopause and perimenopause?

- A change in your menstrual cycle—this is one of the first signs of approaching menopause. You may skip periods or have them closer together.
- Hot flashes (sometimes called hot flushes, or night sweats if they happen at night). This is the most common symptom of menopause.
- Mood disturbances (depression, anxiety).
- Vaginal dryness—the vagina loses its ability to produce wetness during sex.
- Pain during sex—this can happen because the vagina is dry.
- Loss of bladder control—you may have to go to the bathroom more often. You may feel some leaking if you cough or sneeze.
- Skin changes—skin begins to get thinner and drier. This produces wrinkles.
- Lower sex drive—you may feel less interested in having sex.
- Memory loss—you may find that you have trouble remembering things, especially if you are tired or stressed.
- Sleep disturbances (difficulty sleeping, fragmented sleep).

What can you do to relieve symptoms of menopause and perimenopause?

- **To reduce hot flashes:**
  - avoid spicy foods, alcohol and caffeine
  - keep your house comfortably cool, especially at night
  - dress in layers in case you get too warm
  - stop smoking
  - get regular aerobic exercise (like walking). Try to exercise for 30 minutes, 5 times a week
  - maintain a healthy body weight
- **To prevent pain during sex:**
  - use a lubricant (such as K-Y Jelly or Gyne-Moistrin) before having sex
  - use an estrogen cream or moisturizer (such as Replens) every 3 days (or twice a week) in and around the vagina to help relieve dryness
  - any sexual activity will help keep the vagina moist. It doesn't have to be intercourse.

- **To improve bladder control:**
  - try Kegel exercises. Lie on your back with your knees bent. Keep your stomach, back and leg muscles relaxed. Squeeze your pelvic muscles as if you are trying to stop urinating. Hold for a count of 4 to 8 and then relax. Repeat the contracting and relaxing for about 5 minutes, several times daily.
- **For general relief of menopausal and perimenopausal symptoms:**
  - soy supplements have been shown to possibly give some relief from menopause symptoms. There is no proof that other herbal remedies provide relief. For more information, talk to your healthcare provider.
  - weight loss may benefit women who are overweight or obese.

What is hormone therapy?

Hormone therapy involves taking estrogen alone or estrogen combined with another hormone, progestin. Some women have found that hormone therapy can relieve menopause symptoms. However, hormone therapy is not for everyone. Studies indicate that there are also risks to hormone therapy. Your healthcare provider can help you understand the benefits and risks of hormone therapy to find out if it is right for you.

Ask your healthcare provider for information about how to prevent osteoporosis or heart disease after menopause. Your healthcare provider can help you plan a healthy lifestyle.

Chapter 80

Pregnancy and Fertility Testing

Marie Berry, BScPharm, BA, LLB

Pregnancy Testing

For an overview of the female reproductive cycle, see Chapter 76: Contraception.

Once an ovum is fertilized, it may take about 9 days before it is implanted in the endometrial wall. Human chorionic gonadotropin (HCG) is detectable in the blood and urine once the ovum is fertilized and implanted. In healthy women, HCG is a specific marker for pregnancy, because it is produced only by the placenta.

HCG, a glycoprotein produced by the trophoblastic cells of the placenta, maintains the corpus luteum. It replaces luteinizing hormone (LH). HCG can be detected as soon as 6–8 days after conception, and is highest in concentration between 9 a.m. and 12 p.m. Its concentration in the blood doubles about every 2 days, reaching a peak in 60–70 days. It then decreases to a lower level for the rest of the pregnancy. The half-life of HCG is about 5.6 hours. Following parturition it returns to baseline within 10 days. The detection of HCG is the basis of pregnancy testing kits.[1]

Initial pregnancy tests can be performed on urine samples and later confirmed with a blood test. Detectable HCG levels start at 5 mIU/mL during the first week of gestation and rise to a peak of about 100 000 mIU/mL. Blood tests can detect levels as low as 1 mIU/mL and most urine tests are able to detect 20–100 mIU/mL.

Prior to the advent of a biological assay for HCG, pregnancy tests were performed by injecting a woman's urine into a female rabbit. After 5 days, the rabbit was sacrificed and its uterus examined. Since HCG causes swelling of the corpus luteum and of the uterus, a heavy/enlarged rabbit's uterus meant that the woman was most likely pregnant.

In the 1960s, immunoassay technology allowed synthesis of an antibody that combined with HCG to produce a precipitant or change a coloured substrate. The pregnancy testing kits in use today represent the third generation of pregnancy testing technology.

For comparative features of nonprescription products, consult the *Compendium of Products for Minor Ailments*—Home Testing Products: Pregnancy Tests.

First-generation Tests

These tests used polyclonal antibodies, which recognized multiple binding sites on HCG. Unfortunately, these antibodies also reacted with other substances such as LH and follicle-stimulating hormone (FSH), resulting in false-positive results. This generation of tests has been replaced by second- and third-generation tests, which do not require sample collection and preparation, an incubation period or technical skill.

Second-generation Tests

Modern pregnancy tests employ monoclonal antibody technology and are more specific. In second-generation testing kits, the anti-HCG antibody is bound to a solid surface such as a stick, bead or filter paper. If HCG is present, it forms a complex with the antibody to produce a change in colour of a chromogen-reactive enzyme. The HCG becomes sandwiched between the 2 antibodies, one attached to the test surface and the other attached to the colour-producing enzyme.

Second-generation tests can detect HCG as early as the first day of a missed menstrual period and take a shorter time (1–30 minutes) to perform compared with first-generation tests.

Third-generation Tests

The tests available today for home use are third-generation tests (e.g., ClearBlue, First Response) in which the technology is even more refined. One anti-beta-subunit HCG monoclonal antibody is linked to a coloured substrate. If present, HCG binds to this antibody and the resulting complex binds to a second monoclonal antibody bound to a solid surface. The second monoclonal antibody is the alpha-subunit and elicits the colour change. Ease of use and accuracy are significant advantages of third-generation tests, so much so that one American study estimates that one third of women in the US have used third-generation pregnancy tests.[2]

Pregnancy testing kits afford early detection of pregnancy in privacy, and earlier detection can permit earlier prenatal care.[3] They also enable earlier avoidance of harmful chemicals, x-rays, drugs and elective surgery, all of which could potentially harm a developing fetus. The tests are easy to use and readily available with numerous generic versions. They offer speed, convenience and confidentiality, along with economical cost.

Proper Use

It is important to carefully follow the manufacturers' instructions for the specific pregnancy test being used. There may be variations among tests such as the method for collecting the urine, the length of time required to apply urine to the test stick or the symbols used to communicate test results. It is recommended to test at least one day after a missed period and to use the first urine sample of the morning when the HCG levels will be most concentrated. It is advisable to collect the urine midstream to avoid contamination of the sample. In general, urine is either collected in a small plastic cup or directly applied to a testing stick during urination. If urine is collected in a cup, a dropper is used to place a small amount of urine on the test, or the absorbent end of a test stick is placed into the cup for a specified amount of time. If urine is directly applied to a test stick during urination, it is important to place the absorbent end of the stick into the urine stream for the specified amount of time (e.g. 5 seconds). Once the urine has been applied, the test should be placed on a clean, level surface with the result window facing up for the required amount of time indicated in the instructions. Most third-generation tests have control windows to indicate whether the test was performed correctly. Once the specified testing time has elapsed, the control window can confirm whether a successful test has occurred and the test result can be read. A test is considered positive even if the indicator line or symbol is very faint as it confirms HCG was detected in the urine.

False-positive and false-negative results are possible regardless of which generation of test is used. Human error (e.g., holding the wrong end of the test stick in urine stream, exposing the test stick to the urine for less than the required length of time) is usually the cause of erroneous results. The easier a test is to use, the less likely errors will occur.

Timing of the pregnancy test is essential in that accuracy is more closely related to ovulation than to intercourse. Sperm can remain viable in the Fallopian tubes up to 5 days after intercourse and implantation takes an additional 6–12 days after ovulation (and subsequent fertilization). Therefore, false-negative results are possible up to 17 days after intercourse.

Other errors leading to false results include:

- Using an expired testing kit
- Not following the timing recommendations (waving the stick through the urine stream too quickly)
- Testing too early after conception when HCG levels are too low to be detected
- Testing too late (after 60–70 days when HCG levels decline)
- Soap residue, blood or protein in the urine sample
- Cloudy, pink or red urine
- Strong urine odour
- Warm or hot water rinses of the test surface before or after sampling
- Use of fertility drugs containing HCG (note: clomiphene will not affect tests), hormones, corticosteroids
- Ectopic production of HCG by nontrophoblastic tumours
- Conducting the test after missed or incomplete abortion.

Often pregnancy testing kits are purported to be 99% accurate and able to detect pregnancy as early as the first day of a missed period; however, a study showed that of 7 testing kits, only 2 would have detected 95% and 80% of pregnancies on the first day of the missed period.[4] Caution is required when interpreting pregnancy test results.

Fertility Testing

Methods Used to Predict Ovulation

Table 1 compares various methods of predicting the time of ovulation, including prediction methods other than those that are hormone-based.

Table 1: **Methods Used to Predict Ovulation**

Test	Indicators of Ovulation
Basal body temperature	Elevation of basal temperature (0.5°F or 0.28°C) over up to 3 days, lasting at least 11 days, usually continuing to day 1 of menses[5,6]
Chloride ion	Chloride ions levels increase about 6 days prior to ovulation (device is a wrist band with a microcomputer chip which detects chloride ions in perspiration on the skin).[7] This test is not sold in Canada
Cervical mucus	Abundant watery discharge; clear, elastic and stretchable mucus (tested with fingers); changes occur about 3–4 days prior to ovulation[5]
Saliva	Fern-like pattern on glass; changes occur about 3–4 days prior to ovulation (saliva is licked on a slide which then is examined under a microscope)[5]
Endometrial biopsy (late luteal phase)	Histology within 2 days of chronological cycle day based on LH surge[1]
Menstrual cycle history	Most cycles are 26–30 days (range 23–35 days) with ovulation mid-cycle, (e.g., around day 14 for a 28-day cycle). The postovulatory phase is usually more likely to be consistently around 14 days (e.g., in a 35-day cycle, ovulation might occur around day 21)[6]
Midluteal serum progesterone	Values greater than 10 ng/mL[1]
Urinary LH kits (ovulation prediction kits)	Colour change 20–48 h before ovulation;[8] specific time range is product-dependent

Basal Thermometers

For comparative features of nonprescription products, consult the *Compendium of Products for Minor Ailments*—Home Testing Products: Thermometers.

Basal body temperature is the temperature that occurs prior to rising in the morning. It can be taken orally, rectally or vaginally but must be consistently measured the same way and at the same time each day. A basal thermometer measures a more narrow range of temperatures than a fever thermometer (36–38°C or 96–99°F) and is able to detect small fluctuations in the basal temperature. Basal thermometers are easier to read than fever thermometers, and digital versions measuring to 2 decimal points may be even more user friendly.

Electronic basal thermometers combine data about menstrual cycle history with the measured temperatures to provide information about the timing of fertility.

Progesterone is thermogenic; elevated levels cause a rise in body temperature. About 12–24 hours prior to ovulation, a drop in temperature occurs; however, it is not always possible to detect the drop. When ovulation occurs, the corpus luteum releases progesterone, causing a significant rise in temperature that is detectable and lasts for several days. The temperature increase is about 0.5°F or 0.28°C and is measurable by a basal thermometer.[9] This temperature rise occurs over a period of up to 3 days and is usually maintained until the first day of menses—day 1 of the next cycle. It is not the temperature itself that is significant, but the maintained high temperature. A woman records her basal temperatures daily on a graph. With several cycles of data, a pattern may emerge, i.e., the usual day of ovulation in a woman's cycle.[5,6]

To be relevant, the basal body temperature needs to be measured in a consistent manner. Sleep disturbances can affect the temperature, and at least 4 hours of uninterrupted sleep is required before taking the temperature. Air travel, especially with a change in time zones, and jet lag can adversely affect the measurement, as can any factor that may on its own impact temperature, e.g., alcohol consumption, stress, anxiety, or illness, including infections.

Being able to identify a rise in temperature enables a woman to determine when she is most fertile and likely to conceive. Sexual intercourse (ideally every 2 days) during this time will increase the chance of conception. Conversely, a woman will also know when to avoid sexual intercourse if she does not want to conceive. For more information on contraception, see Chapter 76: Contraception.

Some women learn to use symptothermal charting, which combines symptoms (e.g., mucus, pain, breast tenderness, spotting) and basal body temperatures, allowing the fertile period to be more accurately pinpointed.

Ovulation Prediction Kits

For comparative features of nonprescription products, consult the *Compendium of Products for Minor Ailments*—Home Testing Products: Fertility Test Kits.

Ovulation prediction kits are not intended to be used as contraception.

Urine-based Kits

While basal thermometers identify the rise in temperature that accompanies progesterone release, ovulation prediction tests identify the luteinizing hormone (LH) surge that precedes ovulation by measuring its concentration in the urine. Conception is most likely to occur within 36 hours following the LH surge; therefore, a positive ovulation prediction test identifies the most fertile phase of the menstrual cycle.[10]

These tests employ polyclonal and monoclonal antibody technology. One antibody is bound to a test surface and another to an enzyme. If LH is present, it becomes sandwiched between the two antibodies and produces a colour change on the test surface. With no LH in the urine, the second antibody bound to the enzyme is washed away and no colour change occurs. The colour intensity depends upon the amount of LH present.

Most ovulation tests are mixtures of polyclonal and monoclonal antibodies. The polyclonal antibodies may bind with either the alpha- or beta-subunit of LH or even the entire molecule. The monoclonal antibodies are usually specific for the beta-subunit, which is a more accurate identifier of LH.[11]

More recently, tests are beta-subunit–specific antibodies bound to coloured latex particles. The second monoclonal antibody is bound to the test surface. Without LH, the antibody bound to the coloured latex is washed away.

Usually kits contain 5 daily tests that require 3–60 minutes to perform. Using the average length of her cycle, a woman uses a chart to determine the day of her cycle on which she should begin testing. Some test results are compared with baseline colour charts, some to the previous test and others to a control window. These tests are up to 98.3% accurate if performed properly.[12]

Because of its effects on estrogen levels, women taking clomiphene should not start testing for the LH surge until 3 days after taking their last tablet. Otherwise, the test may not accurately indicate the peak fertility time.

Fertility Monitors

Fertility testing technology has advanced to include monitors containing software programs that more specifically pinpoint fertility. These test kits combine the use of monitors with urine testing. The kits contain from 5–20 urine tests and the software program tracks the cycle day, indicating when a urine test should be performed. It usually reports the degree of fertility as low, high or peak.

These advanced tests use monoclonal technology and not only test for LH, but also for estrone-3-glucuronide (E3G), which is a urinary metabolite of estradiol. Estradiol stimulates the secretion of cervical mucus that is favourable for the survival and transport of sperm. The rise in estradiol levels corresponds to the appearance of sperm-supportive cervical mucus. Estradiol levels gradually rise in the early stage of the cycle, reaching a threshold that triggers the LH surge. With these tests, the stick is not read visually, but is inserted into the monitor, which optically reads the test and displays the result.[13]

For all of these kits, urine should be collected at the same time each day, and while some tests are to be done on the first urine in the morning, others can be performed anytime during the day as long as there is a sufficient volume to ensure an effective concentration of LH. Human error accounts for the majority of false readings. The inclusion of test controls and comparison of the results to the previous days' results reduce the chance of errors.

Test results can be affected by tetracycline and other drugs that affect the menstrual cycle such as hormonal contraceptives, fertility treatments that contain HCG or LH and hormone therapy. Pregnancy, breastfeeding, polycystic ovary syndrome and menopause may also affect results.[8] After pregnancy, breastfeeding or discontinuation of hormonal contraceptives or other hormonal therapy, 2 consecutive menstrual cycles are required before a woman can accurately test for LH surge.

Saliva-based Kits

Saliva-based testing detects a fern-like pattern in dried saliva seen under a microscope at a 40× to 60× magnification. Prior to ovulation, estrogen levels rise causing an increase in the salinity of saliva, which produces fern-like patterns when the saliva is dried. Testing is recommended to be performed first thing in the morning before eating, drinking, smoking or brushing the teeth. The saliva sample needs to be dried for at least 5 minutes and bubbles in the sample should be avoided. While the fern-like patterns are usually seen 3–4 days prior to ovulation, daily testing is sometimes recommended to detect changes. Note that not all women's saliva produces a fern-like pattern, and not all women are able to recognize this pattern.

Proper Use

The choice of a fertility testing method or methods depends upon personal preference, motivation of the woman or couple, physical factors (e.g., regularity of the menstrual cycle) and/or the complexity of the testing method. While some studies of accuracy have shown urinary LH tests to be superior to other fertility testing methods,[8] factors such as human error, variability in menstrual cycles and concurrent medical conditions can have a significant impact on the accuracy of any method.

Home diagnostic kits give an approximate time of ovulation and an indication of when a woman may be more fertile. Each kit has a chart or graph that can be used to determine, based on the woman's cycle, when testing should begin. These instructions should be followed for best results.

Couples using home ovulation predictor kits and/or basal body temperature charts to detect ovulation should be instructed in the interpretation of the results. Intercourse should begin before the expected day of ovulation and should occur at approximately 2-day intervals. This timing takes advantage of the fact that sperm survive for up to 5 days in the female reproductive tract, especially in good cervical mucus. Because sperm reserves of the male require at least 2 days for replenishment, more frequent intercourse may result in small volumes and a slightly lower sperm count. The use of artificial lubricants (e.g., K-Y jelly) during intercourse may interfere with fertility because they decrease sperm motility.

Methods Used to Detect Male Infertility

For comparative features of nonprescription products, consult the *Compendium of Products for Minor Ailments*—Home Testing Products: Fertility Test Kits.

Male infertility is defined as any condition in which the male adversely affects the chances of achieving successful pregnancy with his fertile female partner, and it is responsible for approximately 30–40% of infertility cases. While there are many physiological causes of male infertility, it is generally related to sperm production and quality, or ejaculation. Diagnostic evaluation begins with history, physical examination and semen analysis.

Semen analysis examines characteristics such as sperm count, morphology and motility. Sperm count refers to the amount of sperm in the ejaculate with the normal range defined as 20–150 million sperm/mL of semen.[14] Home sperm count tests use the bottom of this range, 20 million sperm/mL, as the threshold for their results. A positive result indicates the sperm count is above 20 million sperm/mL, and a negative result indicates that the count is below 20 million sperm/mL.[15,16]

Home sperm tests are immunodiagnostic devices, employing monoclonal antibodies that recognize the spermatid and sperm-specific acrosomal protein SP-10. SP-10 is readily released from the sperm's acrosomal compartment with mild detergents and remains soluble in aqueous solutions, making it available for detection by monoclonal antibodies.[15]

To perform the test, men are advised to wait at least 48 hours, but not more than 7 days, after their last ejaculation to collect their semen sample. For testing, semen is ejaculated directly into a collection cup and allowed to stand for 20–60 minutes to allow it to liquefy (it is too thick to be tested immediately after ejaculation). A pipette is then used to stir the semen and draw a sample which is added to a detergent-containing buffer solution. The mixture is gently agitated and allowed to stand for 2 minutes before being applied directly to the sperm test assay device. Test results are read 7 minutes after the semen mixture is applied to the assay. The test contains a control line and a test line. A test is positive if any line at all appears at the test position, regardless of how dark or faint it may be. If no line appears in the control position, the test did not run correctly and the results are not valid.[16]

Human error at any stage in the testing process can impact the validity of the results. Some common causes of error include testing a sample collected less than 48 hours after previous ejaculation; not collecting the entire ejaculate, especially the initial drops; not waiting for the sample to liquefy (minimum 20 minutes, up to 3 hours); not adding the correct amount of semen to the buffer solution; adding solid material from the sample to the buffer solution; not adding the correct number of drops of the sperm mixture to the test device; applying the sperm mixture to the incorrect area on the test device; or reading the test incorrectly due to poor lighting or vision.[16]

As male infertility cannot be diagnosed on the basis of sperm count alone, the role of the home sperm count test is limited to that of a front-line self-diagnostic tool to direct men to a fertility specialist. The test may assist couples concerned about their fertility in deciding whether to seek comprehensive clinical evaluation of the fertility status of the male partner. While a negative result may indicate infertility, it is important to appreciate that a positive result cannot be interpreted as confirmation of fertility.

References

1. Stanford JB, White GL, Hatasaka H. Timing intercourse to achieve pregnancy: current evidence. *Obstet Gynecol* 2002;100:1333-41.
2. Pray WS, Pray GE. Detecting pregnancy and ovulation with home test kits. *US Pharm* 2012;37:12-5.
3. Gannon K. Who is most apt to turn to a home pregnancy test? *Drug Topics* 1992;136:46.
4. Cole LA, Sutton-Riley JM, Khanlian SA et al. Sensitivity of over-the-counter pregnancy tests: comparison of utility and marketing messages. *J Am Pharm Assoc (2003)* 2005;45:608-15.
5. Pyper CM. Fertility awareness and natural family planning. *Eur J Contracept Reprod Health Care* 1997;2:131-46.
6. Moghissi KS. Accuracy of basal body temperature for ovulation detection. *Fertil Steril* 1976;27:1415-21.
7. Lennard J. Advanced technology for fertility prediction. *US Pharm* 2006;12:49-54.
8. Eichner SF, Timpe EM. Urinary-based ovulation and pregnancy: point-of-care testing. *Ann Pharmacother* 2004;38:325-31.
9. Downs KA, Gibson M. Basal body temperature graph and the luteal phase defect. *Fertil Steril* 1983;40:466-8.
10. Corsan GH, Ghazi D, Kemmann E. Home urinary luteinizing hormone immunoassays: clinical applications. *Fertil Steril* 1990;53:591-601.
11. Engle JP. Ovulation predictors. *Am Drug* 1993;207:55.
12. When the test really counts: part two: the fertility window. *Consum Rep* 2003;68:48-50.
13. Miller PB, Soules MR. The usefulness of a urinary LH kit for ovulation prediction during menstrual cycles of normal women. *Obstet Gynecol* 1996;87:13-7.
14. Essential Evidence Plus. John Wiley & Sons, Inc. *Infertility (male)*. Available from: www.essentialevidenceplus.com. Accessed September 17, 2015. Subscription required.
15. Coppola MA, Klotz KL, Kim KA et al. SpermCheck Fertility, an immunodiagnostic home test that detects mormozoospermia and severe oligozoospermia. *Hum Reprod* 2010;25:853-61.
16. SpermCheck Fertility. *Instructions for use. Home sperm test for male fertility.* Available from: www.spermcheck.com/wp-content/uploads/2012/05/SCF_US-FNL-INSERT.pdf. Accessed September 17, 2015.

Chapter 81
Premenstrual Syndrome

Thomas E.R. Brown, BScPhm, PharmD

CPhA acknowledges the contribution of Katrina Mulherin as a previous author of this chapter.

Pathophysiology

Definition

The term premenstrual syndrome (PMS) refers to the cyclic recurrence of physical and/or cognitive (behavioural) symptoms during the luteal phase of the menstrual cycle (after ovulation), that ameliorate upon onset of menses.[1] Premenstrual dysphoric disorder (PMDD) is a severe subtype of PMS that includes significant mood changes and impairment of functioning.[1] For a more complete discussion of the menstrual cycle see Chapter 76: Contraception or Chapter 77: Dysmenorrhea.

PMS symptoms occur in 90% of women of reproductive age at some point in life,[1] whereas PMDD affects 3–8% of women.[1] The main focus of this chapter is PMS.

Etiology

The etiology of PMS has not been fully elucidated.[2,3] Several theories have been proposed involving fluctuations in hormonal levels during the menstrual cycle, dysregulation of neurotransmitter systems and nutritional deficiencies.

Increased sensitivity to normal fluctuations in sex steroid hormones (estradiol and progesterone) during the menstrual cycle has been proposed as a possible etiologic factor in PMS.[2,4] A study of premenstrual women demonstrated that the occurrence of symptoms was due to an abnormal response to normal hormonal fluctuations.[5] Because ovarian sex hormones can affect the synthesis, release, reuptake and inactivation of neurotransmitters,[6] fluctuations in these hormones may lead to PMS or PMDD in susceptible women.[4]

Serotonin is a neurotransmitter that plays a role in modulating mood and behaviour.[7] Studies have shown that women with PMS have lower whole blood serotonin concentrations and decreased platelet uptake of serotonin during the late luteal phase of the menstrual cycle, compared with control subjects.[7] Decreased serotonergic neurotransmission may be associated with depressed mood, irritability, anger, aggression, poor impulse control and appetite disturbances.[7]

Although evidence for serotonin abnormalities in PMS is the most convincing, abnormalities in the catecholaminergic, gamma-aminobutyric acid (GABA) and opioid neurotransmitter systems have been observed in women with PMS.[2,4,8] Additionally, the association between negative mood and the luteal phase of the menstrual cycle has been questioned in a systematic review of 47 studies collecting prospective data on mood and menstrual cycles.[9]

Risk Factors

A case-control study of over 3000 American women aged 27–44 found higher doses of vitamin D lowered the risk of developing PMS. Specifically, women with median daily **vitamin D** intake of 706 IU had a relative risk of experiencing PMS of 0.59 compared with women with median daily intake of 112 IU.[10] A subsequent case-control study of 186 women aged 18–30 found no relationship between low plasma levels of late luteal phase 25-hydroxyvitamin D_3 and PMS, but similar to the first study, found a lower risk of PMS in women who consumed ≥100 IU/day of vitamin D.[11] Research to date does not address whether vitamin D monotherapy is effective in treating PMS. Deficiencies in certain nutrients such as calcium, magnesium, manganese, vitamin B_6, vitamin E and linoleic acid have been reported in PMS.[4] However, consistent excess or deficiency in these dietary factors has not been clearly documented in women with PMS as compared with control subjects.[12]

PMS is twice as prevalent in identical twins compared with fraternal twins, suggesting a genetic predisposition to PMS.[2,4]

Evidence suggests that high body mass index,[13] stress[14] and traumatic life events[15] may be risk factors for experiencing PMS. Low parity, oral contraceptive use, menstrual cycle characteristics and socioeconomic or lifestyle variables are not consistently associated with the development of PMS.[4]

Clinical Presentation

PMS is frequently a diagnosis of exclusion, as there is no currently accepted diagnostic test for this condition.[4,16,17] Indeed, some clinicians challenge the very existence of PMS.[16] The differential diagnosis may include anemia, diabetes, thyroid disorders, chronic fatigue syndrome, endometriosis, polycystic ovaries, adverse effects from oral contraceptives, perimenopause, fibrocystic breast changes and various psychiatric disorders.[4,16] These conditions should be considered before a firm diagnosis of PMS is made.

A diagnosis of PMS is generally agreed upon if symptoms:[16]

- are present during the luteal phase of the menstrual cycle
- reach their peak shortly before the beginning of menstruation and remit at the onset of menses or shortly thereafter
- are severe enough to interfere with daily functioning and interpersonal relationships
- are absent during the follicular phase of the menstrual cycle.

The diagnosis of PMS is confirmed through prospective monitoring of a woman's symptoms during at least 2 menstrual cycles.[4,16,18] A daily symptom calendar can be used to determine whether the woman's symptoms are cyclical and are confined to the luteal phase.

Table 1: **Symptoms of Premenstrual Syndrome**

Cognitive/Behavioural	Physical
Aggression	Acne
Anger	Appetite change
Anxiety	Bloating, fluid retention, oliguria
Depression	Breast pain or swelling
Fatigue	Constipation
Forgetfulness	Dizziness or vertigo
Hostility	Fatigue
Irritability	Headache
Lethargy	Hot flashes
Mood lability	Muscle aches
Panic attacks	Nausea and vomiting
Poor concentration	Pelvic heaviness or pressure
Reduced coping skills	Weight gain

Over the last several decades, research into PMS has identified over 100 premenstrual symptoms.[19] Symptoms of PMS can be divided into 2 broad categories: cognitive (or behavioural) and physical (Table 1).[3] The fifth edition of the Diagnostic and Statistical Manual of Mental Disorders (DSM-5) includes PMDD as a formal diagnosis.[20,21] However, debate continues surrounding the potential for pathologizing normal female physiology in establishing diagnoses for PMS and PMDD.[22]

The onset of PMS and related symptoms can occur at any time after puberty[23] with typical onset in the mid-twenties.[1] Women usually seek treatment in their thirties.[4,23] Perimenopausal women can suffer from PMS, but it subsides after menopause.

The number of symptoms required for a diagnosis of PMS is not consistent among different authorities.[16,23] The criteria developed by the American College of Obstetricians and Gynecologists require the presence of at least 1 symptom from a list of specific cognitive and physical symptoms during the 5 days prior to menses and occurring over several cycles. Symptoms must cause social or economic decline in function.[24,25] To prevent overdiagnosis of this condition, it is suggested that the presence of 5 or more symptoms that change in severity throughout the menstrual cycle is appropriate for a diagnosis of PMS.[23]

Goals of Therapy

- Relieve symptoms
- Minimize functional impairment

Healthcare practitioners can support these goals by providing patient education about the pathophysiology of PMS, the proper use of symptom diaries to evaluate symptoms and available treatment options.

Patient Assessment

For a diagnosis of PMS, patients should prospectively report, for at least 2 menstrual cycles, symptoms in the latter half of their cycle. Table 2 presents a sample chart that patients may use to record their symptoms. These complaints should be cyclic in nature, i.e., they should resolve at the start of menses and not be present during the entire menstrual cycle (see Pathophysiology, Clinical Presentation). Refer patients who have severe, debilitating symptoms with a strong affective or psychological component for assessment of possible PMDD (see Table 3). Women with mild to moderate symptoms of PMS often do not seek or require pharmacologic treatment.[1]

Nonpharmacologic Therapy

Figure 1 presents the suggested management of patients with PMS.

Lifestyle Modifications

Relaxation and stress reduction techniques (reflexology, massage, biofeedback) and treatments such as acupuncture and light therapy, although not rigorously studied, can be recommended to women suffering from PMS as a means of promoting a healthy lifestyle and symptom control.[1,26,27] Because symptoms of PMS can include both insomnia and hypersomnia, encourage appropriate sleep hygiene techniques (see Chapter 5: Insomnia).[1,4] Symptom diaries (Table 2) confer a sense of understanding and control of PMS and are recommended for monitoring and improvement in the symptoms themselves.[23]

Data suggest regular moderate exercise has a beneficial effect on the symptoms of PMS[4,23,28] including breast tenderness, fluid retention, stress and depression.[4,28] Encourage women to engage in moderate aerobic activity 3–4 times weekly as a method of alleviating their symptoms.[4]

Table 2: **Sample Monitoring Chart for Premenstrual Symptoms**[a]

Day of Menstrual Cycle	1	2	3	4	5	6	7	8	9	10	11	12	13	14	15	16	17	18	19	20	21	22	23	24	25	26	27	28	29	30	31
Affective or Cognitive Symptoms																															
Aggression																															
Anger																															
Anxiety																															
Depression																															
Fatigue																															
Forgetfulness																															
Hostility																															
Irritability																															
Lack of energy																															
Mood swings																															
Panic attacks																															
Poor concentration																															
Reduced coping skills																															
Physical Symptoms																															
Acne																															
Appetite change																															
Bloating, fluid retention, less urine than usual																															
Breast pain or swelling																															
Constipation																															
Dizziness or vertigo																															
Fatigue																															
Headaches																															
Hot flashes																															
Muscle aches																															
Nausea and vomiting																															
Pelvic heaviness or pressure																															
Weight gain																															

[a] Rate symptoms according to severity (e.g., 3 = severe, 2 = moderate, 1 = mild, 0 = absent).

Table 3: **DSM-5 Diagnostic Criteria for Premenstrual Dysphoric Disorder (PMDD)**

A. In the majority of menstrual cycles, at least five symptoms must be present in the final week before onset of menses, start to *improve* within a few days after the onset of menses and become *minimal* or absent in the week post menses.

B. One (or more) of the following symptoms must be present:

1. Marked affective lability (e.g., mood swings, feeling suddenly sad or tearful, or increased sensitivity to rejection).
2. Marked irritability or anger or increased interpersonal conflicts.
3. Marked depressed mood, feelings of hopelessness or self-deprecating thoughts.
4. Marked anxiety, tension and/or feelings of being keyed up or on edge.

C. One (or more) of the following symptoms must additionally be present, to reach a total of *five* symptoms when combined with symptoms from Criterion B above.

1. Decreased interest in usual activities (e.g., work, school, friends, hobbies).
2. Subjective difficulty in concentration.
3. Lethargy, easy fatigability or marked lack of energy.
4. Marked change in appetite, overeating or specific food cravings.
5. Hypersomnia or insomnia.
6. A sense of being overwhelmed or out of control.
7. Physical symptoms such as breast tenderness or swelling, joint or muscle pain, a sensation of "bloating," or weight gain.

Note: The symptoms in Criteria A–C must have been met for most menstrual cycles that occurred in the preceding year.

D. The symptoms are associated with clinically significant distress or interference with work, school, usual social activities or relationships with others (e.g., avoidance of social activities; decreased productivity and efficiency at work, school or home.)

E. The disturbance is not merely an exacerbation of the symptoms of another disorder, such as major depressive disorder, panic disorder, persistent depressive disorder (dysthymia) or a personality disorder (although it may co-occur with any of these disorders.).

F. Criterion A should be confirmed by prospective daily ratings during at least two symptomatic cycles. **(Note:** The diagnosis may be made provisionally prior to this confirmation.)

G. The symptoms are not attributable to the physiological effects of a substance (e.g., a drug of abuse, a medication, other treatment) or another medical condition (e.g., hyperthyroidism).

Reprinted with permission from the *Diagnostic and Statistical Manual of Mental Disorders*, Fifth Edition, (Copyright ©2013). American Psychiatric Association. All Rights Reserved.

Dietary Modifications

In a study on the effects of caffeine restriction, a large proportion of women who refrained from consuming methylxanthine-containing foods and beverages noted improvement in breast symptoms.[12] Although data are limited, it is reasonable to recommend that women who suffer from PMS limit their intake of caffeine from coffee, tea, chocolate and caffeine-containing soft drinks.[12,29]

Carbohydrate intake may lessen appetite changes and cognitive symptoms.[30] Recommend small, frequent carbohydrate servings to women experiencing these symptoms.

Restricting salt intake in the luteal phase has been suggested as a method of alleviating PMS symptoms of fluid retention, weight gain, bloating and breast swelling and tenderness.[23,25] Although not studied, it is a reasonable recommendation for reducing PMS symptoms.

Pharmacologic Therapy

For comparative ingredients of nonprescription products, consult the *Compendium of Products for Minor Ailments*—Analgesic Products: Internal Analgesics and Antipyretics; Feminine Care Products: Dysmenorrhea and Premenstrual Syndrome Symptom Relief; Vitamin and Mineral Products: Single Entity, Solid Combinations.

The use of prostaglandin inhibitors is based on a theory that PMS results from an excess of prostaglandins.[23] NSAID choices include **ibuprofen** and **naproxen**. Ibuprofen and naproxen are expected to provide symptomatic relief of headache, breast pain and muscle aches experienced during PMS.[4,23] Ibuprofen or naproxen should be started at the onset of pain and used short-term in the lowest effective dose. For more information see Chapter 8: Headache.

A randomized, controlled trial showed that **calcium** 1200 mg daily (in the form of calcium carbonate) was more effective than placebo for reducing symptoms of negative affect, water retention, food cravings and pain in women with PMS. The authors speculated that calcium supplementation might act to replace a calcium deficit, leading to decreased parathyroid hormone secretion and reduced neuromuscular irritability and vascular reactivity.[31] Calcium has the strongest evidence among herbs, vitamins and minerals for its use in PMS (see Table 4).[32,33]

Several small, randomized, placebo-controlled trials have shown **magnesium** to be a promising treatment alternative for premenstrual symptoms such as fluid retention.[4,23] Although the evidence is not definitive for magnesium,[24] if a woman chooses to try this supplement, a dose of 200–400 mg daily throughout the cycle could be recommended.[4] A mild laxative effect has been observed with higher doses of magnesium (see Table 4).[4]

The rationale for using **pyridoxine (vitamin B_6)** in the treatment of PMS stems from the fact that it is a cofactor in the synthesis of dopamine and the metabolism of tryptophan (a serotonin precursor).[12] Vitamin B_6 increases the inhibitory to excitatory amine ratio, which could theoretically alleviate PMS, as several symptoms are thought to represent an excitatory state of the CNS.[12] Some evidence supports the use of vitamin B_6 in the treatment of premenstrual symptoms.[32,34,35,36] A meta-analysis of 9 trials[36] and a systematic review[34] studying the use of vitamin B_6 in PMS concluded that it is likely beneficial in treating premenstrual symptoms and premenstrual depression. Vitamin B_6 can be recommended in doses of 50–100 mg daily.[34,35,36] Doses exceeding 200 mg daily have been associated with peripheral neuropathy (see Table 4).[36]

Although **vitamin E** has been proposed as a potential treatment of PMS, there is no definitive evidence to support its efficacy.[23]

Several combination products include an analgesic as well as **pamabrom** (a diuretic) and/or **pyrilamine** (an antihistamine). Evidence that the addition of these 2 agents offers superior efficacy over an analgesic alone is not available. Most experts believe that if these 2 agents have added benefit, their effects are mild at best.

Oral contraceptives (OCs) containing ethinyl estradiol and various first-, second- and third-generation progestogens have been used to treat PMS but there are few data to support use.[1,25] Psychological response to hormonal fluctuations is thought to be responsible for PMS. OCs halt ovulation but also cause hormonal fluctuations which may explain lack of efficacy for cognitive symptoms.[25] Physical symptoms may improve but adverse effects from OCs are similar to PMS symptoms and patients may find OCs cause more problems.[1] If an OC is used, theoretically, a monophasic preparation might be preferred.[1,25] Initial studies of 4 months of continuous daily ethinyl estradiol 20 µg and levonorgestrel 90 µg for treatment of PMS and PMDD indicates questionable efficacy in short-term trials. The high placebo response suggests little clinical benefit for this treatment.[37]

OCs containing **ethinyl estradiol** 20 or 30 µg plus **drospirenone** 3 mg have been studied in PMS and PMDD. Drospirenone is an antimineralocorticoid progestogen with a similar diuretic effect to spironolactone 25 mg. This diuretic effect, coupled with the reduced hormonal fluctuations seen with monophasic OCs, provides a theoretical basis for its efficacy in PMS. The 20 µg strength of ethinyl estradiol plus drospirenone 3 mg (24/4 preparation where 24 days of active tablets are followed by 4 days of inert tablets) has been approved in the United States for use in women with PMDD who wish to use OCs for contraception. A Cochrane review of drospirenone-containing OCs concluded that drospirenone 3 mg/ethinyl estradiol 20 µg combinations may be effective for endpoints of symptom severity and functional improvement in women with PMDD, but efficacy was not shown beyond 3 months of treatment.[38] Placebo response was high, suggesting little clinically significant effect. No benefit was seen in patients experiencing less severe PMS symptoms.[38] In Canada OCs containing drospirenone (21/7 and 24/4 preparations) are indicated for contraception but not for PMS or PMDD.

Observational studies and systematic reviews have found an increased relative risk of venous thromboembolism (VTE) in women using drospirenone-containing products compared with combination OCs containing levonorgestrel or norgestimate.[39,40,41,42,43,44,45] These findings were supported by population-based, case-control studies in 2 large primary care databases in the United Kingdom.[46] Women who have a family history of VTE or cancer, are on bed rest, or who have other risk factors predisposing to VTE may not be candidates for a drospirenone-containing OC. Given the lack of evidence for sustained clinical benefit for PMDD, consider the risk-benefit ratio of using drospirenone-containing OCs.

Progestogens other than drospirenone require further high-quality trials to determine whether they ameliorate symptoms of PMS.[47]

The SSRIs **citalopram**, **escitalopram**, **fluoxetine**, **paroxetine** and **sertraline** may be effective in treating symptoms of PMS/PMDD.[48] A 2013 Cochrane review examined 31 trials comparing various SSRIs with placebo for effectiveness in PMS and PMDD. SSRIs appeared to have a more defined benefit in women experiencing PMDD than PMS as most of the trials enrolled predominantly women experiencing PMDD. Benefit was seen at low, moderate or high doses whether they were taken continuously or only in the luteal phase of the menstrual cycle. Statistically significant differences in efficacy were apparent, however the degree of clinical significance is questionable. The trials were conducted over a limited 2- to 6-month period and therefore effectiveness beyond 6 months has not been established. Risk of experiencing an adverse effect at a moderate and high SSRI dose was considerable, particularly asthenia and nausea. Notably, the review included predominantly industry-funded trials of low to moderate quality.

The Cochrane review suggested physical symptoms may also be ameliorated by SSRIs; however, it may be that these patients had a mixture of psychological and physical manifestations. An earlier secondary analysis of SSRI effectiveness in PMS and PMDD indicated psychological benefits in PMS and PMDD but not physical relief.[49] Patients with physical symptoms only may not find SSRIs effective.

Other antidepressants such as **clomipramine**, **duloxetine** and **venlafaxine** have also been used in PMS but have comparatively less support than SSRIs for use in this population.[1]

Other therapies include **spironolactone** for breast tenderness and fluid retention, as well as **bromocriptine** for breast tenderness.[1] The dopamine agonist **cabergoline** (0.5 mg daily on day 14 and day 21 of the menstrual cycle) showed similar efficacy to bromocriptine for breast tenderness associated with PMS in a preliminary trial.[50] **GnRH analogues** (e.g., goserelin, leuprolide, nafarelin) and **danazol** (used during luteal phase) are reserved for severe or unresponsive cases of PMS due to their extensive and serious adverse effect profiles.[1]

Natural Health Products

For comparative ingredients of nonprescription products, consult the *Compendium of Products for Minor Ailments*—Herbal and Natural Health Products: Single Entity.

Oil of evening primrose has been shown to be no better than placebo in relief of PMS-related symptoms.[29,51,52] **St. John's wort** has a lack of well-designed trials to support use.[1,53] A Cochrane review found one well-designed trial that supported the use of **jingqianping** granule, a traditional Chinese medicine for increasing the rate of recovery from PMS. However, further study is needed before this remedy can be recommended.[54] **Ginkgo biloba** has been shown to decrease the severity of both physical and psychological symptoms of PMS in a preliminary trial.[55] At this time, there is insufficient evidence to recommend these strategies as appropriate methods of treating PMS.

Chasteberry has been found to have benefit in reducing cyclical breast discomfort and for improving symptoms of PMS overall.[1,32,56,57] However, variances in dosing and study design complicate recommendations. Doses used in trials include 4 mg daily of an extract standardized to 6% of agnuside, 20–40 mg daily of the fruit extract, 40 drops daily of a fluid extract or 35–45 drops 3 times daily of a tincture.[57] Side effects of chasteberry include dizziness, headache, fatigue, dry mouth and mild GI discomfort. A trial comparing chasteberry with fluoxetine found similar efficacy between the 2 treatments.[58]

Monitoring of Therapy

Encourage women to self-monitor their response to various treatment measures by charting their symptoms regularly (Table 2).

Efficacy: Women with unrelenting or progressive symptoms despite drug therapy for 1–3 months (depending on drug and degree of response) should have treatment reassessed.

Safety: Adverse effects of drugs should be screened at appropriate intervals depending on therapy chosen.

Figure 1: **Treatment of Patients with Premenstrual Syndrome (PMS)**

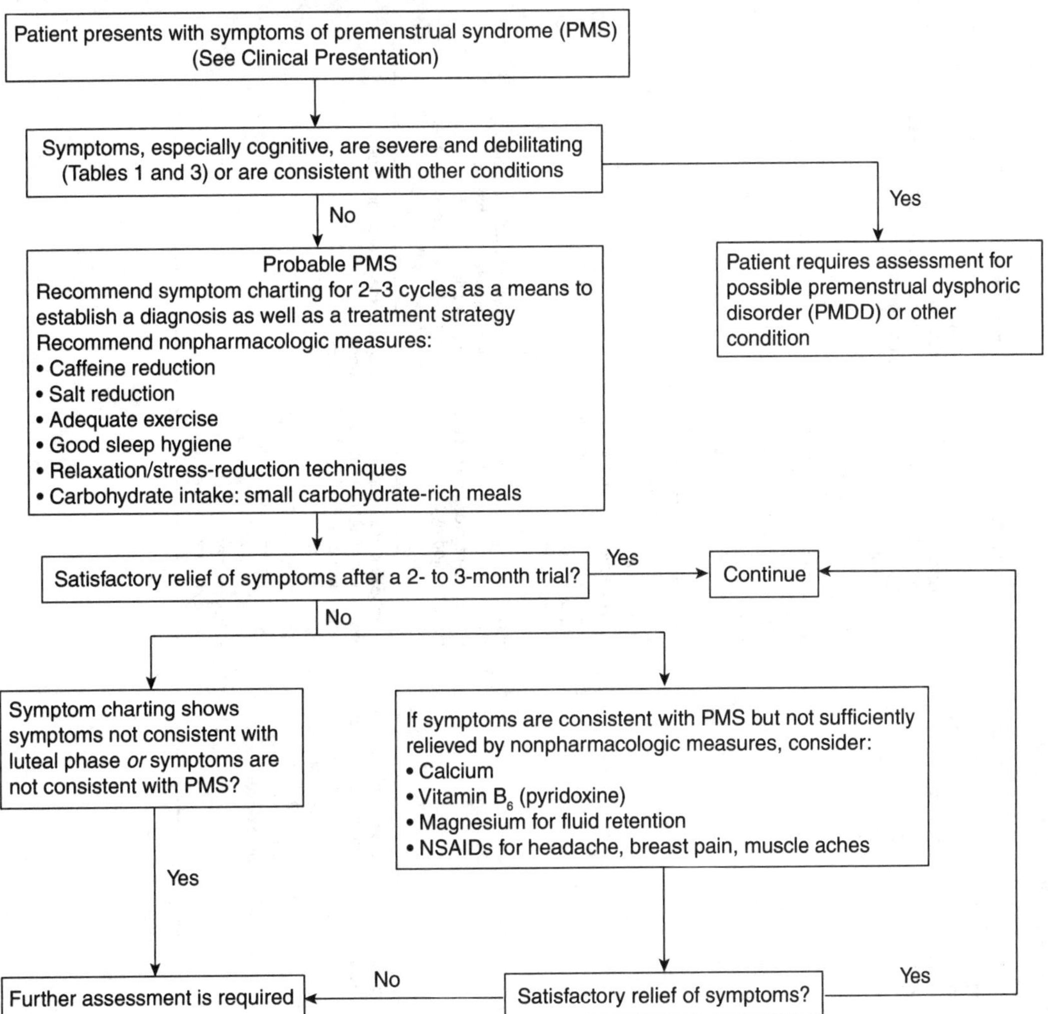

Table 4: Selected Therapies for Premenstrual Syndrome

Class	Drug	Dosage	Adverse Effects	Drug Interactions	Comments	Cost[a]
Minerals	*calcium* Caltrate, generics	1200 mg (elemental calcium) daily in divided doses po	Constipation. Caution in severe renal impairment.	Decreases absorption of bisphosphonates, iron, levothyroxine, phenytoin, phosphate, quinolones, tetracyclines. Antacid effect may alter absorption of other medications; calcium dosing should be separated from other medications by 2 h. May decrease therapeutic effect of calcium channel blockers. May enhance inotropic effects of digoxin and lead to arrhythmias. Thiazide diuretics decrease excretion of calcium and may increase risk of hypercalcemia.	Improvement in mood, water retention, cravings, pain; corroborating trials are required to confirm efficacy.	$$
	magnesium generics	200–400 mg daily po	Diarrhea, asthenia, dizziness.	Magnesium salts decrease GI absorption of drugs dosed concomitantly; dosing should be separated by 2 h.	Good quality evidence is lacking to support use, but may be helpful for fluid retention. Contraindicated in severe renal impairment and heart block.	$
Vitamins	*pyridoxine* (renal symbol) generics	50–100 mg daily po Do not exceed 200 mg/day	Nausea, headache, paresthesia. Sensory neuropathy (ataxia, numbness of hands and feet) has occurred with chronic use of large doses.	Metabolism of levodopa increased; effect prevented when levodopa combined with carbidopa. High doses (80–200 mg/day) may increase metabolism of phenytoin and barbituates. Estrogen therapy increases pyridoxine requirements.	Do not exceed recommended dose.	$

[a] Cost of 30-day supply; includes drug cost only.

(renal symbol) Dosage adjustment may be required in renal impairment.

Legend: $ < $3 $$ $3–6

Resource Tips

Massachusetts General Hospital. MGH Center for Women's Mental Health. *PMS & PMDD*. Available from: www.womensmentalhealth.org/specialty-clinics/pms-and-pmdd/.

U.K. National Health Service. Choices: your health, your choices. *Premenstrual syndrome (PMS)*. Available from: www.nhs.uk/Conditions/Premenstrual-syndrome/Pages/Introduction.aspx.

Suggested Readings

Douglas S. Premenstrual syndrome. Evidence-based treatment in family practice. *Can Fam Physician* 2002;48:1789-97.

Borgelt LM, Gunning K. Disorders related to the menstrual cycle. In: Koda-Kimble MA, Alldredge BK, Corelli RL et al., eds. *Koda-Kimble and Young's applied therapeutics: the clinical use of drugs*. 10th ed. Philadelphia: Wolters Kluwer; Lippincott Williams & Wilkins; 2013. p. 1149-74.

Jarvis CI, Lynch AM, Morin AK. Management strategies for premenstrual syndrome/premenstrual dysphoric disorder. *Ann Pharmacother* 2008;42:967-78.

Jurgens T, Whelan AM. Advising patients on the use of natural health products to treat premenstrual syndrome. *Can Pharm J* 2009;142:228-33.

Laufer LR, Gambone JC. Menstrual cycle-influenced disorders. In: Hacker NF, Gambone JC, Hobel CJ, eds. *Hacker and Moore's essentials of obstetrics and gynecology*. 5th ed. Philadelphia: Saunders;Elsevier; 2010. p. 386-9.

Yonkers KA, O'Brien PM, Eriksson E. Premenstrual syndrome. *Lancet* 2008;371:1200-10.

References

1. Jarvis CI, Lynch AM, Morin AK. Management strategies for premenstrual syndrome/premenstrual dysphoric disorder. *Ann Pharmacother* 2008;42:967-78.
2. Yonkers KA, O'Brien PM, Eriksson E. Premenstrual syndrome. *Lancet* 2008;371:1200-10.
3. Frye GM, Silverman SD. Is it premenstrual syndrome? Keys to focused diagnosis, therapies for multiple symptoms. *Postgrad Med* 2000;107:151-4, 157-9.
4. Frackiewicz EJ, Shiovitz TM. Evaluation and management of premenstrual syndrome and premenstrual dysphoric disorder. *J Am Pharm Assoc (Wash)* 2001;41:437-47.
5. Schmidt PJ, Nieman LK, Danaceau MA et al. Differential behavioural effects of gonadal steroids in women with and in those without premenstrual syndrome. *N Engl J Med* 1998;338:209-16.
6. Pearlstein TB. Hormones and depression: what are the facts about premenstrual syndrome, menopause, and hormone replacement therapy? *Am J Obstet Gynecol* 1995;173:646-53.
7. Rapkin AJ. The role of serotonin in premenstrual syndrome. *Clin Obstet Gynecol* 1992;35:629-36.
8. Pearlstein T, Steiner M. Non-antidepressant treatment of premenstrual syndrome. *J Clin Psychiatry* 2000;61:22-7.
9. Romans S, Clarkson R, Einstein G et al. Mood and the menstrual cycle: a review of prospective data studies. *Gend Med* 2012;9:361-84.
10. Bertone-Johnson ER, Hankinson SE, Bendich A et al. Calcium and vitamin D intake and risk of incident premenstrual syndrome. *Arch Intern Med* 2005;165:1246-52.
11. Bertone-Johnson ER, Cocano-Bedoya PO, Zagarins SE et al. Dietary vitamin D intake, 25-hydroxyvitamin D3 levels and premenstrual syndrome in a college-aged population. *J Steroid Biochem Mol Biol* 2010;121:434-7.
12. Chuong CJ, Dawson EB. Critical evaluation of nutritional factors in the pathophysiology and treatment of premenstrual syndrome. *Clin Obstet Gynecol* 1992;35:679-92.
13. Masho SW, Adera T, South-Paul J. Obesity as a risk factor for premenstrual syndrome. *J Psychosom Obstet Gynaecol* 2005;26:33-9.
14. Deuster PA, Adera T, South-Paul J. Biological, social, and behavioral factors associated with premenstrual syndrome. *Arch Fam Med* 1999;8:122-8.
15. Perkonigg A, Yonkers KA, Pfister H et al. Risk factors for premenstrual dysphoric disorder in a community sample of young women: the role of traumatic events and posttraumatic stress disorder. *J Clin Psychiatry* 2004;65:1314-22.
16. Halbreich U. The diagnosis of premenstrual syndromes and premenstrual dysphoric disorder–clinical procedures and research perspectives. *Gynecol Endocrinol* 2004;19:320-34.
17. Halbreich U, O'Brien PM, Eriksson E et al. Are there differential symptom profiles that improve in response to different pharmacological treatments of premenstrual syndrome/premenstrual dysphoric disorder? *CNS Drugs* 2006;20:523-47.
18. Johnson SR. Clinician's approach to the diagnosis and management of premenstrual syndrome. *Clin Obstet Gynecol* 1992;35:637-57.
19. Pearlstein T, Stone AB. Premenstrual syndrome. *Psychiatr Clin North Am* 1998;21:577-90.
20. Epperson CN, Steiner M, Hartlage SA et al. Premenstrual dysphoric disorder: evidence for a new category for DSM-5. *Am J Psychiatry* 2012;169:465-75.
21. American Psychiatric Association. *Diagnostic and statistical manual of mental disorders: DSM-5*. 5th ed. Washington: American Psychiatric Publishing; 2013.
22. Wakefield JC. DSM-5: proposed changes to depressive disorders. *Curr Med Res Opin* 2012;19:335-43.
23. Wyatt KM, Dimmock PW, O'Brien PM. Premenstrual syndrome. *Clin Evid* 1999;1:286-97.

24. American College of Obstetricians and Gynecologists. Premenstrual syndrome: clinical management guidelines for obstetrician-gynecologists. *ACOG Practice Bulletin* 2000;15:1-9.
25. Dickerson LM, Mazyck PJ, Hunter MH. Premenstrual syndrome. *Am Fam Physician* 2003;67:1743-52.
26. Stevinson C, Ernst E. Complementary/alternative therapies for premenstrual syndrome: a systematic review of randomized controlled trials. *Am J Obstet Gynecol* 2001;185:227-35.
27. Cho SH, Kim J. Efficacy of acupuncture in management of premenstrual syndrome: a systematic review. *Complement Ther Med* 2010;18:104-11.
28. Steege JF, Blumenthal JA. The effects of aerobic exercise on premenstrual symptoms in middle-aged women: a preliminary study. *J Psychosom Res* 1993;37:127-33.
29. Campagne DM, Campagne G. The premenstrual syndrome revisited. *Eur J Obstet Gynecol Reprod Biol* 2007;130:4-17.
30. Sayegh R, Schiff I, Wurtman J et al. The effect of a carbohydrate-rich beverage on mood, appetite, and cognitive function in women with premenstrual syndrome. *Obstet Gynecol* 1995;86:520-8.
31. Thys-Jacobs S, Starkey P, Bernstein D et al. Calcium carbonate and the premenstrual syndrome: effects on premenstrual and menstrual symptoms. Premenstrual Syndrome Study Group. *Am J Obstet Gynecol* 1998;179:444-52.
32. Whelan AM, Jurgens TM, Naylor H. Herbs, vitamins and minerals in the treatment of premenstrual syndrome: a systematic review. *Can J Clin Pharmacol* 2009;16:e407-29.
33. Douglas S. Premenstrual syndrome. Evidence-based treatment in family practice. *Can Fam Physician* 2002;48:1789-97.
34. Williams AL, Cotter A, Sabina A et al. The role for vitamin B-6 as treatment for depression: a systematic review. *Fam Pract* 2005;22:532-7.
35. Kashanian M, Mazinani R, Jalalmanesh S. Pyridoxine (vitamin B6) therapy for premenstrual syndrome. *Int J Gynaecol Obstet* 2007;96:43-4.
36. Wyatt KM, Dimmock PW, Jones PW et al. Efficacy of vitamin B-6 in the treatment of premenstrual syndrome: systematic review. *BMJ* 1999;318:1375-81.
37. Freeman EW, Halbreich U, Grubb GS et al. An overview of four studies of a continuous oral contraceptive (levonorgestrel 90 mcg/ethinyl estradiol 20 mcg) on premenstrual dysphoric disorder and premenstrual syndrome. *Contraception* 2012;85:437-45.
38. Lopez LM, Kaptein AA, Helmerhorst FM. Oral contraceptives containing drospirenone for premenstrual syndrome. *Cochrane Database Syst Rev* 2012;2:CD006586.
39. Lidegaard O, Lokkegaard E, Svendsen AL et al. Hormonal contraception and risk of venous thromboembolism: national follow-up study. *BMJ* 2009;339:b2890.
40. van Hylckama Vlieg A, Helmerhorst FM, Vandenbroucke JP et al. The venous thrombotic risk of oral contraceptives, effects of oestrogen dose and progestogen type: results of the MEGA case-control study. *BMJ* 2009;339:b2921.
41. Parkin L, Sharples K, Hernandez RK et al. Risk of venous thromboembolism in users of oral contraceptives containing drospirenone or levonorgestrel: nested case-control study based on UK General Practice Research Database. *BMJ* 2011;342:d2139.
42. Jick SS, Hernandez RK. Risk of non-fatal venous thromboembolism in women using oral contraceptives containing drospirenone compared with women using oral contraceptives containing levonorgestrel: case-control study using United States claims data. *BMJ* 2011;342:d2151.
43. Gronich N, Lavi I, Rennert G. Higher risk of venous thromboembolism associated with drosperenone-containing oral contraceptives: a population-based cohort study. *CMAJ* 2011;183:E1319-25.
44. Wu CQ, Grandi SM, Filion KB et al. Drospirenone-containing oral contraceptive pills and the risk of venous and arterial thrombosis: a systematic review. *BJOG* 2013;120:801-10.
45. de Bastos M, Stegeman BH, Rosendaal FR et al. Combined oral contraceptives: venous thrombosis. *Cochrane Database Syst Rev* 2014;3:CD010813.
46. Vinogradova Y, Coupland C, Hippisley-Cox J. Use of combined oral contraceptives and risk of venous thromboembolism: nested case-control studies using the QResearch and CPRD databases. *BMJ* 2015;350:h2135.
47. Ford O, Lethaby A, Roberts H et al. Progesterone for premenstrual syndrome. *Cochrane Database Syst Rev* 2012;3:CD003415.
48. Marjoribanks J, Brown J, O'Brien PM et al. Selective serotonin reuptake inhibitors for premenstrual syndrome. *Cochrane Database Syst Rev* 2013;6:CD001396.
49. Freeman EW, Sammel MD, Lin H et al. Clinical subtypes of premenstrual syndrome and responses to sertraline treatment. *Obstet Gynecol* 2011;118:1293-300.
50. Aydin Y, Atis A, Kaleli S et al. Cabergoline versus bromocriptine for symptomatic treatment of premenstrual mastalgia: a randomised, open-label study. *Eur J Obstet Gynecol Reprod Biol* 2010;150:203-6.
51. Khoo SK, Munro C, Battistutta D. Evening primrose oil and treatment of premenstrual syndrome. *Med J Aust* 1990;153:189-92.
52. Collins A, Cerin A, Coleman G et al. Essential fatty acids in the treatment of premenstrual syndrome. *Obstet Gynecol* 1993;81:93-8.
53. Canning S, Waterman M, Orsi N et al. Efficacy of hypericum perforatum (St John's Wort) for the treatment of premenstrual syndrome: a randomized, double-blind, placebo-controlled trial. *CNS Drugs* 2010;24:207-25.
54. Jing Z, Yang X, Ismail KM et al. Chinese herbal medicine for premenstrual syndrome. *Cochrane Database Syst Rev* 2009;(1):CD006414.
55. Ozgoli G, Selselei EA, Mojab F et al. A randomized, placebo-controlled trial of Ginkgo biloba L. in treatment of premenstrual syndromes. *J Altern Complement Med* 2009;15:845-51.
56. Dante G, Facchinetti F. Herbal treatments for alleviating premenstrual symptoms: a systematic review. *J Psychosom Obstet Gynaecol* 2011;32:42-51.
57. Roemheld-Hamm B. Chasteberry. *Am Fam Physician* 2005;72:821-4.
58. Atmaca M, Kumru S, Tezcan E. Fluoxetine versus Vitex agnus castus extract in the treatment of premenstrual dysphoric disorder. *Hum Psychopharmacol* 2003;18:191-5.

Premenstrual Syndrome PMS—What You Need to Know

What is PMS?

PMS is a group of physical and psychological symptoms that affect some women in the last half of their menstrual cycle (leading up to their menstrual period).

What are the symptoms of PMS?

Table 1: **Symptoms of PMS**

Psychological Symptoms	Physical Symptoms
▪ Aggression	▪ Acne
▪ Anger	▪ Changes in appetite (food cravings)
▪ Nervousness	▪ Bloating, fluid retention
▪ Depression	▪ Pain or swelling in breasts
▪ Forgetfulness	▪ Constipation
▪ Sudden mood changes	▪ Dizziness
▪ Panic attacks	▪ Fatigue
▪ Lack of concentration	▪ Headache
▪ Not coping well with stress	▪ Hot flashes
	▪ Muscle aches
	▪ Nausea and vomiting
	▪ Pressure in the pelvic area

What can you do to relieve PMS?

- Try relaxation techniques. Reduce the stress in your life.
- Reduce the amount of caffeine in your diet. This might relieve breast soreness. Caffeine is found in coffee, tea, chocolate and many soft drinks.
- Reducing the amount of salt you eat may reduce bloating.
- Get regular exercise (3–4 times a week). This can help reduce many symptoms of PMS.
- Anti-inflammatory medicines such as ibuprofen and naproxen may help relieve muscle or breast pain and headache. However, some people should not take these medicines. Ask your pharmacist for advice about what medicine is right for you.
- Many women find that a calcium supplement helps to relieve symptoms such as abdominal pain, mood changes, bloating and food cravings. Ask your pharmacist if you should take a supplement of elemental calcium (1200 mg per day in divided doses). If you decide to try calcium, don't take it within 2 hours of any other medications and do not take more than 600 mg for each dose. Take calcium carbonate with a meal.
- A daily vitamin B_6 supplement (50–100 mg daily) may also help. Another name for vitamin B_6 is pyridoxine. **Do not** take more than the recommended dose.
- Chasteberry may help psychological and physical symptoms associated with PMS.

When should you see your healthcare provider?

- If you have severe psychological symptoms.
- If you feel you do not function well when you have PMS.
- If you have tried treating yourself for PMS symptoms but it hasn't worked.

Your healthcare provider may recommend medication to help control your PMS symptoms.

Chapter 82

Prenatal and Postpartum Care

Carla Dillon, BScPharm, ACPR, PharmD

General Principles of Drug Use in Pregnancy and Breastfeeding

The management of common medical conditions during pregnancy and breastfeeding often includes self-medication. It can be a therapeutic challenge to accurately determine the efficacy and safety of management strategies in this patient population. This chapter provides an overview of the assessment and management of some common minor ailments encountered in pregnancy and the postpartum period.

Many women are faced with the dilemma of how to best manage their medical conditions during pregnancy and breastfeeding and few medications are officially approved for use during these times. When treating common medical conditions in a pregnant or breastfeeding woman, the risks and benefits to the patient, fetus and nursing infant must be weighed carefully to help her make an informed decision about medication use. Take care to provide accurate, current and relevant information in a calm, nonalarming manner; provide the perspective that even if a woman does not take any medication during pregnancy, there is a baseline risk of 1–3% for major fetal malformations.[1,2] Table 1 and Table 2 provide some guiding principles for medication use during pregnancy and breastfeeding.

Table 1: **Principles of Recommending Drug Therapy to Pregnant and Breastfeeding Women[3,4,5,6]**

Recommend nonpharmacologic therapy first whenever feasible.
Determine the gestational or infant age. Risk posed by a drug may vary by pregnancy trimester. Premature and newborn infants may be more vulnerable to drug effects.
Consider whether the benefits of drug therapy outweigh the risks.
Choose drugs with published data in pregnancy and breastfeeding over newer drugs with less information.
Choose the most effective agent with the most reassuring safety data in the lowest possible dose for the shortest possible duration.
Choose single entity products to avoid unnecessary drug exposure.
Consider local application of drugs whenever possible to minimize systemic absorption.
Choose drugs with shorter half-lives whenever feasible to minimize medication exposure to the fetus/infant.
Any prolonged use of drug therapy (>3 days) should be approved by a healthcare practitioner.
Reassess if initial therapy for minor ailments fails to provide relief after 3 days.
Whenever feasible, schedule doses when the least amount of drug is anticipated to be in the breast milk (e.g., right after breastfeeding or before the baby is expected to have a long sleep period). Drug diffuses from the milk back to the vascular compartment as plasma drug concentration falls, so that the lowest levels in milk occur just prior to the next dose. Dosing in this manner may not always be practical particularly when breastfeeding young infants who feed frequently and sleep for only short intervals.
If several drugs are equally useful, select the drug that is excreted in breast milk in the lowest concentration with the least effect on the infant.

Table 2: **Myths and Facts Regarding Drug Therapy during Pregnancy and Breastfeeding**[3,4,5,6]

Myths	Facts
"Women who are pregnant should not take any medications." "Women should stop their medications if they become pregnant."	Although only a few medications are specifically indicated for use during pregnancy, many medications are safe for use in pregnancy.[7,8] Uncontrolled medical conditions can often pose a greater risk to a fetus than the treatment medication.[9,10]
"The fetus is only susceptible to teratogenic effects from drug therapy taken during the first 3 months of pregnancy."	The first 3 months of gestation may be the most critical in terms of fetal structural malformations, but functional and behavioural defects are also associated with later exposure. Teratogenic agents are defined as those that are capable of producing structural or functional abnormalities in the embryo or fetus.[11]
"This drug causes malformations in animals, so it should not be used in pregnancy."	Animal data cannot always be extrapolated to human situations,[5] e.g., erythromycin is considered a safe antibiotic to use in pregnancy, but it has been reported to cause malformations in rats,[8] and in contrast, thalidomide was found to be safe in most animal models, but can cause limb defects in human fetuses.[7]
"Due to ease of availability, it can be assumed that nonprescription drug therapies are safe to use in pregnancy and breastfeeding."	Many nonprescription drugs require careful consideration of beneficial vs. harmful effects or have limited safety data in those who are pregnant or breastfeeding.[7,12]
"Due to ease of availability, natural health products can be considered safe in pregnancy and breastfeeding."	In many cases, there is little reliable human data about the safety of natural health products during pregnancy or breastfeeding, e.g., echinacea.[12] Certain herbs such as blue cohosh are specifically contraindicated due to empirical evidence that they can act as abortifacients and cause cardiovascular defects.[13] As with any other medicine, one must weigh the risks and possible benefits of using natural health products during pregnancy. Some natural health products may contain undeclared drugs or contaminants.
"If a drug is excreted in breast milk, it is contraindicated in a breastfeeding mother."	In many cases, only very low concentrations of drugs are present in breast milk and they are still considered safe to use in breastfeeding.[14] In general, taking drugs during breastfeeding poses much less risk to the infant than drug therapy during pregnancy. Healthcare practitioners should consult specific references to determine drug safety in breastfeeding.

Prenatal Nutrition

Key Nutritional Recommendations in Pregnancy

Proper nutrition plays a very important role in a healthy pregnancy. Additional nutrients are needed to meet the needs of the developing fetus (see Table 3).

Table 3: **Key Nutritional Recommendations in Pregnancy**

Nutrient	Role in Pregnancy	Daily Requirement	Nonpharmacologic Therapy	Pharmacologic Therapy	Comments
General	Nutrient requirements are increased due to needs of the growing fetus.		Eat a well-balanced diet. See *Canada's Food Guide*.[15,16,17] If patient is not getting adequate nutrition from diet, recommend dietary counselling.	Prenatal and postpartum vitamin and mineral supplementation. When selecting a multivitamin, the product should contain vitamin B_{12} in addition to the ingredients discussed below.[16,17]	Advise women not to increase the dose of a multivitamin or take more than one multivitamin as high doses of vitamin A (>10 000 IU or >3000 µg RAE per day) can cause birth defects.[16,17]
Calcium	Supports fetal skeletal development. Adequate intake	1000 mg for those 19–50 y (plus **vitamin D** 600 IU);	Eat foods high in calcium, e.g., dairy products and calcium fortified juices.[20]	Supplementation with at least 1000 mg/day is recommended for those with a dietary intake of	May cause or exacerbate constipation. High rate of bone loss during pregnancy and

(cont'd)

Table 3: **Key Nutritional Recommendations in Pregnancy** *(cont'd)*

Nutrient	Role in Pregnancy	Daily Requirement	Nonpharmacologic Therapy	Pharmacologic Therapy	Comments
	reduces the risk of hypertension and pre-eclampsia.[18,19] Maintains maternal stores.	1300 mg for those <19 y (plus **vitamin D** 600 IU)[20,21,22]		less than 600 mg/day, e.g., less than 2 dairy servings/day.[18,19] The upper limit of total daily intake is 2500 mg for those 19–50 y and 3000 mg for those <19 y.[21]	breastfeeding, thus adequate intake is essential for maternal bone health.[20] Calcium-based antacids can have the dual benefits of calcium supplementation and heartburn relief.[20]
Folic acid[a]	Essential for normal development of fetal spine, brain and skull. Reduces the risk of NTDs (e.g., spina bifida, anencephaly).[1,16] Neural tube development occurs early in pregnancy (during wk 3 and 4) when many women may not be aware they are pregnant.[16,17]	0.4 mg[1] See Comments.	Eat foods high in folic acid (e.g., fortified grains, spinach, lentils, chick peas, asparagus, broccoli, peas, brussels sprouts, corn and oranges). Diet alone is unlikely to meet requirement.[1]	Supplementation with 0.4 mg/day, in addition to dietary sources, is recommended for all women with child-bearing potential. Start at least 2–3 months preconception, continuing throughout pregnancy and for 4–6 wk postpartum or as long as breastfeeding continues.[16,23]	Women with moderate risk of NTD[b]: 1 mg daily beginning at least 3 months prior to conception and continuing until 12 wk gestational age, followed by 0.4–1 mg daily until 4–6 wk postpartum or as long as breastfeeding continues.[23] Women with high risk of NTD[c]: 4 mg daily beginning at least 3 months prior to conception and continuing until 12 wk gestational age, followed by 0.4–1 mg daily until 4–6 wk postpartum or as long as breastfeeding continues.[23]
Iodine	Increased requirement as iodine is essential for fetal neurologic development and to maintain maternal metabolism.[24,25]	220–250 µg	Eat foods with iodine, e.g., saltwater seafood, milk. A teaspoon of table salt in Canada contains 380 µg of iodine. Kosher, pickling and sea salt contain much less iodine.[26] Processed foods generally do not use iodized salt.[27,28]	Supplementation with 150 µg/day suggested.[27,29,30] Avoid kelp/seaweed products as they may be contaminated with heavy metals.[27,31]	Sustained iodine intake >500–1100 µg/day should be avoided due to the potential for fetal hypothyroidism.[29]
Iron	Supports normal fetal brain development and builds fetal iron stores in the third trimester. Lowers risk of maternal anemia.[32]	27 mg	Eat foods high in heme iron, e.g., meat, poultry and fish. Eat nonheme iron sources (e.g., fortified food, tofu, lentils, beans) with vitamin C-containing foods. Diet alone is unlikely to meet requirement.[17]	Supplementation with 16–20 mg/day is recommended.[17]	May exacerbate constipation, nausea and vomiting; consider temporary discontinuation in the first trimester[33] or intermittent dosing (e.g., 120 mg once weekly) in those who are not anemic.[34]

[a] For simplicity the term folic acid is used interchangeably with folate. Folic acid is the synthetic form of the B vitamin which is found in fortified foods and supplements. Folate is the natural form found in food.

[b] Moderate risk includes: maternal or paternal personal or family history of other folate-sensitive congenital anomalies (limited to specific anomalies for cardiac, limb, cleft palate, urinary tract, congenital hydrocephaly); maternal or paternal family history of NTD in a first- or second-degree relative; maternal diabetes; maternal kidney dialysis; maternal use of folate-inhibiting medications (carbamazepine, cholestyramine, metformin, methotrexate, phenobarbital, phenytoin, primidone, sulfasalazine, triamterene, trimethoprim, valproic acid); maternal GI malabsorption conditions (e.g., Crohn's disease, active Celiac disease, gastric bypass surgery).[23]

[c] High risk includes: maternal or paternal personal NTD history or a previous NTD pregnancy.[23]

Abbreviations: IU = international units; NTD = neural tube defect; RAE = retinol activity equivalent

Nausea and Vomiting of Pregnancy (NVP)

Pathophysiology

NVP is very common, occurring in about 70% of pregnant women. Approximately one third of pregnant women will experience nausea without vomiting.[35] Despite popular use of the term "morning sickness," NVP persists throughout the day in the majority of cases.[36] NVP usually appears by 4–6 weeks' gestation and disappears by 12–16 weeks; however, it can persist throughout pregnancy in up to 20% of cases.[1,37,38] The nausea and/or vomiting is usually self-limiting and not associated with any adverse fetal outcome.[39] Severe vomiting resulting in significant maternal weight loss may increase the risk of low birth weight babies.[39,40] Even less severe NVP can negatively affect a woman's daily life. It can cause emotional, social and economic problems for the woman and her family.[1,41]

Although it occurs rarely, severe NVP, or hyperemesis gravidarum, may lead to dehydration, malnutrition and weight loss, requiring hospitalization.[1] Hyperemesis gravidarum affects on average 1% of pregnancies and is usually a diagnosis of exclusion.[35,39] Onset is nearly always in the first trimester, usually between weeks 6 and 8.[40] Hyperemesis gravidarum may persist throughout the pregnancy, but usually becomes less extreme as the pregnancy progresses. It tends to recur in subsequent pregnancies, so a previous history makes the diagnosis more likely.[39]

The etiology of NVP is unknown, but it is postulated that multiple factors are involved. Hormonal changes, specifically first trimester elevations of human chorionic gonadotropin (hCG), progesterone and/or estradiol have been implicated. Other proposed causes or contributors include slower gastric emptying, *Helicobacter pylori* infection, psychological predisposition, genetic predisposition, carrying a female fetus and evolutionary adaptation.[1,41,42]

Goals of Therapy

- Reduce incidence and severity of NVP
- Improve functioning and quality of life
- Maintain adequate fetal and maternal nutrition
- Prevent dehydration and significant weight loss
- Reduce the risk of progression to more severe NVP
- Minimize negative fetal effects from treatment

Patient Assessment

Counsel patients with adequate hydration and nutrition despite NVP on nonpharmacologic measures to relieve symptoms. Patients with more severe nausea and vomiting with signs of dehydration or weight loss must be assessed immediately by a healthcare practitioner. The Motherisk Pregnancy-Unique Quantification of Emesis (PUQE-24) scoring system can be used in assessing severity and response to treatment.[43] Information on NVP can also be found in Chapter 36: Nausea and Vomiting.

Nonpharmacologic Therapy

Pregnant women can take many measures to alleviate NVP. Avoiding aggravating factors such as certain smells, fried or spicy food, an empty stomach, stress and fatigue is key. Taking prenatal multivitamins and/or iron supplements after meals or at bedtime is also suggested.[39,42] If the size of the prenatal multivitamin or its iron content is an aggravating factor, consider temporarily stopping the multivitamin, switching to a chewable multivitamin, or switching to multivitamin with no iron or a lower iron content.[33] Intermittent iron supplementation (e.g., once weekly) may also be considered in women who are not anemic[34] (see Table 3). It is important to maintain the recommended intake of folic acid; a folic acid supplement may be needed if the prenatal multivitamin is changed or temporarily discontinued. Detailed information for patients on management of morning sickness is found in Morning Sickness—What You Need to Know.

Acupressure at the Neiguan or P6 point, located 3 finger-widths up from the wrist crease, by use of wrist bands (e.g., Seabands) has been used in the management of nausea and vomiting and appears to be safe in pregnancy.[37,44] This method has shown varying degrees of effectiveness; a short-term study found comparable efficacy to pyridoxine for mild to moderate symptoms.[36,37,44]

Pharmacologic Therapy

For comparative ingredients of nonprescription products, consult the *Compendium of Products for Minor Ailments*—Gastrointestinal Products: Antiemetics; Vitamin and Mineral Products: Single Entity.

Antiemetics are indicated for the treatment of moderate NVP that fails to respond to nonpharmacologic interventions (see Table 8).

The therapy of choice in the management of NVP that is unresponsive to nonpharmacologic measures is Diclectin, a combination delayed-release product containing the first-generation antihistamine **doxylamine** 10 mg and the B vitamin **pyridoxine** 10 mg.[3,37,45,48] It is the only product with Health Canada approval for NVP. Over 33 million pregnant women worldwide have taken delayed-release doxylamine with pyridoxine and it has not been found to increase the risk of teratogenesis or affect neurodevelopment.[2,48,58] To prevent early morning symptoms, 2 Diclectin tablets are taken at bedtime. One additional tablet can be taken in the morning and midafternoon to control daytime nausea. Due to its delayed release, tablets should be taken on a regular basis and not on an as needed basis.[48] Supratherapeutic doses (up to 12 tablets per day) may be needed by some women and appear safe, but evidence is limited to small studies.[38,59] Due to the antihistamine component the most common adverse effect of Diclectin is drowsiness. On discontinuation, Diclectin should be gradually tapered to prevent sudden recurrence of NVP symptoms.[48]

Pyridoxine, also known as vitamin B_6, is a component of Diclectin. In the United States, pyridoxine monotherapy is the recommended first-line pharmacologic option for NVP.[37,60] Pyridoxine can be used in combination with other drug therapies (e.g., dimenhydrinate).[41] Although case reports sparked concern that taking pyridoxine during pregnancy might cause seizures in some newborns, further investigation suggests the infants had an underlying vitamin B_6 deficiency disorder which was unmasked when maternal supplementation was stopped.[54]

Dimenhydrinate is a second-line treatment option but may be preferred when oral drug administration is not possible.[1,39,45] If the patient is vomiting frequently, it can be given orally or rectally 30 or 45 minutes before a dose of Diclectin.[1,41]

Ginger (*Zingiber officinale*) traditionally has been used in many forms (e.g., ginger tea, ginger ale, gingersnaps and powdered ginger root) to alleviate nausea. Powdered ginger root is the form of ginger most commonly used in studies. Small randomized, controlled trials indicate ginger reduces nausea and vomiting of pregnancy and its efficacy is at least comparable to that of dimenhydrinate and pyridoxine.[36,49,50,51,52,61] However, replicating this effect in practice is hindered by the lack of description of the composition of ginger used and lack of standardization of many ginger products.[62] The usual dose is up to 1000 mg per day.[41] Licensed NHP ginger products are available (e.g., Gravol Ginger). Ginger does not appear to be teratogenic and is generally considered safe during pregnancy. However, there are limited data on fetal effects with ginger supplementation.[63,64,65]

Information regarding efficacy and safety is lacking for other traditional remedies such as peppermint, raspberry leaf and chamomile.

Other agents that have been used in the treatment of nausea and vomiting during pregnancy include metoclopramide, ondansetron, phenothiazines (e.g., chlorpromazine, promethazine, prochlorperazine) and methylprednisolone. These agents are used as monotherapy or adjunctive therapy after inadequate response to Diclectin.[41,60] Metoclopramide and phenothiazines are not teratogenic but can cause extrapyramidal effects in the mother, and in the newborn if given near term. Safety data for ondansetron are conflicting. Due to its potential to cause QT prolongation, cleft palate and fetal heart defects, use should be limited to after 10 weeks' gestation. Similarly, methylprednisolone use should be delayed until after 10 weeks' gestation due to possible association with cleft palate.[41]

Allergic Rhinitis during Pregnancy and Breastfeeding

Pathophysiology

Rhinitis affects at least 20% of pregnancies.[66] Common symptoms of allergic rhinitis include nasal itchiness, clear watery rhinorrhea and sneezing.[66] Hormonal changes in pregnancy can worsen nasal symptoms and can induce a form of rhinitis, termed "rhinitis of pregnancy," which presents as congestion and occurs in the absence of other signs of respiratory tract infection or a known allergic cause. Rhinitis of pregnancy occurs in approximately 9% of pregnancies and usually begins later in the pregnancy but can start at any time, with resolution of the syndrome within 1–2 weeks postpartum.[67,68,69,70] More information can be found in Chapter 22: Allergic Rhinitis.

Goals of Therapy

- Relieve symptoms
- Improve functioning and quality of life (e.g., improve sleep)[70]
- Minimize risk of complications such as sinusitis and aggravation of pre-existing asthma

Nonpharmacologic Therapy

The mainstay of nonpharmacologic management of allergic rhinitis during pregnancy is minimizing exposure to allergens, such as pollen, animal dander, dust mites or mold growth, and remaining indoors when necessary. Avoiding exposure to irritants such as cigarette smoke, smog and strong odours is also important. For both allergic and pregnancy-induced rhinitis, nocturnal congestion may be temporarily relieved by elevating the head of the bed and/or use of external nasal dilators (e.g., Breathe Right nasal strips).[70]

Pharmacologic Therapy

For comparative ingredients of nonprescription products, consult the *Compendium of Products for Minor Ailments*—Cough, Cold and Allergy Products.

Therapies for allergic rhinitis and the common cold are outlined in Table 9.

Due to its local application and lack of toxicity, irrigation via **nasal saline** sprays, mists or washes is a recommended sole or adjuvant therapy in providing symptom control to irritated nasal passages during pregnancy.[66,67,68,69,112]

Antihistamines are first-line agents in the treatment of allergic rhinitis.[69] During pregnancy, **first-generation antihistamines** are considered safe; **chlorpheniramine** is considered an agent of choice for allergic rhinitis.[3,67,76] Caution is advised with usual or high-dose first-generation antihistamine therapy near the end of term due to the potential for withdrawal effects in the newborn and retinopathy of prematurity, particularly in low-birth-weight newborns.[67] The second-generation antihistamines **loratadine**, **desloratadine** and **cetirizine** are also considered safe during pregnancy; **fexofenadine** can be considered as an alternative (due to less available safety data).[70,76,80,113,114,115,116] First- or second-generation antihistamines may be used safely during breastfeeding.[76,117,118,119,120] Second-generation antihistamines are sometimes preferred during breastfeeding due to their lower potential to cause adverse effects in the infant, reduced milk production, sedation or anticholinergic effects compared with first-generation antihistamines.[72]

Decongestants can be utilized supplementally for additional symptom relief, if nasal saline fails. Systemic **pseudoephedrine** is generally considered safe to use during pregnancy; however, first-trimester use may cause a small increased risk of abdominal wall and intestinal defects.[12,75,102,104] **Phenylephrine** is more likely than pseudoephedrine to have vasoactive effects such as hypertension and reduced uterine blood flow (though not reported in humans), and is reserved as an alternative to pseudoephedrine.[101,102,103,121,122,123] First-trimester use of phenylephrine has been associated with congenital defects (mostly minor), but further data are required.[103,102] Although **topical decongestants** have lower systemic absorption, evidence is limited regarding use during pregnancy.[12,75,102,108,124,125] First-trimester use of decongestants should be avoided if possible.[70,102,104]

Intranasal **sodium cromoglycate (cromolyn sodium)** is considered a first-line treatment option for allergic rhinitis during pregnancy.[67,69,80] It is well tolerated with few adverse effects and is considered safe in pregnancy and breastfeeding due to minimal absorption across nasal membranes.[6,67,72]

Intranasal corticosteroids are reserved for allergic rhinitis symptoms unresponsive to antihistamines, decongestants and/or sodium cromoglycate.[69] Information regarding the efficacy of intranasal corticosteroids in rhinitis of pregnancy is limited to a single study where no benefit was found.[70,126] **Inhaled** corticosteroids are widely used in the treatment of asthma during pregnancy, particularly **beclomethasone**, **budesonide** and **fluticasone**.[66,67,80] Systemic absorption is minimal; more safety information is available for inhaled/intranasal budesonide.[67,80,127] The majority of data indicate no association with an increased risk of congenital abnormalities with low to moderate doses;[128] however, a small associated risk may exist between intranasal budesonide and cardiac defects, and between inhaled budesonide and orofacial clefts.[96] Minimize exposure when feasible, particularly during the first trimester.[89,96] Data are limited on the safety of intranasal corticosteroids during breastfeeding. They may be excreted into breast milk in small quantities; however, it is unlikely to be clinically significant and they are generally considered compatible with breastfeeding.[6,72,96]

The antileukotrienes **zafirlukast** and **montelukast** have been used in the treatment of allergic rhinitis after other treatments have failed. Harmful effects have not been seen in animal studies but human pregnancy data are limited and use should be limited to cases where the benefit clearly outweighs risk.[67] Safety of these agents in breastfeeding has not been established.[6,67,72]

Allergen immunotherapy can be continued during pregnancy. However, to reduce the risk of a severe allergic reaction, it should not be initiated during pregnancy nor should the strength of the allergen be increased.[67,80] No data are available for safety in breastfeeding; however, it is unlikely to pass into breast milk and it is considered safe to continue breastfeeding.[6]

For more information on further therapy, see Chapter 22: Allergic Rhinitis.

Other Common Conditions in Pregnancy

Table 4 describes the management of some conditions commonly encountered in pregnancy. Many conditions are covered in detail in specific chapters as outlined in the endnotes. See also Appendix V: Pregnancy and Breastfeeding: Self-care Therapy for Common Conditions. Information regarding therapy for depression in pregnancy is discussed in conjunction with therapy of postpartum depression (see Pharmacologic Therapy in Postpartum Depression section).

Table 4: Management of Selected Common Conditions in Pregnancy

Condition	Cause	Nonpharmacologic Therapy	Pharmacologic Therapy[a]	Monitoring of Therapy	Comments
Backache[b], **Headache**[c], **Pelvic pain**	Back muscles under strain due to growing abdomen. Weight of uterus can contribute. Headache commonly results from muscle tension.[129]	Backache, pelvic pain: Relaxation exercises; massage; rest in recumbent position; good posture and lifting techniques; moderate exercise (land- or water-based); pelvic tilts; elevation of one leg while standing; acupuncture.[129,130] Headache: Cool wet cloth to forehead.[129]	**Acetaminophen** is the drug of choice.[5,12] Limit **codeine** to short-term use in pregnancy. High doses of codeine close to term or prolonged use during pregnancy can cause neonatal opiate withdrawal.[87]	Reassess if symptoms are severe or do not improve after 5 days. With codeine, monitor patient for adverse effects such as constipation or drowsiness and reassess if adverse effects are intolerable.	**ASA** (at analgesic doses), **ibuprofen** and **naproxen** have not been associated with congenital malformations in the majority of studies.[131,132,133] However, areas of controversy exist (small, possible increased risk of inhibition of egg implantation,[131] gastroschisis[132] and cardiac defects[134] with first-trimester exposure; premature closure of ductus arteriosus and fetal renal problems with use in the last 8 wk of pregnancy[131] and maternal bleeding during delivery).[12,75,131] Patient must be assessed by appropriate healthcare practitioner immediately if headache is severe and/or associated with blurred vision or nausea/vomiting as this may be a sign of hypertension or preeclampsia.[129,131]
Common Cold[d]	Viral	Bedrest; maintain fluid intake; humidify air; hard candy for a sore throat; saltwater gargle.[12,135]	Many products contain more than 1 ingredient. Use single-ingredient products where possible to minimize exposure to unnecessary drugs. Avoid alcohol-containing products.	Reassess if symptoms are associated with fever, nausea or vomiting.	Avoid use of vitamins and minerals for cold symptoms (e.g., **zinc** lozenges, **vitamin C**) beyond those in prenatal multivitamins as higher doses lack safety information and may exacerbate other pregnancy conditions, e.g., nausea.[12] Avoid **echinacea** due to limited data in pregnancy and lack of standardization of product content.[12]
Constipation[e]	Reduced GI motility due to increased progesterone levels. Other factors: compression of intestines by enlarging uterus, increased water resorption by colon, iron and calcium supplementation and reduced physical activity. Occurs in 10–40% of	Dietary: Eat foods high in fibre, e.g., whole grains, vegetables, fruits, high fibre cereals. Add fibre to diet slowly to prevent bloating and gas.[136,137] The suggested adequate fibre intake during pregnancy is 28 g/day.[138] Increase fluid intake, e.g., 6–8 glasses of water daily.[136,137,139] Lifestyle: Regular moderate exercise.[136,137, 139]	Regular use of **bulk laxatives** such as **psyllium** and/or **stool softeners** such as **docusate**, which are poorly absorbed, can be used for prevention. Since these agents take several days to work, other agents may be needed for acute management. **Docusate** has questionable efficacy.[139] Consider dosage reduction or temporary discontinuation of iron supplements in those without anemia.[140]	Reassess if symptoms do not improve after 5–7 days.	Avoid **mineral oil** and **castor oil** as they may interfere with absorption of fat-soluble vitamins such as vitamin K (could decrease availability to fetus).[141] Castor oil may stimulate uterine contractions and result in bleeding, abortion or uterine rupture.[141,142] **Lactulose** is poorly absorbed and considered compatible with pregnancy; however, its sweet taste may exacerbate nausea. Use of **osmotic laxatives** (e.g., sodium phosphate, magnesium hydroxide) is generally discouraged as other options are less likely to cause

(cont'd)

Table 4: **Management of Selected Common Conditions in Pregnancy** *(cont'd)*

Condition	Cause	Nonpharmacologic Therapy	Pharmacologic Therapy[a]	Monitoring of Therapy	Comments
	pregnancies.[136,137] Can exacerbate nausea.		For acute treatment: **glycerin** suppositories, **PEG**, and **senna**—generally, these agents have limited study data, but are poorly absorbed and considered compatible for as-needed, short-term use during pregnancy.[136,137,143 144]		electrolyte imbalances.[141] Regular use of **osmotic laxatives** such as lactulose or **stimulant laxatives** such as bisacodyl can result in excessive fluid and electrolyte loss; therefore, monitoring, adequate hydration and a balanced diet are important.[137]
Hemorrhoids[f]	Increased venous pressure below the uterus; constipation and associated chronic straining; vessel walls relaxed by progesterone (can lead to swelling).[137,142] Occurs in 25–35% of pregnancies.[142]	Dietary: Prevent constipation and straining, e.g., increase dietary fibre and fluids. Lifestyle: Maintain normal bowel function. Apply ice pack or cold compress to help relieve itching. Keep anal area clean to avoid irritation by cleaning with soap and water after each bowel movement and drying area by dabbing (not wiping). Use a warm water sitz bath for 10–15 min or soak in a warm water bath as needed for comfort. Sit on an air doughnut to relieve discomfort from pressure.[137,142]	Regular use of **bulk laxatives** such as **psyllium** and/or **stool softeners** such as **docusate**) may relieve some discomfort (see constipation above).[137,141,142] Of the rectal agents, external products preferred due to minimal absorption (unless the skin is chafed). Those inserted into rectum may be readily absorbed from rectal mucosa. A skin protectant (e.g., petrolatum) can be used to prevent further skin damage. Although lacking data in pregnancy, short-term use of **topical astringents** (e.g., hamamelis, zinc sulfate) can be used to clean and soothe the hemorrhoid area. **Acetaminophen** may be used for pain relief.[137,142]	Monitor for allergic reactions, which for topical rectal products may resemble hemorrhoid symptoms. Topical astringents can sting and exacerbate symptoms.[141] Reassess if symptoms do not improve after 5–7 days.	Ointments or suppositories containing **topical anesthetics** (e.g., benzocaine, pramoxine), **vasoconstrictors** (e.g., epinephrine) or **hydrocortisone** should be used only under supervision of a healthcare practitioner due to possible systemic absorption with consequent effects on the fetus. Avoid vasoconstrictors in those with hypertension. Reassess if severe pain, protrusion, bleeding or fecal seepage.[137]

Condition	Cause	Nonpharmacologic Therapy	Pharmacologic Therapy[a]	Monitoring of Therapy	Comments
Pigmentary changes (melasma, chloasma, mask of pregnancy)	Cause of this facial skin hyper-pigmentation disorder is unknown. Risk factors include darker skin types, genetic disposition, exposure to UV light, pregnancy, oral hormonal contraceptives and underlying thyroid disorders.[145]	Can be initiated and exacerbated by sun exposure. Avoid excessive exposure to sunlight.[145]	**Broad-spectrum sunscreen** is used in prevention and management.[145] Recommend an SPF of at least 30.[146] Topical **hydroquinone** 2–4% applied BID to the affected areas may be effective. However, data in pregnancy are limited and systemic absorption does occur. Suggest limiting use to severe cases under medical supervision.[147,148] Effectiveness of hydroquinone is enhanced by concurrent use of broad-spectrum sunscreen.[146]	Monitor for skin redness, burning, irritation, unusual skin discolouration.	Usually resolves after pregnancy. However, up to 30% of cases may be persistent.[149] May reoccur and darken with subsequent pregnancies.[150]
Reflux Esophagitis[g]	Decreased pressure or blunted response of the lower esophageal sphincter caused by hormonal changes. Other factors likely contribute. Usually 1st reported in early pregnancy.[151] Predominant symptoms are heartburn and regurgitation which are aggravated by meals and lying down.[136] Occurs in 30–80% of cases.[137]	Dietary: Eat small frequent meals; eat slowly; avoid foods that cause heartburn; eat in an upright position; drink warm milk; avoid oral intake (other than water) within 3 h of going to bed. Lifestyle: Elevate the head of the bed using blocks, or use 2 extra pillows to raise the head; lay on the left side of the body; avoid stooping, bending or assuming other positions that tend to worsen reflux; chew gum.[129,136,137,151]	**Calcium-containing antacids** may be used. Space doses apart from iron-containing supplements. Do not exceed recommended doses. **Magnesium-** or **alginic acid-containing antacids** as well as the H_2 antagonists **ranitidine** and **famotidine** are also safe options.[152] Proton pump inhibitors can be used when other therapies have failed (**omeprazole** is the most studied in pregnancy).[136,137,153,154,155,156]	Monitor for heartburn, regurgitation and nausea as well as other signs and symptoms of heartburn. Reassess if symptoms do not improve after 7 days and/or if a H_2 receptor antagonist is required.	Avoid **ASA** (e.g., Alka-Seltzer). See Backache, Headache, Pelvic Pain row. Avoid **sodium bicarbonate** due to short duration of effect, possible rebound symptoms and metabolic alkalosis with chronic use.[136,143] Avoid **magnesium trisilicate** due to association with fetal nephrolithiasis, hypotonia, respiratory distress and CV impairment.[136,143]

[a] Use the lowest effective dose for the shortest duration possible. Short-acting formulations are generally preferred to minimize fetal exposure time. Avoid alcohol/ethanol-containing liquid formulations. Consider the risk vs. benefit for each individual, including any risk associated with under-treating a maternal condition.
[b] For more information, see Chapter 45: Low Back Pain.
[c] For more information, see Chapter 8: Headache.
[d] For more information, see Chapter 24: Viral Rhinitis, Influenza, Rhinosinusitis and Pharyngitis.
[e] For more information, see Chapter 29: Constipation.
[f] For more information, see Chapter 33: Hemorrhoids.
[g] For more information, see Chapter 31: Dyspepsia and GERD.

Abbreviations: ASA = acetylsalicylic acid; CV = cardiovascular; GI = gastrointestinal; H_2 = histamine 2; NSAID = nonsteroidal anti-inflammatory drug; PEG = polyethylene glycol; PPI = proton pump inhibitor; UV = ultraviolet

Vaccinations during Pregnancy and Breastfeeding

Immunization during pregnancy or breastfeeding can provide the dual benefit of protecting the mother and the fetus/newborn by eliminating the mother as a source of disease transmission as well as transmitting protective levels of maternal antibodies transplacentally or via breast milk. Inactivated or toxoid vaccines can be given to pregnant women when indicated. However, live vaccines are generally contraindicated during pregnancy due to the theoretical risk of transmitting the disease to the fetus. Most vaccines can be given to breastfeeding women with the exception of those vaccines that may pose a risk of transmitting the disease to the infant (e.g., Bacille Calmette-Guérin vaccine, smallpox vaccine, yellow fever vaccine).[157] More information on the use of selected vaccines during pregnancy and breastfeeding can be found in Table 5.

Table 5: **Use of Selected Vaccines during Pregnancy and Breastfeeding**

Vaccine	Use during Pregnancy	Use during Breastfeeding	Comments
Hepatitis A	Recommended when indicated (e.g., close contact with a person with hepatitis A, or travel to an endemic area).[158]		
Hepatitis B	Recommended when indicated (e.g., ongoing exposure risk).[159]		
Influenza (inactivated)	Recommended in all patients at any stage of pregnancy. Associated with reduced maternal and newborn influenza-related morbidity. The risk of influenza-related hospitalization increases with gestation.[160]	Recommended in all patients.[160]	Live attenuated influenza vaccine is not recommended during pregnancy but may be used during breastfeeding when indicated.[160]
Meningococcal conjugate	Recommended when indicated (e.g., travel to a high-risk area, postexposure prophylaxis or during an outbreak).[161]		
Pertussis (acellular)	Recommended in those ≥26 weeks' gestation if not previously vaccinated against pertussis in adulthood, or during local pertussis outbreak, irrespective of immunization history.[162]	Recommended to be given as early as possible postpartum if pertussis vaccine not previously received in adulthood.[162]	Available only as a combination vaccine (Tdap recommended). The greatest morbidity and mortality from pertussis occurs in children <6 months.[162]
Pneumococcal polysaccharide or conjugate	Recommended when indicated (e.g., those with underlying medical conditions such as asthma, diabetes mellitus).[163]		
Tetanus toxoid	Recommended when indicated (postexposure prophylaxis).[164]		

Abbreviations: Td = tetanus diptheria; Tdap = tetanus, diptheria and acellular pertussis

Use of Common Substances/Products during Pregnancy

Information on the use of some common substances/products during pregnancy can be found in Table 6.

Table 6: **Use of Common Substances/Products during Pregnancy**

Substance/ Product	Recommendation in Pregnancy	Comments
Alcohol	Avoid use.[165]	Regular use of alcohol or exposure to high levels of alcohol, can cause fetal harm (fetal alcohol spectrum disorder). The amount of exposure required to cause harm is unclear; therefore, abstinence is recommended.[165,166] The Alcohol and Substance Use Helpline (1-877-327-4636) provides patients and healthcare practitioners with information and counselling on alcohol and recreational substance use during pregnancy and breastfeeding.
Caffeine	Consume ≤300 mg/day.	Conflicting data on the potential for harm (e.g., small for gestational age) with consumption >300 mg/day.[167,168] Average amounts of caffeine in common drinks and foods can be found on the Public Health Agency of Canada's website.[169]
Cigarette smoking	Avoid use and exposure to second-hand smoke.	Associated with a number of negative effects (e.g., spontaneous abortion, preterm labour, small for gestational age, sudden infant death syndrome, childhood respiratory problems). If cessation is unsuccessful after education and behavioural therapy, use of smoking cessation medications should be considered.[170,171,172] Prevention of Gestational and Neonatal Exposure to Tobacco Smoke (PREGNETS) website (www.pregnets.org) provides information and support for those trying to quit smoking during pregnancy and breastfeeding. See also Smoking Cessation.
Hair treatments (e.g., bleaching, colouring, straightening)	Occasional hair treatments unlikely to pose a risk.	Limited human data are available. Based on animal data, minimal systemic absorption and lack of reports of fetal harm, having hair treatments 3–4 times during pregnancy at 6- to 8-wk intervals is unlikely to pose a risk to the fetus.[173,174]

Postpartum Perineal Care and Postepisiotomy Pain

Pathophysiology

The perineum is a diamond-shaped area between the vagina and the anus.[175] A Canadian study found 92% of women who had a vaginal delivery experienced perineal pain on the first day postpartum. A week later 61% reported pain and by 6 weeks postpartum only 7% reported perineal pain.[176] Perineal pain results from trauma to the area as a result of bruising, tearing, episiotomies (enlargement of the vaginal orifice by surgical cutting of the perineum to facilitate delivery) and/or use of a vacuum or forceps to assist delivery.[175,177] The perineum is an extremely tender site for a cut or stitches and women report a wide range of pain, from mild to excruciating.[176] Perineal pain can cause reduced mobility, discomfort during urination or defecation, urinary and fecal incontinence, discomfort while sitting, and sexual dysfunction, and can interfere with providing newborn care.[178,179] The degree and duration of pain are related to the intensity of the trauma. Those who had episiotomies and more extensive tearing (third or fourth degree tears), reported perineal pain at 6 weeks at a rate of 13% and 20% respectively.[176] In contrast, pain resolved within 2.5 weeks for those with an intact perineum or minor tears.[180]

Goals of Therapy

- Relief of perineal pain
- Prevention of complications such as infection

Patient Assessment

When perineal pain is severe or associated with foul-smelling discharge, burning, bleeding or high fever, the patient should be assessed by an appropriate healthcare practitioner immediately.

Nonpharmacologic Therapy

Nonpharmacologic measures to relieve symptoms and help with perineal healing include localized cooling,[178,181] Kegel exercises and rinsing the area with warm water from a perineal squirt bottle after using the toilet. Detailed information for patients on perineum care can be found in Care of the Vaginal Area (Perineum) after Childbirth—What You Need to Know.

Pharmacologic Therapy

For comparative ingredients of nonprescription products, consult the *Compendium of Products for Minor Ailments*—Analgesic Products: Internal Analgesics and Antipyretics; Skin Care Products: Anesthetics.

Short-term relief of perineal pain can be obtained using a local agent (see Table 10). Wipes containing **hamamelis** (witch hazel) may reduce pain and itching.[180] **Topical anesthetic** products containing **lidocaine** are also available but should be used only under the direction of a healthcare practitioner due to the risk of systemic absorption from the area of trauma. The efficacy of topical anesthetics for perineum pain is unclear due to lack of evidence.[187] **Nonopioid analgesics** such as **acetaminophen**, **ibuprofen** and **naproxen sodium** are first-line oral medications for pain in breastfeeding women.[188,189,190] NSAIDs (e.g., ibuprofen, naproxen sodium) may provide similar efficacy to codeine/ acetaminophen products and do not cause constipation.[190] **Opioid analgesics** such as **codeine** were initially considered compatible with breastfeeding; however, depending on ethnicity, 1–29% of the population are ultrarapid metabolizers of CYP2D6, which results in increased conversion of codeine to morphine.[88,89,90,191] A case report in 2006 of an infant death related to ultrarapid metabolism of codeine by the breastfeeding mother sparked concern regarding the safety of codeine use.[191] If a codeine product is deemed necessary, use the lowest effective dose and limit use to a maximum of 4 days if possible. Closely monitor mother and infant for signs of opioid toxicity, e.g., sedation, lethargy and poor milk intake by infant.[88,192]

Postpartum Depression

Pathophysiology

Postpartum blues ("baby blues") is common, occurring in 15–85% of new mothers.[193] Symptoms generally begin sometime in the first week after delivery and may include sadness, insomnia, tearfulness, irritability, fatigue, anxiety and poor appetite. Postpartum blues has only a minimal effect on the mother's ability to function and is transient, resolving spontaneously within 1–2 weeks.[193,194] The cause is unknown, although hormonal changes after delivery are believed to play a role. Postpartum blues usually does not require therapy due to its transient course.

Postpartum depression (PPD) occurs in approximately 13% of new mothers.[195] In contrast to the baby blues, PPD is more disabling; the mother often finds it difficult to take care of her infant and herself. PPD is also more persistent, lasting longer than 2 weeks. The incidence is highest in the first 3 months postpartum with peak onset in the first 4–6 weeks, but may occur anytime in the first 6 months after delivery. The symptoms are the same as for major depressive disorder and can include lowered energy, difficulty concentrating, severe anxiety, feelings of worthlessness or guilt, disturbed sleep and changes in appetite. Maternal attitudes toward the infant are highly variable but can include disinterest, fear of being alone with the infant or excessive intrusiveness that inhibits adequate infant rest.[196] Thoughts of self-harm or suicide can also be present. The etiology may be complex and include biologic and psychosocial factors.[193,194]

PPD may result in the mother feeling too unwell to initiate or maintain breastfeeding. Untreated PPD can also result in impaired child development and is associated with poor cognitive functioning, behavioural inhibition and emotional maladjustment in infants and children.[193]

For more information on depression see Chapter 4: Depression.

Goals of Therapy

- Relieve depressive symptoms
- Identify patients at risk of postpartum depression
- Educate patients on recognizing danger signs

Patient Assessment

Postpartum women should be monitored carefully by their healthcare practitioners. The diagnosis may be difficult to make since changes in sleep, appetite and energy are routine with the arrival of a new baby. The Edinburgh Postnatal Depression Scale is a validated and readily available screening tool consisting of 10 multiple choice questions to be answered by the new mother.[193,194] A brief patient information sheet with a checklist is provided in Postpartum Depression—What You Need to Know. If any of the signs on the checklist apply to a postpartum patient, strongly advise her to seek help by immediately referring her for counselling and/or specialized mental health treatment, and encourage completion of the more specific Edinburgh scale.

Nonpharmacologic Therapy

Psychotherapy may be effective for some women suffering from PPD. Specifically, supportive counselling, cognitive behavioural therapy, interpersonal therapy and psychodynamic therapy have shown benefit.[195] However, psychotherapy may not be an option for some women due to cost, lack of a therapist in the area and difficulty arranging child care to attend sessions.[193] Some women may receive benefit from light therapy, peer support groups and/or regular exercise.

Pharmacologic Therapy

For comparative ingredients of nonprescription products, consult the *Compendium of Products for Minor Ailments*—Herbal and Natural Health Products: Single Entity; Vitamin and Mineral Products: Single Entity.

St. John's wort has been used in the treatment of mild to moderate depression. Information in breastfeeding is conflicting ranging from reports of no adverse effects in infants to reports of jaundice, colic, drowsiness and lethargy.[6,197,198] St. John's wort can interact with many other medications as it induces CYP3A4, including reducing the effectiveness of oral contraceptives.[197] Due to the variability in composition of products and potential for drug interactions, other treatment options are preferred. Use during pregnancy should be avoided as there are insufficient human or animal data.[198,199] If a pregnant woman chooses to use St. John's wort, encourage enrollment in the Motherisk St. John's wort study (1-800-670-6126; www.motherisk.org).

Omega-3 fatty acid supplementation has been investigated for treating depression. Randomized controlled trials have not shown a benefit over placebo in postpartum women; however, studies have been limited by small sample size and variation in the dose of omega-3 used.[193,199] Although omega-3 supplementation cannot presently be recommended for perinatal depression, women should be encouraged to meet dietary intake requirements to aid in normal fetal and infant development.

The safety and efficacy of ***S*-adenosyl-methionine (SAMe)** for treating postpartum depression and depression during pregnancy have not been established; its use should be avoided.[199,200] **Folic acid** has been found to augment antidepressant efficacy, but has not been specifically studied in perinatal depression; doses beyond routine supplementation cannot be recommended (see Table 3).[199]

Women who are breastfeeding may prefer psychotherapy over medication; however, it may be less effective than medication for severe depressive symptoms. PPD generally requires medication and possibly hospitalization to prevent suicide or infanticide. Antidepressants pass into breast milk but usually do not produce adverse effects in the infant. Monitor the infant for irritability, sedation, poor weight gain and change in feeding patterns.[193] The choice of antidepressant should be based on the woman's symptoms and history of antidepressant use. Treat for a minimum of 9 months.[194]

For further information on pharmacotherapy of depression, see Chapter 4: Depression.

Postpartum Contraception

Most healthcare practitioners suggest waiting about 4–6 weeks before resuming intercourse, to allow the woman's body to heal. The uterus and vagina must return to their prepregnancy size, a process that usually occurs more quickly in breastfeeding women.

Many variables such as fatigue, postpartum depression and decreased sex drive can influence this time frame. Many women take much longer before they feel like resuming intercourse; however, surveys indicate a significant number choose to resume intercourse before 6 weeks.[201] Couples need to make individual decisions based on comfort level.

Ovulation usually resumes within 4 weeks after delivery in nonlactating mothers. In breastfeeding mothers, the onset of ovulation is delayed but more variable as it is influenced by the extent of breastfeeding.[201]

The choice of contraceptive method is highly individual. Discussion of the pros and cons of various methods should begin during the last trimester of pregnancy to provide sufficient time to make an informed choice. Contraception should be initiated in the third postpartum week.[201,202] Some long-term contraceptive methods should not be started before 6 weeks postpartum; other options (e.g., barrier methods, progestin-only contraceptives) may need to be used in the interim (see Other Nonhormonal Methods and Hormonal Contraceptives).

Lactational Amenorrhea Method (LAM)

The lactational amenorrhea method (LAM) uses breastfeeding as a contraceptive method. LAM can be as effective as oral contraceptives; however, it is influenced by a number of factors that may make this an impractical method for many women. For LAM to be effective, the mother must breastfeed at regular intervals (no greater than 4 hours during the day or 6 hours at night) and must exclusively breastfeed (supplemental food should be no greater than 5–10% of total feedings).[203] Expressing milk by pump is less vigorous than suckling and may reduce the efficacy of LAM. Even with full breastfeeding and adequate milk production, frequent suckling is believed to be necessary to achieve the full contraceptive effect of LAM.[204] After 6 months or when menstruation resumes, the risk of ovulation increases and thus the efficacy of LAM declines.[203] Some suggest an additional form of contraception be started in the third postpartum month.[201]

Other Nonhormonal Methods

Barrier methods include male and female condoms, sponges, diaphragms and cervical caps, all supplemented by spermicides. Male condoms can be used almost immediately postpartum and can be a good short-term option for those waiting for initiation of a more long-term method. Lubricated condoms can help offset vaginal dryness experienced by some women postpartum.[202]

Diaphragm and cervical cap fitting or refitting should be performed 6–8 weeks after delivery, to allow for completion of uterine involution.[201] The sponge may have a higher failure rate among women who have delivered a child than among women who have not, even with perfect use.[202,205] To decrease the risk of toxic shock syndrome, contraceptive sponges, cervical caps and diaphragms should not be used while there is continued postpartum bleeding.[201,202] The lower effectiveness of barrier methods compared with intrauterine and hormonal options should be considered when choosing a method.[206]

A copper intrauterine device (IUD) can be inserted between 10 minutes and 48 hours postpartum. If this window is missed, wait until >4 weeks postpartum (due to risk of expulsion).[207,208] Although there may be a small increased risk of uterine perforation if IUD insertion occurs while breastfeeding or if <36 weeks postpartum,[209] benefits are considered to outweigh risks.[207,208] Copper IUDs have no known effect on lactation.[201,202,206]

For more information on barrier contraceptive devices, see Chapter 76: Contraception.

Hormonal Contraceptives

For more information on hormonal therapy, consult the *Compendium of Therapeutic Choices*: Contraception

Postpartum use of combination **estrogen-progestin contraceptives** is restricted due to increased risk of venous thromboembolism (VTE) and possible negative effects on breastfeeding.[210] However, after 6 weeks postpartum an estrogen-progestin contraceptive can be initiated.[203,210]

The risk of VTE postpartum is estimated to be 22- to 84-fold greater than that of nonpregnant, nonpostpartum females.[211] This risk steadily declines postpartum and within 6 weeks most women have returned to their pre-pregnancy risk.[201,211] As estrogen-progestin contraceptives independently increase risk of VTE, it is recommended to delay their initiation until more than 6 weeks postpartum.[203,210] Earlier use (>3 weeks postpartum) may be considered in select, low-risk women.[210]

Whether to initiate combined estrogen-containing contraceptives in those who are breastfeeding is an area of controversy. Estrogen has the potential to reduce lactation; however, studies in this area are generally of poor quality and data are lacking with the low-dose estrogen products.[202,212] It is recommended to wait at least until breastfeeding is well established (at least 4–6 weeks postpartum).[202,203,210]

Progestin-only contraceptives (oral **progestin**, **medroxyprogesterone** depot injection and **levonorgestrel** intrauterine device) are generally initiated 4–6 weeks postpartum in breastfeeding women. This time frame is based on the paucity of high-quality data for earlier use and the theoretical concern that neonates are unable to effectively metabolize progestins in breast milk.[202,203,210,213] However, due to the lack of evidence of negative effects on breastfeeding or infant growth and development, guidelines indicate use of progestin-only contraceptives can be considered earlier than 30 days postpartum.[210,213,214,215,216] Although there may be a small increased risk of uterine perforation if IUD insertion occurs while breastfeeding or if <36 weeks postpartum,[209] benefits are considered to outweigh risks.[207,208]

Drug Therapy during Breastfeeding

Nearly all drugs will be present in breast milk to some degree following maternal ingestion.[6] Many lists of drugs that are acceptable to ingest during breastfeeding have been developed, but they differ and are based on subjective interpretation of data. Most of the published data come from single case reports, and reports of drug concentration in breast milk are often based on single dose measurements, not accounting for effects of drug accumulation.[11] Therefore, it is difficult to interpret the clinical significance of this information. Additionally, a drug's effect on milk production is an important consideration. Refer to Table 1 for general principles of drug therapy during breastfeeding.

Table 7 outlines some information pertaining to common medication use during breastfeeding. See also Appendix V: Pregnancy and Breastfeeding: Self-care Therapy for Common Conditions.

Table 7: **Common Medications Usually Considered Compatible with Breastfeeding**[a]

Drug Class	Comments
Acid suppressors	Limited data available. **Calcium-containing antacids** are preferred as they have the additional benefit of replacing maternal calcium lost during breastfeeding. **Magnesium-containing antacids**, **alginic acid** and **sucralfate** are poorly absorbed thus unlikely to produce effects in a breastfed infant.[151] H_2-antagonists are considered compatible; **famotidine** is preferred as it concentrates in breast milk to a lesser degree than **ranitidine** or **cimetidine** and has more safety data than **nizatidine**.[6,7,72] Data on maternal use of **omeprazole** (and other PPIs) during breastfeeding are very limted.[217] Some experts suggest that since these medications are excreted in low amounts into breast milk and are extremely acid labile and therefore likely to be destroyed in the stomach before infant absorption could occur, they are not expected to cause any adverse effects in breastfed infants.[6,219,220]
Analgesics	**Acetaminophen** is the drug of choice.[6,218] Like acetaminophen, **ibuprofen** is routinely used to treat infant fevers. Ibuprofen is compatible with breastfeeding with low levels passing into breast milk.[6] Other options include **ASA**, **codeine** and **naproxen**. ASA is excreted into breast milk; however, no cases of Reye's syndrome from breast milk exposure have been documented.[6,185] **Codeine**, although compatible in most cases, can produce serious toxicity in infants whose mothers are ultrarapid metabolizers of CYP2D6.[88,188,192] More data are available for ibuprofen than naproxen sodium. Ibuprofen has a slightly shorter half-life than naproxen sodium—2 h vs. 10 h.[185] See also: Pharmacologic Therapy in Postpartum Perineal Care and Postepisiotomy Pain section.
Antidiarrheals	**Bulk-forming agents** (e.g., **psyllium**) and **attapulgite** are not absorbed. **Loperamide** and **bismuth** have minimal GI absorption, and are unlikely to affect a breastfed infant.[6] Salicylate is absorbed from bismuth subsalicylate; however, there are no documented reports of Reye's syndrome in infants exposed to salicylates via breast milk.[6]
Antihistamines	See Table 9. First- and second-generation antihistamines can be used.[6,72,80] First-generation antihistamines may cause sedation and irritability in the infant and reduce milk production due to their anticholinergic effects.
Decongestants	See Table 9. **Saline nasal spray** is the drug of choice. No data available for medicated nasal sprays but due to minimal systemic absorption are preferred over oral agents.[218] Oral **pseudoephedrine** is considered safe in breastfeeding; however, it may reduce milk production and cause irritability in the infant.[6,218]
Laxatives	**Bulk-forming agents** are preferred for preventing constipation as they are not absorbed.[218] **Glycerin suppositories** can be used for acute constipation. GI absorption is minimal for **bisacodyl**, **docusate**, **PEG** and **lactulose** and they are unlikely to affect a breastfed infant.[6,218] Senna and cascara have been associated with loose stools or diarrhea in some breastfed infants.[6,218] Avoid mineral oil and castor oil due to the potential to reduce absorption of fat-soluble vitamins.
Vitamins and minerals	Appropriate when used in normal doses. In addition to **folic acid** supplementation before and during pregnancy, it is recommended that women continue daily supplementation with a multivitamin containing folic acid 0.4–1 mg for 4–6 wk postpartum, or as long as breastfeeding continues.[1] **Calcium** supplementation may be needed to achieve the recommended intake (<19 y = 1300 mg/day, 19–50 y = 1000 mg/day) and replace maternal calcium stores which are transferred into breast milk. **Vitamin D** intake should be 600 IU/day during breastfeeding.[20,21,22] **Iodine** requirement is increased during breastfeeding (i.e., 250–290 µg/day).[26,29] Supplementation with 150 µg/day is recommended.[25,29]

[a] See Table 1 for general principles of drug therapy during breastfeeding.

Abbreviations: ASA = acetylsalicylic acid, aspirin; H_2 = histamine 2; IU = international units; PEG = polyethylene glycol; PPI = proton pump inhibitor

Suppression of Lactation

For women who are unable to breastfeed or choose not to, suppression of lactation may be desired. Without suckling stimulation, lactation will gradually cease. However, women may experience leakage, engorgement and/or pain before lactation ends.[221] These symptoms begin 1–4 days postpartum and peak by day 3–5, with some women still experiencing pain at day 14.[222]

Nonpharmacologic Therapy

Despite lack of evidence, the following nonpharmacologic methods are routinely used to reduce the discomfort associated with lactation suppression:

- Wearing a well-fitting, supportive bra (recommended over breast binding which is associated with more breast leakage, tenderness and pain)[223]
- Expressing milk gently (by hand or pump) just enough to relieve pressure but not fully emptying the breast. A warm shower or compress helps induce milk letdown to facilitate expression.[221] Those who have experienced loss of a child may find comfort in donating their expressed milk if a milk bank is readily available
- Placing ice packs or cold cabbage leaves in the bra to reduce pain and swelling.[221]

Pharmacologic Therapy

Nonprescription analgesics are used to reduce pain.[221] In 1988 the US FDA recommended against the routine use of pharmacologic therapies (other than analgesics) for lactation suppression.[222] **Bromocriptine** and **estrogen** are not recommended due to lack of evidence of efficacy and safety concerns including risk of seizures, MI or severe hypotension with bromocriptine[224,225] and venous thromboembolism with estrogens postpartum.[224]

Table 8: **Drug Therapy for Nausea and Vomiting of Pregnancy**[a]

Class	Drug	Dosage	Adverse Effects	Monitoring of Therapy	Comments	Cost[b]
Antihistamine Antiemetics	*dimenhydrinate* Gravol Preparations, generics	50–100 mg Q4–6H PRN po or pr (maximum 200 mg/day when used concurrently with Diclectin 4 tablets/day)[37,45]	Sedation, anticholinergic effects, e.g., dry mouth, constipation.[46] No known teratogenic effects.[47]	Monitor patient for signs and symptoms of sedation and anticholinergic effects, e.g., dry mouth, constipation. Reassess if nausea and vomiting not improved after 3 days or adverse effects are intolerable.	Can also be given parenterally. Minimal data on efficacy.	$
Antihistamine/ vitamin combination	*doxylamine delayed-release/pyridoxine 10 mg/10 mg* Diclectin	1 tablet in the morning and afternoon and 2 tablets at bedtime[41]	Sedation, anticholinergic effects e.g., dry mouth, constipation.[48]	Monitor patient for sedation and anticholinergic effects. Reassess if nausea and vomiting not improved after 3 days or adverse effects intolerable.	Considered drug of choice. Use on a regular rather than PRN basis. Up to 12 tablets/day can be used in some cases. Taper on discontinuation.[48]	$$$
Natural Health Products	*ginger* Gravol Ginger, others	250 mg QID or 500 mg BID po (maximum 1000 mg/day)[41,49,50,51]	Belching[52]	Reassess if nausea and vomiting not improved in 5 days.	Onset of action is up to 3 days. Dose based on powdered ginger root. Products may not be standardized.	$
Vitamins	*pyridoxine* ◗ generics	10 mg or 25 mg Q8H po Preliminary data suggest doses up to 200 mg/day can be safely used in pregnancy[53]	No known teratogenic effects in doses used for nausea and vomiting.[54] High doses (especially >1000 mg/day) have been associated with neuropathy.[55]	Refer to physician if nausea and vomiting not improved in 3 days.	Has reduced nausea and vomiting in small RCTs.[56,57] Consider other sources of pyridoxine in total dose (e.g., Diclectin, prenatal vitamin).	$

[a] To be used only on the advice of a healthcare practitioner.

[b] Cost of 1-day supply; includes drug cost only.

◗ Dosage adjustment may be required in renal impairment.

Legend: $ <$2 $$ $2–4 $$$ $4–6

Table 9: Selected Drug Therapy for Allergic Rhinitis and the Common Cold in Pregnancy and Breastfeeding

Class	Drug[a,b]	Dosage	Maternal Adverse Effects	Monitoring of Therapy	Comments	Cost[c]
Antihistamines, first-generation[d]	*brompheniramine* No single-entity products. Component of many cough/cold products: Dimetapp, Robitussin, generics	4 mg Q4–6H po (maximum 24 mg/day)	Sedation (less than with diphenhydramine), anticholinergic effects, including mucosal drying, which may inhibit lactation.[71]	Monitor mother for sedation and anticholinergic effects, e.g., dry mouth.[71] Monitor breastfeeding infant for signs of irritability, excessive crying and altered sleep.[6,72] If infant experiences these effects or if mother's symptoms do not improve after 1 wk, reassess.	**Pregnancy:** Limited data. Initial data suggested a possible congenital defect association but this was not seen in subsequent studies.[73,74] If possible, avoid in last 2 wk of pregnancy due to possible neonate withdrawal and increased risk of retinopathy of prematurity.[1,66,73,75] **Breastfeeding:** Limited data. Irritability, excessive crying and disturbed sleeping have been reported in a breastfed infant.[6,72,73] Small, occasional doses unlikely to cause adverse effects.[72]	$
	chlorpheniramine Chlor-Tripolon, generics	4 mg Q4–6H po (maximum 24 mg/day)	See brompheniramine.	See brompheniramine.	**Pregnancy:** Considered safe in pregnancy/drug of choice.[3,76] Most data support no increased risk of congenital effects. If possible, avoid in last 2 wk of pregnancy due to possible neonatal withdrawal and increased risk of retinopathy of prematurity.[12,66,75,77] **Breastfeeding:** Very limited data. Sedation or irritability possible in the infant.[6,72] Small occasional doses unlikely to cause adverse effects.[72]	$
	diphenhydramine Benadryl Preparations, generics	25–50 mg Q4–6H po (maximum 300 mg/day)	Sedation, anticholinergic effects, including mucosal drying, which may inhibit lactation.[71]	See brompheniramine.	**Pregnancy:** Most data support no increased risk of congenital effects in pregnant women. Considered compatible with pregnancy.[3,78] If possible, avoid in last 2 wk of pregnancy due to possible neonatal withdrawal and increased risk of retinopathy of prematurity. Avoid use	$

(cont'd)

Table 9: **Selected Drug Therapy for Allergic Rhinitis and the Common Cold in Pregnancy and Breastfeeding** *(cont'd)*

Class	Drug[a,b]	Dosage	Maternal Adverse Effects	Monitoring of Therapy	Comments	Cost[c]
					with temazepam as animal data suggest an increased risk of stillbirth.[12,75,78] **Breastfeeding:** Very limited data. Excreted into breast milk. Sedation or irritability possible in the infant.[6,72,78]	
Antihistamines, second-generation[e]	*cetirizine* Reactine, generics	5–10 mg once daily po	Preferred by patients due to ease of administration and because it is nonsedating in most patients.[69] Sedation and anticholinergic effects, including mucosal drying, which may inhibit lactation but less common than with first-generation antihistamines.[71]	See brompheniramine.	**Pregnancy:** Considered safe in pregnancy, although more safety data are available for first-generation antihistamines.[3,70,76,79,80] **Breastfeeding:** Likely excreted in human breast milk in small amounts. BSACI considers drug of choice for urticaria; however, very limited specific data available and no data for hydroxyzine (the parent compound).[6,72,79,81] Approved in children >2 y. Theoretically less likely to cause sedation or irritability in an infant than first-generation antihistamines.	$
	desloratadine Aerius, generics	5 mg once daily po	Preferred by patients due to ease of administration and because it is nonsedating.[69] Sedation and anticholinergic effects, including mucosal drying, which may inhibit lactation but less common than with first-generation antihistamines.[71]	See brompheniramine.	**Pregnancy:** Animal data and human data for the parent compound (loratadine) suggest it is safe, but no human data are available with desloratadine.[76,82] **Breastfeeding:** No specific data available, but loratadine levels in breast milk are very small and AAP classifies the parent compound (loratadine) compatible with breastfeeding.[6,72,82] Theoretically less likely to cause sedation or irritability in an infant than first-generation antihistamines.	$

Class	Drug[a,b]	Dosage	Maternal Adverse Effects	Monitoring of Therapy	Comments	Cost[c]
	fexofenadine Allegra	120 mg daily po (given as 60 mg BID or as 120 mg once daily)	See desloratadine.	See brompheniramine.	**Pregnancy:** Animal data suggest possible concerns. Very limited human data available.[76,83,84] Considered an alternative agent to those with better and/or more safety data. **Breastfeeding:** Likely excreted into breast milk in small amounts. AAP classifies it as compatible with breastfeeding. However, no specific data are available. Limited data available for the parent compound (terfenadine).[6,72,83] Theoretically less likely to cause sedation or irritability in an infant than first-generation antihistamines.	$
	loratadine Claritin, Claritin Liquid Capsules, generics	10 mg once daily po	See desloratadine.	See brompheniramine.	**Pregnancy:** Considered safe in pregnancy, although more safety data are available for first-generation antihistamines.[3,70,76,80,85] **Breastfeeding:** Small amounts excreted in human breast milk.[6,72] Approved in children >2 y.[86] AAP and BSACI classifies it as compatible with breastfeeding.[81,85] Theoretically less likely to cause sedation or irritability in an infant than first-generation antihistamines.	$

(cont'd)

Table 9: **Selected Drug Therapy for Allergic Rhinitis and the Common Cold in Pregnancy and Breastfeeding** *(cont'd)*

Class	Drug[a,b]	Dosage	Maternal Adverse Effects	Monitoring of Therapy	Comments	Cost[c]
Antitussives[f]	*codeine* generics	10–20 mg Q4–6H PRN po (maximum 120 mg/day)[87]	Sedation, constipation, palpitations, and dizziness.[88]	Use under healthcare practitioner supervision. Should not exceed 4 days in a breastfeeding mother. Closely monitor breastfeeding infants for sedation, lethargy, grey skin and poor milk intake: refer to appropriate healthcare practitioner if these symptoms develop.[6,72,89,90] In most cases, there is consistency between CNS depression in mother and infant. If the mother is symptomatic (e.g., somnolent, groggy), the infant should be examined for signs of CNS depression.[89]	**Pregnancy:** Data do not suggest risk of birth defects.[88,91] If possible, avoid use in the first trimester. Avoid long-term use or high doses close to term (risk of neonatal opiate withdrawal).[88] **Breastfeeding:** Indicated for nonproductive cough.[87] Mothers who are ultrarapid metabolizers of CYP2D6 have increased conversion of codeine to morphine which resulted in death of a breastfed infant. Although a minority of the population are rapid metabolizers of 2D6, caution is warranted; use the lowest effective dose for 4 days or less, or use alternative treatment options.[6,72,89,90]	$
	dextromethorphan Benylin DM, Robitussin DM, generics	10–20 mg Q4H or 30 mg Q6–8H po (maximum 120 mg/day)[92]	Minimal	Monitor infant for sedation.[6] If symptoms do not improve after 1 wk, reassess.	Choose ethanol-free products. **Pregnancy:** Considered safe in pregnancy. Most data support no increased risk of congenital effects.[12,75,93] **Breastfeeding:** Indicated for nonproductive cough.[92] No data in human breastfeeding, but considered probably safe.[6,72,93]	$

Class	Drug[a,b]	Dosage	Maternal Adverse Effects	Monitoring of Therapy	Comments	Cost[c]
Corticosteroids, intranasal[g]	*mometasone furoate* Nasonex	2 sprays in each nostril once daily Reduce to 1 spray in each nostril once daily if possible	Nasal irritation, sore throat.[94]	Monitor mother for nasal irritation, sore throat and reduced milk supply. Monitor breastfeeding infant for reduction in feeding, growth, weight gain.[72,95]	**Pregnancy:** Avoid use in first trimester if possible.[96] No human data. Considered probably compatible with pregnancy based on low systemic bioavailability and safety of other inhaled corticosteroids in asthma.[97] **Breastfeeding:** No human data. Considered probably compatible based on minimal maternal systemic absorption via intranasal route.[72,95,97]	$$$
	triamcinolone acetonide Nasacort Allergy 24HR	2 sprays in each nostril once daily Reduce to 1 spray in each nostril once daily if possible	See mometasone.	Monitor mother for nasal irritation, sore throat and reduced milk supply. Monitor breastfeeding infant for reduction in feeding, growth, weight gain.[72,98]	**Pregnancy:** Avoid use in first trimester if possible.[96] Considered compatible with pregnancy based on data with inhaled form and safety of other inhaled corticosteroids in asthma.[99] **Breastfeeding:** Considered compatible based on minimal maternal systemic absorption via intranasal route.[72,99]	$$

(cont'd)

Table 9: **Selected Drug Therapy for Allergic Rhinitis and the Common Cold in Pregnancy and Breastfeeding** *(cont'd)*

Class	Drug[a,b]	Dosage	Maternal Adverse Effects	Monitoring of Therapy	Comments	Cost[c]
Decongestants, oral[h]	*phenylephrine* No single entity products. Component of many cough/cold products: Dimetapp, Robitussin, others	10 mg Q4H po (maximum 60 mg/day) Efficacy at currently recommended oral dosages has been questioned[100]	Signs and symptoms of adrenergic stimulation; palpitations, increased blood pressure, nervousness, insomnia and dizziness.[100] May reduce milk production.	If mother's adverse effects intolerable or symptoms do not improve after 1 wk, ressess. Monitor infants for signs and symptoms of adrenergic stimulation, e.g., irritability, excessive crying, altered sleep patterns.[6]	**Pregnancy:** Limited evidence of possible association with endocardial cushion defect with first trimester use, however absolute risk minimal.[101,102] Potentially can reduce uterine blood flow.[70,75,103] If possible, avoid use, particularly in the first trimester.[70,102] **Breastfeeding:** Although oral bioavailability is low, it may be excreted into breast milk in small amounts. No data in human breastfeeding are available. May reduce milk production.[6,72] Not preferred as alternatives with better and/or more safety data exist.	$
	pseudoephedrine ❸ Eltor 120, Sudafed, generics	30–60 mg Q4–6H po (maximum 240 mg/day)	See phenylephrine.	If mother's adverse effects intolerable or symptoms do not improve after 1 wk, reassess. Monitor infants for signs and symptoms of adrenergic stimulation, e.g., irritability, excessive crying, altered sleep patterns.[6,72,104,105]	**Pregnancy:** Generally considered safe in pregnancy. Some sources recommend avoidance of pseudoephedrine during the first trimester based on a single, small study showing increased risk of gastroschisis,[106] however, a subsequent, larger study from the same group did not show increased risk.[102] **Breastfeeding:** Excreted in breast milk in small amounts but AAP classifies it as compatible with breastfeeding. Irritability has been reported in breastfed infants. Avoid in mothers with insufficient milk production.[6,72,105]	$

Class	Drug[a,b]	Dosage	Maternal Adverse Effects	Monitoring of Therapy	Comments	Cost[c]
Decongestants, topical[i]	*oxymetazoline* Claritin Allergy Decongestant, Dristan Long Lasting Nasal Mist, generics	Use lowest effective dose according to manufacturer's instructions	Local burning and stinging, sneezing and dryness of nasal mucosa. Use sparingly (maximum 3–5 days) to minimize tolerance or rebound congestion.[12]	If symptoms not improved after 3–5 days refer to physician.[12] Monitor infants for signs and symptoms of adrenergic stimulation, e.g., irritability, excessive crying, altered sleep patterns.[6]	**Pregnancy:** Generally considered safe in pregnancy;[75,80] however, data on safety are limited and conflicting.[102,107] No adverse effects reported with single dose use.[108] Using higher than the recommended dose may reduce uterine blood flow.[109] **Breastfeeding:** No data in human breastfeeding. Preferred over oral agents due to presumed low systemic absorption.[4,6,72]	$
	sodium chloride (normal saline) Hydrasense, Rhinaris, Salinex, generics	Spray into nostrils as needed	Well tolerated.	If symptoms not improved after 1 wk, reassess.	**Pregnancy:** Drug of choice. Safety well established.[66,69] **Breastfeeding:** Drug of choice. Safety well established.	$
	xylometazoline Balminil, Otrivin, generics	Use lowest effective dose according to manufacturer's instructions	See oxymetazoline.	See oxymetazoline.	See oxymetazoline.	$

(cont'd)

Table 9: Selected Drug Therapy for Allergic Rhinitis and the Common Cold in Pregnancy and Breastfeeding *(cont'd)*

Class	Drug[a,b]	Dosage	Maternal Adverse Effects	Monitoring of Therapy	Comments	Cost[c]
Mast cell stabilizers	*sodium cromoglycate* Rhinaris CS Anti-allergic	1 spray in each nostril 6 times daily Reduce to BID–TID after adequate response[110]	Nasal irritation, sneezing, cough, unpleasant taste.[110]	Monitor breastfeeding infant for irriatbility, insomnia, diarrhea, constipation and weight gain.[6]	**Pregnancy:** Considered compatible with pregnancy.[111] **Breastfeeding:** No data. Considered compatible due to low systemic absorption.[6,72,111]	$$

[a] Consider the risk vs. benefit for each individual, including any risk associated with undertreating a maternal condition.

[b] Use the lowest effective dose for the shortest duration possible. Short-acting formulations are generally preferred to minimize fetal/infant exposure time. Avoid alcohol/ethanol-containing liquid formulations.

[c] Cost of smallest available pack size; includes drug cost only.

[d] May reduce rhinorrhea, sneezing, nasal itch and congestion via antihistamine and anticholinergic effects.

[e] May reduce rhinorrhea, sneezing, nasal itch and congestion via antihistamine effects.

[f] Relief of cough through centrally mediated cough suppression. A combination of a first-generation antihistamine and a decongestant is recommended for coughs due to postnasal drip, i.e., upper airway cough syndrome.

[g] Other corticosteroid nasal products are available on prescription. For more information see Chapter 22: Allergic Rhinitis.

[h] Relief of congestion through vasoconstriction of respiratory mucosa.

[i] Relief of congestion through vasoconstriction of respiratory mucosa or osmotic effect (normal saline).

Dosage adjustment may be required in renal impairment.

Abbreviations: AAP = American Academy of Pediatrics; BSACI = British Society for Allergy and Clinical Immunology; CNS = central nervous system; CYP = cytochrome P450; NVP = nausea and vomiting of pregnancy

Legend: $ <$10 $$ $10–20 $$$ $20–30

Table 10: Selected Drug Therapy for Perineal Care and Postepisiotomy Pain[a]

Class	Drug	Dosage	Adverse Effects	Drug Interactions	Comments	Cost[b]
Analgesics	*acetaminophen* Atasol Preparations, Tylenol, generics	325–650 mg Q4–6H PRN po (maximum 4000 mg/day)[182]	Minimal.	Acetaminophen has been reported to increase INR in warfarin-treated patients.[183] Check INR if acetaminophen ≥2 g/day is used for ≥3 consecutive days. Adjust warfarin dosage as required.	If pain not relieved after 2 days, further assessment required. Considered safe in breastfeeding mothers. Amount in breast milk significantly less than pediatric therapeutic dose.[6]	$
	ibuprofen Advil, Advil Liqui-Gels, Motrin, Motrin IB, Motrin Liquid Gels, generics	200–400 mg Q6–8H PRN po (maximum dose for self–care: 1200 mg/day)[184]	GI effects (e.g., nausea, heartburn), dizziness.[184]	Warfarin: Increased anticoagulant effect. Antihypertensives: possible reduction in antihypertensive effect which may require additional antihypertensive therapy. Lithium may interfere with sodium/water balance. Monitor lithium levels when NSAID added. Increased risk of GI bleeding with SSRIs.	If pain not relieved after 2 days, further assessment required. Considered safe in breastfeeding mothers. Amount in breast milk significantly less than pediatric therapeutic dose.[6]	$
	naproxen sodium Aleve, generics	220–440 mg/day PRN po in 1 or divided doses (maximum dose for self–care: 440 mg/day)	See ibuprofen.	See ibuprofen.	See ibuprofen. Considered safe in breastfeeding. However, more data available for ibuprofen, and ibuprofen has a shorter half-life.[6,185]	$
Local agents	*hamamelis* Tucks Medicated Pads	Use as needed for comfort	Contact dermatitis.[186]		May reduce itching and pain. If pain not relieved after 2 days, recommend a trial of oral analgesic.	$$$/40 pads

[a] See Table 1 for general principles of drug therapy during breastfeeding.

[b] Cost of 1-day supply unless otherwise specified; includes drug cost only.

Legend: $ <$2 $$ $2–4 $$$ $4–6

Resource Tips

LactMed (a database, from the U.S. National Library of Medicine, of drugs and other chemicals to which breastfeeding mothers may be exposed. Includes information on the levels of such substances in breast milk and infant blood, and the possible adverse effects in the nursing infant). Available from: toxnet.nlm.nih.gov/cgi-bin/sis/htmlgen?LACT.

Lalonde A, Schuurmans N, Senikas V. *Healthy beginnings: giving your baby the best start, from preconception to birth.* Available from: www.sogc.org/healthybeginnings/index.html.

Motherisk (a Canadian clinical, research and teaching program dedicated to antenatal drug, chemical and disease risk counselling). Motherisk Helpline: 416-813-6780. Available from: www.motherisk.org.

Motherisk. Alcohol and Substance Use Helpline: 1-877-327-4636. Available from: www.motherisk.org/prof/alcohol.jsp.

Motherisk. Nausea and Vomiting of Pregnancy (NVP) Helpline: 1-800-436-8477. Available from: www.motherisk.org/prof/morningSickness.jsp.

Organization of Teratology Information Specialists. MotherToBaby. *Fact Sheets*. Available from: www.mothertobaby.org/otis-fact-sheets-s13037.

Public Health Agency of Canada. *The healthy pregnancy guide*. Available from: www.phac-aspc.gc.ca/hp-gs/guide/index-eng.php.

Society of Obstetricians and Gynaecologists of Canada. Available from: www.sogc.org.

Suggested Readings

Briggs GG, Freeman RK. *Drugs in pregnancy and lactation: a reference guide to fetal and neonatal risk*. 10th ed. Philadelphia: Wolters Kluwer; 2014.

Exposure to psychotropic medications and other substances during pregnancy and lactation: a handbook for health care providers (a Canadian resource developed by the Centre for Addiction and Mental Health and the Motherisk Program). Available from: www.camh.ca/en/education/about/camh_publications/Pages/exposure_psychotropic_meds_pregnancy.aspx.

Ferreira E, Martin B, Morin C. *Grossesse et allaitement: guide thérapeutique*. 2nd ed. Montréal: CHU Sainte-Justine; 2013.

Hale TW, Rowe HE. *Medications and mothers' milk: a manual of lactational pharmacology*. 16th ed. Plano: Hale Publishing; 2014.

Society of Obstetricians and Gynaecologists of Canada. *Clinical practice guidelines* [multiple topics]. Available from: sogc.org/clinical-practice-guidelines/.

References

1. Gill SK, Einarson A. The safety of drugs for the treatment of nausea and vomiting of pregnancy. *Expert Opin Drug Safety* 2007;6:685-94.
2. CPS online. Ottawa: Canadian Pharmacists Association; 2014. *Diclectin* [product monograph]. Available from: www.e-therapeutics.ca. Accessed April 26, 2015. Subscription required.
3. CPS online. Ottawa: Canadian Pharmacists Association; 2015. *Drug use during pregnancy*. Available from: www.e-therapeutics.ca. Accessed May 2, 2015. Subscription required.
4. CPS online. Ottawa: Canadian Pharmacists Association; 2015. *Drug use during breastfeeding*. Available from: www.e-therapeutics.ca. Accessed May 2, 2015. Subscription required.
5. Koren G, Pastuszak A, Ito S. Drugs in pregnancy. In: Koren G, ed. *Maternal-fetal toxicology: a clinician's guide*. 3rd ed. New York: Marcel Dekker; 2001. p. 37-56.
6. Hale TW, Rowe HE. *Medications and mothers' milk: a manual of lactational pharmacology*. 16th ed. Plato: Hale Publishing; 2014.
7. Briggs GG, Freeman RK. *Drugs in pregnancy and lactation: a reference guide to fetal and neonatal risk*. 10th ed. Philadelphia: Wolters Kluwer; 2014.
8. Matsui D, Rieder MJ, Bologa M et al. Drugs and chemicals most commonly used by pregnant women. In: Koren G, ed. *Maternal-fetal toxicology: a clinician's guide*. 3rd ed. New York: Marcel Dekker; 2001. p. 37-56.
9. Geist R, Koren G. Maternal disorders leading to increased reproductive risks. In: Koren G, ed. *Maternal-fetal toxicology: a clinician's guide*. 3rd ed. New York: Marcel Dekker; 2001. p. 697-732.

10. Menezes EV, Yakoob MY, Soomro T et al. Reducing stillbirths: prevention and management of medical disorders and infections during pregnancy. *BMC Pregnancy Childbirth* 2009;9:S4.
11. Buhimschi CS, Weiner CP. Medications in pregnancy and lactation: part 1. Teratology. *Obstet Gynecol* 2009;113:166-88.
12. Wigle PR, McNeal SM, Tibbs K. Pregnancy and OTC cough, cold, and analgesic preparations. *US Pharm* 2006;31:33-47.
13. Dugoua JJ, Perri D, Seely D et al. Safety and efficacy of blue cohosh (Caulophyllum thalictroides) during pregnancy and lactation. *Can J Clin Pharmacol* 2008;15:e66-73.
14. Taddio A, Ito S. Drugs and breast-feeding. In: Koren G, ed. *Maternal-fetal toxicology: a clinician's guide*. 3rd ed. New York: Marcel Dekker; 2001. p. 177-232.
15. Health Canada. *Eating well with Canada's food guide*. Available from: www.hc-sc.gc.ca/fn-an/food-guide-aliment/index-eng.php. Accessed May 2, 2015.
16. Allain-Doiron A, Gruslin A, Innis SM et al. *Prenatal nutrition guidelines for health professionals: folate*. Ottawa: Health Canada; 2009. Available from: www.hc-sc.gc.ca/fn-an/nutrition/prenatal/index-eng.php. Accessed May 2, 2015.
17. Allain-Doiron A, Gruslin A, Innis SM et al. *Prenatal nutrition guidelines for health professionals: iron*. Ottawa: Health Canada; 2009. Available from: www.hc-sc.gc.ca/fn-an/nutrition/prenatal/index-eng.php. Accessed May 2, 2015.
18. Magee LA, Pels A, Helewa M et al. Diagnosis, evaluation, and management of the hypertensive disorders of pregnancy: executive summary. *J Obstet Gynaecol Can* 2014;36:416-41.
19. Hofmeyr GJ, Lawrie TA, Atallah AN et al. Calcium supplementation during pregnancy for preventing hypertensive disorders and related problems. *Cochrane Database Syst Rev* 2014;6:CD001059.
20. Thomas M, Weisman SM. Calcium supplementation during pregnancy and lactation: effects on the mother and the fetus. *Am J Obstet Gynecol* 2006;194:937-45.
21. Health Canada. Food and Nutrition. Dietary reference intakes. *Reference values for elements*. Ottawa: Health Canada. Available from: www.hc-sc.gc.ca/fn-an/nutrition/reference/table/ref_elements_tbl-eng.php. Accessed May 2, 2015.
22. Ross AC, Taylor CL, Yaktine AL et al. Institute of Medicine. *Dietary reference intakes for calcium and vitamin D*. Washington: The National Academies Press; 2011. Available from: books.nap.edu/openbook.php?record_id=13050. Accessed October 28, 2014.
23. Wilson RD; Genetics Committee, Wilson RD et al. Pre-conception folic acid and multivitamin supplementation for the primary and secondary prevention of neural tube defects and other folic acid-sensitive congenital anomalies. *J Obstet Gynaecol Can* 2015;37:534-52.
24. Delange F. Iodine requirements during pregnancy, lactation and the neonatal period and indicators of optimal iodine nutrition. *Public Health Nutr* 2007;10:1571-80.
25. Zimmermann MB. The effects of iodine deficiency in pregnancy and infancy. *Paediatr Perinat Epidemiol* 2012;26:108-17.
26. Dietitians of Canada. *Food sources of iodine*. February 28, 2014. Available from: www.dietitians.ca/Nutrition-Resources-A-Z/Factsheets/Minerals/Food-Sources-of-Iodine.aspx. Accessed March 9, 2016.
27. Council on Environmental Health, Rogan WJ, Paulson JA et al. Iodine deficiency, pollutant chemicals, and the thyroid: new information on an old problem. *Pediatrics* 2014;133:1163-6.
28. Pearce EN, Andersson M, Zimmermann MB. Global iodine nutrition: where do we stand in 2013? *Thyroid* 2013;23:523-8.
29. Stagnaro-Green A, Abalovich M, Alexander E et al. Guidelines of the American Thyroid Association for the diagnosis and management of thyroid disease during pregnancy and postpartum. *Thyroid* 2011;21:1081-125.
30. National Health and Medical Research Council (Australia). *Iodine supplementation for pregnant and breastfeeding women*. NHMRC Public Statement. January 2010. Available from: www.nhmrc.gov.au/guidelines/publications/new45. Accessed August 19, 2014.
31. Natural Medicines Comprehensive Database. Stockton: Therapeutic Research Faculty. *Kelp (Bladderwrack)*. Available from: naturaldatabase.therapeuticresearch.com. Accessed August 19, 2014. Subscription required.
32. Pena-Rosas JP, De-Regil LM, Garcia-Casal MN et al. Daily oral iron supplementation during pregnancy. *Cochrane Database Syst Rev* 2015;7:CD004736.
33. Gill SK, Maltepe C, Koren G. The effectiveness of discontinuing iron-containing prenatal multivitamins on reducing the severity of nausea and vomiting of pregnancy. *J Obstet Gynaecol* 2009;29:13-6.
34. Pena-Rosas JP, De-Regil LM, Dowswell T et al. Intermittent oral iron supplementation during pregnancy. *Cochrane Database Syst Rev* 2012;7:CD0099997.
35. Einarson TR, Piwko C, Koren G. Quantifying the global rates of nausea and vomiting of pregnancy: a meta analysis. *J Popul Ther Clin Pharmacol* 2013;20:e171-83.
36. Matthews A, Haas DM, O'Mathuna DP et al. Interventions for nausea and vomiting in early pregnancy. *Cochrane Database Syst Rev* 2014;3:CD007575.
37. Einarson A, Maltepe C, Boskovic R et al. Treatment of nausea and vomiting in pregnancy: an updated algorithm. *Can Fam Physician* 2007;53:2109-11.
38. Boskovic R, Einarson A, Maltepe C et al. Diclectin therapy for nausea and vomiting of pregnancy: effects of optimal dosing. *J Obstet Gynaecol Can* 2003;25:830-3.
39. ACOG (American College of Obstetrics and Gynecology) Practice Bulletin: nausea and vomiting of pregnancy. *Obstet Gynecol* 2004;103:803-14.
40. Agrawal JR, Friedman S. Gastrointestinal & biliary complications of pregnancy. In: Greenberger NJ, Blumberg RS, Burakoff R, eds. *Current diagnosis & treatment: Gastroenterology, hepatology & endoscopy*. New York: McGraw-Hill; 2009.
41. Maltepe C. Surviving morning sickness successfully: from patient's perception to rational management. *J Popul Clin Pharmacol* 2014;21:e555-64.
42. Badell ML, Ramin SM, Smith JA. Treatment options for nausea and vomiting during pregnancy. *Pharmacotherapy* 2006;26:1273-87.
43. Ebrahimi N, Maltepe C, Bournissen FG et al. Nausea and vomiting of pregnancy: using the 24-hour Pregnancy-Unique Quantification of Emesis (PUQE-24) scale. *J Obstet Gynaecol Can* 2009;31:803-7.
44. Jamigorn M, Phupong V. Acupressure and vitamin B6 to relieve nausea and vomiting in pregnancy: a randomized study. *Arch Gynecol Obstet* 2007;276:245-9.
45. Arsenault MY, Lane CA, MacKinnon CJ et al. The management of nausea and vomiting of pregnancy. *J Obstet Gynaecol Can* 2002;24:817-31.
46. UpToDate. *Drug monograph: dimenhydrinate* Available from: www.uptodate.com. Accessed May 2, 2015. Subscription required.
47. Dimenhydrinate monograph. In: Briggs GG, Freeman RK. *Drugs in pregnancy and lactation: a reference guide to fetal and neonatal risk*. 10th ed. Philadelphia: Wolters Kluwer; 2014. p. 411-2.

48. Madjunkova S, Maltepe C, Koren G. The delayed-release combination of doxylamine and pyridoxine (Diclegis®/Diclectin®) for the treatment of nausea and vomiting of pregnancy. *Paediatr Drugs* 2014;16:199-211.
49. Borrelli F, Capasso R, Aviello G et al. Effectiveness and safety of ginger in the treatment of pregnancy-induced nausea and vomiting. *Obstet Gynecol* 2005;105:849-56.
50. Pongrojpaw D, Somprasit C, Chanthasenanont A. A randomized comparison of ginger and dimenhydrinate in the treatment of nausea and vomiting in pregnancy. *J Med Assoc Thai* 2007;90:1703-9.
51. Ensiyeh J, Sakineh MA. Comparing ginger and vitamin B6 for the treatment of nausea and vomiting in pregnancy: a randomised controlled trial. *Midwifery* 2009;25:649-53.
52. Viljoen E, Visser J, Koen N et al. A systematic review and meta-analysis of the effect and safety of ginger in the treatment of pregnancy-associated nausea and vomiting. *Nutr J* 2014;13:20.
53. Shrim A, Boskovic R, Maltepe C et al. Pregnancy outcome following use of large doses of vitamin B6 in the first trimester. *J Obstet Gynaecol* 2006;26:749-51.
54. Pyridoxine monograph. In: Briggs GG, Freeman RK. *Drugs in pregnancy and lactation: a reference guide to fetal and neonatal risk.* 10th ed. Philadelphia: Wolters Kluwer; 2014. p. 1174-8.
55. Natural Medicines Comprehensive Database. Stockton: Therapeutic Research Faculty. *Monograph: pyridoxine.* Available from: naturaldatabase.therapeuticresearch.com. Accessed May 2, 2015. Subscription required.
56. Vutyavanich T, Wongtra-ngan S, Ruangsri R. Pyridoxine for nausea and vomiting of pregnancy: a randomized, double-blind, place-controlled trial. *Am J Obstet Gynecol* 1995;173:881-4.
57. Sahakian V, Rouse D, Sipes S et al. Vitamin B6 is effective therapy for nausea and vomiting of pregnancy: a randomized, doubled-blind placebo-controlled study. *Obstet Gynecol* 1991;78:33-6.
58. Nulman I, Koren G. Diclectin for morning sickness: long-term neurodevelopment. *Can Fam Physician* 2011;57:193-4.
59. Atanackovic G, Navioz Y, Moretti ME et al. The safety of higher than standard dose of doxylamine-pyridoxine (Diclectin) for nausea and vomiting of pregnancy. *J Clin Pharmacol* 2001;41:842-5.
60. Niebyl JR, Briggs GG. The pharmacologic management of nausea and vomiting of pregnancy. *J Fam Pract* 2014;63:S31-7.
61. Chittumma P, Kaewkiattikun K, Wiriyasiriwach B. Comparison of the effectiveness of ginger and vitamin B6 for treatment of nausea and vomiting in early pregnancy: a randomized double-blind controlled trial. *J Med Assoc Thai* 2007;90:15-20.
62. Schwertner HA, Rios DC, Pascoe JE. Variation in concentration and labeling of ginger root dietary supplements. *Obstet Gynecol* 2006;107:1337-43.
63. Ginger monograph. In: Briggs GG, Freeman RK. *Drugs in pregnancy and lactation: a reference guide to fetal and neonatal risk.* 10th ed. Philadelphia: Wolters Kluwer; 2014. p. 623.
64. Natural Medicines Comprehensive Database. Stockton: Therapeutic Research Faculty. *Monograph: ginger.* Available from: naturaldatabase.therapeuticresearch.com. Accessed April 26, 2015. Subscription required.
65. Chandra K, Einarson A, Koren G. Taking ginger for nausea and vomiting during pregnancy. *Can Fam Physician* 2002;48:1441-2.
66. Scadding GK, Durham SR, Mirakian R et al. BSACI guidelines for the management of allergic and non-allergic rhinitis. *Clin Exp Allergy* 2008;38:19-42.
67. Incaudo GA, Takach P. The diagnosis and treatment of allergic rhinitis during pregnancy and lactation. *Immunol Allergy Clin North Am* 2006;26:137-54.
68. Blaiss MS. Management of rhinitis and asthma in pregnancy. *Ann Allergy Asthma Immunol* 2003;90:16-22.
69. Bousquet J, Khaltaev N, Cruz AA et al. Allergic Rhinitis and its Impact on Asthma (ARIA) 2008 update (in collaboration with the World Health Organization, GA(2)LEN and AllerGen). *Allergy* 2008;63:8-160.
70. Namazy JA, Schatz M. Diagnosing rhinitis during pregnancy. *Curr Allergy Asthma Rep* 2014;14:458.
71. Antihistamines (systemic) monograph. In: *USP DI. Drug information for the health care professional.* 27th ed. Montvale: Micromedex Thomson Healthcare; 2007. p. 333-50.
72. Drugs and Lactation Database (LactMed). Bethesda: U.S. National Library of Medicine; 2009. Available from: toxnet.nlm.nih.gov/cgi-bin/sis/htmlgen?LACT. Accessed May 2, 2015.
73. Brompheniramine monograph. In: Briggs GG, Freeman RK. *Drugs in pregnancy and lactation: a reference guide to fetal and neonatal risk.* 9th ed. Philadelphia: Wolters Kluwer; 2015. p. 161-2.
74. Seto A, Einarson T, Koren G. Evaluation of brompheniramine safety in pregnancy. *Reprod Toxicol* 1993;7:393-5.
75. Erebara A, Bozzo P, Einarson A et al. Treating the common cold during pregnancy. *Can Fam Physician* 2008;54:687-9.
76. So M, Bozzo P, Inoue M et al. Safety of antihistamines during pregnancy and lactation. *Can Fam Physician* 2010;56:427-9.
77. Chlorpheniramine monograph. In: Briggs GG, Freeman RK. *Drugs in pregnancy and lactation: a reference guide to fetal and neonatal risk.* 10th ed. Philadelphia: Wolters Kluwer; 2011. p. 252-9.
78. Diphenhydramine monograph. In: Briggs GG, Freeman RK. *Drugs in pregnancy and lactation: a reference guide to fetal and neonatal risk.* 10th ed. Philadelphia: Wolters Kluwer; 2014. p. 414-6.
79. Cetirizine monograph. In: Briggs GG, Freeman RK. *Drugs in pregnancy and lactation: a reference guide to fetal and neonatal risk.* 10th ed. Philadelphia: Wolters Kluwer; 2014. p. 238-9.
80. Gilbert C, Mazzotta P, Loebstein R et al. Fetal safety of drugs used in the treatment of allergic rhinitis: a critical review. *Drug Saf* 2005;28:707-19.
81. Powell RJ, Du Toit GL, Siddique N et al. BSACI guidelines for the management of chronic urticaria and angio-oedema. *Clin Exp Allergy* 2007;37:631-50.
82. Desloratadine monograph. In: Briggs GG, Freeman RK. *Drugs in pregnancy and lactation: a reference guide to fetal and neonatal risk.* 10th ed. Philadelphia: Wolters Kluwer; 2014. p. 374-5.
83. Fexofenadine monograph. In: Briggs GG, Freeman RK. *Drugs in pregnancy and lactation: a reference guide to fetal and neonatal risk.* 10th ed. Philadelphia: Wolters Kluwer; 2014. p. 543-4.
84. Craig-McFeely PM, Acharya NV, Shakir SA. Evaluation of the safety of fexofenadine from experience gained in general practice use in England in 1997. *Eur J Clin Pharmacol* 2001;57:313-20.
85. Loratadine monograph. In: Briggs GG, Freeman RK. *Drugs in pregnancy and lactation: a reference guide to fetal and neonatal risk.* 10th ed. Philadelphia: Wolters Kluwer; 2014. p. 818-9.
86. CPS online. Ottawa: Canadian Pharmacists Association; 2014. *Claritin* [product monograph]. Available from: www.e-therapeutics.ca. Accessed May 4, 2015. Subscription required.

87. AHFS Drug Information. Bethesda: American Society of Health-System Pharmacists; 2009. *Codeine (antitussives)* [product monograph]. Available from: online.statref.com. Accessed November 19, 2009. Subscription required.
88. Codeine monograph. In: Briggs GG, Freeman RK. *Drugs in pregnancy and lactation: a reference guide to fetal and neonatal risk.* 10th ed. Philadelphia: Wolters Kluwer; 2014. p. 329–31.
89. Motherisk. Toronto: The Hospital for Sick Children; 1999-2009. *Motherisk News: Motherisk advisory for codeine use during breastfeeding.* Available from: www.motherisk.org. Accessed May 11, 2015.
90. Madadi P, Koren G, Cairns J et al. Safety of codeine during breastfeeding: fatal morphine poisoning in the breastfed neonate of a mother prescribed codeine. *Can Fam Physician* 2007;53:33-5.
91. Babb M, Koren G, Einarson A. Treating pain during pregnancy. *Can Fam Physician* 2010;56:25,27.
92. Dextromethorphan (systemic) monograph. In: *USP DI. Drug information for the health care professional.* 27th ed. Montvale: Micromedex Thomson Healthcare; 2007. p. 1057-60.
93. Dextromethorphan monograph. In: Briggs GG, Freeman RK. *Drugs in pregnancy and lactation: a reference guide to fetal and neonatal risk.* 10th ed. Philadelphia: Wolters Kluwer; 2014. p. 385-6.
94. CPS online. Ottawa: Canadian Pharmacists Association; 2014. *Corticosteroids: Eye, Ear, Nose* [CPhA monograph]. Available from: www.e-therapeutics.ca. Accessed May 2, 2015. Subscription required.
95. Mometasone monograph. In: Hale TW, Rowe HE. *Medications and mothers' milk: a manual of lactational pharmacology.* 16th ed. Plato: Hale Publishing; 2014.
96. Budesonide monograph. In: Briggs GG, Freeman RK. *Drugs in pregnancy and lactation: a reference guide to fetal and neonatal risk.* 10th ed. Philadelphia: Wolters Kluwer; 2014. p. 162-4.
97. Mometasone monograph. In: Briggs GG, Freeman RK. *Drugs in pregnancy and lactation: a reference guide to fetal and neonatal risk.* 10th ed. Philadelphia: Wolters Kluwer; 2014. p. 936-7.
98. Triamcinolone monograph. In: Hale TW, Rowe HE. *Medications and mothers' milk: a manual of lactational pharmacology.* 16th ed. Plato: Hale Publishing; 2014.
99. Triamcinolone monograph. In: Briggs GG, Freeman RK. *Drugs in pregnancy and lactation: a reference guide to fetal and neonatal risk.* 10th ed. Philadelphia: Wolters Kluwer; 2014. p. 1399-400.
100. AHFS Drug Information. Bethesda: American Society of Health-System Pharmacists; 2009. *Phenylephrine hypochloride* [product monograph]. Available from: online.statref.com. Accessed November 19, 2009. Subscription required.
101. Rothman KJ, Fyler DC, Goldblatt A et al. Exogenous hormones and other drug exposures of children with congenital heart disease. *Am J Epidemiol* 1979;109:433-9.
102. Yau WP, Mitchell AA, Lin KJ et al. Use of decongestants during pregnancy and the risk of birth defects. *Am J Epidemiol* 2013;178:198-208.
103. Phenylephrine monograph. In: Briggs GG, Freeman RK. *Drugs in pregnancy and lactation: a reference guide to fetal and neonatal risk.* 10th ed. Philadelphia: Wolters Kluwer; 2014. p. 1110.
104. Pseudoephedrine (systemic) monograph. In: *USP DI. Drug information for the health care professional.* 27th ed. Montvale: Micromedex Thomson Healthcare; 2007. p. 2451-5.
105. Pseudoephedrine monograph. In: Briggs GG, Freeman RK. *Drugs in pregnancy and lactation: a reference guide to fetal and neonatal risk.* 10th ed. Philadelphia: Wolters Kluwer; 2014. p. 1168-70.
106. Werler MM, Mitchell AA, Shapiro S. First trimester maternal medication use in relation to gastroschisis. *Teratology* 1992;45:361-7.
107. Oxymetazoline monograph. In: Briggs GG, Freeman RK. *Drugs in pregnancy and lactation: a reference guide to fetal and neonatal risk.* 10th ed. Philadelphia: Wolters Kluwer; 2014. p. 1041-2.
108. Rayburn WF, Anderson JC, Smith CV et al. Uterine and fetal Doppler flow changes from a single dose of a long-acting intranasal decongestant. *Obstet Gynecol* 1990;76:180-2.
109. Baxi LV, Gindoff PR, Pregenzer GJ et al. Fetal heart rate changes following maternal administration of a nasal decongestant. *Am J Obstet Gynecol* 1985;153:799-800.
110. Pendopharm. *Rhinaris* [product monograph]. Available from: pendopharm.com/products/key-products/rhinaris/.
111. Cromolyn sodium monograph. In: Briggs GG, Freeman RK. *Drugs in pregnancy and lactation: a reference guide to fetal and neonatal risk.* 10th ed. Philadelphia: Wolters Kluwer; 2014. p. 332-3.
112. Demoly P, Piette V, Daures JP. Treatment of allergic rhinitis during pregnancy. *Drugs* 2003;63:1813-20.
113. Moretti ME, Caprara D, Coutinho CJ et al. Fetal safety of loratadine use in the first trimester of pregnancy: a multicenter study. *J Allergy Clin Immunol* 2003;111:479-83.
114. Diav-Citrin O, Shechtman S, Aharonovich A et al. Pregnancy outcome after gestational exposure to loratadine or antihistamines: a prospective controlled cohort study. *J Allergy Clin Immunol* 2003;111:1239-43.
115. Kallen B, Olausson PO. No increased risk of infant hypospadias after maternal use of loratadine in early pregnancy. *Int J Med Sci* 2006;3:106-7.
116. Schwarz EB, Moretti ME, Nayak S et al. Risk of hypospadias in offspring of women using loratadine during pregnancy: a systematic review and meta-analysis. *Drug Saf* 2008;31:775-88.
117. Ito S, Blajchman A, Stephenson M et al. Prospective follow-up of adverse reactions in breast-fed infants exposed to maternal medication. *Am J Obstet Gynecol* 1993;168:1393-9.
118. Findlay JW, Butz RF, Sailstad JM et al. Pseudoephedrine and triprolidine in plasma and breast milk of nursing mothers. *Br J Clin Pharmacol* 1984;18:901-6.
119. Lucas BD, Purdy CY, Scarim SK et al. Terfenadine pharmacokinetics in breast milk in lactating women. *Clin Pharmacol Ther* 1995;57:398-402.
120. Hilbert J, Radwanski E, Affrime MB et al. Excretion of loratadine in human breast milk. *J Clin Pharmacol* 1988;28:234-9.
121. Heinonen OP, Slone D, Shapiro S. *Birth defects and drugs in pregnancy.* Littleton: Publishing Sciences Group; 1977.
122. Zierler S, Rothman KJ. Congenital heart disease in relation to maternal use of Bendectin and other drugs in early pregnancy. *N Engl J Med* 1985;313:347-52.
123. Cottle MK, Van Petten GR, van Muyden P. Effects of phenylephrine and sodium salicylate on maternal and fetal cardiovascular indices and blood oxygenation in sheep. *Am J Obstet Gynecol* 1982;143:170-6.
124. Aselton P, Jick H, Milunsky A et al. First-trimester drug use and congenital disorders. *Obstet Gynecol* 1985;65:451-5.
125. Jick H, Holmes LB, Hunter JR et al. First-trimester drug use and congenital disorders. *JAMA* 1981;246:343-6.

126. Ellegard EK, Hellgren M, Karlsson NG. Fluticasone propionate aqueous nasal spray in pregnancy rhinitis. *Clin Otolaryngol Allied Sci* 2001;26:394-400.
127. Yawn B, Knudtson M. Treating asthma and comorbid allergic rhinitis in pregnancy. *J Am Board Fam Med* 2007;20:289-98.
128. Gregersen TL, Ulrik CS. Safety of bronchodilators and corticosteroids for asthma during pregnancy: what we know and what we need to do better. *J Asthma Allergy* 2013;15:117-25.
129. Lalonde A, Schuurmans N, Senikas V. *Healthy beginnings: giving your baby the best start, from preconception to birth*. 4th ed. Mississauga: John Wiley & Sons Canada; 2009.
130. Liddle SD, Pennick V. Interventions for preventing and treating low-back and pelvic pain during pregnancy. *Cochrane Database Syst Rev* 2015;9:CD001139.
131. Ostensen ME, Skomsvoll JF. Anti-inflammatory pharmacotherapy during pregnancy. *Expert Opin Pharmacother* 2004;5:571-80.
132. Kozer E, Nikfar S, Costei A et al. Aspirin consumption during the first trimester of pregnancy and congenital anomalies: a meta-analysis. *Am J Obstet Gynecol* 2002;187:1623-30.
133. Cleves MA, Savell VH, Raj S et al. Maternal use of acetaminophen and nonsteroidal anti-inflammatory drugs (NSAIDs), and muscular ventricular septal defects. *Birth Defects Res A Clin Mol Teratol* 2004;70:107-13.
134. Ofori B, Oraichi D, Blais L et al. Risk of congenital anomalies in pregnant users of non-steroidal anti-inflammatory drugs: a nested case-control study. *Birth Defects Res B Dev Reprod Toxicol* 2006;77:268-79.
135. Upper respiratory infection. In: *ACP Pier* and *AHFS DI Essentials*. Available from: online.statref.com. Accessed November 21, 2009. Subscription required.
136. Keller J, Frederking D, Layer P. The spectrum and treatment of gastrointestinal disorders during pregnancy. *Nat Clin Pract Gastroenterol Hepatol* 2008;5:430-43.
137. Wigle P, Kim K, King A et al. OTC medications for GI disorders in pregnancy. *US Pharm* 2006;31:50-71.
138. Health Canada. Food and Nutrition. Dietary reference intakes. *Reference values for macronutrients*. Ottawa: Health Canada. Available from: www.hc-sc.gc.ca/fn-an/nutrition/reference/table/ref_macronutr_tbl-eng.php. Accessed May 5, 2015.
139. Canadian Agency for Drugs and Technologies in Health. Rapid Response Report: Summary with Critical Appraisal. *Dioctyl sulfosuccinate or docusate (calcium or sodium) for the prevention or management of constipation: a review of the clinical effectiveness*. June 26, 2014. Available from: www.cadth.ca/media/pdf/htis/jul-2014/RC0561%20Stool%20Softeners%20Final.pdf. Accessed October 27, 2014.
140. Gill SK, Maltepe C, Koren G. The effectiveness of discontinuing iron-containing prenatal multivitamins on reducing the severity of nausea and vomiting of pregnancy. *J Obstet Gynaecol* 2009;29:13-6.
141. Alonso-Coello P, Guyatt G, Heels-Ansdell D et al. Laxatives for the treatment of hemorrhoids. *Cochrane Database Syst Rev* 2005;(4):CD004649.
142. Staroselsky A, Nava-Ocampo AA, Vohra S et al. Hemorrhoids in pregnancy. *Can Fam Physician* 2008;52:189-90.
143. Mahadevan U, Kane S. American Gastroenterological Association Institute medical position statement on the use of gastrointestinal medications in pregnancy. *Gastroenterology* 2006;131:278-82.
144. Trottier M, Erebara A, Bozzo P. Treating constipation during pregnancy. *Can Fam Physician* 2012;58:836-8.
145. Sheth VM, Pandya AG. Melasma: a comprehensive update part I. *J Am Acad Dermatol* 2011;65:689-97.
146. Sheth VM, Pandya AG. Melasma: a comprehensive update part II. *J Am Acad Dermatol* 2011;65:699-714.
147. Bozzo P, Chua-Gocheco A, Einarson A. Safety of skin care products during pregnancy. *Can Fam Physician* 2011;57:665-7.
148. Hydroquinone monograph. In: Briggs GG, Freeman RK. *Drugs in pregnancy and lactation: a reference guide to fetal and neonatal risk*. 10th ed. Philadelphia: Wolters Kluwer; 2014. p. 668-9.
149. Skin disease in pregnancy and puerperium. In: Gabbe SG. *Obstetrics: normal and problem pregnancies*. 6th ed. Philadelphia: Elsevier/Saunders; 2012.
150. Light-related diseases and disorders of pigmentation. In: Habif TP. *Clinical dermatology: a color guide to diagnosis and therapy*. 5th ed. Edinburgh: Mosby; 2010.
151. Ali RA, Egan LJ. Gastroesophageal reflux disease in pregnancy. *Best Pract Res Clin Gastroenterol* 2007;21:793-806.
152. Matok I, Gorodischer R, Koren G et al. The safety of H(2)-blockers use during pregnancy. *J Clin Pharmacol* 2010;50:81-7.
153. Ali RA, Egan LJ. Gastroesophageal reflux disease in pregnancy. *Best Pract Res Clin Gastroenterol* 2007;21:793-806.
154. Matok I, Levy A, Wiznitzer et al. The safety of fetal exposure to proton-pump inhibitors during pregnancy. *Dig Dis Sci* 2012;57:699-705.
155. Majithia R, Johnson DA. Are proton pump inhibitors safe during pregnancy and lactation? Evidence to date. *Drugs* 2012;72:171-9.
156. Law R, Maltepe C, Bozzo P et al. Treatment of heartburn and acid reflux associated with nausea and vomiting during pregnancy. *Can Fam Physician* 2010;56:143-4.
157. Part 3: Vaccination of specific populations: Immunization in pregnancy and breastfeeding. In: Public Health Agency of Canada. *Canadian immunization guide*. Evergreen ed. Available from: www.phac-aspc.gc.ca/publicat/cig-gci/p03-04-eng.php. Accessed August 17, 2014.
158. Part 4: Active vaccines: Hepatitis A vaccine. In: Public Health Agency of Canada. *Canadian immunization guide*. Evergreen ed. Available from: www.phac-aspc.gc.ca/publicat/cig-gci/p04-hepa-eng.php. Accessed October 20, 2014.
159. Part 4: Active vaccines: Hepatitis B vaccine. In: Public Health Agency of Canada. *Canadian immunization guide*. Evergreen ed. Available from: www.phac-aspc.gc.ca/publicat/cig-gci/p04-hepbeng.php. Accessed October 20, 2014.
160. Public Health Agency of Canada. An Advisory Committee Statement (ACS). National Advisory Committee on Immunization (NACI). *Statement on seasonal influenza vaccine for 2014-2015*. July 2014. Available from: www.phac-aspc.gc.ca/naci-ccni/flu-grippe-eng.php. Accessed August 17, 2014.
161. Part 4: Active vaccines: Meningococcal vaccine. In: Public Health Agency of Canada. *Canadian immunization guide*. Evergreen ed. Available from: www.phacaspc.gc.ca/publicat/cig-gci/p04-meni-eng.php. Accessed October 20, 2014.
162. Public Health Agency of Canada. An Advisory Committee Statement (ACS). National Advisory Committee on Immunization (NACI). *Update on pertussis vaccination in pregnancy*. February 2014. Available from: www.phac-aspc.gc.ca/naci-ccni/acs-dcc/2014/pvip-vcpg_0214-eng.php. Accessed August 17, 2014.
163. Part 4: Active vaccines: Pneumococcal vaccine. In: Public Health Agency of Canada. *Canadian immunization guide*. Evergreen ed. Available from: www.phac-aspc.gc.ca/publicat/cig-gci/p04-pneu-eng.php. Accessed August 17, 2014.
164. Part 4: Active vaccines: Tetanus toxoid. In: Public Health Agency of Canada. *Canadian immunization guide*. Evergreen ed. Available from: www.phac-aspc.gc.ca/publicat/cig-gci/p04-tet-eng.php. Accessed October 20, 2014.
165. Carson G, Cox LV, Crane J et al. Alcohol use and pregnancy consensus clinical guidelines. *J Obstet Gynaecol Can* 2010;32:S1-31.

166. Public Health Agency of Canada. The Healthy Pregnancy Guide: Alcohol and Pregnancy. Available at: http://www.phac-aspc.gc.ca/hp-gs/guide/03_ap-ag-eng.php. Accessed April 20, 2016.
167. Morgan S, Koren G, Bozzo P. Is caffeine consumption safe during pregnancy? *Can Fam Physician* 2013;59:361-2.
168. Hoyt AT, Browne M, Richardson S et al. Maternal caffeine consumption and small for gestational age births: results from a population-based case-control study. *Matern Child Health J* 2014;18:1540-51.
169. Public Health Agency of Canada. *Healthy pregnancy: Caffeine and pregnancy.* Available from: www.phac-aspc.gc.ca/hp-gs/know-savoir/caffeine-eng.php.
170. Organization of Teratology Information Specialists. MotherToBaby. Fact Sheet. *Cigarette smoking and pregnancy.* June 2014. Available from: mothertobaby.org/fact-sheets/cigarette-smoking-pregnancy/pdf/. Accessed March 9, 2016.
171. Specific populations: Pregnant and breastfeeding women. 2011. In: CAN-ADAPTT. *Canadian smoking cessation guideline.* Available from: www.nicotinedependenceclinic.com/English/CANADAPTT/Guideline/Pregnant%20and%20Breastfeeding%20Women/Home.aspx. Accessed April 20, 2016.
172. Cressman AM, Pupco A, Kim E et al. Smoking cessation therapy during pregnancy. *Can Fam Physician* 2012;58:525-7.
173. Bozzo P, Chua-Gocheco A, Einarson A. Safety of hair products during pregnancy. *Can Fam Physician* 2011;57:665-7.
174. Organization of Teratology Information Specialists. MotherToBaby. Fact Sheet. *Hair treatments and pregnancy.* May 2014. Available from: mothertobaby.org/fact-sheets/hair-treatments-pregnancy/pdf/. Accessed August 20, 2014.
175. Chou D, Abalos E, Gyte GM et al. Drugs for perineal pain in the early postpartum period: generic protocol. *Cochrane Database Syst Rev* 2009;(3):CD007734.
176. Macarthur AJ, Macarthur C. Incidence, severity, and determinants of perineal pain after vaginal delivery: a prospective cohort study. *Am J Obstet Gynecol* 2004;191:1199-204.
177. Carroli G, Mignini L. Episiotomy for vaginal birth. *Cochrane Database Syst Rev* 2009;(1):CD000081.
178. East CE, Begg L, Henshall NE et al. Local cooling for relieving pain from perineal trauma sustained during childbirth. *Cochrane Database Syst Rev* 2012;5:CD006304.
179. Hedayati H, Parsons J, Crowther CA. Rectal analgesia for pain from perineal trauma following childbirth. *Cochrane Database Syst Rev* 2003;(3):CD003931.
180. Moore W, James DK. A random trial of three topical analgesic agents in the treatment of episiotomy pain following instrumental vaginal delivery. *J Obstet Gynaecol* 1989;10:35-9.
181. Petersen MR. Review of interventions to relieve postpartum pain from perineal trauma. *MCN Am J Matern Child Nurs* 2011;36:241-5.
182. CPS online. Ottawa: Canadian Pharmacists Association; 2012. *Acetaminophen* [CPhA monograph]. Available from: www.e-therapeutics.ca. Accessed April 20, 2016. Subscription required.
183. Lopes RD, Horowitz JD, Garcia DA et al. Warfarin and acetaminophen interaction: a summary of the evidence and biologic plausibility. *Blood* 2011;118:6269-73.
184. CPS online. Ottawa: Canadian Pharmacists Association; 2009. *Advil* [product monograph]. Available from: www.e-therapeutics.ca. Accessed April 20, 2016. Subscription required.
185. Spigset O, Hagg S. Analgesics and breast-feeding: safety considerations. *Paediatr Drugs* 2000;2:223-38.
186. Natural Medicines Comprehensive Database. Stockton: Therapeutic Research Faculty. *Monograph: witch hazel.* Available from: naturaldatabase.therapeuticresearch.com. Accessed May 5, 2015. Subscription required.
187. Hedayati H, Parsons J, Crowther CA. Topically applied anaesthetics for treating perineal pain after childbirth. *Cochrane Database Syst Rev* 2005;(2):CD004223.
188. Canadian Agency for Drugs and Technologies in Health. Rapid Response Report. *Peri-partum pain management: safety and guidelines.* Ottawa: CADTH; 2011. Available from: https://www.cadth.ca/media/pdf/htis/sept-2011/RB0406_Peri-partum_Pain_Management_final.pdf Accessed April 20, 2016.
189. Chou D, Abalos E, Gyte GM et al. Paracetamol/acetaminophen (single administration) for perineal pain in the earlypostpartum period. *Cochrane Database Syst Rev* 2010;(3):CD008407.
190. Nauta M, Landsmeer ML, Koren G. Codeine-acetaminophen versus nonsteroidal anti-inflammatory drugs in the treatment of post-abdominal surgery pain: a systematic review of randomized trials. *Am J Surg* 2009;198:256-61.
191. Koren G, Cairns J, Chitayat D et al. Pharmacogenetics of morphine poisoning in a breastfed neonate of a codeine-prescribed mother. *Lancet* 2006;368:704.
192. Madadi P, Moretti M, Djokanovic N et al. Guidelines for maternal codeine use during breastfeeding. *Can Fam Physician* 2009;55:1077-8.
193. Pearlstein T, Howard M, Salisbury A et al. Postpartum depression. *Am J Obstet Gynecol* 2009;200:357-64.
194. Goeser AL. Postpartum depression. *US Pharm* 2008;33:16-20.
195. Shaw E, Kaczorowski J. Postpartum care–what's new? *Curr Opin Obstet Gynecol* 2007;19:561-7.
196. American Psychiatric Association. *Diagnostic and statistical manual of mental disorders: DSM-IV-TR* . 4th ed. Washington: APA; 2000.
197. Natural Medicines Comprehensive Database. Stockton: Therapeutic Research Faculty. *Monograph: St. John's wort.* Available from: naturaldatabase.therapeuticresearch.com. Accessed May 5, 2015. Subscription required.
198. St. John's wort monograph. In: Briggs GG, Freeman RK. *Drugs in pregnancy and lactation: a reference guide to fetal and neonatal risk.* 10th ed. Philadelphia: Wolters Kluwer; 2014. p. 1282-4.
199. Freeman MP. Complementary and alternative medicine for perinatal depression. *J Affect Disord* 2009;112:1-10.
200. Natural Medicines Comprehensive Database. Stockton: Therapeutic Research Faculty. *Monograph: S-adenosyl-methionine (SAMe).* Available from: naturaldatabase.therapeuticresearch.com. Accessed May 5, 2015. Subscription required.
201. Speroff L, Mishell DR. The postpartum visit: it's time for a change in order to optimally initiate contraception. *Contraception* 2008;78:90-8.
202. Kennedy KI, Trussel J. Postpartum contraception and lactation. In: Hatcher RA, Trussell J, Nelson AL et al., eds. *Contraceptive technology.* 19th rev. ed. New York: Ardent Media; 2007.
203. King J. Contraception and lactation. *J Midwifery Womens Health* 2007;52:614-20.
204. Valdes V, Labbok MH, Pugin E et al. The efficacy of the lactational amenorrhea method (LAM) among working women. *Contraception* 2000;62:217-9.
205. Kuyoh MA, Toroitich-Ruto C, Grimes DA et al. Sponge versus diaphragm for contraception: a Cochrane review. *Contraception* 2003;67:15-8.
206. Berens P, Labbok M; Academy of Breastfeeding Medicine. ABM Clinical Protocol #13: Contraception during breastfeeding, revised 2015. *Breastfeed Med* 2015;10:3-12.

207. World Health Organization (WHO). Medical eligibility criteria for contraceptive use. Fifth edition 2015. Available at: http://www.ncbi.nlm.nih.gov/pubmed/26447268

208. Black A, Guilbert E, Costescu D et al. Canadian contraception consensus (part 3 of 4): Chapter 7–Intrauterine contraception. Available at: http://www.ncbi.nlm.nih.gov/pubmed/27032746

209. Heinemann K, Reed S, Moehner S et al. Risk of uterine perforation with levonorgestrel-releasing and copper intrauterine devices in the European Active Surveillance Study on Intrauterine Devices. *Contraception* 2015;91:274-9.

210. Centers for Disease Control and Prevention (CDC). Update to CDC's U.S. medical eligibility criteria for contraceptive use, 2010: revised recommendations for the use of contraceptive methods during the postpartum period. *MMWR Morb Mortal Wkly Rep* 2011;60:878-83.

211. Jackson E, Curtis KM, Gaffield ME. Risk of venous thromboembolism during the postpartum period: a systematic review. *Obstet Gynecol* 2011;117:691-703.

212. Kapp N, Curtis KM. Combined oral contraceptive use among breastfeeding women: a systematic review. *Contraception* 2010;82:10-6.

213. Centers for Disease Control and Prevention (CDC). U.S. medical eligibility criteria for contraceptive use, 2010. *MMWR Morb Mortal Wkly Rep* 2010;59(RR-4):1-86.

214. Kapp N, Curtis K, Nanda K. Progestogen-only contraceptive use among breastfeeding women: a systematic review. *Contraception* 2010;82:17-37.

215. American College of Obstetricians and Gynecologists. ACOG Practice Bulletin No. 121: Long-acting reversible contraception: implants and intrauterine devices. *Obstet Gynecol* 2011;118:184-96.

216. American College of Obstetrics and Gynecology. Special report from ACOG. Breastfeeding: maternal and infant aspects. *ACOG Clinical Review* 2007;12:1S-16S.

217. Marshall JK, Thompson AB, Armstrong D. Omeprazole for refractory gastroesophageal reflux disease during pregnancy and lactation. *Can J Gastroenterol* 1998;12:225-7.

218. Masters KP, Trompeter J. Breast-feeding and OTC medications. *US Pharm* 2007;32:8-12.

219. Ferreira E, Martin B, Morin C. *Grossesse et allaitement: guide thérapeutique*. 2nd ed. Montréal: CHU Sainte-Justine; 2013.

220. Majithia R, Johnson DA. Are proton pump inhibitors safe during pregnancy and lactation? Evidence to date. *Drugs* 2012;72:171-9.

221. Moore DB, Catlin A. Lactation suppression: forgotten aspect of care for the mother of a dying child. *Pediatr Nurs* 2003;29:383-4.

222. Spitz AM, Lee NC, Peterson HB. Treatment for lactation suppression: little progress in one hundred years. *Am J Obstet Gynecol* 1998;179:1485-90.

223. Swift K, Janke J. Breast binding... is it all that it's wrapped up to be? *J Obstet Gynecol Neonatal Nurs* 2003;32:332-9.

224. Oladapo OT, Fawole B. Treatments for suppression of lactation. *Cochrane Database Syst Rev* 2012;9:CD005937.

225. CPS online. Ottawa: Canadian Pharmacists Association; 2013. *Bromocriptine* [CPhA monograph]. Available from: www.e-therapeutics.ca. Accessed april 20, 2016. Subscription required.

Drugs and Pregnancy or Breastfeeding—What You Need to Know

Women who are pregnant or breastfeeding must be very careful about taking any kind of medicine. Some nonprescription drugs and natural health products can cause problems for the baby and/or affect milk production.

Before considering any nonprescription drug or natural remedy, talk to your healthcare provider. They will be able to tell you how the medicine will affect the baby.

- Discuss the risks and benefits of taking any medication or natural remedy before you take it.
- Minimize the amount of medication you might pass on to your baby by asking your healthcare provider about other kinds of products instead of pills (examples—nose spray, ointment).
- Not all natural health products are safe for pregnant and breastfeeding mothers. Just because it says "natural" does not mean it is safe.
- If you are taking medication while breastfeeding, take it right after a feeding or when the baby goes down for a long nap. Leave as much time as possible between when you take the medicine and when you feed the baby.

Morning Sickness—What You Need to Know

Nausea and vomiting are **completely normal** during the first 12 weeks of a pregnancy (12 weeks after your last period). Morning sickness can happen at any time of the day, not just in the morning. **Remember:** Morning sickness usually gets better as your pregnancy progresses!

Suggestions to help you manage nausea or vomiting:

- Avoid smells that make you feel nauseated.
- Eat crackers or dry toast before you get out of bed in the morning.
- Eat any food that looks and smells appealing to you. You may find that bland foods will bother you less.
- Avoid foods that are fatty, fried or spicy.
- Eat 5 or 6 small meals each day instead of eating 3 large meals. Eating large meals or having an empty stomach can worsen nausea. Add a source of protein such as nuts, seeds or dairy to each meal if possible.
- Drink small amounts of fluid regularly between meals.
- Avoid lying down right after eating.
- Take your prenatal vitamins or iron supplements after meals, never on an empty stomach.
- Iron supplements or prenatal vitamins which contain higher amounts of iron can make nausea and vomiting worse. You may stop these supplements for a while and continue to take folic acid alone or in a multivitamin that does not contain iron.
- Heartburn, gas and constipation can make nausea worse. Talk to your pharmacist about ways to manage these problems.
- Products that contain ginger may help to settle your stomach. Talk to your pharmacist about safe use of ginger products.
- Avoid warm places and dress in layers so you can remove some clothing if feeling too warm. Being too hot can make you feel sick.
- Try to get a lot of rest and reduce your stress.
- Try eating at times of the day when nausea is less severe.
- Talk to your healthcare provider about trying acupressure.

Are there safe medications for nausea and vomiting?

Several medications have been proven safe to treat nausea during pregnancy. They do not increase the risk of birth defects. If you find your nausea or vomiting is not reduced by any of the suggestions above, talk to your healthcare provider. They can tell you about safe and effective medications for nausea.

When should you see your healthcare provider?

Pregnant women who have severe vomiting require special treatment to prevent dehydration. See your healthcare provider right away if you have any of the following symptoms:

- Your vomiting does not respond to any type of treatment.
- You are losing weight, or not gaining weight as you should be.
- Diarrhea.
- Fever or body temperature above 39°C.

- You vomit any amount of blood or find coffee ground–like material in the vomitus.
- You cannot keep fluids down and you feel very thirsty or faint when you get up from lying down. This may mean you are dehydrated.

For more information:

- Call the University of Toronto's Motherisk program toll-free helpline at **1-800-436-8477**. They can answer your questions or concerns about nausea and vomiting in pregnancy. They also have an excellent web site with information about morning sickness and many other issues. Go to www.motherisk.org.
- You can learn more about healthy eating during pregnancy from your local public health department or at http://www.healthyparentshealthychildren.ca/starting-off-healthy/eating-during-pregnancy/.

Care of the Vaginal Area (Perineum) after Childbirth—What You Need to Know

After delivering a baby, many women feel soreness or pain in the external vagina and surrounding area (perineum) due to an episiotomy (incision) or tearing during delivery.

Suggestions to relieve symptoms and help with healing:

- Avoid touching the area.
- Change sanitary pads at least every 4–6 hours. Do not use tampons for postpartum bleeding.
- Use a perineal squirt bottle to pour warm water over the perineal area after going to the bathroom.
- Use a sitz bath (warm water, either in the bathtub or a special sitz bath that fits over the toilet seat) after bowel movements.
- Always pat the area dry from front to back to avoid bringing germs from the rectum into the vaginal area.
- To reduce swelling, apply a cold gel pack several times during the first 12–24 hours. Apply the gel pack for 10–20 minutes at a time. Try resting on your side with the gel pack between your legs.
  - You can also wet and freeze a clean maxi-pad or newborn diaper, or wrap an ice pack in a towel and use any of these instead of an gel pack.
- Avoid constipation by eating fibre-rich foods and drinking plenty of water.
- Use a pillow when sitting.
- Avoid standing or sitting for long periods, as this can further strain the perineum.
- Do Kegel exercises to increase circulation and help promote healing. Kegel exercises are small squeezing movements of the vaginal muscles, similar to when you try to stop urinating. Try holding the contraction for up to 8 seconds, then relax. Repeat the contracting and relaxing several times a day.
- Get plenty of rest with your feet up to take pressure off the area.
- Use medicated wipes (such as Tucks) to cleanse and soothe the area.
- Ask your healthcare provider about using acetaminophen, ibuprofen or naproxen sodium for pain.

When should you see your healthcare provider?

See your healthcare provider if you have severe pain, a foul-smelling discharge or a high fever.

Postpartum Depression—What You Need to Know

What is postpartum depression?

Postpartum depression is different from "the baby blues" that many new mothers get after their baby is born. The baby blues usually starts within the first week after childbirth and goes away within 2 weeks. Postpartum depression can occur anytime within the first 6 months after the baby is born, lasts longer than 2 weeks and severely interferes with daily life.

What are the signs of postpartum depression?

Read through the statements below. They are all signs of postpartum depression. If you or anyone you know has any of these signs, seek medical help right away.

- □ My baby blues have not gone away after 2 weeks.
- □ I don't feel like my usual self.
- □ I have strong feelings of sadness or guilt.
- □ I have strong feelings of hopelessness or helplessness.
- □ I often feel very anxious or worried.
- □ I can't sleep, even when I am tired.
- □ I sleep all the time, even when my baby is awake.
- □ I am not able to eat, even when I am hungry.
- □ I am not able to eat because I am never hungry or because I feel sick.
- □ I worry about the baby too much; I'm obsessed with the baby.
- □ I don't worry about the baby at all; it's almost like I don't care.
- □ I am having anxiety or panic attacks.
- □ I feel angry toward the baby.
- □ I think about hurting myself or the baby.

What is the treatment for postpartum depression?

A woman who has postpartum depression needs to see a healthcare provider right away. Don't wait. The healthcare provider may recommend medication, counselling or both to help manage postpartum depression.

The information in this handout is adapted with permission from *Healthy beginnings: giving your baby the best start, from preconception to birth*. 4th ed. Ottawa: Society of Obstetricians and Gynaecologists of Canada, 2009. Available from: www.sogc.org/healthybeginnings/index.html.

Chapter 83

Urinary Incontinence

Cheryl A. Sadowski, BSc(Pharm), PharmD

Urinary incontinence has traditionally been defined as the involuntary loss of urine.[1] However, the term lower urinary tract symptoms (LUTS) is used to describe the broader spectrum of symptoms that can occur with or without incontinence, which can increase morbidity in many individuals.[1,2,3]

LUTS can be broadly classified into storage or voiding symptoms and can be acute or chronic.[4,5] Storage symptoms include daytime frequency, nocturia and urgency. These are often attributable to an overactive bladder, the primary focus of this chapter. Voiding symptoms are associated with benign prostatic hyperplasia, urinary obstruction, poorly contractile bladder or sphincter dysfunction, leading to urinary hesitancy, slow stream, incomplete bladder emptying and dribbling (see Chapter 75: Benign Prostatic Hyperplasia and Associated Lower Urinary Tract Symptoms).

The main types of urinary incontinence include: urge, stress, mixed (urge and stress), overflow, and functional (inability to toilet) incontinence.[4,6,7] Worldwide, LUTS are very common (14% of men and >30% of women) and will become more so as the population ages.[8] In the Canadian Urinary Bladder Survey (CUBS), 43% of men and 57% of women report one or more LUTS.[9] The mean age of men was only 44 years and of women 45 years.

In addition to the over $1 billion/year spent on the treatment of LUTS in Canada, the economic impact (e.g., work disruptions) and psychosocial issues (e.g., stigma, embarrassment, isolation, anxiety and depression) can be very costly.[8,10,11,12,13,14,15] LUTS are associated with medical complications (e.g., skin breakdown, pressure ulcers, increased frequency of urinary tract infections, increased rate of falls and fractures).[16,17,18] It appears that urinary urgency has the greatest impact on quality of life, although all forms of LUTS have also been associated with decreased quality of life, affecting recreational activities, sexual activities and daily life.[11,19,20]

Pathophysiology

The lower urinary tract includes the bladder and urethra and has 2 functional phases—storage and voiding. During the storage phase, the detrusor muscle relaxes and the urethral sphincter tightens. The voiding phase, also known as the micturition cycle, starts when the mechanoreceptors in the bladder wall are stimulated as the bladder volume approaches 250 mL (this volume varies by individual, from 150–600 mL). The cortical centre is then alerted and if the individual is in an appropriate setting, the detrusor muscle contracts while the sphincter opens in a coordinated fashion to allow urine to flow.

The bladder is innervated by the autonomic nervous system (Figure 1). The sympathetic system causes relaxation of the detrusor muscle and tightening of the sphincter. Conversely, the parasympathetic system causes contraction of the detrusor and relaxation of the sphincter. In a "fight or flight" response, when the sympathetic system is dominant, the body shuts down the urinary tract to divert blood and attention to other urgent issues.

While LUTS are not necessarily a normal part of aging, older adults are more susceptible to these symptoms due to changes in physiology such as decreased bladder capacity, increased post-void residual volume and increased spontaneous bladder muscle contractions.[21,22] The pathophysiology depends on the type of incontinence (Table 1). Some medications are associated with causing or exacerbating urinary incontinence (Table 2).[23,24,25]

Figure 1: **Innervation of Bladder Structures**

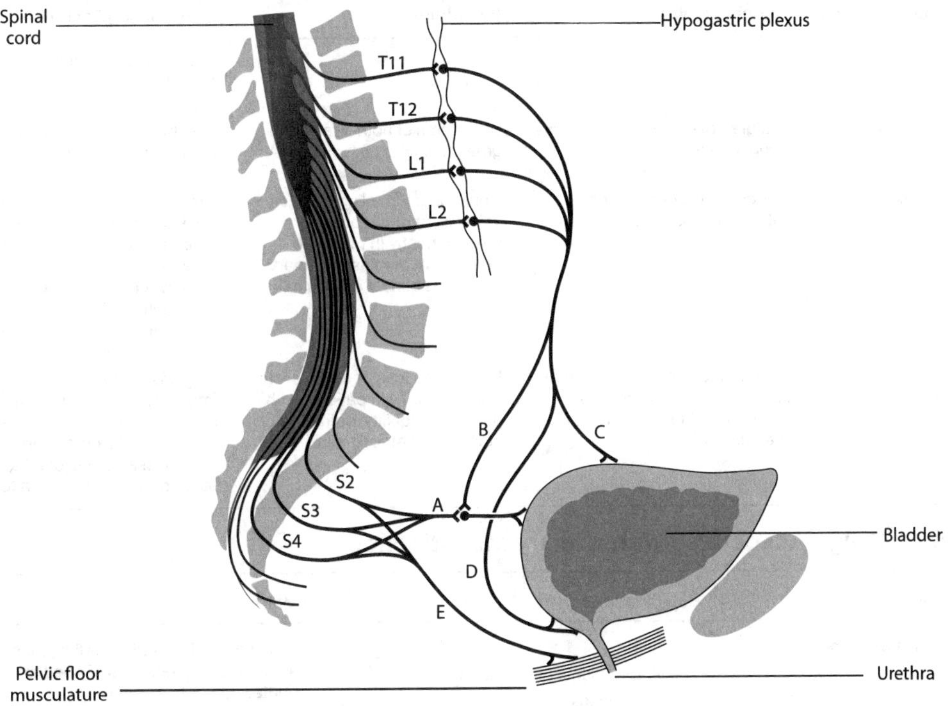

A: Detrusor muscle contraction due to parasympathetic activity B: Detrusor muscle relaxation due to inhibition of parasympathetic activity C: Bladder relaxation due to beta-adrenergic sympathetic activity D: Bladder neck/sphincter contraction due to alpha-adrenergic sympathetic activity E: Pelvic floor muscle contraction due to voluntary somatic activity

Table 1: **Types of Urinary Incontinence**

Type of Incontinence	Pathophysiology	Symptoms	Contributing Factors
Stress incontinence	Loss of bladder neck support (weak pelvic floor muscle) and/or intrinsic urethral sphincter deficiency; more common in women.	Urine loss triggered by activities that cause a rise in intra-abdominal pressure such as coughing, sneezing, jumping, lifting, exercise, shouting. Variable volumes of urine lost.	Pregnancy, childbirth, pelvic organ prolapse, postmenopausal atrophic changes, pelvic surgery (e.g., prostate surgery), obesity, smoking, medications (see Drugs Associated with Urinary Incontinence).
Urge incontinence ("overactive bladder")	Involuntary contractions due to instability of detrusor muscle (or hyper-reflexia of detrusor muscle due to neurologic disorder). Results in inability to suppress contractions; more common in older individuals and those with neurologic conditions (e.g., multiple sclerosis, spinal cord injury).	Involuntary loss of urine due to inability to postpone voiding when the urge is first perceived. Symptoms include frequency, nocturia enuresis. Can be triggered by cues such as running water or opening the door to the bathroom. Variable volumes of urine lost.	Age; dementia; obesity; postmenopausal atrophic changes; prostate surgery; neurologic damage associated with conditions such as diabetes, stroke, multiple sclerosis, Parkinson disease; bladder irritants such as infection, stones, concentrated urine from inadequate fluid intake; constipation; medications (see Drugs

(cont'd)

Table 1: **Types of Urinary Incontinence** *(cont'd)*

Type of Incontinence	Pathophysiology	Symptoms	Contributing Factors
			Associated with Urinary Incontinence).
Mixed stress/urge incontinence	Features of both stress and urge incontinence.	Symptoms of both stress and urge incontinence.	Combination of stress and urge incontinence factors.
Overflow incontinence	Bladder outlet obstruction or detrusor hypoactivity.	Continuous dribbling of small volumes of urine; occurs predominantly in men with prostatic hyperplasia. Urinary bladder is almost always full.	Prostatic hyperplasia, bladder neck contracture, urethral stricture, constipation, diabetes, neurologic problems, medications (see Drugs Associated with Urinary Incontinence).
Functional incontinence	Genitourinary system is normal, but the patient is physically unable to get to or use the toilet in time.	Patient has loss of urine; occurs predominantly in patients with physical disability, dementia or other psychiatric illness.	Cognitive and/or physical impairment; psychological and/or environmental barriers (e.g., lap belts or trays in a geri-chair, locked areas of a facility, stairs required to reach a toilet).

Table 2: **Drugs Associated with Urinary Incontinence**

Urinary Symptom	Medications	Mechanism
Functional incontinence	Alcohol Antidepressants (if sedating) Antipsychotics Muscle relaxants Opioids Sedative-hypnotics	Loss of central micturition reflex; manifests as decreased awareness of need to urinate.
	Cholinergic agonists (e.g., bethanechol) Cholinesterase inhibitors (e.g., donepezil, galantamine, rivastigmine)	Increased urinary frequency associated with detrustor muscle contractions.
Overflow incontinence	Alpha-agonists (e.g., decongestants, midodrine, pseudoephedrine) Anticholinergics Calcium channel blockers Opioids	Urinary retention resulting from impaired detrusor contractility or urethral sphincter tightening. Opioids also cause constipation, which increases parasympathetic discharge.
Stress incontinence	ACE inhibitors Alpha-antagonists (e.g., tamsulosin, terazosin) Cholinergic agonists (e.g., bethanechol) Cholinesterase inhibitors (e.g., donepezil, galantamine, rivastigmine)	Decreased urethral sphincter tone. ACE inhibitors may cause cough, which increases intra-abdominal pressure.
All types of urinary incontinence	Diuretics (e.g., furosemide) Glucocorticoids (systemic) NSAIDs (e.g., celecoxib) Thiazolidinediones	Increased urinary output and detrusor contractions. Fluid retention leading to nocturnal enuresis.

Goals of Therapy

- Eliminate or reduce frequency of incontinence episodes
- Eliminate or reduce severity of symptoms
- Prevent complications:
  - urinary tract infections
  - skin breakdown
  - falls
  - catheterization
- Improve quality of life for patient and caregivers

Patient Assessment

The key areas of patient assessment are bladder history, previous pelvic surgery, medical history (including medication history), physical examination and laboratory investigations.[3,26,27,28,29,30] A full assessment requires medical workup with a physical examination, laboratory data and possibly urodynamic and cystoscopic evaluations.[31]

Bladder History

A number of questionnaires and structured instruments have been designed to determine whether LUTS are problematic for individuals. The basic 3 items are if, when, and how urinary symptoms occur.[26] Some experts have recommended starting the interview or approaching patients with the following case-finding questions:[32,33,34]

- Do you ever leak urine/water when you do not want to?
- Do you ever leak urine/water when you cough, laugh or exercise?
- Do you leak urine/water on the way to the bathroom?
- Do you ever use pads, tissues, or cloth in your underwear to catch urine/water?
- Do you use pads or protective garments?
- How often do you leak urine?

Bladder or voiding diaries can also be helpful in documenting a patient's particular symptom pattern and response to therapy. Table 3 presents a reliable and validated sample diary for patients to use. A 3-day diary collection of data is recommended to assess the situation.[3,35]

Table 3: **Sample Voiding Diary**

Date	Time of day	Intake of Liquids		Bathroom: Urine Volume S = small M = moderate L= large	Accidental Leaks S = small M = moderate L= large	Did you feel a strong urge to go? Y = yes N = no	What activity were you doing when you had the urge to go?	Pad/ Absorbable Product Use
		Type	Volume					

Medical History

- Gynecologic and obstetric history
- History of pelvic surgery
- Bowel history
- Comorbid conditions, e.g., diabetes, stroke, arthritis, Parkinson disease
- Sensory impairments, e.g., vision
- Functional status and mobility
- Current and recently used medications (see Table 2)

Physical Examination

A thorough physical exam is required to rule out modifiable contributing factors. Assessment should include:

- Abdominal examination (e.g., bladder distension)
- Pelvic/gynecologic functions (e.g., cystocele, prolapse)
- Rectal function (e.g., tone, fullness)
- Prostate evaluation (e.g., size, consistency, symmetry, tenderness)
- Neurologic function (e.g., sensory and motor)
- Musculoskeletal function (e.g., mobility)

Investigations

- Urinalysis
- Urine culture
- Bladder scan to assess postvoid residual volume

If further workup is required:[36]

- Serum metabolic profile, e.g., electrolytes, glucose
- Urodynamic (uroflowmetry, cystometry, pressure flow studies) and cystoscopic evaluations

Nonpharmacologic Therapy

For comparative features of nonprescription products, consult the *Compendium of Products for Minor Ailments*—Incontinence Products: Devices.

Nonpharmacologic interventions are considered first-line therapies and should be continued when pharmacologic treatments are employed. The advantage of these measures is that they are often easy to use, do not cause side effects and are less expensive than pharmacologic agents. Table 4 discusses nonpharmacologic interventions.[37,38,39,40,41,42,43,44,45]

The choice of a first- vs. second-line approach is patient specific. A patient may choose an intervention that is easy to implement, more readily accessible, or one that allows for treatment without any devices prior to purchasing any products.

For each type of LUTS, it is appropriate to present the patient with the options and then to aid the patient in deciding on the best method of treatment. Often patients will fare better with a combination of multiple nonpharmacologic treatments or a combination of nonpharmacologic and pharmacologic interventions.

Table 4: Nonpharmacologic Therapy for Urinary Incontinence

Intervention	Type of Urinary Incontinence	Description	Benefits	Drawbacks
Timed voiding	Urge or mixed	Start with voiding every 30 min, then eventually increase the interval between voiding by 30 min until the individual can control the bladder for up to 3-h intervals.	▪ No financial cost ▪ Does not require a lot of training	▪ Patient still is toileting frequently at the beginning ▪ Life schedule can centre around toileting ▪ Takes many weeks or months to achieve control
Bowel management	Urge or overflow	Relieving constipation decreases parasympathetic activity (decreased involuntary bladder contraction) or can reduce pressure on the bladder caused by stool impaction.	▪ Decreased constipation	▪ Requires treatment by diet or with laxative medications. Caution with additional fluid intake that can aid constipation but worsen incontinence
Electrical stimulation (e.g., posterior tibial nerve, sacral, intravaginal)	Urge, stress or mixed	Brief electrical impulses are administered via needles or surface electrodes to inhibit detrusor overactivity, or to strengthen the pelvic floor. The probe may be inserted into the anus or vagina.	▪ Device can be used independently by the patient	▪ Invasive ▪ May be expensive if therapy is not covered by health plan ▪ Requires cleaning ▪ Benefit is lost after treatment cessation
Biofeedback exercises	Urge, stress or mixed	A vaginal or rectal probe detects contractions and sends an auditory or visual signal telling the patient how strong the contractions are.	▪ Can be used independently at home	▪ Costly ▪ Delay from time of use to full benefit is realized
Pelvic floor muscle training (Kegel exercises)	Urge, stress or mixed	The individual contracts the pelvic floor, as if to hold in flatus or interrupt urinary flow, for 5 seconds, then relaxes for 10 seconds. Exercises are increased starting at 30 times per day. The goal is to hold the tensions for 10 seconds, then relax for 20 seconds, repeating up to 100 times per day. Can also be combined with biofeedback.	▪ Little cost and time required ▪ Can be done even if mobility is a concern	▪ Can be distracting if client attempts to complete this while doing other activities ▪ Like any activity involving skeletal muscles, this takes up to 6 wk to show benefit. Can cause myalgia if exercises are overdone or done improperly
Vaginal weights, vaginal cones	Stress	Tampon-shaped weights are inserted into and held in the vagina for short periods of time. Gradually the time is extended and the weight is increased.	▪ Discreet ▪ Does not require counting and timing like Kegel exercises	▪ Weights must be purchased ▪ If weight is too heavy it can fall out ▪ May be distracting or uncomfortable if not properly inserted ▪ Requires cleaning ▪ Like any activity involving skeletal muscles, this takes up to 6 wk to show benefit

(cont'd)

Table 4: **Nonpharmacologic Therapy for Urinary Incontinence** *(cont'd)*

Intervention	Type of Urinary Incontinence	Description	Benefits	Drawbacks
Physiotherapy (pelvic floor exercises)	Urge, stress or mixed	A physiotherapist may work with the patient to continue exercises beyond Kegel exercises to improve pelvic floor strength.	▪ Exercises can often be done independently by the patient	▪ Like any activity involving skeletal muscles, this takes up to 6 wk to show benefit
Surgical procedures for women: ▪ Suburethral sling (e.g., tension-free vaginal tape, transobturator tape, synthetic mesh tape) ▪ Open retropubic colposuspension ▪ Bladder neck needle suspension ▪ Laparoscopic colposuspension	Stress	Repositioning of the bladder neck and urethra to the normal anatomic positions.	▪ Most surgeries are minimally invasive	▪ Most types of surgery have effects that last for many years ▪ Women who plan to have more children are not eligible for surgery in most cases, as the pregnancy would negate the surgical intervention
Surgical procedures for men: inflatable implant	Stress	Usually used in men after prostatectomy, implant is inflated near the bladder neck to lift it into correct anatomical position.	▪ Minimally invasive ▪ Immediate results	▪ Balloon may become damaged and require replacement
Pessary	Stress	A product is inserted into the vagina and fitted by a specialist so that the pessary supports the bladder and urethra through the vaginal wall, while preventing prolapse of the vagina or cervix.	▪ Can be inserted and left for extended periods of time ▪ Patient does not feel the device if inserted properly	▪ Can cause erosions or vaginal infections if not fitted or cleaned properly ▪ Can interfere with sexual intercourse
Bulking agents	Stress	A bulking agent (e.g., autologous fat, ethylene vinyl chloride, collagen, or silicone) is injected around the bladder neck to provide better support and positioning of the bladder and urethra.	▪ Minimally invasive ▪ Results are immediate	▪ Product may disperse and procedure may have to be repeated ▪ Long term effects of injections are unknown
Weight management if BMI >25 kg/m^2	Stress	Weight loss in overweight individuals can reduce pressure on the lower abdomen.	▪ Other risk factors improve, e.g., reduced risk of diabetes, improved blood pressure control	▪ Lifestyle interventions may be difficult to implement
Catheterization	Overflow	A Foley catheter (indwelling catheter), or in-and-out catheterization can be done to bypass an obstruction.	▪ The patient can control voiding if he/she independently conducts in-and-out catheterization ▪ Accurate measures of urine volume,	▪ Catheters increase the risk of urinary and bladder infections ▪ Mobility ▪ Embarrassment due to urine bag (for indwelling catheter)

(cont'd)

Table 4: **Nonpharmacologic Therapy for Urinary Incontinence** *(cont'd)*

Intervention	Type of Urinary Incontinence	Description	Benefits	Drawbacks
			content, etc., can be taken	▪ Some urine leakage may still occur around the catheter
Restriction of irritants (e.g., reduction in alcohol and caffeine intake)	Urge	Caffeine and alcohol are diuretics and direct bladder irritants.	▪ Benefit can be noticed immediately	▪ Lifestyle changes are often the most difficult to implement
Fluid intake management	Urge	Ensuring consumption of 6–8 glasses of water/day to prevent dehydration and concentrated urine, which is a bladder irritant; avoiding fluids in the evening. Some individuals may require restriction of fluids to prevent excessive urine production.	▪ Ensures urine that is not concentrated and irritating	▪ Individuals have difficulty implementing fluid intake when they deal with LUTS ▪ Other conditions, such as heart failure, may contraindicate a certain volume of fluid intake
Urethral plugs, urethral caps, penile clamps	Stress, overflow	The product blocks the urethra to prevent dribbling.	▪ Can be applied by the patient	▪ May cause irritation and skin erosion ▪ May increase urinary tract infections
Commodes or urinals	All	The device is placed at the bedside or convenient to the individual to allow for voiding when moving to a toilet is not an option.	▪ Easy access, usually at the bedside ▪ Allows for independence in voiding if mobility is a concern	▪ Odour ▪ Embarrassment ▪ Some individuals still require assistance to transfer onto the commode or to use the urinal
Environmental modification	All	Installing a higher toilet or toilet seat, adding grab bars, or clearing the way for easy access to the toilet.	▪ Improved safety in the environment ▪ Decreased risk of falls	▪ Some interventions can be costly ▪ Can be noticeable which can be associated with social stigma
Adaptive clothing	All	Wear easy to remove clothing. Choose clothing that can be easily cleaned and can accommodate insertion of pads or absorbable products.	▪ Improved mobility and comfort	▪ Can be costly to purchase different clothes ▪ May require a change in style of clothing
Alarms	All	An alarm can be used to alert someone for scheduled toileting, or can be used in the underwear or bedpad to detect wetness.	▪ Can allow patient to manage toileting independently	▪ Expensive ▪ Invasive ▪ Alarm can let others know there is a health problem
Absorptive products (pads, guards, liners, undergarments, underwear, etc.)	All	The product is worn to absorb urine leakage.	▪ Allow the patient to function independently ▪ Large selection of products available for different needs	▪ Costly ▪ Numerous types requiring healthcare practitioner to direct to the appropriate product ▪ Odour if not used properly

Pharmacologic Therapy

Urge Incontinence

For further discussion of pharmacologic therapy for urge incontinence, consult the *Compendium of Therapeutic Choices*: Urinary Incontinence in Adults.

Some patients may self-treat with anticholinergic medications, such as **dicyclomine**, **dimenhydrinate**, **diphenhydramine** or **scopolamine**. However, these medications are not recommended for the management of urge incontinence due to the availability of safer and more effective alternatives.

The most common medications used for the treatment of urge incontinence have antimuscarinic properties to reduce the responsiveness of the detrusor muscle to parasympathetic impulses. Such agents include **darifenacin**, **fesoterodine**, **oxybutynin**, **solifenacin**, **tolterodine** and **trospium**. These drugs reduce incontinence episodes, improve continence and often improve quality of life.[46,47,48,49,50] However, some patients may not tolerate the increased incidence of side effects (e.g., constipation, blurred vision, dry mouth) when using relatively less selective products (oxybutynin, tolterodine, trospium).[51,52,53,54,55,56,57] Due to toxicity and lack of approved indication for LUTS, tricyclic antidepressants should not be used.

Botulinum toxin (onabotulinumtoxinA) injection into the detrusor muscle is approved for the management of urinary incontinence.[58,59] For troublesome nocturia in younger patients (<65 years of age), **desmopressin** at bedtime may be of benefit but may increase the risk of hyponatremia.[60,61] The evidence is controversial regarding estrogen, but it appears that **intravaginal estrogen** may reduce urinary urgency in some postmenopausal women with vaginal atrophy or dysuria and urge incontinence.[62,63]

Stress Incontinence

This type of urinary incontinence is not usually treated pharmacologically. First-line treatment focuses on pelvic floor muscle training (see Table 4).

Estrogen therapy is ineffective and should not be used to manage this type of urinary incontinence.[46,64] Although **duloxetine** reduces the frequency of urinary incontinence episodes and improves quality of life compared with placebo, it is associated with increased adverse effects (e.g., nausea, diarrhea, headache, dizziness, fatigue, dry mouth, liver toxicity, suicidal ideation).[62] Duloxetine is not licensed in Canada for the management of stress urinary incontinence.

Mixed Stress/Urge Incontinence

When a patient exhibits symptoms suggestive of both urge and stress incontinence, treatment could be directed at the predominant type or both types.

Overflow Incontinence

For further discussion of pharmacologic therapy for overflow incontinence, consult the *Compendium of Therapeutic Choices*: Urinary Incontinence in Adults.

Bethanechol is a cholinergic agonist that increases parasympathetic activity, increasing bladder contractions and relaxing sphincters. This medication can be used for bladder stimulation when it has been confirmed that an obstruction is not present. The side effects are consistent with cholinergic agonism and include diarrhea, nausea, hypersalivation and lacrimation. Alpha-blockers (nonselective: **doxazosin**, **prazosin**, **terazosin**; selective: **alfuzosin**, **tamsulosin**) may be helpful in treating overflow incontinence in cases of benign prostatic hyperplasia or sphincter hyperspasticity.

Monitoring of Therapy

Monitoring involves the following general parameters and recording how bothersome they are:

- Improvement in symptoms, e.g., nocturia, dysuria, hesitancy, urgency
- Number of episodes of incontinence or severity of LUTS/day
- Number of micturitions/day
- Volume of urine/micturition
- Number of absorptive products used
- Urinary flow parameters

When starting pharmacologic therapy, the healthcare practitioner should monitor the patient on a weekly basis for the first month then monthly for the next 3 months then once or twice yearly. This ensures that side effects due to medication use are addressed promptly and informs the healthcare practitioner if the medication is beneficial in reducing symptoms of urinary incontinence. Voiding diaries are useful patient tools for monitoring the efficacy of interventions (see Table 3) and the patient should be encouraged to monitor symptoms daily until symptom control in achieved.

Resource Tips

Bladder and Bowel Foundation (UK). Available from: www.bladderandbowelfoundation.org.

Canadian Continence Foundation. Available from: www.canadiancontinence.ca.

Canadian Nurse Continence Advisors. Available from: www.cnca.ca.

Canadian Urological Association. Available from: www.cua.org.

Canadian Women's Health Network. Available from: www.cwhn.ca.

Overactive Bladder Support Sites:

Peeing Problem. Available from: peeingproblem.ca/en.

The Powder Room. Available from: www.powderroom.ca/en.

The Society of Obstetricians and Gynaecologists of Canada. Available from: www.sogc.org.

Urology Nurses of Canada. Available from: www.unc.org.

Suggested Readings

Frank C, Szlanta A. Office management of urinary incontinence among older patients. *Can Fam Physician* 2010;56:1115-20.

Hersh L, Salzman B. Clinical management of urinary incontinence in women. *Am Fam Physician* 2013;87:634-40.

Larsen B, Post GJ. LUTS: a practical guide to alleviating lower urinary tract symptoms. *JAAPA* 2013;26:26-30.

Polland A, Mock S, Dmochowski RR. Emerging treatments for urinary incontinence. *Expert Opin Emerg Drugs* 2014;19:281-90.

Wagg AS. Antimuscarinic treatment in overactive bladder: special considerations in elderly patients. *Drugs Aging* 2012;29:539-48.

Wood LN, Anger JT. Urinary incontinence in women. *BMJ* 2014;349:g4531.

References

1. Abrams P, Cardozo L, Fall M et al. The standardisation of terminology of lower urinary tract function: report from the Standardisation Sub-committee of the International Continence Society. *Neurourol Urodyn* 2002;21:167-78.
2. Chapple CR, Wein AJ, Abrams P et al. Lower urinary tract symptoms revisited: a broader clinical perspective. *Eur Urol* 2008;54:563-9.

3. Bettez M, Tu le M, Carlson K et al. 2012 update: guidelines for adult urinary incontinence collaborative consensus document for the Canadian Urological Association. *Can Urol Assoc J* 2012;6:354-63.
4. Vella M, Robinson D, Staskin D. A reappraisal of storage and voiding dysfunction. *Curr Urol Rep* 2012;13:482-7.
5. Testa A. Understanding urinary incontinence in adults. *Urol Nurs* 2015;35:82-6.
6. Guzzo TJ, Drach GW. Major urologic problems in geriatrics: assessment and management. *Med Clin North Am* 2011;95:253-64.
7. Thirugnanasothy S. Managing urinary incontinence in older people. *BMJ* 2010;341:c3835.
8. Milsom I, Coyne KS, Nicholson S et al. Global prevalence and economic burden of urgency urinary incontinence: a systematic review. *Eur Urol* 2014;65:79-95.
9. Herschorn S, Gajewski J, Schulz J et al. A population-based study of urinary symptoms and incontinence: the Canadian Urinary Bladder Survey. *BJU Int* 2008;101:52-8.
10. Coyne KS, Sexton CC, Thompson CL et al. Impact of overactive bladder on work productivity. *Urology* 2012;80:97-103.
11. Riss P, Kargl J. Quality of life and urinary incontinence in women. *Maturitas* 2011;68:137-42.
12. Milsom I, Kaplan SA, Coyne KS et al Effect of bothersome overactive bladder symptoms on health-related quality of life, anxiety, depression, and treatment seeking in the united states: results from EpiLUTS. *Urology* 2012;80:90-6.
13. Vrijens D, Drossaerts J, van Koeveringe G et al. Affective symptoms and the overactive bladder—a systematic review. *J Psychosom Res* 2015;78:95-108.
14. Heintz PA, DeMucha CM, Deguzman MM et al. Stigma and microaggressions experienced by older women with urinary incontinence: a literature review. *Urol Nurs* 2013;33:299-305.
15. Abrams P, Smith AP, Cotterill N. The impact of urinary incontinence on health-related quality of life (HRQoL) in a real-world population of women aged 45-60 years: results from a survey in France, Germany, the UK and the USA. *BJU Int* 2015;115:143-52.
16. Brown JS, Vittinghoff E, Wyman JF et al. Urinary incontinence: does it increase risk for falls and fractures? Study of Osteoporotic Fractures Research Group. *J Am Geriatr Soc* 2000;48:721-5.
17. Gray M, Beeckman D, Bliss DZ et al. Incontinence-associated dermatitis: a comprehensive review and update. *J Wound Ostomy Continence Nurs* 2012;39:61-74.
18. Foley AL, Loharuka S, Barrett JA et al. Association between the Geriatric Giants of urinary incontinence and falls in older people using data from the Leicestershire MRC Incontinence Study. *Age Ageing* 2012;41:35-40.
19. Bartoli S, Aguzzi G, Tarricone R. Impact on quality of life of urinary incontinence and overactive bladder: a systematic literature review. *Urology* 2010;75:491-500.
20. Chen J, Sweet G, Shindel A. Urinary disorders and female sexual function. *Curr Urol Rep* 2013;14:298-308.
21. Wagg A. Urinary incontinence in older people: an overview. *Medicine* 2013;41:20-3.
22. Scemons D. Urinary incontinence in adults. *Nursing* 2013;43:52-60.
23. Ouslander JG. Management of overactive bladder. *N Engl J Med* 2004;350:786-99.
24. Holroyd-Leduc JM, Straus SE. Management of urinary incontinence in women: scientific review. *JAMA* 2004;291:986-95.
25. Wagg AS. Antimuscarinic treatment in overactive bladder: special considerations in elderly patients. *Drugs Aging* 2012;29:539-48.
26. Frank C, Szlanta A. Office management of urinary incontinence among older patients. *Can Fam Physician* 2010;56:1115-20.
27. Gibbs CF, Johnson TM, Ouslander JG. Office management of geriatric urinary incontinence. *Am J Med* 2007;120:211-20.
28. Holroyd-Leduc JM, Tannenbaum C, Thorpe KE et al. What type of urinary incontinence does this woman have? *JAMA* 2008;299:1446-56.
29. Larsen B, Post GJ. LUTS: a practical guide to alleviating lower urinary tract symptoms. *JAAPA* 2013;26:26-30.
30. Gormley EA, Lightner DJ, Faraday M et al. Diagnosis and treatment of overactive bladder (non-neurogenic) in adults: AUA/SUFU guideline amendment. *J Urol* 2015;193:1572-80.
31. Cameron AP, Heidelbaugh JJ, Jimbo M. Diagnosis and office-based treatment of urinary incontinence in adults. Part one: diagnosis and testing. *Ther Adv Urol* 2013;5:181-7.
32. Carlson C, Merel SE, Yukawa M. Geriatric syndromes and geriatric assessment for the generalist. *Med Clin North Am* 2015;99:263-79.
33. Smith A, Bevan D, Douglas HR et al. Management of urinary incontinence in women: summary of updated NICE guidance. *BMJ* 2013;347:f5170.
34. Sampselle CM, Wyman JF, Thomas KK et al. Continence for women: a test of AWHONN's evidence-based practice protocol in clinical practice. Association of Women's Health Obstetric and Neonatal Nurses. *J Obstet Gynecol Neonatal Nurs* 2000;29:18-26.
35. Jimenez-Cidre MA, Lopez-Fando L, Esteban-Fuertes M et al. The 3-day bladder diary is a feasible, reliable and valid tool to evaluate the lower urinary tract symptoms in women. *Neurourol Urodyn* 2015;34:128-32.
36. Borrie MJ, Valiquette L. Managing adults with urinary incontinence. Clinical practice guidelines. *Can Fam Physician* 2002;48:114-6.
37. Occhino JA, Siegel SW. Sacral nerve modulation in overactive bladder. *Curr Urol Rep* 2010;11:348-52.
38. Dumoulin C, Glazener C, Jenkinson D. Determining the optimal pelvic floor muscle training regimen for women with stress urinary incontinence. *Neurourol Urodyn* 2011;30:746-53.
39. Dumoulin C, Hay-Smith EJ, Habée-Séguin G. Pelvic floor muscle training versus no treatment, or inactive control treatments, for urinary incontinence in women. *Cochrane Database Syst Rev* 2014;5:CD005654.
40. Price N, Dawood R, Jackson SR. Pelvic floor exercise for urinary incontinence: a systematic literature review. *Maturitas* 2010;67:309-15.
41. Dmochowski RR, Blaivas JM, Gormley EA et al. Update of AUA guideline on the surgical management of female stress urinary incontinence. *J Urol* 2010;183:1906-14.
42. Jonsson Funk M, Levin PJ, Wu JM. Trends in the surgical management of stress urinary incontinence. *Obstet Gynecol* 2012;119:845-51.
43. Novara G, Artibani W, Barber MD et al. Updated systematic review and meta-analysis of the comparative data on colposuspensions, pubovaginal slings, and midurethral tapes in the surgical treatment of female stress urinary incontinence. *Eur Urol* 2010;58:218-38.
44. Kleeman SD, Karram MM. The tension-free vaginal tape procedure. *Urol Clin North Am* 2012;38:39-45.
45. Bash KL. Review of vaginal pessaries. *Obstet Gynecol Surv* 2000;55:455-60.
46. Anger JT, Scott VC, Kiyosaki K et al. Development of quality indicators for women with urinary incontinence. *Neurourol Urodyn* 2013;32:1058-63.
47. Robinson D, Cardozo L. New drug treatments for urinary incontinence. *Maturitas* 2010;65:340-7.
48. Cipullo LM, Cosimato C, Filippelli A et al. Pharmacological approach to overactive bladder and urge urinary incontinence in women: an overview. *Eur J Obstet Gynecol Reprod Biol* 2014;174:27-34.
49. Reynolds WS, McPheeters M, Blume J et al. Comparative effectiveness of anticholinergic therapy for overactive bladder in women: a systematic review and meta-analysis. *Obstet Gynecol* 2015;125:1423-32.

50. Shamliyan T, Wyman JF, Ramakrishnan R et al. Benefits and harms of pharmacologic treatment for urinary incontinence in women: a systematic review. *Ann Intern Med* 2012;156:861-74.
51. Madhuvrata P, Cody JD, Ellis G et al. Which anticholinergic drug for overactive bladder symptoms in adults. *Cochrane Database Syst Rev* 2012;1:CD005429.
52. Swinburn P, Lloyd A, Ali S et al. Preferences for antimuscarinic therapy for overactive bladder. *BJU Int* 2011;108:868-73.
53. Oefelein MG. Safety and tolerability profiles of anticholinergic agents used for the treatment of overactive bladder. *Drug Saf* 2011;34:733-54.
54. Chapple C, Khullar V, Gabriel Z et al. The effects of antimuscarinic treatments in overactive bladder: a systematic review and meta-analysis. *Eur Urol* 2005;48:5-26.
55. Andersson KE. Antimuscarinics for treatment of overactive bladder. *Lancet Neurol* 2004;3:46-53.
56. Staskin DR. Overactive bladder in the elderly: a guide to pharmacologic management. *Drugs Aging* 2005;22:1013-28.
57. Gibson W, Athanasopoulos A, Goldman H et al. Are we shortchanging frail older people when it comes to the pharmacological treatment of urgency urinary incontinence? *Int J Clin Pract* 2014;68:1165-73.
58. Duthie JB, Vincent M, Herbison GP et al. Botulinum toxin injections for adults with overactive bladder syndrome. *Cochrane Database Syst Rev* 2011;(12):CD005493.
59. Yokoyama T, Chancellor MB, Oguma K et al. Botulinum toxin type A for the treatment of lower urinary tract disorders. *Int J Urol* 2012;19:202-15.
60. Raskolnikov D, Friedman FM, Etwaru DJ et al. The evaluation and management of persistent nocturia. *Curr Urol Rep* 2014;15:439.
61. Ebell MH, Radke T, Gardner J. A systematic review of the efficacy and safety of desmopressin for nocturia in adults. *J Urol* 2014;192:829-35.
62. Shamliyan TA, Kane RL, Wyman J et al. Systematic review: randomized, controlled trials of nonsurgical treatments for urinary incontinence in women. *Ann Intern Med* 2008;148:459-73.
63. Cody JD, Jacobs ML, Richardson K et al. Oestrogen therapy for urinary incontinence in post-menopausal women. *Cochrane Database Syst Rev* 2012;10:CD001405.
64. Hersh L, Salzman B. Clinical management of urinary incontinence in women. *Am Fam Physician* 2013;87:634-40.

Urinary Incontinence—What You Need To Know

What is urinary incontinence?

- It means that you leak urine (pee) when you do not want to.

What are the different types of urinary incontinence?

There are 4 main types:

- Stress (most common): you are not able to hold in urine when you cough, sneeze, laugh, jump or run.
- Urge (also known as overactive bladder): your bladder is forcing out urine when you do not want to urinate.
- Mixed: you have symptoms of both stress incontinence and urge incontinence
- Overflow: bladder is too full and leaks some urine.

Who will develop urinary incontinence?

- Both men and women can have overactive bladder.
- Women more commonly develop stress symptoms because pregnancy and childbirth affect the muscles that hold up the bladder.
- Some men develop stress symptoms after surgeries.
- Men develop overflow symptoms when their prostates become larger.
- All forms of urinary incontinence are more common in older adults.

What are the goals of treatment?

- Reduce your symptoms and improve your quality of life
- Prevent urinary infections
- Prevent skin damage and ensure that you do not fall

What are some nondrug measures I can use?

- Scheduled toileting for overactive bladder.
- Pelvic floor muscle training (Kegel exercises) for stress incontinence.
- Catheters for overflow symptoms.

There are also surgical treatments and inserts that can be considered.

For all types of symptoms:

- Monitor the amount of fluid you consume (6–8 glasses of fluids/day). Too much or too little fluid can be associated with incontinence.
- Avoid caffeine.
- Lose weight if you are overweight.
- Wear easy-to-remove clothing.
- Prevent constipation.

Medications

Medications are available for most forms of urinary incontinence. Try nondrug measures first and continue using them even if you start a medication.

Chapter 84
Vaginal Symptoms, Hygiene and Infections

Laura-Lynn Pollock, BSc(Pharm), NARTC, Dip AC

Vaginal Physiology

The vagina is a fibromuscular structure that connects the external genitalia, or vulva, with the internal cervix and uterus. It provides a channel for the removal of menstrual discharge, and the transverse folds or rugae of the vaginal wall allow the flexibility of size and shape that are required for sexual intercourse and childbirth.

Normal vaginal length is variable but is usually between 8 cm and 10 cm. The vagina is positioned at a 45° angle, upwards and posteriorly. It is in close proximity to the bladder, urethra, perineum and rectum (Figure 1).[1]

Figure 1: Female Reproductive System

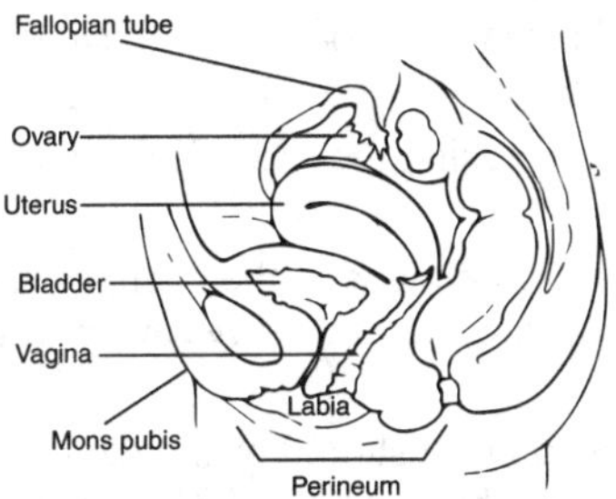

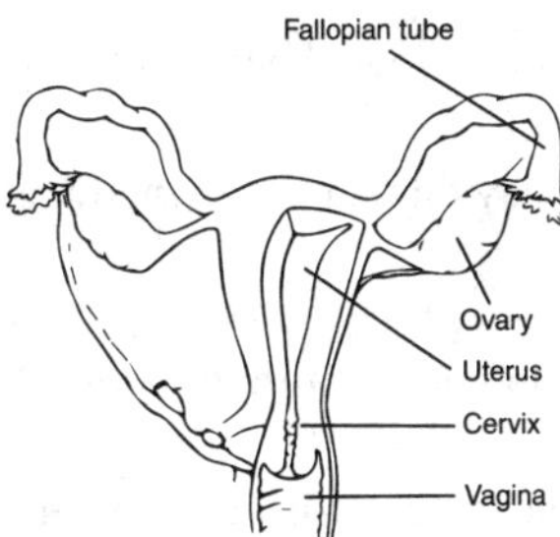

A healthy vaginal environment is maintained by balancing many host factors including bacterial flora, hormonal influences and the epithelial cells lining the vaginal wall. Estrogen induces the maturation of the epithelial cells and stimulates the proliferation of epithelial basal cells. It also increases the cells' ability to store glycogen, which is subsequently metabolized to lactic acid by the vaginal bacterium *Lactobacillus vaginalis*, making the vagina acidic with a pH of 3.5–5.5. The nonpathogenic lactobacilli thrive in the acidic environment while the proliferation of more troublesome microflora is controlled.[2,3]

Normal vaginal discharge varies in quantity, consistency and appearance throughout the menstrual cycle. This discharge can be due to mucus production of the cervical glands, a transudate from the capillaries of the vaginal walls and/or from other sources such as the uterus. Monthly hormone fluctuations are responsible for the changing characteristics of the discharge. Sometimes the discharge is pasty, white and scanty. Around the time of ovulation it is wet and slippery with the consistency of uncooked egg white. There may be no apparent discharge on the days immediately after menses has stopped. Vaginal discharge contributes to the health of the vagina and helps to maintain the pH and normal microflora. It should not cause irritation, burning or itching.[3,4]

A mild odour may occur when vaginal discharge combines with secretions from glands in the vulvar area. This odour should not be unpleasant or cause concern. Causes of unusual or unpleasant odour, genital irritation or itching may include poor hygiene, allergic or sensitivity reactions to products used, vaginal infections or a forgotten tampon.[3,4,5,6]

Genital Hygiene

Proper genital hygiene can be achieved very simply. The perineal area should be washed daily using warm water and mild soap. The outer labia should be gently separated and the clitoral area cleaned and rinsed. This area can be sensitive to perfumes and harsh ingredients in some soaps, so only mild products should be used. After cleansing, the perineal area should be rinsed well with warm water to remove soap residue.

The vagina cleanses itself naturally through its secretions and does not require further cleansing.[1,5]

Normal genital hygiene does not require the use of specialized commercial products; however, a number of products are marketed for just that purpose including vaginal douches, genital towelettes, cleansers and feminine deodorant sprays. Genital hygiene products are used by women of all ages. Women often initiate use of these products in their teens and continue into adulthood. Common reasons for their use include menstrual hygiene, to reduce vaginal odour or vaginal irritation and for hygiene related to sexual activity.[7,8,9,10]

Vaginal Douching

Douching is a process of instilling fluid into the vagina and flushing the cavity.

There are no substantiated benefits to routine douching and it can be associated with significant adverse outcomes:

- Douching may disrupt the normal vaginal environment, increasing the risk of irritation or infection[11,12,13]
- Douching may play a role in the development of ascending infections of the genital tract (e.g., salpingitis and pelvic inflammatory disease), ectopic pregnancy and possibly cancer of the cervix[11,12,13]
- Douching postcoitally is not an effective contraceptive method. It should be avoided until at least 6 hours after intercourse if a vaginal spermicide has been used, because douching can decrease the effectiveness of the spermicide
- Douching should also be avoided within 24 hours prior to a vaginal examination as this may hinder detection of a vaginal infection.

Despite the possible adverse outcomes, douching is still used by women for a variety of reasons. To decrease potential risks, it is important to provide sound advice to these women to help prevent adverse effects. The use of suitable solutions and appropriate technique are important safety factors. Douching should be avoided during pregnancy unless recommended by a healthcare practitioner. Douching is never recommended as a contraceptive method or as a treatment for suspected vaginal infections.[7,8,9,10]

Examples of douching solutions include:

- Plain warm water (simple and least likely to be harmful)
- Vinegar and water (available commercially or can be made at home by adding 15–30 mL vinegar to 1 L of warm water; produces transient decrease in vaginal microflora, similar to flushing with saline)[13]
- Commercially available products containing perfumes, astringents, anti-infectives or proteolytics (these ingredients do not increase effectiveness and can be irritating).

Instillation of the solution is by means of a vaginal syringe. There are two basic kinds of syringes—the fountain syringe and the bulb syringe. The fountain syringe consists of a piece of tubing attached to a bag (similar to a hot water bottle). A rounded plastic nozzle on the end of the tubing is inserted into the vagina. Gravity creates the flow of the solution. The bulb syringe has no tubing; the vaginal tip is attached directly to a small bag or bottle. The fluid is forced out of the bulb by squeezing the device or by the inward pressure exerted by the distended walls of the bulb.

Proper technique is essential for safe douching. The pressure used to instill the solution should be gentle, not forceful. Too much pressure may cause reflux of the solution (and possibly of bacteria) into the uterus and increase the risk of pelvic infection.

Correct technique is outlined in Vaginal Douching—What You Need to Know.

Other Genital Hygiene Products

Genital towelettes (e.g., Tucks) are premoistened disposable wipes that are generally safe for occasional use. They contain ingredients such as perfumes, astringents, emollients and anti-infectives and can be irritating or cause allergic reactions. Mild soap and warm water is preferred for daily cleansing.

Genital washes (e.g., Summer's Eve) are liquid cleansers designed for daily use on the external genitalia. They provide no additional benefit over mild soap and water, but there is no significant risk to their use.

Genital deodorant sprays (e.g., Summer's Eve FDS) contain ingredients such as perfumes and propellants and are marketed to reduce genital odour. Their use is not recommended. They can mask the odour of infections and cause treatment delays. Their use is associated with a high incidence of irritation and allergic reactions. If used, they must not be applied to the inside of the vagina.

Vaginal Dryness

Pathophysiology

It is common to have periods of time when vaginal lubrication is decreased. Low estrogen levels during perimenopause or menopause, in the postpartum period, during breastfeeding and immediately following menses may result in vaginal dryness. Tampons and certain medications can contribute to decreased vaginal lubrication.

Medications associated with decreased vaginal lubrication include:[14,15,16,17]

- Antiarrhythmics
- Antidepressants
- Antihistamines
- Antihypertensives
- Chemotherapy
- Combined hormonal contraceptives

This decreased lubrication may be transient, or it may be long term, as is often the case for peri- or postmenopausal women.[1,4,18] For more information, see Chapter 79: Menopause and Perimenopause.

Reduced estrogen levels cause thinning of the vaginal tissue, loss of collagen support, increased vaginal pH and reduced production of vaginal lubrication even when sexual arousal has occurred. These changes are associated with a number of vaginal symptoms, including:[14,15,16,17]

- abnormal bleeding
- discharge
- dyspareunia (pain during sexual intercourse)
- pruritus
- slow production of lubrication with sexual arousal
- vaginal dryness.

Goals of Therapy

- Provide lubrication to vaginal tissue
- Decrease symptoms associated with vaginal dryness
- Increase level of comfort during sexual intercourse

Patient Assessment

The majority of women seeking advice and relief from vaginal dryness are in peri- or postmenopause. Approximately 15% of perimenopausal and 29–57% of postmenopausal women experience symptoms of vaginal dryness due to urogenital atrophy.[14,18] It is reasonable to recommend a trial of nonprescription vaginal lubricants or moisturizers to women with mild to moderate symptoms.[15,16,17] Vaginal estrogen therapy is more effective than lubricants and moisturizers for vaginal atrophy; therefore, women with severe vaginal dryness or those who have been unresponsive to nonprescription measures should be referred to an appropriate healthcare practitioner for assessment.[19]

Nonpharmacologic Therapy

Some relief from vaginal dryness may result from increasing blood flow to the pelvic region through sexual stimulation. Any form of sexual excitement may help restore vaginal moisture. Intercourse is not necessary to achieve this effect and should be avoided if it is painful.[14,18]

Pharmacologic Therapy

For comparative ingredients of nonprescription products, consult the *Compendium of Products for Minor Ailments*—Feminine Care Products: Vaginal Lubricants; Herbal and Natural Health Products: Single Entity.

First-line options consist mainly of vaginal lubricants and moisturizers. The promotion of condoms for safe sex has been a catalyst for the increased use and development of products that enhance vaginal lubrication. Nonmedicated, water-based products are safe for external and internal application. For vaginal dryness, dyspareunia and for comfort during condom use, **vaginal lubricants** can be applied to the penis (on the outside of a condom if one is worn) and the opening of the vagina during intercourse. The lubricants may be water-based (e.g., K-Y Liquid/Jelly, AstroGlide), silicone-based (e.g., Astroglide X Silicone Liquid) or oil-based (e.g., mineral oil, olive oil), but oil-based lubricants must not be used with latex condoms. Specialty lubricants (flavoured, scented) are also available and some may contain ingredients such as methyl salicylate that can provide a warm, stimulating sensation when applied. These additional ingredients may increase the risk of sensitivity reactions to the products. Vaginal lubricants are short-acting and require frequent re-application.[14,15,16,17,18]

Bioadhesive **vaginal moisturizers**, including polycarbophil gels (e.g., Replens) and hyaluronic acid gels (e.g., Gynatrof), attach to the vaginal epithelium and provide water and electrolytes to the cells.

Other vaginal moisturizers contain less adherent but equally effective ingredients such as pectin.[20] Moisturizers have a longer duration of action (2–3 days) than lubricants and are used on a regular basis, not immediately prior to intercourse. Most women will gain maximum relief from symptoms if a vaginal moisturizer is applied every 3 days, but they can be applied more or less frequently if needed.[16,17,19,20] Oil-based products should be avoided because they can be irritating, difficult to remove, and can damage condoms, diaphragms and cervical caps.

Hormonal supplementation with **estrogens** and **progestogens** is an option (see Chapter 79: Menopause and Perimenopause). Supplementation can be in the form of systemic hormone therapy or by vaginal application of estrogen. Estrogen replacement reverses the vaginal changes seen with menopause and relieves symptoms. Vaginal estrogen provides localized benefits with less systemic absorption/effects compared with oral therapy. Concurrent progestogen supplementation is generally not required with low doses of vaginal estrogen.[21] Careful use of systemic hormone supplementation may be of benefit if there are a number of menopausal symptoms to treat, but it is sometimes necessary to apply estrogen vaginally to relieve vaginal symptoms even if the woman is also using systemic hormones.[14,19,22,23] Topical formulations include cream, vaginal tablets or ring-shaped devices that are inserted into the vagina and deliver estrogen over an extended period. For further discussion of pharmacologic therapy for menopause, consult the *Compendium of Therapeutic Choices*: Menopause.

Two small, short-term studies comparing the effects of vaginal application of bioadhesive polymers and estrogen creams on atrophic vaginal changes demonstrated significant improvement in vaginal symptoms with the use of both therapies.[24,25] However, hormonal therapy (conjugated estrogen and dienestrol creams) was significantly superior to bioadhesive polymers for most parameters measured. Similar results were seen in a systematic review that examined vaginal estrogen and nonhormonal vaginal moisturizers for genitourinary symptoms of menopause. Patients with 2 or more symptoms of vulvovaginal atrophy were substantially more improved using vaginal estrogens, but those with just 1 symptom or only minor complaints had similar symptom resolution with either estrogen or nonhormonal moisturizer.[26]

Natural Health Products

Black cohosh has been used in the management of menopausal symptoms including vaginal dryness, although evidence of efficacy is lacking.[27,28] It can cause nausea and headache and is contraindicated in pregnancy and breastfeeding. The usual dose is 3–6 mL per day of a 1:5 tincture in 60% ethanol, or 500–1000 mg dried root or rhizome 2–3 times daily. Black cohosh should be used with caution in women already taking estrogen and there is concern about its ability to potentiate the action of antihypertensive drugs.[28,29,30] Hepatotoxicity after the use of black cohosh supplements has been reported, but analysis revealed that authentic black cohosh was not present in the supplement in most cases. It is still unclear whether there is any connection between black cohosh ingestion and liver toxicity but caution is recommended.[31]

Vulvovaginal Candidiasis

Pathophysiology

The healthy vagina is host to a number of microorganisms including lactobacilli, streptococci, staphylococci, *Gardnerella vaginalis*, *Candida albicans* (and other *Candida* species), anaerobes and *Ureaplasma urealyticum*. The types and numbers of organisms vary due to such factors as age, sexual history, contraceptive method, pregnancy, menstruation, antibiotic use, vaginal trauma (e.g., surgery) and even tampon use.[3,22,32]

Normally, the organisms live in balance in the vaginal environment without adverse effects. When this harmony is disrupted, overproduction of host organisms or colonization by acquired pathogens can occur. These changes set the stage for the development of vaginitis.[32,33,34]

Vaginitis describes a group of conditions that have similar symptoms but a variety of causes (see Table 1).[33,35,36] Treatment for vaginitis is specific to the cause, so the correct diagnosis is important. Self-treatment is recommended for candidiasis only.

Table 1: **Common Causes of Vaginitis**

Cause	Common Symptoms	Vaginal pH
Vulvovaginal candidiasis	Severe pruritus of vulva and vaginal areas Stinging/burning "Cottage cheese" discharge	<4.5
Atrophy	Vaginal discharge Spotting Soreness, burning	7
Bacterial vaginosis[a]	"Fishy" odour Creamy discharge (yellow/grey)	5–6
Trichomoniasis	Frothy, wet discharge Pruritus possible	≥6

[a] Bacterial vaginosis, the most common cause of vaginitis, is a polymicrobial infection involving deficiency of lactobacilli and overgrowth of anaerobes, often (but not always) including *G. vaginalis*.[36]

Goals of Therapy

- Relieve symptoms
- Cure the infection
- Prevent recurrence
- Prevent misdiagnosis and delayed treatment of another condition

Patient Assessment

The decision to recommend treatment for vulvovaginal candidiasis must be made with care. Other forms of vaginitis or sexually transmitted diseases (which can have similar symptoms)[37] and allergic or adverse reactions must be ruled out.

Further evaluation may be required if the patient:[33,34,36,37]

- is prepubertal—vulvovaginal candidiasis is not common in this group and should be assessed
- presents with vaginal symptoms for the first time
- has an underlying illness such as diabetes
- is pregnant
- has a recurrence of vulvovaginal candidiasis within 2 months of the last episode (complicated cases may require alternative drug therapy)
- is immunosuppressed
- is at risk of a sexually transmitted infection (STI), e.g., history of unprotected intercourse, multiple partners, casual sexual encounters.

Potential predisposing factors for vulvovaginal candidiasis include:[32,33,36]

- Chemical irritants, e.g., antiseptics, deodorants, soaps
- Diabetes mellitus
- Diet
- Immunocompromised conditions, e.g., HIV/AIDS
- Medications, e.g., antibiotics, chemotherapy, corticosteroids, hormone therapy, oral contraceptives, tamoxifen
- Menses
- Pregnancy
- Stress
- Synthetic undergarments
- Tight-fitting clothing

Women who have symptoms of vulvovaginal candidiasis and have had a previous diagnosis of candidiasis may be candidates for self-treatment. An assessment approach is outlined in Figure 2.

Nonpharmacologic Therapy

Although there is no specific nonpharmacologic therapy for vulvovaginal candidiasis, preventive measures are suggested for women wishing to avoid recurrences.

After bacterial vaginosis, *Candida* is the second most common cause of vaginitis. Many women experience recurrent or resistant infections and may wish to control their symptoms by using preventive measures. These include modifying potential predisposing factors where possible. There is a lack of evidence to support the use of preventive measures such as clothing and dietary modifications but these may be worth trying in recurrent, resistant cases and generally do not cause adverse outcomes.[33,36]

Good genital hygiene measures are important, to keep the tissue healthy and free from irritation. Vaginal deodorants, douches, harsh soaps and perfumed products for genital use should be avoided, as irritation or allergic reactions may occur. The regular use of products such as panty liners has not been shown to promote the occurrence of vulvovaginal candidiasis.[38]

Tight clothing and synthetic underwear should be avoided, to minimize the development of warm, moist, irritated skin where *Candida* can proliferate. Cotton underwear and loose-fitting undergarments and pants are recommended.[39]

Dietary modifications have been tried with varying success. Although there is not a clear association between *Lactobacillus* in the gut and vulvovaginal candidiasis, consumption of yogurt with active *Lactobacillus* may decrease the incidence of recurrent infections.[40,41] However, data are inconsistent[42] and more studies are required before this is recommended.

Severe dietary restrictions such as yeast-free and sugar-free diets can be tried but are difficult to follow and no data support their efficacy.[32]

Pharmacologic Therapy

Table 3 outlines treatment options for uncomplicated vulvovaginal candidiasis.

For comparative ingredients of nonprescription products, consult the *Compendium of Products for Minor Ailments*—Feminine Care Products: Anti-infectives for Vaginal Fungal Infections.

After the woman has been assessed to verify the likelihood of vulvovaginal candidiasis, self-treatment can be considered. Simple cases (women with a history of diagnosed vaginal candidiasis and no complicating medical conditions who experience infrequent, mild to moderate symptoms)[32,33] can be treated with nonprescription vaginal antifungals. Short-course therapy (1–3 days) is effective and convenient and may increase adherence due to its simplicity; however, results are not achieved more quickly than longer course treatment (6–7 days). If successful, symptoms resolve within 7 days of beginning treatment.

Several vaginal antifungal products are available. Effectiveness rates (70–90%) are similar among antifungal agents and products.[37,49,50] Selection is determined by length of therapy desired, dosage form preferred and the woman's previous experience. Vaginal antifungals are as effective as oral antifungals for uncomplicated vulvovaginal candidiasis.[50]

Providing directions to ensure correct use and adherence with the chosen regimen is important. The intravaginal product is usually administered at bedtime to increase contact time with vaginal tissue and should be continued through menses if it commences during therapy. The complete course of treatment should be used even if symptoms resolve before completion of the doses. If vulvar symptoms are significant, a topical antifungal can be used adjunctively.

Single-dose oral therapy with **fluconazole** 150 mg is an effective option with high patient acceptability and adherence; however, it has not been shown to be superior to vaginal antifungal therapy for uncomplicated cases of vulvovaginal candidiasis.[50] Oral fluconazole is well tolerated but it can cause side effects such as nausea, abdominal discomfort and headache. A single dose of oral fluconazole 150 mg may be considered as an alternative to topical azoles in women who are pregnant,[45] and may also be used in women who are breastfeeding as amounts excreted into breast milk result in lower exposure than with neonatal fluconazole doses.[46]

Boric acid 600 mg capsules inserted intravaginally (*not taken orally*) once or twice daily for 14 days have also shown variable success in the treatment of resistant vaginal candidiasis and may be an option for women who do not respond to other therapies.[43,48,51,52,53]

Probiotics, such as *Lactobacillus* capsules, have been used orally and sometimes vaginally during courses of oral antibiotic therapy, in an attempt to normalize the vaginal flora and prevent vaginal candidiasis.[54] This measure has had little success in decreasing vaginal candidiasis. If a woman wishes to use such a bacterial replacement while taking antibiotics it will not interfere with therapy but the combination will likely not reduce the occurrence of vulvovaginal candidiasis.[54,55]

A small study using probiotics in combination with oral antifungal therapy showed a significant benefit for treating vulvovaginal candidiasis.[56] More research is needed to confirm this result; however, there is no reason to avoid the combination and there may be possible therapeutic benefits.

Patient preference will play a significant role in the final choice of therapy. If nonprescription therapy is ineffective, the patient requires further examination and evaluation. More extensive therapy may be required.

Generally, the woman's sexual partner is not treated for candidal infection; however, in resistant or recurrent vaginal infection it may be appropriate to recommend that the male partner use antifungal cream on his penis daily for 7 days while the woman is receiving treatment.[34] Refraining from sexual intercourse is also recommended during treatment of resistant or recurrent vaginal infection.

Women with persistent symptoms that have not responded to self-treatment and women with severe symptoms or complications (e.g., diabetes, pregnancy, immunosuppression, HIV infection and risk of other STIs) require further assessment. Persistent cases may respond better to a longer course of therapy (6, 7 or 14 days) or a change in the antifungal product. Complicated cases must be treated individually.[36]

More extensive therapy may be required for persistent or recurrent cases of vaginal candidiasis or for women with a greater tendency to develop candidiasis, e.g., immunocompromised patients. Therapy options include switching to an alternative vaginal antifungal agent or longer courses of oral fluconazole or intravaginal antifungal therapy.[32,33,36,43]

For more information on pharmacologic management of vulvovaginal candidiasis, consult the *Compendium of Therapeutic Choices*: Sexually Transmitted Infections.

Prophylaxis of Vulvovaginal Candidiasis

Prophylactic therapy is sometimes prescribed for women with recurrent candidiasis. Single-dose daily or weekly treatments of oral or topical therapy can help reduce recurrence of candidiasis. Resistance is a concern with prophylactic azole treatment, so it should only be used in women with a persistent problem and under the supervision of an appropriate healthcare practitioner. Vaginal boric acid capsules have also been used monthly, e.g. 300 mg vaginally for 5 days at the beginning of each menstrual cycle.[43]

Prevention of Resistance

Reports of azole-resistant candidiasis are of concern.[33,36,37,50] Self-treatment of vaginal infections is among the speculated, yet unproven, causes; misdiagnosis and inappropriate or incomplete courses of therapy may also be contributing to this resistance. Although not substantiated, it is a reminder that the correct diagnosis and appropriate product use is important for proper self-treatment with vaginal antifungals. *Candida glabrata* is one of the organisms found in resistant cases. *C. glabrata* tends to be found in older women who have used azole therapy and who have a complicating underlying illness such as diabetes.[48] Women with recurrent symptoms of vaginitis may require further evaluation and therapy.[36]

Monitoring of Therapy

Monitoring may be difficult for the healthcare practitioner, as women with vaginal candidiasis are often otherwise healthy individuals who may not be regular clients. Ensure that the woman understands that symptoms should resolve within 7 days of the start of treatment, no matter which regimen is used. She should also know what to do in case of adverse effects or unsuccessful treatment (see Table 2).

Table 2: **Monitoring of Therapy for Vulvovaginal Candidiasis**

Symptoms	Monitoring	Endpoint of Therapy	Actions
Vulvovaginal itching and burning, dyspareunia, discharge	Patient: Daily for 7–10 days Healthcare practitioner: After 7 days or next pharmacy visit	Eradication of symptoms	If symptoms still present 1 wk after start of therapy, patient requires further evaluation and therapy.
Increased irritation (may indicate adverse reaction to product or inappropriate therapy)	As above	As above	Increased severity of symptom(s) should be assessed promptly; discontinue therapy and ensure patient receives further evaluation by appropriate healthcare practitioner.

Toxic Shock Syndrome

Pathophysiology

Toxic shock syndrome (TSS) is a severe, life-threatening condition resulting from toxin-producing strains of *Staphylococcus aureus*. Menstrual TSS became a significant concern with the introduction of hyperabsorbable tampons in the late 1970s. These products had the ability to act as a reservoir for *S. aureus*. Since the removal of these products from the market, the rate of TSS has decreased but it still poses a risk to some women. The prevalence of menstrual TSS is 1–5 per 100 000 women of menstrual age per year. It primarily affects young women (15–25 years of age) who use tampons during menses. Studies have demonstrated that many women have antibodies that protect them from experiencing a reaction to the toxin-producing *S. aureus*; however, some women have little innate protection.[57]

Tampon use is a major risk factor for the development of menstrual TSS. Other risk factors include the use of diaphragms, cervical caps and contraceptive sponges.[58]

TSS can evolve clinically in rapid fashion, with a healthy woman becoming very ill in less than 12 hours.

Criteria for diagnosis include:[58,59]

- Temperature >38.9°C
- Hypotension
- Rash with subsequent desquamation, particularly on the hands and feet
- Involvement of at least 3 of the following systems: GI (vomiting, profuse diarrhea), muscular (severe myalgia), mucous membranes (hyperemia), kidney (renal insufficiency), liver (increased enzymes), blood (thrombocytopenia) and CNS (disorientation, confusion).

If left untreated, TSS can be fatal.

The role of the healthcare practitioner is to:

- Educate patients about signs and symptoms of TSS and how to avoid it
- Know how to ask key questions to identify possible TSS, so that it will be evident when urgent referral for medical care is necessary[60]
- Assess patients for possible TSS.

Patient Assessment

If a young woman presents with symptoms including fever, rash, vomiting, profuse diarrhea, dizziness and/or faintness, TSS should be among the diagnoses considered. Ask the patient how the onset of illness relates temporally to her menstrual period, whether she uses tampons and what contraceptive method she uses. If symptoms are consistent with TSS and can be temporally associated with the use of tampons, a diaphragm, cervical cap or contraceptive sponge, the intravaginal product should be removed immediately and she should be referred for immediate medical attention. Treatment of TSS includes aggressive fluid replacement and iv antibiotic therapy.[58,59]

Prevention

Risk reduction is the key to minimizing the occurrence of TSS that is associated with menstruation and/or contraceptive devices. Advise women on proper use of tampons and barrier contraceptives that are associated with an increased risk of TSS (see Toxic Shock Syndrome—What You Need to Know).

Figure 2: **Assessment of Patients with Vulvovaginal Candidiasis**

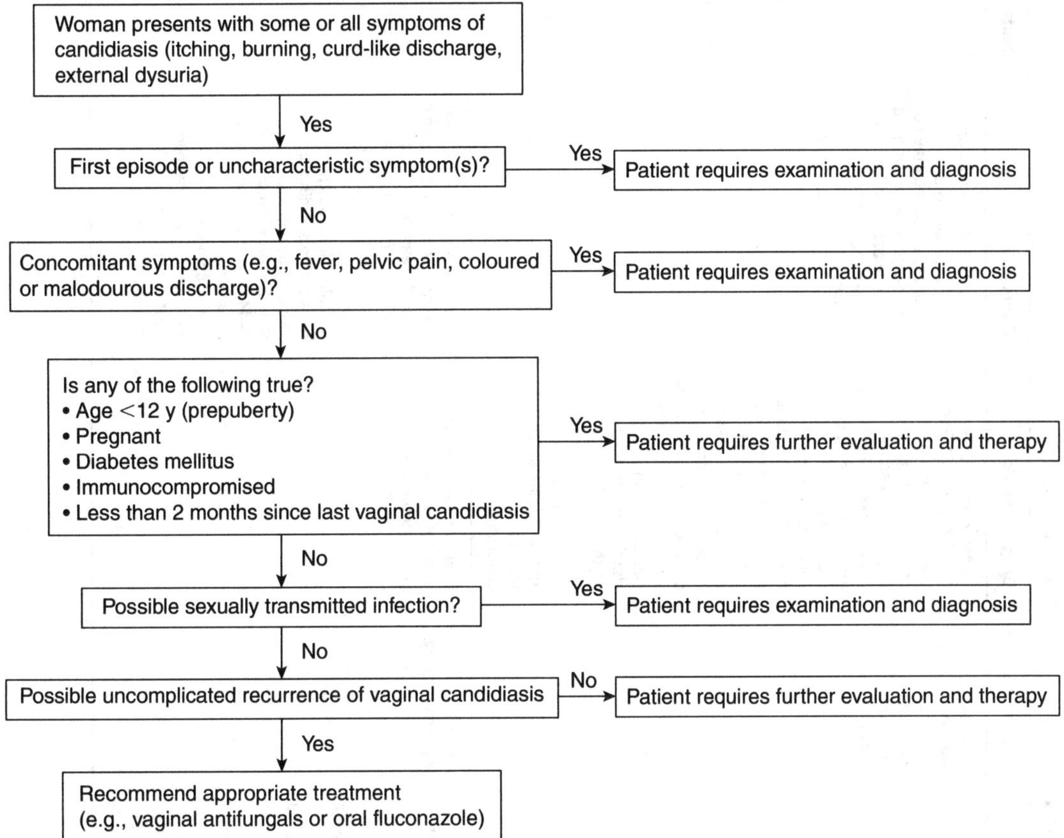

Table 3: **Treatment Options for Uncomplicated Vulvovaginal Candidiasis**[43]

Class	Drug	Dosage	Adverse Effects	Drug Interactions	Comments	Cost[a]
Azole antifungals, oral	*fluconazole* Diflucan One, CanesOral, generics	Uncomplicated infection: 150 mg po as a single dose Recurrent infection:[b] 150 mg every 72 h po × 3 doses; then 150 mg weekly po × 6 months[c]	Headache, nausea, abdominal pain, diarrhea, dyspepsia, dizziness.	Inhibitor of CYP2C9, CYP2C19 and CYP3A4. Decreases serum concentration of clopidogrel's active metabolites and enhances the QT_c-prolonging effect of dronedarone, fluoroquinolones, macrolides, methadone, pimozide, quinine, tricyclic antidepressants and ziprasidone. Decreases metabolism of atorvastatin, benzodiazepines (monitor for increased toxic effects), calcium channel blockers, clarithromycin, colchicine, erythromycin, fentanyl, lovastatin, phenytoin, phosphodiesterase-5 inhibitors, simvastatin, solifenacin and sulfonylureas.	Do not use in girls <12 y.[44] A *single* dose of oral fluconazole 150 mg may be considered as an alternative to topical azoles in women who are pregnant or breastfeeding.[45,46]	$
Azole antifungals, topical	*clotrimazole* Canesten Vaginal, generics	Uncomplicated infection: 200 mg/vaginal tablet: 1 tablet daily pv × 3 days *or* 500 mg/vaginal tablet: 1 tablet pv × single dose *or* 1% vaginal cream: 1 applicatorful daily pv × 7 days *or* 2% vaginal cream: 1 applicatorful daily pv × 3 days *or* 10% vaginal cream: 1 applicatorful pv as a single dose Recurrent infection:[b] intravaginal azole × 7–14 days to achieve mycologic remission, followed by clotrimazole 500 mg/vaginal tablet once monthly × 6 months	Local hypersensitivity.	May diminish therapeutic effect of vaginal progesterone; avoid concomitant use.	Also available as an external cream. External application of topical cream to vulva once or twice daily for up to 7 days may reduce itching and irritation. Menstruation does not necessitate avoiding or stopping treatment. Safe for use in pregnancy; 7–14 days treatment may be necessary. Follow up required if symptoms persist despite treatment or recur within 2 months of onset.	$

Class	Drug	Dosage	Adverse Effects	Drug Interactions	Comments	Cost[a]
	miconazole Monistat, generics	Uncomplicated infection: 100 mg/ovule: 1 ovule daily pv × 7 days *or* 400 mg/ovule: 1 ovule daily pv × 3 days *or* 1200 mg/ovule: 1 ovule pv as a single dose *or* 2% vaginal cream: 1 applicatorful daily pv × 7 days *or* 4% vaginal cream: 1 applicatorful daily pv × 3 days	See clotrimazole.	Topical miconazole may cause increased INRs and bleeding in women taking warfarin. If necessary to use together, consider more frequent INR monitoring, e.g., every 2 days. Caution patient to watch for signs of bleeding. May diminish therapeutic effect of vaginal progesterone; avoid concomitant use.	See clotrimazole.	$
	terconazole Terazol 7, generics	Uncomplicated infection: 0.4% vaginal cream: 1 applicatorful daily pv × 7 days	See clotrimazole.	May diminish therapeutic effect of vaginal progesterone; avoid concomitant use.	Health Canada safety warning: Anaphylaxis and toxic epidermal necrolysis (TEN) have been reported during terconazole therapy. Therapy should be discontinued if anaphylaxis or TEN develops.[47]	$$
Weak acids	*boric acid vaginal capsules*[d]	Recurrent infection:[b] 300–600 mg capsule daily pv × 14 days then maintain with 300 mg capsule pv × 5 days per month beginning the first day of menstrual cycle. Continue for 6 months[c]	Local irritation	None known	Extemporaneously prepared by filling #1 gelatin capsule shell with 300–600 mg boric acid powder USP. NOT to be taken by mouth. Contraindicated in pregnancy. Not first-line therapy, although reported to be >90% effective.[48] Option if first-line agents are unsuccessful or irritating or if infection is resistant.	$$

[a] Cost for specified duration of treatment; includes drug cost only.

[b] Recurrent vulvovaginal candidiasis is defined as 4 or more episodes per year. Treatment for recurrent VVC requires induction therapy followed immediately by maintenance treatment.

[c] Maintenance therapy should continue for 6 months. In cases of recurrence after completed therapy, induction and maintenance treatment should be repeated. Recurrence rates on maintenance treatment are low but can be as high as 50% in women off all therapy.

[d] Extemporaneously compounded preparation.

Dosage adjustment may be required in renal impairment.

Legend: $ <$10 $$ $10–20

Resource Tips

Canadian Women's Health Network. *Keeping your vagina healthy.* Available from: www.rcsf.ca/node/40797.

Our Bodies Ourselves. Available from: www.ourbodiesourselves.org.

Suggested Readings

Boston Women's Health Book Collective. *Our bodies, ourselves*. New York: Simon & Schuster; 2011.

Nurbhai M, Grimshaw J, Watson M et al. Oral versus intra-vaginal imidazole and triazole anti-fungal treatment of uncomplicated vulvovaginal candidiasis (thrush). *Cochrane Database Syst Rev* 2007;4:CD002845.

van Schalkwyk J, Yudin MH; Infectious Disease Committee et al. Vulvovaginitis: screening for and management of trichomoniasis, vulvovaginal candidiasis, and bacterial vaginosis. *J Obstet Gynaecol Can* 2015;37:266-74.

Watson C, Calabretto H. Comprehensive review of conventional and non-conventional methods of management of recurrent vulvovaginal candidiasis. *Aust N Z J Obstet Gynaecol* 2007:47:262-72.

References

1. Alcamo IE, Krumhardt B. The female reproductive system. In: *Barron's anatomy and physiology: the easy way.* 2nd ed. Hauppauge: Barron's Educational Series; 2004. p. 492-500.
2. Newton ER, Piper JM, Shain RN et al. Predictors of the vaginal microflora. *Am J Obstet Gynecol* 2001;184:845-55.
3. Donders GG, Bosmans E, Dekeersmaecker A et al. Pathogenesis of abnormal bacterial vaginal flora. *Am J Obstet Gynecol* 2000;182:872-8.
4. Boston Women's Health Book Collective. Our female bodies: sexual anatomy, reproduction, and the menstrual cycle. In: *Our bodies, ourselves*. New York: Simon & Schuster; 2011. p. 3-29.
5. Boston Women's Health Book Collective. Intro to sexual health. In: *Our bodies, ourselves*. New York: Simon & Schuster; 2011. p. 30-43.
6. Boston Women's Health Book Collective. Sexually transmitted infections. In: *Our bodies, ourselves*. New York: Simon & Schuster; 2011. p. 274-307.
7. Brotman RM, Klebanoff MA, Nansel T et al. Why do women douche? A longitudinal study with two analytic approaches. *Ann Epidemiol* 2008;18:65-73.
8. Rosenberg MJ, Phillips RS, Holmes MD. Vaginal douching. Who and why? *J Reprod Med* 1991;36:753-8.
9. McKee MD, Baquero M, Anderson MR et al. Vaginal douching among Latinas: practices and meaning. *Matern Child Health J* 2009;13:98-106.
10. Grimley DM, Annang L, Foushee HR et al. Vaginal douches and other feminine hygiene products: women's practices and perceptions of product safety. *Matern Child Health J* 2006;10:303-10.
11. Zhang J, Thomas AG, Leybovich E. Vaginal douching and adverse health effects: a meta-analysis. *Am J Public Health* 1997;87:1207-11.
12. Ness RB, Soper DE, Holley RL et al. Douching and endometritis: results from the PID evaluation and clinical health (PEACH) study. *Sex Transm Dis* 2001;28:240-5.
13. Onderdonk AB, Delaney ML, Hinkson PL et al. Quantitative and qualitative effects of douche preparations on vaginal microflora. *Obstet Gynecol* 1992;80:333-8.
14. Palacios S. Managing urogenital atrophy. *Maturitas* 2009;63:315-8.
15. Bachmann GA, Notelovitz M, Kelly SJ et al. Long term nonhormonal treatment of vaginal dryness. *Clin Prac Sexual* 1992;8:3-8.
16. Product Information. *Replens*. Mississauga: Church & Dwight Co; 2016.
17. Hendrix SL. Nonestrogen management of menopausal symptoms. *Endocrinol Metab Clin North Am* 1997;26:379-90.
18. Kelly S. Coping with vaginal dryness. *Clin Prac Sexual* 1992;8:1-4.
19. Pinkerton JV, Stovall DW, Kightlinger RS. Advances in the treatment of menopausal symptoms. *Womens Health (Lond Engl)* 2009;5:361-84.
20. Caswell M, Kane M. Comparison of the moisturization efficacy of two vaginal moisturizers: pectin versus polycarbophil technologies. *J Cosmet Sci* 2002;53:81-7.
21. North American Menopause Society. The 2012 hormone therapy position statement of: the North American Menopause Society. *Menopause* 2012;19:257-71.
22. Reife CM. Office gynecology for the primary care physician, part 1: vaginitis, the Papanicolaou smear, contraception, and postmenopausal estrogen replacement. *Med Clin North Am* 1996;80:299-319.
23. Al-Baghdadi O, Ewies AA. Topical estrogen therapy in the management of postmenopausal vaginal atrophy: an up-to-date overview. *Climacteric* 2009;12:91-105.
24. LE. Comparative study: Replens versus local estrogen in menopausal women. *Fertil Steril* 1994:61:178-80.
25. Bygdeman M., Swahn ML. Replens versus dienestrol cream in the symptomatic treatment of vaginal atrophy in postmenopausal women. *Maturitas* 1996;23:259-63.
26. Rahn DD, Carberry C, Sanses TV et al. Vaginal estrogen for genitourinary syndrome of menopause: a systematic review. *Obstet Gynecol* 2014;124:1147-56.
27. Leach MJ, Moore V. Black cohosh (Cimicifunga spp) for menopausal symptoms. *Cochrane Database Syst Review* 2012;9:CD007244.
28. Natural Medicines Comprehensive Database. *Black cohosh*. Available from: www.naturaldatabase.com. Subscription required.
29. McKenna DJ, Jones K, Humphrey S et al. Black cohosh: efficacy, safety, and use in clinical and preclinical applications. *Altern Ther Health Med* 2001;7:93-100.

30. Hardy ML. Herbs of special interest to women. *J Am Pharm Assoc (Wash)* 2000;40:234-42.
31. Black cohosh products and liver toxicity: update. *Canadian Adverse Reaction Newsletter* 2010;20:1-2. Available from: www.hc-sc.gc.ca/dhp-mps/medeff/bulletin/carn-bcei_v20n1-eng.php#_Black_cohosh_products. Accessed April 27, 2016.
32. Sobel JD, Faro S, Force RW et al. Vulvovaginal candidiasis: epidemiologic, diagnostic, and therapeutic considerations. *Am J Obstet Gynecol* 1998;178:203-11.
33. Sobel JD. Vulvovaginitis. When Candida becomes a problem. *Dermatol Clin* 1998;16:763-8.
34. Hay RJ. The management of superficial candidiasis. *J Am Acad Dermatol* 1999;40:S35-42.
35. Wiesenfeld HC, Macio I. The infrequent use of office-based diagnostic tests for vaginitis. *Am J Obstet Gynecol* 1999;181:39-41.
36. Nyirjesy P. Chronic vulvovaginal candidiasis. *Am Fam Physician* 2001;63:697-702.
37. Ferris DG, Dekle C, Litaker MS. Women's use of over-the-counter antifungal medications for gynecological symptoms. *J Fam Pract* 1996;42:595-600.
38. Farage M, Bramante M, Otaka Y et al. Do panty liners promote vulvovaginal candidiasis or urinary tract infections? A review of the scientific evidence. *Eur J Obstet Gynecol Reprod Biol* 2007;132:8-19.
39. Mayo Clinic. Diseases and Conditions. *Yeast infection (vaginal): prevention.* Available from: www.mayoclinic.org/diseases-conditions/yeast-infection/basics/prevention/con-20035129. Accessed April 29, 2016.
40. Hilton E, Isenberg HD, Alperstein P et al. Ingestion of yogurt containing Lactobacillus acidophilus as prophylaxis for candidal vaginitis. *Ann Intern Med* 1992;116:353-7.
41. Van Kessel K, Assefi N, Marrazzo J et al. Common complementary and alternative therapies for yeast vaginitis and bacterial vaginosis: a systematic review. *Ostet Gynecol Surv* 2003;58:351-8.
42. Shalev E, Battino S, Weiner E et al. Ingestion of yogurt containing Lactobacillus acidophilus compared with pasteurized yogurt as prophylaxis for recurrent candidal vaginitis and bacterial vaginosis. *Arch Fam Med* 1996;5:593-6.
43. van Schalkwyk J, Yudin MH; Infectious Disease Committee et al. Vulvovaginitis: screening for and management of trichomoniasis, vulvovaginal candidiasis, and bacterial vaginosis. *J Obstet Gynaecol Can* 2015;37:266-74.
44. Pfizer Canada Inc. *Diflucan 150* [product monograph]. Available from: www.pfizer.ca/sites/g/files/g10017036/f/201410/DIFLUCAN%282%29.pdf. Accessed April 27, 2016.
45. Molgaard-Nielsen D, Pasternak B and Hviid A. Use of oral fluconazole during pregnancy and the risk of birth defects. *N Engl J Med* 2013;369:830-9.
46. U.S. National Library of Medicine. Drugs and Lactation Database (LactMed). *Fluconazole* CASRN: 86386-73-4. Available from: toxnet.nlm.nih.gov/newtoxnet/lactmed.htm. Accessed April 27, 2016.
47. Government of Canada. Healthy Canadians. *TERAZOL 7 Vaginal Cream 0.4% (terconazole); TERAZOL 3 Dual-Pak—Vaginal Cream 0.8%/ Vaginal Ovules 80 mg (terconazole)—Risk of anaphylaxis and toxic epidermal necrolysis—For health professionals*. Available from: www.healthycanadians.gc.ca/recall-alert-rappel-avis/hc-sc/2014/39911a-eng.php. Accessed April 27, 2016.
48. Jovanovic R, Congema E, Nguyen HT. Antifungal agents vs. boric acid for treating chronic mycotic vulvovaginitis. *J Reprod Med* 1991;36:593-7.
49. Management of patients who have vaginal infections. In: Centers for Disease Control and Prevention. *Sexually transmitted diseases treatment guidelines, 2006*. Available from: www.cdc.gov/std/treatment/2006/rr5511.pdf. Accessed April 27, 2016.
50. Nurbhai M, Grimshaw J, Watson M et al. Oral versus intra-vaginal imidazole and triazole anti-fungal treatment of uncomplicated vulvovaginal candidiasis (thrush). *Cochrane Database Syst Rev* 2007;4:CD002845.
51. Ray D, Goswami R, Dadhwal V et al. Prolonged (3-month) mycological cure rate after boric acid suppositories in diabetic women with vulvovaginal candidiasis. *J Infect* 2007;55:374-7.
52. Sobel JD, Chaim W. Treatment of Torulopsis glabrata vaginitis: retrospective review of boric acid therapy. *Clin Infect Dis* 1997;24:649-52.
53. Watson C, Calabretto H. Comprehensive review of conventional and non-conventional methods of management of recurrent vulvovaginal candidiasis. *Aust N Z J Obstet Gynaecol* 2007;47:262-72.
54. Martinez RC, Seney SL, Summers KL et al. Effect of Lactobacillus rhamnosus GR-1 and Lactobacillus reuteri RC-14 on the ability of Candida albicans to infect cells and induce inflammation. *Microbiol Immunol* 2009;53:487-95.
55. Sobel JD, Wiesenfeld HC, Martens M et al. Maintenance fluconazole therapy for recurrent vulvovaginal candidiasis. *N Engl J Med* 2004:351:876-83.
56. Martinez RC, Franceschini SA, Patta MC et al. Improved treatment of vulvovaginal candidiasis with fluconazole plus probiotic Lactobacillus rhamnosus GR-1 and Lactobacillus reuteri RC-14. *Lett Appl Microbiol* 2009:48:269-74.
57. Parsonnet J, Hansmann MA, Delaney ML et al. Prevalence of toxic shock syndrome toxin 1-producing Staphylococcus aureus and the presence of antibodies to this superantigen in menstruating women. *J Clin Microbiol* 2005;43:4628-34.
58. Goodman B. Body: toxic shocker. *Health* 2005;2:70.
59. Waldvogel F. Staphylococcus aureus (including toxic shock syndrome). In: Mandell GL, Bennett JE, Dolin R, eds. *Mandell, Douglas and Bennett's principles and practice of infectious diseases*. 4th ed. New York: Churchill Livingstone; 1995. p. 1765-7.
60. Issa NC, Thompson RL. Staphylococcal toxic shock syndrome. Suspicion and prevention are keys to control. *Postgrad Med* 2001;110:55-6, 59-62.

Genital Hygiene for Women—What You Need to Know

Tips for good genital hygiene:

- Wash the area around the outside of the vagina daily with warm water and mild soap. Rinse well.
- The inside of the vagina cleanses itself naturally. It is not necessary to douche (rinse out) the inside of the vagina. Douching is not recommended.
- A mild genital odour is normal. You can keep the normal odour to a minimum by washing the genital area each day.

Signs of a possible problem:

You shower, bathe or wash every day but find that you have:

- itching or irritation in the genital area
- an unusual or unpleasant odour
- discomfort (burning, stinging) with sexual intercourse

You may have forgotten to remove a tampon or you may have an infection. See your healthcare provider.

Genital Deodorant Sprays—What You Need to Know

You do not need to use genital deodorant sprays to keep the genital area clean. A daily shower or bath with a mild soap is all that you need. However, if you do decide to use a genital deodorant spray, follow the instructions below.

- Apply the spray to the external genital area only.
- Apply the spray lightly. The propellants in the spray can cause an irritation if you use too much.
- Shake the spray can before using it.
- Hold the can at least 20 cm (8 inches) from your genital area.
- Stop using the spray if it causes burning, irritation or itching. Wash the area with warm water and mild soap. If symptoms don't improve, see your healthcare provider.
- **Do not** spray inside the vagina.
- **Do not** use the spray on irritated or broken skin.
- **Do not** use the spray before sexual intercourse. The spray can irritate the penis or vagina.
- **Do not** insert tampons right after you use the spray.
- **Do not** use the spray when you're wearing menstrual pads. It may cause irritation.

Toxic Shock Syndrome—What You Need to Know

What is toxic shock syndrome?

Toxic shock syndrome (TSS) is a life-threatening infection caused by bacteria that produce deadly toxins. Women who use tampons, contraceptive sponges, diaphragms or cervical caps have a higher risk of developing TSS. A person who has TSS needs immediate medical attention.

What are the symptoms of TSS?

People with TSS can suddenly become very sick, with symptoms such as:

- High fever
- A rash that looks like a sunburn
- Low blood pressure (shock)
- Dizziness or fainting
- Vomiting
- Diarrhea
- Confusion

What you can do to lower your risk of TSS:

- Use sanitary pads instead of tampons during your period, especially overnight.
- If you use tampons, use the lowest absorbency that meets your needs. Change tampons 4–6 times a day and never wear one longer than 8 hours at once.
- Do not use contraceptive sponges, diaphragms or cervical caps during your period.
- If you recently had a baby, do not use tampons for postpartum bleeding. Do not use contraceptive sponges, diaphragms or cervical caps while you are still bleeding. Have a diaphragm or cervical cap refitted 6–8 weeks after you have a baby.

When should you see your healthcare provider?

If you have the symptoms described above and think you might be at risk of TSS, see your healthcare provider right away. TSS is very dangerous. If it is not treated quickly it can be fatal.

Vaginal Douching—What You Need to Know

Some people think that douching keeps a woman's vagina clean and smelling fresh. Some people think that douching can prevent pregnancy. Both of these ideas are wrong!

- You do not need to douche to keep your vagina clean. The vagina has its own natural cleaning system.
- Douching does not work as birth control. You need to use birth control pills or another method to prevent pregnancy.

Douching is not routinely recommended. Talk to your healthcare provider before using a douche.

Is there a safe way to douche?

Find out when it is safe to douche and how to do it properly. Ask your healthcare provider.

Do Not:

- **Do not** douche if you think you have a vaginal infection. Signs of a vaginal infection are irritation around the genitals or an unusual odour. See your healthcare provider to find out if you have a vaginal infection. You will need treatment to cure it.
- **Do not** douche for at least 24 hours before having a vaginal examination.
- **Do not** douche if you are pregnant unless your healthcare provider tells you it is okay.
- **Do not** douche within 6 hours after having sex if you used a vaginal spermicide. Douching can prevent the spermicide from working.

Do:

- Avoid douching or use a douche only occasionally.
- Avoid perfumed products.
- Wash reusable douching equipment with hot water and soap every time you use it.
- Learn how to douche safely. Follow the instructions below.

How do you use a douche safely?

To start:

- If you are using a fountain syringe: Fill the bag with solution. Clamp off the tubing and hang the bag about 30 cm (1 foot) above your hips when you are sitting down. Don't hang it higher than recommended. The pressure will be too high.
- If you are using a bulb syringe: Fill the bag or bottle with solution.

To use the douche:

- Lie on your back in the bathtub with your knees bent.
- Gently insert the plastic tip into the vagina. Slip it in as far as it will go comfortably.
- Release the clamp on the fountain syringe or gently squeeze the bulb syringe to start the flow of fluid into the vagina.
- When enough fluid is inside, you will have a mild feeling of fullness in the pelvic area. Putting in too much fluid or using too much pressure can push fluid into the uterus. This could cause irritation or infection.
- Gently remove the plastic tip from the vagina. Use 1 hand to hold the labia (on either side of the opening to the vagina) together. This will keep the fluid from flowing out of the vagina.

- Release the labia after 1 minute and let the fluid come out.
- Dispose of the douching equipment. If it is reusable, wash it with soap and hot water.

Vaginal Yeast Infection—What You Need to Know

What is a vaginal yeast infection?

A vaginal yeast infection is caused by a group of fungi called *Candida*. Yeast are tiny organisms that live in small numbers on the skin and inside the vagina. The inside of the vagina is usually too acidic for a lot of yeast cells to grow, but if the conditions change, yeast cells may begin to multiply.

Things such as your menstrual period, pregnancy, diabetes, antibiotics and birth control pills can change the environment inside of the vagina so that yeast cells can grow more easily. Moisture and irritation of the vagina may also make it easy for yeast to grow.

What are the signs of a yeast infection?

A yeast infection can be uncomfortable but it is usually not serious. You may have any of the following symptoms:

- Itching and burning in the vagina and around the vulva (the skin that surrounds your vagina)
- A white discharge from the vagina that looks like cottage cheese
- Pain during sexual intercourse
- Swelling of the vulva (you may not be able to notice this)

Vaginal yeast infections are very common. However, the symptoms are similar to other more serious conditions (e.g., some sexually transmitted infections—STIs). Your healthcare provider can tell you if you have a yeast infection or not. See your healthcare provider if:

- you have never had a yeast infection before
- you have diabetes or a weak immune system
- you are pregnant
- you are not sure if you have a yeast infection

Treating yourself for a yeast infection when you have another kind of infection can make the problem worse.

What is the treatment for a yeast infection?

If you have a yeast infection, your healthcare provider may recommend medication that you can buy without a prescription. The treatment will only work if you have a vaginal yeast infection.

Nonprescription medicine for a yeast infection may be a cream or an ovule (tablet) that is inserted inside the vagina using a special applicator. You can also use the cream on the external skin to help reduce itching. The cream will only work if the irritation is caused by the same infection. Another type of treatment is a capsule that you take by mouth. Make sure you know the right way to take your medicine.

How to get the most from the treatment:

- Read the directions completely before using the medication.
- Use the medication exactly as recommended by your healthcare provider.
- If you use medication that you insert into the vagina, use it at bedtime to make sure it stays inside the vagina.
- Continue treatment even if your period starts.

- Use menstrual pads or panty liners to absorb leakage or if your period starts. **Do not** use tampons. They will absorb the medication and decrease its effectiveness.
- Finish all the treatment even if your symptoms go away before it is finished.
- Wash reusable applicators with water and soap after each use. Throw out disposable applicators after 1 use.
- **Do not** share applicators with anyone else.
- Shower or bathe every day to keep the genital area clean.

How to feel more comfortable:

- Wear loose-fitting, cotton underwear and pants.
- Wear pantyhose with a cotton crotch piece.
- Avoid tight-fitting clothes.

Is it okay to have sex while using the treatment?

- Sex is not recommended during your treatment. Your partner could become infected.
- The medicine used in the vagina to treat a yeast infection can decrease the effectiveness of spermicides, condoms, diaphragms and cervical caps. These birth control methods will not work as well during a treatment and for up to 3 days afterward.

When should you see your healthcare provider?

- Before using any nonprescription treatment for the first time. You must be sure that you have a yeast infection before using any medicine.
- If you still have symptoms 7 days after the treatment.
- If the symptoms get worse during treatment.

What can you do to avoid getting another infection?

- Reduce the amount of sugar in your diet.
- Eat unsweetened yogurt.
- Wear cotton underwear.
- Don't wear pantyhose or tights every day.
- Wipe from front to back after using the toilet. This helps to keep bacteria out of your vagina.
- Change out of a wet bathing suit or damp clothes as soon as you can.
- Avoid coloured or perfumed toilet paper, bubble bath, feminine hygiene sprays and deodorant sanitary pads or tampons.

Chapter 85
Dental Conditions

Michelle Bourassa, BPharm, MSc, DMD

This chapter describes the recommended therapy for several dental conditions: dentin hypersensitivity (sensitive teeth), cracked tooth syndrome, postendodontic discomfort, acute alveolar osteitis (dry socket), pulpal inflammation (pulpitis), necrotic pulp, apical periodontitis and periradicular abscess.

For patient assessment, see Figure 1. For an illustration of tooth anatomy, see Chapter 88: Teething, Figure 1.

Dentin Hypersensitivity
Pathophysiology

Dentin is composed of tubules containing fluid that is in contact with the pulp. External stimuli disturb or cause movement of this fluid, thereby activating the nociceptive receptors in the pulp and leading to the perception of pain.[1,2,3,4]

Dentin hypersensitivity, also known as sensitive teeth, is characterized by sharp pain of short duration arising from exposed dentin in response to various stimuli, which cannot be ascribed to any other dental defect or pathology. Stimuli are generally chemical (e.g., acid), thermal (e.g., cold or hot drinks or food, exposure to air), mechanical (e.g., toothbrush, probe, fingernails) or osmotic (e.g., sugar, gel) in nature. Dentin hypersensitivity may be the result of root denudation (exposure) due to gingival recession from toothbrush abrasion. Exposed dentin secondary to the loss of enamel in the crown area or at the radicular level may be another cause of dentin hypersensitivity. Consumption of acidic foods and beverages combined with vigorous tooth brushing with an abrasive toothpaste can lead to progressive erosion. Other causes of dentin hypersensitivity include periodontal disease or surgery, erosion or abfraction (a noncarious lesion) occurring at the cementoenamel junction on the lingual or buccal side of the tooth.

The prevalence of dentin hypersensitivity falls between 4% and 74% of adults.[5] Dentin hypersensitivity is encountered more often in young individuals with root exposure due to rapid gingival recession. Maxillary teeth seem to be more frequently affected, and the buccal surface is the site most often involved.[6]

Prevention

Prevention plays an important role in managing this condition.[1,3,4,7,8] If dentin hypersensitivity occurs, advise patients to brush their teeth properly, to limit their intake of acidic foods and beverages, and to avoid brushing within 2 hours of consuming acidic foods and beverages.[5] Rinsing with water following intake of acidic foods or drinks may also be beneficial. Encourage regular periodontal exams, with supportive therapy when indicated.

Treatment

Evidence is insufficient to permit the development of evidence-based guidelines for the treatment of dentin hypersensitivity. The following recommendations are based on clinical experience.[9]

Chemical or physical blockade of the patent dentinal tubules can prevent movement of the fluid they contain. Physical blockade can be achieved with the application of fluoride varnishes, sealants, resins, glass ionomer cements or soft tissue grafts. Chemical desensitization occurs when pulpal nociceptor activity is blocked or the tubules are occluded with a protein precipitate, a crystallized oxalate deposit or potassium formulations.

Desensitizing toothpastes exert their effect chemically and are the mainstay of treatment of this condition. Recommend the use of a desensitizing toothpaste that contains potassium salts, oxalate salts, citrate salts, strontium salts, stannous fluoride or arginine, applied with a soft or ultra-soft toothbrush. Several commercially available products have received the Canadian Dental Association (CDA) seal of approval (e.g., Sensodyne products, Colgate sensitive products, Crest Pro-health products).[10,11] Advise patients that it may take up to 2 weeks to achieve benefit from a desensitizing agent.[4]

Dental professionals may also apply highly concentrated fluoride preparations (varnishes or solutions) or oxalate salt preparations, which often provide pain relief soon after administration. In resistant or recurrent cases, the dentist may employ physical techniques to achieve a fast and more sustained resolution of the pain.

For comparative ingredients of nonprescription products, consult the *Compendium of Products for Minor Ailments*—Dental Products: Dentifrices.

Cracked Tooth Syndrome

Pathophysiology

Sudden pain that occurs on biting and ceases after the pressure is withdrawn is a classic sign of a cracked tooth.[3,12,13] The pain may be sharp, intense and of short duration, and may occur when eating or when biting on an object (e.g., pencil). Although the usual stimulus is biting, some patients experience sensitivity to thermal changes (particularly cold) or upon exposure to sweets.[14] The pain may originate from the pulp or the periodontium.

A cracked tooth can occur as a result of trauma, extensive filling, or when an intact tooth with an opposing cusp is occluding against a marginal ridge or a foreign body such as a lingual barbell typically worn by individuals with tongue piercings.

Treatment

Various restorative techniques are used to treat cracked teeth.[15] The prognosis depends on the type and the extent of the crack. A poor prognosis is associated with fractures occurring below the level of the alveolar bone; in these cases extraction is usually required.

Postendodontic Discomfort

Pathophysiology

Discomfort following endodontic treatment (root canal) is common. A root canal is a procedure used to eliminate pulpal and periapical diseases. Root canals involve mechanical and biochemical debridement and treatment of the canal system of the affected tooth. The apical extrusion of debris produced during the procedure may lead to apical periodontitis.

Treatment

Usually the pain is mild and requires no medication, or can be relieved by mild analgesics (e.g., **acetaminophen, ibuprofen**).[2,3] The results of a systematic review suggest that the combination of acetaminophen and ibuprofen were most effective for acute pain relief.[16] The discomfort generally subsides within a few days. On occasion, an acute periapical abscess may occur, causing swelling and pain. Advise the patient to consult a dentist immediately. Appropriate treatment includes draining the abscess through the canal or by incision, and **NSAIDs** or a combination of analgesics for pain control. If signs of systemic infection are present, the patient may require oral antibiotic therapy.

For more information regarding analgesics for dental pain and antibacterial regimens for orofacial infections, consult the *Compendium of Pharmaceuticals and Specialities*: Drugs in Dentistry.

Acute Alveolar Osteitis ("Dry Socket")

Pathophysiology

Approximately 1–4% of patients undergoing surgical extraction of an impacted third molar (wisdom tooth) will experience a painful complication known as acute alveolar osteitis.[3,17] In this condition, the healing process is delayed and the bone of the socket is exposed and extremely sensitive. The moderate to severe pain that generally develops 1–3 days after the procedure is usually dull and throbbing, and often radiates to the ear. The extraction site may have a foul odour and impart a bad taste in the mouth. Regional lymphadenitis may be seen in some patients. Although rare, fever may accompany this condition and is self-limiting if untreated. The etiology is not completely understood but increased fibrinolytic activity at the surgical site is suspected. Some risk factors have been identified such as gender (female more than male), site of extraction, traumatic extractions, age and smoking.[18]

Treatment

If patients experience acute alveolar osteitis, advise them to consult a dentist as soon as possible. Treatment generally consists of gentle irrigation of the site with normal saline followed by the insertion of an iodoform gauze soaked with **eugenol** for pain relief. The dressing may be changed every second to third day for 3–6 days if the pain persists.

Even without intervention, the patient would not have any sequelae other than pain throughout the healing period. Provide patients with adequate systemic analgesia such as an **NSAID**, **acetaminophen with codeine** or another opioid or opioid combination if more appropriate. The results of a systematic review suggest that the combination of acetaminophen and ibuprofen were most effective for acute pain relief.[16]

For more information regarding analgesics for dental pain, consult the *Compendium of Pharmaceuticals and Specialities*: Drugs in Dentistry.

Pulpal Inflammation (Pulpitis)

The initial presentation of pulpitis is usually reversible; if untreated it may progress to an irreversible pulpitis. Reversibility may be preserved if the cause is rapidly removed. Common causes include:[2,8]

- Caries
- Recent or faulty restoration (filling)
- Trauma
- Exposed tubules
- Periodontal scaling

Pathophysiology

When the pulp is exposed to a noxious stimulus, an inflammatory reaction is induced with classic manifestations of:

- Vasodilation
- Increased intracellular tissue pressure
- Increase in cellular infiltrates
- Increased levels of mediators such as prostaglandins and neuropeptides

Although initially reversible (enough reparative cells remain in the pulp to allow recovery), the condition could continue to degenerate and may require endodontic therapy to stop the process.[2,3,7,8,19,20] The main symptom of reversible pulpitis is sensitivity or mild pain of brief duration after exposure to cold, sweets and sometimes heat. The pain subsides upon removal of the stimulus. There is no spontaneous pain nor pain on biting. Usually a cause can be identified on dental examination. The type of insult and the patient's age are important factors that affect whether the pulp can recover. With aging, the ability of the pulp to repair itself diminishes.

With irreversible pulpitis, the pain can occur spontaneously and it may be more prolonged on exposure to the initial stimulus. Irreversible pulpitis results from significant pulpal injury (e.g., from caries, trauma or cumulative effect of multiple restorations) and does not respond to removal of the causative factor.[2,7]

Treatment

Reversible pulpitis is treated by correcting the cause.[2,3,7,8,21] If patients experience discomfort following a recent restoration or periodontal scaling, reassure them that the symptoms should diminish and disappear over a 3-month period. Symptomatic treatment (e.g., **desensitizing toothpaste**) may help, and symptoms should be monitored. If the discomfort worsens or lasts longer than 3 months, the patient should seek dental advice.

Caries is treated by removing the decay and placing a filling to occlude the dentinal tubules (see Chapter 88: Teething). If the cavity is extensive and the exposed pulp is carious, the pulpitis is classified as irreversible. In these cases the treatment of choice is a root canal.

In some cases, extraction may be necessary. Pain is usually controlled with nonprescription analgesics (e.g., **acetaminophen**, **ibuprofen** or **naproxen sodium**), but may require prescription doses of **NSAIDs**.[3,21] The results of a systematic review suggest that the combination of acetaminophen and ibuprofen were most effective for acute pain relief.[16]

There is insufficient evidence to support the benefits of antibiotics for irreversible pulpitis.[22]

For comparative ingredients of nonprescription products, consult the *Compendium of Products for Minor Ailments*—Analgesic Products: Internal Analgesics and Antipyretics.

Pulp Necrosis

Pathophysiology

Pulp necrosis may result when inflamed pulp degenerates further; causes are the same as those seen with irreversible pulpitis. At this stage, the reparative potential of the pulp is totally absent and the pulp lacks viable tissue. Inflammation of the periapical tissue may be associated with pulp necrosis.[2,8]

Often, the patient has had a previous episode of symptoms related to irreversible pulpitis. Necrotic pulp does not respond to stimuli such as cold or heat. The patient may feel spontaneous dull and throbbing pain that worsens on lying down or that is stimulated by biting. The latter suggests inflammation of the periapical tissues.[2,8]

Treatment

The appropriate treatment options are extraction or endodontic therapy (root canal). An **NSAID** or mild **analgesic** may be prescribed by the dentist for a few days for possible postoperative pain or discomfort.[2] The results of a systematic review suggest that the combination of acetaminophen and ibuprofen were most effective for acute pain relief.[16]

Acute Apical Periodontitis

Pathophysiology

Acute apical periodontitis is moderate to severe inflammation of the periodontal tissues located near the apex of a tooth. Although it is most frequently associated with a pulpal condition (reversible or irreversible inflamed or necrotic pulp), nonpulpal causes have been identified such as trauma or bruxism (grinding or clenching the upper and lower teeth together, often while sleeping). The periapical tissues show a marked inflammatory response with vasodilation and polymorphonuclear lymphocyte infiltration.[2,21]

Treatment

Acute apical periodontitis is treated by tooth extraction or endodontic therapy. If endodontic treatment is chosen, canal debridement and drainage should be performed by a dentist on an emergency basis. Generally, the drainage provides partial to complete relief of the pain. Some discomfort may persist for a few days and can be managed with a mild **analgesic** or an **NSAID**. The results of a systematic review suggest that the combination of acetaminophen and ibuprofen were most effective for acute pain relief.[16] In more severe cases, an opioid analgesic may be required, but use should be limited to a short period of time.[2,21]

For more information regarding analgesics for dental pain, consult the *Compendium of Pharmaceuticals and Specialties*: Drugs in Dentistry.

Chronic Apical Periodontitis

Pathophysiology

Chronic apical periodontitis is a type of granuloma with inflammation around the tooth's root tip. Some patients may be completely asymptomatic and unaware of the problem while others may experience mild sensitivity on biting or percussion (i.e., the dentist may test by tapping on the tooth).[2,21] The condition is usually a low-grade, long-standing response to canal bacteria and irritants and presents as apical radiolucency on x-ray, which is often when the condition is discovered. The cause is usually necrotic pulp, but chronic apical periodontitis may be associated with other conditions including central giant cell granuloma or cemental dysplasia.[2,21]

Treatment

Chronic apical periodontitis can be treated with the same modalities as necrotic pulp (extraction or root canal). Analgesics can relieve some potential post-procedural discomfort and usually antibiotics are not indicated.[2,21]

Acute Periradicular Abscess

Pathophysiology

Acute periradicular abscess (also known as apical abscess) is an infection resulting from bacterial invasion of the ligament space, surrounding the root and/or apex of the tooth. Patients experience severe pain when biting or palpating the affected tooth.[2] In severe cases, the patient may present with fever, swelling of the tissues adjacent to the tooth, and tenderness of the cervical and submandibular lymph nodes.[23]

Treatment

The gold standard of therapy is to remove the cause of infection and involves primarily establishing drainage through the root canal by a dentist on an emergency basis.[2,8,21] If swelling is severe, drainage of pus through the fluctuant tissue may be required. Consider antibiotic therapy if the patient demonstrates signs of systemic infection or is immunocompromised.

If swelling increases, incision and drainage may be required. If extraoral (i.e., outside the mouth) swelling occurs, the patient requires an immediate dental consultation. If a dentist is not available, the patient should seek medical assistance. Treatment with an antibiotic (e.g., amoxicillin or penicillin, clindamycin, moxifloxacin or a combination of metronidazole with amoxicillin) is required.[2,23,24] If not treated promptly, the infection may spread to surrounding tissues and structures, spread throughout the body and serious complications may arise. Severe cases have required drainage of extraoral pus.[24,25]

For more information regarding antibacterial regimens for orofacial infections, consult the *Compendium of Pharmaceuticals and Specialties*: Drugs in Dentistry.

Suppurative Apical Periodontitis or Chronic Periradicular Abscess

Pathophysiology

Suppurative apical periodontitis (also known as chronic periradicular abscess) refers to an apical lesion that has established drainage through a sinus tract.[8,26] The patient may report a “gumboil” or a foul taste in the mouth. The culprit tooth is usually asymptomatic. Gentle pressure on the gum may expel pus from the fistula.[8,24,26] The cause of this condition is usually necrotic pulp.

Treatment

The usual treatment of suppurative apical periodontitis is tooth extraction or a root canal procedure. Analgesics can relieve potential postprocedural discomfort and antibiotics are not usually indicated.[2]

Figure 1: **Assessment of Patients with Dental Conditions**

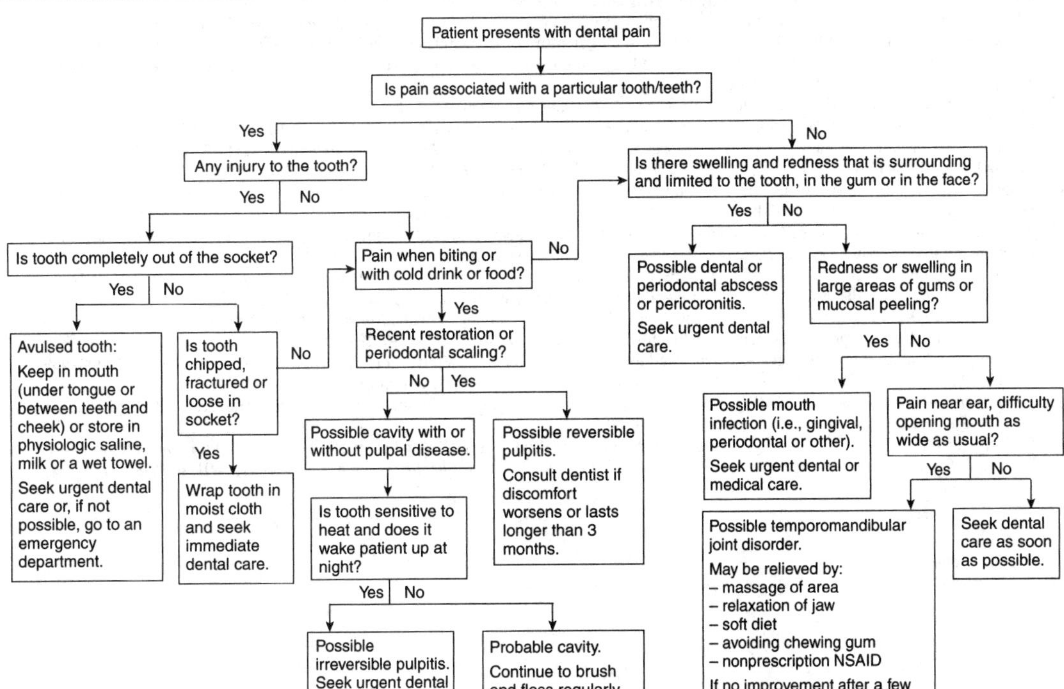

Resource Tips

American Dental Association. *Mouth Healthy: A-Z topics*. Available from: www.mouthhealthy.org.

Canadian Dental Association. *Your oral health*. Available from: www.cda-adc.ca/en/oral_health/index.asp.

Suggested Readings

Miglani S, Aggarwal V, Ahuja B. Dentin hypersensitivity: recent trends in management. *J Conserv Dent* 2010;13:218-24.

Rossman LE, Hasselgren G, Wolcott JF. Diagnosis and management of orafacial dental pain emergencies. In: Cohen S, Hargreaves KM, eds. *Pathways of the pulp*. 9th ed. St. Louis: Mosby Elsevier; 2006. p. 40-58.

References

1. West NX. Dentine hypersensitivity: preventive and therapeutic approaches to treatment. *Periodontol 2000* 2008;48:31-41.
2. Berman LH, Hartwell GR. Diagnosis. In: Cohen S, Hargreaves KM, eds. *Pathways of the pulp*. 9th ed. St. Louis: Mosby Elsevier; 2006. p.2-39.
3. Holland GR. Management of dental pain. In: Lund JP, ed. *Orofacial pain: from basic science to clinical management*. Chicago: Quintessence Pub.; 2001. p. 211-20.
4. Somerman M. Desensitizing agents. In: *ADA/PDR guide to dental therapeutics*. 5th ed. Chicago: American Dental Association; 2009. p. 339-50.
5. Miglani S, Aggarwal V, Ahuja B. Dentin hypersensitivity: recent trends in management. *J Conserv Dent* 2010;13:218-24.
6. Splieth CH, Tachou A. Epidemiology of dentin hypersensitivity. *Clin Oral Investig* 2013;17:S3-8.
7. Bender IB. Pulpal pain diagnosis–a review. *J Endod* 2000;26:175-9.

8. Rossman LE, Hasselgren G, Wolcott JF. Diagnosis and management of orafacial dental pain emergencies. In: Cohen S, Hargreaves KM, eds. *Pathways of the pulp*. 9th ed. St. Louis: Mosby Elsevier; 2006. p. 40-58.
9. Al-Sabbagh M, Harrison E, Thomas MV. Patient-applied treatment of dentinal hypersensitivity. *Dent Clin North Am* 2009;53:61-70.
10. Davies M, Paice EM, Jones SB et al. Efficacy of desensitizing dentifrices to occlude dentinal tubules. *Eur J Oral Sci* 2011;119:497-503.
11. Maldupa I, Brinkmane A, Rendeniece I et al. Evidence based toothpaste classification, according to certain characteristics of their chemical composition. *Stomatologija* 2012;14:12-22.
12. Lynch CD, McConnell RJ. The cracked tooth syndrome. *J Can Dent Assoc* 2002;68:470-5.
13. Banerje S, Mehta SB, Millar BJ. Cracked tooth syndrome. Part 1: aetiology and diagnosis. *Br Dent J* 2010;208:459-63.
14. Mathew S, Thangavel B, Mathew CA et al. Diagnosis of cracked tooth syndrome. *J Pharm Bioallied Sci* 2012;4:S242-4.
15. Lubisich EB, Hilton TJ, Ferracane J. Cracked teeth: a review of the literature. *J Esthet Restor Dent* 2010;22:158-67.
16. Moore RA, Wiffen PJ, Derry S et al. Non-prescription (OTC) oral analgesics for acute pain- an overview of Cochrane reviews. *Cochrane Database Syst Rev* 2015;11:CD010794.
17. Noroozi AR, Philbert RF. Modern concepts in understanding and management of the "dry socket" syndrome: comprehensive review of the literature. *Oral Surg Oral Med Oral Pathol Oral Radiol Endod* 2009;107:30-5.
18. Kolokythas A, Olech E, Miloro M. Alveolar osteitis: a comprehensive review of concepts and controversies. *Int J Dent* 2010;2010:249073.
19. Germain L. Differential diagnosis of toothache pain. Part 1, odontogenic etiologies. *Dent Today* 2012;31:92-7.
20. McClannahan SB, Baisden MK, Bowles WR. Endodontic diagnostic terminology update. *Northwest Dent* 2011;90:25-7.
21. Carrotte P. Endodontics: Part 3. Treatment of endodontic emergencies. *Br Dent J* 2004;197:299-305.
22. Fedorowicz Z, van Zuuren EJ, Farman AG et al. Antibiotic use for irreversible pulpitis. *Cochrane Database Syst Rev* 2013;12:CD004969.
23. Siqueira JF, Rocas IN. Microbiology and treatment of acute apical abscesses. *Clin Microbiol Rev* 2013;26:255-73.
24. Baumgartner JC, Hutter JW, Siquiera JF. Endodontic microbiology and treatment of infections. In: Cohen S, Hargreaves KM, eds. *Pathways of the pulp*. 9th ed. St. Louis: Mosby Elsevier; 2006. p. 580-609.
25. Furst IM, Ersil P, Caminiti M. A rare complication of tooth abscess–Ludwig's angina and mediastinitis. *J Can Dent Assoc* 2001;67:324-7.
26. Roberts G, Scully C, Shotts R. Dental emergencies. In: Scully C, ed. *ABC of oral health*. London: BMJ Books; 2001. p. 35-8.

Urgent Tooth Problems—What You Need to Know

See your dentist immediately if you have any of the following problems:

- A cracked or chipped tooth
- A tooth that is knocked out or loose
- A tooth that is sensitive to cold or heat or biting, or that wakes you up at night with pain
- Swelling and redness around one tooth, in the gums or even in the face
- Peeling gums

What to do until you see the dentist:

Cracked or chipped tooth

- Keep the tooth pieces in a moist cloth and take them with you to see the dentist.

Tooth knocked out or loose

- If the whole tooth is loose or out of its socket, keep it in your mouth, under your tongue or between your teeth and cheek.
- You can also store the tooth in milk, a wet towel or a saline solution. Make saline solution by adding 1.25 mL (one-quarter teaspoon) of table salt to 250 mL (1 cup) of water. If nothing else is available, immerse the tooth in your saliva, and store it in a container.
- If you can't see a dentist right away, go to a medical emergency department.

Chapter 86
Oral Hygiene, Dental Plaque and Caries

Michelle Bourassa, BPharm, MSc, DMD

Dental Plaque

Pathophysiology

Dental plaque is defined as a gelatinous deposit that adheres to the tooth surfaces, fillings or dental prostheses and is not removed by rinsing with water. Plaque is composed of aerobic and anaerobic bacteria in a matrix of bacterial or salivary glycoproteins and dextrans. Dental plaque is also referred to as "biofilm".[1,2] Deposition of plaque may occur on all surfaces of the teeth and may be recognizable within 24 hours. The area with the highest predilection for accumulation of plaque is the interproximal space of the molars and premolars, followed by the interproximal space of the anteriors and finally by the facial surfaces of the molars and premolars. Other areas of accumulation are the gingival margins along with pits and fissures.[2] For an illustration of dental anatomy, see Chapter 88: Teething, Figure 1.

When freshly cleaned teeth are exposed to saliva, a layer of salivary glycoproteins adheres to the surface of the teeth. Oral microorganisms can attach to the glycoproteins or to the tooth enamel itself. Sticky dextrans and levans produced by the bacteria constitute the matrix that permits colonization and aggregation of more bacteria. Initially, plaque is made of gram-positive cocci and rods; with time, gram-negative rods and spirochetes join the existing microorganisms and the volume of plaque increases.[3]

Dental plaque can be divided into 2 types based on its location relative to the gum (supragingival or subgingival). Supragingival plaque is usually white to yellow in colour. When present in small amounts, it can be detected around the collar of the tooth with a probe or disclosing solution. When the volume is large, the eye can easily identify it.[3,4]

Subgingival plaque is a key factor in the development of periodontal diseases. On the tooth surface of subgingival plaque, the initial constituents and stages of plaque formation may be the same as for supragingival plaque. The plaque surface adjacent to the gingiva is, however, somewhat different. The structure appears less dense; the matrix is reduced and bacteria are more free.

Microbiology of Plaque

The microbiology of dental plaque varies greatly on an individual basis and from one area to another in the same mouth. Gram-positive bacteria predominate and are mainly from the *Streptococcus* and *Actinomyces* species. Gram-negative organisms such as *Veillonella* and *Neisseria* are also found, to a lesser extent. Facultative anaerobic streptococci represent a significant proportion of bacteria encountered in plaque. The types and relative amounts of microorganisms evolve with time, eventually producing an ecologic environment favouring anaerobes.[3,5,6,7] With progression of periodontal disease, anaerobic gram-negative bacilli become more dominant.[3,4]

Consequences of Plaque

The presence of plaque plays an important role in 2 pathologic processes in the mouth, the development of caries (cavities) and periodontal diseases.[4,5,8,9] Therefore, effective removal of supragingival dental plaque on a continuous daily schedule is essential to dental and periodontal health throughout life.[10] Subgingival plaque can be removed only with a professional cleaning.

Cariogenic Effect

Dietary sucrose increases plaque formation and the resulting plaque is more cariogenic. Studies have shown that ingestion of sucrose favours the colonization and aggregation of microorganisms on teeth and prosthetic devices. *Streptococcus mutans* and lactobacilli play a primary role in cariogenic plaque. They act by metabolizing sucrose into an acid that causes demineralization of the enamel and, with time, tooth decay.[5,8]

Periopathogenic Effect

To initiate and maintain periodontal disease, plaque has to be present at the tooth surface. The pathogenic role of dental plaque is described in Chapter 87: Periodontal Conditions: Gingivitis and Periodontitis.

Calculus

Dental calculus (tartar) is defined as the calcification of existing plaque deposits on the teeth or any other hard surface in the mouth (fillings, fixed or removable prostheses).[3] It can be located supragingivally or subgingivally. When visible, it has a yellowish colour that may be darkened by dietary or exogenous pigmentation (e.g., coffee, tea, red wine, smoking). Its formation starts in areas close to the salivary gland openings, i.e., lingual (tongue) side of the lower incisors and the buccal (cheek) side of the upper molars. When located under the margin of the gingiva, the calculus often takes on a dark colour and is very adherent to the cementum of the tooth.

The surface of the calculus is usually rough and favours plaque retention, subsequently leading to irritation and periodontal inflammation.

The presence of dental plaque is a prerequisite for calculus formation. In most patients, calcification occurs within 48 hours in newly formed plaque. The amount of calculus being formed varies greatly from one individual to another, and depends on many factors such as the composition of saliva and the concentration of certain enzymes. Therefore, control of calculus formation begins with controlling plaque formation. Calculus requires removal by a professional, with ultrasonic, sonic or sharp instruments. In contrast, supragingival plaque can be controlled with good oral hygiene.

Plaque Control

Mechanical Methods

Mechanical removal of plaque may be achieved by brushing the teeth after every meal and at bedtime, and by flossing once a day, preferably at bedtime. Plaque removal is more effective when toothpaste is used;[8,9] fluoride-containing toothpaste is recommended for caries prevention. In some patients, tools such as interproximal or interspace single-tufted brushes, dental sticks (wood or plastic), handles with a rubber tip or wide spongy floss (e.g., Superfloss) may be helpful for removing plaque from areas difficult to access with a toothbrush and floss.[2,9,11] These devices can also be useful for patients with orthodontic braces, dental implants, wide spaces between teeth or fixed dental prostheses such as bridge work.

Irrigating devices (e.g., dental water flosser, irrigation syringe) can also be useful for patients with bridges or orthodontic appliances, after oral surgery, or for patients who do not have good manual dexterity. They can remove food debris and possibly some plaque.[12] Therefore, they can be recommended as adjunctive devices only. Some studies suggest that a greater reduction of gingival inflammation may result from subgingival irrigation with chlorhexidine by the dentist.[13,14]

Table 1 presents a nonexhaustive list of devices and their role in removing plaque.

Table 1: **Dental Cleaning Devices**[9,15,16]

Device	Role
Toothbrush	Removes plaque from buccal (cheek) and lingual (tongue) sides and occlusal (biting) surfaces of the teeth
Dental floss	Removes plaque from interproximal surfaces (between the teeth)
Interdental brush, interproximal brush Toothpick Rubber tip	Removes plaque from concave root surfaces when attachment loss (detachment of the gingiva due to bone loss) is present, and from other difficult-to-reach areas
Stimulator (rod curved at one end with a sharp rubber tip)	Removes plaque by applying contouring pressure to hyperplastic gingival papillae (noninflammatory enlargement of the gingivae)[11]

Tooth Brushing

The most recommended tooth brushing technique is the sulcular method, which focuses on removal of the plaque adjacent to and within the sulcus (see Chapter 88: Teething).[8,14,16] It is a very effective method for the removal of plaque, particularly from the gingival area of the tooth and gingival crevice (sulcus). The minimum brushing time required to effectively remove plaque is 2–3 minutes.[8,15,17] The tongue should be brushed as well. The technique is described in detail in the patient information section at the end of the chapter.

Toothbrushes

A suitable toothbrush is one with soft or extra-soft, flexible, rounded bristles that can penetrate into the gingival crevice to effectively remove plaque without causing trauma to soft and hard tissues. It should also be small enough to easily reach all areas of the mouth.[13,14,16] Toothbrush replacement is recommended every 3 months, or as soon as the bristles start to splay.[16] Studies have found no consistent superiority of one manual toothbrush over another for either plaque removal or gingival inflammation reduction.[2,15]

Mechanical/powered toothbrushes simulate manual tooth brushing in various ways, such as side-to-side or circular motion. A Cochrane systematic review found that powered toothbrushes are superior to manual toothbrushes at removing plaque and reducing gingival inflammation, and are not more likely to cause injuries to gingivae. Long-term benefits of this for dental health are unclear.[10,18] The use of a mechanical brush may be beneficial when manual technique has failed, for patients with limited dexterity or for patients with orthodontic appliances.[2,13,15]

Dentifrices

Dentifrices (toothpastes, gels, pastes) aid in:[17]

- Minimizing the accumulation of plaque and tartar
- Strengthening the enamel against caries (fluoride-containing products)
- Cleaning the teeth by removing food debris and some stains
- Freshening the mouth.

Dentifrices contain various combinations of the ingredients found in Table 2.[19]

Toothpaste with an attractive appearance and flavour encourages prolonged and regular use.[17] The market is overwhelmed with toothbrushes and toothpastes. Products that have obtained the Canadian Dental Association (CDA) seal meet the needs of most patients. Particular needs should be discussed with the patient's dentist or dental hygienist.

For comparative ingredients of nonprescription products, consult the *Compendium of Products for Minor Ailments*—Dental Products: Dentifrices.

Table 2: **Ingredients of Toothpastes**[2,19]

Ingredients	Role	Comments
Detergents, e.g., sodium lauryl sulfate, sodium-N-lauryl sarcosinate	Foaming action may increase the solubility of plaque during brushing	Adverse effects (e.g., development of aphthous ulcers) in small percentage of patients may necessitate switching to a toothpaste without these agents.
Flavouring agents, e.g., xylitol, sweetening agents	Improve palatability	Xylitol, in combination with fluoride in toothpaste, may also decrease tooth decay.[20]
Humectants, e.g., glycerol, propylene glycol, sorbitol	Prevent toothpaste from drying out	
Thickening agents, e.g., mineral colloids, natural gums, seaweed colloids, synthetic celluloses	Stabilize the formulation	
Abrasive agents, e.g., calcium carbonate, dehydrated silica gels, hydrated aluminum oxides, magnesium carbonate, phosphate salts	Remove debris and residual stains; whiten teeth	May cause burning sensation, drying of mucous membranes, taste alteration, gingival abrasion or enamel erosion. Tooth powders contain about 95% abrasives compared with 20–40% in toothpastes and gels.
Peroxides, sodium triphosphate	Whiteners	May work by breaking down pigments that accumulate on or in the tooth enamel. Some stains cannot be removed by toothpastes containing these whiteners, e.g., tetracycline staining, mottling.
Pyrophosphates, zinc citrate	Prevent supragingival calculus (tartar) formation. Do not affect subgingival or existing calculus.	Mechanism not established. One hypothesis is the reduction of crystal growth on the tooth surface through chelation of cations.
Stannous fluoride, triclosan, zinc citrate	Prevent gingival inflammation	Reduce plaque accumulation through antibacterial and anti-inflammatory activity.[21] Stannous fluoride (and other toothpaste ingredients) may interact with chlorhexidine mouthwash, rendering both agents less effective. Use them 30 min apart.
Fluoride	Reduces caries formation	At a concentration of 1000–1100 ppm, fluoride makes enamel more resistant to demineralization. Excess amounts can cause fluorosis (see Caries: Fluoride).

Flossing

Dental floss and tape, waxed or unwaxed, are equally effective for cleaning proximal surfaces. Individual factors such as contacts (where 2 adjacent teeth come together), restorations, tooth alignment and manual dexterity determine the type of floss used. The floss should slip easily between the teeth and pass the margin of the fillings without tearing and becoming lodged in the interproximal spaces. Unwaxed floss is suitable for most people; if it does not slide easily between the teeth, a waxed floss can be used. For persistent problems with tearing or fraying, brands such as Glide, Colgate Total or Eez-Thru can be tried.

Floss-holding devices have proven effective for some patients who have difficulty guiding the floss with their fingers.[14]

Flossing should be performed every 24 hours along with brushing at least twice a day to prevent plaque formation and subsequent caries and gingival inflammation.[2,22]

Chemotherapeutic Methods

Mouthwashes

In addition to plaque removal through brushing and flossing, chemical plaque control agents may be desirable in some circumstances, and the use of a mouthwash has shown some benefits.[23] A number of commercially available mouthwashes may be good adjuncts to help control the development of supragingival plaque and reduce subsequent gingivitis (Table 3). Oxygenating agents (e.g., hydrogen peroxide, carbamide peroxide) are not recommended because of lack of efficacy and potential adverse effects such as chemical burns of oral mucosa, decalcification of teeth and black hairy tongue.

For comparative ingredients of nonprescription products, consult the *Compendium of Products for Minor Ailments*—Mouth Products: Mouthwashes.

Table 3: **Mouthwashes**[19,23,24]

Active Ingredient(s)	Plaque and Gingivitis Reduction	Comments
Cetylpyridinium chloride 0.05% e.g., Cepacol	Moderate	Less effective than chlorhexidine. May cause staining of teeth.
Chlorhexidine 0.12% e.g., Peridex	High	Gold standard. Requires prescription. Limit use to once or twice daily; prolonged use may cause tooth staining, taste disturbances and discoloration of tongue. Other adverse effects include local irritation or allergic reactions.
Essential oils (thymol, menthol, eucalyptol and methyl salicylate), e.g., Listerine	High	Use for 30 seconds twice daily; high alcohol content in some products; may cause burning sensation, bitter taste or mucosal drying; not recommended for children because of alcohol content.

Care of Prostheses

Any removable prosthesis should be cleaned after eating and before going to bed. Plaque and tartar can accumulate on artificial teeth as on natural ones. A denture brush or a soft toothbrush may be used to clean the prosthesis using a denture cleaner or mild soap. The gums and the remaining teeth should be cleaned carefully as well, with a soft toothbrush. For patients who wear a partial denture, special attention should be paid to cleaning the teeth under the denture's metal clasps as plaque may become trapped, increasing the risk of tooth decay.[25] The toothbrush is not sufficient to remove debris; therefore, immersing the device in a commercial denture cleaning solution is helpful.[26,27,28] The patient should soak the dentures for 15 minutes once daily in the cleaning solution, then brush them. Dentures with metal parts are not compatible with all cleaning solutions; some solutions (e.g., sodium hypochlorite) may cause corrosion of the metal. Household products should be avoided because they are too abrasive for use on acrylic resin surfaces. Dentures should be cleaned over a basin filled with water so that if they are accidentally dropped, the water will prevent breakage.

In spite of proper cleaning techniques, calculus may build up on some prostheses. Calculus should be removed in the dental office with an ultrasonic cleaner.

Dentures should not be worn at night unless recommended by the dentist. They should be placed in a container and soaked (completely covered) in lukewarm water to prevent dehydration and subsequent dimensional change.

If the patient is not able to brush the dentures after the midday meal, they should at least thoroughly rinse the dentures and mouth.

A Health Canada advisory in February 2010 alerted denture wearers to serious health risks associated with excessive use of zinc-containing denture adhesives. Zinc is absorbed systemically when small amounts of zinc-containing adhesives are swallowed during normal use. When these adhesives are applied too frequently or in excessive quantity, over-exposure to zinc can lead to copper deficiency with possible blood dyscrasias and/or neurologic symptoms. Caution patients to use adhesives only according to the manufacturers' instructions and to consult their physician if they may have been exposed to excessive amounts of zinc through overuse of these products.

Implants should be brushed and flossed carefully every day. All sides of the implant should be brushed, and floss used with caution where the implant meets the gum line.[25,29,30] Interdental brushes with nylon-coated core wire may be helpful for maintaining dental implants.[31] Advise patients to avoid using brushes with hard and/or metal components, which can scratch the surface and allow for calculus deposits to form.

Caries

Dental Caries

Dental caries is a localized and progressive dissolution and destruction of the calcified tissues of the teeth resulting from an infectious process.[8,32]

Bacteria from dental plaque (predominantly *S. mutans* and lactobacilli) are capable of producing organic acids from the metabolism of dietary carbohydrates as well as from proteolytic enzymes. In response to the decrease in pH at the tooth surface, calcium and phosphate ions diffuse out of the enamel, and demineralization takes place. With an increase in pH, the process may be reversed. With time, disintegration of the mineral component of enamel and dentin occurs, with subsequent formation of a cavity on either the enamel surface or root surface.

Patients with xerostomia (dry mouth) have a higher risk and incidence of caries (see Chapter 91: Dry Mouth).[33]

Early Childhood Caries

Any preschool-age child presenting with one or more decayed, missing (due to caries) or filled tooth surfaces in a primary tooth is considered to have early childhood caries (ECC), a complex and chronic disease. To reduce the risk of ECC, the Canadian Dental Association recommends dental assessments for infants within 6 months of the first tooth erupting and at least by the age of 1 year.[34] Healthcare practitioners who identify children with ECC should refer them to a dental professional for further assessment and care.

Enamel Caries

Initially, the lesion appears as a white spot due to demineralization of the enamel. With repeated exposure to acid, the surface changes from smooth to rough and may become stained. If left untreated, pitting and then cavitation occurs.[8]

Arrested Caries

Under favourable conditions, the lesional process in the enamel may stop, become inactive and may even regress. Most of the time, arrested enamel caries have an opaque or dark appearance.[8]

Dentin Caries

In the dentin, demineralization is followed by bacterial invasion. Dentin has the ability to produce secondary dentin in an attempt to protect the pulp, but its proximity to the pulp also represents a risk of bacterial invasion into the tooth structure.[8]

Susceptible Sites

The sites on the tooth where plaque can accumulate are more prone to decay: pits and fissures (occlusal surface for the posteriors and palatal surface for the anteriors), smooth enamel surfaces that shelter cariogenic biofilm (proximal and cervical areas), and the root surface. Susceptibility is also dependent upon host factors such as the volume and composition of the saliva.[8,32]

Caries Prevention

Prevention of caries can be achieved by:[8,32]

- Protecting the teeth or strengthening the tooth structures
- Reducing the amount of substrate available to the bacteria
- Removing plaque and calculus through mechanical or chemical procedures.

A combination of the following interventions can facilitate the goals of caries prevention:[8,32,33,34,35]

- Dental assessment of infants within 6 months of eruption of first tooth and no later than 1 year of age
- Regular professional dental care
- Good, regular oral hygiene methods:
  - daily mouth cleaning or tooth brushing for all infants, including those who are breastfed[36]
- Diet low in sugar and dietary acids
- Topical and/or systemic fluorides
- Optimize salivary flow.

Caries Treatment

Depending on caries risk and incidence, some therapeutic modalities may be recommended:[8,35,37,38]

- Modification of the diet in order to limit the substrate, e.g., favouring a noncariogenic diet and limiting exposure to sucrose
- Modification of microflora, e.g., antibacterial mouthwash, topical fluoride
- Plaque disruption, i.e., good oral hygiene involving brushing, flossing, use of other aids
- Modification of tooth surface, e.g., topical or systemic fluoride, smoothing of tooth surface
- Stimulation of salivary flow, e.g., sugarless gum, xylitol-containing gum, saliva substitutes, medications
- Restoration of tooth surfaces, e.g., sealing of pits and fissures at risk of caries, restoration of cavitated lesions, correction of defects.

Pits and Fissures Sealants

The Canadian Dental Association supports the appropriate use of selective sealants based on an individual caries risk assessment and diagnosis by the dentist, along with nutritional counselling, good oral hygiene optimal fluoride exposure and regular dental exams.[25,39]

Role of Saliva

Saliva plays various protective roles against tooth decay:[6,8,33]

- Acts as a reservoir of calcium, phosphate and fluoride ions and therefore favours remineralization
- Contains IgA, lysozyme and peroxidase, which provide some antibacterial action
- Decreases plaque accumulation and helps eliminate food debris
- At high flow rates it has an alkaline pH, which helps buffer against organic acids.

Fluoride

The use of fluoride to prevent and control dental caries is well documented, safe and effective.[35,40,41,42] Systemic fluoride improves the crystallinity and decreases the acid solubility of enamel formed in the pre-eruptive phase of tooth development. In addition, it may affect tooth anatomy and reduce the risk of caries associated with pits and fissures in the teeth. Locally administered fluoride benefits the enamel by reducing demineralization and promoting remineralization of early caries. The resulting remineralized enamel has improved resistance to acid attack. In the presence of fluoride, acid production by bacteria in plaque is decreased, as is the synthesis of extracellular polysaccharides.[8,24]

The addition of fluoride to drinking water is recognized as a cost-effective public health measure.[35] In areas where the water is not fluoridated, supplemental oral fluoride may be considered.[25,42,43]

For caries prevention in children, the monitored use of fluoridated dentifrice is recommended until the child is able to expectorate the dentifrice, which is around the age of 6 years.[25,35,40] For a child between 3 and 6 years old, a pea-sized amount on the toothbrush is recommended; for a child younger than 3, only a rice grain–sized amount of toothpaste should be used and the teeth should be brushed by an adult. To minimize the risk of fluorosis, it is important for the caregiver to ensure the child does not swallow the toothpaste. A nonfluoridated dentifrice may be considered until the age of 3.[40] In some cases, based on the individual child's risk of caries, professionally applied fluoride may be indicated. For children considered at high risk of caries, home protocols may be recommended by the dentist on an individual basis.[35,42]

CDA does not recommend the routine use of fluoride supplements before the eruption of the first permanent tooth. In individual cases where the benefits outweigh the risk of dental fluorosis, practitioners may recommend supplements to young children at appropriate doses. To minimize the risk of dental fluorosis, all other sources of fluoride should be carefully assessed to ensure that total fluoride intake does not exceed 0.05–0.07 mg/kg body weight.[35]

After the eruption of the first permanent tooth the risk of dental fluorosis is decreased and fluoride supplement in the form of lozenges or chewable tablets could be considered as the fluoride would be delivered locally (intra-orally). Lozenges and chewable tablets should be used preferentially over drops for their local action. A lozenge or chewable tablet containing 1 mg of fluoride delivers the same amount of fluoride as 1 g (average amount used) of a 1000 ppm fluoride toothpaste.[35]

Excessive amounts of fluoride may result in dental fluorosis, which typically manifests as white specks on the child's teeth. It is a permanent cosmetic alteration of the enamel; there is no evidence that it affects the health of the child. It affects mainly younger children.[33] To minimize the risk of fluorosis, the total daily dose of fluoride should not exceed 0.05–0.07 mg/kg of body weight.[42]

Fluoride mouthwashes could be recommended to patients at high risk of developing caries, as a preventive measure. The CDA does not recommend this measure for patients under 6 years of age.[35]

Other forms of fluoride may be applied professionally (fluoride gels, foams and varnishes) in infants and adult patients at high risk of developing caries.[35,41,42]

For most Canadians the other forms of fluoride supplements (chewable tablets, lozenges, drops) are not recommended. They may be indicated for high-risk individuals in nonfluoridated communities when fluoride is not obtained in other forms (toothpaste) and after a careful analysis of the total amount from all other sources has been completed.[35]

Children who may be at higher risk of caries due to orthodontic or prosthodontic appliances or reduced salivary function, or children with high caries activity, should be considered for fluoride supplements.[40]

Gastric distress, headache and weakness have been reported in cases of excessive ingestion. Allergic reactions such as rash and other idiosyncratic reactions have been rarely reported.[40] When taken as directed, no adverse effects have been reported.[40]

To prevent overdoses, no more than 120 mg of fluoride should be dispensed per household at one time.[40]

Fluoride tablets should be taken with a glass of water or juice. Calcium from milk or other dairy products may bind with fluoride causing both to be poorly absorbed.[40]

Resource Tips

Canadian Dental Association. Available from: www.cda-adc.ca.

Perry DA. Plaque control for the periodontal patient. In: Newman MG, Takei HH, Klokkevold PR et al., eds. *Carranza's clinical periodontology.* 11th ed. St. Louis: Saunders; 2012. p. 452-60.

Suggested Readings

Ritter AV, Eidson RS, Donovan TE. Dental caries: etiology, clinical characteristics, risk assessment, and management. In: Heymann HO, Swift EJ, Ritter AV, eds. *Sturdevant's art and science of operative dentistry.* 6th ed. St. Louis: Elsevier/Mosby; 2013. p. 41-88.

References

1. Flemmig TF. Periodontitis. *Ann Periodontol* 1999;4:32-8.
2. Claydon NC. Current concepts in toothbrushing and interdental cleaning. *Periodontol 2000* 2008;48:10-22.
3. Manson JD, Eley BM. The oral environment in health and disease. In: Manson JD, Eley BM, eds. *Outline of periodontics*. 4th ed. Oxford: Wright; 2000. p. 26-33.
4. McHugh WD. Dental plaque: thirty years on. In: Newman HN, Wilson M, eds. *Dental plaque revisited : oral biofilms in health and disease : proceedings of a conference held at the Royal College of Physicians, London, 3-5 November 1999*. Cardiff: BioLine; 1999. p. 1-4.
5. Rolla G, Waaler SM, Kjaerheim V. Concepts in dental plaque formation. In: Busscher HJ, Evans LV, eds. *Oral biofilms and plaque control.* Australia: Harwood Academic; 1998. p. 1-17.
6. Marsh PD, Bradshaw DJ. Microbial community aspects in dental plaque. In: Busscher HJ, Evans LV, eds. *Oral biofilms and plaque control.* Australia: Harwood Academic; 1998. p. 43-55.
7. Jones CG. Chlorhexidine: is it still the gold standard? *Periodontol 2000* 1997;15:55-62.
8. Ritter AV, Eidson RS, Donovan TE. Dental caries: etiology, clinical characteristics, risk assessment, and management. In: Heymann HO, Swift EJ, Ritter AV, eds. *Sturdevant's art and science of operative dentistry.* 6th ed. St. Louis: Elsevier/Mosby; 2013. p. 41-88.
9. Perry DA. Plaque control for the periodontal patient. In: Newman MG, Takei HH, Klokkevold PR et al., eds. *Carranza's clinical periodontology.* 11th ed. St. Louis: Saunders; 2012. p. 452-60.
10. Perry DA. Plaque control for the periodontal patient. In: Carranza FA, Newman M G, Takei HH et al., eds. *Carranza's clinical periodontology.* 10th ed. St. Louis: Saunders Elsevier; 2006. p. 728-48.
11. West NX, Moran JM. Home-use preventive and therapeutic oral products. *Periodontol 2000* 2008;48:7-9.
12. Gorur A, Lyle DM, Schaudinn C et al. Biofilm removal with a dental water jet. *Compend Contin Educ Dent* 2009;30:1-6.
13. Forgas L. Plaque control. In: Fedi PF, Vernino AR, Gray JL, eds. *The periodontic syllabus*. 4th ed. Philadelphia: Lippincott Williams & Wilkins; 2000. p. 75-85.

14. Wilson TG, Kornman KS. Treating plaque-associated gingivitis. In: Wilson TG, Kornman KS, eds. *Fundamentals of periodontics*. Chicago: Quintessence Pub.; 1996. p. 319-47.
15. Handcock EB, Newell DH. Preventive strategies and supportive treatment. *Periodontol 2000* 2001;25:59-76.
16. Manson JD, Eley BM. Prevention of periodontal disease. In: Manson JD, Eley BM, eds. *Outline of periodontics*. 4th ed. Oxford: Wright; 2000. p. 132-44.
17. Forward GC, James AH, Barnett P et al. Gum health product formulations: what is in them and why? *Periodontol 2000* 1997;15:32-9.
18. Yaacob M Worthington HV, Deacon SA et al. Powered versus manual toothbrushing for oral health. *Cochrane Database Syst Rev* 2014;6:CD002281.
19. Mariotti AJ, Burrell KH. Mouthrinses and dentifrices. In: American Dental Association. *ADA guide to dental therapeutics*. 2nd ed. Chicago: ADA Pub.; 2000. p. 211-29.
20. Riley P, Moore D, Ahmed F et al. Xylitol-containing products for preventing dental caries in children and adults. *Cochrane Database Syst Rev* 2015;3:CD010743.
21. Riley P, Lamont T. Triclosan/copolymer containing toothpastes for oral health. *Cochrane Database Syst Rev* 2013;12:CD010514.
22. Sambunjak D, Nickerson JW, Poklepovic T et al, Flossing for the management of periodontal diseases and dental caries in adults. *Cochrane Database System Rev* 2011;12:CD008829.
23. Stoeken JE, Paraskevas S, van der Weijden GA. The long-term effect of a mouthrinse containing essential oils on dental plaque and gingivitis: a systematic review. *J Periodontol* 2007;78:1218-28.
24. Jackson RJ. Metal salts, essential oils and phenols–old or new? *Periodontol 2000* 1997;15:63-73.
25. Canadian Dental Association. Available from: www.cda-adc.ca. Accessed December 2015.
26. Gornitsky M, Paradisl I, Landaverde G et al. A clinical and microbiological evaluation of denture cleansers for geriatric patients in long-term care institutions. *J Can Dent Assoc* 2002;68:39-45.
27. Nishi Y, Seto K, Kamashita Y et al. Examination of denture-cleaning methods based on the quantity of microorganisms adhering to a denture. *Gerodontology* 2012;29:e259-66.
28. de Souza RF, de Freitas Oliveira Paranhos H, Lovato da Silva CH et al. Interventions for cleaning dentures in adults. *Cochrane Database Syst Rev* 2009;7:CD007395.
29. McGivney GP, Castlebeery DJ, eds. *McCracken's removable partial prosthodontics*. 9th ed. St. Louis: Mosby; 1995. p. 442-3.
30. American Dental Association. Available from: www.ada.org. Accessed December 2015.
31. Todescan S, Lavigne S, Kelekis-Cholakis A. Guidance for the maintenance care of dental implants: clinical review. *J Can Dent Assoc* 2012;78:c107.
32. Manton DJ, Drummond BK, Kilpatrick N. Dental caries. In: Cameron AC, Widmer RP, eds. *Handbook on pediatric dentistry.* 3rd ed. Edinburgh: Mosby Elsevier; 2008. p. 39-52.
33. Bourassa M, Perusse R. Making their mouths water: general principles for treating xerostomia patients. *Canadian J Restorative Dentistry Prosthodontics* 2008;1:24-7.
34. Canadian Dental Association. *CDA position on early childhood caries*. Ottawa (ON): CDA. Available from: www.cda-adc.ca/_files/position_statements/earlyChildhoodCaries.pdf. Accessed December 2015.
35. Canadian Dental Association. *CDA position on use of fluorides in caries prevention*. Available from: www.cda-adc.ca/_files/position_statements/fluoride.pdf. Accessed December 2015.
36. Canadian Dental Association. *CDA position on breastfeeding and early childhood caries*. Ottawa (ON): CDA. Available from: www.cda-adc.ca/_files/position_statements/BreasfeedingandECC.pdf. Accessed December 2015.
37. Deshpande A, Jadad AR. Impact of polyol-containing chewing gums on dental caries: a systematic review of original randomized controlled trials and observational studies. *J Am Dent Assoc* 2008;139:1602-14.
38. Splieth CH, Alkilzy M, Schmitt J et al. Effect of xylitol and sorbitol on plaque acidogenesis. *Quintessence Int* 2009;40:279-85.
39. Beauchamp J, Caufield PW, Crall JJ et al. Evidence-based clinical recommendations for the use of pit-and-fissure sealants: a report of the American Dental Association Council on Scientific Affairs. *J Am Dent Assoc* 2008;139:257-68.
40. Burrel KH, Chan JT. Systemic and topical fluorides. In: American Dental Association. *ADA guide to dental therapeutics*. 2nd ed. Chicago: ADA Pub.; 2000. p. 230-41.
41. American Dental Association Council on Scientific Affairs. Professionally applied topical fluoride: evidence-based clinical recommendations. *J Am Dent Assoc* 2006;137:1151-9.
42. Brearley Meser L, Mekertichian K. Fluoride modalities. In: Cameron AC, Widmer RP, eds. *Handbook on pediatric dentistry.* 3rd ed. Edinburgh: Mosby Elsevier; 2008. p. 53-69.
43. Tubert-Jeannin S, Auclair C, Amsallem E et al. Fluoride supplements (tablets, drops lozenges or chewing gums) for preventing dental caries in children. *Cochrane Database Syst Rev* 2011;12:CD007592.

Healthy Teeth and Gums—What You Need to Know

Dental Checkups

- See your dentist and hygienist at least once a year, or as often as they recommend.
- Infants should be brought to the dentist for the first visit within 6 months of the eruption of the first tooth or by the age of 1 year.

Brushing your Teeth

- Brush your teeth after each meal and before going to bed.
- Use a toothpaste that you like and that has the seal of the Canadian Dental Association (CDA). Your dentist or hygienist may also recommend a toothpaste.
- Replace your toothbrush with a new one every 3 months or sooner if the bristles are frayed.
- Make sure you use a toothbrush with soft or ultra-soft bristles.

How to Brush Properly

- Place your brush at a 45° angle to your teeth. The bristles should reach the place where the gum and the teeth meet.
- Move your brush in a gentle circle, starting at the gum and moving towards the top of the tooth. Do not scrub your gums hard. You could damage them and your gums could recede.
- Use this gentle circle technique to clean each tooth on the cheek side and the tongue side. For the tongue side of the front teeth, use the tip of your toothbrush. Finish by cleaning the chewing surface of each tooth.
- Brush for a minimum of 2 minutes to make sure your teeth are clean.

Flossing

- Flossing is very important because it removes plaque that you can't reach with your toothbrush, which is about ⅓ of the tooth surface.
- Flossing every day helps keep your gums healthy. It also prevents tartar from forming on your teeth. Tartar is like hardened plaque. You can't remove it yourself. Only your dentist or hygienist can do it.

How to Floss Properly

- Take about 40–50 cm (16–20 inches) of floss (about the length between your hand and your shoulder).
- Wrap each end around your middle fingers, leaving about 8–10 cm (3–4 inches) between your hands.
- Hold the floss between your thumb and index finger of each hand, leaving about 2.5–5 cm (1–2 inches) in between.
- To clean the teeth of the lower jaw, use the index fingers of both hands to guide the floss between the teeth.
- For the upper jaw, use the index finger of one hand and the thumb of the other to guide the floss. **Never** snap the floss into the gums.
- Slide the floss between your teeth and when it reaches the gum line, wrap it into a "C" shape around the tooth and move it *gently* under the gum line.
- Holding the floss tightly against the tooth, glide it up and down 2 or 3 times.

- Floss both sides of each tooth. Don't forget the back of your last upper and lower molars.
- Change to a new section of the floss as it wears.
- For a better result, brush your teeth *after* flossing.

Mouthwash

If your dentist prescribes a mouthwash for you called chlorhexidine (Peridex), this is how you should use it:

- Brush your teeth carefully.
- Rinse your mouth well with water to remove any toothpaste that is still in your mouth.
- Measure the amount of mouthwash prescribed.
- Swish it in your mouth for 30 seconds, then spit it out.
- Repeat these steps as often as your dentist recommends.
- Do not use the mouthwash for more than the number of days your dentist recommended. It can cause dark stains on your teeth and fillings if you use it for too long.

Chapter 87

Periodontal Conditions: Gingivitis and Periodontitis

Michelle Bourassa, BPharm, MSc, DMD

Pathophysiology

Periodontal disease includes any pathologic process involving the periodontium, the tissues supporting the teeth including the cementum, periodontal ligament, alveolar bone and gingiva (see Chapter 88: Teething).[1] Periodontal diseases are divided into 2 categories: gingivitis and periodontitis. Gingivitis is inflammation of the gingiva whereas periodontitis also involves the loss of connective tissue attachment and leads to the resorption of the tooth-supporting bone.[2] Plaque is the most common cause of gingivitis and periodontitis. Plaque (also referred to as biofilm) is composed of aerobic and anaerobic bacteria in a matrix of bacterial or salivary glycoproteins and dextrans.[3,4] Many local and systemic factors influence the periodontal inflammatory response to plaque (see Table 1).[1,5,6,7,8]

Table 1: **Factors Influencing Periodontal Inflammatory Response**[1,5,6,7,8]

Local Factors	Systemic Factors
Quality of oral hygiene	Aging
Anatomic factors, e.g., root morphology, position of tooth in arch, root proximity	Endocrine imbalance (diabetes)
Iatrogenic factors, e.g., dental procedures, restorative material, dentures, implants (peri-implantitis)[9]	Hematologic disorders
Traumatic injury, e.g., toothbrush abrasion, food impaction, fingernail scratch, orthodontics	Emotional or psychological stress
Chemical injury, e.g., ASA tablets applied to the gum[5]	Medications
Smoking	Genetic disorders
	Neoplasms, leukemia, multiple myeloma
	Nutritional deficiencies

Pathogenesis of Periodontal Disease

Plaque or biofilm accumulate at the gingival or supragingival level.[1,7,10,11] If not disrupted, it matures microbiologically, and an inflammatory reaction can be initiated. The tissue reaction produces intermediate products that serve as nutrients for gram-negative anaerobic bacteria. Concomitantly, the inflammation and bacterial enzymes increase tissue permeability, allowing high molecular weight products from the bacteria to penetrate the superficial tissues. Eventually, a balance between the bacterial challenge and the host response is achieved, resulting in a chronic inflammatory process known as gingivitis.

Little is known about what causes the shift from stable, chronic gingivitis to periodontitis. The induction and progression of periodontitis most likely involves disruption in the balance between the bacteria and the host defenses. The bacterial population may change, or host defenses could be transiently or permanently altered by such things as psychological stress, viral infection or smoking. Figure 1 illustrates progressive changes in the development of periodontitis.

In the chronic state, gram-negative bacteria are found in the diseased sites. The predominant gram-negative organisms are *Aggregatibacter actinomycetemcomitans, Porphyromonas gingivalis, Prevotella intermedia, Tannerella forsythensis* (previously *Bacteroides forsythus*), *Campylobacter rectus, Treponema denticola* and *Fusobacterium nucleatum*; many others may also be present.[7] These bacteria produce factors that may be responsible for tissue destruction and alteration of host defenses. Clinical signs of the disease may be partially explained by the normal inflammatory and immune processes detected in the periodontal tissues. The accumulation of bacteria induces the entry of chemotactic products into the tissue and stimulates the migration of inflammatory and immune cells, e.g., polymorphonuclear cells, macrophages and lymphocytes. Dental plaque located supragingivally is a reservoir for bacteria that can migrate subgingivally to form a biofilm in the gingival crevice.[12]

Based on antibody patterns, there appears to be local control of the response. After prolonged exposure to endotoxins, the protective effect of the antibodies tends to decline. Destruction of supragingival plaque through frequent professional cleaning and good oral hygiene has been associated with a beneficial effect on the subgingival bacterial population in moderately deep pockets.[12] In addition, dental interventions such as scaling and root planing have been shown to reactivate the antibodies and provide better protection. Enzymes such as collagenases from the polymorphonuclear cells and fibroblasts, along with inflammatory mediators (e.g., interleukin-1-b and prostaglandin E_2) may be potentially destructive to the connective tissues and bone. When inflammation is allowed to become chronic, the epithelial cells in the junctional epithelium tend to migrate toward the apex.

Figure 1: Progressive Changes in Periodontal Conditions

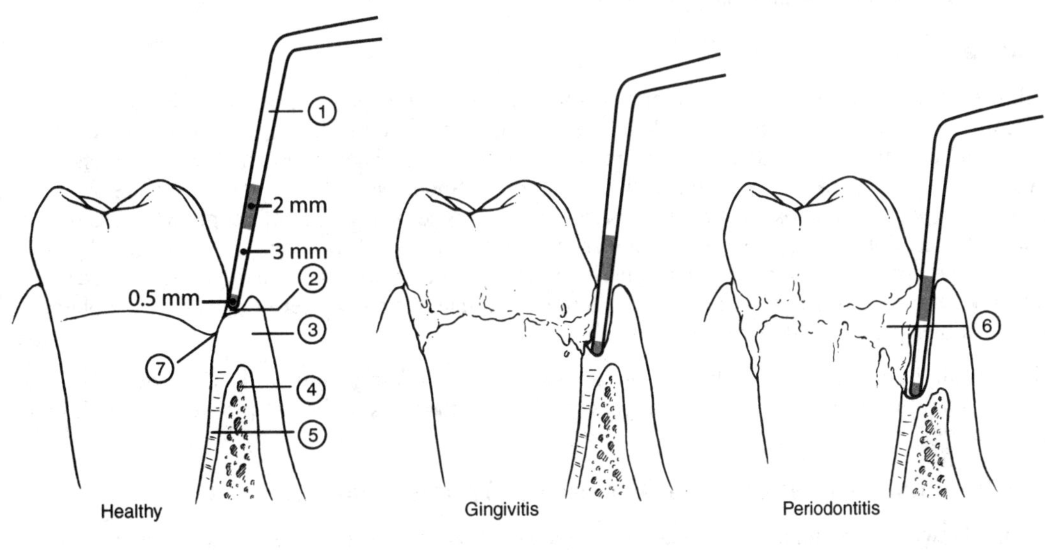

1. periodontal probe
2. sulcus
3. gingiva
4. bone
5. periodontal ligament
6. calculus ± plaque
7. cementoenamel junction

Prevalence

Gingivitis

Gingivitis is the most common form of periodontal diseases. Gingival inflammation in one or more sites of the mouth can be seen in most people.[1,13]

The prevalence and severity of gingivitis vary significantly with age.[8] In an epidemiological study of the U.S. population, gingivitis was detected in early childhood, increased in frequency and severity in adolescence and tended to decrease in frequency in adult groups.[12] In young children, the gingiva around the deciduous teeth seems to be resistant to plaque-induced inflammation.

From the age of 5 or 6 years to puberty, gingivitis is reported very frequently. In fact, chronic gingivitis has been found in 80% of children under the age of 12 and in almost 100% at the age of 14. The incidence of inflammation peaks at around age 12 for girls and age 14 for boys. It seems that the gingival tissue reacts more severely to plaque deposition at puberty than after puberty.[14]

In a group of teens 15–19 years, 79% of subjects showed some gingival inflammation.[15] The prevalence of gingivitis was 54% in the 19–44 age group and declined to 44% at age 45–64 and to 36% in subjects 65 years or older. In most cases the gingivitis was limited to a few teeth.[14,15]

Acute necrotizing ulcerative gingivitis has a low prevalence in rich countries and a higher one in poorer countries, often affecting malnourished children.[14] In western countries, it is usually seen in the 16–30 age group.

Periodontitis

A survey conducted in 2000 in Americans reported a prevalence of moderate to severe periodontitis in 4.2% of an adult population.[1]

In children, periodontal disease is often associated with systemic conditions such as juvenile diabetes mellitus, Down syndrome and many others.[14]

Risk Factors

Both prevalence and severity of periodontal disease increase with age and it seems to become clinically significant in the fourth decade of life.[8,14] For all age groups, the disease seems to be 1.5 times more prevalent in men than in women. People with African background had twice the risk of having periodontal pockets, compared with Caucasians.[16] Socioeconomic status is also a contributing factor, since pockets and loss of attachment are seen in a higher percentage of people with less than a Grade 12 education and in people with a lower income.[7,15,17] Genetic variation may explain why, in equal age groups, the transition from gingivitis to periodontitis appears to be earlier and the disease more severe in Asians than in Europeans.[8,14] Studies estimate the risk of periodontitis in a smoker to be 2.5–7 times greater than in nonsmokers.[7,18]

It is difficult to reliably predict who will progress from gingivitis to periodontitis. Considerable variations have been found in the clinical presentation and the rates of disease progression of chronic periodontitis.[14]

Consequences of Periodontal Disease on Systemic Health

The link between periodontal disease and systemic health is not as established as previously believed;[19] investigations to determine a clearer relationship are underway.[1] The following conditions are being studied:

- Coronary heart diseases
- Adverse pregnancy outcome

- Poor glycemic control in patients with diabetes[20]
- Stroke
- Hyperlipidemia
- Rheumatoid arthritis
- Left ventricular hypertrophy
- Obesity
- Pulmonary infection
- Mortality in the elderly
- Blood cancers, kidney cancer, pancreatic cancer

Goals of Therapy

- Reduce etiologic factors to reduce or eliminate inflammation
- Prevent progression of periodontal disease
- Restore and maintain optimal gingival and periodontal health
- Motivate the patient to maintain a rigorous oral hygiene routine

Patient Assessment

Periodontal disease is assessed and managed by dentists, dental hygienists and periodontists. Encourage patients to maintain good oral hygiene and to see their dentist regularly. The recommended frequency varies according to the needs of each patient, but is never less than once yearly.

Gingivitis

Gingivitis is inflammation of the gingiva. There are many subtypes of gingivitis (Table 2), but they share the following characteristics:[1,21,22,23]

- Discoloration of gingival tissue (red or red-blue)
- Signs of inflammation such as: bleeding on brushing or gentle probing; swelling or puffiness; loss of stippling of the gingiva (surface becomes smoother); loss of gingival tone; firm and leathery texture of the gingival tissue
- The gingival margin is located at or coronal to the cementoenamel junction. Pseudo-pockets may be encountered if swelling or hyperplasia is present
- Probing depths are between 1 and 3 mm or more if swelling is present (Figure 1)
- Pain is uncommon

Periodontitis

Periodontitis usually involves progression of gingivitis to include apical migration of the junctional epithelium, attachment loss, loss of bone and pocketing.[17,23,25] The usual clinical findings are:

- Discoloration of gingival tissue (red or red-blue), or it may appear normal
- Signs of inflammation such as: bleeding on brushing or probing; smooth, shiny gingival surface; loss of stippling of the gingiva; suppuration on occasion; exposed root surface(s)
- The gingival margin may be located anywhere relative to the cementoenamel junction
- Probing depths are in the range of 4 mm or more (Figure 1)
- Occasional pain

Table 2: **Classification of Periodontal Diseases**[22,24]

1. Gingival diseases
   a. Dental plaque-induced gingival diseases
      i. Gingivitis associated with dental plaque only
      ii. Gingival diseases modified by systemic factors
         A. Associated with the endocrine system
         B. Associated with blood dyscrasias
      iii. Gingival diseases modified by medications
         A. Gingival hyperplasia (cyclosporine, phenytoin, calcium channel blockers)
         B. Oral contraceptive-associated gingivitis
      iv. Gingival diseases modified by malnutrition
   b. Non-plaque-induced gingival lesions
      i. Gingival diseases of specific bacterial origin
      ii. Gingival diseases of viral origin
      iii. Gingival diseases of fungal origin
      iv. Gingival lesions of genetic origin
      v. Gingival manifestations of systemic conditions
         A. Mucocutaneous disorders
         B. Allergic reactions
      vi. Traumatic lesions
      vii. Foreign body reactions
      viii. Not otherwise specified
2. Chronic periodontitis[a]
3. Aggressive periodontitis[a]
4. Periodontitis as a manifestation of systemic disease
   a. Associated with hematological disorders
   b. Associated with genetic disorders
   c. Not otherwise specified
5. Necrotizing periodontal diseases
   a. Necrotizing ulcerative gingivitis
   b. Necrotizing ulcerative periodontitis
6. Abscesses of the periodontium
   a. Gingival abscess
   b. Periodontal abscess
   c. Pericoronal abscess (see Chapter 88: Teething)
7. Periodontitis associated with endodontic lesions
8. Developmental or acquired deformities and conditions
   a. Localized tooth-related factors that modify or predispose to plaque-induced gingival diseases/periodontitis
   b. Mucogingival deformities and conditions around teeth
   c. Mucogingival deformities and conditions on edentulous ridges
   d. Occlusal trauma

[a] May be generalized or localized.

Nonpharmacologic Therapy

Gingivitis

The most common form of gingivitis is plaque-induced gingivitis.[17,26,27] The other forms of gingivitis are very rare; consult specialized references for more information.

Plaque control is the gold standard of treatment for gingivitis induced by dental plaque. See Chapter 86: Oral Hygiene, Dental Plaque and Caries.

Periodontitis

Periodontitis is treated by dental professionals. The progression of most periodontal diseases can be delayed or stopped if the treatment plan achieves the following objectives:[1,17,21,26,28,29]

- Removal of the causative factors
- Reduction or elimination of all pockets and establishment of a normal sulcus depth
- Restoration of physiologic gingival and bone architecture
- Establishment of a functional occlusion by occlusal adjustment and restorative procedure
- Maintenance of periodontal health through adequate plaque control by the patient and regular visits to the dentist for close follow up and early intervention, in case of recurrence.

To achieve these objectives, the following interventions may be required:

- Phase I
    - Scaling and root planing
    - Removal of overhanging restorations and other plaque retentive areas
    - Extraction of tooth or teeth
    - Preliminary occlusal adjustment (selective grinding of teeth to establish a stable bite) and odontoplasty (modification of tooth contours)
    - Patient motivation and instruction in proper oral hygiene procedures
    - Evaluation of the results
- Phase II
    - Surgical treatment. This phase includes all procedures designed to reduce or eliminate pockets by resecting or relocating the gingival margin. It may also include the correction of alveolar bone defects and mucogingival defects.
- Phase III
    - Restorative treatment. When indicated, this step involves completion of occlusal adjustment, operative dentistry, replacement of missing tooth or teeth by fixed and/or removable prostheses, placement of dental implants and permanent splinting.
- Phase IV
    - Maintenance treatment. Patients must continue maintenance therapy for their lifetime. Patients who have been diagnosed with moderate to advanced periodontitis may require maintenance recalls as often as every 3 months. The interval between recall appointments is dictated by the level of disease control achieved by the patient at home.

Pharmacologic Therapy

Gingivitis

If plaque control cannot be achieved manually (e.g., due to lack of dexterity) or in patients who are systemically compromised or post-operative, topical antimicrobial products may be used as an adjunct to regular plaque control measures. The Canadian Dental Association has approved several mouth rinses to help in plaque control and reduction of gingivitis. More information about these products and information for patients on proper brushing, flossing and use of **chlorhexidine mouthwash**, can be found in Chapter 86: Oral Hygiene, Dental Plaque and Caries.

Periodontitis

Dental Office Procedures

The effectiveness of scaling and root planing may be slightly increased when combined with irrigation of the crevice with a antimicrobial agent such as **chlorhexidine** or **povidone-iodine** irrigation solution;[30,31,32] however, they may stain the teeth. Iodine derivatives are rarely used in modern practice; they are contraindicated in pregnant or nursing women, in patients with sensitivity to iodine, and those at risk of hypothyroidism.[33]

Chlorine-releasing agents (e.g., sodium hypochlorite, chlorine dioxide chloramines-T) have also been employed in periodontal therapy, although evidence for their long-term efficacy and safety is lacking.[34]

Topical Antibacterials

As an adjunct to tooth brushing and flossing, some dental practitioners recommend the use of **chlorhexidine 0.12% mouthwash** to reduce levels of periodontal pathogens in saliva. Chlorhexidine has shown efficacy vs. broad spectrum bacteria, good adherence to tooth surfaces and oral mucosa, and a low potential for irritation. It should be used under the supervision of a dentist and for a limited period of time, due to the potential for reversible staining of the teeth and irreversible staining of fillings associated with prolonged use.[30,31,33,35] Patient information on the proper use of chlorhexidine mouthwash can be found in Chapter 86: Oral Hygiene, Dental Plaque and Caries.

Triclosan is available as a toothpaste and has shown moderate efficacy in vivo.[36] Commercially available toothpastes containing triclosan may reduce gingival inflammation and bleeding.[37] Anti-infective agents may also be placed subgingivally in vehicles that will allow slow release of the agent into the periodontal pocket. Agents studied include chlorhexidine chips,[38] tetracycline fibres, doxycycline gel,[39] minocycline gel and metronidazole gel. Only **doxycycline gel** (Atridox) is currently available in Canada. Studies have shown little benefit when these products were used as adjuncts to mechanical therapy.[40,41] They are not recommended as single therapy.[17,42,43,44]

Systemic Antibacterials

Patients with plaque-induced gingivitis or chronic periodontitis usually respond well to mechanical periodontal therapy. While little additional benefit is expected from the use of a topical anti-infective agent, some patients may benefit from adjunctive systemic antibacterial therapy.[30,44,45] The goal of antimicrobial therapy is to destroy subgingival microorganisms that remain after local treatment. The best candidates for systemic therapy are patients with continuing loss of periodontal attachment despite appropriate local therapy, refractory periodontitis, early onset periodontitis, medical conditions predisposing to periodontitis, or acute or severe periodontal infections, e.g., periodontal abscess, acute necrotizing gingivitis/periodontitis.[30,45]

The adult oral dosages of antibacterials commonly prescribed for treatment of periodontitis are presented in Table 3.

The optimal agent and dosage regimen, especially for refractory periodontitis, remain unclear. The selection of an agent and dosage regimens have been established empirically rather than through systematic research.

The adult oral dosages of antibacterials commonly prescribed for treatment of acute periodontal abscesses are presented in Table 4. The benefits of systemic antibiotics for periodontal abscesses are unclear;[46] therefore, patient selection for therapy should be considered on a case-by-case basis.[47]

Monitoring of Therapy

- To prevent progression to periodontitis and even eliminate gingivitis, encourage patients with gingivitis to adhere to the oral hygiene regimen recommended by their dentist. Evidence suggests that toothbrushing in addition to flossing regularly reduces gingivitis.[48]
- Encourage patients who are undergoing treatment for periodontitis to keep their scheduled dental appointments and to adhere to prescribed therapy.
- Monitor the patient's use of chlorhexidine mouthwash to help minimize staining due to prolonged use.

Information for the Patient

See Chapter 86: Oral Hygiene, Dental Plaque and Caries.

Table 3: **Antibacterial Regimens for Periodontitis**[43,45,47]

Class	Drug	Dosage	Adverse Effects	Drug Interactions	Cost[a]
Fluoroquinolones	*ciprofloxacin* Cipro, Ciprofloxacin, other generics	500 mg BID po × 8 days	Abdominal pain, nausea, vomiting, photosensitivity, dizziness, headache, drowsiness, insomnia, diarrhea, pseudomembranous colitis. Potential adverse effects on developing cartilage; avoid in children and in pregnancy.	Concomitant iron, antacids, sucralfate reduce absorption of fluoroquinolones; increased INR with warfarin. Consider alternative in patients taking CYP1A2 substrates (e.g., duloxetine, clozapine, cyclobenzaprine), due to inhibition of CYP1A2 by ciprofloxacin. Avoid combining with highest-risk QT_c prolonging agents (e.g., amiodarone, escitalopram, fluoxetine).	$
Lincosamides	*clindamycin* Dalacin C, generics	300 mg TID po × 8 days	Diarrhea, *C. difficile* infection.	Absorption of clindamycin decreased by kaolin. Absorption of erythromycin decreased by clindamycin.	$
Macrolides	*azithromycin* Zithromax, generics	500 mg daily po × 4–7 days	Infrequent GI disturbance.	May increase concentration of colchicine, dabigatran, warfarin; dose adjustments and/or close clinical monitoring are recommended. Increased risk of rhabdomyolysis with simvastatin, atorvastatin. Avoid combining with highest-risk QT_c prolonging agents (e.g., amiodarone, escitalopram, fluoxetine).	$$
Nitroimidazoles	*metronidazole* generics	500 mg TID po × 8 days 250 mg TID po × 8 days in combination with amoxicillin 500 mg TID po × 8 days in combination with ciprofloxacin	GI upset, urethral burning, discolouration of urine (dark or reddish brown).	Disulfiram-like reaction with alcohol may occur during treatment. Increased concentration of warfarin, dose adjustments and/or close clinical monitoring are recommended. Avoid combining with highest-risk QT_c prolonging agents (e.g., amiodarone, escitalopram, fluoxetine).	$$
Penicillins	*amoxicillin* Amoxicillin, other generics	500 mg TID po × 8 days	Usually well tolerated. Hypersensitivity reactions (ranging from minor rashes to anaphylactic shock). Nausea, vomiting, diarrhea.	Penicillins may increase serum concentration of methotrexate, and decrease serum concentration of the active metabolite of mycophenolate. Tetracyclines may decrease the therapeutic effect of penicillins.	$

Class	Drug	Dosage	Adverse Effects	Drug Interactions	Cost[a]
Tetracyclines	*doxycycline* generics	100–200 mg once daily po × 21 days	GI effects; yeast overgrowth; photosensitivity; may increase risk of azotemia; pseudotumor cerebri; contraindicated in pregnant women.	Serum concentrations of tetracyclines may be reduced by antacids, calcium, magnesium and iron salts, carbamazepine, chronic alcohol ingestion, phenobarbital and phenytoin. Methotrexate concentrations may be increased by tetracyclines. Avoid combining with retinoic acid derivatives due to increased risk of pseudotumor cerebri.	$$
	minocycline generics	100–200 mg once daily po × 21 days	See doxycycline.	See doxycycline.	$$$

[a] Cost of specified course of treatment; includes drug cost only.

Dosage adjustment may be required in renal impairment.

Legend: $ < $15 $$ $15–30 $$$ $30–45

Table 4: **Antibacterial Regimens for Acute Periodontal Abscesses**[43,45,47]

Class	Drug	Dosage[a]	Adverse Effects	Drug Interactions	Comments	Cost[b]
Lincosamides	*clindamycin* Dalacin C, generics	Loading dose of 600 mg po, followed by 300 mg QID po	Diarrhea, *C. difficile* infection.	Absorption of clindamycin decreased by kaolin, absorption of erythromycin decreased by clindamycin.	To be considered in patients with allergy to beta-lactam antibacterials.	$$
Macrolides	*azithromycin* Zithromax, generics	Loading dose of 1 g po, followed by 500 mg daily po	Infrequent GI disturbance.	May increase concentration of colchicine, dabigatran, warfarin; dose adjustments and/or close clinical monitoring are recommended. Increased risk of rhabdomyolysis with simvastatin, atorvastatin. Avoid combining with highest-risk QT_c prolonging agents (e.g., amiodarone, escitalopram, fluoxetine).	To be considered in patients with allergy to beta-lactam antibacterials.	$$$
Nitroimidazoles	*metronidazole* generics	250 mg TID po	GI upset, urethral burning, discolouration of urine (dark or reddish brown).	Disulfiram-like reaction with alcohol may occur during treatment. Increased concentration of warfarin, dose adjustments and/or close clinical monitoring are recommended. Avoid combining with highest-risk QT_c prolonging agents (e.g., amiodarone, escitalopram, fluoxetine).	May be used as monotherapy or in combination with amoxicillin or ciprofloxacin.	$
Penicillins	*amoxicillin* ❥ Amoxicillin, other generics	Loading dose of 1 g po, followed by 500 mg TID po	Usually well tolerated. Hypersensitivity reactions (ranging from minor rashes to anaphylactic shock). Nausea, vomiting, diarrhea.	Penicillins may increase serum concentration of methotrexate, and decrease serum concentration of the active metabolite of mycophenolate. Tetracyclines may decrease the therapeutic effect of penicillins.		$$

[a] Treat for 3 days, then evaluate patient to determine whether further antibiotic therapy or dosage adjustment is required.

[b] Cost of 3-day supply; includes drug cost only.

❥ Dosage adjustment may be required in renal impairment.

Legend: $ < $3 $$ $3–6 $$$ $6–9

Resource Tips

American Academy of Periodontology. *Patient resources*. Available from: www.perio.org/patient-resources.

Canadian Dental Association. Available from: www.cda-adc.ca.

Suggested Readings

Cummins D. Vehicles: how to deliver the goods. *Periodontol 2000* 1997;15:84-99.

Dentino A, Lee S, Mailhot J et al. Principles of periodontology. *Periodontol 2000* 2013;61:16-53.

Flemmig TF. Periodontitis. *Ann Periodontol* 1999;4:32-7.

Kinane DF. Causation and pathogenesis of periodontal disease. *Periodontol 2000* 2001;25:8-20.

Slots J; Research, Science and Therapy Committee. Systemic antibiotics in periodontics. *J Periodontol* 2004;75:1553-65.

References

1. Dentino A, Lee S, Mailhot J et al. Principles of periodontology. *Periodontol 2000* 2013;61:16-53.
2. Armitage GC; Research, Science and Therapy Committee of the American Academy of Periodontology. Diagnosis of periodontal diseases. *J Periodontol* 2003;74:1237-47.
3. Flemmig TF. Periodontitis. *Ann Periodontol* 1999;4:32-8.
4. Claydon NC. Current concepts in toothbrushing and interdental cleaning. *Periodontol 2000* 2008;48:10-22.
5. Socransky SS, Haffajee AD. The bacterial etiology of destructive periodontal disease: current concepts. *J Periodontol* 1992;63:322-31.
6. Socransky SS, Haffajee AD. Evidence of bacterial etiology: a historical perspective. *Periodontol 2000* 1994;5:7-25.
7. Socransky SS, Haffajee AD. Dental biofilms: difficult therapeutic targets. *Periodontol 2000* 2002;28:12-5.
8. Tessier JF, Baehni PC. Epidémiologie et étiologie des maladies parodontales. In: Bercy P, ed. *Parodontologie: du diagnostic à la pratique*. Paris: De Boeck Université; 1996. p. 25-35.
9. Smeets R, Henningsen A, Jung O et al. Definition, etiology, prevention and treatment of peri-implantitis—a review. *Head Face Med* 2014;10:34.
10. Kornman KS. The pathogenesis of periodontal diseases: an overview. In: Wilson TG, Kornman KS, eds. *Fundamentals of periodontics*. Chicago: Quintessence Pub.; 1996. p. 1-45.
11. Teughels W, Quirynen M, Jakubovics N. Periodontal microbiology. In: Newman MG, Takei HH, Klokkevold PR et al., eds. *Carranza's clinical periodontology*. 11th ed. St-Louis: Saunders Elsevier; 2012. p. 232-70.
12. Burt B; Research, Science and Therapy Committee of the American Academy of Periodontology. Position paper: epidemiology of periodontal diseases. *J Periodontol* 2005;76:1406-19.
13. Ronderos M, Michalowicz B. Epidemiology of periodontal diseases and risk factors. In: Rose LF, ed. *Periodontics: medicine, surgery, and implants*. St. Louis: Elsevier Mosby; 2004.
14. Manson JD, Eley BM. Epidemiology of pariodontal disease (the size of the problem). In: Manson JD, Eley BM, eds. *Outline of periodontics*. 4th ed. Oxford: Wright; 2000. p. 119-31.
15. Brown LJ, Loe H. Prevalence, extent, severity and progression of periodontal disease. *Periodontology 2000* 1993;2:57-71.
16. Oliver RC, Brown LJ, Loe H. Variations in the prevalence and extent of periodontitis. *J Am Dent Assoc* 1991;122(6):43-8.
17. Pihlstrom BL, Ammons WF. Treatment of gingivitis and periodontitis. Research, Science and Therapy Committee of the American Academy of Periodontology. *J Periodontol* 1997;68:1246-53.
18. Muller HP, Stadermann S, Heinecke A. Longitudinal association between plaque and gingival bleeding in smokers and non-smokers. *J Clin Periodontol* 2002;29:287-94.
19. Li C, Lv Z, Shi Z et al. Periodontal therapy for the management of cardiovascular disease in patients with chronic periodontitis. *Cochrane Database Syst Rev*. 2014;8:CD009197.
20. Simpson TC, Weldon JC, Worthington HV et al. Treatment of periodontal disease for glycaemic control in people with diabetes mellitus. *Cochrane Database Syst Rev* 2015;11:CD004714.
21. Wilson TG, Kornman KS. The periodontium in health and disease. In: Wilson TG, Kornman KS, eds. *Fundamentals of periodontics*. Chicago: Quintessence Pub.; 1996. p. 281-3.
22. Armitage GC. Development of a classification system for periodontal diseases and conditions. *Ann Periodontol* 1999;4:1-6.
23. Gray J. Plaque-related periodontal diseases: pathogenesis. In: Fedi PF, Vernino AR, Gray JL, eds. *The periodontic syllabus*. 4th ed. Philadelphia: Lippincott Williams & Wilkins; 2000. p. 31-40.
24. American Academy of Periodontology Task Force Report on the Update to the 1999 Classification of Periodontal Diseases and Conditions. *J Periodontol* 2015;86:835-8.
25. Flemmig TF. Periodontitis. *Ann Periodontol* 1999;4:32-8.
26. Pihlstrom BL. Periodontal risk assessment, diagnosis and treatment planning. *Periodontology 2000* 2001;25:37-58.
27. Jackson RJ. Metal salts, essential oils and phenols–old or new? *Periodontology 2000* 1997;15:63-73.
28. Gray J. Host defenses and periodontal disease. In: Fedi PF, Vernino AR, Gray JL, eds. *The periodontic syllabus*. 4th ed. Philadelphia: Lippincott Williams & Wilkins; 2000. p. 51-69.
29. Carranza FA, Takei HH. The treatment plan. In: Newman MG, Takei HH, Klokkevold PR et al, eds. *Carranza's clinical periodontology*. 11th ed. St-Louis: Saunders Elsevier; 2012. p. 384-6.
30. Slots J, Jorgensen MG. Efficient antimicrobial treatment in periodontal maintenance care. *J Am Dent Assoc* 2000;131:1293-304.
31. Jorgensen MG, Slots J. Practical antimicrobial periodontal therapy. *Compend Contin Educ Dent* 2000;21:111-4, 116, 118-20.

32. Eberhard J, Jepsen S, Jervoe-Storm PM et al. Full-mouth treatment modalities (within 24 hours) for chronic periodontitis in adults. *Cochrane Database Syst Rev* 2015;4:CD004622.
33. Slots J. Primer for antimicrobial periodontal therapy. *J Periodontal Res* 2000;35:108-14.
34. Galvan M, Gonzalez S, Cohen CL et al. Periodontal effects of 0.25% sodium hypochlorite twice-weekly oral rinse. A pilot study. *J Periodont Res* 2014;49:696-702.
35. Addy M, Moran JM. Clinical indications for the use of chemical adjuncts to plaque control: chlorhexidine formulations. *Periodontology 2000* 1997;15:52-4.
36. Barnett ML. The role of therapeutic antimicrobial mouthrinses in clinical practice: control of supragingival plaque and gingivitis. *J Am Dent Assoc* 2003;134:699-704.
37. Riley P, Lamont T. Triclosan/copolymer containing toothpastes for oral health. *Cochrane Database Syst Rev* 2013;12:CD010514.
38. Ciancio SG. Local delivery of chlorhexidine. *Compend Contin Educ Dent* 1999;20:427-32.
39. Garrett S. Local delivery of doxycycline for the treatment of periodontitis. *Compend Contin Educ Dent* 1999;20:437-40, 442, 444.
40. Hanes PJ, Purvis JP. Local anti-infective therapy: pharmacological agents. A systematic review. *Ann Periodontol* 2003;8:79-98.
41. Bonito AJ, Lux L, Lohr KN. Impact of local adjuncts to scaling and root planing in periodontal disease therapy: a systematic review. *J Periodontol* 2005;76:1227-36.
42. Cummins D. Vehicles: how to deliver the goods. *Periodontol 2000* 1997;15:84-99.
43. Ciancio S, Mariotti A. Antiinfective therapy. In: Newman MG, Takei HH, Klokkevold PR et al., eds. *Carranza's clinical periodontology.* 11th ed. St-Louis: Saunders Elsevier; 2012. p. 482-91.
44. Smiley CJ, Tracy SL, Abt E et al. Evidence-based clinical practice guideline on the nonsurgical treatment of chronic periodontitis by means of scaling and root planing with or without adjuncts. *J Am Dent Assoc* 2015;146:525-35.
45. Slots J; Research, Science and Therapy Committee. Systemic antibiotics in periodontics. *J Periodontol* 2004;75:1553-65.
46. Cope A, Francis N, Wood F et al. Systemic antibiotics for symptomatic apical periodontitis and acute apical abscess in adults. *Cochrane Database Syst Rev* 2014;6:CD010136.
47. Herrera D, Alonso B, de Arriba L et al. Acute periodontal lesions. *Periodontology 2000* 2014;65:149-77.
48. Sambunjak D, Nickerson JW, Poklepovic T et al. Flossing for the management of periodontal diseases and dental carries in adults. *Cochrane Database Syst Revi* 2011;12:CD008829.

Chapter 88

Teething

Michelle Bourassa, BPharm, MSc, DMD

Pathophysiology

The normal primary dentition (also called deciduous or milk teeth) is composed of a total of 20 teeth, divided as follows: 4 incisors, 2 canines (cuspids) and 4 molars on each arch. The complete permanent (adult) dentition includes a total of 32 teeth: 4 incisors, 2 canines, 4 premolars and 6 molars in each arch.[1,2,3] Figure 1 represents the normal anatomy of an adult molar and its related structures.

Figure 1: Anatomy of a Molar

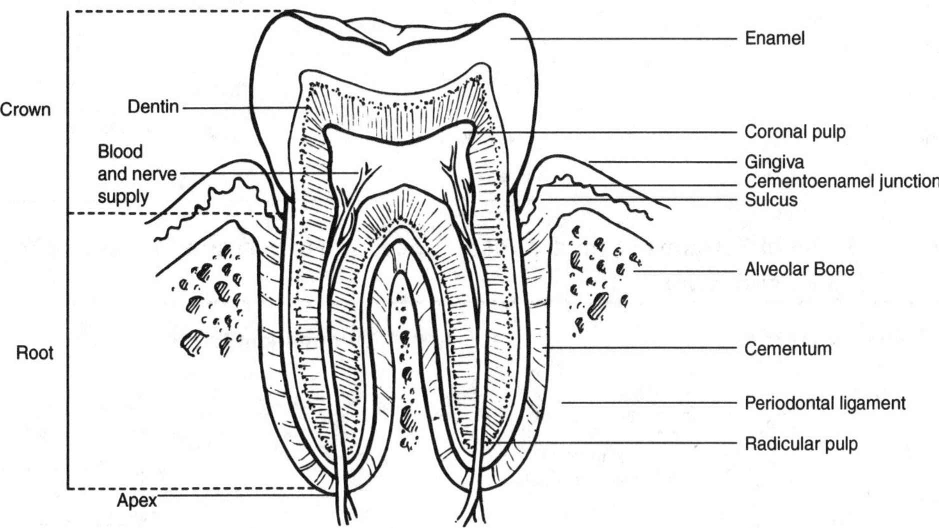

Table 1 presents the usual age range for tooth eruption. Figure 2 depicts the normal primary and permanent dentition.

Primary Teeth

The eruption of the primary teeth is accompanied by signs and symptoms in about two-thirds of infants.[4,5] Usually the symptoms are transient. They may appear up to 4 days prior to the emergence of the tooth. The peak in incidence and severity is usually on the day of eruption or 1 or 2 days before. These symptoms generally resolve within 3 days after eruption.[4,5]

Table 1: **Usual Tooth Eruption Times**[1,2,3]

Teeth	Upper (maxillary)	Lower (mandibular)
Primary		
Central incisors	7–12 months	6–10 months
Lateral incisors	9–13 months	7–16 months
Canines (cuspids)	16–22 months	16–23 months
First molars	13–19 months	12–18 months
Second molars	25–33 months	20–31 months
Permanent		
Central incisors	7–8 y	6–7 y
Lateral incisors	8–9 y	7–8 y
Canines (cuspids)	11–12 y	9–10 y
First premolars	10–11 y	10–12 y
Second premolars	10–12 y	11–12 y
First molars	6–7 y	6–7 y
Second molars	12–13 y	11–13 y
Third molars ("wisdom teeth")	17–21 y	17–21 y

Figure 2: **Occlusal Surface of Primary Teeth (upper and lower) and Permanent Teeth (upper and lower)**

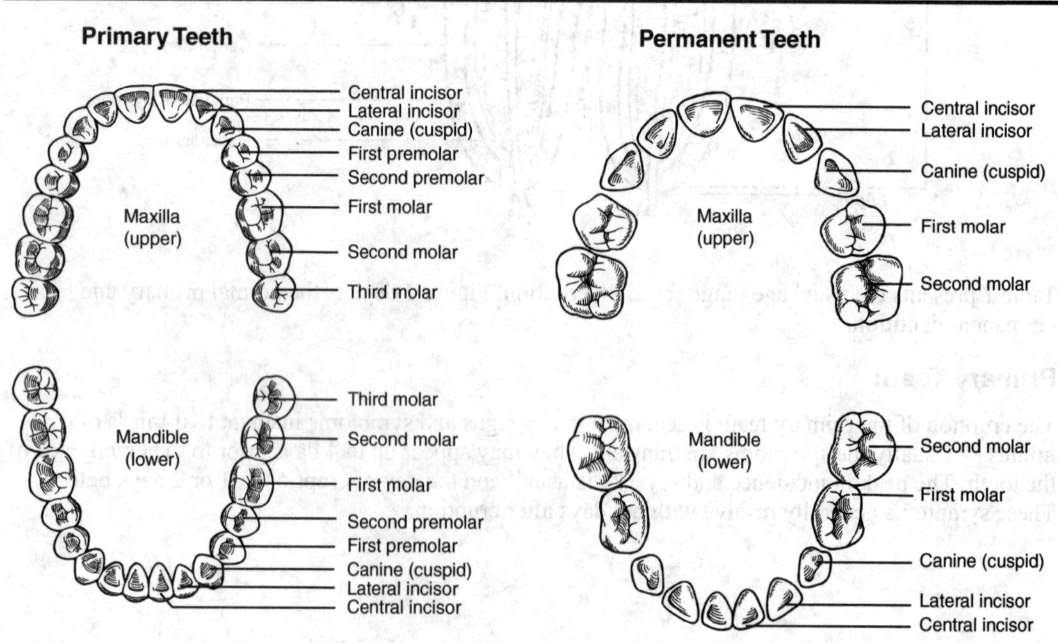

For a few days prior to eruption, the gum overlying the tooth may show signs of inflammation such as redness, irritation, swelling and tenderness. The child may have a greater tendency to rub the gum by biting their fingers, lip, toys or some other object. This action induces more salivation and drooling, which can cause some facial irritation or skin rash. The local inflammation may be sufficient to explain the irritability of the child, which may manifest as agitation, restlessness, crying and insomnia. A meta-analysis reported the most common symptoms associated with primary tooth eruption as: gingival irritation (87%), irritability (68%), and drooling (56%).[6] Other reported symptoms include a decrease in appetite for solid food, increased thirst, mild increase in body temperature (up to 37.7°C),[7] loose stools, ear rubbing and nasal congestion.[5,6,8,9]

Symptoms associated with an erupting tooth may coincide with an infectious process. Do not overlook the possibility of infection particularly when more severe symptoms are present. Fever, diarrhea, vomiting or symptoms of upper respiratory tract infection require assessment; do not presume they are caused by teething.[1,2,4,5,10]

Permanent Teeth

The eruption of a permanent tooth may be associated with the same gingival manifestations as with primary teeth, but the symptoms are usually much less pronounced. There may be local inflammation on the gum over and around the erupting tooth, from a few days prior to emergence of the tooth, to a few days after eruption.[11] Part of the gingiva may overlie the usually distal portion of the surface of the tooth for a relatively long period of time before completely receding. This part of the mucosa is called the operculum. Usually no symptoms result from its presence, but it can be problematic, particularly around the third molars, in the presence of mechanical trauma or plaque. Severe inflammation and marked swelling might then be seen at the operculum. This condition is called pericoronitis and is most often seen in teenagers and young adults. The patient may present with localized or diffuse pain, swelling and/or trauma at the operculum, bad breath and a foul taste in the mouth. When pus is present, the condition is called pericoronal abscess, and immediate dental or medical attention is recommended because the infection may spread into the oropharyngeal area and medially to the base of the tongue.[12] Swelling may extend to the adjacent tissue, and the patient may experience limitation in opening the mouth, lymphadenopathy and low-grade fever.[5,11,13,14,15]

Delayed Tooth Eruption

There is a wide range in eruption times of primary and permanent teeth, due to individual variation (see Table 1). Developmental age is more important than chronological age in assessing delays in eruption. In an otherwise healthy child, a delay of up to 6 months if a primary tooth is involved or up to 12 months in the case of a permanent tooth is usually of no clinical significance.[16,17] Delays can be caused by local factors such as the presence of a tooth in the erupting path, insufficient space in the arch or a dental infection. Rarely, systemic conditions or iatrogenic factors such as chemotherapy or radiotherapy of the head and neck can delay tooth eruption. Table 2 summarizes the possible causes of delayed tooth eruption. Consult a dentist when delays of more than 12 months are encountered.

Eruption Cysts

Occasionally, a localized, dome-shaped, fluctuant, bluish, swollen area, sometimes surrounded by inflammation, appears on the gum overlying the crown of an erupting tooth. The space is filled with tissue, fluid and blood. This condition is called an eruption cyst and is more often seen over erupting molars. Eruption cysts may be encountered in the first and second decades and there is no gender predilection.[8,10,20]

Table 2: **Causes of Delayed Tooth Eruption**[10,17,18,19]

Systemic Causes (infrequent)	Local Causes	Iatrogenic Causes
Down syndrome	Lack of arch space	Chemotherapy
Cleidocranial dysplasia	Ankylosis of the predecessor	Radiotherapy of the head and neck
Congenital hypopituitarism	Premature loss of the predecessor	
Congenital hypothyroidism	Cysts	
Gaucher's disease	Supernumerary teeth (extra teeth)	
Osteoporosis		
Ectodermal dysplasia		
Hypovitaminosis D		

Goals of Therapy

- Minimize pain, irritability and sleep disruption associated with teething pain
- Prevent complications through involvement of medical or dental professionals when indicated for systemic illness, eruption cysts, delayed tooth eruption, pericoronitis or pericoronal abscess

Patient Assessment

Table 3 lists circumstances in which referral to a dentist or physician is indicated.

Table 3: **When to Refer Patients with Teething Problems**

Condition	Recommendation
Pericoronitis	Dental consultation as soon as possible
Pericoronal abscess	Urgent dental or medical consultation
Delays of over 6 months in a primary tooth eruption or 12 months in a permanent tooth eruption	Dental consultation as soon as possible
Suspected systemic illness in a young child, e.g., fever, vomiting, diarrhea, symptoms of upper respiratory infection	Medical consultation when appropriate (these symptoms are not normally associated with teething)
Eruption cysts that do not spontaneously drain, or that cause discomfort and/or interfere with feeding	Dental consultation as soon as possible

Treatment of Teething Pain

Nonpharmacologic Therapy

Local measures can help minimize a child's discomfort during tooth eruption.[1,2,8,10] Something hard, smooth and clean may be given to the child to bite and chew on, such as a frozen facecloth. Safe teethers, cooled in the refrigerator before use, can be very effective in reducing the local symptoms. They should not have any small parts that could break off and cause the child to choke. The Canadian Dental Association recommends rubbing the back of a small, cold spoon on the gum (see Resource Tips).[1] Avoid long-term contact with very cold items. Do not place anything in the child's mouth that could be a choking hazard. Teething biscuits are not recommended because of their sugar content.

Pharmacologic Therapy

For comparative ingredients of nonprescription products, consult the *Compendium of Products for Minor Ailments*—Analgesic Products: Internal Analgesics and Antipyretics; Dental Products: Topical Analgesics for Teething.

For teething pain in infants that is not relieved by nonpharmacologic measures, oral analgesics, such as **acetaminophen** or **ibuprofen**, can be used at the usual analgesic doses (see Table 4).[1,8,10] Systemic analgesics should never be rubbed on the gum.

Although their use is controversial, topical anesthetic agents (**benzocaine** 7.5–10% in a gel formulation) may be applied in a thin layer to the affected gum using a cotton swab or finger, up to 4 times daily.[8,10] The duration of action is 30–45 minutes. Because of concern about disabling the gag reflex if the child swallows the anesthetic, it is recommended that the caregiver wait for an hour before feeding the child, if a local anesthetic has been applied to the gum. Methemoglobinemia is an uncommon but serious adverse effect that has been reported with the use of benzocaine applied to the oral mucosa.[21,22,23] This condition affects oxygen delivery to tissues and is characterized by bluish discoloration of the skin, nausea and fatigue, and can progress to stupor, coma and death. Avoid using benzocaine in patients with hemoglobin or enzyme abnormalities that affect oxygen transport.

Treatment of Pericoronitis or Pericoronal Abscess

These conditions require a dental consultation for appropriate treatment. They can be treated by the dentist with careful debridement of the area with curettage, followed by irrigation with physiologic **saline** solution, **chlorhexidine** 0.12% solution or **hydrogen peroxide** 3%. Some cases require surgical removal of the operculum, extraction of the involved tooth, or extraction or selective grinding of the opposing tooth.[14]

When systemic manifestations or extensive swelling are present, an antibacterial agent targeting gram-negative anaerobes (e.g., **penicillin**, **amoxicillin/clavulanate**, **clindamycin** or **metronidazole**) is usually prescribed along with irrigation and extraction.[9,24,25]

Analgesics (e.g., **acetaminophen** or **ibuprofen**) may be used to control the pain and decrease the fever when present. The patient may be instructed to rinse at home with lukewarm salt water (about one-half teaspoon of table salt in a cup of warm water) every 2–3 hours for 2–3 days.[13,15]

For more information regarding drug therapy for dental conditions, consult the *Compendium of Pharmaceuticals and Specialties*: Drugs in Dentistry.

Treatment of Eruption Cysts

Eruption cysts usually rupture spontaneously. In rare cases, marsupialization (surgical excision of a small amount of gum tissue from the roof of the cyst) under local anesthesia may be indicated if significant discomfort or interference with feeding occurs.[1,18,20]

Table 4: **Pediatric Analgesic Doses for Teething Pain**

Class	Drug	Dosage	Adverse Effects	Cost[a]
Analgesics	*acetaminophen* Atasol Preparations, Tempra, Tylenol, generics	10–15 mg/kg/dose Q4–6H po or pr PRN for symptom management; maximum 75 mg/kg/day Do not exceed adult dose	Uncommon with infrequent use and recommended dose. Chronic use and overdose associated with hepatotoxicity, nephropathy. Potential for toxicity enhanced if concurrent dehydration, prolonged fasting, diabetes mellitus, obesity, concomitant viral infection or family history of hepatotoxic reaction.	$
NSAIDs	*ibuprofen* Advil Pediatric Drops, Motrin Children's, generics	Children ≥6 months: 5–10 mg/kg/dose Q6–8H po PRN for symptom management; maximum 40 mg/kg/day Do not exceed adult dose Children <6 months: 5 mg/kg/dose Q8H	Uncommon with infrequent use and recommended dose. GI intolerance and bleeding. Skin rash, allergic reactions, tinnitus. Reduced renal function, acute renal failure, sodium and water retention. Dehydration enhances risk of renal toxicity.	$

[a] Cost of 1-day supply; available without prescription.

Legend: $ <$2

Resource Tips

American Dental Association. Available from: www.ada.org.

Canadian Dental Association. Available from: www.cda-adc.ca.

Suggested Readings

Massignan C, Cardoso M, Porporatti AL et al. Signs and symptoms of primary tooth eruption: a meta-analysis. *Pediatrics* 2016;137(3):1-19.

Ramos-Jorge J, Pordeus IA, Ramos-Jorge ML et al. Prospective longitudinal study of signs and symptoms associated with primary tooth eruption. *Pediatrics* 2011;128:471-6.

Twetman S, Garcia-Godoy F, Goepferd SJ. Infant oral health. *Dent Clin North Am* 2000;44:487-505.

References

1. Canadian Dental Association. *Dental development.* Available from: www.cda-adc.ca/en/oral_health/cfyt/dental_care_children/development.asp. Accessed February 4, 2016.
2. Pinkham JR. The dynamics of change. In: Pinkham JR, ed. *Pediatric dentistry: infancy through adolescence.* 4th ed. St. Louis: Elsevier Saunders; 2005. p. 166-205.
3. Cameron AC, Widmer RP, Street N et al. Eruption dates of teeth. In: Cameron AC, Widmer RP, eds. *Handbook of pediatric dentistry.* 3rd ed. New York: Mosby Elsevier; 2008. p. 453-55.
4. Macknin ML, Piedmonte M, Jacobs J et al. Symptoms associated with infant teething: a prospective study. *Pediatrics* 2000;105:747-52.
5. Ramos-Jorge J, Pordeus IA, Ramos-Jorge ML et al. Prospective longitudinal study of signs and symptoms associated with primary tooth eruption. *Pediatrics* 2011;128:471-6.
6. Massignan C, Cardoso M, Porporatti AL et al. Signs and symptoms of primary tooth eruption: a meta-analysis. *Pediatrics* 2016;137(3):1-19.
7. Jaber L, Cohen IJ, Mor A. Fever associated with teething. *Arch Dis Child* 1992;67:233-4.
8. Parkin SF. Some oral and dental diseases of childhood. In: Parkin SF, ed. *Notes on paediatric dentistry.* Oxford: Wright; 1991. p. 170-82.
9. Wake M, Hesketh K, Lucas J. Teething and tooth eruption in infants: a cohort study. *Pediatrics* 2000;106:1374-9.
10. Noren J, Koch G, Rasmussen P. Disturbances in tooth development and eruption. In: Koch G, ed. *Pedodontics, a clinical approach.* 1st ed. Copenhagen: Munksgaad; 1991. p. 250-74.
11. Nowak A, Crall J. Prevention of dental disease. In: Pinkham JR, ed. *Pediatric dentistry infancy through adolescence.* 2nd ed. Philadelphia: W.B. Saunders; 1994. p. 192-208.
12. Meng HX. Periodontal abscess. *Ann Periodontol* 1999;4:79-83.
13. Peterson LJ. Principles of management of impacted teeth. In: Peterson LJ, ed. *Contemporary oral and maxillofacial surgery.* 2nd ed. St. Louis: Mosby; 1993. p. 225-60.
14. Holland GR. Management of dental pain. In: Lund JP, ed. *Orofacial pain: from basic science to clinical management.* Chicago: Quintessence Pub.; 2001. p. 211-20.
15. Abrams H, Jasper SJ. Diagnosis and management of acute periodontal problems. In: Falace DA, ed. *Emergency dental care: diagnosis and management of urgent dental problems.* Philadelphia: Lea & Febiger; 1995. p. 132-50.
16. Aldred MJ, Crawford JM, Cameron AC et al. Dental anomalies. In: Cameron AC, Widmer RP, eds. *Handbook of pediatric dentistry.* 3rd ed. New York: Mosby Elsevier; 2008. p. 217-77.
17. Karp JM. Delayed tooth emergence. *Pediatr Rev* 2011;32:e4-17.
18. Vaysse F, Noirrit E, Bailleul-Forestier I et al. [Eruption and teething complications]. *Arch Pediatr* 2010;17:756-7. [French].
19. Huber KL, Suri L, Taneja P. Eruption disturbances of the maxillary incisors: a literature review. *J Clin Pediatr Dent* 2008;32:221-30.
20. Aldred MJ, Cameron AC. Paediatric oral medicine and pathology. In: Cameron AC, Widmer RP, eds. *Handbook of pediatric dentistry.* 3rd ed. New York: Mosby Elsevier; 2008. p. 169-216.
21. Moos DD, Cuddeford JD. Methemoglobinemia and benzocaine. *Gastroenterol Nurs* 2007;30:342-5.
22. Government of Canada. Healthy Canadians. *Benzocaine sprays with methemoglobinemia. Notice to hospitals—Health Canada issued important safety information on benzocaine sprays.* November 23, 2006. Available from: healthycanadians.gc.ca/recall-alert-rappel-avis/hc-sc/2006/14393a-eng.php.
23. U.S. Food and Drug Administration. *FDA Drug Safety Communication: Reports of a rare, but serious and potentially fatal adverse effect with the use of over-the-counter (OTC) benzocaine gels and liquids applied to the gums or mouth.* April 7, 2011. Available from: www.fda.gov/Drugs/DrugSafety/ucm250024.htm.
24. Sixou JL, Magaud C, Jolivet-Gougeon A et al. Evaluation of the mandibular third molar pericoronitis flora and its susceptibility to different antibiotics prescribed in France. *J Clin Microbiol* 2003;41:5794-7.
25. Canadian Dental Association. *What is pericoronitis and how is it treated?* May 27, 2013. Available from: www.oasisdiscussions.ca/2013/05/27/pc-2/. Accessed December 2015.

Teething Pain—What You Need to Know

A baby's first tooth begins to poke through the gums at about 6 months of age. The baby will continue to get teeth over a number of months until there are 20 teeth. About two-thirds of infants will experience some discomfort when teeth come in.

What are the symptoms of teething?

When a baby is teething, you may notice any of these symptoms:

- Redness, swelling or tenderness in the gum at the spot where the tooth is coming in
- Irritable behaviour, restlessness, crying, not sleeping well
- Less hungry for solid food, more thirsty than usual
- Drooling, rubbing the gum

Symptoms of teething **do not** include:

- Fever (above 37.7°C or 100°F)
- Diarrhea
- Common cold symptoms
- Vomiting

If your baby has any of these symptoms, **do not** assume they are caused by teething. See your doctor if necessary.

What you can do to relieve the pain:

- Give the child a cool, safe object to chew on, such as a safe teether or a frozen facecloth. Make sure the object can't break into small pieces that could cause choking. Avoid liquid-filled teethers if the child already has one or more teeth. The teeth could puncture the teether and break off a small piece that could choke the child.
- Rub the gums gently with the back of a cool, small spoon or with a clean finger.
- Give a pain-relieving medicine such as acetaminophen or ibuprofen in the right dose for the child. Your pharmacist can help select a product and tell you how to use it. Do not give ASA (aspirin, acetylsalicylic acid) to a child.
- Although local anesthetics such as benzocaine gel can be rubbed on the gum with a cotton swab, they only numb the area for 30–45 minutes. The local anesthetic may interfere with swallowing if it goes down the child's throat. If you choose to use a benzocaine product, wait for an hour after applying it before you feed the child. Use a very small amount, no more than 4 times a day. Ask your pharmacist to help you select the right product for your child. Stop using the product and seek medical attention if the child has difficulty breathing, gray or bluish skin color, headache, confusion or weakness.

What you should *not* do for teething pain:

- **Do not** give the child teething biscuits. They may contain sugar, which is bad for the teeth and gums.
- **Do not** rub oral pain relievers such as acetaminophen or ibuprofen directly on the gums.

If a blister develops where the tooth is coming in, do not try to break it. These little blisters are not dangerous and they almost always open and drain on their own. You may want to see your dentist if the blister does not go away or if it seems to be causing pain or interfering with feeding.

Chapter 89
Aphthous Ulcers (Canker Sores)

Adeline T. Chau Markarian, BSc(Pharm), ACPR

Aphthous ulcers (aphthous stomatitis, canker sores) and recurrent aphthous ulcers (recurrent aphthous stomatitis) are an inflammatory and noninfectious oral problem of unknown etiology.[1,2] These ulcers are the most prevalent oral lesions in the general population with a frequency of 5–25% and a 3-month recurrence rate of 50%.[1] The first occurrence is usually between the ages of 10 and 20 years with more than one-third of school-aged children experiencing these oral lesions.[3,4] Aphthous ulcers that start in adult age tend to be associated with other systemic conditions or tend to have definable predisposing factors.[5] With age, the frequency and severity of aphthous ulcers tend to decrease.[5] Women, patients under the age of 40 years, individuals with a family history of aphthous ulcers and those in middle and upper-middle class socioeconomic groups have a higher frequency of aphthous ulcers than the general population.[5,6,7]

Pathophysiology

The etiology of aphthous ulcers is unknown but probably multifactorial with local trauma and stress thought to be the most likely precipitating factors.[1,2,5] Allergies, genetic predisposition, nutritional deficiencies, preservatives, foods (e.g., chocolate, coffee, peanuts, cereals, almonds, strawberries, cheese, tomatoes and wheat flour), systemic disease, hormonal changes and some medications (e.g., NSAIDs) may also play a role.[1,2,5,6] Patients with aphthae may have considerable pain which leads to difficulty eating, speaking and swallowing.[1,2,6] Persistent and recurring ulcers can result in weight loss and a decrease in quality of life.[1]

There are 3 types of aphthous ulcers: minor, major and herpetiform. The most common are minor aphthae, occurring in 70–87% of cases.[1,6]

Minor aphthae appear as recurrent, small, round or oval, clearly defined, painful ulcers with shallow necrotic centres, raised margins and erythematous halos. See Aphthous Ulcer (Canker Sore) in Photo Section. They are usually smaller than 1 cm in diameter and have a whitish grey pseudomembrane. Lesions may appear as single or multiple ulcers (1–5 ulcers) usually on movable oral mucosa including the mucosa of the lips and cheeks, the floor of the mouth, the underside of the tongue and the soft palate.[1,6] Minor aphthae heal spontaneously without scarring within 7–10 days but heal more slowly than other oral wounds.[5] A vague localized feeling of discomfort may precede the actual appearance of the lesion by a few days.[6]

Major aphthae (Sutton's disease or periadenitis mucosa necrotica recurrens) are less common, occurring in 7–20% of affected patients and are more severe than minor aphthae. Although similar in appearance to minor aphthae, they are larger, exceeding 1 cm in diameter, deeper and appear in larger numbers (1–10 ulcers).[1] These aphthae involve the mucosa overlying minor salivary glands and can be found on the lips, soft palate and throat.[5] They often scar and can persist for weeks to months causing significant difficulty swallowing.[1] They are frequently found in patients infected with human immunodeficiency virus (HIV).

Herpetiform aphthous ulcers are the least common, representing 5–10% of cases. They appear as multiple small clusters of pinpoint ulcers, 2–3 mm in diameter and 10–100 in number but they may coalesce into widespread, irregular lesions. These ulcers may last 7–30 days and have the potential to scar. Women tend to be affected more often with herpetiform aphthous ulcers and these ulcers usually have a later age of onset than minor and major aphthae.[6]

Goals of Therapy

Infrequent, minor aphthous ulcers:

- Control local pain
- Reduce duration of ulcers
- Restore normal oral function
- Ensure adequate food and fluid intake
- Decrease frequency and severity of recurrences

Patient Assessment

When evaluating a patient with symptoms suggestive of aphthous ulcers, consider other conditions with oral ulcerative manifestations. These include infections (viral, treponemal, fungal), autoimmune diseases (e.g., Behçet's syndrome, inflammatory bowel disease, lupus erythematosus), hematologic diseases (cyclic neutropenia) and neoplasms (squamous cell carcinoma). Patients with iron or vitamin deficiencies (e.g., vitamins B_1, B_2, B_6, B_{12} or folic acid) or gastrointestinal diseases (e.g., ulcerative colitis, Crohn's disease or celiac disease) may also present with aphthae-like ulcers.[5] Alternative diagnoses to aphthous ulcers include primary or secondary oral herpes simplex infections, chickenpox, hand-foot-mouth disease and periodic fever, aphthous stomatitis, pharyngitis and adenitis syndrome (PFAPA). Patients with white thickened patches on the mucosa of the cheeks, gums or tongue may have leukoplakia, a precancerous lesion associated with the use of tobacco products[8] (see Leukoplakia in Photo Section).

Aphthous ulcers normally are not preceded by fever or vesicles and occur almost exclusively on movable oral mucosa (inside of the cheeks and lips, tongue, floor of mouth and soft palate). When patients present with a mouth lesion that is not easily distinguished as an aphthous ulcer or have additional symptoms, such as fever, skin lesions, uveitis, genital ulceration, recurrent bloody or mucous diarrhea, head/neck adenopathy or malar rash, they may be suffering from some other type of lesion or a systemic disorder and should be assessed further (Figure 2).[2] Figure 1 illustrates the structures of the oral cavity.

Prevention

Several well-recognized factors may contribute to the development and duration of aphthous ulcers.

Local Trauma

If accidental self-biting leads to the development of aphthous ulcers, advise the patient to chew carefully and slowly, using extra caution or avoiding sharp-edged foods such as hard candy, hard toast, crackers or potato chips.[6] Teeth, dental procedures and devices can also cause trauma and aphthous ulcers. Patients should consult with their dentist if their teeth or dental appliances have sharp points. Taking care while brushing teeth gently with a soft toothbrush and the early replacement of toothbrushes to prevent injury from "splayed" bristles can also help prevent trauma to the oral mucosa.[5] **Sodium lauryl sulfate** (SLS), commonly found in toothpastes, may interfere with the ulcer healing process and may worsen pain of existing ulcers.[9,10] Patients with SLS-related adverse reactions should use toothpastes that do not contain this detergent.[6,11]

Figure 1: **Anatomy of the Mouth**

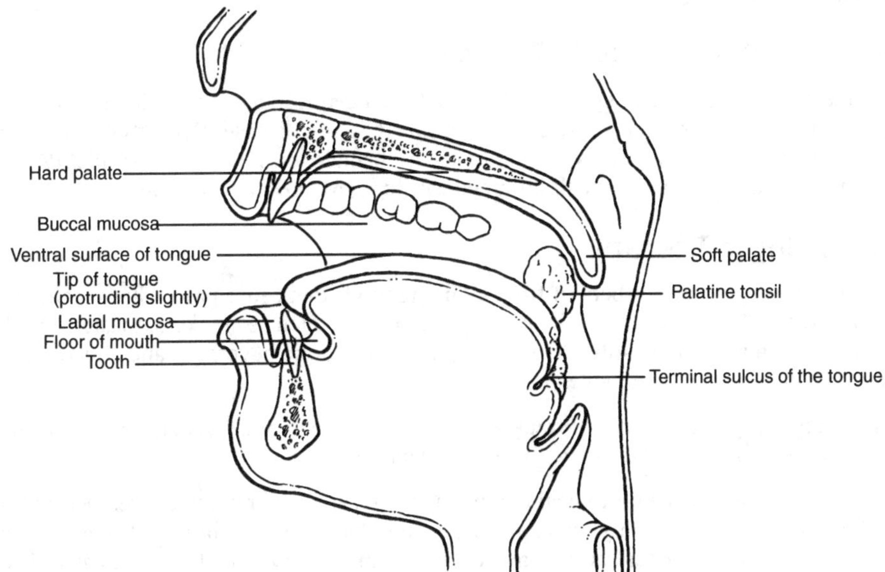

Emotional and Environmental Stress

Stress may precede 60% of initial ulcers and may be involved in 21% of recurrent cases.[1] Frequency of aphthous ulcers is 3 times greater in medical and dental students than in the general population.[1] Relaxation and imagery training may significantly reduce aphthous ulcers.[1]

Nutritional Deficiencies

Deficiencies involving iron, zinc, folic acid and vitamins B_1, B_2, B_6 and B_{12} are more common in patients with aphthous ulcers than in people without aphthous ulcers.[1] Treatment with sublingual **cyanocobalamin** 1000 µg daily for 6 months may shorten ulcer episodes, reduce number of ulcers per month and diminish level of pain even in patients not deficient in vitamin B_{12}.[6,12] Vitamin B_{12} ointment may also provide some analgesic benefit as adjunctive therapy after 2 days of treatment.[13] **Calcium** and **vitamin C** may be deficient in patients with aphthous ulcers. Hematologic screening in children and in patients with a history of ulcers exceeding 6 months may detect these deficiencies.[6,11] Patients with nutritional deficiencies respond well to replacement therapy.[1]

Allergies

Oral hypersensitivity reactions to various food additives, essential oils, mints and dental materials and antibodies to cow's milk and wheat protein have been observed in patients with recurrent aphthous ulcers (RAU).[1] Strict elimination diets involving cow's milk or glutens may resolve or improve RAU.[1] If an allergic or hypersensitivity reaction is suspected, referral to specialist care is warranted.

Drug-related Causes

It has been suggested that patients with RAU have a higher medication intake than those without RAU.[14] Medications associated with RAU include ACE inhibitors, antiarrhythmic medications, beta-blockers, NSAIDs and opioid analgesics.[6,14,15] Although the mechanism is not well understood, drug-related aphthous ulcers usually resolve once the medication is discontinued.[15] Smoking appears to offer a protective effect by producing keratinization of the oral mucosa, although smoking is a risk factor for other oral lesions including leukoplakia.[2,14,15] Nicotine-containing products also tend to decrease the frequency of RAU.[5]

Treatment of Underlying Systemic Disease

Identification and treatment of certain systemic diseases have been associated with improvement of RAU. These systemic conditions include Sweet's syndrome, Crohn's disease, Behçet's disease, various types of neutropenia, pernicious anemia, systemic lupus erythematosus, HIV infection, PFAPA syndrome and mouth and genital ulcers with inflamed cartilage (MAGIC) syndrome.[5]

Nonpharmacologic Therapy

All patients with aphthous ulcers can benefit from avoiding foods that cause pain. These include foods that are hard, crusty, sharp, spicy, salty, acidic or difficult to chew, such as crackers, toasted bread, potato chips, pickles, tomatoes, nuts, citrus fruits and juices. Alcoholic beverages and chocolate may also cause pain and should be avoided when ulcers are present.[6]

Patients should address any sources of oral trauma such as ill-fitting dentures, sharp/broken teeth or using harsh toothpastes containing the detergent sodium lauryl sulfate.

Chemically cauterizing the ulcers with topical compounds (e.g., silver nitrate, hydrogen peroxide) is painful and should be administered only under specialist care due to the possibility of causing local necrosis and delaying healing. Cauterization may decrease pain severity after 1 day but has little effect on speed of healing.[2,16,17]

Encourage patients to maintain regular daily oral hygiene, which includes twice-daily brushing and flossing the teeth and a professional dental cleaning at least every 6 months (see Chapter 86: Oral Hygiene, Dental Plaque and Caries).[6] Aphthae can be cleansed by rinsing the mouth with salt and water (2.5–5 mL table salt per 250 mL warm water) several times daily, especially after meals. There is no evidence to suggest that other cleansing rinses (e.g., sodium perborate or half-strength hydrogen peroxide diluted to 1.5%) provide an advantage over saline rinses.[5]

Pharmacologic Therapy

Patients with major or herpetiform aphthous ulcers, RAU or who have severe pain, difficulty eating, drinking, chewing and swallowing require further evaluation and more extensive drug therapy.

The efficacy of treatment options for aphthous ulcers is mainly anecdotal as few well-designed studies are available.[15] Treatment is therefore empirical and nonspecific and the choice of agent will depend on severity of pain, number of ulcers, frequency of episodes and patient's tolerance to treatment.[15,18]

The American Academy of Oral Medicine recommends topical agents as first-line therapy (see Table 3).[15]

Topical Therapy

For comparative ingredients of nonprescription products, consult the *Compendium of Products for Minor Ailments*—Mouth Products: Cold Sores and Canker Sores.

Protectants

Placing a mucosal adherent agents such as **hydroxypropyl cellulose** or **carboxymethyl cellulose** over the ulcer may provide temporary pain relief and protection.

Local Anesthetics

Infrequent minor aphthous ulcers resolve on their own and may require only short-term pain management. Patients seeking temporary pain relief can apply a product containing a topical anesthetic such as **benzocaine** or **lidocaine**.[16] The duration of action of topical anesthetics is relatively short (20–45 minutes) and these agents may be used with oral analgesics and protectants to provide longer pain relief.

Gels, ointments and pastes can be applied directly to the ulcer using a cotton-tipped swab, such as a Q-tip, 4 times a day, before meals and at bedtime, for up to 1 week.[4] To maximize effectiveness, remind patients to dry the affected mucosa prior to drug application and avoid eating, drinking and speaking for 30 minutes after each application.[6]

Local anesthetics should be used with caution in children under 2 years of age. Increased absorption of benzocaine in infants and young children has led to methemoglobenemia. The use of excessive amounts can lead to choking from difficulty swallowing and to being burned from hot food.

Gel formulations have a high alcohol content and may cause an initial stinging or burning on application which can be distressing to children. Applying ice before using a gel may help prevent this side effect or another dosage form may be selected.[4]

For painful ulcers, **benzydamine 0.15%** topical solution containing ethanol 10% could be used as a rinse every 3 hours on as-needed basis. The solution should not be swallowed and ingestion of food or hot liquids while the mouth is numb should be avoided to minimize the risk of burning the mouth or biting the tongue or cheeks.[19]

Local Anti-inflammatories

Topical corticosteroids (e.g., **clobetasol**, **fluocinonide**, **triamcinolone**) are useful in relieving pain due to their anti-inflammatory properties.[6] Topical corticosteroids are not effective for preventing ulcer recurrence or frequency.[20] Nevertheless, their efficacy can improve if they are started during the early phase of ulceration, when lymphocyte activity is at its maximum.

Establishing effective topical delivery of these agents is a problem because they are readily rubbed or washed away within the mouth. Using the more potent corticosteroids and compounding them with a mucosal adherent improves delivery. **Triamcinolone in Orabase** is available commercially and corticosteroid ointment formulations mix well with equal parts of Orabase, providing better adherence to the oral mucosa.[4] In addition, patients should be advised not to eat or drink for 30 minutes following application. Oropharyngeal candidiasis is a potential side effect and patients should be monitored for the development of this condition when using topical corticosteroids (see Chapter 93: Oral Candidiasis).[6]

Dexamethasone ointment can reduce pain and ulcer size when applied to the affected areas 3 times daily after meals for 5 days. Serum concentration of dexamethasone is not detectable after applications.[21,22] When compared with triamcinolone acetonide in Orabase, dexamethasone ointment may show faster healing of ulcers with similar speed of pain reduction.[23]

Local Antibiotics

Tetracycline 5% or **minocycline** 0.2% mouthwashes may significantly reduce the pain, ulcer size and duration of RAU as compared with placebo.[16,24] The usual dosage is tetracycline 250 mg or minocycline 10 mg 4 times a day for 10 days, administered as a solution that is retained in the mouth for 1–2 minutes then expectorated. Tetracycline is chemically unstable in aqueous solution but can be neutralized with a specific base (see Table 1).[16] Using these oral rinses for more than 5 days may predispose patients to oral fungal infections, skin reactions, sore throat or stained teeth.[1,6] Another concern with frequent or prolonged use is the development of bacterial resistance. Benefits of this treatment should be weighed against its risks.

Topical application of **penicillin G** troches (50 mg 4 times daily) may reduce pain as well as lessen the size, severity, duration and frequency of ulcers.[25]

Table 1: **Preparation and Use of Chemically Stable Tetracycline Suspension**

Tetracycline mouthwash 5% (w/v)
Ingredients:
Tetracycline hydrochloride 5 g Methyl-4-hydroxybenzoate 0.1 g Sodium citrate 6.5 g Propylene glycol 0.6 g Sorbitol solution 70% (non-crystallizable) 65.5 g Tragacanth 0.5 g Purified water to 118.2 g
Preparation:
1. Dissolve methyl-4-hydroxybenzoate in propylene glycol. 2. Dissolve sodium citrate in purified water. 3. Mix dry tragacanth and tetracycline hydrochloride. Mix equal part of sorbitol solution and form a gel with the rest of sorbitol solution. 4. Add sodium citrate solution in portions and stir. 5. Add propylene glycol with the dissolved methyl-4-hydroxybenzoate and stir. Expiration: 6 months
Mode of application: Shake before use. Apply 5 mL of the suspension for 5 min in the mouth cavity up to 5 times daily and for intensive therapy, the same dose to be used for 10–15 min.

Reproduced with permission from Altenburg A, Zouboulis CC. Current concepts in the treatment of recurrent aphthous stomatitis. *Skin Therapy Lett* 2008;13(7):1-4.
Original source: Neues Rezeptur-Formularium for compounded medication: Rezepturhinweise: Tetracyclinhydrochlorid in zahnärztlichen Anwendungen und Mundspülungen. Govi-Verlag Pharmazeutischer Verlag Eschborn (2005).

Systemic Therapy

For comparative ingredients of nonprescription products, consult the *Compendium of Products for Minor Ailments*—Analgesic Products: Internal Analgesics and Antipyretics.

All systemic therapies lack convincing efficacy data.[26] These agents are not generally recommended or required but they may be considered for severe cases of major RAU that are unresponsive to all topical therapies.[1,6] With all systemic medications, aphthous ulcers may recur after discontinuation of therapy.

Acetaminophen may be recommended for pain relief using dosages based on the age or weight of the patient. NSAIDs should be avoided as these agents may cause aphthous ulcers and worsen these lesions.[1,2,5]

Colchicine 1–2 mg daily may induce complete remission and reduce the duration and frequency of ulcers after 3 months of therapy. Symptomatic response may be durable over several years.[27]

Montelukast 10 mg daily for 1 month followed by alternate day dosing for the second month may reduce pain, time to healing and number of new aphthous lesions.[28]

Dapsone can be used for oral and genital aphthous ulcers. It acts as both an antibiotic and an anti-inflammatory agent. Recommended dose is 100–150 mg daily and can be given with ascorbic acid 500 mg daily to prevent hematologic side effects (hemolysis, methemoglobinemia and agranulocytosis). Upon discontinuation of treatment, rapid relapse is common.[6] In patients with complex aphthosis, weak evidence suggests that a combination of both colchicine (up to 1.8 mg/day) and dapsone (up to 125–150 mg/day) may also be effective.[29]

Pentoxifylline 400 mg 3 times daily may reduce pain severity and size of ulcers.[20] This oral anti-TNF agent has few adverse effects (nausea) and can be used in patients with multiple comorbidities or with contraindications to more aggressive treatments. However, it should not be used in pregnant women.[6]

For patients who do not respond to colchicine or pentoxifylline, systemic corticosteroids can be used for acute exacerbations.[16] **Prednisolone**, or its equivalent, can be given at 10–30 mg daily for up to 1 month to shorten the ulcer's duration. Longer treatments are not recommended as new lesions cannot be avoided and long-term adverse effects may occur, such as depression, hyperglycemia, lipodystrophy, moon facies and osteopenia/osteoporosis.[6] Of note, oral corticosteroids are considered safe medications for pregnant patients.

Weak evidence suggests that the anti-TNF agent **infliximab** may be an effective treatment option for patients with severe recurrent oral ulcers who do not respond to other therapies. Infliximab leads to rapid healing of the lesions within a few days after the first dose with no recurrence for 6–8 weeks.[6] The usual dose is 5 mg/kg body weight at variable frequencies.

Thalidomide is an anti-TNF agent with limited use for this indication due to its severe side effects profile (neuropathy, abdominal discomfort, fatigue). This agent is used for the treatment of major aphthae in HIV-positive patients (200 mg/day), but may also be effective for the treatment of major aphthae and orogenital ulcers (50 mg/day). Thalidomide may induce complete remission as early as 14 days of starting treatment but causes adverse effects in the majority of patients.[18] This agent should not be used in pregnant women due to its teratogenicity.[17]

Anecdotal Therapies

Therapies that have been suggested for aphthous ulcers but have received little or no evaluation are listed in Table 2. Some of these products may interact with other medicines or even cause aphthous ulcers; therefore, they should be avoided.[7]

Table 2: **Anecdotal Therapies for Aphthous Ulcers (Not Recommended)**

2-octyl cyanoacrylate (tissue adhesive)	Levamisole	Sucralfate suspension as mouth rinse
Acidophilus	Licorice, deglycyrrhizinated	Testosterone, subcutaneous
Acyclovir	L-Lysine	Thiamine
Agrimony	Mixtures[a]	Tormentil
Calendula	Nicotine patches and chewable tablets	Vitamin B complex
Caraway	Oak bark	Vitamin C
Cranesbill	Oral contraceptives	Witch hazel
Cyclosporine A	Prostaglandin E2 gel	Zinc lozenges
Echinacea	Raw egg	
Helium-neon lasers	Sage	

[a] Various combinations, e.g. 1 part prednisolone syrup 15 mg/5 mL or dexamethasone elixir 0.5 mg/5 mL, 2 parts diphenhydramine elixir 12.5 mg/5 mL, 3 parts doxycycline 25 mg/5 mL or minocycline 50 mg/5 mL, 6 parts lidocaine 2% viscous; used as rinse or applied to ulcer.

Monitoring of Therapy

Advise patients and monitor for potential side effects and complications of treatment. For example, oral corticosteroid use can lead to oral candidiasis, and antimetabolites and alkylating agents can cause hematologic suppression. The patient should monitor ulcer pain daily. Healthcare practitioners should monitor patients for ulcer pain every 3 days for the first week then 1 week later. If the ulcer worsens or is still present after 14 days of self-care, patient may require further assessment and treatment. An oral ulcer is considered chronic if it lasts longer than 2 weeks.[30]

Figure 2: **Assessment of Patients with Aphthous Ulcers**

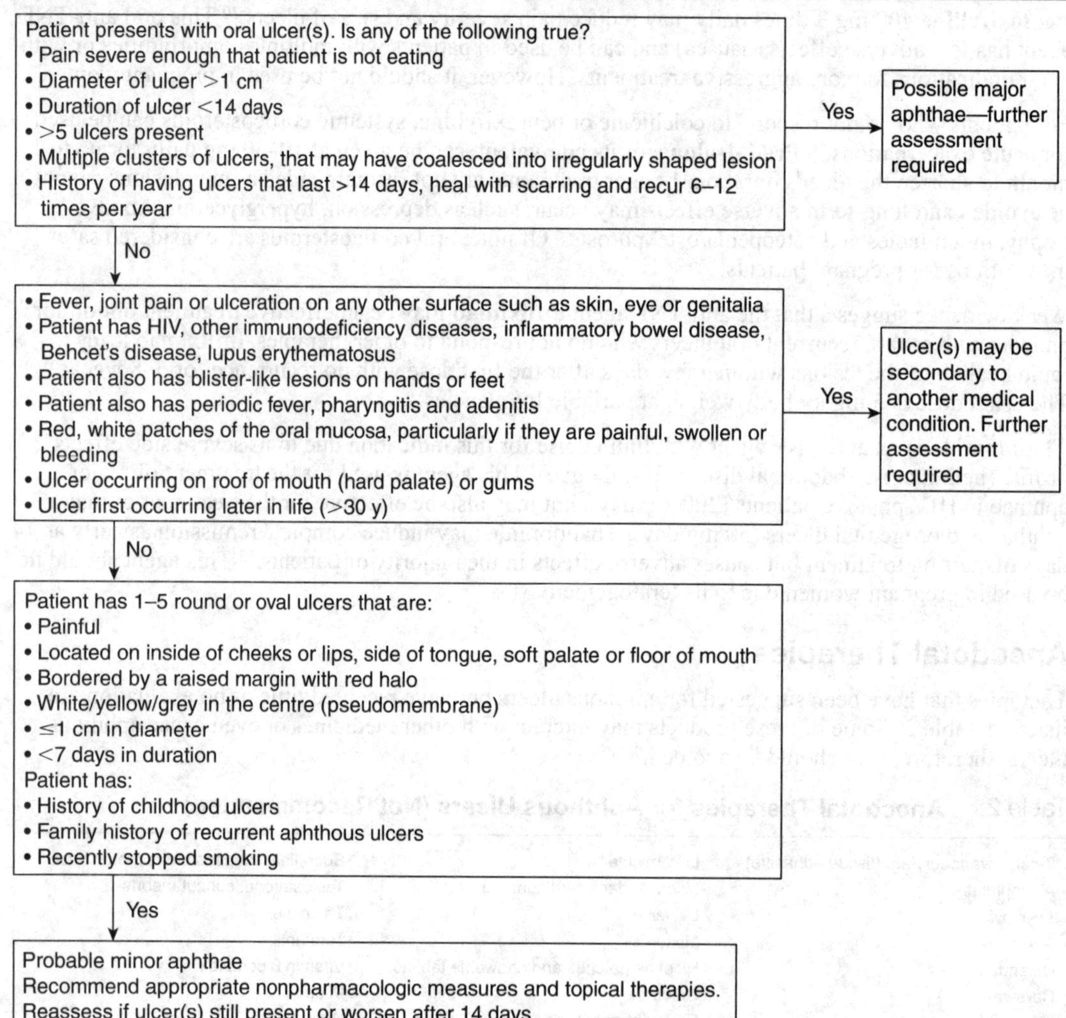

Patient presents with oral ulcer(s). Is any of the following true?
• Pain severe enough that patient is not eating
• Diameter of ulcer >1 cm
• Duration of ulcer <14 days
• >5 ulcers present
• Multiple clusters of ulcers, that may have coalesced into irregularly shaped lesion
• History of having ulcers that last >14 days, heal with scarring and recur 6–12 times per year
Yes
Possible major aphthae—further assessment required
No
• Fever, joint pain or ulceration on any other surface such as skin, eye or genitalia
• Patient has HIV, other immunodeficiency diseases, inflammatory bowel disease, Behcet's disease, lupus erythematosus
• Patient also has blister-like lesions on hands or feet
• Patient also has periodic fever, pharyngitis and adenitis
• Red, white patches of the oral mucosa, particularly if they are painful, swollen or bleeding
• Ulcer occurring on roof of mouth (hard palate) or gums
• Ulcer first occurring later in life (>30 y)
Yes
Ulcer(s) may be secondary to another medical condition. Further assessment required
No
Patient has 1–5 round or oval ulcers that are:
• Painful
• Located on inside of cheeks or lips, side of tongue, soft palate or floor of mouth
• Bordered by a raised margin with red halo
• White/yellow/grey in the centre (pseudomembrane)
• ≤1 cm in diameter
• <7 days in duration
Patient has:
• History of childhood ulcers
• Family history of recurrent aphthous ulcers
• Recently stopped smoking
Yes
Probable minor aphthae
Recommend appropriate nonpharmacologic measures and topical therapies.
Reassess if ulcer(s) still present or worsen after 14 days

Table 3: Topical Therapies for Aphthous Ulcers

Class	Drug	Dosage	Adverse Effects	Comments	Cost[a]
Anesthetics	*benzocaine* Anbesol, Kank-A, Orajel, others	Apply to affected area in the mouth up to QID	Application site burning, edema, erythema, pruritus, rash, stinging, tenderness, urticaria. Rarely methemoglobinemia signs and symptoms (e.g., respiratory distress and cyanosis).	May be useful to apply to sores before eating so mastication could be less painful.	$
	benzydamine 0.15% Pharixia, generics	Rinse mouth with 15 mL TID–QID as needed; do not swallow	Burning, cough, dry mouth, headache, nausea, numbness, sedation, stinging, vomiting.	Dose should be held in the mouth for about 30 seconds for best effect.	$$
	lidocaine Xylocaine Viscous, generics	See benzocaine.	See benzocaine.	See benzocaine.	$
Anti-inflammatories	*triamcinolone acetonide* Oracort	Dab on the ulcers up to TID	Local irritation, sticky or pasty sensation in the mouth.	To avoid a granular gritty sensation do not rub or spread the paste when applying to the lesions. If using multiple times daily, it is preferable to apply after eating.	$$
Protectants	*carboxymethyl cellulose* Orabase Paste	Use as often as needed particularly after eating	Sticky or pasty sensation in the mouth.	Coat the involved area of the mouth with a thin film. Hold in position until it becomes sticky. Do not rub it in.	$

[a] Cost of smallest available pack size; includes drug cost only.

Legend: $ < $10 $$ $10–20

Resource Tips

Mayo Clinic. Diseases and Conditions. *Canker sore*. Available from: www.mayoclinic.com/health/canker-sore/DS00354.

U.S. National Library of Medicine; National Institutes of Health. MedlinePlus. *Canker sore*. Available from: www.nlm.nih.gov/medlineplus/ency/article/000998.htm.

Suggested Readings

Altenburg A, Zouboulis CC. Current concepts in the treatment of recurrent aphthous stomatitis. *Skin Therapy Lett* 2008;13:1-4.

Belenguer-Guallar I, Jiménez-Soriano Y, Claramunt-Lozano A. Treatment of recurrent aphthous stomatitis. A literature review. *J Clin Exp Dent* 2014;6:e168-74.

Messadi DV, Younai F. Aphthous ulcers. *Dermatol Ther* 2010;23:281-90.

References

1. Barrons RW. Treatment strategies for recurrent oral aphthous ulcers. *Am J Health Syst Pharm* 2001;58:41-50.
2. McBride DR. Management of aphthous ulcers. *Am Fam Physician* 2000;62:149-54, 160.
3. Mayo Clinic. Diseases and Conditions. *Canker sore*. Available from: www.mayoclinic.com/health/canker-sore/DS00354. Accessed February 25, 2016.
4. Flaitz CM, Baker KA. Treatment approaches to common symptomatic oral lesions in children. *Dent Clin North Am* 2000;44:671-96.
5. Scully C, Gorsky M, Lozada-Nur F. The diagnosis and management of recurrent aphthous stomatitis: a consensus approach. *J Am Dent Assoc* 2003;134:200-7.
6. Messadi DV, Younai F. Aphthous ulcers. *Dermatol Ther* 2010;23:281-90.
7. Sawair FA. Recurent aphthous stomatitis: do we know what patients are using to treat the ulcers? *J Alternat Complement Med* 2010;16:651-5.
8. For the dental patient. Common mouth sores and patches. *J Am Dent Assoc* 2002;133:391.
9. Shim YJ, Choi JH, Ahn HJ et al. Effect of sodium lauryl sulfate on recurrent aphthous stomatitis: a randomized controlled clinical trial. *Oral Dis* 2012;18:655-60.
10. Healy CM, Paterson M, Joyston-Bechal S et al. The effect of a sodium lauryl sulfate-free dentifrice on patients with recurrent oral ulceration. *Oral Dis* 1999;5(1):39-43.
11. Bailey J, McCarthy C, Smith RF et al. Clinical inquiry. What is the most effective way to treat recurrent canker sores? *J Fam Pract* 2011;60:621-32.
12. Volkov I, Rudoy I, Freud T et al. Effectiveness of vitamin B12 in treating recurrent aphthous stomatitis: a randomized, double-blind, placebo-controlled trial. *J Am Board Fam Med* 2009;22:9-16.
13. Liu HL, Chiu SC. The effectiveness of vitamin B12 for relieving pain in aphthous ulcers: a randomized, double-blind, placebo-controlled trial. *Pain Manag Nurs* 2015;16:182-7.
14. Boulinguez S, Reix S, Bedane C et al. Role of drug exposure in aphthous ulcers: a case-control study. *Br J Dermatol* 2000;143:1261-5.
15. Femiano F, Lanza A, Buonaiuto C et al. Guidelines for diagnosis and management of aphthous stomatitis. *Pediatr Infect Dis J* 2007;26:728-32.
16. Altenburg A, Zouboulis CC. Current concepts in the treatment of recurrent aphthous stomatitis. *Skin Therapy Lett* 2008;13:1-4.
17. Altenburg A, El-Haj N, Micheli C et al The treatment of chronic recurrent oral aphthous ulcers. *Dtsch Arztebl Int* 2014;111:665-73.
18. Chattopadhyay A, Shetty KV. Recurrent aphthous stomatitis. *Otolaryngol Clin North Am* 2011;44:79-88.
19. Lalla RV, Schubert MM, Bensadoun RJ et al. Anti-inflammatory agents in the management of alimentary mucositis. *Support Care Cancer* 2006;14:558-65.
20. Bruce A, Rogers RS. New and old therapeutics for oral ulcerations. *Arch Dermatol* 2007;143:519-23.
21. Belenguer-Guallar I, Jiménez-Soriano Y, Claramunt-Lozano A. Treatment of recurrent aphthous stomatitis. A literature review. *J Clin Exp Dent* 2014;6:e168-74.
22. Liu C, Zhou Z, Liu G et al. Efficacy and safety of dexamethasone ointment on recurrent aphthous ulceration. *Am J Med* 2012;125:292-301.
23. Al-Na'mah ZM, Carson R, Thanoon IA. Dexamucobase: a novel treatment for oral aphthous ulceration. *Quintessence Int* 2009;40:399-404.
24. Gorsky M, Epstein J, Rabenstein S et al. Topical minocycline and tetracycline rinses in treatment of recurrent aphthous stomatitis: a randomized cross-over study. *Dermatol Online J* 2007;13(2):1.
25. Zhou Y, Chen Q, Meng W et al. Evaluation of penicillin G potassium troches in the treatment of minor recurrent aphthous ulceration in a Chinese cohort: a randomized, double-blinded, placebo and no-treatment-controlled, multicenter clinical trial. *Oral Surg Oral Med Oral Pathol Oral Radiol Endod* 2010;109(4):561-6.
26. Brocklehurst P, Tickle M, Glenny AM et al. Systemic interventions for recurrent aphthous stomatitis (mouth ulcers). *Cochrane Database Syst Rev* 2012;9:CD005411.
27. Fontes V, Machet L, Huttenberger B et al. [Recurrent aphthous stomatitis: treatment with colchicine. An open trial of 54 cases]. *Ann Dermatol Venereol* 2002;129:1365-9. [French].
28. Femiano F, Buonaiuto C, Gombos F et al. Pilot study on recurrent aphthous stomatitis (RAS): a randomized placebo-controlled trial for the comparative therapeutic effects of systemic prednisone and systemic montelukast in subjects unresponsive to topical therapy. *Oral Surg Med Oral Pathol Oral Radiol Endod* 2010;109:402-7.
29. Lynde CB, Bruce AJ, Rogers RS. Successful treatment of complex aphthosis with colchicine and dapsone. *Arch Dermatol* 2009;145:273-6.
30. Munoz-Corcuera M, Esparza-Gomez G, Gonzales-Moles MA et al. Oral ulcers: clinical aspects. A tool for dermatologists. Part I. Acute ulcers. *Clin Exp Dermatol* 2009;34:289-94.

Canker Sores—What You Need to Know

To help your canker sore feel better:

- Avoid foods that hurt—foods that are hard, crusty, sharp, spicy, salty, acidic or hard to chew. Examples are: crackers, potato chips, pickles, oranges, lemons, tomatoes and fruit juices.
- Take care to keep your teeth and gums clean but be careful not to hurt the canker sore. Brush your teeth using a *soft* toothbrush twice a day and use dental floss once a day. Use a new *soft* toothbrush if your old one has splayed or broken bristles that can hurt your mouth or the canker sore.
- Rinse your mouth with 1/2–1 teaspoonful (2.5–5 mL) of table salt dissolved in 1 cup of warm water several times a day to help soothe the canker sore. Use this rinse after meals to remove bits of food that may bother the canker sore. Be sure to spit out the salt water after rinsing.
- Most mouthwashes for bad breath have a high alcohol content and using them will make the canker sore sting. Don't use these mouthwashes when you have a canker sore.
- A canker sore should get better on its own in 10–14 days. Your pharmacist may suggest you use an ointment with an anesthetic in it to help the pain for a short time. You may use this 4 times a day for no longer than 14 days. Put a small amount of anesthetic ointment on the canker sore, using a cotton-tipped swab (Q-tips), before eating meals and before going to bed.
- Your pharmacist may suggest that you cover the canker sore with a small amount of Orabase or Zilactin to help lessen the pain.
- You may use a nonprescription pain medicine such as acetaminophen to help reduce the pain. Your pharmacist can help you choose a pain medicine that is right for you and tell you how to take it.

To help prevent canker sores:

- If you sometimes bite the inside of your cheek and a canker sore appears at that spot, take extra care while chewing. Chew your food slowly and try not to talk while you are chewing.
- If you have any teeth or dental work with sharp points, see your dentist so that the sharp points can be made less irritating.
- Most toothpastes have an ingredient called sodium lauryl sulfate. Some people have fewer canker sores when they use a toothpaste that does not have this ingredient in it. Your pharmacist can suggest a toothpaste, if you want to try this approach.

You should see a doctor or dentist if:

- The canker sore is still there after 14 days.
- If the canker sore has gotten larger or if more canker sores have developed.
- The pain is not controlled when using the medication recommended, and you have difficulty chewing or swallowing.
- If you also feel sick, have a fever, pain in the joints, irritated eyes or many, watery bowel movements.

Chapter 90

Cold Sores (Herpes Labialis)

James S. Conklin, BSc(Pharm), ACPR

Pathophysiology

Two herpes simplex viruses (HSV) are most relevant to cold sores: herpes simplex-1 (HSV-1) and herpes simplex-2 (HSV-2). HSV-1, which is most commonly transmitted via saliva, causes the majority of oral herpes infections; HSV-2, which is present in genital secretions, causes the majority of genital herpes infections.[1,2] However, orogenital contact may cause a primary infection of either type in either the oral or genital region.[1,2] Both HSV-1 and HSV-2 can cause primary or recurrent infections. When symptomatic, and involving the oral region, a first infection is known as primary herpes gingivostomatitis. Although not inevitable, 20–40% of patients who experience a primary herpes infection develop subsequent recurrent herpes infections caused by reactivation of HSV that remains latent in neural ganglion cells.[1,2] Recurrences in the oral region most commonly affect the vermilion border of the lips and are known as herpes labialis, cold sores or fever blisters[2,3] (see Cold Sore in Photo Section). Less commonly, recurrences appear on the palate, chin or oral mucosa.[2]

Primary HSV-1 infection occurs in approximately one-third of school-aged children[4] and serological evidence of HSV-1 infection is evident in up to 80% of adolescents and adults.[1,2] Babies generally acquire anti-HSV antibodies from their mothers, which protect them from infection until around 6 months of age.[3]

The incidence of infection with HSV-2 increases after sexual activity begins, with risk factors including being female, a history of sexually transmitted disease and multiple sexual partners.[3,5,6]

Goals of Therapy

- Reduce any discomfort, including pain or itching
- Reduce viral shedding
- Reduce the duration of lesions
- Reduce the severity of the episode
- Prevent secondary bacterial infection
- Prevent recurrences

Patient Assessment

Primary HSV infections are frequently subclinical, or cause symptoms difficult to differentiate from upper respiratory tract infections.[2,7,8] Symptomatic infections may be characterized by malaise, fever, chills, muscle aches, lymphadenopathy and multiple crops of painful vesicles or blisters and ulcerative erosions on the tongue, palate, gingiva, buccal mucosa and lips, occurring 1–26 days after inoculation.[1,2] The lesions rupture readily, leaving small ulcers covered with a pseudomembrane and surrounded by erythema.[5] This primary infection lasts 1–3 weeks without scarring.[6] Constitutional symptoms may last 10–14 days.[2] Oral shedding of the virus may continue up to 23 days.[6] In severe primary episodes, discomfort may interfere with eating and drinking to the point of dehydration.[2] Some patients go on to have recurrent infections, typically 1–6 episodes per year, while others never experience a second episode.[2] A first episode in a patient already seropositive for HSV is termed a nonprimary initial infection, and these infections tend to be less severe.[2]

A prodromal tingling, itching or burning sensation in the location of the eruption may occur 2–24 hours before the appearance of the vesicles in 60% of patients.[2,5,6] The lesion then appears over 1–2 days.[6] Papules on an erythematous base usually become vesicles within hours and then break open, leaking a clear, sticky fluid, and subsequently progress through the stages of ulceration, crusting, and healing over 72–120 hours.[2,6] Time to full healing without scarring may take up to 7–10 days.[5,6] Generally there are no systemic symptoms and patients complain only of the unsightly appearance and pain, and sometimes itching. In a quarter of recurrent cases, the infection heals before blisters or ulcers can form.[1]

Patients who are immunosuppressed by disease or drug therapy are at higher risk of recurrences of HSV. This includes those receiving immunosuppressive cancer chemotherapy or drugs to suppress rejection of organ transplantation, and those with acquired immunodeficiency syndrome (AIDS). Atopic individuals may develop a rapidly progressing HSV cutaneous infection.

Refer immunocompromised patients or those with frequent, persistent, recurrent or swollen oral lesions to an appropriate healthcare practitioner for assessment (Figure 1).

Prevention

Common stressors that can precipitate recurrences include emotional stress, dental extraction, fever, hormonal factors, hyperthermia, menstruation, physical trauma or surgery, sun exposure (UV light) and upper respiratory infection.[1,2,5,9]

Prophylactic treatment prior to dental procedures may be indicated to prevent a recurrence.[10]

Protecting affected areas from sun exposure, especially while at the beach and on ski hills, will likely reduce the frequency of cold sore recurrences.[6,7,11] A **sunscreen** with an SPF of 30 or higher should be applied to the lips and face 30 minutes prior to exposure.

Reducing stress (e.g., eating well, getting enough sleep and exercise, relaxation) may also help prevent recurrences in individuals for whom stress is a known trigger.[5,7]

Avoid spread of cold sores to other parts of the body and to other people by frequent hand washing and avoiding skin-to-skin contact with others until after the blister has dried up and crusted over.

Nonpharmacologic Therapy

Advise patients to keep the lesion clean with gentle washing using a mild soap and water. This can also be accomplished by soaking the area with cool, tap-water compresses.[12] Patients should avoid excessive touching of the lesion and should wash their hands frequently to prevent autoinnoculation and spread of HSV.

Heat application is a treatment yet to be evaluated through randomized research. Devices in the shape of a lipstick have been marketed for use on areas where prodromal symptoms are felt. It is postulated that the high temperature (50 degrees Celsius) blocks replication of the virus and the resultant formation of blisters.[1] More evidence is required before such devices could be recommended for the treatment of cold sores.

Pharmacologic Therapy

Although oral HSV infections in immunocompetent patients are self-limiting, antivirals and analgesics can be recommended for primary or recurrent infections. Topical protectants are also available to help prevent cracking and excessive drying of the HSV lesions (e.g., **allantoin**, **calamine**, **cocoa butter**,

petrolatum, zinc oxide).[13] Table 1 presents nonprescription medications commonly used to manage cold sores. For further discussion of pharmacologic therapy for cold sores, consult the *Compendium of Therapeutic Choices*: Herpesvirus Infections.

For comparative ingredients of nonprescription products, consult the *Compendium of Products of Minor Ailments*—Analgesic Products: Internal Analgesics and Antipyretics; Mouth Products: Cold Sores and Canker Sores; Skin Care Products: Anesthetics, First Aid.

Analgesics

Systemic analgesics such as **acetaminophen**, **ibuprofen** or **naproxen** can be recommended to control moderate to severe pain for a period not exceeding 3 days. Topical products containing anesthetics such as **benzocaine**, **camphor**, **lidocaine**, **menthol**, **phenol**, **pramoxine**, or **prilocaine** may be useful in relieving mild pain for a relatively short period of time. See Table 1 for commonly used doses.

Antivirals

The topical antiviral **docosanol** is used for the treatment of cold sores and prevents the virus from spreading to healthy cells. It should be applied to the HSV lesions multiple times daily at the first sign of pain, itching, burning, redness or tingling. This medication is most helpful when used early in the course of an outbreak and may decrease the duration of painful symptoms and time to healing by 1–3 days.

Several other antiviral agents including **acyclovir**, **famciclovir** and **valacyclovir** have been studied for either the treatment or prophylaxis of cold sores. Not all of these drugs have an official indication for cold sores in the general population. Valacyclovir and famciclovir (prodrugs of acyclovir and penciclovir, respectively) are designed to increase the bioavailability of their active forms.[2] Generally speaking, these antiviral agents have few toxic effects because they are converted by viral thymidine kinase to active drug only once they are inside virally infected cells.[2]

Three differing approaches to antiviral treatment may be used: intermittent episodic therapy (IET), chronic suppressive therapy (CST) or intermittent suppressive therapy (IST).[2]

IET is the treatment of isolated, acute episodes of HSV at the first clinical sign or symptom. For initial primary infections, evidence supports the use of acyclovir, valacyclovir and famciclovir.[18,19,20,21,22] Prompt initiation of treatment is more efficacious, but does not decrease recurrences.[2] IET for recurrent infections is effective if begun within 48 hours of an outbreak.[2] Evidence supports the use of oral acyclovir, valacyclovir, famciclovir and **acyclovir 5% cream** with or without topical **hydrocortisone**.[23,24,25,26,27,28,29] Overall, topical treatments appear to be less effective than systemic treatments.[2]

CST is not indicated for most patients with HSV infection, but may be appropriate for the 5–10% of patients who experience frequent recurrences (≥6 per year), who also experience disfigurement, difficulty swallowing or severe pain, have prolonged episodes, or are particularly distressed.[2] Evidence supports the use of oral acyclovir and valacyclovir.[22,24,30,31]

IST is appropriate when recurrences can be anticipated based on known precipitating factors (see Prevention section below), particularly in situations where decreasing viral shedding will decrease the likelihood of infecting seronegative individuals.[2] Specific dosing guidelines are not available for IST, but extrapolation of data from CST studies is thought to be appropriate.[2] Oral acyclovir has been shown to have some effect on preventing sunlight-induced recurrences but data for topical acyclovir cream are conflicting (possibly due to poor penetration from site of application).[32,33,34,35]

Corticosteroids

Corticosteroids are not routinely recommended for use in oral inflammation caused by viruses, as they may mask the spread of infection and suppress the normal immune response. However, their topical use (e.g., fluocinonide 0.05%, hydrocortisone 1%) in conjunction with antivirals may be helpful.[36]

Natural Health Products

There is some evidence that a cream of **lemon balm** (*Melissa officinalis*) containing 1% of a 70:1 leaf extract, applied to the site of a cold sore during the prodromal stage, reduces the number and size of lesions, although the overall severity of the outbreak is not lessened.[37,38] Lemon balm is usually applied 2–4 times daily from first sign of prodrome to a few days after the lesions have healed.[37,38,39]

Lysine, one of the essential amino acids, is marketed in oral and topical dosage forms for prevention and treatment of cold sores. Evidence regarding the effectiveness of lysine for this indication varies. Some studies suggest its efficacy in prevention is dose dependent. Studies using lower dosages (e.g., 624 mg daily) did not show benefit whereas 6 of 7 studies using doses ranging from 750–4000 mg daily support its use to decrease the frequency of recurrences, and to reduce the severity and time to healing.[8,40,41] Large amounts of nitrogen are produced through the metabolism of lysine. Persons with renal or hepatic disease may have difficulty eliminating this nitrogen and therefore its use as a supplement is contraindicated in these patients. Lysine can increase the absorption and decrease the elimination of calcium.[40,41] Topical application of lysine in a combination product also containing zinc oxide and 14 other ingredients seemed to decrease symptoms and duration of cold sores when applied every 2 hours.[42]

Other Therapies

Limited evidence from a single small study suggests that **zinc sulfate** 22.5 mg twice daily for 4 months may reduce the occurrence of cold sores as well as the duration of lesions during an episode.[8]

There is no published evidence regarding the safety and effectiveness of **heparin** in the treatment of cold sores, although it is an ingredient in frequently recommended products.

Caustic substances such as **silver nitrate** may create further damage and should not be applied to cold sores.

Highly astringent topical ingredients such as **tannic acid** are not recommended for treatment of cold sores. They have the potential to cause excessive drying of the area with resultant fissuring, discomfort and potential bacterial superinfection.[12,13] In addition, the herpes virus may be fractionated by astringents thereby causing resistant strains to emerge.[13]

Monitoring of Therapy

Cold sores are expected to resolve within 2 weeks. If nonpharmacologic and pharmacologic treatments do not relieve the discomfort, the lesions spread, or the patient develops symptoms of systemic illness (e.g., fever, malaise, swollen glands), further evaluation is indicated. If application of a product containing a local anesthetic causes increased erythema and edema in the area of the lesion, contact dermatitis should be suspected and the product discontinued.

Figure 1: **Assessment of Patients with Cold Sores**

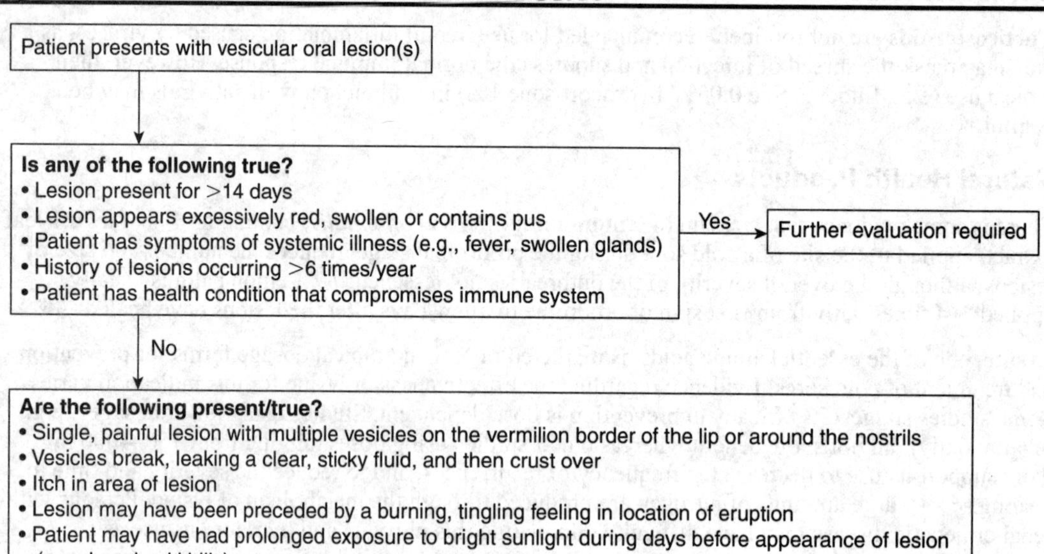

Patient presents with vesicular oral lesion(s)
Is any of the following true?
• Lesion present for >14 days
• Lesion appears excessively red, swollen or contains pus
• Patient has symptoms of systemic illness (e.g., fever, swollen glands)
• History of lesions occurring >6 times/year
• Patient has health condition that compromises immune system
Yes
Further evaluation required
No
Are the following present/true?
• Single, painful lesion with multiple vesicles on the vermilion border of the lip or around the nostrils
• Vesicles break, leaking a clear, sticky fluid, and then crust over
• Itch in area of lesion
• Lesion may have been preceded by a burning, tingling feeling in location of eruption
• Patient may have had prolonged exposure to bright sunlight during days before appearance of lesion (e.g., beach, ski hills)
• Duration >7 days
Yes
Probable cold sore (herpes labialis)
• Recommend pharmacologic and nonpharmacologic treatment (see Table 1)
• Provide patient information
• If lesions spread, pharmacologic treatment does not relieve discomfort, local anesthetics cause erythema and edema or patient develops symptoms of systemic illness, refer to an appropriate healthcare practitioner for further evaluation

Table 1: **Nonprescription Drug Therapy For Cold Sores[a]**

Class	Drug	Dosage	Adverse Effects	Drug Interactions	Comments	Cost[b]
Analgesics, Oral	*acetaminophen* Atasol Preparations, Tempra, Tylenol, generics	**Adults and children >12 y:** 10–15 mg/kg Q4–6H po, not to exceed 4000 mg/24 h **Children <12 y:** 10–15 mg/kg Q4–6H po/pr as needed for symptom management; maximum 75 mg/kg/day. Do not exceed adult dose	Nausea, rash; chronic use of high doses may produce significant liver and renal toxicity.	Increased risk of hepatotoxicity with excessive alcohol intake (>3 drinks/day). Acetaminophen may increase INR in warfarin-treated patients; check INR if acetaminophen dose exceeds 2 g/day for ≥3 consecutive days. Adjust warfarin dosage as required.	Should not be used for >3 days. Intended for pain relief.	$
	ibuprofen Advil, Motrin, generics	**All age groups:** 5–10 mg/kg Q6–8H po, not to exceed 3 doses/day Maximum dose for self-care: 1200 mg/day	Dizziness, headache, lightheadedness, dyspepsia, nausea, heartburn, abdominal pain.	Increased risk of bleeding with anticoagulants (e.g., warfarin) or antiplatelet drugs (e.g., clopidogrel). May decrease effect of antihypertensives. May decrease renal clearance of lithium; monitor lithium levels. Increased risk of GI bleeding when used with SSRIs or corticosteroids.	See acetaminophen.	$
	naproxen sodium Aleve, generics	**Adults and children >12 y:** 220 mg Q8–12H po, not to exceed 440 mg/day	See ibuprofen.	See ibuprofen.	See acetaminophen.	$

(cont'd)

Table 1: **Nonprescription Drug Therapy For Cold Sores**[a] *(cont'd)*

Class	Drug	Dosage	Adverse Effects	Drug Interactions	Comments	Cost[b]
Analgesics, Topical	*benzocaine* Anbesol, Orajel, others	**Adults and children >2 y:** Apply to affected area for 1–5 h then remove	Application site numbness and tingling. Allergic contact dermatitis.	No significant drug interactions.	May offer temporary relief of pain and itching. More likely to cause sensitization than lidocaine. Available as liquid, gel or cream in various strengths.	$$
	camphor/menthol/ phenol Blistex, Blistex Lip Medex, others	**Adults and children >2 y:** Apply to affected area 3–4 times daily	Mild tingling, cool feeling. May leave a white residue on skin. Camphor at a concentration >3% and menthol >1% can cause irritation and inflammation and are therefore contraindicated in treatment of cold sores.	No significant drug interactions.	Offer temporary relief of pain and itching associated with cold sores.	$
	lidocaine Maxilene, generics	**Adults and children >2 y:** Apply to affected area for 1–5 h then remove	See benzocaine.	No significant drug interactions.	May offer temporary relief of pain and itching. May be less sensitizing than benzocaine. Available as liquid, gel or cream in various strengths.	$$

Class	Drug	Dosage	Adverse Effects	Drug Interactions	Comments	Cost[b]
	lidocaine/prilocaine 2.5% EMLA Cream	**Adults and children >2 y:** Apply to affected area for 1–5 h then remove	See benzocaine.	No significant drug interactions.	Application times longer than 5 h have no added benefit since the analgesic effectiveness dissipates over time. May reduce the duration of symptoms and the duration of eruptions by about half.[14,15] May offer temporary relief of pain and itching.	$$
	pramoxine Gold Bond Medicated Anti-Itch, Polysporin Itch Relief, others	**Adults and children >2 y:** Apply to affected area for 1–5 h then remove	Burning or stinging at site of application.	No significant drug interactions.	Local anesthetics with a non-ester, non-amide structure (e.g., pramoxine) are thought to be the least sensitizing.[14,15] Cross-sensitization with other local anesthetics is unlikely.	$$
Antivirals, Topical	*docosanol 10%* Abreva	**Adults and children >12 y:** Apply to the affected area at the first sign of pain, itching, burning, redness or tingling every 3 h for 5–10 days	Mild and infrequent stinging sensation.	No significant drug interactions.	Inhibits fusion between the plasma membrane and the herpesvirus envelope leading to blocking viral entry into the cell.[16,17] Most effective if used early in the course of an outbreak before a large number of host cells are infected. May decrease duration of painful symptoms and time to healing by 17–79 h.[16,17]	$$$

[a] For more information on antiviral therapy for HSV infection, consult the *Compendium of Therapeutic Choices*: Herpesvirus Infections

[b] Cost of smallest available pack size or 3-day supply; includes drug cost only.

Legend: $ < $5 $$ $5–10 $$$ $10–15

Resource Tips

GlaxoSmithKline. *Valtrex*. Available from: www.valtrex.com.

Herpes-Coldsores (HC) Support Network. *Herpes-coldsores*. Available from: www.herpes-coldsores.com.

MayoClinic. Diseases and Conditions. *Cold sore*. Available from: www.mayoclinic.org/diseases-conditions/cold-sore/basics/definition/con-20021310.

MedicineNet. *Cold sores (non-genital herpes simplex infections)*. Available from: www.medicinenet.com/herpes_simplex_infections_non-genital/article.html.

U.S. Centers for Disease Control and Prevention. Available from: www.cdc.gov.

Suggested Readings

Cernik C, Gallina K, Brodell RT. The treatment of herpes simplex infections: an evidence-based review. *Arch Intern Med* 2008;168:1137-44.

Cunningham A, Griffiths P, Leone P et al. Current management and recommendations for access to antiviral therapy of herpes labialis. *J Clin Virol* 2012;53:6-11.

Drugge JM, Allen PJ. A nurse practitioner's guide to the management of herpes simplex virus-1 in children. *Pediatr Nurs* 2008;34:310-8.

Gilbert SC. Management and prevention of recurrent herpes labialis in immunocompetent patients. *Herpes* 2007;14:56-61.

Opstelten W, Neven AK, Eekhof J. Treatment and prevention of herpes labialis. *Can Fam Physician* 2008;54:1683-7.

References

1. Opstelten W, Neven AK, Eekhof J. Treatment and prevention of herpes labialis. *Can Fam Physician* 2008;54:1683-7.
2. Cernik C, Gallina K, Brodell RT. The treatment of herpes simplex infections: an evidence-based review. *Arch Intern Med* 2008;168:1137-44.
3. Greenberg MS. Herpesvirus infections. *Dent Clin North Am* 1996;40:359-68.
4. Flaitz CM, Baker KA. Treatment approaches to common symptomatic oral lesions in children. *Dent Clin North Am* 2000;44:671-96.
5. Birek C. Herpesvirus-induced diseases: oral manifestations and current treatment options. *J Calif Dent Assoc* 2000;28:911-21.
6. Emmert DH. Treatment of common cutaneous herpes simplex virus infections. *Am Fam Physician* 2000;61:1697-706,1708.
7. Nadelman CM, Newcomer VD. Herpes simplex virus infections. New treatment approaches make early diagnosis even more important. *Postgrad Med* 2000;107:189-195, 199-200.
8. Drugge JM, Allen PJ. A nurse practitioner's guide to the management of herpes simplex virus-1 in children. *Pediatr Nurs* 2008;34:310-8.
9. Guerriere-Kovach PM, Brodell RT. Recurrent herpes simplex virus infection. Suppressive, reactive, and preventive antiviral regimens. *Postgrad Med* 2000;107:139-40,143,147.
10. Miller CS, Cunningham LL, Lindroth JE et al. The efficacy of valacyclovir in preventing recurrent herpes simplex virus infections associated with dental procedures. *J Am Dent Assoc* 2004;135:1311-8.
11. Raborn GW, Martel AY, Grace MG et al. Herpes labialis in skiers: randomized clinical trial of acyclovir cream versus placebo. *Oral Surg Oral Med Oral Pathol Oral Radiol Endod* 1997;84:641-5.
12. Covington TR, ed. *Nonprescription drug therapy: guiding patient self-care*. St. Louis: Facts & Comparisons; 2002.
13. Pray WS. *Nonprescription product therapeutics*. 2nd ed. Baltimore: Lippincott Williams & Wilkins; 2006.
14. Cassuto J. Topical local anaesthetics and herpes simplex. *Lancet* 1989;1:100-1.
15. Kaminester LH, Pariser RJ, Pariser DM et al. A double-blind, placebo-controlled study of topical tetracaine in the treatment of herpes labialis. *J Am Acad Dermatol* 1999;41:996-1001.
16. Habbema L, DeBoulle K, Roders GA et al. n-Docosanol 10% cream in the treatment of recurrent herpes labialis: a randomised, double-blind, placebo-controlled study. *Acta Derm Venereol* 1996;76:479-81.
17. Sacks SL, Thisted RA, Jones TM et al. Clinical efficacy of topical docosanol 10% cream for herpes simplex labialis: a multicenter, randomized, placebo-controlled trial. *J Am Acad Dermatol* 2001;45:222-30.
18. Arduino PG, Porter SR. Oral and perioral herpes simplex virus type 1 (HSV-1) infection: review of its management. *Oral Dis* 2006;12:254-70.
19. Nikkels AF, Pierard GE. Treatment of mucocutaneous presentations of herpes simplex virus infections. *Am J Clin Dermatol* 2002;3:475-87.
20. Amir J, Harel L, Smetana Z et al. Treatment of herpes simplex gingivostomatitis with aciclovir in children: a randomised double blind placebo controlled study. *BMJ* 1997;314:1800-3.
21. Chauvin PJ, Ajar AH. Acute herpetic gingivostomatitis in adults: a review of 13 cases, including diagnosis and management. *J Can Dent Assoc* 2002;68:247-51.
22. Rooney JF, Straus SE, Mannix ML et al. Oral acyclovir to suppress frequently recurrent herpes labialis. A double-blind, placebo-controlled trial. *Ann Intern Med* 1993;118:268-72.
23. Spruance SL, Bodsworth N, Resnick H et al. Single-dose, patient-initiated famciclovir: a randomized, double-blind, placebo-controlled trial for episodic treatment of herpes labialis. *J Am Acad Dermatol* 2006;55:47-53.

24. Spruance SL, Stewart JC, Rowe NH et al. Treatment of recurrent herpes simplex labialis with oral acyclovir. *J Infect Dis* 1990;161:185-90.
25. Spruance SL, Jones TM, Blatter MM et al. High-dose, short-duration, early valacyclovir therapy for episodic treatment of cold sores: results of two randomized, placebo-controlled, multicenter studies. *Antimicrob Agents Chemother* 2003;47:1072-80.
26. Chacko M, Weinberg JM. Famciclovir for cutaneous herpesvirus infections: an update and review of new single-day dosing indications. *Cutis* 2007;80:77-81.
27. Spruance SL, Nett R, Marbury T et al. Acyclovir cream for treatment of herpes simplex labialis: results of two randomized, double-blind, vehicle-controlled, multicenter clinical trials. *Antimicrob Agents Chemother* 2002;46:2238-43.
28. Chon T, Nguyen L, Elliott TC. Clinical inquiries. What are the best treatments for herpes labialis? *J Fam Pract* 2007;56:576-8.
29. Fiddian AP, Yeo JM, Stubbings R et al. Successful treatment of herpes labialis with topical acyclovir. *Br Med J (Clin Res Ed)* 1983;286:1699-701.
30. Gilbert SC. Suppressive therapy versus episodic therapy with oral valacyclovir for recurrent herpes labialis: efficacy and tolerability in an open-label, crossover study. *J Drugs Dermatol* 2007;6:400-5.
31. Baker D, Eisen D. Valacyclovir for prevention of recurrent herpes labialis: 2 double-blind, placebo-controlled studies. *Cutis* 2003;71:239-42.
32. Spruance SL, Hamill ML, Hoge WS et al. Acyclovir prevents reactivation of herpes simplex labialis in skiers. *JAMA* 1988;260:1597-9.
33. Nelson MA. Stopping the spread of herpes simplex: a focus on wrestlers. *Phys Sportsmed* 1992;20:117-27.
34. Leflore S, Anderson PL, Fletcher CV. A risk-benefit evaluation of aciclovir for the treatment and prophylaxis of herpes simplex virus infections. *Drug Saf* 2000;23:131-42.
35. Vander Straten M, Carrasco D, Lee P et al. A review of antiviral therapy for herpes labialis. *Arch Dermatol* 2001;137:1232-5.
36. Arain N, Paravastu SC, Arain MA. Effectiveness of topical corticosteroids in addition to antiviral therapy in the management of recurrent herpes labialis: a systematic review and meta-analysis. *BMC Infect Dis* 2015;15:82.
37. Koytchev R, Alken RG, Dundarov S. Balm mint extract (Lo-701) for topical treatment of recurring herpes labialis. *Phytomedicine* 1999;6:225-30.
38. Natural Medicines Comprehensive Database. *Lemon balm*. Available from: www.naturaldatabase.com. Accessed February 8, 2016. Subscription required.
39. Wolbling RH, Leonhardt K. Local therapy of herpes simplex with dried extract from Melissa officinalis. *Phytomedicine* 1994;1:25-31.
40. Tomblin FA, Lucas KH. Lysine for management of herpes labialis. *Am J Health Syst Pharm* 2001;58:298-300,304.
41. Natural Medicines Comprehensive Database. *Lysine*. Available from: www.naturaldatabase.com. Accessed February 8, 2016. Subscription required.
42. Singh BB, Udani J, Vinjamury S et al. Safety and effectiveness of an L-lysine, zinc, and herbal-based product on the treatment of facial and circumoral herpes. *Altern Med Rev* 2005;10:123-7.

Cold Sores—What You Need To Know

What is a cold sore?

A cold sore is a small blister that usually appears on the outer edge of the lip or near the nostrils. Cold sores may appear one at a time or in little groups. Sometimes they are filled with fluid. They usually crust over and form a scab before they go away. They may last a week or 2 and usually don't need any special treatment.

What causes cold sores?

Cold sores are caused by a virus called herpes simplex. They are spread by contact with a person who has the virus. Cold sores are most contagious from the time they first appear until they get dry and crusty.

Once the herpes virus is in your body, you may get cold sores occasionally for the rest of your life. Some people find that bright sunlight or stress can trigger their cold sores.

How to take care of a cold sore?

- Wash gently with mild soap and water to keep the cold sore clean.
- Avoid touching the cold sore with your fingers.
- Wash your hands often with soap and water to avoid getting an infection in the cold sore. Washing your hands also helps stop the spread of the virus.
- Always use your own towel. **Do not** let other people use your towel.
- Use an ointment (such as Vaseline) on the cold sore to keep it from cracking and drying. This helps prevent infection.
- Ask your healthcare provider for information about ointments that contain an anesthetic. The anesthetic may help stop the pain and itching for a short time. Stop using the ointment once the scab falls off.
- The best way to apply an ointment is with a clean, cotton-tipped swab (Q-Tip). If you use your finger, be sure to wash your hands before and after.
- If the cold sore is very painful, you may use a pain medicine such as acetaminophen, ibuprofen or naproxen. Ask your healthcare provider which medicine is best for you.

What can you do to prevent cold sores from spreading?

To stop the virus from spreading:

- **Do not** have skin-to-skin contact with young children, people with eczema, cancer or AIDS or anyone who has had an organ transplant while you have a cold sore.
- **Do not** share forks, spoons, drinking containers, razors or towels while you have a cold sore.
- **Do not** kiss others while you have a cold sore.

You should see a healthcare provider if:

- The cold sore gets worse or the skin around it gets red; you may have an infection.
- The skin around the cold sore becomes red and swollen after using an anesthetic ointment (stop using the ointment).
- The cold sore does not go away after 14 days of care.
- The cold sore spreads or you feel sick with a fever or swollen glands.

- You get cold sores often (6 or more in a year). Your healthcare provider may prescribe medicine to help decrease the number.

How to keep cold sores from coming back?

- Protect yourself from bright sunlight—some people get cold sores at the beach or when skiing. Apply sunscreen (minimum SPF 30) on lips and face 30 minutes before going out into the sun. Wearing a hat with a wide brim can also help.
- Take good care of yourself—some people find that they get cold sores when they are tired and stressed. If this happens to you, try to reduce the stress in your life or learn how to deal with it better. Regular exercise, getting enough sleep and eating well can help.

Chapter 91
Dry Mouth

Victoria Kletas, BScPharm, MSc

Pathophysiology

Dry mouth, also known as xerostomia, is a common symptom usually associated with salivary hypofunction resulting in reduced quantity or altered quality of saliva. It has been estimated that a 50 percent reduction in salivary secretion needs to occur before xerostomia becomes apparent.[1] However, xerostomia and hyposalivation are not synonymous since xerostomia (a subjective feeling) may exist in the presence of normal salivary flow (an objective measure) and some patients may not complain of xerostomia even in the presence of demonstrated hyposalivation. Xerostomia affects about one in every 4–5 adults. It can occur at any age but is more prevalent in older individuals, affecting 25% of women and 16% of men.[2] Rates in institutionalized elderly people may be as high as 50%.[3]

Xerostomia is not a disease, but a manifestation secondary to a medical condition, a drug or radiation to the salivary glands (head and neck area) in cancer patients.[4] Following radiation therapy, the degree of permanent xerostomia depends on the volume of salivary gland included in the fields of radiation and the total radiation dose. Radiation causes a change to secretory cells resulting in a reduction of salivary output and increased viscosity of the saliva.[5]

Xerostomia can be a component of graft-versus-host disease following bone marrow transplantation.[2,6] Mouth breathing due to dyspnea, nasal obstruction or delivery of oxygen via nasal prongs can be a major cause of dry mouth in the terminally ill.[7]

Individuals infected with HIV may sometimes experience salivary and parotid gland enlargement leading to xerostomia.[4] The risk of dry mouth is also increased by smoking or chewing tobacco and the intake of caffeine-containing beverages.[8] Patients undergoing hemodialysis or with poorly controlled diabetes may also be at risk of xerostomia.[9,10]

Sjögren's syndrome, a chronic inflammatory autoimmune disease, is a common cause of dry mouth.[11] It is characterized by lymphocytic infiltration of salivary and lacrimal glands and, in addition to xerostomia, results in blurred vision, decreased lacrimal function, recurrent eye and mouth infections, difficulty swallowing, dry nasal passages, dry throat, and smell and taste alterations.[11,12] Other systemic diseases that can cause xerostomia are listed in Table 1.

Saliva has various protective functions which include maintaining the neutral pH of the mouth, promoting remineralization of teeth, coating the teeth and lubricating the oral mucosa, providing local antimicrobial activity and assisting in the taste mechanism.[6] The loss of saliva's protective functions can affect all of the mouth's functions and may increase the risk of developing *Candida* infection and dental caries.[13] It can also lead to a lack of efficacy of certain medications (e.g., sublingual nitroglycerin or lorazepam). Table 2 lists potential complications of dry mouth that may affect a person's general well-being and quality of life.[2]

Consider xerostomia if a patient is having difficulty eating dry foods such as crackers,[4] or if lipstick adheres to the front teeth in women.[14] On examination, the mucosa may be dry and sticky, with the saliva appearing stringy or foamy. Dental caries may be found at the cervical margin (neck of teeth) or incisal margins (the tips) of the teeth.[4] The mucosa may appear erythematous due to overgrowth of

Candida albicans, with patches commonly affecting the hard or soft palate and dorsal surface of the tongue.

Goals of Therapy

- Prevent complications of dry mouth such as dental caries, poor nutrition, fungal infection
- Relieve symptoms and improve mouth comfort

Table 1: **Systemic Conditions that can Cause or are Associated with Dry Mouth**

Autoimmune diseases	**Neurologic disorders**	**Miscellaneous**
Celiac disease	Bell's palsy	Absent or malformed salivary glands
Rheumatoid arthritis	Parkinson's disease	Alcoholic cirrhosis
Scleroderma	**Psychiatric disorders**	Bone marrow transplantation
Sjögren's syndrome	Alzheimer's disease	Dehydration
Systemic lupus erythematosus	Anxiety	Hypertension
Endocrine disorders	Depression	Nephritis
Addison's disease	**Viral infections**	Nutritional deficiencies
Diabetes mellitus	Hepatitis C	Primary biliary cirrhosis
Hyperlipidemia	HIV infection	
Hypothyroidism	Mumps	
Genetic diseases		
Cystic fibrosis		
Down syndrome		

Table 2: **Potential Complications of Dry Mouth**

Avoidance of some foods that are difficult to chew and swallow	Inhibition of taste sensation
Decreased ability to chew and swallow	Oral infections, e.g., candidiasis, gingivitis
Decreased nutritional status	Tooth loss
Impaired ability or willingness to talk	Wearing dentures becomes uncomfortable or impossible
Increased dental caries	

Patient Assessment

Help patients evaluate their condition by referring to Figure 1. Patients may have differing perceptions of whether or not their mouths are dry. Some have sufficient saliva flow, but complain of dry mouth. Others have true xerostomia, yet do not recognize that their mouths are dry. Encourage patients to conduct a daily mouth examination and check for any red or white patches, ulcers or tooth decay. If anything unusual is found, or if patients are complaining of dry mouth, further assessment is warranted to find the underlying cause.

Difficulty eating (e.g., mouth feels dry while eating, patient has difficulty swallowing food and needs to sip water to swallow dry food), is suggestive of salivary hypofunction as the cause of dry mouth.[6] The continuous presence of dry mouth symptoms during the day is associated with more significant salivary hypofunction than if there is gradual onset of symptoms over the course of the day. Symptoms of dry mouth that occur only at night are usually not associated with salivary hypofunction because salivary function normally approaches zero during sleep.[6] Sleep apnea, nasal congestion and breathing through one's mouth may cause exacerbation of nighttime symptoms of dry mouth.

Patients may experience regional or generalized mucosal pain, often described as "burning," or they may describe the inability to eat acidic or spicy foods, leading them to make changes in their diet.[6] This can be suggestive of chronic atrophic candidiasis, secondary to dry mouth. Patients with chronic atrophic candidiasis frequently also have angular cheilitis, seen as "cracks" in the corners of the mouth. Such patients require formal diagnosis and treatment and appropriate referral is recommended (see Chapter 93: Oral Candidiasis).

One of the more common causes of xerostomia (especially in the elderly) is medications. Many classes of drugs can cause dry mouth including adrenergic agonists, anticholinergics, antidepressants, antiemetics, antihistamines, antiparkinson agents, antipsychotics, benzodiazepines, decongestants, opioids and urinary antispasmodics.[15,16,17] The drug effects on quantity and quality of saliva are generally not permanent. Drugs that cause significant dry mouth in more than 10% of patients are listed in Table 3.[17,18]

Table 3: **Drugs Causing Significant Dry Mouth in >10% of Patients**

Adrenergic agonists	nortriptyline	**Benzodiazepines**
isoproterenol	paroxetine	alprazolam
pseudoephedrine	phenelzine	chlordiazepoxide
Alpha-adrenergic receptor agonists	trimipramine	clonazepam
clonidine	venlafaxine	clorazepate
Antiarrhythmics	**Antiemetics**	diazepam
propafenone	nabilone	flurazepam
Anticholinergics	prochlorperazine	lorazepam
atropine sulfate	**Antihistamines**	oxazepam
belladonna	chlorpheniramine	temazepam
benztropine mesylate	diphenhydramine	**Biologic response modulators**
glycopyrrolate	**Antiparkinson agents**	interferon alfa-2a
ipratropium bromide	selegiline	interferon alfa-2b
scopolamine	trihexyphenidyl	**Ergot alkaloids**
Antidepressants	**Antipsychotics**	ergotamine
amitriptyline	loxapine	**NSAIDs**
amoxapine	olanzapine	**Opioid analgesics**
bupropion	**Antispasmodics**	**Retinoic acid derivatives**
clomipramine	dicyclomine	isotretinoin
desipramine	flavoxate	**Skeletal muscle relaxants**
doxepin	oxybutynin	cyclobenzaprine

Assess the ability of patients with dry mouth to swallow solid dosage forms and assist in exploring alternative options.

Nonpharmacologic Therapy

Whenever possible, treatment should be directed towards the underlying cause of dry mouth. However, since most systemic illnesses causing dry mouth are not curable, management is usually directed towards treatment and prevention of complications and symptomatic control of dry mouth.

Dental Care

Inform patients they are at increased risk of dental caries because of their decreased saliva,[6] and advise them to visit their dentist and dental hygienist for regular checkup and practice regular brushing and flossing of the teeth. Remind patients with xerostomia to avoid sugary or acidic foods or beverages, to help prevent dental caries.

Salivary Flow Stimulation

If the patient's salivary glands are still functioning, physiologic stimulation of saliva flow can be accomplished through masticatory or gustatory stimuli.[6] Encourage patients to chew sugarless gum or suck on sugarless hard candies as needed throughout the day. These substances are sweetened using an alcohol sugar such as xylitol, mannitol, maltitol, lactitol or erythritol, and do not promote dental caries.[19] Labels should be carefully read to ensure the product does not contain simple sugars such as glucose, fructose, sucrose, lactose and maltose, which are cariogenic.[19]

Water Consumption

For general good health it is important that people have sufficient fluid intake. However, unless xerostomia is due to dehydration, patients should not assume that drinking large volumes of water will overcome oral dryness. Frequent small sips of water during the day and sucking on ice chips will help relieve oral symptoms. Lemon juice should be avoided since it depletes the salivary glands of saliva and may erode tooth enamel.[20] The use of **saliva substitutes** may be more convenient for patients during the day or those awakened at night with dry mouth symptoms. Frequent intake of water at night can lead to nocturia and interrupted sleep.

Pharmacologic Therapy

For comparative ingredients of nonprescription product, consult the *Compendium of Products for Minor Ailments*—Mouth Products: Dry Mouth.

Saliva Substitutes

Artificial saliva products can help to replace moisture and lubricate the mouth. They are formulated to mimic natural saliva, but not to stimulate salivary gland production.[21] Artificial saliva substitutes cannot replace all the functions of saliva and their action is short-lived due to swallowing.[6,22] Use has not been shown to prevent caries or oral candidiasis; therefore, they must be considered as replacement therapy rather than a cure.[2,6] These products come in a variety of formulations including solutions, sprays, patches, gels and lozenges and are most convenient for patients to use while travelling or talking and to prevent nocturia from increased fluid intake during the night. They are most useful when used immediately before bedtime or speaking.[23] They contain agents to optimize viscosity, such as hydroxymethylcellulose or carboxymethylcellulose, as well as electrolytes and flavouring (see Table 4).[2] There are limited data to suggest superiority of any of the products; therefore, selection should be based on availability and personal preference.[23] For cracked lips that may be sore, suggest using **petroleum jelly**.[20]

Moi-Stir, available as a spray or swabs, contains electrolytes normally present in saliva, including the chloride salts of calcium, magnesium, potassium and sodium, as well as sodium phosphate dibasic. **Mouth Kote** is a mouth moisturizer composed of yerba santa, water, xylitol, sorbitol and citric acid. **Yerba santa** (*Eriodictyon californicum*) is said to have expectorant properties and is used as a flavouring agent.[24,25]

OraMoist patch is composed of synthetic polymers, xylitol and enzymes such as glucose oxidase and lysozyme. The patch adheres to the hard palate or the inside of the cheeks and dissolves over a period of 2–4 hours.

Oral Balance gel is an oral moisturizer containing a synthetic polymer, polyglycerylmethacrylate, and the salivary enzymes lactoperoxidase and glucose oxidase. In patients with dry mouth secondary to radiation of the salivary glands, it afforded more relief to patients with severe xerostomia than to those with moderate xerostomia.[26] The duration of its moistening effect averaged 1 hour during the daytime and more than 4 hours during the night.[26]

The **Biotene** line of dry mouth products, including toothpaste, mouthwash and gum, contain salivary enzymes, lactoperoxidase, glucose oxidase and lysozyme, the goal being to replace the missing salivary enzyme activity in patients with salivary hypofunction. Patients with dry mouth due to radiation therapy for head and neck cancer have anecdotally reported improvement in their oral symptoms with the use of these products.[27,28] Patients with xerostomia following radiation therapy preferred the taste and consistency of Biotene toothpaste and Oral Balance gel over commercial toothpastes and carboxymethylcellulose gel, but symptom improvement did not reach statistical significance.[27]

Sialogogues

Anethole trithione stimulates the parasympathetic nervous system and increases the secretion of acetylcholine. While it has been used for many years in the treatment of chronic xerostomia, reports differ as to its efficacy. Further research is needed to establish its safety and efficacy for this indication.[29,30]

Another sialogogue is the cholinergic agonist **pilocarpine**.[6,31] It stimulates the exocrine glands with a duration action of 3–5 hours.[32] The lowest effective and tolerated dose should be used for maintenance therapy. Salivary secretion is maximally stimulated approximately 1 hour after administration of pilocarpine. No tolerance to the secretagogue effects of pilocarpine has been reported, nor has long-term improvement in baseline salivary function been found. Increased salivary output is transient, dose-related and consistent.[33] Pilocarpine is effective in patients with Sjögren's syndrome and in those who develop xerostomia while receiving radiation therapy for head or neck cancer.[33] Pilocarpine administered as a mouthwash, by diluting pilocarpine eye drops in water to make a 1–2% pilocarpine solution, has been used effectively to increase salivary flow without any systemic side effects.[34] Its use to treat medication-induced xerostomia is not a Health Canada–approved indication. Use of pilocarpine is contraindicated in patients with uncontrolled asthma or when miosis is undesirable (e.g., acute iritis, angle-closure glaucoma).[23]

Dental Care

The use of fluoride is very important in preventing dental caries in patients with xerostomia. It is applied professionally by the dentist or hygienist and maintained by the patient through daily use of high-fluoride–containing toothpastes (e.g., Prevident) or mouth rinses (e.g., Oral B Fluoride 0.05%, alcohol-free). Sodium fluoride rinses 0.05% used twice daily have been effective in preventing demineralization of enamel in patients with xerostomia while receiving radiation therapy.[35] Patients should avoid use of commercial mouth rinses containing alcohol since alcohol has a drying effect on the oral mucosa.[23]

Monitoring of Therapy

Reassess patients advised to practice appropriate self-care for dry mouth after 1 week. If they are achieving improved mouth comfort through increased intake of fluids and use of sugarless candy and are practicing good dental hygiene, encourage them to continue these measures. Encourage them to seek the advice of a dentist on the care of their teeth and for evaluation of the cause of their dry mouth when appropriate. Evaluate patient acceptance of a saliva substitute (taste, dosage form, degree of comfort attained). Advise patients who are not achieving mouth comfort with one product to try another.[22] If mouth complications arise (e.g., oral candidiasis) or the dryness worsens, further evaluation by a healthcare practitioner is necessary.

If pilocarpine has been prescribed, monitor the patient for excessive cholinergic side effects such as sweating and flushing. If no improvement in mouth discomfort is noted after 1 week of use, dosage adjustment may be necessary.

Figure 1: Assessment of Patients with Dry Mouth

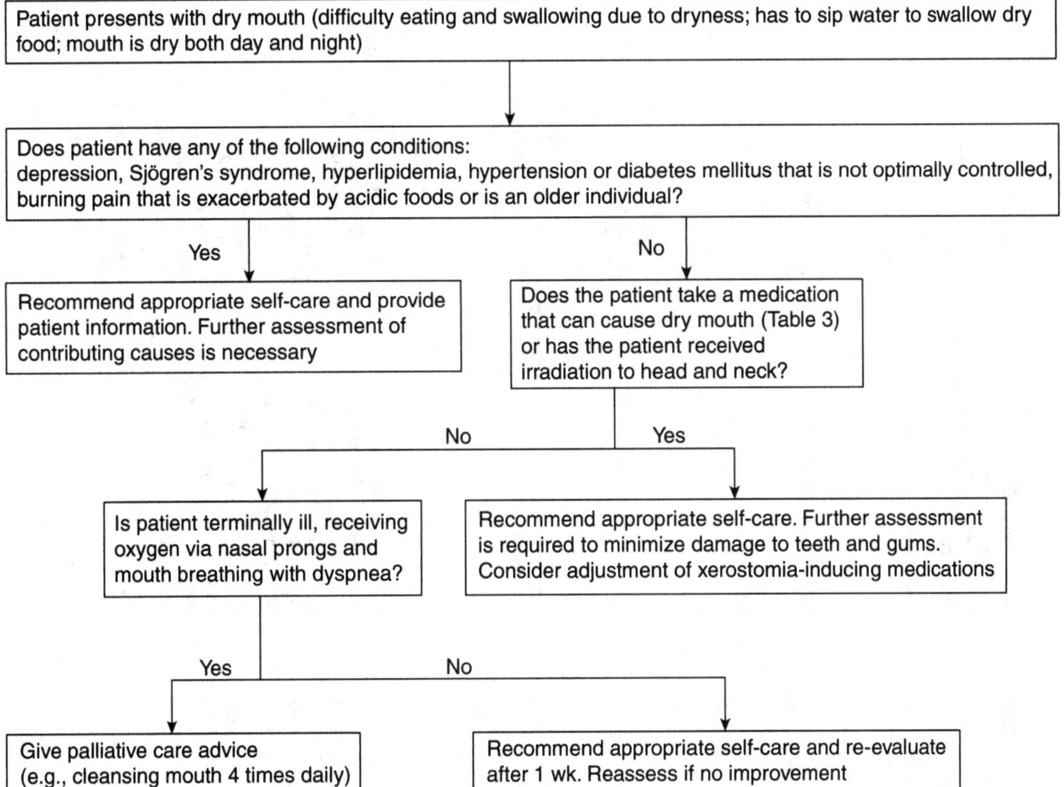

Patient presents with dry mouth (difficulty eating and swallowing due to dryness; has to sip water to swallow dry food; mouth is dry both day and night)
Does patient have any of the following conditions:
depression, Sjögren's syndrome, hyperlipidemia, hypertension or diabetes mellitus that is not optimally controlled, burning pain that is exacerbated by acidic foods or is an older individual?
Yes
No
Recommend appropriate self-care and provide patient information. Further assessment of contributing causes is necessary
Does the patient take a medication that can cause dry mouth (Table 3) or has the patient received irradiation to head and neck?
No
Yes
Is patient terminally ill, receiving oxygen via nasal prongs and mouth breathing with dyspnea?
Recommend appropriate self-care. Further assessment is required to minimize damage to teeth and gums. Consider adjustment of xerostomia-inducing medications
Yes
No
Give palliative care advice (e.g., cleansing mouth 4 times daily)
Recommend appropriate self-care and re-evaluate after 1 wk. Reassess if no improvement

Table 4: **Pharmacologic Therapy for Dry Mouth**

Class	Drug	Dosage	Adverse Effects	Drug Interactions	Comments	Cost[a]
Saliva Substitutes	*electrolyte solution* Moi-Stir	Spray 1–2 puffs into mouth PRN	No known significant adverse effects.	No known significant drug interactions.	Safe to swallow.	$
	polyglycerylmethacrylate/lactoperoxidase/ glucose oxidase Biotene Oral Balance	Apply gel onto tongue and spread thoroughly inside the mouth PRN	See electrolyte solution.	See electrolyte solution.	See electrolyte solution.	$
	xylitol/ polyvinylpyrrolidone/ glucose oxidase/ lysozyme OraMoist	Attach one patch to the hard palate or the inside of the cheeks Q2–4H PRN	Patch may not dissolve completely, necessitating manual removal. May cause burning and irritation at application site. Leaves sticky residue in mouth.	See electrolyte solution.	Some users may not like the taste.	$
	yerba santa Mouth Kote	Spray 3–5 puffs into mouth PRN; swirl in mouth for 10 s then spit	See electrolyte solution.	See electrolyte solution.	See electrolyte solution.	$
Sialogogues	*anethole trithione* Sialor	25 mg TID po before meals	Diarrhea, urine discolouration. Contraindicated in patients with jaundice or biliary tract obstruction.	See electrolyte solution.	Requires several days of treatment to show efficacy.	$$
	pilocarpine Salagen	5–10 mg TID po Reduce starting and maintenance doses in patients with hepatic impairment	Asthenia, chills, conjunctivitis, dizziness, headache, hyperhidrosis, myalgia, nausea, pruritus, rash, rhinitis, skin flushing, tachycardia, taste perversion, tremor, vomiting.	May cause cardiac conduction disturbance if taken concomitantly with beta-blockers. May cause additive effects when taken with drugs exhibiting parasympathomimetic activity. May antagonize anticholinergic effects of anticholinergic drugs. Inhibits CYP2A6 and therefore may affect the pharmacokinetics of CYP2A6 substrates.	May require up to 12 wk of treatment to show dry mouth symptom improvement. An extemporaneous preparation of a pilocarpine 1–2% mouthwash has been used to increase salivary flow. Its use to treat medication-induced xerostomia is not a Health Canada–approved indication.	$$$

[a] Cost of smallest available pack size or 30-day supply of tablets; includes drug cost only.

Legend: $ < $50 $$ $50–100 $$$ $100–150

Resource Tips

Mayo Clinic. Diseases and Conditions. *Dry mouth*. Available from: www.mayoclinic.com/health/dry-mouth/HA00034.

National Institute of Dental and Craniofacial Research. *Dry mouth (xerostomia)*. Available from: www.nidcr.nih.gov/OralHealth/Topics/DryMouth.

Sjögren's Syndrome Foundation. Available from: www.sjogrens.org. Offers useful resources for people with Sjögren's syndrome, including management of dry mouth. Contact them for information concerning *The Moisture Seekers* newsletter.

Suggested Readings

Delli K, Spijkervet FK, Kroese FG et al. Xerostomia. *Monogr Oral Sci* 2014;24:109-25.

Furness S, Worthington HV, Bryan G et al. Interventions for the management of dry mouth: topical therapies. *Cochrane Database Syst Rev* 2011;12:CD008934.

Pinna R, Campus G, Cumbo E et al. Xerostomia induced by radiotherapy: an overview of the physiopathology, clinical evidence, and management of the oral damage. *Ther Clin Risk Manag* 2015;11:171-88.

Plemons JM, Al-Hashimi I, Marek CL et al. Managing xerostomia and salivary gland hypofunction: executive summary of a report from the American Dental Association Council on Scientific Affairs. *J Am Dent Assoc* 2014;145:867-73.

Villa A, Connell CL, Abati S. Diagnosis and management of xerostomia and hyposalivation. *Ther Clin Risk Manag* 2014;11:45-51.

References

1. Dawes C. Physiological factors affecting salivary flow rate, oral sugar clearance, and the sensation of dry mouth in man. *J Dent Res* 1987;66:648-53.
2. Holmes S. Xerostomia: aetiology and management in cancer patients. *Support Care Cancer* 1998;6:348-55.
3. Glazar I, Urek MM, Brumini G et al. Oral sensorial complaints, salivary flow rate and mucosal lesions in the institutionalized elderly. *J Oral Rehabil* 2010;37:93-9.
4. Greenspan D. Xerostomia: diagnosis and management. *Oncology (Williston Park)* 1996;10:7-11.
5. Bartels CL. *Xerostomia. Helping patients with dry mouth*. Available from: www.oralcancerfoundation.org/dental/xerostomia.htm. Accessed February 3, 2016.
6. Daniels TE, Wu AJ. Xerostomia–clinical evaluation and treatment in general practice. *J Calif Dent Assoc* 2000;28:933-41.
7. Sweeney MP, Bagg J, Baxter WP et al. Oral disease in terminally ill cancer patients with xerostomia. *Oral Oncol* 1998;34:123-6.
8. Filshie J, Rubens CN. Complementary and alternative medicine. *Anesthesiol Clin* 2006;24:81-111, viii.
9. Bossola M, Tazza L. Xerostomia in patients on chronic hemodialysis. *Nat Rev Nephrol* 2012;8:176-82.
10. Napeñas JJ, Brennan MT, Fox PC. Diagnosis and treatment of xerostomia (dry mouth). *Odontology* 2009;97:76-83.
11. Dyke S. Clinical management and review of Sjögren's syndrome. *Int J Pharm Compound* 2000;4:338-41.
12. Pray SW. Help for patients with dry mouth. *US Pharm* 2000;25:16, 19-22.
13. Korsten MA, Rosman AS, Fishbein S et al. Chronic xerostomia increases esophageal acid exposure and is associated with esophageal injury. *Am J Med* 1991;90:701-6.
14. Zunt S. Evaluation of the dry mouth patient. *Alpha Omegan* 2007;100:203-9.
15. American Dental Association. *ADA guide to dental therapeutics*. 1st ed. Chicago: ADA Publishing; 1998.
16. Sreebny LM, Schwartz SS. A reference guide to drugs and dry mouth. *Gerodontology* 1986;5:75-99.
17. Wynn RL, Meiller TF. Drugs and dry mouth. *Gen Dent* 2001;49:10-2, 14.
18. Sreebny LM, Schwartz SS. A reference guide to drugs and dry mouth–2nd edition. *Gerodontology* 1997;14:33-47.
19. Hayes C. The effects of non-cariogenic sweeteners on the prevention of dental carries: a review of the evidence. *J Dent Educ* 2001;65:1106-9.
20. Taubert M, Davies EM, Back I. Dry mouth. *BMJ* 2007;334:534.
21. Flynn AA. Counseling special populations on oral health care needs: *Am Pharm* 1993;NS33:33-9.
22. Wynn RL, Meiller TF. Artificial saliva products and drugs used to treat xerostomia. *Gen Dent* 2000;48:630-6.
23. Guggenheimer J, Moore PA. Xerostomia: etiology, recognition and treatment. *J Am Dent Assoc* 2003;134:61-9.
24. Natural Medicines Comprehensive Database. *Yerba santa*. Available from: naturaldatabase.therapeuticresearch.com. Accessed February 6, 2016. Subscription required.
25. *Yerba santa monograph*. In: Review of natural products. St. Louis: Facts and Comparisons; 1991.
26. Regelink G, Vissink A, Reintsema H et al. Efficacy of a synthetic polymer saliva substitute in reducing oral complaints of patients suffering from irradiation-induced xerostomia. *Quintessence Int* 1998;29:383-8.
27. Epstein JB, Emerton S, Le ND et al. A double-blind crossover trial of Oral Balance gel and Biotene toothpaste versus placebo in patients with xerostomia following radiation therapy. *Oral Oncol* 1999;35:132-7.

28. Warde P, Kroll B, O'Sullivan B et al. A phase II study of Biotene in the treatment of postradiation xerostomia in patients with head and neck cancer. *Support Care Cancer* 2000;8:203-8.
29. Ferguson MM. Pilocarpine and other cholinergics drugs in the management of salivary gland dysfunction. *Oral Surg Oral Med Oral Pathol* 1993;75:186-91.
30. Hamada T, Nakane T, Kimura T et al. Treatment of xerostomia with the bile secretion-stimulant drug anethole trithione: a clinical trial. *Am J Med Sci* 1999;318:146-51.
31. Vivino FB, Al-Hashimi I, Khan Z et al. Pilocarpine tablets for the treatment of dry mouth and dry eye symptoms in patients with Sjögren syndrome: a randomized, placebo-controlled, fixed-dose, multicentre trial. P92-01 Study Group. *Arch Intern Med* 1999;159:174-81.
32. Salagen tablets. In: *Physicians' desk reference*. 51st ed. Montvale: Medical Economics Books; 1997. p. 1546-7.
33. Fox PC, Alkinson JC, Macynski AA et al. Pilocarpine treatment of salivary gland hypofunction and dry mouth (xerostomia). *Arch Intern Med* 1991;151:1149-52.
34. Bernardi R, Perin C, Becker FL et al. Effect of pilocarpine mouthwash on salivary flow. *Braz J Med Biol Res* 2002;35:105-10.
35. Meyerowitz C, Featherstone JD, Billings RJ et al. Use of an intra-oral model to evaluate 0.05% sodium fluoride mouth rinse in radiation-induced hyposalivation. *J Dent Res* 1991;70:894-8.

Dry Mouth—What You Need to Know

A dry mouth is not pleasant and it can cause problems. Your teeth may decay more easily and eating may be difficult.

If you have a dry mouth, visit your dentist and your doctor. They can help find out why your mouth is dry. Your dentist can help you protect your teeth from cavities while your mouth is dry.

What can you do to relieve dry mouth?

- Sip water often during the day.
- Avoid or cut down on drinks that contain caffeine (such as coffee, tea and cola). Caffeine causes your mouth to become drier.
- **Do not** use tobacco or alcohol. They both dry out your mouth.
- Chew sugar-free gum or suck on sugar-free candy during the day. This will help keep the mouth moist and won't cause cavities.
- Keep your teeth and gums clean. Brush your teeth twice a day with a soft toothbrush, and floss between teeth once a day.
- To help prevent cavities, use toothpaste that contains fluoride or rinse with a mouthwash that contains fluoride.
- An artificial saliva product may help make your mouth feel more moist. Ask your pharmacist about products to use at night or when you are bothered by dryness. Artificial saliva does not protect your teeth like real saliva. Tell your dentist if you are using one of these products.
- If you have a hard time swallowing your medicine in tablet or capsule form, ask your pharmacist if the same medicine can be taken as a liquid. Some people find it easier to swallow capsules and tablets if they sip some water first, then swallow the capsule or tablet using a full glass of water.
- Use a humidifier or vaporizer in your house to help keep the air moist.
- If you have a hard time eating food, try sipping water during your meal. Choose soft or puréed foods when you can.

Chapter 92

Halitosis

Shirin Abadi, BSc(Pharm), ACPR, PharmD, MBA, FCSHP

Halitosis, bad breath, fetor ex ore, fetor oris and oral malodor are all terms used to describe unpleasant or offensive odours emitted in the exhaled breath. In its simplest form, bad breath may be related to substances ingested such as herbs, spices, garlic, onion, tobacco or alcohol. With a reported prevalence as high as 50%, halitosis can be of great concern to many patients.[1] Given the growing interest, the diagnosis and treatment of halitosis are being incorporated into routine dental care, and specialized dental and multidisciplinary clinics are being set up solely for the treatment of patients with halitosis.[2]

Pathophysiology

Halitosis can be broadly classified into 3 main categories (Figure 1). Genuine halitosis occurs when oral malodor is truly present. Pseudohalitosis occurs when oral malodor is of concern to the patient, but is not perceived by others. Halitophobia occurs when the patient believes halitosis is present, despite having received treatment for genuine halitosis or pseudohalitosis, while lacking any physical or social evidence for the presence of bad breath.[1]

Figure 1: **Classification of Halitosis**

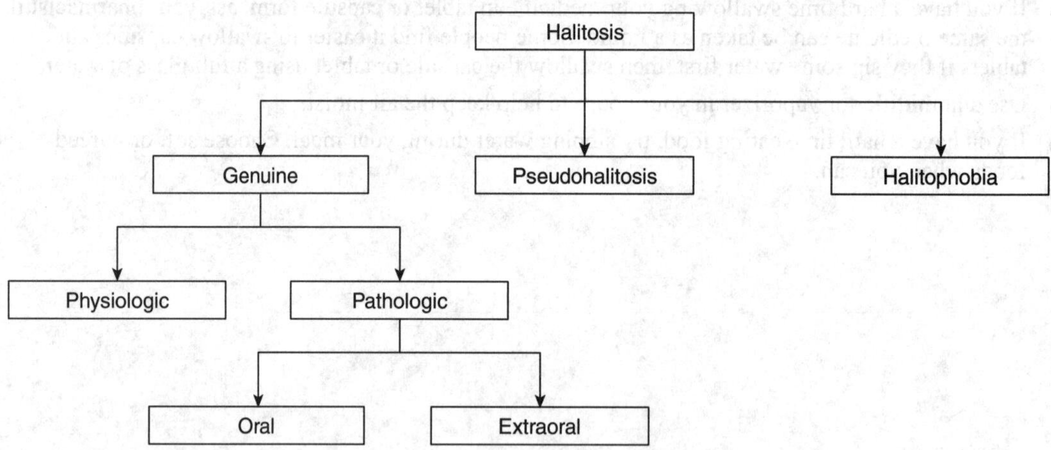

Physiologic halitosis arises from the putrefactive process, the decomposition of organic matter by microorganisms within the mouth, especially at the back of the tongue. The major elements in the production of oral malodor are volatile sulphur compounds (VSC), primarily hydrogen sulfide, methyl mercaptan and dimethyl sulfide (breakdown products of methionine and cysteine), as well as indole and skatole (breakdown products of tryptophan) and cadaverine (breakdown product of lysine).[3] Halitosis usually occurs when there is a shift from gram-positive to gram-negative anaerobic proteolytic bacteria such as *Porphyromonas gingivalis*, *Fusobacterium nucleatum*, *Prevotella intermedia* and spirochetes.[3] Gram-positive anaerobic bacteria such as *Solobacterium moorei* may also be involved in the initial stages of the production of bad breath.[3] Ingestion of systemic antibiotics or regular use of an antibacterial mouthwash can put the patient at risk of overgrowth of anaerobic, odoriferous bacteria or fungi that can be a source of bad breath. Other contributing factors to bad breath include decreased salivary flow, reduced carbohydrate substrate and increased pH.[3,4,5] The oral cavity is the main source of halitosis in most healthy individuals.[5]

Pathologic halitosis is caused by disease or malfunction of the oral tissues (e.g., gingivitis, dental abscess or jaw osteonecrosis), and includes halitosis due to periodontal disease and xerostomia (dry mouth). Xerostomia may be due to a number of factors, including insufficient water intake, breathing through the mouth, medication use (e.g., anticholinergic agents), excessive use of alcohol-based mouthwash, radiation therapy, chronic medical conditions (e.g., depression), smoking and regular caffeine intake. Extraoral pathologic halitosis refers to malodor originating from sources other than the mouth. These may include the nasal, paranasal and laryngeal regions, the upper digestive tract and the lungs, or disorders in any other body system (e.g., diabetes mellitus, hepatic cirrhosis, uremia, malignancy or internal bleeding). Nasal malodor is the most common origin of extraoral halitosis, and may be due to a nasal infection (e.g., sinusitis), problems affecting airflow or mucous secretions (e.g., polyps, postnasal drip) or craniofacial anomalies (e.g., cleft palate).[3]

Pseudohalitosis and halitophobia may have a psychological component, which require the expert advice of a mental health specialist for appropriate management.

There is no reliable way for people to properly assess their breath odour other than organoleptic (human nose) assessments. Some people have a lifelong concern with having bad breath, while at the other extreme, others do not seem to notice that their breath is offensive. Also, the perception of oral malodour differs among members of different cultures.[4,6]

Goals of Therapy

- Identify and resolve causes of halitosis
- Eliminate or minimize signs and symptoms of halitosis
- Encourage safe and effective oral hygiene and regular dental care
- Prevent recurrences and complications
- Improve self-confidence and quality of life

Patient Assessment

Evaluate patients seeking help for bad breath based on their personal, dental and medical history (Figure 2). Information collected should include the patient's specific symptoms and complete medication history, the types of food ingested, tobacco use and alcohol and caffeine intake, as well as whether there are any specific times during which bad breath is most noticeable. Certain foods (e.g., garlic) are known to cause bad breath, and tobacco and alcohol use may also contribute to halitosis. Most people have bad breath upon awakening. Irregular eating can also lead to hunger ketosis and bad breath. Poor dental hygiene, as well as pain and discomfort in the mouth and oral cavity, may signify pathology that requires treatment. Assess patients who wear dentures to determine proper denture hygiene. The long-term use of mouthwashes with alcohol content or antibacterial agents may also contribute to halitosis. For patients experiencing frequent dry mouth, it is important to identify and treat its cause (see Chapter 91: Dry Mouth). Patients with halitosis, pseudohalitosis or halitophobia complicated by other medical conditions or symptoms require further assessment.

Nonpharmacologic Therapy

The oral cavity is the source of bad breath in the majority of patients, and good oral hygiene along with the treatment of any periodontal or oral disease is necessary to relieve the problem. Encourage patients to visit a dental care professional for assessment of oral diseases and for removal of dental plaque and accumulated bacteria on the dorsum of the tongue and in the periodontal pockets. Encourage tooth brushing with a soft-bristled toothbrush at least twice a day, and flossing daily.[7]

A clean tongue is a healthy pink colour. A whitish haze on the tongue can indicate bacterial or fungal buildup.[8] Cleaning the tongue along with other oral hygiene measures may be helpful in decreasing physiologic halitosis.[8,9] Tongue cleaning can be accomplished through the use of a soft, small-headed, child-size toothbrush, or by using a specially designed tongue cleaner or tongue scraper.[10] The tongue is stroked from the back to the tip with the brush or cleaner, then the mouth is rinsed with water. The posterior portion of the tongue is the most important area to clean, but care should be taken not to induce gagging.

It is also important for patients to understand that they should not be overzealous in their cleaning, to avoid causing damage to and bleeding from the tongue's surface. Tongue scrapers must be used cautiously and adult toothbrushes are not recommended for tongue cleaning.[1] Cleaning the tongue with either a cleaner or a scraper may reduce VSC levels more than by cleaning with a toothbrush.[8] However, this reduction in VSC levels may not be long-lasting.[8]

Drinking plenty of fluids and cleaning the mouth after consuming dairy products, meat or fish are adjunctive measures for treating bad breath.[11] Saliva has many functions in keeping the mouth healthy, including lubrication, oxygenation, buffering and antimicrobial action. Increasing saliva flow and tongue action help decrease bad breath; chewing sugarless gum and munching on fibrous vegetables, such as raw carrots and celery, can help accomplish this.[8,12]

Pharmacologic Therapy

Mouthwash

Mouthwashes may supplement oral hygiene. Regular use of a mouthwash may reduce bad breath but single-use mouthwashes may have only a short-term benefit.[13] Most commercial mouthwashes mask odours and provide antiseptic properties for a relatively short time (less than 30 minutes).[5] Rinsing with water is of little help because water offers no antiseptic properties and can wash away saliva, which does have these properties.[8] The action of mouthwashes is optimized when deeply gargled (in addition to rinsing) prior to going to bed. Residues of the oral rinse may remain in the mouth longer during sleep as the individual is not eating or drinking; this is also the time when bacterial activity is at its highest due to decreased salivary flow.[14] The quality of the available evidence supporting the effectiveness of mouthwashes is low, due to sparse data and various methodological flaws (e.g., diversity in the baseline characteristics of the participants and the methods used to assess outcomes).[15]

Chlorhexidine gluconate 0.12% mouthwash appears to be effective in reducing oral malodor by exerting its antibacterial activity on supragingival plaque and the tongue.[15] Its side effects include tooth staining and taste disturbances.[15,16,17] Chlorhexidine mouthwashes are not recommended to be used for more than one week and should be discontinued if mouth ulcers are present.[3]

Regular use of **cetylpyridinium**-containing mouthwashes may reduce bad breath at 2 weeks, while the regular use of **sodium chlorite**-containing mouthwashes may reduce bad breath at 4 weeks.[13] Sodium chlorite is not commercially available in Canada.

Chlorine dioxide and **zinc**-containing mouthwashes (e.g., zinc lactate 0.14%, zinc chloride) may be effective in neutralizing odoriferous sulphur compounds.[15,18,19,20,21] Zinc-containing mouthwashes may be more effective at concentrations ≥1%.[17] However, chlorine dioxide and zinc lactate are not commercially available in Canada.

Mouthwashes containing **essential oils** (e.g., eucalyptol) may be successful in reducing moderate malodor.[16] A potential role may exist for agents such as triclosan, hydrogen peroxide, dehydroascorbic acid, sodium bicarbonate, iminium, allylpyrocatechol, L-trifluoromethionine and medications used for

Helicobacter pylori eradication.[17] Further large, well-designed, randomized controlled trials that examine the long-term use of mouthwashes are required to identify the role of these agents in the management of halitosis.

Combination mouthwashes, such as those containing chlorhexidine and cetylpyridinium chloride, chlorhexidine and zinc, or chlorhexidine, cetylpyridinium chloride and zinc, have demonstrated enhanced effectiveness on VSC levels in clinical trials.[15] It is thought that chlorhexidine and cetylpyridinium may exert a synergistic antimicrobial effect against VSC-producing bacteria, and zinc may transform volatile sulphur compounds into non-odoriferous breakdown products.[15] However, well-designed trials are needed to further establish the safety and efficacy of these combination products, which are not commercially available in Canada. There are currently no other pharmacologic therapies with an established role for the treatment of bad breath available in Canada, unless bad breath is caused by decreased salivary flow (see Chapter 91: Dry Mouth).

For comparative ingredients of nonprescription products, consult the *Compendium of Products for Minor Ailments*—Mouth Products: Mouthwashes.

Natural Health Products

Chlorophyll, parsley, menthol and **mint** have been known as breath fresheners for many years. ***Garcinia mangostana*** (mangosteen) may also play a role in reducing VSC levels.[15] However, there is insufficient reliable evidence supporting regular use of these products for the management of halitosis.[15,17,22]

For comparative ingredients of nonprescription products, consult the *Compendium of Products for Minor Ailments*—Herbal and Natural Health Products: Combinations, Single Entity.

Monitoring of Therapy

After 1 week of practising good oral hygiene including gentle cleaning of the tongue, the patient should see an improvement in their bad breath and this routine should be continued. If the patient's tongue hurts or bleeds following cleaning, or if tongue cleaning causes excessive gagging, it is likely that further instruction on tongue cleaning is required. Dentists and dental hygienists may be better situated to give these instructions.

Mouthwashes containing antibacterial agents such as chlorhexidine and cetylpyridinium may stain the teeth.[15] Zinc-containing mouthwashes may cause a metallic taste in the mouth. Products containing alcohol may cause dryness with long-term use, which can exacerbate bad breath. Monitor the duration of use of these products when possible, and discourage the use of products containing alcohol or antibacterial agents.

Figure 2: Assessment of Patients with Halitosis

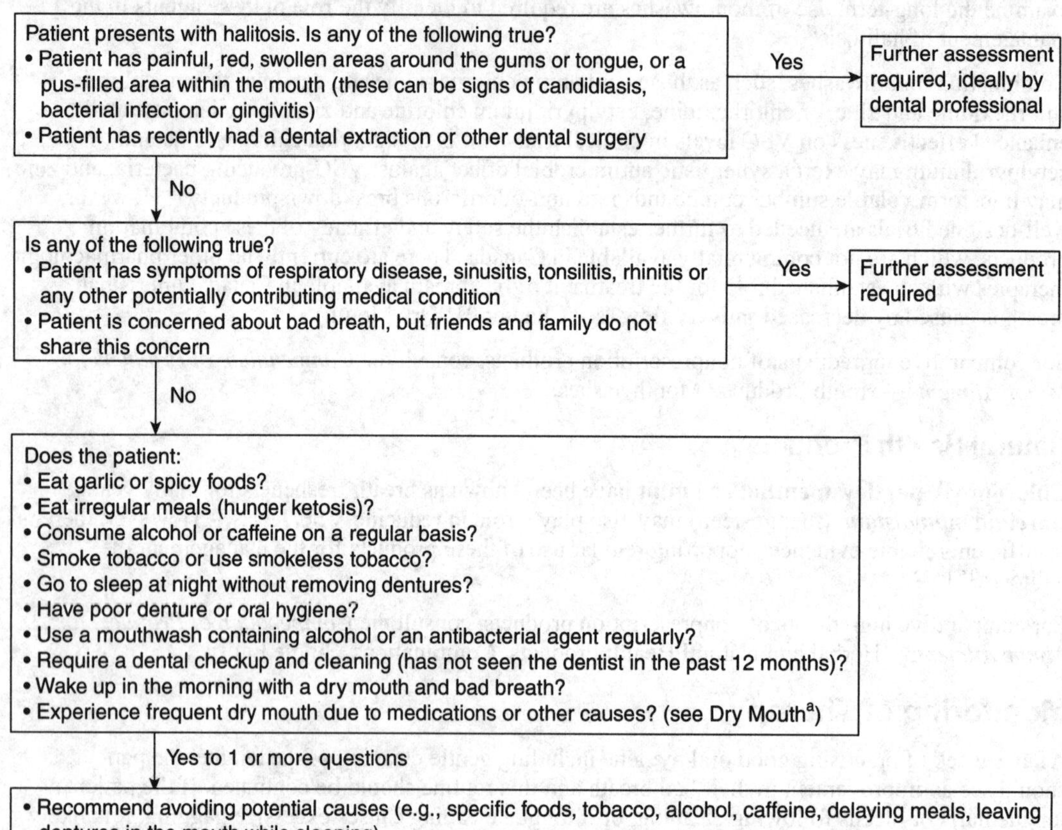
Patient presents with halitosis. Is any of the following true?
• Patient has painful, red, swollen areas around the gums or tongue, or a pus-filled area within the mouth (these can be signs of candidiasis, bacterial infection or gingivitis)
• Patient has recently had a dental extraction or other dental surgery
Yes
Further assessment required, ideally by dental professional
No
Is any of the following true?
• Patient has symptoms of respiratory disease, sinusitis, tonsilitis, rhinitis or any other potentially contributing medical condition
• Patient is concerned about bad breath, but friends and family do not share this concern
Yes
Further assessment required
No
Does the patient:
• Eat garlic or spicy foods?
• Eat irregular meals (hunger ketosis)?
• Consume alcohol or caffeine on a regular basis?
• Smoke tobacco or use smokeless tobacco?
• Go to sleep at night without removing dentures?
• Have poor denture or oral hygiene?
• Use a mouthwash containing alcohol or an antibacterial agent regularly?
• Require a dental checkup and cleaning (has not seen the dentist in the past 12 months)?
• Wake up in the morning with a dry mouth and bad breath?
• Experience frequent dry mouth due to medications or other causes? (see Dry Mouth[a])
Yes to 1 or more questions
• Recommend avoiding potential causes (e.g., specific foods, tobacco, alcohol, caffeine, delaying meals, leaving dentures in the mouth while sleeping)
• Recommend practising good oral hygiene (which includes good denture hygiene, if applicable) and having regular dental checkups
• Recommend cleaning the tongue gently with a soft child-size toothbrush
• If the patient wishes to try a mouth rinse, recommend a product containing cetylpyridinium, zinc or essential oils, or any combination of these ingredients with the lowest available alcohol content, at bedtime for a 1-wk trial. Chlorhexidine mouth rinses may also be provided through a prescription. Advise about potential side effects (e.g., tooth staining with chlorhexidine and cetylpyridinium)
• Discourage long-term use of mouth rinses with high alcohol content or antibacterial agents
• If medication is the likely cause of dry mouth and resulting bad breath, assess for potential adjustment of medication and rule out other possible causes
• Provide a patient information sheet[b] with helpful reminders for the patient to follow

[a] See Chapter 91: Dry Mouth.
[b] See Bad Breath—What You Need to Know.

Resource Tips

American Academy of Family Physicians. Family Doctor. *Halitosis*. Available from: familydoctor.org/familydoctor/en/diseases-conditions/halitosis.html.

Mayo Clinic. Diseases and Conditions. *Bad breath*. Available from: www.mayoclinic.org/diseases-conditions/bad-breath/basics/definition/con-20014939.

Yaegaki K, Coil JM. Examination, classification, and treatment of halitosis; clinical perspectives. *J Can Dent Assoc* 2000;66:257-61.

Suggested Readings

Bollen CM, Beikler T. Halitosis: the multidisciplinary approach. *Int J Oral Sci* 2012;4:55-63.

Fedorowicz Z, Aljufairi H, Nasser M et al. Mouthrinses for the treatment of halitosis. *Cochrane Database Syst Rev* 2008;(4):CD006701.

Rösing CK, Loesche W. Halitosis: an overview of epidemiology, etiology and clinical management. *Braz Oral Res* 2011;25:466-71.

Scully C, Greenman J. Halitology (breath odour: aetiopathogenesis and management). *Oral Dis* 2012;18:333-45.

Van den Broek AM, Feenstra L, de Baat C. A review of the current literature on management of halitosis. *Oral Dis* 2008;14:30-9.

References

1. Yaegaki K, Coil JM. Examination, classification, and treatment of halitosis; clinical perspectives. *J Can Dent Assoc* 2000;66:257-61.
2. Bollen CM, Beikler T. Halitosis: the multidisciplinary approach. *Int J Oral Sci* 2012;4:55-63.
3. UpToDate. Rosenberg M. *Bad breath.* Available from: www.uptodate.com. Accessed March 3, 2016. Subscription required.
4. Scully C, Greenman J. Halitology (breath odour: aetiopathogenesis and management). *Oral Dis* 2012;18:333-45.
5. Messadi DV. Oral and nonoral sources of halitosis. *J Calif Dent Assoc* 1997;25:127-31.
6. Eli I, Baht R, Koriat H et al. Self-perception of breath odor. *J Am Dent Assoc* 2001;132:621-6.
7. Weinberg. MA. Halitosis: the "bad breath" syndrome. *US Pharm* 2001;26:46, 48, 51-52, 57.
8. Van der Sleen MI, Slot DE, Van Trijffel E et al. Effectiveness of mechanical tongue cleaning on breath odour and tongue coating: a systematic review. *Int J Dent Hyg* 2010;8:258-68.
9. Outhouse TL, Al-Alawi R, Fedorowicz Z et al. Tongue scraping for treating halitosis. *Cochrane Database Syst Rev* 2006;(2):CD005519.
10. Seemann R, Kison A, Bizhang M et al. Effectiveness of mechanical tongue cleaning on oral levels of volatile sulfur compounds. *J Am Dent Assoc* 2001;132:1263-7.
11. Carlson-Mann L. The use of tongue cleaners in the treatment of halitosis. *Probe* 1998;32:114-5.
12. Reingewirtz Y, Girault O, Reingewirtz N et al. Mechanical effects and volatile sulfur compound-reducing effects of chewing gums: comparison between test and base gums and a control group. *Quintessence Int* 1999;30:319-23.
13. Scully C, Porter S. Halitosis. *Clin Evid (Online)* 2008.pii:1305.
14. Rosenberg M. Clinical assessment of bad breath: current concepts. *J Am Dent Assoc* 1996;127:475-82.
15. Fedorowicz Z, Aljufairi H, Nasser M et al. Mouthrinses for the treatment of halitosis. *Cochrane Database Syst Rev* 2008;(4):CD006701.
16. Loesche WJ. The effects of antimicrobial mouthrinses on oral malodor and their status relative to US Food and Drug Administration regulations. *Quintessence Int* 1999;30:311-8.
17. Van den Broek AM, Feenstra L, de Baat C. A review of the current literature on management of halitosis. *Oral Dis* 2008;14:30-9.
18. Borden LC, Chaves ES, Bowman JP et al. The effect of four mouthrinses on oral malodor. *Compend Contin Educ Dent* 2002;23:531-6, 538, 540.
19. Kozlovsky A, Goldberg S, Natour I et al. Efficacy of a 2-phase oil: water mouthrinse in controlling oral malodor, gingivitis, and plaque. *J Periodontol* 1996;67:577-82.
20. Rassameemasmaung S, Sirikulsathean A, Amornchat C et al. Effects of herbal mouthwash containing the pericarp extract of Garcinia mangostana L on halitosis, plaque and papillary bleeding index. *J Int Acad Periodontol* 2007;9:19-25.
21. Winkel EG, Roldan S, Van Winkelhoff AJ et al. Clinical effects of a new mouthrinse containing chlorhexidine, cetylpyridinium chloride and zinc-lactate on oral halitosis. A dual-centre, double-blind, placebo-controlled study. *J Clin Periodontol* 2003;30:300-6.
22. Natural Medicines Comprehensive Database. Stockton: Therapeutic Research Facility; 2009. Available from: naturaldatabase.therapeuticresearch.com. Accessed March 3, 2016. Subscription required.

Bad Breath—What You Need to Know

What causes bad breath?

The most common cause of bad breath is a problem with your teeth or gums. If you have not seen a dentist or a dental hygienist recently, make an appointment. They can find out if your teeth or gums are causing bad breath.

Another cause of bad breath is dry mouth. It can cause problems with your teeth and with eating. Many medications can cause dry mouth. If you have this problem, please talk to your pharmacist.

Nose and throat problems, and some other diseases, can also cause bad breath. If you think you may have a condition that could be causing bad breath, please talk to your healthcare provider.

Things you can do to help stop bad breath:

- Take good care of your teeth and gums. Brush your teeth at least twice a day using a soft toothbrush. Replace your toothbrush at least every 3 months. Floss between your teeth at least once a day.
- To remove bacteria, brush the back of your tongue gently using a soft child-size toothbrush. Ensure that you are using the right tongue-cleaning procedure by asking your dentist or dental hygienist.
- Visit the dentist and dental hygienist regularly; once a year is good, every 6 months is better.
- You can try using a mouthwash at bedtime. Mouthwashes are unlikely to provide long-lasting relief. They work for a longer period of time if you swish them in your mouth for 30 seconds and gargle for 30 seconds before spitting and if you do not eat or drink for at least 30 minutes after using them.
- Avoid regular use of mouthwashes containing alcohol or antibacterial agents. The alcohol in the mouthwash can make your mouth dry, and your breath worse. The antibacterial agent in the mouthwash can lead over time to the excessive growth of resistant bacteria or microbes that can cause bad breath.
- Some mouthwashes contain an ingredient that may stain your teeth, such as chlorhexidine and cetylpyridinium. Check with your pharmacist before choosing a mouthwash.
- If you wear removable dentures:
  - Rinse dentures with water after meals to remove loose food debris
  - Brush dentures with lukewarm water, soap or a denture paste, using a denture brush or a regular soft toothbrush at least twice a day to remove plaque and food debris and to help prevent stains
  - Brush your gums and any natural teeth using a separate soft toothbrush at least 2 times a day
  - Take dentures out at bedtime; clean and store them appropriately
- If you wear removable braces, it is also important to keep them clean. Ask your dentist for directions on how best to keep your braces clean.
- Avoid using tobacco and regular alcoholic and caffeinated beverages. They can cause bad breath.
- Eat regular meals, including breakfast, and avoid long periods of hunger.
- Snack on foods that require lots of chewing, such as raw celery and carrot sticks. Chewing causes saliva to flow and helps keep your breath fresh.
- Chew sugarless gum. This will also cause saliva to flow.
- Consume fewer substances associated with bad breath, such as garlic and spicy foods.
- Drink plenty of fluids during the day.

Chapter 93
Oral Candidiasis

Karen Wlock, BScPharm

Pathophysiology

Candida organisms are fungi that normally live as commensals in the human oral cavity.[1] It is estimated that up to 60% of healthy, immunocompetent adults carry *Candida* species as part of their normal oral flora.[2,3] However, when the normal flora is compromised (e.g., by weakened host defence mechanisms), *Candida* overgrowth and direct tissue invasion may occur, leading to the development of opportunistic disease.[1,3] Oral candidiasis, also known as oral thrush, oral candidosis, or moniliasis, is a mucocutaneous opportunistic infection caused by *Candida* species. Host factors are believed to play a more significant role than the virulence of *Candida* in the pathogenesis of disease.[1]

Oral candidiasis is often denoted as a "disease of the diseased" since it selectively occurs in individuals with weakened host defence mechanisms.[1,4] Oral candidiasis is the most common fungal infection found in both immunocompetent and immunocompromised populations, with prevalence greatest among infants and the elderly.[5,6] Xerostomia, experienced by 30–77% of palliative care cancer patients secondary to cancer treatment and medications administered for symptom relief, predisposes these individuals to oral candidiasis.[7]

The high incidence of oral candidiasis in humans can be explained by a multiplicity of predisposing factors (Table 1).

Table 1: Risk Factors for Developing Oral Candidiasis

Disease States	Medications
Addison's disease	Broad-spectrum antibiotics
Anemia (due to iron, folic acid or vitamin B_{12} deficiency)	Cytotoxic chemotherapy
Diabetes mellitus	Immunosuppressive drugs
Human immunodeficiency virus (HIV) infection and AIDS	Inhaled corticosteroids
Hypothyroidism	**Other**
Leukemia	Infancy and childhood (due to an underdeveloped immune system)
Xerostomia (dry mouth): may be caused by anticholinergic drugs, radiation therapy, dental appliances	Local mucosal trauma
	Poor dental or denture hygiene (particularly in the elderly)
	Pregnancy
	Smoking tobacco

C. albicans, reported to account for up to 80% of *Candida* species isolated from the oral cavity, is considered the major cause of oral candidal infections.[1,3,8] Other *Candida* species that cause infection to a lesser extent include *C. glabrata*, *C. tropicalis*, *C. krusei* and *C. dubliniensis*.[1,9]

The human immunodeficiency virus (HIV) pandemic has contributed greatly to the resurgence of oral candidal infections in humans.[9] Up to 90% of HIV-infected individuals are expected to develop oral candidiasis at some point during their disease and, because of this trend, oral candidal infection is often used as a clinical marker to predict HIV disease progression.[4,9,10]

Goals of Therapy

- Resolve infection or reduce acute candidal overgrowth to a level which can be controlled by the host's defences and thereby prevent complications (e.g., progression to esophageal candidiasis).[11]
- Prevent recurrences by managing any underlying risk factors (e.g., use of inhaled corticosteroids, poor dental hygiene, uncontrolled diabetes mellitus) and instituting antifungal prophylaxis if warranted (e.g., in high-risk patients with HIV/AIDS or advanced cancer).

Patient Assessment

Candidal infections are often associated with predisposing factors; therefore, a thorough medical/dental history is required to identify and manage any underlying conditions that may be contributing to the infection. In addition, physical examination of the lesions and a description of the signs and symptoms are paramount to an accurate diagnosis and the differentiation between the various clinical presentations (see Figure 1). Diagnosis of any form of oral candidiasis is based on clinical recognition of typical lesions. Microbiologic tests (e.g., smears, stains and cultures) can be used when doubts regarding diagnosis exist or resistance to an antifungal agent is suspected. Various test methods for identifying the fungal species are available.[12] Empiric therapy with an antifungal medication is often reasonable when the diagnosis is uncertain.

Candidiasis in the oropharyngeal region may be localized (primary oral candidiasis) or may be a manifestation of generalized candidal infection (secondary oral candidiasis).[9,13] Primary oral candidiasis may present as several clinical variants, including acute pseudomembranous (thrush), erythematous or hyperplastic candidiasis. Symptoms vary, and clinical presentation may range from no symptoms at all to a burning sensation painful enough to interfere with swallowing and oral food intake, anorexia and weight loss, nutritional deficiency and decreased quality of life.[3,14]

It is noteworthy that oral candidiasis may appear with more than one group of symptoms simultaneously.[15,16]

Acute pseudomembranous candidiasis, commonly known as thrush, is characterized by creamy, whitish-yellow, elevated plaques (pseudomembranes) on the mucosal lining of the mouth, most frequently on the tongue, soft palate and inner cheek.[2,9,15] The plaques are easily wiped off with a tongue blade, exposing a raw, erythematous base that is not usually painful.[1] Although typically an acute infection, pseudomembranous candidiasis can persist for up to several months or years, especially in patients receiving inhaled or intraoral topical corticosteroids or in HIV-infected individuals. This form of candidiasis is most commonly diagnosed in the first few weeks of an infant's life, in elderly patients and in those with underlying malignancies or HIV infection.[1,16]

Erythematous candidiasis, or atrophic candidiasis, can develop from pseudomembranous candidiasis as plaques are shed, exposing the underlying erythematous lesions. These lesions vary in size, and are accompanied by inflammation of the surrounding tissues. Erythematous lesions can be found on the palate and on the tongue, where they can cause depapillation and dekeratinization.[15] This form of candidiasis often follows the use of broad-spectrum antibiotics (e.g., tetracycline) or the use of inhaled corticosteroids[8] and is the most common variant in HIV infection.[9,15,16]

Hyperplastic candidiasis, or candidal leukoplakia, is a less common form of oral candidiasis predominantly seen in smokers and males over 30 years of age.[9] It is characterized by chronic, discrete lesions that appear as small, translucent white plaques or larger, opaque lesions on the tongue, palate or inner cheek.[1,9] The white plaques cannot be easily wiped off as in the pseudomembranous variant.[3,9] Leukoplakias are considered to be premalignant; therefore, biopsy is recommended.[3,9]

Candida-associated lesions include denture stomatitis and angular cheilitis.[9] Denture stomatitis presents as chronic red, edematous lesions on the denture-bearing mucosa of denture wearers.[1] Although patients are usually symptomless, some experience mild soreness, burning or tingling beneath the denture. Approximately 50% of complete denture wearers experience denture stomatitis.[15] Commonly associated with denture stomatitis is angular cheilitis, a mixed bacterial-fungal infection characterized by sore, erythematous fissuring at the angles of the mouth.[9,15,16] Angular cheilitis may also be a sign of vitamin B_{12}, folic acid or iron deficiency.[3]

Nonpharmacologic Therapy

The development of thrush associated with inhaled corticosteroids (ICS) is rare; the risk can be reduced by the use of a spacer device with metered dose inhalers. Rinsing the mouth and gargling with water after using an ICS or reducing the dose of the ICS when appropriate can also be helpful in preventing recurrent episodes of oral candidiasis.

To aid in healing and prevention of oral candidiasis or angular cheilitis associated with wearing dentures, advise patient to:

- remove dentures overnight
- wear dentures for no longer than 6 hours during the day, to allow the gums to heal and to reduce inflammation
- keep dentures clean and soak them in disinfectant solution when not in use
- clean the gums, tongue and affected mucosa with a soft toothbrush
- review proper fitting of dentures with an oral health practitioner
- stop smoking.

Patients with oral candidiasis due to dry mouth caused by medication may benefit from a medication review and assessment; a reduction in dose or stopping the offending agent may be helpful. Keeping the mouth moist by taking frequent sips of water may also be helpful.

If patients with diabetes experience recurrent oral candidiasis, review diabetes control and refer to an appropriate healthcare practitioner.

If an infant is experiencing thrush, advise parents to keep all toys and feeding bottles/nipples sterilized, to prevent autoinfection and recurrence. If the mother is breastfeeding and also experiencing candidal infection of the nipples, refer her to an appropriate healthcare practitioner for education regarding proper latching and for possible dual pharmacologic treatment of mother and baby.

Pharmacologic Therapy

Elimination of the underlying factor(s) responsible for the opportunistic infection may be sufficient to allow the microflora to return to normal. However, in the majority of cases treatment with an antifungal agent is necessary.[1] Inadequately treated or refractory oral candidiasis can be of particular concern in immunocompromised or myelosuppressed patients, as an initially localized infection may lead to regional (e.g., oropharyngeal to esophageal) or systemic (life-threatening candidemia) spread of the microorganism.[17]

The pharmacologic agents most commonly used for the treatment of oral candidiasis fall into 3 major categories (see Table 2): polyenes (**nystatin**), azoles (**fluconazole**, **itraconazole**, **posaconazole**) and echinocandins (**anidulafungin**, **caspofungin**, **micafungin**).[3,9,18] The echinocandins are administered parenterally, therefore, these agents are rarely used for uncomplicated disease.

Topical nystatin oral suspension is the most commonly used treatment for oral candidiasis,[4,9] and is recommended for initial episodes and mild disease.[19] Nystatin is well tolerated and does not interact with other medications because it is largely not absorbed from the GI tract when administered orally.

Azoles are recommended as second-line agents due to the emergence of azole-resistant *Candida* strains.[9] Resistance of fungi to polyenes is rare. *C. glabrata* and *C. krusei* are innately less susceptible to azoles, and *C. albicans* can acquire azole resistance. Oral **fluconazole** is the most commonly recommended azole, and is recommended for the treatment of moderate to severe disease.[19] In cases of recurrent infections (e.g., patients with HIV/AIDS), fluconazole is considered the drug of choice for episodic treatment and chronic suppression of oral candidiasis.[9,10,19,20] However, in cases of fluconazole resistance, oral **itraconazole** or **posaconazole** can be equally effective alternatives.[9,21,22,23]

Historically, **gentian violet** in 1% aqueous or USP (containing 10% alcohol) solution was applied locally for the treatment of oral candidiasis.[24] However, this agent causes mucosal irritation, ulceration and staining, making it difficult to determine therapeutic progress and decreasing adherence.[24] The safety of gentian violet is also questionable, as it has been linked to carcinogenicity in animal studies.[24,25]

Evidence is insufficient to support **probiotic** therapy in the treatment or prevention of intraoral candidiasis. However, 1 intervention study suggests that probiotic strains of lactobacilli and propionibacteria may be effective in lowering oral *Candida* levels in the elderly.[26] More clinical trials are required to determine the role of probiotics in oral candidiasis therapy, especially with respect to dosing and antibiotic-induced disease.[27]

There is insufficient evidence to support the use of natural health products in the treatment of oral candidiasis.[28]

For comparative ingredients of nonprescription products, consult the *Compendium of Products of Minor Ailments*—Skin Care Products: Antifungals.

Monitoring of Therapy

Since the majority of risk factors for developing a candidal infection are associated with immunocompromised states, it is important to monitor susceptible individuals for signs and symptoms of infection so that early treatment can be instituted and the infection can be resolved before spreading.

Monitor patients taking broad-spectrum antibiotics, undergoing chemotherapy or radiation therapy or those who take corticosteroids orally or by inhalation for signs and symptoms of oral candidiasis. If identified in a patient, prompt evaluation by an appropriate healthcare practitioner is necessary. Once antifungal treatment is initiated, advise the patient to monitor symptoms on a daily basis during treatment and for up to 2 weeks after clearing of symptoms to ensure the infection has completely resolved.

Figure 1: **Assessment of Patients with Oral Candidiasis**

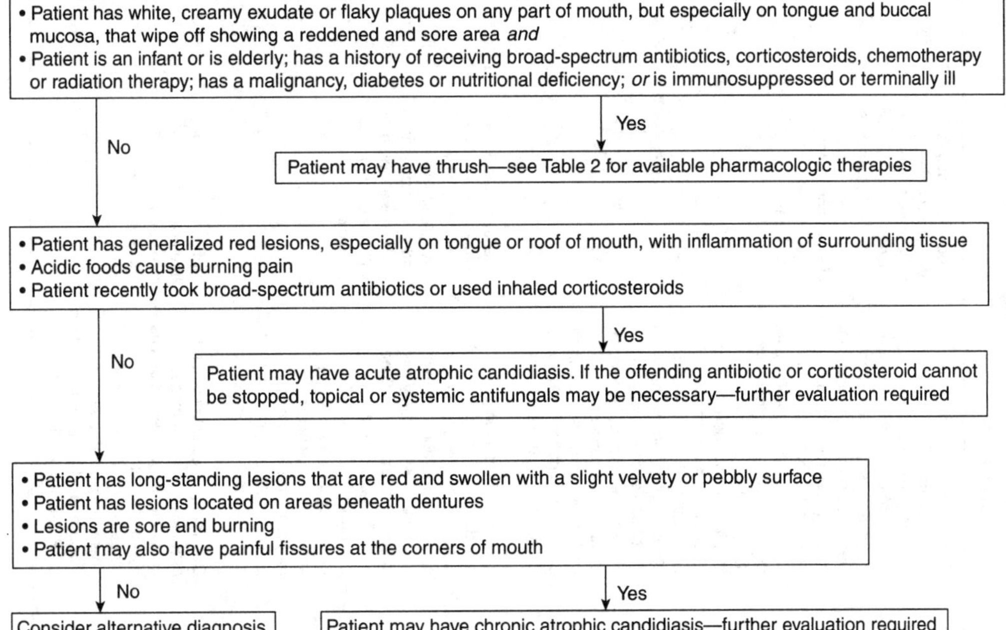

• Patient has white, creamy exudate or flaky plaques on any part of mouth, but especially on tongue and buccal mucosa, that wipe off showing a reddened and sore area *and*
• Patient is an infant or is elderly; has a history of receiving broad-spectrum antibiotics, corticosteroids, chemotherapy or radiation therapy; has a malignancy, diabetes or nutritional deficiency; *or* is immunosuppressed or terminally ill
Yes
No
Patient may have thrush—see Table 2 for available pharmacologic therapies
• Patient has generalized red lesions, especially on tongue or roof of mouth, with inflammation of surrounding tissue
• Acidic foods cause burning pain
• Patient recently took broad-spectrum antibiotics or used inhaled corticosteroids
Yes
No
Patient may have acute atrophic candidiasis. If the offending antibiotic or corticosteroid cannot be stopped, topical or systemic antifungals may be necessary—further evaluation required
• Patient has long-standing lesions that are red and swollen with a slight velvety or pebbly surface
• Patient has lesions located on areas beneath dentures
• Lesions are sore and burning
• Patient may also have painful fissures at the corners of mouth
No
Yes
Consider alternative diagnosis
Patient may have chronic atrophic candidiasis—further evaluation required

Table 2: Pharmacologic Therapy for Oral Candidiasis

Class	Drug	Dosage	Adverse Effects	Drug Interactions	Comments	Cost[a]
Antifungals, Azole	*fluconazole* Diflucan, generics	Treatment: 100–200 mg daily po × 7–14 days Preventive therapy for recurrent infections: 100–200 mg 3 times weekly po	Abdominal pain, diarrhea, nausea, vomiting	Rifampin enhances fluconazole metabolism which may necessitate increased fluconazole dose when these 2 drugs are used concomitantly. Decrease dosage of midazolam and triazolam if these drugs are used with fluconazole. Monitor for increased prothrombin time in patients receiving concomitant fluconazole and warfarin. Monitor for increased phenytoin plasma concentration with concomitant fluconazole use. Monitor for hypoglycemia when fluconazole is used with sulfonylureas (e.g., glyburide). Monitor for increased cyclosporine levels and serum creatinine in patients receiving fluconazole and cyclosporine.	Recommended for the treatment of moderate to severe disease. In HIV/AIDS patients, fluconazole is considered the drug of choice for treatment of oral candidiasis.	$
	itraconazole Sporanox Capsules, Sporanox Oral Solution	Capsules: 100–200 mg daily po after a meal × 2–4 wk Solution: 200 mg daily po on empty stomach × 1–3 wk	Abdominal pain, constipation, diarrhea, dyspepsia, heart failure, hepatotoxicity, hypokalemia, nausea, peripheral neuropathy, pruritus, pulmonary edema, rash, urticaria, vomiting.	Itraconazole is mainly metabolized through CYP3A4. Other substances that either share this metabolic pathway or modify CYP3A4 activity may influence the pharmacokinetics of itraconazole. Similarly, itraconazole may modify the pharmacokinetics of other substances that share this metabolic pathway because itraconazole is a potent CYP3A4 and P-glycoprotein inhibitor.	The itraconazole oral solution should be swished in the oral cavity and swallowed and advise patient not to rinse mouth with water after swallowing.	$$
	posaconazole Posanol	100 mg BID po oral suspension after a meal on the first day then 100 mg once daily after a meal × 13 days	Diarrhea, headache, nausea.	Contraindicated with cisapride, ergot alkaloids, pimozide, quinidine, sirolimus and statins. Avoid concomitant administration with cimetidine, phenytoin and rifabutin. Posaconazole is metabolized via UDP glucuronidation and is a	Not used as a first-line agent. May be considered for resistant cases.	$$$$

Class	Drug	Dosage	Adverse Effects	Drug Interactions	Comments	Cost[a]
				substrate for P-glycoprotein. Therefore, inhibitors or inducers of these clearance pathways may affect posaconazole plasma concentrations. Posaconazole concentrations are unlikely to be altered by inhibitors of CYP450 enzymes. Posaconazole is a strong inhibitor of CYP3A4; may raise plasma levels of drugs metabolized through this enzyme pathway.		
Antifungals, Polyenes	*nystatin* generics	Swish & swallow 100 000 to 500 000 units QID po × 7–14 days	Diarrhea, GI irritation, nausea, rash, urticaria, vomiting.	No clinically significant drug interactions. GI absorption of nystatin is insignificant.	Nystatin's relatively short contact time with the oral mucosa, high clearance from the oral cavity and requirement for frequent applications potentially limit its usefulness.	$

[a] Cost for specified duration of treatment; includes drug cost only.

Dosage adjustment may be required in renal impairment.

Legend: $ <$100 $$ $100–200 $$$ $200–300 $$$$ $300–400

Resource Tips

Canadian Paediatric Society. Caring for Kids. *Thrush*. Available from: www.caringforkids.cps.ca/handouts/thrush.

Suggested Readings

Pappas PG, Kauffman CA, Andes D et al. Clinical practice guidelines for the management of candidiasis: 2009 update by the Infectious Diseases Society of America. *Clin Infect Dis* 2009;48:503-35.

Pienaar ED, Young T, Holmes H. Interventions for the prevention and management of oropharyngeal candidiasis associated with HIV infection in adults and children. *Cochrane Database Syst Rev* 2010;(11):CD003940.

Rhodus NL. Treatment of oral candidiasis. *Northwest Dent* 2012;91:32-3.

Samaranayake LP, Keung Leung W, Jin L. Oral mucosal fungal infections. *Periodontol 2000* 2009;49:39-59.

Worthington HV, Clarkson JE, Khalid T et al. Interventions for treating oral candidiasis for patients with cancer receiving treatment. *Cochrane Database Syst Rev* 2010;(7):CD001972.

References

1. Farah CS, Ashman RB, Challacombe SJ. Oral candidosis. *Clin Dermatol* 2000;18:553-62.
2. Gonsalves WC, Chi AC, Neville BW. Common oral lesions: part I. Superficial mucosal lesions. *Am Fam Physician* 2007;75:501-7.
3. Muzyka BC. Oral fungal infections. *Dent Clin North Am* 2005;49:49-65.
4. Ellepola AN, Samaranayake LP. Oral candidal infections and antimycotics. *Crit Rev Oral Biol Med* 2000;11:172-98.
5. Giannini PJ, Shetty KV. Diagnosis and management of oral candidiasis. *Otolaryngol Clin North Am* 2011;44:231-40.
6. Vazquez JA, Sobel JD. Mucosal candidiasis. *Infect Dis Clin North Am* 2002;16:793-820.
7. Wilberg P, Hjermstad MJ, Ottesen S et al. Oral health is an important issue in end-of-life cancer care. *Support Care Cancer* 2012;20:3115-22.
8. Krol DM, Keels MA. Oral conditions. *Pediatr Rev* 2007;28:15-22.
9. Samaranayake LP, Keung Leung W, Jin L. Oral mucosal fungal infections. *Periodontol 2000* 2009;49:39-59.
10. Patton LL, Bonito AJ, Shugars DA. A systematic review of the effectiveness of antifungal drugs for the prevention and treatment of oropharyngeal candidiasis in HIV-positive patients. *Oral Surg Oral Med Oral Pathol Oral Radiol Endod* 2001;92:170-9.
11. Anibal PC, de Cássia Orlandi Sardi J, Peixoto IT et al. Conventional and alternative antifungal therapies to oral candidiasis. *Braz J Microbiol* 2010;41:824-31.
12. Coronado-Castellote L, Jiménez-Soriano Y. Clinical and microbiological diagnosis of oral candidiasis. *J Clin Exp Dent* 2013;5:e279-86.
13. Axell T, Samaranayake LP, Reichart PA et al. A proposal for reclassification of oral candidosis. *Oral Surg Oral Med Oral Pathol Oral Radiol Endod* 1997;84:111-2.
14. Sharon V, Fazel N. Oral candidiasis and angular cheilitis. *Dermatol Ther* 2010;23:230-42.
15. Appleton SS. Candidiasis: pathogenesis, clinical characteristics, and treatment. *J Calif Dent Assoc* 2000;28:942-8.
16. Fotos PG, Lilly JP. Clinical management of oral and perioral candidosis. *Dermatol Clin* 1996;14:273-80.
17. Laudenbach JM, Epstein JB. Treatment strategies for oropharyngeal candidiasis. *Expert Opin Pharmacother* 2009;10:1413-21.
18. Bartlett JG, Auwaerter PG, Pham PA. *The ABX guide to diagnosis & treatment of infectious diseases*. 1st ed. Montvale: Thomson PDR; 2005. p. 537.
19. Pappas PG, Kauffman CA, Andes D et al. Clinical practice guidelines for the management of candidiasis: 2009 update by the Infectious Diseases Society of America. *Clin Infect Dis* 2009;48:503-35.
20. Pons V, Greenspan D, Lozada-Nur F et al. Oropharyngeal candidiasis in patients with AIDS: randomized comparison of fluconazole versus nystatin oral suspensions. *Clin Infect Dis* 1997;24:1204-7.
21. Vazquez JA, Skiest DJ, Nieto L et al. A multicenter randomized trial evaluating posaconazole versus fluconazole for the treatment of oropharyngeal candidiasis in subjects with HIV/AIDS. *Clin Infect Dis* 2006;42:1179-86.
22. Graybill JR, Vazquez J, Darouiche RO et al. Randomized trial of itraconazole oral solution for oropharyngeal candidiasis in HIV/AIDS patients. *Am J Med* 1998;103:33-9.
23. Phillips P, De Beule K, Frechette G et al. A double-blind comparison of itraconazole oral solution and fluconazole capsules for the treatment of oropharyngeal candidiasis in patients with AIDS. *Clin Infect Dis* 1998;26:1368-73.
24. Hoppe JE. Treatment of oropharyngeal candidiasis and candidal diaper dermatitis in neonates and infants: review and reappraisal. *Pediatr Infect Dis J* 1997;16:885-94.
25. Littlefield NA, Blackwell BN, Hewitt CC et al. Chronic toxicity and carcinogenicity of gentian violet in mice. *Fundam Appl Toxicol* 1985;5:902-12.
26. Hatakka K, Ahola AJ, Yli-Knuuttila H et al. Probiotics reduce the prevalence of oral candida in the elderly–a randomized controlled trial. *J Dent Res* 2007;86:125-30.
27. Meurman JH. Probiotics: do they have a role in oral medicine and dentistry? *Eur J Oral Sci* 2005;113:188-96.
28. Ferreira GL, Pérez AL, Rocha ÍM et al. Does scientific evidence for the use of natural products in the treatment of oral candidiasis exist? A systematic review. *Evid Based Complement Alternat Med* 2015;2015:147804.

Oral Candidiasis—What You Need to Know

What is oral candidiasis?

Oral candidiasis is an infection in the mouth or throat, caused by Candida, a yeast-like fungus. It is also commonly referred to as thrush. Thrush usually appears as whitish or yellowish patches on the tongue or inside the cheeks.

Who can get thrush?

- Healthy newborn babies and infants who suck on pacifiers
- People who wear dentures
- People who have dry mouth—this is more common for older people
- People who have certain diseases (e.g., diabetes mellitus, leukemia and hypothyroidism, HIV/AIDS)
- People who take certain medications (for example, antibiotics, corticosteroids)
- People who have had chemotherapy or radiation therapy

What can you do to prevent thrush?

- Tell your pharmacist, dentist or doctor if you have a dry mouth. They can suggest ways to decrease this problem.
- Don't use a mouthwash that contains a lot of alcohol. If you use a mouthwash that contains alcohol over a long period of time, it can cause your mouth to become dry.
- If you wear dental appliances or dentures, take them out at night and disinfect them.
- If you use an inhaled corticosteroid, rinse your mouth with water after using it. Ask your pharmacist about using a spacer with your inhaler. A spacer can help decrease the chance of getting thrush.

What should you do if you have thrush?

- See your healthcare provider. You will need medication to treat this infection.
- When the infection has cleared up, throw out your old toothbrush and start using a new one.
- If you wear dentures, soak them in a special solution (hypochlorite 0.1%) until the infection is cleared up. Ask your healthcare provider for information about this solution.

Appendix I
Complementary and Alternative Therapies

Cynthia Richard, BScPh, PhD
Paul A. Spagnuolo, BSc, MSc PhD

CPhA acknowledges the contribution of Janet Webb as a previous author of this chapter.

The promotion of wellness to prevent disease and enhance quality of life has engaged individuals in proactive self-care. Greater public awareness about the importance of attaining and maintaining wellness has been accompanied by a remarkable increase in the use of unconventional therapies in patient self-care. These therapeutic approaches bring with them terminologies and philosophies that can be confusing to those trained in the conventional medical sciences typically practised in North America. A vital step in better understanding these approaches is recognition of the extent of use by Canadians, user demographics, reasons for use and patterns of use, all of which continue to evolve. Appreciating the diversity of treatments and the philosophies behind them, finding objective evidence to support or not support their use and the efforts to integrate validated therapies into patient care are challenges facing Canada's healthcare practitioners.

Definitions

Increased human mobility and improved global communication have led to increased awareness of and exposure to previously unfamiliar therapies, and a greater exploration of these treatments by North Americans. Use has surged in developed nations, where these treatments are better known as complementary and alternative medicine (CAM).[1] It is challenging to define the spectrum of CAM approaches. As Western medicine becomes experienced with certain practices, the approaches become standard treatment and are no longer considered complementary or alternative. The National Center for Complementary and Integrative Health (NCCIH) in the United States defines CAM as a group of diverse medical and healthcare systems, practices and products that are not generally considered part of conventional medicine. Conventional medicine (also called Western or allopathic medicine) is medicine as practiced by holders of M.D. (medical doctor) and D.O. (doctor of osteopathic medicine) degrees and by allied health professionals, such as physical therapists, psychologists and registered nurses. The boundaries between CAM and conventional medicine are not absolute, and specific CAM practices may become widely accepted with time.[2]

Although the terms "complementary" and "alternative" medicine are often used interchangeably, they are considered distinct.[2] **Alternative medicine** is used in place of Western medicine (e.g., using herbs rather than conventional pharmaceuticals to treat a condition), whereas **complementary medicine** is used in combination with Western medicine. **Integrative medicine** combines conventional Western medicine and those complementary treatments for which there is sound evidence of effectiveness and safety, but does not replace conventional therapy (e.g., massage and guided imagery to ease pain).[2,3]

Prevalence

Although surveys of CAM use provide inconsistent findings because the definition of CAM varies (e.g., some include prayer in the definition, some only include supplements), they can still be useful to identify trends and patterns.[4] A 2010 survey of Canadians on the use of natural health products (NHPs) found that 73% of Canadians used NHPs (including vitamins).[5] Between 1990 and 1997 in the United States, the use of herbal products increased by 380% and high-dose vitamin use increased by 130%.[6]

A 2012 survey of Americans revealed approximately 33% of adults and 12% of children had used CAM (excluding vitamins and minerals) in the preceding 12 months.[7,8] Dietary supplements (including fish oil, glucosamine/chondroitin, melatonin and probiotics) were the most commonly used complementary health measures, followed by deep breathing techniques. From 2002 to 2012, there was an increase in the use of yoga and tai chi in adults. A survey performed in 2005 in the United Kingdom revealed that 29% of respondents taking prescription drugs had used CAM in the preceding 12 months. The most commonly used therapies were massage, acupuncture, aromatherapy and herbal medicine.[9] General trends include higher prevalence rates of CAM in Western regions, women, those with higher levels of education and income and, importantly, in those with chronic conditions.[7,8,10,11,12,13,14,15]

Certain populations are more likely to use CAM therapies. Surveys undertaken in various regions of Canada have demonstrated high use of CAM therapies by ethnic Chinese Canadians.[16,17,18] First Nations communities also maintain traditional healing practices as demonstrated by a study in Nova Scotia, which found 66% of attendees to a clinic used Mi'kmaq medicine in addition to Western medicine, and of these 92.4% did not discuss this use with their physician.[19]

A survey of Canadians revealed that 12% of the general population visited a CAM practitioner in the previous 12 months. Percentages for patients with specific conditions were: 15% for asthma, 19% for migraine, and 8% for diabetes. Surveyors hypothesized that patients with adequate control of their disease were less likely to seek alternatives.[15] This theory is supported by an analysis of consultations with alternative healthcare practitioners (massage therapy, acupuncture, homeopathic/naturopathic treatment) in Ontario. Women with chronic conditions (fibromylagia, chronic fatigue, high blood pressure, and chemical sensitivities) were more likely to seek a CAM provider if they felt their healthcare needs were not being met.[20]

It is estimated that 57–80% of cancer patients use one or more CAM interventions.[21] The incidence of lifetime use of a CAM product/therapy or visit to a CAM therapist was found to have increased in randomly selected breast cancer survivors in Ontario from 67% in 1998 to 82% in 2005, with 41% of respondents in 2005 reporting use of CAM to manage their cancers.[22] A survey examining the use of herbal remedies by cancer patients in the United Kingdom found that usage increased with time since diagnosis.[23] The use of CAM by pediatric cancer patients since diagnosis was 20–60% in the majority of studies included in a systematic review.[24] Other studies have found similar CAM usage in Canadian pediatric patients in cardiology and neurology clinics.[25,26]

Chronic, difficult-to-treat conditions prompt patients to seek alternatives, and those facing devastating diseases turn to CAM when conventional treatments have been exhausted (although most patients with life-threatening conditions do not use CAM exclusively).

Safety

Although Canadian consumers desire reliable information on CAM, they often base their choices on potentially unreliable or unsubstantiated sources. While scientific evidence and advice from healthcare practitioners affect their choices, patients give strong consideration to the treatment's "naturalness", perceived lack of side effects, and advice from friends and family when deciding to use CAM treatments.[27,28] Claims by unscrupulous manufacturers and distributors can mislead and confuse consumers with pseudoscientific jargon and rhetoric.[29,30] In Canada, although NHPs require premarket approval and evidence to support efficacy, safety and quality and must meet labelling standards, verbal claims are often made by health food store personnel despite lack of supporting evidence.[31] A lack of knowledge of basic safety issues such as herb-drug interactions and contraindications increases the risks of an adverse outcome when such personnel provide advice.[32] Of additional concern is the lack of accreditation or standards for some CAM practitioners in Canada.[33]

A 2010 survey of Canadians regarding NHPs demonstrated increasing public awareness regarding NHP safety issues with physicians and pharmacists the most preferred NHP information sources.[5] Nonetheless, many Canadian consumers are reluctant to discuss NHP usage with conventional healthcare practitioners, fearing lack of support in their decisions to choose NHPs and doubt regarding the consumer's values and beliefs.[34] It has been estimated that less than 1% of those who use NHPs disclose this information to their pharmacist.[35] Case reports have highlighted that using a stepwise approach to conducting a medication history can identify NHP use and prevent unnecessary harm.[36] This approach is recommended as part of Best Possible Medication History (BPMH) guidelines.[37]

When assessing the safety of CAM therapies, in addition to potential harm caused directly by the therapies themselves, practitioners must also consider indirect harm that may arise from choosing less effective CAM treatments over conventional methods that have proven efficacy.[38] For example, patients may choose a CAM treatment over surgery and chemotherapy for cancer treatment, and this may contribute to disease progression. Factors such as the severity and acuteness of the illness, safety and efficacy of the desired CAM treatment, and toxicity associated with conventional treatment must be considered in the risk-benefit analysis of CAM vs. conventional medical treatment.

Evidence

While there may be evidence to support certain CAM treatments, there is often a gap between published randomized controlled trials (RCTs) finding CAM to be of little or no effect, and anecdotal reports of clinical benefit by CAM practitioners and their patients.[39] Pharmacists are well placed to discuss CAM options with patients, especially NHP selection, but many feel ill equipped to provide reliable information based on sound research.[40,41] This leads to frustration at the pharmacy, as less than half of patients surveyed thought that their pharmacist provided useful information about complementary therapies.[42] In direct contrast to drug therapy where research precedes marketing approval, a lack of regulatory oversight in CAM has seen these therapies become embedded and diversified before clinical trials are conducted.[31,39,40,43,44] For example, an assessment of published RCTs of herbal interventions found quality of the reports to be unsatisfactory, reinforcing the need for adoption of established reporting standards.[45] The Consolidated Standards of Reporting Trials (CONSORT) group has developed an Herbal Medicinal Intervention extension to their RCT reporting guidelines, addressing factors such as naming of the products, details of product composition and quality testing.[46] Similar guidelines have been developed for reporting of acupuncture interventions and nonpharmacologic treatment interventions.[47,48]

Mainstream medicine has historically overlooked, ignored or rejected CAM, citing lack of convincing evidence, flawed methodology and bias in CAM research, but increasing use by patients demands greater understanding by practitioners as well as better quality research. Many conventional medicine practitioners claim that benefits from CAM treatment are due only to placebo effect; indeed, factors that may be part of CAM such as the degree of individualization, time spent with the practitioner, and physical interventions (such as acupuncture) are associated with a stronger placebo response.[49,50] For health professionals to adopt any evidence into clinical practice they must be aware of research results, be able to assess and interpret research findings, then apply the evidence into clinical practice.[51] Because CAM does not have a tradition of reliance on double-blinded, randomized, controlled trials that inform modern evidence-based medicine, there are obstacles to this approach, as there are with many nonpharmacologic treatment interventions (see Table 1). Application of scientific research findings into clinical practice by both conventional and CAM practitioners can be haphazard and inconsistent.[60] Schools that teach CAM therapies do not have a tradition of research or research infrastructure, so in certain areas of practice (traditional Chinese medicine) investigators are not familiar enough with clinical trial methodology to perform research that satisfies Western reviewers.

Developing an evidence base for CAM therapies is a well-recognized challenge being addressed internationally. To promote standards of practice in CAM, the World Health Organization has developed training benchmarks to ensure practitioners have adequate knowledge, skills and awareness of appropriate usage and safety in a variety of CAM practices, including traditional Chinese medicine, Ayurveda, naturopathy, osteopathy and others.[61] Additionally, the Cochrane group involved in CAM is distributing guidelines on trial design and reporting standards to CAM practitioners, with a particular focus on traditional Chinese medicine.[58] The NCCIH within the National Institutes of Health has invested US $2 billion to support CAM research.[51] Education programs are underway both to educate CAM practitioners on clinical research methodology[58] and to introduce conventional healthcare practitioners to CAM, to promote open dialogue with patients.[62,63] A recent survey of Canadian regulated CAM schools (including schools of chiropractic, naturopathy, massage therapy and acupuncture) indicated that research methods and evidence-based healthcare training were offered by 81% and 91% of the schools respectively.[64] In addition, suggested core competencies in pharmacy students include the ability to access and critically appraise sources of information related to NHPs and the ability to educate patients on the safety and effectiveness of NHPs.[65]

Despite the challenges, high-quality RCTs in CAM can be designed[66] and do exist.[59] In Canada, collaborative projects to gather CAM evidence include the Canadian Institute of Natural and Integrative Medicine (www.cinim.org), and IN-CAM (the Canadian Interdisciplinary Network for Complementary and Alternative Medicine Research) (www.incamresearch.ca). IN-CAM also provides high-quality reviews of CAM therapies and natural health products (www.camline.ca). Systematic reviews are being used to gather and synthesize evidence and to identify potential areas of research. Cochrane Complementary Medicine is a group dedicated to producing and disseminating systematic reviews of RCTs in numerous CAM areas (acupuncture, massage, chiropractic, homeopathy, herbal medicine, mind-body therapy). Although not without challenges (considering the heterogeneity of CAM therapies), nearly 800 systematic reviews involving CAM were listed in the Cochrane Library in 2015. Cochrane reviews of CAM treatments for specific conditions are made readily available as plain language summaries.[67]

Table 1: **Challenges with Research Involving CAM**

Locating published evidence[44,52,53,54]

- lack of consistent CAM terminology and indexing headings
- publication bias in high-impact journals
  - foreign language
  - journal reviewers may be unfamiliar with CAM methods
- many CAM journals are not included in conventional databases (PubMed)

Methodology and research design issues[39,43,44,55,56,57,58,59]

- heterogeneity of products and practices
  - lack of standardization of biologic products hampers reproducibility
  - individualization of treatment approaches makes effects of treatment difficult to measure
- difficulties with blinding (e.g., acupuncture)
- expectation bias and placebo effect
- lack of appropriate animal models for some areas of CAM, such as those involving nonpharmacologic treatment interventions
- lack of funding for large CAM trials

Integrative Medicine

Integrative initiatives are fostering closer collaboration between conventional and CAM practitioners, to deliver a more comprehensive approach to patient care. Integration can occur on different levels—as individual practitioners combine therapies (e.g., physicians performing acupuncture), or in integrative clinics and institutions where conventional and CAM practitioners work together.[68] Collaboration and communication between conventional and CAM practitioners will improve monitoring of adverse effects, identify potential therapeutic benefits of an integrative approach and foster progress through research.[69] Additionally, working in a collaborative integrated environment positively affects job satisfaction and personal growth of Canadian practitioners.[70] In Alberta, the CAM in UME Project (Complementary and Alternative Medicine Issues in Undergraduate Medical Education) is a medical education initiative to facilitate educating undergraduate medical education students about issues related to patients' use of CAM (www.caminume.ca). The project does not teach medical students to practice complementary therapy, but to be prepared to practice medicine in an environment where CAM may be used by their patients in combination with conventional treatments.[63] Other Canadian examples of initiatives to promote integrative medicine include CARE (Complementary and Alternative Research and Education), which is an academic pediatric integrative medicine program at the University of Alberta (www.CARE.ualberta.ca), and InspireHealth, an integrative cancer care program with several centres in British Columbia (www.inspirehealth.ca).

With the increasing use of CAM therapies, and the integration into mainstream medical practice, healthcare practitioners must become familiar with relevant terminology. The following provides definitions and brief descriptions of categories of CAM and therapeutic modalities that healthcare practitioners may encounter in this evolving area.

Categories of CAM

The National Center for Complementary and Integrative Health in the United States groups CAM therapies into 5 major categories (see also Table 2 and Table 3).

Alternative Medical Systems[2]

These are complex and comprehensive systems of treatment, encompassing both theory and practice, which have developed outside the sphere of conventional medicine. Some have been in use for thousands of years (e.g., traditional Chinese medicine) while others have been developed more recently (e.g., homeopathy). These include traditional Chinese medicine, Ayurveda, homeopathy and naturopathic medicine (see Definition of Therapeutic Modalities).

Mind-body Interventions[2,72,73,74]

These therapies utilize the brain or mind to influence body function (see Table 2). The concept that the mind can influence illness is integral in the healing approaches of traditional Chinese and Ayurvedic medical systems.[71] Evidence from RCTs and systematic reviews suggest a connection between the nervous system and other body systems (e.g., the immune, autonomic and endocrine systems), which may be activated to promote self-healing and well-being. Observed positive psychological effects and enhanced quality of life may be of particular use for individuals with chronic conditions and in need of palliative care. The connection between the mind and body has been explored in the use of support groups for cancer patients (now considered mainstream therapy) and in the effect of exercise on altered mood (e.g., increased endorphins to combat depression). In pediatrics, hypnosis, guided imagery and biofeedback have been used effectively to manage pain, anxiety, stress and sleep disorders.[59] Mind-body interventions are considered low risk.

Natural Product–Based Therapies[2,75]

Also known as biologically-based practices, this describes the use of natural/biologic products, which can be derived from plants (e.g., herbs) or animals (e.g., shark cartilage), and also includes vitamins, minerals, fatty acids, amino acids, proteins, prebiotics, probiotics, whole diets and functional foods (see Table 2). Orthomolecular and megavitamin therapies are in this category.

Manipulative and Body-based Methods[2,76,77,78]

These manual therapies (e.g., chiropractic and massage therapy) involve manipulation or movement of the body (see Table 2). Some methods propose that bodily function depends on proper body alignment, and that misalignment or asymmetry results in illness, possibly at a site distant from the distortion. Correction of body symmetry optimizes the balance between the sensory and motor nervous systems.[76] Restoration of structural imbalance to improve blood and lymph flow is one of the proposed mechanisms by which these therapies facilitate the body's ability to heal itself.[76]

Energy Therapies[2]

These methods seek to manipulate energy fields (biofields) within or surrounding the body (see Table 2). In traditional Chinese Medicine this is referred to as qi (pronounced "chee") which is the vital life force that circulates through the body in invisible pathways termed "meridians". In Ayurveda these life forces are referred to as doshas. The underlying theory maintains that the universe is permeated with a "life force" or "vital energy" that also surrounds and pervades the human body.[79] Imbalance or blockages of the energy may result in disease, and therapy is aimed at correcting these problems. For treatment of a condition, a close, cooperative participation between the practitioner and the patient is required. Therapeutic touch, reiki and qigong are examples of energy therapies.

Table 2: **Major Groupings of Selected Common CAM Approaches[2,71]**

CAM Category	Examples
Alternative medical systems	Ayurvedic medicine Traditional Chinese medicine Homeopathy Naturopathy Japanese traditional medicine Tibetan traditional medicine
Mind-body interventions	Aromatherapy Biofeedback Hypnosis Imagery Relaxation techniques Meditation Tai chi Yoga
Natural product–based therapies	Herbalism Nutrition therapy (includes diet therapy, dietary supplements) Hydrotherapy
Manipulative and body-based methods	Chiropractic manipulation Craniosacral massage Massage Osteopathic manipulation Reflexology Rolfing Tui Na
Energy therapies	Acupuncture, Acupressure, Moxibustion Magnetic therapy Qigong Reiki Therapeutic touch

Table 3: **Examples of Delivery Methods for CAM**[2,71]

CAM Delivery Method	Examples
Treatments primarily self-administered	Herbal remedies Nutritional supplements Health foods Meditation Magnetic therapy
Treatments administered by provider	Acupuncture Massage therapy Reflexology Chiropractic manipulation Osteopathic manipulation
Treatments self-administered under periodic supervision or guidance by provider	Ayurveda Biofeedback Homeopathy Hydrotherapy Nutritional therapy Tai chi

Definition of Therapeutic Modalities

Acupressure

Acupressure is a manual therapy that applies deep pressure to certain acupuncture points.[76,80] It is theorized that different noxious stimuli, including emotional trauma, cause energy to accumulate in particular pressure points situated along the channels or meridians through which qi flows. Application of pressure by the practitioner improves flow of qi, causing a release and dissipation of tension, alleviation of disease and relief of pain.[76] It has been studied for the treatment of nausea of pregnancy, headache, backache, stroke, pain associated with chemotherapy and traumatic brain injury.[80,81] Application of pressure to a particular point on the inside of the wrist has been promoted to alleviate motion sickness, however there is limited evidence to support its efficacy.[82]

Acupuncture

Acupuncture can describe either a therapeutic discipline or a technique, which can vary with different traditional approaches and is now practiced by both conventional and CAM practitioners.[83] Needles of various sizes, but commonly having a shaft of 25 mm and a diameter of 0.25 mm, are inserted at specific points on the body to regulate the flow of qi along chosen meridians.[84,85] In a more conventional approach, these acupuncture points are termed "trigger points," which correspond to areas of increased sensitivity that can produce referred pain in a characteristic manner.[86] Anatomically, these points often correspond to peripheral nerve junctions and may be involved in pain transmission. The technique itself involves the insertion of several needles (usually 4–10), and may vary with respect to angle and depth of insertion, length of time retained (often 10–30 minutes), manipulation methods (e.g., twirling, electrical current) and frequency of treatment.[86] Variations on needle therapy include Shiatsu, moxibustion, acupressure and electric currents. Areas of interest in acupuncture treatment include pain management, including postoperative dental pain, headache, substance abuse, nausea, asthma, urticaria and stroke rehabilitation.[81,86,87,88,89] Neural pathways, neurotransmitters and hormonal factors are believed to be affected by acupuncture.[90] Research supports the use of acupuncture in pain secondary to temporomandibular dysfunction, fibromyalgia, osteoarthritis, low back pain and idiopathic headache,[91,92] including recurrent headache in children.[21,59] Systematic reviews have concluded acupuncture is an option for chronic pain,[93] migraine prophylaxis[94] and tension-type headache.[95]

Applied Kinesiology

This diagnostic technique used by chiropractors and other practitioners is distinct from kinesiology, and uses acupressure points and muscle strength testing to identify health and nutritional problems.[75,96] Practitioners assert that weakness in particular muscles corresponds to specific illnesses or deficiencies which can be corrected by manipulation or supplements.

Aromatherapy

Aromatherapy is a treatment method using volatile (essential) oils derived from plants whose fragrance or odour is deemed an integral part of therapy.[97] The oils are extracted from plants, diluted with vegetable oil then often applied to the skin by massage, or they can be delivered in steam for inhalation of the scent.[80] When applied externally, the fragrance, the massage itself and the dermal absorption of the constituents are all deemed beneficial,[98] although a psychological component cannot be ruled out.[72] In the United Kingdom, aromatherapy has been used in conventional settings such as hospices, palliative care units, cancer units and pediatric units.[97]

Ayurveda

Ayurveda is a major medical system that originated in India and possibly dates back as much as 5000 years.[2,80,99,100] It is a complex system of theory and practice, which considers the body, mind and spirit, and attempts to achieve harmony and balance between them. It is believed that the body is a miniature representation of the universe. The same elements that form the universe form the human body; when the elements are out of balance (i.e., imbalance within the body or between the body and the environment), ill health results. Patient assessment includes physical examination as well as consideration of mental and social factors. Treatment choices include manipulation, diet, yoga, meditation, purification to rid the body of toxins (possibly involving vomiting, purgation or enemas) and rejuvenation therapies to build the body's strength. Herbal therapies are employed, as well as minerals and metals, which might include heavy metals. As with other herbal therapies, the safety of Ayurvedic herbs may be questionable as lead poisoning has occurred following the use of Ayurvedic remedies brought into Canada.[101]

Biofeedback

Biofeedback is a system that permits a patient to regulate body function (e.g., heart rate, blood pressure, degree of muscle contraction) by receiving feedback signals from instruments monitoring a particular physiological function (e.g., brain waves), and to adjust the physiologic process accordingly.[80] It may be effective for varied conditions including irritable bowel, bladder disorders, asthma, headache, post-traumatic stress disorder, cardiac arrhythmias and hypertension.[75,96]

Chinese Herbal Medicine

Chinese herbal medicine is an integral part of Chinese medicine, which encompasses use of animal parts and minerals in addition to plant material.[84,102] Substances can be categorized according to their properties, which include heat clearing, wind dispelling or blood rectifying. The use of medicinal substances can be complex, with specific combinations selected based on their compatibility and complementary/synergistic effects.[103] Typical combinations contain 2–40 herbs in differing amounts, and the combination will be adjusted during the course of treatment according to the clinical presentation.[102] They are usually consumed as a decoction (simmered tea) but also may be dispensed in solid dosage forms or used externally. Be aware that some imported herbal products may contain contaminants or be otherwise adulterated.

Chiropractic

Chiropractic is a body-manipulation therapy aimed at correcting misalignment within the musculoskeletal system.[78] Chiropractors apply a variety of manoeuvres, such as sharp thrusts, to the spine, pelvis and limbs in order to adjust alignment and correct disorders.[104] Although formerly advocated for treating a wide variety of complaints, today it is limited primarily to treating musculoskeletal disorders. There is evidence for its use in acute low back pain and in tension-type and migraine headache.[78,96] While rare, stroke or vertebral artery dissection have followed manipulation of the neck, although causation has not been established.[78]

Craniosacral Therapy

Craniosacral therapy is a manual technique in which gentle pressure is applied to the skull to adjust and normalize rhythmic pulsations of the cerebrospinal fluid.[105,106] It has been purported to relieve pain (e.g., headache) and vertigo.

Cupping and Bleeding

This is a component of Chinese medicine in which a warm glass or bamboo cup is placed on the skin. As it cools, the suction created draws blood and lymph to the skin surface. It is used to assist circulation and to remove "cold and damp" which are considered external causes of disease.[84,105] Arab healers believed that cupping would relieve a variety of ailments, from toothache to elephantiasis.[85]

Dietary Supplements

This term has various interpretations. In the United States it is defined by the *Dietary Supplement Health and Education Act* (1994) as a product intended to supplement the diet which may contain one or more dietary ingredients including vitamins, minerals, amino acids, herbs or other botanicals and other substances.[107] It is an oral dosage form (pill, tablet, capsule or liquid) and must be labelled as a dietary supplement. Its intended use is to resolve a nutritional deficiency or to improve or sustain the function of the body. If used to diagnose, prevent, treat or cure a disease it is considered a drug, and not a dietary supplement. The Act does not require proof of efficacy or safety or standardization.[107] The accepted regulatory term in Canada is Natural Health Product (NHP), which is defined differently (see Natural Health Products).

Functional Foods

According to Health Canada, "a functional food is similar in appearance to, or may be, a conventional food, is consumed as part of a usual diet and is demonstrated to have physiological benefits and/or reduce the risk of chronic disease beyond basic nutritional functions".[108] Functional foods are developed through various means, including fortification with vitamins and/or minerals beyond mandatory requirements, addition of bioactive ingredients, and enhancement of bioactive components through processes such as plant breeding and special livestock feeding.[109] Examples of foods that are thought to have benefit by supplying biologically active ingredients are eggs enriched with omega-3 fatty acids, cereals containing oat bran and tomatoes rich in lycopene.[110] Exemptions in the Food and Drugs Regulations have allowed some functional foods to carry health claims; for example, margarines containing plant sterols may claim to reduce cholesterol on their labels.[111]

Functional Medicine

Functional medicine is a patient-centred care model that integrates conventional and CAM practices, and considers the interplay between environment, lifestyle, genetic and mind-body factors, and their influence on the health of an individual. Nutrition, diet and exercise are strategies emphasized in disease prevention; conventional diagnostic and treatment methods are combined as necessary with CAM therapies in treatment.[112]

Herbalism

Herbalism is an approach that uses plant-based medicines as substitutes for pharmaceuticals, and as vehicles to optimize health and wellness. The WHO has taken the position that, in the absence of opposing scientific evidence, the traditional and historical use of herbal remedies provides evidence of their efficacy and safety;[113,114] they also published a document to guide quality control in herbal medicines.[115] Medical herbalism has been a sustained therapeutic approach in numerous countries, including Western nations such as Germany where modern pharmacology and herbalism successfully coexist.[1] The entire plant kingdom, including moss, algae and fungi may be utilized (although some herbal traditions also use animal parts, insects, metals, rocks or shells).[116] The basis of herbalism is the belief that the physiological response to a plant will be different than the response to an individual chemical component of the plant.[105] Growing conditions and collection and storage methods will also affect response, as will the expectations of the patient and the cultural significance of the plant (which may contribute to increased placebo response).

Holistic Medicine

This is an approach that takes into account the body, mind and spirit of an individual, as well as their interaction, to maintain health and well-being.[105,117] Some argue that competent physicians have always done this, and that it is not the exclusive domain of CAM practitioners.[3] What might be termed a holistic approach, the practice of involving multidisciplinary teams (physicians, spiritual healers and psychological counsellors) has been successfully incorporated into conventional medical practices.[118,119]

Homeopathy

Homeopathy is an alternative medical system, dating back to the early nineteenth century, based on the philosophy that the body has an innate ability to heal itself, and that "like cures like".[77,83,120,121] It teaches that symptoms are manifested when the body attempts to heal itself or to correct an imbalance. The presenting symptoms guide therapy. The premise is that a substance that produces a specific pattern of symptoms in a healthy person will, when given in homeopathic doses, help fight an illness with identical symptomatology. Homeopathic remedies are chosen based on the mental and emotional state of the patient, in addition to the physical. Therapies are highly individualized and, in general, should be made only by a trained homeopath. The closest match between the symptoms of the individual and the remedy is attempted, recognizing that different people will exhibit different symptom patterns. There are more than 2000 homeopathic substances, which are derived from plants, minerals, metals, animal products and even diseased tissues. The substances are prepared in serial dilutions, which are vigorously shaken with each dilution, which is believed to increase potency. Potencies are typically noted as X or C, indicating 1:10 dilutions, or 1:100 dilutions, respectively (e.g., 6X will denote 6 dilutions of 1:10). The goal of the dilution process is that no molecules of the original substance exist in the final preparation. Paradoxically, the greater the dilution, the higher the potency. Preparations of highest potency are reserved for use under the direction of a homeopath. In North America, asthma, headache, depression, allergies, psychosocial problems and skin conditions are among the most frequent conditions treated by homeopaths. In the United Kingdom, homeopathy is often used in children to treat minor self-limiting conditions.[122] Homeopathic medicines are regulated as natural health products in Canada, and authorized products are identified by an eight-digit Homeopathic Medicine Number (DIN-HM).[123] The WHO has developed a document addressing safety issues in homeopathic remedies.[124]

Hydrotherapy

Hydrotherapy includes a multitude of diverse applications including baths, saunas, douches, immersion, wraps and colonic irrigation, where water is used as the main tool of the therapeutic intervention.[85,125]

Hypnotherapy

Hypnotherapy is used to induce a state of relaxation by selective attentional focusing using imagery or distraction, where intrusive thoughts can be ignored.[21,75,126] It includes a suggestive component where therapeutic goals can be introduced (e.g., a pain-free state). It is possible to maintain the behaviour once the hypnotic state has been terminated. Muscle relaxation, altered perception and cognitive distraction are possible mechanisms.[126] It has been used with some success in smoking cessation and has been found useful in coping with pain, distress and anxiety in children with cancer undergoing bone marrow aspiration.[21]

Imagery

Imagery involves the use of directed mental images to promote changes in attitudes or behaviour, relieve symptoms or to encourage physical healing. The process may be guided by a practitioner or patients can be instructed in its application. It is often used for alleviation of stress and its sequelae including insomnia. It is thought to reduce the need for the use of analgesics in cancer patients.[21]

Iridology

Iridology is a discredited method of diagnosis which examines changes in the iris to determine state of health.[72,80]

Magnet Therapy

Magnet therapy involves the application of magnets to treat disorders by influencing ionic currents in the body causing stimulation of cells and enhanced blood flow.[55,106] It is not to be confused with magnetic healing, which was a form of hypnosis. Unipolar or bipolar magnets are fastened into clothing, worn like jewelry (e.g., bracelets), held in place against the skin by adhesive or used in bedding. They have been promoted to treat musculoskeletal complaints such as chronic low back pain, muscle pain in postpolio syndrome and neuropathic pain in diabetes, although a systematic review did not support their use for pain relief.[55]

Massage Therapy

Massage therapy is a manipulative method that uses a variety of manual techniques (stroking, kneading, friction, vibration) applied to soft tissues.[76,78] Human touch itself is considered to be a beneficial part of massage. It is used in traditional medical systems including Ayurveda and Chinese medicine. Massage is used to promote relaxation, relieve muscle tightness, alleviate pain, reduce anxiety and promote sleep. It is used to promote the growth and development of premature infants[59] and might benefit patients suffering from anxiety and chronic cancer pain.[21] It should not be used in patients with deep vein thrombosis, advanced osteoporosis, fractures or where skin is compromised.[78]

Meditation

Meditation is one of the most commonly used mind-body interventions to induce relaxation and a sense of calm.[96] It is a self-directed practice that involves a conscious mental process of becoming aware of one's thoughts and achieving mastery over them. It is becoming increasingly recommended in Western conventional medicine as it has been shown to reduce symptoms of anxiety.[127] Functional magnetic resonance imaging has shown that meditation can activate areas of the brain involved in attention and in the control of the autonomic nervous system. It is an element of different traditional medical systems including Chinese medicine and Ayurveda as a component of yoga, qigong and tai chi. Preliminary evidence has found that some meditation techniques alter blood flow in the brain, lower blood pressure, slow respiratory rate, improve immune function, help with coping strategies and provide a positive emotional state.[75,96,126]

Moxibustion

Moxibustion is a component of Chinese medicine that involves the burning of dried and powdered leaves of *Artemesia vulgaris*.[84] It can be burned in very small amounts directly on the skin, on a mediating substance placed between the burning material and the skin surface or on the handle of an acupuncture needle. It is believed that the burning substance has the ability to enter the meridians and affect the flow of qi. Moxibustion is used in combination with acupuncture for a wide variety of conditions.

Natural Health Products

Natural health products (NHPs) have been regulated in Canada since 2004.[123] According to Health Canada, the definition of a natural health product includes both function and substance.[128] Function captures substances for use in the diagnosis, treatment, mitigation or prevention of disease/disorder; restoring, correcting or modifying organic functions in a manner which maintains or promotes health. Acceptable substances include materials derived from plants, algae, bacteria, fungi and non-human animals; these include vitamins and minerals, herbal remedies, homeopathic medicines, traditional medicines like traditional Chinese medicines, probiotics, and other products like amino acids and essential fatty acids. Numerous exclusions are listed such as antibiotics, blood products, tobacco, injectables, biologics, cannabis and others. Natural health products must be safe for use as patient self-selected products and are available for purchase without the consultation of a healthcare practitioner. Premarket authorization is required for sale. Manufacturers must provide evidence that products are safe, effective and of high quality before obtaining a product license, although the type of evidence varies depending on whether the product has a traditional use claim (supported by traditional evidence) or a modern use claim (typically supported by randomized controlled trials).[128,129,130]

Contamination is a frequent problem with imported NHPs due to lack of rigorous manufacturing standards. In particular, many Chinese herbal products are the subject of Health Canada warnings for containing undeclared medications, bacteria and fungi; most of these are not authorized for sale in Canada.[131,132,133] Practitioners should be reminded to recommend only natural health products that are authorized for sale in Canada, as indicated by a Natural Product Number (NPN), Homeopathic Medicine Number (DIN-HM), or Exemption Number (EN).

Naturopathic Medicine

Naturopathic medicine is a system of treatment, defined by a broad scope of practice, that emphasizes the healing power of nature, and which draws from a wide variety of therapeutic approaches.[125,134,135] The use of nutrition, herbs and natural products is fundamental, with treatments borrowed from Chinese medicine, homeopathy, herbalism, Ayurveda and manual therapies. As it does not identify with one particular mode of therapy, it is generally defined by its approach. This includes core principles of preventive medicine, treatment of the whole person and determination of the cause of the disease. Treatment combinations are individualized for each patient, in an effort to aid self-healing and restore normal body function, rather than attempt to focus on the treatment of symptoms. Interventions include natural products, nutritional counselling, acupuncture, naturopathic manipulation, traditional Chinese medicine, homeopathy and many others.[135]

Nutraceutical

Health Canada defines a nutraceutical as "a product isolated or purified from foods that is generally sold in medicinal forms not usually associated with food. A nutraceutical is demonstrated to have a physiological benefit or provide protection against chronic disease".[108] From a legal standpoint, these products are regulated as natural health products in Canada. The concentrated dosage forms can deliver ingredients in amounts exceeding those found in food.[29] Examples include omega-3 fatty acids derived from marine sources and isoflavones isolated from soy, sold in capsule form.

Orthomolecular Therapy

Orthomolecular therapy is a term derived from the Greek word "orthos," meaning straight or correct, and was first used by Linus Pauling in 1968 to describe the treatment of disease with large quantities of nutrients, especially vitamins.[80] It is similar to megavitamin therapy but minerals, amino acids, hormones and metabolic intermediates can also be administered. The amounts of nutrients administered may be 20–600 times the recommended daily intake.

Osteopathic Medicine

Osteopathic medicine is a system that originated as a manipulative method, but has evolved into mainstream medicine in the United States where practitioners receive a Doctor of Osteopathy (DO) degree and restrict themselves to conventional medicine.[76,104,136] Underlying principles are based on an appreciation of the connection between the body's tissues, fluids and systems; treatment is aimed at restoring integrity of structures and improving interactions of the body's systems. Osteopaths perform various practices which include manual techniques that combine manipulation and massage therapy, such as thrusting (similar to chiropractic methods) and lymphatic drainage and craniosacral therapy (similar to massage therapy). Osteopathic methods attempt to correct symmetry, motion restriction, tissue texture changes and tenderness. In countries other than the United States, such as Great Britain, osteopaths earn Bachelor of Science degrees and have practices similar to that of chiropractors.

Qigong

Qigong is an energy therapy that is a major branch of Chinese medicine and is aimed at manipulating qi.[84] It involves a wide variety of activities to balance, regulate and harness qi in order to promote health, longevity, healing and spiritual development. An internal form has the patient acting alone using exercise, breathing or relaxation methods. In the external form, a practitioner projects his or her qi into the patient via their hands, the use of needles or visualization. In healthy volunteers, it has been shown to reduce cortisol levels, and might be of use to relieve stress.[126] Other potential benefits include hypertension and respiratory disease.[75] Qigong may also improve quality of life for cancer patients.[137]

Reflexology (Zone Therapy)

Reflexology is a manual technique in which the practitioner applies deep pressure using their fingers and thumbs on the patient's feet.[76,98] Different zones on the feet are thought to correspond to areas on the body (equated with meridians) and application of pressure is thought to enhance the flow of energy in the body. Reflexology has been applied for the relief of symptoms associated with chronic conditions such as asthma, headache, and bladder or bowel problems, and to patients suffering stroke, brain injury or spinal cord injury.[81]

Reiki

Reiki is an energy therapy developed in the mid-nineteenth century whereby practitioners channel the universal life energy (i.e., reiki) through meditation and prayer from their own body to the patient's, to promote healing.[76,79] Reiki has been used in the treatment of fibromyalgia, pain, cancer and depression, as well as for overall well-being, but research has not confirmed usefulness for any condition.[138]

Relaxation

Relaxation employs various techniques, approaches and modes of practice.[75,96] Most involve repetitive action (focus on a word, sound, phrase, muscular activity), and adopting a passive attitude toward intruding thoughts with a return to focus. It has been studied in anxiety, depression, pain and irritable bowel syndrome.[96]

Rolfing

Rolfing is a manipulation method that uses deep muscle massage to correct distortions in the body.[76,79] It teaches that distortions in posture reflect a withdrawal response to past emotional and physical trauma, and restoring correct posture with manipulation will release the traumas, resulting in a feeling of lightness and well-being.

Shiatsu

Shiatsu is a Japanese massage technique in which pressure is applied to specific points on the body likened to acupuncture points.[76,80,139] It may be combined with passive stretching to optimize the effect. It has been likened to acupressure in technique, but is used more for prevention of illness than treatment.

Tai chi

Tai chi is a series of precise, focused slow-moving postures accompanied by controlled breathing and a calm, relaxed mind, which involves physical and mental discipline.[126] It is used to unite body and mind and promote balance in life. Limited evidence demonstrates a lowering of blood pressure and heart rate and a reduction in stress. Tai chi may be useful in osteoarthritis of the knee,[140] prevention of falls in the elderly,[141] and improving balance in patients with mild to moderate Parkinson's disease.[142]

Therapeutic Touch

Therapeutic touch is an energy therapy developed in the late 1960s in which providers move their hands above the surface of a patient's body in an attempt to correct imbalance in the patient's energy field and facilitate healing.[76,80,143] Practitioners believe that their hands can transfer energy from themselves to a patient to achieve energy balance within the patient. It is a popular treatment for pain, anxiety, Alzheimer's dementia and stress; therapeutic touch is also used to improve well-being of cancer patients.[96]

Traditional Chinese Medicine

Traditional Chinese medicine, also known as traditional Oriental medicine, is a comprehensive and major medical system, dating back to 3000 BC, which comprises many traditions, philosophies and approaches to treatment.[77,80,83,102,144] It is based on fundamental concepts that include a balance between yin and yang (opposing yet complementary phenomena that exist simultaneously throughout the universe and the body) and unimpeded flow of qi (the vital force or energy which circulates through the body in invisible pathways termed "meridians"). Health problems may reflect a lack of harmony within an individual, or between individuals and their environment, resulting in a blockage in the flow of qi and an imbalance of yin and yang. Diagnosis of the patient involves a multitude of techniques in addition to taking a medical history, which include assessing temperament, examining the tongue and properties of the pulse and noting qualities of speech and breath. The practitioner evaluates how illness manifests itself in the patient, and then treats the person, not the disease. Treatments are highly individualized, and employ various methods, to target the deep cause of the disease rather than only symptoms.[102] Chosen methods of therapy include diet, herbal therapy, acupuncture, moxibustion, cupping and bleeding, tui na and qigong.

Traditional Medicine

The WHO defines traditional medicine as "the sum total of the knowledge, skills, and practices based on the theories, beliefs, and experiences indigenous to different cultures, whether explicable or not, used in the maintenance of health as well as in the prevention, diagnosis, improvement or treatment of physical and mental illness".[145]

Tui Na

Tui Na is a manipulative practice within Chinese medicine, which involves trained practitioners manipulating soft tissues and joints.[76,84] Attention is given to the flow of qi along meridians, and acupuncture points are stimulated. It is commonly used in orthopedic and neurological applications, and can be used in situations where acupuncture is considered inappropriate (e.g., pediatrics).

Yoga

Yoga is one of the top CAM modalities used in North America and is intended to promote relaxation and achieve balance in mind, body and spirit through the use of physical postures, breathing exercises, meditation and a philosophical approach.[96,146] The numerous schools of yoga incorporate these components in varying proportions.[75,96,146] Possible benefits include rejuvenation, awareness, self-realization, stress reduction, increased strength and improved flexibility. It is advocated as a way to increase the mind's flexibility and resilience when faced with stress. Limited research suggests yoga may help with various conditions including asthma,[96] hypertension,[96] depression,[147] pain[148] and anxiety; and it may also improve overall fitness, strength and flexibility.[146] It should be noted that individuals with certain medical conditions (glaucoma, hypertension, severe osteoporosis) could be at risk with some postures.

Summary

Increasing focus on self-care has led patients to explore CAM therapies as means of improving their health and well-being. As primary healthcare practitioners, pharmacists are at the forefront and are often the most trusted practitioners when it comes to consulting on CAM modalities. Understanding the nature of CAM, the history and terminology, and the potential benefits and limitations, will improve the pharmacist-patient relationship and can significantly improve the health of the patient. While, in general, there is limited scientific evidence to support the use of CAM modalities to improve disease outcome, there is evidence to suggest their utility in improving health quality. It is important for pharmacists to be aware patients are participating in these practices and to engage patients to better understand the nature of their CAM practices. This open-minded approach will enable a more comprehensive approach to the patient's overall health.

Suggested Readings

Deng GE, Frenkel M, Cohen L et al. Evidence-based clinical practice guidelines for integrative oncology: complementary therapies and botanicals. *J Soc Integr Oncol* 2009;7:85-120.

Kemper KJ, Vohra S, Walls R et al. American Academy of Pediatrics. The use of complementary and alternative medicine in pediatrics. *Pediatrics* 2008;122:1374-86.

Monti DA, Sufian M, Peterson C. Potential role of mind-body therapies in cancer survivorship. *Cancer* 2008;112:2607-16.

Rogovik AL, Vohra S, Goldman RD. Safety considerations and potential interactions of vitamins: should vitamins be considered drugs? *Ann Pharmcother* 2010;44:311-24.

Siow YL, Gong Y, Au-Yeung KK et al. Emerging issues in traditional Chinese medicine. *Can J Physiol Pharmacol* 2005;83:321-34.

Tachjian A, Maria V, Jahangir A. Use of herbal products and potential interactions in patients with cardiovascular diseases. *J Am Coll Cardiol* 2010:55:515-25.

Vogel JH, Bolling SF, Costello RB et al. Integrating complementary medicine into cardiovascular medicine. A report of the American College of Cardiology Foundation Task Force on Clinical Expert Consensus Documents (Writing Committee to Develop an Expert Consensus Document on Complementary and Integrative Medicine). *J Am Coll Cardiol* 2005;46:184-221.

References

1. WHO Congress on Traditional Medicine and the Beijing Declaration. *WHO Drug Info* 2009;23:8-11.
2. National Center for Complementary and Integrative Health. *Complementary, alternative, or integrative health: what's in a name?* Bethesda: NCCIH, National Institutes of Health. Available from: nccih.nih.gov/health/integrative-health. Accessed April 21, 2016.
3. Ernst E. Disentangling integrative medicine. *Mayo Clin Proc* 2004;79:565-6.
4. Barnes PM, Powell-Griner E, McFann K et al. Complementary and alternative medicine use among adults: United States, 2002. *Adv Data* 2004;343:1-19.
5. Health Canada. Ipsos-Reid. *Natural health product tracking survey—2010 final report.* January 2011. Available from: www.hc-sc.gc.ca/dhp-mps/prodnatur/index-eng.php. Accessed April 21, 2016.
6. Eisenberg DM, Davis RB, Ettner SL et al. Trends in alternative medicine use in the United States, 1990-1997: results of a follow-up national survey. *JAMA* 1998;280:1569-75.
7. Clarke TC, Black LI, Stussman BJ et al. Trends in the use of complementary health approaches among adults: United States, 2002-2012. *Natl Health Stat Report* 2015;79:1-16.
8. Black LI, Clarke TC, Barnes PM et al. Use of complementary health approaches among children aged 4-17 years in the United States: National Health Interview Survey, 2007-2012. *Natl Health Stat Report* 2015;78:1-19.
9. Hunt KJ, Coelho HF, Wider B et al. Complementary and alternative medicine use in England: results from a national survey. *Int J Clin Pract* 2010;64:1496-502.
10. Park J. Health reports: use of alternative health care, 2003. Ottawa: Statistics Canada. *The Daily* 2005 Mar 15. Available from: www.statcan.gc.ca/daily-quotidien/050315/dq050315-eng-htm. Accessed April 21, 2016.
11. Statistics Canada. CANSIM. Canadian Community Health Survey. Table 105-0462. *Contact with alternative health care providers in the past 12 months, by age group and sex, household population aged 12 and over, Canada, provinces, territories, health regions (June 2005 boundaries) and peer groups, *terminated* every 2 years*. Available from: www5.statcan.gc.ca/cansim/a26?lang=eng&id=1050462. Accessed April 21, 2016.
12. McFarland B, Bigelow D, Zani B et al. Complementary and alternative medicine use in Canada and the United States. *Am J Public Health* 2002;92:1616-8.
13. Miller MF, Bellizzi KM, Sufian M et al. Dietary supplement use in individuals living with cancer and other chronic conditions: a population-based study. *J Am Diet Assoc* 2008;108;483-94.
14. Ernst E. The public's enthusiasm for complementary and alternative medicine amounts to a critique of mainstream medicine. *Int J Clin Pract* 2010;64:1472-4.
15. Metcalfe A, Williams J, McChesney J et al. Use of complementary and alternative medicine by those with a chronic disease and the general population—results of a national population based survey. *BMC Complement Altern Med* 2010;10:58.
16. Quan H, Lai D, Johnson D et al. Complementary and alternative medicine use among Chinese and white Canadians. *Can Fam Physician* 2008;54:1563-9.
17. Lai D, Chappell N. Use of traditional Chinese medicine by older Chinese immigrants in Canada. *Fam Pract* 2007;24:56-64.
18. Roth MA, Kobayashi KM. The use of complementary and alternative medicine among Chinese Canadians: results from a national survey. *J Immigr Minor Health* 2008;10:517-28.
19. Cook SJ. Use of traditional Mi'kmaq medicine among patients at a First Nations community health centre. *Can J Rural Med* 2005;10:95-9.
20. Williams AM, Kitchen P, Eby J. Alternative health care consultations in Ontario, Canada: a geographic and socio-demographic analysis. *BMC Complement Altern Med* 2011;11:47.
21. Deng G, Cassileth BR. Integrative oncology: complementary therapies for pain, anxiety, and mood disturbance. *CA Cancer J Clin* 2005;55:109-16.
22. Boon HS, Olatunde F, Zick SM. Trends in complementary/alternative medicine use by breast cancer survivors: comparing survey data from 1998 and 2005. *BMC Womens Health* 2007;7:4.
23. Damery S, Gratus C, Grieve R et al. The use of herbal medicines by people with cancer: a cross-sectional survey. *Br J Cancer* 2011;104:927-33.
24. Bishop FL, Prescott P, Chan YK et al. Prevalence of complementary medicine use in pediatric cancer: a systematic review. *Pediatrics* 2010;125:768-76.
25. Adams D, Whidden A, Honkanen M et al. Complementary and alternative medicine: a survey of its use in pediatric cardiology. *CMAJ Open* 2014;2:E217-24.
26. Galicia-Connolly E, Adams D, Bateman J et al. CAM use in pediatric neurology: an exploration of concurrent use with conventional medicine. *PLoS One* 2014;9:e94078.
27. Tsui T, Boon H, Boecker A et al. Understanding the role of scientific evidence in consumer evaluation of natural health products for osteoarthritis an application of the means end chain approach. *BMC Complement Altern Med* 2012;12:198.
28. Boon H, Kachan N, Boecker A. Use of natural health products: how does being "natural" affect choice? *Med Decis Making* 2013;33:282-97.

29. Hollander JM, Mechanick JI. Complementary and alternative medicine and the management of the metabolic syndrome. *J Am Diet Assoc* 2008;108:495-509.
30. Cohen PA. DMAA as a dietary supplement ingredient. *Arch Intern Med* 2012;172:1038-9.
31. Koren G, Oren D, Rouleau M et al. Comparison of verbal claims for natural health products made by health food stores staff versus pharmacists in Ontario, Canada. *Can J Clin Pharmacol* 2006;13:e251-6.
32. Edwards L, Jefferies S, Healy B et al. What risk to consumers face when seeking medical advice from health food stores? *N Z Med J* 2011;124:81-8.
33. Vogel L. "Hodge-podge" regulation of alternative medicine in Canada. *CMAJ* 2010;182:E569-70.
34. Walji R, Boon H, Barnes J et al. Consumers of natural health products: natural-born pharmacovigilantes? *BMC Complement Altern Med* 2010;10:8.
35. Wu CH, Wang CC, Kennedy J. Changes in herb and dietary supplement use in the U.S. adult population: a comparison of the 2002 and 2007 National Health Interview Surveys. *Clin Ther* 2011;33:1749-58.
36. Necyk C, Barnes J, Tsuyuki RT et al. How well do pharmacists know their patients? A case report highlighting natural health product disclosure. *Can Pharm J* 2013;146:202-9.
37. Ontario College of Pharmacists. Best possible medication history guidelines for medication reconciliation. *Pharmacy Connection* 2007. Available from: www.ocpinfo.com/library/practice-related/download/Best%20Possible%20Medication%20History.pdf. Accessed April 21, 2016.
38. Adams KE, Cohen MH, Eisenberg D et al. Ethical considerations of complementary and alternative medical therapies in conventional medical settings. *Ann Intern Med* 2002;137:660-4.
39. Fonnebo V, Grimsgaard S, Walach H et al. Researching complementary and alternative treatments–the gatekeepers are not at home. *BMC Med Res Methodol* 2007;7:7.
40. Kwan D, Hirschkorn K, Boon H. U.S. and Canadian pharmacists' attitudes, knowledge, and professional practice behaviors toward dietary supplements: a systematic review. *BMC Complement Altern Med* 2006;6:31.
41. Walji R, Boon H, Barnes J et al. Reporting natural health product related adverse drug reactions: is it the pharmacist's responsibility? *Int J Pharm Pract* 2011;19:383-91.
42. Braun LA, Tiralongo E, Wilkinson JM et al. Perceptions, use and attitudes of pharmacy customers on complementary medicines and pharmacy practice. *BMC Complement Altern Med* 2010;10:38.
43. Sirois FM. Motivations for consulting complementary and alternative medicine practitioners: a comparison of consumers from 1997-8 and 2005. *BMC Complement Altern Med* 2008;8:16.
44. Shekelle PG, Morton SC, Suttorp MJ et al. Challenges in systematic reviews of complementary and alternative medicine topics. *Ann Intern Med* 2005;142:1042-7.
45. Gagnier JJ, Moher D, Boon H et al. Randomized controlled trials of herbal interventions underreport important details of the intervention. *J Clin Epidemiol* 2011;64:760-9.
46. Gagnier JJ, Boon H, Rochon P et al. Recommendations for reporting randomized trials of herbal interventions: explanation and elaboration. *J Clin Epidemiol* 2006;59:1134-49.
47. MacPherson H, Altman DG, Hammerschlag R et al. Revised STandards for Reporting Interventions in Clinical Trials of Acupuncture (STRICTA): extending the CONSORT statement. *PLoS Med* 2010;7:e1000261.
48. Boutron I, Moher D, Altman DG et al. Extending the CONSORT statement to randomized trials of nonpharmacologic treatment: explanation and elaboration. *Ann Intern Med* 2008;148:295-309.
49. Teixeira MZ, Guedes CH, Barreto PV et al. The placebo effect and homeopathy. *Homeopathy* 2010;99:119-29.
50. Hróbjartsson A and Gøtzsche PC. Placebo interventions for all clinical conditions. *Cochrane Database Syst Rev* 2010;1:CD003974.
51. Tilburt JC, Curlin FA, Kaptchuk TJ et al. Alternative medicine research and clinical practice: a US national survey. *Arch Intern Med* 2009;169:670-7.
52. Pilkington K. Searching for CAM evidence: an evaluation of therapy-specific search strategies. *J Altern Complement Med* 2007;13:451-9.
53. Cogo E, Sampson M, Ajiferuke I et al. Searching for controlled trials of complementary and alternative medicine: a comparison of 15 databases. *Evid Based Complement Alternat Med* 2011;2011:858246.
54. Bubela T, Koper M, Boon H et al. Media portrayal of herbal remedies versus pharmaceutical clinical trials: impacts on decision. *Med Law* 2007;26:363-73.
55. Pittler MH, Brown EM, Ernst E. Static magnets for reducing pain: systematic review and meta-analysis of randomized trials. *CMAJ* 2007;177:736-42.
56. Kaptchuk TJ. The placebo effect in alternative medicine: can the performance of a healing ritual have clinical significance? *Ann Intern Med* 2002;136:817-25.
57. Mason S, Tovey P, Long AF. Evaluating complementary medicine: methodological challenges of randomised controlled trials. *BMJ* 2002;325:832-4.
58. Manheimer E, Berman B. Producing and disseminating systematic reviews: a summary of the CAM-related work presented at the 13th international Cochrane Colloquium. *J Altern Complement Med* 2006;12:193-6.
59. Kemper KJ, Vohra S, Walls R et al. American Academy of Pediatrics. The use of complementary and alternative medicine in pediatrics. *Pediatrics* 2008;122:1374-86.
60. Jonas WB. Scientific evidence and medical practice: the "drunkard's walk". *Arch Intern Med* 2009;169:649-50.
61. World Health Organization. Essential Medicines and Health Products Information Portal. Available from: apps.who.int/medicinedocs/en/. Accessed April 21, 2016.
62. Nedrow AR, Heitkemper M, Frenkel M et al. Collaboration between complementary and alternative medicine health professionals: four initiatives. *Acad Med* 2007;82:962-6.
63. Complementary and Alternative Medicine Issues in Undergraduate Medical Education. CAM in UME Project. Available from: www.caminume.ca/. Accessed April 21, 2016.
64. Toupin April K and Gaboury I. A survey of Canadian regulated complementary and alternative medicine schools about research, evidence-based health care and interprofessional training, as well as continuing education. *BMC Complement Altern Med* 2013;13:374.
65. Byrne A, Boon H, Austin Z et al. Core competencies in natural health products for Canadian pharmacy students. *Am J Pharm Educ* 2010;74:45.
66. Vohra S, Surette S, Mittra D et al. Pediatric integrative medicine: pediatrics' newest subspecialty? *BMC Pediatr* 2012;12:123.

67. Cochrane Complementary Medicine. Available from: www.cam.cochrane.org/. Accessed April 21, 2016.
68. Andrews JG, Boon H. CAM in Canada: places, practices, research. *Complement Ther Clin Pract* 2005;11:21-7.
69. Riva JJ, Krawchenko IE, Lam JM et al. Chiropractors and pharmacists in a family health team: unlikely allies in the collaborative management of pregnancy-related low back pain. *Can Pharm J* 2011;144:62-5.
70. Gaboury I, Lapierre LM, Boon H et al. Interprofessional collaboration within integrative healthcare clinics through the lens of the relationship-centered care model. *J Interprof Care* 2011;25:124-30.
71. Wieland LS, Manheimer E, Berman BM. Development and classification of an operational definition of complementary and alternative medicine for the Cochrane Collaboration. *Altern Ther Health Med* 2011;17:50-9.
72. Ernst E. The role of complementary and alternative medicine. *BMJ* 2000;321:1133-5.
73. Dacher E. The development of an integrated medical model: toward a postmodern medicine. In: Micozzi MS, ed. *Fundamentals of complementary and alternative medicine*. 2nd ed. New York: Churchill Livingstone; 2001. p. 57-71.
74. Gordon JS. Mind-body medicine: overview. In: Fontanarosa PB, ed. *Alternative medicine: an objective assessment*. Chicago: American Medical Association; 2000. p. 154-6.
75. Vogel JH, Bolling SF, Costello RB et al. Integrating complementary medicine into cardiovascular medicine. A report of the American College of Cardiology Foundation Task Force on Clinical Expert Consensus Documents (Writing Committee to Develop an Expert Consensus Document on Complementary and Integrative Medicine). *J Am Coll Cardiol* 2005;46:184-221.
76. Coughlin P. Manual therapies. In: Micozzi MS, ed. *Fundamentals of complementary and alternative medicine*. 2nd ed. New York: Churchill Livingstone; 2001. p. 100-27.
77. Micozzi MS. Translational issues in conventional and complementary medicine. In: Micozzi MS, ed. *Fundamentals of complementary and alternative medicine*. 2nd ed. New York: Churchill Livingstone; 2001. p. 9-17.
78. National Center for Complementary and Integrative Health. *Chiropractic: in depth*. Bethesda: NCCIH, National Institutes of Health. Available from: nccih.nih.gov/health/chiropractic/introduction.htm. Accessed April 21, 2016.
79. Hurwitz WL. Energy medicine. In: Micozzi MS, ed. *Fundamentals of complementary and alternative medicine*. 2nd ed. New York: Churchill Livingstone; 2001. p. 238-56.
80. Cassileth BR. *The alternative medicine handbook: the complete reference guide to alternative and complementary therapies*. New York: Norton; 1998.
81. Diamond BJ, Shiflett SC, Schoenberger NE et al. Complementary/alternative therapies in the treatment of neurologic disorders. In: Spencer JW, Jacobs JJ, eds. *Complementary/alternative medicine: an evidence-based approach*. St. Louis: Mosby; 1999. p. 170-207.
82. Kronenberg F, Murphy PA, Wade C. Complementary/alternative therapies in select populations: women. In: Spencer JW, Jacobs JJ, eds. *Complementary/alternative medicine: an evidence-based approach*. St. Louis: Mosby; 1999. p. 341-62.
83. Cassidy CM. Social and cultural context of complementary and alternative medicine systems. In: Micozzi MS, ed. *Fundamentals of complementary and alternative medicine*. 2nd ed. New York: Churchill Livingstone; 2001. p. 18-42.
84. Ergil KV. Chinese medicine. In: Micozzi MS, ed. *Fundamentals of complementary and alternative medicine*. 2nd ed. New York: Churchill Livingstone; 2001. p. 303-44.
85. Oumeish OY. The philosophical, cultural, and historical aspects of complementary, alternative, unconventional, and integrative medicine in the Old World. *Arch Dermatol* 1998;134:1373-86.
86. Vickers A, Zollman C. ABC of complementary medicine. Acupuncture. *BMJ* 1999;319:973-6.
87. NIH Consensus Conference. Acupuncture. *JAMA* 1998;280:1518-24.
88. LaRiccia PL. Acupuncture: overview. In: Fontanarosa PB, ed. *Alternative medicine: an objective assessment*. Chicago: American Medical Association; 2000. p. 448-50.
89. Chen CJ, Yu HS. Acupuncture treatment of urticaria. *Arch Dermatol* 1998;134:1397-9.
90. Cooper EL. eCAM: a closer look at clinical analyses. *Evid Based Complement Alternat Med* 2009;6:279-81.
91. Berman BM. Integrative approaches to pain management: how to get the best of both worlds. *BMJ* 2003;326:1320-1.
92. Berman BM, Langevin HM, Witt CM et al. Acupuncture for low back pain. *N Engl J Med* 2010;363:454-61.
93. Vickers AJ, Cronin AM, Maschino AC et al. Acupuncture for chronic pain: individual patient data meta-analysis. *Arch Intern Med* 2012;172:1444-53.
94. Linde K, Allais G, Brinkhaus B et al. Acupuncture for migraine prophylaxis. *Cochrane Database Syst Rev* 2009;1:CD001218.
95. Linde K, Allais G, Brinkhaus B et al. Acupuncture for tension-type headache. *Cochrane Database Syst Rev* 2009;1:CD007587.
96. Natural Medicines. Somerville: Therapeutic Research Center. Available from: naturalmedicines.therapeuticresearch.com. Accessed April 21, 2016. Subscription required.
97. Stevensen CJ. Aromatherapy. In: Micozzi MS, ed. *Fundamentals of complementary and alternative medicine*. 2nd ed. New York: Churchill Livingstone; 2001. p. 146-58.
98. Vickers A, Zollman C. ABC of complementary medicine. Massage therapies. *BMJ* 1999;319:1254-7.
99. Zysk KG, Tetlow G. Traditional ayurveda. In: Micozzi MS, ed. *Fundamentals of complementary and alternative medicine*. 2nd ed. New York: Churchill Livingstone; 2001. p. 345-65.
100. Lad DV. Ayurvedic medicine. In: Jonas WB, Levin JS, eds. *Essentials of complementary and alternative medicine*. Philadelphia: Lippincott Williams & Wilkins; 1999. p. 200-15.
101. Gair R. Heavy metal poisoning from Ayurvedic medicines. *B C Med J* 2008;50:105.
102. Siow YL, Gong Y, Au-Yeung KK et al. Emerging issues in traditional Chinese medicine. *Can J Physiol Pharmacol* 2005;83:321-34.
103. Koo J, Arain S. Traditional Chinese medicine for the treatment of dermatologic disorders. *Arch Dermatol* 1998;134:1388-93.
104. Vickers A, Zollman C. ABC of complementary medicine. The manipulative therapies: osteopathy and chiropractic. *BMJ* 1999;319:1176-9.
105. Jonas WB, Levin JS, eds. *Essentials of complementary and alternative medicine*. Philadelphia: Lippincott Williams & Wilkins; 1999.
106. Spencer JW, Jacobs JJ, eds. *Complementary/alternative medicine: an evidence-based approach*. St. Louis: Mosby; 1999.
107. National Institutes of Health. Office of Dietary Supplements. *Dietary supplements: background information*. Available from: ods.od.nih.gov/factsheets/DietarySupplements-HealthProfessional. Accessed April 21, 2016.
108. Health Canada. Therapeutic Products Programme and the Food Directorate from the Health Protection Branch. *Policy paper–Nutraceuticals/functional foods and health claims on foods*. Available from: www.hc-sc.gc.ca/fn-an/label-etiquet/claims-reclam/nutra-funct_foods-nutra-fonct_aliment-eng.php. Accessed April 21, 2016.

109. Agriculture and Agri-Food Canada. *Functional foods and natural health products*. Available from: www.agr.gc.ca/eng/industry-markets-and-trade/statistics-and-market-information/by-product-sector/functional-foods-and-natural-health-products/functional-foods-and-natural-health-products-canadian-industry/?id=1170856376710. Accessed April 21, 2016.
110. Jones PJ. Clinical nutrition: 7. Functional foods–more than just nutrition. *CMAJ* 2002;166:1555-63.
111. Health Canada. *Plant sterols and blood cholesterol lowering*. Available from: www.hc-sc.gc.ca/fn-an/label-etiquet/claims-reclam/assess-evalu/phytosterols-eng.php. Accessed April 21, 2016.
112. The Institute for Functional Medicine. *What is functional medicine?* Available from: www.functionalmedicine.org. Accessed April 21, 2016.
113. McGuffin M, Hobbs C, Upton R, eds. *American Herbal Products Association's botanical safety handbook*. Boca Raton: CRC Press; 1997.
114. World Health Organization. Regional Office for the Western Pacific. *Research guidelines for evaluating the safety and efficacy of herbal medicines*. Manila: WHO; 1993.
115. World Health Organization. *Quality control methods for herbal materials*. Geneva: WHO; 2011. Available from: apps.who.int/medicinedocs/documents/h1791e/h1791e.pdf.
116. Meserole L. Western herbalism. In: Micozzi MS, ed. *Fundamentals of complementary and alternative medicine*. 2nd ed. New York: Churchill Livingstone; 2001. p. 128-45.
117. Astin JA. Why patients use alternative medicine: results of a national study. *JAMA* 1998;279:1548-53.
118. Watkins AD. Psychoneuroimmunology. In: Micozzi MS, ed. *Fundamentals of complementary and alternative medicine*. 2nd ed. New York: Churchill Livingstone; 2001. p. 200-14.
119. Zollman C, Vickers A. ABC of complementary medicine. Complementary medicine in conventional practice. *BMJ* 1999;319:901-4.
120. Jacobs J, Moskowitz R. Homeopathy. In: Micozzi MS, ed. *Fundamentals of complementary and alternative medicine*. 2nd ed. New York: Churchill Livingstone; 2001. p. 87-99.
121. Vickers A, Zollman C. ABC of complementary medicine. Homoeopathy. *BMJ* 1999;319:1115-8.
122. Erlewyn-Lajeunesse M. Homeopathic medicines for children. *Arch Dis Child* 2012;97:135-8.
123. Health Canada. *About natural health products*. Available from: hc-sc.gc.ca/dhp-mps/prodnatur/about-apropos/cons-eng.php. Accessed April 21, 2016.
124. World Health Organization. *Safety issues in the preparation of homeopathic medicines*. Geneva: WHO; 2009. Available from: www.who.int/medicines/areas/traditional/Homeopathy.pdf.
125. Pizzorno JE, Snider P. Naturopathic medicine. In: Micozzi MS, ed. *Fundamentals of complementary and alternative medicine*. 2nd ed. New York: Churchill Livingstone; 2001. p. 159-92.
126. Monti DA, Sufian M, Peterson C. Potential role of mind-body therapies in cancer survivorship. *Cancer* 2008;112:2607-16.
127. Chen KW, Berger CC, Manheimer E et al. Meditative therapies for reducing anxiety: a systematic review and meta-analysis of randomized controlled trials. *Depress Anxiety* 2012;29:545-62.
128. Health Canada. Drugs and Health Products. *Pathway for licensing natural health products making modern health claims*. Available from: www.hc-sc.gc.ca/dhp-mps/prodnatur/legislation/docs/modern-eng.php. Accessed April 21, 2016.
129. Health Canada. Natural Health Products Directorate. *Product licensing guidance document*. Available from: hc-sc.gc.ca/dhp-mps/alt_formats/hpfb-dgpsa/pdf/prodnatur/license-licence_guide-eng.pdf. Accessed April 21, 2016.
130. Health Canada. Drugs and Health Products. *Pathway for licensing natural health products used as traditional medicines*. Available from: www.hc-sc.gc.ca/dhp-mps/prodnatur/legislation/docs/tradit-eng.php. Accessed April 21, 2016.
131. Government of Canada. Healthy Canadians. *101 Zhangguang Gold 101 super effective hair growth agent and 101 Zhangguang Fabao 101D Doctor Zhao's Chinese traditional herbal hair care formula*. Available from: www.healthycanadians.gc.ca/recall-alert-rappel-avis/hc-sc/2010/13825a-eng.php. Accessed April 21, 2016.
132. Government of Canada. Healthy Canadians. *Fat Burner No. 1 (Qian Mei Yin Zi): unauthorized Chinese herbal weight loss product may pose serious health risks*. Available from: healthycanadians.gc.ca/recall-alert-rappel-avis/hc-sc/2010/13463a-eng.php. Accessed April 21, 2016.
133. Government of Canada. Healthy Canadians. *Nine bacterial and fungal contaminated herbal products and teas*. Available from: www.healthycanadians.gc.ca/recall-alert-rappel-avis/hc-sc/2008/13946a-eng.php. Accessed April 21, 2016.
134. Murray MT, Pizzorno JE. Naturopathic medicine. In: Jonas WB, Levin JS, eds. *Essentials of complementary and alternative medicine*. Philadelphia: Lippincott Williams & Wilkins; 1999. p. 304-21.
135. Verhoef MJ, Boon HS, Mutasingwa DR. The scope of naturopathic medicine in Canada: an emerging profession. *Soc Sci Med* 2006;63:409-17.
136. Goodman H. Osteopathy. In: Jonas WB, Levin JS, eds. *Essentials of complementary and alternative medicine*. Philadelphia: Lippincott Williams & Wilkins; 1999. p. 289-303.
137. Oh B, Butow P, Mullan B et al. Impact of medical Qigong on quality of life, fatigue, mood and inflammation in cancer patients: a randomized controlled trial. *Ann Oncol* 2010;21:608-14.
138. National Center for Complementary and Integrative Health. *Reiki: in depth*. Bethesda: NCCIH, National Institutes of Health. Available from: nccih.nih.gov/health/reiki/introduction.htm. Accessed April 21, 2016.
139. Field T. Massage therapy. In: Jonas WB, Levin JS, eds. *Essentials of complementary and alternative medicine*. Philadelphia: Lippincott Williams & Wilkins; 1999. p. 383-91.
140. Hochberg MC, Altman RD, April KT et al. American College of Rheumatology 2012 recommendations for the use of nonpharmacologic and pharmacologic therapies in osteoarthritis of the hand, hip, and knee. *Arthr Care Res* 2012;64:465-74.
141. Tousignant M, Corriveau H, Roy PM et al. The effect of supervised Tai Chi intervention compared to a physiotherapy program on fall-related clinical outcomes: a randomized clinical trial. *Disabil Rehabil* 2012;34:196-201.
142. Li F, Harmer P, Fitzgerald K et al. Tai chi and postural stability in patients with Parkinson's disease. *N Engl J Med* 2012;366:511-9.
143. Rosa L, Rosa E, Sarner L et al. A close look at therapeutic touch. In: Fontanarosa PB, ed. *Alternative medicine: an objective assessment*. Chicago: American Medical Association; 2000. p. 202-11.
144. Lao L. Traditional Chinese medicine. In: Jonas WB, Levin JS, eds. *Essentials of complementary and alternative medicine*. Philadelphia: Lippincott Williams & Wilkins; 1999. p. 216-32.
145. World Health Organization. *Traditional medicine: definitions*. Available from: www.who.int/medicines/areas/traditional/definitions/en/. Accessed April 21, 2016.
146. National Center for Complementary and Integrative Health. *Yoga for health*. Bethesda: NCCIH, National Institutes of Health. Available from: nccih.nih.gov/health/yoga/introduction.htm. Accessed April 21, 2016.

147. Ravindran AV, Lam RW, Filteau MJ et al. Canadian Network for Mood and Anxiety Treatments (CANMAT) clinical guidelines for the management of major depressive disorder in adults. V. Complementary and alternative medicine treatments. *J Affect Disord* 2009;117:S54-64.
148. Büssing A, Osterman T. Lüdtke R et al. Effects of yoga interventions on pain and pain-associated disability: a meta-analysis. *J Pain* 2012;13:1-9.

Appendix II
Home Testing

Marie Berry, BScPharm, BA, LLB

Home diagnostic devices are used for early diagnosis, to determine whether a certain therapy is effective, to monitor a medical condition, and for screening. Their advantages include confidentiality, convenience, relatively immediate results and an increased understanding of a condition. Considered by some to be the "ultimate house call",[1] home diagnostic devices are meant to augment appropriate medical care. Home testing involves individuals in their health. Advances in technology have increased ease of use and accuracy.

Home testing does not replace appropriate medical care and professional counselling, and there are potential pitfalls. The privacy afforded by home testing can contribute to misinformation, avoidance of treatment and even misdiagnosis, all of which may adversely affect health. Some home diagnostic devices may be inaccurate or inconsistent or test for conditions that may not be appropriate for home testing, e.g., metabolic hormone tests.

This chapter addresses home tests for blood pressure, cholesterol, menopause, drug detection, alcohol use, blood coagulation, celiac disease and urine, and some miscellaneous tests. Two commonly used home testing measures (blood glucose devices and pregnancy/fertility tests) are discussed in Chapter 26: Diabetes Care Devices and Chapter 80: Pregnancy and Fertility Testing.

Blood Pressure

For comparative features of nonprescription products, consult the *Compendium of Products for Minor Ailments*—Home Testing Products: Electronic Blood Pressure Monitors.

Hypertension is asymptomatic, but is a leading risk factor for morbidity and mortality.[2] It is estimated that 1 in 5 Canadian adults have hypertension. One-third of those with hypertension have uncontrolled blood pressure and one-fifth are unaware that they have hypertension. Of those patients who are aware of their hypertension only 64% are adequately treated (BP<140/90) with medication.[3]

Home blood pressure monitoring enables an individual to evaluate whether a new drug or treatment is working, to chart their course (which may act as motivation for adherence), and to identify "white coat" hypertension. The Canadian Hypertension Education Program (CHEP) Guidelines suggest that the use of home blood pressure monitoring on a regular basis should be considered in people with diabetes, suspected nonadherence, demonstrated white-coat effect, and blood pressure controlled in the office but not at home (masked hypertension).[4]

Home blood pressure monitoring should never be considered for self-diagnosis of hypertension. If the blood pressure is elevated with home blood pressure readings, medical advice should be sought for a definitive diagnosis of hypertension.[5]

Electronic Blood Pressure Monitors

Electronic blood pressure monitors are oscillometric, i.e., they measure blood pressure by analyzing small changes in cuff pressure.[6,7] The pressure in the inflated cuff changes as blood moves through expanding and contracting blood vessels. Most electronic monitors have a liquid crystal diode display which makes reading the blood pressure numbers easy. Pulse readings are often provided along with blood pressure readings. Accuracy can be a problem with electronic models. If the reading is consistently too high or too low, it may still be used to evaluate trends, but if the monitor reads too high one time and too low the next, readings have no value. Once purchased, electronic models should be compared in accuracy with blood pressure readings done by a healthcare practitioner. This comparison should be repeated periodically. Both the British Hypertension Society and the Association for the Advancement of Medical Instrumentation have formulated validation standards that indicate whether a particular model is accurate.[8] The Canadian Hypertension Society endorses electronic models that meet the validation standards of these organizations. A heart with a check mark logo appears on the endorsed models.[9]

The proper technique for using blood pressure monitors is important, and should be checked from time to time to ensure no bad habits have developed.[5,10,11] The blood pressure reading should be taken under the same circumstances and at approximately the same time of day. Blood pressure changes with daily cycles, and is typically the lowest during sleep. Activities that can raise blood pressure include public speaking (10 mm Hg), strenuous exercise (60–70 mm Hg), sexual activity (up to 100 mm Hg in men and 80 mm Hg in women) and competitive video gaming (20 mm Hg).[12,13]

Principles of accurate blood pressure measurement include:

- Patient should not exercise within the preceeding 30 minutes
- Ensure the right cuff size is chosen. Cuff size is based on the measurement of the upper arm. For people with thin arms less than 23 cm, there are small cuffs. An adult cuff ranges from 23–33 cm; a large from 33–43 cm. There are also cuff sizes for children
- Cigarettes, caffeine and decongestant medications should be avoided for about an hour before the blood pressure measurement is taken
- Sitting in a chair in a warm, calm environment with both feet on the floor, ankles not crossed, is recommended. The arm in which the blood pressure is to be measured should rest on a firm surface such as a table, palm up, and at the level of the heart. Bulky clothing can interfere with the reading and should be removed. Cuff is placed mid-arm, at heart level, with the bottom of the cuff 3 cm from the fold of the elbow
- The bladder and bowels should be emptied prior to the reading
- Talking while measuring blood pressure will affect the reading
- It is recommended that 2 or 3 readings be taken at one time, resting for about 5 minutes between each reading. The readings can be compared and averaged. Keeping a log of blood pressure readings will reflect what is normal for an individual and the effect of various activities or medications on blood pressure readings.

Electronic models that work on the wrist or finger have been developed; however, their use should be discouraged as they are not as accurate as devices that work on the upper arm.[4] Table 1 provides blood pressure targets for selected patients being treated for hypertension.

Cholesterol

For comparative features of nonprescription products, consult the *Compendium of Products for Minor Ailments*—Home Testing Products: Cholesterol Test Kits.

Elevated cholesterol levels increase the risk of coronary heart disease and stroke. It is estimated that 40% of Canadians have high cholesterol. In-office screening of high-risk individuals and lowering cholesterol levels with diet or medication reduce mortality and morbidity.[15,16]

Cholesterol home tests screen only for elevated total cholesterol; it should be noted that the 2012 Canadian Cardiovascular Society guidelines for diagnosis and treatment of dyslipidemia do not include cholesterol home tests as a method of screening.[15] These tests use an optical reader to determine total cholesterol in a blood sample. A drop of blood is drawn using a lancet and placed on a test strip. Most test strips do not require wiping, but rather use capillary action to move the blood sample to the optical reader.

Table 1: **Blood Pressure Targets in Treated Patients**[14]

Setting	Target SBP/DBP (mm Hg)
Home[a]	<135/85
Office	
General patient population (including those with chronic kidney disease)	<140/90
Isolated systolic hypertension	Age ≤80 y: SBP<140
	Age >80 y: SBP <150
Diabetes	<130/80

[a] Measured by a validated home blood pressure monitor.

Abbreviations: DBP = diastolic blood pressure; SBP = systolic blood pressure

The test strip is impregnated with a reagent that reacts with cholesterol in the blood sample to produce a colour change. The optical reader uses light absorption to determine the degree of colour change, and thus the cholesterol content of the sample. The results are expressed digitally on a liquid crystal diode display.

Test results take 3–15 minutes, depending upon the device, and represent total cholesterol. Home tests do not distinguish among low-density lipoproteins (LDL), high-density lipoproteins (HDL) and triglycerides. To obtain a breakdown of the cholesterol fractions a laboratory procedure is required.

A record of results may be useful for observing trends in an individual's cholesterol over time and under various conditions. This may provide an impetus for healthy lifestyle choices.

Menopause

For comparative features of nonprescription products, consult the *Compendium of Products for Minor Ailments*—Home Testing Products: Menopause Test Kits.

Home diagnostic tests for menopause look for a constantly high level of follicle-stimulating hormone (FSH). During a normal menstrual cycle FSH levels vary, rising as an ovum matures in the ovaries and falling after the release of the ovum at midcycle. With decreasing ovarian function closer to menopause, the body produces less estrogen, causing FSH levels to remain constantly high. However, the Canadian Consensus Conference on Menopause, 2006 indicates that the measurement of FSH alone is not indicative of menopause.[17]

The test is an immunochromatographic one-step test that uses enzyme-linked-immunosorbent serologic assay (ELISA) to detect FSH in urine. A positive result is indicated by a colour change, and 2 positive tests taken a week apart indicate a constantly high level of FSH consistent with menopause. Therefore, if the first test is positive, it should be repeated 1 week later.

A control is built into the test to ensure the test itself is working; however, damaged or expired test material should not be used. The test should be performed using the first urine of the morning because it has the highest concentration of FSH. This also ensures the 2 tests are performed at about the same time each day, minimizing the effect of diurnal variation.

Oral contraceptives and hormone supplements can cause false-negative results by decreasing levels of FSH. During pregnancy FSH levels are elevated, and an undetected pregnancy will result in a false-positive result, as will ovarian or pituitary tumors, which increase FSH levels. Many incorrect results are due to human error—damaging the absorbent end of the test wand, using too small or too large a urine sample, turning the wand upside down after sampling, reading the results too early or too late.

Home tests alone are not diagnostic of menopause, and other criteria such as cessation of menstrual periods need to be considered.[18] Menopause home tests do not indicate the presence or absence of fertility, and should never be the basis of a contraceptive decision. Menopause occurs over months and years, thus menopause home test kits are limited in that they capture FSH levels only in a general quantitative way at a specific time.

Multiple Drug Detection

Some drugs are abused, are potentially addictive, can impair cognitive functioning and/or are the subject of workplace drug screening. These drugs can result in health complications and self-harm. Of special concern are marijuana, phencyclidine (PCP), methamphetamine, cocaine and opiates such as heroin.[19,20,21]

Home drug detection kits are urine tests that use ELISA technology. Drugs can be detected for 3–30 days after use, depending upon the drug and its usage. Other drug detection kits use hair or saliva samples which usually require mailing to a testing laboratory, sometimes located in the United States.

- **Marijuana** can be detected up to 2–8 days after last use; however, with chronic use it can be detected up to 20–30 days after last use. False-positive results have been associated with hemp-containing foods (usually labelled as such), NSAIDs (ibuprofen and naproxen) and the proton pump inhibitor omeprazole. It is not clear whether other members of these drug classes have the same effect. Second-hand marijuana smoke does not usually cause false-positive results.[22]
- **Phencyclidine** can be detected up to 3–7 days after the last dose, and 14–30 days after the last dose with chronic use. Dextroamphetamine, diphenhydramine and ketamine can cause false-positive results.[22]
- **Methamphetamine** can be detected 3–4 days after the last dose, and numerous drugs are associated with false-positive results: amantadine, amphetamine, bupropion, chlorpromazine, desipramine, dextroamphetamine, ephedrine, labetalol, methylamphetamine or ecstasy, pseudoephedrine, phenylephrine, selegiline and trazodone.[22]
- **Cocaine** can be detected up to 8 days after the last dose. Topical anesthetics and coca leaf teas can cause false-positives.[22]
- **Opiates** can be detected up to 4 days after the last dose, depending upon the compound ingested. Dextromethorphan, poppy seeds, quinine, quinolone antibiotics and rifampin can cause false-positive results.[23,24]

Adding products like bleach, alum, oxidizing agents and goldenseal will result in a negative test; however, the test will detect that the urine has been tampered with.[25,26]

Alcohol

Alcohol use and intoxication can cause loss of alertness, impairment of judgment, coma and death. It is implicated in automobile accidents and birth defects. After consumption, alcohol is excreted through the liver and kidneys with 1–5% excreted by evaporation through the breath.

Urine and blood laboratory tests are able to determine alcohol levels; however, home tests measure alcohol found in the breath. The breath is exhaled onto a test substrate housed in a tube. A colour change indicates the presence of alcohol, but often not the quantity of alcohol. Some home tests are intended to be carried on a key chain to be used prior to using a car key.

Breathalyzer tests used by law enforcement agencies also measure alcohol in the breath. These tests utilize an infrared spectroscopic analysis which extrapolates the amount of alcohol detected to a blood alcohol level. Alcohol vapour captured in a chamber will absorb a certain wave frequency when light is beamed through it. The more alcohol present, the more light is absorbed (and thus prevented from reaching a receptor). A computer chip translates the receptor information into a blood alcohol level. Breathalyzers used by law enforcement agencies are accurate and can be expensive. Various less-expensive home versions are available using the same technology,[27] but accuracy may vary from product to product.

Blood Coagulation

For comparative features of nonprescription products, consult the *Compendium of Products for Minor Ailments*—Home Testing Products: Blood Coagulation Monitors.

Home blood coagulation monitors measure prothrombin time (PT) and calculate the International Normalized Ratio (INR).[28] Individuals use home blood coagulation tests in conjunction with a coagulation clinic and/or laboratory testing in order to adjust their own anticoagulant dosage. The variability of INR results has been reported to be 15%;[29] however, this is similar to the variability in laboratory-obtained results.

These monitors use a whole blood sample applied to a cartridge, where it is drawn by capillary action into a channel coated with dried thromboplastin. When the thromboplastin has been rehydrated by the blood sample, coagulation begins. The mixture will continue to move along the channel until a blood clot forms. A laser photometer detects cessation of flow as a change in light scattering, resulting in a PT measurement that is then used to calculate the INR. Results take about 2 minutes. With INR readings above the therapeutic range, home monitors appear to be less accurate. Home monitoring is not recommended in patients with antiphospholipid syndrome, but may be less invasive and better accepted than laboratory procedures in children requiring anticoagulation.

Individuals using home blood coagulation monitors require training, the ongoing support of a coagulation centre and education on using dosage adjustment guidelines. Record keeping is paramount as is continuing evaluation of correct technique and accuracy of the monitor. If individuals are considering home coagulation monitoring, it is important that they work with either their family physician and/or coagulation clinic as well as their pharmacist. The cost of the monitor and testing supplies may limit their use. Some private insurance plans may cover associated costs.[29]

Celiac Disease

For comparative features of nonprescription products, consult the *Compendium of Products for Minor Ailments*—Home Testing Products: Celiac Disease Test Kits.

Celiac disease occurs largely in Caucasians of Northern European ancestry and is an autoimmune disease. Estimated prevalence is 1 in 100 North Americans. With exposure to gliadin and related gluten proteins found in grains such as wheat, barley and rye, the intestinal enzyme transglutaminase modifies the gluten proteins which in turn trigger the body's immune response. The result is damage to the epithelia and villi of the small intestine, causing the associated symptoms, such as diarrhea, flatulence, weight loss and weakness.

Although present even in childhood, celiac disease may not manifest until the fourth decade of life or even later. There is a familial tendency and with a diagnosis of celiac disease, it is usually recommended that family members are also tested. Biopsy of the small intestine, genetic testing for a specific HLA-DQ2 gene (which the vast majority of affected people have) and serological testing for specific IgA antibodies to transglutaminase are used to diagnose the disease.

A home self-test using ELISA technology is available for detection of the antibody to transglutaminase. The test uses a blood sample and includes a control; however, data on the accuracy of these tests are limited, and they cannot be used to confirm or exclude a diagnosis of celiac disease. Patients with symptoms of celiac disease should consult an appropriate healthcare practitioner for a definitive diagnosis and to address potential complications including other related immune diseases. A gluten-free diet is the recommended treatment for celiac disease (see Chapter 41: Special Diets).[30]

Dip-and-read Urine Tests

For comparative features of nonprescription products, consult the *Compendium of Products for Minor Ailments*—Home Testing Products: Urine Glucose and Ketone Test Kits.

Dip-and-read urine tests are used for a variety of conditions such as pregnancy and fertility (see Chapter 80: Pregnancy and Fertility Testing); however, these home diagnostic tests are also used to test for pH, proteins, glucose, ketones and other substances.[31]

Dip-and-read urine tests for protein usually detect albumin, but may not detect other proteins. False-positive results may be caused by excessive exercise, cold exposure, pregnancy, fever, urinary tract infections, diabetes, and even changes in posture. If a dip-and-read urine test is positive for protein, medical attention should be sought since there are numerous potential causes including kidney disease, heart disease, certain types of cancer, rheumatoid arthritis and lupus.[32]

Glucose dip-and-read urine tests were used to monitor control of diabetes; however, these have been replaced by blood glucose monitors. Ketones are the result of the breakdown of fat and are detected in poorly controlled diabetes and in some diets, e.g., the Atkins diet.[33]

Urine is usually acidic, with a pH ranging from 4.5–5. Ingestion of proteins or acidic foods can increase the acidity of urine, and dip-and-read pH tests are used to confirm high-dietary protein intake in patients on high-protein diets. Kidney disease, urinary tract infections and vomiting are associated with elevated urinary pH; diabetic ketoacidosis, diarrhea and starvation lead to lower urinary pH.

Dip-and-read urine tests are considered semiquantitative in that the test colour is compared with a colour chart which represents a range of values.

With dip-and-read urine tests, technique is important:

- Collect urine in a clean sample bottle
- Wash hands before collecting the sample and clean the genital area
- Collect a midstream sample—begin urinating into the toilet, pause, then urinate into the sample bottle until a sufficient sample is obtained, and if needed finish urinating into the toilet
- Completely immerse the test area of the dip-and-read urine test in the collected sample
- Shake off any excess urine and read the test according to the directions
- If the urine sample is not being used immediately, it should be stored in the refrigerator and allowed to warm to room temperature prior to testing.[34]

Fecal Occult Blood Testing

Diagnostic tests for fecal occult blood are not available without a requisition from a qualified healthcare practitioner. They are often ordered for people at risk of colorectal cancer: over age 50, personal history of inflammatory bowel disease, polyps or colorectal cancer, or family history of colorectal cancer. Colorectal cancer is the third most common cause of cancer in Canada with a mortality rate as high as 60%. Early detection is vital to improved survival, and proper use of these tests is essential.

Since patients may perform these tests at home, the following information may be helpful:[35,36,37]

- A blood loss of 0.5–0.75 mL causes the stool to appear dark red or black and tarry; these tests detect even smaller or occult amounts
- Fecal occult blood testing can differentiate between blood and other substances causing stool discolouration, such as dietary intake of beets
- Increased dietary fibre is recommended, to encourage any lesions to bleed and improve accuracy of the test
- Some foods may interfere with the test and are to be avoided for 48–72 hours prior to testing: artichokes, broccoli, cantaloupe, grapefruit, horseradish, melons, mushrooms, parsnips, radishes, red or rare meat, turnips, vitamin C enriched foods
- Some drugs can cause inaccurate results: colchicine, corticosteroids, iron, NSAIDs including ASA, reserpine, warfarin; medical recommendations are usually required regarding these drugs prior to testing
- Some physical conditions can affect test results: anal fissures, bleeding gums, diarrhea, diverticulitis, hemorrhoids, menstruation, nosebleed, peptic ulcer disease, proctitis and ulcerative colitis. Testing may need to be postponed until these conditions are managed
- Stool samples are retrieved from the toilet bowl, thus the toilet bowl must be free of chemicals such as toilet bowl cleaners, disinfectants and deodorizers
- Since cancerous lesions may bleed intermittently, 3 consecutive stool samples are usually recommended to minimize the chance of a false-negative.

Examples of Other Home Diagnostic Tests

Although numerous home diagnostic devices are advertised extensively and available via the Internet (see Table 2), many more sensitive and specific tests are available through healthcare practitioners at little or no cost (e.g., a laboratory "cholesterol test" measures a complete lipid panel at no expense to the patient).

Before purchase of a home diagnostic test, the following should be considered:

- The diagnosis or measurement should be relevant to overall health, e.g., the pH of urine may have no affect on health
- The measurement should provide useful information, e.g., elevated FSH levels are not diagnostic of menopause; elevated PSA levels are not diagnostic of prostate cancer
- The testing kit should be appropriate for home use, e.g., home cholesterol tests may be misinterpreted
- Bogus, contaminated, and counterfeit home diagnostic devices do exist and should be avoided. Healthcare practitioners, the Consumers Union and Health Canada provide information about home testing and recalls of kits
- Some home diagnostic tests are performed entirely at home; others are collection kits with collected samples mailed to a testing laboratory, sometimes located in the United States. Attention should be paid to the location of the testing laboratory, because collected samples may degrade in transit. Confidentiality should be assured for any collected samples sent to a testing laboratory
- A good understanding of how to interpret or act on the results of a home diagnostic test is essential for safe use

- Home diagnostic tests that could be potentially dangerous should be avoided, e.g., allergy testing, in which a potential allergen is used
- Simpler, more straightforward alternatives may be available, e.g., using plastic wrap for skin cancer test kits rather than the transparent sheet that is provided in the kit (see Table 2)
- Home testing for infections should always be performed in conjunction with appropriate medical attention.[38]

With time, technological changes may make some of these home tests more viable.

An evolving area of home testing is the use of apps for computers and mobile phones. Mental health assessments, diabetes monitoring, exercise activity, weight loss and food intake are some examples. As with all home tests, these home testing apps do not replace care provided by healthcare practitioners.

Table 2: **Additional Home Diagnostic Tests**

Home Diagnostic Test	Mechanism	Comments[a]
Allergy testing[39]	Uses a challenge with a substance that could potentially cause an allergy.	Allergy testing needs to be performed with medical supervision in the event that an allergic reaction results.
Alzheimer's disease[40,41]	Uses a scent challenge with various odours; in some cases changes in smell sensation is indicative of Alzheimer's disease.	Other causes of changes in smell sensation can cause false-positives, e.g., nasal congestion; a subjective test; an alternative is the Mini Mental Test.
Helicobacter pylori[42]	A test for the gram-negative bacterium responsible for peptic ulcer disease; an immunochromatographic assay for antibodies to the bacteria using a blood sample and ELISA technology.	Fails to identify whether the infection is current since antibodies may persist for 6 or more months; false-negatives occur when antibody levels are low.
Hepatitis[43]	A test for antibodies to the virus; different assays are able to identify different viruses, e.g., A, B, C.	Uses a blood sample; must be mailed to a testing laboratory, usually located in the United States.
Human immunodeficiency virus[44,45,46]	A test for the antibodies to the virus using ELISA technology; with early detection, precautions can be taken to prevent transmission of the infection.	Uses a blood sample; false-negatives result with testing too early or too late—antibodies take 2–8 wk to develop and in late disease antibody production is low; false-positives occur in multiparous women, those with autoimmune diseases, recently vaccinated people and those with a history of multiple blood transfusions. A 2009 Health Canada Advisory warned against using these tests—see www.healthycanadians.gc.ca/recall-alert-rappel-avis/hc-sc/2009/13392a-eng.php.
Influenza[47]	A nasal swab used in a 3-step procedure to detect antigens to influenza A and B.	Appropriate medical consultation is preferred.
Male fertility[48,49]	A test for quality and quantity of sperm.	Uses a reagent to stain the sperm in the sample; resulting colour is compared with a quantitative colour chart.
	A test for DHEA and/or testosterone.	Uses a saliva sample.
Metabolic hormones, e.g., **cortisol**, **thyroid**[50]	A test for 1 or more metabolic hormones depending upon the testing capacity of the kit purchased.	Uses a saliva sample.

(cont'd)

Table 2: **Additional Home Diagnostic Tests** *(cont'd)*

Home Diagnostic Test	Mechanism	Comments[a]
Prostate cancer[51,52]	A test for prostate specific antigen (PSA) which is elevated in prostate cancer.	Uses a blood sample for in-home detection; benign prostate hyperplasia, prostatitis, autoimmune disease or sexual activity within 48 h of testing may produce false-positives; some rapidly growing tumors do not elevate PSA levels.
Skin cancer[53]	A test for changes in appearance of skin growths.	Uses a transparent sheet that is placed on the skin and any growths are traced; changes over time are noted.
Streptococcal infections[54]	A throat swab is tested using ELISA technology for bacterial antigens. Throat and ear examination kits with fully illustrated guide books.	Both are difficult to use with uncooperative children.
Tobacco use[55]	A test for nicotine or cotinine, a nicotine metabolite; cotinine can be detected up to 4 days after tobacco has been used.	Uses a saliva or urine sample for in-home testing; testing of a hair sample provides results of up to 90 days after tobacco has been used; however, the hair sample must be mailed to a testing laboratory, usually located in the United States.
Urinary tract infections[56]	A urine dip test for nitrites produced by gram-negative bacteria from nitrates, or for leukocyte esterase, indicating the presence of leukocytes in the urine.	False-negative results may be caused by vegetarian diets, tetracycline, high intake of vitamin C.
Vaginal infections[57]	A test strip worn as a "panty liner" which detects the pH of vaginal secretions by a colour change.	Normal pH of vaginal secretions is 4–4.5; bacterial and trichomonas infections raise the pH to 5–6: inaccurate results occur with sweating, during menstruation, less than 1 day before or 5 days after a menstrual period, within 48 h of intercourse or douching, with menopause and within 72 h of applying a vaginal product such as a contraceptive cream.

[a] Availability of these tests may vary: most are not available for direct purchase in Canada and must be obtained and/or analyzed via laboratories in the United States.

Potential Home Diagnostic Testing Problems

Many home tests focus on health conditions that are represented by national health organizations, e.g., the Canadian Diabetes Association. These organizations may have information and/or guidelines regarding the test, including the accuracy and appropriateness of use. Human error is the primary reason for failure or erroneous results when home testing.

Care in preparing, administering and interpreting the results is needed:

- Note the accuracy of the test as well as the substance for which the test is designed (e.g., cholesterol tests measure only total cholesterol and do not provide a lipid profile)
- Read all directions and identify all test components prior to testing
- Check the kit expiry date; do not use an expired test kit
- A clean, undisturbed, well-lit area is ideal for testing; test surfaces should not be touched, and hands should be washed prior to testing to reduce potential contamination
- If the test equipment or monitor uses batteries, make sure they are charged
- Directions for sample collection, including the best time of day for collection, should be followed carefully and any timing should be done accurately with a timer, watch or clock with a minute hand

- If the test uses a control and it fails, results are invalid and should not be used
- Interpretation of the results is essential; e.g., the meaning of a positive or negative result, and when to seek medical attention
- The calibration of monitors should be checked on a routine basis
- If testing is ongoing (e.g., blood pressure), keep a log or diary
- If the subject resists the test procedure (e.g., taking a blood or urine sample or throat swab) the sample may not be adequate and the result inaccurate
- The required manual dexterity and eyesight is also essential
- Human error can occur at each step of a test; tests with fewer steps have less potential for human error
- Many manufacturers have toll-free telephone numbers and websites that are useful resources
- Home diagnostic tests offered via the Internet may not be recognized as accurate, may not be approved for use in Canada, or may require sending a sample to a central laboratory in a manner that degrades the sample.

References

1. Lewis C. Home diagnostic tests: the ultimate house call? *FDA Consum* 2001;35:18-22.
2. Bromfield S, Muntner P. High blood pressure: the leading global burden of disease risk factor and the need for worldwide prevention programs. *Curr Hypertens Rep* 2013;15:134-6.
3. Statistics Canada. *Blood pressure of Canadian adults, 2009 to 2011*. Available from: www.statcan.gc.ca/pub/82-625-x/2012001/article/11714-eng.htm. Accessed October 29, 2015.
4. Canadian Hypertension Education Program (CHEP). Hypertension Canada. *2015 CHEP recommendations for the management of hypertension. Diagnosis & Assessment*. Available from: guidelines.hypertension.ca/diagnosis-assessment/.
5. Chan AH, Campbell NR, Lewanczuk RZ et al. 2008 Canadian Hypertension Education Program guidelines for the management of hypertension by pharmacists. *Can Pharm J (Ott)* 2008;141:327-31.
6. van Egmond J, Lenders JW, Weernick E et al. Accuracy and reproducibility of 30 devices for self-measurement of arterial blood pressure. *Am J Hypertens* 1993;6:873-9.
7. Rotch AL, Dean JO, Kendrach MG et al. Blood pressure monitoring with home monitors versus mercury sphygmomanometer. *Ann Pharmacother* 2001;35:817-22.
8. Bultemeier NC, White JR, Campbell RK. Home monitoring of blood pressure. *US Pharm* 2001;26:81-90.
9. Hypertension Canada. *Devices endorsed by Hypertension Canada*. Available from: hypertension.ca/en/devices-endorsed-by-hypertension-canada. Accessed October 29, 2015.
10. King DS et al. Educating patients on hypertension and blood pressure monitoring. *Drug Topics* 1998;142:1.
11. Hypertension Canada. *Measuring blood pressure the right way* [poster]. Available from: www.hypertension.ca/images/2013_EducationalResources/2013_MeasureBPPoster_EN_HCP1040.pdf. Accessed April 12, 2016.
12. National High Blood Pressure Education Program Working Group report on ambulatory blood pressure monitoring. *Arch Intern Med* 1990;150:2270-80.
13. Pickering TG, James GD, Boddie C et al. How common is white coat hypertension? *JAMA* 1988;259:225-8.
14. Canadian Hypertension Education Program (CHEP). Hypertension Canada. *2015 CHEP online guidelines*. Available from: guidelines.hypertension.ca. Accessed October 29, 2015.
15. Genest J, McPherson R, Frohlich J et al. 2009 Canadian Cardiovascular Society/Canadian guidelines for the diagnosis and treatment of dyslipidemia and prevention of cardiovascular disease in the adult–2009 recommendations. *Can J Cardiol* 2009;25:567-79.
16. Expert Panel on Detection, Evaluation, and Treatment of High Blood Cholesterol in Adults. Executive summary of The Third Report of The National Cholesterol Education Program (NCEP) Expert Panel on Detection, Evaluation, And Treatment of High Blood Cholesterol in Adults (Adult Treatment Panel III). *JAMA* 2001;285:2486-97.
17. Belisle S, Blake J, Basson R et al. Canadian consensus conference on menopause, 2006 update. *J Obstet Gynaecol Can* 2006;28:S7-S94.
18. American Association of Clinical Endocrinologists. Medical guidelines for clinical practice management of menopause. *Endocr Pract* 1999;5:355-66.
19. Woelfel JA. Drug abuse urine tests: false-positive results. *Pharmacist's Letter/Prescriber's Letter* 2005;21:210314.
20. Tests for drugs of abuse. *Med Lett Drugs Ther* 2002;44:71-3.
21. Macdonald DI. Diagnosis and treatment of adolescent substance abuse. *Curr Probl Pediatr* 1989;19:389-94.
22. Colbert DL. Drug abuse screening with immunoassays: unexpected cross-reactivities and other pitfalls. *Br J Biomed Sci* 1994;51:136-46.
23. Daher R., Haidar JH, Al-Amin H. Rifampin interference with opiate immunoassays. *Clin Chem* 2002;48:203-4.
24. Selavka CM. Poppy seed ingestion as a contributing factor to opiate-positive urinalysis results: the Pacific perspective. *J Forensic Sci* 1991;36:685-96.
25. Eskridge KD, Guthrie SK. Clinical issues associated with urine testing of substances of abuse. *Pharmacotherapy* 1997;17:497-510.
26. Floren AE. Urine drug testing and the family physician. *Am Fam Physician* 1994;49:1441-7.
27. Rush BR, Powell LY, Crowe TG et al. Early intervention for alcohol use: family physicians' motivations and perceived barriers. *CMAJ* 1995;152:863-9.
28. Riley RS, Rowe D, Fisher LM. Clinical utilization of the international normalized ratio (INR). *J Clin Lab Anal* 2000;14:101-14.

29. Canadian Agency for Drugs and Technology. *Point-of-care testing of the International Normalized Ratio (INR) for patients taking warfarin or other vitamin K antagonists*. Available from www.cadth.ca/point-care-testing-international-normalized-ratio-inr-patient-taking-warfarin-or-other-vitamin-k. Accessed April 14, 2016.

30. Canadian Celiac Association. *Blood testing for celiac disease*. Available from: www.celiac.ca. Accessed October 29, 2015.

31. Arinzon Z, Peisakh A, Shuval I et al. Detection of urinary tract infection (UTI) in long-term care setting: is the multireagent strip an adequate diagnostic tool? *Arch Gerontol Geriatr* 2009;48:227-31.

32. Deville WL, Yzermans JC, van Duijn NP et al. The urine dipstick test useful to rule out infections. A meta-analysis of the accuracy. *BMC Urol* 2004;4:4.

33. Atkins Nutritionals. Denver, Colorado. Available from: www.atkins.com. Accessed October 29, 2015.

34. Cook JD, Strauss KA, Caplan YH et al. Urine pH: the effects of time and temperature after collection. *J Anal Toxicol* 2007;31:486-96.

35. Allison JE. Colon cancer screening guidelines 2005: the fecal occult blood test option has become a better FIT. *Gastroenterology* 2005;129:745-8.

36. Mandel JS, Bond JH, Church TR et al. Reducing mortality from colorectal cancer by screening for fecal occult blood. Minnesota Colon Cancer Control Study. *N Engl J Med* 1993;328:1365-71.

37. Finley RS, Lindley CM, LaCivita CL et al. Solid tumors. In: Young LY, Koda-Kimble MA, eds. *Applied therapeutics: the clinical use of drugs*. 6th ed. Vancouver: Applied Therapeutics; 1995. p. 93-1 to 93-30.

38. Terrie Y. At home diagnostic tests: a growing trend. *Pharmacy Times* 2009;3:10050. Available from: www.pharmacytimes.com. Accessed October 29, 2015.

39. U.S. National Library of Medicine; National Institutes of Health. MedlinePlus. *Allergy testing—skin*. Available from: www.nlm.nih.gov/medlineplus/ency/article/003519.htm. Accessed October 29, 2015.

40. Wilson RS, Schneider JA, Arnold SE et al. Olfactory identification and incidence of mild cognitive impairment in older age. *Arch Gen Psychiatry* 2007;64:802-8.

41. Bassuk SS, Murphy JM. Characteristics of the Modified Mini-Mental State Exam among elderly persons. *J Clin Epidemiol* 2003;56:622-8.

42. Veldhuyzen van Zanten SJ, Flook N, Chiba N et al. An evidence-based approach to the management of uninvestigated dyspepsia in the era of Helicobacter pylori. Canadian Dyspepsia Working Group. *CMAJ* 2000;162:S3-23.

43. U.S. Food and Drug Administration. *Vaccines, blood & biologics*. Available from: www.fda.gov/biologicsbloodvaccines/default.htm. Accessed October 29, 2015.

44. Hardy A. Rapid HIV home testing. *US Pharm* 2006;7:49052.

45. Wright AA, Katz IT. Home testing for HIV. *N Engl J Med* 2006;354:437-40.

46. Demeter LM, Reichman RC. Detection of human immunodeficiency virus infection. In: Mandell GL, Bennett JE, Dolin R, eds. *Mandell, Douglas, and Bennett's principles and practice of infectious diseases*. 5th ed. Philadelphia: Churchill Livingstone; 2000. p. 1369-74.

47. Rapid diagnostic tests for influenza. *Med Lett Drugs Ther* 1999;41:121-2.

48. Small DR, Collins JA, Wilson EH et al. Interpretation of semen analysis among infertile couples. *CMAJ* 1987;136:829-33.

49. Winters SJ. Current status of testosterone replacement therapy for men. *Arch Fam Med* 1999;8:257-63.

50. American Association of Clinical Endocrinologists. *My endocrine disorder*. Accessed August 31, 2009.

51. Pienta KJ, Esper PS. Risk factors for prostate cancer. *Ann Intern Med* 1993;118:793-803.

52. Prostate cancer. In: The Canadian Task Force on Preventive Health Care. *The Canadian Guide to clinical preventive health care*. 1994. Available from: canadiantaskforce.ca/files/guidelines/1994-red-brick-en.pdf. Accessed October 29, 2015.

53. National Cancer Institute. *Skin cancer screening—health professional version (PDQ)*. Available from: www.cancer.gov/types/skin/hp/skin-screening-pdq. Accessed October 29, 2015.

54. Strep throat. *US Pharm* 2007 Oct;11264. Available from: www.uspharmacist.com. Accessed October 29, 2015.

55. Okuyemi KS, Ahluwalia JS, Harris KJ. Pharmacotherapy of smoking cessation. *Arch Fam Med* 2000;9:270-81.

56. Panesar K. Urinalysis: a guide for pharmacists. *US Pharm* 2009 June. Available from: www.uspharmacist.com. Accessed October 29, 2015.

57. Fem-V: an at-home diagnostic test for vaginal infections. *Pharmacist's Letter/Prescriber's Letter* 2006;22:220503.

Appendix III
Information for the Traveller

Mark Kearney, BSc(Pharm), MSc

Today's travellers seem to be exposed to more risks than they ever have in the past. A number of factors, ranging from an aging population to global warming, have contributed to this situation. Ease of travel has contributed to the development of areas of the world that were once considered exotic and remote. While the presence of resorts at these destinations supports the comfort of the traveller, they can give the traveller a false sense of security with regard to the health risks that may be present. Canada has an aging population with the financial means and the desire to travel. However, they are more likely to be on treatment for chronic medical conditions and are less likely to receive optimal benefit from vaccinations, two factors that leave them at increased risk for travel-related illnesses.

Generally speaking, any traveller to a tropical destination or developing country should receive a pre-travel assessment from a healthcare practitioner certified in travel health. The assessment will identify current risks for the traveller based on their destination and the type of activities they are planning, and it will inform them of the required and recommended vaccines that can help them reduce their risks to diseases.

Information provided in this chapter focuses on nonprescription medications and healthcare advice to assist the patient in reducing their health risks. Patients may also need help to determine their pre-travel needs for vaccinations and other related prescription products. To assess their needs, key information will be required, including their destination, the type of activities they intend to do, an up-to-date vaccination history and a list of their current medications.

Online references can support travellers in making informed decisions about their travel health needs, including the need to seek a pre-travel assessment from a qualified healthcare practitioner. Those who frequently assist travellers seeking pre-travel information will find it beneficial to make themselves familiar with online references provided within this chapter.

Travel First Aid Kits

First aid kits designed for various types of travel can be purchased from camping equipment stores. Basic first aid kits can be purchased from the Canadian Red Cross or from Saint John Ambulance. Alternatively, first aid kits can be prepared by purchasing the necessary supplies from a pharmacy. The contents of these kits will vary depending on the destination and remoteness and type of travel. A partial list of medications and supplies that could be included in a first aid kit can be found in Table 1. Items for the first aid kit should be organized in a sealed plastic bag or a plastic box.

Medications

Analgesics: Acetaminophen is effective for the relief of mild to moderate pain and the reduction of fever (see Chapter 7: Fever). Ibuprofen or naproxen will effectively relieve pain and fever and help in controlling inflammation.

Antacids: An antacid (e.g., calcium carbonate, aluminum and magnesium hydroxide) is effective in the relief of indigestion and heartburn (see Chapter 31: Dyspepsia and GERD).

Antidiarrheals: Both loperamide and bismuth subsalicylate are effective in the management of mild travellers' diarrhea.[1] Bismuth subsalicylate can also be used as a preventive agent.[2] More severe symptoms (e.g., with cramps, bloody diarrhea or fever) require antibiotic therapy (see Chapter 30: Diarrhea).

Antihistamines: Antihistamines can be used to treat minor allergic reactions (see Chapter 22: Allergic Rhinitis and Chapter 55: Atopic, Contact, and Stasis Dermatitis). Certain antihistamines (e.g., dimenhydrinate) are useful to control symptoms associated with motion sickness[3] (see Chapter 36: Nausea and Vomiting).

Antiseptics: Clean water can be used to wash minor cuts or abrasions. If the risk of infection is high cleanse the area with hydrogen peroxide 3% or isopropyl alcohol 70% to prevent skin infections (see Chapter 68: Minor Cuts and Wounds).

Decongestants: Oral pseudoephedrine is useful in adults for relieving congested eustachian tubes during descent of an aircraft.[4] Topical decongestants are generally not useful for this purpose[4] (see Chapter 18: Complications Affecting the Ear: Ear Piercing, Foreign Bodies and Barotrauma).

Emergency contraception: Oral levonorgestrel is available without a prescription at pharmacies and can be used by female travellers to significantly reduce the risk of pregnancy in instances of contraceptive method failure (e.g., broken condom), unprotected consensual intercourse or in cases of sexual assault[5,6] (see Chapter 76: Contraception).

Insect repellents: Insect repellents containing DEET (N, N-diethyl-m-toluamide) or icaridin are effective against a variety of mosquitoes, ticks, fleas, chiggers and flies. Preparations containing soybean oil 2% and p-menthane 3,8 diol (PMD; oil of lemon eucalyptus) are also effective. See Personal Protection Against Vectors, below.

Laxatives: A laxative on its own or in combination with a stool softener (see Chapter 29: Constipation) may be helpful for constipation arising from factors associated with travel (e.g., dietary changes, dehydration).

Table 1: **Travel First Aid Kits**

Category	Items		
Medications	Analgesic	Decongestant	Oral rehydration salts
	Antacid	Emergency contraception	Sunscreen
	Antidiarrheal	Corticosteroid cream	Topical antibiotic cream/ ointment
	Antihistamine	Insect repellent	Topical antifungal cream
	Antiseptic agent	Laxative	Topical antipruritic lotion
First aid supplies	Adhesive bandages	Ice pack	Sterile gauze
	Adhesive tape	Safety pins	Thermometer
	Fine tweezers	Scissors	Moleskin
	Paper and pencil	Latex or vinyl gloves	Triangular bandages
	Matches and candle	Syringes and needles	

Oral rehydration salts: Oral rehydration salts prevent dehydration due to travellers' diarrhea (see Chapter 30: Diarrhea). Alternatively, sports drinks, diluted 1:1 with potable water offer an alternative means of rehydration.[7]

Corticosteroid creams: Hydrocortisone 0.5% or 1% cream is useful in various skin conditions such as mild dermatitis and pruritus. Hydrocortisone lotion is more effective in treating larger areas. Clobetasone 0.05% is slightly more potent than hydrocortisone and also available without a prescription for the treatment of similar conditions[8] (see Chapter 55: Atopic, Contact, and Stasis Dermatitis).

Sunscreens: Sunscreen with a SPF of 30 or greater and UVA blockers (e.g., mexoryl, parsol) helps prevent sunburn (see Chapter 72: Prevention and Treatment of Sun-induced Skin Damage).

Topical antibiotic creams or ointments: Topical antibiotic (e.g., polymyxin B/gramicidin/bacitracin) can be used on superficial wounds likely to become infected (see Chapter 68: Minor Cuts and Wounds).

Topical antifungal creams: Antifungal cream (e.g., clotrimazole, miconazole) can be used to treat topical *Candida* infections associated with heat and humidity[9] (see Chapter 65: Fungal Skin Infections).

Topical antipruritic lotions: Lotions containing local anesthetics and antipruritics provide temporary relief of itchiness associated with mild allergic reactions[10] (see Chapter 55: Atopic, Contact, and Stasis Dermatitis and Chapter 67: Insect Bites and Stings).

For comparative features or ingredients of nonprescription products, consult the *Compendium of Products for Minor Ailments*.

Jet Lag

Jet lag presents with symptoms of malaise, fatigue, disruption of sleep-wake cycles, irritability and impaired cognitive performance, which result from rapidly crossing multiple time zones and attempting to follow the time schedule at the new destination.[11] Typically, these symptoms are more severe when travelling eastward than westward.[11] This is because it is easier to adjust by extending the day rather than shortening it.[11,12,13] As a general rule, it takes 1 day to acclimatize for every hour of time difference at the new destination.

Nonpharmacologic methods of minimizing jet lag symptoms include:[11,12]

- If travelling for 2 days or less, follow the time schedule at the point of departure vs. the time schedule at the destination
- In cases of extended travel, adjust sleep and awakening times by 1 hour each day for several days prior to departure in an attempt to coincide with the time change at the final destination[13]
- Exposure to bright light in the early morning (5:00 a.m. to 11:00 a.m.) will advance the internal clock, and exposure in the evening (10:00 p.m. to 4:00 a.m.) will delay it. Eastward travellers should seek light in the morning and westward travellers should seek light in the evening[13,14]
- Plan to arrive at new destination in the early evening (destination time) when possible
- Anticipate the new time zone. Sleep on the plane if the arrival is in the morning and stay awake if arrival time is in the evening
- Be well rested prior to travel
- Stay well hydrated during the flight by drinking plenty of fluid; avoid in-flight alcohol and caffeine
- Exercise during the flight by stretching and walking; this is particularly helpful when the traveller wants to remain awake
- Exposure to outdoor daylight at the destination may help in resetting the circadian rhythm
- Remain active during daylight hours on arrival at the destination and adopt local mealtimes
- Plan on sleeping the same amount in a 24-hour period as when at home.

Endogenous **melatonin** is produced in the pineal gland.[11,15,16] It is normally secreted at nighttime, between the hours of 9:00 p.m. and 8:00 a.m. Melatonin acts on the internal clock governing circadian rhythms, such as sleeping and body temperature. When these rhythms are disrupted, as with jet lag, sleep disturbances can occur. Several studies show that exogenous melatonin is effective in alleviating the symptoms of jet lag at doses of 3–5 mg daily.[15] Timing of the administration appears to be important. Melatonin taken in advance of departure may actually worsen the symptoms of jet lag compared to melatonin taken nightly starting after arrival at the destination.[16] It may be more effective to take a lower dose (0.5 mg) of melatonin later in the night when crossing multiple time zones on westward trips so as to avoid overlap with endogenous secretion.[14] Dosage form also appears to be important. Sustained-release preparations seem to be less effective than immediate-release formulations.[15] In studies melatonin was effective when taken for 3–5 days after arrival,[15,16] but can be continued until symptoms of jet lag (e.g., daytime fatigue) subside.[17] Travellers should be aware that short-term use of melatonin can cause abdominal cramps, dizziness, drowsiness, headache, irritability, nightmares and transient depressive symptoms, but the incidence of these adverse reactions is low.[15]

High-altitude Illness

Travellers to destinations at altitudes above 2000 metres are at risk of altitude-induced illness.[18] This term encompasses acute mountain sickness (AMS), high-altitude cerebral edema (HACE) and high-altitude pulmonary edema (HAPE).[19] Symptoms of AMS typically occur within the first 48 hours after reaching a new altitude, especially with rapid ascent. The symptom of HACE and HAPE results from the extravascular movement of fluid in the brain and lungs. HACE is the end-stage of AMS and can be fatal. The progression to HACE from mild AMS ranges from 12 hours to 3 days. HAPE can occur without pre-existing AMS and accounts for most deaths from high-altitude illness.[19] Symptoms for each type of altitude illness are listed in Table 2.

While there are individual variations in susceptibility, the risk of illness increases directly with the rate of ascent, the altitude at which one sleeps and the altitude reached.[21] At altitudes between 2000 and 3500 metres, 9–34% will experience symptoms of AMS. Above 4000 metres, 42% will experience these symptoms.[18]

Gradual, step-wise ascent is the best method of prevention. Travellers should heed the following:

- Ascend slowly and avoid direct transport to altitudes above 3000 metres
- Spend 1 or 2 nights at 2500–3000 metres before going higher
- Above 3000 metres, sleeping altitude should not be increased by more than 300–400 metres per night with a rest day (a second night at the same altitude) for every 1000 metres of altitude gained[21]
- Plan day trips to higher elevation with a return to a lower sleeping altitude to accelerate acclimatization.[21]

Travellers should avoid alcohol, sedative-hypnotics and heavy exertion at high altitude.[21] In addition, prophylaxis with **acetazolamide** 125 mg po twice daily is indicated for rapid ascents (24 hours or less) to >3000 metres and rapid increases in sleeping altitude (e.g., 1000-metre increase in altitude within 24 hours). Acetazolamide 250 mg po twice daily can also treat AMS if started early enough after symptoms appear.[18] **Dexamethasone** 4 mg po twice daily for up to 10 days may be used to prevent symptoms, but does not improve acclimatization and should be used in combination with temporary descent so as to facilitate acclimatization.[18,21]

Treatment of AMS includes rest and acclimatization at the same altitude. This may take between 12 hours and 4 days. Simple analgesics, e.g., **ibuprofen** 200 mg po every 6 hours, may help treat headache. Descent of at least 500 metres is indicated if AMS is severe, if symptoms progress during acclimatization or if symptoms of HACE or HAPE occur.[21] For more information, see Suggested Readings.

Table 2: **Clinical Presentation of Variants of High-altitude Illness (Lake Louise Consensus)[20]**

Acute Mountain Sickness	High-altitude Cerebral Edema	High-altitude Pulmonary Edema
In the setting of a recent gain in altitude, the presence of headache and at least one of the following symptoms: ▪ gastrointestinal (anorexia, nausea or vomiting) ▪ fatigue or weakness ▪ dizziness or lightheadedness ▪ difficulty sleeping	In the setting of a recent gain in altitude, either: ▪ the presence of a change in mental status and/or ataxia in a person with AMS, or ▪ the presence of both mental status changes and ataxia in a person without AMS	In the setting of a recent gain in altitude, the presence of the following: Symptoms—at least 2 of: ▪ dyspnea at rest ▪ cough ▪ weakness or decreased exercise performance ▪ chest tightness or congestion Signs—at least 2 of: ▪ crackles or wheezing in at least 1 lung field ▪ central cyanosis ▪ tachypnea ▪ tachycardia

Abbreviations: AMS = acute mountain sickness

Heat and Cold-induced Illnesses

Heat Illnesses

Trips to warmer climates put travellers at risk for heat-induced illness, typically classified as heat exhaustion or heat stroke. Heat exhaustion occurs when the core body temperature rises to between 37°C and 40°C. Heat stroke occurs at core temperatures greater than 40°C, although elevated temperature is not required for diagnosis. It may take up to 10 days for the thermoregulatory system to fully adapt to increased demands placed on it by high temperatures and humidity.[22] See Chapter 9: Heat-related Disorders for a discussion of the signs and symptoms of various heat-related illnesses and their management.

Travellers can take steps to prevent heat-related illnesses including the following:

- Avoid long periods of strenuous physical activity during the first few weeks after arrival at a warm destination
- Maintain adequate hydration and electrolyte intake (see Fluid Requirements)
- Avoid alcohol.

Be especially cautious if taking medications that increase the risk of heat-related illnesses, such as amphetamines, anticholinergics, antiepileptics (e.g., topiramate), antipsychotics, beta-blockers, calcium channel blockers, diuretics, MAOIs and sympathomimetics.[23]

Cold Illnesses

Cold illnesses involve either changes in core body temperature (hypothermia) or localized cold-induced tissue injury (e.g., frostbite).

Hypothermia is defined as a core body temperature of less than 35°C. It can be further classified as mild (core body temperature >32°C and <35°C), moderate (core temperature 28–32°C) or severe (core temperature <28°C).

Frostbite is defined as tissue necrosis resulting from localized hypothermia of peripheral tissues.[24] More details can be found in Chapter 63: Frostbite.

Certain medical conditions (e.g., hypothyroidism, diabetes, peripheral neuropathy, autonomic neuropathy, peripheral vascular disease) and use of medications/substances (e.g., alcohol, antipsychotics, clonidine, meperidine, nicotine/tobacco, sedatives) predispose travellers to cold illnesses. Environmental factors such as wind and moisture can increase the risk of cold illnesses.[25]

In general, medical treatment should be sought immediately for cold-related illnesses as inappropriate rewarming can cause complications. For mild hypothermia, external rewarming (e.g., blankets) is usually sufficient if the affected person is able to generate heat through shivering. Moderate to severe hypothermia is considered a medical emergency.[25] For more information, see Suggested Readings.

Personal Protection Against Vectors

A vector is an organism that plays a role in the transmission of a pathogen between humans or from animal to human.[26] Vectors include fleas, tsetse flies, sand flies, ticks and certain freshwater snails. Mosquitoes are also important vectors. The *Anopheles* mosquito is responsible for transmission of malaria, and the *Aedes* mosquito transmits the dengue and chikungunya viruses. In addition, the *Aedes* mosquito transmits Zika virus, which is a developing concern for travellers. Consult recommended references (see Travel Health Information Resources) for appropriate precautions when travelling to areas where Zika may be present.

A traveller's risk of exposure to a vector depends on the destination, the type and location of accommodations, the duration of the visit and the type of travel planned.

Risk reduction measures include sleeping in well-screened or air-conditioned areas, sleeping under mosquito nets (preferably insecticide-treated), wearing clothing that provides good coverage (e.g., long sleeves, trousers, socks) and using insect repellents. In regions where schistosomiasis (transmitted by freshwater snails) is endemic, contact with freshwater (e.g., lakes, slow running streams) should be avoided.[27] When hiking in tick endemic areas, closed-toed footwear should be worn and pants should be tucked into socks. Additionally, hikers should check for burrowing ticks on the skin after each trek.[28,29]

Screens and mosquito nets should have a mesh size of 1.5 mm or less and should be checked regularly for holes. Mosquito nets impregnated with insecticides (e.g., permethrin) are significantly more effective in preventing malaria than nets without insecticide. Impregnated nets also deter entry by vectors smaller than the mesh size of the net (e.g., sandflies) and are safe for use by children and pregnant women. Permethrin-treated nets remain effective even after laundering. All mosquito nets should either reach the floor all around the bed or be tucked under the mattress. In areas with high pyrethroid resistance, there may be some benefit to combining treated nets with non-pyrethroid insecticide sprays.[30]

Insect Repellents

Repellents containing **diethyltoluamide** (DEET) offer prolonged protection against mosquitoes and other biting insects. **Icaridin** offers similar levels of protection.[31] Repellents containing 2% **soybean oil** are also effective for shorter durations of exposure (90–200 minutes).[32,33]

The duration of effect of insect repellents varies according to a number of factors, including the concentration of repellent and amount applied, temperature and, possibly, wind conditions.[28] It is decreased by sweating, washing and abrasion. Health Canada recommends using a repellent containing DEET or icaridin (picaridin).[31] Various concentrations of DEET and icaridin are available and these vary in their duration of effect.[31] Using a formulation containing more than 30% DEET is not recommended, since the duration of effect is not lengthened above this concentration but the risk of toxicity may be increased.[31] In children aged 6 months to 1 year, a product containing DEET 10% or less should be applied daily. DEET 10% can be applied 3 times a day in children aged 2–12 years.[31] In

Canada, DEET and icaridin products are not recommended for use in children under 6 months of age. In areas where malaria and other insect-borne diseases are endemic, the risk of severe disease outweighs any risk from properly applied products.[31] DEET has been shown to cross the placenta. However, although there are few formal studies, there is no evidence that the use of DEET by pregnant or breastfeeding women poses a health hazard to unborn babies or children who are breastfeeding.[34] See Chapter 67: Insect Bites and Stings for more information on available insect repellents.

Correct Application of Insect Repellents[28,31]

- Test for allergy before using a repellent for the first time by applying to a small patch of skin. Reactions are rare and have typically been reported to occur within 15–30 minutes of application with concentrations of DEET higher than those available on the Canadian market.[35,36]
- Apply sparingly to exposed skin, including the face, wrists, ankles and neck. To apply to the face, dispense repellent into the hands, rub the hands together, then apply to face, taking care to avoid the mouth, eyes and nose.
- Health Canada recommends that sunscreen be applied at least 20 minutes prior to the application of DEET-containing insect repellent if both are to be applied to the same area.[37]
- Wash hands after application to avoid inadvertent transfer of repellent to eyes, mouth and nose.
- Do not apply to broken or inflamed skin.
- Do not apply to children's hands or face.
- DEET may be applied to clothing made from cotton or wool. It may damage acetate, rayon, spandex, nylon and other synthetic materials. Do not apply DEET under clothes.

Malaria

Up to 30 000 travellers from industrialized countries contract malaria each year[38] and fatalities have been reported in North America in returning travellers. The Centers for Disease Control provides an excellent online resource to help travellers determine whether their itinerary includes areas where malaria is endemic (wwwnc.cdc.gov/travel/). Advise travellers to make an appointment at a travel clinic to discuss options for chemoprophylaxis, and to take precautions to prevent insect bites (see Personal Protection Against Vectors).

Uncomplicated malaria typically presents with “flu-like” symptoms (fever, chills, sweats, myalgia, and headache) that may recur at intervals of 48–72 hours. Gastrointestinal symptoms (nausea, vomiting) may also be present, but are more common in children versus adults. However, this cyclical pattern is rarely seen in the most severe form of malaria, caused by *P. falciparum*. Symptoms of severe *P. falciparum* malaria usually occur about 10–12 days after infection and include jaundice, impaired consciousness, prostration, abnormal bleeding and convulsions. Without prompt treatment, respiratory and renal failure, shock, coma and death can occur within 3–7 days. Symptoms caused by other malaria species may appear from 14 days to many months after infection and are typically not life-threatening. Travellers should be advised to seek immediate medical attention if a persistent or cyclical fever develops within a year after returning from a malaria risk area.[39]

Dengue Virus

Dengue virus has become a significant international health concern. The World Health Organization (WHO) estimates that 50–100 million infections, 500 000 dengue hemorrhagic fever cases and 22 000 deaths occur globally each year. Children are more likely to require hospitalization and are more likely to die from the disease than adults.[40] Dengue is the leading cause of systemic febrile illness and the second-most common cause of hospitalization among travellers returning from the Caribbean, South America, South Central Asia and Southeast Asia.[41] Local transmission of dengue virus has been reported in Southern Europe and the Mediterranean and the presence of dengue virus has been confirmed in 36 countries previously thought to be dengue-negative, including the state of Florida.[41,42] Dengue viruses are transmitted to humans through the bites of infective female *Aedes* mosquitoes or via exposure to dengue-infected blood.

Dengue fever (DF) is a severe, flu-like illness but seldom causes death. The incubation period is typically 4–7 days (range 3–14 days). Many travellers infected with dengue virus are asymptomatic. DF is defined clinically by an acute febrile illness with 2 or more of the following symptoms:[41]

- Headache
- Retro-orbital pain
- Muscle or joint pain
- Rash
- Hemorrhagic manifestation or leukopenia

The rash usually appears as the fever subsides, and lasts 2–4 days. The rash is either macular or maculopapular and generalized, often confluent with small patches of normal skin, and it may become scaly and itchy.

Approximately 1% of patients with DF develop dengue hemorrhagic fever (DHF) as the initial fever subsides (usually 3–7 days following onset). Sequential exposure to different strains of the dengue virus is believed to increase the risk of DHF.[43] Without treatment, the fatality rate of DHF is approximately 5%.[44] For more information, see Suggested Readings.

There is currently no vaccine or medication to protect against dengue. As the *Aedes* mosquito is most active during the daytime, precautions against insect bites should be taken during daylight hours whenever travelling to areas of risk for dengue fever (see Personal Protection Against Vectors).

Chikungunya Virus

Chikungunya is a viral disease spread through the bite of an infected *Aedes* mosquito. Symptoms of the disease typically begin within 3–12 days of exposure and can mimic dengue fever.

Symptoms include:

- Fever
- Headache
- Arthritis-like joint pain or swelling
- Rash

Chikungunya infection is usually not fatal, but joint pain may persist for months to years or cause chronic disability.

Until recently, chikungunya outbreaks have been confined to Africa, the Americas, Asia, the Pacific Islands and the Indian subcontinent. However, local transmission of the virus was reported for the first time in Southern Europe in 2007 and on the Caribbean island of Saint Martin in December 2013. Since 2013, local transmission of the virus has been reported on many other islands in the Caribbean, and in Central and South America, Mexico and Florida.[45] In the first half of 2015, over 10 000 cases of chikungunya were confirmed in South and Central America and the Caribbean.[46] In 2014, the Public Health Agency of Canada reported an increase in travel-related chikungunya cases reported in Canada.[47] For more information, see Suggested Readings.

There is no vaccine or medication to protect against chikungunya and no treatment. Precautions against insect bites should be taken during daylight hours whenever travelling to areas of risk for chikungunya (see Personal Protection Against Vectors).

Travelling with Medication

When travelling, all regularly used medications, as well as any emergency or intermittent-use items (e.g., asthma inhalers, nitroglycerin sprays, epinephrine injectors), should be packed in carry-on luggage. Travellers are advised to take extra amounts of each medication as well as a list of all medications (use the generic or chemical name) in case of emergency. Most pharmacies can prepare a list of current prescription medications, provided those medications were filled at the same pharmacy.

Medication should be stored in the original, labelled container to avoid problems at borders and to facilitate drug identification in case of emergency. Consider placing silica packs in medication vials if extended travel is planned in hot, humid environments.

Travellers who must bring syringes and needles to administer injectable medications (e.g., insulin, low molecular weight heparin) should carry a letter from their physician authorizing such possession, which should be presented at customs. When an itinerary includes significant changes in altitude (above 2000 metres), pressure in vials for injection must be equalized. To do this, insert the needle of an empty syringe (without the plunger) into the upright vial for several seconds. Then proceed with the usual withdrawal and injection procedures.[48]

Insulin is stable at room temperature for 30 days. Insulin that will not be used within that time period or any medication that requires refrigeration must be kept cool for the duration of travel. This can be accomplished using a cooler or a chilled thermos. The medication should then be refrigerated once the destination is reached.

All nonprescription liquid medications, creams or ointments must be purchased in volumes of 100 mL or less to be allowed through airport security in carry-on luggage, and must be placed in a clear, 1 L resealable plastic bag. This volume limit does not apply to prescription medications.

If tablets or capsules might experience rough handling (e.g., backpacking), blister packing may prevent breakage. Alternatively, placing cotton wool in the prescription vial may be helpful.

Before travelling, people who use controlled drugs or nonprescription codeine preparations should check with embassies or consulates of the destination country and any country through which the person will travel en route. Regulations vary, and what is legal in Canada may not be permitted in another country.

Travellers requiring oxygen therapy during air travel should contact the airline in advance.[12]

Most airlines will accommodate travellers with special diets if informed at least 24 hours in advance.

Venous Thromboembolism Prophylaxis

Long-distance travel is associated with a risk of venous thromboembolism (VTE) estimated at 0.1–4.8 cases per million travellers.[49] The incidence of VTE is highest in the first 2 weeks after travel, gradually decreasing to normal 8 weeks afterwards.[50]

The magnitude of this risk depends on a variety of factors:

- Type of travel: factors such as a hypobaric environment and decreased oxygen tension may put air travellers at greater risk of VTE than other forms of travel[51,52]
- Duration of travel: flights over 4 hours are associated with a two-fold increased risk of VTE while flights greater than 8 hours show the strongest association with VTE occurrence[50,53,54]
- Frequency of travel: frequent flying (multiple flights greater than 4 hours within an 8-week period) increases the risk for VTE[50]

- Pre-existing individual risk factors: previous VTE, cancer, pregnancy, advanced age, recent surgery, leg fractures and factor V Leiden or other genetic clotting disorders all increase risk for VTE[50,53,54]
- Medication use: use of oral contraceptive or estrogen-based hormone replacement therapy has been shown to increase the risk of VTE as could other medications that promote clotting (e.g., tranexamic acid)[49,50,53]
- Immobility during travel can increase the risk of VTE[51,54]
- Extremes of height and weight: travellers shorter than 162 cm or taller than 185 cm and travellers with a BMI >30 kg/m^2 are at increased risk of VTE.[50,53]

Seventy to 90% of travellers experiencing VTE have one or more of the pre-existing individual risk factors listed above.[49] Travellers at high risk of VTE (e.g., cancer, recent surgery, hypercoaguable disorder, obesity) should be assessed by a qualified healthcare practitioner. Recommendations to prevent VTE among high-risk travellers on long flights include:

- Maintain adequate hydration (avoiding alcohol will help)[54]
- Contract the muscles in the calves regularly or get up out of the seat often. Sit in an aisle seat if feasible[54]
- Wear below-knee graduated compression stockings, providing 15–30 mm Hg of pressure at the ankle.[54]

ASA does not appear to reduce the risk of travel-related VTE and is not recommended as prophylaxis in high-risk travellers.[55]

Travel Clinics

It is recommended that when travelling outside Canada or the United States, travellers should plan a pre-trip visit to their healthcare practitioner or a travel clinic at least 4–6 weeks before their trip. This is important, as there are specific vaccination requirements that vary depending on the planned destination. Travel clinics also provide other services such as assessment of malaria risk and need for expanded medical kits as well as advice on personal protection against vectors. Travel clinics are available across Canada. For a full listing, visit the Public Health Agency of Canada web site at www.phac-aspc.gc.ca/ and click on the "Travel Health" link.

Travel Health Information Resources

Travellers seeking English-speaking physicians can inquire with hotel receptions, tour companies or Canadian embassies. The International Association for Medical Assistance to Travellers (IAMAT) will supply a directory of English-speaking physicians in 125 countries and territories (Table 3).[56] IAMAT physicians have agreed to provide services with set fee schedules.[56] Membership in IAMAT is free of charge although a small donation is requested to help support its work. A variety of commercial databases and Internet sources are available for travel information. Even among reputable websites, conflicting information can be found, and careful consideration by the user is needed. Selected useful websites for travel information are listed in Table 4. In addition, travellers may contact Global Affairs Canada for information on safety and security considerations (1-800-267-6788 or www.international.gc.ca).

Table 3: **Summary of International Association for Medical Assistance to Travellers (IAMAT) Services**

- Membership card—entitles bearer to services and fixed IAMAT rates
- World directory—a directory of English-speaking physicians in 125 countries and territories who have agreed to a set payment schedule
- Traveller clinical record—a passport-size record completed by one's doctor prior to departure
- World immunization chart—provides information on preventive measures
- World malaria risk chart and protection guide—a guide to malaria prophylaxis
- World schistosomiasis risk chart and information brochure—provides information on preventive measures against schistosomiasis
- World climate chart—summary of climate in any part of the world

IAMAT CANADA: 2162 Gordon Street, Guelph, Ontario N1L 1G6
Tel.: 519-836-0102
Fax: 519-836-3412
www.iamat.org

67 Mowat Ave., Suite 036, Toronto, Ontario M6K 3E3
Tel.: 416-652-0137

Table 4: **Web Sites for Travel Medicine Recommendations for the Health Care Practitioner**

Web Site	URL	Description
Centers for Disease Control and Prevention (CDC)	wwwnc.cdc.gov/travel/	US recommendations; Yellow Book: Health information for international travel
Committee to Advise on Tropical Medicine and Travel (CATMAT)	www.phac-aspc.gc.ca/tmp-pmv/catmat-ccmtmv/index-eng.php	International travel health information for health professionals
Public Health Agency of Canada	www.phac-aspc.gc.ca	Regularly updated including information on outbreaks and a list of clinics providing travel health services in Canada
World Health Organization (WHO)	www.who.int	General travel advice; country-specific malaria risk and antimalarial recommendations

Water Concerns for Travellers

Safe drinking water is essential for travellers to foreign countries, as well as for backpackers within Canada, who rely on water from streams, ponds, rivers and lakes.

Fluid Requirements

To function optimally, males require an average intake of 3 L of water a day and women require an average of 2.2 L.[57] Fluid is replenished by consuming water, other beverages and solid foods. Because it is difficult to measure the total amount of fluid obtained by eating food, it is recommended that only fluids be counted toward meeting the daily requirement. Physical exertion increases fluid loss and more fluids should be consumed. Processed bottled water or other bottled beverages are preferable sources of fluids, but not always accessible while travelling. If bottled beverages are used, the seals on the bottles should be checked to ensure they have not been refilled with unprocessed liquids. Otherwise, the methods listed below should be used to treat water prior to consumption.

Unsafe Water

Drinking unsafe water may result in acute infections within hours or days, marked by vomiting, diarrhea, fever, malaise and/or abdominal pain. Diseases contracted by drinking contaminated water may be of viral, bacterial or protozoal origin and include amebiasis (*E. histolytica*), cholera, cryptosporidiosis, *E. coli* enteritis, giardiasis (*G. lamblia*), hepatitis A, *Shigella* enteritis and typhoid fever.[58,59] A survey of travellers showed that young people were more likely to experience gastrointestinal illness.[60] Except for *E. coli*, cholera, typhoid and hepatitis A, vaccines are not available to protect travellers against most of these diseases. Simple precautions to minimize the risk of infection are described in Chapter 30: Diarrhea.

Water treatment methods outlined in this chapter are directed at preventing infectious illnesses from bacteria, viruses and protozoa. However, environmental contaminants (e.g., copper, mercury, lead, pesticides, herbicides) may also exist in water that has not been processed for human consumption. It is best to verify with a local guide whether the drinking water source is suitable for humans.

While physical appearance is not a reliable indicator of safety, turbidity may not only indicate contamination, but may also interfere with disinfection.[59] Cloudy water should be strained through a filter.[29,58,59,61] It can then be boiled or chemically treated with iodine. Once purified, water should be stored in clean, covered containers to reduce the chance of recontamination. Water treated with chlorine or iodine remains drinkable for several days without refrigeration. Water treated by other means should be consumed within 2 days.[59]

Recommended Water Treatment Methods

Heat

Boiling water is the most reliable, and therefore the preferred, method of purifying water for drinking.[59] Boiling eliminates bacteria, viruses and protozoa. Water should be boiled vigorously for 1 minute then allowed to cool to room temperature.[59] At altitudes greater than 2000 metres above sea level, water should be boiled for 3 minutes, or boiled for 1 minute then chemically treated with iodine.[29] Boiled water may taste flat; adding a pinch of salt or oxygenating the water by pouring the water back and forth between two clean containers can improve the taste.[29]

Table 5: **Iodine Products for Water Purification[29,59]**

Iodination	Procedure
Tincture of iodine 2% solution[a]	Add 5 drops (0.25 mL) per L of clear water, or 10 drops (0.5 mL) per L of cold (<5°C) or cloudy water. Mix thoroughly and let stand for at least 30 min before drinking. Very cold or cloudy water should be allowed to stand several hours before use, if possible.
Saturated iodine solution[b]	Add 12.5 mL per L of water and let stand for 15–20 min; add 20 mL per L and let stand for at least 20 min if cold or cloudy water.
Tetraglycine hydroperiodide[b]	Add 1 tablet per L of room temperature water and wait 15 min before use. Use 2 tablets per L of cold or turbid water and wait 20 min.

[a] Available in first aid kits and from pharmacies.
[b] Available at camping equipment stores and drug wholesalers.

Iodination

Iodination is recommended only for short-term use (<2 weeks) if boiling is not feasible.[29,58,59,61] Contact time of the iodine in water should be extended if the water is very cold or cloudy. Ideally, to remove protozoal cysts such as *G. lamblia* and *Cryptosporidium*, water should be first poured through a filter with an absolute pore size of one micrometre or less, then iodinated to kill viruses and bacteria.[29,58,59,61] Iodination should be used with caution in children and avoided in pregnant women and travellers with thyroid disease.[29,58,59,61] Prolonged ingestion of iodine may lead to hypothyroidism or hyperthyroidism, goitre, hypersensitivity, iodism or poisoning, which is manifested by corrosion of the GI tract, metallic taste, vomiting and abdominal pain.[62] Iodine also crosses the placenta and is excreted into breast milk.[62] Iodine may stain and imparts an unpleasant taste to the water; palatability can be improved by adding a vitamin C tablet or powdered drink crystals prior to consumption. Table 5 lists iodine products appropriate for water purification and describes their use.

Chlorine

Treatment of water with **chlorine bleach** is not as reliably effective as iodine. Chlorine treatment alone may not kill some enteric viruses, *G. lamblia* and *E. histolytica* cysts and Cryptosporidium species.[29] If chlorine is used, add 2 drops (0.1 mL) household chlorine bleach to 1 L water (4 drops if water is cloudy), mix and let stand 30 minutes (longer if water is very cold).[59] Another product, **chlorine dioxide**, does kill *Giardia* effectively and has moderate effectiveness against *Cryptosporidia*.[63] Chlorine dioxide does not have an unpleasant taste, but is appropriate for only short-term use.

Filters

Water treatment devices such as filters, micro filters or portable iodine-impregnated resin devices are available from camping equipment stores. Filters or micro filters are available with small pore sizes (0.1–0.3 micrometre). They may remove protozoa, *G. lamblia* cysts and large bacteria, but will not remove viruses.[29] Filtration alone is therefore inadequate to purify water. Although filtration is not mandatory, it complements heating or iodine treatment, if it is used first to remove large particles.

Filters with iodine-impregnated resins are more effective against bacteria than protozoa and viruses. The contact time with the iodine in the filter is too short to kill *Giardia* in cold water, *Cryptosporidium* and some viruses.[3]

Suggested Readings

Centers for Disease Control and Prevention. *2016 Yellow book.* Atlanta: U.S. Department of Health and Human Services, Public Health Service; 2016. Available from: wwwnc.cdc.gov/travel/page/yellowbook-home.htm.

Government of Canada. *Travel health kit.* Available from: travel.gc.ca/travelling/health-safety/kit.

World Health Organization. Poumerol G, Wilder-Smith A, eds. *International travel and health 2012.* Geneva: WHO Press; January 1, 2012 and 2014 and 2015 updates. Available from: www.who.int/ith/en/.

References

1. DuPont HL, Ericsson CD, Farthing MJ et al. Expert review of the evidence base for self-therapy of travelers' diarrhea. *J Travel Med* 2009;16:161-71.
2. Rao G, Aliwalas MG, Slaymaker E et al. Bismuth revisited: an effective way to prevent travelers' diarrhea. *J Travel Med* 2004;11:239-41.
3. Grant E, Grant P. Miscellaneous injuries and first aid equipment. *Pharm J* 1997;258:476-8.
4. Jones JS, Sheffield W, White LJ et al. A double-blind comparison between oral pseudoephedrine and topical oxymetazoline in the prevention of barotrauma during air travel. *Am J Emerg Med* 1998;16:262-4.
5. Mikolajczyk RT, Stanford JB. Levonorgestrel emergency contraception: a joint analysis of effectiveness and mechanism of action. *Fertil Steril* 2007;88:565-71.
6. Raymond E, Taylor D, Trussell J et al. Minimum effectiveness of the levonorgestrel regimen of emergency contraception. *Contraception* 2004;69:79-81.
7. DuPont HL, Ericsson CD. Prevention and treatment of traveler's diarrhea. *N Engl J Med* 1993;328:1821-7.
8. Goustas P, Cork MJ, Higson D. Eumovate (clobetasone butyrate 0.05%) cream: a review of clinical efficacy and safety. *J Dermatolog Treat* 2003;14:71-85.
9. Kyle AA, Dahl MV. Topical therapy for fungal infections. *Am J Clin Dermatol* 2004;5:443-51.
10. Burkhart CG, Burkhart HR. Contact irritant dermatitis and anti-pruritic agents: the need to address the itch. *J Drugs Dermatol* 2003;2:143-6.

11. Committee to Advise on Tropical Medicine and Travel. Travel statement on jet lag. *Can Commun Dis Rep* 2003;29:4-8.
12. Bettes TN, McKenas DK. Medical advice for commercial air travelers. *Am Fam Physician* 1999;60:801-8, 810.
13. Waterhouse J, Reilly T, Atkinson G et al. Jet lag: trends and coping strategies. *Lancet* 2007;369:1117-29.
14. Sack, RL. Clinical practice. Jet lag. *N Engl J Med* 2010;362:440-7.
15. Herxheimer A, Petrie KJ. Melatonin for the prevention and treatment of jet lag. *Cochrane Database Syst Rev* 2002;(2):CD001520.
16. Petrie K, Dawson AG, Thompson L et al. A double-blind trial of melatonin as a treatment for jet lag in international cabin crew. *Biol Psychiatry* 1993;33:526-30.
17. Buscemi N, Vandermeer B, Hooton N et al. Efficacy and safety of exogenous melatonin for secondary sleep disorders and sleep disorders accompanying sleep restriction: meta-analysis. *BMJ* 2006;332:385-93.
18. Schoene RB. Illnesses at high altitude. *Chest* 2008;134:402-16.
19. Hackett PH, Roach RC. High-altitude illness. *N Engl J Med* 2001;345:107-14.
20. Hackett PH, Oelz O. The Lake Louise consensus on the definition and quantification of altitude illness. In: Sutton JR, Coates G, Houston CS, eds. *Hypoxia and mountain medicine: proceedings of the 7th International Hypoxia Symposium held at Lake Louise, Canada, February 1991*. 1st ed. Oxford: Pergamon Press; 1992. p. 327-30.
21. Committee to Advise on Tropical Medicine and Travel (CATMAT). Statement on high-altitude illnesses. An Advisory Committee Statement (ACS). *Can Commun Dis Rep* 2007;33:1-20.
22. Goodyer L. Environmental hazards. *Pharm J* 2001;266:577-80.
23. Barrow MW, Clark KA.. Heat-related illnesses. *Am Fam Physician* 1998;58:749-56, 759.
24. Golant A, Nord RM, Paksima N et al. Cold exposure injuries to the extremities. *J Am Acad Orthop Surg* 2008;16:704-15.
25. Biem J , Koehncke N, Classen D et al. Out of the cold: management of hypothermia and frostbite. *CMAJ* 2003;168:305-11.
26. Vectors of diseases. Hazards and risks for travellers: Part I. *Can Commun Dis Rep* 2001;27:128-32.
27. Vectors and diseases. Hazards and risks for travellers: Part III. *Can Commun Dis Rep* 2001;27:146-8.
28. Goodyer L. Bite avoidance. *Pharm J* 2000;265:298-304.
29. Centers for Disease Control and Prevention. *2016 Yellow book*. Atlanta: U.S. Department of Health and Human Services, Public Health Service; 2016. Available from: wwwnc.cdc.gov/travel/page/yellowbook-home.htm. Accessed November 24, 2015.
30. Lines J, Kleinschmidt I. Is malaria control better with both treated nets and spraying? *Lancet* 2015;385:1375-7.
31. Committee to Advise on Tropical Medicine and Travel (CATMAT). Statement on Personal Protective Measures to Prevent Arthropod Bites *Can Commun Dis Rep* 2012;38:1-18.
32. Lindsay LR, Surgeoner GA, Heal JD. *Evaluation of Bite Blocker as a repellent against spring Aedes spp. mosquitoes*. Guelph: Department of Environmental Biology, University of Guelph; 1996.
33. Fradin MS, Day JF. Comparative efficacy of insect repellents against mosquito bites. *N Engl J Med* 2002;347:13-8.
34. Koren G, Matsui D, Bailey B. DEET-based insect repellents: safety implications for children and pregnant and lactating women. *CMAJ* 2003;169:209-12.
35. von Mayenburg J, Rakoski J. Contact urticaria to diethyltoluamide. *Contact Dermatitis* 1983;9:171.
36. Vozmediano JM, Armario J, Gonzalez-Cabrerizo A. Immunologic contact urticaria from diethyltoluamide. *Int J Dermatol* 2000;39:876-7.
37. Government of Canada. *Insect repellents*. Available from: healthycanadians.gc.ca/product-safety-securite-produits/pest-control-products-produits-antiparasitaires/pesticides/about-au-sujet/insect_repellents-insectifuges-eng.php. Accessed October 16, 2015.
38. Kain KC, Shanks GD, Keystone JS. Malaria chemoprophylaxis in the age of drug resistance. I. Currently recommended drug regimens. *Clin Infect Dis* 2001;33:226-34.
39. Hellgren U. Approach to the patient with malaria. In: Keystone JS et al. *Travel medicine*. St. Louis: Mosby Elsevier; 2004. p. 169-74.
40. Centers for Disease Control and Prevention. *Dengue Homepage. Epidemiology*. Available from: www.cdc.gov/dengue/epidemiology/index.html. Accessed July 2, 2015.
41. World Health Organization. *Dengue and severe dengue*. Available from: www.who.int/mediacentre/factsheets/fs117/en/. Accessed January 22, 2016.
42. Brady OJ, Gething PW, Bhatt S et al. Refining the global spatial limits of dengue virus transmission by evidence-based consensus. *PLoS Negl Trop Dis* 2012;6:e1760.
43. Leong AS, Wong KT, Leong TY et al. The pathology of dengue hemorrhagic fever. *Semin Diagn Pathol* 2007;24:227-36.
44. Halstead SB. Dengue. *Lancet* 2007;370:1644-52.
45. World Health Organization. *Chikungunya*. Available from: www.who.int/mediacentre/factsheets/fs327/en/. Accessed July 2, 2015.
46. Pan American Health Organization. *Chikungunya*. Available from: www.paho.org/hq/index.php?Itemid=40931. Accessed July 2, 2015.
47. Public Health Agency of Canada. *Chikungunya: Global update*. Available from: phac-aspc.gc.ca/tmp-pmv/notices-avis/notices-avis-eng.php?id=120. Accessed November 10, 2015.
48. Traveling with insulin. In: Gulledge J, Beard S. *Diabetes management: clinical pathways, guidelines, and patient education*. 1st ed. Gaithersburg: Aspen Publishers; 1999. p. 157.
49. Lapostolle F, Surget V, Borron SW et al. Severe pulmonary embolism associated with air travel. *N Engl J Med* 2001;345:779-83.
50. Kuipers S, Cannegieter SC, Middeldorp S et al. The absolute risk of venous thrombosis after air travel: a cohort study of 8,755 employees of international organisations. *PLoS Med* 2007;4:e290.
51. Chee YL, Watson HG. Air travel and thrombosis. *Br J Haematol* 2005;130:671-80.
52. Bendz B, Rostrup M, Sevre K et al. Association between acute hypobaric hypoxia and activation of coagulation in human beings. *Lancet* 2000;356:1657-8.
53. Cannegieter SC, Doggen CJ, van Houwelingen HC et al. Travel-related venous thrombosis: results from a large population-based case control study (MEGA study). *PLoS Med* 2006;3:e307.
54. Kahn SR, Lim W, Dunn AS et al. Prevention of VTE in nonsurgical patients: antithrombotic therapy and prevention of thrombosis, 9th ed: American College of Chest Physicians Evidence-Based Clinical Practice Guidelines. *Chest* 2012;141:e195S-e226S.
55. Cesarone MR, Belcaro G, Nicolaides AN et al. Venous thrombosis from air travel: the LONFLIT3 study–prevention with aspirin vs low-molecular-weight heparin (LMWH) in high-risk subjects: a randomized trial. *Angiology* 2002;53:1-6.
56. International Association for Medical Assistance to Travelers. *Medical services and the international traveler*. Guelph: Foundation for the Support of International Medical Training, Inc.; 1982.
57. Water. In: Institute of Medicine (U.S.). Panel on Dietary Reference Intakes for Electrolytes and Water. *Dietary reference intakes for water, potassium, sodium, chloride, and sulfate*. Washington: National Academies Press; 2005. p. 73.

58. Government of Canada. *Travellers' diarrhea.* Available from: travel.gc.ca/travelling/health-safety/diseases/diarrhea. Accessed January 22, 2016.
59. Health Canada. Environmental and Workplace Health. *Drinking water away from home.* Available from: www.hc-sc.gc.ca/ewh-semt/pubs/water-eau/home-foyer-eng.php. Accessed January 22, 2016.
60. Rack J, Wichmann O, Kamara B et al. Risk and spectrum of diseases in travelers to popular tourist destinations. *J Travel Med* 2005;12:248-53.
61. Backer HD. Water disinfection for travellers. In: Centers for Disease Control and Prevention; Brunette GW, ed. *CDC health information for international travel 2010.* Atlanta: U.S. Department of Health and Human Services, Public Health Service; 2010.
62. Backer H, Hollowell J. Use of iodine for water disinfection: iodine toxicity and maximum recommended dose. *Environ Health Perspect* 2000;108:679-84.
63. Korich DG, Mead JR, Madore MS et al. Effects of ozone, chlorine dioxide, chlorine, and monochloramine on Cryptosporidium parvum oocyst viability. *Appl Environ Microbiol* 1990;56:1423-8.

Appendix IV
Medical Devices and Aids to Daily Living

Marie Berry, BSc(Pharm), BA, LLB

Medical devices and aids to daily living (also called assistive devices) are an integral part of the contemporary home healthcare market. It is a growing segment of health care. In 2012, estimates placed the size of the Canadian medical device market at approximately $6.8 billion.[1] The market itself is broad and, in addition to traditional items such as medical equipment, includes first aid and wound care products, sports medicine items, incontinence aids, palliative care products and diagnostic equipment.

Several factors have combined to create this expanded market—longer life expectancies, technological advances and economies involved in modern health care.

The Canadian population is living longer because of advances in medical knowledge and technology. Over time, more elderly people will be living in their homes, requiring medical and assistive devices to carry on their day-to-day living.

Improved technology enables individuals to stay at home or to go home earlier from hospital, and also permits earlier diagnosis and self-care management.

In general, treatment in hospitals is expensive, and both medical and assistive devices allow less costly home-based treatment. Patients are discharged earlier from hospital with home recovery, and not-for-admission or "day" surgery is more common.

The use of medical and assistive devices has economic advantages and provides an improved quality of life by reducing or even eliminating a person's disability. Orthopedic patients (e.g., those with hip replacements or fractures) can be more mobile and independent during postoperative recovery periods. Individuals with brain damage (e.g., from trauma or stroke) or cerebrovascular disease (e.g., vascular dementia) can be better equipped to support daily living and self-care management. Patients with rheumatoid arthritis, amyotrophic lateral sclerosis (ALS) or multiple sclerosis (MS) are better equipped to manage their diseases. Patients with amputations can return home to await rehabilitation programs. Caregivers use medical and assistive devices to facilitate the care they provide.

Medical Devices

Medical devices include a wide range of items. The legal definition is any article, instrument, apparatus or contrivance, including any component, part or accessory thereof, manufactured, sold or represented for use in the diagnosis, treatment, mitigation or prevention of a disease, disorder or abnormal physical state or its symptoms.[2] The definition also includes devices that could be used to restore, correct or modify a body function or body structure, to diagnose pregnancy, and to care for pregnant individuals and their offspring. It is a broad definition and at one time included products intended for animal use; however, the *Medical Devices Regulations* address products for human use only.[3]

In general terms, a medical device is any item of equipment, product or system that is ready-made, customized or adapted and used to maintain or improve functional capabilities of people with a permanent disability or a temporary impairment or physical limitation. When choosing a medical or assistive device, several factors need to be considered. The physical, cognitive and emotional characteristics of the person for whom the piece of equipment is intended affect the choice. For example, a self-propelled wheelchair may increase mobility; however, if the individual does not have the physical strength or endurance to propel it, an electrical model may be a better choice. The nature of the activity needs to be considered, e.g., whether the medical or assistive device is to be used at work, at home or in a social setting. Considerations include the social and cultural context, and whether the device is to be used in an institution or by the individual or caregiver. The degree of complication of the technology involved in the equipment is also a factor.

While a broad range of medical devices are listed in Table 1, this appendix focuses specifically on home safety equipment, mobility aids, patient comfort aids, respiratory aids and home intravenous equipment. Diagnostic tests intended for home use, wound care products, incontinence aids and ostomy products are discussed elsewhere (see Chapter 26: Diabetes Care Devices, Chapter 37: Ostomy Care, Chapter 60: Dressings, Chapter 80: Pregnancy and Fertility Testing, Chapter 83: Urinary Incontinence and Appendix II: Home Testing).

Home Safety Equipment

Home safety equipment is durable medical equipment that is able to withstand day-to-day wear and is intended for in-home use. At one time, high quality equipment was available only in hospital or institutional settings, but today such equipment is intended for in-home use, either by the individual alone or with the assistance of a caregiver. Home safety equipment can be divided into 2 groups that represent the majority of these types of devices: equipment for bathroom safety and equipment for mobility.

An area of growth is equipment designed for use by bariatric patients. In 2013, about 36% of Canadian adults were considered overweight and 26% obese.[4] Bariatric equipment is generally indicated for individuals with a body mass index (BMI) of greater than 30. The majority of standard equipment such as wheelchairs, walkers or bath chairs is intended for individuals weighing up to 250 pounds. Bariatric equipment is wider, made from heavy-duty material and is intended for people weighing more than standard equipment can support. The weight-carrying capacity is usually listed on the equipment.

Equipment for Bathroom Safety

Half of all falls involving Canadian seniors occur at home, with stairs and bathrooms posing the greatest risk.[5] Getting into or out of the bathtub presents a risk and bath oil and bubble bath increase risk by making tubs more slippery.

Showers are an alternative, but some individuals have difficulty standing in a shower. Chairs designed to be used in the shower are an option. Something as simple as a bath mat with suction cups reduces the risk of falls. Bathtub and shower grab bars and poles, along with tub rails, make a bathroom safer.[6] Hand-held or portable shower nozzles facilitate washing while standing or sitting.

Shampoo Trays and Caps

For people confined to bed or in a wheelchair, shampoo trays make washing hair possible. Rinse-free shampoo caps are now being used in and out of hospital to allow cleaning of the hair without the use of running water.

Inflatable Bathtubs

Inflatable vinyl tubs fit over a bed and come with a hand-held shower and hose, making bathing in bed a possibility.

Table 1: **Medical Devices**

Category	Examples	
Home safety equipment	Bathroom safety: ▪ bath rails and poles ▪ bed pans and urinals ▪ commodes ▪ shower chairs ▪ transfer benches	Mobility and transfer: ▪ walkers and canes ▪ wheelchairs
Home diagnostic tools[a]	Blood glucose monitors Blood pressure monitors Cholesterol testing kits	Ovulation testing kits Pregnancy testing kits
Patient comfort aids[b]	Adjustable beds Back, neck and limb braces Cushions	Elastic compression stockings Pressure therapy Pillows
Respiratory aids[c]	Asthma nebulizers Nasal irrigation devices Peak flow meters	Spacers for inhalers Vaporizers, humidifiers
Wound care products[d]	First aid products Specialized dressings	Surgical bandages
Incontinence aids[e]	Bedwetting alarm systems Drainage bags Protectors and sheaths	Under pads Undergarments Urinary catheters
Surgical sundries	Ear plugs Gloves Manicure accessories	Medicine measuring devices Personal hygiene products
Sports and orthopedic products[f]	Belts Braces Hot/cold therapy	Massagers Supports
Home intravenous products	Accessories such as tubing, infusion pumps, needles, syringes	
Sensory aids	Hearing aids	Magnifying glasses

[a] For more information on home diagnostic tools, see Chapter 26: Diabetes Care Devices, and Appendix II: Home Testing.
[b] For more information on features of patient comfort aids, consult the *Compendium of Products for Minor Ailments*—Musculoskeletal Produts: Supports, Braces, Wraps and Elastic Bandages.
[c] For comparative features of peak flow meters, consult the *Compendium of Products for Minor Ailments*—Respiratory Proucts: Peak Flow Meters.
[d] For comparative features of wound care products, consult the *Compendium of Products for Minor Ailments*—Skin Care Products: First aid, Dressings.
[e] For more information on incontinence aids, see Chapter 83: Urinary Incontinence.
[f] For more information on features of sports and orthopedic products, consult the *Compendium of Products for Minor Ailments*—Musculoskeletal Produts: Supports, Braces, Wraps and Elastic Bandages.

Bath Boards/Bathtub Transfer Benches

Bathtub transfers are the greatest cause of anxiety in individuals with permanent or temporary physical limitations, as this is when most falls occur. Requiring assistance in a bathtub transfer may be a sign of lost independence and privacy to some individuals.

Bath boards sit across the tub and usually have handgrips. They are ideal for storing soap and sponges within easy reach and for helping to maintain stability when stepping out of the bathtub. Bath boards are anchored to the inside tub edges with adjustable clamps/grips. The board is the same height as the tub edge and allows the individual to sit on the edge and slide across the board for a sit-down shower or sponge bath.

Transfer benches straddle the bathtub with 2 legs outside the tub and 2 legs inside the tub. The individual sits on the seat outside the bathtub, much like they would in a chair. While seated they can move their legs 1 at a time over the bathtub edge and into the bathtub, pulling themselves over to the portion of the seat positioned above the bath water. See Figure 1.

Figure 1: Use of Bathtub Transfer Bench

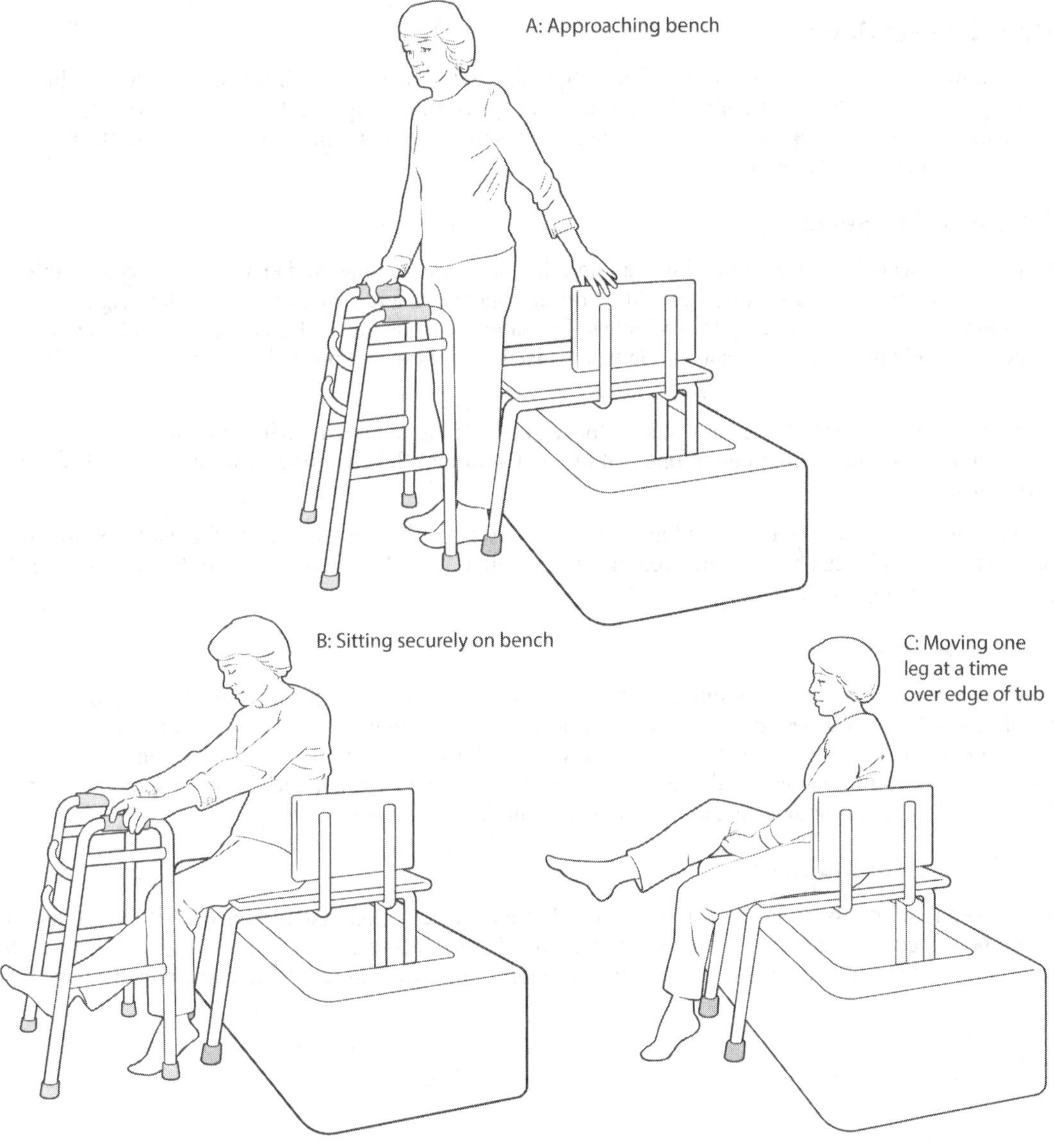

Transfer benches have adjustable heights but are not suitable for deep designer bathtubs. Several trial runs while fully clothed and without bath water are recommended, to adjust the bench to the correct height. The sitting surfaces must be slippery enough so that the transfer is easy, but not so slippery that someone may slide off the surface, especially when it is wet. Transfer benches and boards usually have water drainage holes in the seat surface to prevent the seat from becoming too slippery.

Transfer benches should be easy to clean and if not permanent, they should be light and easy to position. Suction cups and/or rubber tips limit movement of the equipment during transfers. Most have side grab bars and backrests. They should be adjustable so that a person can enter the tub from either the right or the left.

Bath/Shower Seats

Bath/shower seats have 4 legs set inside the tub or shower, allowing an individual to sit down while bathing. Some have backrests, and all have suction cups or rubber tips on the legs to prevent them from slipping. Suction-cup legs, adjustable leg heights, back support, and nonslip, easy-to-clean surfaces are desirable features.

Raised Toilet Seats

Raised toilet seats facilitate sitting down and getting up from the toilet and enable more comfortable transfers from wheelchair to toilet seat. Most raised toilet seats add 4 inches to the toilet height, although some are adjustable up to 6.5 inches. For safety reasons, raised toilet seats should attach directly to the toilet bowl by means of clamps. Raised toilet seats are portable and can be used when travelling.

Some raised toilet seats have a cut-out area for leg positioning in patients with limited range of movement at the hip or other conditions that prevent a normal flexed sitting position (e.g., following hip-replacement surgery).

Raised toilet seats may have attached hand grips. A safety bar can be attached to the wall next to the toilet and hand rails can be used on a regular-height toilet. A trial run will help with the appropriate placement. See Figure 2.

Miscellaneous

Assistive devices such as wash mitts, wash sponges (some have a pocket for a bar of soap), long-handled scrubbing brushes/sponges and tap turners make bathing easier and may help prevent falls. The toilet tissue dispenser should be within easy reach. Various toilet assistive devices enable individuals with limited manual dexterity to use toilet tissue and clean themselves. Splashguards can be attached to any commode seat that sits higher than the toilet bowl.

Equipment for Mobility

Decreased mobility for an individual may mean limited participation in activities of daily living and/or being housebound, bedridden or even institutionalized. Also, decreased mobility has associated health risks such as thromboembolism. Equipment for mobility includes canes, walkers and wheelchairs.

Figure 2: **Raised Toilet Seat With Cut-out For Leg Positioning**

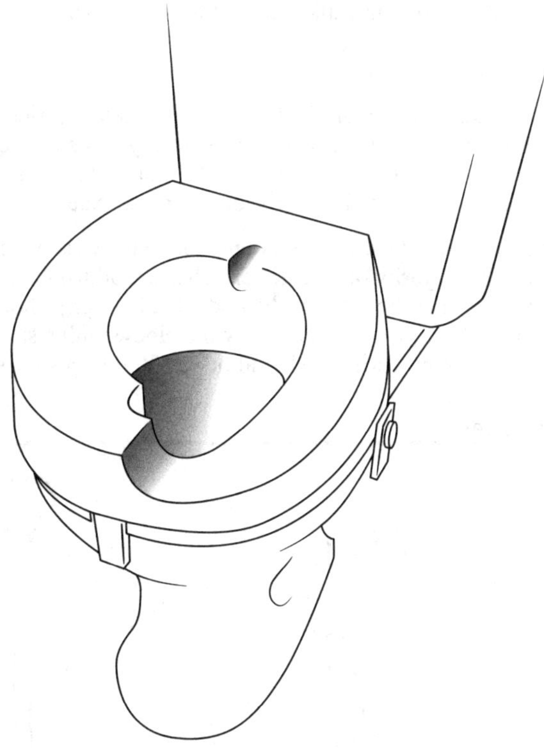

Canes and Walkers

Canes and walkers increase safety and confidence with mobility by reducing instability. Aluminum canes and walkers are lightweight and adjustable, thus easily manoeuvred and ideal for individuals who, because of age or disease, do not have optimal muscle strength. Wooden canes are often heavier and must be cut to adjust the length.

Canes and walkers should be measured to ensure a correct fit.[7] The distance from the top of a cane or walker handle to the ground should equal the distance from the wrist crease to the ground, when the arm is straight down at the side. The measurement should be performed with the individual standing erect and wearing everyday shoes. If the cane is too short, the user will lean forward. If it is too long they will lean backward. Adjustable and telescopic canes enable an individual to find the correct fit. Walkers are measured in a similar manner, and most are adjustable.

A cane handle should afford an easy yet firm grip. A swan's neck handle is easier for balancing, and many handles have moulded grips. Metal and wooden cane tips or walker feet tend to slip. Rubber tips are required to help prevent slips and falls, and are replaceable. A flip-back ice-gripping tip can be attached to the tip of a cane for extra stability in winter. Quad bases (4 legs) add balance to canes and different sized bases are available for stability. Although canes are most comfortably held in the dominant hand, holding the cane in the hand contralateral to the weak or injured side will provide the most balance.

Walkers may have wheels on 2 or 4 legs, and the wheels may be permanent or removable. Some walkers feature a handbreak which will lock the rear wheels. Walker accessories include tote bags, baskets, trays and attached seats. A folding walker eases transportation.

Crutches

Crutches are used as mobility aids and support for knee, leg, or ankle injuries. They may be required on a short- or long-term basis, depending upon whether the injury heals or is ongoing. There are 2 broad categories: forearm or elbow crutches, which are used more often on a long-term basis, and axillary or underarm crutches, which are mainly for short-term use. See Figure 3.

Forearm crutches have handgrips and the crutches extend above the wrist where they are secured by a cuff or collar at the forearm. The majority of forearm crutches are adjustable; however, the appropriate fit is needed. With the arms relaxed at the sides of the body, the handgrip should be level with the wrist. The cuffs should fit around the forearm just below the elbow with a space of 1–2 inches to allow the elbow to bend. The flex in the elbow ideally should be 15–30 degrees for stability and comfort.

Figure 3: **Styles of Crutches**

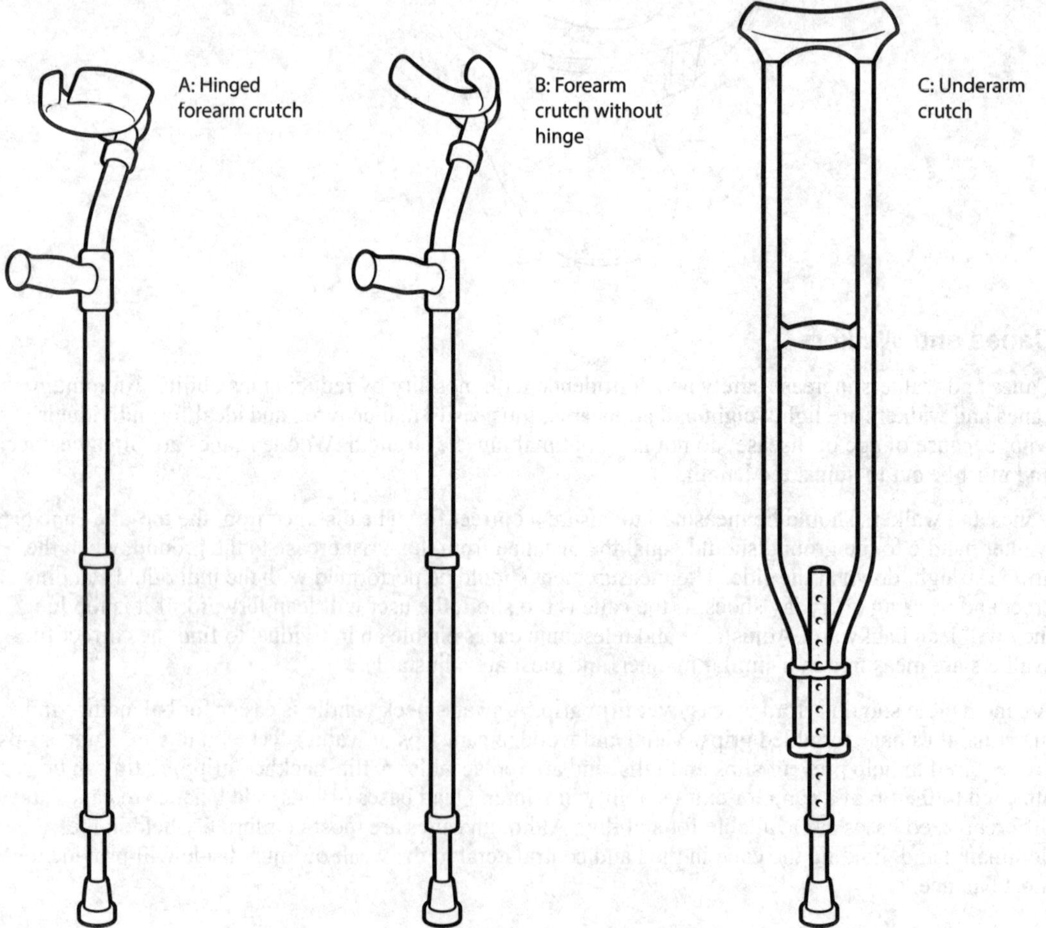

Axillary (underarm) crutches provide support for a lower body injury. The arm pads should not be tight against the axilla, but rather there should be space enough for 2 or 3 fingers or about 1–1.5 inches between the arm pad and the axilla. The handgrip should be adjusted so that with hands in place the arm is flexed about 15–30 degrees. Most crutches are adjustable to ensure proper fit.

If one crutch is used it should be used opposite the injury; however, with 2 crutches it is important to remember to move the crutches first, then the body. Forearm crutches are more difficult to learn to use, but they enable the user to be mobile on various surfaces and are ideal for more active individuals with a chronic injury.

Various handgrips are available. Some have extra padding or gel covers and others have ergonomic design. Forearm crutches have a variety of cuffs for comfort and durability. Some forearm crutches have hinged cuffs allowing the crutch to drop away when the wearer reaches for an object. See Figure 4. The arm pads of axillary crutches are also available with a variety of padding for comfort.

Figure 4: **Hinged Forearm Crutch**

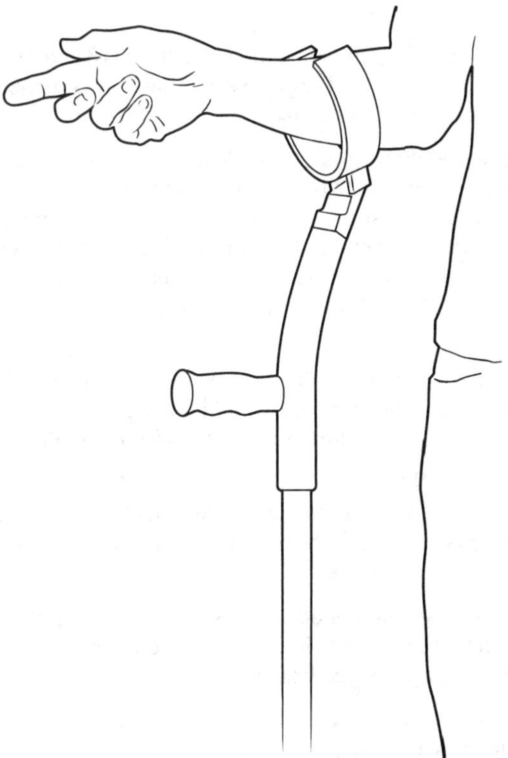

Tips for using crutches:

- Good posture is key for proper fit and use. Slouching over crutches leads to muscle strain and pain. Leaning too far in front of or behind the crutches results in instability and increased risk of falls.
- Nonskid shoes can help prevent falls when using crutches.
- When learning to use crutches, practice is important for preventing falls and increasing mobility.

- Balance, coordination, and upper body strength are needed for using crutches. While forearm crutches provide greater mobility, they also require more balance, coordination, and upper body strength. Axillary crutches may be a better option for a first-time user.
- Crutch tips are usually rubber and slip resistant. They should be inspected regularly for wear and replaced if worn.
- Wooden and metal crutches are both available. Metal crutches, especially aluminum, are lighter and more durable.
- When carrying several items, a backpack is recommended to avoid interference with crutch use.
- Routine inspection is needed to ensure screws or fasteners are not loose and crutch tips or pads are not worn.

Wheelchairs

Wheelchairs should provide comfortable and functional mobility.[8] Consider the everyday routine of the individual before choosing a wheelchair because the choice can vary depending on activities (e.g., going to work, participating in sports). More than one wheelchair may be required to perform different activities.

The method of propulsion of the wheelchair may be independent or assisted by another person. Independent propulsion refers not only to propelling wheels or hand rims manually, but also to the use of electrical controls with the hand, mouth, legs or feet.

Positioning of an individual in a wheelchair should provide adequate balance and support. The buttocks should bear equal loads, with adequate back support. Ideally, the shoulder should align vertically with the elbows, with the arms resting at right angles. The knees and ankles should be at right angles as well. When the individual's centre of gravity is ahead of the wheelchair axle the wheelchair is more stable, while propulsion is easier when the centre of gravity is over the axle. People with severe disabilities may not be able to achieve the ideal position, and adaptation of the chair may be needed.

Wheelchair seat dimensions should fit with body dimensions. A chair that is too large or too small does not function well for the user. The seat and back should not sag. To ensure proper positioning, seat height and individual requirements, the patient should be assessed while sitting in the chair.

The environment in which the chair will be used is a key factor.[9] If the chair is to be used indoors, its size and manoeuvrability must be considered as well as the architectural features of the building or room in question. Measure doorways and check the turning axis of the chair to ensure the wheelchair fits through doorways, both at home and at work.

Wheelchairs used outdoors should be able to negotiate uneven ground, slopes and curbs. This is a major limitation of wheelchairs in that they were designed to function on man-made surfaces, and perform poorly outdoors (e.g., in the park, on the beach).

Wheelchairs used for leisure activities may require high-performance features and should be easy to transport. Appearance and styling may be important. Certain sports (e.g., basketball, track) require specialized wheelchairs that are light and durable with easy manoeuvrability.

When travelling by car, close access to the car seat eases transferring between chair and car. Lightweight chairs with detachable or swing-away armrests and footrests make transfers and transportation easier. Transporter wheelchairs are lightweight and foldable, intended for occasional use such as shopping in a mall or moving through an airport.

Wheelchair accessories can increase comfort and mobility, and can reduce health risks. Wheelchair cushions reduce pressure sores and support the head. Harnesses and seat belts provide support and increase safety. Trays, bags, stump boards, umbrellas and rain hoods, pushing gloves and cuffs, portable ramps, padding, specialized cushions and transfer boards are other examples of wheelchair accessories.

Wheelchair manufacturers use different terms to describe the same features. Check with the manufacturer to clarify the terms and descriptions.

Table 2 summarizes considerations involved in selecting a wheelchair.

Table 2: **Selecting a Wheelchair**

Features	Options/Considerations	
Frame	Amputee Indoor or outdoor use	Regular, lightweight or bariatric construction Style Tilting, reclining or standing
Seat height/depth	Standard Hemiplegic or low seat	Bariatric Variable
Arm rests	Fixed Removable Swing-away	Full length Desk length Wrap-around
Backrest	Height Reclining	Sectional, adjustable, contoured
Footrests/legrests	Fixed Pivoting or swing-away	Removable Elevated
Propulsion	Regular drive One-handed drive	Foot propulsion Electrical
Wheels	Spokes Composite Quick-release axle Caster width/diameter	Pneumatic, semi-pneumatic or solid tires Wheel locks Anti-tip devices
Esthetics	Upholstery and frame colour	Individual's self-image, personality and preferences
Capabilities of chair	Home Work Leisure/sports School	Community Outdoor vs. indoor Terrain
Fit	Seating and postural needs Range of motion	Size, weight, endurance, cognitive and perceptual status of user
Cost	Availability of funding Life expectancy of the wheelchair	In the case of children, changes in size

Patient Comfort Aids

Patient comfort aids include pressure therapy, pillows, cushions, elastic compression stockings and back, neck and limb braces. Some of these devices are used therapeutically as well as for comfort. Pharmacies may facilitate the supply of larger equipment such as adjustable beds.

Elastic Compression Stockings

Elastic compression stockings are also known as surgical or support stockings or hose. In the simplest form, support stockings are intended to relieve tired, aching legs and prevent swelling of feet, ankles and legs. Individuals who stand or sit for long periods of time or older individuals with compromised venous return are ideal candidates for these stockings. Compression stockings may be prescribed for medical conditions such as varicose veins, lymphedema, venous eczema and ulceration, deep vein thrombosis, and post-thrombotic syndrome.[10]

Elastic compression stockings decrease superficial venous pressure, increase the upward flow in unoccluded deep and superficial veins and raise local interstitial pressure. Compression of the leg also prevents some edema. They are designed to give gradual support with the most pressure exerted at the ankle, less at the calf and the least at the thigh.[11] Stockings provide varying compression, ranging from 12–60 mm Hg at the ankle. No single standard classification of compression is used. The most common is: low or class 1 of less than 20 mm Hg; medium or class 2 of 20–30 mm Hg; and high or class 3 of >30 mm Hg.

A correct fit requires accurate measurements of the nonedematous leg, first thing in the morning. To ensure effective compression, the stocking should be washed and dried according to the manufacturer's directions and replaced every 2–3 months. They are intended to be removed at night and put on in the morning before beginning daily activities. Manual dexterity is needed to put on or remove the stockings, and devices are available to assist with this.

Compression stockings are available as pantyhose or socks (above or below the knee), with open or closed toes and in various colours. See Figure 5. The required compression and affected leg area should be the starting point in selection.

Figure 5: **Compression Stocking Styles**

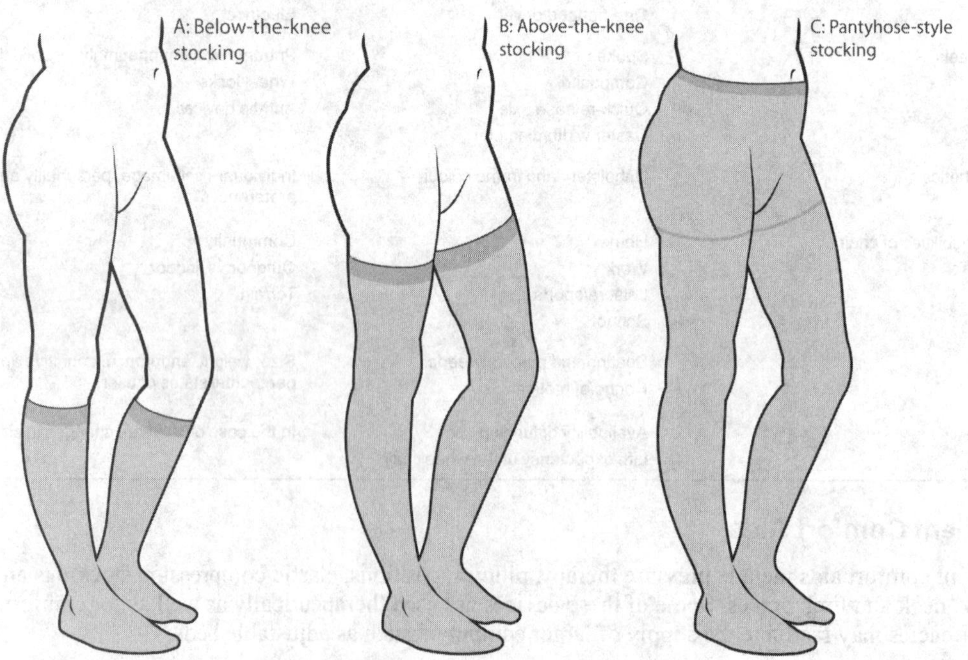

Antiembolism stockings are worn by the nonambulatory individual, to prevent venous emboli caused by inactivity. They provide less support and are not suitable for ambulatory individuals.

Nontherapeutic elastic stocking are widely available and often used by air travellers or by people who feel they have “tired legs”. Precise measurements are not needed and the compression is usually uniform.

Proper fit is essential to ensure comfort and effectiveness. Ill-fitting stockings may be the reason an individual discontinues wearing them. Some stockings, especially ones with high compression, may be esthetically unappealing for some wearers and they may not be worn. The most common reasons for not being able to wear compression stockings include: skin damage (especially seeping, open wounds), allergy to any of the stocking components, extensive leg edema or a malformed leg, a history of peripheral artery disease, and marked impairment of sensation in the leg.

Respiratory Aids

Peak Flow or PEF Meters

Along with established predictive value of respiratory symptoms, peak flow meters help predict and prevent exacerbations in a chronic pulmonary condition such as asthma. They allow home monitoring of a patient's lung function and titration of medication but it is important that use of a peak flow meter be linked to an action plan. Use of peak flow meters is contentious and the Canadian Thoracic Society notes that most people do not require monitoring of peak expiratory flow (PEF). Home monitoring may be suitable for adult patients who are poor perceivers of airway obstruction and by patients with severe asthma; however, in many cases, monitoring of symptoms may be sufficient.[12]

Peak flow meters measure the peak expiratory flow (PEF) rate, or the speed of air that can be forced out after the lungs are fully inflated. PEF meters consist of a mouthpiece with a gauge, an indicator and a scale. There are usually 2 mouthpieces to accommodate either children or adults.

After a complete exhalation, the individual inhales as deeply as possible, places the meter in the mouth and blows out as hard and fast as possible. The final position of the indicator on the scale is the PEF measured in litres per minute. Three consecutive readings are taken, and the highest of the 3 is recorded. Children as young as 4 years are able to perform this test.

While it is recommended that daily measurements be taken at 12-hour intervals, (e.g., 7 a.m. and 7 p.m.), measurements should be taken at times that are convenient and clinically significant for the individual. Measurements are recorded in a log or graph and many meters come with a graph. A note is made if inhaled corticosteroids or beta-agonists are used either before or after the test. These values are compared to “predicted normal” values depending on age, race, gender, height and weight. A better approach is comparison to the individual's personal best which is the highest PEF recorded over a 2- to 3-week period during which asthma is under control.

A zoning system is usually used to make the test reading relevant for the patient. One frequently used zoning system is based on traffic lights. A result in the green zone correlates to 80–100% of the individual's personal best, yellow 60–80%, and red <60%. In the yellow zone, medication may have to be re-evaluated, and in the red zone a bronchodilator is immediately required. If a reading appears in the red zone twice within a 48-hour period, medical attention should be sought.

Problems that can cause false readings include the wrong size of mouth piece, the indicator not being at the bottom of the scale before the test is begun, fingers blocking part of the mouthpiece opening and atmospheric pressure effects. To ensure accuracy of peak flow meters, individuals should be encouraged to take their meter to appointments with healthcare practitioners, to compare the readings with spirometry results.

Vaporizers/Humidifiers

Vaporizers use heat to disperse moisture in the air, which increases the temperature of the space in which they are used. Steam or spills from vaporizers can cause burns. Humidifiers require no heat. They increase humidity by physically dispersing water droplets in the air.

The use of distilled water prevents some mineral buildup in humidifiers; however, vaporizers require some minerals in the water to produce vapour. Regular cleaning of humidifiers and vaporizers is essential to remove debris and limit microbial growth, thus reducing the risk of infection and allergic reactions. Medication should not be added to humidifiers and if used with vaporizers, should only be placed in the medication cup (not the water reservoir).

Nasal Irrigation Devices

Nasal irrigation devices are used to remove excess mucous from nasal cavities. Also termed nasal lavage or douching, nasal irrigation can be useful as an adjunct to oral therapy in treating the symptoms of rhinosinusitis and chronic sinusitis. Various devices are available, for example the neti pot (see Figure 6), but all use the technique of pouring saline into one nostril and allowing it to drain through the other nostril. Gravity and tilting the head facilitate the procedure.

Figure 6: **Neti Pot**

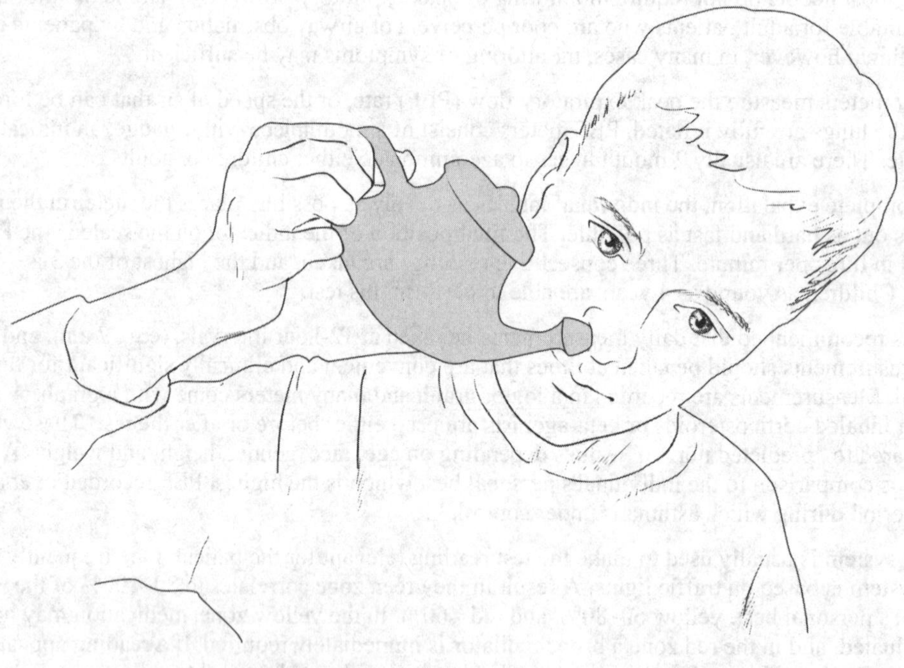

Oxygen Therapy

Ambulatory and hospice patients may require oxygen therapy. With the available technology (e.g., face masks, nasal cannulae, oxygen concentrators, tracheal or endotracheal tubes), oxygen therapy is more portable.

Oxygenated water and ozone therapy are touted as beneficial; however, both are expensive and lack evidence supporting their effectiveness.

Continuous Positive Airway Pressure Machines

Continuous positive airway pressure (CPAP) machines are used to treat obstructive sleep apnea-hypopnea syndrome. Individuals affected by the syndrome experience cessation of breathing (apnea) or shallow breathing (hypopnea) during sleep, which affects the quality and quantity of sleep and results in daytime drowsiness. A mask fits over the face and the CPAP machine maintains an air pressure in the mask that is slightly greater than the surrounding air, which promotes normal breathing. Adherence to CPAP therapy is low; the machine itself is cumbersome, and other potential factors include sleep disturbance and claustrophobia. Education, correct fit of the mask, and air humidification of the bedroom may increase use.

One symptom of obstructive sleep apnea-hypopnea syndrome is snoring. Various devices are available to reduce snoring along with the sleep apnea-hypopnea. Oral appliances reposition the mouth allowing improved breathing and adhesive nasal strips applied to the bridge of the nose open nasal passages.

Home Intravenous Programs

Patients with chronic illness and serious infections may require long hospitalizations away from family, friends and work; however, they might be well enough to reside at home if they were able to obtain the required medication. Home intravenous programs have been developed to meet this need.[13]

Examples of therapies that can be administered through home intravenous programs include:

- Antibiotic therapy for diseases such as infective endocarditis, septic arthritis, cystic fibrosis and osteomyelitis
- Chemotherapy for conditions such as breast cancer, Hodgkin's disease, leukemia or testicular cancer
- Parenteral nutrition for patients with short bowel syndrome, inflammatory bowel disease, chronic intractable diarrhea or chronic idiopathic intestinal obstruction syndrome.

The majority of home intravenous programs involve antibiotics.[14] Other potential therapies include parenteral nutrition, chemotherapy, analgesia, clotting factors for hemophilia, fluid therapy, and biologics (e.g., infliximab, natalizumab, rituximab).

Home intravenous programs represent one of the fastest growing segments of the home health care market. Several factors are responsible:

- More reliable equipment (e.g., better catheters, home infusion pumps)
- Increased patient awareness and involvement
- Cost savings
- Home health support from healthcare practitioners.

To succeed with a home intravenous program, a patient and their family must feel comfortable with the technology and skill required. The patient must have adequate cognitive function and no psychosis or drug addiction problems, both of which can adversely impact adherence (see Table 3).

Table 3: **Criteria for Candidates of Home Intravenous Programs**

Positive Criteria	Negative Criteria
Medical stability	Substance abuse
Manageable infection/disease	Impaired vision
Adherence to program	Home without running water, electricity, refrigeration
Sufficient cognitive function	
Venous access	

Most home intravenous patients have a venous catheter to which tubing and a prepared intravenous drug are attached. The drug infusion takes place over a specified period of time and is accomplished either by gravity or with the use of a pump. The catheter chosen may be a short peripheral line, midline or central line (e.g., Broviac, Hickman or Groshong) depending on duration of therapy, the need for blood sampling, age of the patient, drug properties (e.g., vesicant) and other factors.[14] A heparin lock may be used.

Subcutaneous infusion pumps are implanted devices used to infuse medication, blood products, fluids or nutrition. The pump appears as a raised area under the skin surface. There is a port with a self-sealing silicone rubber septum through which a Huber needle is inserted. The medication enters the body through tubing attached to the Huber needle.

Analgesic pumps are portable external devices that pump analgesic medications, typically morphine, through tubing and into a small needle placed in the subcutaneous tissue. The pump controls the flow of medication and is usually programmed to provide a set dose per time period. The pump can also be used manually with the patient having some control over dosage, but the pump is programmed to provide a limited quantity per time period. The pump is hung outside the tub when showering or bathing and placed under the pillow or hung on a hook when sleeping. Avoid exposing the pump to humidity, heat or freezing.

Parenteral nutrition bypasses the GI tract completely and is infused into the circulation. With total parenteral nutrition (TPN) there may be a loss of GI function, thus returning to orally provided nutrition may be problematic.

Complications

Phlebitis, infiltration and infection at the catheter site are the most common problems. Air emboli, dislodged catheters, migrating ports, catheter leaks and occlusion can also occur. Prepared intravenous solutions must be stored carefully, most often in the refrigerator and sometimes in the freezer.

Aids to Daily Living (Assistive Devices)

The term "aids to daily living" refers to assistive devices that make day-to-day life easier for both individuals and caregivers by facilitating performance of personal care tasks (e.g., clothing with Velcro closures, handle grips for cutlery, wheelchairs and canes). Assistive devices can enable an individual to avoid institutionalization.[15]

Assistive devices are often recommended by occupational therapists who evaluate and recommend adaptations that enable an individual's daily living activities to continue. Mastering the correct technique for using an assistive device can enable individuals to relearn an old skill, perform an old task in a new manner, or use equipment to perform a task.[16] The emphasis is on simplifying tasks, planning ahead, organizing the task, sitting and resting regularly when possible, and using correct body mechanics. Table 4 lists some common aids to daily living.

Table 4: **Examples of Aids to Daily Living**

Dishes	Partitioned; lip or raised edge; suction cup fixed on base; heated; food guards.
Cups	Easy-to-hold handles; detachable handles; attached straws and/or spouts; nose cut outs; weighted bases; insulated; holders to stabilize.
Utensils	Plastic coated spoons; weighted handles; easy to hold grips; swivel utensils; extension handles; specialized handles for odd angles; foam tubing to increase grip; putty to create a customized grip.
Kitchen	Electric and manual knives and peelers with easy-to-hold handles; cutting boards with nails to hold food for cutting; cutting boards with corner guards; easy-to-use and hold can and jar openers.
Home accessories	Doorknob and tap turners and grippers; easy-grip scissors; long reach sponge mops, dusters and vacuums; reading lights and magnifiers; book holders; reachers.
Personal care	Extension combs and brushes; handle grippers for toothbrushes; zipper pulls; elastic shoelaces; sock and pantyhose aids; button hooks; adaptive clothing.
Communications	Games, stickers and communication boards; pen grips; computer accessories.
Recreation	Playing card holders and shufflers; large size edition of games; knitting needle holders; hand cuffs and mobile bridges for pool cues.

Tips for Using Medical and Assistive Devices

To gain the most benefit from medical and assistive devices, they should be used correctly:

- Measurements must be accurate to ensure a correct fit. Read the directions carefully and be sure the correct units are used (e.g., if the manufacturer lists sizes in inches, do the measurement in inches).
- With any medical or assistive device that requires assembly, read the instructions carefully. One option is to have it pre-assembled.
- All directions for use should be thoroughly understood prior to use of any medical or assistive device. If ambiguities exist, they should be clarified.
- Most medical and assistive devices provide the manufacturer's contact information, such as a toll-free number or website. Keeping this information handy makes it easier to investigate problems or ask questions.

References

1. Industry Canada. Canadian Life Science Industries. *Medical devices. Medical device industry profile 2013.* Available from: www.ic.gc.ca/eic/site/lsg-pdsv.nsf/eng/h_hn01736.html. Accessed April 28, 2016.
2. Canada. Department of Justice. *Food and Drugs Act*, R.S. 1985, c. F-27, section 2.
3. Canada. Department of Justice. *Medical Devices Regulations*, SOR/98-282, section 1.
4. Statistics Canada. *Body composition of adults, 2012 to 2013.* 2014. Available from: www.statcan.gc.ca/pub/82-625-x/2014001/article/14104-eng.htm. Accessed March 23, 2015.
5. Public Health Agency of Canada. *The facts: seniors and injury in Canada.* 2011. Available from: www.phac-aspc.gc.ca/seniors-aines/publications/public/injury-blessure/safelive-securite/chap2-eng.php. Accessed May 14, 2015.
6. Chase CA, Mann K, Wasek S et al. Systematic review of the effect of home modification and fall prevention programs on falls and the performance of community-dwelling older adults. *Am J Occup Ther* 2012;66:284-91.
7. Bradley SM, Hernandez CR. Geriatric assistive devices. *Am Fam Physician* 2011;84:405-11.
8. Minkel JL. Seating and mobility considerations for people with spinal cord injury. *Phys Ther* 2000;80:701-9.
9. Tomlinson JD. Managing maneuverability and rear stability of adjustable manual wheelchairs: an update. *Phys Ther* 2000;80:904-11.
10. Lim CS, Davies AH. Graduated compression stockings. *CMAJ* 2014;186:E391-8.
11. Agu O, Hamilton G, Baker D. Graduated compression stockings in the prevention of venous thromboembolism. *Br J Surg* 1999;86:992-1004.
12. Lougheed MD, Lemiere C, Dell SD et al. Canadian Thoracic Society asthma management continuum—2010 consensus summary for children six years of age and over, and adults. *Can Respir J* 2010;17:15-24.
13. Laupland KB, Valiquette L. Outpatient parenteral antimicrobial therapy. *Can J Infect Dis Med Microbiol* 2013;24:9-11.
14. Moore D, Bortolussi R. Home intravenous therapy: accessibility for Canadian children and youth. *Paediatr Child Health* 2011;16:105-14.
15. Finlayson M, Havixbeck K. A post-discharge study on the use of assistive devices. *Can J Occup Ther* 1992;59:201-7.
16. Pedretti LW, Zoltan B. *Occupational therapy: practice skills for physical dysfunction.* 3rd ed. St. Louis: Mosby; 1990.

Appendix V

Pregnancy and Breastfeeding: Self-care Therapy for Common Conditions

Myla E. Moretti, MSc, PhD

Pregnancy and Breastfeeding: Self-care Therapy for Common Conditions

Table 1: Pregnancy and Breastfeeding: Self-care Therapy for Common Conditions

For comparative ingredients of nonprescription products, consult the *Compendium of Products for Minor Ailments.*

Indication	Self-care Drugs of Choice in Pregnancy	Alternatives in Pregnancy	Self-care Drugs of Choice in Breastfeeding	Alternatives in Breastfeeding	Comments
Acne See also Chapter 54: Acne.	*benzoyl peroxide*[1,2]		*benzoyl peroxide*[2]		Topical tretinoin is believed to be nonteratogenic and systemic bioavailability is low; however, continuing use in pregnancy may not be warranted.[3]
Allergic Rhinitis See also Chapter 22: Allergic Rhinitis and Chapter 82: Prenatal and Postpartum Care.	Second-generation antihistamines: *cetirizine*[4,5,6] *loratadine*[7,8,9,10,11] First generation antihistamines: *brompheniramine*,[12] *chlorpheniramine*, *doxylamine*, *diphenhydramine*, *pheniramine*[13,14,15,16]	*desloratadine*, *fexofenadine*[17,18,19]	First- or second-generation antihista-mines[20,21,22,23]		See Nasal Congestion if antihistamine alone is inadequate.
Backache/ headache/ fever/pain See also Chapter 7: Fever, Chapter 8: Headache, Chapter 45: Low Back Pain and Chapter 82: Prenatal and Postpartum Care.	*acetaminophen*[15,16,24,25,26] (with or without codeine[16])	*ASA*[15,27,28,29,30,31,32,33,34,35] *ibuprofen*, *naproxen* See comments	*acetaminophen* *ASA*, *codeine*, *ibuprofen*, *naproxen*		Avoid NSAIDs in the third trimester.[36,37,38] Limit codeine to short-term use in pregnancy. Limit codeine in breastfeeding to short-term use (<4 days) in patients for whom safer effective treatments are unavailable. Discontinue codeine if either mother or infant displays signs of toxicity.[24,39]
Chest Congestion See also Chapter 21: Acute Cough,	*guaifenesin*[15,16,27]		*guaifenesin*		No data on excretion into milk; however, not expected to pose a risk to suckling infant.

(cont'd)

Table 1: **Pregnancy and Breastfeeding: Self-care Therapy for Common Conditions** *(cont'd)*

For comparative ingredients of nonprescription products, consult the *Compendium of Products for Minor Ailments.*

Indication	Self-care Drugs of Choice in Pregnancy	Alternatives in Pregnancy	Self-care Drugs of Choice in Breastfeeding	Alternatives in Breastfeeding	Comments
Chapter 82: Prenatal and Postpartum Care.					
Cold Sores See also Chapter 90: Cold Sores (Herpes Labialis).					No nonprescription therapy of choice; prescription therapy may be preferred.[a]
Conjunctivitis, allergic See also Chapter 12: Assessment of Patients with Eye Conditions and Chapter 13: Conjunctivitis.	See Comments				Though absorption of many nonprescription eye drops is minimal, prescription products may have more evidence of safety in pregnancy.
Conjunctivitis, infectious See also Chapter 12: Assessment of Patients with Eye Conditions and Chapter 13: Conjunctivitis.	See Comments				Though absorption of many nonprescription eye drops is minimal, prescription products may have more evidence of safety in pregnancy.
Constipation See also Chapter 29: Constipation and Chapter 82: Prenatal and Postpartum Care.	Bulk-forming agents: *psyllium*, *bran* Stool softeners: *docusate*	See Comments	*magnesium hydroxide* Bulk-forming agents: *psyllium*, *bran* Stool softeners: *docusate*, *bisacodyl*	*senna*	Glycerin suppositories and polyethylene glycol (PEG) are acceptable for short-term use in acute constipation during pregnancy. Senna and other stimulants may induce uterine contractions and bowel dependence—only short-term use is advised.
Cough See also Chapter 21: Acute Cough and Chapter 82: Prenatal and Postpartum Care.	*dextromethorphan*[15,16,40,41] *codeine*		*dextromethorphan*	*codeine*	No data on excretion of dextromethorphan into milk; however, not expected to pose a risk to suckling infant. Limit codeine to short-term use in pregnancy. Limit codeine in breastfeeding to patients for whom safer effective treatments are unavailable and limit to short-term use (<4 days). Discontinue codeine if either mother or infant displays signs of toxicity.[24,39]

(cont'd)

Table 1: **Pregnancy and Breastfeeding: Self-care Therapy for Common Conditions** *(cont'd)*

For comparative ingredients of nonprescription products, consult the *Compendium of Products for Minor Ailments.*

Indication	Self-care Drugs of Choice in Pregnancy	Alternatives in Pregnancy	Self-care Drugs of Choice in Breastfeeding	Alternatives in Breastfeeding	Comments
Dandruff See also Chapter 58: Dandruff and Seborrheic Dermatitis.	*coal tar preparations*, *pyrithione zinc*		*coal tar preparations*, *pyrithione zinc*		Not studied in human pregnancy or lactation; however, systemic absorption is expected to be negligible.
Dermatitis See also Chapter 55: Atopic, Contact, and Stasis Dermatitis.	See Comments		Nonprescription topical corticosteroids (if used on nipple or areola, wipe off prior to feeding). Water-based products preferred.		Though nonprescription topical corticosteroids are probably safe, appropriate medical assessment is recommended to identify potential pregnancy-specific dermatologic conditions.
Diarrhea See also Chapter 30: Diarrhea.	*attapulgite/kaolin + pectin*[27] *psyllium*[15,16,27,42] See Comments	*bismuth subsalicylate*,[27] *loperamide*[27,43]	*attapulgite/kaolin + pectin*[27] *psyllium*[15,16,27,42] *loperamide*[27,43]		Avoid salicylate-containing compounds in the third trimester.
Fungal Infections, mouth See also Chapter 93: Oral Candidiasis.					No nonprescription therapy of choice.[a] Patient requires further assessment and/or treatment.
Fungal Infections, nails See also Chapter 64: Fungal Nail Infections (Onychomycosis).					No nonprescription therapy of choice.[a] Patient requires further assessment and/or treatment.
Fungal Infections, skin See also Chapter 65: Fungal Skin Infections.	*clotrimazole*, *miconazole*, *nystatin* (topical) See Comments		*clotrimazole*, *miconazole*, *nystatin* (topical)		Though these topical antifungal agents are considered safe, further assessment is recommended to identify potential pregnancy-specific dermatologic conditions.
Fungal Infections, vaginal See also Chapter 84: Vaginal Symptoms, Hygiene and Infections.	*clotrimazole* (topical, vaginal) *miconazole* (topical, vaginal)[44,45,46]	*fluconazole* 150 mg single dose	*clotrimazole* (topical, vaginal) *miconazole* (topical, vaginal)[47]	*fluconazole* 150 mg single dose	Patient requires further assessment and/or treatment if symptoms persevere after nonprescription treatment.
Gingivitis/ periodontitis See also Chapter 87: Periodontal Conditions:	See Comments		See Comments		No nonprescription therapy of choice.[a] Consult dentist for a diagnosis and

(cont'd)

Table 1: Pregnancy and Breastfeeding: Self-care Therapy for Common Conditions (cont'd)

For comparative ingredients of nonprescription products, consult the *Compendium of Products for Minor Ailments.*

Indication	Self-care Drugs of Choice in Pregnancy	Alternatives in Pregnancy	Self-care Drugs of Choice in Breastfeeding	Alternatives in Breastfeeding	Comments
Gingivitis and Periodontitis.					appropriate treatment recommendations.
Hemorrhoids See also Chapter 33: Hemorrhoids, Chapter 82: Prenatal and Postpartum Care.	Bulk-forming agents: *psyllium, bran* Stool softeners: *docusate* Topical: *zinc oxide*	See Comments	Bulk-forming agents: *psyllium, bran* Stool softeners: *docusate* Topical: *zinc oxide*	See Comments	No safety data available for nonprescription topical hemorrhoid products; however, because of the small doses and limited systemic absorption, they can be safely used for symptom relief if bulk-forming agents and stool softeners are inadequate.
Influenza See also Chapter 24: Viral Rhinitis, Influenza, Rhinosinusitis and Pharyngitis.					Treat symptoms and hydration as necessary, see individual symptoms.
Insect Bites and Stings See also Chapter 67: Insect Bites and Stings.	Treatment with ice may be sufficient	*diphenhydramine* (oral or topical) Nonprescription topical corticosteroids	Treatment with ice may be sufficient	*diphenhydramine* (oral or topical) Nonprescription topical corticosteroids	Patient requires further assessment and/or treatment if symptoms are severe or do not resolve within 7 days. Topical diphenhydramine can cause allergic contact dermatitis.
Insect Repellents See also Chapter 67: Insect Bites and Stings.	See Comments		See Comments		Use products with <30% DEET when protective clothing is not sufficient.
Lice See also Chapter 69: Parasitic Skin Infections: Lice and Scabies.	*permethrins*[48,49] *pyrethrins with piperonyl butoxide*		*permethrins*, *pyrethrins with piperonyl butoxide*		Not studied in lactation; however, systemic absorption is expected to be negligible.
Nasal Congestion See also Chapter 22: Allergic Rhinitis and Chapter 82: Prenatal and Postpartum Care.	*pseudoephedrine*[31,32,52,53] See Comments *saline* nasal spray/ drops	Topical nasal decongestants: *oxymetazoline*, *xylometazoline*[15,42,52] *phenylephrine*[16,33,54,56]	*saline* nasal spray/ drops Topical nasal decongestants: *oxymetazoline*, *xylometazoline*[15,42,52]	*pseudoephedrine* (See Comments)	Some sources recommend avoidance of pseudoephedrine during the first trimester based on a single, small study showing increased risk of gastroschisis;[30] however, a recent larger study from the same group did not show increased risk.[55] Though not reported in humans, phenylephrine is more likely than pseudoephedrine to produce vasoactive effects such as hypertension and

(cont'd)

Table 1: **Pregnancy and Breastfeeding: Self-care Therapy for Common Conditions** *(cont'd)*

For comparative ingredients of nonprescription products, consult the *Compendium of Products for Minor Ailments.*

Indication	Self-care Drugs of Choice in Pregnancy	Alternatives in Pregnancy	Self-care Drugs of Choice in Breastfeeding	Alternatives in Breastfeeding	Comments
					reduced uterine blood flow. There may be a risk of decreased milk production with pseudoephedrine in women whose lactation is not well established or who have low milk supply.
Nausea and Vomiting See also Chapter 36: Nausea and Vomiting and Chapter 82: Prenatal and Postpartum Care.	*doxylamine/ pyridoxine*[57]	*dimenhydrinate*[16,58,59,60]	*dimenhydrinate*		Doxylamine 10 mg/ pyridoxine 10 mg (delayed-release combination product) is available on prescription.
Pharyngitis See also Chapter 24: Viral Rhinitis, Influenza, Rhinosinusitis and Pharyngitis.	*acetaminophen*, *ASA*,[15,27,35] *codeine*, *ibuprofen* See comments	*naproxen* See Comments	*acetaminophen*, *ASA*, *codeine*, *ibuprofen*, *naproxen*		Short-term use for pain relief is safe. Avoid NSAIDs in third trimester. Limit codeine to short-term use in pregnancy. Limit codeine in breastfeeding to short-term (<4 days) use in patients for whom safer effective treatments are unavailable. Discontinue codeine if either mother or infant displays signs of toxicity.[24,39] Patient requires further assessment as bacterial infection may require prescription treatment.
Pigmentary changes (chloasma, melasma) See also Chapter 72: Prevention and Treatment of Sun-induced Skin Damage.		*hydroquinone* See Comments		*hydroquinone* See Comments	Minimal human data do not suggest teratogenic risk;[50] however, as treatment is cosmetic only, use should be avoided. Systemic absorption does occur.[51] Sunscreen use can help to prevent or minimize pigmentary changes.
Pinworms See also Chapter 39: Pinworms.	See Comments		See Comments		Published safety data exist only for prescription agents and therefore they are preferred for this indication. However, there are no published reports of adverse outcomes in pregnancy or breastfeeding

(cont'd)

Table 1: **Pregnancy and Breastfeeding: Self-care Therapy for Common Conditions** *(cont'd)*

For comparative ingredients of nonprescription products, consult the *Compendium of Products for Minor Ailments.*

Indication	Self-care Drugs of Choice in Pregnancy	Alternatives in Pregnancy	Self-care Drugs of Choice in Breastfeeding	Alternatives in Breastfeeding	Comments
					associated with pyrantel pamoate.
Reflux Esophagitis See also Chapter 31: Dyspepsia and GERD and Chapter 82: Prenatal and Postpartum Care.	*alginic acid compounds, aluminum, calcium and magnesium antacids, famotidine, omeprazole*[61,62,63] *ranitidine*		*alginic acid compounds, aluminum, calcium and magnesium antacids, famotidine, omeprazole*[64] *ranitidine*		
Rhinorrhea See also Chapter 22: Allergic Rhinitis, Chapter 24: Viral Rhinitis, Influenza, Rhinosinusitis and Pharyngitis and Chapter 82: Prenatal and Postpartum Care.	First-generation antihistamines: *brompheniramine*[12], *chlorpheniramine, doxylamine, diphenhydramine, pheniramine*[13,14,15,16]		First-generation antihistamines[20,21,22,23]		
Scabies See also Chapter 69: Parasitic Skin Infections: Lice and Scabies.	*permethrins*[48,49]		*permethrins*		Not studied in lactation; however, systemic absorption is expected to be negligible.
Smoking Cessation See also Chapter 6: Smoking Cessation.	*nicotine replacement* (patch, gum, inhaler)		*nicotine replacement* (patch, gum, inhaler)		Nicotine replacement has not been well studied in pregnancy or lactation but would provide less toxin exposure for the patient than cigarette smoke. The addition of counselling may improve cessation success rate.
Viral Rhinitis See also Chapter 24: Viral Rhinitis, Influenza, Rhinosinusitis and Pharyngitis.	See Nasal Congestion See Rhinorrhea				
Warts, common or plantar See also Chapter 52: Plantar Warts and Chapter 73: Viral Skin Infections: Common and Flat Warts.	*salicylic acid* preparations[15,27,28,29,30,31,32,33,34,35]		*salicylic acid* preparations		Avoid salicylates in the third trimester.

[a] For many conditions only prescription treatments have been studied. This does not mean that nonprescription therapy is unsafe, but there is no evidence available on which to base a recommendation at this time. For further information on prescription treatment, consult the *Compendium of Therapeutic Choices*.

References

1. Rothman KF, Pochi PE. Use of oral and topical agents for acne in pregnancy. *J Am Acad Dermatol* 1988;19:431-42.
2. Leachman SA, Reed BR. The use of dermatologic drugs in pregnancy and lactation. *Dermatol Clin* 2006;24:167-97, vi.
3. Kaplan YC, Ozsarfati J, Etwel F et al. Pregnancy outcomes following first-trimester exposure to topical retinoids: a systematic review and meta-analysis. *Br J Dermatol* 2015;173:1132-41.
4. Einarson A, Bailey B, Jung G et al. Prospective controlled study of hydroxyzine and cetirizine in pregnancy. *Ann Allergy Asthma Immunol* 1997;78:183-6.
5. Wilton LV, Pearce GL, Martin RM et al. The outcomes of pregnancy in women exposed to newly marketed drugs in general practice in England. *Br J Obstet Gynaecol* 1998;105:882-9.
6. Weber-Schoendorfer C, Schaefer C. The safety of cetirizine during pregnancy. A prospective observational cohort study. *Reprod Toxicol* 2008;26:19-23.
7. Moretti ME, Caprara D, Coutinho CJ et al. Fetal safety of loratadine use in the first trimester of pregnancy: a multicenter study. *J Allergy Clin Immunol* 2003;111:479-83.
8. Diav-Citrin O, Shechtman S, Aharonovich A et al. Pregnancy outcome after gestational exposure to loratadine or antihistamines: a prospective controlled cohort study. *J Allergy Clin Immunol* 2003;111:1239-43.
9. Gilbert C, Mazzotta P, Loebstein R et al. Fetal safety of drugs used in the treatment of allergic rhinitis: a critical review. *Drug Saf* 2005;28:707-19.
10. Kallen B, Olausson PO. No increased risk of infant hypospadias after maternal use of loratadine in early pregnancy. *Int J Med Sci* 2006;3:106-7.
11. Schwarz EB, Moretti ME, Nayak S et al. Risk of hypospadias in offspring of women using loratadine during pregnancy: a systematic review and meta-analysis. *Drug Saf* 2008;31:775-88.
12. Seto A, Einarson T, Koren G. Evaluation of brompheniramine safety in pregnancy. *Reprod Toxicol* 1993;7:393-5.
13. Seto A, Einarson T, Koren G. Pregnancy outcome following first trimester exposure to antihistamines: meta-analysis. *Am J Perinatol* 1997;14:119-24.
14. McKeigue PM, Lamm SH, Linn S et al. Bendectin and birth defects: I. A meta-analysis of the epidemiologic studies. *Teratology* 1994;50:27-37.
15. Aselton P, Jick H, Milunsky A et al. First-trimester drug use and congenital disorders. *Obstet Gynecol* 1985;65:451-5.
16. Heinonen OP, Shapiro S, Slone D. *Birth defects and drugs in pregnancy.* Littleton: Publishing Sciences Group; 1977.
17. Schatz M, Petitti D. Antihistamines and pregnancy. *Ann Allergy Asthma Immunol* 1997;78:157-9.
18. Schick B, Hom M, Librizzi R et al. Terfenadine (Seldane) exposure in early pregnancy. *Teratology* 1994;49:417.
19. Loebstein R, Lalkin A, Addis A et al. Pregnancy outcome after gestational exposure to terfenadine: a multicenter, prospective controlled study. *J Allergy Clin Immunol* 1999;104:953-6.
20. Ito S, Blajchman A, Stephenson M et al. Prospective follow-up of adverse reactions in breast-fed infants exposed to maternal medication. *Am J Obstet Gynecol* 1993;168:1393-9.
21. Findlay JW, Butz RF, Sailstad JM et al. Pseudoephedrine and triprolidine in plasma and breast milk of nursing mothers. *Br J Clin Pharmacol* 1984;18:901-6.
22. Lucas BD, Purdy CY, Scarim SK et al. Terfenadine pharmacokinetics in breast milk in lactating women. *Clin Pharmacol Ther* 1995;57:398-402.
23. Hilbert J, Radwanski E, Affrime MB et al. Excretion of loratadine in human breast milk. *J Clin Pharmacol* 1988;28:234-9.
24. Rebordosa C, Kogevinas M, Horvath-Puho E et al. Acetaminophen use during pregnancy: effects on risk for congenital abnormalities. *Am J Obstet Gynecol* 2008;198:178.e1-7.
25. Streissguth AP, Treder RP, Barr HM et al. Aspirin and acetaminophen use by pregnant women and subsequent child IQ and attention decrements. *Teratology* 1987;35:211-9.
26. Smith J, Taddio A, Koren G. Drugs of choice for pregnant women. In: Koren G, ed. *Maternal-fetal toxicology: a clinician's guide.* 2nd ed. New York: Marcel Dekker; 1994. p. 115-28.
27. Briggs GG, Freeman RK, Yaffe SJ. *Drugs in pregnancy and lactation: a reference guide to fetal and neonatal risk.* 9th ed. Philadelphia: Wolters Kluwer Health; Lippincott Williams & Wilkins; 2011.
28. Barry WS, Meinzinger MM, Howse CR. Ibuprofen overdose and exposure in utero: results from a postmarketing voluntary reporting system. *Am J Med* 1984;77:35-9.
29. Slone D, Siskind V, Heinonen OP et al. Aspirin and congenital malformations. *Lancet* 1976;1:1373-5.
30. Werler MM, Mitchell AA, Shapiro S. First trimester maternal medication use in relation to gastroschisis. *Teratology* 1992;45:361-7.
31. Torfs CP, Katz EA, Bateson TF et al. Maternal medications and environmental exposures as risk factors for gastroschisis. *Teratology* 1996;54:84-92.
32. Werler MM, Sheehan JE, Mitchell AA. Maternal medication use and risks of gastroschisis and small intestinal atresia. *Am J Epidemiol* 2002;155:26-31.
33. Zierler S, Rothman KJ. Congenital heart disease in relation to maternal use of Bendectin and other drugs in early pregnancy. *N Engl J Med* 1985;313:347-52.
34. Werler MM, Mitchell AA, Shapiro S. The relation of aspirin use during the first trimester of pregnancy to congenital cardiac defects. *N Engl J Med* 1989;321:1639-42.
35. Zierler S. Maternal drugs and congenital heart disease. *Obstet Gynecol* 1985;65:155-65.
36. Levin DL. Effects of inhibition of prostaglandin synthesis on fetal development, oxygenation, and the fetal circulation. *Semin Perinatol* 1980;4:35-44.
37. Alano MA, Ngougmna E, Ostrea EM et al. Analysis of nonsteroidal antiinflammatory drugs in meconium and its relation to persistent pulmonary hypertension of the newborn. *Pediatrics* 2001;107:519-23.
38. Stuart MJ, Gross SJ, Elrad H et al. Effects of acetylsalicylic-acid ingestion on maternal and neonatal hemostasis. *N Engl J Med* 1982;307:909-12.
39. Madadi P, Koren G, Cairns J et al. Safety of codeine during breastfeeding: fatal morphine poisoning in the breastfed neonate of a mother prescribed codeine. *Can Fam Physician* 2007;53:33-5.
40. Einarson A, Lyszkiewicz D, Koren G. The safety of dextromethorphan in pregnancy: results of a controlled study. *Chest* 2001;119:466-9.

41. Martinez-Frias ML, Rodriguez-Pinilla E. Epidemiologic analysis of prenatal exposure to cough medicines containing dextromethorphan: no evidence of human teratogenicity. *Teratology* 2001;63:38-41.
42. Jick H, Holmes LB, Hunter JR et al. First-trimester drug use and congenital disorders. *JAMA* 1981;246:343-6.
43. Einarson A, Mastroiacovo P, Arnon J et al. Prospective, controlled, multicentre study of loperamide in pregnancy. *Can J Gastroenterol* 2000;14:185-7.
44. Czeizel AE, Toth M, Rockenbauer M. No teratogenic effect after clotrimazole therapy during pregnancy. *Epidemiology* 1999;10:437-40.
45. Rosa FW, Baum C, Shaw M. Pregnancy outcomes after first-trimester vaginitis drug therapy. *Obstet Gynecol* 1987;69:751-5.
46. Adetoro OO. Tioconazole in the management of recurrent vaginal candidosis during pregnancy in Ilorin, Nigeria. *Curr Ther Res Clin Exp* 1987;41:647-50.
47. Drugs and Lactation Database (LactMed). Bethesda: U.S. National Library of Medicine. Available from: toxnet.nlm.nih.gov/cgi-bin/sis/htmlgen?LACT. Accessed December 22, 2015.
48. Kennedy D, Hurst V, Konradsdottir E et al. Pregnancy outcome following exposure to permethrin and use of teratogen information. *Am J Perinatol* 2005;22:87-90.
49. Mytton OT, McGready R, Lee SJ et al. Safety of benzyl benzoate lotion and permethrin in pregnancy: a retrospective matched cohort study. *BJOG* 2007;114:582-7.
50. Mahé A, Perret JL, Ly F et al. The cosmetic use of skin-lightening products during pregnancy in Dakar, Senegal: a common and potentially hazardous practice. *Trans R Soc Trop Med Hyg* 2007;101:183-7.
51. Wester RC, Melendres J, Hui X et al. Human in vivo and in vitro hydroquinone topical bioavailability, metabolism, and disposition. *J Toxicol Environ Health A* 1998;54:301-17.
52. Rayburn WF, Anderson JC, Smith CV et al. Uterine and fetal Doppler flow changes from a single dose of a long-acting intranasal decongestant. *Obstet Gynecol* 1990;76:180-2.
53. Pentel P. Toxicity of over-the-counter stimulants. *JAMA* 1984;252:1898-903.
54. Rothman KJ, Fyler DC, Goldblatt A et al. Exogenous hormones and other drug exposures of children with congenital heart disease. *Am J Epidemiol* 1979;109:433-9.
55. Yau WP, Mitchell AA, Lin KJ et al. Use of decongestants during pregnancy and the risk of birth defects. *Am J Epidemiol* 2013;178:198-208.
56. Cottle MK, Van Petten GR, van Muyden P. Effects of phenylephrine and sodium salicylate on maternal and fetal cardiovascular indices and blood oxygenation in sheep. *Am J Obstet Gynecol* 1982;143:170-6.
57. Bishai R, Mazzotta P, Atanackovic G et al. Critical appraisal of drug therapy for nausea and vomiting of pregnancy: II. Efficacy and safety of diclectin (doxylamine-B6). *Can J Clin Pharmacol* 2000;7:138-43.
58. Michaelis J, Michaelis H, Gluck E et al. Prospective study of suspected associations between certain drugs administered during early pregnancy and congenital malformations. *Teratology* 1983;27:57-64.
59. Miklovich L, van den Berg BJ. An evaluation of the teratogenicity of certain antinauseant drugs. *Am J Obstet Gynecol* 1976;125:244-8.
60. Nelson MM, Forfar JO. Associations between drugs administered during pregnancy and congenital abnormalities of the fetus. *Br Med J* 1971;1:523-7.
61. Nikfar S, Abdollahi M, Moretti ME et al. Use of proton pump inhibitors during pregnancy and rates of major malformations: a meta-analysis. *Dig Dis Sci* 2002;47:1526-9.
62. Erichsen R, Mikkelsen E, Pedersen L et al. Maternal use of proton pump inhibitors during early pregnancy and the prevalence of hypospadias in male offspring. *Am J Ther* 2012;21:254-9.
63. Matok I, Levy A, Wiznitzer A et al. The safety of fetal exposure to proton-pump inhibitors during pregnancy. *Dig Dis Sci* 2012;57:699-705.
64. Marshall JK, Thompson AB, Armstrong D. Omeprazole for refractory gastroesophageal reflux disease during pregnancy and lactation. *Can J Gastroenterol* 1998;12:225-7.

Appendix VI
Nutritional Supplements

L. Maria Gutschi, BScPhm, PharmD

Vitamins and **minerals** cannot usually be synthesized in the body but occur naturally in certain foods. They are essential in small quantities for normal body metabolism, functioning as cofactors within enzyme systems required for the function of life. Some vitamins such as A and D serve in hormonal or epigenetic pathways. If steady intakes are not met, deficiency diseases occur, which can sometimes lead to death. However, excess intake can result in toxicities, even at doses which were generally thought to be safe. Most individuals in North America ingest sufficient vitamins and minerals in their diets to prevent deficiency diseases; a small number may be at risk and require supplementation of particular nutrients for identified deficiencies. Insufficient vitamin D levels may be common in Canadians due to our northern climate since it is derived primarily from exposure to sunlight.

Nutritional supplements are defined as consumable health products that contain a nutrient or group of nutrients (vitamins, minerals, protein, carbohydrates, fats and oils) which occur naturally in food and which are required for normal functioning of the body. They are intended to supplement but not substitute for a healthy diet. Nutrient supplementation can contribute to overall health and vitality, providing sufficient vitamins, minerals and other nutrients for prevention of deficiency diseases. Although preliminary studies may suggest that nutrient supplementation prevents or reduces risk of chronic disease, a benefit is yet to be proven by large trials in most cases. Additionally, long-term nutrient supplementation may be harmful.

Chronic intake of some drugs can affect or interact with vitamins and minerals. Depending on the nature of interaction, it may be necessary to avoid combination therapy, or drug therapy may necessitate supplementation.

Dietary Reference Intakes for Nutrients

The Dietary Reference Intakes (DRIs) are a comprehensive set of nutrient reference values for healthy populations that can be used for assessing and planning diets.[1,2] Established cooperatively by Canada and the United States, DRIs are derived from scientific data and provide a range of values from optimal to maximum based on indicators of good health, prevention of chronic disease and evaluation of the possible adverse effects of excess intake. The DRI encompasses the reference values described below.

The Estimated Average Requirement (EAR) is the median usual intake value that is estimated to meet the requirement of half the healthy individuals in a life-stage and gender group. At this level of intake, the other half of the individuals in the specified group would not have their needs met. The EAR is based on a specific criterion of adequacy, derived from a careful review of the literature. Reduction of disease risk is considered along with many other health parameters in the selection of that criterion. The EAR is used to calculate the Recommended Dietary Allowance (RDA).[1,2] RDA is defined as the average daily dietary intake level thought to be sufficient to meet the nutrient requirement of nearly all (97–98%) healthy individuals in a particular life stage and gender group.[2]

The Adequate Intake (AI) is a recommended average daily nutrient intake level based on observed/experimentally determined estimates of nutrient intake by a group (or groups) of apparently healthy people who are assumed to be maintaining an adequate nutritional state. The AI is used when there are insufficient data to establish the estimated average requirement on which to base the RDA of a nutrient. It is expected to meet or exceed the needs of most people in the age, gender or life-stage group.[2] A diet with nutrient content below 10% of the EAR is considered the threshold for inadequate intake.[3] Nutritional deficiency refers to an inadequate supply of a particular nutrient that results in illness or disease and is corrected by supplementation of the deficient nutrient. Nutritional deficiency may be the result of inadequate dietary intake or impairment of digestion, absorption, transport or metabolism.

Table 1 provides selected DRIs for common nutrients. Table 2 provides information on the roles, food sources, deficiency states and toxicity related to excess intake of the **fat-soluble vitamins** (A, D, E and K). Table 3 provides information on the roles, food sources, deficiency states and toxicity related to excess intake of the **water-soluble vitamins**: thiamine (B_1), riboflavin (B_2), niacin (B_3), pantothenic acid (B_5), biotin (B_7), folic acid (B_9), cyanocobalamin (B_{12}) and ascorbic acid (C). Choline, while not a vitamin, is an essential nutrient usually grouped with the B-complex vitamins. Table 4 provides information on selected **essential minerals**. Macrominerals (with requirements measured in mg to g per day) include calcium, magnesium, phosphorous, potassium and sodium while microminerals (with requirements measured in μg to mg per day) include copper, chromium, fluoride, iodine, iron, manganese, molybdenum, selenium, vanadium and zinc.

Goals of Therapy

- Identify and correct any nutritional deficiencies (Table 5)
- Tailor supplementation to individual and specific diets
- Ensure excess is not consumed and limit antioxidant supplementation
- Ensure no significant drug-nutrient interactions (Table 6)
- Assess benefit vs. risk in individual patients for prevention or treatment of disease (Table 7)

Indications for General Preventive Supplementation

A benefit from micronutrient supplementation is unlikely for most of the general adult population;[4] encourage consumption of whole foods such as fruits, vegetables, whole grains, legumes, nuts and fish as these may contain other important nutrients required for optimal health (e.g., phytochemicals such as flavonoids, isothiocyanates, isoflavones, saponins) and have been shown to decrease risk of chronic disease and mortality.[5,6] Clarity regarding the potential mortality benefit of supplementation with specific nutrients (e.g., vitamin D and omega-3 fatty acids/fish oils) awaits more evidence from prospective randomized controlled trials.[7] Most Canadians have adequate intake of micronutrients although deficiencies in vitamin A, vitamin C, vitamin D, calcium, magnesium, zinc and folate have been identified in high-risk groups (e.g., those at the lowest level of income and/or education).[8] See Table 5 for a discussion of common deficiencies. Certain groups of individuals may require specific preventive supplementation.

Conditions with increased requirements:

- Pregnancy and breastfeeding
  - **folic acid**: pregnant and breastfeeding women require a folic acid supplement in addition to a diet of folate-rich foods. The recommended supplemental dosage is based upon the female's or male partner's risk for a neural tube defect or other folic acid–sensitive congenital anomaly:[9]
    - low risk: 0.4 mg/day beginning at least 2–3 months before conception and continuing until 4–6 weeks postpartum or as long as breastfeeding continues
    - moderate risk: 1 mg/day beginning at least 3 months before conception and continuing until 12 weeks' gestational age; then 0.4–1 mg/day until 4–6 weeks postpartum or as long as breastfeeding continues

    - high risk: 4 mg/day beginning at least 3 months before conception and continuing until 12 weeks' gestational age; then 0.4–1 mg/day until 4–6 weeks postpartum or as long as breastfeeding continues
  - **calcium**: (intake from dietary sources recommended but many people do not ingest enough) 1300 mg/day for women ≤18 years; 1000 mg/day for those ≥19 years[2]
  - **vitamin D**: 600 IU/day;[2] consider 2000 IU/day for pregnant women during winter months[10]
  - **iron**: if supplementation required, recommended dosage is 27 mg/day.[2,11] Routine iron supplementation during pregnancy in nonanemic women (hemoglobin >130 g/L) may not be without adverse effects[12] and 16 mg/day total supplementation is proposed.[13] Intermittent iron supplementation (± folic acid) may be an alternative for preventing gestational anemia in nonanemic women with adequate antenatal care. Intermittent supplementation is less likely to result in adverse events such as nausea and GI disturbances compared with a daily regimen, and results in similar maternal and infant outcomes.[14] Additionally, the risk of high hemoglobin concentrations may be reduced. The most commonly used intermittent dosing schedule is 120 mg weekly elemental iron, given on 1 day of the week in 2 divided doses. This regimen is not recommended for women who are anemic at the start of their pregnancy.[14]
- Drug-nutrient interactions (see Table 6).

Conditions with risk of inadequate intake:

- Very low calorie diet (<800 kcal/day), either voluntary or involuntary (overall insufficient intake)
- Exclusion diets—lack intake of certain foods, e.g., whole grains, deeply coloured vegetables and fruits, fortified cereals, animal-source foods
  - vegan diets:[15,16] vitamin B_{12}, vitamin D, calcium, omega-3 fatty acids (EPA/DHA), iron and zinc
  - lacto-ovo vegetarian diets:[15,17] omega-3 fatty acids (EPA/DHA), iron and zinc
- Chronic substance abuse (in particular for alcohol abuse): vitamin C, vitamin B_1, folic acid, vitamin B_6 and vitamin B_2 (riboflavin)[1]
- Poverty, social isolation, institutionalization:[18] vitamin A, vitamin C, magnesium, calcium, folic acid, vitamin B_{12} and vitamin D
- At-risk elderly (possibly due to polypharmacy, poor oral health, functional limitations, depression, dementia, social isolation): encourage increased oral intake to manage insufficient micronutrient intake.[19,20] Vitamin B_{12} deficiency (primarily due to chronic food-cobalamin malabsorption and to a lesser extent pernicious anemia)[21] and vitamin D deficiency are common in this group and may require supplementation
  - routine vitamin and mineral supplementation may be associated with increased mortality in elderly women, particularly supplemental iron.[22] Supplementation is not associated with a decreased risk of infections in elderly persons living at home[23]
- Children with severely restricted eating patterns.[24,25]

Conditions with risk of malabsorption:

- Bariatric surgery: vitamins A, D, K, B_1, B_{12}, C and folic acid; calcium, copper, iron, selenium, and zinc. Patients require routine supplementation with vitamins and minerals for 2 years or more, with doses higher than those provided by nonprescription supplements[26,27]
- GI diseases known to cause malabsorption or maldigestion (e.g., lactose intolerance, gluten-sensitive enteropathy, food allergies): fat-soluble vitamins, vitamin B_{12}, vitamin K, zinc, iron, calcium
- Swallowing, chewing or dental problems.

Table 1: Daily Dietary Reference Intakes for Vitamins and Selected Minerals[1,2]

Age, Gender or Life Stage	Vitamins													Minerals				
	A (IU)	B_1 (mg)	B_2 (mg)	B_3 (mg)	Panto-thenic Acid[a] (B_5) (mg)	B_6 (mg)	Biotin[a] (B_7) (µg)	Folate[b] (B_9) (µg)	B_{12} (µg)	C (mg)	D (IU)	E (mg)	K[a] (µg)	Ca[a] (mg)	Fe (mg)	F[a] (mg)	Se (µg)	Zn (mg)
0–6 months[a]	1333	0.2	0.3	2	1.7	0.1	5	65	0.4	40	400	4	2	200	0.27	0.01	15	2
7–12 months[a]	1667	0.3	0.4	4	1.8	0.3	6	80	0.5	50	400	5	2.5	260	11[c]	0.5	20	3[c]
1–3 y	1000	0.5	0.5	6	2	0.5	8	150	0.9	15	600	6	30	700	7	0.7	20	3
4–8 y	1333	0.6	0.6	8	3	0.6	12	200	1.2	25	600	7	55	1000	10	1	30	5
9–13 y	2000	0.9	0.9	12	4	1.0	20	300	1.8	45	600	11	60	1300	8	2	40	8
14–18 y Male	3000	1.2	1.3	16	5	1.3	25	400	2.4	75	600	15	75	1300	11	3	55	11
14–18 y Female	2333	1.0	1.0	14	5	1.2	25	400[d]	2.4	65	600	15	75	1300	15	3	55	9
14–18 y Pregnancy	2500	1.4	1.4	18	6	1.9	30	600[d]	2.6	80	600	15	75	1300	27	3	60	12
14–18 y Breastfeeding	4000	1.4	1.6	17	7	2.0	35	500	2.8	115	600	19	75	1300	10	3	70	13
19–50 y Male	3000	1.2	1.3	16	5	1.3	30	400	2.4	90	600	15	120	1000	8	4	55	11
19–50 y Female	2333	1.1	1.1	14	5	1.3	30	400[d]	2.4	75	600	15	90	1000	18	3	55	8
19–50 y Pregnancy	2567	1.4	1.4	18	6	1.9	30	600[d]	2.6	85	600	15	90	1000	27	3	60	11
19–50 y Breastfeeding	4333	1.4	1.6	17	7	2	35	500	2.8	120	600	19	90	1000	9	3	70	12
51–70 y Male	3000	1.2	1.3	16	5	1.7	30	400	2.4	90	600	15	120	1000	8	4	55	11
51–70 y Female	2333	1.1	1.1	14	5	1.5	30	400	2.4	75	600	15	90	1200	8	3	55	8
≥71 y Male	3000	1.2	1.3	16	5	1.7	30	400	2.4	90	800	15	120	1200	8	4	55	11
≥71 y Female	2333	1.1	1.1	14	5	1.5	30	400	2.4	75	800	15	90	1200	8	3	55	8

[a] RDA unknown; values represent AI.
[b] As dietary folate equivalents DFE (1 DFE = 1 µg folate from food = 0.5 µg folic acid supplement taken on an empty stomach = 0.6 µg from a fortified food or a supplement consumed with food).
[c] Value represents RDA.
[d] All women capable of becoming pregnant should take a supplement of 400 µg of folic acid daily, in addition to the amount of folate found in a healthy diet; this supplement should continue until a pregnancy is confirmed and prenatal care begins. The critical time for neural tube formation is shortly after conception.

Abbreviations: AI = adequate intake; Ca = calcium; F = fluoride; Fe = iron; RDA = recommended dietary allowance; Se = selenium; Zn = zinc

Table 2: **Fat-soluble Vitamins**[1,2,28]

Nutrient	Role and Sources	Deficiency State	Toxicity	Prevention of Toxicity
vitamin A (retinol)	Required for vision, bone growth, reproduction, cell division, cell differentiation. Regulates immune system and gene transcription. Food sources (preformed vitamin A): Liver, fish oils, whole milk, eggs, fortified food products. Food sources (provitamin A): Leafy green vegetables, orange and yellow vegetables, tomato products, fruits.	▪ Deficiency rare, but inadequate intake of retinol reported in 35% of Canadians ≥19 years of age[2] ▪ Abnormal visual adaptation to darkness:[29,30] – Changes in conjunctiva called Bitot spots – Severe deficiency causes blindness ▪ Dry skin, hair and eyes[29,30] ▪ Broken fingernails ▪ Decreased resistance to infections (diarrhea and measles)[29,30] ▪ Papillary hyperkeratosis of the skin[29,30] ▪ Patients/populations at risk of Vitamin A deficiency:[1] – recent immigrants or refugees from developing countries with high incidence of vitamin A deficiency or measles – patients with Crohn's disease – patients with celiac disease – patients with pancreatic diseases	TUL: 10 000 IU/day. Teratogenic at doses >10 000 IU/day. Hepatotoxic. High intake of preformed vitamin A through diet or supplementation may be associated with osteoporosis and fracture risk;[31] can occur subclinically without signs or symptoms of hypervitaminosis at total doses of 5000 IU/day; risk may be highest in those with low vitamin D intake.[32]	Avoid supplementation of preformed vitamin A (retinol) in populations not at risk for deficiency. Encourage dietary intake from vegetables and fruits as there is no evidence of increased osteoporosis risk from dietary intake.
beta-carotene	Food sources (carotenoids): Coloured fruits and vegetables.		No TUL established for dietary beta-carotene.[33] Oral beta-carotene supplements increase risk of first-time nonfatal MI, increase risk of CV mortality[34,35] in adult male smokers; increase risk of lung cancer diagnosis and death in patients at high risk.[35] Vitamin A and beta-carotene supplementation, singly or combined, increase risk of overall mortality.[33]	No RDA established, but 3–6 mg/day recommended. Supplementation with beta-carotene not generally required but may be used for patients/populations at risk of vitamin A deficiency (see Vitamin A) High serum concentrations of alpha-carotene (also found in yellow-orange and dark green vegetables) are associated with decreased risk of mortality.[36] Lycopene, lutein and zeaxanthin are carotenoids which do not have vitamin A activity but have health promoting activity.

Nutrient	Role and Sources	Deficiency State	Toxicity	Prevention of Toxicity
vitamin D (D_3: cholecalciferol D_2: ergocalciferol)	Modulates transcription of >50 genes in cell differentiation, immunity, insulin secretion, hypertension. Required for calcium metabolism. Food sources: Salmon, sardines, tuna and fish oils, fortified milk/orange juice, some mushrooms. Sunlight (activates 7-dehydrocholesterol in the skin).	▪ Insufficiency and deficiency common in Canadians (see Table 5) ▪ Children:[37] – Rickets (costochondral beading, epiphyseal enlargement, bowed legs, persistently open anterior fontanelle) ▪ Adults:[37] – Osteomalacia/osteoporosis	TUL: 4000 IU/day. Hypercalcemia, hypercalciuria, reversible renal impairment, GI symptoms. Single yearly high doses (500 000 IU orally or 300 000 IU IM) have been associated with increased risk of falls and fracture rates especially in the first months post-dose.[38] 400 IU/day plus 2 g/day of calcium was associated with small increased risk of nephrolithiasis.[39] Persons with primary hyperparathyroidism, sarcoidosis, tuberculosis and lymphoma may have increased risk of hypercalcemia with supplementation.	Cholecalciferol (vitamin D_3) most useful in primary care. Avoid large single doses (10 000 IU or more). Total amounts of vitamin D ingestion from various supplements should be recorded/monitored.
vitamin E (α-tocopherol)	Required as an antioxidant for protection from damaging effects of free radicals. Food sources: Nuts, seeds, vegetable oils, egg yolk, wheat germ, fortified or enriched grain products.	▪ Children:[40] – Hemolytic anemia in premature infants and newborns – Hyporeflexia – Spinocerebellar and retinal degeneration ▪ Adults (rare):[40] – Overt deficiency syndromes in adults have never been described	TUL: 1000 mg (1500 IU)/day. GI upset at doses of 200–800 mg/day, antiplatelet effects and bleeding at 800–1200 mg/day. Other toxicity can occur at 1200 mg/day (emotional disturbances, thrombophlebitis, lipid and thyroid effects, gonadal dysfunction).[41] Intervention trials have not supported the hypothesis that vitamin E decreases CV risk[42,43] or prevents cancer.[42,44] Vitamin E supplementation: ▪ showed a small increased risk of heart failure in people at high risk of CVD[44] ▪ may increase risk of death from any cause at doses >400 IU/day[45] ▪ has no significant effect on the incidence or number of days of respiratory infections or antibiotic use[46] ▪ may increase risk of prostate cancer[47]	Little or no supplementation in patients with a history of stroke, CABG surgery, MI or those at risk of prostate cancer. Limit vitamin E supplementation for others to <400 IU/day. Ensure no significant drug-nutrient interactions which can increase bleeding risk (see Table 6).
vitamin K	Required for blood clotting and bone formation. Food sources: Green leafy vegetables, vegetable oils.	▪ Neonates (common):[48,49] – prolonged bleeding and prothrombin time, hemorrhagic manifestations in newborns ▪ Adults (uncommon):[49] – unexpected or excessive bleeding	TUL has not been determined.	Single ingredient oral supplements are not available in Canada. Excess intake of vitamin K from food sources may interfere with the effect of vitamin K antagonist anticoagulants, e.g., warfarin.

(cont'd)

Table 2: **Fat-soluble Vitamins**[1,2,28] *(cont'd)*

Nutrient	Role and Sources	Deficiency State	Toxicity	Prevention of Toxicity
		▪ Risk factors: – alcohol abuse – general malnutrition – malabsorption states – disseminated intravascular coagulation – parencymal liver disease – polycythemia vera		

Abbreviations: AI = adequate intake, established when evidence is insufficient to develop an RDA; is set at a level assumed to ensure nutritional adequacy; CABG = coronary artery bypass graft; CV = cardiovascular; CVD = cardiovascular disease; RDA = recommended dietary allowance, i.e., average daily level of intake sufficient to meet the nutrient requirements of nearly all (97–98%) healthy individuals; TUL = tolerable upper limit, i.e., maximum average daily intake likely to cause no risk of adverse health effects

Table 3: **Water-soluble Vitamins**[1,2,28]

Nutrient	Role and Sources	Deficiency State	Toxicity	Prevention of Toxicity
vitamin B_1 (thiamine)	Required coenzyme for mitochondrial enzymes involved in critical roles in the production of energy from food. Food sources: Wide variety of foods including cereals (rice, wheat), legumes, nuts, wheat germ, pork.	▪ Beriberi (wet): – High-output cardiac failure – Palpitations, weakness, SOB ▪ Beriberi (dry): – Peripheral neuropathy (burning feet syndrome) – Absent knee jerk and deep tendon reflexes – Progressive weakness and muscle atrophy ▪ Sensory disturbances occur first followed by motor disturbances ▪ Wernicke syndrome (CNS involvement occurs in alcohol abusers): – Confusion – Ataxia – Nystagmus ▪ Risk factors: – Malabsoption/malnutrition – Prolonged dieting – Weight loss surgery – Alcohol abuse – Long-term diuretic use; heart failure[50] – Dialysis[51] ▪ Treatment with thiamine as the initial test is used to diagnose deficency	TUL has not been determined.	
vitamin B_2 (riboflavin)	Integral component of flavoenzymes required for redox reactions and metabolism of carbohydrates, fats and proteins. Food sources: Wide variety of foods including fortified cereals, milk and milk products, meat, eggs, nuts.	▪ Deficiency rarely found in isolation. Signs/ symptoms include: – Cheilosis – Angular stomatitis – Glossitis – Seborrheic dermatitis – Corneal vascularization	TUL has not been determined.	

(cont'd)

Table 3: **Water-soluble Vitamins**[1,2,28] *(cont'd)*

Nutrient	Role and Sources	Deficiency State	Toxicity	Prevention of Toxicity
		– Photophobia ▪ Riboflavin deficiency may predispose pregnant women to preeclampsia ▪ Risk factors: – Alcohol abuse – Hypothyrodism or adrenal insufficiency – Lactose intolerance – Malabsorptive states – Pregnancy and lactation – End stage renal disease, dialysis[51]		
vitamin B_3 (niacin, nicotinic acid, niacinamide)	Required to produce hemoglobin and to increase its oxygen-carrying capacity. Helps maintain blood glucose levels in normal range. Food sources: Wide variety of foods including beans, meats, cereals, vegetables.	▪ Pellagra: – Dermatitis (thick scaly pigmented rash in areas exposed to sunlight) – Diarrhea and inflammation of mouth and tongue (glossitis) – Dementia (apathy, disorientation, memory loss) – Also: ○ Sensitivity to sunlight ○ Aggressiveness ○ Insomnia ○ Weakness ○ Ataxia ▪ Risk factors: – Diets high in corn and low in protein – Anorexia nervosa or obesity – Dialysis[51] – Homelessness – Alcoholism – HIV/AIDS	TUL: 35 mg/day Prostaglandin-mediated flushing occurs in doses >30 mg/day (itching, increased intracranial blood flow, headache). Use of large doses (>3 g/day) may cause elevated liver enzyme levels and is a risk factor for jaundice and hepatotoxicity (more common with sustained-release formulations), GI symptoms, impaired glucose tolerance.	Limit routine supplementation to <30 mg/day. Treatment of lipid disorders requires larger doses and should be monitored by a clinician.
vitamin B_5 (pantothenic acid)	Component of coenzyme A which is required to produce energy from food. Food sources: Liver, kidney, yeast, egg yolk, legumes, broccoli.	▪ Deficiency exceptionally rare	TUL has not been determined.	

Nutrient	Role and Sources	Deficiency State	Toxicity	Prevention of Toxicity
vitamin B_6 (pyridoxine)	Has role in production of >100 enzymes required for chemical reactions, e.g., glycogen phosphorylation. Food sources: Fortified cereals, poultry, potatoes, spinach, avocados, bananas, nuts.	▪ Severe deficiency uncommon ▪ Inadequacy associated with: – Microcytic anemia – Seborrhoeic skin lesions, – Convulsions – Irritability, nervousness, insomnia – Peripheral neuropathy (distal limb numbness appears early, distal limb paresthesia or burning foot syndrome occurs later) ▪ Pyridoxine neuropathy occurs in both deficiency and toxicity states ▪ Deficiency also leads to hyperhomocysteinemia ▪ Risk factors: – Sickle cell disease – Malnutrition and malabsorption – Dialysis – Rheumatoid arthritis – Treatment with isoniazide, hydralazine, pyrazinamide – Alcohol abuse	TUL: 100 mg/day Sensory neuropathy with progressive ataxia can occur with high-dose supplementation (100–500 mg/day); reversible upon discontinuation. Supplementation to reduce hyperhomocysteinemia and subsequent atherosclerosis has been disappointing.	Avoid high-dose supplementation.
vitamin B_7 (biotin)	Required for mammalian carboxylase enzymes. Food sources: Egg yolks, liver, yeast, bananas, grapefruit, watermelon, most vegetables.	▪ Deficiency exceptionally rare	TUL has not been determined.	
folic acid (folate)[a]	Required for new cell growth formation and maintenance, especially during periods of rapid growth. Food sources: Legumes (cooked kidney, pinto, fava beans), green leafy vegetables (spinach), liver, fortified flour (mandatory in Canada), fortified breakfast cereals, oranges.	▪ Megaloblastic anemia ▪ Adverse fetal outcomes: – Neural tube defects – Orofacial clefts – Cardiovascular malformations ▪ Risk factors: – Anorexia nervosa – Malabsorption	TUL: 1000 µg/day Doses >1500 µg/day can cause irritability, confusion, exacerbation of seizure frequency, precipitate or exacerbate vitamin B_{12} deficiency. Potential increase in CV risk and colon cancer[52,53] and chronic high doses may	Studies demonstrate mixed results regarding unmetabolized folic acid or intracellular folate and increased cancer and CV risk;[52,56] more study is required to delineate risk-benefit profile. Avoid supplements unless higher folate need is identified (e.g., pregnancy, breastfeeding, methotrexate use).

(cont'd)

Table 3: **Water-soluble Vitamins**[1,2,28] *(cont'd)*

Nutrient	Role and Sources	Deficiency State	Toxicity	Prevention of Toxicity
		– Alcohol abuse – Hyperthyroidism – Pregnancy and lactation – Dialysis[51]	increase risk of solid cancers.[54] Increased rate of cognitive decline in elderly who take large doses is possibly related to low vitamin B_{12} levels.[55]	Limit total supplement intake to ≤0.4 mg/day. Emphasize foods high in folate (e.g., green leafy vegetables, fruits) as intake from foods is not associated with adverse effects.
vitamin B_{12} (cyanocobalamin)	Required for red blood cell formation, DNA synthesis and neurological function. Food sources: Meat, fish, shellfish, eggs, poultry, fortified cereals.	▪ Pernicious anemia ▪ Neurologic deterioration: – Peripheral neuropathy – Cognitive impairment ▪ Deficiency common in Canada[57] (see Table 6)	TUL has not been determined.	
choline	Although not a vitamin, choline is an essential nutrient for structural integrity of cell membranes, cholinergic neurotransmission, and lipid and cholesterol transport and metabolism. Accelerates synthesis and release of acetylcholine. Food sources: Milk, liver, eggs, peanuts; small amounts are synthesized in humans from phospholipids. Dietary sources provide approximately 730–1040 mg/day of choline, mostly as lecithin (phosphatidylcholine).[58]		TUL: 3.5 g/day Ingestion of 7.5 g/day may cause hypotension. Cholinergic signs (sweating and diarrhea) and a fishy body odour may occur with doses of 10–16 g/day.[58]	
vitamin C (ascorbic acid)	Required for collagen formation, *l*-carnitine and protein synthesis. Maintains integrity of skin, connective tissue, bone, blood vessel walls and dentine. Required for wound healing and recovery from burns. Vitamin C is an important physiological antioxidant and regenerates other antioxidants including vitamin E. Food sources: Fruits (especially citrus), vegetables (peppers).	▪ Chronic severe deficiency results in scurvy (rare) ▪ Early presentation: – Malaise and lethargy – Irritability – Dry mouth and eyes ▪ Skin changes include perifollicular hemorrhages, corkscrew hairs ▪ Purpura/ecchymoses seen on legs or buttocks ▪ Splinter hemorrhages	TUL: 2 g/day Several grams taken at once can cause nausea, vomiting, esophagitis and heartburn, flushing and diarrhea. Sleep disturbances and fatigue have also been reported. Long-term ingestion of 2 g/day may precipitate urate or oxalate stones in the urinary tract and increase risk of nephrolithiasis.[59]	Limit supplementation to <2 g/day.

Nutrient	Role and Sources	Deficiency State	Toxicity	Prevention of Toxicity
		▪ Bleeding gums, friability, tooth loss ▪ Anemia and high output heart failure seen late in the disease ▪ Fractures, bleeding into muscles and joints ▪ Risk factors: – Receiving only cow's milk during first year of life – Alcoholism – Elderly – Low income – Smoking – Increased need in pregnancy and lactation, thyrotoxicoses, burns, insulin deficiency – Dialysis[51] – Anorexia nervosa or anorexia due to cancer or HIV infection – Fad diets or severely restricted eating patterns ▪ Depletion can occur within 1–3 months; fatal if untreated but prevention requires only 35 mg/day		

[a] Folate refers to the form found naturally in foods; folic acid is the synthetic form used in fortified foods and supplements.

Abbreviations: AI = adequate intake, established when evidence is insufficient to develop an RDA; is set at a level assumed to ensure nutritional adequacy; CV = cardiovascular; RDA = recommended dietary allowance, i.e., average daily level of intake sufficient to meet the nutrient requirements of nearly all (97–98%) healthy individuals; SOB = shortness of breath; TUL = tolerable upper limit, i.e., maximum average daily intake likely to cause no risk of adverse health effects

Table 4: **Selected Macro- and Microminerals**[1]

Nutrient	Sources	Toxicity	Management
calcium	Food sources: Dairy products, calcium-set tofu, fortified foods, kale and related greens (broccoli, bok choy, cabbage). Deficiency not uncommon in selected patient groups in Canada (see Table 5).	TUL: 2500 mg/day Studies demonstrated mixed results concerning increased risk of cardiac events, particularly MI, if excess calcium supplementation is used with or without vitamin D.[60,61,62,63,64] Calcium intake of >2 g/day (dietary or supplement) may be associated with increased risk of prostate cancer.[65] More trials required to determine if there is a risk of calcium supplementation, especially in persons with adequate dietary calcium intake.	Typical diet provides 500–1000 mg elemental calcium/day; avoid total amounts (from diet and oral supplements) >1.2 g/day. Ensure adequate vitamin D intake.
iron[a]	Food sources (heme iron from hemoglobin): Meat, poultry, fish. Deficiency not uncommon in selected patient groups in Canada (see Table 5).	TUL: 45 mg/day Excess iron is stored in tissues and organs, e.g., liver, heart and may lead to cirrhosis, heart failure. Iron is extremely toxic in overdose; accidental poisoning/death has occurred in children with ingestion of as little as 200 mg.[66]	Avoid supplementation unless prescribed for known or suspected iron deficiency or for increased need. Absorption of nonheme iron, e.g., from plant sources, may be influenced by enhancers (ascorbic or malic acid) or inhibitors (polyphenols, phytates, soy protein).
magnesium	Food sources: Green leafy vegetables; nuts, seeds, whole grains, foods high in fibre.	TUL: 350 mg/day Acute: doses of >5 g are associated with hypotension, nausea, vomiting, facial flushing leading to muscle weakness, breathing difficulties, cardiac arrythmias (plasma levels >1.74–2.61 mmol/L). Chronic: high doses from supplementation/medications may cause diarrhea, nausea, cramping.	Average intake is generally less than recommended, however low dietary intake does not generally result in symptomatic magnesium deficiency. Toxicity risks increased with impaired renal function.
potassium	Food sources: Fruits and vegetables, especially tropical fruits, baked potatoes with skin.	TUL has not been determined for healthy adults. Doses >11 g as a single dose may lead to hyperkalemia in persons who are not accustomed to high intakes even if there is normal kidney function. Acute or chronic renal failure, excessive aldosterone secretion and medications (e.g., potassium-sparing diuretics, ACEIs, ARBs, SMX/TMP) increase risk of hyperkalemia.	Routine supplementation of potassium is not recommended.

Nutrient	Sources	Toxicity	Management
selenium	Food sources: Organ meats, seafood; plant sources dependent on selenium content of soil. Average diet provides approximately 100 µg/day.	TUL: 400 µg/day Selenosis (hair and nail brittleness and loss, gastrointestinal upset, garlic breath odour, fatigue, irritability and mild neuropathy) is rare.[1] Cases were reported in 13 subjects taking supplements which, due to a manufacturing error, contained 27.3 mg (27 300 µg) per tablet.[67]	
zinc	Food sources: Shellfish, red meat, nuts, legumes.	TUL: 40 mg/day Acute: Nausea, vomiting, anorexia, abdominal cramps. Chronic: Doses 150–450 mg/day affect copper status, alter iron function, decrease immune function, decrease HDL. Doses >80 mg/day as used in the AREDS study have been associated with significant increase in genitourinary hospitalizations.[68]	Avoid high-dose supplementation. Monitor persons on high doses of zinc for treatment of macular degeneration for genitourinary effects (urinary retention, UTI, urinary lithiasis).

[a] RDAs are given as doses of elemental iron. Requirements are 1.8 times higher in vegetarians due to the lower bioavailability of iron from a vegetarian diet.

Abbreviations: AI = adequate intake, established when evidence is insufficient to develop an RDA; is set at a level assumed to ensure nutritional adequacy; ARB = angiotensin II receptor blocker; AREDS = Age-Related Eye Disease Study; HDL = high-density lipoprotein; RDA = recommended dietary allowance, i.e., average daily level of intake sufficient to meet the nutrient requirements of nearly all (97–98%) healthy individuals; SMX/TMP = sulfamethoxazole/trimethoprim; TUL = tolerable upper limit, i.e., maximum average daily intake likely to cause no risk of adverse health effects; UTI = urinary tract infection

Table 5: **Supplementation to Prevent or Treat Common Deficiency States**

Deficiency	Patient Groups Affected	Recommendations
vitamin D (cholecalciferol) Adequate levels:[a] >50 nmol/L Deficiency (<25 nmol/L) may be associated with muscle pain, bone pain Suboptimal levels (25–75 nmol/L) may be associated with:[69,70] ▪ Decreased bone health, osteoporosis ▪ Increased CV risk ▪ Muscle weakness and falls ▪ Increased risk of cognitive decline in the elderly,[71] schizophrenia,[72] type I diabetes, depression, cancer (colon, possibly breast and prostate), cancer mortality, multiple sclerosis Evidence from observational studies suggests an association between low serum vitamin D and all-cause and cardiovascular mortality.[73,74] Large randomized controlled trials are required to determine whether vitamin D supplementation mitigates this risk.[75,76] Measurement of vitamin D levels is not routinely required[b] unless high risk of deficiency or concerns regarding toxicity[77]	Approximately 10% of Canadians have inadequate levels for bone health and are at risk for rickets or osteomalacia; 60% have levels <75 nmol/L,[78] the suggested level needed for overall health and disease prevention. Patient groups at increased risk of deficiency/suboptimal levels include:[69] ▪ Dark-skinned individuals ▪ Lack of sunlight due to northern latitude, use of occlusive clothing, staying indoors (e.g., elderly, obese or institutionalized persons) ▪ Medication-induced (see Table 6). Modest decrease in overall mortality, primarily seen in elderly women who are institutionalized or in dependent care.[79]	Health Canada RDA (Table 1) differs from those of other groups: Osteoporosis Canada[80] recommends routine vitamin D supplementation for all Canadian adults year round: ▪ Adults 19–50 y (including pregnant or breastfeeding women): 400–1000 IU daily ▪ Adults >50 y and those at high risk:[c] 800–2000 IU daily International Osteoporosis Foundation[81] ▪ Older adults: 800–1000 IU/day ▪ Obese, limited sun exposure, non-European populations: 2000 IU/day Canadian Cancer Society[82] ▪ Adults during fall and winter months: 1000 IU/day ▪ Adults ≥ 50 y, dark skin or little sun exposure: 1000 IU/day all year round Canadian Pediatric Society[83] ▪ Pregnancy and breastfeeding: Consider 2000 IU/day, especially during winter months[d] Maintenance range: 400–2000 IU/day Evidence and safety supports use of 800–1000 IU/day in Canadians. For severe deficiency (levels <25 nmol/L), consider bolus dosing followed by maintenance: ▪ 2000–4000 IU of D_3 daily for 8–20 wk *or* ▪ 600 000 IU of D_2 over 8 wk (e.g., 50 000 IU weekly for 8–12 wk)[69] Optimal form of vitamin D and regimen for bolus dosing for severe deficiency have not been established. Appropriate vitamin D levels may improve dietary absorption of calcium.[69,84]
vitamin B_{12} Pernicious anemia occurs in 2–4% of US population; overall rate of vitamin B_{12} insufficiency is estimated at 1.5–15%[85]	Persons with macrocytosis or neurologic symptoms. Persons >60 y (marginal depletion reported to be >20%).[86] Persons with gastric, ileal, pancreatic, Crohn's, or celiac disease. Chronic use of PPIs, metformin or H_2 receptor antagonists. Exclusion diets.[87]	Encourage persons at risk of vitamin B_{12} deficiency to consume foods high in vitamin B_{12}. Malabsorption of vitamin B_{12} from food is the main cause of deficiency in the elderly. Consider 1000 µg/day orally for persons taking drugs known to deplete vitamin B_{12} stores.

Deficiency	Patient Groups Affected	Recommendations
calcium	Postmenopausal women.[88] Vegans or those who limit dairy product intake (e.g., due to lactose intolerance). Persons with anorexia or excess exercise leading to amenorrhea.[89]	In postmenopausal women, ≤400 IU vitamin D and ≤1000 mg of calcium supplements provided no benefit for the primary prevention of fractures;[90] high quality evidence for the benefit of higher doses of vitamin D is lacking but 800–2000 IU/day is often recommended.[88] Excess calcium supplementation should be avoided (limit to ≤1200 mg/day from all sources).[88] Calcium carbonate should be taken with food to improve absorption; calcium citrate can be taken without food and is more readily absorbable. Avoid doses >500 mg elemental calcium at one time. Constipation, gas or bloating may be managed with smaller, more frequent dosing, or differing formulations or salts. Vegans and others who limit dairy intake can also obtain adequate dietary calcium through foods such as beans, tofu, nuts, fortified nut or soy beverages, blackstrap molasses, and a variety of vegetables including low-oxalate greens (e.g., bok choy, broccoli, Chinese cabbage, collards, and kale).[15,91]
iron	Female adolescents, women with heavy menstrual losses. Those at high risk of malabsorption (e.g., Crohn's or celiac disease). Patients with renal failure, especially those on dialysis. Persons who engage in intense aerobic exercise; female and vegetarian/vegan athletes; distance runners may also be at risk.[66]	Adult men and postmenopausal women should not take a supplement unless evaluated, as deficiency is rare and supplementation may be harmful.[22] Vegetarians/vegans should consider consuming nonheme sources of iron together with foods high in vitamin C (e.g., citrus fruits) to improve absorption.

[a] Evidence of the relationship between disease due to vitamin D insufficiency and 25-hydroxyvitamin D levels is evolving.
[b] Excludes patients with conditions such as osteoporosis, rickets, osteopenia, malabsorption syndromes and renal disease or those taking drugs that affect vitamin D metabolism.
[c] High-risk adults are those with osteoporosis, multiple fractures or conditions affecting vitamin D absorption.
[d] The effectiveness of this regimen and possible side effects should be checked with periodic assays for 25(OH)D and calcium.

Abbreviations: CV = cardiovascular; IU = international unit; PPI = proton pump inhibitor; RDA = recommended dietary allowance; SPF = sun protection factor

Table 6: **Clinically Significant Drug–Nutritional Supplement Interactions**[41,92]

Supplement	Drug	Interaction	Management
beta-carotene, vitamin A	Hepatotoxic drugs (acetaminophen, carbamazepine, isoniazid, methotrexate)	May increase risk of liver disease.	Avoid combination.
	Retinoids (isotretinoin, acitretin, etretinate, tazarotene)	Additive toxic effects.	Avoid combination.
	Warfarin	Increased risk of vitamin A toxicity and bleeding.	Avoid combination.
calcium	Diuretics	Possible hypocalcemia (with loop diuretics) or hypercalcemia (with thiazides).	May require calcium supplementation with loop diuretics.
	Fluoroquinolones, tetracyclines, bisphosphonates, glucocorticoids	Decreased absorption, possible decreased efficacy, risk of treatment failure.	Separate calcium doses at least 4 h apart from bisphosphonates; consider temporarily discontinuing supplementation while receiving fluoroquinolones or tetracyclines. Normal dairy intake is unlikely to decrease efficacy.
folic acid	Methotrexate (low-dose)	Increased folate requirements to prevent GI and liver toxicity.	Supplement with 1–5 mg/day; avoid on days when methotrexate ingested.
	Phenytoin	Folic acid may be a cofactor in phenytoin metabolism, decrease serum phenytoin levels with large doses of folic acid and potential increase in seizure frequency.	Avoid folic acid supplements >1 mg/day.
iron	Allopurinol	Increased iron storage in liver.	Avoid combination.
	Bisphosphonates, fluoroquinolones, levothyroxine, levodopa, tetracyclines	Form insoluble complexes with iron.	Separate doses at least 2 h apart. Avoid iron and levodopa combination.
	PPIs,[93] H_2 antagonists	Decrease absorption of nonheme iron, retard clinical response to iron supplementation.	May require change to heme iron formulation if iron-deficiency anemia occurs on chronic PPI therapy. Separate doses at least 2 h apart.
magnesium	Bisphosphonates, tetracyclines	Forms insoluble complexes; results in reduced absorption.	Separate doses by at least 2 h.

Supplement	Drug	Interaction	Management
	Diuretics	Loop/thiazide diuretics: Possible magnesium depletion. Potassium-sparing diuretics: Reduced magnesium excretion.	Regular monitoring of magnesium levels required.
	PPIs[94]	Chronic long-term use of PPIs may cause hypomagnesemia. Possibly accompanied by hypocalcemia and hypokalemia.	Periodic monitoring suggested. Supplements may be required.
niacin	Antihyperglycemic agents	Impairs glucose tolerance in a dose-dependent manner.	Doses >4 g/day may increase plasma glucose by an average of 16% and HbA_{1c} by 21%; increased requirements for antihyperglycemic agents may be necessary.
	Carbamazepine	Niacin 60–80 mg/day may increase carbamazepine levels.	Monitor carbamazepine levels, avoid niacin supplementation.
	Statins	Increased risk of myopathies.	Monitor signs and symptoms, use lowest dose possible.
pyridoxine (vitamin B_6)	Antiepileptic drugs (phenytoin, phenobarbital)	Can decrease phenytoin and phenobarbital serum levels by increasing metabolism.	Discontinue pyridoxine or increase dose of antiepileptic drug.
	Isoniazid	Acts as an antagonist and can induce peripheral neuropathy.	Supplementation recommended but limit pyridoxine to 10–50 mg/day.
	Levodopa	Decreased anti-parkinson effect.	Avoid supplementation; consider treatment with levodopa/carbidopa combination.
vitamin B_{12}	H_2 blockers	Possible decreased vitamin B_{12} levels but evidence is conflicting.	
	Metformin	10–30% of patients who take metformin may have decreased vitamin B_{12} absorption.	Supplementation of crystalline vitamin B_{12} may be required.
	PPIs[93]	Reduce absorption (probably by inhibiting intragastric proteolysis and the release of vitamin B_{12} from food).	Supplementation of crystalline vitamin B_{12} may be required, especially in the elderly or if on PPI >10 y.
vitamin D	Antiepileptic drugs (carbamazepine, phenytoin, phenobarbital)	Increased vitamin D metabolism to inactive compounds and decreased calcium absorption.	Supplementation may be required.

(cont'd)

Table 6: Clinically Significant Drug–Nutritional Supplement Interactions[41,92] *(cont'd)*

Supplement	Drug	Interaction	Management
	Cholestyramine, colestipol, orlistat	Decreased absorption.	Supplementation may be required.
	Corticosteroids	Can impair vitamin D metabolism; long-term use can contribute to development of osteoporosis as corticosteroids also inhibit calcium absorption.	Supplementation may be required.
	Rifampin	Increased vitamin D metabolism.	Supplementation may be required.
vitamin E	Warfarin, ASA, NSAIDs	May increase risk of bleeding.	Limit vitamin E dose to ≤200 IU/day and monitor INR.

Abbreviations: HbA_{1c} = hemoglobin A_{1c}; INR = International Normalized Ratio; PPI = proton pump inhibitor

Table 7: **Evidence-based Supplementation to Prevent or Treat Disease**

Disease/Condition	Supplement	Evidence of Benefit/Risk	Recommendations
Age-related macular degeneration	*antioxidants plus copper and zinc*	May be beneficial; data primarily from AREDS[95] in patients with age-related macular degeneration (AMD). The addition of lutein and zeaxanthin or omega-3 fatty acids to the original AREDS formula did not demonstrate reduced risk of progression of AMD.[96]	Discuss supplementation with specialist/family physician since data are not available for other patient groups. Beta-carotene–containing formulations are no longer recommended for prevention of AMD progression because of an increased risk of lung cancer.[96] Lutein and zeaxanthin may be a suitable replacement for beta-carotene in the original AREDS formulation.
Cardiovascular disease, primary prevention	*omega-3 fatty acids*	Benefits of fatty fish/omega-3 fatty acid supplementation have been questioned.[97,98] Definitive benefits to be determined in upcoming trials.	2 servings weekly of low-mercury fish (tuna, sardines, salmon) recommended. May consider supplementation to provide 1 g/day of EPA+DHA[a] in those who do not consume fish. Persons with sensitivity to finned fish appear to tolerate fish oil supplements;[99] alternatively a DHA supplement derived from algae may be used for vegetarians, vegans or those with severe allergies.
	vitamin D	Supplementation in older patients (>70 y) with isolated systolic hypertension did not improve blood pressure, despite baseline low 25-hydroxyvitamin D levels.[100] Dosing of 100 000 IU/3 months may be a study limitation.	Vitamin D supplementation is unlikely beneficial for primary prevention of cardiovascular disease.
	folic acid	Folic acid in combination with enalapril appears to reduce the risk of first stroke in persons with hypertension but without established CVD.[101]	Persons with the lowest baseline folate levels benefitted the most. Applicability to the Canadian population with mandatory folic acid fortification program is uncertain.
Cardiovascular disease, secondary prevention	*B vitamins (folic acid, vitamin B_6, vitamin B_{12}) and antioxidants*	No benefit seen on CV events with B vitamins and potential harm from antioxidants.[102,103,104,105]	Avoid routine use.
	omega-3 fatty acids	Modest reduction in CV mortality and hospitalization in patients with mild to severe HF and reduced EF.[106] No benefit seen if post-MI patients optimally treated[107] or given low doses.[108] Lack of benefit seen when initiated after acute phase of CV event.[102]	1 g/day (EPA+DHA).[a,109] Formulation of omega-3 acid ethyl esters used in trials (Omacor/Lovanza) is not yet available in Canada. Routine supplementation with omega-3 fatty acid capsules no longer recommended for secondary prevention of MI, but is unlikely to cause harm;[110]

(cont'd)

Table 7: **Evidence-based Supplementation to Prevent or Treat Disease** *(cont'd)*

Disease/Condition	Supplement	Evidence of Benefit/Risk	Recommendations
		Lack of benefit for prevention of recurrent AF.[111]	≥2 servings of oily fish weekly as part of a Mediterranean diet for secondary prevention of MI also unlikely to harm.[110] Monitor INR if on warfarin.
Cancer prevention, colon	*folic acid*	1 mg/day in high-risk patients with polyps not effective in reducing colon cancer[112] and may increase risk. Supplementation in the general population does not appear to be beneficial.[113]	Avoid supplementation for cancer prevention especially in those at high risk; increasing folate from dietary sources may be beneficial.
	calcium, vitamin D	Additional studies are needed on use of calcium, vitamin D before these can be routinely recommended.	
	antioxidants		Avoid antioxidant supplementation.[33,114]
Cancer prevention, other	*vitamin E*	Long-term vitamin E supplementation does not prevent cancer.[115] Supplementation increases risk of prostate cancer by 17%; effect is apparent by the third year of supplementation.[47]	Limit or avoid vitamin E supplementation, especially in those at high risk (e.g., smokers). Avoid in males, especially those >60 y.
	selenium	Selenium supplementation does not prevent cancer.[47]	Limit supplementation for primary prevention of cancer.
	B vitamins (*folic acid*, *vitamin* B_6, *vitamin* B_{12})	Vitamin B supplementation does not decrease overall risk of breast cancer.[116]	Limit supplementation for primary prevention of breast cancer.
	beta-carotene	Beta-carotene supplements increase risk of gastric and lung cancer at doses of 20–30 mg/day and at any dose in patients at high risk (smokers, asbestos exposure).[105,117]	Avoid beta-carotene, retinol especially in those at high risk (smokers); supplement with foods high in alpha-carotenes.[36]
	vitamin D	Benefit of vitamin D for cancer prevention awaiting clarification from definitive trials as data are conflicting (possible increased risk of pancreatic cancer with high vitamin D levels).[118]	Canadian Cancer Society recommends: ▪ Adults during fall and winter months: 1000 IU/day ▪ Adults ≥ 50 y, dark skin or little sun exposure: 1000 IU/day all year round[82]
Cancer prevention, secondary, skin	*niacinamide*	High-risk patients (i.e., ≥ 2 nonmelanoma skin cancers in previous 5 y) had significant reduction in the rate of development of new skin cancers.[119]	500 mg niacinamide (vitamin B_3) twice daily; not niacin.[119] Rebound effect seen if treatment discontinued.[119]

Disease/Condition	Supplement	Evidence of Benefit/Risk	Recommendations
Childhood development (cognitive and visual)	*omega-3 fatty acids*	Maternal supplementation with omega-3 fatty acids during pregnancy did not result in significant differences in cognitive or visual development.[120,121] Supplementation of formula-fed infants with omega-3 fatty acids may improve cognitive development.[122]	More studies required.
Cognitive decline	*B vitamins (folic acid, vitamin B_6, vitamin B_{12}) and antioxidants*	Supplementation with B vitamins[123] or antioxidants (vitamin C, vitamin E, beta-carotene)[124] does not prevent cognitive decline.	Avoid high-dose vitamin B and antioxidant supplementation.
	omega-3 fatty acids/fish oil	Insufficient data to recommend omega-3 fatty acid supplementation to prevent cognitive decline.	A possible decreased risk with fish consumption has been seen in observational trials.[124]
Diabetes	*omega-3 fatty acids*	Omega-3 fatty acids lower triglycerides and VLDL but have no effect on glycemic control; LDL levels may increase insignificantly. Insufficient data to make recommendations for diabetes prevention.[125]	Awaiting controlled clinical trial data to support observational data.
	vitamin D	Risk of type 1 diabetes may be decreased in children who were supplemented—may prevent type 1 diabetes.[126]	No change to current recommendations until RCT evidence is available. Data are insufficient to recommend vitamin D for primary prevention of type 2 diabetes or for glycemic control.
	B vitamins (folic acid, vitamin B_6, vitamin B_{12})	High-dose vitamin B therapy (folic acid, vitamin B_6 and vitamin B_{12}) did not slow progression of diabetic nephropathy and increased risk of vascular events.[127]	Avoid supplementation.
Gout	*vitamin C*	Vitamin C supplementation (median dose of 500 mg per day) modestly decreased serum uric acid levels in healthy patients,[128] but a small RCT did not show any urate-lowering effects in patients with gout.[129]	Limit doses to <2 g/day. More study required to determine optimal dose and effect on clinical outcomes (number of gouty attacks).
Headache	*omega-3 fatty acids*	Dietary intervention of increased n-3 EPA and DHA and decreased n-6 LA intake decreased the number and intensity of headaches and increased quality of life.[132]	Unknown if supplementation will result in similar outcomes. Larger confirmatory trials needed before recommendation can be made. For more information, see Chapter 8: Headache.
Heart failure	*omega-3 fatty acids*	May be considered in those with mild to moderate heart failure.[130] Those with preserved EF >40% may not benefit.	1 g daily of EPA+DHA.[a] The formulation of omega-3 acid ethyl esters used in trials (Omacor/Lovanza) is not available in Canada.

(cont'd)

Table 7: **Evidence-based Supplementation to Prevent or Treat Disease** *(cont'd)*

Disease/Condition	Supplement	Evidence of Benefit/Risk	Recommendations
			Monitor for increased bleeding if on warfarin. Doses >3 g/day may be associated with bleeding.
	coenzyme Q_{10}	Supplementation has no effect on exercise capacity or LV function in patients with heart failure despite increased blood levels.[131]	Higher quality studies required to determine if there are benefits on morbidity or mortality when added to current standard of care.
Mood disorders (major depressive disorder)	*B vitamins (folic acid, vitamin B_6 and vitamin B_{12})*	Limited data suggest potential benefit, especially in women when used as adjunctive therapy.[133] Supplemental B vitamins may increase rates of remission with antidepressant therapy in middle-aged and older adults.[134] Supplemental vitamin B_6, B_{12} and folic acid decrease risk of depression after stroke or TIA.[135] Short-term folic acid augmentation as monotherapy may not provide benefit.[136,137]	Supplementation with vitamin B_6 25 mg, vitamin B_{12} 500 µg and folic acid 2 mg daily may be considered as adjuvant therapy in patients receiving antidepressants, or for stroke patients at risk of depression. Balance potential benefit of folic acid supplementation with long-term risk. Uncertain whether benefit occurs in those with or without folate deficiency.
	omega-3 fatty acids/fish oil	Data primarily as adjunctive therapy at doses of 1–4 g/day; EPA alone or with DHA appears to show greater benefits.[a,133] Fish oil supplementation during pregnancy does not reduce risk of postpartum depression and has not been shown to improve neurodevelopment in offspring.[121,138,139]	More studies required. For more information, see Chapter 4: Depression.
	selenium	Insufficient evidence for the use of selenium to prevent postpartum depression.[139]	More studies required.
Pain, chronic or neuropathic	*vitamin D*	One trial has shown a beneficial effect of supplementation with vitamin D in chronic pain conditions.[140]	Recommendation regarding use of vitamin D to decrease incidence of chronic pain awaits high quality trial evidence.[141]
Pregnancy-related conditions and pregnancy outcomes	*calcium*	Oral calcium may prevent pre-eclampsia and decrease risk of death or complications related to hypertension.[142]	1 g daily in divided doses may be beneficial, especially for women with low baseline calcium intake or at high risk of pre-eclampsia.
	folic acid	There is strong evidence to suggest that prophylactic therapy with folic acid, prior to and during pregnancy, reduces the risk of fetal neural tube defects. Preconception supplementation with folic acid significantly reduces the risk of neonate being small for gestational age.[143]	0.4 mg/day via a daily multivitamin is recommended for all women of child-bearing potential.[9] SOGC makes specific supplementation recommendations based upon risk of neural tube defects:[9]

Disease/Condition	Supplement	Evidence of Benefit/Risk	Recommendations
			▪ Low-risk: Supplement 0.4 mg/day beginning at least 2–3 months before conception and continuing until 4–6 weeks postpartum or as long as breastfeeding continues ▪ Moderate-risk: Supplement 1 mg/day beginning at least 3 months before conception and continuing until 12 weeks' gestational age; then supplement 0.4–1 mg/day until 4–6 weeks postpartum or as long as breastfeeding continues ▪ High-risk: Supplement 4 mg/day beginning at least 3 months before conception and continuing until 12 weeks' gestational age; then supplement 0.4–1 mg/day until 4–6 weeks postpartum or as long as breastfeeding continues.
	magnesium	Magnesium supplementation during pregnancy does not reduce risk of perinatal mortality, small-for-gestational-age newborns or maternal pre-eclampsia.[144]	No evidence to recommend supplementation.
	vitamin D	Observational studies suggest an association between maternal vitamin D levels and offspring birthweight, bone mass and serum calcium concentrations. More studies are required to provide evidence of benefit of supplementation during pregnancy.[145]	Consider recommending 2000 IU/day for pregnant women during winter months.[83]
Psychotic disorders/ schizophrenia	*omega-3 fatty acids/fish oil*	May be beneficial for early prevention in persons at ultra-high risk of psychosis.[146] May allow decreased antipsychotic doses, but its use for treatment of schizophrenia remains experimental.[147] Little evidence of benefit for manic symptoms of bipolar disorder.[148]	Requires confirmatory trials.
	folic acid	Supplementation improved negative symptoms in patients with specific gene variants (*FOLH1*).[149]	Folic acid 2 mg and vitamin B_{12} 400 µg may be beneficial in those with *FOLH1* gene variants.
Respiratory conditions	*vitamin C*	Limited evidence that vitamin C may decrease pneumonia incidence and decrease respiratory symptoms; benefits seen in those at high risk of or known to have malnutrition/insufficient intake.[150]	Vitamin C prophylaxis may have a small, but consistent effect on the duration of symptoms of the common cold. Children in particular may benefit.[151]

(cont'd)

Table 7: **Evidence-based Supplementation to Prevent or Treat Disease** *(cont'd)*

Disease/Condition	Supplement	Evidence of Benefit/Risk	Recommendations
		Vitamin C supplementation halves the risk of a common cold in persons who are under extreme physical stress for short periods of time (e.g., marathon runners, skiers, soldiers in subarctic conditions). No benefit seen for duration or severity of cold.[151] Vitamin C prophylaxis is not beneficial in reducing incidence of the common cold in the general population.[151]	
	zinc	Zinc lozenges may reduce the duration of the common cold when administered within 24 hours of onset of symptoms.[152]	Zinc lozenges ≥75 mg/day for the duration of the cold is the recommended dose.
Rheumatologic conditions	*omega-3 fatty acids/fish oil*	Supplementation with fish oil as adjunct to DMARD therapy may significantly increase the remission rate in early RA.[153]	5.5 g/day of EPA+DHA[a] in liquid form. Monitor for GI disturbances, burping; potential increased risk of bleeding.
	vitamin D	Supplementation with vitamin D 2000 IU improved inflammatory and hemostatic markers as well as disease activity in patients with SLE and vitamin D insufficiency.[154]	Vitamin D supplementation may be beneficial, but larger trials required before routine supplementation can be recommended.
Triglyceridemia	*omega-3 fatty acids*	Efficacy appears similar to fibrates.[155]	2–4 g/day of EPA+DHA[a] supplements in capsule form. Monitor for GI disturbances, burping; potential increased risk of bleeding.

[a] EPA and DHA are essential fatty acids found in cold water fish.

Abbreviations: AF = atrial fibrillation; AREDS = Age-Related Eye Disease Study; CVD = cardiovascular disease; DHA = docosahexaenoic acid; DMARD = disease-modifying antirheumatic drug; EF = ejection fraction; EPA = eicosapentaenoic acid; FOLH1 = folate hydrolase 1; HF = heart failure; INR = international normalized ratio; LA = linoleic acid; LDL = low-density lipoprotein; LV = left ventricular; RA = rheumatoid arthritis; RCT = randomized controlled trial; SLE = systemic lupus erythematosus; SOGC = Society of Obstetricians and Gynaecologists of Canada; TIA = transient ischemic attack; VLDL = very-low-density lipoprotein

References

1. Institutes of Medicine of the National Academies. *Dietary Reference Intakes (DRIs): recommended dietary allowances and adequate intakes, vitamins and elements*. Available from: www.iom.edu/Activities/Nutrition/SummaryDRIs/~/media/Files/Activity%20Files/Nutrition/DRIs/RDA%20and%20AIs_Vitamin%20and%20Elements.pdf. Accessed January 14, 2016.
2. Health Canada. *Dietary reference intakes tables*. Available from: www.hc-sc.gc.ca/fn-an/nutrition/reference/table/index-eng.php. Accessed January 14, 2016.
3. Health Canada. *Do Canadian adults meet their nutrient requirements through food intake alone?* Available from: www.hc-sc.gc.ca/fn-an/surveill/nutrition/commun/art-nutr-adult-eng.php#n8. Accessed January 14, 2016.
4. McCormick DB. Vitamin/mineral supplements: of questionable benefit for the general population. *Nutr Rev* 2010;68(4):207-13.
5. Sofi F, Cesari F, Abbate A et al. Adherence to Mediterranean diet and health status: meta-analysis. *BMJ* 2008;337:a1344.
6. Ford ES, Bergmann MM, Kroger J et al. Healthy living is the best revenge: findings from the European Prospective Investigation into Cancer and Nutrition-Potsdam Study. *Arch Intern Med* 2009;169(15):1355-62.
7. VITAL Study. *The VITamin D and OMEGA-3 TriaL (VITAL)*. Available from: www.vitalstudy.org/. Accessed January 14, 2016.
8. Tarasuk V, Fitzpatrick S, Ward H. Nutrition inequities in Canada. *Appl Physiol Nutr Metab* 2010;35(2):172-9.
9. Wilson RD; Genetics Committee, Audibert F et al. Pre-conception folic acid and multivitamin supplementation for the primary and secondary prevention of neural tube defects and other folic acid-sensitive congenital anomalies. *J Obstet Gynaecol Can* 2015;37(6):534-52.
10. Vitamin D supplementation: recommendations for Canadian mothers and infants. *Paediatr Child Health* 2007;12(7):583-98.
11. Pena-Rosas JP, De-Regil LM, Dowswell T et al. Daily oral iron supplementation during pregnancy. *Cochrane Database Syst Rev* 2012;12:CD004736.
12. Ziaei S, Norrozi M, Faghihzadeh S et al. A randomized placebo-controlled trial to determine the effect of iron supplementation on pregnancy outcome in pregnant women with hemoglobin > or = 13.2 g/dl. *BJOG* 2007;114(6):684-8.
13. Cockell KA, Miller DC, Lowell H. Application of the Dietary Reference Intakes in developing a recommendation for pregnancy iron supplements in Canada. *Am J Clin Nutr* 2009;90(4):1023-8.
14. Pena-Rosas JP, De-Regil LM, Dowswell T et al. Intermittent oral iron supplementation during pregnancy. *Cochrane Database Syst Rev* 2012;7:CD009997.
15. Craig WJ, Mangels AR, American Dietetic Association. Position of the American Dietetic Association: vegetarian diets. *J Am Diet Assoc* 2009;109(7):1266-82.
16. Dietitians of Canada. *Healthy eating guidelines for vegans*. Available from: www.dietitians.ca/getattachment/c8c30477-aad8-4283-9164-079855fabb6d/FACTSHEET-Guidlines-for-Vegans.pdf.aspx. Accessed January 14, 2016.
17. Dietitians of Canada. *Healthy guidelines for lacto-ovo vegetarians*. Available from: www.dietitians.ca/getattachment/fcf61129-526a-4c5b-964b-b297d9c6f513/FACTSHEET-Guidelines-Lacto-Ovo.pdf.aspx. Accessed January 14, 2016.
18. Kirkpatrick SI, Tarasuk V. Food insecurity is associated with nutrient inadequacies among Canadian adults and adolescents. *J Nutr* 2008;138 (3):604-12.
19. Marian M, Sacks G. Micronutrients and older adults. *Nutr Clin Pract* 2009;24(2):179-95.
20. Mucci E, Jackson SH. Nutritional supplementation in community-dwelling elderly people. *Ann Nutr Metab* 2008;52(Suppl 1):33-7.
21. Andres E, Loukili NH, Noel E et al. Vitamin B12 (cobalamin) deficiency in elderly patients. *CMAJ* 2004;171(3):251-9.
22. Mursu J, Robien K, Harnack LJ et al. Dietary supplements and mortality rate in older women: the Iowa Women's Health Study. *Arch Intern Med* 2011;171(18):1625-33.
23. Avenell A, Campbell MK, Cook JA et al. Effect of multivitamin and multimineral supplements on morbidity from infections in older people (MAVIS trial): pragmatic, randomised, double blind, placebo controlled trial. *BMJ* 2005;331(7512):324-9.
24. Sobotka SA, Deal SB, Casper TJ et al. Petechial rash in a child with autism and Trisomy 21. *Pediatr Ann* 2014;43(6):224-6.
25. Kitcharoensakkul M, Schulz CG, Kassel R et al. Scurvy revealed by difficulty walking: three cases in young children. *J Clin Rheumatol* 2014;20(4):224-8.
26. Shankar P, Boylan M, Sriram K. Micronutrient deficiencies after bariatric surgery. *Nutrition* 2010;26(11-12):1031-7.
27. Schweitzer DH, Posthuma EF. Prevention of vitamin and mineral deficiencies after bariatric surgery: evidence and algorithms. *Obes Surg* 2008;18(11):1485-8.
28. Linus Pauling Institute. Oregon State University. Micronutrient Research for Optimal Health. Micronutrient Information Center. Available from: lpi.oregonstate.edu/infocenter/. Accessed January 14, 2016.
29. National Institutes of Health. Office of Dietary Supplements. *Vitamin A: fact sheet for health professionals*. Available from: ods.od.nih.gov/factsheets/VitaminA-HealthProfessional/#en5. Accessed January 14, 2016.
30. Medscape. Drugs & Diseases. *Vitamin A deficiency*. Available from: emedicine.medscape.com/article/126004-overview. Accessed January 14, 2016.
31. Feskanich D, Singh V, Willett WC et al. Vitamin A intake and hip fractures among postmenopausal women. *JAMA* 2002;287(1):47-54.
32. Caire-Juvera G, Ritenbaugh C, Wactawski-Wende J et al. Vitamin A and retinol intakes and the risk of fractures among participants of the Women's Health Initiative Observational Study. *Am J Clin Nutr* 2009;89(1):323-30.
33. Bjelakovic G, Nikolava D, Gluud LL et al. Mortality in randomized trials of antioxidant supplements for primary and secondary prevention: systematic review and meta-analysis. *JAMA* 2007;297(8):842-57.
34. Tornwall ME, Virtamo J, Korhonen PA et al. Effect of alpha-tocopherol and beta-carotene supplementation on coronary heart disease during the 6-year post-trial follow-up in the ATBC study. *Eur Heart J* 2004;25(13):1171-8.
35. Omenn GS, Goodman GE, Thornquist MD et al. Effects of a combination of beta carotene and vitamin A on lung cancer and cardiovascular disease. *N Engl J Med* 1996;334(18):1150-5.
36. Li C, Ford ES, Zhao G et al. Serum {alpha}-carotene concentrations and risk of death among US adults: the third National Health and Nutrition Examination Survey Follow-up Study. *Arch Intern Med* 2011;171(6):507-15.
37. National Institutes of Health. Office of Dietary Supplements. *Vitamin D: fact sheet for health professionals*. Available from: ods.od.nih.gov/factsheets/VitaminD-HealthProfessional/. Accessed January 14, 2016.
38. Sanders KM, Stuart AL, Williamson EJ et al. Annual high-dose oral vitamin D and falls and fractures in older women: a randomized controlled trial. *JAMA* 2010;303(18):1815-22.
39. Jackson RD, LaCroix AZ, Gass M et al. Calcium plus vitamin D supplementation and the risk of fractures. *N Engl J Med* 2006;354(7):669-83.
40. National Institutes of Health. Office of Dietary Supplements. *Vitamin E: fact sheet for health professionals*. Available from: ods.od.nih.gov/factsheets/VitaminE-HealthProfessional/. Accessed January 14, 2016.

41. Rogovik AL, Vohra S, Goldman RD. Safety considerations and potential interactions of vitamins: should vitamins be considered drugs? *Ann Pharmacother* 2010;44(2):311-24.
42. Lee IM, Cook NR, Gaziano JM et al. Vitamin E in the primary prevention of cardiovascular disease and cancer: the Women's Health Study: a randomized controlled trial. *JAMA* 2005;294(1):56-65.
43. Sesso HD, Buring JE, Christen WG et al. Vitamins E and C in the prevention of cardiovascular disease in men: the Physicians' Health Study II randomized controlled trial. *JAMA* 2008;300(18):2123-33.
44. Lonn E, Bosch Y, Yusuf S et al. Effects of long-term vitamin E supplementation on cardiovascular events and cancer: a randomized controlled trial. *JAMA* 2005;293(11):1338-47.
45. Miller ER, Pastor-Barriuso R, Dalal D et al. Meta-analysis: high-dosage vitamin E supplementation may increase all-cause mortality. *Ann Intern Med* 2005;142(1):37-46.
46. Meydani SN, Leka LS, Fine BC et al. Vitamin E and respiratory tract infections in elderly nursing home residents: a randomized controlled trial. *JAMA* 2004;292(7):828-36.
47. Klein EA, Thompson IM, Tangen CM et al. Vitamin E and the risk of prostate cancer: the Selenium and Vitamin E Cancer Prevention Trial (SELECT). *JAMA* 2011;306(14):1549-56.
48. Crowther CA, Crosby DD, Henderson-Smart DJ. Vitamin K prior to preterm birth for preventing neonatal periventricular haemorrhage. *Cochrane Database Syst Rev* 2010;(1):CD000229.
49. National Institutes of Health. Office of Dietary Supplements. *Vitamin K: fact sheet for health professionals*. Available from: ods.od.nih.gov/factsheets/VitaminK-HealthProfessional/. Accessed January 14, 2016.
50. DiNicolantonio JJ, Niazi AK, Lavie CJ et al. Thiamine supplementation for the treatment of heart failure: a review of the literature. *Congest Heart Fail* 2013;19(4):214-22.
51. Clase CM, Ki V, Holden RM. Water-soluble vitamins in people with low glomerular filtration rate or on dialysis: a review. *Semin Dial* 2013;26(5):546-67.
52. Sauer J, Mason JB, Choi SW. Too much folate: a risk factor for cancer and cardiovascular disease? *Curr Opin Clin Nutr Metab Care* 2009;12(1):30-6.
53. Cole BF, Baron JA, Sandler RS et al. Folic acid for the prevention of colorectal adenomas: a randomized clinical trial. *JAMA* 2007;297(21):2351-9.
54. Ebbing M, Bonaa KH, Nygard O et al. Cancer incidence and mortality after treatment with folic acid and vitamin B12. *JAMA* 2009;302(19):2119-26.
55. Morris MC, Evans DA, Bienias JL et al. Dietary folate and vitamin B12 intake and cognitive decline among community-dwelling older persons. *Arch Neurol* 2005;62(4):641-5.
56. Vollset SE, Clarke R, Lewington S et al. Effects of folic acid supplementation on overall and site-specific cancer incidence during the randomised trials: meta-analyses of data on 50 000 individuals. *Lancet* 2013;381(9871):1029-36.
57. Caring for Kids New to Canada. Medical Conditions. *Vitamin B12 deficiency.* Available from: www.kidsnewtocanada.ca/conditions/b12. Accessed January 14, 2016.
58. Linus Pauling Institute. Oregon State University. Micronutrient Information Center. *Choline*. Available from: lpi.oregonstate.edu/infocenter/othernuts/choline/. Accessed January 14, 2016.
59. Taylor EN, Stampfer MJ, Curhan GC. Dietary factors and the risk of incident kidney stones in men: new insights after 14 years of follow-up. *J Am Soc Nephrol* 2004;15(12):3225-32.
60. Bolland MJ, Grey A, Avenell A et al. Calcium supplements, with or without vitamin D and risk of cardiovascular events: reanalysis of the Women's Health Initiative limited access data set and meta-analysis. *BMJ* 2011;342:d2040.
61. Lewis JR, Calver J, Zhu K et al. Calcium supplementation and the risks of atherosclerotic vascular disease in older women: results of a 5-year RCT and a 4.5-year follow up. *J Bone Miner Res* 2011;26(1):35-41.
62. Michaelsson K, Melhus H, Warensjo Lemming E et al. Long term calcium intake and rates of all cause and cardiovascular mortality: community based prospective longitudinal cohort study. *BMJ* 2013;346:f228.
63. Xiao Q, Murphy RA, Houston DK et al. Dietary and supplemental calcium intake and cardiovascular disease mortality: the National Institutes of Health-AARP diet and health study. *JAMA Intern Med* 2013;173(8):639-46.
64. Langsetmo L, Berger C, Kreiger N et al. Calcium and vitamin D intake and mortality: results from the Canadian Multicentre Osteoporosis Study (CaMos). *J Clin Endocrinol Metab* 2013;98(7):3010-8.
65. Aune D, Navarro Rosenblatt DA, Chan DS et al. Dairy products, calcium and cancer risk: a systematic review and meta-analysis of cohort studies. *Am J Clin Nutr* 2015;101(1):87-117.
66. Office of Dietary Supplements, National Institutes of Health. *Iron: dietary supplement fact sheet* . Available from: ods.od.nih.gov/factsheets/Iron-HealthProfessional/. Accessed January 14, 2016.
67. Centers for Disease Control and Prevention. *CDC alert on adverse effects associated with consuming "Total Body Formula" and "Total Body Mega Formula"*. Available from: dhhs.ne.gov/publichealth/han%20Documents/advisory041408.pdf. Accessed January 14, 2016.
68. Johnson AR, Munoz A, Gottlieb JL et al. High dose zinc increases hospital admissions due to genitourinary complications. *J Urol* 2007;177(2):639-43.
69. Holick MF. Vitamin D deficiency. *N Engl J Med* 2007;357(3):266-81.
70. Stone S, Regier L, Jensen B. *Vitamin D: therapeutic overview & evaluation of evidence for current claims*. Saskatoon Health Region: RxFiles; Dec 2010. Available from: www.rxfiles.ca. Subscription required.
71. Llewellyn DJ, Lang IA, Langa LM et al. Vitamin D and risk of cognitive decline in elderly persons. *Arch Intern Med* 2010;170(13):1135-41.
72. McGrath JJ, Burne TH, Feron F et al. Developmental vitamin D deficiency and risk of schizophrenia: a 10-year update. *Schizophr Bull* 2010;36(6):1073-8.
73. Schöttker B, Jorde R, Peasey A et al. Vitamin D and mortality: meta-analysis of individual participant data from a large consortium of cohort studies from Europe and the United States. *BMJ* 2014;348:g3656.
74. Khaw KT, Luben R, Wareham N. Serum 25-hydroxyvitamin D, mortality, and incident cardiovascular disease, respiratory disease, cancers, and fractures: a 13-y prospective population study. *Am J Clin Nutr* 2014;100(5):1361-70.
75. Bjelakovic G, Gluud LL, Nikolova D et al. Vitamin D supplementation for prevention of mortality in adults. *Cochrane Database Syst Rev* 2014;1:CD007470.
76. Chowdhury R, Kunutsor S, Vitezova A et al. Vitamin D and risk of cause specific death: systematic review and meta-analysis of observational cohort and randomised intervention studies. *BMJ* 2014;348:g1903.

77. Ontario Health Technology Advisory Committee. OHTAC recommendation. *Clinical utility of vitamin D testing*. Available from: www.hqontario.ca/english/providers/program/ohtac/tech/recommend/rec_vitamin%20d_201002.pdf. Accessed January 14, 2016.
78. Langlois K, Green-Finestone L, Little J et al. Vitamin D status of Canadians as measured in the 2007 to 2009 Canadian Health Measures Survey. *Health Rep* 2010;21(1):47-55.
79. Bjelakovic G, Gluud LL, Nikolova D et al. Vitamin D supplementation for prevention of mortality in adults. *Cochrane Database Syst Rev* 2011;(7):CD007470.
80. Osteoporosis Canada. *High dose vitamin D supplementation does not improve muscle function and may increase the risk of falls*. Available from: www.osteoporosis.ca/wp-content/uploads/Vit-D-Rapid-Response-Jan-6-2016.pdf. Accessed January 14, 2016.
81. Dawson-Hughes B, Mithal A, Bonjour JP et al. IOF position statement: vitamin D recommendations for older adults. *Osteoporos Int* 2010;21(7):1151-4.
82. Canadian Cancer Society. *Vitamin D*. Available from: www.cancer.ca/en/prevention-and-screening/live-well/vitamin-d/?region=on. Accessed January 14, 2016.
83. Vitamin D supplementation: recommendations for Canadian mothers and infants. *Paediatr Child Health* 2007;12(7):583-9.
84. Heaney RP. Vitamin D and calcium interactions: functional outcomes. *Am J Clin Nutr* 2008;88(2):541S-544S.
85. National Institutes of Health. Office of Dietary Supplements. *Vitamin B12: fact sheet for health professionals*. Available from: ods.od.nih.gov/factsheets/VitaminB12-HealthProfessional/#h5. Accessed January 14, 2016.
86. Allen LH. How common is vitamin B-12 deficiency? *Am J Clin Nutr* 2009;89(2):693S-6S.
87. Hudson B. Vitamin B-12 deficiency. *BMJ* 2010;340:c2305.
88. Papaioannou A, Morin S, Cheung AM et al. 2010 clinical practice guidelines for the diagnosis and management of osteoporosis in Canada: summary. *CMAJ* 2010;182(17):1864-73.
89. Health Canada. *Vitamin D and calcium: updated Dietary Reference Intakes*. Available from: www.hc-sc.gc.ca/fn-an/nutrition/vitamin/vita-d-eng.php. Accessed January 14, 2016.
90. Moyer VA; U.S. Preventive Services Task Force. Vitamin D and calcium supplementation to prevent fractures in adults: U.S. Preventive Services Task Force recommendation statement. *Ann Intern Med* 2013;158(9):691-6.
91. Osteoporosis Canada. *Calcium: an important nutrient that builds stronger bones*. Available from: www.osteoporosis.ca/osteoporosis-and-you/nutrition/calcium-requirements/. Accessed January 14, 2016.
92. Sulli MM, Ezzo DC. Drug interactions with vitamins and minerals. *US Pharm* 2007;1:42-55.
93. McColl KE. Effect of proton pump inhibitors on vitamins and iron. *Am J Gastroenterol* 2009;104(Suppl 2):S5-9.
94. Mouchantaf R. Proton pump inhibitors: hypomagnesemia accompanied by hypocalcemia and hypokalemia. *Can Adverse React Newsl* 2011;21(3):1-2. Available from: www.hc-sc.gc.ca/dhp-mps/alt_formats/pdf/medeff/bulletin/carn-bcei_v21n3-eng.pdf. Accessed January 14, 2016.
95. Age-Related Eye Disease Study Research Group. A randomized, placebo-controlled, clinical trial of high-dose supplementation with vitamins C and E, b-carotene, and zinc for age-related macular degeneration and vision loss: AREDS report no. 8. *Arch Ophthalmol* 2001;119(10):1417-36.
96. Age-Related Eye Disease Study 2 Research Group. Lutein + zeaxanthin and omega-3 fatty acids for age-related macular degeneration: the Age-Related Eye Disease Study 2 (AREDS2) randomized clinical trial. *JAMA* 2013;309(19):2005-15.
97. Hooper L, Thompson RL, Harrison RA et al. Omega 3 fatty acids for prevention and treatment of cardiovascular disease. *Cochrane Database Syst Rev* 2004;(4):CD003177.
98. Risk and Prevention Study Collaborative Group, Roncaglioni MC, Tombesi M et al. n-3 fatty acids in patients with multiple cardiovascular risk factors. *N Engl J Med* 2013;368(19):1800-8.
99. Mark BJ, Beaty AD, Slavin RG. Are fish oil supplements safe in finned fish-allergic patients? *Allergy Asthma Proc* 2008;29(5):528-9.
100. Witham MD, Price RJ, Struthers AD et al. Cholecalciferol treatment to reduce blood pressure in older patients with isolated systolic hypertension: the VitDISH randomized controlled trial. *JAMA Intern Med* 2013;173(18):1672-9.
101. Huo Y, Li J, Qin X et al. Efficacy of folic acid therapy in primary prevention of stroke among adults with hypertension in China: the CSPPT randomized clinical trial. *JAMA* 2015;313(13):1325-35.
102. Galan P, Kesse-Guyot E, Czernichow S et al. Effects of B vitamins and omega 3 fatty acids on cardiovascular diseases: a randomised placebo controlled trial. *BMJ* 2010;341:c6273.
103. Kris-Etherton PM, Lichtenstein AH, Howard BV et al. Antioxidant vitamin supplements and cardiovascular disease. *Circulation* 2004;110(5):637-41.
104. Myung SK, Ju W, Cho B et al. Efficacy of vitamin and antioxidant supplements in prevention of cardiovascular disease: systematic review and meta-analysis of randomised controlled trials. *BMJ* 2013;346:f10.
105. Fortmann SP, Burda BU, Senger CA et al. Vitamin and mineral supplements in the primary prevention of cardiovascular disease and cancer: an updated systematic evidence review for the U.S. Preventive Services Task Force. *Ann Intern Med* 2013;159(12):824-34.
106. Marik PE, Varon J. Omega-3 dietary supplements and the risk of cardiovascular events: a systematic review. *Clin Cardiol* 2009;32(7):365-72.
107. Rauch B, Schiele R, Schneider S et al. OMEGA, a randomized, placebo-controlled trial to test the effect of highly purified omega-3 fatty acids on top of modern guideline-adjusted therapy after myocardial infarction. *Circulation* 2010;122(21):2152-9.
108. Kromhout D, Giltay EJ, Geleijnse JM et al. n-3 fatty acids and cardiovascular events after myocardial infarction. *N Engl J Med* 2010;363(21):2015-26.
109. McKelvie RS, Moe GW, Ezekowitz JA et al. The 2012 Canadian Cardiovascular Society heart failure management guidelines update: focus on acute and chronic heart failure. *Can J Cardiol* 2013;29(2):168-81.
110. National Institute for Health and Care Excellence. *Myocardial infarction: cardiac rehabilitation and prevention of further MI*. Available from: www.nice.org.uk/guidance/cg172/chapter/1-recommendations. Accessed January 14, 2016.
111. Macchia A, Grancelli H, Varini S et al. Omega-3 fatty acids for the prevention of recurrent symptomatic atrial fibrillation: results of the FORWARD (randomized trial to assess efficacy of PUFA for the maintenance of sinus rhythm in persistent atrial fibrillation). *J Am Coll Cardiol* 2013;61(4):463-8.
112. Cole BF, Baron JA, Sandler RS et al. Folic acid for the prevention of colorectal adenomas: a randomized clinical trial. *JAMA* 2007;297(21):2351-9.
113. Cooper K, Squires H, Carroll C et al. Chemoprevention of colorectal cancer: systematic review and economic evaluation. *Health Technol Assess* 2010;14(32):1-206.
114. Wilkins T, Reynolds PL. Colorectal cancer: a summary of the evidence for screening and prevention. *Am Fam Physician* 2008;78(12):1385-92.

115. Lonn E, Bosch J, Yusuf S et al. Effects of long-term vitamin E supplementation on cardiovascular events and cancer: a randomized controlled trial. *JAMA* 2005;293(11):1338-47.
116. Zhang SM, Cook NR, Albert CM et al. Effect of combined folic acid, vitamin B6, and vitamin B12 on cancer risk in women: a randomized trial. *JAMA* 2008;300(17):2012-21.
117. Druesne-Pecollo N, Latino-Martel P, Norat T et al. Beta-carotene supplementation and cancer risk: a systematic review and metaanalysis of randomized controlled trials. *Int J Cancer* 2010;127(1):172-84.
118. World Health Organization. International Agency for Research on Cancer. *Vitamin D and cancer.* Available from: www.iarc.fr/en/publications/pdfs-online/wrk/wrk5/Report_VitD.pdf. Accessed January 15, 2016.
119. Chen AC, Martin AJ, Choy B et al. A phase 3 randomized trial of nicotinamide for skin-cancer chemoprevention. *N Engl J Med* 2015;373(17):1618-26.
120. Gould JF, Smithers LG, Makrides M. The effect of maternal omega-3 (n-3) LCPUFA supplementation during pregnancy on early childhood cognitive and visual development: a systematic review and meta-analysis of randomized controlled trials. *Am J Clin Nutr* 2013;97(3):531-44.
121. Makrides M, Gibson RA, McPhee AJ et al. Effect of DHA supplementation during pregnancy on maternal depression and neurodevelopment of young children: a randomized controlled trial. *JAMA* 2010;304(15):1675-83.
122. Jiao J, Li Q, Chu J et al. Effect of n-3 PUFA supplementation on cognitive function throughout the life span from infancy to old age: a systematic review and meta-analysis of randomized controlled trials. *Am J Clin Nutr* 2014;100(6):1422-36.
123. van der Zwaluw NL, Dhonukshe-Rutten RA, van Wijngaarden JP et al. Results of 2-year vitamin B treatment on cognitive performance: Secondary data from an RCT. *Neurology* 2014;83(23):2158-66.
124. Plassman BL, Williams JW, Burke JR et al. Systematic review: factors associated with risk for and possible prevention of cognitive decline in later life. *Ann Intern Med* 2010;153(3):182-93.
125. Hartweg J, Perera R, Montori V et al. Omega-3 polyunsaturated fatty acids (PUFA) for type 2 diabetes mellitus. *Cochrane Database Syst Rev* 2008;(1):CD003205.
126. Zipitis CS, Akobeng AK. Vitamin D supplementation in early childhood and risk of type 1 diabetes: a systematic review and meta-analysis. *Arch Dis Child* 2008;93(6):512-7.
127. House AA, Eliasziw M, Cattran DC et al. Effect of B-vitamin therapy on progression of diabetic nephropathy: a randomized controlled trial. *JAMA* 2010;303(16):1603-9.
128. Juraschek SP, Miller ER, Gelber AC. Effect of oral vitamin C on uric acid: a meta-analysis of randomized clinical trials. *Arthritis Care Res (Hoboken)* 2011;63(9):1295-306.
129. Stamp LK, O'Donnell JL, Frampton C et al. Clinically insignificant effect of supplemental vitamin C on serum urate in patients with gout: a pilot randomized controlled trial. *Arthritis Rheum* 2013;65(6):1636-42.
130. Howlett JG, McKelvie RS, Arnold JM et al. Canadian Cardiovascular Society Consensus Conference guidelines on heart failure, update 2009: diagnosis and management of right-sided heart failure, myocarditis, device therapy and recent important clinical trials. *Can J Cardiol* 2009;25(2):85-105.
131. Madmani ME, Solaiman AY, Tamr Agha K et al. Coenzyme Q10 for heart failure. *Cochrane Database Syst Rev* 2013;9:CD008684.
132. Ramsden CE, Faurot KR, Zamora D et al. Targeted alteration of dietary n-3 and n-6 fatty acids for the treatment of chronic headaches: a randomized trial. *Pain* 2013;154(11):2441-51.
133. Freeman MP, Fava M, Lake J et al. Complementary and alternative medicine in major depressive disorder: the American Psychiatric Association Task Force Report. *J Clin Psychiatry* 2010;71(6):669-81.
134. Almeida OP, Ford AH, Hirani V et al. B vitamins to enhance treatment response to antidepressants in middle-aged and older adults: results from the B-VITAGE randomised, double-blind, placebo-controlled trial. *Br J Psychiatry* 2014;205(6):450-7.
135. Almeida OP, Marsh K, Alfonso H et al. B-vitamins reduce the long-term risk of depression after stroke: the VITATOPS-DEP trial. *Ann Neurol* 2010;68(4):503-10.
136. Bedson E, Bell D, Carr D et al. Folate Augmentation of Treatment–Evaluation for Depression (FolATED): randomised trial and economic evaluation. *Health Technol Assess* 2014;18(48):vii-viii, 1-159.
137. Fava M, Mischoulon D. Folate in depression: efficacy, safety, differences in formulations, and clinical issues. *J Clin Psychiatry* 2009;70(Suppl 5):12-7.
138. Mozurkewich EL, Clinton CM, Chilimigras JL et al. The Mothers, Omega-3, and Mental Health Study: a double-blind, randomized controlled trial. *Am J Obstet Gynecol* 2013;208(4):313.e1-9.
139. Miller BJ, Murray L, Beckmann ML et al. Dietary supplements for preventing postnatal depression. *Cochrane Database Syst Rev* 2013;10:CD009104.
140. Knutsen KV, Brekke M, Gjelstad S et al. Vitamin D status in patients with musculoskeletal pain, fatigue and headache: a cross-sectional descriptive study in a multi-ethnic general practice in Norway. *Scand J Prim Health Care* 2010;28(3):166-71.
141. Straube S, Derry S, Moore RA et al. Vitamin D for the treatment of chronic painful conditions in adults. *Cochrane Database Syst Rev* 2010;(2):CD007771.
142. Hofmeyr GJ, Lawrie TA, Atallah AN et al. Calcium supplementation during pregnancy for preventing hypertensive disorders and related problems. *Cochrane Database Syst Rev* 2014;6:CD001059.
143. Hodgetts V, Morris R, Francis A et al. Effectiveness of folic acid supplementation in pregnancy on reducing the risk of small-for-gestational age neonates: a population study, systematic review and meta-analysis. *BJOG* 2015;122(4):478-90.
144. Makrides M, Crosby DD, Bain E et al. Magnesium supplementation in pregnancy. *Cochrane Database Syst Rev* 2014;4:CD000937.
145. Harvey NC, Holroyd C, Ntani G et al. Vitamin D supplementation in pregnancy: a systematic review. *Health Technol Assess* 2014;18(45):1-190.
146. Amminger GP, Schafer MR, Papageorgiou K et al. Long-chain omega-3 fatty acids for indicated prevention of psychotic disorders: a randomized, placebo-controlled trial. *Arch Gen Psychiatry* 2010;67(2):146-54.
147. Joy CB, Mumby-Croft R, Joy LA. Polyunsaturated fatty acid supplementation for schizophrenia. *Cochrane Database Syst Rev* 2006;(3):CD001257.
148. Montgomery P, Richardson AJ. Omega-3 fatty acids for bipolar disorder. *Cochrane Database Syst Rev* 2008;(2):CD005169.
149. Roffman JL, Lamberti JS, Achtyes E et al. Randomized multicenter investigation of folate plus vitamin B12 supplementation in schizophrenia. *JAMA Psychiatry* 2013;70(5):481-9.
150. Hemila H, Louhiala P. Vitamin C for preventing and treating pneumonia. *Cochrane Database Syst Rev* 2013;8:CD005532.
151. Hemila H, Chalker E. Vitamin C for preventing and treating the common cold. *Cochrane Database Syst Rev* 2013;1:CD000980.

152. Singh M, Das RR. Zinc for the common cold. *Cochrane Database Syst Rev* 2013;6:CD001364.
153. Proudman SM, James MJ, Spargo LD et al. Fish oil in recent onset rheumatoid arthritis: a randomized, double-blind controlled trial within algorithm-based drug use. *Ann Rheum Dis* 2015;74(1):89-95.
154. Abou-Raya An About-Raya S, Helmii M. The effect of vitamin D supplementation on inflammatory and hemostatic markers and disease activity in patients with systemic lupus erythematosus: a randomized placebo-controlled trial. *J Rheumatol* 2013;40(3):265-72.
155. Kris-Etherton PM, Harris S, Apel LJ et al. Fish consumption, fish oil, omega-3 fatty acids, and cardiovascular disease. *Circulation* 2002;106 (21):2747-57.

Glossary of Abbreviated Terms

5-ASA	5-aminosalicylic acid
AC	before meals
ACE	angiotensin-converting enzyme
ACEI	angiotensin-converting enzyme inhibitor
ADL	activities of daily living
AIDS	acquired immunodeficiency syndrome
AMD	age-related macular degenration
aPTT	activated partial thromboplastin time
ARB	angiotensin receptor blocker
ASA	acetylsalicylic acid
AST	aspartate transaminase
AUC	area under the concentration curve
BCG	bacillus Calmette-Guérin
BID	twice daily
BMD	bone mineral density
BMI	body mass index
BMR	basal metabolic rate
BP	blood pressure
BPH	benign prostatic hyperplasia
BUN	blood urea nitrogen
C&S	culture and sensitivity
CABG	coronary artery bypass graft
cAMP	cyclic adenosine monophosphate
CBC	complete blood count
CBT	cognitive behavioral therapy
CCB	calcium channel blocker
cfu/L	colony-forming units/litre
cGMP	cyclic guanosine monophosphate
CHD	coronary heart disease
CK	creatine kinase
ClCr	creatinine clearance
CMV	cytomegalovirus
CNS	central nervous system
COPD	chronic obstructive pulmonary disease
CPAP	continuous positive airway pressure
CPK	creatine phosphokinase
CPR	cardiopulmonary resuscitation
CRP	C-reactive protein
CSF	cerebrospinal fluid
CT	computed tomography
DEET	diethyltoluamide
DNA	deoxyribonucleic acid
DPI	dry powder inhaler
DVT	deep vein thrombosis
ECG	electrocardiogram
EEG	electroencephalogram
EMLA	eutetic mixture of local anesthetics
ENT	ear, nose and throat
EPS	extrapyramidal symptoms
ESR	erythrocyte sedimentation rate
FDA	Food and Drug Administration (USA)
FEV	forced expiratory volume
FSH	follicle-stimulating hormone
GERD	gastroesophageal reflux disease
GFR	glomerular filtration rate
GI	gastrointestinal
GnRH	gonadotropin-releasing hormone
GTT	glucose tolerance test
h	hour(s)
H2RA	H2-receptor antagonist
Hb	hemoglobin
HbA_{1c}	glysolated hemoglobin
HCG	human chorionic gonadotropin
HDL-C	high-density lipoprotein cholesterol
HEPA	high efficiency particulate air
HF	heart failure
HIV	human immunodeficiency virus
HPV	human papilloma virus
HRQOL	health-related quality of life
HRT	hormone replacement therapy
HS	bedtime
IBW	ideal body weight
ICU	intensive care unit
im, IM	intramuscular
INR	International Normalized Ratio
IOP	intraocular pressure
IU	international unit
IUD	intrauterine device
IUS	intrauterine system
iv, IV	intravenous
J	joule
LCD	liquor carbonis detergens
LDL-C	low-density lipoprotein cholesterol
LFT	liver function test
LH	luteinizing hormone
LMWH	low-molecular-weight heparins
MAC	mycobacterium avium complex

MAO monoamine oxidase
MAOI monoamine oxidase inhibitor
MDI metered-dose inhaler
MI myocardial infarction
min minute(s)
MRI magnetic resonance imaging
MRSA methicillin-resistant *S. aureus*
MS multiple sclerosis
MSSA methicillin-sensitive *S. aureus*
NAPRA National Association of Pharmacy Regulatory Authorities
NG nasogastric
NIH National Institutes of Health
NNT number needed to treat
NPT nocturnal penile tumescence
NRT nicotine replacement therapy
NS normal saline
NSAIDs nonsteroidal anti-inflammatory drugs
NYHA New York Heart Association
OA osteoarthritis
OC oral contraceptive
OR odds ratio
OTC over-the-counter, nonprescription
PABA para-aminobenzoic acid
PC after meals
PID pelvic inflammatory disease
PMDD premenstrual dysphoric disorder
PMS premenstrual syndrome
po, PO by mouth
PPI proton pump inhibitor
pr, PR rectally
PRN when necessary
PSA prostate specific antigen
PT prothrombin time
PTSD post-traumatic stress disorder
pv, PV vaginally
PTT partial thromboplastin time
Q4H every four hours
QHS each bedtime
QID four times daily
RA rheumatoid arthritis
RBC red blood cell
RCT randomized control trial
RICE rest, ice, compression, elevation
RR relative risk
s second(s)
SAMe S-adenosyl-L-methionine
SaO_2 oxygen saturation
sc, SC subcutaneous
SIADH syndrome of inappropriate antidiuretic hormone
sl, SL sublingual
SNRI serotonin and norepinephrine reuptake inhibitor
SOGC Society of Obstetricians and Gynaecologists of Canada
SPF sun protection factor
SSRI selective serotonin reuptake inhibitor
STI sexually transmitted infection
TCA tricyclic antidepressant
TID three times daily
TSH thyroid-stimulating hormone
USP United States Pharmacopoeia
UTI urinary tract infection
UVA ultraviolet-A
UVB ultraviolet-B
UVC ultraviolet-C
WBC white blood cell
WHO World Health Organization
wk week(s)
y year(s)

Index

A

B

C

E

F

G

I

J

K

L

M

N

O

P

Q

R

S

T

U

V

W

X

Y

Z